# GASTROINTESTINAL ONCOLOGY

*Edited by*

James L. Abbruzzese, M.D., F.A.C.P.
Douglas B. Evans, M.D., F.A.C.S.
Christopher G. Willett, M.D.
Cecilia Fenoglio-Preiser, M.D.

OXFORD
UNIVERSITY PRESS
2004

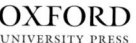

# OXFORD
## UNIVERSITY PRESS

Oxford  New York
Auckland  Bangkok  Buenos Aires  Cape Town  Chennai
Dar es Salaam  Delhi  Hong Kong  Istanbul  Karachi  Kolkata
Kuala Lumpur  Madrid  Melbourne  Mexico City  Mumbai
Nairobi  São Paulo  Shanghai  Singapore  Taipei  Tokyo  Toronto

Copyright © 2004 by Oxford University Press, Inc.

Published by Oxford University Press, Inc.
198 Madison Avenue, New York, New York, 10016
http://www.oup-usa.org

Oxford is a registered trademark of Oxford University Press

Library of Congress Cataloging-in-Publication Data
Gastrointestinal oncology / [edited] by James Abbruzzese . . . [et al.].
p. ; cm.
Includes bibliographical references and index.
ISBN 0-19-513372-2 (cloth)
1. Gastrointestinal system—Cancer.
I. Abbruzzese, James L.
[DNLM: 1. Digestive System Neoplasms.
WI 149 G25744 2003]
RC280.D5 G3782 2003    616.99′43—dc21    2002034602

2 4 6 8 9 7 5 3 1

Printed in the United States of America
on acid-free paper

# Preface

In recent years, tremendous progress has been made in our understanding of the pathobiology and molecular biology of gastrointestinal cancers. Yet, despite this progress, the clinical management of these diverse and challenging neoplasms remains difficult. This is particularly true once these cancers metastasize. Numerically, cancer affecting the gastrointestinal tract is the most common of all human malignancies, affecting patients worldwide with varying frequencies. For example, in developed countries colorectal cancers are extremely common whereas hepatocellular cancer predominates in other areas of the world. Interestingly, the specific regions of the gastrointestinal tract that are most prone to malignant transformation have changed during the course of the twentieth century. Through the early decades distal gastric adenocarcinomas were extremely common, becoming much less prevalent since the 1940s. However, more recently we have witnessed the rise of proximal gastric and gastroesophageal junction adenocarcinomas. These rapidly evolving events challenge both our understanding of gastrointestinal carcinogenesis and our strategies for diagnosis and treatment.

Clinical advances in the management of these diverse neoplasms now frequently rely on collaborative interactions among a wide variety of cancer specialists including surgical, radiation, and medical oncologists, gastroenterologists, radiologists, and pathologists. Increasingly, however, there is the recognition that more rapid progress in the management of these cancers will require earlier interventions. To facilitate efforts in prevention, early diagnosis, and therapy of gastrointestinal cancer, closer interactions between clinical scientists and basic researchers will be needed. In this spirit, the first part of this text introduces a series of concepts and topics that are important to gastrointestinal malignancies in general. These topics include epidemiologic principles, prevention, screening, familial gastrointestinal cancers, developmental and molecular biology, pathobiology, general therapeutic principles, emerging therapies, and palliative care. The second part of the book covers each of the specific cancers affecting the human gastrointestinal tract. Where sufficient information exists, each of these chapters is introduced by a series of state-of-the-art discussions outlining our current understanding of the pathobiology and molecular biology relevant to each cancer. Subsequent sections describe the multidisciplinary management of specific clinical situations emphasizing the integrated contribution of each medical specialist to the diagnosis, staging, and treatment of that specific gastrointestinal malignancy. It is hoped that by organizing the treatment-related chapters around clinical scenarios the reader will be able to readily find the information necessary to effectively manage the complex clinical situations encountered by patients with gastrointestinal malignancies.

We anticipate that this book will serve to provide information useful to physicians and scientists engaged in the care of patients and study of these malignancies, as well as medical professionals, medical students, and allied health professionals interested in learning more about the biology and clinical behavior of gastrointestinal cancers. Beyond this aim, we hope that this book will stimulate the rapid translation and dissemination of basic science discoveries into novel clinical strategies that will provide significant benefit to our patients.

*Houston, Texas*                        J.L.A.
*Houston, Texas*                       D.B.E.
*Boston, Massachusetts*          C.G.W.
*Cincinnati, Ohio*                    C.F.-P.

# Contents

# Contents

# Gastrointestinal Oncology

# Contributors

JAMES L. ABBRUZZESE, M.D., F.A.C.P.
*Professor and Chair*
*Department of Gastrointestinal Medical Oncology*
*UT M. D. Anderson Cancer Center*
*Houston, TX*

EDDIE K. ABDALLA, M.D.
*Service de Chirurgie Digestive*
*Hopital Beaujon*
*Clichy Cedex, France*

S. NICHOLAS AGOFF, M.D.
*Acting Assistant Professor, Cytopathology*
*University of Washington Medical Center/*
*Harborview Medical Center*
*Seattle, WA*

STEVEN A. AHRENDT, M.D.
*Associate Professor*
*Department of Surgery*
*University of Rochester Medical Center*
*Rochester, NY*

JAFFER A. AJANI, M.D.
*Professor, Department of Gastrointestinal Medical Oncology*
*UT M. D. Anderson Cancer Center*
*Houston, TX*

YASSER AL-ANTABLY, M.D.
*Department of Medicine/Gastroenterology*
*Kaiser Permanente*
*Sacramento Medical Center*
*Sacramento, CA*

CHRISTOPHER I. AMOS, Ph.D.
*Professor*
*Department of Epidemiology*
*UT M. D. Anderson Cancer Center*
*Houston, TX*

NADIR ARBER, M.D., M.H.A.
*Associate Professor of Medicine and Gastroenterology*
*Head, Gastrointestinal Oncology Unit*
*Department of Gastroenterology*
*Tel Aviv "Sourasky" Medical Center*
*Tel Aviv University*
*Tel Aviv, Israel*

RICHARD J. ASPINALL, M.B., B.S., M.R.C.P.
*Clinical Research Fellow*
*Imperial Cancer Research Fund*
*Molecular Oncology Unit*
*Imperial College School of Medicine*
*Hammersmith Hospital*
*London, U.K.*

JEAN-PIERRE AYOUB, M.D.
*CHUM (Centre Hospitalier Universitaire de Montréal)*
*University of Montreal*
*Notre Dame Hospital*
*Montreal, Quebec*
*Canada*

MARK W. BABYATSKY, M.D.
*Assistant Professor of Medicine*
*Director of Gastrointestinal Research*
*Mount Sinai School of Medicine*
*New York, NY*

ULYSSES J. BALIS, M.D.
*Assistant Professor of Pathology*
*Harvard Medical School*
*Department of Pathology*
*Massachusetts General Hospital*
*Boston, MA*

ROBERT S. BENJAMIN, M.D.
*Professor and Chair, Department of*
*Department of Sarcoma Medical Oncology*
*UT M. D. Anderson Cancer Center*
*Houston, TX*

AL B. BENSON, III, M.D.
*Professor of Medicine*
*Division of Hematology and Oncology*
*Northwestern University*
*Chicago, IL*

JORDAN D. BERLIN, M.D.
*Assistant Professor of Medicine*
*Clinical Director, Gastrointestinal Oncology*
*Ingram Cancer Center*
*Division of Hematology/Oncology*
*Vanderbilt University*
*Nashville, TN*

RUSSELL S. BERMAN, M.D.
*Assistant Professor*
*Department of Surgery (Oncology)*
*New York University*
*New York, NY*

MALCOLM M. BILIMORIA, M.D.
*Department of Surgery*
*Evanston Hospital*
*Evanston, IL*

RONALD BLEDAY, M.D.
*Section Chief, Division of Colorectal Surgery*
*Brigham and Women's Hospital*
*Associate Professor of Surgery*
*Harvard Medical School*
*Boston, MA*

GEORGE R. BLUMENSCHEIN, M.D.
*Assistant Professor*
*Department of Thoracic/Head & Neck*
*Medical Oncology*
*UT M. D. Anderson Cancer Center*
*Houston, TX*

RANDALL E. BRAND, M.D.
*Evanston-Northwestern Healthcare System*
*Glenview, IL*

DEAN E. BRENNER, M.D.
*Professor*
*Department of Internal Medicine*
*Department of Pharmacology*
*University of Michigan Medical School*
*Ann Arbor, MI*

EDUARDO BRUERA, M.D.
*Professor and Chair*
*Department of Palliative Care*
*& Rehabilitation Medicine*
*UT M. D. Anderson Cancer Center*
*Houston, TX*

FERNANDO CABANILLAS, M.D.
*Clinical Professor*
*Department of Lymphoma*
*UT M. D. Anderson Cancer Center*
*Houston, TX*

NORMAN J. CARR, M.B., B.S., M.R.C.Path.
*Consultant Histopathologist*
*Department of Cellular Pathology*
*Southampton General Hospital*
*Southampton, U.K.*

KENNETH J. CHANG, M.D.
*Head, Gastrointestinal Oncology*
*Director, Interventional Endoscopy Center*
*Associate Professor of Medicine*
*University of California, Irvine*
*Chao Family Comprehensive Cancer Center*
*Orange, CA*

CHUSILP CHARNSANGAVEJ, M.D.
*Professor and Deputy Division Head for Research*
*Department of Diagnostic Radiology*
*Division of Diagnostic Imaging*
*UT M. D. Anderson Cancer Center*
*Houston, TX*

PAUL J. CHIAO, Ph.D.
*Assistant Professor*
*Department of Surgical Oncology*
*UT M. D. Anderson Cancer Center*
*Houston, TX*

MICHAEL A. CHOTI, M.D., F.A.C.S.
*Assistant Professor, Surgery*
*The Johns Hopkins School of Medicine*
*Johns Hopkins Hospital*
*Baltimore, MD*

ROBERT R. CIMA, M.D.
*Instructor in Surgery*
*Harvard Medical School*
*Associate Surgeon*
*Brigham and Women's Hospital*
*Division of General Surgery*
*Boston, MA*

JEFFREY W. CLARK, M.D.
*Assistant Professor of Medicine*
*Harvard Medical School*
*Massachusetts General Hospital*
*Department of Medicine (Hematology/Oncology)*
*Boston, MA*

DANIEL G. COIT, M.D., F.A.C.S.
*Chief, Gastric & Mixed Tumor Service*
*Memorial Sloan-Kettering Cancer Center*
*New York, NY*

JANICE N. CORMIER, M.D.
*Assistant Professor*
*Department of Surgical Oncology*
*UT M. D. Anderson Cancer Center*
*Houston, TX*

GILBERT J. COTE, Ph.D.
*Associate Professor*
*Department of Endocrine Neoplasia & Hormonal Disorders*
*UT M. D. Anderson Cancer Center*
*Houston, TX*

STEVEN A. CURLEY, M.D.
*Professor, Department of Surgical Oncology*
*Chief, Gastrointestinal Tumor Surgery*
*UT M. D. Anderson Cancer Center*
*Houston, TX*

PETER V. DANENBERG, Ph.D.
*Professor of Biochemistry and Molecular Biology*
*University of Southern California*
*Keck School of Medicine*
*USC/Norris Comprehensive Cancer Center*
*Los Angeles, CA*

AHMED ELSAYEM, M.D.
*Assistant Professor*
*Department of Palliative Care & Rehabilitation Medicine*
*UT M. D. Anderson Cancer Center*
*Houston, TX*

DOUGLAS B. EVANS, M.D., F.A.C.S.
*Professor, Department of Surgical Oncology*
*UT M. D. Anderson Cancer Center*
*1515 Holcombe Boulevard*
*Houston, TX 77030*

SCOTT J. EVANS, M.D.
*Lutheran Medical Center*
*Department of Medical Imaging*
*Wheatridge, CO*

CECILIA FENOGLIO-PREISER, M.D.
*MacKenzie Professor and Director of*
*Pathology and Laboratory Medicine*
*College of Medicine*
*University of Cincinnati*
*Cincinnati, OH*

ELLIOT K. FISHMAN, M.D.
*Professor, Department of Radiology*
*Johns Hopkins University*
*School of Medicine*
*Baltimore, MD*

CHARLES S. FUCHS, M.D., M.P.H.
*Associate Professor of Medicine*
*Harvard Medical School*
*Department of Medical Oncology*
*Dana-Farber Cancer Institute*
*Boston, MA*

ROBERT F. GAGEL, M.D.
*Division Head Ad Interim,*
*Division of Internal Medicine*
*Professor, Department of Endocrine Neoplasia and Hormonal*
*    Disorders*
*UT M. D. Anderson Cancer Center*
*Houston, TX*

LAURIE E. GASPAR, M.D.
*Professor and Chair*
*Department of Radiation Oncology*
*University of Colorado Health Sciences Center*
*Anschutz Cancer Pavilion*
*Aurora, CO*

ANDREW Q. GIAP, M.D.
*Clinical Instructor*
*Division of Gastroenterology*
*Department of Medicine*
*University of California*
*Irvine, California*

JONATHAN N. GLICKMAN, M.D., Ph.D.
*Assistant Professor of Pathology*
*Harvard Medical School*
*Department of Pathology*
*Brigham & Women's Hospital*
*Boston, MA*

JOHN R. GOFFIN, M.D.
*Medical Oncology*
*Visiting Clinical Associate*
*Dana Farber Cancer Institute*
*Boston, MA*

MICHAEL GOGGINS, M.D.
*Assistant Professor of Pathology, Medicine, and Oncology*
*Johns Hopkins Medical Institutions*
*Baltimore, MD*

JOE W. GRISHAM, M.D.
*Kenan Professor*
*Department of Pathology and Laboratory Medicine*
*University of North Carolina at Chapel Hill*
*School of Medicine*
*Chapel Hill, NC*

JOSE G. GUILLEM, M.D., M.P.H.
*Associate Attending Surgeon*
*Memorial Sloan-Kettering Cancer Center*
*New York, NY*

MANAL M. HASSAN, M.D., M.P.H., Ph.D.
*Assistant Professor*
*Department of Gastrointestinal Medical Oncology*
*UT M. D. Anderson Cancer Center*
*Houston, TX*

ERNEST T. HAWK, M.D., M.P.H.
*Chief, Gastrointestinal and Other Cancer Research Group*
*National Cancer Institute/Division of Cancer Prevention*
*Bethesda, MD*

ANA OLIVEIRA HOFF, M.D.
*Clinical Endocrinologist*
*Albert Einstein Hospital*
*Sao Paulo, Brazil*

PAULO M. HOFF, M.D., F.A.C.P.
*Center for Clinical Studies in Cancer (NECC)*
*Albert Einstein Hospital*
*Sao Paulo, Brazil*

KAREN M. HORTON, M.D.
*Assistant Professor of Radiology*
*Johns Hopkins Hospital*
*Baltimore, MD*

JANUSZ JANKOWSKI, M.D., Ph.D., F.R.C.P. (Edin)
*Reader in Medicine/Consultant Gastroenterologist*
*Department of Medicine and Institute for Cancer Research*
*University of Birmingham*
*Birmingham*
*U.K.*

MARINA E. JEAN, M.D.
*Cincinnati, OH 45208*

J. MILBURN JESSUP, M.D., F.A.C.S.
*Professor, Department of Oncology*
*Georgetown University Medical Center*
*Lombardi Cancer Center*
*Washington, DC*

XIAOLONG JIAO, M.D.
*Attending Thoracic Surgeon*
*Department of Thoracic Surgery*
*Hubei Cancer Hospital*
*Wuhan, Hubei*
*P.R. China*

CHRISTOPHER JOHNNIDES, M.D.
*General Surgery Resident*
*Allegheny General Hospital*
*Pittsburgh, PA*

NANCY B. KIVIAT, M.D.
*Professor of Pathology*
*Department of Pathology*
*University of Washington*
*Harborview Medical Center*
*Seattle, WA*

MARK J. KRASNA, M.D.
*Professor of Surgery*
*Head, Division of Thoracic Surgery and*
*Director of Thoracic Oncology*
*The University of Maryland Medical Center*
*Baltimore, MD*

MATTHEW H. KULKE, M.D.
*Assistant Professor of Medicine*
*Harvard Medical School*
*Department of Medical Oncology*
*Dana-Farber Cancer Institute*
*Boston, MA*

SANDEEP LAHOTI, M.D.
*Gastroenterologist*
*Medical Clinic of Houston*
*Houston, TX*

GREGORY Y. LAUWERS, M.D.
*Associate Professor of Pathology*
*Harvard Medical School*
*Director, Gastrointestinal Pathology Service*
*Department of Pathology*
*Massachusetts General Hospital*
*Boston, MA*

NICHOLAS R. LEMOINE, M.D., Ph.D., F.R.C.Path.
*Professor of Molecular Pathology*
*Imperial Cancer Research Fund*
*Molecular Oncology Unit*
*Imperial College School of Medicine*
*Hammersmith Hospital*
*London, U.K.*

DONGHUI LI, Ph.D.
*Assistant Professor*
*Department of Gastrointestinal Medical Oncology*
*UT M. D. Anderson Cancer Center*
*Houston, TX*

PAUL J. LIMBURG, M.D., M.P.H.
*Assistant Professor of Medicine*
*Mayo Medical School*
*Division of Gastroenterology*
*Head, Colorectal Neoplasia Interest Group*
*Mayo Foundation*
*Rochester, MN*

REGINALD V. N. LORD, F.R.A.C.S.
*Assistant Professor of Surgery*
*University of Southern California*
*Keck School of Medicine*
*Los Angeles, CA*

ANDREW M. LOWY, M.D.
*Assistant Professor*
*Chief, Surgical Oncology*
*University Of Cincinnati Medical Center*
*Cincinnati, OH*

HENRY T. LYNCH, M.D.
*Chairman, Department of*
*Preventive Medicine/Public Health*
*Hereditary Cancer Institute*
*Creighton University School of Medicine*
*Omaha, NE*

PATRICK M. LYNCH, J.D., M.D.
*Associate Professor, Department of*
*Gastrointestinal Medicine and Nutrition*
*UT M. D. Anderson Cancer Center*
*Houston, TX*

PAUL F. MANSFIELD, M.D.
*Associate Professor*
*Department of Surgical Oncology*
*UT M. D. Anderson Cancer Center*
*Houston, TX*

ROBERT J. MAYER, M.D.
*Professor of Medicine,*
*Harvard Medical School*
*Director, Center for Gastrointestinal Oncology*
*Department of Medical Oncology*
*Dana-Farber Cancer Institute*
*Boston, MA*

CORNELIUS McGINN, M.D.
*Assistant Professor*
*University of Michigan Medical School*
*Department of Radiation Oncology*
*University of Michigan Health System*
*Ann Arbor, MI*

DIANA MEDGYESY, M.D.
*Medical Oncology*
*Rocky Mountain Cancer Center*
*Fort Collins, CO*

WILSON MERTENS, M.D.
*Medical Director, Cancer Center*
*Baystate Medical Center*
*Springfield, MA*

BRUCE D. MINSKY, M.D.
*Department of Radiation Oncology*
*Memorial Sloan-Kettering Cancer Center*
*New York, NY*

STEVEN F. MOSS, M.D., M.R.C.P.
*Associate Professor of Medicine*
*Brown University School of Medicine*
*Division of Gastroenterology*
*Department of Medicine*
*Rhode Island Hospital*
*Providence, RI*

GEORGE MUTEMA, M.D., Ph.D.
*Assistant Professor of Clinical Medicine*
*Department of Pathology and Laboratory Medicine*
*University of Cincinnati*
*College of Medicine*
*Cincinnati, OH*

ALFRED I. NEUGUT, M.D., Ph.D.
*Professor of Medicine and Public Health (Epidemiology)*
*College of Physicians & Surgeons*
*Head, Cancer Prevention and Control*
*Herbert Irving Comprehensive Cancer Center*
*Columbia University*
*New York, NY*

AMY NOFFSINGER, M.D.
*Assistant Professor of Pathology and Laboratory Medicine*
*College of Medicine*
*University of Cincinnati*
*Cincinnati, OH*

ROBERT D. ODZE, M.D., F.R.C.P.(C)
*Associate Professor of Pathology*
*Harvard Medical School*
*Director, Gastrointestinal Pathology Service*
*Brigham and Women's Hospital*
*Boston, MA*

KIRANPREET S. PARMAR, M.D.
*4434 Amboy Road*
*Staten Island, NY 10312*

SHREYASKUMAR R. PATEL, M.D.
*Associate Professor*
*Department of Sarcoma Medical Oncology*
*UT M. D. Anderson Cancer Center*
*Houston, TX*

YEHUDA Z. PATT, M.D.
*Professor of Oncology*
*University of Maryland*
*Greenebaum Cancer Center*
*Baltimore, MD*

THOMAS G. PAULSON, Ph.D.
*Programs in Gastrointestinal Oncology and Cancer Biology*
*Divisions of Human Biology and Public Health Sciences*
*Fred Hutchinson Cancer Research Center*
*Department of Medicine (Gastroenterology Division)*
*University of Washington*
*Seattle, WA*

PETER W. T. PISTERS, M.D., F.A.C.S.
*Associate Professor*
*Department of Surgical Oncology*
*UT M. D. Anderson Cancer Center*
*Houston, TX*

JAMES PLUDA, M.D.
*Investigational Drug Branch*
*Cancer Therapy Evaluation Program (CTEP)*
*National Cancer Institute*
*Rockville, MD*

RAPHAEL E. POLLOCK, M.D., Ph.D.
*Head, Division of Surgery*
*Professor and Chairman,*
*Department of Surgical Oncology*
*UT M. D. Anderson Cancer Center*
*Houston, TX*

GEOFFREY PORTER, M.D.
*QEII Health Sciences Center*
*Halifax, Nova Scotia, Canada*

BARBARA PRO, M.D.
*Assistant Professor*
*Department of Lymphoma*
*UT M. D. Anderson Cancer Center*
*Houston, TX*

JOE B. PUTNAM, JR., M.D.
*Professor and Deputy Chairman*
*Department of Thoracic and Cardiovascular Surgery*
*UT M. D. Anderson Cancer Center*
*Houston, TX*

DAVID RABEN, M.D.
*Associate Professor*
*Department of Radiation Oncology*
*University of Colorado Health Sciences Center*
*Anschutz Cancer Pavilion*
*Aurora, CO*

ISAAC RAIJMAN, M.D., F.A.C.P.
*Clinical Associate Professor*
*Director of Endoscopy*
*University of Texas*
*Houston Health Science Center*
*Houston, TX*

ASIF RASHID, M.D., Ph.D.
*Associate Professor*
*Department of Pathology*
*UT M. D. Anderson Cancer Center*
*Houston, TX*

PAVAN REDDY, M.D.
*Lecturer, Department of Internal Medicine*
*Hematology/Oncology*
*Comprehensive Cancer Center*
*University of Michigan Health System*
*Ann Arbor, MI*

RAYBURN REGO, M.D.
*Gastroenterologist*
*St John's Health Systems*
*Mountain View, MO*

BRIAN J. REID, Ph.D., M.D.
*Programs in Gastrointestinal Oncology and Cancer Biology*
*Divisions of Human Biology and Public Health Sciences*
*Fred Hutchinson Cancer Research Center*
*Departments of Medicine (Gastroenterology Division) and*
 *Genetics*
*University of Washington*
*Seattle, WA*

JASON M. ROBKE, M.D.
*General Surgery Resident*
*Allegheny General Hospital*
*Pittsburgh, PA*

MARK S. ROH, M.D.
*Chair, Department of Surgery, and*
*Director, Division of Surgical Oncology,*
*Allegheny General Hospital*
*Professor, Human Oncology, and*
*Professor, Surgery,*
*Drexel University College of Medicine*
*Pittsburgh, PA*

MACE L. ROTHENBERG, M.D.
*Professor of Medicine,*
*Vanderbilt University Medical Center*
*Ingram Professor of Cancer Research and*
*Director, Phase I Drug Development Program*
*Vanderbilt-Ingram Cancer Center*
*Nashville, TN*

MELANIE ROYCE, M.D.
*Assistant Professor*
*Department of Breast Medical Oncology*
*UT M. D. Anderson Cancer Center*
*Houston, TX*

MACK T. RUFFIN, IV, M.D.
*Associate Professor*
*Department of Family Medicine*
*University of Michigan Health System*
*Ann Arbor, MI*

LEONARD B. SALTZ, M.D.
*Associate Attending Physician*
*Department of Medicine*
*Gastrointestinal Oncology Service*
*Memorial Sloan-Kettering Cancer Center*
*New York, NY*

ANTONIA R. SEPULVEDA, M.D., Ph.D.
*Assistant Professor of Pathology*
*University of Pittsburgh Medical Center*
*UPMC Presbyterian Hospital*
*Department of Pathology*
*Pittsburgh, PA*

HAIM SHIRIN, M.D.
*Division of Gastroenterology*
*Department of Medicine*
*Edith Wolfson Medical Center*
*Holon, Israel*

IMAD SHUREIQI, M.D.
*Assistant Professor*
*Department of Clinical Cancer Prevention*
*UT M. D. Anderson Cancer Center*
*Houston, TX*

JOHN M. SKIBBER, M.D.
*Associate Professor*
*Department of Surgical Oncology*
*UT M. D. Anderson Cancer Center*
*Houston, TX*

WILLIAM SMALL, JR., M.D.
*Assistant Professor*
*Division of Radiation Oncology*
*Robert H. Lurie Comprehensive*
*Cancer Center of Northwestern University*
*Chicago, IL*

DAVID L. SMITH, M.D.
*Clinical Fellow*
*Department of Surgical Oncology*
*UT M. D. Anderson Cancer Center*
*Houston, TX*

THOMAS C. SMYRK, M.D.
*Transplant Center/Pathology*
*Mayo Clinic*
*Rochester, MN*

LESLIE H. SOBIN, M.D., F.R.C.Path.
*Chief, Division of Gastrointestinal Pathology*
*Armed Forces Institute of Pathology*
*Washington, D.C.*

ROGER D. SOLOWAY, M.D.
*Marie B. Gale Centennial*
*Professor of Medicine*
*Division of Gastroenterology*
*Department of Internal Medicine*
*The University of Texas*
*Medical Branch at Galveston*
*Galveston, TX*

STUART JON SPECHLER, M.D.
*Chief, Division of Gastroenterology*
*Dallas VA Medical Center*
*Dallas, TX*

IRA J. SPIRO, M.D., Ph.D.*
*(Dr. Spiro is deceased-his last address is shown)*
*Department of Radiation Oncology*
*Massachusetts General Hospital*
*Boston, MA*

*Deceased

MARGARET R. SPITZ, M.D., M.P.H.
*Professor and Chair*
*Department of Epidemiology*
*UT M. D. Anderson Cancer Center*
*1515 Holcombe Boulevard*
*Houston, TX*

GRANT STEMMERMANN, M.D.
*Professor, Department of Pathology and Laboratory Medicine*
*University of Cincinnati*
*College of Medicine*
*Cincinnati, OH*

FLORIAN M. STRASSER, M.D.
*Clinical Fellow*
*Department of Palliative Care*
*& Rehabilitation Medicine*
*UT M. D. Anderson Cancer Center*
*Houston, TX*

LI-KUO SU, Ph.D.
*Assistant Professor*
*Department of Molecular and Cellular Oncology*
*UT M. D. Anderson Cancer Center*
*Houston, TX*

EIICHI TAHARA, M.D., Ph.D., F.R.C.Path.
*Professor Emeritus, Hiroshima University*
*Chairman, Hiroshima Cancer Seminar Foundation*
*Hiroshima*
*Japan*

MARK S. TALAMONTI, M.D., F.A.C.S.
*Professor and Chief, Surgical Oncology*
*Department of Surgery*
*Northwestern University*
*The Feinberg School of Medicine*
*Chicago, IL*

MARGARET A. TEMPERO, M.D.
*Deputy Director*
*University of California San Francisco*
*Comprehensive Cancer Center*
*San Francisco, CA*

LARISSA K. F. TEMPLE, M.D., F.R.C.S.(C)
*Department of Surgery/Colorectal Service*
*Memorial Sloan-Kettering Cancer Center*
*New York, NY*

PAULA M. TERMUHLEN, M.D.
*Assistant Professor, Department of Surgery*
*Wright State University*
*Kettering Medical Center*
*Kettering, OH*

CHRIS TSELEPIS, M.D.
*Department of Medicine and Cancer Research*
*University of Birmingham*
*Birmingham, U.K.*

JEAN-NICOLAS VAUTHEY, M.D.
*Professor*
*Department of Surgical Oncology*
*UT M. D. Anderson Cancer Center*
*Houston, TX*

JAYE L. VINER, M.D.
*Program Director*
*Gastrointestinal and Other Cancer Research Group*
*Division of Cancer Prevention*
*National Cancer Institute, NIH*
*Bethesda, MD*

IRVING WAXMAN, M.D.
*Director of Endoscopy and*
*Professor of Clinical Medicine*
*University of Chicago*
*Chicago, IL*

CHRISTOPHER G. WILLETT, M.D.
*Associate Professor of Radiation Oncology*
*Harvard Medical School*
*Director of Intraoperative Radiation Therapy*
*Department of Radiation Oncology*
*Massachusetts General Hospital*
*Boston, MA*

HENRY Q. XIONG, M.D.
*Assistant Professor*
*Department of Gastrointestinal Medical Oncology*
*UT M. D. Anderson Cancer Center*
*Houston, TX*

JAMES C. YAO, M.D.
*Assistant Professor*
*Department of Gastrointestinal Medical Oncology*
*UT M. D. Anderson Cancer Center*
*Houston, TX*

# Part I

# General Principles

# Chapter 1

# Epidemiological Principles for the Study of Gastrointestinal Cancers

CHRISTOPHER I. AMOS AND MARGARET R. SPITZ

This chapter discusses some of the general principles and designs used in epidemiological studies of gastrointestinal cancers, with an emphasis on molecular and genetic epidemiological methods. These newer methods have come to play an important role in understanding the etiology of gastrointestinal cancers, yet textbook discussions of these methods are limited. Also, because of the importance and difficulty of measuring dietary intake, we shall include a short section describing some of the major dietary assessment tools. We close the chapter with a section discussing informed consent for epidemiological studies.

## Measures of Risk

Epidemiological studies cannot be designed as controlled experiments in which a potential risk factor is introduced into a population. Therefore, epidemiological studies are observational, and the results measure associations between risk factors and disease outcomes. Associations can be useful for classifying individuals into risk sets, regardless of whether a causal relationship between the disease and its correlate can be established. Typical measures of risk include the absolute risk, relative risk, and odds ratio. Here we briefly describe the main risk measures; much more detail can be found in standard epidemiological reference texts such those by Rothman and Sander[1] (1998) or by Selvin (1996).[2]

*Absolute risk* is the most easily interpreted risk measure; it is usually specified in terms of risk per time unit per individual. Using the cells defined by Table 1–1, the absolute risk among exposed individuals per unit time is $a/(a + c)$. The *relative risk* is the risk for disease among individuals who have been exposed to a risk factor, divided by the risk for disease among individuals who have not been exposed to that risk factor. From Table 1–1, the relative risk from an exposure is: $[a/(a + c)]/[b/(b + d)]$. The *odds ratio* is the ratio of the probabilities of exposure among the diseased persons to the probability of exposure among the nondiseased persons, divided by the probability of nonexposure among the diseased persons divided by the probability of nonexposure among the nondiseased persons. From Table 1–1, this ratio is $[a/b]/[c/d]$. When the frequency of cases in a population is low, the odds ratio approximates the relative risk. For relative risks greater than 1, the odds ratio overestimates the relative risk, but the odds ratio is nearly unbiased when studying uncommon events such as the risk of developing specific cancers.

Odds ratios are used to estimate relative risks for several reasons. In case–control studies, if the frequency of disease is not well established in the target population but is nevertheless uncommon, the odds ratio gives a nearly unbiased estimate of the relative risk. Also, commonly used tools for analysis of data such as logistic regression readily provide an estimate of the odds ratio. However, for common diseases (i.e., those that occur in more than 10% of the population), the odds ratio substantially overestimates the relative risk.

## Assessing Causality in Epidemiological Studies

Because epidemiological studies are usually observational by design, unmeasured variables can affect the results and interpretation of the studies. A variable is called a *confounder* if it is correlated with both the disease presence and with one or more of the predictors that are being studied. When confounders can be measured, they must be included in the analysis, as their inclusion reduces bias and increases the precision of risk estimates.

To establish a causal relationship between a risk factor and a disease outcome, Hill[3] suggested evaluating the following characteristics of the association: *(1)* strength, *(2)* consistency, *(3)* specificity, *(4)* temporality, *(5)* biologic gradient, *(6)* plausibility, *(7)* coherence, *(8)* experimental evidence, and *(9)* analogy. By

**Table 1-1** Parameters for calculating risk in epidemiological studies

|  | *Exposed* | *Not Exposed* |  |
| --- | --- | --- | --- |
| Diseased | $a$ | $b$ | $a + b$ |
| Not diseased | $c$ | $d$ | $c + d$ |
|  | $a + c$ | $b + d$ |  |

strength of the association, we mean that causal associations should be stronger than noncausal associations.

*Consistency,* the second of Hill's postulates for showing causality, means that different studies having similar designs should lead to similar observations. Provided the individuals included in each study have similar characteristics, any fluctuation in risk estimates across studies should reflect chance variation. Larger studies should provide a more reliable estimate of the risk associated with an exposure. Unfortunately, epidemiological studies cannot be duplicated exactly because the same study subjects will not be selected into different studies. Questionnaires and other protocols for data collection often differ between studies, and this lack of standardization can be a source of variability. In addition, some characteristics of the study subjects may vary between studies. When important potential confounders are not included in the analyses they can affect the consistency of results across studies. Thus, it is important that methods for data collection and analysis are standardized when confirmatory studies are planned. To ensure that studies can be duplicated, each study must maintain protocol documents that include a careful description of the study population, the control population (if applicable) and its selection, and all of the questionnaires, data collection tools, and laboratory assays that were used. Whenever possible, standardized questions (e.g., those used in national healthy surveys) are recommended to ensure consistency of data with data from other sources. Emphases on layout, logical sequence, and user-friendly format are important. The Co-operative Family Registry for Colorectal Cancer has assembled an extensive set of questionnaires relevant to colorectal cancer. These can be obtained through request from the National Institutes of Health, at the URL http://www.infosystems.epi.uci.edu/contacts.htm#cfrbccs. The design issues relevant to collecting genetic and epidemiological data for studying colorectal cancer have been thoroughly described by Haile and co-workers.[4]

The other postulates from Hill[3] require less explanation. By *temporality,* we mean that causal events must precede the disease outcome. Studies designed to study the etiology of a disease usually focus on studies of newly incident cases. The prevalent cases of disease reflect both the incidence of the disease as well as the lethality of the disease, so that interpreting results from prevalent cases can be difficult. *Biological gradient* means that higher levels of exposure should be associated with higher risk. Sometimes a threshold effect may be anticipated in which levels of exposure beyond a certain level do not increase risk beyond that of the threshold value. Some of Hill's attributes are infrequently available (experimental evidence) or may not be very helpful for establishing causality (specificity, coherence, and analogy).

## Basic Designs of Epidemiological Studies

### Cohort Studies

*Prospective* cohort studies are performed by identifying a group of subjects, interviewing them, and collecting samples and/or data from them at baseline and then following them forward in time. The advantage of this design is that one can easily establish temporal relationships between events and causes, and biases relating to incomplete recall of exposures are minimized. In addition, both absolute risk and relative risk measures of disease can be estimated.[5] Another advantage may be the availability of prediagnostic specimens, if these are collected as a part of the design. The disadvantages of this design include the difficulty of maintaining follow-up with the study subjects and potential inefficiency if the disease outcome of interest is rare or infrequent in the study population. One approach to limit the cost of the prospective cohort design is to set up the cohort and then conduct laboratory analyses only for study subjects who become affected with the disease of interest along with a matched set of study subjects who do not become affected. This type of design is called a *nested case–control* design because it is a case–control study nested within a cohort.[6]

*Retrospective* cohort designs are conducted by identifying a set of study subjects at the present time and then tracing their histories into the past. This design provides estimates of absolute and relative risk, and it is usually easier to collect data using this design than for a prospective cohort study. However, the retrospective design is more subject to biases that can occur if the study subjects are required to recall past exposures. In addition, biases can develop in cohort studies if the current study subjects reflect a biased sampling from the target population. This design is often used for family studies, in which a person is asked to provide information about the time to onset for cancer or other diseases for his/her relatives. In this case, the relatives form a retrospective cohort.[7]

### Case-Control Studies and Control Selection

Epidemiologists often use case–control studies because they are relatively easy to conduct. The case population is sampled according to a predetermined protocol. The gold standard is population-based case ascertainment.[8] This generally requires a rapid case-ascertainment system tied to an incident cancer registry. If one is planning phenotypic or functional assays, patients should be enrolled as soon as possible after diagnosis and before treatment is initiated.[9]

Controls must be selected to be comparable with the cases,[10] but selecting a suitable control population is challenging since identifying the characteristics that ensure comparability with the case population is not easily accomplished. To avoid selection biases, the controls have to be sampled from the control population according to a well-controlled scheme. For example, when cases are referred to a population-based registry, the controls should be randomly sampled from other members of that population. Often, controls are matched according to criteria that are known to be related to the disease risk. Matching minimizes the variability among subjects attributable to known risk factors that may not be of interest and hence increases the efficiency of a study to detect novel associations.[11] For matching, controls are often grouped into strata with the cases according to demographic characteristics such as age, ethnicity, and gender. In this case, controls are not matched specifically with cases so that the subsequent analysis is performed unconditionally with respect to matching of cases with specific controls. In the unconditional analyses, the effects of the stratifying variables are included in the analysis as confounders, so that effects from other potential predictors can be accurately assessed. Sometimes, tight matching of controls to cases is performed. In this case, the analysis is usually performed using a conditional analysis in which each case is matched to its control or set of controls.[1,2]

The comparison population should ideally be comparable to the patient population in terms of socioeconomic status and other unmeasured determinants. There are several methods of accruing controls. One is to use random-digit telephone dialing, but when it is necessary to obtain blood samples from each participant, one must anticipate a low response rate from this method. In addition, because of the frequent use of Caller ID devices, at least one-fourth of residential subscribers are able to screen out unfamiliar callers. As a result, there may be an increased potential for sample bias if this approach is used. Using sibling controls could lead to overmatching from the standpoint of the genetic profile. Use of peer controls is a convenient and inexpensive approach that to some extent controls for age, ethnicity, social class, and lifestyle factors. However, this approach does not work in studies of patients with recently diagnosed, potentially lethal diseases.[12] A popular method for selecting controls has been to use data tapes from the Department of Public Safety Driver and Motor Vehicle Bureau, but because older adults may no longer have driver's licenses, this approach might exclude potential controls. Furthermore, several states have passed legislation banning distribution of lists of registered drivers with names and addresses.

A tradeoff may be necessary between epidemiological rigor and feasibility. While population-based studies are the gold standard for epidemiological case–control research, one may be unable to conduct population-based studies for practical reasons, for example, when studying very rare diseases for which the catchment population would be prohibitively large or for studying diseases that are very rapidly lethal. Population-based external control data are readily available from a variety of sources. The Surveillance, Epidemiology and End-Results registries[13] (SEER) (http://seer.cancer.gov/Publications/) provide extensive data from several very large population-based registries. This data resource, however, does not currently include data concerning environmental or lifestyle-related exposures. SEER data are useful for evaluating the similarity of one's case population to population-based attributes. Moreover, statistical methods can be applied to embed one's case–control study into the larger population-based registry, provided the control group can be represented by the population that is covered by one of the SEER registries.[14] The Connecticut tumor registry[15] has been in existence for a century and so forms an excellent external control that can allow for secular trends in the risks for cancer for the historical cohort design often used in family studies. Finally, the American Cancer Society (http://www2.cancer.org/research/) has also assembled two very large cohorts of subjects who were healthy at enrollment.[16] In summary, constructing an optimal design for an epidemiological study requires careful attention to the sources of study subjects. In general, avoiding bias is easier when using a cohort study, but prospective cohort studies are prohibitively expensive and often inefficient for studies of biomarkers. Case–control studies are cost-effective, but selection of adequate controls and minimizing of sources of bias are difficult design issues.

## Case–Control Studies for Evaluating Screening Efficacy

Controlled randomized trials are the gold standard for measuring the ability of a screening modality to reduce mortality. These trials are costly. Case–control studies can also be used to evaluate the efficacy of screening tests. The case–control design is less costly, but owing to its retrospective nature and lack of randomization, case–control studies may be more prone to bias.[17] In such screening studies, cases would be persons who have developed advanced disease or died from cancer. According to Weiss and Lazovich,[18] controls should be chosen to represent the screening experience of the population at risk of developing cancer. In practice, it is often desirable to obtain screening histories from persons newly diagnosed with cancer. Those subjects who develop progressive disease or die will become the "cases," and controls can be chosen to represent the screening experience of the underlying population from which the incident cases arose, generally a source population composed of nondiseased and diseased, non-case subjects.

Exposure in this instance is the screening test. It is important to separate true screening from tests performed because of the presence of symptoms. The cases and controls must have similar risk for "exposure," i.e., to be screened. Therefore, it is usual that the exposure period ends when the case subject is diagnosed. Weiss[19] stresses that the analysis must focus explicitly on screening during the premalignant phase. This requires an estimate of the duration of the occult invasive but asymptomatic phase and identifiable premalignancy (polyp).

## Genetic Epidemiological Designs

Genetic epidemiological methods are designed to characterize the familial and genetic risk for disease and to identify and characterize the causative genetic factors. Genetic factors are important determinants of risk for a minority of cancers occurring through the digestive tract, and it is therefore useful to understand some of the methods that are used in genetic epidemiology. Genetic epidemiological methods for gene characterization of cancer susceptibility have been reviewed by Thomas,[20] and methods for gene discovery have been reviewed by Schaid and co-workers.[21]

### Assessing Familiality and Segregation Analysis

As mentioned above, a commonly used tool in genetic epidemiology is the historical cohort design. In this design, families are selected through an index case or proband. Information is then collected from relatives of the proband about their current age, age at onset for cancer(s), and age at death. Data from many cancers are reliably collected from first-degree relatives but may not be very reliable for more distant relatives.[22,23] Where feasible, information about epidemiological risk factors can be collected. Proxy questionnaires must be collected from the deceased relatives, thus limiting the extent of epidemiological data that can be reliably collected from the relatives. In some cases, information about the proband may help to define risk strata for the relatives. The *kin–cohort* design[24,25] is a version of the historical cohort method in which mutation data and other information from the proband is used to construct penetrance estimates for the mutations. Specifically, the age to onset among first-degree relatives of mutation-positive probands is compared with the age to onset among first-degree relatives of mutation-negative probands. This approach can efficiently estimate *penetrance,* which is the probability of developing a disease, given one's underlying, inferred genotype. However, to estimate risks accurately from family studies, ascertainment corrections, which allow for the selection process by which subjects were accrued into the study, must be applied.[26,27]

*Segregation analysis* is an alternative approach for estimating the penetrance of genetic factors predisposing for cancer. Segregation analyses seek to identify the relationship between an individual's genotype and the resulting phenotype. Inheritance of genetic factors results in a specific form of genotype dependence among family members. Although the genotypes at a disease locus cannot usually be directly measured, the inheritance of disease within families can be compared with that expected under specific genetic models. In segregation analysis, we search for the model that most closely approximates the observed familial data. The models evaluated by classic segregation analyses include a major genetic factor, environmental effects that may be correlated among family members, and polygenic effects.[28,29] These polygenic effects model the inheritance of many independent genetic factors, each having small effects. Fitting mixed major gene and polygenic models to large pedigrees is computationally difficult, and alternative strategies have been developed. An excellent approach is to replace the exact numerical integrations with an approximation of the cumulative normal distribution; this approach has been implemented by Sandra Hasstedt in her program PAP.[30] The regressive model[31,32] evaluates the dependence from familial influences by a sequential conditioning argument. Conditional on the major-gene influences, the affection of a relative can also affect an individual's risk for affection in this modeling strategy. This approach can easily accommodate effects from epidemiological risk factors and provides an excellent approximation to data from complex pedigrees.

Segregation analyses usually assume that only a single major genetic factor is modeled, because trying to fit multiple genetic factors is technically difficult, and the parameters corresponding to effects from multiple genetic factors may not be jointly identifiable. Recent studies using Monte Carlo Markov chain methods[33] have been able to jointly model effects from several unlinked genetic loci, each having a different impact on the age to onset for disease.

## Linkage Analysis

Genetic linkage studies are implemented once evidence for major-gene inheritance has been provided and a genetic model has been defined by segregation analysis. In *linkage studies,* the coinheritance of inferred disease susceptibility with genetic markers is evaluated. The results of linkage studies can provide definitive evidence for major-gene effects upon disease susceptibility and can also indicate the gene's approximate location for subsequent positional-cloning strategies. The observations in a linkage study consist of the disease status and marker values of related individuals in families, and families are the sampling units. The unit of analysis becomes the separable meiotic events from which the recombination events can be identified. Parametric linkage studies can be implemented without exact knowledge of the genetic model characterizing disease risk without risk of increased false-positive evidence for linkage.[34] In this case, an approximate model can be specified. Greenberg et al.[35] showed that performing analysis under either a recessive or dominant model can lead to reasonable power for a number of different genetic models. Alternatively, model-free methods can be applied.[36] Model-free methods including age-specific risks for disease have recently been developed.[37,38]

## Risk Assessment and Molecular Epidemiology

Traditional epidemiological research relies on measures of "external exposure" (usually self-reported) in defining disease exposure associations. Such an approach to this classical epidemiology is limited in its capability to evaluate factors beyond age, gender, and ethnicity that affect host susceptibility to carcinogenic exposure. Once carcinogen-induced genetic and epigenetic

events began to be elucidated either by genetic epidemiological studies or from analysis of mouse models, knowledge of the molecular etiology of cancer rapidly began to accrue. The newer molecular epidemiology paradigm represents the confluence of sophisticated advances in molecular biology with field-tested epidemiological methodology. There is now increasing interest in the use of biomarkers in cancer epidemiology to enhance exposure assessment, gain insight into disease mechanisms, understand susceptibility, and refine risk assessment.

Vineis and Caporaso[39] have categorized molecular epidemiological studies into three categories: *(1)* markers of interindividual differences in susceptibility; *(2)* measures of internal exposures (including dose to the target tissue—DNA; and *(3)* early biological effects of exposure (e.g., cytogenetic damage, mutations).

## Markers of Interindividual Differences in Susceptibility

Any factor that influences carcinogen absorption, distribution, or accumulation in the target tissue will affect cancer susceptibility. The challenge in quantitative human risk assessment of carcinogenic exposures is to account for this interindividual variation in susceptibility that may occur at any phase of carcinogenesis. There is a rapidly expanding body of literature suggesting that genetically determined factors abrogate the effects of environmental carcinogens and that this biologic variability may occur at any phase of the multistage carcinogenic process. Evaluation of these differences is part of the broad field of ecogenetics, the study of genetically determined differences in response to environmental agents.

For example, the dose of carcinogens to which a target tissue is exposed is modulated by genetic polymorphisms in the enzymes responsible for activation and detoxification of these carcinogens. Genetic differences in these pathways are an important source of interindividual difference in susceptibility. These polymorphisms, although generally associated with weak effect on the risks for cancer, are frequent in the population, and therefore the associated attributable risks may be fairly high. An individual's cancer risk is therefore likely to be defined by the balance between metabolic activation and detoxification of xenobiotic compounds, as well as by the efficiency of DNA repair. It is most likely that multiple susceptibility factors jointly determine the manner in which environmental or lifestyle factors influence cancer susceptibility. Study of susceptibility to common cancers and widely prevalent exposures may provide further insights into the basic mechanisms of carcinogenesis.

Common cancers are unlikely to be caused by a single explanatory gene or gene–environmental interaction. A single genetic variant may not have a strong effect but, in conjunction with other variants, may shift the risk profile in an unfavorable direction. Multiple susceptibility factors must therefore be accounted for to evaluate the effect of gene–environmental interactions on common cancer risks.

## Markers of Internal Exposure

The net effect of exogenous carcinogen exposure and inherited traits for absorption, metabolism, and DNA repair is the carcinogen–DNA adduct.[40] This interrelationship between susceptibility markers and measurements of biologically effective dose, such as nitrosamine–DNA adducts, is the focus of considerable interest and may be useful for estimating the risk attributable to germline mutations.[40] DNA–carcinogen adducts are reaction products, often formed during the biotransformation of chemical carcinogens by xenobiotic metabolizing enzymes to reactive intermediates that are electrophilic and can therefore bind covalently to DNA. DNA adducts can be removed by DNA repair processes; however, chronic exposure often leads to steady-state accumulation in a target tissue. The biological potential of a given DNA adduct depends on many factors, including its mutagenic potential, reparability, location within a target gene, and, of course, the nature of the target gene. In general, however, the steady-state levels of specific DNA–carcinogen adducts in target tissues during chronic exposure are the net result of exposure and of rates of absorption, metabolism, and repair.

### Markers of Biologic Effects of Exposure

An example of markers of the biologic effects of carcinogen exposure would include *p53* mutation analysis. Mutations in the *p53* tumor suppressor gene are the most common genetic alterations identified in human cancer, and such mutations can be used as "fingerprints" of specific exposures in molecular epidemiology.[39,41] Distinct differences in the mutational frequency and type are found in different tumor types and are attributed in part to the effects of specific mutagens. The distribution of mutations along the *p53* gene is nonrandom and is characterized by several mutational hot spots, especially at codons 157, 248, and 273, corresponding to amino acids within the DNA binding domain of p53.[42]

### Diet Assessment in Epidemiological Studies

A variety of dietary instruments are available to assess dietary intake. The commonly used food frequency questionnaires (FFQ) are often self-administered and assess the usual frequency of consumption from a list of foods over a specified time. The two most commonly used semiquantitative questionnaires are the Block Health Habits and History[43] and the Willett[44] questionnaire. Semiquantitative questionnaires ask how often foods are used in terms of a specified unit of consumption. Both questionnaires have been extensively evaluated for their validity and reproducibility.

The full-length Block questionnaire[43] was designed to include foods representing at least the top 90% of nutrient intake from the National Health and Nutrition Examination Survey data set. A shorter 60-item version includes foods representing the top 80% of nutrient intake. The Block questionnaire requests estimates of consumption daily, weekly, monthly, yearly, or never/rarely. Portion sizes are small, medium, or large. Scannable versions are also available. The Willett questionnaire[44] has one standard portion size for each food item, and respondents indicate their relative frequency of consumption using nine different alternatives (ranging from never to six or more times a day). For each instrument, daily nutrient intakes are estimated by multiplying frequency responses by specified portion size and nutrient values.

A comparison of these two instruments[45,46] showed that the Block instrument had an overall underestimation bias but was more successful in estimating an individual's proportional intake of energy from fat and carbohydrates than the Willett. The Willett instrument was better at classifying vitamin A and calcium intakes. Both instruments are continually undergoing revision. For assessing the influence of nutritional factors in the etiology of gastrointestinal malignancies, a section on food preparation and doneness should be added to assess intake of heterocyclic amines.[47]

Measurement error is often quite high for data collected from dietary instruments. Commonly used statistical methods such as logistic regression assume that predictors such as dietary measures reflect minimal measurement error. Generally, failing to allow for measurement error during the analysis leads to attenuation of effects and risk estimates towards the null hypothesis of no effect. Methods to allow for measurement error in dietary surveys have been developed by several groups.[48–50] Allowing for measurement error during the analysis corrects for the attenuation in risk estimates attributable to an exposure but does not generally affect hypothesis testing.

### Informed Consent for Epidemiological Studies

In the past, epidemiologists were able to utilize only "surrogate" or indirect markers of inherited susceptibility (such as family history). Now, specific gene mutations are being incorporated into epidemiological studies, raising issues of ethical, legal, and psychological concerns for study participants. These concerns are not the same for all genes being evaluated. For example, highly penetrant genes (such as *FAP*), although rare in the population, are associated with high absolute risks of colon cancer for carriers of the mutation. The implications associated with finding such mutations in study participants are substantial. Low-risk susceptibility genotypes, by contrast, are associated with low relative and absolute risks but may have high population-attributable risks (because of their high prevalence). It is far less likely that these low relative risks individually would affect clinical decision making or result in potential for discrimination.[51] It has been suggested that specimens be made anonymous, for complete protection of privacy for study subjects. However, this leads to a loss of vital information and may lead to inaccuracies. For example, follow-up studies that assess survivorship of subjects become impossible when samples are labeled anonymously.

Many ethical issues in the conduct of studies remain unresolved. For example, is it necessary to recontact subjects who participated in earlier studies to again obtain consent to conduct additional analyses on stored samples? Is such recontacting even feasible? Hunter and Caporaso[51] proposed a level of consent that should be proportional to the degree of risk involved. Thus, less stringent consent procedures may be appropriate for "low-risk" susceptibility genotypes. They also recommended a clear distinction between "the testing of hypotheses about potential genetic influences on disease in research studies [e.g., evaluating gene–environmental interactions] and the use of genetic testing in clinical settings."[51]

Investigators collecting sensitive information such as genetic test results and information on illicit drug use behavior or sexual behavior can apply for a certificate of confidentiality.[52] The certificate of confidentiality protects the investigator from discovery of patient records as a part of legal proceedings but has not yet undergone a legal challenge related to epidemiological studies. Current standards of many Institutional Review Boards do not require specific consent for the collection of nonsensitive lifestyle and environmental exposure information. However, informing subjects about the potential uses of their information is prudent and IRB review may facilitate future studies.

### References

1. Rothman KJ, Sander G. Modern Epidemiology, 2nd ed. Lippincott-Raven; Philadelphia, 1998.
2. Selvin S. Statistical Analysis of Epidemiologic Data, 2nd ed. Oxford University Press, New York, 1996.

3. Hill AB. The environment and disease. Association or causation? Proc R Soc Med 58:295–300, 1965.

4. Haile RW, Siegmund KD, Gauderman WJ, et al. Study-design issues in the development of the University of Southern California Consortium's colorectal cancer family registry. J Natl Cancer Inst Monogr 26:89–93, 1999.

5. Langholz B, Rothman N, Wacholder S, et al. Cohort studies for characterizing measured genes. J Natl Cancer Inst Monogr 29:39–42, 1999.

6. Wacholder S. Practical considerations in choosing between the case–cohort and nested case–control designs. Epidemiology 2:155–158, 1991.

7. Amos CI, Rubin L. Major gene analysis for disease and disorders of complex etiology. Exp Clin Immunogenet 12:141–155, 1995.

8. Zhao LP, Hsu L, Davidov O, et al. Population-based family study designs: an interdisciplinary research framework for genetic epidemiology. Genet Epidemiol 14:365–388, 1997.

9. Caporaso N, Rothman N, Wacholder S. Case–control studies of common alleles and environmental factors. J Natl Cancer Inst Monogr 26:31–38, 1999.

10. Wacholder S, McLaughlin JK, Silverman DT, et al. Selection of controls in case–control studies. I. Principles. Am J Epidemiol 135:1019–1028, 1992.

11. Stürmer T, Brenner H. Potential gain in efficiency and power to detect gene–environment interactions by matching in case–control studies. Genet Epidemiol 18:63–80, 2000.

12. Takeshima Y, Seyama T, Bennett WP, et al. *p53* mutations in lung cancers from non-smoking atomic-bomb survivors. Lancet 342:1520–1521, 1993.

13. Surveillance, Epidemiology and End Results (SEER) Program. Public Use Data (1973–1998), National Cancer Institute, DCCPS, Surveillance Research Program, Cancer Statistics Branch, released April 2001.

14. Wacholder S. The case–control study as data missing by design: estimating risk differences. Epidemiology 7:144–150, 1996.

15. State of Connecticut Department of Public Health. Cancer Incidence in Connecticut 1980–1996. 1999, pp. 1–36.

16. Thun MJ, Calle EE, Rodriguez C, Wingo PA. Epidemiological research at the American Cancer Society. Cancer Epidemiol Biomarkers Prev 9:861–868, 2000.

17. Cronin KA, Weed DL, Connor RJ, et al. Case–control studies of cancer screening: theory and practice [review]. J Natl Cancer Inst 90:498–504, 1998.

18. Weiss NS, Lazovich D. Case–control studies of screening efficacy: the use of persons newly diagnosed with cancer who later sustain an unfavorable outcome. Am J Epidemiol 143:319–322, 1996.

19. Weiss NS. Case–control studies of the efficacy of screening tests designed to prevent the incidence of cancer [commentary]. Am J Epidemiol 149:1–4, 1999.

20. Thomas DC. Design of gene characterization studies: an overview. J Natl Cancer Inst Monogr 26:17–24, 1999.

21. Schaid DJ, Buetow K, Weeks DE, et al. Discovery of cancer susceptibility genes: study designs, analytic approaches, and trends. J Natl Cancer Inst Monogr 26:1–26, 1999.

22. Airewele G, Adatto P, Cunningham J, et al. Family history of cancer in patients with glioma: a validation study of accuracy. J Natl Cancer Inst 90:543–544, 1998.

23. Love RR, Evans AM, Josten DM. The accuracy of patient reports of a family history of cancer. J Chronic Dis 38:289–293, 1985.

24. Gail MH, Pee D, Carroll R. Kin-cohort designs for gene characterization. J Natl Cancer Inst Monogr 26:55–60, 1999.

25. Wacholder S, Hartge P, Struewing, et al. The kin–cohort study for estimating penetrance. Am J Epidemiol 148:623–630, 1998.

26. Langholz B, Ziogas A, Thomas DC, Faucett C, Huberman M, Goldstein L. Ascertainment bias in rate ratio estimation from case–sibling control studies of variable age-at-onset diseases. Biometrics 55:1129–1136, 1999.

27. Olson JM, Cordell HJ. Ascertainment bias in the estimation of sibling genetic risk parameters. Genet Epidemiol 18:217–235, 2000.

28. Lalouel JM, Rao DC, Morton NE, et al. A unified model for complex segregation analysis. Am J Hum Genet 35:816–826, 1983.

29. Elston RC, Stewart J. A general model for the genetic analysis of pedigree data. Hum Hered 21:523–542, 1971.

30. Hasstedt SJ. A variance components/major locus likelihood approximation to quantitative data. Genet Epidemiol 8:113–125, 1991.

31. Bonney GE. Regressive logistic models for familial disease and other binary traits. Biometrics 42:611–625, 1986.

32. Demenais FM. Regressive logistic models for familial diseases. A formulation assuming an underlying liability model. Am J Hum Genet 49:773–785, 1991.

33. Daw EW, Payami H, Memens EJ, et al: The number of trait loci in late-onset Alzheimer's diseases. Am J Hum Genet 66:196–204, 2000.

34. Williamson JA, Amos CI. On the asymptotic behavior of the estimate of the recombination faction under the null hypothesis of no linkage when the model is misspecified. Genet Epidemiol 7:309–318, 1990.

35. Greenberg DA, Abreu P, Hodge SE. The power to detect linkage in complex disease by means of simple LOD-score analyses. Am J Hum Genet 63:870–879, 1998.

36. Whittemore AS. Genome scanning for linkage: an overview. Am J Hum Genet 59:704–716, 1996.

37. Li H, Thompson EA, Wijsman EM. Semiparametric estimation of major gene effects for age of onset. Genet Epidemiol 15:279–298, 1998.

38. Siegmund KD, Todorov AA. Linkage analysis for diseases with variable age of onset. Hum Hered 50:205–210, 2000.

39. Vineis P, Caporaso N. Tobacco and cancer epidemiology and the laboratory. Environ Health Perspect 103:156–160, 1995.

40. Shields PG. Pharmacogenetics: detecting sensitive populations. Environ Health Perspect 102:81–87, 1994.

41. Rothman N, Stewart WF, Schulte PA. Incorporating biomarkers into cancer epidemiology: a matrix of biomarker and study design categories. Cancer Epidemiol Biomarkers Prev 4:301–311, 1995.

42. Smith LE, Denissenko MF, Bennett WP, et al. Targeting of lung cancer mutational hotspots by polycyclic aromatic hydrocarbons. J Natl Cancer Inst 92:803–811, 2000.

43. Block G, Hartman AM, Dreser CM, et al. A data-based approach to diet questionnaire design and testing. Am J Epidemiol 124:453–469, 1986.

44. Willett WC, Reynolds RD, Cottrell-Hoehner S, et al. Validation of a semiquantitative food questionnaire; comparison with a 1-year diet record. J Am Diet Assoc 87:43–47, 1987.

45. Caan BJ, Slattery ML, Potter J, et al. Comparison of the Block and the Willett self-administered semiquantitative food frequency questionnaires with an interviewer-administered dietary history. Am J Epidemiol 148:1137–1147, 1998.

46. Wirfalt AK, Jeffery RW, Elmer PJ. Comparison of food frequency questionnaires: the reduced Block and Willett questionnaire differ in ranking on nutrient intakes. Am J Epidemiol 124:1148–1156, 1998.

47. Sinha R, Kulldorff M, Chow WH, et al. Dietary intake of heterocyclic amines, meat-derived mutagenic acitivty, and risk of colorectal adenomas. Cancer Epidemiol Biomarkers Prev 10:559–562, 2001.

48. Carroll RJ, Freedman L, Pee D. Design aspects of calibration studies in nutrition, with analysis of missing data in linear measurement error models. Biometrics 53:1440–1457, 1997.

49. Spiegelman D, McDermott A, Rosner B, et al. Regression calibration method for correcting measurement-error bias in nutritional epidemiology. Am J Clin Nutr 65(4 Suppl):1179S–1186S, 1997.

50. Wong MY, Day NE, Bashir SA, et al. Measurement error in epidemiology: the design of validation studies I: univariate situation. Stat Med 18:2815–2829, 1999.

51. Hunter D, Caporaso N. Informed consent in epidemiologic studies involving genetic markers. Epidemiology 8:596–599, 1997.

52. Earley CL, Strong LC. Certificates of confidentiality: a valuable tool for protecting genetic data. Am J Hum Genet 57:727–731, 1995.

# Chapter 2

# Prevention and Screening Principles Relevant to Gastrointestinal Malignancies

IMAD SHUREIQI, PAVAN REDDY, MACK T. RUFFIN, IV, AND DEAN E. BRENNER

Strategies for the prevention of any disease can be categorized as primary, secondary, or tertiary. *Primary prevention strategies* aim to reduce the incidence of disease and generally target the entire population without symptoms or disease. For gastrointestinal cancers, primary prevention strategies include diet or dietary supplements, smoking cessation, hepatitis B vaccine, avoidance or elimination of environmental carcinogens, and risk reduction.

*Secondary prevention strategies*, i.e., early detection or screening, aim to reduce disease-specific mortality and the duration and severity by finding the disease in an asymptomatic phase and instituting treatment early. For gastrointestinal cancers, secondary prevention strategies are the fecal occult blood test, digital rectal examination, flexible sigmoidoscopy, colonoscopy, air contrast barium enema, upper endoscopy, chemoprevention for individuals at high risk for cancer development.

*Tertiary prevention strategies* deal with patients with symptomatic disease. Tertiary prevention strategies in cancer focus on reducing the incidence of recurrence or on the early detection of recurrence and would include therapeutic vaccines.

This chapter has two aims. First, we will review the scientific approach to developing evidence for validating primary and secondary prevention services. Second, we will review the relevant data on primary and secondary prevention strategies for gastrointestinal cancers.

## Primary Prevention

The goal of primary prevention is to prevent the development of a disease. Primary prevention is directed at individuals susceptible to a particular disease and is used to reduce the incidence of that disease and its sequelae. The causes or risk factors for a disease must be established for primary prevention to be feasible.

Thus observational studies aimed at eliciting the risk factors and/or etiology of a specific disease are needed to develop primary prevention strategies.

Once various risk factors or causes of a specific disease have been well defined, then interventions to eliminate the risk can be developed and tested. Interventions include chemoprevention for asymptomatic individuals identified by risk assessment. A randomized controlled trial with the primary outcome of interest being prevention of the disease is the gold standard. As outlined below, other levels of evidence can be considered. Classic examples of well-accepted primary prevention strategies for cancer are smoking cessation and hepatitis B vaccines.

## Secondary Prevention

In contrast to primary prevention, secondary prevention with screening involves testing asymptomatic individuals to detect early subclinical disease. Determining the benefit and advisability of cancer screening is a difficult task that requires detailed investigation before widespread recommendations can be supported. The key criteria that should be considered before screening is adopted areas are as follows:

1. The disease should be a serious health problem imposing a significant burden of suffering on the population.
2. The target population should be clearly defined and have a reasonable disease prevalence.
3. The target population should be accessible.
4. The screening test should have acceptable performance sensitivity, specificity, and positive predictive value.
5. The test should be acceptable to the target population.
6. An effective treatment for the target cancer should be available, with evidence that early treatment alters the natural course of the disease.
7. A reasonable expectation should exist that individuals will have a positive screening test.

Several levels of evidence can be used to support a given position on cancer screening. As with primary prevention, a well-designed and carefully performed randomized controlled trial is the gold standard for developing a secondary prevention strategy; such a trial, however, is not practical or available for all screening procedures. Therefore, the following levels of evidence for validation of a secondary prevention maneuver have been established[1]:

1. Evidence from at least one randomized controlled trial
2. Evidence from controlled trials that use allocation methods other than randomization
3. Evidence from well-designed cohort or case–control studies, preferably from more than one research center or research group
4. Evidence from multiple time series with or without intervention
5. Dramatic results in uncontrolled experiments
6. Opinions of respected authorities

In developing and interpreting data on screening and research design, investigators and clinicians should be aware of two important issues: lead time bias and length bias. Individuals who participate in screening programs may harbor cancer and have the cancer detected earlier than it would have been in the absence of screening. Therefore, survival duration (a typical measure of importance to most physicians and patients) is automatically lengthened for cancers detected by screening, even if the individual does not live longer. This is lead time bias and makes survival time an invalid end point for determining the efficacy of a screening procedure. The screening procedure and subsequent early treatment must clearly alter the natural course of a disease to be considered beneficial.

Cancer screening is most likely to detect individuals who have longer periods of asymptomatic, subclinical disease. This overrepresentation of longer-duration preclinical disease introduces a bias that makes the screening procedure appear more effective. Individuals with more indolent or dormant preclinical disease have a far more favorable outcome than do individuals with shorter preclinical phases, unrelated to early detection.

Chemoprevention can also be a secondary prevention strategy when it is linked to identifying populations with precancerous disease, usually by screening. One example of chemoprevention is the use of nonsteroidal anti-inflammatory agents in populations with adenomatous colorectal polyps.

## Esophageal Cancer

Cancer of the esophagus is fatal with a short survival for most individuals diagnosed. It is the ninth most common cancer in the world, with approximately 300,000 new cases diagnosed every year.[2] Two major histologic types of esophageal cancer predominate—squamous cell carcinoma and adenocarcinoma. Squamous cell carcinoma is the predominant histologic type worldwide, with a unique geographic distribution suggesting important environmental and genetic contributions to its pathogenesis. The incidence of adenocarcinoma of the esophagus is rapidly rising among white men in first-world countries[3–6] and has recently surpassed the incidence of squamous cell carcinoma of the esophagus in the United States.[7] Because of the important differences in incidence, geographic distribution, and pathogenesis, the two main histologic types are discussed separately.

### Squamous Cell Carcinoma

#### Burden of suffering

The incidence rates of squamous cell carcinoma of the esophagus are very low in North Africa and West Africa and very high among black males in South and North America.[8] In Linxian populations (Henan Province of China), esophageal cancer occurs at an annual incidence rate of 161 new cases per 100,000 males and 103 new cases per 100,000 females. The north central and east central provinces of Shanxi, Henan, and Jiangsu have similarly high incidences, whereas southern provinces, such as Yunnan, Hunan, or Guangdong, have much lower incidences.[8] High incidences among both males and females are reported in populations of largely Turkic origin surrounding the eastern shore of the Caspian Sea (Turkmenistan, Kazakhstan, and bordering regions of northeast Iran).[8] In Europe, a high incidence is reported primarily in males of specific counties in Brittany and in the main whisky-distilling areas of Scotland.[8] In the United States, from 1950 to 1980, the mortality rates from squamous cell carcinoma of the esophagus increased among African Americans but the rate remained unchanged among Caucasians.[4,7,9] In Latin America, incidence rates have remained stable except in S o Paulo, Brazil, where the incidence among males and females has increased greatly. Latin American incidence rates are highest in Uruguay.[8]

#### Primary prevention strategies

In the United States and Western Europe, 90% or more of the risk of squamous cell carcinoma of the esophagus has been attributed to chronic alcohol and tobacco exposure; in other parts of the world, dietary and other environmental factors play larger roles.[4,9] Because smoking and alcohol are generally commingled factors, the effect of each upon carcinogenesis is difficult to discern. Tobacco-associated carcinogens may be delivered via chewing tobacco, by swallowing (e.g., betel juice),[10] or by inhaling smoke. A recent population-based study in Denmark found a moderate intake of wine does not increase the risk of squamous cell carcinoma of the esophagus, whereas a moderate intake of beer (7–21 glasses per week) considerably increased the risk after adjustment for smoking.[11] A parametric function devised by Breslow and Day[12] suggests that the risk of esophageal cancer rises exponentially with increasing alcohol consumption but rises linearly with increased tobacco smoking. Large population-based studies published to date[13,14] suggest that the lower risk in former smokers appears to be partially due to lower alcohol consumption.[8] Recently published data from a small case–control study in Spain suggest that withdrawal from either habit significantly reduces esophageal cancer risk whereas exposure to both synergistically enhanced risk, especially in women.[15]

The high-risk region of Henan Province of northern China is one of the most intensively studied regions for squamous cell carcinoma of the esophagus. Consumption of pickled vegetables, moldy foods, or foods contaminated with polycyclic aromatic hydrocarbons, silica fiber, or the fungus *Fuariarum moniliformis*[16–18] and work-related exposure to combustion products (by chimney sweeps, waster incinerator workers, bus-garage workers, and vulcanization workers)[19] or to metal dust, especially beryllium, have been cited as important risk factors.[20] Nutritional deficiencies, particularly in iron, zinc, selenium, and B complex and C vitamins, appear to play roles in carcinogenesis.[21,22] However, the precise carcinogenesis mechanisms and relative importance of each of these nutrients in the carcinogenesis process have yet to be unraveled. A diet deficient in fresh vegetables is an important risk factor for esophageal cancer.[23,24]

The role of infectious agents such as the human papillomavirus (HPV) upon risk and transformation in the esophagus is unclear. The use of highly sensitive polymerase chain-reaction (PCR) based methods, while enhancing the detection of HPV DNA in esophageal tissue or cellular samples, has not clarified whether HPV plays a pivotal carcinogenic role. For example, recent studies using different degenerate PCR approaches in two laboratories documented HPV DNA in 17% of 117 carcinomas studied and in 42% of 117 cytologic scrapings. Only 2% of the HPV DNA detected were the high-risk types HPV 16, 18, and 33.[25] Using in situ hybridization of paraffin-embedded samples, HPV DNA sequences were detected in 8% of 36 samples.[26]

Thermal injury appears to be important in the risk for esophageal cancer. In high-incidence regions of South America, maté, a hot beverage of *Ilex paraguayensis*, is drunk through a metal tube that brings hot liquid onto the posterior portion of the tongue, and the liquid is rapidly swallowed. The hot drink alone or the component of the maté combined with other risk variables such as alcohol intake or smoking may be responsible for the high incidence of esophageal cancer in this population.[27,28] Studies from other geographic areas appear to support this hypothesis. An increased risk of esophageal cancer has been demonstrated in Japanese who drink hot green tea,[24] Puerto Ricans who drink hot coffee,[22] and residents of the Eastern Caspian[29] and China areas who drink hot tea.[30]

A genetic susceptibility has been demonstrated by the association of esophageal cancer and keratosis palmaris et plantaris in two Liverpool families,[8] and by case–control studies in high-incidence areas. For example, the incidence (47%) of esophageal cancer in Turkoman patients with a positive family history is higher than the incidence (2%) in non-Turkoman patients living in the same region of northern Iran.[31] In China, the standardized mortality ratio of esophageal cancer among first-degree relatives of patients with esophageal cancer was 2.4. Pairwise association between parents, but not between siblings, suggests that environmental factors play a larger role in adults than in children.[32]

Specific inherited genetic mutations associated with such familial aggregations have not been discovered to date; however, a number of clues are emerging. The $p16^{INK4a}$ and $p15^{INK4b}$ genes, which encode cyclin-dependent kinase inhibitors localized to 9p21, might be altered and are common inactivation targets in esophageal cancers from Henan, China.[33] Glutathione-*S*-transferase M1- and T1-positive genotypes have a fourfold risk of developing esophageal cancer in Linxian (Henan Province) families.[34] Also, *p53* mutations in esophageal cancers in southern China have hot spots in exon 5, codon 176, whereas *p53* mutations are more evenly distributed in exons 5–8 in northern China.[35]

In first-world countries, the most important primary prevention strategy for squamous cell carcinoma of the esophagus has been the control of cigarette smoking and alcohol abuse. Approaches to control of alcohol and tobacco use have not been separately demonstrated to reduce the incidence of esophageal squamous cell carcinoma, although reduced exposure to both alcohol and tobacco markedly reduces esophageal cancer.[13,14] In third-world countries, diet enhancement and reduction of the consumption of burning hot beverages have reduced the odds ratio of chronic esophagitis, a precancerous condition. Diet enhancement includes supplementing meals with micronutrients and increasing the intake of fresh vegetables and fruits.[30]

### Secondary prevention strategies

Secondary prevention strategies consist of cytologic evaluation for the detection of precancerous lesions in high-risk subjects and chemopreventive interventions with micronutrient supplements.

The low prevalence (0.2%) of esophageal dysplasia in postmortem studies suggests that there is no role for routine screening for esophageal dysplasia or squamous cell esohageal tumors in the United States. In high-incidence areas such as northern China, local resources limit routine endoscopic screening, but cytologic screening of this population has detected dysplasia in 18% to 28% of subjects tested and has detected cancer in 0.7% to 3% of subjects tested.[8,36] A small biopsy study of 175 samples stained with proliferation markers (Ki-67 and proliferating cell nuclear antigen) demonstrated increased staining as the epithelia progressed from normal to basal cell hyperplasia to dysplasia.[37]

Cytologic screening may be useful for selecting individuals with dysplasia who might benefit from chemopreventive intervention. Although changes in histologic classification have differed between and within trials over time, the data appear to support continued evaluation and eventual adaptation of cytologic examination as a screening tool in very high–risk regions, assuming that the cost and standardized pathology are more clearly defined than published data suggest.

A number of nutritional chemoprevention trials were conducted in China's Henan Province. Treatment with a combination of riboflavin, retinol, and zinc reduced the prevalence of esophageal micronucleated cells.[38,39] The effects of this combination on the dysplastic precursor lesions were not evident.[40] A U.S. National Cancer Institute (NCI) study of multiple vitamin and mineral supplements in 3318 high-risk Chinese subjects in Henan Province found little overall difference in the cumulative risk of esophageal cancer, but a significant increase was found in reversion to nondysplastic cytology in the treated group.[41] In a larger cohort of 29,584 subjects in the same region, the NCI used a one-half replicate of a 2 × 4 factorial experimental design that tested the effects of four combinations of nutrients: retinol and zinc; riboflavin and niacin; vitamin C and molybdenum; and β-carotene, vitamin E, and selenium. After 5.25 years, there was little overall difference in the cumulative risk of esophageal cancer between those receiving vitamin or micronutrient supplements and those receiving a placebo. Supplementation with β-carotene, vitamin E, and selenium reduced the esophageal cancer prevalence by 42%.[42,43] Although these trials demonstrated that nutrition plays a crucial role in esophageal carcinogenesis, it is unclear how applicable these repletion trials are to different populations of the world, such as those in first-world countries. To date, no comparative data in different genetic, cultural, or socioeconomic populations have been generated to verify these interesting and potentially important insights.

There are no secondary prevention strategies with data to support a recommendation for populations in the United States or other first-world countries, regardless of the burden of squamous cell esophageal cancer.

### Future goals and research issues

The geographic distribution of squamous cell carcinoma of the esophagus and the strong association between this disease and nutritional and environmental factors suggest that nutritional interventions, as described in the reports of research in China, are likely to play major roles in the control of this disease. In the United States, efforts to control smoking and alcohol consumption might also reduce the incidence of this disease. Chemopreventive interventions in the United States or other first-world countries may, in the future, be focused on nutritional repletion in lower socioeconomic groups, particularly those with smoking and alcoholism problems. Familial risk in the United States, such as that suggested by the research in China and Great Britain, appears to be minimal. The focus of research efforts should be on primary preventive interventions.

## Adenocarcinoma of the Esophagus

### Burden of suffering

In the 1950s and 1960s, the vast majority of esophageal cancers were squamous cell carcinomas.[44] Adenocarcinoma of the esophagus was considered such an uncommon tumor that some authorities questioned its very existence. For the past two decades, however, the incidence of adenocarcinoma of the esophagus and esophagogastric junction has increased at a rate exceeding that for any other cancer in the United States.[5,7,45] Today, adenocarcinomas make up more than 50% of all esophageal malignancies in this country.[7]

Esophageal adenocarcinomas develop in patients with Barrett's esophagus at the rate of approximately 1 cancer per 125 patient-years of follow-up.[6,45,46] Expressed as cases per 100,000 patients, the annual incidence rate for esophageal cancer in patients with Barrett's esophagus is approximately 800 cases per 100,000 individuals. For comparison, the annual incidence of lung cancer in men over age 65 in the general population is approximately 500 cases per 100,000 individuals. Cancer incidence rates also can be expressed as the percent of a population that develops cancer each year. For adult patients with Barrett's esophagus, the annual rate of cancer development is approximately 0.8%. By any yardstick, therefore, a substantial risk exists for esophageal cancer to develop in patients with Barrett's esophagus.[4–6,45–48]

### Primary prevention strategies

Most patients with Barrett's esophagus have severe, chronic gastroesophageal reflux disease as defined by weak lower-esophageal sphincter pressure, decreased amplitude of contractions in the distal esophagus, increased acid exposure, increased bile acid exposure, and the presence of a hiatal hernia.[49,50] Additional risk factors include a high body mass index and smoking.[51] Alcohol does not appear to be a risk factor.

The average age at which Barrett's esophagus is diagnosed is 55 years. For unknown reasons, Barrett's esophagus occurs primarily in Caucasian males.[47,49,52] In most cases, the diagnosis of Barrett's esophagus is established by the examination of biopsy specimens obtained during endoscopic evaluation of the esophagus.[53] Endoscopically, columnar epithelium in the esophagus can be readily identified by its characteristic red color and velvet-like texture. These features contrast sharply with the pale, glossy appearance of the adjacent squamous epithelium. Endoscopists ordinarily suspect that Barrett's esophagus is present when they see long segments of columnar epithelium extending up the esophagus well above the esophagogastric junction. The diagnosis is confirmed when biopsy specimens from these long segments contain any of three types of columnar epithelia.[54] Esophageal adenocarcinomas arise from dysplastic regions of Barrett's columnar, intestinal type metaplasia.[47,52] The reported prevalence rates of adenocarcinoma among patients with Barrett's esophagus range from 0% to 46.5%, with an average rate of about 10%.[47,52] The risk of developing esophageal adenocarcinoma for patients with Barrett's esophagus is approximately 40-fold that for patients without Barrett's esophagus.[52]

The reason for the rapid increase in the incidence of esophageal adenocarcinoma remains unclear. Familial aggregations of gastroesophageal reflux symptoms have been documented in patients with Barrett's esophagus.[49,55] Furthermore, recent data have suggested that *Helicobacter pylori* (*H. pylori*) infections with cagA-positive strains may protect against the development of Barrett's esophagus.[56] If this is so, then *H. pylori* eradication may actually enhance the risk of esophageal cancer.[49]

Adenocarcinoma of the gastric cardia and esophagogastric junction is associated with Barrett's esophagus in approximately 40% of cases.[57] Ascertaining the origin of an adenocarcinoma involving the esophagus, esophagogastric junction, and gastric cardia is difficult. Thus, the relationship between columnar metaplasia and tumor of the gastroesophageal junction and gastric cardia is unclear. Recent data from Sweden suggest that the relationship between adenocarcinoma of the gastric cardia and gastroesophageal reflux disease is relatively weak (odds ratio [OR], 2.0, 95% confidence interval [CI], 1.4–2.9) compared with the relationship between esophageal adenocarcinoma and gastroesophageal reflux disease (OR, 7.7; 95% CI, 5.3–11.4).[58]

Dysplasia in Barrett's esophagus is an ominous finding. A number of studies suggest that high-grade dysplasia in this condition often progresses rapidly to malignancy. For example, Hameeteman and colleagues described eight patients with high-grade dysplasia in Barrett's esophagus, five of whom had invasive cancer detected within 1 year of the discovery of the high-grade dysplastic changes.[59] In a more recent study by Levine and colleagues, high-grade dysplasia in 7 (24%) of 29 patients progressed to invasive cancer during a follow-up period of 2 to 46 months,[60,61] and Drewitz and colleagues found that 4 of 4 patients who developed adenocarcinoma of the esophagus after a diagnosis of Barrett's esophagus had dysplasia.[62] Furthermore, of patients who have undergone esophageal resection on the basis of endoscopic findings of only high-grade dysplasia in Barrett's esophagus, approximately one-third have been found to have an inapparent malignancy in the resected specimen.[61,63] These cancers were missed by the endoscopist preoperatively because of biopsy sampling error. For these reasons, many authorities recommend esophageal resection for patients found to have high-grade dysplasia in Barrett's esophagus.[61,64] Unfortunately, the mortality rate for esophageal resection is approximately 4% to 10%, and there can be substantial long-term morbidity for those who survive the surgery.[47,61]

Although few data are available on the frequency with which low-grade dysplasia progresses to high-grade dysplasia, available studies suggest that the rate is similar to that with which high-grade dysplasia progresses to adenocarcinoma. For example, in one study that included five patients with low-grade dysplasia who eventually developed adenocarcinoma in Barrett's esophagus, all five patients progressed from low-grade to high-grade dysplasia within a period of 5 years.[59] Unlike with dysplastic colonic polyps, which are removed colonoscopically as soon as they are detected, esophageal resection is generally not recommended for patients with low-grade dysplasia.[64]

Neoplastic progression in Barrett's esophagus is associated with a multistep process of genomic instability and clonal evolution leading to the appearance of aneuploid cells with multiple molecular abnormalities.[65] Since Barrett's esophagus is thought to arise in most cases from chronic esophageal reflux, one might conclude that changes in lifestyle (e.g., changes in food intake or in positioning during sleep) combined with aggressive medical care (e.g., drug treatment with inhibitors of gastric acid secretion) might reduce or eliminate the progression of Barrett's esophagus. The effectiveness of lifestyle changes or of drug treatment alone or in combination in reducing the incidence of Barrett's esophagus or esophageal cancer has not been prospectively studied, and the data on several possible risk factors are inconsistent and inconclusive. Thus, one cannot make uniform recommendations regarding primary preventive strategies.

## Secondary prevention strategies

Secondary prevention of esophageal adenocarcinoma consists of early detection followed by management of Barrett's esophagus. Management consists of medical management, surveillance, ablation, and chemoprevention interventions. There are no data related to the early detection of Barrett's esophagus, since the endoscopic and cytologic early detection studies have focused on populations at risk for squamous cell cancer of the esophagus. Most Barrett's esophagus is currently detected by endoscopy performed to evaluate symptoms.

Medical management, consisting of food-intake changes, positioning during sleep, and aggressive acid reduction with potent proton pump inhibitors, which are sometimes administered at higher-than-standard doses over as long as 4 years, has led to total reversal of Barrett's esophagus (intestinal metaplasia) in only 1 of 175 reported cases.[66] These data reflect the preponderance of data regarding multiple acid-suppressive regimens, indicating that medical therapy is ineffective in promoting the reversal of columnar to squamous epithelium.[67]

Most investigators recommend endoscopic surveillance of low-grade esophageal dysplasia every 6 to 12 months.[47,49,68] Once the likelihood of dysplasia is eliminated, endoscopic surveillance is recommended every 2 to 3 years, although rigorous randomized trials documenting the efficacy of surveillance as a means of decreasing death caused by esophageal adenocarcinoma have not been performed.[49,69]

Recent studies have shown that ablative technology such as Nd:YAG laser, argon laser, photodynamic therapy, and multipolar electrocoagulation removes metaplastic and dysplastic Barrett's epithelia. However, insufficient data about the relative efficacy of these modalities are available to define their role in the treatment of metaplasia, low-grade dysplasia, or both.[67] Two reports have noted that the deep biopsies of squamous mucosa in previously metaplastic areas treated with ablative therapies may show columnar cells beneath the squamous epithelium.[67]

The use of pharmacologic approaches to reverse proliferative, precancerous lesions such as those in Barrett's esophagus is an attractive, new secondary preventive maneuver. Sampliner and Garewal administered 13-*cis*-retinoic acid at a dose of 1 mg/kg/day to 16 patients. Only 11 of the16 patients completed 6 weeks of treatment because of unacceptable toxicity. Barrett's metaplasia was not reversed in any of these 11 patients.[70] Gerner and colleagues treated eight patients with difluoromethylornithine (DFMO), a polyamine inhibitor, 1.5 g/m$^2$/day with the goal of determining whether treatment changes the ornithine decarboxylase and polyamine levels in Barrett's mucosa. No data were provided as to whether DFMO induced pathologic or gross changes in the Barrett's mucosa.[71]

## Future goals and research issues

Key clinical questions regarding the efficacy of endoscopic surveillance and the usefulness of aggressive medical and ablative methods remain to be addressed. The pivotal barrier to successful assessment of the efficacy of these and other potential secondary or primary preventive strategies lies in a lack of sufficiently robust surrogate end points that reliably predict future emergence of malignant clones. As noted above, emerging evidence of a multistep molecular carcinogenesis process may be harnessed to predict those lesions with a high potential to progress to transformation and invasion. Such molecular end points may be also used to assess the efficacy of interventions designed to prevent progression or reverse premalignant lesions such as those in Barrett's esophagus.

# Gastric Cancer

## Burden of Suffering

Gastric cancer has shown a marked decline in its incidence and mortality rate over the last six decades. Yet gastric cancer remains the second most common cause of cancer-related death worldwide,[2] and the most common cause of cancer-related death in low socioeconomic groups. With over 50% of the world's population living at or below the poverty line, the burden imposed by gastric cancer in this vulnerable segment of the population is enormous. The incidence of gastric cancer varies greatly worldwide. The incidence rates are high in Japan, parts of Latin America, and Eastern Europe, while they are low in the United States, United Kingdom, and Canada.[2]

In the United States, there has been a remarkable decline in the incidence of gastric cancer over the last several decades. In 1930, gastric cancer was the leading cause of cancer death in American men.[72] Over the last seven decades, the age-adjusted death rates dropped from 37 to 5 per 100,000 person-years in males and from 28 cases to 2 per 100,000 person-years in females.[73] Despite the overall decline, however, data from SEER have revealed a steady increase in the proximal and esophagogastric junctional adenocarcinoma since 1976, at a rate exceeding even that of melanoma.[4] Recent data showed the continuing upward trend in white males.[7] Similar trends of increases have been reported from Europe.[3] Furthermore, adenocarcinoma of the gastric cardia has been associated with 40% of Barrett's esophagus cases.[49]

The overall 5-year survival rate from gastric cancer has improved from 11% to 17% in whites and 8% to 18% in blacks from 1960 to 1989. Yet, gastric cancer has the fifth poorest 5-year survival rate among all cancers. The 5-year survival rate for patients with advanced gastric cancer continues to remain dismal, with 3% for stage IV disease and 13% for stage III disease in the United States[74] and only a shade better at 9% for stage III and IV disease in Japan.[75] The overall improved survival rates are at least partially due to early diagnosis and treatment.

In the United States, the incidence of gastric cancer is higher in African Americans than whites,[7] and is highest in Asian Americans. The incidence rate for Asian Americans, however, is lower than for the population of Japan or Southeast Asia. A steady increase in the rate of adenocarcinoma of the gastric cardia region in American white males is now being observed.[7] Based on the SEER data from 1973 to 1990, the age-adjusted incidence of stomach cancer per 100,000 individuals is 11.7 in blacks and 6.2 in whites. Gastric carcinoma is predominantly a disease of the aged, showing a steep increase in incidence after age 55, and is also more prevalent in men than in women.[76]

Multiple studies from different countries have consistently found an association between gastric cancer and poverty, based on either income[77] or education.[78] Interestingly, no consistent association between gastric cancer and either occupation or industrial exposure has been observed. Since the first report by Haenszel in 1961, several studies have shown that the incidence rates of gastric cancer in migrant populations to the United States are lower, more in tune with the overall trend of incidence in the United States. These data suggest that environmental factors play a dominant role in the etiology of stomach cancer.[79,80]

## Primary Prevention

Several environmental factors, including cigarette smoking, alcohol consumption, radiation exposure, and intake of nitrate and related compounds, salted foods, carbohydrates, and fruits and vegetables have been studied in relation to stomach cancer. In addition, several antecedent conditions; including *H. pylori* infection, chronic atrophic gastritis, gastric polyps, gastrectomy, and genetic factors, are associated with stomach cancer. Primary prevention can potentially target these risk factors.

### Environmental factors

The association between cigarette smoking and either stomach cancer or the development of precancerous lesions is equivocal. Heavy use of cigarettes has been linked to an increased risk of stomach cancer.[78,81] Other investigators have found a positive association between cigarette smoking and stomach cancer, but a dose–response effect was not observed.[82–84] In other studies, however, no clear association between smoking and gastric cancer development has been demonstrated.[85,86] Studies of the relationship between alcohol intake and gastric cancer have been inconclusive.[83,87,88] Similar to results seen with cigarette smoking, there has been no dose–response effect demonstrated.

Ionizing radiation exposure, especially in the atomic bomb survivors in Japan, has been associated with an elevated incidence of gastric cancer.[89] An increased risk has been shown among patients with ankylosing spondylitis treated with X-ray.[90] The risk of stomach cancer increases as the age at exposure to irradiation decreases.[91]

A large number of studies from multiple countries have confirmed the association between diet and the development of stomach cancer.[92] Foods rich in nitrite compounds and their secondary amines, *N*-nitrosoamines, have been implicated as the major culprits, although some epidemiologic data have been inconsistent. Two thorough reviews on this topic have been published.[93,94]

Smoked and salted foods have been incriminated as increasing the risk of gastric cancer, whereas fruits and vegetables have been found to reduce the risk.[92] In the United States, salt intake has decreased dramatically since the early 1900s,[95] paralleled with a decrease in stomach cancer mortality rates. Urinary salt excretion and the consumption of salted fish and vegetables have been correlated with stomach cancer rates in different regions of Japan.[96] In addition, high salt concentrations can injure the gastric mucosa and facilitate absorption of known carcinogens. The data from dietary case–control studies have been inconsistent while the preponderance studies have found that salted foods and cured meats increased the risk for stomach cancer[76]; other studies have not reported similar results. While quantitative metabolic differences may contribute to the conflicting results, most observers consider salted foods a risk for stomach cancer.

Accompanying the decline in stomach cancer has been a 50% reduction in carbohydrate consumption in the United States.[95] A variety of dietary case–control studies have consistently reported a high carbohydrate intake associated with increased risk for stomach cancer.[76] Unlike the intake of nitrates, salt, and carbohydrates, the intake of fresh fruits and vegetables is consistently inversely associated with stomach cancer.[76] These findings are remarkable, given the inaccuracies in measuring an individual's intake. Care must be taken not to assume that a single micronutrient linked to a diet high in fresh fruits and vegetables is responsible for the protective effect. Additionally, the widespread availability of refrigeration since the 1900s has lessened the need for salting, smoking, or pickling and has promoted the availability and consumption of fresh fruits and vegetables.

### Antecedent conditions

An overwhelming amount of evidence links *H. pylori* infection to gastric carcinoma.[97–99] A multinational study by the Eurogast Study Group of 17 populations in Europe, the United States, and Japan revealed a direct association between gastric cancer and *H. pylori* seropositivity.[100] A recent meta-analysis of all the data showed a relative risk (RR) as high as 9 for developing gastric cancer associated with *H. pylori*.[101] Another recent study from Sweden reported that *H. pylori* infection may lead to gastric cancer or duodenal ulcer, but seldom both in the same patient. This suggests that the development of a duodenal ulcer may offer protection against cancer development and also implies that *H. pylori*–induced mechanisms of ulcer and cancer development may be mutually exclusive.[102] Studies have also demonstrated higher rates of *H. pylori* infection at an early age in regions endemic for gastric cancer and in low socioeconomic groups.[103,104] Even though a large number of people harbor *H. pylori* infection, not all of them develop gastric cancer. This evidence indicates that *H. pylori* infection is insufficient to cause gastric cancer alone. However, chronic *H. pylori* infection may be a requisite component of the gastric carcinogenesis process.[105]

Chronic atrophic gastritis lesions are closely linked to gastric cancer.[106] The prevalence of atrophic gastritis is highest in regions of the world that have high rates of gastric cancer.[107,108] Atrophic gastritis is found in 80%–90% of patients with gastric cancer, whereas approximately 10% of patients with chronicatrophic gastritis develop gastric carcinoma.[109] Atrophic gastritis associated with pernicious anemia and *H. pylori* has also been associated with gastric cancer,[110,111] but so far, few data are available on identifying, screening, and intervening for patients with atrophic gastritis or on the prevention of gastric cancer in the patients.

Patients with gastric adenomatous polyps but not with hyperplastic polyps are at an increased risk for developing gastric carcinoma.[112] The risk is directly proportional to the size of the polyp.[113] Even though a recent Italian study suggests the necessity of strict follow-up after polypectomy,[114] the evidence that a polypectomy reduces the risk of gastric cancer or that surveillance provides any benefit is inconclusive.

Distal gastrectomy for benign disorders, particularly peptic ulcer disease, is associated with an increased risk for gastric cancer.[115,116] A meta-analysis by Tersmette and colleagues on the risk of gastric stump cancer indicates that the relative risk remains low for up to 20 years after gastrectomy and then increases to the range of 1.5 to 3.[117] Because of the absence of any prospective data and the low postgastrectomy relative risk for transformation, routine surveillance screening has not been recommended.[118]

Several observational studies and numerous case reports have suggested an association between iatrogenic achlorhydria and gastric cancer, but the evidence is not convincing.

Gastric carcinoma has been observed to cluster in families, the Napolean Bonaparte family probably being the most famous example.[119] Gastric cancer has occurred with greater frequency in people with blood type A,[120] patients with hereditary nonpolyporis colorectal cancer HNPCC-II,[121] and in the first-degree relatives of patients with stomach cancer.[122] Researchers have identified several oncogenes that are activated, (c-*myc*, c-*erb2B*, c-*erbA* and K-*ras*) and silenced tumor suppressor genes (*p53*, *APC*). Recently, Gong and colleagues reported that a K-*ras* mutation associated with atrophic gastritis may predict the earliest detectable event prior to development of gastric cancer.[123]

### Primary Prevention

The central focus of primary prevention for stomach cancer is diet. A diet with at least 12% of caloric intake from protein to balance carbohydrate intake is advisable. It is also advisable to reduce the intake of foods altered by salting, smoking, pickling, or other chemical preservatives.[124] Agricultural methods can be modified to reduce the nitrate content of vegetables. The dramatic decreases in the burden of stomach cancer in the United States are linked to the dietary changes associated with improved transport of fresh produce, wide availability of fresh or frozen meat, and home refrigeration and freezing. Enhanced technology with its associated changes in the quality of the food supply highlights the power of primary prevention.

### Secondary Prevention

Observations dating from 1938 indicate a very favorable prognosis in cases in which gastric carcinoma is confined to the mucosa or submucosa.[125,126] Survival rates greater than 90% in patients diagnosed with early-stage disease have prompted screening of asymptomatic patients in countries that have a high incidence of gastric cancer, such as Japan, Chile, and Venezuela.[125] The percentage of resected cancers that are diagnosed as early-stage gastric cancer is about 10% to 20% in most Western nations and about 40% in Japan,[127] probably reflecting the effect of mass screening introduced in 1957 in Japan.[128] These percentages may overestimate the incidence of early-stage disease in the community because most of the data have been taken from surgical cohorts. The long-term prognosis for patients with surgically resected early-stage gastric cancer is excellent, with 90% and 85% 10-year survival rates being reported from Japan[129] and the West,[130] respectively. A French study reported a 20-year survival rate of 50%, even when all causes of mortality were included.[131] Thus, a compelling amount of evidence indicates that early diagnosis and treatment substantially improve survival rates in populations with high incidence rates of stomach cancer.

Widespread screening and intervention with endoscopy has been found to be beneficial in Japan,[75] although preliminary data from a more recent study seem to contradict this finding.[132] Also, a case–control study from Latin America, which also has a high incidence of gastric cancer, failed to show benefit to widespread screening.[133] Several reports have described regression of pre-neoplastic changes[134,135] in the gastric mucosa from eradication of *H. pylori*, although a few did not.[136]

The cost-effectiveness of screening and treatment for *H. pylori* infection to prevent gastric cancer was evaluated by Parsonnet and colleagues,[137] and the results were recently confirmed by Fendrick and colleagues.[138] Screening for and eradication of *H. pylori* prevented only 30% of attributable cancers; it would cost a total of $1 billion, with a cost-effectiveness of $25,000 per year per life saved. Cost-effectiveness of screening in childhood was even less. The strategy of serologic testing to identify specific strains of *H. pylori*, such as cag A, and post-treatment urea breath tests were of little value and were cost-prohibitive.[138] These studies underscore the fact that generalized population screening is not cost-effective. Better risk stratification and better preventive measures such as vaccines[139] need evaluation.

Screening may be beneficial only in high-risk populations. Characteristics of the populations at increased risk for stomach cancer are male gender, age 60 years and older, low socioeconomic status, family history of gastric cancer, a history of known precursor antecedents, and ionizing radiation to the stomach region. Even though the studies done so far have not shown that screening a population for *H. pylori* is cost-effective, a new multicenter randomized controlled study (called PRISMA) on the eradication of *H. pylori* to prevent stomach cancer is underway in Europe. The results of this study should help determine the benefit of *H. pylori* screening.

Chemoprevention offers another potentially cost-effective method of gastric cancer prevention. Results of the Linxian study[42] of ascorbic acid for the chemoprevention of gastric cancer have been disappointing. The study failed to show benefit of this chemoprevention possibly because *H. pylori* was not eradicated or because the intervention was done at the wrong time. For instance, recent data from Sweden suggest that chemopreventive intervention may be more beneficial if initiated early in the carcinogenesis process.[140] Other recent data from Seattle suggest the probable chemopreventive benefit from aspirin or nonsteroidal agents in reducing the risk of gastric cancer.[141] Until better chemopreventive agents are rigorously documented to slow human carcinogenesis clinically, the World Health Organization's recommendation to eat more fruit and vegetables to reduce the risk of gastric cancer remains an appropriate standard.[142] The most tangible results in the high-risk population may come from using a chemopreventive agent with *H. pylori* eradication.

## Pancreatic Cancer

### Burden of Suffering

Exocrine pancreatic cancer makes up 95% of pancreatic cancers; therefore, this section will focus on cancer prevention for exocrine pancreatic cancer,[143] which remains a highly lethal cancer that contributes to cancer death at a level disproportionate to its incidence. Pancreatic cancer ranks thirteenth in incidence and ninth in mortality for both sexes combined worldwide.[144] In the United States, pancreatic cancer is the fourth most common cause of cancer death, while it ranks eighth and tenth in incidence in females and males, respectively.[73] Pancreatic cancer is usually diagnosed at an unresectable, late-stage cancer.[145] Ninety-eight percent of cases diagnosed cause death at median survival after diagnosis is less than 1 year,[146] which explains the reason for its mortality rank exceeding its incidence rank.

### Primary Prevention

The cause(s) of pancreatic cancer remains unknown. Nevertheless, there are several risk factors for the disease that are amenable to primary prevention. Additionally, these risk factors define subgroups of the population who may benefit from a secondary prevention as in the case of patients with familial pancreatic cancer.

#### Smoking

Cigarette smoking is the most consistently identified risk factor for pancreatic cancer, with several case–control studies having shown this association.[147–152] Additionally, large prospective studies have confirmed that cigarette smoking increases pancreatic cancer risk. For example, in a study of 167,767 subjects who were followed for a total of 2,116,229 person-years, smoking increased pancreatic cancer risk 2.5-fold (95% CI, 1.7–3.6).[153] In a study of 35,000 Swedish subjects who were followed for 365,500 person-years, cigarette smoking was also associated with an increased risk of pancreatic cancer.[154] In 1986 the International Agency for Research on Cancer (IARC) concluded that smoking is a cause of pancreatic cancer.[155]

Smoking was strongly associated with an increased risk for pancreatic cancer in a number of other population-based studies.[156–160] Therefore, the most significant step that could be taken to prevent pancreatic cancer would be to eliminate cigarette smoking.

## Dietary risk factors

It is rational to rank diet high among the potential risk factors for pancreatic cancer, since the pancreas is intimately related to digestion and absorption. For example, studies of immigrant populations to Australia have shown that the incidence of pancreatic cancer reflected changes in dietary habits.[161,162] Many epidemiologic studies have indicated that fruits and vegetables help protect against pancreatic cancer.[151,163–167] Micronutrients, such as folic acid and pyroxidine, might also have protective effects against pancreatic cancer.[147] Other case–control studies have shown that various dietary ingredients such as fat or refined sugar, methods for food preparation (e.g., grilling, wood-fire cooking), and increased calorie intake might increase the risk of pancreatic cancer.

Various biases, such as selection and recall biases, can affect the results of these case–control studies. Also, the results of some of these studies are conflicting, as in the case of the association between fat intake and the risk of pancreatic cancer. Numerous nutrient studies provide little insight into the relationship between diet and pancreatic cancer. In general, meat, animal protein, and fat appear to be associated with an increased risk. Vegetables and fruit, along with the related micronutrients, are associated with decreased risk.[148,168,169]

## Coffee

Epidemiologic data conflict regarding the association between coffee consumption and pancreatic cancer risk. Five case–control studies have shown that coffee consumption is associated with an increase in the risk of pancreatic cancer.[164,170–173] Coffee consumption was also associated with a twofold (95% CI, 1.08–4.3) increase in the risk of pancreatic cancer in a prospective study of 33,976 postmenopausal women in Iowa between 1986 and 1994.[174]

Several case–control studies showed no significant association between coffee consumption and pancreatic cancer.[148,150,175–177] Additionally, large cohort studies have supported the lack of the association between coffee consumption and pancreatic cancer risk.[157,160] Therefore, the association between coffee intake and pancreatic cancer remains unconfirmed. The increased risk associated with coffee consumption may result from residual confounding with cigarette smoking or from other sources of confounding or bias.

## Alcohol

Early case–series[178] and ecologic[179] studies suggested that alcohol consumption increased the risk of pancreatic cancer. However, other ecologic studies[180–182] found no relationship between alcohol consumption and pancreatic cancer incidence. The early cohort studies were generally null or inconclusive.[183–186]

In a review of the literature in 1986, Velema and colleagues[187] argued that the evidence of a causal association between pancreatic cancer and total alcohol consumption of any specific type of alcohol was weak. Subsequent studies have reported no consistent associations. In the Iowa women's study, the risk of pancreatic cancer was increased with alcohol intake.[174] In a cohort of 9353 individuals who were followed for 7.7 years, the risk of pancreatic cancer increased with a history of alcoholism (standardized incidence ratio [SIR] = 1.5; CI, 0.9–2.3).[188]

In contrast, investigators in a large case–control study of 486 pancreatic cancer patients and 2109 control subjects found no significant association between alcohol intake at average consumption levels for the U.S. population and pancreatic cancer.

The possibility of an increased risk with heavy alcohol intake could not be ruled out.[189] The association between high alcohol intake and pancreatic cancer risk still persists, but is likely to be important only in smokers.

## Occupational exposure

Some studies suggest that certain occupational exposures increase the risk of developing pancreatic cancer.[190] One large case–control study found a positive association between formaldehyde exposure and pancreatic cancer risk.[191] Another case–control study of 451 patients with pancreatic cancer and 1552 control subjects randomly selected in Shanghai suggested that exposure to metal, textile dusts, electric magnetic fields, or certain chemicals increases the risk of pancreatic cancer.[192] A study of 2238 Danes working in sulfide mills showed that these workers had an increased risk for pancreatic cancer.[193] Likewise, another study showed that workers in areas where vinyl resins and polyethylene were processed had a higher risk of pancreatic cancer.[194] DDT and two of its derivatives (DDD and ethylan) were associated with an increased risk of pancreatic cancer in a nested study in a cohort of 5886 workers in chemical plants.[195]

Exposure to agents such as acrylamide, however, has not been found to increase the risk of pancreatic cancer.[196] Similarly, no increased risk of pancreatic cancer was found in relation to exposure to styrene, toluene, or xylene in a study of 5301 Finnish workers who were monitored for approximately 20 years.[197] No common element in the list of possible occupations is linked to pancreatic cancer. It is important to emphasize that, in addition to the published results mentioned above, an unknown but very large number of cohorts have been examined and yielded negative results. These findings have not been published, highlighting that many of the positive findings are likely due to chance.

## Diabetes

Evidence suggests that diabetes mellitus is associated with a moderate increase in the risk of pancreatic cancer. In vitro, insulin receptors enhance the proliferation of pancreatic cells.[198] Two case–control studies have shown that diabetes increases pancreatic cancer risk,[149,199] whereas a third large case–control study failed to show this association.[200]

Many large prospective studies have demonstrated an association between diabetes and increased pancreatic cancer risk. In one large prospective study of 1,089,586 men and women,[201] diabetes moderately increased the risk of pancreatic cancer during 12 years of follow-up. In a second study of 109,581 hospitalized diabetic patients in Denmark, the SIR for pancreatic cancer was 2.1-fold the expected incidence for the general population (95% CI, 1.9–2.4) during a follow-up period of 1–4 years.[202] A third large cohort study of 51,008 diabetic patients in Sweden found a moderate but significant increase in pancreatic cancer risk (RR = 1.4; 95% CI, 1.2–1.7).[203] The risk of pancreatic cancer was also increased in other large cohort studies of diabetic patients.[157,204] The preponderance of evidence indicates that diabetes mellitus is associated with a moderate increase in pancreatic cancer risk.

## Chronic pancreatitis

The concept of chronic pancreatitis being a predisposing factor to pancreatic cancer is supported by a large number of epidemiologic studies. One large, retrospective study was a U.S. Veterans Administration study in which the incidence of previous pancreatitis was compared between 2639 patients with pancreatic cancer and a matched control group of 7774 subjects without pancreatic cancer.[205] The study showed that pancreatic cancer patients were more likely than the control subjects to have a history of pancreatitis.

A Swedish population-based study also found that pancreatitis was associated with an increased risk of pancreatic cancer. The risk decreased with time; however, raising questions regarding the causal relationship between chronic pancreatitis and cancer.[206] Moreover, this study was not limited to chronic pancreatitis, and its results cannot definitively rule out the possibility that chronic pancreatitis contributes to the development of pancreatic cancer. Other studies, including several case-control studies[176,207,208] and two cohort studies, have supported this association.

A cohort of 174 patients with chronic pancreatitis who were followed for 14 years had a significant increase in the incidence of pancreatic cancer.[209] In another prospective study, the incidence of pancreatic and nonpancreatic cancers in 246 patients with chronic pancreatitis was higher than that expected for the general population.[210] These data are further corroborated by findings from a retrospective multinational cohort study of 2015 subjects with chronic pancreatitis.[211] In this study, chronic pancreatitis was associated with an increased incidence of pancreatic cancer over time, which reached 1.8% after 10 years and 4% after 20 years.

Similarly, epidemiologic data from Japan showed an increased risk of pancreatic cancer in patients with chronic pancreatitis.[160] Other studies have demonstrated that patients with chronic pancreatitis and hereditary pancreatitis have an increased risk of developing pancreatic cancer.[212–216] Therefore, evidence indicates that chronic pancreatitis is a significant risk factor for pancreatic cancer.

### Hereditary risk factors

A family history of pancreatic cancer increases the risk for the disease,[209,217] and in rare instances pancreatic cancer cases aggregate in families.[218] Furthermore, an estimated 10% of pancreatic cancer cases are hereditary.[146] The risk of pancreatic cancer is increased with some familial cancer syndromes, such as that associated with a mutation in the *BRCA2* gene[219–221] and an estimated 7% of patients with sporadic pancreatic cancer have a *BRCA2* germline mutation.[222]

Other hereditary cancer syndromes, such as familial polyposis coli syndrome, are associated with an increased risk of pancreatic cancer.[223,224] Furthermore, a germline mutation of *p16* is associated with increased risks of melanoma and pancreatic cancer, as shown in studies of members of melanoma-prone families with a *p16M* mutation.[172,225]

Finally, patients with hereditary pancreatitis are also at an increased risk of pancreatic cancer, as discussed earlier in this section. With improvements in genetic testing to identify individuals at high risk, the challenge is to develop adequate methods for screening and prevention in these patients. A recent report suggested that surveillance for dysplasia in patients with familial pancreatic cancer is possible with the combination of clinical data and endoscopic retrograde cholangiopancreatography (ERCP).[146]

### Other risk factors

Various other risk factors for pancreatic cancer have been proposed. Some data suggest that cholelithiasis is one of these factors.[226] However, in a large case–control study, no increase in pancreatic cancer risk was found with a history of cholelithiasis or cholecystectomy.[227]

A history of testicular cancer has also been suggested as a risk factor in large epidemiologic studies. In one study of 29,000 men who survived testicular cancer, these patients had an increased risk for developing pancreatic cancer.[228] A second study of 6187 Danish men with a history of testicular cancer who were followed for 59,000 person-years also showed a peak incidence of pancreatic cancer 10 to 19 years after having testicular cancer.[229]

In one study, patients diagnosed with malignant melanoma at an age younger than 50 years were also found to have an increased risk for developing pancreatic cancer.[230]

## Chemoprevention

Animal models suggest that chemoprevention is feasible in pancreatic cancer. Studies in rat models have shown that a putative chemopreventive agent such as vitamin C, green tea polyphenols, or selenium as a diet supplement inhibited pancreatic tumorigenesis in animals.[231–234] Secondary analyses of the α-tocopherol β-carotene (ATBC) cancer prevention study showed that β-carotene, α-tocopherol, or a combination of the two was ineffective in preventing pancreatic cancer.[235]

Studies designed to clinically evaluate chemoprevention for pancreatic cancer are scarce. This is likely because of the relatively low incidence of the disease compared with other, more common malignancies such as breast or colon cancer; the difficulty with defining groups who are at risk; a lack of effective screening methods; and a lack of surrogate biomarkers for chemoprevention studies. Chemoprevention studies that use cancer incidence end points are very difficult to conduct because of the relatively low incidence of the disease. Moreover, biomarkers predictive of risk, pre-neoplasia, or early invasive cancer have not been validated. Without such biomarkers, early-phase chemoprevention trials will be difficult to initiate.

## Secondary Prevention

The value of screening for pancreatic cancer is still undefined since no effective, accurate method is available to identify the disease at an early stage. In addition, the efficacy of prophylactic pancreatectomy for precancerous lesions such as atypical intraductal hyperplasia is unconfirmed.[146] Thus, the whole concept of secondary prevention through early diagnosis and subsequent treatment is without supporting evidence. Several lines of evidence support the concept that atypical ductal hyperplasia can progress into invasive carcinoma.[236] Atypical ductal hyperplasia is estimated to precede the development of invasive cancer by a mean of 6 years.[146] If we had the ability to detect this precancerous stage for pancreatic cancer, we would significantly improve the value of screening in this disease.[236]

Currently, in most cases, pancreatic cancer is diagnosed in advanced stages, which is likely a major contributor to the poor prognosis of the disease. Pancreatectomy is the only potentially curative treatment modality that is available[237] (see Chapter 32 for more details). Unfortunately, pancreatectomy is performed in only 10% to 20% of pancreatic cancer cases worldwide.[237] Likewise, in a recent report from the U.S. National Data Base collected on 100,313 patients diagnosed with pancreatic cancer between 1989 and 1995, pancreatectomy was performed in only 9% of patients.[145]

The likely cause for the low utilization of this procedure is that a large proportion of patients present with unresectable disease. Even for patients who are examined for resection, pancreatectomy is performed in a small percentage of cases, as shown in a Scandinavian study of a cohort of 330 pancreatic cancer patients, only 29% of whom had resectable disease at the time of surgical exploration.[238]

The importance of early detection is demonstrated in the 5-year survival rates, which were three to four times higher for patients who had undergone a pancreatectomy than patients who had unresectable disease.[145] Furthermore, disease stage is important, even in patients who undergo resection. In a study from Johns Hopkins Hospital, the 5-year survival rates in 201 patients who underwent resection were 36% for patients with stage I and II disease vs. 14% for patients with stage III disease.[239] In another study, the 5-year survival rate was greatly impacted by the resected tumor's size, with a 41% survival rate in cases with tumors measuring 2 cm or less compared with a 21% survival rate in cases with larger tumors.[240] Thus, the ability to detect the disease at a very early stage is crucial to improving survival.

Exocrine pancreatic cancer arises in the pancreatic ductal epithelium in what appears to be a multistep carcinogenesis process similar to what is observed in other cancers, such as colon cancer[241,242] (see Chapter 30 for more details). Initially, the epithelial cells transform from cuboidal to columnar to form what is called "flat hyperplasia."[241] In the next step, *atypical ductal hyperplasia* (also known as *pancreatic dysplasia* or *ductal papillary hyperplasia*), cells develop atypical cellular and nuclear morphologic changes in addition to epithelial architectural changes.[241] To date, no studies have been done to determine if these precancerous stages can be detected or whether the course of the disease can be altered in this phase.

Many genetic mutations accumulate during the multistep progression of pancreatic cancer. This accumulation in genetic mutations leads to the activation of oncogenes and the inactivation of suppressor genes,[241] which are thought to play a role in pancreatic carcinogenesis. One of the most commonly observed mutations is the K-*ras* mutation, the rate of which increases during the multistep progression of pancreatic cancer. It is identified in more than 90% of pancreatic cancer cases.[241]

A K-*ras* mutation has been detected in the bile, pancreatic juice, and stool samples from patients with pancreatic cancer and ductal hyperplasia,[146,243,244] and it might become a biomarker that can be used for future prevention studies. To date, no studies using these genetic mutations as screening procedures have been done.

Unfortunately, pancreatic cancer has no specific clinical signs or symptoms in its early stages.[237] Furthermore, efforts to develop a diagnostic modality have focused more on accurate staging and the identification of patients who would most benefit from pancreatectomy than on use of the modality in early detection. For example, contrast-enhanced spiral computed tomography (CT) is considered one of the best modalities currently available for pancreatic diagnostic imaging. However, this modality has limited ability to detect pancreatic tumors measuring less than 1 cm,[237] and the test is more accurate in predicting which tumors are not resectable than in predicting those that are.[245]

Thus, effective methods for screening are lacking, and efforts have recently been redirected to evaluate the efficacy of a variety of proposed diagnostic methodologies as screening tools for pancreatic cancer in high-risk populations.[246] One recent study evaluated the effectiveness of screening and the predicative value of some screening tools in patients with a family history of pancreatic cancer.[146] In that study of 14 patients, pancreatic dysplasia was used an end point. Spiral CT and tumor markers (CEA and CA19-9 levels) had low sensitivities for detecting pancreatic dysplasia. Seven of these patients were referred for pancreatectomy because of a suspicion of pancreatic dysplasia (atypical ductal hyperplasia). In these seven patients, dysplasia was found at the time of surgery.[146] In 3/7 patients with pancreatic dysplasia, a K-*ras* mutation was detected by analyses of pancreatic juice. No patient in the study was reported to have developed pancreatic cancer. However, the follow-up period has been relatively short (12 to 30 months for the group that had surgery and 8 to17 months in the group that had no surgery).

The long-term effects and predictive value of pancreatectomy in patients with pancreatic dysplasia or the value of detecting dysplasia in patients with pancreatic cancer remain unknown.[146] Total pancreatectomy is associated with significant morbidity (e.g., brittle diabetes); therefore, the overall benefit-to-risk ratio needs to be adequately assessed before making recommendations for the population at large. Further development of screening and intervention tools is badly needed.

## Future Direction

It is obvious that the field of chemoprevention for pancreatic cancer is still in the very early stages of development. Better methods for screening and early detection are needed. Chemoprevention seems to be feasible, based on preclinical models; however, clinical development of putative effective agents has yet to be started. The increase in our ability to identify subjects at high risk for this incurable disease further underscores the great need to address issues surrounding the development of effective screening and chemoprevention for pancreatic cancer.

## Biliary Tract Cancer

### Burden of Suffering

Biliary cancer is a relatively rare but fatal disease.[247] In the United States, approximately 7500 new cases are diagnosed each year; nearly 5000 of these are gallbladder cancers, and the rest are bile duct cancers.[248] Biliary cancer accounts for 1% of the total cancer deaths in the United States.[73] Incidence rates vary worldwide, with the highest rates occurring in Latin American countries, such as Peru. Very high rates are also seen in Eastern European regions, such as Poland and Hungary. Very low rates have been observed in the United States, the United Kingdom, and the Indian subcontinent.[249]

Marked differences in the incidence rates of biliary tract cancer among various races and ethnic groups in the same geographic area have been observed. For example, Native American Indians, Hispanic Americans, and Alaskan natives have higher incidence rates in the United States.[250,251] The highest incidence rates have been observed in the Maori population of New Zealand, people of Polish ethnicity in Europe, and in the Miyagi Japanese.[252–254]

As with most epithelial cancers, the risk of biliary cancer increases with increasing age, with peak incidence in the sixth and seventh decades; an exception is in Native American women, for whom incidence peaks at a younger age.[252] Biliary cancer is one of the few cancers that show a female preponderance. However, in certain ethnic groups (e.g., Japanese), the incidence is similar in both sexes.[255]

Globally there appears to be a downward trend in the mortality and incidence rates of biliary tract cancer. This may partially be due to an increase in the number of cholecystectomies.[256,257]

## Primary Prevention

Numerous common, benign conditions are known to be risk factors for the development of biliary tract cancer. Understanding the risks posed by these conditions, modifying these risks, and screening the appropriate populations are imperative to reducing the burden placed by this fatal disease.

Cholelithiasis is among the most common gastrointestinal disorders. It has long been observed to be overwhelmingly associated with gallbladder carcinoma. Gallbladder cancer has been noted to be high in the population subgroup that has a high incidence of gallstones.[258] The association is directly proportional to the size of the stones.[259,260] Furthermore, pooled analysis from a study conducted by the International Agency for Research on Cancer suggests that the association is stronger in symptomatic patients.[261]

Lew and colleagues, in the landmark clinical trial published in 1979, first observed that obese women exhibited a higher mortality from the biliary cancers during a 13-year follow-up.[262] This was subsequently observed in many trials. The recently published SEARCH data also reveal a similar association.[261]

Several studies have reported a strong association between diet and biliary cancer.[263–265] An inverse relationship with biliary cancer occurrence was seen with fruit, vegetable, and fiber intake.[261,266] A direct correlation was seen between the incidence of biliary cancer and total calorie and sugar intake.[261] Data regarding animal protein have been less clear.

An association between fecundity and biliary cancer has been reported by multiple studies. A higher incidence of biliary cancer is seen in multiparous women, young primiparous women, and in females with early menarche and late menopause.[267–269] However, no clear association with oral contraceptive pills has been demonstrated.[252]

Biliary cancer has been observed to be more common with certain infections. Chronic typhoid infection has been associated with gallbladder carcinoma.[270,271] Infections with certain parasites, such as *Opisthorchis viverrini* in Southeast Asia and *Opisthorchis sinensis* in Japan, Korea, and Vietnam, have been associated with greater incidence of cholangiocarcinoma.[270,272]

A number of mutations in oncogenes (such as K-*ras*, c-*myc*, c-*neu*, c-*erb-b2*) and in tumor suppressor genes (e.g., *p53*, *bcl-2*) have been described in biliary cancers. However, little is known about the role of these genes in the development, prognosis, or surveillance of biliary cancers.[273] Nonetheless, the higher susceptibility of particular ethnic minorities clearly points toward genetic risk factors, which are probably activated by an environmental insult.

Primary sclerosing cholangitis,[274] cigarette smoking,[261] congenital anomalies, biliary adenomas,[273] and heavy-metal exposure[275] have all been shown to be associated with an increased risk for developing biliary carcinoma.

There is no evidenced-based recommendation for primary prevention that can be made for populations at average or increased risk for the disease.

## Secondary Prevention

In spite of all the technical and biologic advances of recent years, a major improvement in the survival rates of patients with biliary cancer is unlikely to be achieved by treating advanced-stage biliary cancers. The maximum tangible impact can be made only by effective prevention strategies. Because biliary cancer is not a globally rampant or an endemic disease, mass screening is likely to be expensive and of little value. Although it is a rare disease, biliary cancer is uniformly fatal, and hence screening high-risk populations may be cost-effective.

Symptoms from biliary tract cancer tend to develop very late if the tumor is in the gallbladder but occur relatively early if the tumor arises from other areas in the tract.[273] Gallbladder tumors remain confined to the gallbladder for a prolonged period of time without giving rise to any specific symptoms, thus offering an opportunity to treat at a limited stage but at the same time making it hard to detect early.[276] Most gallbladder cancers are detected at an advanced stage because of a paucity of specific symptoms earlier.[277] Because cure rates of limited disease are reasonable, early suspicion, rapid diagnosis, and prompt surgical resection will reduce the overall mortality rate associated with the disease.

The natural history of gallbladder cancer and the various well-documented risk factors offer a unique scope for developing effective and valid preventive measures, by targeting high-risk populations. More studies need to be done to better delineate and stratify target populations, to identify cost-effective screening methods such as tumor marker assays, and noninvasive radiographic techniques.

On the basis of available data, it would seem logical that prophylactic cholecystectomy would be effective. But so far, no convincing evidence of gain of life expectancy from prophylactic cholecystectomy has been observed.[278] This is probably secondary to the lack of appropriate stratification of patients, combined with the relatively low incidence of the disease in the populations studied. Native American Indian women with gallstones should probably be a target population in a future, well-designed study.

Data on sonographic screening are also not sufficiently conclusive to recommend routine screening of any particular population. Given all the data available to date, the best strategy to adopt is to recommend a healthy lifestyle and diet. Clearly, much can and needs to be done in terms of prevention. Chemopreventive strategy, especially in high-risk groups, such as those with primary sclerosing cholangitis or cholelithiasis, may be one of the better ways of preventing this fatal disease.

## Future Directions

Future leads into the prevention of biliary tract cancer are likely to come from research that addresses nutritional, metabolic, hormonal, and genetic determinants of gallstones. By linking risk factors for the development of gallstones, it should be possible to clarify the origins of biliary tumors and develop effective preventive strategies.

## Liver Cancer

### Burden of Suffering

A number of tumor types occur in the liver, but except for primary hepatocellular carcinoma (HCC), all are very rare. Hepatocellular carcinoma, by contrast, is one of the most common tumors in the world today and is occurring with increasing frequency in the United States.[279] It is one of the three most common causes of cancer mortality in the world, accounting for 250,000 to 1,000,000 deaths annually.

About 80% of HCCs are etiologically associated with chronic infection with hepatitis B virus (HBV).[280] On the basis of sev-

has a better prognosis than small bowel cancer in the general population.[310] Familial adenomatous polyposis syndrome is associated with a marked increase in the risk of duodenal adenocarcinoma (RR = 33; 95% CI, 13–681) and ampullary adenocarcinoma (RR = 124; 95% CI, 34–317).[311] Crohn's disease is associated with a marked increase in small bowel cancer by approximately 86-fold.[312] In patients with Crohn's disease, small bowel cancer tends to occur with a more distal distribution and at younger ages and has a worse prognosis.[313]

In one recent study, no association was found between alcohol or tobacco and the risk of small bowel cancer.[314] Because the disease is rare, no clinical reports exist on measures of primary or secondary prevention for small bowel cancer.

## Colon Cancer

### Burden of Suffering

Colorectal carcinoma is one of the most common cancers in the world. The disease incidence rates rank third among cancers in males and second among cancers in females worldwide.[144] In the United States, colorectal cancer ranks third in cancer incidence in both sexes.[73] The incidence rates are higher in developed countries than in developing countries; for example, the incidence rate of colorectal cancer is 20-fold higher in Australia than in middle Africa.[144] Dietary habits probably cause this marked variation in colorectal cancer incidence. This is based on studies of immigrant populations to the United States and Australia, where dietary changes in these populations were reflected in changes in colorectal cancer incidence rates.[161,315]

The U.S. colorectal cancer mortality rates decreased steadily between 1990 and 1995 by an average of 1.5% per year.[316] This decrease was not likely caused by advances in the treatment of metastatic disease, which remains incurable, with a slight improvement in survival duration despite chemotherapy.[317] Likewise, adjuvant chemotherapy is unlikely to be the cause for this improvement despite the modest improvement (approximately 4% to 13%) in survival rates for stage III colon cancer with adjuvant therapy, because cases of stage III disease represent only 25% of all cases.[318,319]

In contrast, the incidence rates of colorectal cancer in the United States decreased by 2.3% annually between 1990 and 1995.[316] This decrease in incidence rates is more likely to be the major contributor to the reduction of colon cancer mortality for the same period. This underscores the importance of prevention as the means of controlling the mortality rates for colorectal cancer.

### Primary Prevention

The cause(s) of colorectal cancer remains unknown. However, a variety of risk factors have been identified: age, family history, environmental factors, and prior colonic disease (e.g., colonic polyps, cancer, or inflammatory bowel disease). These risk factors help to identify subgroups within the general population that are at increased risk for developing colorectal cancer, allowing the level of surveillance to be tailored to the risk profile. Predication of the risk profile is also crucial to direct the development of current and future chemoprevention to the populations with the greatest need. In addition, modifiable risk factors are amenable to primary prevention.

### Diet

A large number of preclinical studies (in vitro and animal studies) support the notion that increased fat intake promotes colonic

carcinogenesis. Studies in animal carcinogenesis models for colon cancer have shown that dietary fats, polyunsaturated fatty acids (PUFAs) in particular, enhance colonic carcinogenesis in animals.[320,321] In these models, the position of the first unsaturated function from the methyl terminal group (the n function) can alter PUFAs' procarcinogenic effects. The PUFAs with n-6 function, such as linoleic acid and arachidonic acid, promote colonic carcinogenesis, whereas the corresponding n-3 PUFAs, such as fish oil, lack that effect or have opposite effects in the same animal models.[322]

In contrast to findings in preclinical studies, the association between fat intake and colon cancer is less supported by currently available clinical data. Although many (12 of 13) ecological studies have supported this association between fat intake and the risk of colon cancer, most large case–control and cohort studies show no association.[323]

In some of the studies in which no association with total fat intake was found, other potential links between colon cancer and dietary fats were found, such as the source of fat or the type of fat in relation to family history. For example, in the Nurses' Health Study, colon cancer risk was higher with red meat than with white meat intake.[324] In another large cohort study, subgroup analyses revealed a possible interaction between hereditary colon cancers and fat intake.[325]

Epidemiologic studies are limited by a variety of biases. Correlational or ecologic studies are unable to control for confounding factors because the exposure measures represent average exposure rather than actual individual exposures. Case–control and cohort studies may be limited by recall biases. Interventional studies will be less prone to these types of weakness, but when designed with an end point of cancer incidence, will require 10 to 20 years and enormous resources to finish because colorectal cancer develops over a long period in the general population. Therefore, interventional studies have used colonic adenomatous polyp incidence as a surrogate end point.

In one of these interventional studies (the Australian Polyp Prevention Project), 424 patients with a history of resected polyps were randomized to either a regular diet or to a diet lower (25% reduction) in fat, rich in fiber, and supplemented with β-carotene. The interventional diet lowered the incidence of large (>1 cm) adenomatous polyps, although the overall incidences of adenomas were similar in the two groups at 4 years of follow-up.[326] In the second study, 201 subjects were randomized to either a low-fat (<50 g), high-fiber diet (50 g) or a regular Western diet.[327] No significant risk reduction was detected (RR = 1.2; 95% CI, 0.6–2.2). Therefore, except for ecologic studies, clinical studies have yet to confirm the preclinical findings that link fat consumption and colorectal cancer.

Several lines of evidence suggest that dietary fiber might have a protective effect against colon cancer. Many retrospective epidemiologic studies have shown that high fiber intake reduces the risk of colon cancer.[328] Data pooled for meta-analyses from 37 observational epidemiologic studies, as well as 16 case–control studies, showed that dietary fiber has a protective effect (RR = 0.57; 95% CI, 0.5–0.64).[329]

Nevertheless, one large, prospective cohort study, the Nurses' Health Study, showed no protective effects from dietary fibers.[330] Several randomized interventional studies have also evaluated the possible effect of dietary fiber. In one study, the Toronto Polyp Prevention Trial, no benefit was found. However, several other interventional studies, such as the Health Professionals' Study, the Familial Adenomatous Polyposis Trial, and the Australian Polyp Prevention Project (large adenomas), have demonstrated that dietary fibers have a possible protective effect against colon cancer.[331a] More recently, two very large randomized studies showed that high fiber diets had no effects on the risk of colorectal adenoma recurrence.[331b,c] Thus, the protective effects of fiber seem to be unlikely.

Evidence suggests that tea and coffee consumption might reduce the risk of colorectal cancer.[332,333]

### Environmental exposures

A variety of studies support the concept that environmental factors can influence the risk of colon cancer.[334] Studies have shown that environmental and genetic factors can interact to affect the risk of colorectal carcinoma.[325,335] Environmental exposure in the colon would be expected to occur mainly through ingested substances (e.g., dietary substances and medications). Nevertheless, dietary factors are difficult to study because of the large variations in human diets and the complexity of dietary ingredients.

Increased leisure time has a protective effect against colon cancer, as shown in several case–control studies,[336,337] a population–case–referent study,[338] and large prospective observational studies.[339–341] Fewer studies have shown that occupational physical activities have similar protective effects.[342,343]

Similarly, exercise reduces the risk of developing colonic adenoma, as shown in case–control and observational studies.[344–346] The cause for the protective effect remains unclear; however, several mechanisms have been proposed, including the following:

1. A reduction in the colonic transient time results in a reduction in the colonic mucosa exposure to fecal carcinogens.[339]
2. A reduction of hyperinsulinemia, a condition associated with an increase in the risk of colon cancer, results in reduced risk. Also, colon cancers express receptors for insulin-like growth factors.[347–353]
3. A reduction in prostaglandin levels and modulation of bile acid metabolism.[340]

The preponderance of epidemiologic evidence indicates that alcohol consumption contributes to colon tumorigenesis. In eight of nine epidemiologic studies that include case–control and large, prospective observational studies, alcohol use increased the risk of colon cancer.[354–361] Likewise, several epidemiologic studies have shown that alcohol consumption promotes the development of colonic polyps.[344,360,362–365]

The relationship between smoking and colon cancer remains controversial, with some but not all studies showing an association. Several studies have shown that smoking increases the risk of developing colonic adenomas.[366–368] In one case–control study of 779 patients with colorectal cancer and 2315 randomly chosen control subjects, a history of smoking increased the risk of colorectal cancer in women.[369] Several other studies, however, found no association between smoking and the risk of colorectal cancer, including a large case–control study of 1953 patients with colorectal cancer and 4154 control subjects[370] and a second study of 1584 patients and 2879 control subjects.[371] Additionally, two large, prospective, observational studies have shown no association between smoking and colorectal cancer. One Swedish study of 135,000 male construction workers followed for 20 years found no association between smoking and colorectal cancer (RR = 0.98; 95% CI, 0.82–1.17 for colon cancer and RR = 1.16; 95% CI, 0.94–1.44 for rectal cancer among current smokers).[372] Similarly, a Norwegian study of 28,000 subjects who were followed for 26 years did not detect an increase in colorectal cancer risk with smoking.[156] Therefore, the association between smoking and colon cancer remains unconfirmed.

### Family history

A family history of colon cancer increases the individual's risk of developing the disease.[373] The two best-known hereditary colon cancer syndromes are familial adenomatous polyposis (FAP) and hereditary nonpolyposis colon cancer (HNPCC) (see Chapter 54 for more details).

It is estimated that approximately 20% to 30% of colorectal cancers are familial,[374] and approximately 10% of cases have defined hereditary cancer syndromes. This increase in risk varies from being quite high, as in families with hereditary bowel cancer syndromes (e.g., FAP and hereditary nonpolyposis colon cancer), to being minimally increased in cases in which the family history involves only distant relatives.[375]

Familial adenomatous polyposis is an autosomal dominant disease[376] that affects multiple systems. The disease is characterized by the development of a very large number of polyps (>100) at a very young age (the second decade of life). If left untreated, it leads to the development of colorectal cancer in almost all patients in the fourth decade of life.[373,377]

Hereditary nonpolyposis colon cancer is a hereditary cancer syndrome characterized by an autosomal dominant inheritance pattern that leads to the development of colon cancer at an early age (mean, 45 years) and to other extracolonic cancers (especially endometrial, ovarian, gastric, small bowel, and urinary tract).[378] In contrast to FAP, HNPCC is somewhat difficult to distinguish clinically. Therefore, clinical criteria (Amsterdam criteria) were developed in the early 1990s to clinically detect HNPCC: three relatives in two successive generations, at least one of whom developed colorectal cancer before the age of 50, with one being a first-degree relative to one of the other two.[379] The Amsterdam criteria were, however, found to have a low sensitivity for the detection of HNPCC, and therefore newer criteria with higher sensitivity have been developed (e.g., the Bethesda guidelines,[380] and the newer International Collaborative Group on HNPCC criteria[381]).

Subjects with HNPCC are at a very high risk for developing colorectal cancer with or without extracolonic tumors (Lynch I and II syndromes). Colorectal cancers in patients with HNPCC are characterized by young age of onset, more proximal colon location than sporadic cancers, increased risk of metachronous and synchronous colorectal cancers, and faster transformation rates of colonic adenomas into colonic cancers.[378,382]

Hamartomatous polyposis syndromes (e.g., Peutz-Jeghers syndrome and juvenile polyposis) are hereditary syndromes associated with the development of hamartomas in the large and small intestine. These syndromes are associated with an increased risk of colorectal cancer. This increase in risk is not as well defined and is believed to be less than that observed with HNPCC and FAP.[383]

### Prior colon diseases

Chronic inflammatory bowel diseases such as ulcerative colitis and Crohn's disease increase the risk of colorectal cancer.[384] This increased risk is related to the duration of the inflammatory disease, age of onset, and the degree of dysplasia.[384–387] The cancers associated with these diseases are usually flat and infiltrating, commonly developing from an area of precancerous dysplasia rather than from polyps.[383] Colonoscopy, with multiple biopsies for dysplasia detection, is recommended every 1 to 2 years, starting at 8 years from the onset of inflammatory bowel disease and at 12 to 15 years from the onset of left-sided colitis.[375]

Patients with a history of colon cancer have a risk of metachronous colon cancer that has been estimated to be between 0.5% and 3.6%. The cumulative annual incidence was estimated in a study of 5476 patients to be around 0.35%.[388] Patients with a history of adenomatous polyps are also at an increased risk for developing colorectal cancer.[389,390] Patients with a history of colon cancer and adenomatous polyps are considered to have a moderately increased risk by American Cancer Society (ACS) criteria and require increased surveillance.[375] The ACS recommends that patients with adenomas or carcinoma have a full colonoscopy performed at the time of diagnosis. A colonoscopy is to be repeated 1 year after a curative resection of a colorectal cancer. In cases of adenoma or carcinoma, a colonoscopy or a double-contrast barium enema or flexible sigmoidoscopy if the rectosigmoid is not well visualized on barium enema is recommended after 3 years, and then every 5 years.[375]

There are numerous potential primary preventive strategies for colorectal cancer, but no evidenced-based recommendation can currently be made. A diet high in fruit and vegetables would be a reasonable step toward colorectal cancer prevention and would provide numerous other health benefits.

## Secondary Prevention

### Natural history and pathogenesis

Colorectal cancer develops in a chronic multistep process, which allows the opportunity for early detection and treatment interventions. Several lines of evidence indicate that colonic adenoma is a precancerous step that precedes colorectal carcinoma.[391] The prevalence patterns in the general population and the anatomic distribution patterns are similar for adenoma and carcinoma, and carcinoma is usually associated with adenoma. Additionally, the removal of colonic adenomas is very effective in preventing the development of colon cancer,[389] a result that has become one of the major incentives for recommending periodic screening for colonic carcinoma.

The aberrant crypt focus (ACF) has emerged as an early morphologic stage for colonic carcinogenesis and a precursor to both colonic adenoma and carcinoma. Initially, Bird and colleagues described ACF as large, thick crypts recognized with methylene blue staining of the colon in mice treated with a colonic carcinogen, azoxymethane.[392] The ACF, especially the dysplastic type, were later recognized as precancerous lesions on the basis of their temporal association with chemically induced colon cancer in animals.[393] Studies in patients with colonic adenoma and carcinoma suggest ACF to be an earlier step in colonic carcinogenesis than either adenoma or carcinoma of the colon in human.[394]

The morphologic precancerous conditions of colon adenoma and ACF are preceded and accompanied by submorphologic cellular changes. Many functional genetic mutations occur as colon carcinogenesis evolves.[395] These mutations are thought to accumulate in a sequence in which the loss of several tumor suppressor genes precedes the activation of oncogenes that allow the malignant transformation.[396,397]

It has been estimated that approximately 6% of the U.S. population will develop colorectal cancer within their lifetime.[375] Thus, screening for colorectal cancer is recommended for the general population starting at the age of 50.[375] Unfortunately, screening for colorectal cancer remains underused, as reflected in the high proportions of patients who present with late-stage disease.

According to the National Cancer Data Base report on colon cancer cases from U.S. hospital cancer registries between 1988 and 1993, 45.7% of patients were diagnosed with stage III or IV disease.[398] Of concern is that the ratio of early-stage to late-stage disease was higher in patients 60 years or older (ratio of 1.1–1.4) than in patients aged less than 60 years (ratio of 0.8–0.9).[398]

Therefore, screening and primary prevention of colorectal cancer are important public health goals.

Surgical resection remains the primary curative treatment in colon cancer, and the cure rates depend on the stage of disease; thus, the detection of early-stage disease leads to better cure rates.[399,400] Moreover, because colonic adenomas are precancerous lesions for colonic cancer, the removal of polyps can drastically reduce the incidence of colorectal cancer, as demonstrated in the National Polyp Prevention Study.[389,390]

A variety of screening methods are available that can detect the disease in early stages, and some of these methods detect even precancerous lesions (e.g., polyps). Indeed, data are available to show the success of these screening methods to various degrees in reducing the morbidity and mortality rate from colon cancer. Chemoprevention is a promising new strategy to prevent colorectal cancer that is attracting increasing interest. It is hoped that through the use of different prevention strategies, the incidence of and mortality from this common cancer will be markedly decreased.

## Screening Methods

Only a small percentage of tumors occur within the reach of the digital rectal examination. In a study of 1500 patients reported in 1977 accurately diagnosed, 10% of all colorectal tumors were by digital rectal examination.[401] The sensitivity of the digital rectal examination improves with the addition of fecal occult blood (FOB) testing, as demonstrated in a retrospective study of patients who underwent a colonoscopy for the evaluation of a positive FOB test by digital rectal examination and had no gastrointestinal symptoms. Adenoma or carcinoma was found in 28% of these patients.[402] Digital rectal examination is part of the routine physical examination and it is likely to continue to contribute to the detection of colon tumors, especially with the addition of FOB testing to the examination.

Several very large randomized studies have demonstrated that screening with FOB testing reduces the mortality rate from colorectal cancer (Table 2–2). The reduction ranged from 33% with annual screening[403] to 15% with biannual screening.[404] These differences in mortality reduction reflect the variability in the frequency and type of FOB testing used in the different studies.

The specificity and sensitivity of FOB testing for colorectal cancer detection vary considerably depending on the technique used for testing.[407] Rehydration of FOB cards has been shown to increase sensitivity while lowering the positive predictive value.[403] This improvement in the sensitivity has helped to improve detection rates; the rate of negative colonoscopies, however, increased as well. In fact, one of the criticisms of the Minnesota study[403] was the high rate of colonoscopies in this cohort. This was interpreted by some investigators to mean that the benefit of screening should be attributed mainly to colonoscopy instead of to the FOB test.

A reduction in colorectal cancer mortality rates was shown despite the colorectal cancer incidence in these studies remaining similar between the observation and the intervention arm (Table 2–2). The percentage of patients diagnosed with earlier stages of colon cancer was higher in all of these studies (Table 2–2). This downstaging of the disease at the time of diagnosis is a likely cause for the reduction in colorectal mortality rates in screened patients. Thus, FOB screening benefits patients by detecting colorectal cancer at earlier stages rather than by lowering the incidence of the disease by detecting colonic adenoma.

**Table 2–2** Controlled clinical trials of screening by fecal occult blood tests

| Reference | Subjects Completing Test n (% total) | Sensitivity (%) | PPV* | Decrease in Mortality Rate from Colorectal Cancer (%) | Patients with Dukes' Stage A and B | |
|---|---|---|---|---|---|---|
| | | | | | Screened (%) | Control (%) |
| Mandel et al., 1993[403] | 4300 (76) | 81 | 5.6 | 30 | 65 | 33 |
| | 20,000 (76) | 94 | 2.2 | | | |
| Kronborg et al., 1996[405] | 20,672 (67) | 33 | 17 | 18 | 56 | 48 |
| Hardcastle et al., 1996[404] | 75,253 (60) | 67 | 10.2 | 15 | 90 | 40 |
| Kewenter et al., 1994[406] | 4436 (67) | 22 | 4.8 | N/A[†] | 65 | 33 |
| | 16,911 (62) | 84 | 5 | | | |

*Positive predicative value for detecting colorectal cancer.

[†]Data are not matured enough to show any effect of screening on mortality from colorectal cancer.

This would be expected, given that FOB screening has much higher sensitivity for cancer than for adenomas.[408]

One advantage of FOB screening is that it is more convenient, thus the compliance rates in the general population are likely to be higher than for invasive methods (e.g., flexible colonoscopy).[409] The improvement in cure rates from FOB screening is partial (≤30%; see Table 2–3). The cure rates for colorectal cancer can be further improved if more cases are detected in stage I and can reach 100% if the disease is detected in precancerous stages (i.e., adenoma). All of these factors argue for the need for complementary or alternative methods to FOB testing to achieve better success rates.

Flexible sigmoidoscopy covers only a part of the colon and allows the detection of only half of all colorectal neoplasias.[383] However, with the shift in the location of lesions to the right side of the colon, the adequacy of this screening modality has been questioned.[410] Although this modality has been advocated as being more convenient than colonoscopy, it is estimated that only 30% of eligible patients undergo flexible sigmoidoscopy.[411]

Nevertheless, flexible sigmoidoscopy has been shown to reduce colorectal cancer mortality rates in retrospective studies. A case–control study has shown that rigid sigmoidoscopies decrease the odds ratio of colorectal cancer mortality from tumors within the reach of the scope.[412] Two other case–control studies have suggested that use of screening sigmoidoscopy reduces colorectal cancer mortality rates.[413,414] Nevertheless, data from randomized controlled studies to support these findings are still lacking.

In an attempt to improve the effectiveness of this screening modality, sigmoidoscopy has been combined with the FOB test for screening. In a randomized study of 12,479 patients from New York City, the addition of FOB testing lowered the mortality rate of colorectal cancer. Patients who underwent the combined screening were discovered with earlier-stage disease and survived longer.[390]

The effectiveness of the barium enema study as a screening method is influenced to a large degree by the marked variability in its accuracy. Double-contrast barium enema has a higher sensitivity than single contrast, but the sensitivity for double-contrast barium enema varies widely, from 50% to 80% for polyps smaller than 1 cm, 70% to 90% for polyps larger than 1 cm, and 55% to 85% for Dukes' stage A or B colon cancers.[383] The sensitivity of the barium enema study for detecting colorectal cancer is lower than that of colonoscopy, as shown in a retrospective analysis of 2193 consecutive colorectal cancer cases.[415]

The double-contrast barium enema study has been combined with sigmoidoscopy to improve sensitivity of the barium enema by better visualization of the rectosigmoid area. In one Swedish study, the sensitivity of this combined method was 97.6% for carcinoma and 99% for adenoma.[416] The current guidelines for screening average-risk and moderate-risk populations allow screening colonoscopy to be used instead of the double-contrast enema combined with flexible sigmoidoscopy in cases where the rectosigmoid region is not well visualized by the latter methods.[375]

Colonoscopy is considered to be the most accurate method for screening, and is the only method of screening that permits both the full visualization of the colon and the removal of precancerous lesions.[383] The risk of serious complications with colonoscopy, however, is higher than with less invasive procedures. Nevertheless, the value of colonoscopy in reducing the incidence of colorectal cancer was clearly shown in the National Polyp Project Study.[389] Screening colonoscopy is now recommended by the ACS, especially for high-risk groups.

## Chemoprevention

Colorectal cancer has been one of the primary targets for the clinical development of chemoprevention with agents such as nonsteroidal anti-inflammatory drugs (NSAIDs) and calcium.

Many preclinical studies have demonstrated that NSAIDs inhibit colon carcinogenesis in vitro,[417,418] and inhibit chemically or genetically induced intestinal carcinogenesis in rodent models.[419–427] The molecular mechanism responsible for the chemopreventive activity of NSAIDs remains unknown. Hypothesized mechanisms of actions have included the cyclooxygenase (COX) suppression of immune function,[428] cellular oxidative stress,[428,429] and apoptosis regulation.[430–432] Non–COX mediated mechanisms have also been postulated and include the suppression of nuclear factor (NF)-κB activation,[433] inhibition of Ap-1 activity,[434] enhancement of apoptosis,[435,436] and inhibition of angiogenesis.[437]

The COXs mediate the conversion of arachidonic acid, a common polyunsaturated fatty acid, to prostaglandins. COX-1 is a constitutive enzyme that produces $PGE_2$ for various physiologic functions, whereas COX-2, with a few exceptions, is a predominantly inducible enzyme that is up-regulated during pathologic events, such as inflammation and tumorigenesis.

Several lines of evidence suggest that the formation of $PGE_2$ via COX-2 contributes to colonic carcinogenesis. First, the amount of $PGE_2$—but not that of other prostaglandins—is higher in colon tumors than in the normal colonic mucosa. $PGE_2$ promotes the proliferation of transformed colonic cells in some preclinical models.[438] This increase in $PGE_2$ is likely mediated by COX-2 during colon tumorigenesis because COX-2, but not COX-1, is up-regulated in human colon adenomas and cancers.[439] Furthermore, selective COX-2 inhibition suppresses colonic carcinogenesis in animals.

The NSAIDs have properties other than COX-2 inhibition that are likely to contribute to their chemopreventive effects, such as lipoxygenase modulation, protein kinase C (PKC) inhibition, NF-κB activation, PPAR-γ activation,[440] and PPAR-δ inhibition.[441] Moreover, NSAIDs that are incapable of inhibiting COX-2 suppress colon carcinogenesis in rats,[442–444] and NSAIDs inhibit colon cancer cell growth in vitro by inducing apoptosis[444] independently of COX inhibition. Even agents that selectively target COX-2 might exert their chemopreventive effects through mechanisms that are independent of COX inhibition (e.g., apoptotic effects).[445]

Arachidonic acid can form other active metabolites through various lipoxygenase enzymes (e.g., the 5, 8, 12, or 15 lipoxygenases). The predominance of lipoxygenase products over prostaglandins in the colonic epithelium[446] and the possible role of lipoxygenase products in colon carcinogenesis[447] may reflect additional or alternative arachidonic acid metabolic pathways that might be modulated by NSAIDs.[447–449] A variety of clinical evidence suggests that the chronic administration of NSAIDs re-duces the risk of colon cancer. Seven large retrospective studies have shown that NSAIDs reduce the risk of developing colorectal cancer by 40% to 50%[450–456] (Table 2–3). Four of five large, prospective, observational studies have shown a similar benefit[361,457–460] (Table 2–4).

In the Nurses' Health Study, the reduction in risk was statistically significant only when aspirin was taken for 20 years or more (RR = 0.56; 95% CI, 0.36–0.90).[361] One observational study of elderly patients showed that use of aspirin increases the risk of colon cancer;[460] on further follow-up in the same study, the increased risk became nonsignificant in women.[453] This study has been criticized because it lacked follow-up data on aspirin intake, which is likely to be important given the high likelihood of substantial aspirin intake in an elderly population.

A prospective randomized study, the Physicians' Health Study (PHS), failed to confirm the benefit of NSAIDs in protecting against colon cancer.[463] The PHS involved 22,071 healthy male physicians between the ages of 40 and 84 years who were randomized to one of four treatment arms (aspirin, β-carotene, both, or placebo) in a $2 \times 2$ factorial design.[464] The aspirin arm was ended after 5 years to allow any study participant to take aspirin because of its demonstrated benefit in preventing myocardial infarctions. Analyses at 5 and 12 years of observation showed no benefit of aspirin as a colorectal cancer preventive.[463,464]

The PHS is less likely than other published population-based studies to have had the biases associated with retrospective or

**Table 2–3** Retrospective studies of nonsteroidal anti-inflammatory drugs and colon cancer

| Reference | NSAIDs | OR (95% CI) for Colorectal Cancer with Treatment | Patient Characteristics | Comments |
|---|---|---|---|---|
| Rosenberg et al., 1991[454] | NSAIDs | 0.5 (0.4–0.8) | 1326 patients with colorectal cancer and 4891 control subjects | Hospital-based |
| Kune et al., 1988[452] | ASA | 0.53 | 715 colorectal cancer patients and 727 age- and gender-matched control subjects | Population-based |
| Sug et al., 1993[456] | ASA | 0.33 (0.72–0.15) compared with screening clinic visitors, 0.44 (1.1–0.18) compared with hospital controls | 490 patients with colon cancer, 340 with rectal cancer, and 212 with polyps Control subjects: 524 hospitalized patients without cancer or GI disease and 1138 healthy visitors to the screening clinic | OR for colonic polyp also decreased with ASA use |
| Muscat et al., 1994[450] | NSAIDs | 0.64 (0.42–0.97) for males, 0.32 (0.18–0.57) for females | 511 colorectal cancer patients, 500 age- and gender-matched control subjects | Hospital-based case–control study |
| Peleg et al., 1994[451] | ASA and NSAIDs | 0.52 (0.39–0.91) to 0.08 (0.01–0.59), depending on duration of ASA use; 0.34 (0.15–0.77) for NSAIDs use ≥350 days | 97 cases with 388 age- and gender-matched control subjects | |
| Collet et al., 1999[461] | NSAIDs | 0.57 (0.36–0.89) for colon cancer, 0.26 (0.11–0.61) for rectal cancer | Case–control study nested in a nonconcurrent cohort linkage study | Significant effects required exposure of 11–15 years |
| Smalley et al., 1999[455] | NSAIDs (non-ASA) | 0.49 (0.24–1) | 104,217 aged 65 years or older (population database retrospective cohort study) | Benefit was higher for right-sided colon cancers |

ASA, aspirin; CI, confidence interval; NSAIDs, nonsteroidal anti-inflammatory drugs; OR, odds ratio.

**Table 2-4** Prospective observational studies of nonsteroidal anti-inflammatory drugs and colorectal cancer

| Reference | NSAIDs | OR (95% CI) for Colorectal Cancer with Treatment | Patient Characteristics | Comments |
|---|---|---|---|---|
| Giovannucci et al., 1995[361] | ASA | 0.56 (0.36–0.9) | Large cohort of nurses | Benefit was seen after 20 years of consistent use of aspirin |
| Schreinemacher and Everson, 1994[458] | ASA | 0.35 (0.17–0.73), younger men | 2668 subjects aged 25–74 followed for an average of 12.4 years | |
| Giovannucci et al., 1994[459] | ASA | 0.68 (0.52–0.92) | 47,900 physicians | |
| Thun et al., 1991[457] | ASA and other NSAIDs | Men 0.6 (0.4–0.89); women 0.58 (0.37–0.9) | Nested case–control, 598 patients and 3058 matched control subjects | Study was nested in a prospective study of 662,424 adults |
| Paganini-Hill, 1994[462] | ASA | 1.5 (1.1–2.2) | 13,987 (cohort of resident of retirement community; median age, 73) | RR further decreased with further follow-up (RR in women, 1.01) |

ASA, aspirin; CI, confidence interval; NSAIDs, nonsteroidal anti-inflammatory drugs; OR, odds ratio.

observational studies (e.g., recall bias); however, the randomized portion of the study lasted only 5 years, and then the study essentially became observational. After the end of the aspirin randomization, most (71%) of the participants chose to take aspirin regularly. This imbalance in treatment arms could have decreased the statistical power of the follow-up analysis to detect an effect.[463]

The relatively short follow-up period may have affected the ability of the PHS to reveal a chemopreventive benefit for aspirin. The benefit in the Nurses' Health Study required 20 years of chronic aspirin use. A newly reported case–control study has demonstrated the need for extended NSAID use (at least 11 to 15 years) to reduce the risk of colorectal cancer.[461]

Several issues must therefore be addressed before NSAIDs can be recommended as chemopreventive agents in common medical practice. First, the benefit of these agents in colorectal cancer prevention must be prospectively confirmed. Although several epidemiologic studies have demonstrated potential benefit from NSAIDs, large randomized, confirmatory studies designed to evaluate these issues are still lacking. In the absence of predictive biomarkers, long and costly studies that might last for 20 years or more will be needed to document beneficial preventive outcomes. Second, NSAID agents and effective doses with acceptable side-effect profiles for long-term use must be selected. The agent or agents to be selected need to be effective and have the fewest side effects from chronic (possibly decades-long) administration. Finally, the patient populations who will benefit from this type of chemoprophylaxis must be defined. As genetic testing methods for hereditary colon diseases improve, increasing numbers of individuals will be identified as being susceptible to colorectal cancer and will require preventive measures.

As an example, selective COX-2 inhibitors have been selected for chemoprevention clinical studies because of the demonstrated preclinical activity of these agents in suppressing colon tumorigenesis[421] and the premise of fewer side effects with COX-2 selectivity. Prospective trials of NSAIDs and COX-2 inhibitors as colorectal chemopreventive agents in humans have focused on reduction in adenoma recurrence as a surrogate end point for reduction in colorectal cancer occurrence.[465,466] Prospective polyp reduction trials are currently ongoing in the United States and Europe. While a selective COX-2 inhibitor, celecoxib, caused a

modest reduction in colonic adenoma recurrence and growth in human familial polyposis subjects,[466] sulindac, a COX-1 and COX-2 inhibitor, had no effect in a similar cohort.[467a] Aspirin moderately reduced recurrence rates of sporadic colorectal adenomas for the 81 mg/day dose but not for the 325 mg/day dose in a large randomized study.[467b] Results from other randomized studies of sporadic colorectal adenoma risk and NSAIDs are expected in the near future.

Several lines of evidence suggest the potential role of a dietary calcium supplement in colorectal cancer chemoprevention. Calcium supplementation inhibits colonic carcinogenesis in animal studies.[468,469] Calcium supplements also reduce colonic cell proliferation rates and promote differentiation in humans.[470,471]

One proposed mechanism for this effect is that calcium binds deoxycholic acid and neutralizes its pro-proliferative effects.[472–474] In a case–control study of 3428 subjects in Taiwan, high calcium levels in drinking water had a protective effect against colon cancer.[475] In a recent review of currently available epidemiologic data from 20 published studies, Martinez and colleagues found that the protective effects of calcium against colon cancer are weak at best.[476] Still, the role of calcium in colon cancer prevention has been further supported by the results of a recent randomized study in which calcium supplementation reduced adenoma recurrence in patients with a recent history of colonic adenoma.[477]

Vitamin supplementation, especially folic acid, reduces the risk of colorectal cancer. Intake of fruit and vegetables, natural sources of vitamins, protects against colon cancer, as shown in large number of epidemiologic studies.[478,479]

Fewer studies have examined the relationship between vitamin D and colon cancer.[476] The limited data available suggest that vitamin D provides protective effects that deserve further investigation. Vitamin $D_3$ supplementation has been shown to have anticarcinogenic effects in animals.[480,481]

Although fruits and vegetables contain ingredients that might have protective effects, multivitamin supplementation has also been shown to have a protective effect against colon cancer, as in a recent case–control study (OR, 0.49).[482] More specifically, folate inhibits colonic carcinogenesis in animals[483] and reduces the risk for developing colonic adenomas.[484]

Hormone replacement therapy has shown protective effects against colorectal cancer in several epidemiologic studies. In meta-analyses of 19 studies published by 1996, hormone replacement therapy resulted in a 15% reduction in the relative risk of colorectal cancer (RR = 0.85; 95% CI, 0.73–0.99).[485] Findings from the Nurses' Health Study later supported these findings, showing also a risk reduction with the use of hormone replacement therapy that disappeared within 5 years of cessation of treatment.[486]

In conclusion, various promising agents for chemoprevention are currently under clinical investigation, but more data are required to recommend the use of these agents in clinical practice.

## Future Directions

The encouraging recent trend in reduced incidence and mortality rates from colorectal cancer is likely to continue because of improvements in early detection and prevention. Nevertheless, colorectal cancer remains a major cause of cancer death in the United States and throughout the world. More improvement in the utilization of screening modalities is needed. New tools to diagnose hereditary colon cancer are expected to improve our ability to tailor screening according to the individual's risk profile. New and promising chemopreventive agents are under active clinical development. The future is likely to hold more improvement in reducing the mortality and morbidity rates from this common malignancy.

## References

1. U.S. Preventive Services Task Force. Guide to Clinical Preventive Services: Report of the U.S. Preventive Services Task Force, 2nd ed. Williams & Wilkins, Baltimore, 1996.
2. Parkin D, Pisani P, Ferlay J. Estimates of the worldwide incidence of eighteen major cancers in 1985. Int J Cancer 54:594–606, 1993.
3. Powell J, McConkey C. Increasing incidence of adenocarcinoma of the gastric cardia and adjacent sites. Br J Cancer 62:440–443, 1990.
4. Blot W, Devesa S, Kneller R, Fraumeni JJ. Rising incidence of adenocarcinoma of the esophagus and gastric cardia. JAMA 265:1287–1289, 1991.
5. Blot W, Devesa S, Fraumeni JJ. Continuing climb in rates of esophageal adenocarcinoma: an update. JAMA 270:1320–1325, 1993.
6. Blot W. Esophageal cancer trends and risk factors. Semin Oncol 21:403–410, 1994.
7. Devesa S, Blot W, Fraumeni J. Changing patterns in the incidence of esophageal and gastric carcinoma in the United States. Cancer 83:2049–2053, 1998.
8. Munoz N, Day N. Esophageal cancer. In: Schottenfeld D, Fraumeni J (eds): Cancer Epidemiology and Prevention. Oxford University Press, New York, 1998, pp 681–706.
9. Fraumeni J, Blot W. Geographic variation in esophageal cancer mortality in the United States. J Chron Dis 30:759–767, 1977.
10. Jussawalla D. Epidemiological assessment of aetiology of oesophageal cancer in greater Bombay. Presented at the International Seminar on Epidemiology of Oesophageal Cancer, Bangalore, India, 1971.
11. Gronbaek M, Becker U, Johansen D, et al. Population-based cohort study of the association between alcohol intake and cancer of the upper digestive tract. BMJ 317:844–847, 1998.
12. Breslow N, Day N. Statistical Methods in Cancer Research. The Analysis of Case–Control Studies. International Agency for Research on Cancer, Lyon, 1980.
13. Rogot E, Murray J. Smoking and causes of death among U.S. veterans: 16 years of observation. Publ Health Rep 95:213–222, 1980.
14. Rogot E, Murray J. Cancer mortality among nonsmokers in an insured group of U.S. veterans. J Natl Cancer Inst 65:1163–1168, 1980.
15. Castellsague X, Monoz N, DeStefani E, et al. Independent and joint effects of tobacco smoking and alcohol drinking on the risk of esophageal cancer in man and women. Int J Cancer 82:657–664, 1999.
16. Roth M, Strickland K, Wang G, et al. High levels of carcinogenic polycyclic aromatic hydrocarbons present within the food from Linxian, China may contribute to that region's high incidence of oesophageal cancer. Eur J Cancer 34:757–758, 1998.
17. Syndenham E, Thiel P, Marasas W, et al. Natural occurrence of some fusarium mycotoxins in corn from low and high esopyhageal cancer

prevalence areas of the Transkei, Southern Africa. J Agric Food Chem 38:1900–1903, 1990.
18. O'Neill C, Jordan P, Bhatt T, Newman R. Silica and esophageal cancer. Ciba Found Symp 121:214–230, 1986.
19. Gustavsson P, Evanoff B, Hogstedt C. Increased risk of esophageal cancer among workers exposed to combustion products. Arch Environ Health 48:243–245, 1993.
20. Yu M, Garabrant D, Peters J, Mack T. Tobacco, alcohol, diet, occupation, and carcinoma of the esophagus. Cancer Res 48:3843–3848, 1988.
21. IRAC/Iran Study Group. Esophageal cancer studies in the Caspian littoral of Iran: results of population studies. A prodrome. J Natl Cancer Inst 59:1127–1138, 1977.
22. Martinez I. Factors associated with cancer of the esophagus, mouth, and pharynx in Puerto Rico. J Natl Cancer Inst 42:1069–1094, 1969.
23. Herbert J, Landon J, Miller D. Consumption of meat and fruit in relation to oral and esophageal cancer: a cross-national study. Nutr Cancer 19:169–179, 1993.
24. Hirayma T. An epideiological study of cancer of the oesophagus in Japan, with special reference to the combined effect of selected environmental factors. Presented at the International Seminar on Epidemiology of Oseophageal Cancer, Bangalore, India, 1971.
25. de Villiers E, Lavergne D, Chang F, et al. An interlaboratory study to determine the presence of human papillomavirus DNA in esophageal carcinoma from China. Int J Cancer 81:225–228, 1999.
26. Chang F, Syrjanen S, Wang L, Shen Q, Syrjanen K. p53 overexpression and human papillomavirus (HPV) infection in oesophageal squamous cell carcinomas derived from a high-incidence area in China. Anticancer Res 17:709–715, 1997.
27. Vassallo A, Correa P, De Stefani E, et al. Esophageal cancer in Uruguay: a case–control study. J Natl Cancer Inst 75:1005–1009, 1985.
28. Victoria C, Munoz N, Day N, et al. Hot beverages and oesophgeal cancer in southern Brazil: a case–control study. Int J Cancer 39:710–716, 1987.
29. Ghadirian P. Thermal irritation and esophageal cancer in northern Iran. Cancer 60:1909–1914, 1987.
30. Wahrendorf J, Chang-Claude J, Qui S, et al. Precursor lesions of oesophageal cancer in adolescents in a high-risk population in China. Lancet 2:1239–1241, 1989.
31. Ghadirian P. Familial history of esophageal cancer. Cancer 56:2112–2116, 1985.
32. Chang-Claude J, Becher H, Blettner M, et al. Familial aggregation of oesophageal cancer in a high incidence area in China. Int J Epidemiol 26:1159–1165, 1997.
33. Xing E, Nie Y, Wang L, Yang G, Yang C. Aberrant methylation of p16$^{INK4a}$ and deletion of p15$^{INK4b}$ are frequent events in human esophageal cancer in Linxian, China. Carcinogenesis 20:77–84, 1999.
34. Lin D, Tang Y, Lu S. Glutathione S-transferase M1, T1 genotypes and the risk of esophageal cancer: a case–control study. Chin J Epidemiol 19:195–199, 1998.
35. Lung M, Chan W, Zong Y, et al. p53 mutational spectrum of esophageal carcinomas from five different geographical locales in China. Cancer Epidemiol Biomarkers Prev 5:277–284, 1996.
36. Shen O, Liu SF, Dawsey SM, et al. Cytologic screening for esophageal cancer: results from 12,877 subjects in a high-risk population in China. Int J Cancer 54:185–188, 1993.
37. Wang L, Zhou Q, Yang C. Esophageal and gastric cardia epithelial cell proliferation in northern Chinese subjects living in high-incidence area. J Cell Biochem 28–29 Suppl:159–165, 1997.
38. Munoz N, Hayashi M, Lu J, et al. Effect of riboflavin, retinol, and zinc on micronuclei of buccal mucosa and of esophagus: a randomized double-blind intervention study in a high-risk population in China. J Natl Cancer Inst 79:687–691, 1987.
39. Wahrendorf J, Munoz N, Lu J, et al. Blood, retinol and zinc riboflavin status in relation to precancerous lesions of the esophagus: findings from a vitamin intervention trial in the People's Republic of China. Cancer Res 48:2280–2283, 1988.
40. Munoz N, Wahrendorf J, Lu J, et al. No effect of riboflavine, retinol and zinc on prevalence of precancerous lesions of esophagus: a randomized double-blind intervention study in a high-risk population of China. Lancet ii:111–114, 1985.
41. Mark S, Liu S, Li J, et al. The effect of vitamin and mineral supplementation on esophageal cytology: results from the Linxian Dysplasia Trial. Int J Cancer 57:162–166, 1994.
42. Blot W, Li J, Taylor P, et al. Nutrition intervention trials in Linxian, China: supplementation with specific vitamin/mineral combinations, cancer incidence and disease specific mortality in the general population. J Natl Cancer Inst 85:1483–1492, 1993.

43. Taylor P, Li B, Dawsey S, et al. Prevention of esophageal cancer: the nutrition intervention trials in Linxian, China. Linxian Nutrition Intervention Trials Study Group. Cancer Res 54:2029s–2031s, 1994.

44. Puestow C, Gillesby W, Guynn V. Carcinoma of the esophagus. Arch Surg 70:662–669, 1955.

45. Cameron A. Epidemiology of columnar-lined esophagus and adenocarcinoma. Gastroenterol Clin North Am 26:487–496, 1997.

46. Spechler S. The frequency of esophageal cancer in patients with Barrett's esophagus. Acta Endoscop 22:541–544, 1992.

47. Spechler S. Barrett's esophagus. Semin Oncol 21:431–437, 1994.

48. Spechler S, Zeroogian J, Antonioli D, Wang H, Goyal R. Prevalence of metaplasia at the gastro-oesophageal junction. Lancet 344:1533–1536, 1994.

49. Sampliner R. Adenocarcinoma of the esophagus and gastric cardia: is there progress in the face of increasing cancer incidence? Ann Intern Med 130:67–69, 1999.

50. Lieberman D, Oehlke M, Helfand M, et al. Risk factors for Barrett's esophagus in community-based practice. Am J Gastroenterol 92:1293–1287, 1997.

51. Brown L, Swanson C, Gridley G, et al. Adenocarcinoma of the esophagus: role of obesity and diet. J Natl Cancer Inst 87:104–109, 1995.

52. Spechler SJ, Goyal RK. Barrett's esophagus. N Engl J Med 315:362–371, 1986.

53. Bozymski E. Barrett's esophagus: endoscopic characteristics. In: Spechler S, Goyal R (eds): Barrett's Esophagus: Pathophysiology, Diagnosis, and Management. Elsevier Science Publishing, New York, 1985, pp 113–120.

54. Paull A, Trier J, Dalton M, et al. The histologic spectrum of Barrett's esophagus. N Engl J Med 295:476–480, 1976.

55. Romero Y, Cameron A, Locke G, et al. Familial aggregation of gastroesophageal reflux in patients with Barrett's esophagus and esophageal adenocarcinoma. Gastroenterology 113:1449–1456, 1997.

56. Vicari J, Peek R, Falk G, et al. The seroprevalence of cagA-positive *Helicobacter pylori* strains in the spectrum of gastroesophageal reflux disease. Gastroenterology 115:50–57, 1998.

57. Clark G, Smyrk T, Burdiles P, Hoeft S, Peters J. Is Barrett's metaplasia the source of adenocarcinomas of the cardia? Arch Surg 129:609–614, 1994.

58. Lagergren J, Bergstrom R, Lindgren A, Nyren O. Symptomatic gastroesophageal reflux as a risk factor for esophageal adenocarcinoma. N Engl J Med 340:825–831, 1999.

59. Hameeteman W, Tytgat G, Houthoff H, van den Tweel J. Barrett's esophagus: development of dysplasia and adenocarcinoma. Gastroenterology 96:1249–1256, 1989.

60. Levine D, Haggitt R, Blount P, et al. An endoscopic biopsy protocol can differentiate high-grade dysplasia from early adenocarcinoma in Barrett's esophagus. Gastroenterology 105:40–50, 1993.

61. Levine D. Management of dysplasia in the columnar-lined esophagus. Gastroenterol Clin North Am 26:613–634, 1997.

62. Drewitz D, Sampliner R, Garewal H. The incidence of adenocarcinoma in Barrett's esophagus: a prospective study of 170 patients followed 4.8 years. Am J Gastroenterol 92:212–215, 1997.

63. Altorki N, Sunagawa M, Little A, Skinner D. High-grade dysplasia in the columnar-lined esophagus. Am J Surg 161:97–100, 1991.

64. Dent J, Bremner C, Collen M, Haggitt R, Spechler S. Working party report to the World Congresses of Gastroenterology, Sydney 1990: Barrett's oesophagus. J Gastroenterol Hepatol 6:1–22, 1991.

65. Barrett M, Sanchez C, Galipeau P, et al. Allelic loss of 9p21 and mutation of CDKN2/p16 gene develop as early lesions during neoplastic progression in Barrett's esophagus. Oncogene 13:1867–1873, 1996.

66. Sampliner R. Ablative therapies for the columnar-lined esophagus. Gastroenterol Clinics North Am 26:685–694, 1997.

67. Bozymski E, Shaheen N. Barrett's esophagus: acid suppression but no regression. Am J Gastroenterol 92:556–557, 1997.

68. Spechler S. Endoscopic surveillance for patients with Barrett's esophagus: does the cancer risk justify the practice? Ann Intern Med 106:902–904, 1987.

69. Morales T, Sampliner R. Barrett's esophagus: update on screening, surveillance, and treatment. Arch Intern Med 159:1411–1416, 1999.

70. Fennerty B, Sampliner R, Garewal H. Esophageal ulceration associated with 13-cis-retinoic acid therapy in patients with Barrett's esophagus. Gastrointest Endosc 35:442–443, 1989.

71. Gerner E, Garewal H, Emerson S, Sampliner R. Gastrointestinal tissue polyamine contents of patients with Barrett's esophagus treated with α-difluoromethylornithine. Cancer Epidemiol Biomarkers Prev 4:325–330, 1994.

72. Haenszel W. Variation in incidence and mortality from stomach cancer

73. Jemal A, Thomas A, Murray T, Thun M. Cancer statistics, 2002. CA Cancer J Clin 52:23–47, 2002.

74. Wanebo HJ, Kennedy BJ, Chmiel J, et al. Cancer of the stomach. A patient care study by the American College of Surgeons. Ann Surg 218:583–592, 1993.

75. Maruyama K, Okabayashi K, Kinoshita T. Progress in gastric cancer surgery in Japan and its limits of radicality. World J Surg 11:418–425, 1987.

76. Nomura A. Stomach cancer. In: Shottenfeld D, Fraumeni JJ (eds): Cancer Epidemiology and Prevention, 2nd ed. Oxford University Press, New York, 1996, pp 707–724.

77. Jedrychowski W, Boeing H, Wahrendorf J, et al. Vodka consumption, tobacco smoking and risk of gastric cancer in Poland. Int J Epidemiol 22:606–613, 1993.

78. You WC, Blot WJ, Chang YS, et al. Diet and high risk of stomach cancer in Shandong, China. Cancer Res 48:3518–3523, 1988.

79. Haenszel W. Cancer mortality among foreign born in the U.S. J Natl Cancer Inst 26:37–132, 1961.

80. Gregorio DI, Flannery JT, Hansen H. Stomach cancer patterns in European immigrants to Connecticut, United States. Cancer Causes Control 3:215–221, 1992.

81. McLaughlin J, Hrubec Z, Blot W, Fraumeni JJ. Stomach cancer and cigarette smoking among U.S. veterans 1954–1980. Cancer Res 50:3804, 1990.

82. Hoshiyama Y, Sasaba T. A case–control study of stomach cancer and its relation to diet, cigarette, and alcohol consumption in Saitama Prefecture, Japan. Cancer Causes Control 3:441–448, 1992.

83. Nomura A, Grove JS, Stemmermann GN, Severson RK. A prospective study of stomach cancer and its relation to diet, cigarettes, and alcohol consumption. Cancer Res 50:627–631, 1990.

84. Kato I, Tominaga S, Matsumoto K. A prospective study of stomach cancer among rural Japanese populations: a 6-year survey. Jpn J Cancer Res 83:568–575, 1992.

85. La Vecchia C, Negri E, Descarli A, D'Avanzo B, Franceschi S. A case-control study of diet and gastric cancer in Northern Italy. Int J Cancer 40:484–489, 1987.

86. Wynder E, Kmet J, Dungal N, et al. An epidemiological investigation of gastric cancer. Cancer 16:1461–1496, 1963.

87. Chyou PH, Nomura AM, Hankin JH, Stemmermann GN. A case–cohort study of diet and stomach cancer. Cancer Res 50:7501–7504, 1990.

88. Hansson L, Baron J, Nyren O, et al. Tobacco, alcohol and the risk of gastric cancer: a population-based case–control study in Sweden. Int J Cancer 57:26–31, 1994.

89. Nakamura K. Stomach cancer in atomic-bomb survivors. Lancet 2:866–867, 1977.

90. Court Brown W, Doll R. Mortality from cancer and other causes after radiotherapy for ankylosing spondylitis. BMJ 2:1327–1332, 1965.

91. Kohn N, Fry R. Radiation carcinogenesis. N Engl J Med 310:504–509, 1984.

92. Fuchs C, Mayer R. Gastric carcinoma. N Engl J Med 333:32–41, 1995.

93. Mirvish S. The etiology of gastric cancer. Intragastric nitrosamide formation and other theories. J Natl Cancer Inst 71:629–647, 1983.

94. Forman D. Dietary exposure to *N*-nitroso compounds and the risk of human cancer. Cancer Surv 6:719–738, 1987.

95. Hartman P. Putative mutagens and carcinogens in foods. I. Nitrate/nitrite ingestion and gastric cancer mortality. Environ Mutagen 5:111–121, 1983.

96. Tsugana S, Akabane M, Inami T, et al. Urinary salt excretion and stomach cancer mortality among four Japanese populations. Cancer Causes Control 2:165–168, 1991.

97. Nomura A, Stemmermann GN, Chyou PH, et al. *Helicobacter pylori* infection and gastric carcinoma among Japanese Americans in Hawaii. N Engl J Med 325:1132–1136, 1991.

98. Forman D, Newell DG, Fullerton F, et al. Association between infection with *Helicobacter pylori* and risk of gastric cancer: evidence from a prospective investigation. BMJ 302:1302–1305, 1991.

99. Parsonnet J, Friedman GD, Vandersteen DP, et al. *Helicobacter pylori* infection and the risk of gastric carcinoma. N Engl J Med 325:1127–1131, 1991.

100. Eurogast. The Eurogast Study Group: international association between *Helicobacter pylori* and gastric cancer. Lancet 341:1359–1362, 1993.

101. Forman D, Webb P, Parsonnet J. *H. pylori* and gastric cancer [letter]. Lancet 343:243–244, 1994.

102. Hansson LE, Nyren O, Hsing AW, et al. The risk of stomach cancer in patients with gastric or duodenal ulcer disease. N Engl J Med 335:242–249, 1996.

with particular reference to the U.S. J Natl Cancer Inst 21:213–262, 1958.

103. Scheiman JM, Cutler AF. *Helicobacter pylori* and gastric cancer. Am J Med 106:222–226, 1999.
104. Graham DY, Malaty HM, Evans DG, et al. Epidemiology of *Helicobacter pylori* in an asymptomatic population in the United States. Effect of age, race, and socioeconomic status. Gastroenterology 100: 1495–1501, 1991.
105. Parsonnet J. *Helicobacter pylori* and gastric cancer. Gastroenterol Clin North Am 22:89–104, 1993.
106. Correa P. Human gastric carcinogenesis: a multistep and multifactorial process—First American Cancer Society Award Lecture on Cancer Epidemiology and Prevention. Cancer Res 52:6735–6740, 1992.
107. Correa P, Haenszel W, Cuello C, et al. Gastric precancerous process in a high-risk population: cross-sectional studies. Cancer Res 50:4731–4736, 1990.
108. Imai T, Kubo T, Watanabe H. Chronic gastritis in Japanese with reference to high incidence of gastric carcinoma. J Natl Cancer Inst 47:179–195, 1971.
109. You WC, Blot WJ, Li JY, et al. Precancerous gastric lesions in a population at high risk of stomach cancer. Cancer Res 53:1317–1321, 1993.
110. Hsing AW, Hansson LE, McLaughlin JK, et al. Pernicious anemia and subsequent cancer. A population-based cohort study. Cancer 71:745–750, 1993.
111. Nightingale TE, Gruber J. *Helicobacter* and human cancer. J Natl Cancer Inst 86:1505–1509, 1994.
112. Ming S, Goldman H. Gastric polyps: a histogenetic classification and its relation to cancer. Cancer 18:721–726, 1965.
113. Nakamura T, Nakano G. Histopathological classification and malignant change in gastric polyps. J Clin Pathol 38:754–764, 1985.
114. Papa A, Cammarota G, Tursi A, et al. Histologic types and surveillance of gastric polyps: a seven year clinico-pathological study. Hepatogastroenterology 45:579–582, 1998.
115. Caygill CP, Hill MJ, Kirkham JS, Northfield TC. Mortality from gastric cancer following gastric surgery for peptic ulcer. Lancet 1:929–931, 1986.
116. Stalnikowicz R, Benbassat J. Risk of gastric cancer after gastric surgery for benign disorders. Arch Intern Med 150:2022–2026, 1990.
117. Tersmette AC, Offerhaus GJ, Tersmette KW, et al. Meta-analysis of the risk of gastric stump cancer: detection of high-risk patient subsets for stomach cancer after remote partial gastrectomy for benign conditions. Cancer Res 50:6486–6489, 1990.
118. Dubrow R. Gastric cancer following peptic ulcer surgery [editorial; comment]. J Natl Cancer Inst 85:1268–1270, 1993.
119. Sokoloff B. Predisposition of cancer in Bonaparte family. Am J Surg 40:673–678, 1938.
120. Haenszel W, Kurihara M, Locke FB, Shimuzu K, Segi M. Stomach cancer in Japan. J Natl Cancer Inst 56:265–274, 1976.
121. Lynch HT, Smyrk TC, Watson P, et al. Genetics, natural history, tumor spectrum, and pathology of hereditary nonpolyposis colorectal cancer: an updated review. Gastroenterology 104:1535–1549, 1993.
122. La Vecchia C, Negri E, Franceschi S, Gentile A. Family history and the risk of stomach and colorectal cancer. Cancer 70:50–55, 1992.
123. Gong C, Mera R, Bravo JC, et al. K-ras mutations predict progression of preneoplastic gastric lesions. Cancer Epidemiol Biomarkers Prev 8:167–171, 1999.
124. National Academy of Sciences. The Health Effects of Nitrate, Nitrite, and N-nitroso Compounds. National Academy Press, Washington, DC, 1981, pp 1–544.
125. Everett SM, Axon AT. Early gastric cancer in Europe. Gut 41:142–150, 1997.
126. Saeki J. Mitteil Med Gessellsch Tokyo 52:191, 1938.
127. Nishi M, Ishihara S, Nakajima T, et al. Chronological changes of characteristics of early gastric cancer and therapy: experience in the Cancer Institute Hospital of Tokyo, 1950–1994. J Cancer Res Clin Oncol 121:535–541, 1995.
128. Shimizu S, Tada M, Kawai K. Early gastric cancer: its surveillance and natural course. Endoscopy 27:27–31, 1995.
129. Yamazaki H, Oshima A, Murakami R, Endoh S, Ubukata T. A long-term follow-up study of patients with gastric cancer detected by mass screening. Cancer 63:613–617, 1989.
130. Guadagni S, Reed PI, Johnston BJ, et al. Early gastric cancer: follow-up after gastrectomy in 159 patients. Br J Surg 80:325–328, 1993.
131. Moreaux J, Bougaran J. Early gastric cancer. A 25-year surgical experience. Ann Surg 217:347–355, 1993.
132. Shizuyo I, Hiroshi H, Chisato N, et al. Evaluation of a screening program on reduction of gastric cancer mortality in Japan: preliminary results from a cohort study. Prev Med 29:102–106, 1999.
133. Pisani P, Oliver WE, Parkin DM, Alvarez N, Vivas J. Case–control study of gastric cancer screening in Venezuela. Br J Cancer 69:1102–1105, 1994.
134. Genta RM, Lew GM, Graham DY. Changes in the gastric mucosa following eradication of *Helicobacter pylori*. Mod Pathol 6:281–289, 1993.
135. Uemura N, Mukai T, Okamoto S, et al. Effect of *Helicobacter pylori* eradication on subsequent development of cancer after endoscopic resection of early gastric cancer. Cancer Epidemiol Biomarkers Prev 6:639–642, 1997.
136. Sung J, Lin S. Effects of Curry *Helicobacter pylori* on precancerous gastric lesions: one-year follow-up of a prospective randomized study in China. Gastroenterology 114, 1998.
137. Parsonnet J, Harris RA, Hack HM, Owens DK. Modelling cost-effectiveness of *Helicobacter pylori* screening to prevent gastric cancer: a mandate for clinical trials. Lancet 348:150–154, 1996.
138. Fendrick AM, Chernew ME, Hirth RA, et al. Clinical and economic effects of population-based *Helicobacter pylori* screening to prevent gastric cancer. Arch Intern Med 159:142–148, 1999.
139. Tsugawa M, Shachter R. Cost-effectiveness of vaccine development for *Helicobacter pylori* using Institute of Medicine model. Gastroenterology 114, 1998.
140. Hansson LE, Nyren O, Bergstrom R, et al. Nutrients and gastric cancer risk. A population-based case–control study in Sweden. Int J Cancer 57:638–644, 1994.
141. Farrow DC, Vaughan TL, Hansten PD, et al. Use of aspirin and other nonsteroidal anti-inflammatory drugs and risk of esophageal and gastric cancer. Cancer Epidemiol Biomarkers Prev 7:97–102, 1998.
142. National Research Council. Diet and Health Implication for Reducing Chronic Disease Risk. Academy Press, Washington, DC, 1990.
143. Evans DB, Abbruzzese JL, Rich TA. Cancer of the pancreas. In: Vincent T, DeVita J, Hellman S, Rosenberg S (eds): Cancer: Principles and Practice of Oncology. Lippincott-Raven, Philadelphia, 1997, pp 1054–1087.
144. Parkin DM, Pisani P, Ferlay J. Global cancer statistics. CA Cancer J Clin 49:33–64, 1999.
145. Sener SF, Fremgen A, Menck HR, Winchester DP. Pancreatic cancer: a report of treatment and survival trends for 100,313 patients diagnosed from 1985 to 1995, using the National Cancer Database. J Am Coll Surg 189:1–7, 1999.
146. Brentnall TA, Bronner MP, Byrd DR, Haggitt RC, Kimmey MB. Early diagnosis and treatment of pancreatic dysplasia in patients with a family history of pancreatic cancer. Ann Intern Med 131:247–255, 1999.
147. Stolzenberg-Solomon RZ, Albanes D, Nieto FJ, et al. Pancreatic cancer risk and nutrition-related methyl-group availability indicators in male smokers. J Natl Cancer Inst 91:535–541, 1999.
148. Norell SE, Ahlbom A, Erwald R, et al. Diet and pancreatic cancer: a case–control study. Am J Epidemiol 124:894–902, 1986.
149. Lee CT, Chang FY, Lee SD. Risk factors for pancreatic cancer in Orientals. J Gastroenterol Hepatol 11:491–495, 1996.
150. Wynder EL, Dieck GS, Hall NE. Case–control study of decaffeinated coffee consumption and pancreatic cancer. Cancer Res 46:5360–5363, 1986.
151. Fernandez E, La Vecchia C, Decarli A. Attributable risks for pancreatic cancer in northern Italy. Cancer Epidemiol Biomarkers Prev 5:23–27, 1996.
152. Partanen TJ, Vainio HU, Ojajarvi IA, Kauppinen TP. Pancreas cancer, tobacco smoking and consumption of alcoholic beverages: a case–control study. Cancer Lett 116:27–32, 1997.
153. Fuchs CS, Colditz GA, Stampfer MJ, et al. A prospective study of cigarette smoking and the risk of pancreatic cancer. Arch Intern Med 156:2255–2260, 1996.
154. Ogren M, Hedberg M, Berglund G, Borgstrom A, Janzon L. Risk of pancreatic carcinoma in smokers enhanced by weight gain. Results from 10-year follow-up of the Malmo Preventive Project Cohort Study. Int J Pancreatol 20:95–101, 1996.
155. Tobacco Smoking, Vol. 38. International Agency for Research on Cancer, Lyon, France, 1986.
156. Engeland A, Andersen A, Haldorsen T, Tretli S. Smoking habits and risk of cancers other than lung cancer: 28 years' follow-up of 26,000 Norwegian men and women. Cancer Causes Control 7:497–506, 1996.
157. Hiatt RA, Klatsky AL, Armstrong MA. Pancreatic cancer, blood glucose and beverage consumption. Int J Cancer 41:794–797, 1988.
158. Neugut A, Jacobson J, Ahsan H, et al. Incidence and recurrence rates of colorectal adenomas: a prospective study. Gastroenterology 108:402–408, 1995.
159. Moolgavkar SH, Stevens RG. Smoking and cancers of bladder and pancreas: risks and temporal trends. J Natl Cancer Inst 67:15–23, 1981.
160. Ohyanagi H, Okumura S, Yamamoto M, et al. Epidemiological studies on pancreatic cancer [in Japanese]. Gan To Kagaku Ryoho 12:189–199, 1985.

161. McMichael AJ, McCall MG, Hartshorne JM, Woodings TL. Patterns of gastro-intestinal cancer in European migrants to Australia: the role of dietary change. Int J Cancer 25:431–437, 1980.

162. Faivre J, Bedenne L, Arveux P, Klepping C. Descriptive epidemiology of cancer of the pancreas [in French]. Bull Cancer 77:39–46, 1990.

163. Olsen GW, Mandel JS, Gibson RW, Wattenberg LW, Schuman LM. Nutrients and pancreatic cancer: a population-based case–control study. Cancer Causes Control 2:291–297, 1991.

164. Bueno de Mesquita HB, Maisonneuve P, Runia S, Moerman CJ. Intake of foods and nutrients and cancer of the exocrine pancreas: a population-based case–control study in The Netherlands. Int J Cancer 48:540–549, 1991.

165. Ji BT, Chow WH, Gridley G, et al. Dietary factors and the risk of pancreatic cancer: a case–control study in Shanghai China. Cancer Epidemiol Biomarkers Prev 4:885–893, 1995.

166. Mills PK, Beeson WL, Abbey DE, Fraser GE, Phillips RL. Dietary habits and past medical history as related to fatal pancreas cancer risk among Adventists. Cancer 61:2578–2585, 1988.

167. Lyon JL, Slattery ML, Mahoney AW, Robison LM. Dietary intake as a risk factor for cancer of the exocrine pancreas. Cancer Epidemiol Biomarkers Prev 2:513–518, 1993.

168. Kalapothaki V, Tzonou A, Hsieh CC, et al. Nutrient intake and cancer of the pancreas: a case–control study in Athens, Greece. Cancer Causes Control 4:383–389, 1993.

169. Farrow DC, Davis S. Diet and the risk of pancreatic cancer in men. Am J Epidemiol 132:423–431, 1990.

170. Lyon JL, Mahoney AW, French TK, Moser R Jr. Coffee consumption and the risk of cancer of the exocrine pancreas: a case–control study in a low-risk population. Epidemiology 3:164–170, 1992.

171. Clavel F, Benhamou E, Auquier A, Tarayre M, Flamant R. Coffee, alcohol, smoking and cancer of the pancreas: a case–control study. Int J Cancer 43:17–21, 1989.

172. Goldstein AM, Fraser MC, Struewing JP, et al. Increased risk of pancreatic cancer in melanoma-prone kindreds with *p16INK4* mutations. N Engl J Med 333:970–974, 1995.

173. Goto R, Masuoka H, Yoshida K, Mori M, Miyake H. A case–control study of cancer of the pancreas [in Japanese]. Gan No Rinsho Spec No Feb:344–350, 1990.

174. Harnack LJ, Anderson KE, Zheng W, et al. Smoking, alcohol, coffee, and tea intake and incidence of cancer of the exocrine pancreas: the Iowa Women's Health Study. Cancer Epidemiol Biomarkers Prev 6:1081–1086, 1997.

175. Farrow DC, Davis S. Risk of pancreatic cancer in relation to medical history and the use of tobacco, alcohol and coffee. Int J Cancer 45:816–820, 1990.

176. Kalapothaki V, Tzonou A, Hsieh CC, et al. Tobacco, ethanol, coffee, pancreatitis, diabetes mellitus, and cholelithiasis as risk factors for pancreatic carcinoma. Cancer Causes Control 4:375–382, 1993.

177. Zatonski WA, Boyle P, Przewozniak K, et al. Cigarette smoking, alcohol, tea and coffee consumption and pancreas cancer risk: a case–control study from Opole, Poland. Int J Cancer 53:601–607, 1993.

178. Dorken V. Einige Daten bei 280 Patienten mit Pankreaskrebs. Gastroenterologia 102:47–77, 1964.

179. Hinds M, Kolonel I, Lee J, et al. Association between cancer incidence and alcohol/cigarette consumption among five ethnic groups in Hawaii. Br J Cancer 41:929–940, 1980.

180. Blot W, Fraumeni JJ, Stone B. Geographic correlates of pancreas cancer in the United States. Cancer 42:373–380, 1978.

181. Kono S, Ikeda M. Correlation between cancer mortality and alcoholic beverage in Japan. Br J Cancer 40:449–455, 1979.

182. Sarles H. An international survey on nutrition and pancreatitis. Digestion 9:389–403, 1973.

183. Halkulinen T, Lehtinaki L, Lehtonen M, et al. Cancer mortality among two male cohorts with increased alcohol consumption in Finland. J Natl Cancer Inst 52:1711–1713, 1974.

184. Klatsky A, Friedman G, Siegelaub A. Alcohol and mortality: a ten-year Kaiser-Permanente experience. Ann Intern Med 95:139–145, 1981.

185. Monson R, Lyon J. Proportional mortality among alcoholics. Cancer 36:1077–1079, 1975.

186. Jensen O. Cancer morbidity and causes of death among Danish brewery workers. Int J Cancer 23:454–463, 1979.

187. Velema J, Walker A, Gold E. Alcohol and pancreatic cancer, insufficient epidemiologic evidence for a causal relationship. Epidmiol Rev 8:28–41, 1986.

188. Adami HO, McLaughlin JK, Hsing AW, et al. Alcoholism and cancer risk: a population-based cohort study. Cancer Causes Control 3:419–425, 1992.

189. Silverman DT, Brown LM, Hoover RN, et al. Alcohol and pancreatic cancer in blacks and whites in the United States. Cancer Res 55:4899–4905, 1995.

190. Lin RS, Kessler II. A multifactorial model for pancreatic cancer in man. Epidemiologic evidence. JAMA 245:147–152, 1981.

191. Kernan GJ, Ji BT, Dosemeci M, et al. Occupational risk factors for pancreatic cancer: a case–control study based on death certificates from 24 U.S. states. Am J Ind Med 36:260–270, 1999.

192. Ji BT, Silverman DT, Dosemeci M, et al. Occupation and pancreatic cancer risk in Shanghai, China. Am J Ind Med 35:76–81, 1999.

193. Rix BA, Villadsen E, Lynge E. Cancer incidence of sulfite pulp workers in Denmark. Scand J Work Environ Health 23:458–461, 1997.

194. Selenskas S, Teta MJ, Vitale JN. Pancreatic cancer among workers processing synthetic resins. Am J Ind Med 28:385–398, 1995.

195. Garabrant DH, Held J, Langholz B, Peters JM, Mack TM. DDT and related compounds and risk of pancreatic cancer. J Natl Cancer Inst 84:764–771, 1992.

196. Marsh GM, Lucas LJ, Youk AO, Schall LC. Mortality patterns among workers exposed to acrylamide: 1994 follow-up. Occup Environ Med 56:181–190, 1999.

197. Anttila A, Pukkala E, Riala R, Sallmen M, Hemminki K. Cancer incidence among Finnish workers exposed to aromatic hydrocarbons. Int Arch Occup Environ Health 71:187–193, 1998.

198. Fisher WE, Boros LG, Schirmer WJ. Insulin promotes pancreatic cancer: evidence for endocrine influence on exocrine pancreatic tumors. J Surg Res 63:310–313, 1996.

199. Talamini G, Bassi C, Falconi M, et al. Alcohol and smoking as risk factors in chronic pancreatitis and pancreatic cancer. Dig Dis Sci 44:1303–1311, 1999.

200. O'Mara BA, Byers T, Schoenfeld E. Diabetes mellitus and cancer risk: a multisite case–control study. J Chron Dis 38:435–441, 1985.

201. Calle EE, Murphy TK, Rodriguez C, Thun MJ, Heath CW Jr. Diabetes mellitus and pancreatic cancer mortality in a prospective cohort of United States adults. Cancer Causes Control 9:403–410, 1998.

202. Wideroff L, Gridley G, Mellemkjaer L, et al. Cancer incidence in a population-based cohort of patients hospitalized with diabetes mellitus in Denmark. J Natl Cancer Inst 89:1360–1365, 1997.

203. Adami HO, McLaughlin J, Ekbom A, et al. Cancer risk in patients with diabetes mellitus. Cancer Causes Control 2:307–314, 1991.

204. Morris DV, Nabarro JD. Pancreatic cancer and diabetes mellitus. Diabet Med 1:119–121, 1984.

205. Bansal P, Sonnenberg A. Pancreatitis is a risk factor for pancreatic cancer. Gastroenterology 109:247–251, 1995.

206. Ekbom A, McLaughlin JK, Karlsson BM, et al. Pancreatitis and pancreatic cancer: a population-based study. J Natl Cancer Inst 86:625–627, 1994.

207. Fernandez E, La Vecchia C, Porta M, et al. Pancreatitis and the risk of pancreatic cancer. Pancreas 11:185–189, 1995.

208. La Vecchia C, Negri E, D'Avanzo B, et al. Medical history, diet and pancreatic cancer. Oncology 47:463–466, 1990.

209. Rocca G, Gaia E, Iuliano R, et al. Increased incidence of cancer in chronic pancreatitis. J Clin Gastroenterol 9:175–179, 1987.

210. Ammann RW, Knoblauch M, Mohr P, et al. High incidence of extrapancreatic carcinoma in chronic pancreatitis. Scand J Gastroenterol 15:395–399, 1980.

211. Lowenfels AB, Maisonneuve P, Cavallini G, et al. Pancreatitis and the risk of pancreatic cancer. International Pancreatitis Study Group. N Engl J Med 328:1433–1437, 1993.

212. Chari ST, Mohan V, Pitchumoni CS, et al. Risk of pancreatic carcinoma in tropical calcifying pancreatitis: an epidemiologic study. Pancreas 9:62–66, 1994.

213. Augustine P, Ramesh H. Is tropical pancreatitis premalignant? Am J Gastroenterol 87:1005–1008, 1992.

214. Gates LK Jr, Ulrich CD 2nd, Whitcomb DC. Hereditary pancreatitis. Gene defects and their implications. Surg Clin North Am 79:711–722, vii–viii, 1999.

215. Whitcomb DC, Applebaum S, Martin SP. Hereditary pancreatitis and pancreatic carcinoma. Ann NY Acad Sci 880:201–209, 1999.

216. Lowenfels AB, Maisonneuve P, DiMagno EP, et al. Hereditary pancreatitis and the risk of pancreatic cancer. International Hereditary Pancreatitis Study Group. J Natl Cancer Inst 89:442–446, 1997.

217. Silverman DT, Schiffman M, Everhart J, et al. Diabetes mellitus, other medical conditions and familial history of cancer as risk factors for pancreatic cancer. Br J Cancer 80:1830–1837, 1999.

218. Hruban RH, Petersen GM, Goggins M, et al. Familial pancreatic cancer. Ann Oncol 10:69–73, 1999.

219. Thorlacius S, Olafsdottir G, Tryggvadottir L, et al. A single *BRCA2* mutation in male and female breast cancer families from Iceland with varied cancer phenotypes. Nat Genet 13:117–119, 1996.

220. Gayther SA, Ponder BA. Mutations of the *BRCA1* and *BRCA2* genes and the possibilities for predictive testing. Mol Med Today 3:168–174, 1997.

221. Berman DB, Costalas J, Schultz DC, et al. A common mutation in *BRCA2* that predisposes to a variety of cancers is found in both Jewish Ashkenazi and non-Jewish individuals. Cancer Res 56:3409–3414, 1996.

222. Goggins M, Schutte M, Lu J, et al. Germline *BRCA2* gene mutations in patients with apparently sporadic pancreatic carcinomas. Cancer Res 56:5360–5364, 1996.

223. Giardiello FM, Offerhaus GJ, Lee DH, et al. Increased risk of thyroid and pancreatic carcinoma in familial adenomatous polyposis. Gut 34:1394–1396, 1993.

224. Flanders TY, Foulkes WD. Pancreatic adenocarcinoma: epidemiology and genetics. J Med Genet 33:889–898, 1996.

225. Bullock GJ, Green JL, Baron PL. Impact of p16 expression on surgical management of malignant melanoma and pancreatic carcinoma. Am J Surg 177:15–18, 1999.

226. Schattner A, Fenakel G, Malnick SD. Cholelithiasis and pancreatic cancer. A case–control study. J Clin Gastroenterol 25:602–604, 1997.

227. Gullo L. Risk of pancreatic and periampullary cancer following cholecystectomy. Ann Oncol 10:127–128, 1999.

228. Travis LB, Curtis RE, Storm H, et al. Risk of second malignant neoplasms among long-term survivors of testicular cancer. J Natl Cancer Inst 89:1429–1439, 1997.

229. Moller H, Mellemgaard A, Jacobsen GK, Pedersen D, Storm HH. Incidence of second primary cancer following testicular cancer. Eur J Cancer 5:672–676, 1993.

230. Schenk M, Severson RK, Pawlish KS. The risk of subsequent primary carcinoma of the pancreas in patients with cutaneous malignant melanoma. Cancer 82:1672–1676, 1998.

231. Woutersen RA, Appel MJ, Van Garderen-Hoetmer A. Modulation of pancreatic carcinogenesis by antioxidants. Food Chem Toxicol 37:981–984, 1999.

232. Majima T, Tsutsumi M, Nishino H, Tsunoda T, Konishi Y. Inhibitory effects of beta-carotene, palm carotene, and green tea polyphenols on pancreatic carcinogenesis initiated by N-nitorsobis(2-oxopropyl)amine in Syrian golden hamsters. Pancreas 16:13–18, 1998.

233. Roebuck BD, MacMillan DL, Bush DM, Kensler TW. Modulation of azaserine-induced pancreatic foci by phenolic antioxidants in rats. J Natl Cancer Inst 72:1405–1410, 1984.

234. Longnecker DS, Curphey TJ, Kuhlmann ET, Roebuck BD. Inhibition of pancreatic carcinogenesis by retinoids in azaserine-treated rats. Cancer Res 42:19–24, 1982.

235. Rautalahti MT, Virtamo JR, Taylor PR, et al. The effects of supplementation with alpha-tocopherol and beta-carotene on the incidence and mortality of carcinoma of the pancreas in a randomized, controlled trial. Cancer 86:37–42, 1999.

236. Brat DJ, Lillemoe KD, Yeo CJ, Warfield PB, Hruban RH. Progression of pancreatic intraductal neoplasias to infiltrating adenocarcinoma of the pancreas. Am J Surg Pathol 22:163–169, 1998.

237. Worthington TR, Williamson RC. The continuing challenge of exocrine pancreatic cancer. Compr Ther 25:360–365, 1999.

238. Bakkevold KE, Arnesjo B, Kambestad B. Carcinoma of the pancreas and papilla of Vater—assessment of resectability and factors influencing resectability in stage I carcinomas. A prospective multicentre trial in 472 patients. Eur J Surg Oncol 18:494–507, 1992.

239. Yeo CJ, Cameron JL, Lillemoe KD, et al. Pancreaticoduodenectomy for cancer of the head of the pancreas. 201 patients. Ann Surg 221:721–731; discussion 731–723, 1995.

240. Onoyama H, Kamigaki T, Yamamoto M, Saitoh Y. Treatment and present status of pancreatic cancer [in Japanese]. Gan To Kagaku Ryoho 19:2304–2310, 1992.

241. Hilgers W, Kern SE. Molecular genetic basis of pancreatic adenocarcinoma. Genes Chromosomes Cancer 26:1–12, 1999.

242. Sakorafas GH, Tsiotou AG. Multi-step pancreatic carcinogenesis and its clinical implications. Eur J Surg Oncol 25:562–565, 1999.

243. Abbruzzese JL, Evans DB, Raijman I, et al. Detection of mutated c-Ki-ras in the bile of patients with pancreatic cancer. Anticancer Res 17:795–801, 1997.

244. Caldas C, Hahn SA, Hruban RH, et al. Detection of K-ras mutations in the stool of patients with pancreatic adenocarcinoma and pancreatic ductal hyperplasia. Cancer Res 54:3568–3573, 1994.

245. Phoa SS, Reeders JW, Rauws EA, et al. Spiral computed tomography for preoperative staging of potentially resectable carcinoma of the pancreatic head. Br J Surg 86:789–794, 1999.

246. Levin B. An overview of preventive strategies for pancreatic cancer. Ann Oncol 10:193–196, 1999.

247. Henson D, Albores S, Corle D. Carcinoma of the gall bladder; types, stages, grade and survival rates. Cancer 70:1493–1497, 1992.

248. Landis SH, Murray T, Bolden S, Wingo PA. Cancer statistics, 1998 [published errata appear in CA Cancer J Clin 1998;48:192 and 1998;48(6):329]. CA Cancer J Clin 48:6–29, 1998.

249. Parkin D, Muir C, Whalen S. Cancer Incidence in Five Continents, Vol. VI. IARC Sci (Ed Publ. No. 120). International Agency for Research on Cancer, Lyon, 1992.

250. Trapido E, Chen F, Davis K, Lewis N, MacKinnon J. Cancer among Hispanic males in south Florida. Arch Intern Med 154:177–185, 1994.

251. Boss L, Lanier A, Dohan P, Bender T. Cancer of gall bladder and biliary tract in Alaskan natives. J Natl Cancer Inst 69:1005–1007, 1982.

252. Fraumeni J, Devesa S, McLaughlin J, Stanford J. Biliary tract cancer. In: Schottenfeld D, Fraumeni J (eds): Cancer Epidemiology and Prevention, 2nd ed. Oxford University Press, Oxford, 1997, pp 794–805.

253. Strom B, Soloway R, Rios-Dolenz J, et al. Risk factors for gall bladder cancer. Cancer 76:1747–1756, 1995.

254. Zatonski W, LaVecchia C, Przewozniak K, et al. Risk factors for gall bladder cancer: a Polish case–control study. Int J Cancer 51:707–711, 1992.

255. Lowenfels A, Boyle P, Maisonneuve P, Zatonski W. Epidemiology of gall bladder cancer. Hepatogastroenterology 46:1529–1532, 1999.

256. Diehl A. Increased cholecytectomy rate after the introduction of laparoscopic cholecystectomy. JAMA 271:501–505, 1994.

257. Diehl A, Beral V. Cholectyectomy and changes in mortality from gall bladder cancer. Lancet 2:187–189, 1981.

258. Lowenfels A, Lindstrom C, Conway M. Gall stones and risk of gall bladder cancer. J Natl Cancer Inst 75:77–80, 1985.

259. Diehl A. Gall stone size and risk of gall bladder cancer. JAMA 250:2323–2326, 1983.

260. Lowenfels A, Walker A, Althaus D, Townsend G, Domellof L. Gall stone growth, size and risk of gall bladder cancer: an interracial study. Int J Epidemiol 18:50–54, 1989.

261. Zatonski W, Lowenfels A, Boyle P, et al. Case–control study of the SEARCH program of IARC. J Natl Cancer Inst 89:1132–1138, 1997.

262. Lew EA, Garfinkel L. Variations in mortality by weight among 750,000 men and women. J Chron Dis 32:563–576, 1979.

263. Boing H, Martinez L, Frentzel-Beyme R, Oltersdorf L. Regional nutritional patterns and cancer mortality in Federal Republic of Germany. Nutr Cancer 7:121–130, 1985.

264. Pixley F, Mann J. Dietary factors in etiology of gall stones: a case–control study. Gut 29:1511–1515, 1988.

265. Maclure KM, Hayes KC, Colditz GA, et al. Weight, diet, and the risk of symptomatic gallstones in middle-aged women. N Engl J Med 321:563–569, 1989.

266. Negri E, LaVecchia C. Vegetable and fruit consumption and cancer risk. Int J Cancer 48:350–354, 1991.

267. Lambe M, Trichopoulos D, Hsieh C, et al. Parity and cancers of gall bladder and extrahepatic biliary tract. Int J Cancer 54:941–944, 1993.

268. La Vecchia C, Negri E, Franceschi S, Parazzini F. Long-term impact of reproductive factors on cancer risk. Int J Cancer 57:215–219, 1993.

269. Moerman C, Berns M, Bueno de Mesquita H, Runia S. Reproductive history and cancer of biliary tract in women. Int J Cancer 57:146–153, 1994.

270. Watanapa P. Cholangiocarcinoma in patients with opisthorchiasis. Br J Surg 83:1062–1064, 1996.

271. Nath G, Singh H, Shukla V. Chronic typhoid carriage and carcinoma of gall bladder. Eur J Cancer Prev 6:557–559, 1997.

272. Shin HR, Lee CU, Park HJ, et al. Hepatitis B and C virus, *Clonorchis sinensis* for the risk of liver cancer: a case–control study in Pusan, Korea. Int J Epidemiol 25:933–940, 1996.

273. de Groen PC, Gores GJ, LaRusso NF, Gunderson LL, Nagorney DM. Biliary tract cancers. N Engl J Med 341:1368–1378, 1999.

274. Kornfeld D, Ekbom A, Ihre T. Survival and risk of cholangiocarcinoma in patients with primary sclerosing cholangitis. A population-based study. Scand J Gastroenterol 32:1042–1045, 1997.

275. Shukla V, Prakash A, Tripathi B, Reddy D, Singh S. Biliary heavy metal concentration in cancer of gall bladder: case–control study. BMJ 317:1288–1289, 1998.

276. Roa I, Araya J, Villaseca M, et al. Preneoplastic lesions and gall bladder cancer: an estimate of period required for progression. Gastroenterology 111:232–236, 1996.

277. Chijiwa K, Tanaka M. Cancer of gall bladder: an appraisal of surgical resection. Surgery 115:751–756, 1994.

278. Moerman CJ, Bueno-de-Mesquita HB. The epidemiology of gallbladder cancer: lifestyle-related risk factors and limited surgical possibilities for prevention. Hepatogastroenterology 46:1533–1539, 1999.

279. El-Serag H, Mason A. Rising incidence of hepatocellular carcinoma in the United States. N Engl J Med 340:745–750, 1999.

280. World Health Organization. Report of WHO meeting. Prevention of Liver Cancer. World Health Organization, Geneva, 1983.

281. London W, McGlynn K. Liver cancer. In: Schottenfeld D, Fraumeni J (eds): Cancer Epidemiology and Prevention. Oxford University Press, New York, 1996, pp 772–793.

282. Moradpour D, Wands J. Hepatic oncogenesis. In: Zakim D, Boyer T (eds): Hepatology: A Textbook of Liver Disease. W.B. Saunders, Philadelphia, 1996, pp 1490–1512.

283. Beasley RP, Hwang LY, Lin CC, Chien CS. Hepatocellular carcinoma and hepatitis B virus. A prospective study of 22,707 men in Taiwan. Lancet 2:1129–1133, 1981.

284. Alter MJ, Kruszon-Moran D, Nainan OV, et al. The prevalence of hepatitis C virus infection in the United States, 1988 through 1994. N Engl J Med 341:556–562, 1999.

285. Heintges T, Wands JR. Hepatitis C virus: epidemiology and transmission. Hepatology 26:521–526, 1997.

286. Alter MJ, Hadler SC, Judson FN, et al. Risk factors for acute non-A, non-B hepatitis in the United States and association with hepatitis C virus infection. JAMA 264:2231–2235, 1990.

287. Schreiber GB, Busch MP, Kleinman SH, Korelitz JJ. The risk of transfusion-transmitted viral infections. The Retrovirus Epidemiology Donor Study. N Engl J Med 334:1685–1690, 1996.

288. Castells L, Vargas V, Gonzalez A, et al. Long interval between HCV infection and development of hepatocellular carcinoma. Liver 15:159–163, 1995.

289. IARC. Hepatitis viruses. In: IARC Monographs on the Evaluation of Carcinogenic Risks to Humans, Vol. 59. World Health Organization, Lyon, France, 1994, pp 45–221.

290. IARC. Some naturally occurring substances: food items and constituents, heterocyclic aroamic amine and mycotoxins. In: IARC Monographs on the Evaluation of Carcinogenic Risks to Humans, Vol. 56. Lyon, France, World Health Organization, 1993, p 245.

291. Ozturk M. p53 mutation in hepatocellular carcinoma after aflatoxin exposure. Lancet 338:1356–1359, 1991.

292. Dufour M. Chronic liver disease and cirrhosis. In: Everhart J (ed): Digestive Diseases in the United United States: Epidemiology and Impact, Vol. 94-1447. Government Printing Office, Washington, DC, 1994, pp 615–646.

293. Margolis HS, Alter MJ, Hadler SC. Hepatitis B: evolving epidemiology and implications for control. Semin Liver Dis 11:84–92, 1991.

294. Edmunds W, Medley G, Nokes D, Hall A, Whittle H. The influence of age on the development of the hepatitis B carrier state. Proc R Soc Lond B Biol Sci 253(1337);197–201, 1993.

295. Mast E, Mahoney F, Alter M, Margolis H. Progress toward elimination of hepatitis B virus transmission in the United States. Vaccine 16 (Suppl): S48–S51, 1998.

296. Mast E, Williams I, Alter M, Margolis H. Hepatitis B vaccination of adolescent and adult high-risk groups in the United States. Vaccine 16 (Suppl): S27–S29, 1998.

297. Mast EE, Alter MJ, Margolis HS. Strategies to prevent and control hepatitis B and C virus infections: a global perspective. Vaccine 17:1730–1733, 1999.

298. Mahoney FJ, Stewart K, Hu H, Coleman P, Alter MJ. Progress toward the elimination of hepatitis B virus transmission among health care workers in the United States. Arch Intern Med 157:2601–2605, 1997.

299. Bolondi L, Gaiani S, Casali A, Serra C, Piscaglia F. Screening for the early diagnosis of hepatocellular carcinoma: cost-effectiveness analysis [in Italian]. Radiol Med (Torino) 94:4–7, 1997.

300. Heyward WL, Lanier AP, McMahon BJ, et al. Early detection of primary hepatocellular carcinoma. Screening for primary hepatocellular carcinoma among persons infected with hepatitis B virus. JAMA 254:3052–3054, 1985.

301. Izzo F, Cremona F, Ruffolo F, et al. Outcome of 67 patients with hepatocellular cancer detected during screening of 1125 patients with chronic hepatitis. Ann Surg 227:513–518, 1998.

302. Larcos G, Sorokopud H, Berry G, Farrell GC. Sonographic screening for hepatocellular carcinoma in patients with chronic hepatitis or cirrhosis: an evaluation. AJR Am J Roentgenol 171:433–435, 1998.

303. McGlynn K, London WT, Hann HW, Sharrar RG. Prevention of primary hepatocellular carcinoma in Asian populations in the Delaware Valley. Prog Clin Biol Res 216:237–246, 1986.

304. Pateron D, Ganne N, Trinchet JC, et al. Prospective study of screening for hepatocellular carcinoma in Caucasian patients with cirrhosis. J Hepatol 20:65–71, 1994.

305. Zoli M, Magalotti D, Bianchi G, et al. Efficacy of a surveillance program for early detection of hepatocellular carcinoma. Cancer 78:977–985, 1996.

306. McMahon BJ, London T. Workshop on screening for hepatocellular carcinoma. J Natl Cancer Inst 83:916–919, 1991.

307. Di Bisceglie AM, Rustgi VK, Hoofnagle JH, Dusheiko GM, Lotze MT. NIH conference. Hepatocellular Carcinoma. Ann Intern Med 108:390–401, 1988.

308. Chow JS, Chen CC, Ahsan H, Neugut AI. A population-based study of the incidence of malignant small bowel tumours: SEER, 1973–1990. Int J Epidemiol 25:722–728, 1996.

309. Howe JR, Karnell LH, Menck HR, Scott-Conner C. Adenocarcinoma of the small bowel: review of the National Cancer Data Base, 1985–1995. Cancer 86:2693–2706, 1999.

310. Rodriguez-Bigas MA, Vasen HF, Lynch HT, et al. Characteristics of small bowel carcinoma in hereditary nonpolyposis colorectal carcinoma. International Collaborative Group on HNPCC. Cancer 83:240–244, 1998.

311. Offerhaus GJ, Giardiello FM, Krush AJ, et al. The risk of upper gastrointestinal cancer in familial adenomatous polyposis. Gastroenterology 102:1980–1982, 1992.

312. Greenstein AJ, Sachar DB, Smith H, Janowitz HD, Aufses AH Jr. A comparison of cancer risk in Crohn's disease and ulcerative colitis. Cancer 48:2742–2745, 1981.

313. Collier PE, Turowski P, Diamond DL. Small intestinal adenocarcinoma complicating regional enteritis. Cancer 55:516–521, 1985.

314. Negri E, Bosetti C, La Vecchia C, et al. Risk factors for adenocarcinoma of the small intestine. Int J Cancer 82:171–174, 1999.

315. Haenszel W, Kurihara M. Studies of Japanese migrants. I. Mortality from cancer and other diseases among Japanese in the United States. J Natl Cancer Inst 40:43–68, 1968.

316. Wingo PA, Ries LA, Rosenberg HM, Miller DS, Edwards BK. Cancer incidence and mortality, 1973–1995: a report card for the U.S. Cancer 82:1197–1207, 1998.

317. Benson AB 3rd. Therapy for advanced colorectal cancer. Semin Oncol 25:2–11, 1998.

318. Dube S, Heyen F, Jenicek M. Adjuvant chemotherapy in colorectal carcinoma: results of a meta-analysis. Dis Colon Rectum 40:35–41, 1997.

319. Figueredo A, Fine S, Maroun J, Walker-Dilks C, Wong S. Adjuvant therapy for stage III colon cancer after complete resection. Provincial Gastrointestinal Disease Site Group [published erratum appears in Cancer Prev Control 1997; 1: 351]. Cancer Prev Control 1:304–319, 1997.

320. Nigro ND, Bull AW, Boyd ME. Inhibition of intestinal carcinogenesis in rats: effect of difluoromethylornithine with piroxicam or fish oil. J Natl Cancer Inst 77:1309–1313, 1986.

321. Broitman SA, Vitale JJ, Vavrousek-Jakuba E, Gottlieb LS. Polyunsaturated fat, cholesterol and large bowel tumorigenesis. Cancer 40:2455–2463, 1977.

322. Phinney S. Metabolism of exogenous and endogenous arachidnoic acid in cancer. Adv Exp Med Biol 399:87–94, 1996.

323. Giovannucci E, Goldin B. The role of fat, fatty acids, and total energy intake in the etiology of human colon cancer. Am J Clin Nutr 66:1564S–1571S, 1997.

324. Willett W, Stampfer M, Colditz G, Rosner B, Speizer F. Relation of meat, fat, and fiber intake to the risk of colon cancer in a prospective study among women. N Engl J Med 323:1664–1672, 1990.

325. Slattery ML, Potter JD, Duncan DM, Berry TD. Dietary fats and colon cancer: assessment of risk associated with specific fatty acids. Int J Cancer 73:670–677, 1997.

326. MacLennan R, Macrae F, Bain C, et al. Randomized trial of intake of fat, fiber, and beta carotene to prevent colorectal adenomas. The Australian Polyp Prevention Project. J Natl Cancer Inst 87:1760–1766, 1995.

327. McKeown-Eyssen GE, Bright-See E, Bruce WR, et al. A randomized trial of a low-fat high fiber diet in the recurrence of colorectal polyps. Toronto Polyp Prevention Group [published erratum appears in J Clin Epidemiol 1995;48:i]. J Clin Epidemiol 47:525–536, 1994.

328. Reddy BS, Hedges AR, Laakso K, Wynder EL. Metabolic epidemiology of large bowel cancer: fecal bulk and constituents of high-risk North American and low-risk Finnish population. Cancer 42:2832–2838, 1978.

329. Trock B, Lanza E, Greenwald P. Dietary fiber, vegetables, and colon cancer: critical review and meta-analyses of the epidemiologic evidence. J Natl Cancer Inst 82:650–661, 1990.

330. Fuchs CS, Giovannucci EL, Colditz GA, et al. Dietary fiber and the risk of colorectal cancer and adenoma in women. N Engl J Med 340:169–176, 1999.

331a. Macrae F. Wheat bran fiber and development of adenomatous polyps: evidence from randomized, controlled clinical trials. Am J Med 106:38S–42S, 1999.

331b. Schatzkin A, Lanza E, Corle D, et al. Lack of effect of a low-fat, high-fiber diet on the recurrence of colorectal adenomas. Polyp Prevention Trial Study Group. N Engl J Med 342:1149–1155, 2000.

331c. Alberts DS, Martinez ME, Roe DJ, et al. Lack of effect of a high-fiber cereal supplement on the recurrence of colorectal adenomas. Phoenix Colon Cancer Prevention Physicians' Network. N Engl J Med 342: 1156–1162, 2000.

332. Inoue M, Tajima K, Hirose K, et al. Tea and coffee consumption and the risk of digestive tract cancers: data from a comparative case–referent study in Japan. Cancer Causes Control 9:209–216, 1998.

333. Tavani A, Pregnolato A, La Vecchia C, et al. Coffee and tea intake and risk of cancers of the colon and rectum: a study of 3,530 cases and 7,057 controls. Int J Cancer 73:193–197, 1997.

334. Slattery ML, Edwards SL, Boucher KM, Anderson K, Caan BJ. Lifestyle and colon cancer: an assessment of factors associated with risk. Am J Epidemiol 150:869–877, 1999.

335. Mahmoud NN, Dannenberg AJ, Bilinski RT, et al. Administration of an unconjugated bile acid increases duodenal tumors in a murine model of familial adenomatous polyposis. Carcinogenesis 20:299–303, 1999.

336. Tang R, Wang JY, Lo SK, Hsieh LL. Physical activity, water intake and risk of colorectal cancer in Taiwan: a hospital-based case–control study. Int J Cancer 82:484–489, 1999.

337. White E, Jacobs EJ, Daling JR. Physical activity in relation to colon cancer in middle-aged men and women. Am J Epidemiol 144:42–50, 1996.

338. Gerhardsson de Verdier M, Hagman U, Steineck G, Rieger A, Norell SE: Diet, body mass and colorectal cancer: a case–referent study in Stockholm. Int J Cancer 46:832–838, 1990.

339. Gerhardsson M, Floderus B, Norell SE. Physical activity and colon cancer risk. Int J Epidemiol 17:743–746, 1988.

340. Martinez ME, Giovannucci E, Spiegelman D, et al. Leisure-time physical activity, body size, and colon cancer in women. Nurses' Health Study Research Group. J Natl Cancer Inst 89:948–955, 1997.

341. Giovannucci E, Rimm EB, Ascherio A, et al. Alcohol, low-methionine—low-folate diets, and risk of colon cancer in men. J Natl Cancer Inst 87:265–273, 1995.

342. Tavani A, Braga C, La Vecchia C, et al. Physical activity and risk of cancers of the colon and rectum: an Italian case–control study. Br J Cancer 79:1912–1916, 1999.

343. Hsing AW, McLaughlin JK, Chow WH, et al. Risk factors for colorectal cancer in a prospective study among U.S. white men. Int J Cancer 77:549–553, 1998.

344. Kahn HS, Tatham LM, Thun MJ, Heath CW Jr. Risk factors for self-reported colon polyps. J Gen Intern Med 13:303–310, 1998.

345. Sandler RS, Pritchard ML, Bangdiwala SI. Physical activity and the risk of colorectal adenomas. Epidemiology 6:602–606, 1995.

346. Giovannucci E, Colditz GA, Stampfer MJ, Willett WC. Physical activity, obesity, and risk of colorectal adenoma in women (United States). Cancer Causes Control 7:253–263, 1996.

347. Gerber M, Corpet D. Energy balance and cancers. Eur J Cancer Prev 8:77–89, 1999.

348. Kono S, Honjo S, Todoroki I, et al. Glucose intolerance and adenomas of the sigmoid colon in Japanese men (Japan). Cancer Causes Control 9:441–446, 1998.

349. Moore MA, Park CB, Tsuda H. Physical exercise: a pillar for cancer prevention? Eur J Cancer Prev 7:177–193, 1998.

350. Hu FB, Manson JE, Liu S, et al. Prospective study of adult onset diabetes mellitus (type 2) and risk of colorectal cancer in women. J Natl Cancer Inst 91:542–547, 1999.

351. Schoen RE, Tangen CM, Kuller LH, et al. Increased blood glucose and insulin, body size, and incident colorectal cancer. J Natl Cancer Inst 91:1147–1154, 1999.

352. Freier S, Weiss O, Eran M, et al. Expression of the insulin-like growth factors and their receptors in adenocarcinoma of the colon. Gut 44: 704–708, 1999.

353. Zou T, Fleisher AS, Kong D, et al. Sequence alterations of insulin-like growth factor binding protein 3 in neoplastic and normal gastrointestinal tissues. Cancer Res 58:4802–4804, 1998.

354. Hirayama T. Association between alcohol consumption and cancer of the sigmoid colon: observations from a Japanese cohort study. Lancet 2:725–727, 1989.

355. Pollack ES, Nomura AM, Heilbrun LK, Stemmermann GN, Green SB. Prospective study of alcohol consumption and cancer. N Engl J Med 310:617–621, 1984.

356. Pickle LW, Greene MH, Ziegler RG, et al. Colorectal cancer in rural Nebraska. Cancer Res 44:363–369, 1984.

357. Chyou PH, Nomura AM, Stemmermann GN. A prospective study of colon and rectal cancer among Hawaii Japanese men. Ann Epidemiol 6:276–282, 1996.

358. Glynn SA, Albanes D, Pietinen P, et al. Alcohol consumption and risk of colorectal cancer in a cohort of Finnish men. Cancer Causes Control 7:214–223, 1996.

359. Murata M, Takayama K, Choi BC, Pak AW. A nested case–control study on alcohol drinking, tobacco smoking, and cancer. Cancer Detect Prev 20:557–565, 1996.

360. Honjo S, Kono S, Shinchi K, et al. The relation of smoking, alcohol use and obesity to risk of sigmoid colon and rectal adenomas. Jpn J Cancer Res 86:1019–1026, 1995.

361. Giovannucci E, Egan K, Hunter D, et al. Aspirin and the risk of colorectal cancer in women. N Engl J Med 333:609–614, 1995.

362. Baron JA, Sandler RS, Haile RW, et al. Folate intake, alcohol consumption, cigarette smoking, and risk of colorectal adenomas. J Natl Cancer Inst 90:57–62, 1998.

363. Kearney J, Giovannucci E, Rimm EB, et al. Diet, alcohol, and smoking and the occurrence of hyperplastic polyps of the colon and rectum (United States). Cancer Causes Control 6:45–56, 1995.

364. Kensler T, Styczynski P, Groopman J, et al. Mechanisms of chemoprotection by oltipraz. J Cell Biochem Suppl 16I:167–172, 1992.

365. Kato I, Tominaga S, Matsuura A, et al. A comparative case–control study of colorectal cancer and adenoma. Jpn J Cancer Res 81:1101–1108, 1990.

366. Nagata C, Shimizu H, Kametani M, et al. Cigarette smoking, alcohol use, and colorectal adenoma in Japanese men and women. Dis Colon Rectum 42:337–342, 1999.

367. Potter JD, Bigler J, Fosdick L, et al. Colorectal adenomatous and hyperplastic polyps: smoking and N-acetyltransferase 2 polymorphisms. Cancer Epidemiol Biomarkers Prev 8:69–75, 1999.

368. Todoroki I, Kono S, Shinchi K, et al. Relationship of cigarette smoking, alcohol use, and dietary habits with sigmoid colon adenomas. Ann Epidemiol 5:478–483, 1995.

369. Newcomb PA, Storer BE, Marcus PM. Cigarette smoking in relation to risk of large bowel cancer in women. Cancer Res 55:4906–4909, 1995.

370. Tavani A, Gallus S, Negri E, et al. Cigarette smoking and risk of cancers of the colon and rectum: a case–control study from Italy. Eur J Epidemiol 14:675–681, 1998.

371. D'Avanzo B, La Vecchia C, Franceschi S, Gallotti L, Talamini R. Cigarette smoking and colorectal cancer: a study of 1,584 cases and 2,879 controls. Prev Med 24:571–579, 1995.

372. Nyren O, Bergstrom R, Nystrom L, et al. Smoking and colorectal cancer: a 20-year follow-up study of Swedish construction workers. Natl Cancer Inst 88:1302–1307, 1996.

373. Ivanovich JL, Read TE, Ciske DJ, Kodner IJ, Whelan AJ. A practical approach to familial and hereditary colorectal cancer. Am J Med 107: 68–77, 1999.

374. Lynch HT, de la Chapelle A. Genetic susceptibility to non-polyposis colorectal cancer. J Med Genet 36:801–818, 1999.

375. Byers T, Levin B, Rothenberger D, Dodd GD, Smith RA. American Cancer Society guidelines for screening and surveillance for early detection of colorectal polyps and cancer: update 1997. American Cancer Society Detection and Treatment Advisory Group on Colorectal Cancer. CA Cancer J Clin 47:154–160, 1997.

376. Burt RW, Bishop DT, Cannon LA, et al. Dominant inheritance of adenomatous colonic polyps and colorectal cancer. N Engl J Med 312: 1540–1544, 1985.

377. Bishop T, Kolodner R. DNA repair disorders and multiple primary cancers. In: Neugut AI, Meadows AT, Robinson E (eds): Multiple Primary Cancers. Lippincott Williams & Wilkins, Philadelphia, 1999, pp 197–212.

378. Lynch HT, Smyrk T. Hereditary nonpolyposis colorectal cancer (Lynch syndrome). An updated review. Cancer 78:1149–1167, 1996.

379. Vasen HF, Mecklin JP, Khan PM, Lynch HT. The International Collaborative Group on Hereditary Non-Polyposis Colorectal Cancer (ICG-HNPCC). Dis Colon Rectum 34:424–425, 1991.

380. Rodriguez-Bigas MA, Boland CR, Hamilton SR, et al. A National Cancer Institute Workshop on Hereditary Nonpolyposis Colorectal Cancer Syndrome: meeting highlights and Bethesda guidelines. J Natl Cancer Inst 89:1758–1762, 1997.

381. Park JG, Vasen HF, Park KJ, et al. Suspected hereditary nonpolyposis colorectal cancer: International Collaborative Group on Hereditary Non-Polyposis Colorectal Cancer (ICG-HNPCC) criteria and results of genetic diagnosis. Dis Colon Rectum 42:710–715; discussion 715–716, 1999.

382. Jass JR, Smyrk TC, Stewart SM, et al. Pathology of hereditary nonpolyposis colorectal cancer. Anticancer Res 14:1631–1634, 1994.

383. Winawer SJ, Fletcher RH, Miller L, et al. Colorectal cancer screening: clinical guidelines and rationale [published errata appear in Gastroenterology 1997;112:1060 and 1998;114:625]. Gastroenterology 112: 594–642, 1997.

384. Gillen CD, Walmsley RS, Prior P, Andrews HA, Allan RN. Ulcerative colitis and Crohn's disease: a comparison of the colorectal cancer risk in extensive colitis. Gut 35:1590–1592, 1994.

385. Mayer R, Wong WD, Rothenberger DA, Goldberg SM, Madoff RD. Colorectal cancer in inflammatory bowel disease: a continuing problem. Dis Colon Rectum 42:343–347, 1999.

386. Snapper SB, Syngal S, Friedman LS. Ulcerative colitis and colon cancer: more controversy than clarity. Dig Dis 16:81–87, 1998.

387. Jain SK, Peppercorn MA. Inflammatory bowel disease and colon cancer: a review. Dig Dis 15:243–252, 1997.

388. Cali RL, Pitsch RM, Thorson AG, et al. Cumulative incidence of metachronous colorectal cancer. Dis Colon Rectum 36:388–393, 1993.

389. Winawer SJ, Zauber AG, Ho MN, et al. Prevention of colorectal cancer by colonoscopic polypectomy. The National Polyp Study Workgroup. N Engl J Med 329:1977–1981, 1993.

390. Winawer SJ, Zauber AG, O'Brien MJ, et al. Randomized comparison of surveillance intervals after colonoscopic removal of newly diagnosed adenomatous polyps. The National Polyp Study Workgroup. N Engl J Med 328:901–906, 1993.

391. Crawford J. The gastrointestinal tract. In: Cotran R, Dumar V, Collins T (eds): Robbins Pathologic Basis of Disease, 6th ed. W.B. Saunders, Philadelphia, 1999, pp 831–832.

392. Bird RP. Observation and quantification of aberrant crypts in the murine colon treated with a colon carcinogen: preliminary findings. Cancer Lett 37:147–151, 1987.

393. McLellan EA, Medline A, Bird RP. Sequential analyses of the growth and morphological characteristics of aberrant crypt foci: putative preneoplastic lesions. Cancer Res 51:5270–5274, 1991.

394. Takayama T, Katsuki S, Takahashi Y, et al. Aberrant crypt foci of the colon as precursors of adenoma and cancer. N Engl J Med 339:177–1284, 1998.

395. Watne AL. Colon polyps. J Surg Oncol 66:207–214, 1997.

396. Vogelstein B, Fearon ER, Hamilton SR, et al. Genetic alterations during colorectal-tumor development. N Engl J Med 319:525–532, 1988.

397. Fearon ER, Vogelstein B. A genetic model for colorectal tumorigenesis. Cell 61:759–767, 1990.

398. Jessup JM, McGinnis LS, Steele GD Jr, Menck HR, Winchester DP. The National Cancer Data Base. Report on colon cancer. Cancer 78:918–926, 1996.

399. Cohen A, Minsky B, Schilsky R. Cancer of the colon. In: Vincent T, DeVita J, Hellman S, Rosenberg S (eds): Cancer: Principles and Practice of Oncology. Lippincott-Raven, Philadelphia, 1997, pp 1144–1184.

400. Obrand DI, Gordon PH. Incidence and patterns of recurrence following curative resection for colorectal carcinoma. Dis Colon Rectum 40:15–24, 1997.

401. Weiss W, Hanak H, Huber A. Clinical value of rectal digital examination in early diagnosis of colorectal cancer [author's transl]. Wien Klin Wochenschr 89:654–660, 1977.

402. Brint SL, DiPalma JA, Herrera JL. Is a Hemoccult-positive rectal examination clinically significant? South Med J 86:601–603, 1993.

403. Mandel JS, Bond JH, Church TR, et al. Reducing mortality from colorectal cancer by screening for fecal occult blood. Minnesota Colon Cancer Control Study [published erratum appears in N Engl J Med 1993; 329:672]. N Engl J Med 328:1365–1371, 1993.

404. Hardcastle JD, Chamberlain JO, Robinson MH, et al. Randomised controlled trial of faecal-occult-blood screening for colorectal cancer. Lancet 348:1472–1477, 1996.

405. Kronborg O, Fenger C, Olsen J, Jorgensen O, Sondergaard O. Randomised study of screening for colorectal cancer with faecal-occult-blood test. Lancet 348:1467–1471, 1996.

406. Kewenter J, Brevinge H, Engaras B, Haglind E, Ahren C. Results of screening, rescreening, and follow-up in a prospective randomized study for detection of colorectal cancer by fecal occult blood testing. Results for 68,308 subjects. Scand J Gastroenterol 29:468–473, 1994.

407. St. John DJ, Young GP, Alexeyeff MA, et al. Evaluation of new occult blood tests for detection of colorectal neoplasia. Gastroenterology 104:1661–1668, 1993.

408. Ransohoff DF, Lang CA. Small adenomas detected during fecal occult blood test screening for colorectal cancer. The impact of serendipity. JAMA 6–78, 1990.

409. Brevinge H, Lindholm E, Buntzen S, Kewenter J. Screening for colorectal neoplasia with faecal occult blood testing compared with flexible sigmoidoscopy directly in a 55–56 years' old population. Int J Colorectal Dis 12:291–295, 1997.

410. Nazarian HK, Giuliano AE, Hiatt JR. Colorectal carcinoma: analysis of management in two medical eras. J Surg Oncol 52:46–49, 1993.

411. Wallace MB, Kemp JA, Meyer F, et al. Screening for colorectal cancer with flexible sigmoidoscopy by nonphysician endoscopists. Am J Med 107:214–218, 1999.

412. Selby JV, Friedman GD, Quesenberry CP Jr, Weiss NS. A case–control study of screening sigmoidoscopy and mortality from colorectal cancer. N Engl J Med 326:653–657, 1992.

413. Newcomb PA, Norfleet RG, Storer BE, Surawicz TS, Marcus PM. Screening sigmoidoscopy and colorectal cancer mortality J Natl Cancer Inst 84:1572–1575, 1992.

414. Muller AD, Sonnenberg A. Prevention of colorectal cancer by flexible endoscopy and polypectomy. A case–control study of 32,702 veterans. Ann Intern Med 123:904–910, 1995.

415. Rex DK, Rahmani EY, Haseman JH, et al. Relative sensitivity of colonoscopy and barium enema for detection of colorectal cancer in clinical practice. Gastroenterology 112:17–23, 1997.

416. Kewenter J, Brevinge H, Engaras B, Haglind E. The yield of flexible sigmoidoscopy and double-contrast barium enema in the diagnosis of neoplasms in the large bowel in patients with a positive Hemoccult test. Endoscopy 27:159–163, 1995.

417. Pollard M, Luckert PH. Treatment of chemically induced intestinal cancers with indomethacin. Proc Soc Exp Biol Med 167:161–164, 1981.

418. Pollard M, Luckert PH. Effect of indomethacin on intestinal tumors induced in rats by the acetate derivative of dimethylnitrosamine. Science 214:558–559, 1981.

419. Oshima M, Dinchuk J, Kargman S, et al. Suppression of intestinal polyposis in Apc$^{D716}$ knockout mice by inhibition of cyclooxygenase 2 (COX-2). Cell 87:803–809, 1996.

420. Kawamori T, Lubet R, Steele V, et al. Chemopreventive effect of curcumin, a naturally occurring anti-inflammatory agent, during the promotion/progression stages of colon cancer. Cancer Res 59:597–601, 1999.

421. Kawamori T, Rao C, Seibert K, Reddy B. Chemopreventive effect of celecoxib, a specific cyclooxygenase-2 inhibitor on colon carcinogenesis. Cancer Res 58:409–412, 1998.

422. Rao C, Rivenson A, Simi B, Reddy B. Chemoprevention of colon cancer by dietary curcumin. Ann NY Acad Sci 125:201–204, 1996.

423. Rao C, Tokumo K, Rigotty J, et al. Chemoprevention of colon carcinogenesis by dietary administration of piroxicam, α-difluoromethylornithine, 16-α-fluoro-5-androsten-17-one, and ellagic acid individually and in combination. Cancer Res 51:4528–4553, 1991.

424. Rao CV, Simi B, Reddy BS. Inhibition of dietary curcumin of azoxymethane induced ornithine decarboxylase, tyrosine, protein kinase, arachidonic acid metabolism and aberrant crypt foci formation in the rat colon. Carcinogenesis 14:2219–2225, 1993.

425. Reddy AChP, Lokesh BR. Studies on the inhibitory effects of curcumin and eugenol on the formation of reactive oxygen species and the oxidation of ferrous iron. Mol Cell Biochem 137:1–8, 1994.

426. Reddy BS, Rao CV, Rivenson A, Kelloff G. Inhibitory effect of aspirin on azoxymethane-induced colon carcinogenesis in F344 rats. Carcinogenesis 14:1493–1497, 1993.

427. Chiu C, McEntee M, Whelan J. Sulindac causes rapid regression of preexisting tumors in Min/+ mice independent of prostaglandin biosynthesis. Cancer Res 57:4267–4273, 1997.

428. Marnett LJ. Aspirin and the role of prostaglandins in colon cancer. Cancer Res 52:5575–5589, 1992.

429. DeRubertis FR, Craven PA. Early alterations in rat colonic mucosal cyclic nucleotide metabolism and protein kinase activity induced by 1,2-dimethylhydrazine. Cancer Res 40:4589–4598, 1980.

430. Howe L, Subbaramaiah K, Chung W, Dannenberg A, Brown A. Transcriptional activation of cyclooxygenase-2 in Wnt-1 transformed mouse mammary epithelial cells. Cancer Res 59:1572–1577, 1999.

431. Tsujii M, DuBois RN. Alterations in cellular adhesion and apoptosis in epithelial cells overexpressing prostaglandin endoperoxide synthase 2. Cell 83:493–501, 1995.

432. Boolbol S, Dannenberg A, Chadburn A, et al. Cyclooxygenase-2 overexpression and tumor formation are blocked by sulindac in a murine model of familial adenomatous polyposis. Cancer Res 56:2556–2560, 1996.

433. Kopp E, Ghosh S. Inhibition of NF-κB by sodium salicylate and aspirin. Science 265:956–958, 1994.

434. Dong Z, Huang C, Brown R, Ma W. Inhibition of activator protein 1 activity and neoplastic transformation by aspirin. J Biol Chem 272: 9962–9970, 1997.

435. Piazza G, Rahm A, Finn T, et al. Apoptosis primarily accounts for the growth-inhibitory properties of sulindac metabolites and involves a mechanism that is independent of cyclooxygenase inhibition, cell cycle arrest, and p53 induction. Cancer Res 57:2452–2459, 1997.

436. Piazza G, Rahm A, Pamukcu R, Ahnen D. Apoptosis fully accounts for the growth inhibitory activity of sulindac. Proc Annu Meet Am Assoc Cancer Res 37:A1902, 1996.

437. Tsujii M, Kawano S, Tsuji S, et al. Cyclooxygenase regulates angiogenesis induced by colon cancer cells [published erratum appears in Cell 1998;94: 271]. Cell 93:705, 1998.

438. Qiao L, Kozoni V, Tsioulias GJ, et al. Selected eicosanoids increase the proliferation rate of human colon carcinoma cell lines and mouse colonocytes in vivo. Biochim Biophys Acta 1258:215–223, 1995.

439. Eberhart CE, Coffey RJ, Radhika A, et al. Up-regulation of cyclooxygenase 2 gene expression in human colorectal adenomas and adenocarcinomas. Gastroenterology 107:1183–1188, 1994.

440. DuBois RN, Gupta R, Brockman J, et al. The nuclear eicosanoid receptor, PPARgamma, is aberrantly expressed in colonic cancers. Carcinogenesis 19:49–53, 1998.

441. He TC, Chan TA, Vogelstein B, Kinzler KW. PPARdelta is an APC-regulated target of nonsteroidal anti-inflammatory drugs. Cell 99:335–345, 1999.

442. Piazza G, Mehta R, Alberts D, et al. Antineoplastic activity of sulindac does not require cyclooxygenase inhibition. Proc Annu Meet Am Assoc Cancer Res 37:A1901, 1996.

443. Piazza GA, Alberts DS, Hixson LJ, et al. Sulindac sulfone inhibits azoxymethane-induced colon carcinogenesis in rats without reducing prostaglandin levels. Cancer Res 57:2909–2915, 1997.

444. Piazza GA, Rahm AL, Krutzsch M, et al. Antineoplastic drugs sulindac sulfide and sulfone inhibit cell growth by inducing apoptosis. Cancer Res 55:3110–3116, 1995.

445. Elder D, Halton D, Hague A, Paraskeva C. Induction of apoptotic cell death in human colorectal carcinoma cell lines by a cyclooxygenase-2 (COX-2)-selective nonsteroidal anti-inflammatory drug: independence from COX-2 protein expression. Clin Cancer Res 3:1679–1683, 1997.

446. Craven PA, DeRubertis FR. Profiles of eicosanoid production by superficial and proliferative colonic epithelial cells and sub-epithelial cells and sub-epithelial colonic tissue. Prostaglandins 32:387–399, 1986.

447. Shureiqi I, Wojno KJ, Poore JA, et al. Decreased 13-S-hydroxyoctadecadienoic acid levels and 15-lipoxygenase-1 expression in human colon cancers. Carcinogenesis 20:1985–1995, 1999.

448. Shureiqi I, Chen D, Lee JJ, et al. 15-LOX-1: a novel molecular target of nonsteroidal anti-inflammatory drug-induced apoptosis in colorectal cancer cells. J Natl Cancer Inst 92:1136–1142, 2000.

449. Shureiqi I, Chen D, Lotan R, et al. 15-Lipoxygenase-1 mediates nonsteroidal anti-inflammatory drug–induced apoptosis independently of cyclooxygenase-2 in colon cancer cells. Cancer Res 60:6846–6850, 2000.

450. Muscat JE, Stellman SD, Wynder EL. Nonsteroidal anti-inflammatory drugs and colorectal cancer. Cancer 74:1847–1854, 1994.

451. Peleg II, Maibach HT, Brown SH, Wilcox CM. Aspirin and nonsteroidal anti-inflammatory drug use and the risk of subsequent colorectal cancer. Arch Intern Med 154:394–399, 1994.

452. Kune GA, Kune S, Watson LF. Colorectal cancer risk, chronic illnesses, operations, and medications: case–control results from the Melbourne Colorectal Cancer Study. Cancer Res 48:4399–4404, 1988.

453. Paganini-Hill A, Hsu G, Ross RK, Henderson BE. Aspirin use and incidence of large bowel cancer in a California retirement community. J Natl Cancer Inst 83:1182–1183, 1991.

454. Rosenberg L, Palmer JR, Zauber AG, et al. A hypothesis: nonsteroidal anti-inflammatory drugs reduce the incidence of large-bowel cancer. J Natl Cancer Inst 83:355–358, 1991.

455. Smalley W, Ray WA, Daugherty J, Griffin MR. Use of nonsteroidal anti-inflammatory drugs and incidence of colorectal cancer: a population-based study. Arch Intern Med 159:161–166, 1999.

456. Suh O, Mettlin C, Petrelli NJ. Aspirin use, cancer, and polyps of the large bowel. Cancer 72:1171–1177, 1993.

457. Thun MJ, Namboodiri MM, Heath CW Jr. Aspirin use and reduced risk of fatal colon cancer. N Engl J Med 328:1593–1596, 1991.

458. Schreinemachers DM, Everson RB. Aspirin use and lung, colon, and breast cancer incidence in a prospective study. Epidemiology 5:138–146, 1994.

459. Giovannucci E, Rimm EB, Stampfer MJ, et al. Aspirin use and the risk for colorectal cancer and adenoma in male health professionals. Ann Intern Med 121:241–246, 1994.

460. Paganini-Hill A, Chao A, Ross R, Henderson B. Aspirin use and chronic diseases a cohort study of the elderly. BMJ 299:1247–1250, 1989.

461. Collet JP, Sharpe C, Belzile E, et al. Colorectal cancer prevention by non-steroidal anti-inflammatory drugs: effects of dosage and timing. Br J Cancer 81:62–68, 1999.

462. Paganini-Hill A. Aspirin and the prevention of colorectal cancer: a review of the evidence. Semin Surg Oncol 10:158–164, 1994.

463. Sturmer T, Glyn R, Lee I, et al. Aspirin use and colorectal cancer: post-

464. Gann PH, Manson JE, Glynn RJ, Buring JE, Hennekens CH. Low-dose aspirin and incidence of colorectal tumors in a randomized trial. J Natl Cancer Inst 85:1220–1224, 1993.

465. Giardiello FM, Hamilton SR, Krush AJ, et al. Treatment of colonic and rectal adenomas with sulindac in familial adenomatous polyposis. N Engl J Med 328:1313–1316, 1993.

466. Steinbach G, Lynch PM, Phillips RK, et al. The effect of celecoxib, a cyclooxygenase-2 inhibitor, in familial adenomatous polyposis. N Engl J Med 342:1946–1952, 2000.

467a. Giardiello FM, Yang VW, Hylind LM, et al. Primary chemoprevention of familial adenomatous polyposis with sulindac. N Engl J Med 346: 1054–1059, 2002.

467b. Baron JA, Cole BF, Sandler RS, et al. A randomized trial of aspirin to prevent colorectal adenomas. NEJM 348:891–899, 2003.

468. Li H, Kramer P, Lubet R, et al. Effects of calcium on azoxymethane-induced aberrant crypt foci and cell proliferation in the colon of rats. Cancer Lett 124:39–46, 1998.

469. Beaty MM, Lee EY, Glauert HP. Influence of dietary calcium and vitamin D on colon epithelial cell proliferation and 1,2-dimethylhydrazine-induced colon carcinogenesis in rats fed high-fat diets. J Nutr 123:144–152, 1993.

470. Holt P, Atillasoy E, Gilman J, et al. Modulation of abnormal colonic epithelial cell proliferation and differentiation by low-fat diary foods: a randomized controlled trial. JAMA 280:1074–1079, 1998.

471. Buset M, Lipkin M, Winawer S, Swaroop S, Friedman E. Inhibition of human colonic epithelial cell proliferation in vivo and in vitro by calcium. Cancer Res 46:5426–5430, 1986.

472. Wargovich M, Eng V, Newmark H. Calcium inhibits the damaging and compensatory proliferative effects of fatty acids on mouse colonic epithelium. Cancer Lett 23:253–258, 1984.

473. Wargovich M, Eng V, Newmark H, et al. Calcium ameliorates the toxic effect of deoxycholic acid on colonic epithelium. Carcinogenesis 4: 1205–1207, 1983.

474. Bartram HP, Kasper K, Dusel G, et al. Effects of calcium and deoxycholic acid on human colonic cell proliferation in vitro. Ann Nutr Metab 41:315–323, 1997.

475. Yang CY, Chiu HF, Chiu JF, Tsai SS, Cheng MF. Calcium and magnesium in drinking water and risk of death from colon cancer. Jpn J Cancer Res 88:928–933, 1997.

476. Martinez ME, Willett WC. Calcium, vitamin D, and colorectal cancer: a review of the epidemiologic evidence. Cancer Epidemiol Biomarkers Prev 7:163–168, 1998.

477. Baron J, Beach M, Mandel J, et al. Calcium supplements for the prevention of colorectal adenomas. N Engl J Med 340:101–107, 1999.

478. Steinmetz KA, Potter JD. Vegetables, fruit, and cancer prevention: a review. J Am Diet Assoc 96:1027–1039, 1996.

479. Willett WC. Micronutrients and cancer risk. Am J Clin Nutr 59:1162S–1165S, 1994.

480. Salim EI, Wanibuchi H, Taniyama T, et al. Inhibition of development of N, N′-dimethylhydrazine-induced rat colonic aberrant crypt foci by pre, post and simultaneous treatments with 24R,25-dihydroxyvitamin D3. Jpn J Cancer Res 88:1052–1062, 1997.

481. Evans SR, Schwartz AM, Shchepotin EI, Uskokovic M, Shchepotin IB. Growth inhibitory effects of 1,25-dihydroxyvitamin D3 and its synthetic analogue, 1alpha,25-dihydroxy-16-ene-23yne-26,27-hexafluoro-19-norcholecalciferol (Ro 25-6760), on a human colon cancer xenograft. Clin Cancer Res 4:2869–2876, 1998.

482. White E, Shanon J, Patterson R. Relationship between vitamin and calcium supplement use and colon cancer. Cancer Epidemiol Biomarkers Prev 6:769–774, 1997.

483. Kim YI, Salomon RN, Graeme-Cook F, et al. Dietary folate protects against the development of macroscopic colonic neoplasia in a dose-responsive manner in rats. Gut 39:732–740, 1996.

484. Giovannucci E, Stampfer M, Colditz G, et al. Folate, methionine, and alcohol intake and risk of colorectal adenoma. J Natl Cancer Inst 85:875–884, 1993.

485. Hebert-Croteau N. A meta-analysis of hormone replacement therapy and colon cancer in women. Cancer Epidemiol Biomarkers Prev 7:653–659, 1998.

486. Grodstein F, Martinez ME, Platz EA, et al. Postmenopausal hormone use and risk for colorectal cancer and adenoma. Ann Intern Med 128: 705–712, 1998.

trial follow-up data from the Physicians Health Study. Ann Intern Med 128:713–720, 1998.

# Chapter 3

# The Role of Inheritance in the Diagnosis and Management of Gastrointestinal Malignancies

PATRICK M. LYNCH

The role of inheritance in causation of cancer can be thought of in many ways. To the genetic epidemiologist, clustering of cancer in families provides a sense of the presence and significance of inherited susceptibility at the population level. The clinician may come to appreciate that critical, more or less obvious physical traits recur predictably within a family and are associated with risk of certain types of malignancy. The modern molecular biologist is now able to perform linkage analysis within cancer-prone families, even in instances where no physical stigmata are present. When linkage is established between the cancer phenotype and specific polymorphic genetic markers, identification and sequencing of the cancer-predisposing gene soon follows and predictive genetic testing becomes possible. Even more subtle characterization of genetic risk is becoming a reality as molecular biologists unravel the complexities of genetically determined variation in the processing of environmental carcinogens.

Other authors in this text will address in greater detail some of the more common inherited gastrointestinal (GI) cancer–predisposing conditions. Most recent effort has been devoted to inherited susceptibility to colorectal cancer. Striking disease phenotypes in familial adenomatous polyposis (FAP) and its non-adenomatous polyposis counterparts, Peutz-Jeghers syndrome (PJS) and juvenile polyposis (JP), have been recognized for many decades. Hereditary nonpolyposis colorectal cancer (HNPCC) has generated tremendous interest in recent years due to its relatively greater prevalence and the discovery of the family of mismatch repair genes that cause it, as well as the novel tumor phenotype involving instability in microsatellite genes. A number of excellent reviews are now available to readers interested in the role of molecular diagnostics in clinical management of FAP and HNPCC.[1–4] This chapter will briefly address the current knowledge of inherited susceptibility to the relatively less common disorders.

## Genetic Counseling, Testing, and Standards of Care

Before commenting on specific GI organ sites, their cancer-predisposing syndromes, and corresponding genes, some introduction to the issues involved in genetic counseling and genetic testing is in order.

The American Society of Clinical Oncology (ASCO) has taken a very strong position on the responsibility of its constituent oncologists in the area of genetic susceptibility evaluation and management.[5] The ASCO stated that oncologists must become competent to perform risk assessment, to identify subjects that would benefit from genetic counseling and testing, and to be familiar with appropriate measures for surveillance and management in such high-risk groups. Specific key points included the following:

1. Affirmation of the need for oncologists to take a family history and to counsel patients regarding familial risk, prevention, and surveillance options, and to recognize families in which genetic *testing* might aid counseling
2. The importance of testing in the context of outcomes evaluations, including establishment of registries to better determine the significance of identified mutations
3. A commitment by ASCO to provision of cancer genetics education for its members
4. The continued need for safeguarding informed consent
5. Support for predisposition testing only in the setting of sufficiently strong family history or early age at onset, when adequate interpretation can be provided and when results have the ability to influence clinical management
6. The recommendation that oncologists should discuss risks and benefits of early cancer detection and prevention measures
7. The importance of laboratory oversight in the interest of maintaining quality control in predisposition testing

8. Endorsement of antidiscrimination legislation in the areas of insurance and employment
9. Equal patient access to genetic testing and related services, to be covered by public and third-party payers
10. Support for research into the psychological impact of genetic testing.

In its position statement, the ASCO was quite specific in naming categories of disease in which genetic testing would be considered standard of care (including *APC* testing in FAP, as well as genetic testing in multiple endocrine neoplasia 2a and 2b, retinoblastoma, and von Hippel–Lindau syndrome). In the case of HNPCC and inherited breast cancer (BRCA), data in support of genetic testing were not as strongly evidence based and the benefit of testing was "presumed but not established." Recognizing that these recommendations are now 3 years old, updated recommendations are likely to be developed in the very near future and would probably consider HNPCC and BRCA testing to be the standard of care for subjects meeting specified clinical and/or laboratory criteria.

Not all involved in formulating the ASCO guidelines regarded genetic testing as an intervention ripe for standard clinical practice. A dissenting minority of the ASCO task force that drafted the 1996 guidelines felt that genetic susceptibility testing, at least for BRCA, should continue to be performed only in the course of "hypothesis-driven research" approved by institutional review boards (IRBs). In essence, the dissenters took the position that insufficient protection existed in the areas of informed consent, privacy and confidentiality, and content and process of genetic counseling in clinical practice not otherwise regulated by IRB-approved protocols. These concerns were also voiced in commentaries by the National Breast Cancer Coalition and the National Action Plan on Breast Cancer.[6] Until a true consensus is reached on the readiness for clinical implementation of genetic testing, legitimate argument may persist as to the standard of care for clinicians. It is interesting to note that reservations expressed by the ASCO dissenters and advocacy groups were limited to testing for breast cancer susceptibility and did not address colorectal cancer susceptibility testing. The controversies over testing for breast cancer and colorectal cancer susceptibility are essentially identical: testing accuracy, mutation-associated disease risk, medical management, counseling and educational needs, and quality of life. Consequently, the difference in response to testing in the two settings appears to have more to do with heightened attention devoted to breast cancer by investigators and advocates alike.

The American Society of Human Genetics (ASHG) adopted a position consistent with the minority ASCO opinion. The ASHG concluded that testing should continue to be investigational and performed only by "appropriately trained health care professionals who have a therapeutic relationship with the patient and are fully aware of the genetic, clinical, and psychological implications of testing."[7]

The American Cancer Society[8] has also taken a strong position on surveillance as well as genetic counseling for FAP and HNPCC. In the case of FAP, recommendations are for "counseling to consider genetic testing and referral to a specialty center," and specifically for endoscopy beginning at puberty and continued every 1–2 years, followed by colectomy at diagnosis of polyps. For HNPCC, surveillance by means of colonoscopy is recommended beginning at age 21 and at 2-year intervals up to age 40, then annually in individuals who are carriers of HNPCC mutations. The same recommendation exists for those with a family history of HNPCC but in whom testing has not been done. This presumably also includes those families in which genetic testing has been done but has not been informative.

Members of the Cancer Genetics Studies Consortium (CGSC) reported a consensus statement for both HNPCC and BRCA surveillance and management, in relation to genetic testing.[9,10] The consortium itself consisted of individuals from institutions participating in a coordinated series of studies of psychosocial parameters surrounding susceptibility testing. Criteria for "quality of evidence" were adopted upon which recommendations were adapted from the U.S. Preventive Services Task Force. Surveillance recommendations were provided for individuals regarded as "carriers" on the basis of genetic testing and for those "at risk" but for whom testing could not be done or is uninformative. Colon surveillance recommendations were similar to those of the American Cancer Society: colonoscopy initiated at age 20–25 and repeated at 1- to 3-year intervals. For endometrial surveillance, transvaginal ultrasound was recommended annually, beginning at age 25–35. Whereas colon surveillance recommendations were based on "multiple time series with and without intervention,"[11] recommendations for endometrial surveillance relied on "expert opinion" only. Recommendations for prophylactic surgical intervention, based on expert opinion, included subtotal colectomy as well as consideration of hysterectomy with oophorectomy. While targeted primarily at individuals with incident tumors, consideration of truly prophylactic surgery was considered appropriate in carefully selected circumstances in individuals known to be carriers of pathologic mutations.

Another panel of experts provided clinical guidelines and a rationale for colorectal cancer screening, which included the approach to FAP and HNPCC.[12] Its report was endorsed by the American Cancer Society, American College of Gastroenterology, American Gastroenterological Association, American Society of Colon and Rectal Surgeons, American Society for Gastrointestinal Endoscopy, Oncology Nursing Society, and Society of American Gastrointestinal Endoscopic Surgeons, among others. For those with a family history of FAP, the panel recommends genetic counseling and consideration of genetic testing. A genetic test to exclude carrier status was only considered informative if a mutation had been identified in another affected family member. For known carriers and those of unknown status, yearly sigmoidoscopy beginning at puberty is recommended. When polyposis is demonstrated, consideration should be given to colectomy. Similar genetic counseling and testing recommendations were made for those with HNPCC. Examination of the entire colon is recommended at 1- to 2-year intervals, beginning between age 20 and 30, and yearly after age 40.

From the variety of views presented here on genetic testing, practitioners can gain an appreciation for the rapidly evolving applications of genetic testing in the clinical setting and the potential for such testing to alter clinical management.

## Esophagus

While rare, the most well-known inherited condition that predisposes to squamous carcinoma of the esophagus is keratosis palmare et plantare. This is a generalized hyperproliferation of squamous epithelium. A number of related cutaneous phenotypes exist, but are not necessarily associated with increased risk of esophageal or other visceral cancer. Several genetic loci associated with tylosis have been identified. The only one definitely associated with squamous carcinoma of the esophagus has been mapped to chromosome 17q. Selection of this chromosome region for linkage analysis stemmed from the recognition of several keratin genes in this region that had been linked to various cutaneous diseases. Linkage was accomplished by means of polymorphic markers D17S785 and D17S1602 in one study[13] and with D17S515 and, again, D17S785 by different investigators.[14] This is the relatively later-onset, or "A," form of the disease. The juvenile-onset, or "B," form does not appear to be associated with esophageal cancer. Reclassification on the basis of differences in cutaneous phenotype has been proposed.[13,15]

## Barrett's Esophagus

Examples of familial aggregation of Barrett's esophagus have been described, but none compellingly denote the presence of a simply inherited predisposition. Familial clustering of reflux esophagitis and of hiatal hernia has also been reported. Simple inheritance has not been demonstrated in such cases either, and the relationship, if any, to Barrett's esophagus must be complex.[16,17]

## Stomach

Gastric cancer has generally been considered an environmental disease, influenced by regional variation in diet and food preparation and preservation. More recently, an infectious etiology has been implicated, with *Helicobacter pylori* contributing to an inflammation–gastritis–metaplasia–dysplasia pathway. Historically, no major genetic contribution has been considered.

For many years, cases of gastric cancer have been observed in patients with FAP, though such tumors are uncommon when compared with those of the colorectum and duodenum. Most reports of gastric cancer in FAP are from Japan, where the incidence is 2.1%.[18] Gastric cancer occurs in well under 1% of Western patients with FAP.[19] Patients with FAP commonly have non-neoplastic fundic gland polyps. These are essentially hyperplastic and confined to the body and fundus of the stomach. They can be very dramatic in appearance because of their tendency to be rather numerous and occasionally large. However, for the most part they have been considered innocuous, once biopsied and found to lack any dysplasia. There has been one report of dysplasia arising in fundic gland polyps and complicated by invasive gastric cancer.[20] Adenomas of the stomach are uncommon, even in FAP, and when they do occur are usually confined to the antrum. Such antral adenomas represent the precursors to most invasive cancer that do occur and, as such, should be sought for and removed in the course of surveillance endoscopy.

Stomach cancer does not appear to be increased in families with BRCA1 and BRCA2.[21] Gastric cancers do occur rather commonly in families with HNPCC[22,23] and are second only to endometrial cancer as extracolonic malignancies in some series. No specific genotype–phenotype correlations have been observed in cancers arising in patients with known mismatch repair gene mutations.[23] Pathologic and molecular evaluation of HNPCC-associated gastric cancers has shown a high proportion of them to have an intestinal or well-differentiated histology and to show evidence of microsatellite instability (MSI).[23] In otherwise unselected series of gastric cancers, conflicting results have been observed regarding an association between familiality and microsatellite instability, with two studies showing higher rates of MSI in those with a positive family history and two showing no such association (summarized in Ottini et al.).[24]

Documentation of a genetic basis for familial clustering of site-specific gastric cancer, not associated with polyposis or other inherited syndromes, has been elusive. Recent excitement has been generated by the discovery of linkage between gastric cancer susceptibility in a New Zealand Maori family and a chromosome 16 locus (D16S752) near the gene for E-cadherin (*CDH1*).[25] A germline mutation in the E-cadherin gene was identified in this same family, a G → T transversion in exon 7. Following this, single-strand conformation polymorphism (SSCP) analysis of eight unrelated gastric families showed pathologic alterations in exons 2, 3, 5, 10, 11, 13, and 15, respectively, and in intron 8.[25,26] The authors proposed the term "hereditary diffuse gastric cancer" (HDGC) to reflect the added observation of diffuse or undifferentiated tumor histology. Richards and colleagues[27] identified *CDH1* mutations in two of eight British families with gastric cancer. The ages at onset were not as young as in the New Zealand series, perhaps contributing to the lower mutation yield. One family included a young patient (age 30) with rectal cancer. This patient was a mutation carrier who had not yet developed stomach cancer. The rectal tumor in this patient did not show loss of heterozygosity (LOH) for the CDH1 locus.

That E-cadherin may be of more generalized importance in gastric cancer is demonstrated by the frequent mutation and loss of the gene in sporadic cases of gastric cancer.[28] E-cadherin is an important cell-adhesion molecule involved in establishing and maintaining cell polarity and differentiation. Its interactions with B-catenin and the APC protein will continue to shed light on the pathogenesis of GI and perhaps other malignancies.[29,30]

## Pancreas

### Multiple Endocrine Neoplasia I

Multiple endocrine neoplasia type 1 (MEN-1) is comprised of neoplasia involving the parathyroid, anterior pituitary, and, of note to this discussion, benign and malignant neuroendocrine tumors of the pancreas and gut. MEN-1 is distinguished from the subtypes of MEN-2 by the spectrum of tumors as well as by the responsible genes. While MEN-2 has been mapped to chromosome 10, specifically the *RET* protooncogene, MEN-1 is associated with a chromosome 11q13 locus, referred to as MEN1.[31–34] Not surprisingly, the *MEN1* gene is a tumor suppressor gene. Consequently, syndrome tumors commonly show LOH. Consistent with Knudson's two-hit hypothesis, the mutated allele received from the diseased parent is constitutionally inactivated, while the normal, wild-type allele inherited from the nondiseased parent becomes somatically inactivated, resulting in complete loss of tumor-suppressor gene function.

The *MEN1* gene has been shown to carry a variety of disease-causing mutations, with most families reported to date exhibiting novel mutations.[35] As such, no simple method such as allele-specific oligonucleotide (ASO) testing is feasible at this time. In addition, no consistent genotype–phenotype correlations have been described. As a consequence of the sequencing of the *MEN1* gene, it has become possible to directly test for germline mutations in individual subjects with multiple endocrine tumors, even when family history is negative or otherwise not amenable to linkage analysis. In a National Institutes of Health (NIH) series of apparently sporadic subjects, *MEN1* gene mutations were found in seven of eight subjects.[35] In another series, it was concluded that as many as 10% of all *MEN1* mutations are spontaneous.[36]

The function of the *MEN1* gene is not known. The gene shows little homology to infrahuman genes of known function. The gene-associated protein is nuclear, like the proteins produced by many other tumor-suppressor genes.[37]

In a recent review from the NIH, several obstacles to widespread predictive testing for *MEN1* mutations were noted. Because many different mutations exist in the gene and many of these are missense mutations, otherwise straightforward testing methods such as the ASO noted above or protein truncation assays cannot be effectively utilized. Demand is likely to be limited because the condition is so rare. Demand is further compounded by the fact that determination of carrier status in a given patient would not greatly facilitate diagnostic or therapeutic (preventative) interventions.

Approaches to diagnosis and treatment of neuroendocrine tumors of the pancreas and intestinal tract that comprise components of the MEN1 syndrome are described in Chapter 65.

### Exocrine Pancreas

Adenocarcinoma arising in the exocrine pancreas carries one of the worst prognoses of common malignancies. Cures, while rare, depend on early detection. Such early detection is uncommon because identification of subjects at increased risk is not usually possible and screening/diagnostic measures are expensive and insensitive for early tumors. Given the grim picture for dealing with pancreatic cancer, it would be ideal to be able to identify subjects at increased risk. Familial pancreatic cancer is uncommon and not well characterized as a clinical entity. Pancreatic adenocarcinoma is an occasional feature of such conditions as FAP and HNPCC. However, its infrequency in each condition is such that no enhanced surveillance for pancreatic cancer has ever been recommended. Occasional families have been described with clustering of pancreatic cancer alone or pancreatic cancer in combination with other tumors that do not fit well into known syndromic classification schemes.

Families with mutations in the melanoma-predisposing gene *p16(supINK4)* have been observed to have a markedly increased risk of pancreatic adenocarcinoma.[38,39] One investigation[38] evaluated 19 families with multiple cases of melanoma and found altered *p16* alleles in 10. In these families, compared with melanoma families lacking pathologic mutations, a 13-fold relative risk of pancreatic cancer was noted. The small number of assessable cases of pancreatic cancer did carry *p16(supINK4)* mutations. Mutations in the gene varied among cases, arguing against the presence of any significant genotype–phenotype correlation. No pancreatic tumors were evaluated for evidence of somatic mutations, although other reports of *p16* mutations (commonly allelic deletions and homozygous deletions) in pancreatic cancer have been described.[40]

In another report, Whelan and colleagues[39] described a family with a mutation in the same *p16* gene, although the term *CDKN2* (for *cyclin-dependent-kinase* inhibitor) was used. Three cases of pancreatic cancer, one squamous cell carcinoma and two adenocarcinoma, were reported. Limited tissue was available in each case for analysis, such as needle biopsy of the pancreatic mass. From the limited, non-neoplastic, stromal tissue, the investigators were able to determine the presence of the germline mutation that had been identified in an index case. Insufficient tumor material was available for studies of LOH at the CDKN2 locus. These cases nicely illustrate the potential for genetic analysis even when scant amounts of tissue are available, but at the same time emphasize the problem in the study of pancreatic cancer of often having *very* little tissue to work with. There has been at least one report of familial pancreatic cancer, not occurring in the context of familial melanoma, in which a germline mutation in *p16* has been observed.[41] However, this was the only family from among 21 kindreds with two or more cases of pancreatic cancer in which a *p16* mutation was identified.

In considering the impact of possible testing for *p16* mutations in familial pancreatic cancer, several vexing issues exist. Such mutations apparently occur in a very small proportion of familial pancreatic cancer. When pancreatic cancer occurs in the context of familial melanoma and a *p16* mutation is identified,

the penetrance or absolute risk for pancreatic cancer remains relatively low, despite the high relative risk noted above. As such, any recommendations for surveillance or intervention are problematic. The cost-effectiveness of existing surveillance measures such as spiral computed tomography (CT) or endoscopic ultrasound has yet to be evaluated, much less demonstrated.

The notion has been advanced of considering prophylactic pancreatectomy for patients at highest risk, namely, those with a family history of pancreatic cancer and abnormalities at endoscopic retrograde cholangiopancreatography (ERCP) and/or endosonography.[42] One such study was done of three pancreatic cancer families without evidence of mutations in *p16*, hereditary pancreatitis gene, or mismatch repair genes. Investigations included spiral CT, endosonography, ERCP, and serum markers (CEA and CA19-9). Of 14 subjects evaluated, 9 had symptoms of pancreatic exocrine or endocrine insufficiency. The most common finding was the presence of small, 1- to 2-mm echogenic foci on endosonography. The ERCP findings consisted of mild ductal irregularities of the type commonly seen in chronic pancreatitis. Pancreatectomies were carried out on the basis of ERCP abnormalities combined with family history. Widespread epithelial dysplasia was present in each case. Spiral CT and serum markers were considered insensitive for the changes found at ERCP and endosonography. Surveillance of the type employed was recommended for those with two or more first-degree relatives with pancreatic cancer, those with one first-degree relative diagnosed before age 50, and those with two or more second-degree relatives if one of them was diagnosed at an early age.

Adenocarcinoma of the pancreas has been described as a sometimes feature of other inherited precancerous syndromes. A germline mutation in the *STK11/LKB1* gene responsible for the PJS has been observed in at least one patient developing pancreatic cancer and intestinal hamartoma in a PJS family. As might be expected, loss of the wild-type allele of the *STK11/LKB1* gene was observed in the pancreas tumor itself. Homozygous deletion or mutation/deletion of this gene was also observed in 4%–6% of sporadic pancreatic and biliary cancers.[43]

There is some controversy over the question of whether pancreatic cancer is integral to the tumor spectrum of either FAP or HNPCC. In one large study of extracolonic tumors in HNPCC, no statistical overrepresentation of pancreatic cancer could be identified.[44] Pancreatic cancers have been described in FAP, but are uncommon.[45] The uncommon occurrence of adenocarcinomas involving the pancreatic ducts proper should not be confused with the very real and substantial risk of periampullary and other duodenal malignancy in subjects with FAP.[46] Strategies for surveillance of the at-risk duodenum in FAP have been devised, with the goal of reducing the risk of duodenal (including periampullary) cancer from its reported frequency of about 4% in FAP.[47]

A variety of tumors have been described in familial breast and breast/ovarian cancer. In one large series of Ashkenazi Jewish subjects with specific *BRCA1* and *BRCA2* mutations, a twofold, but not statistically significant, increase in pancreatic cancer was observed.[21]

### Hemochromatosis and Other Inherited Liver Disease

Hereditary hemochromatosis is a progressive disease in which defects of iron metabolism lead to accumulation of iron pigmentation in the liver and other organs. It is progressive in that it commonly leads to frank cirrhosis of the liver. Its importance to this chapter lies in the fact that it predisposes to hepatocellular carcinoma and great strides have been made in understanding its genetic basis. Hemochromatosis occurs most commonly in northern Europeans, particularly Celtic and Scandinavian populations.

Linkage of hemochromatosis to an HLA locus (HLA-A3) on chromosome 6 was established in 1977.[48] The gene was not cloned until 1996[49] and was found to be a major histocompatibility gene, now referred to as *HFE*.[50] The vast majority of cases have been found to be homozygous for the same missense mutation (G → A at nucleotide 845, resulting in a tyrosine substitution for cysteine), termed *C282Y*. Because it is a rather common allele, as many as 1 in 200 white Americans may be expected to be homozygous carriers and to have iron overload. Another, less common mutation (*H63D*) results in milder iron overload.

Management of hemochromatosis is accomplished most readily by phlebotomy, and is important in preventing complications such as cirrhosis, heart failure, and diabetes. However, there are issues related to prevention and early detection of hepatocellular carcinoma. Ideally, early detection of hemochromatosis itself should be accomplished by screening young adults for iron overload by means of transferring saturation, iron binding capacity, or serum ferritin, along with genetic testing for *C282Y* and *H63D* in those with screening test abnormalities.

The oncologist should be concerned with hemochromatosis because the risk of hepatocellular carcinoma is increased between 23- and 200-fold over that of the general population.[51,52] Hepatoma occurs most commonly in men over age 55 and usually, but not always, in the setting of cirrhosis. In general, clinical presentation and tumor biology are indistinguishable from that encountered in hepatocellular carcinoma complicating alcoholic and viral hepatitis.[53]

$\alpha_1$-Antitrypsin deficiency is an uncommon cause of chronic liver disease and hepatoma. However, as its inheritance has been determined, it is noted for completeness.[54] $\alpha_1$-Antitrypsin is a protease inhibitor, hence the term PI to describe the various genotypes. Normal subjects carry the MM phenotype, while disease is associated with ZZ and SS phenotypes. Hepatoma occurs primarily in subjects with ZZ or MZ phenotypes. Hepatocellular carcinoma has also been observed as a complication of hereditary tyrosinemia. Affected children who do not die early from hepatic insufficiency may go on to develop cirrhosis, which is likely a key factor in pathogenesis.[55]

Wilson's disease is an autosomal recessively inherited disorder of copper metabolism, characterized by ophthalmic, neurologic, and liver disease. The liver disease may manifest as acute and fulminant hepatitis, as chronic active hepatitis, or as cirrhosis.[56] Fortunately, the complication of hepatocellular carcinoma is quite rare and, as such, beyond the scope of this chapter. It is mentioned here because Wilson's disease is always included in the differential diagnosis of cirrhosis and because its genetic basis has been established, namely the *ATP7B* gene on chromosome 13q14.3.[57,58]

## Inflammatory Bowel Disease

Chronic ulcerative colitis (UC) and Crohn's disease (CD) are forms of inflammatory bowel disease (IBD) of uncertain etiology, with theories of causation historically invoking infectious, autoimmune, environmental, and even psychiatric factors. Patients with long-standing UC and CD are at increased risk of colorectal cancer, although the risk does not reach the level seen in carriers of *APC* or mismatch repair gene mutations. Because some subjects with IBD have positive family histories of the same condition, possible inherited susceptibility has long been entertained but not established. Early investigations showed high but not complete concordance for UC and CD among monozygotic twins.[59,60] In one UC case–control study of colorectal cancer familiality, colorectal cancer was reported in 14% of 147 case families vs. only 6.7% of 150 control families ($P = 0.03$).[61] Spurred on by investigations of this kind, other investigators carried out molecular studies to determine whether disease expression was linked to specific genetic loci, with rather complex linkage suggested for loci on chromosomes 16 and 12.[62–65] The rationale for these investigations as well as their limitations have been reviewed by Gusella and Podolsky.[66] Specifically, complex and overlapping UC and CD phenotypes, variation among ethnic groups, and significant environmental interactions have confounded efforts to confirm linkage. Once linkage is demonstrated, investigators have a choice between studying so-called candidate loci in the chromosome region of interest or the more methodical process of demonstrating linkage disequilibrium. Little if any mention has been made of the association between colorectal cancer risk and the presence of alterations in specified IBD loci. This is anticipated to require a more thorough understanding of the nature of such loci, including mutations and polymorphisms in IBD-related genes. Genes involved in mediating inflammation have been investigated. An increased frequency of a promoter region polymorphism in the kinin B1 receptor gene (G$^{-699}$ → C) has been described in CD and UC patients in Quebec.[67] In a series of Japanese CD patients, an increased frequency of selected alleles of the tumor necrosis factor (TNF) gene was identified.[68] It can be anticipated that other genes involved in mediation of inflammation will be similarly investigated in various population groups. As the human genome map becomes more well characterized, such studies will increasingly address, as "candidate genes," those inflammation-mediator genes located near loci in which at least modest genetic linkage has been shown.

## Polymorphic Genes Potentially Associated with Cancer Risk by Means of Differential Metabolism of Carcinogens

Most of the attention in this discussion is devoted to dominant or single gene–determined cancer susceptibility in which significant environmental interaction is not required. However, a variety of polymorphic genes have been identified that may increase or, for that matter, decrease cancer risk by virtue of the manner in which their gene products are involved in the differential metabolism of carcinogenic compounds.

For more than 40 years, individuals have been known to vary, on genetic grounds, in the rapidity of acetylation of such drugs as isoniazid, the so-called rapid and slow acetylator phenotypes.[69] There are now two main acetylator polymorphisms, NAT1 and NAT2. NAT2 is important in the variable metabolism of a number of drugs in addition to isoniazid. The action of NAT1 is less well understood. The genes are located on the short arm of chromosome 8 (8p22),[70] a region commonly involved in LOH in human tumors.[71] In rodent models, variation in metabolism of aromatic and heterocyclic amines has been observed and has in turn been correlated with tumor or premalignant phenotypes. In one Syrian hamster investigation, differential NAT2-dependent expression of aberrant crypt foci was observed in response to 3,2′-dimethyl-4-aminobiphenyl.[72] In human studies of the genetic epidemiology of NAT allelotypes and gastrointestinal tumors, results have been mixed. An association has been reported in several studies between NAT1*10 allele and colorectal cancer, with the risk being greatest in those who were NAT2 rapid acetylators.[73,74] Emphasizing the complex interactions between NAT polymorphisms and environmental factors, increased risk was confined to men who were rapid acetylators and who were over age 60 and who, in addition, were consumers of high volumes of red meat.[74] However, data have been inconsistent regarding NAT alleles and colorectal cancer risk. Hein et al. did not find an association between the NAT1*10 allele and adenomas in a large sigmoidoscopy case–control series. There have been several recent reviews of the molecular genetics and epidemiology of NAT.[75]

## Glutathione-*S*-Transferase (GST) Genes and Gastrointestinal Cancer Risk

A family of glutathione transferases, represented by *GSTM1* (chromosome 1p13.3) and *GSTT1* (chromosome 22q11.2), code for enzyme products that are involved in the metabolism of a variety of xenobiotics, chemotherapy drugs, and potential carcinogens. In the case of GSTM1, it is quite common for individuals to be homozygous for deletion of the gene (one-third to two-thirds of the members of many populations) and to therefore express no functional detoxifying enzyme. The homozygous deletion, or null, form of GSTT1 occurs less commonly in whites, but is about as common as the GSTM1 null form in Africans and Asians. Clearly, the very high population frequency of these null phenotypes suggests that the absolute risk of cancer that can be attributed to the genotype in any given individual will be modest.

## Conclusion

A clinician concerned with the treatment of gastrointestinal malignancy need not always understand the underlying cause of the malignancy. Its presence and extent or stage may provide sufficient information on which to base therapy, whether surgery, chemotherapy, radiation, or some combination of these. However, if the question of causation has not arisen earlier, the therapist can expect the astute patient to ask about possible etiologic factors, including inherited susceptibility.

In this chapter, I have provided a brief overview of some of the more common genetic contributions to risk of gastrointestinal cancers (excluding the colon and rectum, which are addressed in Chapter 54). When a patient presents with a malignancy or precancerous lesion in the setting of a family history of the same tumor, the possibility of an inherited risk must be entertained. When history, physical, or tissue findings support the possibility of one of the conditions discussed, the clinician must be prepared to obtain appropriate genetics consultation and/or testing.

## References

1. O'Leary TJ. Molecular diagnosis of hereditary nonpolyposis colorectal cancer. JAMA 282:281–282, 1999.
2. Gebert JF, Dupon C, Kadmon M, et al. Combined molecular and clinical approaches for the identification of families with familial adenomatous polyposis coli. Ann Surg 229:350–361, 1999.
3. Syngal S, Fox EA, Li C, et al. Interpretation of genetic test results for hereditary nonpolyposis colorectal cancer: implications for clinical predisposition testing. JAMA 282:247–253, 1999.
4. Ivanovich JL, Read TE, Ciske DJ, et al. A practical approach to familial and hereditary colorectal cancer. Am J Med 107:68–77, 1999.
5. American Society of Clinical Oncology. Statement of the American Society of Clinical Oncology: genetic testing for cancer susceptibility, adopted on February 20, 1996. J Clin Oncol 14:1730–1736, 1996.
6. Visco FM, Skolnick M, Collins FS. Commentary on the ASCO statement on genetic testing for cancer susceptibility. J Clin Oncol 14:1737, 1996.
7. Anonymous. Statement of the American Society of Human Genetics on genetic testing for breast and ovarian cancer predisposition. Am J Hum Genet 55:i–iv, 1994.
8. Byers T, Levin B, Rothenberger D, et al. American Cancer Society guidelines for screening and surveillance for early detection of colorectal polyps and cancer: update 1997. CA Cancer J Clin 47:154–160, 1997.
9. Burke W, Petersen G, Lynch P, et al. Recommendation for follow-up care of individuals with an inherited predisposition to cancer. I. Hereditary nonpolyposis colon cancer. Cancer Genetics Studies Consortium. JAMA 277:915–919, 1997.
10. Burke W, Daly M, Garber J, et al. Recommendations for follow-up care of individuals with an inherited predisposition to cancer. II. *BRCA1* and *BRCA2*. Cancer Genetics Studies Consortium. JAMA 277:997–1003, 1997.
11. Jarvinen HJ, Meclin J-P, Sistonen P. Screening reduces colorectal cancer rate in families with hereditary nonpolyposis colorectal cancer. Gastroenterology 108:1405–1411, 1995.
12. Winawer SJ, Fletcher RH, Rex D, et al. Colorectal cancer screening and surveillance: clinical guidelines and rationale. Gastroenterology 124:544–560, 2003.
13. Stevens HP, Kelsell DP, Bryant SP. Linkage of an American pedigree with palmoplantar keratoderma and malignancy (palmoplanter ectodermal dysplasia type III) to 17q24. Arch Dermatol 132:640–651, 1996.
14. Risk JM, Field EA, Field JK, et al. Tylosis oesophageal cancer mapped. Nat Genet 8:319–321, 1994.
15. Maillefer RH, Greydanus MP. To B or not to B: is tylosis truly benign? Two North American genealogies. Am J Gastroenterol 94:829–834, 1999.
16. Romero Y, Cameron AJ, Locke GR III, et al. Familial aggregation of gastroesophageal reflux in patients with Barrett's esophagus and esophageal adenocarcinoma. Gastroenterology 113:1449–1456, 1997.
17. Carre IJ, Johnston BT, Thomas PS, Morrison PJ. Familial hiatal hernia in a large five-generation family confirming true autosomal dominant inheritance. Gut 45:649–652, 1999.
18. Utsunomiya J, Maki T, Iwama T. Phenotypic expression of Japanese patients with familial adenomatous polyposis. In: Herrera L, et al. (eds): Familial Adenomatous Polyposis. Alan R. Liss, New York, 1990, pp 101–107.
19. Jagelman DG, DeCosse JJ. Upper gastrointestinal cancer in familial adenomatous polyposis. Lancet 1:1149–1150, 1988.
20. Zwick A, Munir M, Ryan CK, et al. Gastric adenocarcinoma and dysplasia in fundic gland polyps of a patient with attenuated adenomatous polyposis coli. Gastroenterology 113:659–663, 1997.
21. Struewing JP, Hartge P, Wacholder S, et al. The risk of cancer associated with specific mutations of *BRCA1* and *BRCA2* among Ashkenazi Jews. N Engl J Med 336:1401–1408, 1997.
22. Vasen HFA, Offerhaus GJA, den Hartog Jafger FCA, et al. The tumour spectrum in hereditary non-polyposis colorectal cancer: a study of 24 kindreds in The Netherlands. Int J Cancer 46:31–34, 1990.
23. Aarnio M, Salovaara R, Aaltonen LA, et al. Features of gastric cancer in hereditary nonpolyposis colorectal cancer syndrome. Int J Cancer 74:551–555, 1997.
24. Ottini L, Palli D, Falchetti M, et al. Microsatellite instability in gastric cancer is associated with tumor location and family history in a high-risk population from Tuscany. Cancer Res 57:4523–4529, 1997.
25. Guilford P, Hopkins J, Harraway J, et al. E-cadherin germline mutations in familial gastric cancer. Nature 392:402–405, 1998.
26. Guilford PJ, Hopkins JBW, Grady WM, et al. E-cadherin germline mutations define an inherited cancer syndrome dominated by diffuse gastric cancer. Hum Mutat 14:249–255, 1999.
27. Richards FM, McKee SA, Rajpar MH, et al. Germline E-cadherin gene (*CDH1*) mutations predispose to familial gastric cancer and colorectal cancer. Hum Mol Genet 8:607–610, 1999.
28. Becker K-F, Atkinson MJ, Reich U, et al. E-cadherin gene mutations provide clues to diffuse type gastric carcinomas. Cancer Res 54:3845–3852, 1994.
29. Ilyas M, Tomlinson IP, Hanby A, et al. Allele loss, replication errors and loss of expression of E-cadherin in colorectal cancers. Gut 40:654–659, 1997.
30. Ilyas M, Tomlinson IP. The interactions of APC, E-cadherin, and beta-catenin in tumour development and progression. J Pathol 182:128–137, 1997.
31. Mulligan LM, Eng C, Healey CS, et al. Specific mutations of the *RET* protooncogene are related to disease phenotype in MEN 2A and FMTC. Nat Genet 6:70–74, 1994.
32. Larsson C, Skogseid B, Nakamura Y, et al. Multiple endocrine neoplasia type 1 gene maps to chromosome 11 and is lost in insulinoma. Nature 332:85–87, 1988.

33. Guru SC, Agarwal SK, Manickam P, et al. A transcript map for the 2.8-Mb region containing the multiple endocrine neoplasia type 1 locus [letter]. Genome Res 7:725–735, 1997.

34. Chandrasekharappa SC, Guru SC, Manickam P, et al. Positional cloning of the gene for multiple endocrine neoplasia type 1. Science 276:404–407, 1997.

35. Agarwal SK, Kester MB, Debelenko LV, et al. Germline mutations of the *MEN1* gene in familial multiple endocrine neoplasia type 1 and related states. Hum Mol Genet 7:1169–1175, 1997.

36. Bassett JH, Forbes SA, Pannett AA, et al. Characterization of mutations in patients with multiple endocrine neoplasia type 1. Am J Hum Genet 62:232–244, 1998.

37. Guru SC, Goldsmity PK, Burns, AL, et al. Menin, the product of the *MEN1* gene, is a nuclear protein. Proc Natl Acad Sci USA 95:1630–1634, 1998.

38. Goldstein AM, Fraser MC, Struewing JP, et al. Increased risk of pancreatic cancer in melanoma-prone kindreds with *p16(supINK4)* mutations. N Engl J Med 333:970–974, 1995.

39. Whelan AJ, Bartsch D, Goodfellow PJ. Brief report: a familial syndrome of pancreatic cancer and melanoma with a mutation in the *CDKN2* tumor-supressor gene. N Engl J Med 333:975–977, 1995.

40. Caldas C, Hahn SA, da Costa LT, et al. Frequent somatic mutations and homozygous deletions of the *p16 (MTS1)* gene in pancreatic adenocarcinoma. Nat Genet 8:27–32, 1994.

41. Moskulak CA, Hruban RH, Lietman A, et al. Novel germline p16INK4 allele (Asp145Cys) in a family with multiple pancreatic carcinomas. Hum Mutat 12:70–72, 1997.

42. Brentnall TA, Bronner MP, Byrd DR, et al. Early diagnosis and treatment of pancreatic dysplasia in patients with a family history of pancreatic cancer. Ann Intern Med 131:247–255, 1999.

43. Su GH, Hruban RH, Bansal RK, et al. Germline and somatic mutations of the *STK11/LKB1* Peutz-Jeghers gene in pancreatic and biliary cancers. Am J Pathol 1454:1835–1840, 1999.

44. Watson P, Lynch HT. Extracolonic cancer in hereditary nonpolyposis colorectal cancer. Cancer 71:677–685, 1993.

45. Bulow S. Extracolonic manifestations of familial adenomatous polyposis. In: Herrera L, et al. (eds): Familial Adenomatous Polyposis. Alan R. Liss, New York, 1990, pp 109–114.

46. Burt R, Berenson MM, Lee RG, et al. Upper gastrointestinal polyps in Gardner's syndrome. Gastroenterology 86:295–301, 1984.

47. Vasen HF, Bulow S, Myrhoj T, et al. Decision analysis in the management of duodenal adenomatosis in familial adenomatous polyposis. Gut 40:716–719, 1997.

48. Simon M, Bourel M, Genetet B, Fauchet R. Idiopathic hemochromatosis: demonstration of recessive transmission and early detection by family HLA typing. N Engl J Med 297:1017–1021, 1977.

49. Feder JN, Gnirke A, Thomas W, et al. A novel MHC class I–like gene is mutated in patients with hereditary haemochromatosis. Nat Genet 13:399–408, 1996.

50. Bodmer JG, Parham P, Albert ED, et al. Putting a hold on 'HLA-H'. Nat Genet 15:234–235, 1997.

51. Yang Q, McDonnell SM, Khoury M, et al. Hemochromatosis-associated mortality in the United States from 1979 to 1992: an analysis of multiple-cause mortality data. Ann Intern Med 129(11S):946–953, 1998.

52. Neiderau C, Fischer R, Purschel A, et al. Long-term survival in patients with hereditary hemochromatosis. Gastroenterology 110:1107–1119, 1996.

53. Deugnier YM, Guyader D, Crantock L, et al. Primary liver cancer in genetic hemochromatosis: a clinical, pathologic and pathogenetic study of 54 cases. Gastroenterology 104:228–234, 1993.

54. Eriksson S, Carlson J, Velez R. Risk of cirrhosis and primary liver cancer in $\alpha$1-antitrypsin deficiency. N Engl J Med 314:736–739, 1986.

55. Weinberg AG, Mize CE, Worthen HG. The occurrence of hepatoma in the chronic form of hereditary tyrosinemia. J Pediatr 88:434–438, 1976.

56. Sternlieb I. Evolution of the hepatic lesion in Wilson's disease (hepaticolenticular degeneration). In: Popper H, et al (eds): Progress in Liver Disease, Vol. 4. Grune & Stratton, New York, 1972, pp 511–526.

57. Bull PC, Thomas GR, Rommens JM, et al. The Wilson disease gene is a putative copper transporting P-type ATPase similar to the Menkes gene. Nat Genet 5:327–337, 1993.

58. Tanzi RE, Petrukhin K, Chernov J, et al. The Wilson disease gene is a copper transporting ATPase with homology to the Menkes disease gene. Nat Genet 5:344–350, 1993.

59. Tysk C, Lindberg E, Jarnerot G, Floderus-Myrhed B. Ulcerative colitis and Crohn's disease in an unselected population of monozygotic and dizygotic twins: a study of heritability and the influence of smoking. Gut 29:990–996, 1988.

60. Satsangi J, Jewell DP, Rosenberg WM, Bell JI. Genetics of inflammatory bowel disease. Gut 35:696–700, 1994.

61. Nuako KW, Ahlquist DA, Mahoney DW, et al. Familial predisposition for colorectal cancer in chronic ulcerative colitis: a case–control study. Gastroenterology 115:1079–1083, 1998.

62. Hugot JP, Laurent-Puig P, Gower-Rousseau C, et al. Mapping of a susceptibility locus for Crohn's disease on chromosome 16. Nature 379:821–823, 1996.

63. Brant SR, Fu Y, Fields CT, et al. American families with Crohn's disease have strong evidence for linkage to chromosome 16 but not chromosome 12. Gastroenterology 115:1056–1061, 1998.

64. Satsangi J, Parkes M, Louis E, et al. Two-stage genome-wide search in inflammatory bowel disease provides evidence for susceptibility loci an chromosomes 3, 7, and 12. Nat Genet 14:199–202, 1996.

65. Duerr RH, Barmada MM, Zhang L, et al. Linkage and association between inflammatory bowel disease on chromosome 12. Am J Hum Genet 63:95–100, 1995.

66. Gusella JF, Podolsky DK. Inflammatory bowel disease: is it in the genes? Gastroenterology 115:1286–1289, 1998.

67. Bachvarov DR, Landry M, Houle S, et al. Altered frequency of a promoter polymorphic allele of the kin in B1 receptor gene in inflammatory bowel disease. Gastroenterology 115:1045–1048, 1998.

68. Negoro K, Kinouchi Y, Hiwatashi N, et al. Crohn's disease is associated with novel polymorphisms in the 5′-flanking region of the tumor necrosis factor gene. Gastroenterology 117:1062–1068, 1999.

69. Hughes HB, Biehl JP, Jones AP, Schmidt LH. Metabolism of isoniazid in man as related to the occurrence of peripheral neuritis. Am Rev Res Dis 70:266–273, 1954.

70. Blum M, Grant DM, McBride W, et al. Human arylamine *N*-acetyltransferase genes: isolation, chromosomal localization, and functional expression. DNA Cell Biol 9:193–203, 1990.

71. Matas N, Thygesen P, Stacey M, et al. Mapping *AAC1, AAC2,* and *AACP,* the genes for arylamine *N*-acetyltransferases, carcinogen metabolising enzymes on human chromosome 8p22, a region frequently deleted in tumours. Cytogenet Cell Genet 77:290–296, 1997.

72. Feng Y, Wagner RJ, Fretland AJ, et al. Acetylator genotype (NAT2)-dependent formation of aberrant crypts in congenic Syrian hamsters administered 3,2′-dimethyl-4-aminobiphenyl. Cancer Res 56:527–531, 1996.

73. Bell DA, Stephens E, Castranio T, et al. Polyadenylation polymorphism in the *N*-acetyltransferase gene 1 (*NAT1*) increases risk of colorectal cancer. Cancer Res 55:3537–3542, 1995.

74. Chen J, Stampfer MJ, Hough HL, et al. A prospective study of *N*-acetyltransferase genotype, red meat intake, and risk of colorectal cancer. Cancer Res 58:3307–3311, 1998.

75. Hein DW, Doll MA, Fretland AJ, et al. Molecular genetics and epidemiology of the NAT1 and NAT2 acetylation polymorphisms. Cancer Epidemiol Biomarkers Prev 9:29–42, 2000.

# Chapter 4

# Developmental Biology of the Gastrointestinal Tract

## MARK W. BABYATSKY

Advances in molecular techniques have provided tremendous insights into the complex sequence of events that occur during the maturation of an initial hollow tube to the specialized multifunctional gastrointestinal (GI) tract and its appendages. Unique developmental pathways particular to the functional characteristics of the individual digestive organ or set of organs have emerged, particularly through recent gene deletion models of specific developmental factors in mice. The luminal GI tract elaborates, during and following fetal development, a capacity for the constant self-renewal necessary for maintenance of an extensive mucosal barrier and motility, while the liver and pancreas complement each other's roles in nutrient metabolism, slow cell turnover, and capacity for regeneration. Carcinogenesis is often accompanied by dedifferentiation and reversion to a fetal cellular phenotype. This chapter will examine the gross and microscopic differentiation of each of the digestive organs and appendages, as well as recently elucidated mechanisms of control of their structural and functional maturation.

By the fourth week of gestation, the human GI tract can be recognized when infolding creates an endoderm-lined tubular structure extending from the esophagus to anus. The nascent GI tract is joined in its ventral region to the yolk stalk and allantois, which remain outside of the embryo. The alimentary tract can be divided developmentally into foregut, midgut, and hindgut, reflecting roughly those structures supplied by the celiac, superior mesenteric, and inferior mesenteric arteries, respectively. The foregut includes the esophagus, stomach, duodenum (to the level of the ampulla of Vater), liver, pancreas, and biliary tract. The midgut extends from the middle second portion of the duodenum to the proximal transverse colon. The hindgut includes the distal transverse colon and the remaining large intestine to the proximal anal canal.

## Esophagus

The most proximal portion of the digestive tract functions almost exclusively as a conduit for food and salivary secretions from the oropharynx to the stomach. Development of the esophagus subsequently requires less complex mechanisms than the more distal and specialized alimentary organs.

### Structural Development

At 21 days of human gestation, fusion of septa arising from the lateral walls results in division of an initial single tube into the esophagus and upper trachea. This process of septation begins at the carina, extends distally, and is completed by the 5th to 6th weeks of gestation.[1] The esophagus migrates dorsal to the trachea by the end of the second month of gestation. The close relationship between the developing esophagus and trachea contributes to the potential for development of anomalies involving connections between the esophagus and trachea. By the 4th week of gestation, the esophagus can be distinguished from the stomach.[2] The esophagus also extends distally; its mature length relative to other structures is achieved by the 7th week of gestation. Rapid proliferation of the endodermal lining leads to near or actual occlusion of the lumen at approximately the same time. Vacuolization of the endoderm reestablishes the lumen by the 8th week of gestation through a process known as *recanalization*. This sequence of rapid mucosal proliferation, luminal obliteration, and subsequent recanalization is not unique to the esophagus but occurs simultaneously throughout the luminal GI tract. Failure of recanalization can lead to the development of esophageal stenosis or atresia, which may be seen in association with tracheoesophageal fistulae.

Histologically, the esophagus is initially covered by a simple, cuboidal epithelium. A double layer of cuboidal cells along with occasional neuroblasts interspersed in a developing layer of circular muscle can be recognized during the 5th week of gestation.[3] The outer longitudinal muscle layer can first be appreciated by approximately 13 weeks' gestation. The esophageal epithelium becomes ciliated during the 10th week of gestation and is replaced by a stratified squamous epithelium characteristic of the mature esophagus by the 22nd week of gestation.[4] Superficial glands may be found as early as the 18th week of gestation, but the deep mucosal glands characteristic of the mature esophagus are rare before birth and appear to develop postnatally.[5]

The cells that ultimately form the enteric nervous system migrate from the neural crest during the first trimester.[6] By the 8th week of gestation, neuroblasts have matured and become more numerous; synaptic protein and glial supporting tissue can be demonstrated asymmetrically penetrating the outer layers of the poorly differentiated muscular layer.[7] Immunoreactivity for neuropeptides appears during the 11th week of gestation when bombesin and neuropeptide Y can first be detected in the myenteric plexus.[8] The onset of expression of other neuropeptides occurs between the 13th and 18th week of gestation in the myenteric plexus and, in order of appearance, include vasoactive intestinal peptide (VIP), galanin, substance P, somatostatin, met-enkephalin, and calcitonin gene-related peptide (CGRP). Neuronal density peaks at 16–20 weeks of gestation, decreasing to adult levels in the third trimester. However, neuropeptide immunoreactivity increases relative to total nerve area along with the functional increase of esophageal motility throughout gestation (see below). In neonates and adults, the muscle of the proximal esophagus is striated and does not contain peptide-immunoreactive nerves, being derived from the caudal branchial arches and innervated by branches of the vagi. In the mid-esophagus, an intermediate zone exists after birth where neuropeptides are found in the smooth muscle circular layer but not in the longitudinal layer of striated muscle. Neuropeptide immunoreactivity can be detected in both muscle layers in the distal esophagus. The submucous plexus, noted to be virtually absent in the adult human esophagus,[9] is present by 13 to 19 fetal weeks, when protein gene peptide 9.5 (PGP), a generalized neuronal marker, and VIP immunoreactivity can be seen.

## Functional Development

Throughout the GI tract, structural features appear mature by the end of the second trimester, but functional development continues throughout fetal gestation and into postnatal life. Esophageal development generally adheres to this paradigm.

### Swallowing/sucking

Tagged erythrocyte isotope studies[10,11] and ultrasonography[12] demonstrate fetal swallowing as early as the 11th week of gestation. The rate of fetal swallowing of amniotic fluid increases from 13 ml/day at 20 weeks' gestation to 450 ml/day in the presence of a mean amniotic fluid volume of 850 ml at term.[10] The role of swallowing in the regulation of amniotic fluid volume remains unclear,[13] but fetal swallowing is important in GI tract development; fetal sheep[14] and rabbits[15] treated with second-trimester esophageal ligation demonstrate altered enterocyte morphology, including absence of microvilli, glycogen accumulation, and altered lysosomal morphology, similar to changes observed in malnourished infants. Absorption of infused intraamniotic nutrients has been demonstrated in fetal rabbits,[16] indicating that nutrient delivery via the fetal GI tract may be a potential treatment for intrauterine growth retardation. Sucking can be detected as early as 18 to 20 weeks' gestation,[17] although in preterm infants, sucking movements are generally feeble. By 34 to 35 weeks' gestation, a mature nutritive sucking pattern develops.[18] Before neonates can suck effectively, esophageal motility of preterm infants is characterized by poorly propagated, low-pressure biphasic contractions. Even for the first 12 hours following the birth of the full-term infant, swallowing is poorly coordinated, with both a high peristaltic rate and frequent, nonperistaltic, simultaneous contractions throughout the length of the esophagus.[19]

### Lower esophageal sphincter

Ultrasound studies demonstrate the development of a functional lower esophageal sphincter (LES) during the 32nd week of human gestation causing gastric enlargement by reduction of gastroesophageal reflux.[20] The LES pressures increase dramatically during the last trimester[21] and again postnatally.[22,23] Free postnatal gastroesophageal reflux is common and persists in up to 10% of infants for the first year.[24] This functional immaturity in the LES mechanism at birth appears to be shared by other animal species.

## Stomach

### Structural Development

In the 4-week-old embryo, the stomach forms as a fusiform dilatation of the foregut (Fig. 4–1A) in the neck. As the stomach and esophagus grow, the stomach descends into the abdomen by the 7th week of gestation. The gastric walls grow at different rates, yielding a characteristic asymmetric shape as the dorsal border (the forerunner of the greater curvature) grows more rapidly than the ventral border (Fig. 4–1B). During the 6th week of gestation, the stomach undergoes a 90° clockwise rotation along its longitudinal axis so that the dorsal border lies to the left and the ventral border (emerging lesser curvature) moves to the right (Fig. 4–1C). Resulting from this rotation, the left and right vagi largely supply the anterior and posterior areas of the stomach, respectively. Although at the end of the 7th week of gestation the shape of the stomach is suggestive of the adult stomach configuration, the cardia is still moving to the left of midline and the antrum is still moving to the right, so that the near-final shape of the stomach is assumed at 8 to 9 weeks of gestation.[25] The greater curvature, lesser curvature, corpus, antrum, and pylorus can be distinguished by 14 weeks of gestation.

Histologically, the lining of the stomach initially consists of a stratified columnar epithelium comprised of two to three cell layers, first recognized during the 7th week of gestation.[26] Gastric pits increase in number by weeks 10 to 11 of gestation. In the rat, "primitive chief cells" which resemble mature chief cells in ultrastructure but, analogous to mucous neck cells, bind various lectins,[27] are noted from the 16th day of gestation until postnatal day 14. Gastric stem cells, although not yet clearly defined, appear to be located in the mucous neck region, producing the differentiated cell types that migrate toward the surface or base of the pits.[28] Ablation of parietal cells in transgenic mice by diphtheria toxin alter the balance between all of the differentiated cell types, suggesting important developmental interactions between the cell lineages.[29]

Enteroendocrine cells can be detected by the 8th week of human gestation, and the fully differentiated spectrum of endocrine

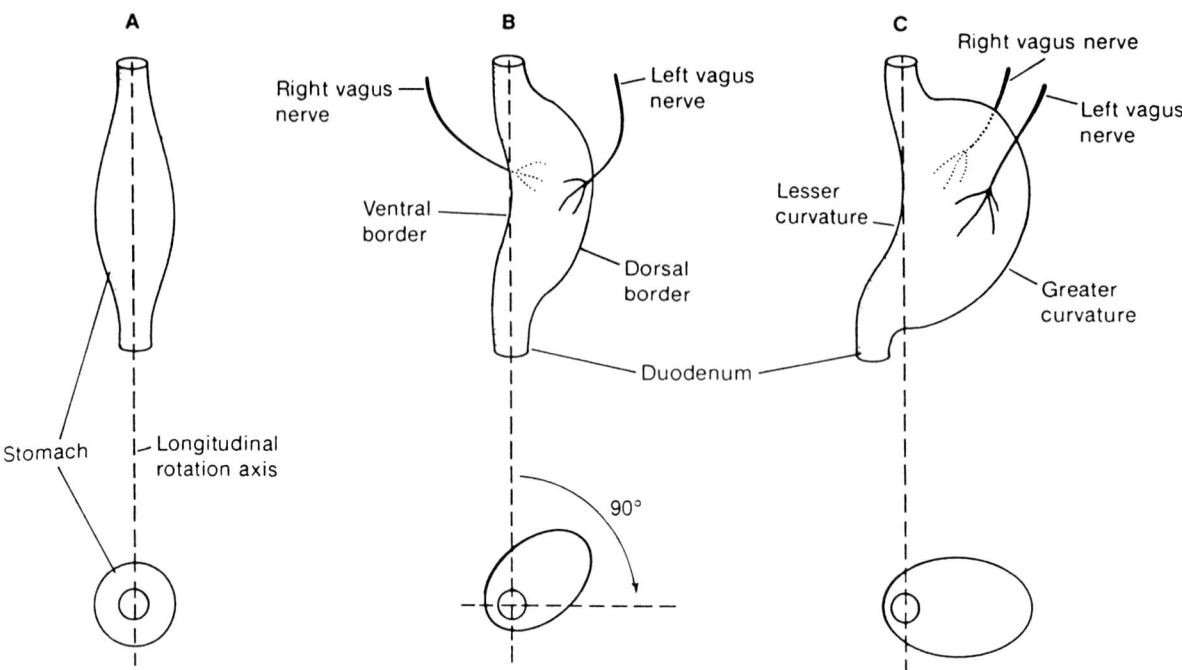

**Figure 4-1** Schematic representation of the positional changes of the stomach. *A:* The stomach at 4 weeks. *B:* Rapid growth of the dorsal border, resulting in asymmetry. *C:* After a 90° clockwise rotation along the longitudinal axis, the left and right nerves supply the anterior and posterior stomach, respectively. (Adapted from Sadler TW, ed. Langman's Medical Embryology. Williams & Wilkins, Baltimore, 1985.)

cell types can be detected by week 10,[30] suggesting a possible role in fetal development of the stomach. Extensive immunohistochemical studies have not been performed in human fetuses, but have been conducted in fetal rats. Substance P, neurokinin A, and CGRP appear first,[31] followed by peptide YY cells, which increase with age, and are frequently colocalized with gastrin G cells after birth.[32] During the first postnatal week, gastrin G cells appear in the gastric antrum while those in the pancreas disappear. Similarly, somatostatin D cells appear throughout the gastric mucosa,[33] although they are detectable in the pancreas and duodenum in mid-gestation.[34] Although earlier studies failed to demonstrate enterochromaffin-like (ECL) cells in the gastric mucosa before birth,[35] studies using highly specific histamine antisera demonstrate histamine-containing cells by mid-gestation, at least in rodents.[36,37]

Tyrosine kinases and phosphatases are two families of important enzymes that have been shown to play key roles in gastric development. Two families of receptor tyrosine kinase genes, *elk/erk* and *esk/TTK,* are expressed at high levels in rat stomach from the 14th to the 16th days of gestation,[38] decreasing following day 18, and undetectable in adult rats. Protein tyrosine phosphatases may be as important as kinases in development. PRL-1 phosphatase expression correlates with terminal differentiation of gastric zymogen cells, and may play roles in the development of other digestive organs, such as the esophagus, liver, and small intestine.[39] Both kinase and phosphatase genes are expressed early in development and reexpressed in a variety of gastric cancers, and are implicated in embryogenesis and carcinogenesis of the stomach.

Muc-1, an epithelial mucin expressed in the mature upper gastrointestinal tract, is also expressed at high levels early in rat gestation.[40] Muc-1 messenger RNA is detected in the stomach by the 10th day of gestation and protein is found by day 12. Initially, Muc-1 lines the luminal border of the gastric mucosa prior to the development of gastric glands, immediately following the initiation of branching and differentiation of the gastric epithelial buds, suggesting a role for mucin in gastric epithelial development. Spasmolytic polypeptide, a member of the trefoil family of peptides,[41] is abundantly expressed in fetal stomach, prior to the expression of gastric hormones such as gastrin or somatostatin, suggesting a role in gastric functional maturation.[42]

## Functional Development

In conjunction with the small intestine, structural features of the stomach are well developed by the end of the second trimester, while functional maturation continues throughout fetal gestation and into postnatal life. However, human gastric functional development is precocious, occurring in advance of the time when the functions are needed. In contrast, most other animal species undergo altricial development: maturation of secretory and enzymatic functions coincide with weaning, a process that takes place during the 3rd week of life.[43] Although precocious and altricial development are different in many respects, much of our knowledge of gastric function has been gained through study of rodent and other animal models.

Neither gastric secretory capacity nor gastric motility are fully developed at birth in either humans or rats. Although the fetal development of gastric motility has not been studied in detail, by the 27th to 28th week of gestation in humans, the gastric antrum only exhibits 20% to 25% of the motility reached by the term infant.[44] The maturation of gastric secretion has been studied in greater detail. The gastric mucosa of most animals, including humans, is capable of secreting some acid before birth.[45] As noted, parietal cells are present prior to the end of gestation. In the rat, basal gastric acid secretion in the rat increases from the 19th to the 21st day of gestation with maximal stimulation by pentagastrin at day 21.[46] However, acid secretion is very low in the neonatal rat and is insensitive to gastrin.[47,48] The pH of gastric contents is nearly neutral in the term rat, remains between pH 5 and 6 on day 10 after birth, falls to pH 4 on day 15, reaching adult levels only after weaning.[49] In humans, production rates for acid are less than 50% of adult values during the first 3 months of life and reach mature levels only after the age of 2 years.[50]

Neonates are relatively insensitive to gastrin and this state is evidenced by neonatal hypergastrinemia in humans,[51] dogs,[52] and rats.[53] Neonatal gastric pH remains at 5.5–7 for the first few days after birth. Recent studies have revealed that the CCK-B receptor, which binds gastrin, is present before birth,[54] suggesting that the receptor is functionally immature. Compared to the acid response to gastrin, early normal gastric acid response to cholinergic stimulation has been demonstrated at birth[55] while the gastric secretory response to histamine[56] is less than that observed after weaning, in a manner similar to that observed for gastrin. Produced by the parietal cell along with hydrochloric acid, intrinsic factor is detectable in the gastric mucosa by the 14th week of gestation in humans and rapidly increases after birth, achieving mature levels by day 10 after birth.[50] The intrinsic factor receptor is expressed coordinately with its ligand and becomes restricted to the ileum at around 25 weeks' gestation.[57] Gastric lipase is expressed as early as 11 weeks of gestation, reaching adult levels by the third postnatal month.[58]

Although mucous neck cells and chief cells are not fully differentiated until 14 days after birth, secretion of pepsinogen and peptic activity can be detected in parallel with acid secretion in the near-term rat stomach. Pepsinogen 1 immunoreactivity can be demonstrated in secretory granules of primitive chief cells of the fundic mucosa in developing mice by the 16th day of gestation.[59] After birth, pepsinogens I and III are present in almost equal amounts in rat fundic mucosa by postnatal day 13, but pepsinogen I levels rise to adult levels after weaning.[60] In humans, pepsinogen secretion is half of adult levels during the first 3 months after birth but rises to adult levels by 2 years of age. The mucous neck cell may be the primary source of pepsinogen in the neonate, but mature chief cells, which appear after birth, soon become the major source of pepsinogen. Gastric pepsinogen secretion also appears to be responsive to cholinergic stimulation at an earlier age than that observed for gastrin or histamine stimulation.

In the rat, concentrations of free cortisone rise immediately before the onset of weaning and reach a peak during the weaning process.[61] In the neonate, injection of adrenocorticotropic hormone (ACTH) or glucocorticoids causes a precocious rise in gastric pepsinogen levels,[62] functional gastrin receptors,[63] an early rise in antral gastrin concentrations, and an earlier induction of acid secretion response to histamine, carbachol, and gastrin stimulation.[64] Furthermore, cortisone administration induces a precocious rise in pepsinogen messenger RNA and a decrease in methylation of the pepsinogen genes, reflecting induction of differentiation of chief cells.[65] Conversely, adrenalectomy delays the rise in antral gastrin levels and development of gastrin receptors by 7 days, although gastrin levels do eventually normalize; this delay can prevented by cortisone administration to the adrenalized rats. Administration of corticosterone following adrenalectomy prevents these maturational delays. Maturational glucocorticoid sensitivity disappears after weaning. Thyroxine also induces a precocious rise in pepsinogen activity, an effect

which is additive to that of corticosterone. Estrogens reduce food intake, acid secretion, serum gastrin levels, and the number of gastrin receptors in the female or castrated male rat.[66]

## Small Intestine/Colon

The ontogeny of small intestine function has received more attention than that of any other part of the GI tract. The developmental, longitudinal, and crypt–villus unit axes found in this highly specialized region of the alimentary canal have afforded the broad use of chimeric, transgenic, and gene deletion studies to understand the complex specialized functions of this rapidly proliferating and differentiating segment. In the colon, recent insights concerning development of the enteric nervous system have provided a unique model for understanding the multigenic complexity of a distinct disease phenotype, Hirschsprung's disease.

### Structural Development

During the 5th week of gestation, the tubular midgut portion of the intestinal tract, which is joined to the yolk sac by the vitelline duct, rapidly elongates, ventrally herniating into the yolk sac. The vitelline duct, which normally becomes obliterated before birth, occasionally persists as a Meckel diverticulum. Between weeks 5 and 10 of gestation, the small intestine extends through the umbilicus as the result of further elongation. During this period of rapid elongation, the midgut rotates 90° around the superior mesenteric artery present in the dorsal mesentery. This rotation brings the proximal midgut to the right and the distal midgut, to the left (Fig. 4–2A). The midgut reenters the abdominal cavity in the 10th week of gestation. During the process in which the midgut reenters the abdomen, it undergoes a further 180° rotation, for a total rotation of 270° (Fig. 4–2B). The proximal jejunum enters first and occupies the left side of the abdomen, and the ileum settles into the right side.

When the midgut reenters the abdominal cavity, the cecal swelling enters last, locating temporarily in the right upper quadrant just caudal to the right lobe of the liver (Fig. 4–2C). Between the 3rd and 5th months of gestation, the cecum descends into the right iliac fossa and becomes fixed to the posterior wall of the abdomen (Fig. 4–2D). As the liver increases in size, the ascending colon and the hepatic flexure become distinct from the transverse colon. The descending colon loses its mesentery and becomes anchored to the abdominal wall, leaving the sigmoid in its more caudal position on a mesentery.

The rectum arises independently from the remaining large intestine as a subdivision of the cloaca, which is separated from the urogenital sinus by the urorectal septum. The urorectal septum reaches the cloacal membrane during the 7th week of gestation, forming the perineum (Fig. 4–3). During the 8th week, the rectum fuses with the colon, and the cloacal membrane forms the anal membrane, which is lost during the 9th week to establish communication with the amniotic space.

The small intestine and colon are initially lined by a simple cuboidal epithelium. Similar to processes described for esophageal and gastric development, epithelial proliferation during weeks 6 and 7 may lead to occlusion of the lumen, especially in proximal areas. At 8 weeks, the epithelium is stratified and heparin sulfate, type IV collagen, and laminin, largely produced by the epithelial cell population, are detectable at the base of the undifferentiated epithelium, forming a basement membrane before terminal differentiation of specialized intestinal epithelium oc-

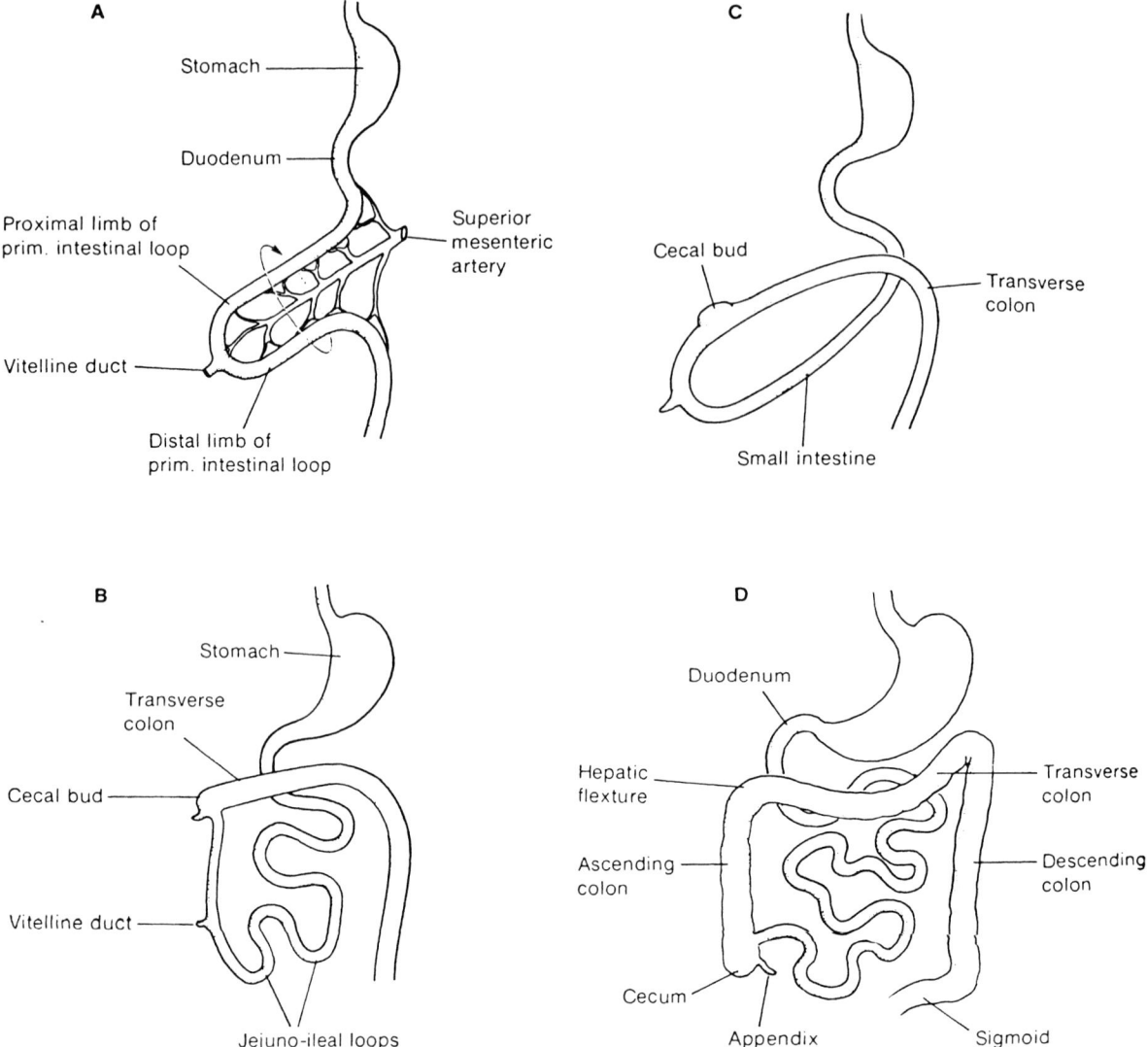

**Figure 4–2** Migration of the intestinal loops. *A:* The intestine after a 90° rotation around the axis of the superior mesenteric artery, the proximal loop on the right and the distal loop on the left. *B:* The intestinal loop after a further 180° rotation. The transverse colon passes in front of the duodenum. *C:* Position of the intestinal loops after reentry into the abdominal cavity. Notice the elongation of the small intestine, with formation of the small intestine loops. *D:* Final position of the intestines after descent of the cecum into the right iliac fossa. (Adapted from Sadler TW, ed. Langman's Medical Embryology. Williams & Wilkins, Baltimore, 1985.)

curs.[67] The lumen is reestablished during weeks 9 and 10, and a simple columnar epithelium is again found by the week 12.

Villi are first recognizable in the proximal intestine, developing in a proximal-to-distant gradient; the process is complete by the end of week 3 of gestation. The mechanism of villus formation in humans is unclear, but in the stratified epithelium of the near-term fetal rat small intestine and colon, secondary lumina are thought to play a crucial role in the formation of the villi.[68] These lumina surround the main lumen and are joined by continuous tight junctions. The secondary lumina enlarge and eventually fuse with the main lumen, leaving a villus outpouching. Crypt formation begins in the 10th to 12th weeks of gestation, and crypts appear in a proximal to distal sequence. Brunner glands appear in weeks 13 and 14.

The four cell types found within the intestinal epithelium are absorptive columnar, goblet, enteroendocrine, and Paneth cells. They appear to arise from a common progenitor cell in the mid-

dle to high part of the crypt. Studies using chimeric and transgenic mice and several cellular markers have demonstrated that the crypts in mature animals are clonal products of single progenitor cells.[69] However, related observations suggest that crypts are polyclonal during initial development and that entrenchment of a single stem cell must be established during development through competitive mechanisms, which remain undefined.

The intestinal tube is initially surrounded by a layer of mesoderm that ultimately forms connective tissue, muscle, and serosa. As in the gastric mucosa, enteroendocrine cells can be detected by the 8th week of gestation, with early differentiation of the various specific cell types. The circular muscle layer can be discerned by week 8; its appearance is followed closely by the emergence of the longitudinal muscle layer. Myenteric (Auerbach's plexus) ganglia can be detected by 9 weeks, followed by the submucosal (Meissner's plexus) by the 13th week. Peyer patches emerge approximately during week 20.

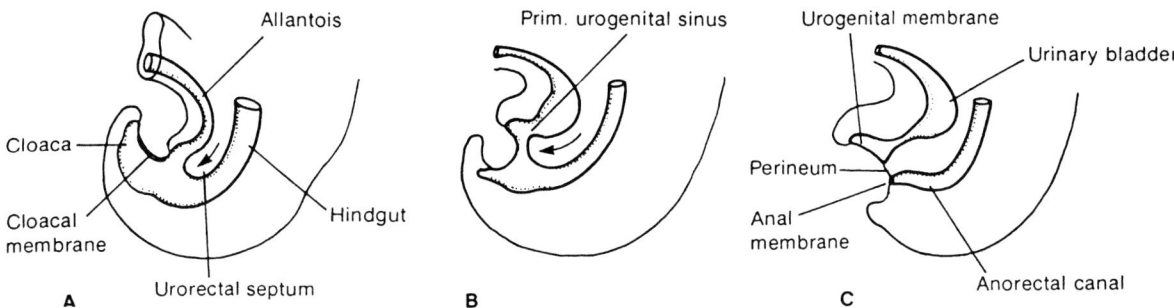

**Figure 4-3** Successive stages of development of the cloacal region. The urorectal septum (*A*) grows toward the cloacal membrane (*B*) to form the perineum (*C*) by week 8 of gestation. (Adapted from Sadler TW, ed. Langman's medical embryology. Williams & Wilkins, Baltimore, 1985.)

## Functional Development of the Small Intestine

The small intestine performs highly specialized functions responsible for most of the digestive and absorptive processes that characterize the most important mission of the luminal GI tract. As such, maturation of these complex functions can be arbitrarily analyzed by specific nutrient groups.

### Carbohydrate digestion and absorption

Lactase-phloridizin hydrolase (LPH) activity can be detected early in the human fetus, measurable by 12 weeks of gestation.[70] A significant increase in this activity occurs after the 24th week, and a late gestational surge is observed throughout the third trimester. In rodents, this burst of activity is observed later, occurring immediately prior to birth, which falls at the time of weaning in association with a change from a diet rich in maternal milk lactose to a laboratory diet rich in sucrose and starch as the primary carbohydrate source. Humans demonstrate high LPH activity at birth, but the decrease in activity does not correlate well temporally with weaning, and humans are the only known species in which LPH activity does not uniformly fall in the postweaning period.

Paradoxically, disaccharidase activities, such as those of sucrase-isomaltase, maltase, and trehalase, which should be physiologically unnecessary before weaning, are already present after 10 weeks of gestation at 60% to 70% of human adult levels (Table 4–1). Glucoamylase, a microvillus enzyme, has similarly been detected as early as the 10th week of gestation. Seventy percent of adult levels are achieved by 26 to 34 weeks of gestation. Salivary amylase can be detected after 20 weeks of gestation, and the level increases with fetal age. Proximal to distal gradients for LPH and other glucosidase activities can be demonstrated after 17 weeks of gestation, with maximal activities in the proximal jejunum and progressively less of these enzymatic activities along the more distal portions of the small intestine.[71]

In contrast to human development, adult levels of disaccharidase activities in rodents is only observed during postnatal weaning.[72] Sucrase-isomaltase and trehalase activities are undetectable before weaning but rise to adult levels by the 4th week of life. This pattern differs from the precocious pattern of human development, in which activity of the α-glucosidases rises during fetal life and reaches adult levels by term.[73]

In all species studied, glucose transporters are present before birth, but fructose transporters appear only in the postnatal period. Uptake of glucose against a concentration gradient is demonstrable in the jejunum and ileum at 11 to 19 weeks of gestation in humans.[74] Active Na-dependent transport can be demonstrated after 19 days of gestation in fetal rat ileum. In the rodent, expression of SGLT1, a Na-dependent glucose transporter, remains unchanged after birth. Mutations of the *SGLT1* gene result in severe glucose/galactose malabsorption and can result in overwhelming diarrhea of the newborn.[75] The longitudinal gradient in the level of glucose transport, well documented in the mature intestine, occurs by 17–20 weeks.[76] The facilitative transporter for glucose, GLUT-2, and that for fructose, GLUT-5, appear in rat fetal intestine prior to villus formation.[77]

After birth, carbohydrate transport levels are genetically programmed to match the species' natural diet.[78] The aldohexose transporters, which take up galactose and glucose with various affinities, demonstrate a shift to glucose transport corresponding to a decrease in dietary galactose in the suckling animal.[79] After weaning, fructose transport capacity rises sharply in rats and rabbits but not in cats; their adult diet continues to contain little fructose. Rats prevented from weaning still undergo the same steep rise in fructose uptake capacity, however, despite continued low fructose intake.[80] It is unclear if the increase in absorptive capacity for hexose transport after birth reflects an increase in the number of transporters or an increased efficiency of the transporters present.

**Table 4-1** Specific activities of disaccharidases in the mid-jejunum of developing human fetuses

| Fetal Age (weeks) | Lactase (μm/g/min) | Sucrase (μm/g/min) | Maltase (μm/g/min) | Isomaltase (μm/g/min) |
|---|---|---|---|---|
| 10–14 | 6.1 ± 2.2 | 52.1 ± 15.1 | 129.2 ± 37.6 | 10.1 ± 2.9 |
| 14–16 | 7.2 ± 3.7 | 62.1 ± 35.0 | 138.7 ± 57.3 | 10.3 ± 5.5 |
| 16–24 | 7.6 ± 2.5 | 80.7 ± 28.0 | 172.1 ± 62.3 | 13.5 ± 4.4 |

Adapted from Antonowicz I, Chang SK, Grand RJ. Development and distribution of lysosomal enzymes and disaccharidases in human fetal intestine. Gastroenterology 67:51, 1974.

## Protein digestion and absorption

Pancreatic trypsin and chymotrypsin activities depend on activation of enterokinase, and thus enterokinase plays an important role in the early stages of protein digestion. Enterokinase activity is only 6% of adult levels at 26 to 30 weeks of gestation and remains at 20% of adult levels even at the time of parturition.[81] Although trypsin can be detected at 20 weeks' gestation, its activity becomes measurable only at 28 weeks, reflecting its activation by enterokinase. Microvillar dipeptidase enzymes, which complete peptide digestion, are detected throughout the length of the small intestine in the 11-week-old fetus.[82] Adult levels of dipeptidase activity have been demonstrated in the 14- to 16-week-old fetus. Concentrations of other microvillar dipeptidases are generally found in a longitudinal gradient with highest levels in the proximal intestine. Leucine aminopeptidase is an exception to this general organization, with distal activity twice that of proximal activity in the 16th week of gestation. Brush border and cytosolic peptidases occur at adult levels in the neonate and aid in proteolysis in neonatal life. Rat microvillar peptidase activity rises dramatically at weaning.[83]

Active amino acid transport has been demonstrated in fetal tissue. The uptake of L-alanine against a concentration gradient has been demonstrated in everted gut sacs from 11- to 19-week-old fetuses.[84] At the time of birth, levels appear to be essentially equivalent to those of the adult. Six different amino acid transporters for neutral and charged amino acids have been demonstrated during the second trimester in the human fetus.[85] In the fetus and neonate, macromolecular transport plays an important role in the digestion of proteins and lipids. In experimental animals, the small intestine epithelium appears to be more permeable to amino acids and peptides in the immediate postnatal period than in the mature intestine. Macromolecular tracers infused into the amniotic fluid or the intestinal lumen late in gestation are absorbed into enterocytes of humans, monkeys, guinea pigs, and rats. This process does not take place by a paracellular pathway; it reflects a high rate of pinocytosis.[86] The rat small intestine is capable of pinocytosis by 19 or 20 days of gestation. This process is extremely active in the first 2 weeks postnatally and decreases dramatically with weaning. The sites of absorption of different proteins vary in the rat. Intact immunoglobulins are transported in the jejunum but not the ileum.[87] Nutritional proteins undergo pinocytosis in the ileum in a nonspecific manner. Pinocytosis of nutritional proteins and immunoglobulins decreases at weaning, although the adult rat can still absorb small amounts of intact protein.[88] In parallel with the extensive use of pinocytosis, enterocytes exhibit high levels of lysosomal proteases, such as cathepsins and other peptidases, during the first 2 weeks postnatally, but these levels fall thereafter. These intracellular enzymes provide a mechanism for protein digestion before the maturation of the mechanisms necessary for production and secretion of pancreatic proteolytic enzymes. Intact proteins are also absorbed in premature and term human infants during the first few months of life.[89] Macromolecules may continue to cross the healthy adult small intestine, but the amounts are extremely low compared with those observed in the newborn. Imperfect barrier function during the first months of life may play an important role in conferring a tolerance of or sensitivity to dietary proteins.

## Lipid digestion and absorption

Lipase has long been detected in pancreatic extracts of human fetuses in the 16th week of gestation.[90] Although levels rise significantly during the third trimester, in week 32 of gestation, lipase activity remains only 50% of term levels, which are themselves only 10% of the levels found in adults. The human neonate also has lingual lipase activity, which rises to adult levels by 2 years of age. The relatively low levels of lipase may explain the presence of unhydrolyzed triglycerides in the feces of neonates. In humans and rats, lingual lipase and maternal milk lipase aid in neonatal fat digestion.[91] Gastric lipase appears as early as 10–13 weeks.[92] Adult distribution of gastric lipase is established by 16 weeks' gestation and appears to be the major determinant of lipolytic activity in gastric aspirates of premature infants. Lingual lipase is produced in the serous glands of the tongue and appears to aid in the digestion of milk triglycerides in neonatal rats, mainly thorough hydrolysis in the stomach.[91] In the rat, lingual lipase exists in small amounts at birth and increases markedly at weaning. Maternal milk lipase also plays a role in fat digestion. The relative importance of these lipases in the economy of dietary lipid remains controversial.

Synthesis of bile acids from cholesterol and conjugation with taurine and glycine can be demonstrated in organ culture in vitro using human liver tissue obtained from fetuses after 15 weeks of gestation.[93] Biliary secretion can be demonstrated as early as the 22nd week of gestation. Bile acid reabsorption occurs in the neonate by passive diffusion throughout the small intestine, but active Na-dependent ileal transport of bile acids does not occur until weaning in rats, rabbits, and humans.[94] Both secretion and reabsorption of bile acids are lower in suckling rats than in adults. Bile acid concentrations are initially too low to facilitate the formation of micelles. In the neonatal period, before the maturation of bile acid secretion and reabsorption and the mature production of pancreatic lipase, the suckling rat's small intestine exhibits increased permeability to lipid, which may be absorbed intact as triglyceride.[95]

The lipoproteins required for chylomicron production are abundant in the small intestine of the suckling rat, and chylomicrons can be formed and presumably transported into lymphatic channels.[96] After weaning, the dietary content of fat decreases, pancreatic lipase activity matures, and fewer large lipid particles are seen in the enterocyte. Ileal bile acid absorption also begins at this time, reaching adult capacity after 1 month in the rat.[97] In human neonates, bile acid synthesis occurs at relatively high levels. However, ileal resorptive mechanisms are not yet mature, and a reduction in the bile acid pool results. In premature infants, this reduction is even more severe (Table 4–2), and 10% to 20% of fat intake in formula-fed premature infants may not be absorbed.[98] During the first 4 to 6 weeks of human life, intraluminal bile acid levels increase as absorptive mechanisms mature, leading to improved lipid absorption.

## Small intestine immune system

The GI tract, particularly the small intestine, contains the largest and most complex immune system of any organ. The gut-

**Table 4–2** Bile salt synthesis in premature and newborn infants

| Age | Cholic Acid Pool (mg/m²) | Cholic Acid Synthesis (mg/m²/d) |
| --- | --- | --- |
| Premature infant | $85 \pm 20$ | $34 \pm 6$ |
| Full-term infant | $290 \pm 36$ | $110 \pm 20$ |
| Adult | $600 \pm 20$ | $190 \pm 25$ |

From Hamosh M. A review. Fat digestion in the newborn: role of lingual lipase and preduodenal digestion. Pediatr Res 13:615, 1979.

associated lymphoid tissue (GALT) encompasses organized aggregates dominated by lymphocytes (Peyer patches) and a diffuse heterogeneous population of lymphocytes, monocytes, or macrophages, and other cells, such as eosinophils and mast cells, of the lamina propria. Lymphocytes designated as intraepithelial lymphocytes are scattered throughout the surface epithelium.

Structures resembling Peyer patches can be demonstrated as early as 11 weeks of human gestation; by 14 weeks, CD4$^+$ and CD8$^+$ lymphocytes can be seen.[99] By the end of the second trimester, Peyer patches histologically resemble the adult structure, indicating that antigen exposure or bacterial colonization are not necessary for their development; however, germinal centers do not form until after birth.[100] Transgenic mice carrying a null mutation for tumor necrosis factor $\alpha$ (TNF-$\alpha$) do not develop Peyer patches or lymph nodes, and splenic organization is markedly abnormal; if the 55 kDa receptor for TNF-$\alpha$ is disrupted, lymph nodes and splenic tissue develop normally, but Peyer patches are still absent, suggesting that the 55 kDa receptor provides specificity for Peyer patch development.[101]

Lamina propria lymphocytes are first detected after 11 weeks of gestation. During fetal life they consist of increasing numbers of scattered T and B cells.[102] IgA- and IgM-producing plasma cells are not found in the lamina propria until after birth and antigenic exposure.[103] Intraepithelial lymphocytes appear between 11 and 12 weeks of gestation.[104] Fetal lamina propria lymphocytes are mostly CD4$^+$, as in the adult lamina propria, while fetal intraepithelial lymphocytes are often CD4$^-$ and CD8$^-$; CD8$^+$ cells become more predominant after birth.[105] Macrophages are present after 12 weeks, but they become much more abundant after birth.[106]

Unlike mature colonic and ileal villus epithelium, fetal intestinal epithelial cells do not express major histocompatibility complex (MHC) class II antigen, suggesting that antigen exposure may be important for induction of MHC class II. In rats, suckling and germ-free animals have fewer intestinal lymphocytes than adults, and weaning, associated with intestinal maturation and increasing bacterial colonization, is also characterized by marked development of the mucosal immune system.[107] Cyclosporine A, an inhibitor of T-lymphocyte activation, retards the normal development of small intestine, but some maturation still occurs at the end of weaning.[108] The natural killer activity of intraepithelial and lamina propria lymphocytes is absent before birth but rises dramatically after weaning.[109]

### Vitamins and minerals

Copper, iron, magnesium, and zinc are absorbed by the suckling rat small intestine in increased amounts, but rates of absorption decline to normal during the weaning period.[110] Lead, cadmium, radium, plutonium, barium, and other toxic heavy metals are also absorbed more easily in the suckling than adult rat. Active transport of calcium occurs throughout the rat small intestine and colon before weaning but appears to depend on mechanisms distinct from those in the mature mucosa. This absorption is uniform throughout the intestine and does not require vitamin D, in contrast to the vitamin D–dependent uptake mechanisms concentrated in the duodenum that appear in the 4th postnatal week.[111]

Human neonates absorb iron, copper, calcium, and zinc well.[112] They also absorb lead more efficiently than adults. Although the mechanisms remain uncertain, these processes can facilitate lead intoxication. Inadequate bone mineralization is a common problem in premature human infants. This is not thought to result from a lack of absorptive capacity but from an insuffi-

cient supply of calcium in maternal or formula milk. Simple calcium supplementation can correct the calcium imbalance.

Vitamin absorption in the newborn has not been extensively studied. Impaired absorption of fat-soluble vitamins is present in neonates and likely reflects the same pattern of impaired absorption of all lipids. Vitamin B$_{12}$ absorption has been demonstrated in the rat neonate.[113] Intrinsic factor receptor activity is detectable throughout the small intestines and colons of human fetuses after 10 to 19 weeks, but it is present only in the distal ileum at the end of fetal development.[114] Folate absorption is impaired in the human neonate and infant, compared within the adult. Biotin transport was found to be higher in the ileum than in the jejunum of suckling rats, equal in both parts of the small intestine in weanlings, and higher in the jejunum than in the ileum of adult rats.[115]

## Regulation of Small Intestinal Maturation

### Role of diet

During weaning, a process that is temporally determined in most species but widely variable in humans, the infant GI tract is exposed to a dramatic change in dietary composition. Maternal milk is high in fat and low in carbohydrate, and a "conventional" diet includes relatively high amounts of carbohydrate and a low fat content. The major carbohydrate source changes from lactose to a more varied mixture, usually sucrose and starch.

Many maturational changes of the small intestine occur at the same time as weaning, suggesting dietary composition as an important factor in digestive tract development. Although this association may be important in the rodent, dietary changes in humans are not essential to the expression of many functional activities that emerge before weaning. LPH exhibits an accelerated surge before parturition, which suggests that the birth process (and possibly hormonal factors related to it), rather than a dietary challenge, regulates expression of this activity. Even in rodents, the importance of dietary components in triggering changes in various activities during weaning may be limited, and it has been found that similar changes occur at almost the same time in rats prevented from weaning.[116] Early weaning can lead to precocious maturation, but premature weaning also elevates glucocorticoid levels, which accelerates intestinal development (see below). Intestinal explants implanted into the kidney, subcutaneous space, or culture in vitro demonstrate a normal pattern of functional maturation, minimizing the importance of diet as crucial for intestinal development.[117] Rat ileum bypassed by surgical implantation at 12 to 14 days of age expresses sucrase-isomaltase and maltase activity at the expected time of weaning.[118] A role for hormones in mediating the temporal pattern of development is implied by the absence of precocious expression of sucrase-isomaltase or maltase in intestinal explants from 6-day-old rats cultured in the absence of hormones.

Although dietary factors are not essential for the temporal sequence of intestinal development, they may modulate the process. High-carbohydrate diets stimulate intestinal glucose transport by increasing the number of glucose transporters along the crypt–villus axis.[119] This induction appears to be specific in that humans or rats fed a diet high in maltose or sucrose exhibit increased maltase or sucrase-isomaltase activity, but not LPH activity.[120] Similarly, feeding lactose appears to increase the level of brush border membrane LPH in rats, and prolonged suckling delays the usual decrease in lactase expression that occurs at weaning.[121] However, high levels of lactase mRNA persist after premature weaning. Furthermore, malnourished suckling rats display delayed patterns of mucosal enzyme development, which can be reversed by refeeding.[122] Bypassed segments maintain high levels of lactase activity, and decreased lactase activity is found in segments of the intestine left in continuity.[118]

Although nutrients in the diet appear to have a limited impact on intestinal maturation, other substances in maternal milk may affect these processes. Pig, rabbit, and dog neonates in their first 24 hours after birth experience greater increases in small intestine weight, size, and DNA or protein content when fed colostrum than when fed an artificial diet.[123] Rat neonates fed colostrum also exhibit higher intestinal DNA content and synthesis, although total intestinal weight was not significantly different from that of neonatal rats fed mature milk.[124] The time frame in which factors in colostrum or breast milk exert an effect on GI tract development varies among animal species.[125] Potential growth factors contained in breast milk include epidermal growth factor (EGF), insulin-like growth factor 1 (IGF-1), and insulin. High concentrations of EGF are found in human, mouse, and rat milk.[126] EGF is found throughout the lumen of the GI tract at higher levels in the intestinal lumen of suckling rats than in that of adult rats. These levels directly correlate with the milk intake, implicating milk as an important source of EGF in the suckling period.[127] IGF-1 is also found in human milk and colostrum, protein bound but released after treatment with acid.[128] Insulin, too, is found in colostrum and milk, and if administered to a neonate mouse, premature development of sucrase-isomaltase activity takes place.[129] Glucocorticoids and thyroxine, which may play important roles in gastrointestinal maturation, are present in human milk, although not in physiologically significant quantities.[130] Formula containing various amounts of corticosterone has been shown to result in intestinal expression of sucrase-isomaltase and maltase activity in adrenalectomized rats only when the formula contains a concentration of corticosterone considerably higher than that found in maternal milk. This concentration produces a serum level similar to that of 18- to 20-day-old control rats, when sucrase-isomaltase and maltase activities are normally expressed.

### Hormones and peptide growth factors

Hormonal and other peptide growth factors may play a more direct role on intestinal maturation than diet. Among these factors, glucocorticoids have been the most thoroughly investigated. Tissue concentrations of free corticosterone rise 48 hours prior to the appearance of the enzymatic changes associated with weaning (Fig. 4–4), suggesting that changes in functional maturation associated with weaning may be mediated, at east in part, by changes in corticosteroid concentration.

Administration of glucocorticoids to rats and mice during the suckling period prematurely decreases pinocytosis, LPH levels, and lysosomal hydrolases and prematurely increases sucrase-isomaltase, maltase, trehalase, peptidase, pancreatic and salivary amylase, pepsinogen, and gastrin receptor levels.[43] Glucocorticoids increase sucrase-isomaltase and LPH messenger RNA levels in rats, although enzyme activities appear also to be regulated by post-transcriptional events.[131] Glucocorticoids also mediate similar enzymatic changes in intestinal neonatal mucosal explants in vitro in the absence of other compounding factors. Age appears to be critical in the influence of glucocorticoids, as they accelerate the rate of cellular proliferation of the suckling rat but not of the adult rat.[132] Glucocorticoid receptor concentration in the intestinal mucosa also peaks at the time of weaning in the rat.[133] Hypophysectomy is associated with decreased intestinal

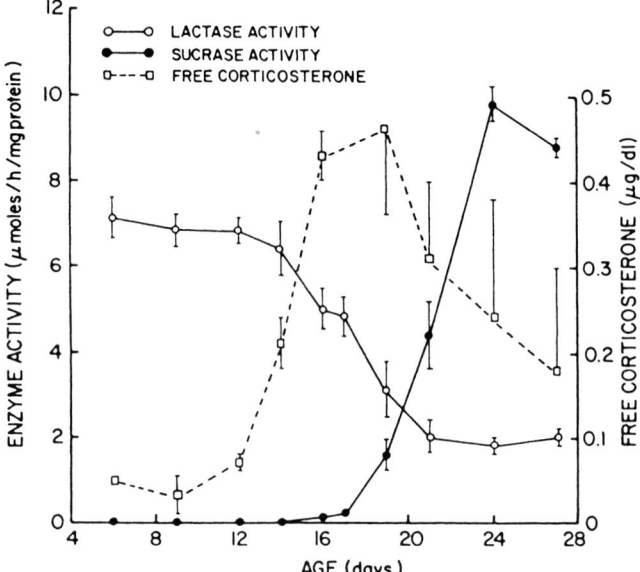

**Figure 4–4** Development of activity of lactase and sucrase in jejunal mucosa compared with free corticosterone in plasma. Values are given as means ± SE for five rats. Absence of error bars indicates SE was smaller than the symbol. (From Henning SJ. Plasma concentrations of total and free corticosterone during development in the rat. Am J Physiol 235:E451, 1978.)

sucrase-isomaltase activity in suckling rats; this can be normalized by administration of cortisone. Glucocorticoid levels rise at 12 to 14 days of age in the rat, but intestinal enzyme levels do not respond to glucocorticoid administration after 16 to 17 days. Similarly, enzyme levels are not stimulated by glucocorticoids in rats adrenalectomized after 17 to 18 days of age.[134] It is noteworthy that, although adrenalectomy slows the rate of enzymatic changes at weaning in the rat, the changes begin at approximately the same time and eventually reach the same levels as those of sham-operated controls.[135] These changes may thus be genetically programmed and glucocorticoids may not be essential. This is supported also by preservation of the normal pattern of intestinal differentiation of fetal intestine transplanted into adult mice.[136,137] Further, gene deletion of corticoid-releasing hormone (CRH) in mice does not alter GI tract development.[138] In humans, prenatal administration of glucocorticoids decreases the incidence of necrotizing enterocolitis in the neonate, presumably by promoting intestinal maturation, including the intestinal mucosal barrier.[139] Glucocorticoids also promote human fetal intestinal maturation in organ culture.[140] Mothers who receive glucocorticoids in late pregnancy have been found to deliver neonates with higher bile salt pool size than neonates of the same age born to mothers who were not treated.[141]

Thyroxine influences intestinal maturation in a similar manner, but directly stimulates glucocorticoid expression, which suggests that the role of thyroxine may simply be through induction of glucocorticoids.[142] Hypothyroidism prevents or delays intestinal maturation and abolishes the developmental rise of corticosterone. The maturational delay in the expected rise in sucrase-isomaltase and related activity in hypothyroid fetuses can be reversed by administration of glucocorticoids without the addition of thyroxine.[133] However, thyroxine may still be important in certain aspects of gastrointestinal maturation. Thyroxine and corticosteroids are synergistic in enhancing expression of small intestine enzymes before weaning in the rat.[143] Administration of cortisone results in only partial restoration of reduced jejunal lactase activity after hypophysectomy; thyroxine fully restores this decline in the absence of any effect on corticosterone levels. Thyroxine ($T_4$) administration alone decreases LPH mRNA levels, increases intestinal alkaline phosphatase, but has no effect on sucrase-isomaltase mRNA levels in rat small intestine.[144]

Colostrum and maternal milk in many animal species, including humans, contains EGF. At weaning, the concentration of EGF in mouse maternal milk decreases, and endogenous sources of EGF increase markedly.[145] EGF may have important trophic effects throughout the GI tract, although the imprecise temporal relation of declining maternal milk EGF concentrations to the augmented production from endogenous sources indicates that EGF is unlikely to play an essential role in the regulation of developmental changes. EGF administered orally increases cell growth in the intestine and pancreas of neonatal rats, even though much of the administered and endogenous growth factor was undoubtedly degraded by proteolytic enzymes.[146] EGF in amniotic fluid is taken up in the small intestine by endocytosis in the 20-day-old rat fetus and has been suggested to play a role in fetal intestinal development.[147] TGF-α, which can also bind to the EGF receptor, is expressed by multiple cells throughout the GI tract and may contribute to fetal gastrointestinal development.[148] Knockout of the EGF receptor gene in mice results in minimal defects in GI tract development and normal structural and functional development of the small intestine, suggesting less of a role of these gut peptides in intestinal maturation.[149]

Gastrin may play a role in GI tract development. It is found in detectable concentrations in fetal plasma and at high levels in neonatal plasma, and is trophic for segments of adult intestine. Antrectomy performed on mid-gestation fetal sheep induces a 70% decrease in plasma gastrin levels, which causes a reduction in crypt and villus density, a decrease in the crypt-to-villus ratio in the distal small intestine, and shorter gastric glands and deeper gastric pits. Furthermore, mice bearing deletions of the gastrin[150] or cholecystokinin-B/gastrin receptor[151,152] genes demonstrate decreased numbers of parietal and enterochromaffin-like cells, resulting in atrophy of the corpus mucosa, particularly in the pit and basal regions.

Bombesin, also known as gastrin-releasing peptide (GRP), stimulates gastric, colonic, and pancreatic cell growth in suckling rats.[153] Parenteral administration of bombesin during the suckling period of rabbits results in hypertrophy of the stomach, small intestine, and colon.[154] Bombesin/GRP has been found in the breast milk of some mammals, which provides a source of this peptide for the neonate in addition to any endogenous production.[155] Administration of bombesin/GRP to fetal sheep induces small intestinal growth.[156]

Exogenous insulin administered to suckling mice causes premature maturation of the small intestine.[157] These effects include precocious cessation of the intestinal macromolecular transport and induction of sucrase-isomaltase and other brush border enzymes in adrenalectomized suckling rats.[158] Endogenous insulin levels rise during the weaning period in the rat, although no clear role has been established for insulin in the maturation of the GI tract. In humans, insulin induces proliferation of small intestinal epithelium of 15- to 17-week-gestation cultured intestinal explants, correlating with the appearance of intestinal insulin receptors, although intestinal enzyme expression is not altered.[159]

Insulin-like growth factor I and II and their receptors are expressed during fetal small intestine development of mammalian species, as are their binding proteins, decreasing in expression after the fetal and neonatal periods.[160] IGF-I induces both cellular proliferation and intestinal disaccharide expression, while IGF-II stimulates intestinal epithelial cell proliferation; its effects on functional maturation remain unknown.

## Transcriptional regulation

Investigations have elucidated transcriptional hierarchies that are responsible for tissue- and cell-specific expression along the length of the entire GI tract. Normal gut tube formation is dependent on reciprocal interactions between the endoderm and the mesoderm.[161,162] Hepatic nuclear factor 3β (HNF-3β), one of the hepatic nuclear factors first described in liver development, plays an important role in early gut endoderm formation,[163] and is capable of inducing transcription of Sonic hedgehog, a segment polarity gene, expressed in the earliest stages of gut formation in the primitive endoderm.[164] Sonic hedgehog, in turn, induces expression of members of the Abd-B class of *Hox* genes during early hindgut formation, perhaps through the induction of mesodermal Bmp-4, a member of the TGF-β superfamily.[165] Targeted deletions of both Sonic hedgehog and Indian hedgehog in mice show multiple phenotypic alterations including gut malrotation, annular pancreas.[166] In addition, gene deletion of Indian hedgehog results in disordered intestinal epithelial cell proliferation and differentiation, while knockout of Sonic hedgehog leads to imperforate anus and a Hirschsprung-like denervation (see Colon section below). *Hox* gene expression in the mesoderm then plays a critical role in the formation of gastrointestinal morphologic boundaries.[167] One member of this family, *Hoxa5*, is expressed in the midgut mesenchyme at the time of remodeling and differentiation. While targeted disruption in mice demonstrates that *Hoxa5* is not essential for small intestine development, functional maturation and region-specific differentiation are significantly altered.[168] Gene deletions of other *Hox* family members should provide more insights into the role of these factors in gastrointestinal regionalization and morphogenesis.

Homeobox genes lying outside of the *Hox* gene clusters also appear to be important in the regulation of differentiation of the digestive tract. Homologs of the *Drosophila* caudal gene play roles in intestinal development. These genes, designated *Cdx1* and *Cdx2* in the mouse, are expressed early in development when endoderm differentiates into columnar epithelium within nascent villi.[169,170] Cdx1 is expressed in the distal gut and Cdx2 is maximally expressed more proximally, with overlap of both in the midgut; Cdx1 is expressed primarily in the crypts, while Cdx2 is predominant in the villi.[171] Developmentally, Cdx2 expression precedes Cdx1 expression in developing mouse intestine as early as day 9.5 of gestation; adult levels are achieved postnatally and do not change with weaning. Null mutation of *Cdx1* in mice results in anterior homeotic transformation of the vertebrae, but no gross intestinal phenotype.[172] Knockout of *Cdx2* leads to early embryonic death; heterozygotes develop polypoid-like lesions of the colon containing areas of esophageal, gastric and small intestinal mucosa, suggesting the importance of *Cdx2* in regional differentiation of the GI tract.[173]

Further complexity of transcriptional regulation of intestinal development has already been recognized through analysis of factors controlling the expression of genes such as *Cdx1* and *Cdx2*. For example, the Wnt/β-catenin signaling pathway induces expression of Cdx1 in rodent embryonic stem cells and endoderm.[174] Tcf-4, a member of the Tcf/Lef-1 (T cell factor/lymphocyte enhancer factor 1) family of transcription factors, mediates the β-catenin transactivation of the *Cdx1* gene through several Tcf-binding motifs located in the Cdx1 promoter. Mice homozygous

## Liver

As noted above, the pancreas and liver share an embryologic origin and, as the major accessory glands to the digestive tract, they share similar properties of slow cell turnover and regenerative capacity. Furthermore, the liver exhibits both endocrine properties, synthesizing many products involved in metabolism, elimination, and influence of distant organs.

### Structural Development

The primordium of the liver is the first of the digestive organs to be grossly and microscopically recognizable. During the 3rd week of gestation, the liver emerges as a thickening of the endodermal epithelium lining the ventral wall near its junction with the yolk sac.[332] This thickening forms a ventral outpouching, the hepatic diverticulum, which becomes hollow, lined by columnar epithelium, and continuous with the portion of the luminal foregut destined to become the duodenum. Studies utilizing embryonic tissue explants have demonstrated that this early differentiation is induced by precardiac mesenchyme.[333] Murine hepatic endoderm cultivated in the absence of precardiac mesenchyme does not further differentiate.[334] Interestingly, FGF1 or FGF2 can replace the inductive properties of cardiac mesoderm and thus play key roles in the early induction of the liver.[335]

The hepatic diverticulum divides into a large cranial diverticulum that becomes the mature liver, and a smaller caudal bud, which will give rise to the gallbladder, common bile duct, and cystic duct. At 6 weeks of human gestation, the liver is bilobed, as the rapidly proliferating lateral walls result in the formation of the right and left lobes of the liver.[336] These irregularly shaped hepatoblasts migrate form the intestinal endoderm to invade the mesenchyme of the septum transversum, which has formed in continuous association with the yolk sac mesoderm, and surround preexisting sinusoids, producing the liver bud.[337] Hepatoblast growth continues in cords between the two vitelline veins and into the capillary network of the septum transversum; hepatoblasts give rise to both the hepatocyte and biliary epithelial cell lineages. These hepatic cords then subdivide the capillaries, leading to the formation of the adult pattern of parenchyma and sinusoids. As the liver grows further and differentiates, the septum transversum gives rise to the hepatic reticuloendothelial system and hematopoietic tissue. During the 6th week of gestation, hematopoiesis commences, contributing to the liver's 10% of total fetal weight at 9 weeks of gestation.

In rodents, endodermal cells are similarly induced to differentiate by precardiac mesenchyme on the 8th day of gestation. The hepatic diverticulum is first recognizable microscopically as a thickening of the ventral floor of the foregut on day 9.5 of mouse gestation, invading the septum transversum over the subsequent day.[337] On day 11, the mesenchyme of the septum transversum induces the cells of the hepatic endoderm to differentiate into hepatoblasts. At approximately the same time, hematopoietic cells migrate to the liver from the yolk sac. By day 12.5 of mouse gestation, the liver is a large organ of varied cell types, of which up to 60% are hematopoietic cells.[338] From days 14 to 16 of rat gestation, hepatoblasts become cuboidal and exhibit the major structural features of the mature hepatocyte, coincident with the appearance of primitive bile canaliculi and both tight and gap junctions that develop between the surfaces of adjacent hepatocytes.[339,340] Mesenchyme is also required for this second phase of cellular differentiation into hepatocytes; candidate molecules most likely derive form the extracellular matrix,

and appear to include $\beta_1$-integrin.[341] Following gestational days 16 to 17, the first mature bile canaliculi appear, although bile secretion does not occur until after birth.[342]

### Functional Development

Liver-specific gene products are expressed at varying points of fetal development and are under transcriptional control of recently defined sets of genes (see below). Albumin, a frequent clinical marker of adult liver biosynthetic capacity, is actually the first specific gene product detected: by in situ hybridization, albumin messenger RNA can be visualized as early as 9.5 days of mouse gestation, prior to cellular assembly into a recognizable liver bud.[343] Alpha fetoprotein expression is detectable by prenatal day 12 in the mouse.[344] By day 16 of gestation, $\alpha$-fetoprotein is near its maximal level while albumin is just beginning to increase.[345] On the same day, transthyretin and transferrin gene expression can first be measured.[346] At birth, $\alpha$-fetoprotein transcription rapidly decreases, while albumin transcription reaches its maximal rate near the time of weaning. Other liver-specific products synthesized maximally at the time of weaning include cytochrome P450, tyrosine aminotransferase, and contrapsin.

A finite set of growth factors has been thought to play major roles in the regulation of fetal development of the liver. By RT-PCR, hepatocyte growth factor (HGF) and its receptor, c-met, are detectable as early as day 14 of rat embryogenesis.[347] Rat fetal hepatocyte cultures derived from fetal liver as early as day 15 of gestation proliferate in response to HGF. HGF and c-met mRNAs are also detectable early in mouse and human fetal liver.[348,349] Targeted disruption of HGF or c-met in mice results in hepatic hypoplasia.[350,351] Although EGF is capable of stimulating DNA synthesis in cultured human fetal hepatocytes,[352] only its homolog, TGF-$\alpha$, is present during fetal development.[353] EGF mRNA expression begins at 2 weeks after birth.[354]

#### Transcriptional regulation

Serving as a paradigm for transcriptional control of mammalian development, a transcriptional hierarchy important in cell differentiation and development was first described in the liver.[355] Most of the genes that determine the hepatocyte phenotype are themselves regulated at the level of transcription,[356] suggesting a cascade of transcriptional regulation important in mammalian development similar to the transcriptional control seen in *Drosophila* development. Expression of $\alpha$-fetoprotein, albumin, carbomoylphosphate synthase, etc., i.e., markers of the hepatocyte phenotype, require distinct sets of transcription factors, although expression of these markers also occurs in extrahepatic tissues, such as embryonic kidney, intestine, and heart. These transcription factors themselves, which are also expressed in extrahepatic tissues, appear to work in various combinations to provide the specific sets of signals required for the genetic program of hepatic differentiation. During early fetal development, the liver-enriched transcription factors are all initially expressed at very high levels in the developing heart and subsequently in the hepatic primordium, which implicates a role for these factors in the induction of precardiac mesenchyme into differentiating hepatocytes.

The first stage of hepatogenesis occurs in the ventral endoderm juxtaposing the developing heart. The HNF-3 family of transcriptions factors, which are closely homologous to *Drosophila forkhead,* have crucial roles in the commitment of these endodermal cells to a hepatic lineage.[357] The HNF-3 family of transcription factors is required for hepatocyte-specific gene expression of many liver-specific genes including transthyretin, $\alpha_1$-antitrypsin, and tyrosine aminotransferase.[358] HNF-3$\beta$ is the first of this family of transcription factors to be expressed in development, originating in the mouse in the anterior portion of the primitive streak at the onset of gastrulation. HNF-3$\alpha$ is expressed later, beginning in the primitive midline endoderm in the region of the invaginating foregut. HNF-3 exerts its effects by marking liver-specific genes such as albumin to be expressed if the potential endoderm encounters appropriate environmental signals, similar as those encountered in the precardiac mesenchyme.[359] These specific genes are marked by HNF-3's modulation of chromatin structure around enhancers of genes expressed in the developing liver.[360] HNF-3 cooperates with another transcription factor, GATA-4, to maximize liver-specific gene enhancers.[361] Targeted disruption of either HNF-3$\beta$ or GATA-4 leads to severely altered foregut morphogenesis as early as day 8.5 of gestation.[362,363]

Another gene critical for the commitment of early foregut endoderm to a hepatic fate is *Hex* (hematopoietically expressed homeobox), expression of which is essential for the earliest stages of liver development.[364] Deletion of *Hex* in mice results in complete absence of the liver, although other GI organs appear to developed normally by 13.5 days of gestation.[365]

Following commitment to a hepatic fate, other factors are important for the further differentiation of these cells into hepatocytes. At very early stages of mammalian development, many of these factors are expressed ubiquitously at low levels throughout the embryo. The HNF-1 family is first expressed in the mouse liver on day 10.5 of gestation and on day 12 in the rat.[366] The HNF-1 binding site is the most liver-specific of the liver-enriched transcription factors, and appears to be critical for liver-specific gene expression. However, expression of HNF-1 is coincident with, i.e., does not precede, the expression of such important liver proteins as $\alpha$-fetoprotein and albumin, which suggests that other factors must be more significant in the initiation of the expression of certain liver-specific genes. C/EBP, thought initially to be a CCAAT enhancer binding protein,[367] is a leucine zipper transcription factor that, like HNF-1, binds to a number of liver-specific genes. Its onset of expression in the rodent is a few days earlier than HNF-1, albumin or $\alpha$-fetoprotein, suggesting a possible role in hepatocyte differentiation.

HNF-6 behaves similarly to the HNF-1 proteins and C/EBP.[368] Inactivation of any of these genes affects liver development only in specific and relatively insignificant ways,[369,370] suggesting that hepatocyte differentiation is governed by the action of multiple factors acting coordinately.

In contrast, gene inactivation of HNF-4$\alpha$, a member of the zinc finger thyroid–steroid hormone receptor superfamily which is normally expressed as early as day 8.5 of mouse gestation,[371] leads to severe disruption of liver differentiation.[372] While disruption of HNF-4$\alpha$ causes early embryonic death due to defects in visceral endoderm function, complementation with HNF-4$\alpha$ containing visceral endoderm produced mice with livers that were morphologically normal, but demonstrated marked downregulation of at least 14 genes important in hepatocyte function. Thus, although HNF-4$\alpha$ is dispensable for early stages of hepatic development, it is required for complete differentiation from hepatoblast to hepatocyte or the development of polarized hepatic epithelium.

Transcriptional control is also important in later-stage proliferation and morphogenesis, often through ultimate activation of the AP-1 transcription factor. Targeted inactivation of *c-jun*,[373] *Hlx*,[374] and *Xbp-1*[375] produces mice with liver hypoplasia. In the c-*jun* knockout, lethal metabolic damage occurs throughout the embryo by day 11 to 15 of gestation. Mutations in the NF-$\kappa$B p65 subunit,[376] I$\kappa$B kinase,[377] or NF-$\kappa$B essential modulator,[378] components of the NF-$\kappa$B signaling pathway, result in normal liver development until day 12.5 of mouse development and subsequent apoptotic deaths of developing hepatocytes and fetal death. The role of NF-$\kappa$B in liver development is to protect against TNF-$\alpha$–mediated apoptosis.[379]

During hepatic development, individual transcription factors often cross-regulate expression of one another and autoregulate expression of their own genes. Many more transcriptional regulators will become apparent in the future. However, recent observations have already shown the complexity of these factors and their roles in liver development. The molecular mechanisms controlling mesenchymal regulation of hepatic morphogenesis need to be further defined.

In conclusion, the GI tract represents a dynamic model for the study of cell and tissue development, growth, and differentiation. Although insights into newly described growth factors and mechanisms of cell-to-cell communications and interactions have allowed much greater understanding of the regulation of intestinal growth and development, the precise signals controlling these processes and the specific pathways of events such as cell migration, adhesion, renewal, extrusion, and transformation require further definition. Understanding of these processes in great detail will be critical for further advancements in our knowledge of the processes involved in neoplasia, and perhaps result in novel and important therapeutic targets.

## References

1. DeNardi FG, Riddell RH. The normal esophagus. Am J Surg Pathol 15:296–309, 1991.
2. Grand RJ, Watkins JB, Torti FM. Development of the human gastrointestinal tract: a review. Gastroenterology 50:790–812, 1976.
3. Smith RB, Taylor IM. Observations of the intrinsic innervation of the human foetal oesophagus between the 10-mm and 140-mm crown–rump length stages. Acta Anat 81:127–145, 1972.
4. Johns BAE. Developmental changes in the oesophageal epithelium in man. J Anat 86:431–449, 1952.
5. Menard D, Arsenault P. Maturation of human fetal esophagus maintained in organ culture. Anat Rec 217:348–354, 1987.
6. Le Douarin NM. The ontogeny of the neural crest in avian embryo chimeras. Nature 286:663–669, 1980.
7. Hitchcock RJI, Pemble MJ, Bishop AE, Spitz L, Polak JM. Quantitative study of the development and maturation of human oesophageal innervation. J Anat 180:175–192, 1992.
8. Hitchcock RJI, Pemble MJ, Bishop AE, Spitz LE, Polak JM. The ontogeny and distribution of neuropeptides in the human fetal and infant esophagus. Gastroenterology 102:840–848, 1992.
9. Smith RB, Taylor IM. Observations on the intrinsic innervation of the human foetal oesophagus between the 10-mm and 140-mm crown–rump length stages. Acta Anat 81:127–138, 1972.
10. Pritchard JA. Fetal swallowing and amniotic fluid volume. Obstet Gynecol 28:606–617, 1966.
11. Abramovich DR. Fetal factors influencing amniotic fluid volume and composition of liquor amnii. J Obstet Gynaecol Br Commonw 77:865–877, 1970.
12. Bowie JD, Clair MR. Fetal swallowing and regurgitation: observation of normal and abnormal activity. Radiology 144:877–878, 1982.
13. Abramovich DR. The volume of amniotic fluid and factors affecting or regulating this. In: Fairweather DVI, Eskes TKAB (eds): Amniotic Fluid. Excerpta Medica, Amsterdam, 1973, pp 29–42.
14. Trehair JF, Harding R. Ultrastructural anomalies in the fetal small intestine indicate that fetal swallowing is important for normal development: an experimental study. Virchows Arch A Pathol Anat 420:305–320, 1992.
15. Phillips JO, Diamond JM, Fonkalsrud EW. Fetal rabbit intestinal malabsorption: implications for transamniotic feeding. J Pediatr Surg 25:909–915, 1990.

16. Phillips JO, Fonkalsrud EW, Mirzayein A, et al. Uptake and distribution of continuously infused intra-amniotic nutrients in fetal rabbits. Obstet Gynecol 45:861–825, 1985.

17. Dumont RC, Rudolph CD. Development of gastrointestinal motility in the infant and child. Gastroenterol Clin North Am 23:655–671, 1994.

18. Crump EP, Gore PM, Horton C. The sucking pattern of preterm infants. Hum Biol 30:128–141, 1958.

19. Daniels H, Devlieger H Casaer P, Callens M, Eggermont E. Nutritive and non-nutritive sucking in preterm infants. J Dev Physiol 8:117–121, 1986.

20. Nagata S, Koyanagi T, Horimoto N, Satoh S, Nakano H. Chronological development of the fetal stomach assessed using real-time ultrasound. Early Hum Dev 22:15–22, 1990.

21. Newell SJ. Development of the lower oesophageal sphincter in the preterm infant. In: Milla PJ (ed): Disorders of Gastrointestinal Motility in Childhood. Wiley, London, 1988, pp 17–41.

22. Boix-Ochoa J, Canals J. Maturation of the lower oesophageal sphincter. J Paediatr Surg 11:749–756, 1976.

23. Gryboski JD, Thayer WR Jr, Spiro HM. Esophageal motility in infants and children. Pediatrics 31:382–398, 1963.

24. Carre IV. The management of gastroesophageal reflux. Arch Dis Child 60:71–75, 1983.

25. Hawass NED, Al-Bawadi MG, Fatani JA, Meshari AA, Edrees YB. Morphology and growth of the fetal stomach. Invest Radiol 26:998–1004, 1991.

26. Nishimura H. Atlas of Human Prenatal Histology. Igaku-Shoin, Tokyo, 1983.

27. Kataoka K, Sakano Y, Miura J. Histogenesis of the mouse gastric mucosa with special reference to type and distribution of proliferative cells. Arch Histol Jpn 47:459–474, 1984.

28. Karam S, Lebond CP. Origin and migratory pathways of the eleven epithelial cell types present in the body of the mouse stomach. Microsc Res Tech 31:193–214, 1995.

29. Li Q, Karam SM, Gordon JI. Diphtheria toxin-mediated ablation of parietal cells in the stomach of transgenic mice. J Biol Chem 271:3671–3676, 1996.

30. Facer P, Bishop AE, Cole GA, et al. Developmental profile of chromogranin, hormonal peptides, and 5-hydroxytryptamine in gastrointestinal endocrine cells. Gastroenterology 97:48–56, 1989.

31. Flatt PR, Swantson-Flatt SK, Bailey CJ, McGregor GP, Conlon JM. Substance P, neurokinin A, and calcitonin gene-related peptide during development of the rat gastrointestinal tract. Regul Pept 33:313–320, 1991.

32. Onolfo JP, Lehy T, Labeille D, Gres L. Growth pattern of the polypeptide-YY cell population in the upper digestive tract of the rat during the perinatal period and after weaning. Cell Tissue Res 258:569–576, 1989.

33. Ekelund M, Hakanson R, Hedenbro J, Rehfeld JF, Sundler F. Endocrine cells and parietal cells in the stomach of the developing rat. Acta Physiol Scand 124:483–497, 1985.

34. Alumets J, Sundler F, Hakanson R. Distribution, ontogeny, and ultrastructure of somatostatin immunoreactive cells in the pancreas and gut. Cell Tissue Res 185:465–479, 1977.

35. Hakanson R, Owman C, Sjoberg N-O. Three different systems of monoamine-storing cells in the gastrointestinal tract of fetal and neonatal rats. Acta Physiol Scand 75:213–220, 1969.

36. Nissinen MJ, Panula P. Distribution of histamine in developing rat tissues. Agents Actions 33:177–180, 1991.

37. Nissinen MJ, Hakanson R, Panula P. Ontogeny of histamine-immunoreactive cells in rat stomach. Cell Tissue Res 267:241–249, 1992.

38. Iwase T, Tanaka M, Suzuki M, et al. Identification of protein-tyrosine kinase genes preferentially expressed in embryo stomach and gastric cancer. Biochem Biophys Res Commun 194:698–705, 1993.

39. Kong W, Swain GP, Li S, Diamond RH. PRL-1 PTPase expression is developmetnally regulated with tissue specific patterns in epithelial tissures. Am J Physiol Gastrointest Liver Physiol 279:G613–G621, 2000.

40. Braga MM, Pemberton LF, Duhig T, Gendler SJ. Spatial and temporal expression of an epithelial mucin, Muc-1, during mouse development. Development 115:427–437, 1992.

41. Thim L. A new family of growth factor–like peptides. FEBS Lett 250:85–94, 1989.

42. Jeffrey GP, Oates PS, Wang TC, Babyatsky MW, Brand SJ. Spasmolytic polypeptide: a trefoil peptide secreted by gastric mucous cells. Gastroenterology 106:436–442, 1994.

43. Henning SJ. Functional development of the gastrointestinal tract. In:

44. Bissett WM, Watt JB, Rivers JPA, et al. The ontogeny of fasting small intestinal motor activity in the human infant. Gut 29:483–496, 1988.

45. Deren JS. Development of structure and function in the fetal and newborn stomach. Am J Clin Nutr 24:144–159, 1971.

46. Garzon B, Ducroc R, Geloso JP. Ontogenesis of gastric acid secretion in fetal rat. Pediatr Res 15:921–925, 1982.

47. Garzon B, Ducroc R, Onolfo JP, Desjeux JF, Geloso JP. Biphasic development of pentagastrin sensitivity in rat stomach. Am J Physiol 242:G111–G115, 1982.

48. Hervatin F, Moreau E, Geloso JP. Development of acid secretory function in the rat stomach: sensitivity to secretagogues and corticosterone. Pediatr Gastroenterol Nutr 9:82–88, 1989.

49. Christie DL. Development of gastric function in the first month of life. In: Lebenthal E (ed): Textbook of Gastroenterology and Nutrition in Infancy. Raven Press, New York, 1981, pp 109–131.

50. Agunod M, Yaganuchi N, Lopez R, et al. Correlative study of hydrochloric acid, pepsin and intrinsic factor in newborns and infants. Am J Dig Dis 14:400–414, 1969.

51. Rogers IM, Davidson DC, Lawrence J, Ardill J, Buchanan KD. Neonatal secretion of gastrin and glucagon. Arch Dis Child 49:197–209, 1974.

52. Mallow MH, Morrisson FH, Denson SE, et al. Neonatal gastric motility in dogs: maturation and response to pentagastrin. Am J Physiol 236:E562–E580, 1979.

53. Johnson LR. Effects of somatostatin and acid on inhibition of gastrin release in newborn rats. Endocrinology 114:743–751, 1984.

54. Lay JM, Jenkins C, Friis-Hansen L, Samuelson LC. Structure and developmental expression of the mouse CCK-B receptor gene. Biochem Biophys Res Commun 272:837–842, 2000.

55. Seidel ER, Johnson LR. Ontogeny of the gastric mucosal muscarinic receptor and sensitivity to carbachol. Am J Physiol 246:G550–G558, 1984.

56. Ackerman SH. Ontogeny of gastric acid secretion in the rat: evidence for multiple response systems. Science 217:75–81, 1982.

57. Schohn H, Gueant JI, Leheup B, et al. Intrinsic factor receptor during fetal development of the human receptor. Biochem J 286:153–156, 1992.

58. Sarles J, Moreau H, Verger R. Human gastric lipase: ontogeny and variations in children. Acta Paediatr 81:511–513, 1992,

59. Kataoka K, Takeoka Y, Furihata C. Immunocytochemical study of pepsinogen 1–producing cells in the fundic mucosa of the stomach in developing mice. Cell Tissue Res 261:211–217, 1990.

60. Furihata C, Saito D, Fujiki H, et al. Purification and characterization of pepsinogens and a unique pepsin from rat stomach. Eur J Biochem 105:43–50, 1980.

61. Henning SJ. Plasma concentrations of total and free corticosterone during development in the rat. Am J Physiol 235:E451–E462, 1978.

62. Ikezaki M, Johnson LR. Development of sensitivity to different secretagogues in the rat stomach. Am J Physiol 244:G165–G173, 1983.

63. Peitsch W, Takeuchi L, Johnson LR. Mucosal gastrin receptor VI. Induction by corticosterone in newborn rats. Am J Physiol 240:G442–G449, 1981.

64. Ichnose M, Miki K, Tatematsu M, et al. Hydrocortisone-induced enhancement of expression and changes in methylation of pepsinogen genes in stomach mucosa of the developing rat. Biochem Biophys Res Commun 172:1086–1093, 1990.

65. Kumegawa M, Takuma T, Hosoda S, Kunii S, Kauda Y. Precocious induction of pepsinogen in the stomach of suckling mice by hormones. Biochem Biophys Acta 543:243–250, 1978.

66. Johnson LR, Peitsch W, Takeuchi K. Mucosal gastrin receptor VIII. Sex-related differences in binding. Am J Physiol 243:G469–G474, 1982.

67. Beaulieu JF, Vachon PH, Chartrand S. Immunolocalization of extracellular matrix components during organogenesis in the human small intestine. Anat Embryol 183:363–369, 1991.

68. Colony PC. Successive phases of human fetal intestinal development. In: Kretchmer N, Minkowki A (eds): Nutritional Adaptation of the Gastrointestinal Tract of the Newborn. Raven Press, New York, 1983, pp 3–44.

69. Gordon JI. Intestinal epithelial differentiation: new insights from chimeric and transgenic mice. J Cell Biol 108:1187–1194, 1989.

70. Antonowicz I, Lebenthal E. Developmental pattern of small intestinal enterokinase and disaccharidase activities in the human fetus. Gastroenterology 72:1299–1303, 1977.

71. James PS, Smith MW, Tivey DR. Single-villus analysis of disacchari-

Johnson LR (ed): Physiology of the Gastrointestinal Tract, 2nd ed. Raven Press, New York, 1987, pp 285–313.

dase expression by different regions of the mouse intestine. J Physiol 401:533–545, 1988.

72. Rubino A, Zimbalatti F, Auricchio S. Intestinal disaccharidase activities in adult and suckling rats. Biochem Biophys Acta 92:305–312, 1964.

73. Mobassaleh M, Montgomery RK, Biller JA, et al. Development of carbohydrate absorption in the fetus and neonate. Pediatrics 75[Suppl]:160–166, 1985.

74. Koldovsky O, Heringova A, Jirsova V, et al. Transport of glucose against a concentration gradient in everted sacs of jejunum and ileum of human fetuses. Gastroenterology 48:185–195, 1965.

75. Turk E, Zabel B, Mundios S, Dyer J, Wright EM. Glucose/galactose malabsorption caused by a defect in the Na+/glucose cotransporter. Nature 350:354–356, 1991.

76. Malo C, Berteloot A. Proximo-distal gradient of Na+-dependent D-glucose transport activity in the brush border membrane vescicles from the human fetal small intestine. FEBS Lett 220:201–205, 1987.

77. Matsumoto K, Takao Y, Akazawa S, et al. Developmental change of facilitative glucose transporter expression in rat embryonal and fetal intestine. Biochem Biophys Res Commun 193:1275–1282, 1993.

78. Buddington RK, Chen JW, Diamond JM. Genetic and phenotypic adaptation of intestinal nutrient transport to diet. J Physiol 393:261–267, 1987.

79. Freeman HJ, Quamme GA. Age-related changes in sodium-dependent glucose transport in rat small intestine. Am J Physiol 251:G208–G217, 1986.

80. Toloza EM, Diamond J. Ontogenetic development of nutrient transporters in rat intestine. Am J Physiol 263:G593–G604, 1992.

81. Antonowicz I, Lebenthal E. Developmental pattern of small intestinal enterokinase and disaccharidase activities in the human fetus. Gastroenterology 72:1299–1303, 1977.

82. Levin RJ, Koldovsky O, Hoskova J, et al. Electrical activity across human foetal small intestine associated with absorption processes. Gut 9:206–213, 1968.

83. Eindberg T. Intestinal dipeptidases: characterization, development, and distribution of intestinal dipeptidases of the human foetus. Clin Sci 30:505–514, 1966.

84. Reisenauer AM, Lee FA, Castillo RO. Ontogeny of membrane and soluble amino-oligopeptidases in rat intestine. Am J Physiol 262:G178–G185, 1992.

85. Malo C. Multiple pathways for amino acid transport in brush border membrane vesicles isolated from the human small intestine. Gastroenterology 100:1644–1650, 1991.

86. Colony PC, Neutra MR. Macromolecular transport in the fetal rat intestine. Gastroenterology 89:294–306, 1985.

87. Walker WA, Isselbacher KJ. Uptake and transport of macromolecules by the intestine. Possible role in clinical disorders. Gastroenterology 67:531–550, 1974.

88. Walker WA, Cornell R, Davenport LM, Isselbacher KJ. Macromolecular absorption. Mechanism of horseradish peroxidase uptake and transport in adult neonatal rat intestine. J Cell Biol 54:195–205, 1972.

89. Eastham EJ, Lichauco T, Grady MI, Walker WA. Antigeneity of infant formulas: role of immature intestine on protein permeability. J Pediatr 93:561–564, 1978.

90. Tachibana T. Physiological investigation of the fetus. 4. Lipase in pancrease. Jpn J Obstet Gynecol 11:92–100, 1928.

91. Hamosh M. Oral lipases and lipid digestion during the neonatal period. In: Lebenthal E (ed): Textbook of Gastroenterology and Nutrition in Infancy. Raven Press, New York, 1981, pp 445–471.

92. Menard D, Monfils S, Tremblay E. Ontogeny of human gastric lipase and pepsin activities. Gastroenterology 108:1650–1656, 1995.

93. De Bell ER, Brown A, Blacklow NR, et al. Organ culture of fetal liver: a new model system. Pediatr Res 7:292A, 1973.

94. Acra SA, Ghishan FK. Active bile salt transport in the ileum: characteristics and ontogeny. J Pediatr Gastroenterol Nutr 10:421–425, 1990.

95. Berendson PB, Blanchette-Mackie EJ. Milk lipid absorption and chylomicron production in the suckling rat. Anat Rec 195:397–414, 1979.

96. Mak KM, Trier JS. Lipoprotein particles in the jejunal mucosa of postnatal developing rats. Anat Rec 194:491–506, 1979.

97. Little JM, Lister R. Ontogenesis of intestinal bile salt absorption in the neonatal rat. Am J Physiol 239:G319–G326, 1990.

98. Watkins JB. Role of bile acids in the development of the enterohepatic curculation. In: Lebenthal E (ed): Textbook of Gastroenterology and Nutrition in Infancy. Raven Press, New York, 1981, pp. 167–191.

99. Insoft RM, Sanderson IR, Walker WA. Development of immune function in the intestine and its role in neonatal diseases. Pediatr Clin North Am 43:551–571, 1996.

100. Spencer J, MacDonald T, Finn T, Isaacson PG. Development of gut associated lymphoid tissue in the terminal ileum of fetal human intestine. Clin Exp Immunol 64:536–543, 1986.

101. Neumann B, Luz A, Pfeffer K, Holzmann B. Defective Peyer's patch organogenesis in mice lacking the 55-kD receptor for tumor necrosis factor. J Exp Med 184:259–264, 1996.

102. MacDonald TT, Spencer J. Ontogeny of the gut-associated lymphoid system in man. Acta Paediatr Suppl 395:3–5, 1994.

103. Brandtzaeg P. Research in gastrointestinal immunology. State of the art. Scand J Gastroenterol 20:137–150, 1985.

104. Orlic D, Lev R. An electron microscopic study of intraepithelial lymphocytes in human fetal small intestine. Lab Invest 37:554–561, 1977.

105. Spencer J, Isaacson P, Walker-Smith J, et al. Heterogeneity of intraepithelial subpopulations in fetal and post-natal intestine. J Pediatr Gastroenterol Nutr 9:173–177, 1989.

106. Harvey J, Jones DB, Wright DH. Differential expression of MHC- and macrophage-associated antigens in human fetal and postnatal intestine. Immunology 69:409–415, 1990.

107. Cummins AG, Steele TW, Labrooy JT, et al. Maturation of the rat small intestine at weaning: changes in epithelial cell kinetics, bacterial flora, and mucosal immune activity. Gut 29:1672–1679, 1988.

108. Cummins AG, Labrooy JT, Shearman DJC. The effect of cyclosporin A in delaying maturation of the small intestine during weaning in the rat. Clin Exp Immunol 75:451–458, 1989.

109. Tice DG. Ontogeny of natural activity in rat small bowel. Transplant Proc 22:2458–2459, 1990.

110. Gallagher ND, Mason R, Foley KE. Mechanisms of iron absorption and transport in neonatal rat intestine. Gastroenterology 64:438–444, 1973.

111. Batt ER, Schachter D. Developmental pattern of some intestinal transport mechanisms in newborn rats and mice. Am J Physiol 216:1064–1068, 1969.

112. Dostal LA, Toverud SV. Effect of vitamin $D_3$ on duodenal calcium absorption in vivo during early development. Am J Physiol 246:G528–G534, 1984.

113. Boass A, Wilson TH. Development of mechanisms for intestinal absorption of vitamin $B_{12}$ in the growing rats. Am J Physiol 204:101–110, 1963.

114. Schohn H, GuJant JL, Leheup B, et al. Intrinsic factor receptor during fetal development of the human intestine. Biochem J 286:153–156, 1992.

115. Said HM, Redah R. Ontogenesis of the intestinal transport of biotin in the rat. Gastroenterology 94:68–72, 1988.

116. Henning SJ. Postnatal development: coordination of feeding, digestion, and metabolism. Am J Physiol 241:G199–G214, 1981.

117. Kendall K, Jumawan J, Koldovsky O. Development of jejunoileal differences of lactase, sucrase, and beta-galactosidase in isografts of fetal rat intestine. Biol Neonate 36:206–214, 1979.

118. Tsuboi KK, Kwong LK, Ford WDA, et al. Delayed ontogenic development in the bypassed ileum of the infant rat. Gastroenterology 80:1550–1556, 1981.

119. Dulue I, Galluser M, Raul F, et al. Dietary control of lactase mRNA distribution along the rat small intestine. Am J Physiol 262:G954–G961, 1992.

120. Raul F, Kedinger M, Simon PM, et al. Comparative in vivo and in vitro effect of mono- and disaccharides on intestinal brush border enzyme activities in suckling rats. Biol Neonate 39:200–207, 1981.

121. Gerraris RP, Villenas SA, Hirayama BA, et al. Effect of diet on glucose transporter site density along the intestinal crypt–villus axis. Am J Physiol 262:G1060–G1068, 1992.

122. Hamilton JR, Guiraldes E, Rossi M. Impact of malnutrition on the developing gut: studies in suckling rats. J Pediatr Gastroenterol Nutr 2[Suppl 1]:S151–S156, 1983.

123. Heird WC, Schwarz SM, Hansen IH. Colostrum-induced enteric mucosal growth in beagle puppies. Pediatr Res 18:512–515, 1984.

124. Berseth CL, Lichtenberger LM, Morriss FH Jr. Comparison of the gastrointestinal growth-promoting effects of rat colostrum and mature milk in newborn rats in vivo. Am J Clin Nutr 37:52–60, 1983.

125. Sheard NF, Walker WA. The role of breast milk in the development of the gastrointestinal tract. Nutr Rev 46:1–8, 1988.

126. Grueters A, Alm J, Laksmaman J, et al. Epidermal growth factor in mouse milk during early lactation: lack of dependency on submandibular glands. Pediatr Res 19:853–856, 1985.

127. Schanders RP, Grimes J, Davis D, et al. EGF content in the gastrointestinal tract of rats: effect of age and fasting on feeding. Am J Physiol 256:G856–G864, 1989.

128. Donovan SM, Odle J. Growth factors in milk as mediators of infant development. Annu Rev Nutr 14:147–167, 1994.

Using a regional colorectal cancer registry, Kee and colleagues[18] reviewed records of 3217 patients in Northern Ireland from 1990 to 1994. The mean follow-up duration from the time of diagnosis was 54 months. The investigators found no improvement in the 2-year mortality rate for patients whose operations were performed by higher-volume surgeons, or in higher-volume hospitals. In fact, their data suggested a trend toward higher mortality rates in institutions in which more than 33 operations were performed per year as compared with those in which fewer than 33 were performed. However, less than 20% of the cases were performed by surgeons who averaged fewer than 10 cases per year, and less than 20% of cases were performed by surgeons with fewer than 13 years' experience.

From 1983 to 1990, Porter and colleagues[19] evaluated 683 cases of patients with rectal cancer who underwent surgery by 52 surgeons from five hospitals in Edmonton, Canada. Five of the surgeons had additional training in colorectal surgery. The follow-up duration was greater than 5 years for 97% of the patients. During the 7-year study period, nearly half of the patients were operated on by surgeons who performed fewer than 21 operations. A higher proportion of low- and mid-level rectal tumors were managed by specialty-trained surgeons; these surgeons were more likely than the non–specialty-trained surgeons to perform a low anterior resection. Despite the fact that the more technically complex operations were performed by the specialty-trained surgeons, multivariate analysis suggested that local recurrence, a particularly strong indicator of surgical technique, was more common in those patients operated on by surgeons who had no additional training (hazard ratio [HR] 2.5; $P < 0.01$) or who had done fewer than 21 cases over the study period (HR 1.8; $P < 0.01$). Similarly, disease-free survival was associated with the level of training (HR 1.5; $P = 0.03$) and surgical experience (HR 1.4; $P < 0.01$).

Schrag and colleagues[20] evaluated records of 27,968 patients with colon cancer from the Surveillance, Epidemiology, and End Results (SEER)–Medicare linked database. All patients were 65 years of age or older and had undergone surgery between 1991 and 1996. The main outcomes evaluated were hospital volume–related 30-day operative mortality rates and 5-year cancer-related mortality rates. The results suggested a positive relationship between hospital volume and survival. The 5-year mortality rate in the low-volume (<3 cases/year) centers (54.8%) was 4.4% higher than that in the very high–volume (>32 cases/year) centers (50.4%). Also, the 30-day mortality was 2% higher in the low-volume centers than in the high-volume centers. The association between hospital volume and survival was concentrated among patients with stage II and III disease and did not change with risk adjustment. The difference in outcomes of patients with stage III disease could not be explained by variations in the use of adjuvant chemotherapy.

Harmon and colleagues[21] from Johns Hopkins Hospital conducted a cross-sectional analysis of patients who had undergone surgical resection for colorectal cancer. The researchers used Maryland state discharge data from 1992 to 1996 and categorized the patients into three groups on the basis of annual case volume per surgeon (low, <5; medium, 5–10; high, >10) and per hospital (low, <40; medium, 40–70; high, >70). The study included 9739 surgical procedures by 812 surgeons at 50 hospitals over 5 years. Their outcome analysis was limited to in-hospital mortality, length of stay, and hospital charges. Because the study was large, they were able to evaluate the effect of both surgeon and hospital volume. The majority of surgeons (81%) and hospitals (58%) were in the low-volume subgroup. The low-volume surgeons operated on 36% of the patients, at an average rate of less than 2 cases per year. The results of the study suggested that higher surgeon volume was associated with a significant improvement in all outcomes measured—in-hospital mortality, length of stay, and hospital charges. The improvement in outcome associated with the medium-volume surgeons who performed surgery in medium- or high-volume hospitals was as great as that associated with the high-volume surgeons, but this result was not seen in low-volume hospitals.

## Esophageal and Hepatic Cancer

Patti and colleagues[22] reviewed discharge abstracts of 1561 patients who had undergone esophagectomy from 1990 to 1994 in 273 hospitals in California. Fifty percent of all patients had undergone surgery in hospitals that averaged fewer than three cases per year. Hospital volume was the most significant independent variable affecting perioperative mortality. The average mortality rate was 4.8% in centers that averaged more than 30 cases over the study period, compared with 16% in hospitals averaging fewer than 30 cases. This difference could not be accounted for by other patient-related factors associated with surgical mortality. Only 17.5% of the patients had undergone surgery in the highest-volume hospitals.

Choti and colleagues[23] evaluated the in-hospital mortality rate associated with hepatic resection in the same manner as that used to study pancreatic surgery mortality rates.[23] More than 43% of the surgical procedures had been performed at their institution, which averaged more than 40 cases per year. The remaining operations had been performed at 35 other hospitals that averaged only 1.5 cases per year. Metastatic disease was the leading indication for surgery followed by primary hepatic malignancy. The in-hospital mortality rate associated with hepatic resection at a single high-volume institution was 1.5%, compared with 7.9% in the remaining (low-volume) hospitals in Maryland.

Glasgow and colleagues[24] used the same database as Patti and colleagues[22] to review all of the discharge abstracts of patients who had undergone major hepatic resection for hepatocellular carcinoma (HCC) in California from 1990 to 1994. Five hundred seven hepatectomies were performed for HCC in 138 hospitals over the 5-year study period. Half of all patients had been operated on at hospitals that averaged six resections over the 5 years; these centers accounted for 88.4% of all the reporting hospitals. The highest-volume hospitals averaged 37 resections and accounted for only 2.9% of the hospitals. Grouped together, the low-volume centers averaged three or fewer resections per year and accounted for over 97% of the hospitals. In the lowest-volume centers, the risk-adjusted mortality rate was 22.7%, compared with 9.4% in the highest-volume centers. The average length of stay was also significantly shorter in the highest-volume hospitals than in the lowest-volume hospitals.

Using the same SEER database as Schrag and co-workers,[20] Begg and colleagues[25] reviewed all 5013 patients in the registry over age 65 who had undergone pancreatectomy, esophagectomy, pneumonectomy, hepatectomy, and pelvic exenteration for cancer diagnosed between 1984 and 1993. These procedures were chosen because they often involved extensive preoperative evaluation and judgment, meticulous surgical technique, and expert postoperative care. The authors demonstrated a decreasing risk of death with increasing hospital operative volume in all procedures for gastrointestinal malignancies that were evaluated. The difference in outcomes could not be accounted for by differences in patient comorbidities, and the investigators found no evidence that high-volume centers cared for a lower-risk subset of patients.

Despite criticisms about their methodology, these studies provide substantial evidence that results of complex surgical procedures are considerably better in facilities where they are performed more frequently. What is not addressed well in these studies is the necessary level of training of the health-care providers involved. It is assumed that the high-volume centers employ surgeons with more advanced training and other health-care professionals important to the delivery of high-quality patient care. With training comes experience and therefore improved outcome. The differences outlined in the above studies are substantial enough that they become important to the public and to referring physicians. The results of the studies add support to the National Cancer Policy Board's recommendation as outlined by Hillner et al.[7] to ensure that patients undergoing technically difficult procedures associated with increased mortality in lower-volume centers receive their care in hospitals with more extensive experience. These data and others support the claim that sufficiently complex oncologic operations should be done by adequately trained surgical oncologists.

## Conclusion

The treatment of gastrointestinal malignancies is entering a new era marked by an emphasis on a greater understanding of the genetic basis of tumor formation and metastasis. Molecular-based diagnostics, sophisticated imaging techniques, and a rapidly expanding array of systemic therapies, including novel treatments based on the molecular profile of the individual tumor, have greatly complicated the care of patients. Exploratory surgery is rarely performed, and elective operations for solid tumors of the gastrointestinal tract are performed with the expectation that they will improve the length and quality of patient survival, with a low risk for major morbidity or mortality. Importantly, surgery is now performed as one part of a carefully developed treatment plan (ideally, one that is protocol based) designed to maximize survival duration while minimizing treatment time and toxicity. The surgeon's responsibility to the patient is much greater than in the past; he or she must combine technical excellence with a complete understanding of the disease and its treatment options.

## References

1. Schweitzer RJ, Edwards MH, Lawrence W. Training guidelines for surgical oncology. Cancer 48:2336–2340, 1981.
2. Evans DB, Lee JE, Charnsangavej C. Unusual pancreatic tumors. In: Cameron JL (ed): Current Surgical Therapy, 6th ed. Mosby-Year Book, Philadelphia, 1998, pp 527–532.
3. Windham TC, Pearson AS, Skibber JM, et al. Significance and management of local recurrences and limited metastatic disease in the abdomen. Surg Clin North Am 80:761–774, 2000.
4. Wolff RA, Abbruzzese JL, Evans DB. Neoplasms of the exocrine pancreas. In: Holland JF, Frei E, Bast RC, Kufe DW, Pollock RE, Weichelbaum RR (eds): Cancer Medicine, 5th ed. B.C. Decker, Ontario, 2000, pp 1436–1464.
5. Longnecker DS, Hruban RH, Adler G, Kloppel G. Intraductal papillary mucinous neoplasms of the pancreas. In: Hamilton SR, Aaltonen LA (eds): World Health Organization Classification of Tumors: Tumors of the Digestive System. IARC Press, Lyon, France, 2000, pp 237–240.
6. Sohn TA, Yeo CJ, Cameron JL, et al. Intraductal papillary mucinous neoplasms of the pancreas: an increasingly recognized clinicopathologic entity. Ann Surg 234:313–322, 2001.
7. Hillner BE, Smith TJ, Desch CE. Hospital and physician volume or specialization and outcomes in cancer treatment: importance in quality of cancer care. J Clin Oncol 18:2327–2340, 2000.
8. Luft HS, Bunker JP, Enthoven AC. Should operations be regionalized? The empirical relation between surgical volume and mortality. N Engl J Med 301:1364–1369, 1979.
9. Steele GD. Is more better? Ann Surg 227:168–169, 1998.
10. Fernandez-del Castillo C, Rattner DW, Warshaw AL. Standards for pancreatic resection in the 1990s. Arch Surg 130:295–300, 1995.
11. Yeo CJ, Cameron JL, Sohn TA, et al. Six hundred fifty consecutive pancreaticoduodenectomies in the 1990's: pathology, complications, and outcomes. Ann Surg 226:248–260, 1997.
12. Birkmeyer JD, Samuel RG, Finlayson RG, et al. Effect of hospital volume on in-hospital mortality with pancreaticoduodenectomy. Surgery 125:250–256, 1999.
13. Lambert LA, Birkmeyer JD. Risks of perioperative mortality with pancreaticoduodenectomy. In: Evans DB, Pisters PWT, Abbruzzese JL (eds): Pancreatic Cancer. Springer-Verlag New York, New York, 2001, pp 201–211.
14. Lieberman MD, Kilburn H, Lindsey M, Brennan MF. Relation of perioperative deaths to hospital volume among patients undergoing pancreatic resection for malignancy. Ann Surg 222:638–645, 1995.
15. Gordon TZ, Burleyson GP, Tielsch JM, Cameron JL. The effects of regionalization on cost and outcome for one general high-risk surgical procedure. Ann Surg 222:211–212, 1995.
16. Hutter MM, Glasgow RE, Mulvihill SJ. Does the participation of a surgical trainee adversely impact patient outcomes? A study of major pancreatic resections in California. Surgery 128:286–292, 2000.
17. Birkmeyer JD, Warshaw AL, Finlayson SRG, Grove MR, Tosteson ANA. Relationship between hospital volume and late survival after pancreaticoduodenectomy. Surgery 126:178–183, 1990.
18. Kee F, Wilson RH, Harper C, et al. Influence of hospital and clinician workload on survival from colorectal cancer: cohort study. BMJ 318 (7195):1381–1385, 1990.
19. Porter GA, Soskolne CL, Yakimets WW, Newman S. Surgeon-related factors and outcome in rectal cancer. Ann Surg 227:157–167, 1998.
20. Schrag D, Cramer LD, Bach PB, Cohen AM, Warren JL, Begg CB. Influence of hospital procedures volume on outcomes following surgery for colon cancer. JAMA 284:3028–3035, 2000.
21. Harmon JW, Tang DG, Gordon TA, et al. Hospital volume can serve as a surrogate for surgeon volume for achieving excellent outcomes in colorectal resection. Ann Surg 230:404–411, 1999.
22. Patti MG, Corvera CU, Glasgow RE, Way LW. A hospital's annual rate of esophagectomy influences the operative mortality rate. J Gastrointest Surg 2:186–192, 1998.
23. Choti MA, Bowman HM, Pitt HA, et al. Should hepatic resections be performed at high-volume referral centers? J Gastrointest Surg 2:11–20, 1998.
24. Glasgow RE, Showstack JA, Katz PP, Corvera CU, Warren RS, Mulvihill SJ. The relationship between hospital volume and outcomes of hepatic resection for hepatocellular carcinoma. Arch Surg 134:30–35, 1999.
25. Begg CB, Cramer LD, Hoskins WJ, Brennan MF. Impact of hospital volume on operative mortality for major cancer surgery. JAMA 280:1747–1751, 1998.

# Chapter 7

# Therapeutic Principles of Gastrointestinal Neoplasia: Radiation Oncology

IRA J. SPIRO AND CHRISTOPHER G. WILLETT

A successful cancer treatment should render the patient free of local, regional, and distant disease. This therapy should have minimal morbidity and maintain the patient's pretreatment functional status. Local therapy alone may be sufficient for patients with very–early stage disease. Conversely, patients with advanced but localized cancer are more frequently treated with multiple modalities, often combining surgery, radiation, and chemotherapy. One important advantage of radiation is that it can include major vessels, nerves, connective tissues, and hollow viscera with relatively low risk of producing complications, thus improving functional and cosmetic outcome.

The mainstay of treatment of gastrointestinal malignancies has been surgery. Over the past 15 years, radiation therapy, frequently in combination with chemotherapy, has played an increasingly important role in the treatment of various gastrointestinal malignancies.

The optimal use of radiation, whether used as a sole treatment modality or as a part of a multimodality program, requires an understanding of the action of radiation from the physical level to the whole-organ level. Generally, there are two strategies to enhance the efficacy of radiation therapy: (1) improve the physical dose distribution so as to increase dose in the tumor relative to normal tissues and (2) increase the differential response to radiation between tumor and normal tissues. The former strategy relates to physical parameters; the latter, to biological ones.

## Physical Aspects of Radiation Therapy

In modern practice, radiation therapy is delivered by linear accelerators. Thoracic, abdominal, and pelvic tumors are most appropriately treated with equipment capable of delivering beam energies in the range of 10 to 25 MV X-rays. Compared with beams delivered by older, lower-energy equipment, these beams offer the relative advantage of lower surface doses with an increased dose at a given depth in tissue. At these high energies, beams also offer sharp lateral field edges with rapid dose fall-off. This characteristic allows for less irradiation of nontarget tissues. Isocentric gantries and patient couches capable of a multitude of movement options allow for an almost infinite choice of beam portals incident on the patient. The ultimate choice of beam energy and treatment technique is based on delivering the highest feasible concentration of dose in the target volume (i.e., the volume judged to contain cancer cells) while minimizing the dose to normal tissues.

To realize this goal, sophisticated high-speed computers plan treatment in three dimensions, using anatomic information obtained from computed tomography (CT) and/or magnetic resonance imaging (MRI). In addition, computer-controlled dynamic treatment systems allow for gantry, collimator (i.e., field border), and couch movement during treatment. In this manner, the high-dose treatment volume is able to conform more accurately to the target volume.[1] Other modern advances include on-line portal imaging systems, which allow for instant verification of the radiation treatment field. Modern radiation oncologists are also increasingly making use of improved patient immobilization devices. In the last several years, more importance has been placed on target organ motion during the "beam on" time. Both three-dimensional treatment planning and sophisticated immobilization systems have provided a greater understanding of how organ motion affects the delivery of radiation dose to a target. One method of dealing with organ motion is to gate the delivery of radiation to the respiratory cycle.

In addition to conventional external beam irradiation, other specialized modalities are available for the treatment of gastrointestinal malignancies. Intraoperative radiation therapy (IORT) is a technique whereby irradiation, usually via an electron beam or low-energy X-rays, is applied directly to a tumor or tumor bed at the time of surgery while critical normal tissues, such as the small bowel, are displaced from the treated region.[2] This modality has been used in the care of patients with rectal cancer, pancreatic cancer, and gastric cancer. Brachytherapy (from the Greek *brachy*, meaning short) implant techniques have also been employed. Brachytherapy became available in the early part of this century, soon after radioactive isotopes were discovered. This type of treatment has been used for patients with esophageal, biliary, pancreatic, rectal, and anal cancer. In general, temporarily dwelling hollow catheters can be placed at the time of surgery or under ultrasound or CT guidance. These catheters can then be remotely loaded with radioactive sources at the time of surgery or later. These techniques allow for high doses of radiation to be delivered to relatively small volumes of tissue. In addition to brachytherapy, there has also been interest in the use of charged-particle (mostly proton) accelerators, which are available at a small number of institutions.[3] Conventional X-rays and protons have similar biological properties and hence similar killing effects. The advantage of protons lies in their superior physical dose distribution. Protons have a defined range in tissue, and dose distributions can be designed that conform more closely to the tumor volume. Because of these unique physical properties, proton therapy may lead to substantial reductions in normal tissue irradiation. Figures 7–1 and 7–2 illustrate a comparison of two treatments plans, one using protons and the other using conventional high-energy X-rays, to treat a patient with a biliary carcinoma (Color Figs. 7–1 and 7–2 in separate color insert). With the proton plan there is substantially less hepatic irradiation than with the X-ray plan.

## Biological and Genetic Considerations

The target for radiation-induced lethality in tumor cells is DNA. Unrepaired or misrepaired double-strand breaks or DNA base damage presumably leads to cell killing. In addition, a number of factors alter the response of tumor cells and normal tissues to radiation. These factors include but are not limited to *(1)* the inherent radiosensitivity of the cells in question, *(2)* the capacity of these cells to repair radiation damage, *(3)* the oxygen and nutrient status of the tumor, *(4)* the position of an individual cell in the cell cycle, and *(5)* the capacity for repopulation. To improve the therapeutic differential between tumor cells and normal tissues, these factors are exploited in part by giving radiation treatments as a series of equal fractions over a number of weeks.

The reasons for some cells (such as seminoma cells) being exquisitely sensitive to radiation while other cells (such as rectal carcinoma cells) require higher doses for control, or for not all patients with a given histology showing equal sensitivity are poorly understood. Clearly, genetic factors must play a role in determining the response of cells to radiation, although the molecular basis for these differences is not yet understood. Recently, there has been wider recognition of the role of programmed cell death, or apoptosis.[4,5] This process of cell death is not linked to mitosis and was first appreciated in lymphocytes, although now it is known to occur to varying degrees in normal and tumor tissues. Of interest is the finding that a normal *p53* gene is required for this process.[6] Tumor cells with mutant *p53* alleles or lacking a normal p53 allele may therefore be more resistant to cell killing if the apoptotic process is not functioning.

For the most part, both normal tissues and tumor cells are capable of repair between doses of radiation. However, while normal tissues may possess a greater capacity for repair, they may

also require more time to do so. Therefore, spacing radiation fractions by at least 6 hours (usually 24 hours) may provide a greater advantage to normal tissues. Even small therapeutic gains, when exponentially expanded over a course of treatment, can become significant. Cells also vary considerably in their radiosensitivity depending on their position in the mitotic cycle. S-phase cells are most radioresistant, while cells in late G2 and mitosis are most radiosensitive.[7] A dose of 200 cGy (1 cGy = rad) will eradicate tumor cells in the most sensitive phases of the cycle, preferentially leaving behind cells in resistant phases. If another dose of radiation is given 24 hours later, some of the cells in resistant phases of the cycle will have moved to more sensitive ones. Late-responding normal tissues, which are not actively cycling, will be preferentially spared by this effect.

The absence of molecular oxygen is an effective radioprotector, and tumor cells at low oxygen tensions are relatively resistant to radiation.[8] This phenomenon can occur because tumor cells can outgrow their blood supply. As well-oxygenated radiosensitive cells within a tumor are killed off, resistant hypoxic cells in the tumor may reoxygenate over time. Fractionated radiotherapy would therefore be more beneficial to normal, well-oxygenated tissues. Repopulation occurs not only in acutely responding normal tissue, such as the gut epithelium, but also in tumors. Moreover, a therapeutic advantage would occur if the rate of repopulation was more rapid in normal tissues than in tumors. In general, it is best to deliver in the shortest possible period of time a course of radiation that will be tolerated by acutely responding normal tissue. Treatment delays beyond this time due to radiotherapy toxicity or elective break will favor tumor proliferation.

## Dose–Response Relationships in Radiation Therapy

The relationship between radiation dose and tumor control probability is shown in Figure 7–3. The delivery of the physical dose to the tumor is controlled by the physical factors discussed above, while the shape of the curve is determined by the biological fac-

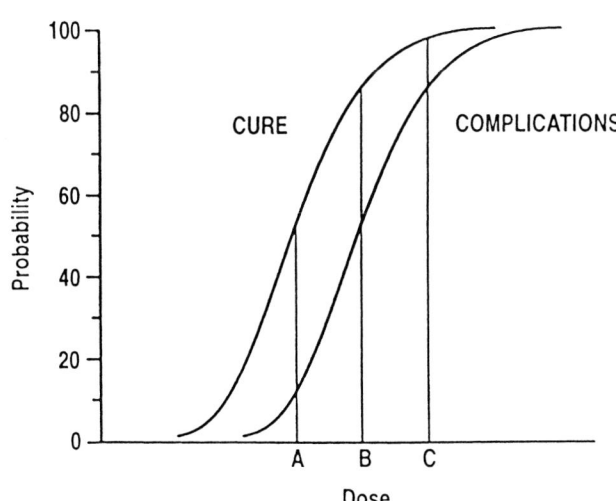

**Figure 7-3** Probability of tumor cure or complications vs. dose. Doses that produce no complications achieve low cure rates (dose A). Doses that achieve high levels of cure produce unacceptably high complication rates (dose C). Intermediate doses are chosen so that the benefits and risks of therapy are well balanced (dose B).

tors. Normal tissues also display similar sigmoidal dose–response curves, although fractionated radiation therapy generally places this curve to the right of the tumor curve. At doses that produce no complications, cure rates are low (Fig. 7–3, dose A), while tumor doses that produce cure rates of greater than 90% may produce unacceptable morbidity (Fig. 7–3, dose C). In general, intermediate doses are chosen so that the benefits and risks of therapy are well balanced (Fig. 7–3, dose B).

The precise number of cells in a tumor that need to be inactivated is also a critical determinant of the probability of tumor control. For example, if a tumor contains $10^8$ clonogenic cells and a dose of 180 cGy reduces tumor cell survival by 50%, then 30 fractions of 180 cGy would reduce survival by $9 \times 10^{-10}$. The probability of tumor control ($P_{control}$) would then be given by the equation:

$$P_{control} = e^- \text{ (cell number } x \text{ surviving fraction)}$$

$$= e^- (10^8 \times 9 \times 10^{-10})$$

$$= 0.91 \text{ or } 91\%$$

Analogy could be made to the small burden of rectal cancer cells remaining after resection. If the cell number were to increase 10-fold from $10^8$ clonogenic cells to $10^9$, or approximately 1 g, then the probability of cure would decrease to:

$$P_{control} = e^- (10^9 \times 9 \times 10^{-10})$$

$$= 0.41 \text{ or } 41\%$$

To achieve the same probability of control, an additional three fractions of radiation would have to be delivered.

## Combined Modality Therapy

Various strategies for increasing the therapeutic gain of radiation treatment have been recommended. Altered radiation fractionation schemes for delivering more than one treatment a day at 4- to 6-hour interfraction intervals are being investigated.[9–12] Such programs may produce an additional benefit for normal tissues and reduce the repopulation of tumor cells during the course of therapy. Strategies that reduce the hypoxic burden in a tumor are also being investigated. These include the use of perfluorocarbons and carbogen as oxygen substitutes and the use of hypoxic cell sensitizers. Normal tissue protection is another means for improving therapeutic gain. Sufhydryl-containing compounds are able to scavenge the hydroxyl radicals produced by radiation, which are thought to mediate radiation injury. Unfortunately, to date, both radioprotectors and hypoxic cell sensitizers have proved to be toxic and offer limited improvement over conventional treatment.

One of the major advances in the treatment of patients with gastrointestinal cancer has been the evolution of combined modality therapy. This includes the use of radiation therapy with surgery, chemotherapy, or both. Surgery is effective in removing bulk disease but would be expected to have a lower therapeutic index for subclinical disease. At doses that produce acceptable normal-tissue injury, radiation therapy is effective at eliminating small tumors and subclinical disease. Combinations of these local treatments can produce better locoregional control and improve survival. In Swedish trials evaluating preoperative irradiation and surgery, the combination improved local control and survival rates when compared to surgery alone.[13] Importantly,

combinations of radiation therapy and chemotherapy in gastrointestinal malignancies have resulted not only in improved local control but also in reductions in distant metastasis rates. In prospective randomized trials in patients with resected stage II and III rectal cancer, the combination of postoperative irradiation and 5-fluorouracil (5-FU)–based chemotherapy improved rates of local control and freedom from distant metastasis, compared with surgery, postoperative irradiation, or postoperative chemotherapy only. Similarly, in patients with advanced esophageal cancer, the combination of radiation therapy and chemotherapy (5-FU and cisplatin) has been shown to improve outcome, compared with radiation therapy only.[14] As combined modality therapy has become established in the management of patients with many different types of gastrointestinal malignancies, innovative efforts in defining the optimal sequence and administration of these modalities have been pursued to further enhance the therapeutic ratio. For example, in patients undergoing adjuvant therapy for stage II and III rectal cancer, the peripheral venous infusion of 5-FU during radiation therapy has resulted in an improved survival rate, compared with 3 consecutive days of bolus administration of 5-FU during the first and last weeks of radiation therapy.[15] With the development of new systemic agents (e.g., taxanes, gemcitabine, irinotecan), antiangiogenesis drugs, and targeted molecular agents (e.g., tyrosine kinase and farnesyl transferase inhibitors), a new era of clinical investigation of combined modality therapy has begun. One of the major goals in the next decade will be the integration of these agents with current modalities in the care of patients with gastrointestinal cancer.

## References

1. Tait DM, Nahum AE, Meyer LC, et al. Acute toxicity in pelvic radiotherapy: a randomized trial of conformal versus conventional treatment. Radiother Oncol 42:121–136, 1997.
2. Gunderson LL, Willett CG, Harrison LB, Calvo FA. Intraoperative Irradiation: Techniques and Results. Humana Press, 1999.
3. Suit HD, Krengli M. Basis for interest in proton beam radiation therapy. In: Amaldi U, Larsson B, Lemoigne Y (eds): Advances in Hadrontherapy. Elsevier Science B.V., Amsterdam, 1997, pp 29–37.
4. Lane DP. A death in the life of p53. Nature 362:786–787, 1993.
5. Clarke AR, Purdie CA, Harrison DJ, et al. Thymocyte apoptosis induced by p53-dependent and independent pathways. Nature 362:849–852, 1993.
6. Lowe SW, Bodis S, McClatchey A, et al. p53 status and the efficacy of cancer therapy in vivo. Science 266:807–810, 1994.
7. Terasima R, Tolmach LJ. X-ray sensitivity and DNA synthesis in synchronous populations of HeLa cells. Science 140:490–492, 1963.
8. Spiro IJ, Ling CC, Stickler R, Gaskill J. Oxygen radiosensitization at low dose rate. Br J Radiol 58:357–363, 1985.
9. Withers HR. Biological basis for altered fractionation schemes. Cancer 55:2086–2095, 1985.
10. Coucke PA, Cuttat JF, Mirimanoff RO. Adjuvant postoperative accelerated hyperfractionated radiotherapy in rectal cancer: a feasibility study. Int J Radiat Oncol Biol Phys 27:885–889, 1993.
11. Coucke PA, Sartorelli B, Cuttat JF, Jeanneret W, Gillet M, Mirimanoff RO. The rationale to switch from postoperative hyperfractionated accelerated radiotherapy to preoperative hyperfractionated accelerated radiotherapy in rectal cancer. Int J Radiat Oncol Biol Phys 32:181–188, 1995.
12. Movsas B, Hanlon A, Lanciano R, et al. Phase I dose escalating trial of hyperfractionated pre-operative chemoradiation for locally advanced rectal cancer. Int J Radiat Oncol Biol Phys 42:43–50, 1998.
13. Swedish Rectal Cancer Trial. Improved survival with preoperative radiotherapy in resectable rectal cancer. N Engl J Med 336:980–987, 1997.
14. Herskovic A, Martz LK, Al-Sarraf M, et al. Combined chemotherapy and radiotherapy compared with radiotherapy alone in patients with cancer of the esophagus. N Engl J Med 326:1593–1598, 1992.
15. O'Connell MJ, Martenson JA, Weiand HS, et al. Improving adjuvant therapy for rectal cancer by combining protracted infusion fluorouracil with radiation therapy after curative surgery. N Engl J Med 331:502–507, 1994.

# Chapter 8

# Therapeutic Principles of Gastrointestinal Neoplasia: Chemotherapy

HENRY Q. XIONG AND JAMES L. ABBRUZZESE

Cytotoxic chemotherapy has constituted a major modality in the treatment of cancer since its first use for cancer patients five decades ago. The clinical use of chemotherapy continues to expand as a result of the continuous discovery of new agents and their increasingly rational use. Chemotherapy can be given as a single agent or in combination with different cytotoxic agents or different treatment modalities, including radiation, vaccines, and novel targeted therapeutics. Chemotherapy is clearly part of the mainstream of treatment for metastatic and recurrent gastrointestinal malignancies. Its role in adjuvant therapy for a number of cancers has been well established, and neoadjuvant chemotherapy is actively being evaluated for the treatment of several gastrointestinal malignancies. As our knowledge of how to combine chemotherapy with other modalities improves and new agents are constantly added, the role of chemotherapy in the treatment of gastrointestinal malignancies will expand further.

## Tumor Cytokinetics, Resistance, and Chemotherapy

The study of cytokinetics has provided much of the theoretical basis for the development of current cytotoxic chemotherapy. Using murine leukemia as a model, Skipper and co-workers[1] discovered two important phenomena. First, tumor growth fits an exponential model. That is, at any given time, cells proliferate at a constant rate. Second, cytotoxic agents kill a fixed fraction of tumor cells regardless of tumor burden, commonly referred to as *log kill*. A treatment that reduces a tumor population from $10^6$ to $10^2$ cells should reduce a population of $10^4$ cells to one. The fraction of cells killed will increase as the dose of the cytotoxic agent increases. Therefore, to achieve maximal log kill, the cytotoxic agent should be used at the maximal tolerated dose, with repeat doses administered as soon as possible. Moreover, each agent

used in combination therapy should add its own log kill to the overall cytotoxic effect. Hence, combinations of different agents at the maximal tolerated doses given for a sufficient number of cycles should achieve the greatest log kill, potentially killing all tumor cells and rendering the patient cured. This reasoning has had a profound influence on the development of single agents as well as combination cytotoxic chemotherapy.

A large body of experimental and clinical evidence has demonstrated that human cancer growth does not follow a purely exponential growth model but instead follows a sigmoid-shaped Gompertzian curve as initially described by Gompertz.[2] Norton and Simon applied the Gompertzian growth model to describe the growth patterns of melanoma and mammary carcinoma.[3] Subsequently, Gompertzian growth has been validated for colorectal cancer as well as a variety of other human cancers.[4–6] As the Gompertzian growth curve predicts, small tumors have the greatest growth fraction, but only yield a small overall increase in cell number since the total cell number is small. At the other extreme, the total cell number is very large but the growth fraction is at a minimum. The decreased growth rate is the result of decreased cell proliferation rather than increased cell death.[7] In the middle portion of the curve, growth reaches a maximum because the product of cell number and proliferating cells reaches maximum. This model, often referred to as the *Norton-Simon model*,[8] has great implications for designing and understanding cytotoxic chemotherapy. According to Gomperztian growth kinetics, chemotherapy administered early in the cancer growth cycle should achieve a greater log kill than that administered at a later stage of cancer growth, because tumor cells proliferate faster at an early stage and proliferating cells are generally more sensitive to chemotherapy. This concept underlies the use of adjuvant therapy and early institution of chemotherapy when tumor burden is minimal and more cells are sensitive to chemotherapy.

However, this model also predicts that regrowth after each cycle of chemotherapy will be at its maximum when tumor burden is minimal, potentially counterbalancing the greater log kill effect and possibly limiting the efficacy of adjuvant or early institution of chemotherapy. Thus, based purely on a kinetic model, without considering biochemically resistant cells, it is challenging to cure cancer. In support of this notion, adjuvant chemotherapy for breast cancer has less effect on overall survival than on disease-free survival.[9] The explanation for this phenomenon is that institution of chemotherapy at an early stage or as an adjuvant therapy reduces tumor burden to a minimum, below that of clinically detectable disease, and thus the disease-free survival is prolonged. However, the residual tumor grows back and eventually becomes clinically evident recurrent or metastatic disease, causing death of the patient due to the physiologic effects of progressive cancer that kills the patient.

The heterogeneity of cancer cell populations and emerging resistance to cytotoxic agents further complicate cancer treatment. Substantial evidence suggests that drug-resistant mutations in tumor cells arise by a mechanism similar to that seen in microbial populations. That is, drug-resistant tumor cells arise spontaneously, independent of the selecting agent.[10] On the basis of this assumption, Goldie and Coldman[11] developed a mathematic model relating the drug sensitivity of a tumor to its spontaneous mutation rate. The model predicts that both the proportion and the absolute number of resistant cells increase with time and depend on the mutation rate and the time when mutation occurs. Moreover, for a given tumor with a non-zero mutation rate, the likelihood of there being at least one resistant cell will be increased from 5% to 95% within 5 doublings or a 2-log increase in tumor cells. Thus the expectation for cure of a tumor is a function of the spontaneous mutation rate of resistance and the size of the tumor at the time chemotherapy is initiated. To cure a cancer, chemotherapy should start at as small a tumor size as possible and should include as many drugs as possible provided there is no cross-resistance. If combination chemotherapy is precluded by overlapping toxicity, an alternating non–cross-resistant-chemotherapy regimen at each cycle would be the most effective strategy.[12] For example, treatments A and B are equally efficacious and non–cross-resistant but cannot be administered concurrently. Therefore, the best way to combine these two regimens will be ABAB, instead of any other fixed combination. In slow-growing tumors, such as most tumors arising from the gastrointestinal tract, the degree of heterogeneity and the extent of multiple levels of drug resistance are much greater than in faster-growing tumors, as predicted by Goldie and Coldman.[13] Thus the chances of eradication of a slow-growing tumor at an advanced stage (not necessarily a clinically advanced stage) by chemotherapy are even smaller.

Gastrointestinal malignancies, which have a wide range of chemosensitivity, are considered to be, as a group, the least sensitive to chemotherapy[14] because of the development of drug resistance. The development of resistance after exposure to one drug often confers resistance to a variety of drugs.[15] The mechanism that accounts for this phenomenon is the development of a multidrug-resistant (MDR) phenotype.[16] This phenotype is due to amplification of the *MDR1* gene, which is a member of the superfamily of genes encoding membrane transport proteins; one of them is P-glycoprotein. P-Glycoprotein acts as a drug efflux pump that actively transports drugs out of tumor cells, thereby preventing cytotoxic agents from reaching an effective intracellular level.[17] Although P-glycoprotein expression is induced upon exposure to drugs in most malignancies, gastrointestinal malignancies have high intrinsic expression of P-glycoprotein, and thus intrinsic resistance to chemotherapy. It has been speculated that P-glycoprotein may have a physiological function in the gastrointestinal tract. Increased expression of MDR1 mRNA and P-glycoprotein has been detected in untreated tumors from the esophagus, stomach, colon, liver, and pancreas.[18–20] The expression of P-glycoprotein in colon cancer has been documented to be a prognostic factor for tumor aggressiveness and resistance to cytotoxic agents.[21] There is less expression of P-glycoprotein in gastric cancers than in colorectal cancers, which may partially account for their differential chemosensitivity (gastric cancer is relatively more chemosensitive than colorectal cancer).[22,23]

P-glycoprotein is not the only mechanism of drug resistance in gastrointestinal malignancies. Another membrane transporter gene, designated *MDR-associated protein* (MRP), has recently been discovered.[24] MRP has a function similar to P-glycoprotein, and its overexpression confers an MDR phenotype similar to that of P-glycoprotein. Intrinsic expression of MRP mRNA was higher in colorectal cancer than in normal colorectal tissue, whereas expression levels were similar in gastric cancer and normal gastric tissue.[25] MRP expression was also detected in several pancreatic cancer cell lines that had little, if any, expression of P-glycoprotein.[26] The clinical significance of MRP expression, however, has not yet been defined.

Glutathione-*S*-transferase (GST) has been identified as a different mechanism that mediates intrinsic and acquired drug resistance. The GST enzymes are involved in an important pathway in detoxification of reactive oxygen species. Elevated intrinsic expression of GST proteins has been detected in colorectal cancer, gastric cancer, and esophageal cancer cell lines.[27–31] Studies on human cancer cell lines suggest that GST and MDR act together, leading to increased drug efflux and metabolism.[32]

In addition to genetic alterations that confer resistance to chemotherapy on tumor cells, physiological conditions and the three-dimensional structure of a solid tumor may affect the efficacy of chemotherapy as well.[33] A solid tumor consists of three components: malignant cells, the extracellular matrix, and the vasculature. The characteristics of the tumor vasculature and extracellular matrix will affect therapeutic agent delivery to the tumor cells as well as the efficacy of the agent. A solid tumor has a heterogeneous perfusion with a well-vascularized periphery and a blood vessel–depleted central necrotic area. Moreover, there are increased transvascular and interstitial pressure gradients in the tumor compared with the surrounding tissue.[34] Therefore, the delivery of a therapeutic agent to tumor cells is adversely affected.

Tissue oxygenation and the pH of a solid tumor may also affect therapeutic response.[35,36] It is well known that tissue radiosensitivity depends on oxygen tension.[37] The influence of oxygenation on the efficacy of cytotoxic agents is more complicated. Some agents, such as doxorubicin, 5-fluorouracil (5-FU), vincristine, and carboplatin, seem to be more toxic to well-oxygenated tumor cells. However, other agents, including mitomycin C and misonidazole, are more toxic to less-oxygenated tumor cells.[38] Moreover, hypoxia slows cell proliferation that may indirectly decrease the efficacy of a cytotoxic agent. By the same mechanism, low pH values may also decrease the efficacy of cytotoxic agents such as doxorubicin and bleomycin.[39]

Study of the mechanism of tumor growth kinetics and resistance has greatly enriched our knowledge of chemotherapy. However, there are only a few active agents against gastrointestinal malignancies because of intrinsic resistance. Much effort should be focused on looking for active new agents. Meanwhile, applying basic knowledge to currently available active agents will optimize their usage.

## Clinical Uses of Chemotherapy

### Adjuvant Chemotherapy

Surgery remains the only possible cure for gastrointestinal malignancies, although recurrence after surgery is a common event, depending on the stage, anatomic site, and lymph node involvement of the tumor. Once recurrent or metastatic disease occurs, chemotherapy or combined modality offers little hope for cure, emphasizing the important role of adjuvant therapy. The development of recurrent or metastatic disease after the primary tumor has been surgically removed is widely believed to be due to the existence of micrometastasis or residual local disease.[40–42] Adjuvant chemotherapy can eradicate the micrometastasis or residual disease, thus increasing the cure rate or prolonging survival. The theoretical advantages of adjuvant chemotherapy are very compelling.[43,44] On the basis of the theory of tumor cytokinetics and drug resistance, a tumor at its early growth (micrometastasis) would be expected to be more sensitive to chemotherapy and less likely to develop resistance to cytotoxic agents. Clinical data have documented the effectiveness of adjuvant chemotherapy in treating tumors arising from the colon,[45] rectum,[45,46] and pancreas[47] but not those from the esophagus,[48] stomach,[48,49] or liver.[50]

The selection of patients for adjuvant chemotherapy is dictated by the risk of recurrence. It is therefore not surprising that patients with a high risk of recurrence benefit most. Studies on colorectal cancer have demonstrated that adjuvant chemotherapy confers a survival advantage for patients with stage III disease, although subsets of patients with stage II disease may benefit as well.[51] Cytotoxic agents used in adjuvant chemotherapy are generally selected from among those that have demonstrated efficacy in the metastatic setting. In most cases where adjuvant therapy shows efficacy in the metastatic setting, it is also highly active against advanced disease. Only a few regimens are active against gastrointestinal malignancies: 5-FU combined with leucovorin or levamisole is used for colon cancer; 5-FU combined with radiation is used for rectal and pancreatic cancer; and gemcitabine has shown superiority over 5-FU for metastatic pancreatic cancer[52] (its use in adjuvant and neoadjuvant settings is a focus of active study).[53] Dose and dose intensity (dose per unit time) are important variables that determine the efficacy of a therapy.[54,55] It has been clearly demonstrated that an increase in dose intensity results in better survival for patients with breast cancer.[56,57] Clinical experience in colorectal cancer also supports the use of high doses of 5-FU and leucovorin.[58,59] The timing of therapy may also affect treatment outcome. Adjuvant therapy is usually initiated 3–6 weeks after surgery to allow sufficient time for recovery. Previous experimental studies suggest that earlier initiation of adjuvant therapy usually results in better outcomes.[60]

Adjuvant chemotherapy is not recommended for esophageal, gastric, or liver cancer except in the context of a clinical trial, since there is no established active regimen so far.

### Neoadjuvant Chemotherapy

Neoadjuvant chemotherapy is a component of a multidisciplinary treatment strategy that involves systemic chemotherapy first, followed by local therapy with either surgery or radiation.[61] The main purpose of neoadjuvant chemotherapy is to downstage the primary tumor, thus rendering it resectable or decreasing the extent of surgery required and hence improving the cosmetic and functional outcome. There are other theoretical benefits to neoadjuvant chemotherapy.[62] Neoadjuvant chemotherapy acts on micrometastasis just as adjuvant chemotherapy does. Treatment is administrated while the primary tumor is present so that response can be assessed and therapy continued only in patients who respond. If the primary tumor responds to the regimen, one can assume that micrometastic disease will also respond. Moreover, patients are more likely to receive the planned dose of chemotherapy on schedule since they will not have the problems often encountered in the adjuvant setting, such as surgery-related complications or delayed recovery. Finally, patients who have progressive disease can be identified and spared unnecessary surgery, or alternative therapy can be initiated sooner.

Neoadjuvant therapy also has potential disadvantages. First, patients who present with a localized tumor but have progressive disease during neoadjuvant therapy may miss the chance for cure by surgery. Second, because of the continued presence of the primary tumor there is a theoretical risk of developing micrometastasis during neoadjuvant therapy that otherwise would have been removed. Third, the precise pathologic stage may be altered, and consequently the information needed to recommend further therapy may be obscured.

Neoadjuvant chemotherapy has been used to treat head and neck cancer, breast cancer, bladder cancer, and sarcoma, since the preservation of organ function and cosmetic considerations are of great concern owing to the location of these tumors. However, its use in gastrointestinal malignancies is still largely experimental, and it is often combined with radiation. Neoadjuvant therapy has been used successfully in patients with rectal cancer with the particular intent to preserve sphincter function as well as decrease local recurrence and improve survival. Several studies reported that neoadjuvant therapy resulted in downstaging of the tumor and therefore in an increase in sphincter-preserving surgery.[63,64] An ongoing clinical trial to evaluate the role of neoadjuvant therapy will likely confirm the positive role of neoadjuvant therapy for sphincter preservation.[65] Clinical studies on both esophageal and gastric cancers found that patients who received neoadjuvant therapy had no greater survival benefit than those who received surgery alone.[66–69] However, patients with gastric cancer who responded to neoadjuvant therapy (24%–38%) did have a survival advantage over those who do not respond,[70] indicating the need for more active neoadjuvant regimens. Clinical studies on pancreatic cancer have demonstrated that neoadjuvant therapy is feasible and safe.[71,72] One study showed that patients who received neoadjuvant chemoradiation and intraoperative radiation had low local recurrence rates.[73] Ongoing studies will establish the role of neoadjuvant therapy for pancreatic cancer.[74]

At the present time, except for rectal cancer, neoadjuvant therapy is not recommended for patients with gastrointestinal malignancies, except within clinical trials.

### Combination Chemotherapy

Studies of tumor growth kinetics and drug resistance, as discussed above, predict that combination chemotherapy is better than single-agent therapy. This is particularly true for hematologic malignancies and germ cell tumors, for which almost all of the curative therapies are combination chemotherapy.[14] However, combination chemotherapy is less successful in gastrointestinal malignancies, simply because of a lack of active single agents. In an ideal combination, the individual agents act synergistically so that the net cytotoxic effect is more than the sum of the individual agents without a simultaneous increase of toxicity. The outcome of combination chemotherapy is determined by many variables, including the activity, cross-resistance, and side-effect profiles of individual agents and their interactions. Of these variables, the activity of individual agents is the major determinant of a successful combination regimen. Generally, an agent achieving a partial response rate of less than 20% when used alone contributes little to combinations other than toxicity.[14]

Dose response is another important factor to consider. A less optimal combination may result from a compromised dose of individual agents used in combination primarily because of concerns about toxicity. Individual agents with different mechanisms of cytotoxicity and drug resistance should be included in combination. Unfortunately, as discussed previously, gastrointestinal malignancies have high intrinsic mutltidrug resistance rates. Only a limited number of single agents have documented activity, which is a major obstacle in designing combination regimens. Overlapping toxicity also limits the development of combinations. The strategy of decreasing the dose of individual agents or prolonging the dose interval to decrease dose-limiting toxicity may also compromise efficacy. When bone marrow suppression is the dose-limiting toxicity, hematopoietic growth factors may be used to overcome toxicity.

Lack of active single agents has been the major reason for failure of combination regimens in treating gastrointestinal malignancies. Although several combination regimens have been studied in pancreatic cancer, none showed better efficacy than 5-FU alone in terms of prolonged survival.[75] Studies on gastric, esophageal, and colorectal cancers have demonstrated similar disappointing results.[76] The recent addition of new agents such as irinotecan, oxaliplatin, and gemcitabine offers investigators the opportunity to develop new combination therapies. Gemcitabine combined with other agents in the treatment of pancreatic cancer is one focus of active study.[74] Irinotecan combined with 5-FU and leucovorin[77] and irinotecan combined with oxaliplatin[78] have shown activity against colorectal cancer.

## Regional Therapy

The goal of regional therapy is to improve drug delivery to tumors confined to an anatomical site, thus increasing efficacy while simultaneously minimizing systemic drug delivery and hence systemic toxicity. Regional therapy, mainly hepatic arterial infusion and intraperitoneal chemotherapy, has been used for gastrointestinal malignancies for many years. Its value, however, is still debatable.[79]

### Hepatic Arterial Infusion

Hepatic arterial infusion (HAI) has several advantages, especially from a pharmacological point of view. Both primary and metastatic hepatic tumors larger than 3 cm depend on the hepatic artery for their blood supply, while normal hepatic tissue obtains its blood supply mainly through the portal vein.[80] The cytotoxic agent delivered through the hepatic artery will not only be concentrated in the hepatic tumor but also be extracted and metabolized by the liver on the first pass, thus producing a lower systemic drug level and less systemic toxicity. Consequently, higher doses of cytotoxic agents can be delivered to tumors through HAI than through systemic therapy. Local drug delivery can further be increased through blocking blood flow. One way of blocking blood flow is to inject drug concurrently with degradable starch microspheres that plug up circulation temporarily; serum amylase gradually degrades the microspheres within 20 to 40 minutes, therefore allowing slow drug release.[81] This technique is frequently referred to as *chemoembolization.* Furthermore, studies have demonstrated that the liver is frequently the first or only site of metastasis from gastrointestinal malignancies, especially colon cancer.[82] Thus the liver is a perfect target for regional therapy.

A number of clinical trials have consistently found that HAI offers higher response rates than systemic therapy for hepatic metastases from colon cancer.[83–86] The response rate is usually more than twice that achieved by systemic therapy: studies of HAI have reported an impressive 50% response, while systemic therapy offered less than 20% response. However, HAI has had less effect on survival because of frequent extrahepatic relapse and progression, resulting in a median survival similar to that following systemic therapy. Hepatic arterial infusion has been used to treat other gastrointestinal cancers, including hepatocellular carcinoma[87–89] and pancreatic cancer.[90–93] A number of clinical trials showed survival benefits for patients with pancreatic cancer treated with HAI compared with systemic therapy. In addition, quality of life generally improved during therapy even if there was no prolongation of survival. However, the available data are not sufficient to justify routine use because of the small number of patients included in the studies. Despite causing minimal systemic toxicity, HAI is associated with local toxicity and complications. Chemical hepatitis and biliary sclerosis are fairly common events, especially when floxuridine (FUDR) is used.[94] Complications related to implantation of implantable pumps, hepatic artery thrombosis, dislocation of catheter tip, and pump dysfunction are occasional events and often associated with surgical expertise.[95]

### Intraperitoneal Chemotherapy

The peritoneal surface and the liver are common anatomic sites for treatment failure after surgical resection.[96–98] Up to 44% of patients who underwent curative resection for colorectal cancer were found to have peritoneal carcinomatosis at a second-look procedure.[97]

The pharmacological rationale for intraperitoneal chemotherapy has been well established.[99] The peritoneal cavity can be thought as a dialysis membrane through which substances pass by virtue of their size, charge, lipid solubility, and molecular weight. The peritoneal clearance of a drug is inversely proportional to its molecular weight. Therefore, large molecules, such as many cytotoxic agents, take longer to clear from the cavity than small ones. Once a drug is cleared from the peritoneal membrane, it will mainly be delivered into the liver through portal circulation. Thus, the liver is also a target of intraperitoneal chemotherapy, although it can be argued that most of the blood supply to hepatic metastases is derived from the hepatic arteries. Intracellular drug concentration after intraperitoneal drug administration depends on diffusion. A drug given in this manner can reach only the top four to six layers of cells in tumor masses.[100] Beyond six cell layers, drug diffusion into tumor masses is minimal and does not offer any advantage over systemic drug administration. Thus, intraperitoneal chemotherapy would appear to benefit patients with microscopic tumors or very small gross nodules on the peritoneal surface. Large nodules

(0.5 cm) would probably not be exposed to adequate drug concentrations. Although the peritoneal cavity is a confined space, the drug distribution is imperfect. To ensure distribution throughout the entire peritoneum, large volumes of solution (enough to cause clinical distention) should be used. Drug distribution is further compromised by adhesions, a natural fibrotic reaction to surgery and plastic catheters.

Despite the sound pharmacological rationale, the efficacy of intraperitoneal chemotherapy has not been sufficiently evaluated in clinical trials since most phase I clinical trials are restricted to small numbers of patients and few phase II studies on established peritoneal carcinomatosis have been published. Sugarbaker and co-workers[101] randomly assigned patients with advanced colorectal cancer to receive 5-FU systemically or intraperitoneally. No difference was found in disease-free interval or survival between the two groups, although patients treated intraperitoneally had a lower incidence of peritoneal carcinomatosis.

Analysis of the mechanism of peritoneal tumor spread has provided the rationale for intraperitoneal chemotherapy as an adjuvant therapy. Intraperitoneal spread of tumor cells can occur prior to surgery by direct tumor invasion or leakage of tumor cells from lymphatics. It can also occur during perioperative mobilization and surgical dissection. Moreover, fibrin entrapment of intraabdominal tumor emboli on a traumatized peritoneal surface and tumor promotion of these entrapped cells through growth factors involved in the wound healing process may also contribute to the intraperitoneal diffusion of the tumor.[102] Thus, the best timing of intraperitoneal chemotherapy would be perioperatively when there is only microscopic residual disease. Moreover, since drug delivered intraperitoneally can penetrate only a few cell layers, it makes sense to use it as an adjuvant therapy. Several clinical trials have shown promising results in patients with resectable gastrointestinal malignancies. Scheithauer and co-workers[103] compared systemic adjuvant chemotherapy with systemic plus intraperitoneal chemotherapy in patients with resected colon cancer. In this clinical trial, patients treated with systemic and intraperitoneal chemotherapy had improved disease-free survival and overall survival, with an estimated 43% reduction in the mortality rate. Yu and colleagues[104] reported that the 5-year survival for patients with stage III stomach cancer who underwent surgery plus adjuvant intraperitoneal chemotherapy was 49% compared with 18% for those who received surgery only. Given these encouraging results, further clinical evaluation is certainly warranted.

## Chemoradiation

Surgery is the only modality that offers a potential cure for gastrointestinal malignancies. However, it is indicated only for patients who present with localized disease, and recurrence is common after curative resection. Patients with locally advanced unresectable but nonmetastatic disease and those who cannot undergo surgery frequently receive definitive radiation therapy. Radiation usually provides temporal local control of disease but plays a limited role in prolonging survival or cure. Chemotherapy used for metastatic diseases or as adjuvant treatment adds limited value in treating gastrointestinal malignancies. Given the limitations of surgery, chemotherapy, and radiation as single modalities, the use of chemotherapy combined with radiation (chemoradiation) has become common in treating gastrointestinal malignancies.

Radiation and chemotherapy have complementary actions.[105,106] Tumor cells develop resistance to chemotherapy and to radiation by similar mechanisms, but generally the two forms of resistance do not overlap. Thus combined radiation with chemotherapy offers the potential to eradicate subpopulations within a tumor that might resist either single modality. Moreover, systemically delivered chemotherapy will affect not only the primary tumor but also established distant metastasis or micrometastasis that would not be accessible to radiation, thus decreasing distant failure. Furthermore, combining chemotherapy with radiation will have a complementary effect on primary tumors. Locally advanced solid tumors have a tendency to develop hypoxic and avascular central areas that are resistant to radiation and inaccessible to chemotherapeutic agents. Fractionated radiation will shrink the tumor and thus might improve vascular access to initially large tumors by chemotherapeutic agents. The remaining tumor cells may proliferate more rapidly in response to radiation damage, thus becoming more vulnerable to chemotherapy because of the increased fraction of proliferating cells. Chemotherapy, by contrast, may improve oxygenation by killing subpopulations of cells and shrinking the tumor, thus enhancing the radiation effect.

Chemotherapy may also function as a radiosensitizer to enhance the radiation effect through a variety of mechanisms. DNA is a critical target of radiation damage, with double-strand DNA breaks being the lethal lesions. This effect is counterbalanced by DNA repair. Therefore, drugs that inhibit DNA repair machinery should enhance the radiation effect. Several drugs, including hydroxyurea, 5-FU, cisplatin, and irinotecan, have been shown to inhibit DNA repair or increase the damage caused by radiation.[107–110] Cells vary in their response to radiation as a function of their phase in the cell cycle, with cells in $G_2/M$ phase being threefold more sensitive than cells in late $S/G_1$ phase.[111] A chemotherapeutic agent that imposes cell-cycle block at $G_2/M$ phase would sensitize the cell population to radiation effect. Studies have shown that the taxanes capable of arresting cells at the $G_2/M$ phase have radiosensitization effects on several tumor cell lines.[112–114] Furthermore, chemotherapeutic agents such as 5-FU, doxorubicin, and paclitaxel can reduce the threshold of cells to the radiation effect. In other words, tumor cells exposed to these drugs are more sensitive to the cytotoxic effect of radiation, resulting in a left shift of the survival curve.[106] Lastly, apoptosis is one of the mechanisms by which cells respond to radiation. Drugs that induce apoptosis, such as paclitaxel and gemcitabine, will enhance the radiation effect.[115,116]

Chemoradiation has been used as adjuvant or neoadjuvant therapy for resectable tumors, definitive therapy for locally advanced but nonmetastatic tumors, and palliation for symptomatic metastatic or recurrent diseases. The efficacy of chemoradiation over radiation or chemotherapy alone has been demonstrated in anal and rectal cancers and pancreatic cancer.[117–120] Its efficacy in gastric and esophageal cancer, however, is less well defined.[66,121–123] 5-FU is the drug most commonly used in combination with radiation to treat gastrointestinal malignancies. Several other chemotherapeutic agents that have demonstrated in vitro efficacy as radiation sensitizers, including taxanes, irinotecan, and gemcitabine, are being actively investigated for the treatment of gastrointestinal malignancies.[124–126]

## Assessment of Response and Toxicity

Assessment of the efficacy of chemotherapy is dictated by the goal of such therapy. The goal of adjuvant chemotherapy is to decrease recurrence and increase cure. Thus the efficacy is measured by overall and relapse-free survival. In addition to the goals mentioned above, the intent of neoadjuvant therapy is also to downstage the primary tumor and to preserve organ function. As-

Prevention of metastatic spread by postoperative immunotherapy with virally modified autologous tumor cells. III. Postoperative activation of tumor-specific CTLP from mice with metastases requires stimulation with the specific antigen plus additional signals. Invasion Metastasis 9:117–33, 1989.

43. Ockert D, Schirrmacher V, Beck N, et al. Newcastle disease virus-infected intact autologous tumor cell vaccine for adjuvant active specific immunotherapy of resected colorectal carcinoma. Clin Cancer Res 2: 21–28, 1996.

44. Patel BT, Lutz MB, Schlas P, Schirrmacher V. An analysis of autologous T-cell anti-tumour responses in colon-carcinoma patients following active specific immunization (ASI). Int J Cancer 51:878–885, 1992.

45. Woodlock TJ, Sahasrabudhe DM, Marquis DM, Greene D, Pandya KJ, McCune CS. Active specific immunotherapy for metastatic colorectal carcinoma: phase I study of an allogeneic cell vaccine plus low-dose interleukin-1 alpha. J Immunother 22:251–259, 1999.

46. Riethmuller G, Schneider-Gadicke E, Schlimok G, et al. Randomized trial of monoclonal antibody for adjuvant therapy of resected Dukes' C colorectal carcinoma. German Cancer CO17-1A Study Group. Lancet 343:1177–1183, 1994.

47. Riethmuller G, Holz E, Schlimok G, et al. Monoclonal antibody therapy for resected Dukes' C colorectal cancer: seven-year outcome of a multicenter randomized trial. J Clin Oncol 16:1788–1794, 1998.

48. Litvinov V, Velders MP, Bakker HA, Flenren GJ, Warnaar SO. Ep-CAM: a human epithelial antigen is a homophilic cell-cell adhesion molecule. J Cell Biol 125:437–446, 1994.

49. Li W, Berencsi K, Basak S, et al. Human colorectal cancer (CRC) antigen CO17-1A/GA733 encoded by adenovirus inhibits growth of established CRC cells in mice. J Immunol 159:763–769, 1997.

50. Basak S, Speicher D, Eck S, et al. Colorectal carcinoma invasion inhibition by CO17-1A/GA733 antigen and its murine homologue. J Natl Cancer Inst 90:691–697, 1998.

51. Takamuku K, Baba K, Arinaga S, Li J, Mori M, Akiyoshi T. Apoptosis in antibody-dependent monocyte-mediated cytotoxicity with monoclonal antibody 17-1A against human colorectal carcinoma cells: enhancement with interferon gamma. Cancer Immunol Immunother 43:220–225, 1996.

52. Wettendorff M, Iliopoulos D, Tempero M, et al. Idiotypic cascades in cancer patients treated with monoclonal antibody CO17-1A. Proc Natl Acad Sci USA 86:3787–3791, 1989.

53. Herlyn D, Wettendorff M, Iliopoulos D, Schmoll E, Schedel I, Koprowski H. Modulation of cancer patients' immune responses by administration of anti-idiotypic antibodies. Viral Immunol 2:271–276, 1989.

54. Tempero MA, Pour PM, Uchida E, Herlyn D, Steplewski Z. Monoclonal antibody CO17-1A and leukapheresis in immunotherapy of pancreatic cancer. Hybridoma 5 (Suppl 1):S133–138, 1986.

55. Ragnhammar P, Fagerberg J, Frodin JE, et al. Effect of monoclonal antibody 17-1A and GM-CSF in patients with advanced colorectal carcinoma—long-lasting, complete remissions can be induced. Int J Cancer 53:751–758, 1993.

56. Austin EB, Robins RA, Baldwin RW, Durrant LG. Induction of delayed hypersensitivity to human tumor cells with a human monoclonal anti-idiotypic antibody. J Natl Cancer Inst 83:1245–1248, 1991.

57. Durrant LG, Buckley TJ, Denton GW, Hardcastle JD, Sewell HF, Robins RA. Enhanced cell-mediated tumor killing in patients immunized with human monoclonal antiidiotypic antibody 105AD7. Cancer Res 54: 4837–4840, 1994.

58. Robins RA, Denton GW, Hardcastle JD, Austin EB, Baldwin RW, Durrant LG. Antitumor immune response and interleukin 2 production induced in colorectal cancer patients by immunization with human monoclonal anti-idiotypic antibody. Cancer Res 51:5425–5429, 1991.

59. Denton GW, Durrant LG, Hardcastle JD, Austin EB, Sewell HF, Robbins RA. Clinical outcome of colorectal cancer patients treated with human monoclonal anti-idiotypic antibody. Int J Cancer 57:10–14, 1994.

60. Fagerberg J, Steinitz M, Wigzell H, Askelof P, Mellstedt H. Human anti-idiotypic antibodies induced a humoral and cellular immune response against a colorectal carcinoma-associated antigen in patients. Proc Natl Acad Sci USA 92:4773–4777, 1995.

61. Somasundaram R, Zaloudik J, Jacob L, et al. Induction of antigen-specific T and B cell immunity in colon carcinoma patients by anti-idiotypic antibody. J Immunol 155:3253–3261, 1995.

62. Herlyn D, Somasundaram R, Zaloudik J, et al. Cloned antigens and anti-idiotypes. Hybridoma 14:159–166, 1995.

63. Gold P, Freedman SO. Demonstration of tumor-specific antigens in human colonic carcinoma by immunological tolerance and absorption techniques. J Exp Med 121:439–462, 1965.

64. Clinical practice guidelines for the use of tumor markers in breast and colorectal cancer. Adopted on May 17, 1996 by the American Society of Clinical Oncology. J Clin Oncol 14:2843–2877, 1996.

65. von Kleist S, King M, and Havemann K. Demonstration of antibodies in patients' sera, directed against nonspecific cross-reacting antigen. J Natl Cancer Inst 61:1385–1391, 1978.

66. Mavligit GM, Gutterman JU, McBride CM, Hersh EM. Cell-mediated immunity to human solid tumors: in vitro detection by lymphocyte blastogenic responses to cell-associated and solubilized tumor antigens. Natl Cancer Inst Monogr 37:167–176, 1973.

67. Williams AF, Barclay AN. The immunoglobulin superfamily—domains for cell surface recognition. Annu Rev Immunol 6:381–405, 1988.

68. Zimmermann W, Ortlieb B, Friedrich R, von Kleist S. Isolation and characterization of cDNA clones encoding the human carcinoembryonic antigen reveal a highly conserved repeating structure. Proc Natl Acad Sci USA 84:2960–2964, 1987.

69. Thompson JA, Pande H, Paxton RJ, et al. Molecular cloning of a gene belonging to the carcinoembryonic antigen gene family and discussion of a domain model. Proc Natl Acad Sci USA 84:2965–2969, 1987.

70. Hostetter RB, Campbell DE, Chi K, et al. Carcinoembryonic antigen enhances metastatic potential of human colorectal carcinoma. Arch Surg 125:300–304, 1990.

71. Moudgil KD, Southwood S, Ametani A, Kim K, Sette A, Sercarz EE. The self-directed T cell repertoire against mouse lysozyme reflects the influence of the hierarchy of its own determinants and can be engaged by a foreign lysozyme. J Immunol 163:4232–4237, 1999.

72. Corman JM, Sercarz EE, Nanda NK. Recognition of prostate-specific antigenic peptide determinants by human CD4 and CD8 T cells. Clin Exp Immunol 114:166–172, 1998.

73. Foon KA, Yannelli J, Bhattacharya-Chatterjee M. Colorectal cancer as a model for immunotherapy. Clin Cancer Res 5:225–236, 1999.

74. Bhattacharya-Chatterjee M, Mukerjee S, Biddle W, Foon KA, Kohler H. Murine monoclonal anti-idiotype antibody as a potential network antigen for human carcinoembryonic antigen. J Immunol 145:2758–2765, 1990.

75. Foon KA, John WJ, Chakraborty M, et al. Clinical and immune responses in resected colon cancer patients treated with anti-idiotype monoclonal antibody vaccine that mimics the carcinoembryonic antigen. J Clin Oncol 17:2889–2895, 1999.

76. Pervin S, Chakraborty M, Bhattacharya-Chatterjee M, Zeytin H, Foon KA, Chatterjee SK. Induction of antitumor immunity by an anti-idiotype antibody mimicking carcinoembryonic antigen. Cancer Res 57:728–734, 1997.

77. Foon KA, Chakraborty M, John WJ, Sherratt A, Kohler H, Bhattacharya-Chatterjee M. Immune response to the carcinoembryonic antigen in patients treated with an anti-idiotype antibody vaccine. J Clin Invest 96: 334–342, 1995.

78. Foon KA, John WJ, Chakraborty M, et al. Clinical and immune responses in advanced colorectal cancer patients treated with anti-idiotype monoclonal antibody vaccine that mimics the carcinoembryonic antigen. Clin Cancer Res 3:1267–1276, 1997.

79. Foon KA, John WJ, Chakraborty M, et al. Clinical and immune responses in surgically resected colorectal cancer (CRC) patients treated with an anti-idiotype (Id) monoclonal antibody that mimics carcinoembryonic antigen (CEA) with or without 5-fluorouracil. Proc Am Soc Clin Oncol 17:435a, 1998.

80. Chatterjee SK, Tripathi PK, Chakraborty M, et al. Molecular mimicry of carcinoembryonic antigen by peptides derived from the structure of an anti-idiotype antibody. Cancer Res 58:1217–1224, 1998.

81. Schlom J. Carcinoembryonic antigen (CEA) peptides and vaccines for carcinoma. In: Kast WM (ed): Peptide-based Cancer Vaccines. Landes Bioscience, Georgetown, TX, 2000, pp 90–105.

82. Kantor J, Irvine K, Abrams S, Kaufman H, DiPietro J, Schlom J. Antitumor activity and immune responses induced by a recombinant carcinoembryonic antigen vaccinia virus vaccine. J Natl Cancer Inst 84: 1084–1091, 1992.

83. Tsang KY, Zaremba S, Nieroda CA, Zhu MZ, Hamilton JM, Schlom Jr. Generation of human cytotoxic T cells specific for human carcinoembryonic antigen epitopes from patients immunized with recombinant vaccinia-CEA vaccine. J Natl Cancer Inst 87:982–990, 1995.

84. Kantor JR, Irvine K, Abrams S, et al. Immunogenicity and safety of a recombinant vaccinia virus vaccine expressing the carcinoembryonic antigen gene in a nonhuman primate. Cancer Res 52:6917–6925, 1992.

85. McAneny D, Ryan CA, Beazley RM, Kaufman HL. Results of phase I trial of a recombinant vaccinia virus that expresses carcinoembryonic antigen in patients with advanced colorectal cancer. Ann Surg Oncol 3:495–500, 1996.

86. Tsang KY, Zhu MZ, Nieroda CA, et al. Phenotypic stability of a cytotoxic T-cell line directed against an immunodominant epitope of human carcinoembryonic antigen. Clin Cancer Res 3:2439–2449, 1997.

87. Marshall JL, Hawkins MJ, Tsang KY, et al. Phase I study in cancer patients of a replication-defective avipox recombinant vaccine that expresses human carcinoembryonic antigen. J Clin Oncol 17:332–337, 1999.

88. Hodge JW, McLaughlin JP, Kantor JA, Schlom J. Diversified prime and boost protocols using recombinant vaccinia virus and recombinant non-replicating avian pox virus to enhance T-cell immunity and antitumor responses. Vaccine 15:759–768, 1997.

89. Disis ML, Bernhard H, Shiota FM, et al. Granulocyte-macrophage colony-stimulating factor: an effective adjuvant for protein and peptide-based vaccines. Blood 88:202–210, 1996.

90. Conry RM, LoBuglio AF, Loechel F, et al. A carcinoembryonic antigen polynucleotide vaccine for human clinical use. Cancer Gene Ther 2: 33–38, 1995.

91. Tanaka F, Fujie T, Tahara K, et al. Induction of antitumor cytotoxic T lymphocytes with a MAGE-3-encoded synthetic peptide presented by human leukocytes antigen-A24. Cancer Res 57:4465–4468, 1997.

92. Kawashima I, Hudson SJ, Tsai V, et al. The multi-epitope approach for immunotherapy for cancer: identification of several CTL epitopes from various tumor-associated antigens expressed on solid epithelial tumors. Hum Immunol 59:1–14, 1998.

93. Barnd DL, Lan MS, Metzgar RS, Finn OJ. Specific, major histocompatibility complex–unrestricted recognition of tumor-associated mucins by human cytotoxic T cells. Proc Natl Acad Sci USA 86:7159–7163, 1989.

94. Andrews CW Jr, Jessup JM, Goldman H, et al. Localization of tumor-associated glycoprotein DF3 in normal, inflammatory, and neoplastic lesions of the colon. Cancer 72:3185-3190, 1993.

95. Nakamori S, Ota DM, Cleary KR, Shirotani K, Irimura T. MUC1 mucin expression as a marker of progression and metastasis of human colorectal carcinoma. Gastroenterology 106:353–361, 1994.

96. MacLean GD, Reddish MA, Koganty RR, Longenecker BM. Antibodies against mucin-associated sialyl-Tn epitopes correlate with survival of metastatic adenocarcinoma patients undergoing active specific immunotherapy with synthetic STn vaccine. J Immunother Emphasis Tumor Immunol 19:59–68, 1996.

97. Akagi J, Nakagawa K, Egami H, Ogawa M. Induction of HLA-unrestricted and HLA-class-II–restricted cytotoxic T lymphocytes against MUC-1 from patients with colorectal carcinomas using recombinant MUC-1vaccinia virus. Cancer Immunol Immunother 47:21–31, 1998.

98. Triozzi PL, Kim JA, Aldrich WA, Young DC, Sampsel JN, Martin EW Jr. Localization of tumor-reactive lymph node lymphocytes in vivo using radiolabeled monoclonal antibody. Cancer 73:580–589, 1994.

99. Kim JA, Bresler HS, Martin EW Jr, Aldrich W, Heffelfinger M, Triozzi PL. Cellular immunotherapy for patients with metastatic colorectal carcinoma using lymph node lymphocytes localized in vivo by radiolabeled monoclonal antibody. Cancer 86:22–30, 1999.

# Chapter 10

# Therapeutic Principles of Gastrointestinal Neoplasia
## Emerging Therapies: Gene Therapy

RICHARD J. ASPINALL AND NICHOLAS R. LEMOINE

If gene therapy is to prove an effective weapon against cancer, then where better to start than in the gastrointestinal tract? Not only are the abdominal viscera collectively the most common site of human malignancy, but cancers of these organs are perhaps the best understood of all. In particular, we now know a great deal about the precise molecular genetics of colonic and pancreatic cancers, and this knowledge opens up a whole range of potential targets for gene therapy approaches. Furthermore, the easy access to most parts of the gastrointestinal tract by endoscopic intubation means that local application of novel therapies is that much easier. In this chapter, we will explain the basic principles of gene therapy and highlight some important areas where these novel treatments are being explored.

## What Is Gene Therapy?

The term *gene therapy* can be applied to any therapeutic procedure in which genes are introduced into human somatic cells. A whole decade has elapsed since the first reported gene therapy study, in which patents with malignant melanoma were treated with retrovirally modified tumor-infiltrating lymphocytes.[1] As occurs with many new technologies, the initial euphoria over gene therapy was followed by some disillusionment as the replacement of defective genes proved more difficult than was at first thought. Gradual improvements in gene delivery technology and advances in our understanding of the molecular pathology of neoplasia are starting to renew our optimism regarding the use of anticancer gene therapy.[2] Most studies to date have used one of two approaches. In vivo gene therapy involves the administration of genes to target tissues within the whole living organism. A more direct method is to use ex vivo gene transfer in which cells (typically of hematological origin) are removed from the body, genetically modified, and reinfused. More recently, a

third option has arisen from the discovery that injected genetic material can evoke potent immune responses, giving rise to the concept of DNA vaccination. With these aims, gene therapy could theoretically be applied to Mendelian monogenetic diseases or to illnesses with a complex multigenetic basis or used to limit the effects of acquired genetic damage (Table 10–1).

The transfer of therapeutic genes is made possible by packaging the nucleic acid into a delivery vehicle or *vector*, which may be either a virus or a plasmid, or the DNA itself may be coated onto synthetic particles that can be fired into the target tissues using a "gene gun." The genetic construct should also contain a regulatory element to control the expression of the relevant gene. The use of tissue-specific promoter sequences is one method by which gene therapy can be targeted to a particular site.

## Vectors and Routes of Delivery

As perhaps the most critical element of any successful gene therapy approach, the choice of vector is all important. There are a number of different methods of delivery available (Table 10–2), although the vast majority of gene therapies use a viral approach.

### Plasmid DNA

In the future, injectable plasmid DNA is likely to be increasingly used in genetic vaccination,[3] a strategy that can evoke potent immune responses against the antigen encoded by the genetic sequence. DNA vaccines are being explored as anticancer immunotherapies[4] and also as a way of increasing the protection against potentially oncogenic infective pathogens such as the hepatitis B and C viruses.[5,6] After injection of the plasmid into skeletal muscle or the subcutaneous tissues, the DNA can be taken up

**Table 10-1** Therapeutic strategies in gene therapy

| Diseases | Examples | Gene Therapy Approach |
|---|---|---|
| Monogenetic diseases | Cystic fibrosis<br>Familial adenomatous polyposis<br>Hereditary hemochromatosis | Gene correction or replacement<br>Mutant RNA repair by ribozymes |
| Complex genetic diseases | Sporadic cancers<br>Inflammatory bowel disease | Gene augmentation—e.g., expression of cytokine genes or suicide genes for prodrug activation<br>DNA vaccination |
| Acquired genetic pathology | Hepatitis B, hepatitis C viruses | Blockade of abnormal genes by antisense oligonucleotides, ribozymes, dominant negative mutants<br>DNA vaccination |

and expressed by antigen-presenting cells or myocytes, under the control of a eukaryotic promoter.

## Liposomal Gene Transfer

Another relatively straightforward technique is to complex the plasmid DNA with cationic liposomes, which increase the efficiency of gene transfer by enhancing the uptake of the plasmid by the relevant cells.[7] Liposomal transfer of therapeutic genes to the gastrointestinal system in vivo has been demonstrated in the esophagus,[8] biliary tract,[9] and pancreas,[10] to give just three ex-

**Table 10-2** Vectors and methods of delivering gene therapy

| Vector | Comments |
|---|---|
| Naked plasmid DNA | Requires the least preparation<br>Particularly effective for delivery into muscle or skin<br>Useful for DNA vaccination studies |
| Liopsomal transfer | DNA complexed with cationic lipid<br>Relatively unstable<br>Relatively inefficient transfection |
| Retroviral vectors | Single-stranded RNA genome<br>After reverse transcription, DNA is stably integrated into genome<br>Requires dividing cells to be effective<br>Possibility of insertional mutagenesis<br>May be limited by sensitivity to lysis by human complement |
| Adenoviral vectors | Linear, double-stranded genome<br>Able to infect a wide range of cell types, which do not need to be actively dividing<br>Episomal (extrachromosomal) situation limits duration of effect<br>Immune response may limit repeated treatments |
| SV40 virus | Stable expression<br>High viral titers<br>Expressed in nondividing cells<br>Little inflammatory or immune response<br>Small size allows easy manipulation, but limits size of transgene insert |
| Intracellular bacteria | Examples include *Salmonella typhimurium* and modified *E. coli* strains<br>Engineered to invade epithelial or antigen-presenting cells and release plasmid DNA into cytosol<br>Particularly effective for genetic vaccination<br>Expression of DNA is relatively short-lived and there is low efficiency for direct transfer to epithelia |

amples. Liposomal DNA complexes are relatively unstable in the circulation, however, and can be susceptible to opsonins, phagocytes, and digestive enzymes. The use of liposomal gene transfer is an effective way of delivering genes to cell cultures, as shown by, for example, the functional transfer of a normal adenomatous polyposis coli (APC) gene into colonic epithelium,[11] but its potency in vivo is much lower. A further limitation of its use is that the expression of the transferred gene is transient, although there can be circumstances in which a short-term effect is desirable.

## Particle Bombardment

Therapeutic DNA can be coated onto microparticles, composed of gold or tungsten, and fired into the tissues with a gene gun. The main advantage of this technique over simple plasmid injection is a much greater potency, with a smaller quantity of DNA required to achieve an equivalent transfection.[12] Gene guns can be used to transfer DNA or RNA to cultured cells or to targeted tissues in vivo, but their main use is in DNA vaccination, delivering nucleic acids to antigen-presenting cells in the skin.[13]

## Adenoviruses

Many different types of adenoviruses have been described, although most gene therapy studies are based on modified versions of adenovirus types 2 and 5c, which have a double-stranded DNA genome of approximately 36 kb.[14] This consists of four early-phase (or E) transcriptional regions, E1–E4, and four late-phase genes, L1–L4. The E1 region encodes transcription factors necessary for the expression of the other genes and viral replication. E3, however, encodes proteins capable of down-regulating certain aspects of the host immune response, such as glycoprotein 19K, which can inhibit transport of major histocompatibility (MHC) class I molecules from the endoplasmic reticulum. The L1–L4 genes encode structural proteins such as hexon, penton, and fiber. Modification of these genes can be used to overcome some of the potential drawbacks of adenoviral vectors (see below), with replication-incompetent E1-deleted mutants being used most commonly.

Recombinant adenoviruses have a number of important advantages that make them useful for gene therapy. They can be prepared at relatively high titers, can direct high levels of gene expression, and are relatively stable in vivo.[15] However, the episomal persistence of the transferred adenoviral genome, while avoiding the risk of insertional mutagenesis, means that the expression of the transgene is usually limited to a few weeks.[16] If given intravenously, over 90% of the adenovirus is taken up by the liver, which can, of course, be an advantage in liver-directed gene therapy but limits the efficacy of this route for targeting other tissues.

Adenoviruses are also relatively immunogenic, with their use being limited by preexisting immunity to the virus or by the immune response generated after repeated courses of adenoviral gene therapy. However, a number of different strategies can be deployed to overcome this immune response, including oral tolerization with adenoviral proteins,[17] transient immunosuppression,[18] and replacement of immunogenic viral domains.[19]

Manipulation of the immune response against adenoviruses may also alter their ability to target specific tissues. It has recently been demonstrated that stable, efficient transduction of the colonic epithelium can be achieved following the intravenous administration of an adenovirus construct, but only if the virus was given to mice who were immunosuppressed.[20] Many investigators have further modified the adenoviral genome and gradually deleted large areas of DNA sequences, leading to the use of so-called gutless adenoviruses that retain just the minimum number of genes necessary for viral packaging and replication.[21]

### Adeno-associated Viruses

The human parvovirus, adeno-associated virus type 2, has a number of features that may make it the basis of a useful gene therapy vector.[22] There is no known human disease association, it generates little or no immune response, and it is capable of stable integration into the host genome. However, the maximum size of the therapeutic gene that may be inserted is limited to around 4 kb maximum, and the somewhat complicated life cycle of the virus reduces the amount of recombinant virus that can be produced experimentally. As a proof of principle, it was recently shown that an adeno-associated virus, administered orally, could direct the persistent expression of a β-galactosidase transgene in small bowel epithelium and could also phenotypically reverse an animal model of lactose intolerance.[23]

### Retroviruses

Retroviruses have a single-stranded RNA genome that, after infection of a mammalian cell, undergoes reverse transcription to DNA that can be stably integrated into the host genome. Those retroviruses used for gene therapy are mainly derived from the Moloney murine leukemia virus (MMLV), and they have been the subject of a relatively large number of clinical studies.[24] MMLV-derived vectors possess a number of positive features, including the ubiquitous expression of receptors for the viral envelope protein, the nonpathogenicity of MMLV infection, and the ability to transfer an insert of up to 8 kb in size. Disadvantages, however, include an inability to infect nondividing cells and the possibility of insertional mutagenesis.

In gastrointestinal oncology, retroviruses have mainly been used for the ex vivo modification of tumor cells as part of immunotherapy protocols.[25] Murine models have shown successful retroviral treatment of hepatocellular carcinoma in vivo by conferring tumor-specific expression of tumor necrosis factor[26] or by the herpes simplex thymidine kinase enzyme rendering the cells sensitive to ganciclovir.[27]

Some investigators have explored lentiviruses as possible gene therapy vectors. A class of complex retroviruses related to the human immunodeficiency virus, lentiviruses appear to have some advantages, such as the ability to both infect and achieve sustained transgene expression in nondividing tissues such as the liver and skeletal muscle.[28] Concerns remain, however, about the possibility of insertional mutagenesis and the relative paucity of animal models for safety testing prior to studies in humans.[29]

### Poxviruses

Among the largest and most complex viruses known, poxviruses have a linear double-stranded DNA genome that consists of around 200 genes. Their large capacity and relative genomic stability make them possible candidates for gene therapy vectors, although the site of the transferred gene is cytoplasmic, rather than being integrated into the host genome.[30] This, together with the possibility of preexisting antiviral immunity, means that gene expression may be relatively transient, although this may leave a therapeutic window sufficient for a prodrug activation approach to be successful.[31]

### Emerging Viral Vectors

In the search for optimal vectors, a number of other viruses have been investigated in addition to the more established candidates above.

Recombinant vectors based on simian virus 40 (SV40) are showing great promise, with a number of advantages such as stable transgene expression, lack of immunogenicity, high transduction efficiency, and a favorable safety profile.[32] However, the size of the transgene that may be carried is limited to less than 5 kb.

Baculoviruses, which normally infect insect hosts, have also been used as the basis for recombinant vector production. They have a double-stranded DNA genome of approximately 131 kb in size and are relatively simple to manufacture, with a presumed lack of pathogenicity to humans. Early experiments have shown that efficient gene transfer into human liver cell lines is possible in vitro,[33] and animal studies are under way.

As we discuss below, the herpes simplex virus (HSV) thymidine kinase gene is commonly exploited as a method of selective prodrug activation when transferred to the target tissue by another viral vector. This approach has also been assessed using modified herpes viruses themselves to infect tumor cells prior to administering ganciclovir. One murine study recently demonstrated long-term survival of animals with intraperitoneal dissemination of pancreatic cancer, following gene therapy with a replication-conditional HSV vector and ganciclovir.[34]

### Intracellular Bacteria

It is well known that gene transfer can naturally occur between phylogenetically remote bacteria, between bacteria and plants, and also between bacteria and yeasts. Recently, a number of investigators have shown that it is possible to achieve functional gene transfer to humans from bacteria capable of intracellular invasion. The possible advantages of bacterial vectors are that they are relatively much more easy to manufacture than viruses and also have the potential to carry very large plasmid inserts.

The key to gene transfer from bacteria is their ability to invade mammalian cells—either spontaneously, as with bacteria such as *Salmonella* or *Shigella*, or by modifying the bacterial genome to express *invasin* genes that enable the bacteria to enter. These agents have been exploited in two main areas.

First, *Salmonella* strains have been used as effective mucosal vectors for DNA vaccination.[35] *Salmonella* mutants that are metabolically dependent on supplemented media ("auxotrophs") are used to carry a plasmid encoding the relevant antigen's DNA sequence under eukaryotic promoter control. After oral administration, the bacteria invade antigen-presenting cells in the gut mucosa. The subsequent lack of their essential metabolic supplements causes the bacteria to die within 24–48 hours, releasing the plasmid into the antigen-presenting cell cytoplasm. Such an approach has been shown to achieve effective gene transfer to dendritic cells and to confer protective antitumor immunity in a murine fibrosarcoma model.[36]

The second area of bacterial vector use is likely to be in transferring genes to epithelial cells. Some in vitro studies have used a modified *E. coli* bacterium, an auxotroph dependent on diaminopimelate supplementation. By engineering this nonpathogenic bacterium to express the *invasin* gene from *Listeria monocytogenes* and the *hly* gene from *Yersinia pseudotuberculosis,* it was possible to design a bacterium that could invade nonphagocytic cells, free itself from the cytoplasmic vesicle, and then die (due to lack of diaminopimelate) while releasing its plasmid DNA into the mammalian cell.[37] These vectors are currently being assessed in a range of tissues in vivo, but they would appear to offer some potential for gene therapy to the gastrointestinal tract in particular.

## Therapeutic Strategies

Cancer cells have proved susceptible to a wide range of gene therapy approaches (Table 10–3). Some of the more common methods applicable to gastrointestinal tumors are discussed below.

### Genetic Prodrug Activation Therapy

Conventional cytotoxic chemotherapy inevitably carries the risk of damaging normal tissues as well as neoplastic cells. A common goal of many gene therapists is to devise methods of selectively delivering chemotherapy to tumors.

Genetic prodrug activation therapy (GPAT) relies on the tumor-specific expression of so-called suicide genes within cancer cells. The different metabolic profile of tumor cells thus enables otherwise nontoxic prodrugs to be activated within the tumor without significant systemic side effects. The presence of

**Table 10–3** Examples of gene therapy–based techniques applicable to cancer treatment

| Procedures | Examples |
| --- | --- |
| Tumor suppressor gene replacement and/or induction of apoptosis | Wild-type *p53* |
| | *p21*<sup>WAF1</sup> |
| | *p16* |
| | Retinoblastoma gene |
| | TNF receptor |
| | Fas-estrogen receptor |
| Blockade of dominant gene expression by antisense s oligonucleotides | K-*ras* |
| | Mutant *p53* |
| | *ERBB2* |
| | *Bcl-2* |
| Genetic prodrug activation therapy | HSV thymidine kinase |
| | *E. coli* cytosine deaminase |
| | *E. coli* uracil phosphoribosyltransferase |
| Immunotherapy | Cytokine gene therapy |
| | Costimulatory molecule gene therapy |
| | Tumor antigen vaccines |
| | Dendritic cell manipulation |

HSV, herpes simplex virus; TNF, tumor necrosis factor.

enzymes produced by the introduced genes can confer sensitivity to antiviral agents or can dramatically increase the therapeutic index of cytotoxic drugs.

Many studies have involved the transfer of the herpes simplex (or varicella zoster) thymidine kinase gene to confer sensitivity to ganciclovir. Others have used *E. coli* cytosine deaminase, which converts nontoxic 5-fluorocytosine into the cytotoxic 5-fluorouracil (5-FU), and advances in pharmacology are providing an increasing choice of prodrug-activating enzymes.[38] For example, the *E. coli* uracil phosphoribosyltransferase enzyme has recently been adenovirally transduced into pancreatic, hepatocellular, colonic, and gastric cancer cell lines and shown to overcome resistance to 5-FU therapy.[39] Clearly, the intention of most GPAT studies is to achieve truly tumor-specific expression of the enzyme construct. This may be achieved by using transduction, targeting, and/or transcription targeting of tumor cells.

*Transduction targeting* preferentially delivers genes by selecting a particular cellular phenotype. With brain tumors, for example, this may be as simple as using a retrovirus to selectively infect dividing cells in the central nervous system. An alternative method of gene delivery is to use ligands that recognize tumor-specific cell surface markers.[40] Hepatocellular carcinoma cells have been selectively targeted in this way using a monoclonal antibody–based vector that recognizes an internalizable membrane glycoprotein.[41]

*Transcription targeting* exploits tumor-specific promoters to drive the expression of the therapeutic gene. As a result, the gene product is preferentially expressed in those cells that bear the transcription factors required to activate the promoter. For example, the amylase promoter can be used to direct expression of an adenoviral construct in the exocrine pancreas.[42]

Malignant cells can be targeted by using the promoter and enhancer elements of tumor-associated genes or oncogenes, such as carcinoembryonic antigen (CEA).[43] In addition to being commonly overexpressed in colorectal cancers, this marker is also increased in around 40% of gastric adenocarcinomas. In view of this, the CEA promoter has recently been used to drive tumor-specific gene expression in gastric cancer cells.[44]

Other investigators have targeted the promoter for the *MUC1* gene, which encodes the polymorphic epithelial mucin[45] overexpressed in some some breast cancers and cholangiocarcinomas. Abnormal expression patterns of *MUC2, MUC4,* and *MUC5* are commonly found in pancreatic adenocarcinomas[46] and could form the basis of similar strategies.

Similarly, the ERBB2 promoter has been exploited to drive the selective expression of suicide genes in cancer cells,[47] and this mechanism has recently been studied in a phase I clinical trial of 5-fluorocytosine treatment of skin metastases in patients with breast cancer.[48] This latter study demonstrated that tumor-specific expression of the cytosine deaminase gene was possible in vivo, without systemic side effects. Further trials are in progress.

Some studies of GPAT directed against hepatocellular carcinomas have used the transcriptional regulatory sequences of the genes for α-fetoprotein or albumin. Given that albumin is consitutively expressed in normal hepatocytes and α-fetoprotein may be expressed by progenitor cells in the liver, there is probably a requirement for more tumor-specific targets.[49]

However, even when GPAT is precisely delivered, the cytotoxic effects are not completely specific. Many investigators have described a "bystander effect," seen when administering a prodrug to a mixed population of transfected and untransfected cells that leads to an unexpectedly high rate of cell death. In one example, transfection of just 10% of a cell population led to more than 50% of cells being killed by the addition of the prodrug.[50]

Different mechanisms have been proposed to explain this phenomenon. In the case of 5-FU generation, the cytotoxic agent itself is able to diffuse into adjacent cells from those killed by activation of the prodrug. With the thymidine kinase/ganciclovir approach, the bystander effect requires direct cell-to-cell contact to occur and it now seems likely that this phenomenon is mediated via intercellular gap junction communications.[51]

## Anti-oncogene Approaches

Activating mutations of oncogenes are a key component of many tumors. For example, constitutively active mutants of the K-*ras* oncogene are found in 80%–90% of pancreatic adenocarcinomas, 40%–60% of colorectal cancers, and 50%–100% of cholangiocarcinomas, and they are a feature of premalignant change in Barrett's esophagus and chronic ulcerative colitis. Consequently, gene therapists are studying ways of down-regulating the actions of this and other oncogenes, in addition to pharmacological approaches that inhibit the activity of the protein product.[52] For example, the growth of cells transformed by the Her-2/*Neu* oncogene can be inhibited by gene therapy that utilizes expression of the adenoviral *E1A* gene, down-regulating the oncogene at a transcriptional level.[53]

Another approach is to use so-called antisense strategies that have also been studied for their ability to block the transcription or translation of viral genes, particularly in patients with chronic hepatitis.[54] This technique uses nucleic acids that are complementary to a particular sequence of DNA or RNA. The hybridization of these oligonucleotides to their target effectively blocks the transcription or translation of the chosen gene.

The most commonly used approaches involve DNA molecules of 15–20 nucleotides in length. The binding of the construct to its mRNA counterpart can either cause steric hindrance of ribosomal 40S subunit binding, block the initiation codon, or result in mRNA cleavage by RNase H, depending on the chosen target site. Alternative methods include manipulating oligonucleotides to irreversibly bind genes prior to transcription (forming a triple helix with loss of gene expression), targeting transcription factors, or using ribozymes to divide RNA sequences.

Antisense technology directed at K-*ras* expression has been shown to reduce tumor growth in a lung cancer model.[55] More recently, the liposome-mediated gene transfer of an antisense K-*ras* construct has been used to treat murine pancreatic cancer in vivo by intraperitoneal injection, resulting in a significant suppression of tumor growth.[10] Antisense oligonucleotides directed against ERBB2 reduce the growth of ERBB2-positive breast cancer cell lines,[56] and this approach might also be applicable to pancreatic cancer, where the mechanism of ERBB2 transformation is similar.

In cholangiocarcinoma cell lines, antisense oligonucleotides against the overexpressed Bcl-2 led to both a reduction in Bcl-2 expression and a significant reduction of the threshold for inducing apoptosis.[57]

Antisense strategies are still evolving, and there continues to be controversy over their true specificity and exact mode of action. For example, oligonucleotides directed against p53 in human pancreatic cancer cell lines have antiproliferative results that are not related to the expression of p53.[58] It has also been suggested that the unmethylated cytosine-phosphate-guanine (CpG) motifs seen in some bacterial DNA-based oligonucleotides can act as immunomodulators and cause increased humoral and cel-

lular immune activation.[59] Such non-antisense mechanisms may explain many of the early successes of antisense therapy.

An alternative strategy is to use ribozymes, enzymes that have a catalytic site itself composed of RNA. Ribozomes are capable of cleaving many target RNA molecules, and their physiological roles include the splicing of RNA precursors and the protective cleavage of RNA produced by pathogenic viruses. They may also be exploited by other viruses as part of their life cycle. Ribozymal therapy has been used to target mutant p53 in lung cancer cells, reducing the level of expression and leading to a slowing of cellular proliferation.[60] The ability to refine and deliver specific ribozymes remains an important challenge for cancer gene therapists.[61]

In an alternative strategy, chimeric RNA–DNA oligonucleotides are being used to correct abnormal gene expression. Early studies have shown that these chimeric molecules are able to direct site-specific gene repair[62] and may potentially be useful in the correction of mutated oncogenes.

## Tumor Suppressor Gene Replacement and Pro-apoptotic Therapies

The concept of tumor suppressor gene (TSG) replacement remains appealing, although there have been few convincing demonstrations of its practical success in vivo. Gastrointestinal malignancies may demonstrate a number of different alterations in TSGs, expressed at disparate time points in tumorigenesis and hence at various locations within the same tumor mass. Consequently, there may only be a narrow "therapeutic window" due to the transient involvement of a defective tumor suppressor mechanism in carcinogenesis. Therefore, it seems unlikely that a single TSG replacement strategy would become the sole therapy for gastrointestinal cancers in vivo, notwithstanding any difficulties in efficient gene delivery to the tumor site. However, these problems may not be insurmountable, and there are many reports of successful TSG replacement strategies in laboratory-based models. The possibility of combining TSG replacement with other gene therapy techniques remains promising.

One of the most frequently studied approaches is that of restoring the normal function of *p53*, a TSG commonly defective in cancers of the gastrointestinal tract and overall the most commonly described genetic abnormality of all human malignancies.[63] Replication-deficient adenoviruses[64] and retroviruses[65] have been used as vectors to carry wild-type *p53*, suppressing growth in a variety of different cancers including pancreatic adenocarcinoma[66] and gastric adenocarcinoma,[67] and the technique is now the subject of clinical trials for the treatment of primary and secondary liver cancers.[15] As mentioned earlier, results in vivo may not necessarily be the same as those seen in the laboratory. For instance, transfection of hepatocellular carcinomas with a *p53*-bearing adenovirus construct failed to reduce tumor growth in one transgenic mouse model.[68] In addition to any direct effect on cellular proliferation, the restoration of *p53* function can markedly increase the sensitivity of a tumor to conventional chemotherapeutic drugs.[69]

The functional replacement of other defective tumor suppressor genes is being explored. For example, *p21^WAF1* transfection of pancreatic tumor cell lines, using a recombinant adenoviral construct can lead to cell cycle arrest at $G_0/G_1$ and significant growth inhibition of the cultured cells.[70]

Other groups have pursued the in vitro restoration of functional *p16* in cancer cells. Increased apoptotic cell death was observed in hepatic, colonic, and non–small cell lung cancer cell lines transfected with *p16* adenoviral constructs, particularly if there was concomitant overexpression of *p53*.[71] Like *p21^WAF1*, *p16* inhibits the effects of cyclin-dependent kinase (CDK) enzymes. Under normal circumstances, the retinoblastoma gene product discourages DNA synthesis and cell division, but this protein can be inactivated by a CDK-mediated phosphorylation. Given that certain digestive tract cancers, such as pancreatic adenocarcinoma, express a functional retinoblastoma protein, a *p16* replacement strategy may be a useful approach. Interestingly, in a rat model of proliferative cholangitis, the direct transfer and overexpression of the retinoblastoma gene to the biliary epithelium using an adenoviral construct led to a significant inhibition of epithelial proliferation.[72] This could potentially be of use in the adjunctive therapy of malignant biliary strictures.

Other strategies to induce tumor cell apoptosis have included transfection with the R55 tumor necrosis factor (TNF) receptor gene, followed by the administration of mutein TNF.[73] An alternative approach has been to transfect pancreatic tumor cell lines with a cDNA encoding a fusion protein of Fas and the ligand-binding region of the estrogen receptor. Following transfection, the addition of estrogens could induce cell death.[74]

## Oncolytic Viruses

While perhaps not gene therapy in the classical sense, selectively replicating adenoviruses such as the ONYX-015 agent have been used to target *p53*-deficient tumors,[75] with cytolytic effects that can augment standard chemotherapy drugs. Initial results from clinical trials in head and neck cancer appear encouraging.[76] Reoviruses are also under investigation for any possible oncolytic effects.

## Immunotherapy

The field of anticancer immunotherapy has received new impetus recently, driven by advances in our understanding of basic immunology and the molecular biology of neoplasia. In many ways, immunological therapies could be considered the ideal cancer therapies: specifically searching for and destroying malignant cells throughout the body while leaving normal tissues unharmed. This clinical potential has yet to be fulfilled, but important advances in the laboratory have given cause for optimism.

Earlier concepts of tumor immunology centered on the immune surveillance hypothesis[77] with the view that discriminating between self and non-self antigens should allow for the recognition and elimination of tumor cells that expressed "foreign" proteins. However, tumor-specific lymphocytes are well described in many malignancies, e.g., in pancreatic adenocarcinoma[78] and in hepatocellular carcinoma quite distinct from the immune response to hepatic viruses.[79] It is clear that, despite being recognized by tumor-specific T lymphocytes, antigenic tumors do evade the immune system, perhaps because the generation of an effective immunological response against a presented antigen requires costimulatory signals to trigger activation, as opposed to tolerance.[80]

According to this "danger" model of immunity, tumor cells that multiply and grow in an apparently healthy way without tissue damage or necrosis are unlikely to be rejected and instead induce tolerance by presenting their tumor antigens to T cells without the costimulatory signals that occur in an inflammatory response. It is hypothesized that even large tumors that develop ischemic necrosis at their centers will still evade the immune system, as any tumor-specific T cells will presumably have already induced tolerance to the large mass of tissue.[81] Many of our current attempts to tip the balance of immunity against tumor cells will still involve combinations of conventional debulking treatments (e.g., surgery, radiotherapy, or chemotherapy) to reduce the tumor burden. Immunotherapy that induces "danger signals" is then more likely to succeed.[82]

Recent work has suggested that an important determinant of generating an antitumor response is the mechanism of cancer cell death. While apoptosis could be considered immunologically silent, nonapoptotic cell death can induce the expression of heat shock proteins, thereby increasing the immunogenicity of the tumor.[83] The mycobacterial vaccine Bacille Calmette-Guerin (BCG) has been used as a successful topical treatment for superficial bladder cancer, presumably reflecting the nonspecific induction of inflammation and development of costimulation. In a study that built on this approach, patients with stage II/III colon cancer were given intradermal vaccinations of irradiated autologous tumor cells mixed with BCG in addition to surgical resection of the tumor. A 5-year follow-up has recently reported a 44% reduction in cancer recurrence.[84]

Other researchers have looked at determining specific tumor "antigens" in particular defining epitopes that may be presented to (and recognized by) T cells via the MHC class I route. Melanoma antigens such as gp100 or tyrosinase have so far provided the greatest number of HLA-A2–presented epitopes for study,[85,86] but there are also a number of possible tumor antigens that associate with digestive tract cancers. Theoretically, this could encompass the protein products of any of the mutant genes described earlier. Examples that have been identified as possible targets for cytotoxic T cells to date include the HLA-A2 restricted epitope of *MUC2*,[87] codon 12 mutants of K-*ras*,[88] and mutated *p53*.[88] Early clinical studies in patients with gastrointestinal cancers have shown that cytotoxic T cells can be generated against cells bearing *ras* mutations after peptide vaccination.[89] In addition to peptides, DNA vaccines have been used to stimulate antitumor immune responses. Examples include DNA vaccination against neu/ERBB2[90] CEA[91] in murine cancer models.

Clinical trials of cytokine therapy in patients with melanoma have shown encouraging results by increasing tumor immunogenicity, but problems with systemic toxicity have prompted the use of gene transfer strategies to express and deliver cytokines at tumor sites. One approach has been the adoptive transfer of cytokine genes (such as interleukin-2) into ex vivo cultured tumor-infiltrating lymphocytes that are then infused back into the patient. An alternative method is to transduce the tumor cells themselves ex vivo with immunostimulatory cytokines such as granulocyte-macrophage colony-stimulating factor (GM-CSF), irradiate them, and return the cells to the host as a cellular vaccine. A clinical trial using this latter approach is now under way in patients with pancreatic cancer.[92]

Inducing tumor cells to express costimulatory molecules on their surface could enable them to activate T cells directly, bypassing the requirement for antigen-presenting cells. Transfection of human tumor cell lines with the B7.1 molecule can invoke cellular immunity in this way.[93]

Elsewhere, attempts are being made to stimulate antitumor immunity with vaccines based on viral or bacterial vectors[4] or by the manipulation of antigen-presenting dendritic cell populations.[94] These cells have a pivotal role in the capture and presentation of antigens to T cells via class I and II MHC molecules, as well as posessing a host of costimulatory and cell-adhesion molecules. Dendritic cell-derived vaccines can be developed ex vivo by pulsing the cells with tumor-derived peptides or transfecting them with the genes for tumor-associated antigens before transfusing them back into the patient. Clinical trials of dendritic cell vaccination are currently in progress for breast cancer, melanoma, B-cell lymphoma, and prostate cancer. Recent work has suggested that the antigen-presenting cytoplasmic vesicles ("exosomes") present within dendritic cells may themselves be able to activate specific CTLs and eradicate established tumors.[95]

### Combination Therapies

As with much of the existing conventional treatment of cancer, many of the novel gene therapy–based methods may be more effective when combined with each other or with more established modalities. Potential examples include the transfection of cells with two different cytokine genes or with two different prodrug activating enzymes or combining cytokine gene transfection with GPAT. As mentioned earlier, using these newer therapies can dramatically alter the responsiveness of cancer cells to existing treatments. For instance, it was recently demonstrated that cholangiocarcinoma cells could be made sensitive to radiotherapy, both in vitro and in vivo, by prior transfection with the cytosine deaminase GPAT gene.[96]

Another group studied a combination of three therapies: a selectively cytopathic adenovirus FGR (similar to ONYX-015), double suicide genes (cytosine deaminase and HSV-1 TK in the same fusion gene construct), and tumor irradiation. Specificity was maintained, in that neither the FGR virus itself nor the suicide genes caused significant toxicity to normal cells. The addition of the double GPAT system enhanced the cytopathic effects of the FGR virus and further increased the tissue sensitivity to radiotherapy.[97]

As discussed above, immunotherapy seems more likely to succeed if the tumor burden is relatively low. In addition to the currently available debulking treatments, combining immunotherapy with antiangiogenic agents such as angiostatin or endostatin, which reduce tumor blood supply, may prove more effective.[98]

### Conclusions

As we learn more about the molecular pathology of gastrointestinal cancers, we will uncover potential targets for therapeutic agents. Anticancer strategies currently make up the vast majority of clinical gene therapy trials, and this position seems unlikely to change in the near future. Although there have been relatively few clinical successes so far, the current status of gene therapy has been likened to the development of recombinant proteins in the 1980s, with agents such as erythropoietin and the interferons having now become established in the clinical arena.[99] The future of gene therapy for gastrointestinal cancers will certainly be interesting,[100] as many of the techniques discussed in this chapter begin to move from the laboratory to the bedside.

### References

1. Rosenberg SA, Aebersold P, Cornetta K, et al. Gene transfer into humans: immunotherapy of patients with advanced melanoma using tumor infiltrating lymphocytes modified by retroviral gene transduction. N Engl J Med 323:570–578, 1990.
2. Aspinall RJ, Lemoine NR. Gene therapy for pancreatic and biliary malignancies. Ann Oncol 10 Suppl 4:188–192, 1999.
3. Donnelly JJ, Ulmer JB, Shiver JW, Liu MA. DNA vaccines. Annu Rev Immunol 15:615–648, 1997.
4. Chen C-H, Wu T-C. Experimental vaccine strategies for cancer immunotherapy. J Biomed Sci 5:231–252, 1998.
5. Davis HL, Schirmbeck R, Reimann J, Whalen RG. DNA-mediated immunization in mice induces a potent MHC class I–restricted cytotoxic T lymphocyte response to the hepatitis B envelope protein. Hum Gene Ther 6:1447–456, 1995.
6. Lagging LM, Meyer K, Hoft D, et al. Immune responses to plasmid DNA encoding the hepatitis C virus core protein. J Virol 69:5859–5863, 1995.
7. Felgner PL, Zelphati O, Liang X. Advances in synthetic gene-delivery system technology. In: Friedmann T (ed): The Development of Human Gene Therapy. Cold Spring Harbor Laboratory Press, Cold Spring Harbor, NY, 1999, pp 241–260.
8. Schmid RM, Weidenbach H, Draenert GF, et al. Liposome mediated gene transfer into the rat oesophagus. Gut 41:549–556, 1997.
9. Uehara T, Honda K, Hatano E, et al. Gene transfer to the rat biliary tract with the HVJ-cationic liposome method. J Hepatol 30:836–842, 1999.
10. Aoki K, Yoshida T, Sugimura TV, Terada M. Liposome-mediated in vivo gene transfer of antisense K-*ras* construct inhibits pancreatic tumor dissemination in the murine peritoneal cavity. Cancer Res 55:3810–3816, 1995.
11. Hargest R, Williamson R. Expression of the APC gene after transfection into a colonic cancer cell line. Gut 37:826–829, 1995.
12. Fynan EF, Webster RG, Fuller, DH, et al. DNA vaccines: protective immunizations by parenteral, mucosal and gene gun innoculations. Proc Natl Acad Sci USA 90:11478–11482, 1993.
13. Condon C, Watkins SC, Celluzzi CM, et al. DNA-based immunization by in vivo transfection of dendritic cells. Nat Med 2:1122–1128, 1996.
14. Ilan Y, Saito H, Thummala NR, Chowdhury NR. Adenovirus-mediated gene therapy of liver diseases. Semin Liver Dis 19:49–59, 1999.
15. Hauses M, Schackert HK. Gene therapy and gastrointestinal cancer: concepts and clinical facts. Langenbecks Arch Surg 384:479–488, 1999.
16. Smith TA, Mehaffey MG, Kayda DB, et al. Adenovirus mediated expression of therapeutic levels of human factor IX in mice. Nat Genet 5:397–402, 1993.
17. Yang Y, Greenough K, Wilson JM. Transient immunoblockade prevents formation of neutralizing antibody to recombinant adenovirus and allows repeated gene transfer to mouse liver. Gene Ther 3:412–420, 1996.
18. Ilan Y, Sauter B, Chowdhury NR, et al. Oral tolerization to adenoviral proteins permits repeated adenovirus-mediated gene therapy in rats with pre-existing immunity to adenovirus. Hepatology 27:1368–1376, 1998.
19. Nabel GJ. Development of optimized vectors for gene therapy. Proc Natl Acad Sci USA 96:324–326, 1999.
20. Brown GR, Thiele DL, Silva M, Beutler B. Adenoviral vectors given intravenously to immunocompromised mice yield stable transduction of the colonic epithelium. Gastroenterology 112:1586–1594, 1997.
21. Schnieder G, Morral N, Parks RJ, et al. Genomic DNA transfer with a high-capacity adenovirus vector results in improved in vivo gene expression and decreased toxicity. Nat Genet 18:180–183, 1998.
22. Kotin RM. Prospects for the use of adeno-associated virus as a vector for human gene therapy. Hum Gene Ther 5:793–801, 1994.
23. During MJ, Xu R, Young D, et al. Peroral gene therapy of lactose intolerance using an adeno-associated virus vector. Nat Med 4:1131–1135, 1998.
24. Crystal RG. Transfer of genes to humans: early lessons and obstacles to success. Science 270:404–410, 1995.
25. Sobol RE, Royston I, Fakhrai H, et al. Injection of colon carcinoma patients with autologous irradiated tumor cells and fibroblasts genetically modified to secrete interleukin-2 (IL-2): a phase-I study. Hum Gene Ther 6:195–204, 1995.
26. Cao G, Kuriyama S, Du P, et al. Complete regression of established murine hepatocellular carcinoma by in vivo tumor necrosis factor α gene transfer. Gastroenterology 112:501–510, 1997.
27. Kuriyama S, Masui K, Kikukawa M, et al. Complete cure of established murine hepatocellular carcinoma is achievable by repeated injections of retroviruses carrying the herpes simplex virus thymidine kinase gene. Gene Ther 6:525–533, 1999.
28. Kafri T, Blomer U, Peterson DA, et al. Sustained expression of genes delivered directly into liver and muscle by lentiviral vectors. Nat Genet 17:314–317, 1997.
29. Shetty K, Wu GY, Wu CH. Gene therapy of hepatic diseases: prospects for the new millenium. Gut 46:136–139, 2000.
30. Moss B. Vaccinia virus: a tool for research and vaccine development. Science 252:1662–1667, 1991.
31. Gnant MF, Noll LA, Irvine KR, et al. Tumor-specific gene delivery using recombinant vaccinia virus in a rabbit model of liver metastases. J Natl Cancer Inst 91:1744–1750, 1999.
32. Strayer DS. Gene therapy using SV40-derived vectors: what does the future hold? J Cell Physiol 181:375–384, 1999.

33. Boyce FM, Bucher NLR. Baculovirus-mediated gene transfer into mammalian cells. Proc Natl Acad Sci USA 93:2348–2352, 1996.

34. Kasuya H, Nishiyama Y, Nomoto S, et al. Intraperitoneal delivery of hrR3 and ganciclovir prolongs survival in mice with disseminated pancreatic cancer. J Surg Oncol 72:136–141, 1999.

35. Darji A, Guzman CA, Gerstel B, et al. Oral somatic transgene vaccination using attenuated S. typhimurium. Cell 91:765–775, 1997.

36. Paglia P, Medina E, Arioli I, et al. Gene transfer in dendritic cells, induced by oral DNA vaccination with Salmonella typhimurium results in protective immunity against a murine fibrosarcoma. Blood 92:3172–3176, 1998.

37. Grillot-Courvalin C, Goussard S, Huetz F, et al. Functional gene transfer from intracellular bacteria to mammalian cells. Nat Biotechnol 16:862–866, 1998.

38. Encell LP, Landis DM, Loeb LA. Improving enzymes for cancer gene therapy. Nat Biotechnol 17:143–147, 1999.

39. Kanai F, Kawakami T, Hamada H, et al. Adenovirus-mediated transduction of Escherichia coli uracil phosphoribosyltransferase gene sensitizes cancer cells to low concentrations of 5-fluorouracil. Cancer Res 58:1946–1951, 1998.

40. Han X, Kasahara N, Kan YW. Ligand-directed retroviral targeting of human breast cancer cells. Proc Natl Acad Sci USA 92:9747–9751, 1995.

41. Mohr L, Schauer JI, Boutin RH, et al. Targeted gene transfer to hepatocellular carcinoma cells in vitro using a novel monoclonal antibody-based gene delivery system. Hepatology 29:82–89, 1999.

42. Dematteo RP, Mcclane SJ, Fisher K, et al. Engineering tissue-specific expression of a recombinant adenovirus: selective transgene transcription in the pancreas using the amylase promoter. J Surg Res 72:155–161, 1997.

43. Osaki T, Tanio Y, Tachibana I, et al. Gene therapy for carcinoembryonic antigen–producing lung cancer cells by cell type specific expression of herpes simplex virus thymidine kinase gene. Cancer Res 54:5258–5261, 1994.

44. Lan KH, Kanai F, Shiratori Y, et al. Tumor-specific gene expresion in carcinoembryonic antigen-producing gastric cancer cells using adenovirus vectors. Gastroenterology 111:1241–1251, 1996.

45. Ring CJ, Martin LA, Blouin P, et al. Use of transcriptional regulatory elements of the MUC1 and ERBB2 genes to drive tumor-selective expression of a prodrug-activating enzyme. Gene Ther 4:1045–1052, 1997.

46. Terada T, Ohta T, Sasaki M, et al. Expression of MUC apomucins in normal pancreas and pancreatic tumors. J Pathol 180:160–165, 1996.

47. Ring CJ, Harris JD, Hurst HC, Lemoine NR. Suicide gene expression induced in tumor cells transduced with recombinant adenoviral, retroviral and plasmid vectors containing the ERBB2 promoter. Gene Ther 3:1094–1103, 1996.

48. Pandha H, Rigg A, Martin LA, et al. Genetic prodrug activation therapy for breast cancer targeted by the ERBB2 promoter: results of a phase I study. J Clin Oncol 17:2180, 1999.

49. Ohguchi S, Nakatsukasa H, Higashi T, et al. Expression of alpha-fetoprotein and albumin genes in human hepatocellular carcinomas: limitations in the application of the genes for targeting human hepatocellular carcinoma in gene therapy. Hepatology 28:599–607, 1998.

50. Freeman SM, Abboud CN, Whartenby KA, et al. The "bystander effect": tumor regression when a fraction of the tumor mass is genetically modified. Cancer Res 53:5274–5283, 1993.

51. Yang L, Chiang Y, Lenz HJ, et al. Intercellular communication mediates the bystander effect during herpes simplex thymidine kinase/ganciclovir-based gene therapy of human gastrointestinal tumor cells. Hum Gene Ther 9:719–728, 1998.

52. Chen Y. Inhibition of K-ras–transformed rodent and human cancer cell growth via induction of apoptosis by irreversible inhibitors of ras endoprotease. Cancer Lett 131:191–200, 1998.

53. Chang JY, Xia W, Shao R, Hung MC. Inhibition of intratracheal lung cancer development by systemic delivery of E1A. Oncogene 13:1405–1412, 1996.

54. Branch AD. A hitchhiker's guide to antisense and nonantisense biochemical pathways. Hepatology 24:1517–1529, 1996.

55. Georges RN, Mukhopadhyay T, Zhang Y, et al. Prevention of orthotopic human lung cancer growth by intratracheal instillation of a retroviral antisense K-ras construct. Cancer Res 53:1743–1746, 1993.

56. Colomer R, Lupu R, Bacus SS, Gelmann EP. ErbB-2 antisense oligonucleotides inhibit the proliferation of breast carcinoma cells with erbB-2 oncogene amplification. Br J Cancer 70:819–825, 1994.

57. Harnois DM, Que FG, Celli A, et al. Bcl-2 is overexpressed and alters the threshold for apoptosis in a cholangiocarcinoma cell line. Hepatology 26:884–890, 1997.

58. Barton CM, Lemoine NR. Antisense oligonucleotides directed against p53 have antiproliferative effects unrelated to effects on p53 expression. Br J Cancer 71:429–437, 1995.

59. Klinman DM, Yamshchikov G, Ishigatsubo Y. Contribution of CpG motifs to the immunogenicity of DNA vaccines. J Immunol 179:97–106, 1997.

60. Cai DW, Mukhopadayay T, Roth JA. Suppression of lung cancer cell growth by ribozyme-mediated modification of p53 pre-mRNA. Cancer Gene Ther 2:199–205, 1995.

61. Thompson JD, Macejak D, Couture L, Stinchcomb DT. Ribozymes in gene therapy. Nat Med 1:277–278, 1995.

62. Yoon K, Cole-Strauss A, Kmiec EB. Targeted gene correction of episomal DNA in mammalian cells mediated by a chimeric RNA–DNA oligonucleotide. Proc Natl Acad Sci USA 93:2071–2076, 1996.

63. Levine AJ. P53, the cellular gatekeeper for growth and division. Cell 88:323–331, 1997.

64. Zhang WW, Fang X, Mazur W, et al. High-efficiency gene transfer and high-level expression of wild-type p53 in human lung cancer cells mediated by recombinant adenovirus. Cancer Gene Ther 1:5–13, 1994.

65. Fujiwara T, Cai DW, Georges RN, et al. Therapeutic effect of a retroviral wild-type p53 expression vector in an orthotopic lung cancer model. J Natl Cancer Inst 86:1458–1462, 1994.

66. Bouvet M, Bold RJ, Lee J, et al. Adenovirus-mediated wild-type p53 tumor suppressor gene therapy induces apoptosis and suppresses growth of human pancreatic cancer. Ann Surg Oncol 5:681–688, 1998.

67. Ohashi M, Kanai F, Ueno H, et al. Adenovirus mediated p53 tumor suppressor gene therapy for human gastric cancer cells in vitro and in vivo. Gut 44:366–371, 1999.

68. Bao JJ, Zhang WW, Kuo MT. Adenoviral delivery of recombinant DNA into transgenic mice bearing hepatocellular carcinomas. Hum Gene Ther 7:355–365, 1996.

69. Fujiwara T, Grimm EA, Mukhopadhyay T, et al. Induction of chemosensitivity in human lung cancer cells in vivo by adenovirus-mediated transfer of the wild-type p53 gene. Cancer Res 54:2287–2291, 1994.

70. Joshi US, Dergham ST, Chen YQ, et al. Inhibition of pancreatic tumor cell growth in culture by p21$^{WAF1}$ recombinant adenovirus. Pancreas 16:107–113, 1998.

71. Sandig V, Brand K, Herwig S, et al. Adenovirally-transfected p16 INK4/CDKN2 and p53 genes cooperate to induce apoptotic tumor cell death. Nat Med 3:313–319, 1997.

72. Terao R, Honda K, Hatano E, et al. Suppression of proliferative cholangitis in a rat model with direct adenovirus-mediated retinoblastoma gene transfer to the biliary tract. Hepatology 28:605–612, 1998.

73. Sato T, Yamauchi N, Sasaki H, et al. An apoptosis-inducing gene therapy for pancreatic cancer with a combination of 55-kDa tumor necrosis factor (TNF) receptor gene transfection and mutein TNF administration. Cancer Res 58:1677–1683, 1998.

74. Kawaguchi Y, Takebayashi H, Kakizuka A, et al. Expression of Fas-estrogen receptor fusion protein induces cell death in pancreatic cancer cell lines. Cancer Lett 116:53–59, 1997.

75. Heise C, Sampson-Joannes A, Williams A, et al. ONYX-015, an E1B gene-attenuated adenovirus, causes tumor-specific cytolysis and antitumor efficacy that can be augmented by standard chemotherapeutic agents. Nat Med 3:639–645, 1997.

76. Kirn D, Hermiston T, McCormick F. ONYX-015: clinical data are encouraging. Nat Med 4:1341–1342, 1998.

77. Burnet FM. The concept of immunological surveillance. Prog Exp Tumor Res 13:1–27, 1970.

78. Qin H, Chen W, Takahashi M, et al. CD4+ T-cell immunity to mutated ras protein in pancreatic and colon cancer patients. Cancer Res 55:2984–2987, 1995.

79. Tabor E: Liver tumors and host defense. Semin Liver Dis 17:351–355, 1997.

80. Fuchs EJ, Matzinger P. Is cancer dangerous to the immune system? Semin Immunol 8:271–280, 1996.

81. Matzinger P. An innate sense of danger. Semin Immunol 10:399–415, 1998.

82. Todryk SM, Chong H, Vile RG, et al. Can immunotherapy by gene transfer tip the balance against colorectal cancer? Gut 43:445–449, 1998.

83. Melcher A, Todryk S, Hardwick N, et al. Tumor immunogenicity is determined by the mechanism of cell death via induction of heat shock protein expression. Nat Med 5:581–587, 1998.

84. Vermorken J, Claessen A, Van Tinteren H, et al. Active specific immunotherapy for stage II and stage III human colon cancer: a randomised trial. Lancet 353:345–350, 1999.

85. Rosenberg SA. The immunotherapy of solid cancers based on cloning

the genes encoding tumor-rejection antigens. Annu Rev Med 47:481–491, 1996.

86. Bohm CM, Hanski ML, Stefanovic S, et al. Identification of HLA-A2-restricted epitopes of the tumor-associated antigen MUC2 recognized by human cytotoxic T cells. Int J Cancer 75:688–693, 1998.

87. Peace DJ, Smith JW, Chen W, et al. Lysis of *ras* oncogene-transformed cells by specific cytotoxic T lymphocytes elicited by primary in vitro immunization with mutated ras peptide. J Exp Med 179:473–479, 1994.

88. McCarty TM, Liu X, Sun JY, et al. Targeting p53 for adoptive T-cell immunotherapy. Cancer Res 58:2601–2605, 1998.

89. Khleif SN, Abrams SI, Hamilton JM, et al. A Phase I vaccine trial with peptides reflecting *ras* oncogene mutations of solid tumors. J Immunother 22:155–165, 1999.

90. Amici A, Venanzi FM, Concetti A: Genetic immunization against *neu/erbB2* transgenic breast cancer. Cancer Immunol Immunother 47: 183–190, 1998.

91. Conry RM, Lobuglio AF, Loechel F, et al. A carcinoembryonic antigen polynucleotide vaccine has in vivo antitumor activity. Gene Ther 2: 59–65, 1995.

92. Jaffee EM, Abrams R, Cameron J, et al. Clinical protocol: a phase I clinical trial of lethally irradiated allogeneic pancreatic tumor cells transfected with the GM-CSF gene for the treatment of pancreatic adenocarcinoma. Hum Gene Ther 9:1951–1971, 1998.

93. Dohring C, Angman L, Spagnoli G, Lanzavecchia A. T-helper and accessory-cell independent cytotoxic responses to human tumor cells transfected with a B7 retorviral vector. Int J Cancer 57:754–759, 1994.

94. Timmerman JT, Levy R. Dendritic cell vaccines for cancer immunotherapy. Annu Rev Med 50:507–529, 1999.

95. Zitvogel L, Regnault A, Lozier A, et al. Eradication of established murine tumors using a novel cell-free vaccine: dendritic cell-derived exosomes. Nat Med 4:594–600, 1998.

96. Pederson LC, Buchsbaum DJ, Vickers SM, et al. Molecular chemotherapy combined with radiation therapy enhances killing of cholangiocarcinoma cells in vitro and in vivo. Cancer Res 57:4325–4332, 1997.

97. Freytag SO, Rogulski KR, Paielli DL, et al. A novel three-pronged approach to kill cancer cells selectively: concomitant viral, double suicide gene and radiotherapy. Hum Gene Ther 9:1323–1333, 1998.

98. Dellabona P, Moro M, Crosti MC, et al. Vascular attack and immunotherapy: a 'two hits' approach to improve biological treatment of cancer. Gene Ther 6:153–154, 1999.

99. Morgan RA, Blaese RM. Gene therapy: lessons learnt from the past decade. BMJ 319:1310, 1999.

100. Vile RG, Russell SJ, Lemoine NR. Cancer gene therapy: hard lessons and new courses. Gene Ther 7:2–8, 2000.

# Chapter 11

# Therapeutic Principles of Gastrointestinal Neoplasia
## Emerging Therapies: Antiangiogenic and Antimetastatic Agents

PAULO M. HOFF, JAMES L. ABBRUZZESE, AND JAMES PLUDA

Despite decades of intensive research, traditional chemotherapeutic agents fail to offer a complete cure for most cancer types. This sad reality is particularly true for metastatic cancers originating in the gastrointestinal tract. However, research has advanced our understanding of the mechanisms by which the cancer cells grow locally and metastasize to distant sites, and has inspired a growing number of researchers to explore novel approaches, including ways to block angiogenesis and metastasis.

The ability of a tumor to invade healthy tissues and to metastasize is the primary hallmark of cancer, and metastasis is the leading cause of death among cancer patients. The cellular events required for invasion also drive angiogenesis. However, a cancer cell can succeed in these processes only in the context of astounding intercellular and intracellular changes, including unregulated tumor growth and upsets in motility and proteolysis.[1] The formation of distant metastases is thus a complex phenomenon, involving sequential steps that produce important tumor–host interactions.[2] Each known step in the complex series of events that facilitate not only cancer cell survival and multiplication but also the generation of distant metastases was painstakingly discovered and independently explored. Attractive targets for novel antitumor therapies continue to emerge as researchers identify the many cellular enzymes and pathways involved in these complex events.

A large body of evidence demonstrates the importance of angiogenesis in the formation and maintenance of cancers and their metastases. This chapter reviews this evidence and describes the novel therapies being developed to prevent angiogenesis and the formation of distant metastases.

## Angiogenesis

*Angiogenesis* is the process involving activation of existing endothelial cells to form new blood vessels. This process is essential for the growth of the primary tumor, since even the most resistant cancer cell depends upon oxygen and nutrients for its survival and proliferation. Although cancer cells in a small tumor can obtain oxygen and nutrients by passive diffusion, this process is inadequate once the tumor grows beyond 1–2 mm in diameter. Disturbing recent evidence suggests that certain types of tumors may be able to form vessels without the participation of true endothelial cells; however, new blood vessels formed from endothelial cells are generally considered essential for tumor growth.[3] As discussed below, this complex process is even more important in the development of distant metastases.

For angiogenesis to occur, endothelial cells must gain access to the tumor site where the new vessel is needed. Tumor cells generate chemical factors that induce localized destruction of the basement membrane in existing vessels closest to the site. Adjacent vascular endothelial cells then migrate through the resulting passage into the surrounding connective tissue. The endothelial cells proliferate, forming a new vessel. Unlike vessels formed physiologically during such natural processes as embryonic development and wound healing,[4] those formed by neoplastic tumors are typically crude, leaky, and dilated, resulting in erratic blood flow.[5] Therefore, the delivery of oxygen and nutrients through tumor blood vessels is faulty, and the clearance of metabolic residues is poor, rendering the environment irrigated by those abnormal vessels acidic[6] and the tumor cells hypoxic.[7] Compared with normal cells, hypoxic cells tend to be more resistant to radiotherapy.[8] Faulty blood vessels in tumors may also increase resistance to chemotherapy by inhibiting the ability of active drug to reach all cancer cells. Unfortunately, the crude vessel network is often sufficiently functional to allow the tumor to grow and metastasize.

Since the early 1970s, researchers[9] have tried to isolate the factor or factors produced by tumors that allow them to form new vessels, grow, and spread to distant sites. Only in the late 1980s

**Table 11–1** Angiogenic growth factors and receptors

| Factor | Receptor |
|---|---|
| Basic fibroblast growth factor (bFGF) | FGFR1-4 |
| Vascular endothelial growth factor (VEGF) | Flk-1/KDR |
| | Flt-1 |
| Placental growth factor (PlGF) | FGFR1-4 |
| Fibroblast growth factor 3 (FGF-3) | FGFr1-4 |
| Fibroblast growth factor 4 (FGF-4) | FGFr1-4 |
| Acidic fibroblast growth factor (aFGF) | FGFr1-4 |
| Epidermal growth factor (EGF) | EGFR |
| Transforming growth factor alpha (TGF-α) | EGFR |
| Hepatocyte growth factor (HGF) | c-MET |
| Tumor necrosis factor α (TNF-α) | TNFR-55 |
| Transforming growth factor β (TGF-β) | TGF-βR I, II, III |
| Thymidine phosphorilase/platelet-derived endothelial cell growth factor (PD-ECGF) | Unclear |
| Angiogenin | Angiogenin receptor |
| Platelet-derived growth factor (PDGF) | PDGFR |
| Granulocyte colony-stimulating factor | G-CSFR |
| Pleiotrophin | Unknown |
| Proliferin | Unknown |
| Interleukin-8 (IL-8) | Unknown |
| Ang-1 | Unidentified |
| Ang-2 | Unidentified |

did Folkman and colleagues[10,11] isolate basic fibroblast growth factor (bFGF), the first well-documented angiogenic growth factor. Since then, the number of known angiogenic growth factors has steadily increased (Table 11–1). Knowledge of the existence and mechanisms of action of these growth factors provides researchers with opportunities to isolate naturally occurring inhibitors targeted to specific steps in angiogenesis or to develop artificial ones.

Researchers have always suspected that routine physiologic processes produce natural inhibitors. Normal cartilaginous tissues, for example, are avascular. Perhaps even more intriguing, some metastases tend to grow faster following surgical removal of the primary tumor, which suggests that the primary tumor produced some kind of inhibitor that limited the growth of the metastases. However, the isolation of an active antiangiogenic compound has proved to be a difficult task. The first hope for success came in the early 1980s, when Folkman and colleagues[12] showed that a combination of steroids and heparin fragments inhibited angiogenesis. Further research facilitated the isolation of angiostatin, a plasminogen fragment with potent antiangiogenic activity,[13] and endostatin, a fragment of type XVIII collagen.[14]

Other investigators are concentrating their efforts on finding an artificial antiangiogenic agent. Thalidomide, for example, a drug that gained notoriety for its teratogenic potential,[15,16] has attracted renewed attention based precisely on its peculiar side effects. This drug is being investigated as an antiangiogenic treatment for cancer.[17,18] Other workers are devoting their efforts to the development of new antiangiogenic agents.

## Metastasis

One of the most frustrating experiences in oncology is the development of metastasis in a patient previously rendered free of disease. Unfortunately, such occurrences are not only common but also highly lethal. The metastatic process usually requires

that the primary tumor secure its own blood supply. Thereafter, the tumor can shed cells directly into the circulation, allowing them to travel to distant sites. However, only a tiny fraction of the cancer cells released into the circulation succeed in forming viable metastatic tumors; indeed, less than 0.01% of circulating tumor cells are thought to survive and form metastases. Sampling blood from the right ventricle of mice, Glaves[19] demonstrated that release of up to $10^8$ viable cancer cells into the circulation during the growth of B16 melanomas and Lewis lung tumors produced an average of less than 100 lung metastases. The same investigator and colleagues[20] sampled blood in the renal veins of 10 patients prior to surgery for renal carcinoma; despite the daily release of a staggering $10^7$–$10^9$ cancer cells into the circulation, some patients showed no evidence of metastasis several months after surgery.

The failure of most cancer cells to form metastases is due to several factors, most still poorly understood. Paget[21] concluded over a century ago that the metastatic spread of a particular type of tumor depended not on chance, but rather on the embedding of adequate "seeds," or cells with metastatic potential, into fertile "soil," or organs in which the cells have a growth advantage. Fidler and colleagues[22,23] extensively studied and confirmed this concept, demonstrating that tumors are biologically heterogeneous, each containing cell subpopulations of varying metastatic potential. For the primary tumor to grow and for cancer cells to gain access to the circulation, angiogenesis is essential.[9,23,24] To form a metastasis, a cell or group of cells must detach from the primary tumor, invade host tissues, enter the circulation, stop at a distant site, undergo extravasation into the target organ, and divide to form a metastatic tumor. During these processes, cancer cells must survive the host immune surveillance system.[25,26]

Most human cells maintain constant contact with an extracellular matrix composed of fibrous elements, proteins, glycosamines, and other molecules. A highly specialized extracellular matrix for epithelial cells is the *basement membrane*, which is composed of laminin, type IV collagen, entactin/nidogen, and heparan sulfate proteoglycan. Small variations in this composition depend on the specific site; for instance, researchers[27] have identified at least seven types of laminin. The extracellular matrix for mesenchymal cells typically comprises interstitial collagens, types I–III elastin, proteoglycans, fibronectin, vitronectin, and other components.[28]

Normal cells cannot survive for long away from their extracellular matrix and soon undergo apoptosis or cell-cycle arrest.[29] However, cancer cells have been known to survive away from an extracellular matrix. The ability of cancer cells to detach from the primary tumor, penetrate the circulation, and survive away from their extracellular matrix for a sufficient period most likely depends on changes in the cell-adhesion molecules (CAMs). These molecules include *integrins,* which are transmembrane receptors for proteins of the extracellular matrix; *cadherins,* which are intercellular adhesion receptors; *adhesion molecules* of the immunoglobulin superfamily, which are involved in cell–cell adhesion; and hyaluronate-binding proteins. The CAMs mediate vital homotypic and heterotypic cellular interactions and also regulate cellular functions during embryogenesis, wound healing, inflammation, hemostasis, bone resorption, apoptosis, cell proliferation, tumor growth, and metastasis.[30–34] Decreased expression of CAMs may initiate cell detachment from the primary tumor.

To form a metastasis, a cell released into the circulation (either blood or lymphatic) must survive without the appropriate extracellular matrix and escape the patient's immune system. Evidence that T lymphocytes[35] and natural killer (NK) cells[36] can inhibit metastasis suggests that cancer cells eliciting immunological responses may be cleared from the circulation before they are able to establish themselves. Potent hemodynamic forces also limit the ability of cancer cells to survive in the circulation. Only a small number of cells survive these natural defense mechanisms and move to the next step in metastasis.

The surviving cancer cells eventually stop circulating, usually after being trapped in a small vessel.[36] During metastasis, the interaction of tumor cells with platelets and white blood cells can form a thrombus, whose exact importance in metastasis remains unclear. Once the cells have been arrested within an organ vessel, they must undergo extravasation to be able to grow as a new tumor. The cell adheres to a denuded basement membrane (in a damaged vessel, for example) or reaches the basement membrane by extending pseudopodia into the endothelial cell junctions or by provoking endothelial cell retraction. The attached cancer cell excretes proteolytic enzymes that initiate digestion of the basement membrane.[37,38] Members of all five classes of proteinases that have been identified—serine, cysteine, threonine, matrix metallo-, and aspartyl—have been implicated in aggressive metastatic growth.[39,40] After the cancer cells undergo extravasation and establish themselves, they begin to proliferate. The presence of specific growth factors, angiogenic factors, and other cytokines determines whether the cells succeed in forming a viable metastasis.

## Antiangiogenic and Antimetastatic Therapies

Inhibition of tumor angiogenesis and metastasis represents a novel target for antitumor therapy. An ideal inhibitor of angiogenesis would be specific for a particular step, aspect, or component of the neovascularization process and display a broad spectrum of antitumor activity. It would lack resistance and be nontoxic. Because antiangiogenic agents may serve as an adjunct to cytotoxic therapy, an ideal inhibitor would be easy to combine with conventional therapies. Ideal antiangiogenic/antimetastatic therapies would also be effective in the adjuvant setting or as maintenance after cytoreduction or curative surgery.

The favorable toxicity profile of these agents raises special considerations for study design. Maximum tolerated dose, the conventional end point of phase I trials of cytotoxic agents, may be inappropriate for antiangiogenic agents, since the effective dose is likely to be significantly lower than the maximum tolerated dose.[41] Some researchers propose alternative end points, such as pharmacologically optimal dose or optimal biologically effective dose, for phase I trials of these agents. Other commonly recommended end points include endothelial cell and tumor cell apoptosis and proliferation rates, as well as the status of their various receptors. Although the need for frequent biopsies, the lack of validated tests, and tumor heterogeneity represent obstacles to the adoption of a new standard phase I methodology for these agents, promising noninvasive studies, such as digital contrast magnetic resonance imaging (MRI), tridimensional ultrasound, positron emission tomography (PET), 3-D single photon emission computed tomography (SPECT), and cine-helical computed tomography (CT) should soon be available.

Even more complicated is the adaptation of phase II trials. The traditional end points of phase II trials—rates of response, times to progression, and survival—may be irrelevant to noncytotoxic agents.[42] The fact that antiangiogenic agents typically produce results only in the long term, after months of therapy, adds to the confusion.[42] Some investigators advocate the use of historical controls, and the use of combinations of test drugs with well-established cytotoxic agents. Other investigators[41,43] propose a complete change in methodology, i.e., proceeding directly from phase I to phase III trials with combinations of antiangiogenic and cytotoxic agents.

The development of phase III trials for antiangiogenic agents is less complex. Antiangiogenic agents tend to display a slower effect, but will nevertheless need to show a survival advantage over conventional therapy to be accepted. In a randomized trial, the antiangiogenic agent could be tested as a single agent or in combination with one or more treatments, such as another antiangiogenic agent, radiotherapy, chemotherapy, or hormonal therapy. Survival is the most rigorous end point, and should be the primary focus of any randomized trial. A less rigorous end point, such as time to disease progression, could serve as an additional end point in randomized trials, provided that placebo is used in the control arm to avoid biases. Patients in the control arm should receive either the standard therapy or no therapy when a standard does not exist.

Recent research[44,45] has identified several agents with antiangiogenic potential. Clinical trials of the first compounds directed at specific cellular targets will yield important information for the research teams striving to starve tumors and prevent metastasis.[44,45] The number of antiangiogenic agents grows ex-

**Table 11-2** Agents that block matrix metalloproteinase breakdown

| Agent | Manufacturer | Mechanism | Stage of Development |
|---|---|---|---|
| Marimastat | British Biotech (Oxford, United Kingdom) | Synthetic inhibitor of matrix metalloproteinases | Phase III |
| Bay 12-9566 | Bayer (West Haven, CT) | Synthetic inhibitor of tumor growth | Development on hold |
| AG3340 | Agouron Pharmaceuticals (La Jolla, CA) | Synthetic inhibitor of matrix metalloproteinases | Phase III |
| Col-3 | Collagenex Pharmaceuticals (Newton, PA) | Synthetic inhibitor of matrix metalloproteinases | Phase I |
| BMS-275291 | Bristol-Myers Squibb (Wallingford, CT) | Synthetic inhibitor of matrix metalloproteinases | Phase I |
| Neovastat | Aeterna (Sainte-Foy, Quebec, Canada) | Naturally occurring inhibitor of matix metalloproteinases | Phase III |
| CGS 27023A | Novartis (Basel, Switzerland) | Synthetic inhibitor of matrix metalloproteinases | Phase I |

**Table 11-3** Agents that directly inhibit endothelial cells

| Agent | Manufacturer | Mechanism | Stage of Development |
|---|---|---|---|
| TNP-470 | TAP Pharmaceuticals (Deerfield, IL) | Analogue of fumagillin; inhibits endothelial cell growth | Phase II |
| Thalidomide | Celgene Corp. (Warren, NJ) | Unknown | Phase II |
| Squalamine | Magainin Pharmaceuticals (Plymouth Meeting, PA) | Extract from shark liver; inhibits sodium-hydrogen exchanger NHE3 | Phase II |
| Combretastatin | Oxigene (Boston, MA) | Induces apoptosis | Phase II scheduled |
| Endostatin | EntreMed (Rockville, MD) | Inhibits endothelial cells | Phase I |

ponentially, and only a handful of even the best-known agents are likely to become widely available. However, the examples of five classes of agents described below demonstrate the range of drugs currently under study.

## Agents That Block Matrix Metalloproteinase (MMP) Breakdown

Table 11–2 describes agents that prevent angiogenesis and metastasis by modulating the ability of the cancer cell to interact with or destroy the matrix. Agents currently in advanced stages of development include marimastat, a synthetic agent that inhibits the activity of MMP-1, -2, -7, and -9. Its dose-limiting toxicity seems to be musculoskeletal, and the agent has reached phase III trials in glioblastoma and pancreatic, small-cell lung, gastric, and breast cancers. Investigators are studying marimastat in combination with various cytotoxic agents. The synthetic agent Bay 12-9566 inhibits the activity of MMP-2, -3, -8, and -9. Dose-limiting toxicities of this orally administered agent are thrombocytopenia, hyperbilirubinemia, and transient elevation of liver enzymes. Phase III trials[46] were halted by Bayer. Another orally administered synthetic agent, AG3340, inhibits the activity of MMP-2, -3, and -13. AG3340 caused a reversible, joint-related toxicity when used at high doses but seems to display a favorable profile when combined with conventional chemotherapeutic agents. Phase III trials[47] in non–small-cell lung, prostate, breast, and brain cancers are in progress.

Investigators continue to introduce synthetic agents with mechanisms of action that interfere with MMP activity. CGS 27023A inhibits the activity of MMP-1, -2, -3, and -9. It is administered orally, and its toxicities include a maculopapular rash, myalgia, arthralgia, and nausea. However, when used at lower doses, CGS 27023A seems to be well tolerated. The tetracycline derivative Col-3 down-regulates expression of MMP-2 and -9. Phase I trials of Col-3 in solid tumors are in progress. Agent BMS-275291, another synthetic MMP inhibitor, is currently undergoing phase I trials in solid tumors.

Naturally occurring MMP inhibitors are also under development. Neovastat acts by inhibiting MMP-2 and may also interfere with the interaction between vascular endothelial growth factor (VEGF) and its receptor. At high doses, neovastat produces gastrointestinal toxicity. The drug is currently undergoing a phase III trial in non–small-cell lung cancer.

## Agents That Directly Inhibit Endothelial Cells

Several agents inhibit angiogenesis by directly interacting with endothelial cells and inhibiting their function or response to outside stimuli (Table 11–3). TNP-470, a synthetic analogue of fumagillin, is given intravenously. Its main toxicity is neurological. It is in the advanced stage of development for use as a single agent and in combination with other therapies.[48,49] Kudelka and colleagues[50] reported that the drug produced complete response in cervical cancer.

Although thalidomide gained notoriety after causing dramatic birth defects in the late 1950s and early 1960s,[15,16] D'Amato and colleagues[18] more recently reported the drug's antiangiogenic potential. Thalidomide, which is being studied worldwide as a treatment for various types of cancer, seems to be particularly active in multiple myeloma.[51] The main side effects of the agent are drowsiness, constipation, and peripheral neuropathy, in addition to its teratogenic potential. Squalamine, an aminosterol extracted from the liver of dogfish sharks, acts by inhibiting the sodium-hydrogen exchanger NHE3. Initial phase I trials are under way.

**Table 11-4** Agents that block activators of angiogenesis

| Agent | Manufacturer | Mechanism | Stage of Development |
|---|---|---|---|
| SU5416 | Sugen (So. San Francisco, CA) | Blocks VEGF receptor | Phase III |
| SU6668 | Sugen (So. San Francisco, CA) | Blocks VEGF and FGF, and PDGF receptor | Phase I |
| PTK787/ZK 22584 | Novartis (Basel, Switzerland) | Blocks VEGF receptor | Phase II |
| Interferon-α | Commercially available | Inhibition of bFGF and VEGF production | Phase III |
| Anti-VEGF antibody | NCI (Bethesda, MD) and Genentech (So. San Francisco, CA) | Monoclonal antibody | Phase II |
| TAS-102 | Taiho Pharmaceuticals (Tokyo, Japan) | Blocks thymidine phosphorylase | Phase I |

**Table 11-5** Agents that inhibit endothelial-specific integrin/survival signaling

| Agent | Manufacturer | Mechanism | Stage of Development |
|---|---|---|---|
| Vitaxin | Ixsys (San Diego, CA) | Antibody directed toward integrin | Phase II |
| EMD 121974 | Merck (Darmstadt, Germany) | Small molecule blocker of integrin | Phase II scheduled |

Combretastatin A-4, also known as CA4P, is a tubulin-binding agent that induces apoptosis of proliferating endothelial cells. The drug is still in a very early stage of development; phase I trials are scheduled to be open soon.

Endostatin, perhaps the best-known antiangiogenic agent, has raised enormous expectations among physicians and patients. This 20 kDa C-terminal fragment of type XVIII collagen specifically inhibits endothelial proliferation and potently inhibits angiogenesis and tumor growth. O'Reilly and colleagues[14] reported that *E. coli*–derived Endostatin caused primary tumors to regress to dormant, microscopic lesions, with no apparent toxicity. Immunohistochemistry revealed blockade of angiogenesis and high but balanced rates of tumor-cell proliferation and apoptosis. Phase I trials have recently been completed in the United States.

### Agents That Block Activators of Angiogenesis

Several agents interact with cellular receptors involved in angiogenesis or with the ligands or signaling pathways of these receptors (Table 11–4). The small-molecule agent SU5416 inhibits VEGF receptor tyrosine kinase[52] and specifically blocks Flk-1.[53] SU5416 is given as an intravenous infusion; the main toxicities are headaches, nausea, and vomiting. Phase II and III trials of SU5416 in combination with other agents in the treatment of several types of tumors are in progress. Another small-molecule agent, SU6668, inhibits VEGF and platelet-derived growth factor (PDGF) and fibroblast growth factor (FGF) receptors. The drug is given orally; initial phase I trials are under way. PTK787/ZK 22584 inhibits VEGF KDR receptor tyrosine kinase and may inhibit the PDGF receptor as well. Phase III trials of this orally administered agent are imminent. Asano and colleagues[54] studied the effect of an antibody directed against VEGF to decrease the availability of ligand to the VEGF receptors. The anti-VEGF antibody is currently in phase II trials in solid tumors. Interferon-α is commercially available and approved for the treatment of different types of cancer, from leukemias to melanoma. Because of its antiangiogenic properties, interferon-α inhibits bFGF and VEGF production.[55,56]

### Agents That Inhibit Endothelial-Specific Integrin/Survival Signaling

The monoclonal antibody Vitaxin is directed against the vitronectin receptor, which mediates several biological processes critical to neointima formation following vessel injury (Table 11–5). Blockade of this receptor may reduce neointima formation by inhibiting smooth muscle cell migration, decreasing transforming growth factor-$\beta_1$ expression, enhancing apoptosis, or reducing neovascularization.[57] Phase I and II trials are under way to assess the use of Vitaxin as an intravenous infusion. EMD 121974 is a chemically synthesized cyclized pentapeptide that blocks integrin receptors. Single-agent phase I trials of EMD 121974 in solid tumors are ongoing.

### Agents with Nonspecific Mechanisms of Action

As we learn more about the mechanisms of action of various agents, the number of agents with antiangiogenic potential tends to increase. Agents that are believed to block angiogenesis include many chemotherapeutic agents, as well as agents with unclear mechanisms of action (Table 11–6). However, the National Cancer Institute is currently conducting phase I and II trials of CAI, which seems to act primarily by inhibiting calcium influx into the cell. Interleukin-12, which seems to up-regulate interferon-δ and other cytokines, is currently being investigated for intravenous and intraperitoneal administration. IM862, an agent currently in phase III trials for the treatment of AIDS-related Kaposi's sarcoma, is another antiangiogenic drug with an unknown mechanism of action.

### Conclusion

As discussed in this chapter, the field of antiangiogenic and antimetastatic agents is rich with opportunities for the development of novel antitumor therapies. The large number of agents currently in clinical trials holds the promise that an effective agent may soon become available for clinical use.

**Table 11-6** Agents with nonspecific mechanisms of action

| Agent | Manufacturer | Mechanism | Stage of Development |
|---|---|---|---|
| CAI | NCI (Bethesda, MD) | Inhibits calcium influx | Phase II |
| Interleukin-12 | Genetics Institute (Cambridge, MA) | Upregulates interferon-δ and IP-10 | Phase II |
| IM862 | Cytran (Kirkland, WA) | Unknown | Phase III |

## References

1. Liotta LA, Steeg PS, Stetler-Stevenson WG. Cancer metastasis and angiogenesis: an imbalance of positive and negative regulation. Cell 64:327–336, 1991.
2. Fidler IJ, Hart IR. Biological diversity in metastatic neoplasms: origins and implications. Science 217:998–1003, 1982.
3. Folkman J. The vascularization of tumors. Sci Am 234:58–64, 1976.
4. Folkman J, Shing Y. Angiogenesis. J Biol Chem 267:10931–10934, 1992.
5. Less JR, Skalak TC, Sevick EM, Jain RK. Microvascular architecture in a mammary carcinoma: branching patterns and vessel dimensions. Cancer Res 51:265–273, 1991.
6. Newell K, Franchi A, Pouyssegur J, Tannock I. Studies with glycolysis-deficient cells suggest that production of lactic acid is not the only cause of tumor acidity. Proc Natl Acad Sci USA 90:1127–1131, 1993.
7. Manz R, Otte J, Thews G, Vaupel P. Relationship between size and oxygenation status of malignant tumors. Adv Exp Med Biol 159:391–398, 1983.
8. Bush RS, Jenkin RD, Allt WE, et al. Definitive evidence for hypoxic cells influencing cure in cancer therapy. Br J Cancer (Suppl) 37:302–306, 1978.
9. Folkman J. Tumor angiogenesis: therapeutic implications. N Engl J Med 285:1182–1186, 1971.
10. Folkman J, Klagsburn M. Angiogenic factors. Science 235:442–447, 1987.
11. Vlodavsky I, Folkman J, Sullivan R, et al. Endothelial cell–derived basic fibroblast growth factor: synthesis and deposition into subendothelial extracellular matrix. Proc Natl Acad Sci USA 84:2292–2296, 1987.
12. Folkman J, Taylor S, Spillberg C. The role of heparin in angiogenesis. Ciba Found Symp 100:132–149, 1983.
13. O'Reilly MS. Angiostatin: an endogenous inhibitor of angiogenesis and of tumor growth. EXS 79:273–294, 1997.
14. O'Reilly MS, Boehm T, Shing Y, et al. Endostatin: an endogenous inhibitor of angiogenesis and tumor growth. Cell 88:277–285, 1997.
15. James WH. Teratogenetic properties of thalidomide. BMJ 5469:1064, 1965.
16. Burgio GR. The thalidomide disaster briefly revisited. Eur J Pediatr 136:229–230, 1981.
17. Konno H, Tanaka T, Baba M, Kanai T, Nakamura S. Antiangiogenic therapy for liver metastasis of gastrointestinal malignancies. J Hepatobiliary Pancreat Surg 6:1–6, 1999.
18. D'Amato RJ, Loughnan MS, Flynn E, Folkman J. Thalidomide is an inhibitor of angiogenesis. Proc Natl Acad Sci USA 91:4082–4085, 1994.
19. Glaves D. Correlation between circulating cancer cells and incidence of metastases. Br J Cancer 48:665–673, 1983.
20. Glaves D, Huben RP, Weiss L. Haematogenous dissemination of cells from human renal adenocarcinomas. Br J Cancer 57:32–35, 1988.
21. Paget S. The distribution of secondary growths in cancer of the breast. Lancet 1:571–573, 1889.
22. Fidler IJ, Kripke ML. Metastasis results from preexisting variant cells within a malignant tumor. Science 197:893–895, 1977.
23. Fidler IJ. Critical determinants of cancer metastasis: rationale for therapy. Cancer Chemother Pharmacol 43(Suppl):S3–S10, 1999.
24. Fidler IJ. Host and tumour factors in cancer metastasis. Eur J Clin Invest 20:481–486, 1990.
25. Schwartz R, Walk A, Toomes H, Schirrmacher V. Assay for the determination of human carcinoma cells in circulating blood. J Cancer Res Clin Oncol 109:122–129, 1985.
26. Schirrmacher V. Cancer metastasis: experimental approaches, theoretical concepts, and impacts for treatment strategies. Adv Cancer Res 43:1–73, 1985.
27. Burgeson RE, Chiquet M, Deutzmann R, et al. A new nomenclature for the laminins. Matrix Biol 14:209–211, 1994.
28. Dedhar S, Hannigan GE, Rak J, Kerbel RS. The extracellular environment and cancer. In: Tannock IF, Hill RP (eds): The Basic Science of Oncology, 3rd ed. McGraw-Hill, New York, 1998, pp 197–218.
29. Boudreau N, Sympson CJ, Werb Z, Bissell MJ. Suppression of ICE and apoptosis in mammary epithelial cells by extracellular matrix. Science 267:891–893, 1995.
30. Agrez MV. Cell adhesion molecules and colon cancer. Aust N Z J Surg 66:791–798, 1996.
31. Streit M, Schmidt R, Hilgenfeld RU, Thiel E, Kreuser ED. Adhesion receptors in malignant transformation and dissemination of gastrointestinal tumors. Recent Results Cancer Res 142:19–50, 1996.
32. Horn S, Moersig W, Moll R, Oelert H, Lorenz J. Expression of cell adhesion molecules in lung cancer cell lines. Exp Toxicol Pathol 48:535–540, 1996.
33. Tuszynski GP, Wang TN, Berger D. Adhesive proteins and the hematogenous spread of cancer. Acta Haematol 97:29–39, 1997.
34. Joseph-Silverstein J, Silverstein RL. Cell adhesion molecules: an overview. Cancer Invest 16:176–182, 1998.
35. Matsui S, Ahlers JD, Vortmeyer AO, et al. A model for CD8$^+$ CTL tumor immunosurveillance and regulation of tumor escape by CD4 T cells through an effect on quality of CTL. Immunology 163:184–193, 1999.
36. Greenberg AH, Egan SE, Jarolim L, Gingras MC, Wright JA. Natural killer cell regulation of implantation and early lung growth of H-ras–transformed 10T1/2 fibroblasts in mice. Cancer Res 47:4801–4805, 1987.
37. Kramer RH, Vogel KG, Nicolson GL. Solubilization and degradation of subendothelial matrix glycoproteins and proteoglycans by metastatic tumor cells. Biol Chem 257:2678–2686, 1982.
38. Nicolson GL. Cancer metastasis. Organ colonization and the cell-surface properties of malignant cells. Biochim Biophys Acta 695:113–176, 1982.
39. Chambers AF, Matrisian LM. Changing views of the role of matrix metalloproteinases in metastasis. J Natl Cancer Inst 89:1260–1270, 1997.
40. Mignatti P, Rifkin DB. Biology and biochemistry of proteinases in tumor invasion. Physiol Rev 73:161–195, 1993.
41. Eckhardt SG, Pluda JM. Development of angiogenesis inhibitors for cancer therapy. Invest New Drugs 15:1–3, 1997.
42. Eckhardt SG. Angiogenesis inhibitors as cancer therapy. Hosp Pract (Off Ed) 34:63–68, 1999.
43. Eisenhauer EA. Phase I and II trials of novel anti-cancer agents: endpoints, efficacy and existentialism. The Michel Clavel Lecture, held at the 10th NCI-EORTC Conference on New Drugs in Cancer Therapy, Amsterdam, 16–19 June 1998. Ann Oncol 9:1047–1052, 1998.
44. Folkman J. Angiogenesis and angiogenesis inhibition: an overview. EXS 79:1–8, 1997.
45. Drummond AH, Beckett P, Brown PD, et al. Preclinical and clinical studies of MMP inhibitors in cancer. Ann NY Acad Sci 878:228–235, 1999.
46. Brown PD. Clinical studies with matrix metalloproteinase inhibitors. APMIS 107:174–180, 1999.
47. Shalinsky DR, Brekken J, Zou H, et al. Broad antitumor and antiangiogenic activities of AG3340, a potent and selective MMP inhibitor undergoing advanced oncology clinical trials. Ann NY Acad Sci 878:236–270, 1999.
48. Figg WD, Pluda JM, Lush RM, et al. The pharmacokinetics of TNP-470, a new angiogenesis inhibitor. Pharmacotherapy 17:91–97, 1997.
49. Kudelka AP, Levy T, Verschraegen CF, et al. A phase I study of TNP-470 administered to patients with advanced squamous cell cancer of the cervix. Clin Cancer Res 3:1501–1505, 1997.
50. Kudelka AP, Verschraegen CF, Loyer E. Complete remission of metastatic cervical cancer with the angiogenesis inhibitor TNP-470 [letter]. N Engl J Med 338:991–992, 1998.
51. [No authors listed] Thalidomide shows promising results in patients with multiple myeloma. Oncology 13:744, 1999.
52. Fong TA, Shawver LK, Sun L, et al. SU5416 is a potent and selective inhibitor of the vascular endothelial growth factor receptor (Flk-1/KDR) that inhibits tyrosine kinase catalysis, tumor vascularization, and growth of multiple tumor types. Cancer Res 59:99–106, 1999.
53. Strawn LM, McMahon G, App H, et al. Flk-1 as a target for tumor growth inhibition. Cancer Res 56:3540–3545, 1996.
54. Asano M, Yukita A, Matsumoto T, Hanatani M, Suzuki H. An anti-human VEGF monoclonal antibody, MV833, that exhibits potent anti-tumor activity in vivo. Hybridoma 17:185–190, 1998.
55. Ellis LM, Fidler IJ. Angiogenesis and metastasis. Eur J Cancer 32A:2451–2460, 1996.
56. Ricketts RR, Hatley RM, Corden BJ, Sabio H, Howell CG. Interferon-alpha-2a for the treatment of complex hemangiomas of infancy and childhood. Ann Surg 219:605–614, 1994.
57. Coleman KR, Braden GA, Willingham MC, Sane DC. Vitaxin, a humanized monoclonal antibody to the vitronectin receptor (alphavbeta3), reduces neointimal hyperplasia and total vessel area after balloon injury in hypercholesterolemic rabbits. Circ Res 84:1268–1276, 1999.

# Part II

## Management of Specific Neoplasms

## Section 1

## Cancer of the Esophagus

# Chapter 12

# Epidemiology and Molecular Epidemiology of Esophageal Cancer

REGINALD V.N. LORD AND PETER V. DANENBERG

The two main histopathologic types of esophageal cancer are squamous cell carcinoma (SCC) and adenocarcinoma. Squamous cell carcinoma is the more prevalent type worldwide, but adenocarcinoma is more prevalent in many Western countries. Both SCC and adenocarcinoma of the esophagus have remarkable epidemiologic features. Squamous cell carcinoma has had the most varied geographical incidence of any cancer for many decades, which suggests the existence of critically important, but largely unclear, environmental and molecular factors. Equally remarkable, there has been a dramatic increase in the incidence of adenocarcinoma of the esophagus in Western countries in recent decades. The precise reasons for this incidence trend are also unclear. Largely reflecting the variability in esophageal SCC incidence, the incidence of esophageal cancer ranges from less than 10 per 100,000 population in Western countries to more than 100 per 100,000 in the Linxian province in China[1] and in areas of central Asia such as the North Gonbad area in Iran.[2] Worldwide, the most recent estimates are that esophageal cancer is the sixth most common cancer in men (212,600 new cases, 4.9% of all cancers) and the ninth most common in women (103,200 new cases, 2.7% of all cancers).[3]

Esophageal cancer is a deadly cancer. The current estimated annual number of deaths due to esophageal cancer for the United States is 12,600, only 500 fewer than the estimated 13,100 new cases of esophageal cancer.[4] Of the new cases, approximately three-quarters will occur in men,[4] and a male predominance is found for esophageal cancer of both histopathologic subtypes throughout the world. In the United States, cancer of the esophagus was the fifth most common site for cancer death in men aged 40–59 in 1999, behind lung and bronchus, colon and rectum, pancreas, and non-Hodgkin's lymphoma.[4] The 5-year relative cancer survival rate, adjusted for normal life expectancy, for esophageal cancer for all races in the United States for the pe-

riod 1989–1996 was 12%.[5] Only cancer of the pancreas (4% 5-year relative survival rate) and cancer of the liver (5% 5-year relative survival rate) have worse survival outcomes. The U.S. esophageal cancer 5-year relative survival rate for the 1989–1995 period was better for whites (13%) than for blacks (9%).[5]

Amid these unfavorable statistics, an encouraging finding is that the 5-year relative cancer survival rates for esophageal cancer have increased by a greater proportion than for any other malignancy: the survival rate of 5% for all races in 1974–1976 increased to 7% in 1980–1982, and a substantial increase, to 12%, was observed for the period 1989–1996.[5] Individual institutions have also reported significant improvements in survival, particularly for patients enrolled in endoscopic surveillance programs.[6–9]

Esophageal cancer thus provides a challenge to identify significant associations or causes for these incidence patterns. This chapter attempts to summarize the critical results of published research, giving more detail for the results for esophageal adenocarcinoma. Primary esophageal cancers other than SCC and adenocarcinoma, all of which are comparatively rare,[10] are not discussed.

## Classification of Adenocarcinoma of the Esophagus

The relationship between esophageal adenocarcinomas that arise within the tubular esophagus and adenocarcinomas found at, or immediately below, the gastroesophageal junction can be confusing. Primary adenocarcinomas of the esophagus are thought to arise in most cases from areas of Barrett's esophagus, the condition in which the normal squamous epithelium of the distal esophagus is replaced by a metaplastic columnar epithelium. The Barrett's epithelium is continuous with the columnar mucosa of the stomach. Malignant change within a clone of Barrett's cells will result in the development of esophageal adenocarcinoma if the clone is located within the tubular esophagus, but if the malignant focus is situated within the distal portion of the Barrett's segment, adjacent to the stomach, then the adenocarcinoma will be located at the gastroesophageal junction.[11]

The common Barrett's esophagus etiology in many or most cases suggests that it is reasonable to group esophageal and gastroesophageal junction adenocarcinomas together. Some molecular findings[12,13] also support the concept that esophageal and gastroesophageal junction adenocarcinomas should be considered together. Especially if Barrett's esophagus is present in the neighboring epithelium, adenocarcinomas arising either in the esophagus or at the junction may be classified as Barrett's-associated adenocarcinomas, or "Barrett's cancers."

Somewhat confusingly, the terms *cardia, gastric cardia,* and *subcardia* are also used for the site of origin of adenocarcinomas arising in the region of the gastroesophageal junction or immediately distal to the junction. Historically, the cardia was located at the gastroesophageal junction. The term *cardiospasm,* for example, was previously used for the disease achalasia, in which there is typically a high-pressure, nonrelaxing lower esophageal sphincter at the physiologic gastroesophageal junction.[14–17] Many studies use this traditional meaning for the location of the cardia, so that adenocarcinoma of the cardia is a synonym for adenocarcinoma of the gastroesophageal junction. Other studies, however, including those that have used the U.S. National Cancer Institute Surveillance, Epidemiology, and End Results (SEER) Program data, include cancers that arise in the most proximal section of the stomach, distal to the gastroesophageal junction, as cardia or "gastric cardia" cancers. Still others use the term *subcardia* to denote tumors in this proximal gastric region.

Unfortunately, there are few anatomic landmarks to distinguish any of these regions. Those landmarks that are present, such as the anatomic gastroesophageal junction located at the proximal extent of the gastric rugal folds,[18] can be obliterated or distorted by tumor. Furthermore, it can be difficult or impossible to determine the exact site of origin of cancers in this area because many tumors are large, involving both the proximal stomach and the distal esophagus, and, perhaps because the tumor has overrun the epithelium from which it arose,[19] there may be no adjacent area of Barrett's esophagus. Additional classification problems arise in patients who do not undergo operative resection, in whom the subsite must usually be determined at endoscopy. Anatomic subsite classification of these tumors at endoscopy can be difficult because of movement in this region, which is tethered to the diaphragm, and because tumor stenosis may prevent examination of the stomach. As a result, it may not be possible to accurately assess the extent of gastric involvement or the likelihood that the tumor is a primary gastric cancer. One study found involvement of the gastroesophageal junction in more than two-thirds of patients with either lower esophageal or cardia cancers,[20] while another study noted that more than 70% of esophageal and gastric cancer registrations at one registry lacked precise anatomic subsite information.[21]

For these reasons, there is probably some inaccuracy in the subsite classification of adenocarcinomas in this region in large studies such as epidemiology studies. It is not possible to be definite about the subsite origin of all tumors classified as esophageal, junctional, cardiac, or gastric, despite the stated ability of some studies to do so. It must therefore be considered that the cardia or junctional adenocarcinoma populations may be significantly different in different studies, and significant heterogene-

ity may be present within these groups even within the same study. These differences can influence study findings. It is likely that the more proximally situated esophageal adenocarcinomas are related to Barrett's esophagus, hiatus hernia, and gastroesophageal reflux disease. In contrast, tumors that arise several centimeters distal to the gastroesophageal junction are significantly less likely to be related to reflux, hernia, or Barrett's esophagus.[22,23] These more distally situated cancers are more likely to be primary gastric cancers, with different epidemiologic[24,25] and genetic profiles compared with those for esophageal adenocarcinomas.

## Incidence

### Adenocarcinoma

Sustained declines in overall, age-adjusted cancer incidence and mortality rates in the United States have been reported in the last several years. In view of this, the increase in the incidence of esophageal adenocarcinoma in Western countries during the last three decades is even more remarkable.[26] The increases in the incidence of adenocarcinoma of the esophagus and gastric cardia among men in the nine areas of the U.S. SEER Program in the period from 1976 to 1987 ranged from 4% to 10% per year, and thus exceeded those of any other type of cancer.[27] The incidence of esophageal and cardia adenocarcinomas continued to rise into the 1990s at a high rate of increase, although other cancers such as prostate cancer (with a rise in incidence due to the more widespread use of screening tests), melanoma, non-Hodgkin's lymphoma, and female lung cancer recorded higher rates of increase for some periods.[28–30]

Similar increases in incidence during the last several decades have been reported from other areas of the United States[31–35] and from other countries or regions, including Australia,[36,37] Canada,[38] Denmark,[39–41] regions of France, Belgium, The Netherlands, and Switzerland,[42–46] New Zealand,[47] Norway,[48] Sweden,[49,50] and areas of the United Kingdom.[21,51–56] Not all European areas have observed an increase in incidence.[57] There is some evidence for an increase in cardia adenocarcinoma in Asian counties, but the incidence of esophageal adenocarcinoma has not changed.[58–62] Gastroesophageal reflux and intestinal metaplasia in the lower esophagus and gastroesophageal junction regions are increasingly prevalent in some parts of Asia,[63,64] suggesting that the incidence of esophageal adenocarcinoma may rise in these areas in the future.

There is a steady increase in the esophageal cancer mortality rates with advancing age in both sexes.[30] Esophageal and cardia adenocarcinomas are rare in children and are very uncommon in persons younger than 30 years.[65–68] The incidence is at least several-fold higher in men than in women.[5,26,69] Adenocarcinoma is also approximately three times more common in whites than blacks in the United States, in contrast to esophageal SCC, which has a higher incidence in blacks.[70] The group with the largest increase in incidence in recent decades has been white men,[27–29,36,49,71] but increases in other groups including women[28,29] and blacks[28,29] have been observed within the past 10 years. The incidence rate for esophageal adenocarcinoma among white men in the United States more than tripled between 1974–1976 and 1992–1994, from 0.7 to 3.2 per 100,000, and adenocarcinoma now exceeds SCC in this population group.[29] The increase during this period was most pronounced in men older than 65 years, among whom there were threefold to fourfold increases, but the rates also doubled among white men less than 65 years old.[29]

The incidence of cardia cancers is also increasing.[26–29,34,49,72] In the United States SEER regions, almost half of all gastric cancers are now gastric cardia cancers.[27,29,30] The rate of increase is lower than that for esophageal adenocarcinoma, however, and in some areas no significant rise in the incidence of cardia cancer has been observed.[36,45,72] Differences in the incidence trends for cardia adenocarcinomas in different regions and in comparison with esophageal adenocarcinoma may partly reflect variability in the inclusion criteria for cardia cancers, as discussed below in the section on the classification of adenocarcinomas. If adenocarcinomas of the gastroesophageal junction or cardia are included with esophageal adenocarcinomas, both white men and white women in western countries are now more likely to develop an adenocarcinoma than an esophageal SCC. In contrast to cancers arising at the gastric cardia, stomach cancer other than adenocarcinoma of the cardia has been falling in incidence in Western societies for more than 50 years.[73–76]

It is likely that the reported rise in esophageal adenocarcinoma is a true phenomenon rather than merely the result of improvements in diagnosis or classification. A confounding factor for this statement is the fact that flexible endoscopy was widely adopted during the period of incidence increase. Flexible endoscopy has improved the clinician's ability to make a precisely localized histopathologic diagnosis. Before the introduction of flexible endoscopy, some esophageal cancers may have been assumed to be SCCs, and adenocarcinomas in the gastroesophageal junction region may have been falsely classified as gastric rather than esophageal cancers. Indeed, some older coding systems classified adenocarcinoma of the distal esophagus as proximal stomach cancers. The significance of these confounding factors is limited, however, by the observation of a gender difference. A gender difference would not be expected if changes in diagnostic and classification methods alone were responsible for the incidence rise.[27,33] Furthermore, a shift in classification of cancers at the distal esophagus to esophageal cancer rather than proximal gastric cancer or gastric cardia cancer would be expected to result in a fall in the incidence rate for gastric cardia cancer, rather than the rise observed in some areas.[30,37,49,52]

## Squamous Cell Carcinoma

Esophageal cancer is the fourth most common cancer in men in less developed regions, where SCC predominates over adenocarcinoma.[3] The estimated variation in esophageal cancer risk between high- and low-incidence areas is 15 times for men and 20 times for women.[3] In high-incidence areas, the rates tend to be high for both men and women. Approximately half of the world's esophageal cancer cases are thought to occur in China, where esophageal cancer is second only to gastric cancer in incidence and the mortality rates for esophageal and gastric cancers are very similar.[1,71] Marked differences in incidence are found in different regions of China. In one area (Linxian), the mortality rate from esophageal cancer has exceeded 100 per 10,000 for both men and women.[1]

The high-incidence Asian or Central Asian "esophageal cancer belt" has probably existed for many centuries.[2,77,78] The belt stretches from eastern Turkey though the east Caspian littoral, Northern Iran and Afghanistan, the region of Kashmir, and the Republics of Kazakhstan, Uzbekistan, and Turkmenistan. Those of Turkic origin are at high risk in these areas. Similarly, those of Mongol origin are at high risk in the high-incidence parts of Siberia.[1] The SCC rates are also high or very high among blacks in the Traskei in South Africa,[79,80] among blacks in regions in North America, and in parts of Normandy and Brittany,[43,81,82] southeast Brazil, Uruguay,[83] and in the Caribbean. A significant fall in incidence has been observed among Chinese in Singapore.[84]

## Risk Factors

### Barrett's Esophagus, Gastroesophageal Reflux Disease, and Adenocarcinoma

The most important risk factor for the development of esophageal adenocarcinoma is the presence of Barrett's esophagus. Although three types of columnar epithelium have traditionally been described in segments of Barrett's esophagus,[85] a widely used current definition for this disease requires that intestinal (also known as specialized) metaplasia be present microscopically within an area of visible columnar mucosa. Intestinal metaplasia is characterized by the presence of mucin-filled goblet cells with an often villiform surface epithelium.[86] The exact mechanisms by which Barrett's esophagus develops in response to gastroesophageal reflux, and even the cellular origin of Barrett's epithelium, remain uncertain. The presence and extent of Barrett's esophagus are associated with the severity and chronicity of the gastroesophageal reflux, as assessed by monitoring acid exposure in the distal esophagus.[87] The development of Barrett's esophagus is also associated with mixed reflux of both duodenal contents (containing bile salts and pancreatic juice) and gastric contents (containing hydrochloric acid and pepsin).[88–90]

It is estimated that at least 700,000 Americans have Barrett's esophagus,[91,92] and visible Barrett's esophagus is found in 4%–12% of patients who undergo upper gastrointestinal endoscopy for the investigation of reflux symptoms such as heartburn, regurgitation, and dysphagia.[93–95] Another 10% or more of those undergoing endoscopy in Western societies have areas of columnar epithelium with intestinal metaplasia that are not visible at endoscopy but are detected by microscopic examination of biopsies from the gastroesophageal junction.[96–101] These areas have been termed *ultrashort segment Barrett's esophagus* or *cardiac mucosa with intestinal metaplasia* (CIM).[102] Similar to the findings for esophageal adenocarcinoma, the incidence of this condition seems to have been increasing in recent decades,[103,104] although precise measurement of this increase is confounded by the concomitant increase in the frequency of endoscopic examination.[105] Barrett's esophagus also shares with esophageal adenocarcinoma a marked male predominance, an increasing incidence with age, and a similar racial distribution.[106]

The calculated risk of adenocarcinoma developing in patients with Barrett's esophagus varies widely in published studies. The estimated annual risk of developing esophageal adenocarcinoma ranges from 0.2% to 2.0%, equivalent to 1 in 441 to 1 in 52 patient-years. These estimates confer between a 30-fold and a 125-fold relative risk for adenocarcinoma for patients with Barrett's esophagus compared with an age-matched general population without Barrett's esophagus.[95,107–114] More recent prospective studies indicate that the risk of adenocarcinoma may be less than previously thought. Drewitz et al.[112] followed 170 patients with Barrett's esophagus for a mean of 57 months or 4.8 years (range 6–156 months), for a total of 834 patient-years. Patients with adenocarcinoma at diagnosis or within 6 months of diagnosis were excluded. Adenocarcinoma developed in four patients, an incidence of 1 per 208 patient-years of follow-up.[112] Similarly, in a study of 136 patients with Barrett's esophagus followed but one that is unsuccessful because of the overwhelming number of growth-stimulatory pathways in adenocarcinomas or the failure of p21 to associate with other cyclins.

## Cyclin-dependent Kinases

At this stage, it is worth discussing the molecular biology of cell cycling in more depth to clarify the subsequent literature on the molecular biology of adenocarcinoma and SCC in the esophagus. As previously discussed, wild-type p53 induces p21 expression. Cyclin-dependent kinases require association with a cyclin for their activity. For example, cyclin D1, which contributes to cell-cycle progression through the $G_1$ phase, associates preferentially with CDK4, CDK6, or proliferating cell nuclear antigen (PCNA).[62] A consequence of the association between cyclin D1 and CDK4 or CDK6 is phosphorylation of the retinoblastoma tumor suppressor gene product pRb.[63] Hyperphosphorylation of pRb leads to its dissociation from transcription factors such as E2F that transcriptionally regulate growth-promoting genes. Hence, one can envisage how wild-type p53, through p21, can keep a check on cell-cycle progression by inhibiting the CDKs and consequently preventing hyperphosphorylation of the pRb, thus maintaining its association with the transcription factors. When CDKs are active, they allow hyperphosphorylation of pRb, which causes the dissociated transcription factor E2F to transcribe S-phase genes, with resultant passage of cells into S phase. Three other proteins that are implicated in the regulation of the transition from $G_1$ to S phase are MDM-2, p16, and p27.

The *MDM-2* (murine double minute 2) gene encodes a 90,000 kDa protein that functions in a negative feedback mechanism regulating the activity of *p53*[64,65] and *Rb* genes.[66,67] Thus, any subsequent amplification and overexpression of the *MDM-2* gene can block the cell-cycle control activity of these two tumor suppressor genes. *MDM-2* interacts physically and functionally with pRb, as with p53, and inhibits pRb's growth-regulatory function. Two very recent studies have examined the role of MDM-2 in esophageal adenocarcinomas.[68,69] Both studies provide evidence of low-level or no *MDM-2* gene amplification, and one of them[68] identified overexpression of MDM-2 in 55% of adenocarcinomas examined, though only in the presence of wild-type p53. One might hypothesize that *MDM-2* is responsible for stabilization of the p53 protein and possible loss of tumor suppressor activity, as also proposed by Oliner et al.[65] Another protein of interest is p16, which maps to 9p21 and has already been described in Table 13–1 as the subject of LOH and mutations in esophageal cancer. This protein forms binary complexes with CDK4 and CDK6, inhibiting their ability to phosphorylate the Rb protein.[70] Hence, loss of the p16 protein would probably result in increased Rb phosphorylation and allow cells to enter into S phase. In terms of p16 expression in esophageal cancer, Takeuchi et al.[71] reported in 1997 that of 111 SCCs of the esophagus, 50% had a complete loss of p16 expression, a finding that would follow from LOH and gene inactivation studies.[34,72–75] When the same tumors were also examined for cyclin D1 expression, 25% exhibited positive expression.

p27 is a CDK inhibitor thats binds to cyclin–CDK complexes and regulates the transition from $G_1$ to S phase. It has been reported to be overexpressed in the presence of growth-inhibitory cytokines such as TGF-β. P27 thus acts as a link between the extracellular environment and the cell cycle.[76–78]

Jiang et al.[79] found a 3- to 10-fold amplification of the cyclin D1 gene in 32% of SCC tumors examined, and 92% showed overexpression of the cyclin D1 protein, observations that are consistent with those from several other studies.[80–84] A study by Arber et al.[85] investigated the overexpression of cyclin D1 in both adenocarcinoma and SCC of the esophagus in parallel. Within the esophagus, 71% of the SCC and 64% of the adenocarcinomas were positive for increased cyclin D1 nuclear staining. Hence overexpression of cyclin D1 was common in both adenocarcinoma and SCC of the esophagus as well as in a number of other human SCC.[86–88] The likely consequence of overexpression of cyclin D1 is increased cellular proliferation as cells enter rapidly into S phase from the $G_1$ phase. This interpretation is supported by evidence from studies by Quelle et al.[89] and Jiang et al.[83] These two groups overexpressed cyclin D1 in cultured cells and reported a shortened $G_1$ phase, resulting in a more rapid entry into S phase and increased cell proliferation.

Matsumoto et al.[81] reported that there is also overexpression of the cyclin D1 partner CDK4 in esophageal SCC. In 43% of tumors overexpressing cyclin D1 there was overexpression of CDK4, although on statistical analysis there was no significant relationship in immunopositivity between cyclin D1 and CDK4. These findings suggest that, although CDKs are catalytic partners of cyclins, in human esophageal SCC these proteins often exhibit dysregulated overexpression. However, Matsumoto et al. postulated that the prognosis of patients with tumors that were cyclin D1 and CDK4 positive may be significantly poorer than that of patients with cyclin D1 negative tumors.

The means by which Rb protein is hyperphosphorylated by the cyclin–CDK complex has also been investigated in the context of esophageal cancer. As noted earlier, LOH of the *Rb* gene is present in both SCC and adenocarcinoma of the esophagus (Table 13–1). A recent immunohistochemical analysis of Rb in SCC of the esophagus revealed different patterns of pRb expression among the tumor samples;[81a] 16 of 56 tumors examined displayed extensive Rb staining (comparable to that to normal epithelia), whereas tumors showed little if any Rb staining. As might be expected, 90% of the tumor samples with Rb LOH expressed little or no pRb. These results suggest that LOH is the main event leading to Rb inactivation. Remarkably, Rb alteration was strongly associated with p53 alteration; in these samples, the tumors that had the most severe Rb inactivation stained intensely for mutant p53. It has already been postulated that aberrant Rb and p53 can deregulate cell-cycle control so that apoptosis is avoided,[90] which can greatly increase the growth advantage of the affected cells and accelerate tumor formation. This hypothesis is supported by a recent study by Hashimoto et al.,[91] who have shown that patients with SCC of the esophagus marked by mutant p53 expression and low Rb expression have a very poor prognosis.

As for *p27* mutation in esophageal SCC, there is evidence from Ohashi et al.[92] that, although there are no genetic aberrations in the gene, there is reduced expression of the protein in such cases. In the cases examined, those patients with low p27 levels had a poorer prognosis than those with normal p27 levels. The process by which p27 is reduced in esophageal SCC seems to be proteosome-mediated degradation.[78] Interestingly, *p27* expression levels and/or activity have been reported to be elevated by TGF-β, which might suggest that at this late stage of carcinogenesis there is no longer signaling via this pathway.

All of the cell-cycling events discussed above that occur in normal esophagus and esophageal cancer are diagrammed in Figure 13–1.

Normal mucosa

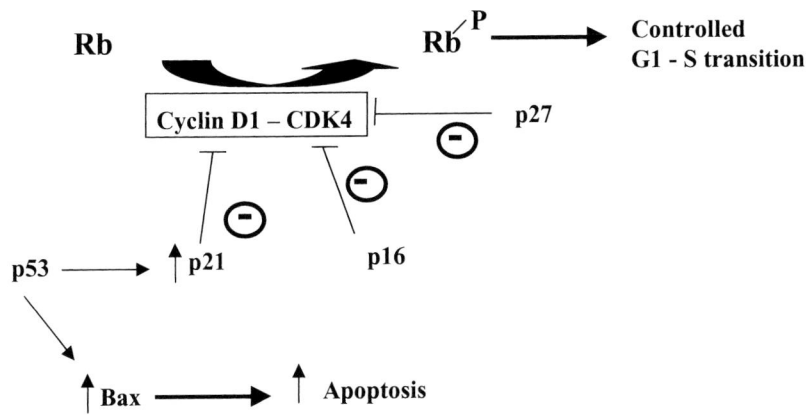

Esophageal cancer

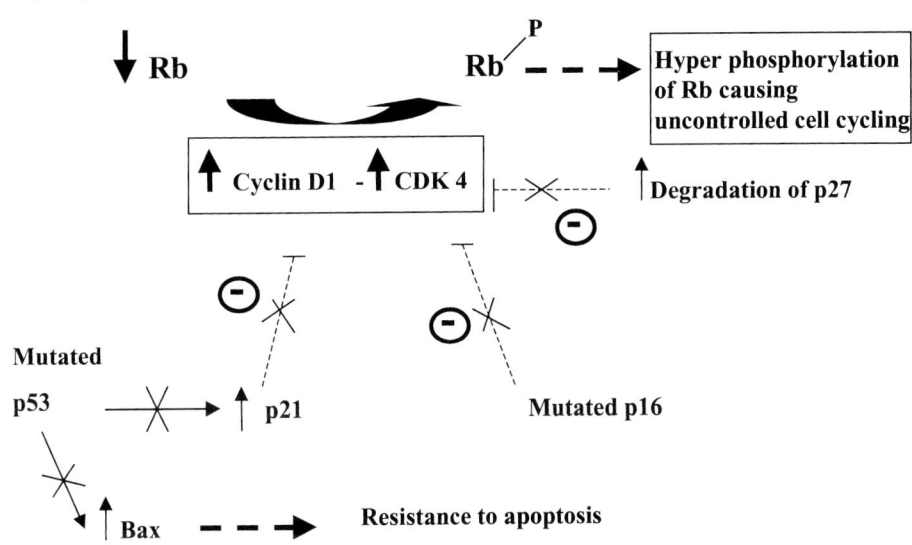

**Figure 13-1** A diagrammatic representation of cell-cycle control in normal esophagus versus esophageal cancer.

## Extracellular Signaling through Receptor-linked Tyrosine Kinases

The intracellular events described above are in many instances initiated by either genetic aberrations or the action of other intracellular signals. Many of these intracellular signals, however, are also generated by an extracellular stimulus. It has long been recognized that a key mechanism for induction of cellular growth and transformation involves extracellular stimuli such as growth factors. Activation of the receptor-linked tyrosine kinase of these growth factors results in the transmission of intracellular signals.[93] Two such receptor-linked tyrosine kinases are the products of oncogenes c-erb-B1 (EGFR) and c-erbB-2, both of which have been implicated in esophageal cancer.[94-99] Amplification or overexpression of either gene has been shown to indicate poor prognosis in several human cancers.[100,101]

Ligands that bind the EGFR and the c-erbB-2 tyrosine kinases have been characterized and shown to promote tumor cell proliferation.[102,103] The ligands for EGFR are transforming growth factor α (TGF-α) and epidermal growth factor (EGF), both of which have been shown to be up-regulated in esophageal adenocarcinoma.[104-106] Interestingly, TGF-α expression is thought to be the more important of the two because it is increased more dramatically than that of EGF, in part because incomplete cleavage of the prepro-TGF-α molecule in dysplastic tissue allows juxtacrine mitogenic stimulation.[104] In addition, the in vivo and in vitro correlations with dysplastic progression and tumorigenic biology are stronger for TGF-α. It is has been postulated that TGF-α overexpression is an early event in the progression of Barrett's metaplasia to adenocarcinoma, thus implicating extracellular signaling in the progression of esophageal cancer.[105-108] Interestingly, Grb7, a ligand for both EGFR and c-erbB-2,[109,110] is laboratory is investigating the possibility that γ-catenin may also be phosphorylated and involved in signaling events.

## Matrix Metalloproteinases

So far, this review has focused on the details of how esophageal cancer grows through genetic instability, increased cell cycling, and evasion of apoptosis, and on the prerequisite modulation of cell adhesion for cells to detach from a primary tumor site and ultimately metastasize. For tumor invasion to occur, there must be degradation of the extracellular matrix and connective tissue surrounding the tumor cells. The matrix metalloproteinases

(MMPs) are a family of enzymes that collectively are able to degrade most components of the extracellular matrix; considerable evidence indicates that individual MMPs have an important role in tumor invasion and metastasis in esophageal cancer.[146–150] A study by Murray et al.[146] found MMP-1, MMP-2, and MMP-9 in esophageal tumors, with MMP-2 and MMP-9 being present in more than 70% of all tumors examined. MMP-1, however, was detected in only 24% of esophageal tumors and its presence was associated with poor prognosis.

The first stage in the invasion process of malignant esophageal cells is the degradation of the basement membrane, the main component of which is type IV collagen. Type IV collagen is

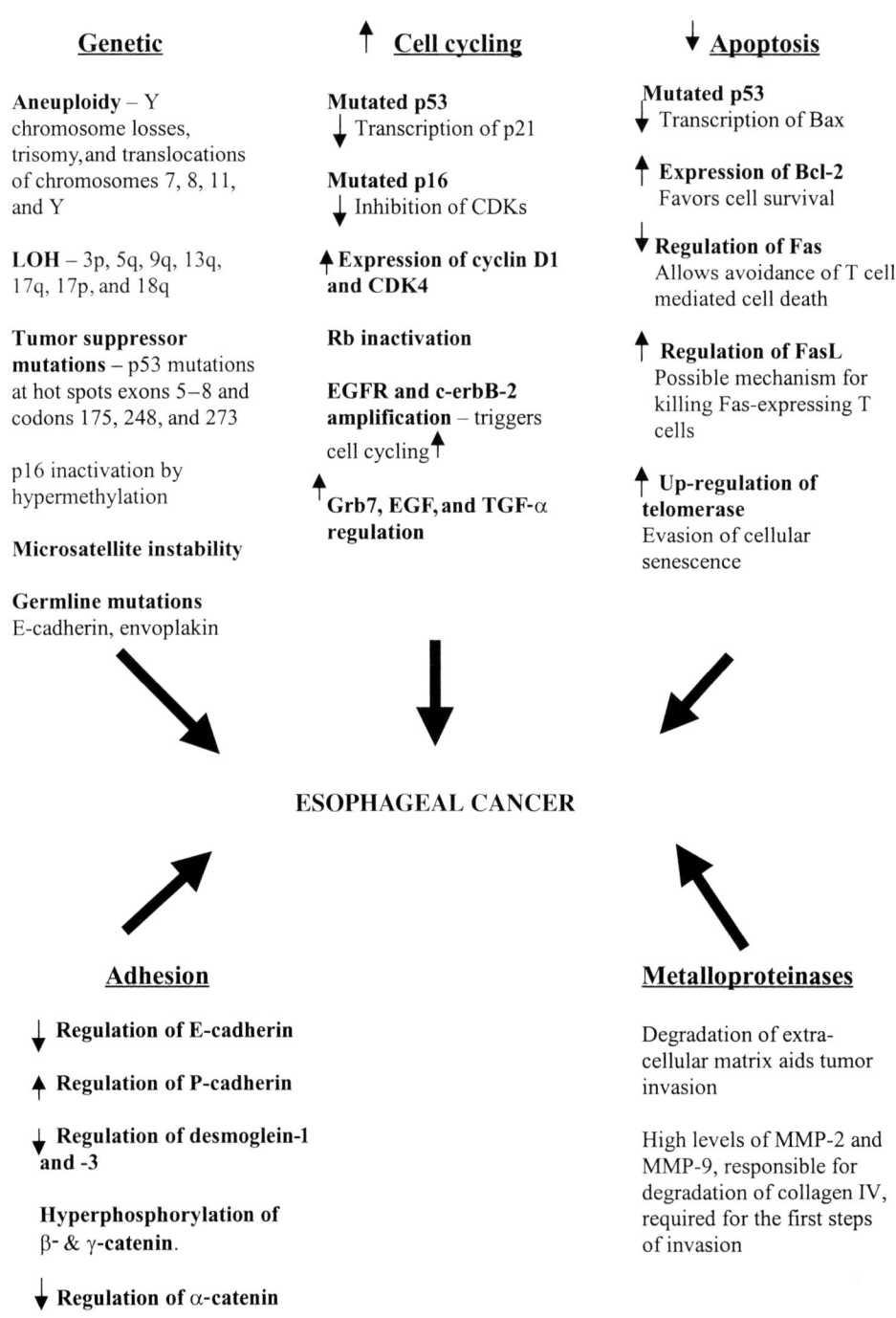

**Figure 13-2**  A summary of the potential molecular events involved in the pathogenesis of esophageal cancer.

most effectively broken down by MMP-2 and MMP-9 hence it is of no surprise that in the esophageal tumors examined high levels of these MMPs were observed. For further invasion to occur, other substrates need to be degraded and the role of other MMPs such as MMP-1 thus becomes evident. Tumors expressing MMP-1 are probably the most aggressive. Immunohistochemical studies performed by Adachi et al.[148] and Yamamoto et al.[146] have revealed high levels of MMP-7 in tumor samples, implicating this protein in the progression of esophageal cancer.

## Convergence in Mechanisms of Molecular Progression

In both SCC and adenocarcinoma, very similar mechanisms of cancer progression are observed. Initially, clonal expansion occurs as a consequence of increased cell cycling due to *p53* mutations, alteration of CDKs, and growth factor stimulation. Subsequently, clonal purification as a consequence of apoptosis of neighboring cells allows "transformed" cells to expand into adjacent tissues. At this point, subtle changes in cell adhesion enable cells to migrate into differentiated compartments while the stem cells in the metaplastic glands bifurcate, resulting in gland fission.[151] The final transition is the invasion of the basement membrane by these cells, primarily through the action of metalloproteinases. The potential molecular events involved in esophageal cancer are depicted in Figure 13–2.

The challenge in future work will be to further delineate the molecular pathology of esophageal cancer and apply findings to precise diagnosis, prognosis, and treatment of patients with this devastating disease.

## References

1. Robaszkiewicz M, Reid BJ, Volant A, Cauvin JM, Rabinovitch PS, Gouerou H. Flow-cytometric DNA content analysis of esophageal squamous cell carcinomas. Gastroenterology 101:1588–1593, 1991.
2. Itakura Y, Sasano H, Mori S, Nagura H. DNA ploidy in human esophageal squamous dysplasias and squamous cell carcinomas as determined by image analysis. Mod Pathol 7:867–873, 1994.
3. Rabinovitch PS, Reid BJ, Haggitt RC, Norwood TH, Rubin CE. Progression to cancer in Barrett's esophagus is associated with genomic instability. Lab Invest 60:65–71, 1989.
4. Garewal HS, Sampliner R, Liu Y, Trent JM. Chromosomal rearrangements in Barrett's esophagus: a premalignant lesion of esophageal adenocarcinoma. Cancer Genet Cytogenet 42:281–286, 1989.
5. Shimada Y, Imamura M, Wagata T, Yamaguchi N, Tobe T. Characterization of 21 newly established esophageal cancer cell lines. Cancer 69:277–284, 1992.
6. Rosenblum-Vos LS, Meltzer SJ, Leana-Cox J, Schwartz S. Cytogenetic studies of primary cultures of esophageal squamous cell carcinoma. Cancer Genet Cytogenet 70:127–131, 1993.
7. Watanabe M, Kuwano H, Tanaka S, Toh Y, Sadanaga N, Sugimachi K. Flow cytometric DNA analysis is useful in detecting multiple genetic alterations in squamous cell carcinoma of the esophagus. Cancer 85: 2322–2328, 1999.
8. Lasko D, Cavenee W, Nordenskjold M. Loss of constitutional heterozygosity in human cancer. Annu Rev Genet 25:281–314, 1991.
9. Montesano R, Hollstein M, Hainaut P. Genetic alterations in esophageal cancer and their relevance to etiology and pathogenesis: a review. Int J Cancer 69:225–235, 1996.
10. Mori T, Yanagisawa A, Kato Y, Miura K, Nishihira T, Mori S, Nakamura Y. Accumulation of genetic alterations during esophageal carcinogenesis. Hum Mol Genet 3:1969–1971, 1994
11. Shibagaki I, Shimada Y, Wagata T, Ikenaga M, Imamura M, Ishizaki K. Allelotype analysis of esophageal squamous cell carcinoma. Cancer Res 54:2996–3000, 1994.
12. Pack SD, Karkera JD, Zhuang Z, Pak ED, Balan KV, Hwu P, Park WS, Pham T, Ault DO, Glaser M, Liotta L, Detera-Wadleigh SD, Wadleigh RG. Molecular cytogenetic fingerprinting of esophageal squamous cell carcinoma by comparative genomic hybridization reveals a consistent pattern of chromosomal alterations. Genes Chromosomes Cancer 25: 160–168, 1999.
13. Rumpel CA, Powell SM, Moskaluk CA. Mapping of genetic deletions on the long arm of chromosome 4 in human esophageal adenocarcinomas. Am J Pathol 154:1329–1334, 1999.
14. Peralta RC, Casson AG, Wang RN, Keshavjee S, Redston M, Bapat B. Distinct regions of frequent loss of heterozygosity of chromosome 5p and 5q in human esophageal cancer. Int J Cancer 23:600–605, 1998.
15. Maesawa C, Tamura G, Suzuki Y, Ogasawara S, Ishida K, Saito K, Satodate R. Aberrations of tumor-suppressor genes (*p53, apc, mcc* and *Rb*) in esophageal squamous-cell carcinoma. Int J Cancer 57:21–25, 1994.
16. Boynton RF, Blount PL, Yin J, Brown VL, Huang Y, Tong Y, McDaniel T, Newkirk C, Resau JH, Raskind WH, Haggitt RC, Reid BJ, Meltzer SJ. Loss of heterozygosity involving the APC and MCC genetic loci occurs in the majority of human esophageal cancers. Proc Natl Acad Sci USA 89:3385–3388, 1992.
17. Muzeau F, Flejou JF, Thomas G, Hamelin R. Loss of heterozygosity on chromosome 9 and *p16* (*MTS1, CDKN2*) gene mutations in esophageal cancers. Int J Cancer 72:27–30, 1997.
18. Aoki T, Mori T, Du X, Nishihira T, Matsubara T, Nakamura Y. Allelotype study of esophageal carcinoma. Genes Chromosomes Cancer 10: 177–182, 1994.
19. Huang Y, Boynton RF, Blount PL, Silverstein RJ, Yin J, Tong Y, McDaniel TK, Newkirk C, Resau JH, Sridhara R, Reid BJ, Meltzer SJ. Loss of heterozygosity involves multiple tumor suppressor genes in human esophageal cancers. Cancer Res 52:6525–6530, 1992.
20. Tarmin L, Yin J, Zhou X, Suzuki H, Jiang HY, Rhyu MG, Abraham JM, Krasna MJ, Cottrell J, Meltzer SJ. Frequent loss of heterozygosity on chromosome 9 in adenocarcinoma and squamous cell carcinoma of the esophagus. Cancer Res 54:6094–6096, 1994.
21. Gonzalez MV, Artimez ML, Rodrigo L, Lopez-Larrea C, Menendez MJ, Alvarez V, Perez R, Fresno MF, Perez MJ, Sampedro A, Coto E. Mutation analysis of the *p53, APC,* and *p16* genes in the Barrett's oesophagus, dysplasia, and adenocarcinoma. J Clin Pathol 50:212–217, 1997.
22. Huang Y, Meltzer SJ, Yin J, Tong Y, Chang EH, Srivastava S, McDaniel T, Boynton RF, Zou ZQ. Altered messenger RNA and unique mutational profiles of p53 and Rb in human esophageal carcinomas. Cancer Res 53:1889–1894, 1993.
23. Meltzer SJ, Yin J, Huang Y, McDaniel TK, Newkirk C, Iseri O, Vogelstein B, Resau JH. Reduction to homozygosity involving p53 in esophageal cancers demonstrated by the polymerase chain reaction. Proc Natl Acad Sci USA 88:4976–4980, 1991.
24. Neshat K, Sanchez CA, Galipeau PC, Blount PL, Levine DS, Joslyn G, Reid BJ. *p53* mutations in Barrett's adenocarcinoma and high-grade dysplasia. Gastroenterology 106:1589–1595, 1994.
25. Swift A, Risk JM, Kingsnorth AN, Wright TA, Myskow M, Field JK. Frequent loss of heterozygosity on chromosome 17 at 17q11.2–q12 in Barrett's adenocarcinoma. Br J Cancer 71:995–998, 1995.
26. Karkera JD, Balan KV, Yoshikawa T, Lipman TO, Korman L, Sharma A, Patterson RH, Sani N, Detera-Wadleigh SD, Wadleigh RG. Systematic screening of chromosome 18 for loss of heterozygosity in esophageal squamous cell carcinoma. Cancer Genet Cytogenet 111:81–86, 1999.
27. Miyake S, Nagai K, Yoshino K, Oto M, Endo M, Yuasa Y. Point mutations and allelic deletion of tumor suppressor gene *DCC* in human esophageal squamous cell carcinomas and their relation to metastasis. Cancer Res 54:3007–3010, 1994.
28. Frankel RH, Bayona W, Koslow M, Newcomb EW. *p53* mutations in human malignant gliomas: comparison of loss of heterozygosity with mutation frequency. Cancer Res 52:1427–1433, 1992.
29. Fearon ER, Vogelstein B. A genetic model for colorectal tumorigenesis. Cell 61:759–767, 1990.
30. Hollstein M, Shomer B, Greenblatt M, Soussi T, Hovig E, Montesano R, Harris CC. Somatic point mutations in the *p53* gene of human tumors and cell lines: updated compilation. Nucl Acids Res 24:141–146, 1996.
31. Hamelin R, Flejou JF, Muzeau F, Potet F, Laurent-Puig P, Fekete F, Thomas G. TP53 gene mutations and p53 protein immunoreactivity in malignant and premalignant Barrett's esophagus. Gastroenterology 107: 1012–1018, 1994.
32. Gleeson CM, Sloan JM, McGuigan JA, Ritchie AJ, Russell SE. Base transitions at CpG dinucleotides in the *p53* gene are common in esophageal adenocarcinoma. Cancer Res 55:3406–3411, 1995.
33. Barrett MT, Sanchez CA, Galipeau PC, Neshat K, Emond M, Reid BJ. Allelic loss of 9p21 and mutation of the *CDKN2/p16* gene develop as

early lesions during neoplastic progression in Barrett's esophagus. Oncogene 13:1867–1873, 1996.

34. Wong DJ, Barrett MT, Stoger R, Emond MJ, Reid BJ. p16INK4a promoter is hypermethylated at a high frequency in esophageal adenocarcinomas. Cancer Res 57:2619–2622, 1997.

35. Powell SM, Papadopoulos N, Kinzler KW, Smolinski KN, Meltzer SJ. APC gene mutations in the mutation cluster region are rare in esophageal cancers. Gastroenterology 107:1759–1763, 1994.

36. Ilyas M, Tomlinson IP. Genetic pathways in colorectal cancer. Histopathology 28:389–399, 1996.

37. Meltzer SJ, Yin J, Manin B, Rhyu MG, Cottrell J, Hudson E, Redd JL, Krasna MJ, Abraham JM, Reid BJ. Microsatellite instability occurs frequently and in both diploid and aneuploid cell populations of Barrett's-associated esophageal adenocarcinomas. Cancer Res 54:3379–3382, 1994.

38. Gleeson CM, Sloan JM, McGuigan JA, Ritchie AJ, Weber JL, Russell SE. Ubiquitous somatic alterations at microsatellite alleles occur infrequently in Barrett's-associated esophageal adenocarcinoma. Cancer Res 56:259–263, 1996.

39. Iwaya T, Maesawa C, Ogasawara S, Tamura G. Tylosis esophageal cancer locus on chromosome 17q25.1 is commonly deleted in sporadic human esophageal cancer. Gastroenterology 114:1206–1210, 1998.

40. Caldos C, Carneiro F, Lynch HT, et al. Familial gastric cancer: overview and guidelines for management [review]. J Med Genet 36:873–880, 1999.

41. Gotz C, Montenarh M. p53: DNA damage, DNA repair, and apoptosis. Rev Physiol Biochem Pharmacol 127:65–95, 1996.

42. Montenarh M. Biochemical properties of the growth suppressor/oncoprotein p53. Oncogene 7:1673–1680, 1992.

43. el-Deiry WS, Tokino T, Velculescu VE, Levy DB, Parsons R, Trent JM, Lin D, Mercer WE, Kinzler KW, Vogelstein B. WAF1, a potential mediator of *p53* tumor suppression. Cell 75:817–825, 1993.

44. Harper JW, Adami GR, Wei N, Keyomarsi K, Elledge SJ. The p21 Cdk-interacting protein Cip1 is a potent inhibitor of G1 cyclin-dependent kinases. Cell 75:805–816, 1993.

45. Miyashita T, Reed JC. Tumor suppressor p53 is a direct transcriptional activator of the human *bax* gene. Cell 80:293–299, 1995.

46. el-Deiry WS, Harper JW, O'Connor PM, et al. WAF1/CIP1 is induced in p53-mediated G1 arrest and apoptosis. Cancer Res 54:1169–1174, 1994.

47. el-Deiry WS, Kern SE, Pietenpol JA, Kinzler KW, Vogelstein B. Definition of a consensus binding site for p53. Nat Genet 1:45–49, 1992.

48. Funk WD, Pak DT, Karas RH, Wright WE, Shay JW. A transcriptionally active DNA-binding site for human p53 protein complexes. Mol Cell Biol 12:2866–2871, 1992.

49. Ramel S, Reid BJ, Sanchez CA, Blount PL, Levine DS, Neshat K, Haggitt RC, Dean PJ, Thor K, Rabinovitch PS. Evaluation of p53 protein expression in Barrett's esophagus by two-parameter flow cytometry. Gastroenterology 102:1220–1228, 1992.

50. Wang DY, Xiang YY, Tanaka M, Li XR, Li JL, Shen Q, Sugimura H, Kino I. High prevalence of p53 protein overexpression in patients with esophageal cancer in Linxian, China and its relationship to progression and prognosis. Cancer 74:3089–3096, 1994.

51. Sarbia M, Bittinger F, Grabellus F, Verreet P, Dutkowski P, Willers R, Gabbert HE. Expression of Bax, a pro-apoptotic member of the Bcl-2 family, in esophageal squamous cell carcinoma. Int J Cancer 73:508–513, 1997.

52. Lam KY, Law S, Tin L, et al. The clinicopathological significance of p21 and p53 expression in esophageal squamous cell carcinoma: an analysis of 153 patients. Am J Gastroenterol 94:2060–2068, 1999.

53. Shiohara M, el-Deiry WS, Wada M, Nakamaki T, Takeuchi S, Yang R, Chen DL, Vogelstein B, Koeffler HP. Absence of *WAF1* mutations in a variety of human malignancies. Blood 84:3781–3784, 1994.

54. Ohashi K, Nemoto T, Eishi Y, Matsuno A, Nakamura K, Hirokawa K. Expression of the cyclin dependent kinase inhibitor p21WAF1/CIP1 in oesophageal squamous cell carcinomas. Virchows Arch 430:389–395, 1997.

55. Seta T, Imazeki F, Yokosuka O, Saisho H, Suzuki T, Koide Y, Isono K. Expression of p53 and p21WAF1/CIP1 proteins in gastric and esophageal cancers: comparison with mutations of the *p53* gene. Dig Dis Sci 43:279–289, 1998.

56. Toh Y, Kuwano H, Sonoda K. Correlation between reduced p21WAF1/CIP1 expression in esophageal carcinomas. Int J Oncol 11:703–708, 1997.

57. Wakasugi E, Kobayashi T, Tamaki Y, Ito Y, Miyashiro I, Komoike Y, Takeda T, Shin E, Takatsuka Y, Kikkawa N, Monden T, Monden M. p21(Waf1/Cip1) and p53 protein expression in breast cancer. Am J Clin Pathol 107:684–691, 1997.

58. Ogawa M, Maeda K, Onoda N, Chung YS, Sowa M. Loss of p21WAF1/CIP1 expression correlates with disease progression in gastric carcinoma. Br J Cancer 75:1617–1620, 1997.

59. Michieli P, Chedid M, Lin D, Pierce JH, Mercer WE, Givol D. Induction of WAF1/CIP1 by a p53-independent pathway. Cancer Res 54:3391–3395, 1994.

60. Parker SB, Eichele G, Zhang P, Rawls A, Sands AT, Bradley A, Olson EN, Harper JW, Elledge SJ. p53-independent expression of p21Cip1 in muscle and other terminally differentiating cells. Science 267:1024–1027, 1995.

61. Hanas JS, Lerner MR, Lightfoot SA, Raczkowski C, Kastens DJ, Brackett DJ, Postier RG. Expression of the cyclin-dependent kinase inhibitor p21(WAF1/CIP1) and p53 tumor suppressor in dysplastic progression and adenocarcinoma in Barrett esophagus. Cancer 86:756–763, 1999.

62. Sherr CJ. Mammalian G1 cyclins. Cell 73:1059–1065, 1993.

63. Dowdy SF, Hinds PW, Louie K, Reed SI, Arnold A, Weinberg RA. Physical interaction of the retinoblastoma protein with human D cyclins. Cell 73:499–511, 1993.

64. Momand J, Zambetti GP, Olson DC, George D, Levine AJ. The mdm-2 oncogene product forms a complex with the p53 protein and inhibits p53-mediated transactivation. Cell 69:1237–1245, 1992.

65. Oliner JD, Pietenpol JA, Thiagalingam S, Gyuris J, Kinzler KW, Vogelstein B. Oncoprotein MDM2 conceals the activation domain of tumour suppressor p53. Nature 362:857–860, 1993.

66. Martin K, Trouche D, Hagemeier C, Sorensen TS, La Thangue NB, Kouzarides T. Stimulation of E2F1/DP1 transcriptional activity by MDM2 oncoprotein. Nature 375:691–694, 1995.

67. Xiao ZX, Chen J, Levine AJ, Modjtahedi N, Xing J, Sellers WR, Livingston DM. Interaction between the retinoblastoma protein and the oncoprotein MDM2. Nature 375:694–698, 1995.

68. Soslow RA, Altorki NK, Yang G, Xie D, Yang CS. mdm-2 expression correlates with wild-type p53 status in esophageal adenocarcinoma. Mod Pathol 12:580–586, 1999.

69. Morgan RJ, Newcomb PV, Hardwick RH, Alderson D. Amplification of cyclin D1 and *MDM-2* in oesophageal carcinoma. Eur J Surg Oncol 25:364–367, 1999.

70. Serrano M, Hannon GJ, Beach D. A new regulatory motif in cell-cycle control causing specific inhibition of cyclin D/CDK4. Nature 366:704–707, 1993.

71. Takeuchi H, Ozawa S, Ando N, Shih CH, Koyanagi K, Ueda M, Kitajima M. Altered *p16/MTS1/CDKN2* and cyclin D1/*PRAD-1* gene expression is associated with the prognosis of squamous cell carcinoma of the esophagus. Clin Cancer Res 3:2229–2236, 1997.

72. Mori T, Miura K, Aoki T, Nishihira T, Mori S, Nakamura Y. Frequent somatic mutation of the *MTS1/CDK4I* (multiple tumor suppressor/cyclin-dependent kinase 4 inhibitor) gene in esophageal squamous cell carcinoma. Cancer Res 54:3396–3397, 1994.

73. Cairns P, Polascik TJ, Eby Y, et al. Frequency of homozygous deletion at *p16/CDKN2* in primary human tumours. Nat Genet 11:210–212, 1995.

74. Merlo A, Herman JG, Mao L, Lee DJ, Gabrielson E, Burger PC, Baylin SB, Sidransky D. 5′ CpG island methylation is associated with transcriptional silencing of the tumour suppressor p16/CDKN2/MTS1 in human cancers. Nat Med 1:686–692, 1995.

75. Suzuki H, Zhou X, Yin J, et al. Intragenic mutations of *CDKN2B* and *CDKN2A* in primary human esophageal cancers. Hum Mol Genet 4:1883–1887, 1995.

76. Toyoshima H, Hunter T. p27, a novel inhibitor of G1 cyclin–Cdk protein kinase activity, is related to p21. Cell 78:67–74, 1994.

77. Sherr CJ, Roberts JM. Inhibitors of mammalian G1 cyclin-dependent kinases. Genes Dev 9:1149–1163, 1995.

78. Pagano M, Tam SW, Theodoras AM, Beer-Romero P, Del Sal G, Chau V, Yew PR, Draetta GF, Rolfe M. Role of the ubiquitin–proteasome pathway in regulating abundance of the cyclin-dependent kinase inhibitor p27. Science 269:682–685, 1995.

79. Jiang W, Zhang YJ, Kahn SM, Hollstein MC, Santella RM, Lu SH, Harris CC, Montesano R, Weinstein IB. Altered expression of the cyclin D1 and retinoblastoma genes in human esophageal cancer. Proc Natl Acad Sci USA 90:9026–9030, 1993.

80. Fujii S, Tominaga O, Nagawa H, Tsuno N, Nita ME, Tsuruo T, Muto T. Quantitative analysis of the cyclin expression in human esophageal cancer cell lines. J Exp Clin Cancer Res 17:491–496, 1998.

81. Matsumoto M, Furihata M, Ishikawa T, Ohtsuki Y, Ogoshi S. Comparison of deregulated expression of cyclin D1 and cyclin E with that of cyclin-dependent kinase 4 (CDK4) and CDK2 in human oesophageal squamous cell carcinoma. Br J Cancer 80:256–261, 1999.

81a. Xing EP, Yang GY, Wang LD, et al. Loss of heterozygosity of the Rb gene correlates with pRb protein expression and associates with p53 alteration in human esophageal cancer. Clin Cancer Res 5:1231–1240, 1999.

82. Tsuruta H, Sakamoto H, Onda M, Terada M. Amplification and overexpression of EXP1 and EXP2/cyclin D1 genes in human esophageal carcinomas. Biochem Biophys Res Commun 196:1529–1536, 1993.

83. Jiang W, Kahn SM, Tomita N, Zhang YJ, Lu SH, Weinstein IB. Amplification and expression of the human cyclin D gene in esophageal cancer. Cancer Res 52:2980–2983, 1992.

84. Morgan RJ, Newcomb PV, Hardwick RH, Alderson D. Amplification of cyclin D1 and MDM-2 in oesophageal carcinoma. Eur J Surg Oncol 25:364–367, 1999.

85. Arber N, Gammon MD, Hibshoosh H, Britton JA, Zhang Y, Schonberg JB, Roterdam H, Fabian I, Holt PR, Weinstein IB. Overexpression of cyclin D1 occurs in both squamous carcinomas and adenocarcinomas of the esophagus and in adenocarcinomas of the stomach. Hum Pathol 30:1087–1092, 1999.

86. Bartkova J, Lukas J, Muller H, Strauss M, Gusterson B, Bartek J. Abnormal patterns of D-type cyclin expression and G1 regulation in human head and neck cancer. Cancer Res 55:949–956, 1995.

87. Callender T, el-Naggar AK, Lee MS, Frankenthaler R, Luna MA, Batsakis JG. PRAD-1 (CCND1)/cyclin D1 oncogene amplification in primary head and neck squamous cell carcinoma. Cancer 74:152–158, 1994.

88. Nakagawa H, Zukerberg L, Togawa K, Meltzer SJ, Nishihara T, Rustgi AK. Human cyclin D1 oncogene and esophageal squamous cell carcinoma. Cancer 76:541–549, 1995.

89. Quelle DE, Ashmun RA, Shurtleff SA, Kato JY, Bar-Sagi D, Roussel MF, Sherr CJ. Overexpression of mouse D-type cyclins accelerates G1 phase in rodent fibroblasts. Genes Dev 7:1559–15571, 1993.

90. Sherr CJ. Cancer cell cycles. Science 274:1672–1677, 1996.

91. Hashimoto N, Tachibana M, Dhar DK, et al. Expression of p53 and RB proteins in squamous cell carcinoma of the esophagus: their relationship with clinicopathologic characteristics. Ann Surg Oncol 6:489–494, 1999.

92. Ohashi Y, Sasano H, Yamaki H, Shizawa S, Shineha R, Akaishi T, Satomi S, Nagura H. Cell cycle inhibitory protein p27 in esophageal squamous cell carcinoma. Anticancer Res 19:1843–1848, 1999.

93. Ullrich A, Schlessinger J. Signal transduction by receptors with tyrosine kinase activity. Cell 61:203–212, 1990.

94. Shiga K, Shiga C, Sasano H, Miyazaki S, Yamamoto T, Yamamoto M, Hayashi N, Nishihira T, Mori S. Expression of c-erbB-2 in human esophageal carcinoma cells: overexpression correlated with gene amplification or with GATA-3 transcription factor expression. Anticancer Res 13:1293–1301, 1993.

95. Yokota J, Yamamoto T, Toyoshima K, Terada M, Sugimura T, Battifora H, Cline MJ. Amplification of c-erbB-2 oncogene in human adenocarcinomas in vivo. Lancet 1:765–767, 1986.

96. Lam KY, Tin L, Ma L. C-erbB-2 protein expression in oesophageal squamous epithelium from oesophageal squamous cell carcinomas, with special reference to histological grade of carcinoma and pre-invasive lesions. Eur J Surg Oncol 24:431–435 1998.

97. Tanaka S, Mori M, Akiyoshi T, Tanaka Y, Mafune K, Wands JR, Sugimachi K. Coexpression of Grb7 with epidermal growth factor receptor or Her2/erbB2 in human advanced esophageal carcinoma. Cancer Res 57:28–31, 1997.

98. Lu SH, Hsieh LL, Luo FC, Weinstein IB. Amplification of the EGF receptor and c-myc genes in human esophageal cancers. Int J Cancer 42:502–505, 1988.

99. al-Kasspooles M, Moore JH, Orringer MB, Beer DG. Amplification and over-expression of the EGFR and erbB-2 genes in human esophageal adenocarcinomas. Int J Cancer 54:213–219, 1993.

100. Nicholson S, Richard J, Sainsbury C, Halcrow P, Kelly P, Angus B, Wright C, Henry J, Farndon JR, Harris AL. Epidermal growth factor receptor (EGFr): results of a 6-year follow-up study in operable breast cancer with emphasis on the node negative subgroup. Br J Cancer 63: 146–150, 1991.

101. Slamon DJ, Godolphin W, Jones LA, et al. Studies of the HER-2/neu proto-oncogene in human breast and ovarian cancer. Science 244:707–712, 1989.

102. Di Marco E, Pierce JH, Aaronson SA, Di Fiore PP. Mechanisms by which EGF receptor and TGF alpha contribute to malignant transformation. Nat Immun Cell Growth Regul 9:209–221, 1990.

103. Stein D, Wu J, Fuqua SA, Roonprapunt C, Yajnik V, D'Eustachio P, Moskow JJ, Buchberg AM, Osborne CK, Margolis B. The SH2 domain protein GRB-7 is co-amplified, overexpressed and in a tight complex with HER2 in breast cancer. EMBO J 13:1331–1340, 1994.

104. Brito MJ, Filipe MI, Linehan J, Jankowski J. Association of transforming growth factor alpha (TGFA) and its precursors with malignant change in Barrett's epithelium: biological and clinical variables. Int J Cancer 60:27–32, 1995.

105. Jankowski J, McMenemin R, Yu C, Hopwood D, Wormsley KG. Proliferating cell nuclear antigen in oesophageal diseases; correlation with transforming growth factor alpha expression. Gut 33:587–591, 1992.

106. Jankowski J, Coghill G, Tregaskis B, Hopwood D, Wormsley KG. Epidermal growth factor in the oesophagus. Gut 33:1448–1453, 1992.

107. Jankowski J, McMenemin R, Hopwood D, Penston J, Wormsley KG. Abnormal expression of growth regulatory factors in Barrett's oesophagus. Clin Sci (Colch) 81:663–638, 1991.

108. Jankowski J. Altered gene expression of growth factors and their receptors during esophageal tumorigenesis. Gastroenterol Clin Biol 18: D40–D45, 1994.

109. Margolis B, Silvennoinen O, Comoglio F, Roonprapunt C, Skolnik E, Ullrich A, Schlessinger J. High-efficiency expression/cloning of epidermal growth factor-receptor-binding proteins with Src homology 2 domains. Proc Natl Acad Sci USA 89:8894–8898, 1992.

110. Stein D, Wu J, Fuqua SA, Roonprapunt C, Yajnik V, D'Eustachio P, Moskow JJ, Buchberg AM, Osborne CK, Margolis B. The SH2 domain protein GRB-7 is co-amplified, overexpressed and in a tight complex with HER2 in breast cancer. EMBO J 13:1331–1340, 1994.

111. Tanaka S, Mori M, Akiyoshi T, Tanaka Y, Mafune K, Wands JR, Sugimachi K. Coexpression of Grb7 with epidermal growth factor receptor or Her2/erbB2 in human advanced esophageal carcinoma. Cancer Res 57:28–31, 1997.

112. Yoshida K, Tsuda T, Matsumura T, Tsujino T, Hattori T, Ito H, Tahara E. Amplification of epidermal growth factor receptor (EGFR) gene and oncogenes in human gastric carcinomas. Virchows Arch B Cell Pathol Mol Pathol 57:285–290, 1989.

113. Chiang PW, Beer DG, Wei WL, Orringer MB, Kurnit DM. Detection of erbB-2 amplifications in tumors and sera from esophageal carcinoma patients. Clin Cancer Res 5:1381–1386, 1999.

114. Kim R, Clarke MR, Melhem MF, Young MA, Vanbibber MM, Safatle-Ribeiro AV, Ribeiro U Jr, Reynolds JC. Expression of p53, PCNA, and c-erbB-2 in Barrett's metaplasia and adenocarcinoma. Dig Dis Sci 42:2453–2462, 1997.

115. Polkowski W, van Sandick JW, Offerhaus GJ, ten Kate FJ, Mulder J, Obertop H, van Lanschot JJ. Prognostic value of Lauren classification and c-erbB-2 oncogene overexpression in adenocarcinoma of the esophagus and gastroesophageal junction. Ann Surg Oncol 6:290–297, 1999.

116. Ozawa S, Ueda M, Ando N, Shimizu N, Abe O. Prognostic significance of epidermal growth factor receptor in esophageal squamous cell carcinomas. Cancer 63:2169–2173, 1989.

117. Suo Z, Su W, Holm R, Nesland JM. Lack of expression of c-erbB-2 oncoprotein in human esophageal squamous cell carcinomas. Anticancer Res 15:2797–2798, 1995.

118. Whittles CE, Biddlestone LR, Burton A, Barr H, Jankowski JA, Warner PJ, Shepherd NA. Apoptotic and proliferative activity in the neoplastic progression of Barrett's oesophagus: a comparative study. J Pathol 187:535–540, 1999.

119. Ohbu M, Saegusa M, Kobayashi N, Tsukamoto H, Mieno H, Kakita A, Okayasu I. Expression of bcl-2 protein in esophageal squamous cell carcinomas and its association with lymph node metastasis. Cancer 79:1287–1293, 1997.

120. Parenti AR, Rugge M, Shiao YH, Ruol A, Ancona E, Bozzola L, Ninfo V. bcl-2 and p53 immunophenotypes in pre-invasive, early and advanced oesophageal squamous cancer. Histopathology 31:430–435, 1997.

121. Patel DD, Bhatavdekar JM, Chikhlikar PR, Patel YV, Shah NG, Ghosh N, Suthar TP, Balar DB. Clinical significance of p53, nm23, and bcl-2 in T3-4N1M0 oesophageal carcinoma: an immunohistochemical approach. J Surg Oncol 65:111–116, 1997.

122. Gratas C, Tohma Y, Barnas C, Taniere P, Hainaut P, Ohgaki H. Upregulation of Fas (APO-1/CD95) ligand and down-regulation of Fas expression in human esophageal cancer. Cancer Res 58:2057–2062, 1998.

123. O'Connell J, Bennett MW, O'Sullivan GC, Collins JK, Shanahan F. Resistance to Fas (APO-1/CD95)-mediated apoptosis and expression of Fas ligand in esophageal cancer: the Fas counterattack. Dis Esophagus 12:83–89, 1999.

124. Bennett MW, O'Connell J, O'Sullivan GC, Brady C, Roche D, Collins JK, Shanahan F. The Fas counterattack in vivo: apoptotic depletion of tumor-infiltrating lymphocytes associated with Fas ligand expression by human esophageal carcinoma. J Immunol 160:5669–5675, 1998.

125. Hughes SJ, Nambu Y, Soldes OS, Hamstra D, Rehemtulla A, Iannettoni MD, Orringer MB, Beer DG. Fas/APO-1 (CD95) is not translo-

cated to the cell membrane in esophageal adenocarcinoma. Cancer Res 57:5571–5578, 1997.

126. Morales CP, Lee EL, Shay JW. In situ hybridization for the detection of telomerase RNA in the progression from Barrett's esophagus to esophageal adenocarcinoma. Cancer 83:652–659, 1998.

127. Takubo K, Nakamura K, Izumiyama N, Mafune K, Tanaka Y, Miyashita M, Sasajima K, Kato M, Oshimura M. Telomerase activity in esophageal carcinoma. J Surg Oncol 66:88–92, 1997.

128. Koyanagi K, Ozawa S, Ando N, Takeuchi H, Ueda M, Kitajima M. Clinical significance of telomerase activity in the non-cancerous epithelial region of oesophageal squamous cell carcinoma. Br J Surg 86: 674–679, 1999.

129. Asai A, Kiyozuka Y, Yoshida R, Fujii T, Hioki K, Tsubura A. Telomere length, telomerase activity and telomerase RNA expression in human esophageal cancer cells: correlation with cell proliferation, differentiation and chemosensitivity to anticancer drugs. Anticancer Res 18:1465–1472, 1998

130. Behrens J, Birchmeier W. Cell–cell adhesion in invasion and metastasis of carcinomas. Cancer Treat Res 71:251–266, 1994.

131. Bailey T, Biddlestone L, Shepherd N, Barr H, Warner P, Jankowski J. Altered cadherin and catenin complexes in the Barrett's esophagus-dysplasia adenocarcinoma sequence: correlation with disease progression and dedifferentiation. Am J Pathol 152:135–144, 1998.

132. Bongiorno PF, al-Kasspooles M, Lee SW, Rachwal WJ, Moore JH, Whyte RI, Orringer MB, Beer DG. E-cadherin expression in primary and metastatic thoracic neoplasms and in Barrett's oesophagus. Br J Cancer 71:166–172, 1995.

133. Shiozaki H, Tahara H, Oka H, Miyata M, Kobayashi K, Tamura S, Iihara K, Doki Y, Hirano S, Takeichi M, Mori T. Expression of immunoreactive E-cadherin adhesion molecules in human cancers. Am J Pathol 139: 17–23, 1991.

134. Kadowaki T, Shiozaki H, Inoue M, Tamura S, Oka H, Doki Y, Iihara K, Matsui S, Iwazawa T, Nagafuchi A, Tsukita S, Mori T. E-cadherin and alpha-catenin expression in human esophageal cancer. Cancer Res 54:291–296, 1994

135. Wijnhoven BP, de Both NJ, van Dekken H, Tilanus HW, Dinjens WN. E-cadherin gene mutations are rare in adenocarcinomas of the oesophagus. Br J Cancer 80:1652–1657, 1999.

136. Krishnadath KK, Tilanus HW, van Blankenstein M, Hop WC, Kremers ED, Dinjens WN, Bosman FT. Reduced expression of the cadherin–catenin complex in oesophageal adenocarcinoma correlates with poor prognosis. J Pathol 182:331–338, 1997.

137. Tamura S, Shiozaki H, Miyata M, Kadowaki T, Inoue M, Matsui S, Iwazawa T, Takayama T, Takeichi M, Monden M. Decreased E-cadherin expression is associated with haematogenous recurrence and poor prognosis in patients with squamous cell carcinoma of the oesophagus. Br J Surg 83:1608–1614, 1996.

138. Swami S, Kumble S, Triadafilopoulos G. E-cadherin expression in gastroesophageal reflux disease, Barrett's esophagus, and esophageal adenocarcinoma: an immunohistochemical and immunoblot study. Am J Gastroenterol 90:1808–1813, 1995.

139. Nakanishi Y, Ochiai A, Akimoto S, Kato H, Watanabe H, Tachimori Y, Yamamoto S, Hirohashi S. Expression of E-cadherin, alpha-catenin,

beta-catenin and plakoglobin inesophageal carcinomas and its prognostic significance: immunohistochemical analysis of 96 lesions. Oncology 54:158–165, 1997.

140. Sanders DS, Bruton R, Darnton SJ, Casson AG, Hanson I, Williams HK, Jankowski J. Sequential changes in cadherin-catenin expression associated with the progression and heterogeneity of primary oesophageal squamous carcinoma. Int J Cancer 79:573–579, 1998.

141. Guilford P, Hopkins J, Harraway J, McLeod M, McLeod N, Harawira P, Taite H, Scoular R, Miller A, Reeve AE. E-cadherin germline mutations in familial gastric cancer. Nature 392:402–405, 1998.

142. Gayther SA, Gorringe KL, Ramus SJ, Huntsman D, Roviello F, Grehan N, Machado JC, Pinto E, Seruca R, Halling K, MacLeod P, Powell SM, Jackson CE, Ponder BA, Caldas C. Identification of germ-line E-cadherin mutations in gastric cancer families of European origin. Cancer Res 58:4086–4089, 1998.

143. Natsugoe S, Mueller J, Kijima F, Aridome K, Shimada M, Shirao K, Kusano C, Baba M, Yoshinaka H, Fukumoto T, Aikou T. Extranodal connective tissue invasion and the expression of desmosomal glycoprotein 1 in squamous cell carcinoma of the oesophagus. Br J Cancer 75:892–897, 1997.

144. Shiozaki H, Iihara K, Oka H, Kadowaki T, Matsui S, Gofuku J, Inoue M, Nagafuchi A, Tsukita S, Mori T. Immunohistochemical detection of alpha-catenin expression in human cancers. Am J Pathol 144:667–674, 1994.

145. Kimura Y, Shiozaki H, Doki Y, Yamamoto M, Utsunomiya T, Kawanishi K, Fukuchi N, Inoue M, Tsujinaka T, Monden M. Cytoplasmic beta-catenin in esophageal cancers. Int J Cancer 84:174–178, 1999.

146. Murray GI, Duncan ME, O'Neil P, McKay JA, Melvin WT, Fothergill JE. Matrix metalloproteinase-1 is associated with poor prognosis in oesophageal cancer. J Pathol 185:256–261, 1998.

147. Shima I, Sasaguri Y, Kusukawa J, Nakano R, Yamana H, Fujita H, Kakegawa T, Morimatsu M. Production of matrix metalloproteinase 9 (92-kDa gelatinase) by human oesophageal squamous cell carcinoma in response to epidermal growth factor. Br J Cancer 67:721–727, 1993.

148. Adachi Y, Itoh F, Yamamoto H, Matsuno K, Arimura Y, Kusano M, Endoh T, Hinoda Y, Oohara M, Hosokawa M, Imai K. Matrix metalloproteinase matrilysin (MMP-7) participates in the progression of human gastric and esophageal cancers. Int J Oncol 13:1031–1035, 1998.

149. Yamamoto H, Adachi Y, Itoh F, Iku S, Matsuno K, Kusano M, Arimura Y, Endo T, Hinoda Y, Hosokawa M, Imai K. Association of matrilysin expression with recurrence and poor prognosis in human esophageal squamous cell carcinoma. Cancer Res 59:3313–3316, 1999.

150. Duncan ME, Richardson JP, Murray GI, Melvin WT, Fothergill JE. Human matrix metalloproteinase-9: activation by limited trypsin treatment and generation of monoclonal antibodies specific for the activated form. Eur J Biochem 258:37–43, 1998.

151. Jankowski JA, Wright NA, Meltzer SJ, Triadafilopoulos G, Geboes K, Casson AG, Kerr D, Young LS. Molecular evolution of the metaplasia–dysplasia–adenocarcinoma sequence in the esophagus. Am J Pathol 154:965–973, 1999.

# Chapter 14

# Pathology and Natural History of Esophageal Cancer

JONATHAN N. GLICKMAN AND ROBERT D. ODZE

Esophageal cancer accounts for about 5%–6% of all malignant tumors of the gastrointestinal tract.[1] Worldwide, squamous cell carcinoma is the most common, although the incidence of adenocarcinoma has increased dramatically in recent years.[2] Esophageal cancers are categorized primarily by their cell of origin (Table 14–1). However, in some tumors (e.g., adenoid cystic carcinoma), the origin is not always known conclusively. The histologic classification used in this chapter is a variation of the one proposed by the World Health Organization (WHO).[3]

## Epithelial Tumors

### Benign Tumors

#### Esophageal squamous papilloma

Esophageal squamous papilloma is the most common benign epithelial tumor of the esophagus.[4] Its incidence ranges from 0.01% to 0.04%, although recent studies suggest that the incidence is probably grossly underestimated.[5] Clinically, papillomas occur in men and women equally, from early childhood to late adult life.[6] Most papillomas are asymptomatic. However, large lesions may cause epigastric pain, dysphagia, or even obstructive symptoms.

Grossly, papillomas appear as small, discrete, sessile, or pedunculated, soft tan-colored lesions that range in size from 0.5 to 2.5 cm. Most papillomas occur in the distal esophagus, but proximal and mid-esophageal lesions are not uncommon, particularly when multiple.[4] In fact, up to 20% of patients have multiple papillomas.

Microscopically, three distinct pathologic types have been described.[4] The exophytic type is composed of elongated finger-like papillary structures. The endophytic type shows a smooth surface contour with an inverted papillomatous proliferation. The least common is the spiked or "verrucoid" type, which has a spiked surface contour, prominent hyperkeratosis, and a distinct granular cell layer. All histologic types show a branched fibrovascular lamina propria core with a mild degree of acute and chronic inflammation. Variable features include koilocytosis, parakeratosis, binucleation, dyskeratosis, and a prominent granular cell layer.

The pathogenesis of squamous papillomas is controversial.[4–9] However, most studies suggest that these lesions probably arise as a result of infection with human papilloma virus (HPV) (type 6, 11, 18, 33, or 35).[4] However, some studies have failed to show an association with HPV and suggest that these lesions may develop as a result of chronic mucosal irritation, perhaps secondary to gastroesophageal reflux disease. The differences in HPV infectivity rates among different studies may be related to differences in methods use to detect HPV and, possibly, infection with novel HPV subtypes.

Esophageal squamous papillomas are considered benign lesions with little or no malignant potential. Rarely, cases may be associated with overlying squamous dysplasia or even squamous cell carcinoma.[10]

### Adenoma

Adenomas of the esophagus are a heterogeneous group of lesions that bear no clinical or pathologic resemblance to adenomas that occur elsewhere in the gastrointestinal system. Adenomas of the esophagus may develop from the submucosal gland or duct system or, more commonly, from metaplastic columnar epithelium in patients with Barrett's esophagus. Adenomas that develop from the submucosal gland/duct system are extremely rare, and fewer than 15 cases have been reported.[11,12] Pathologically, adenomas that develop from the submucosal glands are histologically sim-

**Table 14-1** General classification of esophageal cancer

| *Epithelial Tumors* | *Lymphoma/Leukemia* |
|---|---|
| Benign | Hodgkin's lymphoma |
| Squamous papilloma | Non–Hodgkin's lymphoma |
| Submucosal gland/duct adenoma | B cell |
| Barrett's esophagus–associated polypoid dysplasia | T cell |
| | Anaplastic |
| Malignant | Ki-67 |
| Squamous cell carcinoma | Other |
| Squamous cell carcinoma variants | Leukemia |
|     Basaloid carcinoma | *Mesenchymal Tumors* |
|     Carcinosarcoma | Inflammatory fibrovascular polyp |
|     Verrucous carcinoma | Inflammatory fibroid polyp |
| Adenocarcinoma—Barrett's-associated | Neural (granular cell tumor, schwannoma, neurofibroma, malignant peripheral |
| Adenocarcinoma—non–Barrett's associated |   nerve sheath tumor) |
|     Heterotopia associated | Vascular (hemangioma, angiosarcoma) |
|     Submucosal gland/duct associated | Smooth muscle (leiomyoma, leiomyosarcoma) |
| Adenoid cystic carcinoma | Skeletal muscle (rhabdomyosarcoma) |
| Mixed adenosquamous carcinoma | Adipose tissue (lipoma, liposarcoma) |
|     Composite tumor | Fibrous tissue (fibroma, fibrosarcoma) |
|     Adenosquamous carcinoma | Gastrointestinal stromal tumor (GIST) |
|     Mucoepidermoid carcinoma | Other |
| Other (choriocarcinoma) | *Melanoma* |
| *Endocrine Tumors* | Primary |
| Well differentiated (carcinoid) | Metastasis |
| Moderately differentiated | *Metastasis* |
| Pooly differentiated (small-cell carcinoma) | Lung |
| | Stomach |
| | Breast |
| | Other |

ilar to lesions that arise from the salivary glands.[12] Microscopically, these lesions may show a mixture of tubular, cystic, and papillary growth patterns that may resemble intraductal papilloma of the breast, sialadenoma papiliferum, or pleomorphic adenoma of the salivary gland.

More commonly, adenoma-like lesions may develop in the distal esophagus in patients with Barrett's esophagus.[13] However, in this setting, the tumor is better termed *polypoid dysplasia*, since it has a much higher degree of malignant potential than does the submucosal gland/duct type. Pathologically, polypoid dysplastic lesions in Barrett's esophagus are usually well-defined, sessile, or pedunculated polyps that range in size from 0.5 to 1.5 cm and occur most commonly in the mid- or distal esophagus in areas involved with Barrett's esophagus. Histologically, they are composed of a tubular or tubular-villous proliferation of low and/or high dysplastic epithelium similar to flat dysplasia in Barrett's epithelium. These tumors have a high association with adenocarcinoma, the latter usually occurring within either the polyp or the adjacent nonpolypoid mucosa. Therefore, they should be treated in a manner similar to that for flat dysplasia.[13]

## Malignant Tumors

### Squamous cell carcinoma

**Clinical features** Squamous cell carcinoma is defined as malignant epithelial neoplasm that shows morphologic evidence of squamous (i.e., keratinocyte) differentiation and is the most common malignant tumor of the esophagus, causing an estimated 11,500 deaths in the Unites States in 1997.[14,15] It affects men more commonly than women (male/female ratio: 3–4:1), with a peak incidence in the seventh decade of life. There is a marked geographic and ethnic variation in the incidence of squamous cell carcinoma. High-risk areas include China, Iran, South America, and South Africa.[15] Interestingly, in the United States, which is considered a low-risk region for this tumor, the disease is approximately five times more common in African-American men than in Caucasian men.[16] Common presenting symptoms include dysphagia and weight loss. In addition, a small proportion of patients may present with hypercalcemia secondary to parathyroid hormone-related protein production by the tumor.[17] A minority (up to 3%) of patients with esophageal squamous cell carcinoma also have concurrent head and neck squamous cell carcinoma.[18]

**Pathogenesis** The pathogenesis of squamous cell carcinoma is multifactorial and varies significantly in different regions of the world.[19] Known risk factors in high-incidence areas include consumption of food or water rich in nitrates and nitrosamines and chronic esophagitis, presumably related to particular dietary practices. Additional risk factors, common to both high- and low-risk regions, include smoking, alcohol, lye ingestion, and vitamin deficiency, as well as a variety of other predisposing conditions, such as achalasia, Plummer-Vinson syndrome, and tylosis palmaris et plantaris, a rare autosomal dominant disorder.[20–22]

Human papilloma virus (HPV) infection has been implicated in tumorigenesis, particularly in high-risk areas.[23,24] However, its role in low-risk areas remains controversial. Viral types considered high risk include types 16 and 18.[25] In one study by Togawa and colleagues,[26] tumor samples from various countries were tested for HPV in a single laboratory, and the overall HPV positivity rate was 14%.[26] However, in one study of carcinomas from different regions in the United States, the prevalence of HPV infection by polymerase chain reaction (PCR) analysis was less than 2%.[27] Thus, HPV is likely a causative factor in only a fraction of squamous cell carcinomas.

## Squamous dysplasia/carcinoma in situ

**Pathology** Esophageal squamous cell carcinoma develops through a progression of premalignant, or dysplastic, squamous precursor lesions, as does its counterpart in the skin and cervix. *Dysplasia* is defined as the presence of unequivocal neoplastic cells confined to the epithelium, above the level of the basement membrane (Fig. 14–1). It is commonly graded as low (mild and

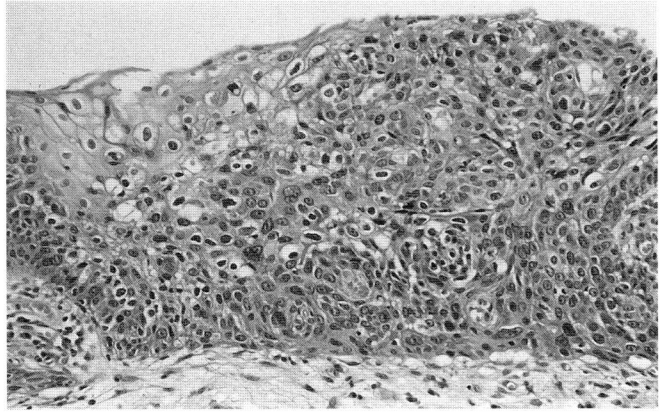

A

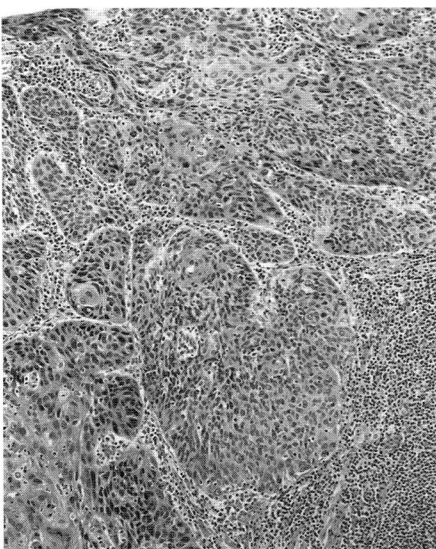

B

**Figure 14-1** *A:* High-power view of squamous mucosa showing high-grade (severe) squamous dysplasia. In the center and right side of the field, the epithelium is composed of large, hyperchromatic cells with pleomorphism, loss of polarity, and significant cellular overlap. The dysplastic cells involve the entire thickness of the epithelium but do not penetrate the underlying lamina propria. *B:* This low-power photograph shows a moderately to well-differentiated invasive squamous cell carcinoma in association with overlying high-grade dysplastic epithelium. The carcinoma shows irregular lobules of malignant-appearing squamoid cells infiltrating the submucosa in association with a marked inflammatory reaction. Focal keratinization is present in the left side of the field.

moderate) or high grade (severe and carcinoma in situ) depending on the extent of involvement of the epithelium and the degree of cytologic atypia of the cells.[15] However, different grading systems are used in different parts of the world, and the criteria for each category have not been standardized.[28] In the western world, most pathologists do not use the term *carcinoma in situ* and consider this finding part of the spectrum of high-grade dysplasia.[15] Dysplasia is found adjacent to squamous cell carcinoma in up to 67% of resected cases, and mapping studies have shown that it is frequently multifocal.[29–31]

Grossly, dysplastic squamous mucosa may appear erythematous, friable, eroded, plaque-like, or nodular.[29] However, in some instances dysplasia may show no gross abnormality. Thus, screening and surveillance of patients with, or at risk for, dysplasia may be challenging for endoscopists. Recently, mucosal staining with Lugol's iodine (which highlights dysplastic squamous epithelium) has been advocated as a means of improving the sensitivity of endoscopic detection of dysplasia.[32] Another potential means of improving detection is exfoliative balloon cytology, a technique often used for screening in China.[33]

Microscopically, dysplasia involves the surface epithelium but may also spread into the esophageal mucosal gland ducts.[34] By convention, *low-grade dysplasia* is defined as neoplastic involvement of the lower one- to two-thirds of the epithelium, whereas *high-grade dysplasia* involves the upper third of the epithelium.[15] Dysplastic cells show nuclear hyperchromasia, pleormorphism, an increased nuclear/cytoplasmic ratio, nuclear overlapping, and an increased mitotic rate. Rarely, dysplastic cells may involve the epithelium in a discontinuous or "pagetoid" pattern.[35] High-grade dysplasia usually shows a higher degree of nuclear atypia and more abundant atypical mitoses than does low-grade dysplasia.

**Natural history** Although dysplasia is a precursor to invasive carcinoma, the time to development of carcinoma varies widely. Furthermore, although it is felt that carcinoma generally progresses through a sequence of changes from low- to high-grade dysplasia and invasive carcinoma, carcinoma may develop directly from low-grade dysplasia. In one study from China, 9% of patients with dysplasia developed invasive carcinoma over a 15-year study period.[33] In another study, 15% of patients with mild (low-grade) dysplasia progressed to severe (high-grade) dysplasia, whereas 30% of those with severe dysplasia developed invasive carcinoma after 8 years of follow-up.[36] Interestingly, dysplasia has also been shown to regress. In such instances, however, the dysplasia may have actually represented an exuberant reactive process, rather than a true neoplastic proliferation. For instance, in one endoscopic study,[37] nearly 40% of dysplastic lesions regressed, 20% remained unchanged, and nearly 40% eventually progressed.

**Management** Management decisions for patients with squamous dysplasia should be made in conjunction with the clinical and endoscopic findings. Dysplasia, whether low or high grade, if associated with a mass lesion, should, in most instances, be considered squamous carcinoma and treated as such. In fact, any mucosal lesion considered high-grade dysplasia should be thoroughly evaluated by endoscopy and multiple biopsies, along with perhaps other imaging studies, such as ultrasonography, to exclude the presence of underlying invasive carcinoma. If no carcinoma is identified, treatment of patients with flat high-grade dysplasia should be individualized; options include continued surveillance, endoscopic ablation, or surgical resection. Patients with low-grade dysplasia should also be evaluated thoroughly to rule out an associated malignancy. However, low-grade dysplasia, in the absence of an underlying carcinoma, may be managed with brush cytology, repeat mucosal biopsies, and continued surveillance. In some cases, it may be difficult to differentiate reactive atypia from true low-grade dysplasia, and thus it is often necessary to repeat biopsies in patients after therapy for the associated inflammation prior to definitive diagnosis and treatment.

### Invasive squamous cell carcinoma

Squamous cell carcinomas are separated into early "superficial" and late "advanced" forms. As a result of aggressive screening protocols, the early superficial type has become more prevalent, representing 15% to 20% of all squamous carcinomas.[15] *Superficial squamous cell carcinoma* is defined as a tumor that shows invasion either confined to the mucosa or infiltrating the submucosa (pT1a and pT1b, respectively).[15,28] In most studies, superficial carcinoma also includes cases with lymph node metastasis, but not distant metastasis.[38–41] Since these tumors are less advanced at the time of diagnosis, a higher proportion of patients are asymptomatic at the time of clinical diagnosis. Grossly, superficial carcinomas may appear entirely normal or as flat, granular, plaque-like or slightly depressed tumors, with or without superficial ulceration.[41] Up to 20% of superficial carcinomas are multifocal.[39,42]

*Advanced squamous cell carcinomas* represent the majority of esophageal cancers and are defined as tumors with extension beyond the submucosa. Grossly, advanced tumors may appear as fungating, infiltrating, ulcerating, and/or stricturing lesions or may show a mixture of these growth patterns.[15] Microscopically, both superficial and advanced squamous cell carcinomas are categorized as well, moderate, or poorly differentiated.[15,38] Well-differentiated lesions show abundant keratinocytes and intercellular bridges, whereas moderately differentiated tumors show a greater degree of cytologic atypia, more mitoses and necrosis, and less keratinocyte formation (Fig. 14–1). Poorly differentiated squamous cell carcinomas typically show no keratinization but often show larger, more bizarre and pleomorphic cells that bear little resemblance to normal squamous cells. The degree of tumor differentiation, as well as the gross pattern of growth, has not been consistently shown to be related to prognosis.

Patients treated preoperatively with chemotherapy and/or radiotherapy often show little or no residual tumor in their resection specimen. Tumor cells, when present, often appear markedly enlarged or bizarre shaped. In some cases, they may be difficult to differentiate from chemotherapy or radiation-induced reactive stromal atypia. In these instances, a cytokeratin immunohistochemical stain may be helpful to differentiate these two conditions (positive in tumor cells, negative in stromal cells). The presence of residual tumor is documented in the American Joint Committee on Cancer (AJCC) TNM classification by the symbol *R* and classified as no residual tumor (R0), microscopic residual tumor (R1), or macroscopic residual tumor (R2).[43] The extent of residual tumor is documented by placing the symbol *y* before the pathologic TNM stage (e.g., ypT1).

Squamous cell carcinoma of the esophagus tends to invade deeply through all layers of the esophageal wall and may spread to adjacent organs such as the trachea, aorta, mediastinum, or pericardium. Intramural metastases are not uncommon.[44] The strongest predictor of prognosis is based on the AJCC TNM pathologic staging system, which is based on a combination of depth of invasion, lymph node metastasis, and distant metastasis (Tables 14–2 and 14–3).[45–47] For instance, patients with submucosal tumors have a 5-year survival rate of approximately 70%,

**Table 14–2** American Joint Committee on Cancer TNM staging system for esophageal carcinomas

| Stage | Description |
|---|---|
| *Primary Tumor (T)* | |
| TX | Primary tumor cannot be assessed |
| T0 | No evidence of primary tumor |
| Tis | Carcinoma in situ/high-grade dysplasia |
| T1 | Tumor invades lamina propria or submucosa |
| T1a | Tumor invades lamina propria |
| T1b | Tumor invades submucosa |
| T2 | Tumor invades muscularis propria |
| T3 | Tumor invades adventitia |
| T4 | Tumor invades adjacent structures |
| *Regional Lymph Nodes (N)* | |
| NX | Regional lymph nodes cannot be assessed |
| N0 | No regional lymph nodes metastasis |
| N1 | Regional lymph node metastasis |
| N1a | 1–3 nodes involved |
| N1b | 4–7 lymph nodes involved |
| N1c | >7 lymph nodes involved |
| *Distant Metastasis (M)* | |
| MX | Distant metastasis cannot be assessed |
| M0 | No distant metastasis |
| M1 | Distant metastasis |
| For Tumors of Lower Thoracic Esophagus | |
| M1a | Metastasis in celiac lymph nodes |
| M1b | Other distant metastases |
| For Tumors of Upper Thoracic Esophagus | |
| M1a | Metastasis in cervical nodes |
| M1b | Other distant metastases |
| For Tumors of Mid-thoracic Esophagus | |
| M1a | Not applicable |
| M1b | Nonregional lymph nodes or other distant metastases |

compared with 40% to 50% for patients with tumors that extend into the muscularis propria, and 20%–30% for patient with tumors that extend beyond the esophageal wall.[48,49]

Lymph node metastasis is an independent predictor of survival.[48,49] Five-year survival rates for patients with superficial carcinoma are close to 80% in high-risk areas and slightly lower in low-risk countries. Similar to patients with early gastric cancer, patients with intramucosal squamous cell carcinoma have lymph node metastasis in less than 10% of cases, whereas pa-

**Table 14–3** TNM stage grouping for esophageal carcinomas

| Stage | T | N | M |
|---|---|---|---|
| Stage 0 | Tis | N0 | M0 |
| Stage I | T1 | N0 | M0 |
| Stage IIA | T2 | N0 | M0 |
| | T3 | N0 | M0 |
| Stage IIB | T1 | N1 | M0 |
| | T2 | N1 | M0 |
| Stage III | T3 | N1 | M0 |
| | T4 | Any N | M0 |
| Stage IV | Any T | Any N | M1 |
| Stage IVA | Any T | Any N | M1a |
| Stage IVB | Any T | Any N | M1b |

T, primary tumor; N, lymph nodes; M, metastasis.

tients with cancers that extend beyond the submucosa show lymph node metastasis in up to 50% of cases.[48,50] Carcinomas originating in the upper and mid-thoracic esophagus are more likely to metastasize to the cervical and upper mediastinal nodes, whereas tumors from the lower third often metastasize to the lower mediastinal or perigastric nodes.[48] The lungs, liver, pleura, and kidneys are the most frequent sites of distant involvement.[51]

Although pathologic stage is the strongest predictor of survival, some studies have also shown an association with tumor differentiation, tumor size, and tumor location.[46,47] However, these factors need to be tested in large prospective studies. Molecular genetic alterations, such as DNA aneuploidy and *p53* mutations, are common in squamous cell carcinoma and, in some studies, have also been correlated with aggressive behavior.[45,52,53]

### Squamous cell carcinoma variants

**Basaloid carcinoma** Basaloid carcinoma of the esophagus is an unusual variant of squamous cell carcinoma that occurs more commonly in the upper aerodigestive tract and represents between 1% and 11% of esophageal squamous cell carcinomas. The clinical and demographic features of patients with this tumor are similar to those of patients with squamous cell carcinoma.[54]

Pathologically, basaloid carcinomas may be large, bulky, fungating tumors that frequently ulcerate and cause stricture formation.[54,55] They develop mostly in the mid- and distal esophagus. Microscopically, basaloid carcinomas often show biphasic or multiphasic differentiation. Thus, it is common to find a mixture of squamous cell carcinoma or adenocarcinoma elements within the tumor. For instance, in a study of 18 basaloid carcinomas, 72% showed areas of squamous cell carcinoma, 50% of which included in situ squamous cell carcinoma.[54] Thus, basaloid carcinomas have been proposed to arise from a multipotential stem cell in the native squamous epithelium. However, others consider basaloid carcinoma simply a poorly differentiated morphologic variant of squamous cell carcinoma.

Basaloid carcinomas are characterized by a solid, cribriform, or trabecular proliferation of oval to round, large, pleomorphic, basaloid cells that contain an open, pale chromatin pattern, small nucleoli, and scant cytoplasm (see Color Fig. 14–2 in separate color insert).[54,55] Basaloid carcinomas often show a prominent hyalin-like stromal matrix, and these may resemble adenoid cystic carcinomas from the salivary glands.

Basaloid carcinoma of the esophagus is considered a highly aggressive variant of squamous cell carcinoma.[54–56] However, recent studies have shown no significant differences in overall survival between these two histologic variants.

**Carcinosarcoma of the esophagus** Carcinosarcoma of the esophagus was first described by in 1865 and represents approximately 2% of all esophageal malignancies.[57] It is defined as a biphasic tumor characterized by the presence of both squamous cell carcinoma (or carcinoma in situ) and spindle cell sarcoma. Several terms have been used to describe this lesion, including polypoid carcinoma of the esophagus, spindle cell carcinoma, and pseudosarcoma.[57–59] Similar to squamous cell carcinoma, carcinosarcoma occurs predominantly in men who are 40–90 years of age. Because of the predominant intraluminal growth pattern, symptoms are usually related to obstruction.

The origin of carcinosarcoma has been the subject of considerable controversy. However, recent immunohistochemical and electron microscopic studies strongly suggest that the spindle cell component probably arises as a result of metaplasia of malignant squamous cells.[60]

Most carcinosarcomas are located in the mid- or distal esophagus and are large polypoid lesions that protrude into the esophageal lumen. Microscopically, the tumor is characterized by a combination of epithelial ("carcinoma") and spindle cell ("sarcoma") elements (Fig. 14–3).[57] In fact, some tumors show only a minimal amount of the epithelial component, which is usually located either at the base of the polyp or at the periphery of the invasive tumor. The sarcomatous component may be heterogeneous and consist of poorly differentiated high-grade spindle-cell sarcoma, or it may show malignant bone, smooth muscle, skeletal muscle, or cartilaginous differentiation.[57,59,61]

The prognosis of carcinosarcoma is poor.[57,58] Roughly 50% of patients have lymph node metastasis at the time of diagnosis. Overall, 5-year survival rates range from 10% to 15%.

**Verrucous carcinoma** Verrucous carcinoma of the esophagus, an extremely rare malignancy,[62] is considered a low-grade, less invasive form of squamous cell carcinoma.[62] Affected patients range in age from 35 to 80 years; similar to squamous cell carcinoma, this cancer is more common in men. Presenting com-

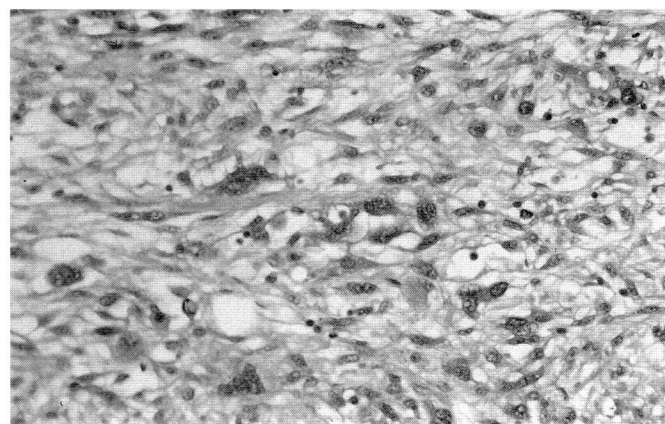

**A**

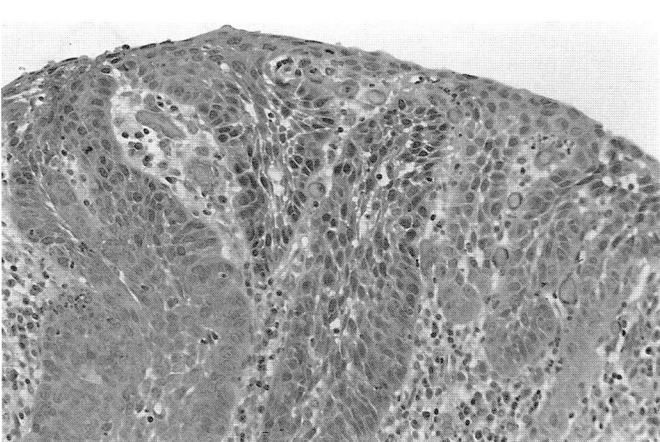

**B**

**Figure 14–3** Polypoid carcinosarcoma of the esophagus. *A:* A high-power view of the sarcomatous component of this neoplasm showing high-grade pleomorphic and bizarre-shaped spindle cells. *B:* High-grade dysplasia is present in the mucosa at the periphery of this tumor and represents the epithelial component of the lesion. The dysplastic epithelium in this case shows irregular buds of neoplastic cells infiltrating the lamina propria with broad pushing margins.

plaints usually consist of a combination of dysphagia, weight loss, coughing, and hematemesis. Unfortunately, these tumors may grow to a large size before the onset of symptoms, thus leading to a long delay in diagnosis.[62,63] A high proportion of cases are associated with chronic caustic injury (such as lye ingestion) achalasia, esophageal diverticular disease, or gastroesophageal reflux disease.[63]

Pathologically, verrucous carcinomas show an exophytic papillary growth pattern and often involve the entire circumference of the esophageal lumen, in contrast to squamous papillomas, which are usually well-localized, discrete, polypoid lesions.[4] Microscopically, verrucous carcinomas typically reveal a very well–differentiated verrucoid, or papillomatous, proliferation of reactive-appearing squamous cells with minimal cytologic atypia, prominent acanthosis, hyperkeratosis, swollen rete pegs, a low mitotic rate, and broad pushing margins. Rarely, lymph node metastasis may be present, but distant metastases have not been reported. Unfortunately, verrucous carcinomas often form fistula tracts with surrounding organs, which is the major cause of morbidity and mortality in affected patients.[62]

### Barrett's esophagus–associated adenocarcinoma

More than 95% of adenocarcinomas arise in association with Barrett's esophagus and form up to 80% of all primary cancers confined to the lower third of the esophagus.[15] In fact, the incidence of esophageal adenocarcinoma has risen dramatically over the past 20 to 30 years.[64–68] Because of the strong association with gastroesophageal reflux disease, the demographic features of patients with adenocarcinoma are similar to those of patients with Barrett's esophagus. These tumors occur most often in white men at a median age of 60 years.[69] Presenting symptoms are similar to those of squamous cell carcinoma and include dysphagia and weight loss as signs typically associated with advanced disease. However, some patients may be asymptomatic or have symptoms related only to their reflux disease. Adenocarcinoma develops through a stepwise progression starting with gastroesophageal reflux disease, which leads to Barrett's esophagus, dysplasia, and, eventually, to adenocarcinoma.[67,70–72]

### Barrett's esophagus

**Clinical features** *Barrett's esophagus* is defined as the metaplastic conversion of squamous epithelium into columnar epithelium. It develops as a result of chronic gastroesophageal reflux disease and is the most important risk factor for the development of adenocarcinoma in affected patients.[72] However, rarely, Barrett's esophagus may develop as a result of lye ingestion, chemotherapy, or severe pancreatic or biliary fluid reflux.[73,74] Familial cases have also been reported but are rare.[75] Approximately 10% of patients with gastroesophageal reflux disease develop Barrett's esophagus.[67,72] This figure is based primarily on autopsy studies, and recent studies suggest that the true prevalence of Barrett's esophagus is probably much greater than previously believed.[76]

**Pathology of Barrett's esophagus** Barrett's esophagus is classified as either long-segment or short-segment type, based on the degree of involvement of the distal esophagus.[72] Patients with columnar metaplasia involving at least 3 cm of esophageal mucosa are considered to have long-segment type, whereas cases with less than 3 cm of involvement are classified as short-segment type. More recently, the definition of either type of Barrett's esophagus has been modified to include only cases with intestinal (goblet cell) metaplasia. Some patients have intestinal metaplasia at the gastroesophageal junction and also have a

slightly irregular squamocolumnar ("Z" line) junction. As a result, they have been referred to as having "ultra-short" Barrett's esophagus.

Endoscopically, Barrett's esophagus is characterized by pink, salmon-colored mucosa, similar in appearance to the normal stomach. Small tongues of gastric-appearing mucosa may be seen to extend for variable lengths proximal to the gastroesophageal junction.

Microscopically, at least three types of epithelium may be present in columnar segments of Barrett's esophagus,[72] although most patients contain a mixture of all types. The fundic type contains epithelium indistinguishable from the gastric corpus (contains oxyntic glands), whereas the junctional type closely resembles the proximal gastric cardia epithelium, consisting of mucous-type glands with overlying mucinous columnar epithelium. The most common and recognizable form of Barrett's esophagus is the specialized or intestinal type, which consists of surface epithelium lined by mucous cells and intestinal-type goblet cells (Fig. 14–4). In the specialized type, the underlying glan-

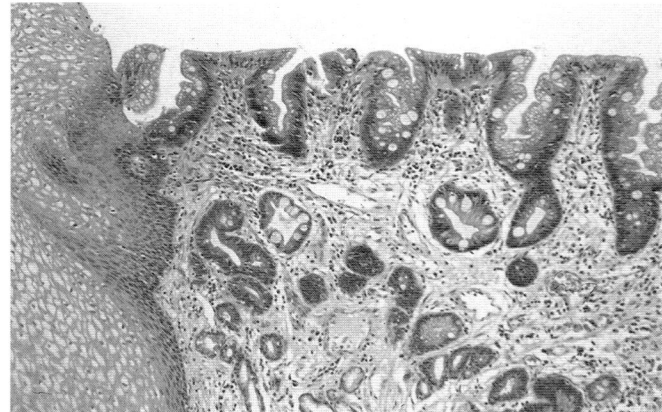

A

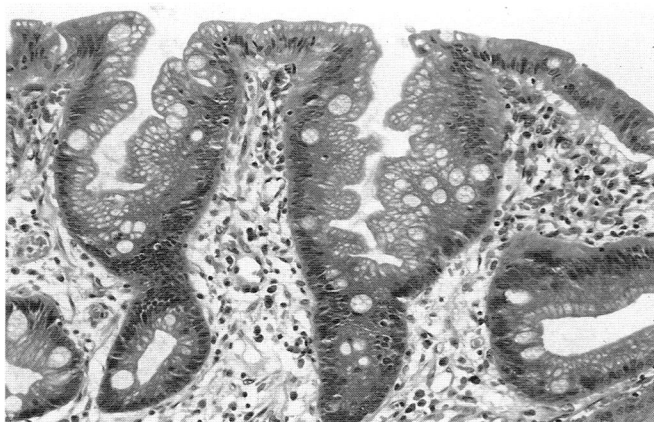

B

**Figure 14–4** *A:* Low-power view of the neosquamocolumnar junction in a patient with long-segment Barrett's esophagus. The squamous epithelium (on the left) forms an abrupt junction with specialized-type columnar epithelium (right side). Under the surface and crypt epithelium, the glands show mixed mucous and intestinal-type cells. *B:* This photograph shows a high-power view of the overlying specialized type epithelium. The cells lining the surface and crypt epithelium are predominantly mucinous, with scattered goblet cells. The crypts are slightly hyperplastic and show mildly increased hyperchromaticity and pseudostratification, but there is no dysplasia.

dular epithelium may show a variety of additional cell types, including goblet cells, mucous cells, Paneth cells, endocrine cells, or pancreatic acinar cells. Recently, a specialized form of "multilayered" epithelium has been identified in patients with Barrett's esophagus.[77] This latter epithelium shows morphologic, cytochemical, and ultrastructural features of both squamous and columnar epithelium and is therefore believed to represent an early or intermediate phase in the conversion of squamous to columnar epithelium.

Up to 25% of the general population may show intestinal metaplasia at the gastroesophageal junction.[78] In these cases, both *Helicobacter pylori* infection and gastroesophageal reflux disease have been proposed as possible etiologic agents[79] Unfortunately, histologic analysis alone is not helpful in determining whether a particular specimen represents short-segment (or ultra-short) Barrett's esophagus and thus correlation with endoscopic findings is necessary. Some investigators[80] have proposed that cytokeratin 7/20 immunostaining may help to differentiate these two conditions, but this is controversial.[81] Similarly, mucin histochemistry is not useful in this differential diagnosis.[82]

**Natural history of Barrett's esophagus** Approximately 8% to 10% of patients with Barrett's esophagus eventually develop adenocarcinoma.[67,83] Patients with Barrett's esophagus have a 30- to 125-fold increased risk of developing adenocarcinoma compared with the general population.[84] However, recent prospective studies suggest that the risk may be exaggerated and that it may be as low as 3% to 5%.[85–89] Both duration and length of Barrett's esophagus have been proposed as risk factors for the development of adenocarcinoma.[90–92] Virtually all adenocarcinomas arise in association with specialized columnar epithelium.[87,93] Alcohol and tobacco use, in addition to a positive family history, may also contribute to malignant progression in Barrett's esophagus.

## Dysplasia in Barrett's esophagus

Dysplasia in Barrett's esophagus, defined as unequivocal neoplastic epithelium without invasion of the lamina propria, is the most important risk factor for development of adenocarcinoma.[67,84,89,94,95] Five to twenty percent of patients with Barrett's esophagus develop dysplasia in the course of their illness.[89,94] Dysplasia is categorized as negative, indefinite, or positive (low or high grade) in a manner analogous to the classification scheme used in inflammatory bowel disease.[96,97] Endoscopically, dysplasia may have no distinguishing features, or it may appear as a slightly raised erythematous and velvety area of mucosa.[98,99] Occasionally, dysplasia may be polypoid.[100] Microscopically, dysplasia may appear villiform or papillary in contour, and contain irregular crowded or branched glands.[95–97] Features of dysplasia include decreased mucin production, nuclear hyperchromasia, pleomorphism, an increased nuclear-to-cytoplasmic ratio, increased mitoses, and nuclear stratification (Fig. 14–5). In general, high-grade dysplasia shows a greater degree of cytologic atypia and architectural complexity than does low-grade dysplasia. However, even among experienced observers, there is an appreciable degree of interobserver variability in the diagnosis of dysplasia, particularly low-grade dysplasia.[95] A diagnosis of indefinite for dysplasia usually applies to cases that show atypical cytologic and/or architectural atypia, but the presence of active inflammation and/or ulceration makes it difficult to differentiate reactive epithelial changes from true dysplasia. Negative for dysplasia refers to reactive changes that are morphologically nondysplastic. By convention, carcinoma in situ is included in the category of high-grade dysplasia. Intramucosal adenocarcinoma is

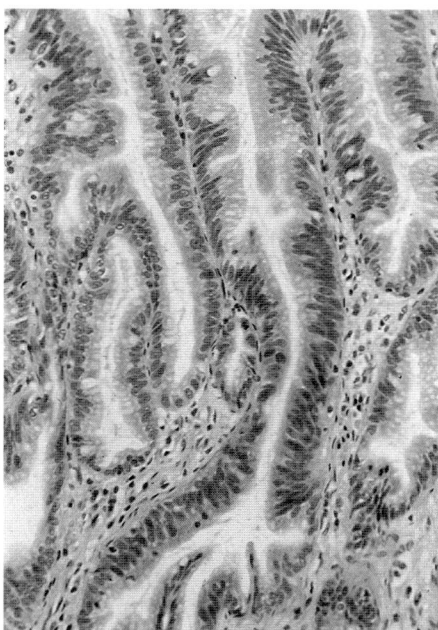

**Figure 14–5** High-power view of a patient with Barrett's esophagus and low-grade dysplasia. The epithelium contains hyperchromatic, pencil-shaped cells with pseudostratification, decreased mucin production, and a lack of surface maturation. The appearance is similar to that of a colonic adenoma.

recognized by the presence of single cells or clusters of cells infiltrating the lamina propria with or without a desmoplastic response. Because of the occasional difficulty in identifying and classifying dysplasia, confirmation of the diagnosis by a pathologist experienced in the evaluation of biopsies from Barrett's patients is essential prior to commencing treatment.

**Natural history of dysplasia** The natural history of dysplasia is poorly understood, primarily because most studies are retrospective, contain insufficient numbers of patients, show a high degree of selection bias, or suffer from a high degree of interobserver variability. In general, low-grade dysplasia usually progresses to high-grade dysplasia and eventually adenocarcinoma. However, it may remain stable for a long period of time or even regress.[84] Progression to carcinoma occurs over a highly variable time period that ranges from 1 to 10 years in prospective studies.[84,99] For cases in which low-grade dysplasia is seen in association with a mass lesion, the risk of concurrent malignancy ranges from 10% to 50%.[101] Patients with flat high-grade dysplasia have a higher association with concurrent adenocarcinoma, up to 30% to 50% of cases in some studies.[95,98,102–105] In cases with a mass lesion, the association with cancer approaches 90% to 100%.[103,105] In two recent prospective studies, 50% to 60% of patients with high-grade dysplasia developed adenocarcinoma within a 5-year follow-up period, compared with 8% to 12% of patients with low-grade dysplasia and 4% of patients with biopsies considered negative or indefinite for dysplasia.[92,94]

A number of adjunctive techniques have been proposed recently as having a possible role in screening for dysplasia or predicting the progression to adenocarcinoma. For instance, DNA content abnormalities (aneuploidy), as measured by flow cytometry, and elevated S-phase fractions increase with progressively higher grades of dysplasia and may be predictive of future development of dysplasia or adenocarcinoma.[94,106] However, the prognostic potential of aneuploidy is controversial. Abnormalities in *p53* and *p16* may also be present early in the evolution of dysplasia and in some studies have been predictive of a poor outcome as well.[107–109]

**Management of dysplasia** The management of patients with dysplasia in Barrett's esophagus is controversial and varies from institution to institution. However, certain principles are fairly uniform (Table 14–4).[110] In patients without dysplasia, endoscopic surveillance with mucosal biopsies is recommended. However, the optimal frequency of endoscopic surveillance is controversial, and current practice ranges from once a year to once every 5 years. Patients with a biopsy considered indefinite or low-grade dysplasia should receive treatment to reduce inflammation (antireflux therapy) prior to repeat endoscopy. In general, follow-up in 3 to 6 months is recommended. If low-grade dysplasia persists after treatment, continued surveillance at an increased frequency is generally recommended. The management of patients with high-grade dysplasia varies from continued surveillance (with an aggressive biopsy protocol) to surgical resection. Newer forms of therapy, such as endoscopic mucosal ablation or photodynamic therapy, may be considered for high surgical risk patients.[111,112] In general, most institutions recommend a surgical resection for patients with high-grade dysplasia, because of the high association with concurrent or subsequent adenocarcinoma.[102–105] Low- or high-grade dysplasia in association with a mass lesion should be considered a strong indication for surgical resection, because of the high association with invasive carcinoma.

### Pathology of Barrett's esophagus–associated adenocarcinoma

Similar to squamous cell carcinoma, adenocarcinoma may appear as a large, exophytic, and ulcerating lesion (see Color Fig. 14–6 in separate color insert). Early carcinomas may show only slight mucosal depression or elevation, with or without surface erosion.[98,99] Microscopically, most adenocarcinomas are intestinal type, composed of a mixture of glands, tubules, and papillary structures.[15,69] They are categorized as well, moderate, or poorly differentiated on the basis of degree of gland formation. Rarely, Paneth cells and/or endocrine cells may be abundant.[113] A small proportion of adenocarcinomas may show mucinous (colloid) features or signet ring–cell morphology.[69,114] It is not uncommon to find areas of squamous or even neuroendocrine differentiation in adenocarcinoma.[113] Dysplasia is found adjacent to adenocarcinoma in 70% to 90% of cases.[69,95] Similar to squamous cell carcinomas, adenocarcinomas are also staged according to the AJCC TNM system (Table 14–2).[43]

**Table 14–4** Management of dysplasia in Barrett's esophagus

| Diagnosis | Management |
| --- | --- |
| Negative for dysplasia | Regular follow-up/surveillance |
| Indefinite for dysplasia | Medical therapy (treat inflammation) |
| | Repeat biopsy after 3–6 months |
| Positive for dysplasia | |
| Low grade | Medical therapy |
| | Continued surveillance at increased frequency |
| High grade | Immediate extensive rebiopsy |
| | Consider surgical resection |
| Low or high grade associated with a mass | Surgical resection |

Because of the expanding popularity of preoperative chemotherapy and/or radiotherapy in the management of patients with adenocarcinoma, it is not uncommon to find little or no residual tumor in the resection specimen after treatment. Similar to squamous cell carcinoma, individual or small clusters of highly unusual, bizarre, and pleomorphic cells may be present within the esophageal wall or associated with extravasated mucin. On occasion, resection specimens may show pools of acellular mucin without malignant cells. The prognostic significance of this finding has not been investigated.

**Natural history and prognosis** Most adenocarcinomas show spread into or through the muscularis propria at the time of clinical presentation.[69,115,116] Advanced tumors may spread directly into the mediastinum, aorta, or the proximal stomach. Metastases to regional lymph nodes are present in 50% to 60% of patients and, as also occurs with squamous cell carcinoma, the likelihood of finding lymph node metastasis is related to the depth of tumor invasion.[69,117,118] For instance, in one study of 32 early adenocarcinomas, none of the tumors that were limited to the mucosa showed lymph node metastasis, compared with 30% of tumors that infiltrated the submucosa.[117] The lungs, liver, pleura, and kidneys, as well as other portions of the gastrointestinal tract, are common sites of distant metastasis. The AJCC TNM pathologic staging system is the most important and prognostically useful method of evaluating patient survival.[116,118] Patients with tumor limited to the mucosa or submucosa have 5-year survival rates of 80% to 100%, compared with 10% to 20% for patients who have tumors that extend beyond the muscularis propria.[69,116–118] Some studies suggest that tumor differentiation or lymphovascular or perineural invasion may be independent predictors of survival, but this has yet to be confirmed in prospective multivariate studies.[118]

### Adenocarcinoma variants

**Non–Barrett's-associated adenocarcinoma** Adenocarcinomas that develop in patients without Barrett's esophagus are extremely rare. They may arise in association with gastric heterotopia or the esophageal submucosal glands.[119,120] Adenocarcinomas that arise in heterotopic gastric mucosa are usually located in the upper third of the esophagus and often show a papillary growth pattern. Adenocarcinomas that develop from the submucosal gland/duct system may resemble ordinary adenocarcinomas or may have a tubular appearance, containing cells that appear similar to the native esophageal glands or ducts.

**Adenoid cystic carcinoma** True adenoid cystic carcinoma of the esophagus is an extremely rare tumor presumably derived from the submucosal glands.[121,122] In fact, the majority of cases previously termed adenoid cystic carcinoma are more likely basaloid carcinomas with adenoid cystic carcinoma–like features.[121] True adenoid cystic carcinomas are distinguished from basaloid carcinomas in that they are more common in women, typically present at an earlier age, show no histologic association with squamous cell carcinoma, and have a much better prognosis. Pathologically, adenoid cystic carcinomas are composed of two distinct cell populations: basaloid and ductal epithelial cells. The basaloid cells in adenoid cystic carcinoma, in contrast to those in basaloid carcinoma, are small and hyperchromatic, show minimal pleomorphism, and have infrequent mitosis. The duct cells usually grow in a trabecular or cribriform pattern. Abundant basement membrane stromal material is usually present surrounding nests of cells and located between epithelial bridges within cribriform spaces. Since very few cases have been reported, the natural history of true adenoid cystic carcinoma is unclear. However, there is evidence to suggest that the prognosis is better than for patients with either squamous cell carcinoma or adenocarcinoma.[121,122]

**Mixed adenocarcinoma/squamous cell carcinoma** Esophageal carcinomas have a high propensity to exhibit multidirectional differentiation.[123] It is not uncommon to find a mixture of cell types in any individual tumor, the most common being a mixture of squamous and glandular elements.[123,124] These tumors have been variously termed composite tumor, adenoacanthoma, adenosquamous carcinoma, and mucoepidermoid carcinoma.[125–127] In a study by Newman and colleagues in 1992,[123] an ultrastructural examination of 43 esophageal carcinomas showed evidence of multidirectional differentiation in 11 cases. Most commonly, the tumors in that study showed a mixture of squamous cell carcinoma and adenocarcinoma. However, some tumors show combined features of small cell carcinoma and basaloid carcinoma. In fact, in rare instances, adenocarcinoma may even show malignant cyto- or syncytiotrophoblastic differentiation simulating the appearance of a placental-type choriocarcinoma.[128] The most widely accepted pathogenetic mechanism for tumors with mixed lines of differentiation is neoplastic transformation of a totipotent primitive stem cell presumably located in the basal region of the squamous epithelium.[123] Another theory is that these tumors develop because of metaplastic differentiation of neoplastic cells, similar to the pathogenesis of carcinosarcoma.

*Adenoacanthoma* is defined as a tumor composed of malignant glandular elements combined with benign squamous epithelium.[126] In contrast, *adenosquamous carcinoma* is the diagnosis when the squamous element is also malignant.[129] The WHO classifies mucoepidermoid carcinoma as a tumor composed of an intimate mixture of squamous and mucin-secreting epithelium, although there is much histologic overlap with adenosquamous carcinoma.[3] The natural history of mixed tumors is similar to that of pure squamous cell carcinoma or pure adenocarcinoma, depending on the predominant cell component.[126]

## Endocrine Tumors

### Carcinoid tumor

Well-differentiated (carcinoid tumor) or moderately differentiated neuroendocrine tumors of the esophagus are extremely rare.[130] However, the gross and microscopic features are similar to those that occur in other parts of the gastrointestinal tract. Because they occur infrequently, little is known about their biologic behavior.

### Small-cell ("oat-cell") carcinoma

The esophagus is the most common extrapulmonary site for poorly differentiated neuroendocrine carcinomas (small-cell carcinoma).[131,132] They comprise 0.5% to 2% of all primary esophageal tumors, occur more often in men than in women, and typically develop in the fifth and sixth decades of life.[131–133] The typical presentation of patients with small-cell carcinoma includes severe weight loss, dysphagia, chest pain, and hematemesis. The pathologic features of esophageal small-cell carcinoma are similar to those that occur in the lung.[132,134] Grossly, most of these cancers develop in the distal esophagus and grow as large

fungating or stricturing lesions that can measure up to 18 cm in size. Histologically, small-cell carcinoma is characterized by a proliferation of small "blue" hyperchromatic cells with inconspicuous or entirely absent nucleoli, prominent individual cell necrosis, a high degree of nuclear molding, and a brisk mitotic rate (Fig. 14–7). Up to 50% of small-cell carcinomas may show focal squamous or glandular differentiation.[132–135] Thus, it is also believed that these tumors probably develop from a multipotential stem cell. However, derivation from neuroendocrine or Merkel cells, which normally reside in the squamous epithelium, has also been proposed.[134,136] By immunohistochemistry, these tumors show chromogranin, synaptophysin, and neuron-specific enolase (NSE) positivity demonstrating the presence of neuroendocrine differentiation. By electron microscopy, numerous dense-core neurosecretory granules are observed.

Overall, small-cell carcinomas are highly aggressive neoplasms that carry an extremely poor prognosis.[133,135] Most patients present with an advanced stage at the time of diagnosis and survive less than 1 year. However, a few patients may survive longer because of a good response to chemotherapy or radiotherapy or both.

### Lymphoma

Fewer than 100 primary esophageal lymphomas have been reported; most have been secondary and have resulted from local extension of gastric disease.[137,138] However, esophageal lymphomas may develop in patients with acquired immunodeficiency syndrome (AIDS) or in patients who are immunosuppressed for other reasons. Pathologically, two-thirds of lymphomas are of the Hodgkin's type.[138] Non-Hodgkin's lymphoma is usually either large-cell or immunoblastic B-cell type, with other types such as T-cell, large-cell anaplastic, or Ki-1 lymphoma occurring rarely. Because of the extreme rarity of primary esophageal lymphomas, it is important that a patient who presents with an esophageal lymphoma be investigated thoroughly for other possible extraintestinal (spleen, liver, lymph node, or bone marrow) primary sources of disease.

### Mesenchymal Tumors

Benign mesenchymal tumors of the esophagus are quite common, whereas malignant tumors (sarcoma) are quite rare.[139,140]

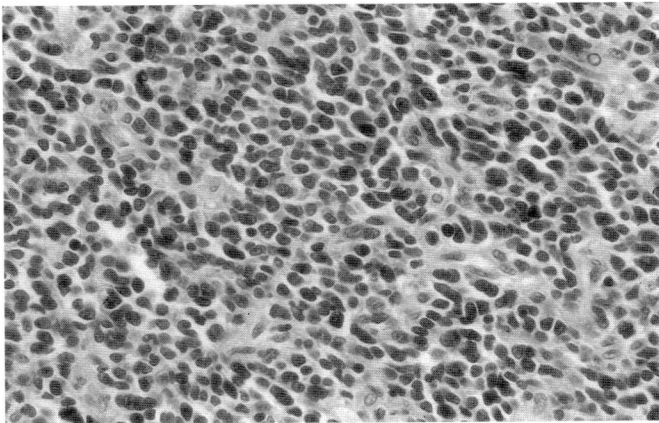

**Figure 14-7** High-power view of a primary esophageal small-cell carcinoma. Similar to those that arise in the lungs, primary esophageal small-cell carcinomas show a proliferation of small, hyperchromatic cells without nucleoli.

The vast majority of benign tumors are granular cell tumors and leiomyomas. Benign vascular tumors, such as hemangioma, are uncommon. Inflammatory fibrovascular polyps are discussed here because the etiology of this lesion (i.e., reactive vs. neoplastic) is unclear.

## Inflammatory fibrovascular polyp

This is an extremely rare, unusual, and rather dramatic lesion that occurs in the upper third of the esophagus and predominantly in elderly men.[141,142] Inflammatory fibrovascular polyps are characteristically large polypoid lesions that may regurgitate into the hypopharynx and cause asphyxia or laryngeal obstruction.[141] Their pathogenesis is unclear. Some investigators regard them as reactive lesions, whereas others believe that they are neoplastic.[141,142] Pathologically, inflammatory fibrovascular polyps are composed of a loose, predominantly myxoid, highly collagenized stroma showing various combinations of fibrous tissue, adipose tissue, smooth muscle tissue, and vascular tissue mixed with lymphoid aggregates, plasma cells, and mast cells. Because of the variety of cell types that may be present in these lesions, many synonyms, such as lipoma, fibroma, and fibrolipoma, have been applied to this tumor.[141–143] Inflammatory fibrovascular polyps are benign tumors with no malignant potential. However, clonality studies have not been performed.

## Granular cell tumor

The esophagus is the second most frequently involved gastrointestinal site (after the tongue) for the development of granular cell tumors. Granular cell tumor is a benign neoplasm of schwann cell origin and is the second most common esophageal mesenchymal tumor (after leiomyoma).[144,145] They may occur sporadically or in patients with such familiar disorders as neurofibromatosis.

Clinically, these tumors occur equally in men and women, usually in early to mid-adult life.[144–146] Because of their small size, granular cell tumors are usually asymptomatic, although large tumors may produce obstructive-type symptoms. In fact, most granular cell tumors are found incidentally at the time of endoscopy for other gastrointestinal complaints.

Grossly, most granular cell tumors occur in the lower esophagus but less commonly arise in the upper and middle esopha-

gus. Up to 20% may be multiple.[147] Endoscopically, they usually appear as smooth, sessile, grayish-white submucosal lesions with discrete borders. Microscopically, they are composed of plump, epithelioid, or spindle cell–shaped "histiocytoid" cells, with finely granular eosinophilic cytoplasm and bland, oval-to-round, eccentrically located nuclei (Fig. 14–8). These tumors characteristically stain positively with periodic acid–schiff stain and with S-100. The eosinophilic granular cytoplasm is due to the presence of numerous autophagic vacuoles and irregularly shaped lysosomes that can be seen by electron microscopy.[145] Overlying pseudoepitheliomatous-reactive hyperplasia of the squamous epithelium may be present and, at times, may be confused with well-differentiated squamous cell carcinoma.

The vast majority of granular cell tumors are benign and remain stable in size with time.[147] However, some may progress slowly. Malignant granular cell tumors are very rare, and their diagnosis is based primarily on the finding of distant metastasis.[148]

## Leiomyoma

Leiomyomas form approximately 0.4% of all esophageal neoplasms and are the most common benign mesenchymal tumor of the esophagus.[139,149] They occur in men slightly more often than in women, usually in mid- to late adult life.[149] Since most leiomyomas are small in size and intramural in location, few cause significant symptoms. In fact, most are detected incidentally at the time of endoscopy.

Leiomyomas may be single or multiple and most often occur in the esophagogastric junctional region.[149] They commonly arise from the inner circular layer of the muscularis propria. The diagnosis is usually made on the basis of evaluation of endoscopic mucosal biopsy tissue but may be suspected on the basis of radiographic imaging studies, which may show a well-circumscribed intramural smooth, round tumor with sharp borders.

Pathologically, most are between 1 and 5 cm in diameter. Endoscopically, they are well-circumscribed, pale, firm lesions that have a whorled appearance on cut section. Microscopically, leiomyomas show a proliferation of bland, relatively hypocellular, spindle-shaped cells arranged in bundles and short fascicles (Fig. 14–9). One unusual form of leiomyoma is referred to as *leiomyomatosis*, which is defined as a series of nodular thickenings of the muscularis that tend to involve the entire esophagus.[150]

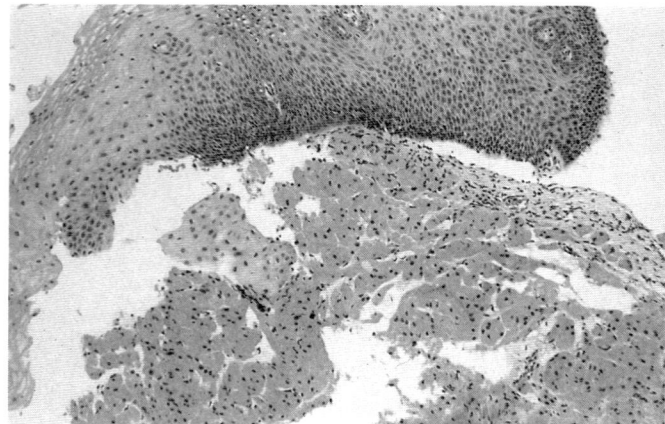

**A**

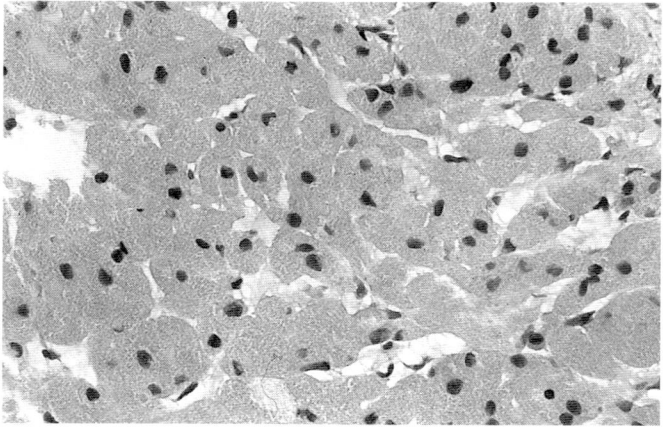

**B**

**Figure 14–8** *A:* Low-power view of an esophageal mucosal biopsy containing a granular cell tumor in the lamina propria beneath the overlying squamous epithelium. *B:* The cells have a histiocytoid appearance and contain eosinophilic granular cytoplasm and small oval to round hyperchromatic nuclei.

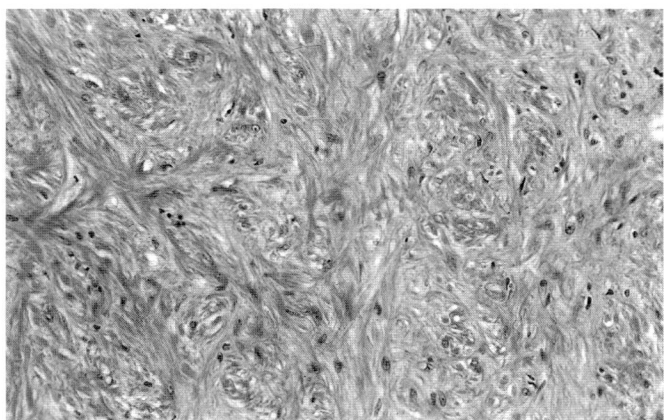

**Figure 14-9** High-power view of a benign leiomyoma of the esophagus. The tumor is composed of a bland proliferation of spindle-shaped cells with eosinophilic cytoplasm, similar in appearance to normal smooth muscle cells, but in an abnormal architectural pattern. The cells are arranged in interlacing thin bundles and fascicles. No mitotic figures are present.

When numerous and small, they may be referred to as "seedling" leiomyomas.[151]

Leiomyomas are benign lesions with no malignant potential. Treatment usually depends on the clinical significance of the tumor and may involve either endoscopic removal or transthoracic enucleation.

## Sarcoma

Primary sarcomas of the esophagus are extremely rare.[140,152,153] In fact, most tumors with a sarcomatous appearance are actually carcinosarcomas. However, individual case reports or small series of leiomyosarcomas, malignant nerve sheath or vascular tumors, and gastrointestinal stromal tumors have been reported.[152,153] A small number of rhabdomyosarcomas, synovial cell sarcomas, osteosarcomas, malignant fibrous histiocytomas, and liposarcomas have also been reported.[153,154]

In one recent report of 17 stromal tumors by Miettinen and colleagues,[152] 12 of these tumors occurred in men with a median age of 63 years.[152] The most common complaint was dysphagia, and all tumors occurred in the distal esophagus. Similar to gastrointestinal stromal tumors that occur elsewhere in the gastrointestinal system, all tumors in this series were CD117 (c-Kit) and CD34 positive by immunohistochemical analysis. The behavior of esophageal stromal tumors is related to the size of the lesion, the degree of mitoses, necrosis, and the presence or absence of infiltrative features.

## Malignant Melanoma

The majority of esophageal malignant melanomas represent metastasis.[155,156] However, primary malignant melanoma forms up to 0.1% of all esophageal malignancies and represents approximately 3% of all melanomas in the body.[156,157] Interestingly, up to 50% of reported cases were described in Japan. Esophageal malignant melanomas are believed to arise from intraepithelial melanocytes that are normally present in up to 20% of the adult population.[158] Clinically, similar to melanomas that develop in other organs, they are often seen in older adults and are slightly

more common in men than in women. Typical symptoms include epigastric pain, dysphagia, and weight loss.

Grossly, esophageal melanomas are usually large, polypoid, fungating, or ulcerating tumors that may develop at any location in the esophagus; however, they are most common in the mid- to distal region. Microscopically, esophageal melanomas resemble those that arise in the skin.[159] They consist of epitheliod and/or spindle-shaped cells arranged in sheets or uniform nests. Cells typically have a large vesicular nucleus with a prominent eosinophilic nucleolus and are often associated with an atypical junctional melanocytic proliferation in the overlying squamous epithelium. Pigmented granules may be present in the in situ or invasive portions of the tumor. The diagnosis is established by finding the typical morphologic features in conjunction with immunohistochemical positivity for S-100 and/or HMB-45 or by demonstration of intracytoplasmic melanosomes by electron microscopy. Because most melanomas of the esophagus are metastatic, a diagnosis of primary melanoma should be made only when an overlying junctional component is present and there is no clinical or radiologic evidence of tumor elsewhere in the body.

Primary esophageal melanomas are highly aggressive tumors that carry a poor prognosis.[157] Unfortunately, most are discovered at an advanced stage. Five-year survival rates of less than 10% have been reported in small series.[157]

## Metastasis

The esophagus is a rather uncommon location for metastasis.[160] Most metastatic tumors are due to direct spread from either an adjacent lung cancer or from cancer of the gastric cardia, larynx, tracheobronchial tree, or thyroid gland.[161] Breast cancer may spread to the esophagus via the intercostal lymphatics (Fig. 14–10).[162] Leukemic cells rarely spread to the esophagus and are usually limited to the mucosa or submucosa when present.[163] As mentioned above, melanoma may spread to the esophagus, and this is usually by a hematogenous route. Metastatic tumors are diagnosed on the basis of a high degree of clinical and pathologic suspicion. Ancillary tests such as cytokeratin 7 (lung cancer, breast cancer, pancreatic cancer), cytokeratin 20 (colon cancer), TTF-1 (lung cancer, thyroid cancer), thyroglobulin (thyroid

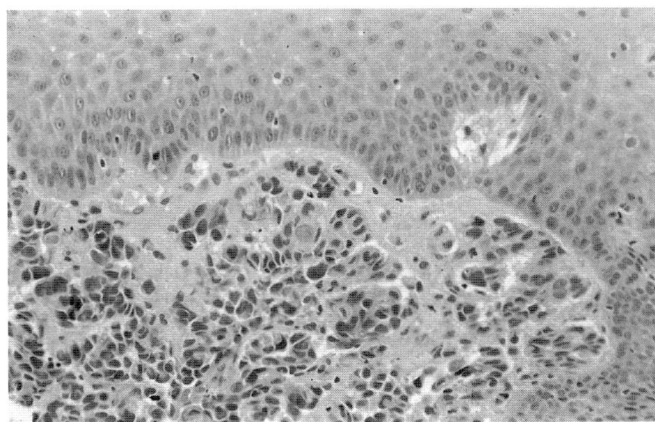

**Figure 14-10** Esophageal mucosal biopsy from a patient with a metastatic, poorly differentiated ductal carcinoma of the breast. In the lamina propria, there are poorly formed glands containing highly atypical cells. By immunohistochemical analysis, these cells were positive for estrogen and progesterone receptor, similar to the patient's primary tumor.

cancer), and ER/PR (breast cancer) may be performed to confirm a specific diagnosis.

## References

1. Parkin DM, Laara E, Muir CS. Estimates of the worldwide frequency of sixteen major cancers in 1980. Int J Cancer 41:184–197, 1988.
2. Yang PC, Davis S. Incidence of cancer of the esophagus in the US by histologic type. Cancer 61:612–617, 1988.
3. Hamilton SR, Aaltonen LA, eds. World Health Organization Classification of Tumors. Pathology and Genetics of Tumors of the Digestive System. IARC Press, Lyon, 2000.
4. Odze R, Antonioli D, Shocket D, et al. Esophageal squamous papillomas, a clinicopathologic study of 38 lesions and analysis of human papillomavirus by the polymerase chain reaction. Am J Surg Pathol 17:803–812; 1993.
5. Orlowska J, Jarosz D, Gugulski A, et al. Squamous cell papillomas of the eosphagus: report of 20 cases and literature review. Am J Gastroenterol 89:434–437, 1994.
6. Carr NJ, Bratthauer GL, Lychy JH, et al. Squamous cell pappillomas of the esophagus: a study of 23 lesions for human papillomavirus by in situ hybridization and the polymerase chain reaction. Hum Pathol 25:536–540, 1994.
7. Talamini G, Capelli P, Zamboni G, et al. Alcohol, smoking and papillomavirus infection and risk factors for esophageal squamous-cell papilloma and esophageal squamous-cell carcinoma in Italy. Int J Cancer 874–878, 2000.
8. Poljak M, Orlowska J, Cerar A. Human papillomavirus infection in esophageal squamous cell papillomas: a study of 29 lesions. Anticancer Res 15:965–970, 1995.
9. Lavergne D, De Villiers EM. Papillomavirus in esophageal papillomas and carcinomas. Int J Cancer 80:680–684, 1999.
10. Waluga M, Hartleb M, Sliwinski ZK, et al. Esophageal squamous-cell papillomatosis complicated by carcinoma. Am J Gastroenterol 95:1592–1593, 2000.
11. Rouse RV, Soetikno RM, Baker RJ, et al. Esophageal submucosal gland duct adenoma. Am J Surg Pathol 19:1191–1196, 1995.
12. Banducci D, Rees R, Bluett MK, et al. Pleomorphic adenoma of the cervical esophagus: a rare tumor. Ann Thorac Surg 44:653–655, 1987.
13. Thurberg BL, Duray PH, Odze RD. Polypoid dysplasia in Barrett's esophagus: a clinicopathologic, immunohistochemical and molecular study of five cases. Hum Pathol 30:745–752, 1999.
14. Parker SL, Tong T, Bolden S, Wingo PA. Cancer statistics 1997. CA Cancer J Clin 47:5–27, 1997.
15. Lewin KJ, Appelman HD. Tumors of the esophagus and stomach. In: Rosai J (ed): Atlas of Tumor Pathology, Third Series, Fascicle 18. Armed Forces Institute of Pathology, Washington, DC, 1996, p 467.
16. Brown LM, Hoover RN, Greenberg RS, et al. Are racial differences in squamous cell esophageal cancer explained by alcohol and tobacco use? J Natl Cancer Inst 86:1340–1345, 1994.
17. Tachimori Y, Watanabe H, Kato H, et al. Hypercalcemia in patients with esophageal carcinoma. The pathophysiologic role of parathyroid hormone–related protein. Cancer 68:2625–2629, 1991.
18. Ina H, Shibuya H, Ohashi I, et al. The frequency of a concomitant early esophageal cancer in male patients with oral and oropharyngeal cancer. Cancer 73:2038–2041, 1994.
19. Ribeiro U, Posner MC, Safatle-Reynolds AV, Reynolds JC. Risk factors for squamous cell carcinoma of the oesophagus. Br J Surg 83:1174–1185, 1996.
20. Streitz JM, Ellis FH, Gibb SP, Heatley GM. Achalasia and squamous cell carcinoma of the esophagus: analysis of 241 patients. Ann Thorac Surg 59:1604–1609, 1995.
21. Meijssen MA, Tilanus HW, van Blankenstein M, et al. Achalasia complicated by oesophageal squamous cell carcinoma: a prospective study in 195 patients. Gut 33:155–158, 1992.
22. Marger RS, Marger D. Carcinoma of the esophagus and tylosis. A lethal genetic combination. Cancer 72:17–19, 1993.
23. Chang F, Syrjanen S, Wang L, Syrjanen K. Infectious agents in the etiology of esophageal cancer. Gastroenterology 103:1336–1348, 1992.
24. Chang F, Syrjanen S, Shen Q, et al. Human papillomavirus involvement in esophageal carcinogenesis in the high-incidence area of China. A study of 700 cases by screening and type-specific in situ hybridization. Scand J Gastroenterol 35:123–130, 2000.
25. Poljak M, Cerar A, Seme K. Human papillomavirus infection in esophageal carcinomas: a study of 121 lesions using multiple broad-spectrum polymerase chain reactions and literature review. Hum Pathol 29:266–271, 1998.
26. Togawa K, Jaskiewicz K, Takahashi H, et al. Human papillomavirus DNA sequences in esophageal squamous cell carcinoma. Gastroenterology 107:128–136, 1994.
27. Turner JR, Shen LH, Crum CP, et al. Low prevalence of human papillomavirus infection in esophageal squamous cell carcinomas from North America: analysis by a highly sensitive and specific polymerase chain reaction–based approach. Hum Pathol 28:174–178, 1997.
28. Rubio CA, Liu FS, Zong Zhao HZ. Histological classification of intraepithelial neoplasias and microinvasive squamous carcinoma of the esophagus. Am J Surg Pathol 13:685–690, 1989.
29. Dawsey SM, Wang GQ, Weinstein WM, et al. Squamous dysplasia and early esophageal cancer in the Linzian region of China: distinctive endoscopic lesions. Gastroenterology 105:1333–1340, 1993.
30. Mandard AM, Mamay J, Gignoux M, et al. Cancer of the esophagus and associated lesions: detailed pathologic study of 100 esophagectomy specimens. Hum Pathol 15:660–669, 1984.
31. Kuwano H, Matsuda H, Matsuoka H, et al. Intra-epithelial carcinoma concomitant with esophageal squamous cell carcinoma. Cancer 59:783–787, 1987.
32. Dawsey SM, Fleischer DE, Wang GQ, et al. Mucosal iodine staining improves endoscopic visualization of squamous dysplasia and squamous cell carcinoma of the esophagus in Linxian, China. Cancer 83:220–231, 1998.
33. Dawsey SM, Yu Y, Taylor PR, et al. Esophageal cytology and subsequent risk of esophageal cancer. A prospective follow-up study from Linxian, China. Acta Cytol 38:183–192, 1994.
34. Tajima Y, Nakanishi Y, Tachimori Y, et al. Significance of involvement by squamous cell carcinoma of the ducts of esophageal submucosal glands. Analysis of 201 surgically resected superficial squamous cell carcinomas. Cancer 89:248–254, 2000.
35. Chu P, Stagias J, West AB, et al. Diffuse pagetoid squamous cell carcinoma in situ of the esophagus: a case report. Cancer 79:1865–1870, 1997.
36. Qui S, Yang G. Precursor lesions of esophageal cancer in high-risk populations in Henan Province, China. Cancer 62:551–557, 1998.
37. Shu YJ, Yuan XQ, Jin SP. Further investigation of the relationship between dysplasia and cancer of the esophagus [in Chinese]. Clin Med J 1:39–41, 1981.
38. Goseki N, Koike M, Yoshida M. Histopathologic characteristics of early stage esophageal carcinoma. Cancer 69:1088–1093, 1992.
39. Kuwano H, Ohno S, Matsuda H, et al. Serial histologic evaluation of multiple primary squamous cell carcinomas of the esophagus. Cancer 61:1635–1638, 1988.
40. Yoshinaka H, Shimazu H, Fukumoto T, Baba M. Superficial esophageal carcinoma: a clinicopathological review of 59 cases. Gastroenterology 86:1413–1418, 1991.
41. Bogomoletz WV, Molas G, Gayet B, Pote: F. Superficial squamous cell carcinoma of the esophagus: a report of 76 cases and review of the literature. Am J Surg Pathol 13:535–546, 1989.
42. Morita M, Kuwano H, Yasuda M, et al. The multicentric occurrence of squamous epithelial dysplasia and squamous cell carcinoma in the esophagus. Cancer 74:2889–2895, 1994.
43. Lee RG, Compton CC. Protocol for the examination of specimens removed from patients with esophageal carcinoma. Arch Pathol Lab Med 121:925–929, 1997.
44. Takubo K, Sasajima K, Yamashita K, et al. Prognostic significance of intramural metastasis in patients with esophageal carcinoma. Cancer 65:1816–1819, 1990.
45. Wang LS, Chow KC, Chi KH, et al. Prognosis of esophageal squamous cell carcinoma: analysis of clinicopathological and biological factors. Am J Gastroenterol 94:1933–1940, 1999.
46. Torres CM, Wang HH, Turner JR, et al. Pathologic prognostic factors in esophageal squamous cell carcinoma: a follow-up study of 74 patients with or without preoperative chemoradiation therapy. Mod Pathol 12:961–968, 1999.
47. Robey-Cafferty SS, El-Naggar AK, Sahin AA, et al. Prognostic factors in esophageal squamous carcinoma. Anat Pathol 95:844–849, 1991.
48. Ando N, Ozawa S, Kitagawa Y, et al. Improvement in the results of surgical treatment of advanced squamous esophageal carcinoma during 15 consecutive years. Ann Surg 232:225–232, 2000.
49. Tajima Y, Nakanishi Y, Oochiai A. Histopathologic findings predicting lymph node metastasis and prognosis of patients with superficial esophageal carcinoma: analysis of 240 surgically resected tumors. Cancer 88:1285–1293, 2000.

50. Holscher AH, Bollschweiler E, Schneider PM, et al. Prognosis of early esophageal cancer. Comparison between adeno- and squamous cell carcinoma. Cancer 76:178–186, 1995.

51. Mandard AM, Chasle J, Marnay M, et al. Autopsy findings in 111 cases of esophageal cancer. Cancer 48:329–335, 1981.

52. Koki Y, Shiozaki H, Tahara H, et al. Prognostic value of DNA ploidy in squamous cell carcinoma of esophagus. Cancer 72:1813–1818, 1993.

53. Tsutsui S, Kuwano H, Mori M, Matsuura H, Sugimachi K. A flow cytometric analysis of DNA content in primary and metastatic lesions of esophageal squamous cell carcinoma. Cancer 70:2586–2591, 1992.

54. Cho KJ, Jang JJ, Lee SS, et al. Basaloid squamous carcinoma of the oesophagus: a distinct neoplasm with multipotential differentiation. Histopathology 36:331–334, 2000.

55. Singh ZN, Ray R, Karak AK, et al. Basaloid-squamous carcinoma, a distinct histopathological entity. Indian J Cancer 33:86–91, 1996.

56. Sarbia M, Verreet P, Bittinger F, et al. Basaloid squamous cell carcinoma of the esophagus. Cancer 79:1872–1878, 1997.

57. Iascone C, Barreca M. Carcinosarcoma and pseudosarcoma of the esophagus: two names, one disease—comprehensive review of the literature. World J Surg 23:153–157, 1999.

58. Lauwers GY, Grand LD, Scott GV, et al. Spindle cell squamous carcinoma of the esophagus: analysis of ploidy and tumor proliferative activity in a series of 13 cases. Hum Pathol 29:863–868, 1998.

59. Kinoshita Y, Tsurumaru M, Udagawa H, et al. Carcinosarcoma of the esophagus with metastases showing osteosarcoma: a case report and review of the literature. Dis Esophagus 11:189–193, 1998.

60. Balercia G, Bhan AK, Dickersin GR. Sarcomatoid carcinoma: an ultrastructural study with light microscopic and immunohistochemical correlation of 10 cases from various anatomic sites. Ultrastruct Pathol 19:249–263, 1995.

61. Nakagawa S, Nishimaki T, Suzuki T, et al. Histogenetic heterogeneity in carcinosarcoma of the esophagus. Report of a case with immunohistochemical and molecular analyses. Dig Dis Sci 44:905–909, 1999.

62. Biemond P, ten Kate FJW, van Blankenstein M. Esophageal verrucous carcinoma: histologically a low-grade malignancy but clinically a fatal disease. J Clin Gastroenterol 13:102–107, 1991.

63. Kavin H, Yaremki L, Valaitis J, et al. Chronic esophagitis evolving to verrucous squamous cell carcinoma: possible role of exogenous chemical carcinogens. Gastroenterology 110:904–914, 1996.

64. Blot WJ, Devesa SS, Kneller RW, et al. Rising incidence of adenocarcinoma of the esophagus and gastric cardia. JAMA 265:1287–1289, 1991.

65. Daly JM, Karnell LH, Menck HR. National Cancer Data Base report on esophageal carcinoma. Cancer 78:1820–1828, 1996.

66. Devesa SS, Blot WJ, Fraumeni JF. Changing patterns in the incidence of esophageal and gastric carcinoma in the United States. Cancer 83: 2049–2053, 1998.

67. Reid BJ. Barrett's esophagus and esophageal adenocarcinoma. Gastroenterology 20:817–834, 1991.

68. Sharma VK, Chockalingam H, Homung CA, et al. Changing trends in esophageal cancer: a 15-year experience in single center. Am J Gastroenterol 93:702–705, 1998.

69. Paraf F, Flejou J-F, Pignon J-P, et al. Surgical pathology of adenocarcinoma arising in Barrett's esophagus. Am J Surg Pathol 19:183–191, 1995.

70. Hamilton SR, Smith RRL, Cameron JL. Prevalence and characteristics of Barrett's esophagus in patients with adenocarcinoma of the esophagus or esophagogastric junction. Hum Pathol 19:942–948, 1988.

71. Cameron AJ, Lomboy CT, Pera M, et al. Adenocarcinoma of the esophagogastric junction and Barrett's esophagus. Gastroenterology 109: 1541–1546, 1995.

72. Spechler SJ, Goyal RK. Barrett's esophagus. N Engl J Med 315:362–371, 1986.

73. Peters FTM, Sleijfer DTT, van Hoff GW, et al. Is chemotherapy associated with the development of Barrett's esophagus? Dig Dis Sci 38: 923–926, 1993.

74. Waring JP, Legrand J, Chinichain A. Duodenogastric reflux in patients with Barrett's esophagus. Dig Dis Sci 35:759–762, 1990.

75. Jochem JV, Fuerst PA, Fromkes JJ. Familial Barrett's esophagus associated with adenocarcinoma. Gastroenterology 102:1400–1402, 1992.

76. Winters C, Spurling TJ, Chobanian SJ, et al. Barrett's esophagus. A prevalent, occult complication of gastroesophageal reflux disease. Gastroenterology 92:118–124, 1987.

77. Glickman JN, Chen YY, Wang H, Antonioli DA, Odze RD. Phenotypic characteristics of a distinctive multilayered epithelium suggest that it is a precursor in the development of Barrett's esophagus. Am J Surg Pathol 25:569–578, 2001.

78. Spechler S. The role of gastric carditis in metaplasia and neoplasia at the gastroesophageal junction. Gastroenterology 117:218–228, 1998.

79. Goldblum JR, Vicari JJ, Falk GW, et al. Inflammation and intestinal metaplasia of the gastric cardia: the role of gastroesophageal reflux and *H. pylori* infection. Gastroenterology 114:633–669, 1998.

80. Ormsby AH, Goldblum JR, Rice TW, et al. Cytokeratin subsets can reliably distinguish Barrett's esophagus from intestinal metaplasia of the stomach. Hum Pathol 30:288–294, 1999.

81. Glickman JN, Wang H, Das KM, et al. Phenotype of Barrett's esophagus and intestinal metaplasia of the distal esophagus and gastroesophageal junction. Am J Surg Pathol 25:87–94, 2001.

82. Chen YY, Wang HH, Antonioli DA, et al. Significance of acid mucin positive nongoblet columnar cells in the distal esophagus and gastroesophageal junction. Hum Pathol 30:1488–1495, 1999.

83. Cameron AJ, Ott BJ, Payne WS. The incidence of adenocarcinoma in columnar-lined (Barrett's) esophagus. N Engl J Med 313:857–859, 1985.

84. Hameeteman W, Tytgat GNJ, Houthoff HJ, van den Tweel JG. Barrett's esophagus: development of dysplasia and adenocarcinoma. Gastroenterology 96:1249–1256, 1989.

85. Tytgat GNJ, Houthoff HJ, van den Tweel JG. Barrett's esophagus: development of dysplasia and adenocarcinoma. Gastroenterology 96: 1249–1256, 1989.

86. Menke-Pluymers MBE, Hop WCJ, Dees J, van Blankenstein M, Tilanus JW. Risk factors for the development of an adenocarcinoma in columnar-lined (Barrett) esophagus. Cancer 72:1155–1158, 1993.

87. Ovaska J, Miettien M, Kivilaakso E. Adenocarcinoma arising in Barrett's esophagus. Dig Dis Sci 34:1336–1339, 1989.

88. O'Connor JB, Falk GW, Richter JE. The incidence of adenocarcinoma and dysplasia in Barrett's esophagus. Am J Gastroenterol 94:2037–2042, 1999.

89. Conio M, Cameron AJ, Romero Y, et al. Secular trends in the epidemiology and outcome of Barrett's oesophagus in Olmsted County, Minnesota. Gut 48:304–309, 2001.

90. Iftikhar SY, James PD, Steele RJ, et al. Length of Barrett's oesophagus: an important factor in the development of dysplasia and adenocarcinoma. Gut 33:1155–1158, 1992.

91. Rudolph RE, Vaughan TL, Storer BE, et al. Effect of segment length on risk for neoplastic progression in patients with Barrett esophagus. Ann Intern Med 132:612–620, 2000.

92. Weston AP, Badr AS, Hassanein RS. Prospective multivariate analysis of clinical, endoscopic, and histological factors predictive of the development of Barrett's multifocal high-grade dysplasia or adenocarcinoma. Am J Gastroenterol 94:3413–3419, 1999.

93. Skinner DB, Walther BC, Riddell RH. Barrett's esophagus: comparison of benign and malignant cases. Ann Surg 198:554–566, 1983.

94. Reid BJ, Levine DS, Longton D, et al. Predictors of progression to cancer in Barrett's esophagus: baseline histology and flow cytometry identify low- and high-risk patient subsets. Am J Gastroenterol 95:1669–1676, 2000.

95. Hamilton SR, Smith RRL. The relationship between columnar epithelial dysplasia and invasive adenocarcinoma arising in Barrett's esophagus. Am J Clin Pathol 87:301–312, 1987.

96. Reid BJ, Haggitt RC, Rubin CE, et al. Observer variation in the diagnosis of dysplasia in Barrett's esophagus. Hum Pathol 19:166–178, 1988.

97. Geisinger KR, Teot LA, Richter JE. A comparative cytopathologic and histologic study of atypia, dysplasia and adenocarcinoma in Barrett's esophagus. Cancer 69:8–17, 1992.

98. Levine DS, Haggitt RC, Blount PL, Rabinovitch PS, Rusch VW, Reid BJ. An endoscopic biopsy protocol can differentiate high-grade dysplasia from early adenocarcinoma in Barrett's esophagus. Gastroenterology 105:40–50, 1993.

99. Robertson CS, Mayberry JF, Nicholson DA, James PD, Atkinson M. Value of endoscopic surveillance in the detection of neoplastic change in Barrett's oesophagus. Br J Surg 75:760–763, 1988.

100. Thurberg BL, Duray PH, Odze RD. Polypoid dysplasia in Barrett's esophagus: a clinicopathologic, immunohistochemical and molecular study of five cases. Hum Pathol 30:745–752, 1999.

101. Ovaska J, Miettien M, Kivilaakso E. Adenocarcinoma arising in Barrett's esophagus. Dig Dis Sci 34:1336–1339, 1989.

102. Altorki NK, Sunagawa M, Little AG, Skinner DB. High-grade dysplasia in the columnar-lined esophagus. Arn J Surg 161:97–99, 1991.

103. Rice TW, Falk GW, Achkar E, Petras RE. Surgical management of high-grade dysplasia in Barrett's esophagus. Am J Gastroenterol 88:1832–1836, 1993.

104. Sampliner RE: High-grade dysplasia in Barrett's esophagus: an evolving clinical dilemma. Am J Gastroenterol 88:1811–1812, 1993.

105. Pera M, Trastek VF, Carpenter HA, Alien MS, Deschamps C, Pairolero PC. Barrett's esophagus with high-grade dysplasia: an indication for esophagectomy. Ann Thorac Surg 54:199–204, 1992.

106. Reid BJ, Blount PL, Rubin CE, Levine DS, Haggitt RC, Rabinovitch PS. Flow-cytometric and histological progression to malignancy in Barrett's esophagus: prospective endoscopic surveillance of a cohort. Gastroenterology 102:1212–1219, 1992.

107. Ramel S, Reid BJ, Sanchez CA, et al. Evaluation of P53 protein expression in Barrett's esophagus by two-parameter flow cytometry. Gastroenterology 10:1220–1228, 1992.

108. Younes M, Levobitz RM, Lechago V, Lechago J. P53 protein accumulation in Barrett's metaplasia, dysplasia, and carcinoma: a follow-up study. Gastroenterology 6:1637–1642, 1993.

109. Jankowski J, Wright NA, Meltzer SJ, et al. Molecular evolution of the metaplasia–dysplasia–adenocarcinoma sequence in the esophagus. Am J Pathol 154:965–973, 1999.

110. Sampliner RE. Practice guidelines on the diagnosis, surveillance, and therapy of Barrett's esophagus. The Practice Parameters Committee of the American College of Gastroenterology. Am J Gastroenterol 93:1028–1032, 1998.

111. Nijhawan PK, Wang KK. Endoscopic mucosal resection for lesions with endoscopic features suggestive of malignancy and high-grade dysplasia within Barrett's esophagus. Gastrointest Endosc 52:328–332, 2000.

112. Gossner L, Stolte M, Sroka R, et al. Photodynamic ablation of high-grade dysplasia and early cancer in Barrett's esophagus by means of 5-aminolevulinic acid. Gastroenterology 114:448–455, 1998.

113. Hamilton K, Chiappori A, Olson S, et al. Prevalence and prognostic significance of neuroendocrine cells in esophageal adenocarcinoma. Mod Pathol 13:475–481, 2000.

114. Chejfec G, Jablokow VR, Gould VE. Linitis plastica carcinoma of the esophagus. Cancer 51:2139–2143, 1983.

115. Streitz JM, Williamson WA, Ellis FH. Current concepts concerning the nature and treatment of Barrett's esophagus and its complications. Ann Thorac Surg 54:586–591, 1992.

116. Menke-Pluymers MBE, Schoute NW, Mulder AH, et al. Outcome of surgical treatment of adenocarcinoma in Barrett's oesophagus. Gut 33:1454–1958, 1992.

117. van Sandick JW, van Lanschot JJ, ten Kate FJ, et al. Pathology of early invasive adenocarcinoma of the esophagus or esophagogastric junction: implications for therapeutic decision making. Cancer 88:2429–2437, 2000.

118. Torres C, Turner JR, Wang HH, et al. Pathologic prognostic factors in Barrett's-associated adenocarcinoma. Cancer 85:520–528, 1999.

119. Lauwers GY, Scott GV, Vauthey JN. Adenocarcinoma of the upper esophagus arising in cervical ectopic gastric mucosa, rare evidence of malignant potential of so-called "Inlet Patch." Dig Dis Sci 43:901–907, 1998.

120. Endoh Y, Miyawaki M, Tamura G, et al. Esophageal adenocarcinoma that probably originated in the esophageal gland duct: a case report. Pathol Int 49:156–159, 1999.

121. Tsang WYW, Chang JKC, Lee KC, et al. Basaloid-squamous carcinoma of the upper aerodigestive tract and so-called adenoid cystic carcinoma of the oesophagus: the same tumour type? Histopathology 19:35–46, 1991.

122. Morisaki Y, Yoshizumi Y, Hiroyasu S, et al. Adenoid cystic carcinoma of the esophagus: report of a case and review of the Japanese literature. Surg Today 26:1006–1009, 1996.

123. Newman J, Antonakopoulos GN, Darnton SJ, et al. The ultrastructure of oesophageal carcinomas: multidirectional differentiation. A transmission electron microscopic study of 43 cases. J Pathol 167;193–198, 1992.

124. Nakagawa S, Nishimaki T, Kanda T, et al. Composite tumor with papillary adenocarcinoma and squamous cell of the esophagus: report of a case. Surg Today 30:364–367, 2000.

125. Nishimaki T, Nakagawa S, Aizawa K, et al. Composite tumor of the esophagus with tripartite differentiation. Dig Dis Sci 42:1041–1046, 1997.

126. Lam KY, Dickens P, Loke SL, et al. Squamous cell carcinoma of the oesophagus with mucin-secreting component (muco-epidermoid carcinoma and adenosquamous carcinoma): a clinicopathologic study and review of literature. Eur J Surg Oncol 20:31–35, 1994.

127. Matsuki A, Nishimaki T, Suzuke T, et al. Esophageal mucoepidermoid carcinoma containing signet-ring cells: three case reports and a literature review. J Surg Oncol 71:54–57, 1999.

128. Kikuchi Y, Tsuneta Y, Kawai T, Aizawa M. Choriocarcinoma of the esophagus producing chorionic gonadotropin. Acta Pathol Jpn 38:489–499, 1988.

129. Ter RB, Govil YK, Leite L, et al. Adenosquamous carcinoma in Barrett's esophagus presenting as pseudoachalasia. Am J Gastroenterol 94:268–272, 1999.

130. Soga J. Esophageal endocrinomas, an extremely rare tumor: a statistical comparative evaluation of 28 ordinary carcinoids and 72 atypical variants. J Exp Clin Cancer Res 17:47–57, 1998.

131. Takubo K, Nakamura K-I, Sawabe M, et al. Primary undifferentiated small cell carcinoma of the esophagus. Hum Pathol 30:216–221,1999.

132. Medgyesy DC, Wolff RA, Putnam JB, et al. Small cell carcinoma of the esophagus, The University of Texas M.D. Anderson Cancer Center experience and literature review. Cancer 88:262–267, 2000.

133. Casas F, Ferrer F, Farrus B, et al. Primary small cell carcinoma of the esophagus, a review of the literature with emphasis on therapy and prognosis. Cancer 80:1366–1372, 1997.

134. Lam KY, Law S, Tung PH, Wong J. Esophageal small cell carcinomas, clinicopathologic parameters, p53 overexpression, proliferation marker, and their impact on pathogenesis. Arch Pathol Lab Med 120:228–233, 2000.

135. Mori M, Matsukuma A, Adachi Y, et al. Small cell carcinoma of the esophagus. Cancer 63:564–573, 1989.

136. Harmse JL, Carey FA, Baird AR, et al. Merkel cells in the human oesophagus. J Pathol 189:176–179, 1999.

137. Taal BG, Van Hererde P, Somers R. Isolated primary oesophageal involvement by lymphoma: a rare cause of dysphagia: two case histories and a review of other published data. Gut 34:994–998, 1993.

138. Ruskone-Fourmetraux A, Aegerter P, Delmer A, et al. Primary digestive tract lymphoma: a prospective multicentric study of 91 patients. Gastroenterology 105:1662–1671, 1993.

139. Plachta A. Benign tumors of the esophagus: review of literature and report of 99 cases. Am J Gastroenterol 38:639–652, 1962.

140. Hatch GF, Wertheimer-Hatch L, Hatch KF. et al. Tumors of the esophagus. World J Surg 24:401–411, 2000.

141. Wu MH, Chuang CM, Tseng YL. Giant intraluminal fibrovascular polyp of the esophagus. Hepatogastroenterology 45:2115–2116, 1998.

142. Goldman N. Fibrovascular polyp of the esophagus. Otolaryngol Head Neck Surg 118:734–735, 1998.

143. Belafsky P, Amedee R, Zimmerman J. Giant fibrovascular polyp of the esophagus. South Med J 92:428–431, 1999.

144. Tada S, Iida M, Yao T, Miyagahara T, Hasuda S, Fujishima M. Granular cell tumor of the esophagus: endoscopic ultrasonographic demonstration and endoscopic removal. Am J Gastroenterol 85:1507–1511, 1990.

145. Fisher ER, Wechsler H. Granular cell myoblastoma—a misnomer. Electron microscopic and histochemical evidence concerning its Schwann cell derivation and nature (granular cell schwannoma). Cancer 15:936–943, 1962.

146. Buley ID, Gatter KC, Kelley PMA, Haryet A, Millard PR. Grandular cell tumor revisited: an immunological and ultrastructural study. Histopathology 12:263–274, 1988.

147. Joshi A, Chandrasoma P, Kiyabu M. Multiple granular cell tumors of the gastrointestinal tract with subsequent development of esophageal squamous carcinoma. Dig Dis Sci 37:1612–1618, 1992.

148. Ross RC, Miller TR, Foote FR. Malignant granular-cell myoblastoma. 5:112–121, 1952.

149. Seremitis MG, Lyons WS, DeGuzman VC, Peabody JW Jr. Leiomyomata of the esophagus: an analysis of 838 cases. Cancer 38:2166–2177, 1976.

150. Kabuto T, Taniguchi K, Iwanaga T, et al. Diffuse leiomyomatosis of the esophagus. Dig Dis Sci 25:388–391, 1980.

151. Takubo K, Nakagawa H, Tsuchiya S, et al. Seedling leiomyoma of the esophagus and esophagogastric junction zone. Hum Pathol 12:1006–1010, 1981.

152. Miettinen M, Sarlomo-Rikala M, Sobin LH, et al. Esophageal stromal tumor: a clinicopathologic immunohistochemical and molecular genetic study of 17 cases and comparison with esophageal leiomyomas and leiomyosarcomas. Am J Surg Pathol 24:211–222, 2000.

153. Perch SJ, Soffen EM, Whittington R, Brooks JJ. Esophageal sarcomas. J Surg Oncol 48:194–198, 1991.

154. Vartio T, Nickels J, Hockerstedt K, Scheinin TM. Rhabdomyosarcoma of the oesophagus. Light and electron microscopic study of a rare tumor. Virchows Arch A 386:357–361, 1980.

155. Lam KY, Law S, Wong J. Malignant melanoma of the oesophagus: clinicopathological features, lack of p53 expression and steroid receptors and a review of the literature. Eur J Surg Oncol 25:168–172, 1999.

156. Schuchter LM, Green R, Fraker D. Primary and metastatic diseases in malignant melanoma of the gastrointestinal tract. Curr Opin Oncol 12: 181–185, 2000.
157. Syrigos KN, Konstadoulakis MM, Ricaniades N, et al. Primary malignant melanoma of the esophagus: report of two cases and review of the literature. In Vivo 13:421–422, 1999.
158. Sharma SS, Venkateswaran S, Chacko A, Mathan M. Melanosis of the esophagus: an endoscopic, histochemical and ultrastructural study. Gastroenterology 100:13–16, 1991.
159. Symmans WF, Grimes MM. Malignant melanoma of the esophagus: histologic variants and immunohistochemical findings in four cases. Surg Pathol 4:222–234, 1991.
160. Anderson MF, Harrell GS. Secondary esophageal tumors. AJR Am J Roentgerol 135:1243–1246, 1980.
161. Antler AS, Ough Y, Pitchumoni CS, et al. Gastrointestinal metastases from malignant tumors of the lungs. Cancer 49:170–172, 1982.
162. Holyoke ED, Nemoto T, Dao TL. Esophageal metastases and dysphagia in patients with carcinoma of the breast. J Surg Oncol 1:97–107, 1969.
163. Dewar GJ, Lim CNH, Michalysyn B. Gastrointestinal complications in patients with acute and chronic leukemia. Can J Surg 24:67–71, 1981.

# Chapter 15

# Clinical Aspects and Management of Esophageal Carcinoma: Diagnostic and Staging Procedures

## MARK J. KRASNA AND XIAOLONG JIAO

Esophageal cancer, a disease described in Chinese historical records at least 2000 years ago, is among the 10 most frequent cancers in the world. The annual incidence reported in Western countries is 3 per 100,000, compared with 140 per 100,000 in an area of Central Asia that is known as the "esophageal cancer belt." Esophageal cancer remains one of the most lethal of all cancers. Once diagnosis is established, prognosis is poor, with a dismal 5-year survival rate of less than 10%. The results of single modality treatment have been poor except with surgery for early esophageal cancer. Recently, neoadjuvant chemotherapy, radiotherapy, and combined chemoradiation therapy have been added to the treatment of this disease in order to enhance local control, increase resectability rates, and improve the disease-free survival. The initial results of these multimodality treatments are encouraging. Since management of esophageal cancer and survival of patients depends on the stage of the disease, accurate staging is vital in the diagnostic evaluation. Recent advances in computed tomography (CT), magnetic resonance imaging (MRI), and position emission tomography (PET) of the esophagus, as well as endoscopic ultrasound (EUS) and minimally invasive thoracoscopic/laparoscopic staging (Ts/Ls) offer new hope for reliable preoperative diagnosis and staging of patients with esophageal cancer.

## Investigations in High-risk Patients

Cytological study is of great value in the screening of asymptomatic persons in high-incidence areas. In China, abrasive balloon cytology is a practical and cost-effective method for screening high-risk patients. It consists of introducing a balloon probe into the gastric cavity of patients, inflating it, and then withdrawing it through the esophagus. Exfoliated esophageal cells are collected by the abrasive balloon surface. This technique has been successful for mass screening in endemic areas such as Henan Province in China and certain regions of Iran.[1–3] However, in the United States and Western Europe, this technique is generally considered to be inappropriate because of the risks linked to esophageal varices or gastric ulcers, which are frequent in these patients. Instead, endoscopic screening for high-risk people who have had long-standing gastroesophageal reflux symptoms with concomitant Barrett's metaplasia is recommended.[4] Recent advances in endoscopic techniques such as staining and fluorescence endoscopy have improved the detection of early lesions of the esophagus.

## Diagnosis and Staging

The most commonly used diagnostic and staging modalities are the barium swallow study, chest radiography (CXR), esophagoscopy, bronchoscopy, gallium scanning, CT, MRI, and EUS. More recent innovations include EUS-guided fine needle aspiration (FNA), thoracoscopic and laparoscopic staging, and PET scanning.

Usually, the first diagnostic method is a barium swallow, followed by endoscopy with biopsy. After histological diagnosis of carcinoma is confirmed, a CT scan of the thorax and abdomen should be obtained to stage the tumor (T), lymph node metastases (N), and distant metastases (M). In some countries, abdominal ultrasound examinations are often performed instead of CT to diagnose liver or celiac lymphatic metastasis.

Chest radiography has a minimal role in the modern diagnosis and staging of esophageal cancer, although it can reveal an abnormal finding in up to 47.5% of the patients with esophageal cancer.[5] However, in some countries, it is still used routinely to identify hilar or mediastinal adenopathy, evidence of pulmonary metastases, secondary pulmonary infiltrates caused by aspiration, and pleural effusion. Bronchoscopy is helpful in determining involvement of the tracheobronchial tree for patients with middle- and upper-thirds diseae.[6-8] Nuclear medicine scans of the liver have only limited use in preoperative assessment. Inculet and colleagues compared CT, liver and spleen scans, and bone scans. They found that nuclear scans only predicted bony metastasis that was not detected by CT scan.[9]

## Endoscopy

Endoscopy remains the method of choice for the confirmation of esophageal cancer. Its use in detection of early lesions is improved by the use of staining techniques. Toluidine blue, a metachromatic stain from the thiazine group, has a particular affinity for RNA and DNA and therefore stains suspect areas in the mucosa, which are richer in nuclei than normal mucosa. It can reveal preinvasive lesions, demonstrate their multicentricity, and locate satellite centers and flat or occult forms of dysplasia or carcinoma in situ. False-negative results can be attributed to submucosal infiltration of the tumor or hyperkeratosis of a lesion that is more easily seen macroscopically since there is often leukoplakia or an exophytic appearance. The sensitivity of toluidine blue staining is 82% and the specificity, 75%.[10,11] Lugol's solution reacts specifically with glycogen in the epithelium, staining normal mucosa brown, whereas inflamed areas, gastric heterotopia, and cancer are not stained. It is easier to use than toluidine blue and produces fewer false-negative results.[12,13] A sensitivity of 46%, a specificity of 90%, a positive predictive value of 26%, and a negative predictive value of 96% were noted for staining with Lugol's solution by Fagundes and co-workers.[14] The dyeing capabilities of methylene blue, which stains absorbent cells, can also be used to identify foci of intestinal metaplasia in Barrett's mucosa during endoscopy. These staining techniques should be used in high-risk patients if the yield of endoscopy is to be improved. Endo and Kawano suggested that three points be included in screening for the detection of mucosal cancer of the esophagus: (1) esophagoscopy for patients with only slight esophageal symptoms; (2) annual endoscopic examination for high-risk populations; and (3) endoscopic staining with Lugol's solution for abnormal findings on conventional endoscopy.[15] Recently, fluorescence endoscopy has been used for the detection of endogenous or exogenous fluorophores associated with malignancy.[16-20] It has a capacity for detecting flat and occult neoplastic areas, and a certain amount of tissue diagnosis is also possible since fluorescent areas are related to neoplasia. The primary objective of fluorescence endoscopy is the detection of dysplasia in Barrett's esophagus.

## Computed Tomography

Although the role of CT in evaluating esophageal cancer has been thoroughly studied, questions regarding its utility still remain. While CT is highly effective in the assessment of mediastinal esophageal carcinomas, it is less helpful in the staging of cervical or gastroesohageal junction carcinomas. At the present time, CT scanning is considered complementary to endoscopy, conventional barium studies, and EUS for the pretreatment evaluation of esophageal neoplasms. It plays a key role in assessing initial tumor bulk for radiation therapy planning and is also useful in monitoring tumor response to the cytoreductive therapy. The CT scan is also very useful in depicting extraesophageal tumor spread to contiguous structures and distant metastases.

A CT scan evaluation is performed using 7- to 10-mm collimation and contiguous slices from the thoracic inlet through the liver to include the upper abdominal lymph node groups. Metastasis to celiac nodes occurs most frequently with distal esophageal neoplasms and is present in nearly one-third of patients with tumors of the proximal esophagus.[21] Either barium or water-soluble oral contrast agents are routinely administered. Adequate distention of the gastroesophageal junction is essential to exclude tumor involvement of this anatomic segment. Intravenous contrast material should be administered by the dynamic bolus technique to ensure optimal opacification of the heart, mediastinal vessels, and liver.

The normal thoracic esophagus is generally well visualized on routine CT scans of the chest and upper abdomen. Wall thickness varies with the degree of luminal distention. The well-distended esophageal wall is less than 3 mm thick; measurements greater than 5 mm are abnormal regardless of the degree of distention. Intraluminal air is seen in 60% of normal patients. The amount of mediastinal fat surrounding the normal esophagus on CT scans depends on body habitus. Mediastinal fat does not usually surround the esophagus on every CT scan section through the thorax; however, absence of fat planes are most often observed where the esophagus is in contact with the aorta, trachea, left main-stem tronchus, and left atrium.

Computed tomography scan staging of esophageal cancer includes assessment of (1) the extent of involvement of the esophageal wall by tumor, (2) tumor invasion of the periesophageal fat and adjacent structures, and (3) metastases to regional nodes or distant organs. The two key prognostic features of esophageal cancer are (1) the depth of tumor infiltration into or through the esophageal wall and (2) the presence or absence of visceral metastasis. Although the thickness of the esophageal wall can often be determined by CT, the individual layers of esophageal wall cannot. T1 and T2 lesions show an esophageal mass thickness between 5 and 15 mm, and T3 lesions show a thickness greater than 15 mm. T4 lesions show invasion of contiguous structures on CT.

The utility of different CT scan criteria in predicting invasion of vital structures has been studied. Specific findings of tracheobronchial invasion include demonstration of a tracheobronchial fistula or extension of tumor into the airway lumen. If an esophageal tumor indents or displaces the adjacent airway, luminal invasion is likely. Thickening of the wall of the tracheobronchial tree also suggests invasion. Simple absence of the fat plane between the aorta and tracheobronchial tree does not indicate invasion because this is a frequent finding in normal individuals. The CT scan is most successful in predicting tracheobronchial involvement, with sensitivities ranging from 31% to 100%, specificities ranging from 86% to 98%, and accuracies from 74% to 97%.[22] Accurate preoperative assessment of aortic invasion is of great importance for planning surgery. Computed tomographic evidence of aortic invasion can be determined by the degree of contact between the esophagus and the aorta. The additional use of intraaortic endovascular sonography can be helpful in detecting aortic invasion. Koda and colleagues compared CT and endovascular sonography in the diagnosis of aortic invasion by esophageal cancer. The sensitivity, specificity, and accuracy of CT was 67%, 92%, and 89%, respectively, while those of intraaortic endovascular sonography were 100%.[23] On CT scan, pericardial invasion is suggested by pericardial thickening adjacent to tumor, pericardial effusion, or inward deformity of the heart with loss of the intervening fat plane at the level of the tumor but with preservation of the fat plane at levels immediately above and below. Although CT is useful in the determination of the extent of local disease, it is not as accurate in the staging of lymph node involvement; it is limited in differentiating between small normal nodes and those nodes invaded by tumor but small in size. It cannot differentiate between hyperplastic and neoplastic nodes. It has been suggested that mediastinal nodes greater than 10 mm in diameter in the short axis should be classified as pathologic and that subdiaphragmatic nodes greater than 8 mm in diameter be considered abnormal. The accuracy of the CT scan in predicting lymph node involvement ranges from 83% to 87% for abdominal lymph nodes but only from 51% to 70% for mediastinal nodes.[22] Computed tomography is very accurate in determining the presence of liver and adrenal gland metastasis.

## Magnetic Resonance Imaging

Magnetic resonance imaging (MRI) offers an alternative to CT for the evaluation of esophageal cancer. However, the practical applications of MRI are limited by the lack of reliable contrast agents for the gastrointestinal tract and the substantially longer imaging time required for this procedure. Its application in esophageal carcinoma has received scant attention.

Several studies compared MRI and CT results with regard to staging and evaluating the resectability of esophageal carcinoma.[24–26] According to these studies, MRI was considered useful for the preoperative diagnosis of esophageal carcinoma. Like CT, MRI is highly accurate for detecting distant metastases of esophageal cancer, especially to the liver, and for determining advanced local spread (T4). However, it is less reliable in defining early infiltration (T1–T3). Magnetic resonance imaging appears to be as sensitive as CT in predicting mediastinal invasion. Quint and co-workers reported an accuracy of 100% for both CT and MRI in predicting tracheobronchial invasion.[27] However, the accuracy for aortic and pericardial invasion decreased to 75% and 88%, respectively, in the latter study.

An advantage of MRI is the ability to accurately determine tumor length by imaging in the coronal and sagittal planes (as opposed to CT, in which the tumor length must be estimated indirectly by adding the single-slice thicknesses),[28] but this information has only limited clinical value. Another advantage of MRI is the loss of signal in the vessels and the air-filled trachea and bronchi, which may provide a clear delineation between the tumor and the aorta and the tracheobronchial tree. Like CT scans, MRI scans are poor at detecting tumors restricted to mucosa or submucosa and also tend to understage the regional lymph nodes.

## Endoscopic Ultrasound

One of the newer modalities used in the staging of esophageal cancer is EUS, which utilizes the technologies of flexible endoscopy and ultrasonic imaging. By virtue of its ability to depict the various layers of the esophageal wall and periesophageal tissues, EUS has proved useful in staging esophageal cancer.[29]

Endoscopic ultrasound seems to be more accurate than CT in diagnosing the early or advanced stage of disease. Tio and collegues found that the accuracy of EUS for T1 and T2 cancer was 85%, vs. 12% for CT. The overall accuracy of EUS was 85%, vs. 59% for CT.[30] Stenosis is a definite limiting factor for EUS. The alternative is to use a small-caliber ultrasound instrument such as an esophagoprobe. If the stenosis is very tight, a catheter echo probe can be inserted via the biopsy channel during routine endoscopy to visualize the depth of tumor invasion and the regional lymph nodes.[31] If the catheter probe is in optimal work-

ing condition and has a high imaging quality, the aorta, left atrium, and azygos vein can be visualized. Gentle maneuvering of the transducer forward and backward is important in assessing the extent of the tumor and in identifying periesophageal lymph nodes. Lymph nodes at a distance of more than 2 cm from the esophageal lumen cannot be imaged because of the very limited penetration depth of ultrasound. For patients with severe stenosis, a nonoptical, wire-guided echoendoscope can markedly reduce the occurrence of incomplete esophageal cancer staging and improve the detection of metastatic disease.[32]

Endoscopic ultrasound is also of help in the assessment of unresectability. The most important findings for unresectability are tumor invasion into the left atrium with loss of smooth flexible movement of the pericardium on real-time EUS, tumor invasion into the wall of the descending aorta or fixation of the tumor on the spinal body, tumor invasion into the pulmonary vein or artery, or both, or tumor invasion into the tracheobronchial system. The latter should be further evaluated by bronchoscopy with transbronchial FNA for confirmation of the diagnosis. This is recommended because tumor invasion into an air-containing organ such as the tracheobronchial system or pleura may be difficult to diagnose by EUS, as air accumulations adjacent to the target of interest may be obscured by artifacts.

With some modifications, EUS can be used to evaluate the depth of infiltration of early-stage esophageal cancer. The soft-balloon method utilizing a condom succeeded in obtaining a clear and reproducible picture by keeping deaerated water in a condom. However, the condom, which covered the endoscope lens, eliminated the usual endoscopic sight. Inoue and colleagues developed a modified method that enables both normal endoscopic observation and ultrasonic probe study with only one insertion of the endoscope.[33]

The use of EUS-guided FNA was reported in the diagnosis of esophageal cancer recurrence after distal esophageal resection in 1989.[34] Later, use of transbronchial needle was introduced, following a modification of the echo endoscope.[35] Curved-array echo endoscopes appear to be more suitable than radial scanning echo endoscopes, since the needle can be visualized along its entire length sonographically during the procedure. Mediastinal lymphadenopathy can be evaluated by FNA, which is often crucial in planning the strategy of treatment, particularly prior to surgery. In a recent study by Reed and co-workers, EUS with FNA was found to be useful in the detection and confirmation of celiac axis lymph nodes metastasis.[36]

Endoscopic ultrasound has been used primarily in staging biopsy-proven cancers. However, it's also useful in the diagnosis of esophageal cancer and should be performed in selected patients with esophageal strictures whose biopsies are negative for malignancy (i.e., those with suspicious endoscopic or radiographic appearance; those with atypical presentations such as profound weight loss, short duration of symptoms, or advanced age; and those who fail to respond to treatment). Faigel and colleagues used EUS in four patients with dysphagia whose endoscopic biopsy results were negative for malignancy and found a large infiltrating tumor invading through the esophageal wall into the surrounding tissues in all cases. These lesions were proved to be esophageal cancer either by surgery or repeat biopsy.[37]

As 50% of patients who undergo surgery for esophageal cancer suffer recurrent disease within 2 years, the value of endosonography for surveillance after surgery has been assessed. Fockens and colleagues performed EUS every 6 months in patients who underwent surgery with curative intent to detect early recurrences before the appearance of symptoms or of macroscopic signs such as a lesion visible at endoscopy or on barium esohpagograms. They reported that the finding of suspicious lymph nodes had an 88% positive predictive value for recurrence and the finding of focal wall thickening or on adjacent mass had a 100% positive predictive value.[38] However, the clinical usefulness of this type of follow-up remains to be evaluated in terms of influence on patient survival.

Since multimodal neoadjuvant treatment for esophageal cancer has been used with increased frequency, restaging of the neoplasm remains fundamental in evaluating the response to therapy and in planning an operation. Many studies have evaluated the role of EUS in this setting.[39–41] In a recent study, Laterza and co-workers reported that the feasibility of EUS before and after neoadjuvant treatment was 71.2% and 83.9%, respectively. The overall accuracy of EUS detecting the wall invasion was 47.9%. The more frequent error was overstaging, especially in patients with complete response and in patients with minimal residual disease. In the assessment of lymph node involvement, EUS showed an overall accuracy of 71.2%. Sensitivity for diagnosing N1 and N0 was 73.7% and 68.6%, respectively. The results suggest that EUS is feasible in most patients after preoperative radiotherapy and chemotherapy, but that its accuracy in T-stage evaluation was worsened by the confounding presence of radiation fibrosis and soft tissue reaction after radiotherapy and chemotherapy.[42] Zuccaro and colleagues studied EUS staging in 59 patients with esophageal cancer before and after preoperative concurrent chemoradiotherapy. The accuracy of EUS in evaluation of T stage after chemoradiotherapy was only 37%, and its sensitivity for N1 disease was only 38%.[43] Since EUS was unable to distinguish postradiation fibrosis and inflammation from residual tumor, the predictive value of EUS after chemoradiotherapy is inadequate for use in clinical decision making.

When EUS is combined with other ultrasonographic techniques, increased accuracy of staging may be expected. According to Natsugoe and colleagues, ultrasonography in patients with superficial esophageal carcinomas is accurate in staging cervical and abdominal lymph nodes. Endoscopic ultrasound is accurate in staging mediastinal lymph nodes. The combined use of ultrasonography and EUS could increase the accuracy of diagnosing nodal lesions of esophageal cancer.[44] Mortensen and co-workers found that the combination of EUS and laparoscopic ultrasonography for pretherapeutic assessment of upper gastrointestinal (GI) tract was superior to the use of CT + ultrasonagraphy, laparoscopy, and EUS. Endoscopic ultrasound + laparoscopic ultrasonography correctly identified all nonresectable patients.[45]

Recently, the principle behind EUS—introducing the an external imaging transducer, such as used in ultrasonography, in combination with an endoscope into the GI tract for higher-resolution imaging—has also been applied to MRI, resulting in a new technique called endoscopic MRI. The magnetic resonance endoscope consists of a nonferrous endoscope with a radiofrequency receiver coil incorporated into its tip. Inui and co-workers first reported their preliminary results of this technique for visualization and staging of gastrointestinal tumors.[46] Sufficient images were obtained in seven of eight esophageal cases (88%) but in only 14 of 24 gastric cases (58%). In patients in whom adequate visualization was achieved, the endoscopic MRI results of local and regional staging were consistent with surgical, histopathological, CT, and/or EUS results in all six esophageal cancer cases and in 89% (T stage) and 56% (N stage) of the nine patients with gastric cancer. Kulling and colleagues studied the accuracy of endoscopic MRI for the local staging of esophageal cancer in 15 patients, and found that endoscopic MRI find-

ings of transmural tumor invasion and nodal status agreed with ultrasonography in 11of 15 cases and in 12 of 15 cases, respectively. Endoscopic magnetic resonance images were inadequate in four cases as a result of motion artifacts. These results show that endoscopic MRI of esophageal cancer in staging local disease is comparable to endosonography.[47] The potential advantage of endoscopic MRI is the three-dimensional (3-D) visualization of lesions, and its combination with conventional magnetic resonance scanning may provide comprehensive staging of esophageal cancer.

A 3-D image can also be obtained with advanced EUS equipment. The 3-D EUS image is reconstructed by composing the radial and linear images obtained by spiral scanning of the ultrasonic probe in the sheath. This system also allows numerous functions (e.g., multifreeze, high-resolution images, measurement, etc.) that can help in making a definitive diagnosis. So far, there are have been only a few preliminary reports. Yoshimoto examined 190 lesions of the esophagus and gastrointestinal tract by 3-D EUS and found that high-resolution images were more precise and finer than those obtained by plain EUS. Three-dimensional EUS contributed more useful and finer images than conventional EUS examinations. Gastrointestinal lesions were generally well displayed and recognizable.[48] Hunerbein and co-workers used a high-resolution radial miniprobe in five patients with esophageal cancer and reconstructed 3-D images from serial transverse sections on a computer workstation. This system accurately visualized the tumor and surrounding structures and improved the assessment of longitudinal tumor infiltration and the spatial relation of the tumor to relevant mediastinal structures.[49]

## Positron Emission Tomography

Positron emission tomography with the glucose analogue 2-[$^{18}$F]fluoro-2-deoxy-D-glucose (FDG) has been used to detect and stage a variety of malignancies. Recent studies have shown PET to be useful in identifying malignant pulmonary nodules and in staging mediastinal disease in non–small cell lung cancer.[50–52] The initial results in the application of PET in the staging of esophageal cancer are also encouraging. Block and co-workers compared CT and PET in staging of patients with esophageal cancer. Among 58 patients, increased FDG uptake was identified at the site of the primary tumor in 56 patients. The PET was positive in all 17 patients with metastatic disease, whereas CT was positive for metastases in only five. Pathologic lymph node metastases were found in 21 patients. These nodes were detected by PET in 11 patients and by CT in six. The results show that PET improved staging and facilitated selection of patients for operation by detecting distant disease not identified by CT alone.[53] In another similar study, Rankin and colleagues reported that both PET and CT are effective in showing the primary tumor and are about equally sensitive in the demonstration of periesophageal nodes, and that PET is probably more sensitive than CT for the detection of distant metastases.[54] Kole and co-workers also reported that PET has a higher sensitivity for nodal and distant metastases and a higher accuracy for determining resectability than CT. They found that the diagnostic accuracy of CT and PET in determining resectability was 65% and 88%, respectively. For CT and PET together the accuracy was 92%. Positron emission tomography and CT together would have decreased ill-advised surgery by 90%.[55] In a study of the role of PET in staging esophageal cancer, Luketich and associates found that for distant metastases, the sensitivity, specificity, and accuracy of PET were 88%, 93%, and 91%, respectively. For local-regional nodal metastases, the sensitivity, specificity, and accuracy were 45%, 100%, and 48%, respectively. These results suggest that PET may improve the ability to detect distant metastases missed by conventional noninvasive staging of esophageal cancer; however, small local-regional nodal metastases cannot be identified by current PET technology.[56] Yet, according to Flanagan and colleagues, PET is superior to CT for predicting local nodal disease and detecting distant metastasis of esophageal cancer.[57]

Another potential use of PET in esophageal cancer is for the detection of responses to chemotherapy and radiotherapy. Historically, clinicians have used tumor shrinkage to assess efficacy, but this may not be the best indicator of response to treatment. FDG-PET imaging can identify changes in glucose uptake, which may prove to be a better indicator of a favorable response to treatment. Many studies have suggested that changes in the uptake of FDG predict tumor response to therapy. Positron emission tomography has been shown to be helpful in classifying responses to chemotherapy and in predicting survival in patients with lung cancer and head and neck cancer.[58–61] At present, the major indication of FDG-PET for digestive cancer is the detection and staging of colorectal cancer recurrences.[62] However, PET could be of value in assessing the response of esophageal cancer to chemoradiation therapy. Couper and colleagues used PET, CT, dysphagia scores, and weight changes for comparison of evidence of response to chemotherapy, and found that changes in tumor FDG uptake were seen in all tumors after chemotherapy. Four patients who demonstrated response by CT had large reductions in FDG uptake after chemotherapy. Two patients with an increase in FDG uptake reported no improvement in dysphagia and continued to lose weight during therapy. The results show that PET may have a role to play in the assessment of patients with upper GI malignancy receiving chemotherapy.[63]

## Minimally Invasive Staging

Many surgical studies show a significant stratification of survival following resection of esophageal cancer based on accurate pathologic staging. Multimodality treatment of this disease has been introduced; however, it is difficult to compare different treatment modalities because of the lack of precise preoperative staging. Preoperative minimally surgical staging in esophageal cancer may solve this problem, just as the successful use of mediastinoscopy has helped in preoperative staging for lung cancer. Such staging in esophageal cancer may separate advanced disease from early local disease. Prognostication in patients with esophageal cancer might enable more appropriate allocation of chemotherapy or radiation therapy, thus reducing the morbidity and mortality associating with treating esophageal cancer.

Murray and associates first reported their experience with minimally invasive surgical staging for esophageal cancer in 1977. They used mediastinoscopy and minilaparotomy prospectively in 30 esophageal cancer patients. Seven were found to have positive lymph nodes by mediastinoscopy, and 16 had celiac lymph nodes identified.[64] Dagnini and co-workers did routine laparoscopy in 369 esophageal cancer patients, and they noted intraabdominal metastases in 14% and celiac lymph node metastases in 9.7%. All these patients with metastasis avoided unnecessary resection.[65] Stein and colleagues assessed the clinical value of diagnostic laparoscopy combined with laparoscopic ultrasound as well as peritoneal lavage in 127 patients with cancer of the esophagus or cardia. Diagnostic laparoscopy with laparoscopic ultrasound revealed previously unknown findings, particularly in patients with locally advanced adenocarcinoma of the distal esophagus or cardia (hepatic metastases in 22% and peritoneal tumor spread or free tumor cells in the abdominal cavity in 25%), whereas the diagnostic gain was low in those patients with squamous cell esophageal cancer. The sensitivity and specificity of laparoscopic ultrasound in predicting positive celiac lymph nodes were 67% and 92%, respectively. These data indicate that diagnostic laparoscopy with laparoscopic ultrasound and peritoneal lavage can provide therapeutically relevant new information in patients with locally advanced adenocarcinoma of the distal esophagus or cardia, but the clinical value in patients with squamous cell esophageal cancer is limited.[66]

With the advances in thoracoscopic (Ts) and laparoscopic (Ls) techniques, Ts/Ls has been used for staging esophageal cancer in some centers.[67] Recent reports show that Ts/Ls staging can correctly predict nodal metastasis for esophageal cancer, just as mediastinoscopy does for lung cancer. Krasna and McLaughlin first described the efficacy of thoracoscopic lymph node staging in esophageal cancer.[68] They further reported their successful experience with combined Ts/Ls for staging disease in the chest and abdomen in a follow-up series from three institutions of the Cancer and Leukemian Group B (CAALGB) with an accuracy of over 90%.[67] A more recent report of 65 patients showed a 94% accuracy with laparoscopy and 91% accuracy with thoracoscopy in esophageal cancer staging.[69] When compared to EUS, Ts/Ls staging is superior in detecting lymph node metastases.[70] Their study also demonstrated that clinical stage evaluation based on noninvasive diagnostic methods including CT, MRI, and EUS may be used to guide surgeons to focus on the suspicious areas for the most high-yield biopsy targets when doing Ts/Ls staging.[71] The main advantage of the Ts/Ls staging procedure is that it provides greater accuracy in evaluation of regional and celiac lymph nodes. Such information is very important in patient stratification and selection of therapy, especially in the setting of new treatment protocols. Furthermore, the histologic status of mediastinal and abdominal lymph nodes is critical for the design of the field for irradiation. It allows for maximizing dose delivery to areas of known disease, while minimizing dose to surrounding sensitive, normal tissue.[72]

Minimally invasive surgical techniques in combination with new molecular diagnostic techniques may improve the ability to stage cancer patients. Kassis and associates used the reverse transcriptase-polymerase chain reaction (RT-PCR) of carcinoembryonic antigen (CEA) mRNA to increase the detection of micrometastases in lymph nodes from esophageal cancer patients with minimally invasive staging. Metastases were present in 29 of 60 lymph nodes sample (48%) when examined histopathologically. Use of RT-PCR identified nodal metastases in 46 of these 60 samples (77%), and RT-PCR detected CEA mRNA in all 29 histologically positive samples and in 17 histologically negative lymph nodes. All lymph nodes from patients with benign disease were negative both histopathologically and by RT-PCR. These results show that RT-PCR is more sensitive than histologic examination in the detection of lymph node metastases in esophageal cancer and can lead to diagnosis of a more advanced stage in some patients.[73] Luketich and colleagues further reported that a positive RT-PCR assay of CEA mRNA with negative histologic findings may have poor prognostic implications.[74] Krasna and associates found that immunohistochemical study of the molecular marker of p53 can also be used for this purpose. In their study, 71.4% of patients with metastasis of thoracoscopy/laparoscopy lymph nodes (Ts/Ls LN) verified by hematoxylin/eosin (H/E) were p53 positive; 14.2% of patients with negative Ts/Ls LN by H/E were p53 positive. In patients with p53-

positive Ts/Ls LN, 23% had a pathologic complete response after chemoradiation with a median survival of 16 months. In patients with p53-negative Ts/Ls LN, 50% had a pathologic complete response with a median survival of 31.5 months ($P = 0.05$). The results suggested that p53 protein overexpression in Ts/Ls LN may not only increase the detection of occult lymphatic metastasis but also predict response to chemoradiation and survival in esophageal cancer patients.[75] Jiao et al. recently reported that immunohistochemistry study of cytokeratin (CK), an antibody to epithelial cells, can also be used to detect occult micrometastasis in Ts/Ls lymph nodes, and patients with positive CK findings tended to have poor survival.[76]

## Other New Diagnostic and Staging Methods

Recent reports on the prognostic value of pleural lavage cytology (PLC) in lung cancer patients without a pleural effusion who undergo surgical resection suggest that a significant number of patients with otherwise early-stage disease will have positive pleural cytology results and a poorer prognosis than patients with negative cytology results. Some authors advocate adding PLC to the TNM staging system of lung cancer.[77–80] So far, however, the literature on PLC has been focused on lung cancer. Jiao and associates recently reported that positivity of PLC in thoracic squamous cell esophageal cancer is also very high (18.8%).[81] Natsugoe and co-workers found that positive PLC correlates with regrowth of residual tumor and poor prognosis in esophageal cancer.[82] Malignant tumor cells were also found in peritoneal lavage fluid from adenocarcinoma of the distal esophagus or cardia.[66] Whether these results suggest an advanced stage of disease is unknown. The clinical and prognostic value of PLC and peritoneal lavage cytology for esophageal cancer needs further study.

Other potential valuable diagnostic and staging tools include detection of occult lymphatic metastasis and circulating or bone marrow tumor cells,[83] serum telemerase activity, cellular proliferation modifications, DNA ploidy analysis, and some molecular markers such as p21, p53, Rb, thymidin synthetase, etc.

## Conclusions

Survival of patients with esophageal cancer treated with current treatment modalities remains low. Early diagnosis, appropriate staging, and, if indicated, preoperative multiple modality treatment followed by surgery may offer the patient a chance for improved survival.[84] Recent advances in CT, MRI, and PET of the esophagus, as well as EUS and minimally invasive Ts/Ls offer new hope for reliable preoperative diagnosis and staging of esophageal cancer. Noninvasive methods such as CT, MRI, PET, and EUS can provide valuable diagnostic and staging information; nonetheless, they should be considered complementary, not competitive modalities. The strength of each modality compensates for the limitations of the other. Minimally invasive Ts/Ls staging is a promising method for staging lymph nodes in esophageal cancer patients. It is hoped that it will be as accurate as mediastinoscopy in staging lung cancer, and that it will help identify the presence or absence of mediastinal invasion, thereby delineating which patients have early local disease amenable to surgical resection and which patients have advanced disease. Such surgical pathologic staging will be especially useful in evaluating and comparing the results of clinical trials of preoperative chemotherapy and/or radiotherapy. In light of the encouraging results of recent multimodality treatment studies on esophageal cancer,[85] the concept of accurate pretreatment staging of esophageal cancer should soon be realized and accepted in the clinic. However, further studies are needed to develop a cost-effective diagnosis and staging protocol for esophageal cancer.

## References

1. Huang GJ. What is the value of abrasive cytology? In: Giuli R (ed): Cancer of the Esophagus: One Hundred and Thirty-Five Questions. S.A. Maloine, Editeur, Paris, 1984, pp 320–324.
2. Huang GJ, Shao LF, Zhang DW, et al. Diagnosis and surgical treatment of early esophageal carcinoma. Chin Med J 94:229–232, 1981.
3. Lightdale CJ, Winawer SJ. Screening diagnosis and staging of esophageal cancer. Semin Oncol 11:101–112, 1984.
4. Sautereau D. Screening for early esophageal cancer: whom and how? Endoscopy 31:325–328, 1999.
5. Lindell MM Jr, Hill CA, Libshitz HI. Esophageal cancer: Radiographic chest findings and their prognostic significance. AJR Am J Roentgenol 133:461–464, 1979.
6. Choi TK, Siu KF, Lam KH, Wang J. Bronchoscopy and carcinoma of the esophagus. I. Findings of bronchoscopy in carcinoma of the esophagus. Am J Surg 147:757–759, 1984.
7. Choi TK, Siu KF, Lam KH, Wang J. Bronchoscopy and carcinoma of the esophagus. II. Findings of bronchoscopy in carcinoma of the esophagus. Am J Surg 147:760–762, 1984.
8. Postlethwait RW: Tracheobronchial invasion by carcinoma of the esophagus. In: DeMeester NR, Skinner DB (eds): Esophageal Disorders; Pathophysiology and Therapy. Raven Press, New York; pp 389–391, 1985.
9. Inculet RI, Keller SM, Dwyer A, Roth JA. Evaluation of noninvasive tests for the preoperative staging of carcinoma of the esophagus: a prospective study. Ann Thorac Surg 40:561–565, 1985.
10. Seitz JF, Monges G, Navarro P, et al. Depistage endoscopique des dysplasies et des cancers infracliniques de l'oesophage. Resultats d'une etude prospective avec coloration vitale par le bleu de toluidine chez 100 patients alcoolo-tabagiques. Gastroenterol Clin Biol 14:15–21, 1990.
11. Fontolliet Ch, Monnier Ph. Giabilite histologique de la coloration vitale au bleu de toluidine. Acta Endosc 21:617–630, 1991.
12. Ban S, Toyonaga A, Harada H, et al. Iodine staining for early endoscopic detection of oesophageal cancer in alcoholics. Endoscopy 30:253–257, 1998.
13. Meyer V, Burtin P, Bour B, et al. Endoscopic detection of early esophageal cancer in a high-risk population: does lugol staining improve videoendoscopy? Gastrointest Endosc 45:480–484, 1997.
14. Fagundes RB, De Barros SGS, Putten ACK, et al. Occult dysplasia is disclosed by lugol chromoendoscopy in alcoholics at high risk for squamous cell carcinoma of the esophagus. Endoscopy 31:281–285, 1999.
15. Endo M, Kawano T. Detection and classification of early squamous cell esophageal cancer. Dis Esophagus 10:155–158, 1997.
16. Bohorfoush AG. Tissue spectroscopy for gastrointestinal diseases. Endoscopy 28:372–380, 1996.
17. Stepp H, Skoka R, Baumgartner R. Fluorescence endoscopy of gastrointestinal diseases: basic principles, techniques and clinical experience. Endoscopy 30:379–386, 1998.
18. Haringsma J, Tytgat GNJ. The value of fluorescence techniques in gastrointestinal endoscopy: better than the endoscopist's eye? The European experience. Endoscopy 30:416–418, 1998.
19. Marcon N, Wilson BE. The value of fluorescence techniques in gastrointestinal endoscopy: better than the endoscopist's eye? The North American experience. Endoscopy 30:419–421, 1998.
20. Vo Dinh T, Panjehpour M, Overholt BF. Laser fluorescence for esophageal cancer and dysplasia diagnosis. Ann NY Acad Sci 838:116–122, 1998.
21. Foley WD. Dynamic hepatic CT. Radiology 170:617–622, 1989.
22. Saunders HS, Wolfman NT, Ott DJ. Esophageal cancer radiologic staging. Radiol Clin North Am 35:281–294, 1997.
23. Koda Y, Nakamura K, Kaminou T, et al. Assessment of aortic invasion by esophageal carcinoma using intraaortic endovascular sonography. AJR Am J Roentgenol 170:133–135, 1998.
24. Takashima S, Takeuchi N, Shiozaki H, et al. Carcinoma of the esophagus: CT vs. MR imaging in determining resectability. AJR Am J Roentgenol 156:297–302, 1991.
25. Sai M. Clinical assessmsnt of esophageal cancer by magnetic resonance imaging. J Tokyo Med Coll 51:292–299, 1993.
26. Hamada H, Yasuda T, Kudou K, et al. Usefulness of magnetic resonance imaging in diagnosis of invasion to the adventitia and lymph node metastasis of esophageal carcinoma. Jpn J Gastroenterol Surg 24:962–967, 1991.

27. Quint LE, Glazer GM, Orringer MB. Esophageal imaging by MR and CT: study of normal anatomy and neoplasms. Radiology 156:727–731, 1985.

28. Nakashima A, Naksshima K, Seto H, et al. Thoracic esophageal carcinoma: evaluation in the sagittal section with magnetic resonance imaging. Abdom Imaging 22:20–23, 1997.

29. Tio TL. Diagnosis and staging of esophageal carcinoma by endoscopic ultrasonography. Endoscopy 30(Suppl 1):A33–A40, 1998.

30. Tio Tl, Blank L, Wijers OB, et al. Staging and prognosis using endosonography in patients with inoperable esophageal carcinoma treated with combined intraluminal and external radiation. Gastrointest Endosc 40:304–310, 1993.

31. Chak A, Canto M, Gerdes H, et al. Prognosis of esophageal cancers preoperatively staged to be locally invasive (T4) by endoscopic ultrasound (EUS): a multicenter retrospective cohort study. Gastrointest Endosc 42:501–506, 1995.

32. Mallery S, Van Dam J. Increased rate of complete EUS staging of patients with esophageal cancer using the nonoptical, wire-guide echoendoscope. Gastrointest Endosc 50:53–57, 1999.

33. Inoue H, Kawano T, Takeshita K, Iwai T. Modified soft-balloon methods during ultrasonic probe examination for superficial esophageal cancer. Endoscopy 30(Suppl 1):A41–A43, 1998.

34. Tio TL, Cohen P, Coene PP, et al. Preoperative TNM classification of esophageal carcinoma by endoscoy and computed tomography. Gastroenterology 96:147–186, 1989.

35. Kim CY, Thomson A, Bandres D, et al. Endoscopic ultrasound–guided fine-needle aspiration biopsy using radial scanning endosconography: results of diagnostic accuracy [abstract]. Gastroenterology A3341, 1997.

36. Reed CE, Mishra G, Sahai AV, et al. Esophageal cancer staging: improved accuracy by endoscopic ultrasound of celiac lymph nodes. Ann Thorac Surg 67:319–321, 1999.

37. Faigel DO, Deveney C, Phillips D, Fennerty MB: Biopsy-negative malignant esophageal stricture: diagnosis by endoscopic ultrasound. Am J Gastroenterol 93:2257–2260, 1998.

38. Fockens P, Manshanden CG, van Lanschot JJ, Obertop H, Tytgat GN. Prospective study on the value of endosonographic follow-up after surgery for esophageal carcinoma. Gastrointest Endosc 46:487–491, 1997.

39. Quirk D, Lynch T, Grossbard M, et al. A prospective study of pre- and post-adjuvant treatment EUS in patients with esophageal cancer. In: American Gastroenterological Association: Proceeding of Digestive Disease Week, Washington, DC, A–844, No. 3370, 1997.

40. Balmain LG, Chong W, Mertz H. Accuracy of endoscopic ultrasound in tumor staging after irradiation and chemotherapy. Gastrointest Endosc 45:AB167, 1997.

41. Boubein LD, DuBrow R, David C, et al. Endoscopic ultrasonography in the quantitative assessment of response to chemotherapy in patients with adencarcinoma of the esophagus and esophagogastric junction. Endoscopy 25:587–591, 1993.

42. Laterza E, Manzoni G, Guglielmi A, et al. Endoscopic ultrasonography in the staging of esophageal carcinoma after preoperative radiotherapy and chemotherapy. Ann Thorac Surg 67:1466–1469, 1999.

43. Zuccaro G Jr, Rice TW, Goldblum J, et al. Endoscopic ultrasound cannot determine suitability for esophagectomy after aggressive chemoradiotherapy for esophageal cancer. Am J Gastroenterol 94:906–912, 1999.

44. Natsugoe S, Yoshinaka H, Morinaga T, et al. Ultrasonographic detection of lymph-node metastases in superficial carcinoma of the esophagus. Endoscopy 28:674–679, 1996.

45. Mortensen MB, Scheel-Hincke JD, Madsen MR, Qvist N, Hovendal C. Combined endoscopic ultrasonography and laparoscopic ultrasonography in the pretherapeutic assessment of resectability in patients with upper gastrointestinal malignancies. Scand J Gastroenterol 31:1115–1119, 1996.

46. Inui K, Nakazawa S, Yoshino J, et al. Endoscopic MRI: preliminary results of a new technique for visualization and staging of gastrointestinal tumors. Endoscopy 27:480–485, 1995.

47. Kulling D, Feldman DR, Kay CL, Hoffman BJ, Reed CE: Local staging of esophageal cancer using endoscopic magnetic resonance imaging: prospective comparison with endoscopic ultrasound. Endoscopy 30:745–749, 1998.

48. Yoshimoto K. Clinical application of ultrasound 3-D imaging system in lesions of the gastrointestinal tract. Endoscoy 30(Suppl 1):A145–148, 1998.

49. Hunerbein M, Gretschel S, Ghadimi BM, Schlag PM. Three-dimensional endoscopic ultrasound of the esophagus. Preliminary experience. Surg Endosc 11:991–994, 1997.

50. Lowe VJ, Naunheim KS. Current role of positron emission tomography in thoracic oncology. Thorax 53:703–712, 1998.

51. Lowe VJ, Fletcher JW, Gobar L, et al. Prospective investigation of positron emission tomography in lung nodules. J Clin Oncol 16:1075–1084, 1998.

52. Graeber GM, Gupta NC, Murray GF. Positron emission tomographic imaging with fluorodeoxyglucose is efficacious in evaluating malignant pulmonary disease. J Thorac Cardiovasc Surg 117:719–727, 1999.

53. Block MI, Patterson GA, Sundaresan RS, et al. Improvement in staging of esophageal cancer with the addition of positron emission tomography. Ann Thorac Surg 64:770–776, 1997.

54. Rankin SC, Taylor H, Cook GJ, Mason R. Computed tomography and positron emission tomography in the pre-operative staging of oesophageal carcinoma. Clin Radiol 53:659–665, 1998.

55. Kole AC, Plukker JT, Nieweg OE, Vaalburg W. Positron emission tomography for staging of oesophageal and gastroesophageal malignancy. Br J Cancer 78:521–527, 1998.

56. Luketich JD, Schauer PR, Meltzer CC, et al. Role of positron emission tomography in staging esophageal cancer. Ann Thorac Surg 64:765–769, 1997.

57. Flanagan FL, Dehdashti F, Siegel BA, et al. Staging of esophageal cancer with 18F-fluorodeoxyglucose positron emission tomography. AJR Am J Roentgenol 168:417–424, 1997.

58. Hebert ME, Lowe VJ, Hoffman, et al. Positron emission tomography in the pretreatment evaluation and follow-up of non–small cell lung cancer patients treated with radiotherapy: preliminary findings. Am J Clin Oncol 19:416–421, 1996.

59. Vansteenkiste JF, Stroobants SG, De Leyn PR, et al. Potential use of FDG-PET scan after induction chemotherapy in surgically staged IIIa-N2 non–small-cell lung cancer: a prospective pilot study. Ann of Oncol 9:1193–1198, 1998.

60. Lowe VJ, Dunphy FR, Varvares M, et al. Evaluation of chemotherapy response in patients with advanced head and neck cancer using [F-18] fluorodeoxyglucose positron emission tomography. Head Neck 19:666–674, 1997.

61. Sakamoto H Nakai Y, Ohashi Y, et al. Monitoring of response to radiotherapy with fluorine-18 deoxyglucose PET of head and neck squamous cell carcinomas. Acta Otolaryngol Suppl 538:254–260, 1998.

62. Paulus P, Hustinx R, Daenen F, et al. Usefulness of $^{18}$FDG positron emission tomography in detection and follow-up of digestive cancers. Acta Gastroenterol Belg 60:278–280, 1997.

63. Couper GW, McAteer D, Wallis F, et al. Detection of response to chemotherapy using positron emission tomography in patients with oesophageal and gastric cancer. Br J Surg 85:1403–1406, 1998.

64. Murray GF Wilcox BR, Stared PIK. The assessment of operability of esophageal carcinoma. Ann Thorac Surg 23:393–346, 1977.

65. Dagnini G, Galdironi MW, Marin G, et al. Laparoscopy in abdominal staging of esophageal carcinoma. Gastrointest Endosc 32:400–402, 1986.

66. Stein HJ, Kraemer SJ, Feussner H, Fink U, Siewert JR. Clinical value of diagnostic laparoscopy with laparoscopic ultrasound in patients with cancer of the esophagus or cardia. J Gastrointest Surg 1:167–173, 1997.

67. Krasna MJ, Reed C, Jaklitsch MT, Cushing D, Sugarbaker D, The Cancer and Leukemia Group B Thoracic Surgeons: Thoracoscopic staging of esophageal cancer: a prospective multiinstitutional trial. Ann Thorac Surg 60:1337–1340, 1995.

68. Krasna MJ, McLaughlin JS. Efficacy and safety of thoracoscopy for diagnosis and treatment of intrathoracic disease: the University of Maryland experience. Surg Laparosc Endosc 4:182–188, 1994.

69. Krasna MJ, Flowers JL, Attar S, McLaughlin J. Combined thoracoscopic/laparoscopic staging of esophageal cancer. J Thorac Cardiovas Surg 111:800–807, 1996.

70. Luketrich JD, Schauer P, Landrenear R, et al. Minimally invasive surgical staging is superior to endoscopic ultrasound in detecting lymph node metastases in esophageal cancer. J Thorac Cardiovasc Surg 114:817–823, 1997.

71. Krasna MJ, Jiao X, Sonett JR, et al. Thoracoscopic/laparoscopic lymph node staging in esophageal cancer: do clinicopathological factors affect the outcome? Ann Thorac Surg 73:1710–1713, 2002.

72. Jiao X, Krasna MJ, Sonett J, et al. Pretreatment surgical lymph node staging predicts results of trimodality therapy in esophageal cancer. Eur J Cardiothorac Surg 19:880–886, 2001.

73. Kassis ES, Nguyen N, Shriver SP, et al. Detection of occult lymph node metastases in esophageal cancer by minimally invasive staging combined with molecular diagnostic techniques. Journal of the Society of Laparoendoscopic Surgeons 2:331–336, 1998.

74. Luketich JD, Kassis ES, Shriver SP, et al. Detection of micrometastases in histologically negative lymph nodes in esophageal cancer. Ann Thorac Surg 66:1715–1718, 1998.

75. Krasna MJ, Mao YS, Sonett J, et al. *P53* gene protein overexpression predicts results of trimodality therapy in esophageal cancer patients. Ann Thorac Surg 68:2021–2025, 1999.

76. Jiao X, Eslami A, Olga I, et al. Immunohistochemistry analysis of micrometastasis in pretreatment lymph node from patients with esophageal cancer. Presented at the 49th Annual Meeting of the Southern Thoracic Surgical Association, Florida, U.S.A. November 7–9, 2002.

77. Kondo H, Naruke T, Tsuchihuya R, et al. Pleural lavage cytology immediately after thoracotomy as a prognostic factor for patients with lung cancer. Jpn J Cancer Res 80:233–237, 1989.

78. Okumura M, Ohshima S, Kotake Y, et al. Intraoperative pleural lavage cytology in lung cancer patients. Ann Thorac Surg 51:599–603, 1991.

79. Buhr J, Berghauser KH, Gonner S, et al. The prognostic significance of tumor cell detection in intraoperative pleural lavage and lung tissue cultures for patients with lung cancer. J Thorac Cardiovasc Surg 113:683–687, 1997.

80. Dresler CM, Fratelli C, Babb J. Prognostic value of positive pleural lavage in patients with lung cancer resection. Ann Thorac Surg 67:1435–1439, 1999.

81. Jiao X, Zhang M, Wen Z, Krasna MJ. Pleural lavage cytology in esophageal cancer without pleural effusions: clinicopathologic analysis. Eur J Cardiovasc Thorac Surg 17:575–579, 2000.

82. Natsugoe S, Shimada M, Nakashima S, et al. Intraoperative pleural lavage in esophageal carcinoma. Ann Surg Oncol 6:305–307, 1999.

83. Jiao X, Krasna MJ. Clinical significance of micrometastasis in lung and esophageal cancer: a new paradigm in thoracic oncology. Ann Thorac Surg 74:278–284, 2002.

84. Krasna MJ, Saum K. New strategies for staging esophageal cancer. In: Franco KL, Putnam JB, (eds): Advanced Therapy In Thoracic Surgery. B.C. Decker, Ontario, 1998, pp 431–440.

85. Krasna MJ, Mao YS. Making sense of multimodality therapy for esophageal cancer. Surg Oncol Clin North Am 8:259–278, 1999.

# Chapter 16

# Clinical Aspects and Management of Esophageal Carcinoma
## Management Options: Potentially Resectable Esophageal Cancer

JOE B. PUTNAM, JR.

Esophageal cancer is an uncommon but deadly disease. In the United States in the year 2000, there were an estimated 12,300 new cases of esophageal carcinoma (9200 men, 3100 women) and 12,100 deaths (9200 men, 2900 women). The major histologic types of esophageal cancer are squamous (epidermoid) carcinoma and adenocarcinoma, with squamous cell carcinoma accounting for the vast majority (98%) of cancers in the upper and middle esophagus. While in the past, squamous carcinoma predominated, today the incidence of adenocarcinoma of the esophagus is gaining in frequency.[1] Worldwide, esophageal cancer still occurs mostly as squamous cell carcinoma, but in the United states and Europe, the incidence of adenocarcinoma in the distal esophagus and at the gastroesophageal junction is increasing dramatically.[2,3] Adenocarcinoma of the esophagus has been frequently classified as a gastric carcinoma. However, esophageal adenocarcinomas arising in Barrett's epithelium are clearly esophageal in origin. Adenocarcinomas arising in the gastric cardia and distal esophagus frequently metastasize to nodal groups in the drainage bed of the esophagus and spread submucosally along the esophagus. The treatment and prognosis of these tumors are similar to those of squamous cancer.

While the incidence of adenocarcinoma of the esophagus has increased rapidly over the past decade in the United States and parts of Western Europe, the incidence of esophageal squamous cell carcinomas has remained relatively constant.[4,5] Analysis of Surveillance, Epidemiology and End Results (SEER) data from 1973 to 1987 on frequency, incidence, staging, and survival for cancers of the esophagus[6] indicates that the incidence of adenocarcinomas of esophagus and gastric cardia increased, whereas incidence rates for esophageal squamous cell carcinoma remained stable and rates for gastric adenocarcinoma decreased. Blacks were noted to have a higher incidence rate than whites for gastric adenocarcinoma and squamous cell carcinoma of the esophagus, and white men had higher incidence rates for adenocarcinomas of the esophagus and gastric cardia than blacks.[7] Risk factors such as alcohol and cigarettes were significant for both histological types, although higher risk was noted for adenocarcinoma in individuals who were in the highest decile of body mass index.[8,9] Ingestion of raw vegetables tended to decrease the risk.[9]

The incidence of adenocarcinoma of the esophagus in whites is higher than in blacks.[10,11] In the United States, the incidence of adenocarcinoma of the esophagus has increased over six- to sevenfold in the past 30 years. From 1976 to 1987 the increases among men ranged from 4% to 10% per year and exceeded those of other cancers during this period. This increase could not be explained by a change in the incidence of gastric cancer or squamous cancer. Excessive and long-term alcohol consumption and smoking increase the risk for developing both squamous cell and adenocarcinoma of the esophagus, and together these risk factors act synergistically. In the United States, the risk of developing adenocarcinoma of the distal esophagus/cardia was increased in patients with a current or former smoking history and consumption of 4 or more ounces of alcohol, and intake of total fat and vitamin A from animal sources was associated with increased risk of esophageal cancer.[5] Patients with Barrett's esophagus have a 30- to 125-fold increased risk for adenocarcinoma of the esophagus compared to a normal population. Patients with a short esophagus and peptic stricture are also at increased risk.

The morbidity associated with dysphagia and the shortened survival of patients with this disease have prompted investigators to consider novel and multiple treatment strategies. About 90% of patients die from the disease; death is usually caused by malnutrition from dysphagia or pneumonia. Palliation of dysphagia and improved survival with radiation therapy or a combination of chemotherapy and radiation therapy have been noted. Surgery and radiation therapy provide good local control; however, these options have traditionally carried high morbidity and mortality, as the disease is frequently advanced at diagnosis. Improvements in surgical technique, staging, and postoperative management have reduced surgical mortality to 5% or less in most series. Even with improvements in palliation of dysphagia with laser, stents, brachytherapy, and, more recently, photodynamic therapy, the overall 5-year survival remains poor at less than 5%. Despite these efforts and improvements in single therapeutic interventions, multidisciplinary therapy appears to provide a survival advantage over single-modality therapy. Phase II and prospective randomized trials to improve survival are under way in numerous centers worldwide.

Previous series examining the role of surgery in the treatment of esophageal carcinoma have generally shown that resectable patients with pathologic node-negative disease have anticipated 5-year survival of up to 40%. Patients with positive lymph nodes, after complete resection, have a 5-year survival of approximately 20%. The technique of esophagectomy does not affect survival.[12] Patients undergoing resection done in clinics where larger numbers of operations are performed by surgeons with more experience have improved results over those undergoing resection in clinics where smaller numbers of operations are conducted by surgeons with less experience.

## Predisposing Conditions

A host of dietary carcinogens, such as elevated levels of nitrates, foods containing fungi (*Geotrichum candidum*, *Fusarium* species, and *Aspergillus* species), rough foods that injure the esophageal mucosa, or thermal injury from drinking boiling hot tea or coffee, and infections (human papillomavirus) are associated with squamous cell carcinoma of the esophagus.[13] Other predisposing conditions are discussed below.

Tylosis is a disease inherited in an autosomal dominant fashion and characterized by hyperkeratosis of the skin of the palms and soles and papillomata of the esophagus. Squamous cell carcinomas of the esophagus develop with a high frequency (40%) in affected families.[14–16]

In patients with achalasia the risk for developing esophageal carcinoma may be 14% to 16% greater than in the normal population risk.[17] These cancers can occur in the thoracic portion of the esophagus corresponding to the air–fluid interface of retained food and liquids. Cancers generally occur late (>17 years average) after the diagnosis is made.[18,19]

Barrett's esophagus is a premalignant condition that may proceed to development of adenocarcinoma of the esophagus[20] and will be discussed later in this chapter.

Caustic burns to the esophagus are increasingly rare; however, squamous cell carcinoma may develop in such patients 40 to 50 years after injury.[21] Three-quarters of all these tumors are located in the middle third of the esophagus.[21,22] Squamous carcinomas arising in lye strictures are responsible for 1% to 4% of esophageal carcinomas.[21,23] Patients with prior history of caustic ingestion should be routinely screened, particularly when the time from injury exceeds 20 years.[22] The low incidence of carcinoma and the potentially high operative morbidity associated with resection of a chronically scarred esophagus argue against casual resection of these strictures. If repeated dilations fail, a bypass may relieve dysphagia in the absence of cancer.

There are reports of cancer of the upper esophagus associated with upper esophageal webs.[24] In 1919 Paterson[25] described a syndrome consisting of dysphagia from an esophageal web combined with iron-deficiency anemia and glossitis. The association of esophageal webs with iron deficiency anemia, glossitis, cheilosis, koilonychia, brittle fingernails, and splenomegaly is referred to as the Plummer-Vinson or Paterson-Kelly syndrome. The condition is premalignant, as approximately 10% of individuals will develop neoplasms of the esophagus or hypopharynx.[24] Treatment of the webs consists of endoscopic disruption. Dilations may be necessary if endoscopic disruption is not successful. Myotomy and resection of the web may be required.

Esophageal cancers may develop as second primary tumors in patients with other primary tumors of the upper aerodigestive tract. This field-type spread results from exposure to a carcinogen such as cigarette smoke. Patients with upper aerodigestive tract cancers develop second primary tumors at the rate of 4% of patients per year.[26,27] In patients with head and neck cancers, one-third of the second primary tumors arise in the esophagus.

Infection by certain microorganisms has been associated with the development of esophageal neoplasms. These microorganisms may act indirectly on the esophageal epithelium by (*1*) forming carcinogens or other products to enhance or attenuate carcinogenesis or (*2*) directly affecting the esophagus itself.[28] Human papilloma virus (HPV) DNA is associated with occurrence of squamous cell carcinoma in Japan; patients with papilloma virus infection have poorer survival than patients not infected.[29] This virus has been noted in almost 50% of squamous cell carcinoma cases from China.[30]

Patients at high risk for gastric carcinoma may have a high incidence of *Helicobacter pylori* infection,[31] although neoplasms involving the cardia may be less likely to have a strong association with *H. pylori* infection. Although most patients with *H. pylori* infection will not develop gastric carcinoma, associated factors in combination with *H. pylori* infection may predispose a patient to carcinogenesis. In one study, over 15% of patients with Barrett's esophagus were noted to be infected with *H. pylori* and all patients (*n* = 9) who were infected also had a chronic inflammatory reaction.[32]

## Anatomy

The esophagus lies between the hypopharynx and the stomach and provides gastrointestinal continuity for normal alimentation. The esophagus itself begins at the cricoid cartilage (topographically at the level of the sixth cervical vertebrae) (Fig. 16–1). The cervical esophagus is about 3–5 cm long and extends to the thoracic inlet, lying just to the left of midline. The thoracic esophagus begins at the thoracic inlet and extends 20 to 25 cm to the gastroesophageal junction or to the esophageal hiatus of the diaphragm. The intrathoracic component of the esophagus is nestled among all major thoracic structures, thus complete resection presents a technical challenge to the surgeon.

During endoscopy, lesions are localized in the esophagus by measuring the distance to the abnormality from the central incisors. By this measure, the esophagus begins about 15 cm from the incisors (at the cricopharyngeus muscle) and terminates at the gastroesophageal junction, 40 cm distally. The thoracic inlet begins about 20 cm from the central incisors (at the level of TI).

The American Joint Committee for Cancer (AJCC) Staging and End Results Reporting has divided the esophagus into four principal regions: the cervical esophagus, extending from the cricopharyngeus to the thoracic inlet approximately 18–20 cm from the incisiors; the upper thoracic esophagus, extending from the thoracic inlet to the level of the tracheal bifurcation (24 cm from incisors); the mid-thoracic esophagus, which is the proxi-

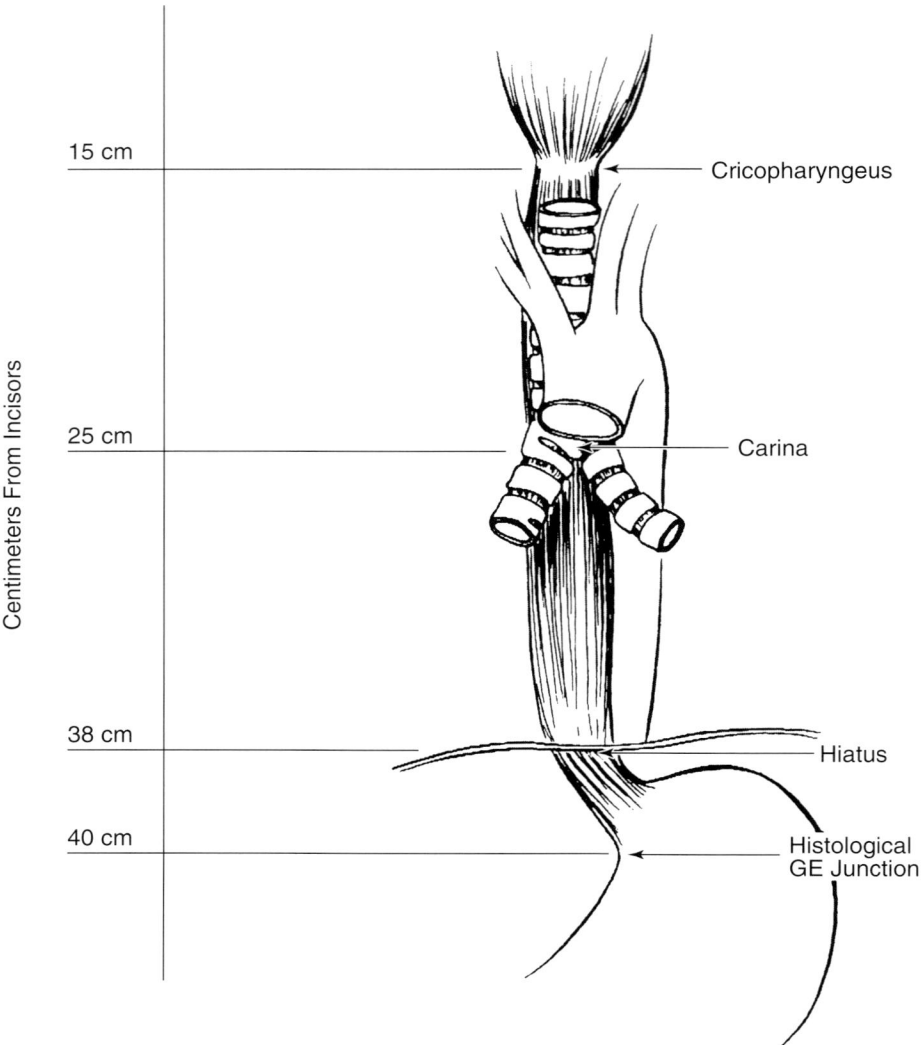

Centimeters From Incisors

15 cm — Cricopharyngeus

25 cm — Carina

38 cm — Hiatus

40 cm — Histological GE Junction

**Figure 16–1** Esophageal anatomy. The esophagus begins at the crico-pharyngeus approximately 15 cm from the incisors. The esophagus and left main-stem bronchus cross at approximately 25 cm. The diaphrag-matic esophageal hiatus occurs at approximately 37 to 38 cm with the distal esophagus joining the stomach at approximately 40 to 41 cm. GE, gastroesophageal.

mal portion of the esophagus between the tracheal bifurcation and the esophagogastric junction with a lower level approximately 32 cm from the incisors; and the lower thoracic esophagus, approximately 8 cm long, which is the distal portion of the esophagus between the tracheal bifurcation and the esophagogastric junction. This includes the intraabdominal portion of the esophagus.[33]

The AJCC standards are based on anatomic and length criteria. Most radiologists and surgeons divide the esophagus into thirds to correspond to the following: the upper third, from the cricopharyngeus to the superior portion of the aortic arch; the middle third, from the superior portion of the aortic arch to the inferior pulmonary vein; and the distal third, from the inferior pulmonary vein to the gastroesophageal junction. This simple anatomic classification is commonly used. About 15% of all esophageal cancers occur in the upper third of the esophagus, 50% in the middle, and 35% in the lower third. The numbers vary from series to series, and some report that the lower-third lesions are the most common, as these are the tumors most amenable to therapy.

The esophagus crosses behind the left main-stem bronchus at its junction with the trachea. Tracheoesophageal fistulas commonly occur here. Topographically, this occurs at the angle of Louis anteriorly, or T4–5, posteriorly (about 23 to 25 cm from the incisors). The arch of the aorta passes in front of and lateral to the esophagus at this level and may produce a shallow depression that pulsates during endoscopy. Histologically, the esophagus has four layers—mucosa, submucosa, muscle coat or muscularis propria, and adventitia. The esophagus, unlike other organs in the gastrointestinal tract, does not have a serosal layer. As a tumor partially obstructs the lumen, the esophagus distends so that tumors may grow to considerable size and involve adjacent structures before symptoms develop.

## Blood Supply

The blood supply to the esophagus is segmental, with three main arterial sources: inferior thyroid artery, the bronchial arteries at the level of the carina, and the left gastric and inferior phrenic artery (Fig. 16–2). Autopsy studies have reported that all the major vascular branches that supply the esophagus divide into minute branches some distance from the esophagus. This capillary network extends into the esophagus and supplies the submucosal area with a rich vascular supply. Because of this rich vascular plexus within the submucosa, the esophagus can be mobilized for a length and remain viable. The transhiatal esophagectomy therefore can be performed without significant hemorrhage as long as the dissection is performed within this 1-cm capillary zone around the esophagus.[34] The blood supply of the cervical esophagus is via the superior and inferior thyroid arteries. There may be small branches supplied from the subclavian artery. The thoracic esophagus is supplied by branches from the aorta to the esophagus just below the level of the carina. The lower esophagus and cardia are supplied by branches from the left gastric artery. The veins from the thoracic esophagus drain into the azygous and hemizygous system and the intercostal veins, which are tributaries of the azygous system.

## Lymphatic Drainage

The lymphatic supply of the esophagus is extensive. A dense network of lymphatic vessels within the mucosa and the submucosa communicate freely with lymphatic channels in the muscular layers of the esophagus and with those that extend through the esophagus into the thoracic nodes. Lymphatic fluids from any portion of the esophagus may travel to any other portion of the esophagus and may spread to any region of the thorax or draining nodal bed. Tumors and lymph from tumors from any portion of the esophagus may spread to any other portion of the esophagus because of the rich lymphatic supply and drainage system. Tumors of any portion of the esophagus may drain into the supraclavicular lymph nodes or into the cervical nodes. A careful physical examination for enlarged lymph nodes must be performed to evaluate the patient for metastases to these nodes. A thorough palpation of both supraclavicular fossae, including the areas behind the sternocleidomastoid muscles and the clavicular heads, may yield significant results to the careful examiner. A histologic diagnosis may be obtained by needle aspiration and cytologic examination or by node excision.[35] A positive result demonstrates systemic spread of the disease and modifies subsequent treatment. Local control of esophageal cancers with surgery or radiation therapy must consider the potential for lymphatic involvement with tumor at the time of treatment. Although lymphatic flow is unpredictable, the pattern of the lymphatic drainage favors a longitudinal spread rather than a circumferential spread.

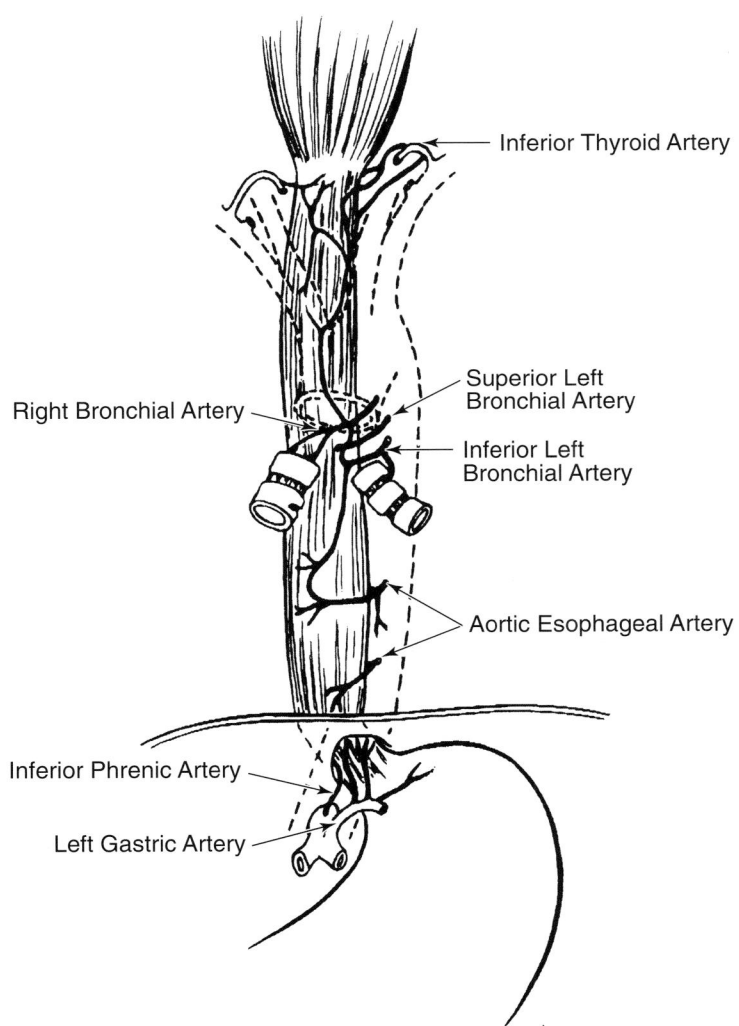

**Figure 16–2** Esophageal arterial supply. The esophageal arterial blood arises from segmental vessels feeding the esophagus in the cervical region, the intrathoracic area, and in the abdomen.

The lymph drains to several regional beds and includes all lymph nodes lying adjacent to that region. For optimal staging of mediastinal lymph nodes, a mediastinal lymph node dissection should include six or more lymph nodes from the major mediastinal lymph node stations. For the upper third of the esophagus, the lymph drains to the scalene, internal jugular, upper cervical, periesophageal, and supraclavicular nodes. For the upper and middle thirds, the lymph drains to the peritracheal, superior mediastinal, hilar, subcarinal, paraesophageal, periaortic, and pericardial regions. For the distal third, the lymph drains to the lesser curvature, left gastric, and celiac axis nodes. For intrathoracic tumors, involvement of more distant nodes, such as cervical or celiac axis nodes, is considered distant metastasis. However, for cervical tumors, supraclavicular and periesophageal nodes superior to the thoracic inlet would be considered regional lymph nodes, and celiac axis lymph nodes would be considered regional lymph nodes for distal esophageal/gastroesophageal junction tumors. For middle-third tumors (entirely intrathoracic, with the gastroesophageal junction lying in the abdomen), celiac axis lymph nodes would usually be considered distant metastases.

As the rich lymphatic drainage of the esophagus is responsible for metastatic spread throughout the entire esophagus, resection of 10 cm of esophagus beyond the tumor is recommended. Because the esophagus is only 20 to 25 cm in the chest, a total esophagectomy is usually required for optimal surgical control. A lesser resection may be performed; however, so-called skip areas without total esophagectomy may increase the risk for local recurrence.[36,37]

## Clinical Presentation

Today, the usual patient who presents with esophageal cancer in the United States is a white man between 55 and 65 years of age with a long-standing history of gastroesophageal reflux, cigarette use, and alcohol intake. Dysphagia is the initial symptom of carcinoma of the esophagus in most patients. Significant weight loss ($\geq$10%) is uncommon. These patients may complain of a vague difficulty in swallowing for the preceding 3 to 6 months or perhaps only once. Specific physical findings are rare, with the exception of cachexia, palpable supraclavicular lymph nodes, or hepatomegaly. Regurgitation of undigested food, retrosternal or epigastric pain, or aspiration pneumonia may be present in advanced lesions along with anemia, hematemesis, melena, cough from a tracheoesophageal fistula, hemoptysis, or problems related to nerve involvement, i.e., Horner's syndrome or paralysis of the recurrent laryngeal nerve.[38-43] Tumors of the esophagus may present with superior vena cava syndrome, but this is rare in the absence of dysphagia. Erosion of the esophagus into the aorta may result in exsanguinating hemorrhage. Other signs of unresectable malignant disease may be found with malignant pleural effusion or malignant ascites. Palpable supraclavicular or cervical lymph nodes should be biopsied to exclude metastases.[35]

Patients with dysphagia should undergo a plain chest roentgenogram (for evaluation of the thorax and mediastinum) and a barium swallow. The gross appearance of a carcinoma of the esophagus is best depicted by an esophagram. Rarely do other lesions present with the characteristic appearance of cancer of the esophagus. Confirmation of the histology of the tumor requires endoscopy with biopsy and brushings of the esophagus.

## Diagnosis

Any patient who complains of dysphagia (and weight loss) must be suspected to have an esophageal carcinoma. A history and physical examination should be performed and a chest X-ray film and a barium swallow obtained. Particular attention should be paid to history of gastroesophageal reflux, alcohol and tobacco abuse, weight loss, and other constitutional symptoms. A barium swallow provides the initial assessment of the extent of disease in the esophagus and may suggest the involvement of other thoracic structures (Fig. 16–3). Blood studies can determine the presence of anemia from chronic blood loss from friable tumors.

Esophagoscopy is required for histologic confirmation and identification of the location of the primary tumor and to determine the presence of intramural metastasis. Flexible and rigid esophagoscopy are appropriate modalities. Intramural metastasis (a negative prognostic factor for survival) may be identified in up to 11% patients. Seventy percent of intramural metastases on the proximal side of the esophageal tumor may be detected during this examination.[37]

All lesions seen at the time of the esophagoscopy must be brushed and then biopsied. This combination of diagnostic procedures (brushing cytology plus biopsy) yields an overall accuracy of 98.8% and exceeds that of biopsy alone (93.9%) or cytology alone (87.9%).[44-46] Benign tumors, such as leiomyomas, may enlarge and create symptoms such as dysphagia, although the tumor may not invade through the mucosa. Biopsies of the normal mucosa are not recommended, as resection of these benign lesions is recommended. Biopsies of this normal mucosa overlying the mass may yield little information and increase the risk of mucosal perforation at resection.

## Screening and Early Detection

In China, mass screening is performed using the "the Chinese balloon" (a long, small-caliber stomach tube with a balloon cov-

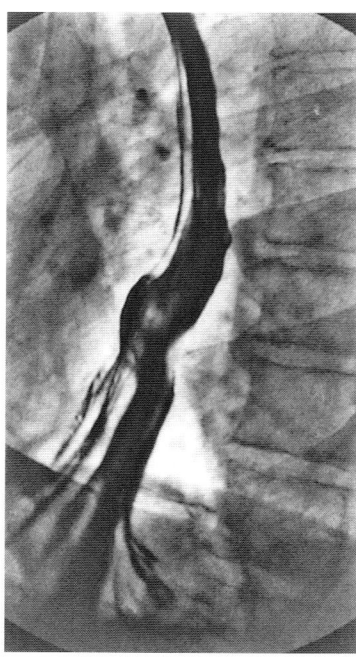

**Figure 16–3** Barium swallow. The barium swallow provides a simple cost-effective radiographic examination of the esophagus with excellent anatomic correlation. In this particular patient, a distal esophageal adenocarcinoma was diagnosed. A hiatal hernia is present and the esophagus is shortened.

ered with nylon netting on the distal end). This balloon is passed into the stomach, inflated, and then withdrawn the entire length of the esophagus; cells for cytologic study are trapped in the nylon net. In the United States, screening for esophageal cancer is not effective in the general population, but patients such as those with lye-induced strictures or Barrett's esophagus, who are at higher risk, should undergo periodic screening with upper endoscopy.

## Staging

The main objectives of clinical staging of esophageal carcinoma are (1) to identify patients who may benefit from definitive treatment of their primary carcinoma; (2) to exclude patients with metastases from surgery, because their survival time is short (about 6 months)[42]; and (3) to assess responses to radiation therapy, chemotherapy, and surgical interventions. Accurate clinical staging of esophageal carcinoma is difficult because of its location deep within the thorax. Because many esophageal cancers are treated with preoperative radiation and chemotherapy, postsurgical evaluation may not accurately define the stage of the initial diagnosed cancer. The TNM staging system for cancer of the cervical and thoracic esophagus is outlined in Table 16–1. Stage grouping is given in Table 16–2.

Esophageal carcinoma commonly metastasizes to the liver,

**Table 16-1** TNM designators

| Stage | Description |
| --- | --- |
| *Primary Tumor (T)* | |
| TX | Primary tumor cannot be assessed |
| T0 | No evidence of primary tumor |
| Tis | Preinvasive carcinoma (carcinoma in situ) |
| T1 | Tumor invades lamina propria or submucosa |
| T2 | Tumor invades muscularis propria |
| T3 | Tumor invades adventitia |
| T4 | Tumor invades adjacent structures |
| *Regional Lymph Nodes (N)* | |
| Cervical esophagus (cervical and supraclavicular lymph nodes) | |
| NX | Regional lymph nodes cannot be assessed |
| N0 | No demonstrable metastasis to regional lymph nodes |
| N1 | Regional lymph nodes contain metastatic tumor |
| Thoracic esophagus (nodes in the thorax, not those of the cervical, supraclavicular, or abdominal areas) | |
| NX | Regional lymph nodes cannot be assessed |
| N0 | No regional lymph node metastasis |
| N1 | Regional lymph node metastasis |
| *Distant Metastasis (M)* | |
| MX | Distant metastasis cannot be assessed |
| M0 | No evidence of distant metastasis |
| M1 | Distant metastasis present |
| Esophageal carcinoma located in the lower thoracic esophagus | |
| M1a | Metastasis in celiac lymph nodes |
| M1b | Nonregional lymph nodes and/or other distant metastasis |
| Esophageal carcinoma located in the upper thoracic esophagus | |
| M1a | Metastasis in cervical lymph nodes |
| M1b | Other distant metastasis[a] |

[a]For tumors of mid-thoracic esophagus use only M1b, since these tumors with metastasis in nonregional lymph nodes have an equally poor prognosis as those with metastasis in other distant sites.

**Table 16-2** Stage groupings for esophageal carcinoma

| Stage | T | N | M |
| --- | --- | --- | --- |
| Stage 0 | Tis | N0 | M0 |
| Stage I | T1 | N0 | M0 |
| Stage IIA | T2 | N0 | M0 |
| | T3 | N0 | M0 |
| Stage IIB | T1 | N1 | M0 |
| | T2 | N1 | M0 |
| Stage III | T3 | N1 | M0 |
| | T4 | Any N | M0 |
| Stage IV | Any T | Any N | M1 |
| Stage IVA | Any T | Any N | M1a |
| Stage IVB | Any T | Any N | M1b |

the peritoneum, as well as the lungs, pleura, or kidney. Patients with metastases should not be subjected to surgical resection as their primary treatment modality. Patients with lymph node involvement have a shortened life expectancy because nodal metastases (even adjacent but separate nodal metastases) often represent systemic spread of tumor beyond the limits of the resection. Excellent palliation of dysphagia may be obtained with surgery in these patients, but improvement in survival rests with better adjuvant therapy. Preoperative clinical staging should include a chest X-ray film, a barium swallow, and computed tomographic (CT) scans of the chest and upper abdomen (to include the liver and adrenals) (Fig. 16–4). Computed tomographic scans of the chest may identify accurately patients whose tumors involve the airways or aorta. Computed tomography is a poor way to detect small (<1 cm) abdominal lymph node metastases or small liver metastases.[47] A bone scan should be obtained in patients with complaints of bone pain, along with plain films of the abnormal areas. A bronchoscopy is mandatory for patients with a middle- or upper-third tumor. Bone scans and bronchoscopy may identify metastases not evident by CT scan.[48] Bronchoscopy should always be done for patients with esophageal carcinoma of the upper or middle third of the esophagus. Direct extension into the trachea may be evaluated with inspection, biopsy, and brushing. Second primary tumors may also be identified. Pulmonary function studies are helpful in assessing the patient's physiologic reserves and ability to tolerate thoracotomy.

Esophageal ultrasound is more accurate than CT staging, particularly in assessing the extent of tumor involvement of the esophageal wall and the presence or absence of enlarged paraesophageal lymph nodes. Transesophageal biopsy under esophageal ultrasound guidance can be performed for histological diagnosis of these enlarged lymph nodes.[49,50] Esophageal ultrasound is inaccurate in evaluating tumor response after esophagectomy.[51,52]

Laparoscopy and thoracoscopy have been proposed as means to evaluate the presence of nodal involvement in patients with esophageal carcinomal. Evaluation of the subdiaphragmatic surface, peritoneum, surface of the liver, and the celiac axis can also be evaluated. A feeding jejunostomy can be placed at the same time in patients who may be eligible for induction therapy. Patients undergoing thoracoscopy with identificaton of intrathoracic metastases may be spared further interventions.[53–55]

Positron emission tomography (PET) scanning, generally using $^{18}$F-deoxyglucose (FDG), for esophageal carcinoma has been evaluated and found to be complementary to other imaging studies.[56] FDG-PET was more accurate (sensitive) for identifying distant nodal metastases than CT and endoscopy combined.[57]

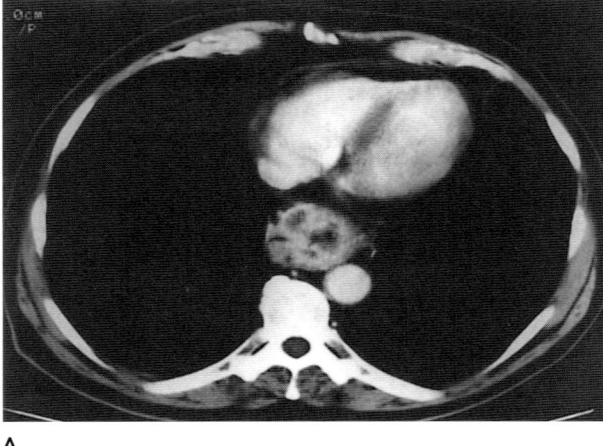
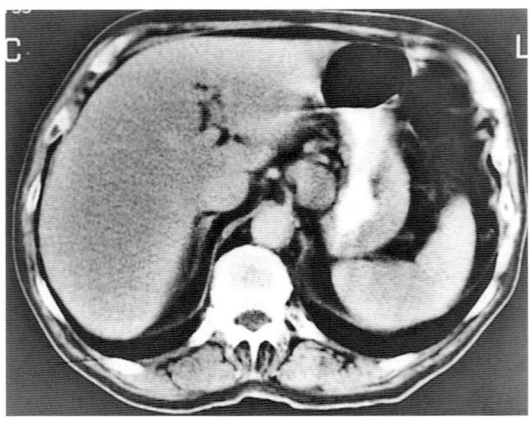

A                                              B

**Figure 16-4** *A:* Computed tomography (CT) of the esophagus. Computed tomography of the chest and upper mediastinum is performed to assist with pretreatment staging. In this patient a large, bulky, distal esophageal adenocarcinoma is identified. No surrounding lymph nodes are noted. Both soft tissue and pulmonary windows are reviewed. The CT scan of the chest should include the upper abdomen to the level of the adrenals. In this fashion, the most significant abdominal organs at risk can be evaluated. A separate abdominal CT scan is not usually necessary. *B:* Computed tomography of the celiac axis. A large celiac axis lymph node is identified. Pretreatment staging in this patient should include histological analysis of this lymph node. The simplest form of evaluation could include fine needle aspiration. Alternatives include laparoscopy with exploration and biopsy.

## Natural History and Patterns of Spread

Esophageal cancers are characterized by extensive local growth, lymph node metastases, and invasion of adjacent structures before becoming more widely disseminated. In patients with early-stage squamous cell carcinoma of the esophagus who are asymptomatic and have in situ carcinoma, 3 to 4 years may pass before advanced cancer develops.[58] Patients with adenocarcinoma may have had Barretts's esophagus associated with years of gastroesophageal reflux and repetitive chemical trauma to the distal esophagus prior to developing esophageal adenocarcinoma. The unique lymphatic drainage of the esophagus and the long interval during which the tumor is asymptomatic account for the extensive involvement of lymph nodes and structures adjacent to the esophagus at the time of diagnosis. The poor prognosis of these patients is influenced by the proximity of the aorta and trachea and the absence of a serosal covering. In one series of 117 patients with esophagectomy and extensive lymph node dissection, mortality was less than 3%. Lymphatic metastases were identified in the neck in 32% of these patients, and in about half of the lymph nodes in the chest and abdomen.[59]

Distant metastases are less often identified when patients present with dysphagia from carcinoma of the esophagus. Autopsies have shown that widespread distant metastases are almost always present at the time of death.[60] Esophageal carcinoma can spread to any viscera or site (liver, lung, pleura, stomach, peritoneum, kidney, adrenal gland, brain, and bone) and is most likely present as subclinical disease when the patient is first diagnosed.[61] Surgery for esophageal carcinoma should focus on both local and systemic control of the disease to provide palliation of dysphagia (local control) and improved survival (systemic control). The risks of esophagectomy (bleeding, infection, leak, death) exceed the benefits in patients with unresectable disease or visceral metastases.

## Second Primary Cancers

Synchronous or metachronous squamous cell carcinomas of the aerodigestive tract occur in 5% to 12% of patients with carcinoma of the esophagus. About half can be found in the head and neck areas. The oral cavity, pharynx, larynx, and lung are the most frequent sites. Oral and pharyngeal cancers are most often associated with cancer of the esophagus, and laryngeal cancers are most often associated with cancer of the lung. Direct laryngoscopy, bronchoscopy, and esophagoscopy may be helpful to exclude synchronous lung or esophageal cancer or both in those patients with head and neck cancers. Most of these second primary cancers are asymptomatic.[62,63]

## Therapy for Cancer of the Esophagus

The two primary local-control modalities for clinically localized cancer of the esophagus are surgery and radiation therapy. Resection alone is the treatment of choice for most early (stage I) lesions. For patients with more advanced localized cancers, neither treatment has been shown definitively to be superior. The low survival rates noted with single-modality therapy have prompted numerous investigations into multimodality therapy, including preoperative radiation therapy, preoperative chemotherapy, and combined preoperative radiation therapy and chemotherapy. Palliation is the primary goal for patients with advanced local cancers or metastases.

### Surgical Therapy for Carcinoma of the Esophagus

With rare exceptions, carcinoma of the esophagus is a systemic disease at diagnosis. In most patients, surgery represents the best chance for cure and the best palliation for dysphagia and local control of their disease. Various methods of esophagectomy have been proposed, but the individual surgeon must evaluate the benefits of a particular approach in treating the patient with esophageal carcinoma. Resection inconsistently results in cure, except in carcinomas in situ or in stage I carcinomas found serendipitously. Katlic and others[64] at the Massachusetts General Hospital examined the outcome of 701 patients with squamous cell carcinoma of the esophagus treated between 1950 and 1979. Tumor location was upper third in 25% of patients, middle third in 52%, and lower third in 23%. Resection was performed in 261 cases (37.2% overall). Postoperative mortality fell from 30% in the 1950s to 10% in the 1970s. Respiratory complications were the predominant cause of death. Five-year survival rates ranged from 7% to 20%. Long-term survival was uncommon and numerous studies have evaluated combined modality therapy to improve palliation and survival in patients with carcinoma of the esophagus.[65–69] Surgeons should strive to achieve certain goals in patients undergoing esophagectomy:

- Obtain optimal local control of the tumor
- Relieve dysphagia
- Achieve an operative mortality of 6% or less
- Minimize hospitalization
- Minimize early and late events associated with surgery (leak, pneumonia, stricture, reflux, etc.)
- Evaluate the results of preoperative induction therapy

Today, operative mortality of less than 6% can be achieved,[70,71] although postoperative events affect significant numbers of patients.[12,69,71]

## Preoperative evaluation of patients with esophageal carcinoma

Any patient who presents with dysphagia and weight loss must be considered as having esophageal carcinoma until this diagnosis is excluded. Patients without evidence of extra regional spread of the disease may be excellent candidates for resection or for various multimodality treatments for carcinoma of the esophagus. Noninvasive studies can be used to evaluate the patient for potential treatment options.

Patients with local or locoregional carcinoma of the esophagus are usually considered suitable candidates for resection of the esophagus and reestablishment of gastrointestinal continuity. Because of the extent of resection, adequate cardiac and pulmonary reserves are needed. Patients for resection involving thoracotomy should have adequate pulmonary reserve and cessation of smoking for a minimum of 2 weeks before surgery. Advanced age alone is not a contraindication for resection.[72–74] Patients with alcoholic cirrhosis or portal hypertension may have abdominal venous varicosities that preclude resection.

A number of studies are required to evaluate the patient for resectability. A history and physical examination may allow the astute clinician the opportunity to assess the patient's physiological fitness for esophagectomy, or it may identify the presence of supraclavicular metastases. The barium swallow and the esophagoscopy provide information about the length of the tumor, circumferential extent of the tumor, and character of the tumor (bleeding, fungating, polypoid, etc.). Patients should have a CT scan of the chest and upper abdomen. Patients with metastases from esophageal carcinoma have a shortened life expectancy, and surgical resection in these patients is usually not justified.[75] Endoscopic ultrasonography of the esophagus has been used to assess the extent of the circumferential involvement of the esophageal carcinoma with the surrounding structures, particularly for tumors of the upper and middle third of the esophagus, and may assist in clinical staging. The length of the esophagus involved by the cancer, infiltration of the cancer into adjacent organs, and involvement of lymph nodes may be assessed by this technique.[52,76–81] Bronchoscopy is mandatory for patients with tumors involving the middle or upper third of the esophagus. Tumor invading the posterior membranous trachea or a tracheoesophageal fistula renders the patient surgically unresectable.

The results of several studies using CT in the assessment of esophageal cancer have been reviewed.[48,82–85] Those using preoperative CT followed by surgical confirmation of stage have shown that CT is best at assessing local extensions of disease and at delineating liver or adrenal metastases. Computed tomography is less accurate in assessing the degree of periesophageal lymph node involvement or adjacent tissue invasion, and CT underestimates the length of the esophageal lesion. Computed tomographic scans are helpful in planning radiation therapy and may be useful in assessing the tumor response to radiation therapy and chemotherapy.

Nuclear magnetic resonance imaging (MRI) is also used to determine the extent of involvement of esophageal cancer with adjacent organs. Although MRI shares many qualities of CT scanning, MRI scans may better asses the relation of the tumor to vascular structures, such as the aorta, or that to the membranous trachea.[50,86]

Endoscopy, with the rigid or flexible esophagoscope, is used to evaluate the mucosal extent of esophageal cancers. Flexible esophagoscopy may evaluate the entire esophagus and is optimal for determining tumors of the distal esophagus that may involve the gastric cardia or proximal stomach. Patients with tumors of the upper or middle esophagus may benefit from rigid or flexible esophagoscopy and bronchoscopy in assessment of the extent of tumor and mobility of the esophagus and trachea, as second malignancies within the aerodigestive tract may be present. Bronchoscopy is not often required in patients with a distal third tumor who have had a normal chest X-ray film and a normal CT scan of the chest. In patients with a middle-third tumor, flexible bronchoscopy may screen for second primary tumors of the tracheobronchial tree. Patients with an upper-third tumor must undergo bronchoscopy because of the intimate relation of the esophagus with the posterior membranous trachea. Rigid bronchoscopy is helpful to evaluate fixation of the posterior membranous trachea. Bulging of the posterior membranous trachea or the left main-stem bronchus or narrowing of the left main-stem bronchus implies abutting tumor. Biopsy and brushings of this area are mandatory.

Patients with distal esophagecal carcinoma and clinically enlarged (>1 cm) or otherwise clinically resectable histologically positive celiac nodes are suitable for surgery. Patients with histologic evidence of extraregional metastases (e.g., middle-third tumor and positive celiac lymph nodes) usually do not benefit from surgery. Resection (separately or en bloc) or biopsy of the celiac and lesser curvature lymph nodes is valuable in planning subsequent therapy and providing prognostic data. Celiac node involvement occurs in 10% of patients with upper esophageal malignancies, and with lower esophageal cancers, the incidence increases at least fivefold.[87]

The presence of metastases (bone, liver, brain, or extensive and unresectable regional nodal metastases) precludes resection for cure. Surgeons who attempt palliative esophageal resection or a bypass of the unresectable esophageal tumor should be experienced and the risk of the procedure should be less than the anticipated 5-year survival rate (e.g., if the 5-year survival rate is 5%, the mortality from the operation should be less than 5%). If the patient has metastases, then palliation should include methods other than resection or bypass. These patients usually have a projected survival of less than 1 year and the advantages of an esophagectomy or bypass are rarely apparent.[75,88]

### Preparation of the patient for surgery

Proper evaluation and preparation of the patient and planning of the operation often make the postoperative course of the esophagectomy stable and predictable. Patients are not permitted to smoke for a minimum of 2 weeks before surgery. Incentive spirometry is begun before surgery and continued throughout the postoperative course to minimize atelectasis. Active patients with a normal electrocardiogram (EKG) may not require further evaluation of cardiac function before surgery. Patients older than 60 years, those with a history of heart disease or abnormal EKG, or those with atherosclerosis may benefit from further cardiovascular evaluation before surgery.

Although patients with squamous cell carcinoma often present with weight loss, patients with distal adenocarcinoma infrequently present with significant weight loss. Presurgical weight loss greater than 10% has a negative impact on subsequent survival. Roth and colleagues[65] noted that patients with a weight loss of less than 10% responded better to chemotherapy and overall did better than patients with a weight loss greater than 10%, implying that those patients who lost less had less advanced disease. Still, there is no evidence that correction of this weight loss before surgery improves prognosis.[40,65]

Other preoperative preparations are helpful. Dental hygiene should be optimized as anaerobic bacteria within the mouth can cause synergistic and perhaps fatal pulmonary or mediastinal infection. Dental work or extraction can precede esophageal resection, or may be performed at the same time as the esophagectomy. Perioperative antibiotics for wound infection prophylaxis and prophylaxis for deep venous thrombosis or pulmonary embolism (such as subcutaneous heparin 5000 U every 8 to 12 hours, or sequential compression devices) are routinely used.

In the operating room, an arterial monitoring catheter and at least two large-bore intravenous lines are placed to provide fluids and blood products. A central line may be used in older patients or those with underlying cardiac dysfunction. An esophagoscopy is always performed by the surgeon before resection or any esophageal manipulation. Flexible or rigid bronchoscopy is performed by the surgeon in the operating room in patients with carcinoma of the middle or upper third of the esophagus.

### Approaches to Esophageal Resection

Esophagectomy for carcinoma of the esophagus poses considerable physiologic and technical challenges. Various techniques are used to resect the esophagus (Table 16–3).[89–92] The stomach is used most commonly to reestablish alimentary tract continuity. The total thoracic esophagectomy (three-field technique—abdomen, chest, neck) and the transthoracic or Lewis procedure (named after Ivor Lewis, a British surgeon) both require thoracotomy and celiotomy. In transhiatal esophagectomy, the entire esophagus is bluntly resected through the esophageal hiatus and the thoracic inlet; a thoracotomy is avoided and a cervical esophagogastrostomy anastomosis is created. The value of a more rad-

**Table 16–3** Types of resection

*Transthoracic [Lewis] Esophagectomy*[89]

Laparotomy and preparation of gastric conduit and node dissection
Right thoracotomy for esophageal mobilization and resection
Intrathoracic anastomosis

*Radical En Bloc Esophagectomy*[301]

Laparotomy and preparation of conduit (colon)
Thoracoabdominal exploration with resection en bloc of
    Thoracic esophagus
    Mediastinal lymph nodes
    Stomach
    Spleen
    Celiac and thoracic lymph nodes

*Total Thoracic Esophagectomy*[91]

Laparotomy and preparation of gastric conduit and node dissection
Neck exploration/mobilization of esophagus (with regional lymph node dissection)
Resection of head of left clavicle to widen thoracic inlet
Retrosternal placement of conduit
Cervical anastomosis
Right thoracotomy for esophageal resection (and regional lymph node dissection)

*Transhiatal Esophagectomy*[100]

Laparotomy and preparation of gastric conduit and node dissection
Left neck exploration and mobilization of cervical esophagus
Transhiatal resection
Posterior mediastinal placement of conduit
Cervical anastomosis

ical operation (sometimes called an *en bloc esophagectomy*), in terms of survival, palliation of symptoms, and reduction in morbidity and mortality,[93] is no greater than that of the transhiatal esophagectomy.[94]

Patients with previous gastric resection may require the colon or jejunum to reestablish gastrointestinal continuity. Blood supply to the colon can be defined by preoperative angiography. Rarely used, but of historical interest, are external skin tubes or external appliances (tubes) that may be interposed for gastrointestinal continuity. Free jejunal graft interposition (15–20 cm) has been used successfully after resection of carcinoma of the upper cervical esophagus or hypopharynx that does not extend past the thoracic inlet. After cervical esophageal resection, proximal and distal anastomoses are completed to stabilize the graft. Vascular access is usually obtained from the external carotid artery and the internal jugular vein. Alternatively, a jejunal conduit may be used, although it must be "supercharged" with a microvascular arterial and venous anastomosis to the neck vessels.

The colon is the second conduit choice for esophageal replacement after the stomach. The blood supply to the colon is not always constant (the left-side vascular supply is more constant than the right side). A preoperative angiogram is valuable in evaluating the vascular anatomy and the segment of colon to by preserved. Complications may occur in up to 35.7% of patients having left colon interposition for esophageal cancer (mortality, 11.9%).[95] Functional results after colon interposition are good to excellent in most patients. Cervical anastomotic leakage (13.5%) remains a significant postoperative event after cervical anastomosis. In another study, 21 of 26 patients had left colon interposition, and 3 patients required reoperation for empyema, ischemia, and subphrenic abscess. No patient had a leak, and the

30-day operative mortality was 4.5%. Functional results were rated as good.[96] The right colon may be mobilized by dividing the ileocolic and right colic arteries and basing the blood supply on the middle colic artery. If the length is not sufficient because of a short ascending colon, the left colon may be preferable. The left colon may have a more consistent blood supply than the right colon. The left colon may be mobilized after dividing the left colic artery and placed in an isoperistaltic position. Branches from the inferior mesenteric artery may be divided to further mobilize the colon. At least 2 cm of mesentery are needed to protect the marginal artery.

## Results After Resection

The operative mortality following esophageal resection and reconstruction has slowly decreased over the past 30 years. The major components of the operation, such as staging, identification of intrathoracic extent and resection of tumor, and reestablishment of alimentary tract continuity, are better defined. Selection of conduit, location and construction of the esophageal conduit, construction of the anastomosis, management of anastomotic leak, and postoperative respiratory compromise have been identified as problems in establishing alimentary tract continuity.[97] Various solutions have been proposed to optimize the resection and minimize risks. In 1945, Sweet proposed a left thoracoabdominal approach for esophagectomy.[98] In 1946, Lewis proposed a combined laparotomy and right thoracotomy.[89,99] The transhiatal or blunt esophagectomy avoids a thoracotomy and places the gastric conuit in the posterior mediastinum.[100,101] Each technique has particular advantages and disadvantages (Table 16–3).[65,102–118]

Factors such as operative volume, hospital size, and cancer specialization affect morbidity, mortality, and hospital use after esophagectomy for cancer. In one study comparing 13 national cancer institutions and 88 community hospitals, complications of care, length of stay, hospital charges, and mortality were affected by the number of esophagectomies performed rather than hospital size or cancer specialization. Mortality was lower in national cancer institution hospitals (4.2% [confidence interval (CI), 2.0%–6.4%] vs. 13.3% [CI, 4.2%–26.2%], $P = 0.05$) and in hospitals performing a large number of esophagectomies (3.0% [CI, 0.09%–5.1%] vs. 12.2% [CI, 4.5%–19.8%], $P < 0.05$). Multivariate analysis revealed that the independent risk factor for operative mortality was the volume of esophagectomies performed (odds ratio [OR], 3.97; $P = 0.03$) and not the number of nonesophageal operations, hospital size, or cancer specialization. Hospitals performing a large number of esophagectomies also showed a tendency toward decreased complications (55% vs. 68%, $P = 0.06$), decreased length of stay (14.7 days vs. 17.7 days, $P = 0.006$), and decreased charges ($39,867 vs. $62,094, $P < 0.005$).[119] The authors noted that improved outcomes and decreased hospital use occurred in hospitals that performed larger numbers of esophagectomies. As with other complex operations, esophagectomy should not be performed by an inexperienced esophageal surgeon.[119]

Age alone is not a contraindication to surgery. Patients older than 70 years benefit from esophageal resection and have a postoperative mortality similar to that of other age groups.[120–123]

Most surgeons develop expertise in and emphasize a single technique of esophagectomy. The decrease in operative mortality reflects refinement in surgical technique due to increased experience in operative and perioperative care in the surgical treatment of carcinoma of the esophagus in various centers throughout the world. Ellis[109] described an 18-year experience with 275 patients who underwent resection, with a 30-day mortality rate of only 2.2%. Intrathoracic esophagogastrostomy was performed in 196 patients, whereas cervical anastomosis was performed in 61 patients (53 of them had a transhiatal esophagectomy). Major complications (e.g., prolonged hospital stay) occurred in 40 patients (14.5%). Tumor stage remained the most important determinant of long-term survival; the actuarial 5-year survival rate was 20.8% for all patients and 23.3% for those patients in whom a curative resection was achieved. Mathisen and colleagues[103] reported on 104 patients with intrathoracic anastomoses after esophagectomy for carcinoma of the esophagus with nonanastomotic leaks. Sixty-four of the patients had a left thoracoabdominal incision, and 40 patients underwent a Lewis esophagectomy. All anastomoses were constructed by the two-layer inverting technique with interrupted silk sutures. Operative mortality was 2.9% (3 patients), and 5% (5 patients) required one to three dilations. Major complications included pneumonia (12 patients, 12%), and reexploration for bleeding (2 patients, 2%). Positive lymph node metastases were identified in 75% of patients, and anastomotic recurrence was documented in 6 patients (6%).[103] Shao et al.[124] reported on 6123 cases of carcinoma of the gastric cardia and esophagus for which the resectability rate was 89.9%. Overall mortality was 3%, and the complication rate was 10.3%. The 5-year survival rate was 36.8%, and 10-year survival rate was 17.2%.

### Transthoracic esophagecomy

In 1946, Lewis[89] proposed a combined laparotomy and right thoracotomy approach that provided excellent exposure for preparation of the gastric conduit and for resection of the esophagus with reanastomosis of the conduit in the chest (Fig. 16–5). In a recent series of 100 patients treated with a combined laparotomy and right thoracotomy, postoperative complications occurred in 27 patients (including pulmonary complications in 11 and anastomotic leak in 9). The 30-day operative mortality was 3%. The 5-year survival rate was 85% for patients with stage I tumors, 34% for patients with stage 11 tumors, and 15% for patients with stage III tumors. Thirty-one patients required postoperative dilations for some degree of dysphagia.[111] In another study of 100 patients who underwent Lewis esophagogastrectomy, 70 patients were cured and 30 were palliated. Operative mortality was 4% and morbidity was 7% (due to anastomotic leakage). Fifteen patients had pulmonary complications. The 3-year survival rate was 25%; it was better in early-stage disease (stage I or II, 68.4%) than in later-stage disease (stage III, 23%).[91] Mitchell[104] had excellent results in a series of 40 esophagogastrectomies performed with laparotomy and right thoracotomy: there was no operative mortality, no anastomotic leak, and no major pulmonary complication.

### Radical en bloc esophagectomy

Radical resection for esophageal cancer provides local control of the neoplasm. Although radical surgery may be considered curative for early-stage disease, surgery cannot completely control systemic spread or wide lymphatic spread in either disease. The survival rate after radical en bloc esophagectomy[93] may be similar to that after transhiatal esophagectomy.[125] DeMeester and colleagues[105] proposed an extended en bloc resection of carcinoma of the esophagus consisting of thoracic esophagectomy, mediastinal lymph node dissection, and gastrectomy with abdominal (celiac) lymph node dissection. Alimentary tract continuity was reestablished using the left colon. Operative mortality

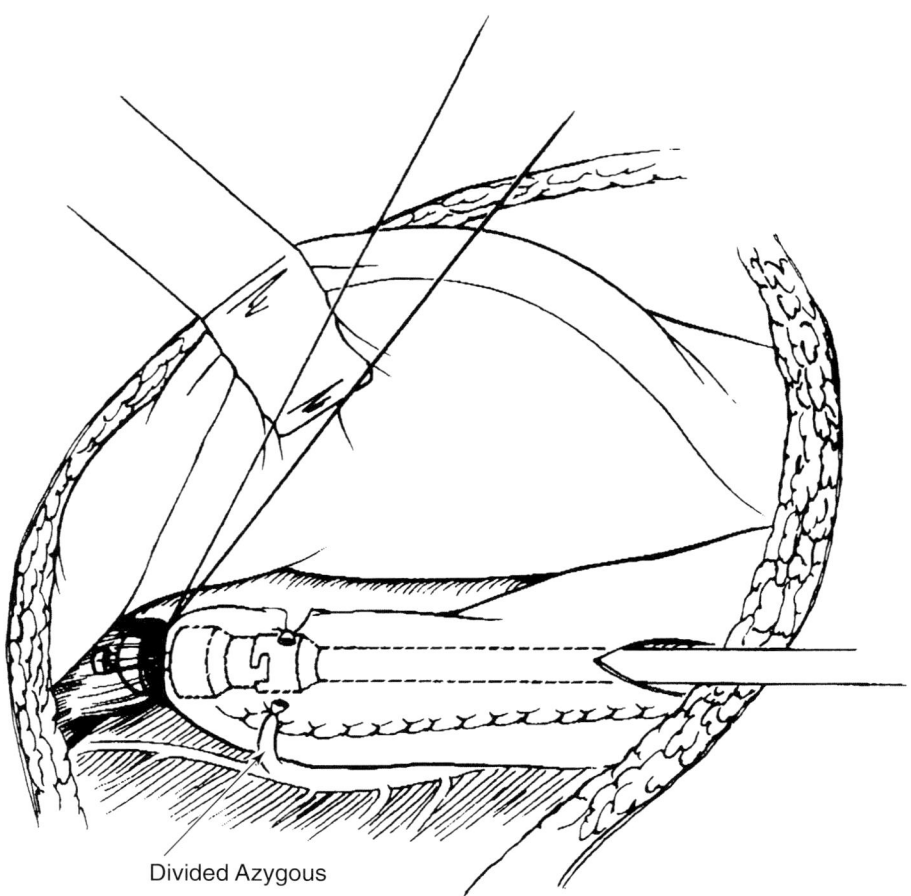

Divided Azygous

**Figure 16–5** Intrathoracic stapled anastomosis. A transthoracic (or Lewis-type) esophagectomy includes celiotomy, creation of a gastric conduit, and abdominal lymph node dissection, followed by thoracotomy, mobilization of the esophagus in the chest, thoracic lymph node dissection, and intrathoracic esophagogastric anastomosis. General surgical goals are a 5-cm distal margin 10-cm proximal margin. The anastomosis should be performed above the level of the azygos vein.

was 7%, and actuarial survival rate was 53% at 5 years (stages I and II). In 111 patients treated with en bloc esophagectomy, operative mortality was 11% and complications occurred in 49 patients (44%). No recurrences were noted after 3 years. Survival was dependent on stage.

Total thoracic esophagectomy

A total thoracic esophagectomy (TTE), as described by Akiyama,[38] consists of laparotomy for mobilization of the stomach or colon with retrosternal placement of the conduit and cervical anastomosis (and right thoracotomy) for esophageal resection. One study compared results of TTE (21 patients) with the Lewis procedure (25 patients),[126] and found that overall operative decreased to 5% as experience was gained. The 5-year survival rate was 20%. No differences in long-term survival were noted between the two groups, but there was better reflux control in patients undergoing TTE.

Transhiatal esophagectomy

Transhiatal esophagectomy (THE) has been proposed as an alternative to transthoracic esophagectomy (TThE) (Fig. 16–6). Critics of THE suggest that the operation is inadequate for cancer. Proponents suggest that THE minimizes pulmonary complications, operative time, and duration of hospitalization while palliating dysphagia. Even with middle-third tumors, operative mortality is similar to that of the transthoracic approach (9%).[127] A substantial learning curve for THE is apparent, as surgeons with less experience have more complications than surgeons with more experience. The anatomy of structures important in performing THE has been described.[128] Orringer reported 100 patients with mortality of 6% after THE and no mortality from anastomotic leaks.[94,125] Complications included pleural entry in two-thirds of the patients, and recurrent laryngeal nerve injury (transient) in 31 patients. Rarely, tracheal laceration (2 patients), chylothorax (2 patients), or anastomotic leak (5 patients, 5%) was noted. In contrast, other investigators describe THE performed in 40 patients with a 30-day mortality rate of 12%. Complications included pleural entry (71%), transient hoarseness (19%), and anastomotic leak (17%). Pulmonary complications occurred in 7% of the patients and caused all six postoperative deaths (11%).[113] Respiratory complications were common in another group of 54 patients after THE (41%).[116] Atrial fibrillation occurred in 26% of patients, and transient recurrent laryngeal nerve palsy occurred in 11%. The overall 3-year survival rate was 10%. All patients had normal swallowing, but 11 had strictures requiring dilation (20%) at some point after surgery.[106] In one literature review, the authors concluded that the cervical anastomotic leak rate may approach 15%.[129]

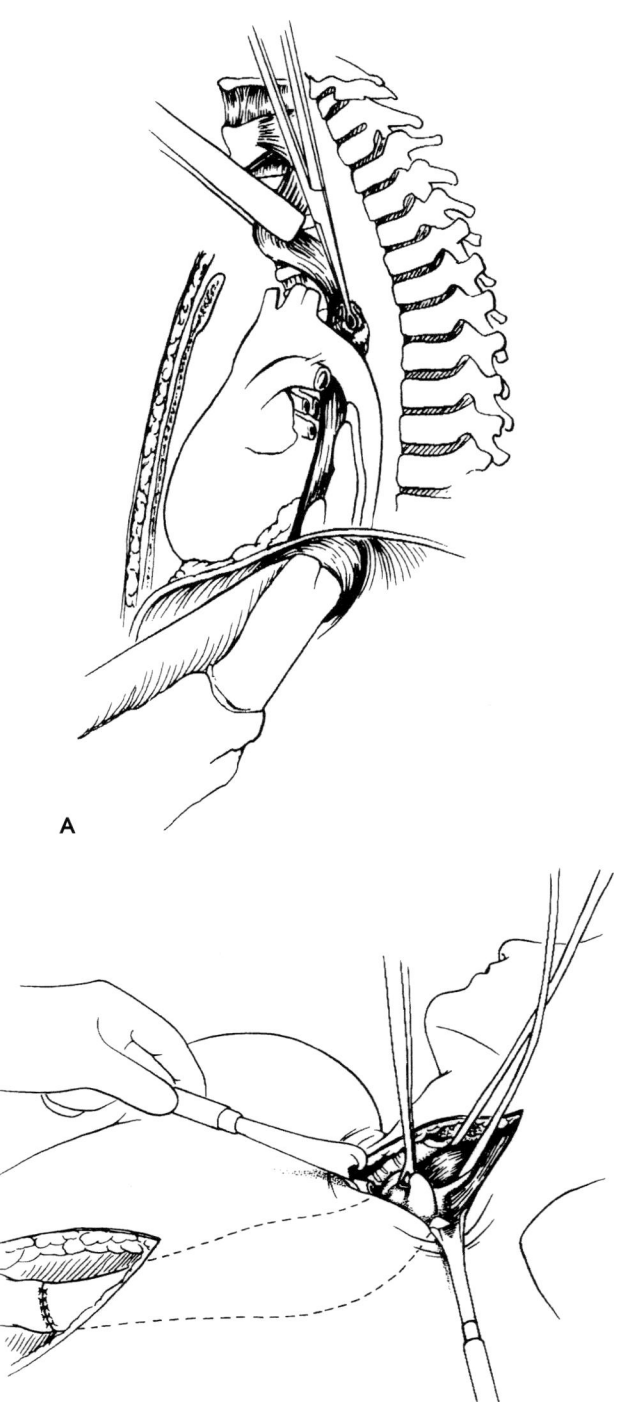

**A**

**B**

**Figure 16-6** *A:* Transhiatal esophagectomy, lateral view. The esophagus may be mobilized via the diaphragmatic esophageal hiatus, and as well as the thoracic inlet (thoracic hiatus). In this manner, a thoracotomy can be avoided. A cervical esophagogastric anastomosis is required. The mobilization of the esophagus requires a posterior dissection to separate the esophagus from the aorta and vertebra. An anterior dissection separates the esophagus from the hiatus, the pericardium, the subcarinal area, and the posterior membranous trachea. Lateral attachments are then identified and either bluntly dissected or identified, ligated, and divided. With the esophagus mobilized, the esophagus is divided in the neck and removed. *B:* Transhiatal esophagectomy, reconstruction. The gastric conduit is brought up to the neck via the posterior mediastinum. A cervical anastomosis is then performed. A pyloromyotomy or pyloroplasty is routinely performed to aid in gastric drainage.

An extensive review of one author's experience in THE has recently been published.[100] In 1085 patients who underwent THE between 1976 and 1998, 74% were performed for cancer and the remainder for benign disease. The operation was performed as intended in 98% of patients. Hospital mortality was 4%. The stomach was the conduit of choice in over 96% of patients. Postoperative events included anastomotic leak (13%), atelectasis/pneumonia (2%), and other events (intrathoracic hemorrhage, recurrent laryngeal nerve paralysis, chylothorax, and tracheal laceration, <1% each). Actuarial survival was similar to that reported for transthoracic esophagectomy. Late functional results were good to excellent in 70% of patients. Refinements included perioperative conditioning, side-to-side stapled cervical esophagogastric anastomosis, and thoracic epidural anesthesis.

Local recurrence of esophageal neoplasms may follow THE.[130,131] Patterns of recurrence in 35 patients were as follows: 13 patients (37%) had no evidence of disease after 18 months; 22 patients (63%) developed recurrent esophageal cancer within 14 months, 13 of whom were asymptomatic; and 11 patients (32%) had local recurrence. Metastatic spread was usually outside the conduit, and CT scans were better than barium studies in detecting the recurrent tumor.[132] Other studies have noted no differences in recurrence rates between transhiatal and transthoracic resection.[12]

### Comparison of transhiatal esophagectomy and transthoracic esophagectomy

Transhiatal esophagectomy and transthoracic esophagectomy have been compared in several studies. In one study, 52 patients underwent TThE and 26 patients underwent THE. Five anastomotic leaks occurred in the THE group, and only one required hospitalization longer than 14 days. Three leaks occurred in patients in the TThE group, and the hospital stays of these three patients were extended by several weeks. Overall morbidity was similar: 3 of the 52 TThE patients (6%) and 2 of the THE patients (8%) died. Transhiatal esophagectomy works as well as TThE without causing significant increases in hospitalization duration, mortality, or morbidity.[107] In another study, TThE was performed in 43 patients and THE was done in 29. The demographics of the two groups were similar. Fewer complications occurred in the THE group (48%) than in the TThE group (86%, $P < 0.05$). There was a better mortality rate in the THE group than in the TThE group (7% vs. 14%, $P < 0.05$), less intraoperative blood loss (1187 ml vs. 2150 ml, $P < 0.05$), and shorter postoperative hospitalization (12.3 days vs. 22.2 days, $P < 0.05$). There was no difference in survival rates.[112]

In a third review, 210 patients with middle or distal esophageal carcinoma underwent resection by THE ($n = 38$) or TThE ($n = 172$).[133] More complications occurred in the THE group, including excessive bleeding and perforation of the esophagus at the tumor in 7 patients (18%) and recurrent laryngeal nerve injury in 5 patients (13%). The survival was better in the TThE group.

In a review of 221 patients, results for TThE ($n = 134$), THE ($n = 42$), or TTE (three-field technique, $n = 45$) were evaluated.[12] Postoperative events requiring additional treatment occurred in 75% of patients with TThE (which included pleural entry and tube thoracostomy), in 69% with THE, and in 80% with TTE. The overall operative mortality rate was 6.8% (15/221). Patients with a cervical anastomosis had a higher leak rate (13%) than those with an intrathoracic anastomosis (6%). Median survival was 22 months (19% 5-year survival) and did not differ substantially by operation type or stage. Patients with adenocarcinoma stages III and IIb showed a trend toward improved survival after TThE despite similar rates of local and distant recurrence. Transthoracic esophagectomy, transhiatal esophagectomy, and total thoracic esophagectomy had similar morbidity, mortality, and recurrence rates. Survival and sites of recurrence reflected disease stage, not the technique of esophagectomy used.[134]

## Left thoracotomy

The left thoracotomy approach has been used for resection of carcinoma of the distal esophagus; resection is hampered, however, by the aortic arch. Pradhan and colleagues[115] examined the left thoracotomy approach in 110 patients. Postoperative mortality was 2.7% and morbidity was caused by respiratory complications, which occurred in 21 patients (19%). Page and colleagues[114] noted the same results in 119 patients, with a perioperative mortality of 8.7% (10 of 115 patients), a leakage rate of 1.7% (2 of 115), and benign stricture in 16 patients (4%).[114] The survival rate at 3 years was 22.1%. This approach compromises the surgeon's ability to completely resect the maximal extent of esophagus. The potential for inadequate resection margins is high.

## Endothoracic endoesophageal resection

In an endothoracic endoesophageal pull-through procedure, the mucosa of the esophagus is cored out with the tumor, theoretically eliminating bleeding, chylothorax, and membranous tracheal injury.[135] In a study of 68 patients, the operative mortality was 13.2% (9 patients). Overall leaks occurred in 13.3% of patients. A gastric conduit was preferred, but the left colon was used if the stomach was not suitable.[136]

## Video-assisted esophagectomy

Video-assisted thoracic surgery (VATS) techniques have been applied to esophagectomy.[137–139] While it is technically possible to perform all mechanical aspects of esophagectomy with VATS techniques,[138] prolonged intraoperative time and the potential for inadequate exploration or staging may have an adverse impact on the patient's operation.[140] A multi-institutional trial of thoracoscopic staging of esophageal cancer via a right thoracoscopy approach and laparoscopic staging of the celiac axis correctly staged 88% of patients.[141] Thoracoscopic staging of esophageal carcinoma may allow patients to be better selected for prospective multimodality trials. At this time, video-assisted esophagectomy, in combination with the open technique, does not appear to confer any added advantages over traditional open approaches to esophageal resection.[142,143]

## Laryngoesophagectomy

Esophageal neoplasms in the cervical esophagus may involve the posterior membranous trachea and the cricopharyngeus muscle. Tumors in the hypopharynx may extend to the cervical esophagus. As most of these patients have squamous cell carcinoma of the esophagus, combined therapy with radiation and chemotherapy are most commonly recommended. In this manner, local control is achieved, vocal cord function is maintained, alimentation is improved, and survival is enhanced. Alternatively in these patients, resection of the larynx and the esophagus is required. An anterior cervical tracheostomy with a gastric or free jejunal graft interposition is performed. When the tumor involves more of the trachea, an anterior mediastinal tracheostomy may be constructed after removal of the breast plate. The esophagus is mobilized by means of a transhiatal approach.[144,145] Laryngoesophagectomy with gastric or jejunal interposition offers the best chance for cure or palliation of advanced hypopharyngeal and laryngeal tumors[146] or for those patients who have recurrence after previous radiation therapy. In one study of 41 patients with squamous cell carcinoma of the esophagus treated with laryngectomy, esophagectomy, and gastric interposition, 21 had undergone previous radiation therapy. Complications included one operative death (2.5%) and anastomotic leaks in nine patients (22%). All nine of these patients had had previous radiation therapy, and three required flap reconstruction. The average postoperative hospital stay was 31 days. The overall 2-year survival rate was 35%. In a study of 42 patients, mortality was 19% and the complication rate was 40%. The length of hospitalization ranged from 23 days (without complications) to 44 days (with complications).[147]

## Special situations

Several unique situations may be faced by the surgeon treating a patient who has undergone a previous esophagectomy. Local recurrence, particularly in the cervical esophagus after chemotherapy radiation, may require a resection with jejunal interposition, or perhaps a gastric interposition with laryngectomy. In this particular situation, the breast plate may have to be divided to gain access to the upper thoracic esophagus. A thoracotomy is not usually needed simply to replace the area of local recurrence in the cervical esophagus.

In some patients, postoperative catastrophes may occur, such as necrosis of the gastric conduit or esophageal perforation with excessive mediastinal and intrathoracic contamination. Resection of the conduit and esophageal diversion (via a cervical end-esophagostomy or an anterior thoracic end-esophagostomy) to facilitate drainage and debridement of this significant esophageal perforation and mediastinal contamination are required. After a period of recovery, which may last for serveral weeks to several months, gastrointestinal continuity should be reestablished. A colon conduit (or a jejunal conduit with a "supercharged" arterial and venous anastomosis in the neck) may be required. As the posterior mediastinal space will be obliterated from the infection, the most likely and suitable position for a conduit would be in the retrosternal space. In creating the retrosternal space, care must be taken to minimize hypertension from cardiac compression and disruption of branches from the internal mammary artery. In patients with significant pleural contamination from the mediastinal floor/pleural infection, small branches from the internal mammary artery to the anterior pleura may be a enlarged and cause postoperative bleeding. Patients who have had previous aortocoronary bypass may have this space obliterated. In these patients, an extrathoracic anterosternal, subcutaneous towel may be necessary.

Particular attention must be paid to creating an optimal environment in the anterior thoracic cervical area. Typically the clavicle–first rib–manubrium junction must be removed. The inferior mesenteric artery may or may not be divided. Through this maneuver, the thoracic inlet, is enlarged, providing the necessary exposure and minimizing future compression of the conduit (Fig. 16–7).

## Postoperative Events

The normal convalesence may be interrupted or prolonged by one or more postoperative events requiring therapy. These events, or possible complications of esophagectomy, have decreased during the past several years. During the past decade, mortality from this procedure dropped from 31% to 6%. The cumulative 5-year survival rate remains unchanged at 21%. Extended resection has

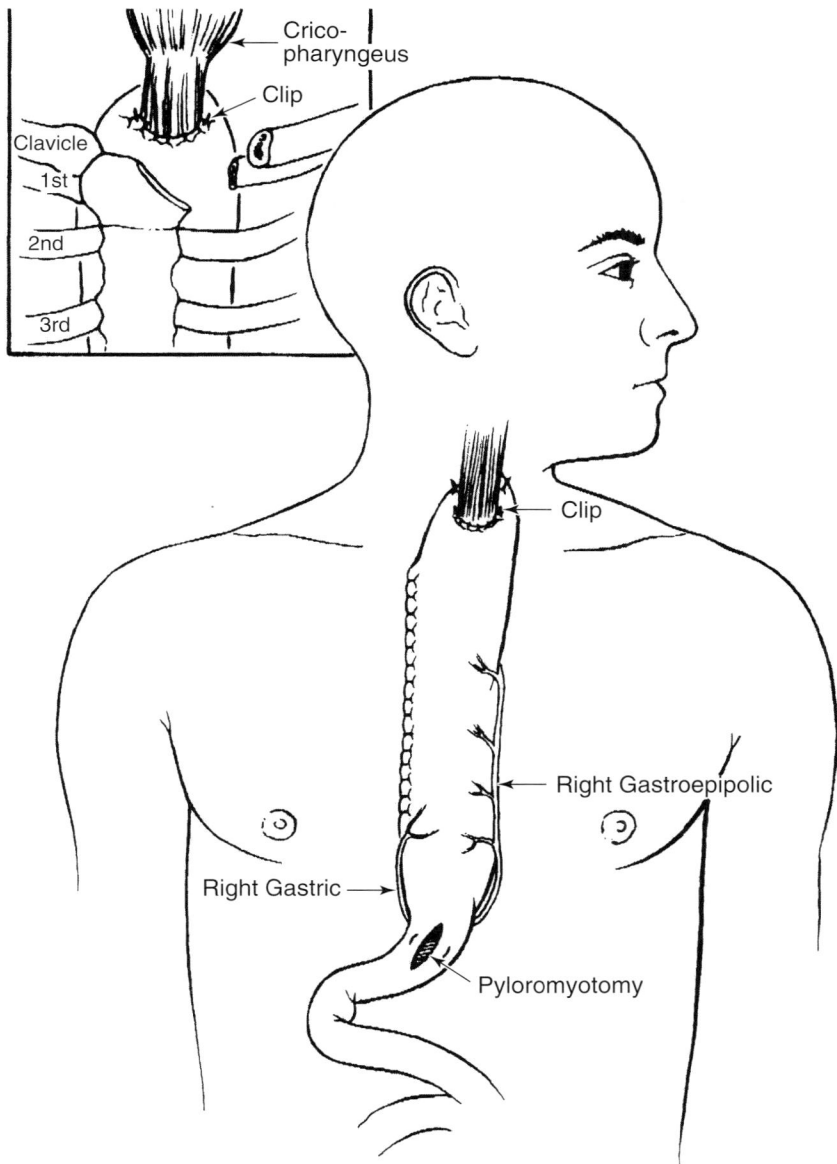

**Figure 16-7** Retrosternal conduit. If the posterior mediastinal route is not available, a retrosternal route is preferred. Removal of the clavicle and manubrium is required. The thoracic inlet is opened so that no pressure is placed on the conduit or on the anastomosis.

no survival advantage over conventional resection or transhiatal esophagectomy in terms of long-term survival.[148] In a study of 202 patients who underwent esophageal resection, 21 patients died in the hospital (10.4%); 14 patients died of multisystem failure. Risk factors were postoperative respiratory failure ($P < 0.001$), emergency reoperation ($P < 0.001$), and leak ($P < 0.01$). Forty-two percent of survivors had complications. Gastric stasis occurred in 8%.[149]

### Anastomosis and anastomotic leak

An anastomotic leak in the chest may be life threatening. Attention to detail and meticulous technique are needed for both hand-sewn and mechanical (stapled) anastomoses.[150] Early anastomotic leak (within 3–4 days) reflects poor technique; however, later anastomotic leaks probably represent tension on the anastomosis or ischemia. In one series, 14 of 242 patients who under-went intrathoracic anastomosis had a leak, and 2 patients died. Hand-sewn anastomoses and single-layer anastomoses were more likely to leak than were mechanical or stapled anastomoses and double-layer suturing.[151] Techniques, locations, and results for various anastomoses were evaluated in 221 patients (122 sutured and 99 stapled). Leaks occurred in 21 sutured anastomoses (17.2%) and in 7 stapled anastomoses (7.1%) ($P < 0.05$). Strictures were more common in the stapled group (13 of 99, 13%) than in the hand-sewn group (2 of 122, 1.6%).[152] The overall mortality rate was 20%. Benign strictures were dilated in 22% of surgical patients.[153]

In one series of 114 consecutive patients who underwent transhiatal esophagectomy, a functional cervical side-to-side esophagogastric anastomosis was created with the assistance of a linear endoscopic stapler. In contrast to the expected cervical anastomotic leak rate of 10% to 15%, among 111 survivors only

3 had significant anastomotic leaks (2.7%). The advantages of this type of mechanical cervical anastomosis include improved patient swallowing, ease of subsequent dilation, and improved patient satisfaction with swallowing.[154]

Differences in cervical or thoracic anastomosis from esophagectomy were examined in a prospective trial.[118] Forty-nine patients underwent laparotomy and right thoracotomy with intrathoracic anastomosis (TA), and 43 patients underwent laparotomy, right thoracotomy, and cervical anastomosis (CA). Anastomotic leak was more frequent after CA (26%) than after TA (4%, $P < 0.002$). Respiratory complications were more frequent with TA than with CA ($P =$ not significant). Thirty-day mortality rates were similar for the two groups (14.3% TA, and 9.3% CA). Strictures occurred in 14% of patients who had TA and in 23% of those who had CA. Duration of survival was related to extent of disease; the 2-year survival rate was 47%, and the 3.5-year survival rate was 30%.[118]

Evaluation for anastomotic leakage should include thin barium, as water-soluble contrast may be insufficient to demonstrate a leak.

### Chylothorax

Chylothorax may occur in 1% to 2% of patients after transthoracic esophagectomy. Mortality is increased if the patient is allowed to drain >10 cc/kg body weight/day of chyle for more than 7 to 14 days. Early bowel rest, no oral intake, and total parenteral nutrition may be of great value in reducing the flow of chyle and allowing the chyle leak to heal. Reoperation may be required if significant drainage persists over 7 to 14 days. Reoperation and ligation of the thoracic duct may prevent wasting, hypoalbuminemia, and leukocyte depletion. Anticipation, identification, and correction of this problem should be undertaken at the initial operation.

### Gastric emptying procedure

Some type of gastric drainage procedure, pyloroplasty or pyloromyotomy, is required. Fok et al.[155] examined over 200 patients in two groups, with and without pyloroplasty. Patients without pyloroplasty had more problems with pulmonary complications, gastric outlet obstruction, and prolonged gastric conduit transit time than patients with pyloroplasty. Either type of drainage procedure is appropriate.[156]

### Pulmonary events

Pulmonary events may be significantly increased after esophagectomy (30%) in some studies, and may be even higher after receiving perioperative chemotherapy and radiation therapy,[157–159] although this has not been observed by some authors.[160] Therapeutic strategies to minimize pneumonia have been developed[161] and include overnight mechanical ventilation, chest physiotherapy, video pharyngoesophagram on postoperative day 6 or 7, and graduated diet after acceptable esophagram.

### Recurrent laryngeal nerve injury

Recurrent laryngeal nerve (RLN) injury (paresis or paralysis) may occur in 1%–3% of all patients having a cervical anastomosis. If a RLN paralysis is suspected and the patient is not aspirating, then reevaluation in 3–6 months may be considered, as nerve function may return or contralateral RLN compensation may occur with improvement of phonation. Otherwise, Teflon injection or other techniques may be considered to create better apposition of the vocal cords.

## Adenocarcinoma of the Esophagus

Adenocarcinoma involving the distal esophagus at the level of the gastroesophageal junction may be described as a gastroesophageal junction tumor. Many of these tumors arise in Barrett's esophagus, a premalignant lesion.[162] Studies examining the results of treatment and survival of these patients often make no distinction between tumors arising from the stomach extending into the esophagus and those arising primarily from the esophagus. The definition of an esophageal adenocarcinoma is a tumor with the epicenter in the esophagus. If the epicenter is specifically at the gastroesophageal junction, this condition should be treated as an esophageal carcinoma.

Primary adenocarcinoma of the esophagus is increasing at a rapid rate. In a series of 163 patients with esophageal cancer seen between 1975 and 1982, 6.7% had a primary adenocarcinoma of the esophagus.[163] This figure is close to that reported from Denmark, in which 6.9% of the esophageal carcinomas were found to be adenocarcinoma.[164] Some studies have shown that esophageal adenocarcinomas accounted for 34% of all esophageal cancers and 60% of tumors confined to the lower third of the esophagus.[165] More recently, rates of adenocarcinoma of the esophagus have increased 4% to 10% per year in contrast to declining rates of adenocarcinoma of the more distal portions of the stomach.[2,166–168] The SEER program noted that the overall incidence of adenocarcinoma (0.4 persons per 100,000) increased more than 74% in the United States in white men between 1973 and 1982, with most of these tumors (79%) arising in the lower third of the esophagus.[167] This disease affects primarily white males[115,127,148,149,152] who have a greater frequency of hiatal hernia (40%) and of smoking and alcohol use.

### Origins of Primary Adenocarcinoma

Adenocarcinoma of the esophagus may arise from three sources: superficial and deep glands of the esophagus, embryonic remnants of glandular epithelium in the esophagus, or metaplastic glandular epithelium. The superficial and deep glands of the esophagus are mucus-secreting cells indistinguishable in appearance from the cardiac glands of the stomach. Secretions from the superficial glands located within the mucosa enter the lumen of the esophagus through ducts lined by a single layer of mucus cells. The terminal portion of the ducts from these glands is lined with squamous cells. The deep esophageal glands are thought to give rise to the mucoepidermoid carcinomas found occasionally in the esophagus.[169]

Primary adenocarcinoma of the esophagus may arise from ectopic islands of columnar epithelium or submucosal glands. These glands may be congenital or may arise from Barrett's esophagus (columnar cell-lined epithelium). Aberrant gastric mucosa, particularly in the upper and middle third of the esophagus, may be Barrett's mucosa and give rise to primary adenocarcinoma.[170]

## Barrett's Esophagus

Barrett's esophagus, or columnar cell–lined esophagus (CLE), may be found in up to 20% of patients undergoing esophagoscopy for esophagitis. The number of these patients who develop adenocarcinoma is unknown but it may be as many as half of all patients.[171] The relation between Barrett's esophagus and adenocarcinoma is not completely clear, but 59% to 86% of all adenocarcinomas of the esophagus may arise in Barrett's mucosa.

Therefore, Barrett's esophagus and adenocarcinoma may have a common etiology.[171–173] Repetitive chemical trauma from reflux may damage the squamous mucosa of the esophagus, which may be replaced by glandular epithelium growing up from the stomach. Submucosal esophageal glands from within the esophagus itself may proliferate and cover the injured esophageal surface.

The natural history of Barrett's esophagus has been studied at length.[90,168,174,175] Once Barrett's esophagus occurs, it is unlikely that it will resolve. Medical or surgical management has little influence on the subsequent development of malignancy. If esophagitis is found in a patient with Barrett's esophagus, it must be corrected and controlled. Routine annual or biannual screening should be performed for all patients with Barrett's esophagus, and any severe dysplasia should be resected.[176] In a study of 241 patients with Barrett's esophagus, the prevalence of adenocarcinoma was 27% (65 patients).[77] Thirty percent of the patients were operated on for adenocarcinoma arising from Barrett's mucosa. In 8 patients, the carcinoma was discovered on routine endoscopy for a incidence of 3.3%, and in 4 other patients, disease progression from Barrett's esophagus to carcinoma was documented. The 65 patients with carcinoma underwent surgery; 61 (94%) had operable disease. The operative mortality rate was 3.3%, and the actuarial 5-year survival rate was 23.7%. Adenocarcinoma occurred in six patients who had previous antireflux surgery; this surgery did not consistently protect against the development of carcinoma in patients with a previous diagnosis of Barrett's esophagus. Surveillance must be continued for life.[175] In another study conducted over 10 years, 76 patients were identified as having Barrett's esophagus.[171] Fifty-six patients (74%) had complications relating to their reflux. Twenty-nine patients had carcinoma (38%). Antireflux surgery was performed in 35 patients. The resolution of Barrett's esophagus in the esophagus of these patients was not well documented.

## Incidence of Adenocarcinoma in Barrett's Esophagus

Numerous investigators have examined the clinical and molecular changes that occur as Barrett's mucosa evolves from minimal or mild dysplasia to severe dysplasia or carcinoma in situ and then to invasive malignancy. Barrett's esophagus is frequently identified at the periphery of the esophageal adenocarcinoma, suggesting that the tumor arises from Barrett's mucosa. However, Barrett's mucosa is not identified in all patients with esophageal adenocarcinoma. On the one hand, the apparent absence of Barrett's mucosa on histologic examination may be related to the overgrowth of adenocarcinoma in all areas previously occupied by the Barrett's mucosa; on the other hand, the neoplasm may arise in an area uninvolved by Barrett's mucosa. In one study conducted over 6 years, 50 patients with Barrett's esophagus were identified.[177] Twelve patients had superficial adenocarcinoma arising in Barrett's esophagus, for a prevalence of 24%. High-grade dysplasia was identified in 6 of the 12 patients, but this diagnosis was later changed to adenocarcinoma. Duhaylongsod and Wolfe[178] examined 16 patients with adenocarcinoma arising in Barrett's esophagus, 34 patients with adenocarcinoma not related to Barrett's esophagus, and 30 patients with Barrett's esophagus without adenocarcinoma. A marked male predominance was noted among those with malignant Barrett's esophagus. Most of the malignancies were located at the gastroesophageal junction. The 4-year survival rate in non–Barrett's adenocarcinoma was 35%, whereas that in Barrett's adenocarcinoma was 60%.[178]

## Management of Barrett's Esophagus

### Medical management

In one prospective randomized study, 67 patients with Barrett's esophagus were followed over 36 months. Medical management (predominantly $H_2$ blockers) did not result in consistent reduction in the extent of Barrett's epithelium over this period. Eighty-two percent of the patients had a change in length of the lesion at <1 cm per year.[179] Omeprazole (20 mg/day) reduced the percentage of time patients had an esophageal pH below 4 and reduced the number of reflux episodes longer than 5 minutes, but it had no effect on acid clearance. In patients with Barrett's esophagus, omeprazole lowered intragastric acidity.[165] Omeprazole may be more effective than $H_2$ blockers (e.g., cimetidine, ranitidine) in causing regression of Barrett's esophagus.[180]

### Surgical management

Resection is the treatment of choice in patients with adenocarcinoma of the esophagus or gastroesophageal junction. Longitudinal spread of tumor along the rich lymphatic plexus is frequent and esophagectomy is required. Surgery is the treatment of choice in patients with Barrett's esophagus who have severe or high-grade dysplasia.[176,181–185] As occult invasive adenocarcinoma may be present even with a preoperative diagnosis of only severe dysplasia, current recommendations are to perform esophagectomy for these patients.

Surgical management of patients with high-grade dysplasia is identical to that for patients with carcinoma in situ. The management of high-grade (or severe) dysplasia was examined in nine patients without evidence of carcinoma who had columnar lining of the esophagus extending from the cardia.[182] Eight patients underwent resection and colon interposition; the other patients had sleeve resection of the cervical esophagus. Multifocal carcinoma was found in three patients, and one patient had microinvasive carcinoma. No carcinoma was found in the remaining four patients. Esophagectomy was indicated in these patients, because 45% had esophageal carcinoma, and the potential for long-term survival is high. In another study in which 88 patients with Barrett's mucosa were identified, 19 underwent resection, including those with high-grade dysplasia (3 patients) or parietal cells in the esophagus (1 patient), those who did not undergo long-term surveillance (2 patients), and those for whom it was not possible to exclude adenocarcinoma preoperatively (2 patients). Five patients were resected for large, penetrating ulcer, a complication of Barrett's esophagus.[186]

## Surveillance for Patients with Barrett's Mucosa

Barrett's esophagus is a potential premalignant condition, and endoscopic surveillance is mandatory. Surveillance for Barrett's mucosa progressing to adenocarcinoma was conducted in 32 patients with Barrett's esophagus.[187] Adenocarcinoma developed in three patients during 166.1 patient years. Dysplasia was found in two of these patients 6 and 15 months before the diagnosis of adenocarcinoma. One patient had adenocarcinoma. Barrett's mucosa was unchanged in all but three patients despite operative or medical treatment over 3 to 12 years. Some investigators suggest that annual screening for Barrett's is not effective. The incidence in one study was one new case in 170 patient-years, and the survival of patients with Barrett's esophagus was not different from an age- and sex-matched control population.[188] Others recommend endoscopic surveillance every 2 years as a better use of resources.[189]

## Palliation Options for Carcinoma of the Esophagus

Therapy directed at palliation of carcinoma of the esophagus must balance the benefits of therapy against the risks of therapy and the "opportunity costs" of a patient with a limited life expectancy who is spending much time receiving therapy with only modest response. Single-agent chemotherapy has a slight response rate (up to 20%) while combination chemotherapy (cisplatin or carboplatin with 5-FU, a taxane, or both) has better response rates (15% to 80%) and median duration of response (7 months), although with substantial toxicity. Overall, the outcome remains poor for these patients. Patients with esophageal carcinoma may be surgically unresectable because of the extent of the tumor locally or metastases distally. These patients require relief from dysphagia and pain. Numerous modalities are available for palliation of symptoms of esophageal obstruction. Obstruction may be treated with simple but repetitive dilation, endoluminal stents, laser ablation of endoesophageal tumor, photodynamic therapy, radiation therapy (external-beam or intraluminal brachytherapy or both), enteral feeding via jejunostomy, pain control, treatment of symptomtatic bleeding from the tumor, and simple dilation. The application of a given method of palliation depends to a great extent on the patient's physical condition and the expertise of the surgeon, oncologist, and radiation therapist. Photodynamic therapy requires using an injectable porphyrin derivative for tumor sensitization, although with a side effect of skin photosensitivity to sunlight for 1month or more.[258]

### Radiation Therapy

#### External-beam irradiation

External-beam irradiation or endoluminal brachytherapy can cause significant tumor reduction with palliation of dysphagia in up to three-quarters of patients.

#### Intraluminal brachytherapy

Patients with symptomatic esophageal carcinoma not amenable to surgical resection and previously treated with external-beam irradiation may be candidates for endoluminal brachytherapy.[259–261] In this procedure, a radioactive bead is placed through a catheter prepositioned through the area to be irradiated. This radioactive source passes through the area in a given amount of time to provide a finite and controlled radiation dose to the local tissues. The depth of penetration of radiation rarely exceeds 2 or 3 cm.[262] Fleischman and colleagues[263] showed that 9 of 10 patients with advanced esophageal cancer treated with intraluminal brachytherapy achieved palliation equivalent to that of external-beam irradiation. Most patients had already experienced failures of other palliative modalities. Most patients treated with single high-dose rate have a very poor prognosis (6 weeks or so; median survival, 4 months).[259] In one large series, there was little morbidity from external doses of 47.5 to 70 Gy in combination with 4 to 10 Gy of endoluminal irradiation given in one to three fractions. Strictures are the most frequently noted post-treatment event. Other post-treatment events include fistula formation, hemorrhage, erosion into adjacent structures (trachea, bronchus, aorta, etc.), pneumonitis, pericarditis, myocarditis, and spinal cord damage.

### Surgery

All surgery for symptomatic carcinoma of the esophagus is palliative in the strictest sense, as tumors have often spread through the lymphatics. Because of the high attendant mortality and morbidity, resection or bypass of unresectable esophageal carcinoma should be carefully considered before being undertaken as a means of palliation.[264,265] Occasionally, patients undergo mobilization of the stomach or conduit and resection of the esophagus only to have remaining gross disease found. In these patients, surgery serves as excellent palliation, and this residual disease may be further controlled by radiation therapy or a combination of radiation therapy and chemotherapy.

The survival rate of patients with metastatic esophageal carcinoma is poor.[266] Despite some advocates of esophageal bypass, most surgeons do not advocate this procedure because of the high attendant morbidity and mortality. Orringer[75] examined the results in 37 patients who underwent gastric bypass for palliation of esophageal carcinomas. Operative mortality was 24% (9 patients), and anastomotic leaks occurred in 19% (7 patients). Only 25% of patients (7 of 28) achieved good palliation. The average survival in patients who left the hospital alive was 5.9 months.

Other groups have examined the value of esophageal bypass alone and in comparison with other modes of palliation. Mannell et al.[264] examined 124 patients who underwent esophageal bypass for unresectable disease. Hospital mortality was 11% (11 patients). Median survival was 5 months and was improved by radiation therapy. Patients who survived the surgery (82%) had complete and lasting palliation of dysphagia. Holting and colleagues[267] studied 71 patients who received surgical palliation (n = 26) or endoscopic laser palliation (n = 45). Survival rates were the same in both groups. The stenosis-free interval was longer in the surgery group (24 weeks), and local reocclusion was more common in the laser group. Hospital mortality was 19%, and complications occurred in 31%.

Segalin and colleagues[268] examined patients treated with bypass, intubation, or laser. Overall mortality was 9.6%, and the 1-year survival rate was 29.1%. Excellent or good results were obtained in 78% of patients. In patients undergoing bypass (n = 49), the mortality rate was 20.4% and the median survival was 6.2 months. Intubation was performed in 254 patients; the 30-day mortality was 10.2% and the median survival 4.0 months. Laser therapy was performed in 50 patients with no operative mortality (median survival, 4.1 months). Surgical treatment alone provided palliation of dysphagia, although with high operative morbidity and mortality. Better palliation may be obtained with intubation or laser.

Cervical esophagostomy (a "spit fistula") and gastrostomy do not palliate any patient with esophageal carcinoma. The cervical esophagostomy stoma is difficult to manage, and results in patients being social outcasts. Eating or drinking is possible, but oral alimentation is not possible.

### Dilation

Simple dilation is less consistently effective in palliating dysphagia from esophageal carcinoma than other modalities. The neoplasm continues to grow and narrow the lumen despite frequent dilations. Lundell et al.[269] examined the palliative effect of repeated endoscopic dilation in 41 patients. Dysphagia recurred in all patients, and most dilations had to be repeated at 4-week intervals. Most patients required three or fewer dilations during their remaining life span. The complication rate (perforation) was low (5%), and only a short hospital stay was required.

### Esophageal Intubation

For many years, tubes of various sorts have been forced through the esophageal lumen partially obstructed with neoplasm in an attempt to relieve dysphagia. Complications from placement of tubes are high (~10%), as is hospital mortality (~10%). Pattison and colleagues[270] examined 71 patients treated with pulsion intubation (11 patients, 15.5% mortality) and traction intubation (6 patients, 15.4% mortality). Mortality is similar in other studies.[271] Esophageal intubation may be helpful in patients with tracheoesophageal fistula to prevent or limit soilage of the tracheobronchial tree.[272]

Kratz and colleagues[273] compared three tubes: Celestin tubes, implanted by laparotomy and traction; Proctor-Livingston tubes, implanted by pulsion with laparotomy for staging; and Atkinson tubes, placed by pulsion. Patients with the Atkinson tube had few complications and a low mortality rate (6% mortality) compared with the other tubes (42% mortality). Patients undergoing laparotomy had an associated 41% hospital death rate.

Several studies have compared intubation with laser therapy for palliation. Most suggest that laser therapy is preferable because of its lower mortality and morbidity rates; survival rates are equivalent.[274,275] Buset and colleagues[276] treated 116 patients by intubation and 28 patients by laser. The morbidity rate for intubation was 13.8% and that for laser was 3.6%; the mortality rate was 4.3% for intubation and 0% for laser. In a prospective and nonrandomized two-center trial, Loizou and colleagues[277] treated 43 patients with laser and 30 patients with intraluminal intubation. Relief of dysphagia (80%) and survival rates (5 to 6 months) were similar between the two groups. Laser-treated patients did better over the remainder of their lives but required more procedures.

## Stents

Metallic expandable stents are being used with some success for the short-term palliative management of unresectable esophagogastric neoplasms.[278] Many devices are available for esophageal intubation. The tube or stent may be introduced with a pusher tube, which is loaded either onto a bougie or over an endoscope and expands after placement. The latter method permits visualization of the obstructed lumen. The success rate is 90% to 97%. Placement of these stents provides an improved ability to swallow, oral alimentation, relief from pulmonary aspiration, independence from physician or hospital for care, and ability to remain in a outpatient environment. Contraindications of stent placement are cancer <2 cm below the cricopharyngeus, limited life expectancy (less than 6 weeks), or uncooperativeness. Complications include perforation, misposition or dislocation, tumor overgrowth from noncovered stents, reflux, stricture, pressure necrosis, food impaction, obstruction, bleeding, and failure of intubation and may occur in 10%–20% of patients. Stents may be as cost-effective as laser and intraluminal brachytherapy.[279] Metal expansile stents may be better than plastic Atkinson tubes in the palliation of dysphagia from unresectable esophageal carcinoma.[280]

## Laser

Laser ablation of obstructive lesions is effective in palliating dysphagia[281–285] and has been shown to have a lower mortality rate and fewer complications than tube insertion. Hahl and colleagues[286] treated 69 patients with laser therapy and 27 patients with esophageal tube insertion. Patients with laser treatment had no fatal complications and had an overall complication risk of 8.7% and a 1-year survival rate of 2%. Patients with tube insertion had a mortality rate of 11% and a complication rate of 48%, and there were no 1-year survivors. The combination of laser

therapy and intubation was not significantly better than laser therapy alone.[275]

Several factors may affect long-term outcome after laser therapy. Predictors of long-term survival include initial tumor length of <6 cm ($P < 0.01$),[274,287] improvement after the initial laser treatment ($P < 0.005$), and an adenocarcinoma histologic type ($P < 0.05$).[274] Reed and colleagues[288] conducted a prospective randomized trial examining esophageal intubation alone ($n = 10$), intubation plus radiation therapy ($n = 8$), and laser ablation plus intubation plus radiation therapy ($n = 9$). Eighty percent of patients who had a tube insertion had complications. Survival was not significantly different between groups.

## Single-Agent Chemotherapy

Although combination chemotherapy is usually recommended, several reviews[200,206,289] have outlined the results of single-agent studies. The cumulative response rate for any one drug is low, on the order of 15% to 30%, and there is no indication of survival benefit.[290–292] Symptomatic improvement is brief. Bleomycin, 5-FU, mitomycin, and cisplatin are the four agents used most often because of their activity as single agents or in combination and their additive or synergistic effects with radiation. Because of the potential for pulmonary toxicity, bleomycin is no longer included in neoadjuvant regimens, having been replaced by 5-FU. Cisplatin may have a reponse rate of up to 21%. Paclitaxel promotes the stabilization of microtubules and is a cycle-specific agent affecting cells in the $G_2$–M phase[293] and enhances radiation effects that may be both concentration- and schedule-dependent.[292,294]

## Combination Chemotherapy

Cisplatin at 100 mg/m$^2$ on day 1 and 5-FU at 1000 mg/m$^2$/day by continuous infusion for 96–120 hours is the regimen most commonly used to treat patients with either squamous or adenocarcinoma histology.[290,295] Somewhat higher response rates, in the 40% to 60% range, are reported from trials administering two to three cycles of cisplatin and 5-FU as neoadjuvant therapy prior to surgery. Attempts to substitute carboplatin for cisplatin have been unsuccessful. A phase II trial of carboplatin and vinblastine from the Memorial group reported no response in 16 patients.[296] These results[297–300] indicate that carboplatin and cisplatin do not have comparable activity in carcinoma of the esophagus. Still, 30% to 40% of patients with recurrent or metastatic carcinoma of the esophagus respond to cisplatin-based combination chemotherapy. Response duration is brief, as the majority of patients achieve only a partial response. Currently, cisplatin and 5-FU should be considered the standard first-line treatment for patients with either squamous cell carcinoma or adenocarcinoma.

## Summary

Esophageal carcinoma is a complex disease with significant morbidity. Surgical morbidity and mortality have gradually been reduced. Survival will depend on accurate pretreatment staging and optimizing patient selection for specific therapy. Earlier diagnosis and an understanding of predisposing conditions may enable some patients to be diagnosed at an earlier (and more treatable) stage. A multidisciplinary approach to treatment, which may include chemotherapy, radiation therapy, and surgery, appears to be the most likely strategy for improvement of local control, systemic control, and survival. Future investigations will be needed to determine the best regimens for multidisciplinary management.

## References

1. Mayer RJ. Overview: the changing nature of esophageal cancer. Chest 103:404S–405S, 1993.
2. Powell J, McConkey CC. Increasing incidence of adenocarcinoma of the gastric cardia and adjacent sites. Br J Cancer 62:440–443, 1990.
3. Blot WJ, Devessa SS, Fraumeni JF. Continuing climb in rates of esophageal adenocarcinoma: an update. JAMA 270:1320, 1993.
4. Brown LM, Silverman DT, Pottern LM, Schoenberg JB, Greenberg RS, Swanson GM, et al. Adenocarcinoma of the esophagus and esophagogastric junction in white men in the United States: alcohol, tobacco, and socioeconomic factors. Cancer Causes Control 5:333–340, 1994.
5. Kabat GC, Ng SK, Wynder EL. Tobacco, alcohol intake, and diet in relation to adenocarcinoma of the esophagus and gastric cardia. Cancer Causes Control 4:123–132, 1993.
6. National Cancer Institute. Cancer Statistics Review 1973–1987. HHS, PHS, National Institutes of Health, Bethesda, MD, 1990.
7. Thomas RM, Sobin LH. Gastrointestinal cancer. Cancer 75(1 Suppl): 154–170, 1995.
8. Brown LM, Swanson CA, Gridley G, Swanson GM, Schoenberg JB, Greenberg RS, et al. Adenocarcinoma of the esophagus: role of obesity and diet. J Natl Cancer Inst 87:104–109, 1995.
9. McKinney A, Sharp L, Macfarlane GJ, Muir CS. Oesophageal and gastric cancer in Scotland 1960–90. Br J Cancer 71:411–415, 1995.
10. Hesketh PJ, Clapp RW, Doos WG, Spechler SJ. The increasing frequency of adenocarcinoma of the esophagus. Cancer 64:526–530, 1989.
11. Blot WJ, Devesa SS, Kneller RW, Fraumeni JF Jr. Rising incidence of adenocarcinoma of the esophagus and gastric cardia. JAMA 265: 1287–1289, 1991.
12. Putnam JBJ, Suell DM, McMurtrey MJ, Ryan MB, Walsh GL, Natarajan G, et al. Comparison of three techniques of esophagectomy within a residency training program. Ann Thorac Surg 57:319–325, 1994.
13. Munoz N, Crespi M. High-risk conditions and precancerous lesions of the oesophagus. In: Sherlock P, Morson BC, Barbaba L, Veronesi U (eds): Precancerous Lesions of the Gastrointestinal Tract. New York: Raven Press, 1983, pp 53–63.
14. Marger RS, Marger D. Carcinoma of the esophagus and tylosis. A lethal genetic combination. Cancer 72:17–19, 1993.
15. Ashworth MT, Nash JR, Ellis A, Day DW. Abnormalities of differentiation and maturation in the oesophageal squamous epithelium of patients with tylosis: morphological features. Histopathology 19:303–310, 1991.
16. Harper PS, Harper RMJ, Howel-Evans AW. Carcinoma of the oesophagus with tylosis. Q J Med 34:317, 1970.
17. Streitz JM Jr, Ellis FH Jr, Gibb SP, Heatley GM. Achalasia and squamous cell carcinoma of the esophagus: analysis of 241 patients. Ann Thorac Surg 59:1604–1609, 1995.
18. MacFarlane SD. Carcinoma of the esophagus. In: Hill L, Kozarek R, McCallum R, Mercer CD (eds): The Esophagus: Medical and Surgical Management. W.B. Saunders, Philadelphia, 1988, pp 237–256.
19. Goldblum JR, Whyte RI, Orringer MB, Appelman HD. Achalasia. A morphologic study of 42 resected specimens. Am J Surg Pathol 18: 327–337, 1994.
20. Stein HJ, Siewert JR. Barrett's esophagus: pathogenesis, epidemiology, functional abnormalities, malignant degeneration, and surgical management [review]. Dysphagia 8:276–288, 1993.
21. Hopkins JRA, Postlethwait RW. Caustic burns and carcinoma of the esophagus. Ann Thorac Surg 194:146–148, 1992.
22. Isolauri J, Markkula H. Lye ingestion and carcinoma of the esophagus. Acta Chir Scand 155:269–271, 1989.
23. Appelqvist P, Salmo M. Lye corrosion carcinoma of the esophagua: a review of 63 cases. Cancer 45:2655–2658, 1980.
24. Shamma MH, Benedict EB. Esophageal webs. N Engl J Med 259:378–384, 1958.
25. Paterson DR. Clinical type of dysphagia. J Laryngol Otol 34:289, 1919.
26. Licciardello JT, Spitz MR, Hong WK. Multiple primary cancer in patients with cancer of the head and neck: second cancer of the head and neck, esophagus, and lung. Int J Radiat Oncol Biol Phys 17:467–476, 1989.
27. Cooper JS, Pajak TF, Rubin P, Tupchong L, Brady LW, Leibel SA, et al. Second malignancies in patients who have head and neck cancer: incidence, effect on survival and implications based on the RTOG experience. Int J Radiat Oncol Biol Phys 17:449–456, 1989.
28. Craddock VM. Aetiology of oesophageal cancer: some operative factors. Eur J Cancer Prev 1:89–103, 1992.
29. Furihata M, Ohtsuki Y, Ogoshi S, Takahashi A, Tamiya T, Ogata T. Prognostic significance of human papillomavirus genomes (type-16,

30. -18) and aberrant expression of p53 protein in human esophageal cancer. Int J Cancer 54:226–230, 1993.
30. Chang F, Syrjanen S, Shen Q, Wang L, Wang D, Syrjanen K. Human papillomavirus involvement in esophageal precancerous lesions and squamous cell carcinomas as evidenced by microscopy and different DNA techniques. Scand J Gastroenterol 27:553–563, 1992.
31. Genta RM, Huberman RM, Graham DY. The gastric cardia in Helicobacter pylori infection. Hum Pathol 25:915–919, 1994.
32. Borhan Manesh F, Farnum JB. Study of Helicobacter pylori colonization of patches of heterotopic gastric mucosa (HGM) at the upper esophagus. Dig Dis Sci 38:142–146, 1993.
33. American Joint Committee on Cancer. Manual for Staging of Cancer. J.B. Lippincott, Philadelphia, 1992, pp 57–61.
34. Liebermann-Meffert DMI, Luescher U, Neff U, Ruedi TP, Allgower M. Esophagectomy without thoracotomy: is there a risk of intramediastinal bleeding? Ann Surg 206:184–192, 1987.
35. van Overhagen H, Lameris JS, Zonderland HM, Tilanus HW, van Pel R, Schutte HE. Ultrasound and ultrasound-guided fine needle aspiration biopsy of supraclavicular lymph nodes in patients with esophageal carcinoma. Cancer 67:585–587, 1991.
36. Watson WL, Goodner JT, Miller TP, et al. Torek esophagectomy: the case against segmental resection for esophageal cancer. J Thorac Cardiovasc Surg 32:347, 1956.
37. Takubo K, Sasajima K, Yamashita K, Tanaka Y, Fujita K. Prognostic significance of intramural metastasis in patients with esophageal carcinoma. Cancer 65:1816–1819, 1990.
38. Akiyama H. Surgery for Cancer of the Esophagus, 1st ed. Williams and Wilkins, Baltimore, 1990.
39. Ojala K, Sorri M, Jokinin K, et al. Symptoms of carcinoma of the oesophagus. Med J Aust 1:384–385, 1982.
40. Pedersen H, Hansen HS, Cederquist C, et al. The prognostic significance of weight loss and its integration in stage grouping of oesophageal cancer. Acta Chir Scand 148:363–366, 1982.
41. Sweet RH. Carcinoma of the esophagus and stomach. JAMA 137:1213–1215, 1948.
42. Stair JM, Brian JE. The spectrum of esophageal carcinoma. J Ark Med Soc 82:107–114, 1982.
43. Duranceau A, Jamieson GG. Malignant tracheoesophageal fistula. Ann Thorac Surg 37:346–354, 1984.
44. Zargar SA, Khuroo MS, Jan GM, Mahajan R, Shah P. Prospective comparison of the value of brushings before and after biopsy in the endoscopic diagnosis of gastroesophageal malignancy. Acta Cytol 35:549–552, 1991.
45. Kobayashi S, Kasugai T. Brushing cytology for the diagnosis fo gastric cancer involving the cardia of the lower esophagus. Acta Cytol 22:155, 1978.
46. Winaiwer SJ, Sherlock P, Belladonn JA, et al. Endoscopic brush cytology in esophageal cancer. JAMA 232:1358, 1975.
47. Becker CD, Barbier P, Porcellini B. CT evaluation of patients undergoing transhiatal esophagectomy for cancer. J Comput Assist Tomogr 10:607–611, 1986.
48. Inculet RI, Keller SM, Dwyer A, Roth JA. Evaluation of noninvasive tests for the preoperative staging of carcinoma of the esophagus: a prospective study. Ann Thorac Surg 40:561–565, 1985.
49. Fukuda M, Hirata K, Natori H. Endoscopic ultrasonography of the esophagus. World J Surg 24:216–226, 2000.
50. Meyenberger C, Fantin AC. Esophageal carcinoma: current staging strategies. Recent Results Cancer Res 155:63–72, 2000.
51. Zuccaro G Jr, Rice TW, Goldblum J, Medendorp SV, Becker M, Pimentel R, et al. Endoscopic ultrasound cannot determine suitability for esophagectomy after aggressive chemoradiotherapy for esophageal cancer. Am J Gastroenterol 94:906–912, 1999.
52. Rice TW, Boyce GA, Sivak MV. Esophageal ultrasound and the preoperative staging of carcinoma of the esophagus. J Thorac Cardiovasc Surg 101:536–543, 1991.
53. Luketich JD, Meehan M, Nguyen NT, Christie N, Weigel T, Yousem S, et al. Minimally invasive surgical staging for esophageal cancer. Surg Endosc 14:700–702, 2000.
54. Krasna MJ, Jiao X. Thoracoscopic and laparoscopic staging for esophageal cancer. Semin Thorac Cardiovasc Surg 12:186–194, 2000.
55. Krasna MJ, Jiao X. Use of minimally invasive surgery in staging esophageal cancer. J Laparoendosc Adv Surg Tech A 10:161–164, 2000.
56. Fukunaga T, Okazumi S, Koide Y, Isono K, Imazeki K. Evaluation of esophageal cancers using fluorine-18-fluorodeoxyglucose PET. J Nucl Med 39:1002–1007, 1998.
57. Lerut T, Flamen P, Ectors N, Van Cutsem E, Peeters M, Hiele M, et al. Histopathologic validation of lymph node staging with FDG-PET scan

in cancer of the esophagus and gastroesophageal junction: a prospective study based on primary surgery with extensive lymphadenectomy. Ann Surg 232:743–752, 2000.

58. Guanrei Y, He H, Sunghong Q, et al. Endoscopic diagnosis of 115 cases of early esophageal carcinoma. Endoscopy 14:157–161, 1982.

59. Isono K, Ochiai T, Okuyama K, Onoda S. The treatment of lymph node metastasis from esophageal cancer by extensive lymphadenectomy. Jpn J Surg 20:151–157, 1990.

60. Mantravadi R, Ladd T, Briele H, et al. Carcinoma of the esophagus: sites of failure. Int J Radiat Oncol Biol Phys 8:1897–1901, 1982.

61. Arbitol A, Straus M, Granklin G, et al. Infusional chemotherapy and cyclic chemotherapy for inoperable esophageal and gastric cardia carcinoma. Am J Clin Oncol 6:195, 1983.

62. Shibuya H, Tahogi M, Horiuchi J, et al. Carcinomas of the esophagus with synchronous or metachronous primary carcinoma in other organs. Acta Radiol Oncol 21:39–43, 1982.

63. Shons AR, McQuarrie DG. Multiple primary epidermoid carcinomas of the upper aerodigestive tract. Arch Surg 120:1007–1009, 1985.

64. Katlic MR, Wilkins EWJr, Grillo HC. Three decades of treatment of esophageal squamous carcinoma at the Massachusetts General Hospital. J Thorac Cardiovasc Surg 99:929–938, 1990.

65. Roth JA, Pass HI, Flanagan MM, Graeber GM, Rosenberg JC, Steinberg S. Randomized clinical trial of preoperative and postoperative adjuvant chemotherapy with cisplatin, vindesine, and bleomycin for carcinoma of the esophagus. J Thorac Cardiovasc Surg 96:242–248, 1988.

66. Whittington R, Coia LR, Haller DG, Rubenstein JH, Rosato EF. Adenocarcinoma of the esophagus and esophago-gastric junction: the effects of single and combined modalities on the survival and patterns of failure following treatment [see comments]. Int J Radiat Oncol Biol Phys 19:593–603, 1990.

67. Orringer MB, Forastiere AA, Perez-Tamayo C, Urba S, Takasugi BJ, Bromberg J. Chemotherapy and radiation therapy before transhiatal esophagectomy for esophageal carcinoma. Ann Thorac Surg 49:348–354, 1990.

68. Roth JA, Ajani JA, Rich TA. Multidisciplinary therapy for esophageal cancer. Adv Surg 23:239–260, 1990.

69. Kelsen DP, Ginsberg R, Pajak TF, Sheahan DG, Gunderson L, Mortimer J, et al. Chemotherapy followed by surgery compared with surgery alone for localized esophageal cancer. N Engl J Med 339(27): 1979–1984, 1998.

70. Millikan KW, Silverstein J, Hart V, Blair K, Bines S, Roberts J, et al. A 15-year review of esophagectomy for carcinoma of the esophagus and cardia. Arch Surg 130:617–624, 1995.

71. Fok M, Law SY, Wong J. Operable esophageal carcinoma: current results from Hong Kong. World J Surg 18:355–360, 1994.

72. Keeling P, Gillen P, Hennessy TP. Oesophageal resection in the elderly. Ann R Coll Surg Engl 70:34–37, 1988.

73. Nishi M, Hiramatsu Y, Hioki K, Kojima Y, Sanada T, Yamanaka H, et al. Risk factors in relation to postoperative complications in patients undergoing esophagectomy or gastrectomy for cancer. Ann Surg 207: 148–154, 1988.

74. Adam DJ, Craig SR, Sang CT, Cameron EW, Walker WS. Esophagectomy for carcinoma in the octogenarian. Ann Thorac Surg 61:190–194, 1996.

75. Orringer MB. Substernal gastric bypass of the excluded esophagus: results of an ill-advised operation. Surgery 96:467–470, 1984.

76. Halvorsen RA Jr, Thompson WM. Primary neoplasms of the hollow organs of the gastrointestinal tract: staging and follow-up. Cancer 67: 1181–1188, 1991.

77. Siewert JR, Holscher AH, Dittler HJ. Preoperative staging and risk analysis in esophageal carcinoma. Hepatogastroenterology 37:382–387, 1990.

78. Tio TL, Coene PP, den Hartog JFC, Tytgat GN. Preoperative TNM classification of esophageal carcinoma by endosonography. Hepatogastroenterology 37:376–381, 1990.

79. Vilgrain V, Mompoint D, Palazzo L, Menu Y, Gayet B, Ollier P, et al. Staging of esophageal carcinoma: comparison of results with endoscopic sonography and CT. Am J Roentgenol 155:277–281, 1990.

80. Tio TL, Cohen P, Coene PP, Udding J, den Hartog JFC, Tytgat GN. Endosonography and computed tomography of esophageal carcinoma Preoperative classification compared to the new (1987) TNM system. Gastroenterology 96:1478–1486, 1989.

81. Tio TL, Coene PP, Schouwink MH, Tytgat GN. Esophagogastric carcinoma: preoperative TNM classification with endosonography. Radiology 173:411–417, 1989.

82. Sharma OP, Subnani S. Role of computerized tomography imaging in staging oesophageal carcinoma. Semin Surg Oncol 5:355–358, 1989.

83. Duignan JP, McEntee GP, OConnell DJ, Bouchier Hayes DJ, OMalley E. The role of CT in the management of carcinoma of the oesophagus and cardia. Ann R Coll Surg Engl 69:286–288, 1987.

84. Salonen O, Kivisaari L, Standertskjold Nordenstam CG, Somer K, Virkkunen P. Computed tomography in staging of oesophageal carcinoma. Scand J Gastroenterol 22:65–68, 1987.

85. Dix BR, Robbins PD, Spagnolo DV, Padovan GL, House AK, Iacopetta BJ. Clonal analysis of colorectal tumors using K-*ras* and *p53* gene mutations as markers. Diagn Mol Pathol 4:261–265, 1995.

86. Chandawarkar RY, Kakegawa T, Fujita H, Yamana H, Hayabuthi N. Comparative analysis of imaging modalities in the preoperative assessment of nodal metastasis in esophageal cancer. J Surg Oncol 61: 214–217, 1996.

87. Guernsey JM, Knudsen DF. Abdominal exploration in the evaluation of patients with carcinoma of the thoracic esophagus. J Thorac Cardiovasc Surg 59:62, 1970.

88. Lerut T, De Leyn P, Coosemans W, Van Raemdonck D, Scheys I, LeSaffre E. Surgical strategies in esophageal carcinoma with emphasis on radical lymphadenectomy. Ann Surg 216:583–590, 1992.

89. Lewis I. The surgical treatment of carcinoma of the esophagus with special reference to a new operation for growth of the middle third. Br J Surg 2:18–31, 1946.

90. Altorki NK, Skinner DB. En bloc esophagectomy: the first 100 patients. Hepatogastroenterology 37:360–363, 1990.

91. Akiyama H, Hiyama M, Hashimoto C. Resection and reconstruction for carcinoma of the thoracic oesophagus. Br J Surg 63:206–209, 1976.

92. Orringer MB, Marshall B, Stirling MC. Transhiatal esophagectomy for benign and malignant disease. J Thorac Cardiovasc Surg 105:265–276; discussion 276–277, 1993.

93. Skinner DB. En bloc resection for neoplasms of the esophagus and cardia. J Thorac Cardiovasc Surg 85:59–71, 1983.

94. Orringer MB. Transhiatal esophagectomy without thoracotomy for carcinoma of the thoracic esophagus. Ann Surg 200:282–288, 1984.

95. Huang MH, Sung CY, Hsu HK, Huang BS, Hsu WH, Chien KY. Reconstruction of the esophagus with the left colon. Ann Thorac Surg 48: 660–664, 1989.

96. Lundell L, Olbe L. Colonic interposition for reconstruction after resection of cancer in the esophagus and gastroesophageal junction. Eur J Surg 157:189–192, 1991.

97. Byth PL, Mullens AJ. Peri-operative care for oesophagectomy patients. Aust Clin Rev 11:45–50, 1991.

98. Sweet RH. Surgical management of carcinoma of the mid thoracic esophagus. N Engl J Med 233:1–7, 1945.

99. Hayes N, Shaw IH, Raimes SA, Griffin SM. Comparison of conventional Lewis-Tanner two-stage oesophagectomy with the synchronous two-team approach [corrected and republished in Br J Surg 1995; 82(3):426]. Br J Surg 82:95–97, 1995.

100. Orringer MB, Marshall B, Iannettoni MD. Transhiatal esophagectomy: clinical experience and refinements. Ann Surg 230:392–400, 1999.

101. Bartels H, Thorban S, Siewert JR. Anterior versus posterior reconstruction after transhiatal oesophagectomy: a randomized controlled trial. Br J Surg 80:1141–1144, 1993.

102. Lozac'h P, Topart P, Etienne J, Charles JF. Ivor Lewis operation for epidermoid carcinoma of the esophagus. Ann Thorac Surg 52:1154–1157, 1991.

103. Mathisen DJ, Grillo HC, Wilkins EW Jr, Moncure AC, Hilgenberg AD. Transthoracic esophagectomy: a safe approach to carcinoma of the esophagus. Ann Thorac Surg 45:137–143, 1988.

104. Mitchell RL. Abdominal and right thoracotomy approach as standard procedure for esophagogastrectomy with low morbidity. J Thorac Cardiovasc Surg 93:205–211, 1987.

105. DeMeester TR, Zaninotto G, Johansson KE. Selective therapeutic approach to cancer of the lower esophagus and cardia. J Thorac Cardiovasc Surg 95:42–54, 1988.

106. Gotley DC, Beard J, Cooper MJ, Britton DC, Williamson RC. Abdominocervical (transhiatal) oesophagectomy in the management of oesophageal carcinoma. Br J Surg 77:815–819, 1990.

107. Hankins JR, Attar S, Coughlin TRJr, Miller JE, Hebel JR, Suter CM, et al. Carcinoma of the esophagus: a comparison of the results of transhiatal versus transthoracic resection. Ann Thorac Surg 47:700–705, 1989.

108. Altorki NK, Skinner DB. En bloc esophagectomy: the first 100 patients. Hepatogastroenterology 37:360–363, 1990.

109. Ellis FH Jr. Treatment of carcinoma of the esophagus or cardia. Mayo Clin Proc 64:945–955, 1989.

110. Mansour KA, Downey RS. Esophageal carcinoma: surgery without preoperative adjuvant chemotherapy. Ann Thorac Surg 48:201–204; 1989.

111. King RM, Pairolero PC, Trastek VF, Payne WS, Bernatz PE. Ivor Lewis esophagogastrectomy for carcinoma of the esophagus: early and late functional results. Ann Thorac Surg 44:119–122, 1987.

112. Goldfaden D, Orringer MB, Appelman HD, Kalish R. Adenocarcinoma of the distal esophagus and gastric cardia: comparison of results of transhiatal esophagectomy and thoracoabdominal esophagogastrectomy. J Thorac Cardiovasc Surg 91:242–247, 1986.

113. Gupta NM. Transhiatal esophagectomy. Acta Chir Scand 156:149–52; 1990.

114. Page RD, Khalil JF, Whyte RI, Kaplan DK, Donnelly RJ. Esophagogastrectomy via left thoracophrenotomy. Ann Thorac Surg 49:763–766, 1990.

115. Pradhan GN, Eng JB, Sabanathan S. Left thoracotomy approach for resection of carcinoma of the esophagus. Surg Gynecol Obstet 168:49–53, 1989.

116. Matthews HR, Steel A. Left-sided subtotal oesophagectomy for carcinoma. Br J Surg 74:1115–1117, 1987.

117. Mannell A, Becker PJ. Evaluation of the results of oesophagectomy for oesophageal cancer. Br J Surg 78:36–40, 1991.

118. Chasseray VM, Kiroff GK, Buard JL, Launois B. Cervical or thoracic anastomosis for esophagectomy for carcinoma. Surg Gynecol Obstet 169:55–62, 1989.

119. Swisher SG, Deford L, Merriman KW, Walsh GL, Smythe R, Vaporicyan A, et al. Effect of operative volume on morbidity, mortality, and hospital use after esophagectomy for cancer. J Thorac Cardiovasc Surg 119:1126–1132, 2000.

120. Muehrcke DD, Kaplan DK, Donnelly RJ. Oesophagogastrectomy in patients over 70. Thorax 44:141–145, 1989.

121. Kuwano H, Morita M, Baba K, Kitamura K, Toh Y, Matsuda H, et al. Surgical treatment of esophageal carcinoma in patients eighty years of age and older. J Surg Oncol 52:36–39, 1993.

122. Thomas P, Doddoli C, Neville P, Pons J, Lienne P, Giudicelli R, et al. Esophageal cancer resection in the elderly. Eur J Cardiothorac Surg 10:941–946, 1996.

123. Naunheim KS, Hanosh J, Zwischenberger J, Turrentine MW, Kesler KA, Reeder LB, et al. Esophagectomy in the septuagenarian. Ann Thorac Surg 56:880–883; discussion 883–884, 1993.

124. Shao LF, Gao ZG, Yang NP, Wei GQ, Wang YD, Cheng CP. Results of surgical treatment in 6,123 cases of carcinoma of the esophagus and gastric cardia. J Surg Oncol 42:170–174, 1989.

125. Orringer MB. Transhiatal esophagectomy without thoracotomy for carcinoma of the esophagus. Adv Surg 19:1–49, 1986.

126. Plukker JT, van Slooten EA, Joosten HJ. The Akiyama procedure in the surgical management of oesophageal cardiacarcinoma. Eur J Surg Oncol 14:33–40, 1988.

127. Hurley JP, Keeling P. Transhiatal oesophagectomy—its role for tumours of the middle third of the intrathoracic oesophagus. Ir Med J 83:23–25, 1990.

128. Strano S, Bremner CG. Transhiatal blunt esophagectomy. Surg Gynecol Obstet 166:541–544, 1988.

129. Bardini R, Bonavina L, Asolati M, Ruol A, Castoro C, Tiso E. Single-layered cervical esophageal anastomoses: a prospective study of two suturing techniques. Ann Thorac Surg 58:1087–1089; discussion 1089–1089, 1994.

130. Forastiere AA, Orringer MB, Perez-Tamayo C, Urba SG, Husted S, Takasugi BJ, et al. Concurrent chemotherapy and radiation therapy followed by transhiatal esophagectomy for local-regional cancer of the esophagus. J Clin Oncol 8:119–127, 1990.

131. Forastiere AA, Orringer MB, Perez-Tamayo C, Urba SG, Zahurak M. Preoperative chemoradiation followed by transhiatal esophagectomy for carcinoma of the esophagus: final report. J Clin Oncol 11:1118–1123, 1993.

132. Becker CD, Barbier PA, Terrier F, Porcellini B. Patterns of recurrence of esophageal carcinoma after transhiatal esophagectomy and gastric interposition. Am J Roentgenol 148:273–277, 1987.

133. Fok M, Siu KF, Wong J. A comparison of transhiatal and transthoracic resection for carcinoma of the thoracic esophagus. Am J Surg 158:414–419, 1989.

134. Goldminc M, Maddern G, Le Prise E, Meunier B, Campion JP, Launois B. Oesophagectomy by a transhiatal approach or thoracotomy: a prospective randomized trial. Br J Surg 1993;80:367–370, 1993.

135. Bumm R, Holscher AH, Feussner H, Tachibana M, Bartels H, Siewert JR. Endodissection of the thoracic esophagus. Technique and clinical results in transhiatal esophagectomy. Ann Surg 218:97–104, 1993.

136. Saidi F, Abbassi A, Shadmehr MB, Khoshnevis Asl G. Endothoracic endoesophageal pull-through operation. A new approach to cancers of the esophagus and proximal stomach. J Thorac Cardiovasc Surg 102:43–50, 1991.

137. Gossot D, Fourquier P, Celerier M. Thoracoscopic esophagectomy: technique and initial results. Ann Thorac Surg 56:667–670, 1993.

138. Liu HP, Chang CH, Lin PJ, Chang JP. Video-assisted endoscopic esophagectomy with stapled intrathoracic esophagogastric anastomosis. World J Surg 19:745–747, 1995.

139. Cuschieri A. Endoscopic subtotal oesophagectomy for cancer using the right thoracoscopic approach. Surg Oncol 2 Suppl 1:3–11, 1993

140. Gamliel Z, Krasna MJ. The role of video-assisted thoracic surgery in esophageal disease. Chest Surg Clin North Am 8:853–870, 1998.

141. Krasna MJ, Reed CE, Jaklitsch MT, Cushing D, Sugarbaker DJ. Thoracoscopic staging of esophageal cancer: a prospective, multiinstitutional trial. Cancer and Leukemia Group B Thoracic Surgeons. Ann Thorac Surg 60:1337–1340, 1995.

142. Kawahara K, Maekawa T, Okabayashi K, Hideshima T, Shiraishi T, Yoshinaga Y, et al. Video-assisted thoracoscopic esophagectomy for esophageal cancer. Surg Endosc 13:218–223, 1999.

143. Gossot D, Cattan P, Fritsch S, Halimi B, Sarfati E, Celerier M. Can the morbidity of esophagectomy be reduced by the thoracoscopic approach? Surg Endosc 9:1113–1115, 1995.

144. Lam KH, Choi TK, Wei WI, Lau WF, Wong J. Present status of pharyngogastric anastomosis following pharyngolaryngo-oesophagectomy. Br J Surg 74:122–125, 1987.

145. Baker JW Jr, Schechter GL. Management of panesophageal cancer by blunt resection without thoracotomy and reconstruction with stomach. Ann Surg 203:491–499, 1986.

146. Kato H, Tachimori Y, Watanabe H, Nakatsuka T, Mashima K, Ebihara S, et al. Mediastinal tracheostomy during esophagectomy for cervicothoracic esophageal carcinoma invading the proximal trachea. J Surg Oncol 55:78–83, 1994.

147. Ujiki GT, Pearl GJ, Poticha S, Sisson GA Sr, Shields TW. Mortality and morbidity of gastric 'pull-up' for replacement of the pharyngoesophagus. Arch Surg 122:644–647, 1987.

148. Muller JM, Zieren U, Wolters U, Pichlmaier H. Results of esophagectomy and gastric bypass for cancer of the esophagus. Hepatogastroenterology 36:522–528, 1989.

149. Griffin S, Desai J, Charlton M, Townsend E, Fountain SW. Factors influencing mortality and morbidity following oesophageal resection. Eur J Cardiothorac Surg 3:419–423, 1989.

150. Urschel JD. Esophagogastrostomy anastomotic leaks complicating esophagectomy: a review. Am J Surg 169:634–640, 1995.

151. Peracchia A, Bardini R, Ruol A, Asolati M, Scibetta D. Esophagovisceral anastomotic leak. A prospective statistical study of predisposing factors. J Thorac Cardiovasc Surg 95:685–691, 1988.

152. McManus KG, Ritchie AJ, McGuigan J, Stevenson HM, Gibbons JR. Sutures, staplers, leaks and strictures. A review of anastomoses in oesophageal resection at Royal Victoria Hospital, Belfast 1977–1986. Eur J Cardiothorac Surg 4:97–100, 1990.

153. Smirniotis V, Morritt GG. EEA stapler in oesophagogastrectomies. Int Surg 75:36–38, 1990.

154. Orringer MB, Marshall B, Iannettoni MD. Eliminating the cervical esophagogastric anastomotic leak with a side-to-side stapled anastomosis. J Thorac Cardiovasc Surg 119:277–288, 2000.

155. Fok M, Cheng SW, Wong J. Pyloroplasty versus no drainage in gastric replacement of the esophagus. Am J Surg 162:447–452, 1991.

156. Law S, Cheung MC, Fok M, Chu KM, Wong J. Pyloroplasty and pyloromyotomy in gastric replacement of the esophagus after esophagectomy: a randomized controlled trial. J Am Coll Surg 184:630–636, 1997.

157. Kolh P, Honore P, Degauque C, Gielen J, Gerard P, Jacquet N. Early stage results after oesophageal resection for malignancy—colon interposition vs. gastric pull-up. Eur J Cardiothorac Surg 18:293–300, 2000.

158. Eguchi R, Ide H, Nakamura T, Hayashi M, Ohta M, Okamoto F, et al. Analysis of postoperative complications after esophagectomy for esophageal cancer in patients receiving neoadjuvant therapy. Jpn J Thorac Cardiovasc Surg 47:552–558, 1999.

159. Scholz J, Steinhofel U, Durig M, Prause A, Bause HW, Hamper K, et al. Postoperative pulmonary complications in patients with esophageal cancer. Clin Invest 71:294–298, 1993.

160. Tabira Y, Okuma T, Kondo K, Yoshioka M, Mori T, Tanaka M, et al. Does neoadjuvant chemotherapy for carcinoma in the thoracic esophagus increase postoperative morbidity? Jpn J Thorac Cardiovasc Surg 47:361–367, 1999.

161. Gillinov AM, Heitmiller RF. Strategies to reduce pulmonary complications after transhiatal esophagectomy. Dis Esophagus 11:43–47, 1998.

162. Rogers EL, Goldkind SF, Iseri OA, Bustin M, Goldkind L, Hamilton SR, et al. Adenocarcinoma of the lower esophagus. A disease primarily of white men with Barrett's esophagus. J Clin Gastroenterol 8:613–618, 1986.

163. Steiger Z, Wilson RF, Leichman L, et al. Primary adenocarcinoma of the esophagus. J Surg Oncol 36:68–70, 1987.

164. Cederquist C, Nielsen J, Berthelsen A, et al. Adenocarcinoma of the esophagus. Acta Chir Scand 146:411, 1980.

165. Wang HH, Antonioli DA, Goldman H. Comparative features of esophageal and gastric adenocarcinomas: recent changes in type and frequency. Hum Pathol 17:482–487, 1986.

166. Lund O, Hasenkam JM, Aagaard MT, Kimose HH. Time-related changes in characteristics of prognostic significance in carcinomas of the oesophagus and cardia. Br J Surg 76:1301–1307, 1989.

167. Yang PC, Davis S. Incidence of cancer of the esophagus in the US by histologic type. Cancer 61:612–617, 1988.

168. Harvey JC, Kagan AR, Hause D, Sachs T, Frankl H. Adenocarcinoma arising in Barrett's esophagus. J Surg Oncol 45:162–163, 1990.

169. Ming SC. Tumors of the esophagus and stomach. Atlas of Tumor Pathology, 2nd series, Fascile 7. Armed Forces Institute of Pathology, Washington, DC, 1973, pp 1–279.

170. Barrett N. The lower esophagus lined by columnar epithelium. Surgery 41:881, 1957.

171. Rosenberg JC, Budev H, Edwards RC, et al. Analysis of adenocarcinoma in Barrett's esophagus utilizing a staging system. Cancer 55:1353–1360, 1985.

172. Molina JE, Lawton BR, Myers WO, et al. Esophagogastrectomy for adenocarcinoma of the cardia. Ann Surg 195:146–151, 1982.

173. Kalish RJ, Clancy PE, Orringer MB, et al. Clinical, espidemiologic and morphologic comparison between adenocarcinomas arising in Barrett's esophageal mucosa and in the gastric cardia. Gastroenterology 86:461–467, 1984.

174. DeMeester TR, Barlow AP. Surgery and current management for cancer of the esophagus and cardia. Curr Probl Cancer 12:243–328, 1988.

175. Streitz JM Jr, Ellis FH Jr, Gibb SP, Balogh K, Watkins E Jr. Adenocarcinoma in Barrett's esophagus. A clinicopathologic study of 65 cases. Ann Surg 213:122–125, 1991.

176. Dent J. Approaches to oesophageal columnar metaplasia (Barrett's oesophagus). Scand J Gastroenterol Suppl 168:60–66, 1989.

177. De Baecque C, Potet F, Molas G, Flejou JF, Barbier P, Martignon C. Superficial adenocarcinoma of the oesophagus arising in Barrett's mucosa with dysplasia: a clinico-pathological study of 12 patients. Histopathology 16:213–220, 1990.

178. Duhaylongsod FG, Wolfe WG. Barrett's esophagus and adenocarcinoma of the esophagus and gastroesophageal junction. J Thorac Cardiovasc Surg 102:36–41, 1991.

179. Sampliner RE, Garewal HS, Fennerty MB, Aickin M. Lack of impact of therapy on extent of Barrett's esophagus in 67 patients. Dig Dis Sci 35:93–96, 1990.

180. Fiorucci S, Santucci L, Farroni F, Pelli MA, Morelli A. Effect of omeprazole on gastroesophageal reflux in Barrett's esophagus. Am J Gastroenterol 84:1263–1267, 1989.

181. Altorki NK, Sunagawa M, Little AG, Skinner DB. High-grade dysplasia in the columnar-lined esophagus. Am J Surg 161:97–99, 1991.

182. Altorki NK, Skinner DB. Adenocarcinoma in Barrett's esophagus. Semin Surg Oncol 6:274–278, 1990.

183. Palley SL, Sampliner RE, Garewal HS. Management of high-grade dysplasia in Barrett's esophagus. J Clin Gastroenterol 11:369–372, 1989.

184. Williamson WA, Ellis FH, Gibb SP, Shahian DM, Aretz HT, Heatley GJ, et al. Barrett's esophagus. Prevalence and incidence of adenocarcinoma. Arch Intern Med 151:2212–2216, 1991.

185. Starnes VA, Adkins RB, Ballinger JG, et al. Barrett's esophagus: a surgical entity. Arch Surg 119:563–567, 1984.

186. Altorki NK, Skinner DB, Segalin A, Stephens JK, Ferguson MK, Little AG. Indications for esophagectomy in nonmalignant Barrett's esophagus: a 10-year experience. Ann Thorac Surg 49:724–726, 1990.

187. Ovaska J, Miettinen M, Kivilaakso E. Adenocarcinoma arising in Barrett's esophagus. Dig Dis Sci 34:1336–1339, 1989.

188. Van der VAH, Dees J, Blankensteijn JD, Van Blankenstein M. Adenocarcinoma in Barrett's oesophagus: an overrated risk. Gut 30:14–18, 1989.

189. Achkar E, Carey W. The cost of surveillance for adenocarcinoma complicating Barrett's esophagus. Am J Gastroenterol 83:291–294, 1988.

190. Ancona E, Ruol A, Castoro C, Chiarion-Sileni V, Merigliano S, Santi S, et al. First-line chemotherapy improves the resection rate and long-term survival of locally advanced (T4, any N, M0) squamous cell carcinoma of the thoracic esophagus: final report on 163 consecutive patients with 5-year follow-up. Ann Surg 226):714–723, 1997.

191. National Comprehensive Cancer Network. Practice Guidelines for Esophageal Cancer. NCCN Proceedings. In press.

192. Lightdale C, Botet J, Brennan M, et al. Endoscopic ultrasonography compared to computerized tomography for peroperative staging of gastric cancer. Gastrointest Endosc 35:154, 1989.

193. Tio TL, Coene PP, Luiken GJ, Tytgat GN. Endosonography in the clinical staging of esophagogastric carcinoma. Gastrointest Endosc 36:S2–S10, 1990.

194. Mandard AM, Chasle J, Marnay J, Villedieu B, Bianco C, Roussel A, et al. Autopsy findings in 111 cases of esophageal cancer. Cancer 48:329–335, 1981.

195. Anderson L, Ladd T. Autopsy findings in squamous cell carcinoma of the esophagus. Cancer 50:1587–1590, 1982.

196. Attah E, Hadju S. Benign and malignant tumors of the esophagus at autopsy. J Thorac Cardiovasc Surg 55:396, 1980.

197. Bosch A, Frias Z, Caldwell WL, Jaeschke WH. Autopsy findings in carcinoma of the esophagus. Acta Radiol Oncol 18:103–112, 1979.

198. Aisner JA, Forastiere AA, Aaroney R. Patterns of recurrence for cancer of the lung and esophagus. Cancer Treat Symp 2:87, 1983.

199. Roth JA, Putnam JBJ. Surgery for cancer of the esophagus. Semin Oncol 21:453–461, 1994.

200. Ajani JA. Contributions of chemotherapy in the treatment of carcinoma of the esophagus: results and commentary. Semin Oncol 21:474–482, 1994.

201. Branchereau S, Calise D, Ferry N. Factors influencing retroviral-mediated gene transfer into hepatocytes in vivo. Hum Gene Ther 5:803–808, 1994.

202. Sugimachi K, Matsuoka H, Ohno S, Mori M, Kuwano H. Multivariate approach for assessing the prognosis of clinical oesophageal carcinoma. Br J Surg 75:1115–1118, 1988.

203. Iizuka T, Isono K, Kakegawa T, Watanabe H. Parameters linked to 10-year survial in Japan of resected esophageal carcinoma. Chest 96:970–971, 1989.

204. Roder JD, Busch R, Stein HJ, et al. Prognostic factors in patients with squamous cell cancer of the esophagus undergoing transthoracic en bloc resection. In: Nabey K (ed): Diseases of the Esophagus. Springer-Verlag, Tokyo, 1993, pp 714–725.

205. Roder JD, Busch R, Fink U, et al. Ratio of invaded to removed lymph nodes as a predictor of survival in squamous cell cancer of the esophagus. Br J Surg 81:410–413, 1994.

206. Flood WA, Forastiere AA. Esophageal cancer. Curr Opin Oncol 7:381–386, 1995.

207. Fink U, Stein HJ, Bochtler H, et al. Neoadjuvant therapy for squamous cell esophageal carcinoma. Ann Oncol 5:S17, 1994.

208. Ilson DH, Kelsen DP. Combined modality therapy in the treatment of esophageal cancer. Semin Oncol 21:493, 1994.

209. Faberberg J, Stockeld D, Lewensohn R. Combined treatment modalities in esophageal cancer: Should chemotherapy be included? Acta Oncol 33:439–450, 1994.

210. Urba S, Orringer M, Turrisi A, et al. A randomized trial comparing transhiatal esophagectomy to preoperative concurrent chemoradiation followed by esophagectomy in locoregional esophageal carcinoma. Proc Clin Oncol 14:199, 1995.

211. Forastiere AA, Heitmiller R, Lee DJ, Abrams R, Zahurak M. A 4-week intensive preoperative chemoradiation program for locoregional cancer of the esophagus [meeting abstract]. Proc Annu Meet Am Soc Clin Oncol 13:A568, 1994.

212. Urba SG, Orringer MB, Turrisi A, Iannettoni M, Forastiere A, Strawderman M. Randomized trial of preoperative chemoradiation versus surgery alone in patients with locoregional esophageal carcinoma. J Clin Oncol 19:305–313, 2001.

213. Ajani JA, Ryan B, Rich TA, McMurtrey M, Roth JA, DeCaro L, et al. Prolonged chemotherapy for localized squamous carcinoma of the oesophagus. Eur J Cancer 28A(4–5):880–884, 1992.

214. Vignoud J, Visset J, Paineau J, et al. Pre-operative chemotherapy in 60 cases of squamous cell carcinoma of the esophagus. In: Proceedings of the Int'l Congress on Neo-Adjuvant Chemotherapy, 1991, 5A.

215. Vignoud J, Visset J, Paineau J, et al. Preoperative chemotherapy in squamous cell carcinoma of the esopahgus: clincal and pathological analysis, 48 cases. Ann Oncol 1:45, 1990.

216. Wright CD, Mathisen DJ, Wain JC, Corillo HC, Hilgenberg AD, Mancure AC, et al. Evolution of treatment strategies for adenocarcinoma of the esophagus and gastroesophageal junction. Ann Thorac Surg 56:1574–1578, 1994.

217. Schlag PM. Randomized trial of preoperative chemotherapy for squamous cell cancer of the esophagus. The Chirurgische Arbeitsgemeinschaft fuer Onkologie der Deutschen Gesellschaft fuer Chirurgie Study Group. Arch Surg 127:1446–1450, 1992.

218. Nygaard K, Hagen S, Hansen HS, Hatlevoll R, Hultborn R, Jakobsen A, et al. Pre-operative radiotherapy prolongs survival in operable esophageal carcinoma: a randomized, multicenter study of pre-operative radiotherapy and chemotherapy. The second Scandinavian trial in esophageal cancer. World J Surg 16:1104–1109, 1992.

**Table 17-3** Schema for definitive and palliative treatment from the American Brachytherapy Society consensus guidelines for brachytherapy of esophageal cancer

| Suggested Scheme for Definitive Treatment | Suggested Scheme for Palliative Treatment |
| --- | --- |
| *External Beam Radiotherapy (EBRT)* | *Recurrence after EBRT or Short Life Expectancy* |
| 45–50 Gy in 1.8–2.0 Gy fx, 5/week with concurrent chemotherapy followed by brachytherapy[a] | Brachytherapy (HDR 10–14 Gy in 1–2 fx or LDR 20–40 Gy in a single course at 0.4–1.0 Gy/hour) |
| Brachytherapy after EBRT and not concurrent with chemotherapy | *No Previous EBRT* |
| HDR: total dose of 10 Gy, 5 Gy/fx, 1 fx/week starting 2–3 weeks following completion of EBRT | EBRT 30–40 Gy in 2–3 Gy fx followed by brachytherapy (HDR 10–14 Gy in 1–2 fx or LDR 20–25 Gy in a single course at 0.4–1.0 Gy/hour) |
| LDR: total dose of 20 Gy single course, 0.4–1.0 Gy/hour starting 2–3 weeks after completion of EBRT | *No Previous EBRT and Life Expectancy >6 Months* |
| | Guidelines similar to those for definitive therapy above |

fx, fractions; HDR, high-dose rate; LDR, low-dose rate; XRT, radiation therapy.

[a]All brachytherapy doses specified 1 cm from mid-source/mid-dwell position. Applicator diameter of 6–10 mm is recommended.

Adapted from Gaspar LE, Nag S, Herskovic A, Mantravadi R, Speiser B. American Brachytherapy Society (ABS) consensus guidelines for brachytherapy of esophageal cancer. Int J Radiat Oncol Bio Phys 38:127–132, 1997.

1 and 5 for a total dose of 40 Gy. The 5-FU was administered as a continuous infusion of 300 mg/m$^2$ for 5 days during radiation weeks 1 and 5 and increased to 1000 mg/m$^2$ during weeks 9 and 13. Carboplatin was given on the first day of each cycle at a dose of 360 mg/m$^2$. Twenty-seven patients were treated, 10 of whom had disease limited to the esophagus. Only one patient was noted to have disease progression in the radiation field.[32]

The EORTC randomized inoperable patients to receive concurrent CDDP or radiotherapy alone. Radiation was delivered at 20 Gy in five fractions two times, separated by a 15-day rest period. A CDDP dose of 100 mg/m$^2$ was given before each radiation cycle and repeated every 21–28 days for a total of six cycles. The overall median survival in the combined-therapy group was 10.5 months. There was a significant improvement in local-regional progression-free survival in the combined-therapy group ($P = 0.015$).

Other combinations of chemotherapy with radiation therapy have been of interest. Izquierdo and colleagues[33] combined sequential CDDP, bleomycin, and radiation therapy to treat unresectable nonmetastatic squamous cell carcinoma of the esophagus. The median survival was 8 months with a 4-year survival rate of 8%. A 64% improvement in dysphagia was noted.[33] More recently, pilot data have been reported on combining continuous CDDP (5–10 mg/m$^2$/day on days 1–5, 8–12, and 15–19) and 5-FU (600 mg/m$^2$ on days 1–5) with external-beam radiation therapy; 79% of patients noted relief of dysphagia.[34] The com-

bination of vinorelbine and external-beam radiation therapy also has been evaluated and found to be feasible.[35]

Paclitaxel with radiotherapy for locally advanced disease has been evaluated. Bernard and co-workers[36] reported on a phase I/II trial combining paclitaxel, 5-FU, and CDDP with radiation (45 Gy) in patients with locally advanced or metastatic disease. The study included some patients whose disease was potentially resectable. Toxicities included one grade 4 neutropenia and one grade 4 mucositis. One patient who underwent surgical resection died postoperatively of a pulmonary embolus. However, no definitive conclusions were reached.[36]

In addition to the use of newer chemotherapeutic agents, intensification of treatment also has been utilized to improve nonsurgical treatment. In Intergroup trial 0122 (five cycles of 5-FU and CDDP, three neoadjuvant and two concurrent with 64.8 Gy of radiation) the treatment-related death rate was 9%, so the regimen was not further developed.[37,38] However, the higher dose of radiation was felt to be tolerable and so formed the basis of Intergroup trial 0123. That trial randomized patients to receive 50.4 Gy or 64 Gy of radiation with concurrent chemotherapy. The chemotherapy consisted of CDDP at a dose of 75 mg/m$^2$ on day 1 and continuous infusion 5-FU at a dose of 1000 mg/m$^2$ on days 1–4 of weeks 1 and 5 during radiation. These cycles were repeated 4 weeks after radiation. This trial was recently closed early because there was no advantage to the patient receiving the higher dose (B. Minsky, personal communication, 1999). There-

**Table 17-4** Results of combined chemotherapy and radiation therapy for inoperable esophageal cancer

| Study | Patients (n) | Chemotherapy Regimen | Radiation Dose | Median Survival (Months) | 1-Year Survival | 2-Year Survival | 3-Year Survival | 5-Year Survival |
| --- | --- | --- | --- | --- | --- | --- | --- | --- |
| Roussel et al.[13] | 78 | MTX | 56.25/2.25 fx | 9 | 31 | — | 12 | — |
| Roussel et al.[14] | 110 | CDDP | 40/4 fx | NS | 47 | 20 | 8 (4 years) | — |
| Seitz et al.[31] | 35 | 5-FU, CDDP | 40/4 fx | 17 | 55 | 41 | — | — |
| Urba and Turrisi[32] | 27 | 5-FU, carboplatin | 40/2 fx, bid | 6 | — | — | — | — |
| Izquierdo et al.[33] | 25 | CCDP, bleomycin | 50–65 | 8 | 25 | — | — | — |

bid, twice a day; fx, dose per fraction; NS, not stated.

fore, if combined-modality treatment is used, concurrent 5-FU, CDDP chemotherapy, and radiotherapy is recommended. The total dose of radiation should be at least 50.4 Gy.

## Palliation of Dysphagia with Combined Chemotherapy and Radiation Therapy

Coia and co-workers[39] published a detailed analysis of swallowing function following combined radiation therapy and chemotherapy. The study included 120 patients treated with different combination regimens. The majority of the evaluable patients (88%) noted improvement in dysphagia, with a median time to initial improvement of 2 weeks. Maximum benefit was seen within 4 weeks in 86% of responding patients. There was significantly more improvement in patients with distal thoracic lesions than in those with tumor of the upper two-thirds of the esophagus (95% vs. 79%). All but two of the patients could swallow at least soft or solid food without dysphagia at the time of maximal improvement.[39]

Long-term swallowing function was assessed in 25 patients who survived for more than 1 year. Three patients developed benign strictures, all of which responded to dilatation. Seventeen patients were asymptomatic, 5 had some dysphagia to solid foods, and 3 could eat only soft foods. Two-thirds of the patients treated with palliative intent only were found to have no significant dysphagia until death or last follow-up examination.[39]

Gill and colleagues[40] treated a series of patients with combined CDDP, 5-FU, and radiation therapy. Complete durable relief of dysphagia within 2–6 weeks was noted in 60% of patients.

## Chemotherapy Alone

The use of chemotherapy alone in patients with locally unresectable nonmetastatic disease is limited. The regimens and outcomes are similar to those in patients with metastatic disease and are summarized in the next chapter.

## Conclusions: Definitive Management

Locally unresectable nonmetastatic esophageal cancer is incurable in the majority of patients. However, aggressive combined therapies do offer a small but real chance of sustained disease control. In addition, sustained relief of dysphagia is an achievable goal in most patients. Patients who can tolerate it should be treated with combined chemotherapy and radiation therapy. The use of a brachytherapy boost is yet to be defined, but the results of some series suggest that it does provide a benefit.

## Endoscopic Palliation

As we have discussed, chemotherapy and radiation therapy are important first-line treatments for patients with unresectable esophageal cancer. Unfortunately, some patients continue to manifest dysphagia after initial therapy or develop recurrent dysphagia. Other patients are poor candidates for either chemotherapy or radiation therapy. A number of alternative therapies have been developed to maintain the ability to swallow. These therapies will be reviewed because they help to improve quality of life.

## Esophageal Dilatation

Esophageal dilatation is critical in the management of esophageal cancer patients. The normal esophageal lumen has a func-

tional diameter of 25 mm. When the lumen's diameter is decreased to less than 18 mm, alterations in diet and in food consistency is necessary; when it is decreased to 13 mm, solid-food dysphagia is noted in all cases. Most malignant strictures can be safely dilated to 16 to 17 mm in several sessions.[41]

Esophageal dilation may, however, increase the risk of perforation, especially when performed during radiotherapy. In 1978, Heit and colleagues[42] reviewed their experience with 26 patients who received 616 dilatations over a 3-year period. Twenty-four patients noted improvements in swallowing. Two hundred twenty-two dilatations were accomplished during radiotherapy, and 60 were accomplished before the placement of esophageal prosthetic tubes. Only 3 complications were noted during the 616 dilatations. There was only one perforation, which was successfully managed conservatively. The perforation rate was thus less than 0.01%. There was no morbidity or mortality associated with dilatation preformed during radiotherapy.[42]

Cassidy and associates[43] reviewed their experience with 151 patients undergoing 1336 dilatations. Three serious complications were noted—two perforations and one hemorrhage (serious complication rate of 1.9%). All three of these complications resulted in death. Dilation was unsuccessful in 15% of patients, and placement of a peroral prosthesis was necessary.[43] Lundell and co-workers[44] reviewed the use of dilatation in 41 patients who underwent 128 dilatations. A prosthetic device was inserted if symptoms persisted, despite dilatations, or if significant complications arose. Perforation occurred in 5% of the dilatations. The interval between dilatations was approximately 4 weeks. Repeat dilatations were done when dysphagia recurred.[44]

It would appear that esophageal dilatation is reasonably safe and provides rapid, albeit temporary, relief of dysphagia in the majority of patients.

## Peroral Prostheses and Stents

Peroral stenting opens the lumen of the esophagus to allow the continuation of oral feeding and management of saliva (Fig. 17–2; Color Fig. 17–3, in separate color insert). Peroral pros-

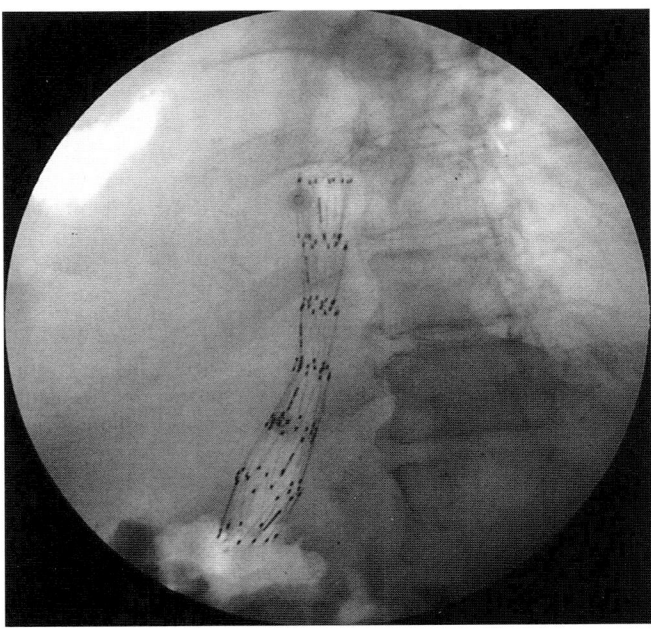

**Figure 17-2** Radiographic view of a deployed esophageal stent.

theses have been made from a number of materials over the years, including animal tusks, coiled silver wire, raw gum latex, plastic, and silicone. Recently, expandable metal stents have replaced plastic and silicone prostheses.[41]

In the initial experience with palliative stenting of the esophagus, the stenting was done at the time of laparotomy. A review of published reports by Johnson and co-workers[45] in 1976 found an overall operative mortality rate of 23% in 189 patients undergoing this procedure.

Improvements in endoscopy and technical improvements in introducers and stents allowed placement without laporotomy. Atkinson and Ferguson[46] used endoscopic placement of a Celestin tube in 13 patients. All patients experienced improvement in swallowing. There was one treatment-related death.[46] A subsequent trial by these same authors noted one death in 25 patients treated with an updated technique.[47] Unrah and Pagliero[48] compared endoscopic pulsion intubation with laparotomy-placed traction intubation. The overall complication rate was 42.9% in the pulsion group vs. 38.5% in the traction group. The hospital mortality rate was 14.3% in the pulsion group and 23.1% in the traction group.[48] Similar mortality rates were noted by Pattison and co-workers.[49] Fugger and colleagues[50] reported an 87% success rate but a 16% associated mortality rate in 95 patients who underwent endoscopic tube implantations. Gasparri and colleagues[51] reported an overall 7.6% mortality rate for 248 endoscopic intubations. They also noted an improvement in mortality when the Dumon-Gilliard type of prosthetic introducer was used.[51]

Although a successfully placed endoscopic tube is highly effective in improving the ability to swallow, the complication rate is high. Recently, the use of self-expanding metallic stents (SEMS) has begun to replace the use of plastic esophageal stents.[52] In a randomized trial in 42 patients, Knyrim and co-workers[53] compared an expandable metallic stent to a plastic prosthesis.[53] Complications were significantly reduced in the patients who received metallic stenting compared to those receiving plastic stenting ($P < 0.001$). Dysphagia and Karnofsky performance status improved significantly and to a similar degree in both treatment groups. The most common cause of recurrent dysphagia was migration in the plastic-stent group and ingrowth or overgrowth in the metal-stent group.[53] A second randomized trial of metallic stents vs. plastic stents noted a significant difference in complication rate (0% vs. 20%) and mortality rate (0% vs. 15.8%) in favor of metallic stents.[54] Segalin and associates[55] reported on 160 consecutive unselected patients treated with esophageal stenting. Approximately half the patients received a traditional Wilson Cook silicone stent positioned with a Dumon-Savary introducer, and half received a self-expanding metallic stent. The hospital morbidity rate was 14.2% in the traditional-stent group and 8% in the metallic-stent group. Dysphagia was improved in 96.8% of patients, with an overall hospital mortality rate of 1.9%.[55] Shields[56] reviewed the literature and noted an overall improvement in procedural mortality rates with metallic stents compared to plastic stents (1% vs. 7%). Ramirez and colleagues[52] surveyed gastroenterologists regarding the use of SEMS. The survey noted higher than expected technical difficulties (e.g., incomplete failure of full stent expansion, failure of deployment, and stent replacement) but a low procedural mortality rate of 0.5%.[52]

There is some debate regarding the safety of stent placement in patients who also are treated with chemotherapy, radiation, or both. Kinsman and co-workers[57] reported that esophageal stent placement after prior radiation and chemotherapy increased the risk of life-threatening complications from 2.5% to 36.4% and

increased mortality from 0% to 23%.[57] This was not seen by other authors,[56,58,59] and it has been suggested that the morbidity and mortality were likely due to the stent barbs that were used.[60] Song and colleagues[59] noted a significant increase in massive bleeding when radiotherapy was employed after stent placement in patients, although bleeding was not noted in the series reported by Segalin and associates.[55] Ludwig and co-workers[61] reported on 40 consecutive patients who underwent mesh stenting. Twelve of these patients also received concurrent chemotherapy and radiation, which significantly improved survival.[61] Raijman and colleagues[62] retrospectively analyzed records of 60 patients who underwent esophageal stenting. Among the patients with no previous chemotherapy or radiotherapy, the life-threatening complication rate was 9.5% compared with 8% in patients with previous chemotherapy, radiation, or both. There was no stent-related mortality.[62]

It appears that esophageal stenting procedures have the ability to improve swallowing and quality of life in selected esophageal cancer patients. Self-expanding metallic stents have been a major improvement over rigid prostheses, owing to their efficacy and improved side-effect profile. The integration of chemotherapy and radiation therapy remains to be fully defined.

## Laser Ablation

Fleischer and co-workers[63] were the first to describe a new technique using a high-power neodymium yttrium-aluminum-garnet (Nd:YAG) laser as an endoscopic approach to palliation of obstructive esophageal cancer. They reported on five patients who underwent 4 to 13 treatments over 8 to 28 days. All patients were able to eat solid food after completion of the therapy, and there were no significant complications.[63]

In an international survey of laser therapy for upper gastrointestinal tumor stenosis, Ell and Demling[64] noted an initial success rate of 83%. This was associated with a low 4.1% complication rate and a 1.0% mortality rate. Ell and Demling reported an 80.6% initial-improvement rate and a 1.6% mortality rate in 62 patients treated in their clinic. The dysphagia-free interval was 3 to 6 weeks.[64] In a study of 308 patients who received laser therapy, Spinelli and colleagues[65] found that 74% showed a decrease in dysphagia. The number of sessions ranged from 1 to 6 with a dysphagia-free interval of 6 to 8 weeks. Prelaser dilatation was accomplished in 31% to 50% of the patients. Complications were noted in 3% of patients, with a 1% mortality rate.[65]

A number of series have compared effects of laser therapy with those of intubation or SEMS placement. Hahl and co-workers[66] reviewed records of 96 patients treated with laser or insertion of an esophageal tube. Intubation was more successful than laser treatment (89% vs. 55%) but also produced a higher mortality rate (12% vs. 0%). Adam and co-workers[67] performed a prospective randomized trial comparing laser therapy with SEMS therapy in 60 patients. The patients who received SEMS therapy experienced significantly better palliation in both the short and long term ($P = 0.003$). All patients treated with laser therapy alone required repeat treatment every 4 to 5 weeks.[67]

In summary, laser therapy improves swallowing in the majority of patients and is associated with a favorable complication rate. In general, more than one application is needed for initial improvement. The palliation is limited, and laser therapy often must be repeated every 4 to 6 weeks. Laser ablation may be helpful in the ablation of polypoid eccentric intraluminal masses prior to stent placement, in prevention of tumor overgrowth or ingrowth after stenting, or in achievement of homeostasis for bleeding.[41]

## Photodynamic Therapy and Chemical Ablation

Photodynamic therapy involves the administration of a chemical photosensitizer that accumulates in higher concentration in neoplastic cells than in normal tissue. After approximately 48 hours, the tissue is exposed to a laser, leading to a chemical reaction that produces oxygen radicals that destroy cells. Lightdale and associates[68] preformed a large randomized trial comparing photodynamic therapy to laser ablation in 236 patients. The response rates at 1 month were 32% in the photodynamic-therapy group and 20% in the laser-therapy group ($P < 0.05$). The improvement in mean dysphagia grade was similar ($-0.75$ in photodynamic-therapy group and $-0.67$ in the laser-therapy group). Time to palliation failure was 74 days in the photodynamic-therapy group and 42 days in the laser-therapy group. There were more mild to moderate complications, including sunburn, following photodynamic therapy.[68]

Endoscopic ethanol tumor injection has been used to produce tumor necrosis. Payne-James and associates[69] reported on 11 patients treated with ethanol injection, six of whom also received dilatation. Ten of 11 patients (91%) improved by at least one dysphagia grade after one treatment, and all patients eventually improved. The mean number of dilatations and injections per patient was 1.2 and 3.3, respectively.[69] Carazzonne and co-workers[70] recently performed a randomized trial of laser therapy vs. intratumoral ethanol injection in 47 patients. There was a much higher incidence of pain with the alcohol injections than with the laser ablation. The success rate was higher in the laser-treated group than in the ethanol-treated group (88% vs. 78%). The mean dysphagia-free intervals for the two groups were 30 and 37 days, respectively.[70]

## Conclusions

The treatment of unresectable nonmetastatic esophageal cancer is a challenging clinical problem for surgeons, medical oncologists, radiation oncologists, and gastroenterologists. Unfortunately, even with aggressive combined-modality therapy, the majority of patients will succumb to their disease. Treatments need to be individualized, with emphasis on maintaining as high a quality of life as possible.

## References

1. Merriam-Webster's Medical Desk Dictionary. Merriam-Webster, Inc., Massachusetts, 1993.
2. Coia LR, Myerson RJ, Tepper JE. Late effects of radiation therapy on the gastrointestinal tract. Int J Radiat Oncol Biol Phys 31:1213–1236, 1995.
3. Bolton JS, Fuhrman GM, Richardson WS. Esophageal resection for cancer. Surg Clin North Am 78:773–794, 1998.
4. Mannell A, Becker PJ, Nissenbaum M. Bypass surgery for unresectable oesophageal cancer: early and late results in 124 cases. Br J Surg 75:283–286, 1988.
5. Segalin A, Little AG, Ruol A, et al. Surgical and endoscopic palliation of esophageal carcinoma. Ann Thorac Surg 48:267–271, 1989.
6. Orringer MB. Substernal gastric bypass of the excluded esophagus: results of an ill-advised operation. Surgery 96:467–470, 1984.
7. Hirai T, Yamashita Y, Mukaida H, et al. Bypass operation for advanced esophageal cancer: an analysis of 93 cases. Jpn J Surg 19:182–188, 1989.
8. van Andel JG, Dees J, Dijkhuis CM, et al. Carcinoma of the esophagus: results of treatment. Ann Surg 190:684–689, 1979.
9. Petrovich Z, Langholz B, Formenti S, Luxton G, Astrahan M. Management of carcinoma of the esophagus: the role of radiotherapy. Am J Clin Oncol 14:80–86, 1991.
10. Okawa T, Kita M, Tanaka M, Ikeda M. Results of radiotherapy for inoperable locally advanced esophageal cancer. Int J Radiat Oncol Biol Phys 17:49–54, 1989.
11. De-Ren S. Ten-year follow-up of esophageal cancer treated by radical radiation therapy: analysis of 869 patients. Int J Radiat Oncol Biol Phys 16:329–334, 1989.
12. Caspers RJL, Welvaart K, Verkes RJ, Hermans J, Leer JWH. The effect of radiotherapy on dysphagia and survival in patients with esophageal cancer. Radiother Oncol 12:15–23, 1988.
13. Roussel A, Jacob JH, Haegele, et al. Controlled clinical trial for the treatment of patients with inoperable esophageal carcinoma: a study of the EORTC Gastrointestinal Tract Cancer Cooperative Group. In: Schlag P, Hohenberger P, Metzger U (eds): Combined Modality Therapy of Gastrointestinal Tract Cancer. Springer-Verlag, Berlin-Heidelberg, 1988, pp 21–29.
14. Roussel A, Haegele P, Paillot B, et al. Results of the EORTC-GTCCG phase III trial of irradiation vs irradiation and CDDP in inoperable esophageal cancer (abstract 583). Proc Am Soc Clin Oncol 13:199, 1994.
15. Herskovic A, Martz K, Al-Sarraf M, et al. Combined chemotherapy and radiotherapy compared with radiotherapy alone in patients with cancer of the esophagus. N Engl J Med 326:1593–1598, 1992.
16. Al-Sarraf M, Martz K, Herskovic A, et al. Progress report of combined chemoradiotherapy versus radiotherapy alone in patients with esophageal cancer: an Intergroup study. J Clin Oncol 15:277–284, 1997.
17. Wara WM, Mauch PM, Thomas AN, Phillips TL. Palliation for carcinoma of the esophagus. Radiology 121:717–720, 1976.
18. O'Rourke IC, Tiver K, Bull C, Gebski V, Langlands AO. Swallowing performance after radiation therapy for carcinoma of the esophagus. Cancer 61:2022–2026, 1998.
19. Gaspar LE, Nag S, Herskovic A, Mantravadi R, Speiser B. American Brachytherapy Society (ABS) consensus guidelines for brachytherapy of esophageal cancer. Int J Radiat Oncol Biol Phys 38:127–132, 1997.
20. International Commission on Radiation Units and Measurements. Dose and Volume Specification for Reporting Intracavitary Therapy in Gynecology: Report 38. Bethesda, MD, International Commission on Radiation Units and Measurements, 1985.
21. Fleischman EH, Kagan R, Bellotti JE, Streeter OE, Harvey JC. Effective palliation for inoperable esophageal cancer using intensive intracavitary radiation. J Surg Oncol 44:234–237, 1990.
22. Fontanesi J, Rodriguez RR, Robinson JC. Intracavitary irradiation as a primary treatment for unresectable esophageal carcinoma. Endocuriether Hypertherm Oncol 5:231–234, 1989.
23. Jager JJ, Pannebakker M, Rijken J, de Vos J, Vismuans FJ. Palliation in esophageal cancer with a single session of intraluminal irradiation. Radiother Oncol 25:134–136, 1992.
24. Sur RK, Singh DP, Sharma SC, et al. Radiation therapy of esophageal cancer: role of high dose rate brachytherapy. Int J Radiat Oncol Biol Phys 22:1043–1046, 1992.
25. Yin WB. Brachytherapy of carcinoma of the esophagus in China, 1970–1974 and 1982–1984. In: Martinez AA, Orton CG, Mould RF (eds): Brachytherapy: HDR and LDR. Nucletron Corp, Columbia, MD, 1990, pp 52–56.
26. Calais G, Dorval E, Louisot P, et al. Radiotherapy with high dose rate brachytherapy boost and concomitant chemotherapy for stages IIB and III esophageal carcinoma: results of a pilot study. Int J Radiat Oncol Biol Phys 38:769–775, 1997.
27. Iwasa M, Ohmori Y, Iwasa Y, et al. Effect of multidisciplinary treatment with high dose rate intraluminal brachytherapy on survival in patients with unresectable esophageal cancer. Digest Surg 15:227–235, 1998.
28. Okawa T, Dokiya T, Nishio M, Hishikawa Y, Morita K. Multi-institutional randomized trial of external radiotherapy with and without intraluminal brachytherapy for esophageal cancer in Japan. Int J Radiat Oncol Biol Phys 45:623–628, 1999.
29. Gaspar LE. Esophageal brachytherapy: a phantom menace? Int J Radiat Oncol Biol Phys 45:549–550, 1999.
30. Gaspar LE, Qian C, Kocha WI, Coia LR, Herskovic A, Graham M. A phase I/II study of external beam radiation, brachytherapy and concurrent chemotherapy in localized cancer of the esophagus (RTOG 92-07): preliminary toxicity report. Int J Radiat Oncol Biol Phys 37:593–599, 1997.
31. Seitz JF, Giovannini M, Padaut-Cesana J, et al. Inoperable nonmetastatic squamous cell carcinoma of the esophagus managed by concomitant chemotherapy (5-fluorouracil and cisplatin) and radiation therapy. Cancer 66:214–219, 1990.
32. Urba SG, Turrisi AT III. Split-course accelerated radiation therapy combined with carboplatin and 5-fluorouracil for palliation of metastatic or unresectable carcinoma of the esophagus. Cancer 75:435–439, 1995.
33. Izquierdo MA, Marcuello E, de Segura GG, et al. Unresectable nonmetastatic squamous cell carcinoma of the esophagus managed by sequential chemotherapy (cisplatin and bleomycin) and radiation therapy. Cancer 71:287–292, 1993.

34. Teruy M, Itoh A, Morita K, et al. A low dose of cisplatin infusion prior to radiation and continuous 5-fluorouracil infusion as a chemoradiation therapy (CRT) for advanced esophageal cancer: results of a pilot study (abstract 1121). Proc Am Soc Clin Oncol 18:292, 1999.

35. Adeni A, Francois E, Conroy T, et al. Phase I study of vinorelbine and concurrent radiation for locally advanced esophageal cancer (abstract 1041). Proc Am Soc Clin Oncol 18:271, 1999.

36. Bernard S, Poole M, Socinski M, et al. Paclitaxel (T) combined with 5-fluorouracil (FU) and cisplatin (P) concomitant with radiotherapy (RT) in locally advanced or metastatic esophageal cancer—preliminary report of a phase I/II trials (abstract 1102). Proc Am Soc Clin Oncol 17:286, 1998.

37. Minsky BD, Neuberg D, Kelsen DP, Pisansky TM, Ginsberg R, Benson A III. Neoadjuvant chemotherapy plus concurrent chemotherapy and high-dose radiation for squamous cell carcinoma of the esophagus: a preliminary analysis of the phase II Intergroup Trial 0122. J Clin Oncol 14:149–155, 1996.

38. Minsky BD, Neuberg D, Kelsen DP, Pisansky TM, Ginsberg RJ, Pajak T. Final report of Intergroup Trial 0122 (ECOG PE-289, RTOG 90-12): phase II trial of neoadjuvant chemotherapy plus concurrent chemotherapy and high-dose radiation for squamous cell carcinoma of the esophagus. Int J Radiat Oncol Biol Phys 43:517–523, 1999.

39. Coia LW, Soffen EM, Schultheiss TE, Martin EE, Hanks GE. Swallowing function in patients with esophageal cancer treated with concurrent radiation and chemotherapy. Cancer 71:281–286, 1993.

40. Gill PG, Denham JW, Jamieson GG, Devitt PG, Yeah E, Olwany C. Patterns of treatment failure and prognostic factors associated with the treatment of esophageal carcinoma with chemotherapy and radiotherapy either as sole treatment or followed by surgery. J Clin Oncol 10:1037–1043, 1992.

41. Boyce HW. Palliation of dysphagia of esophageal cancer by endoscopic lumen restoration techniques. Cancer Control 6:73–83, 1999.

42. Heit HA, Johnson LF, Siegel SR, Boyce HW. Palliative dilation for dysphagia in esophageal carcinoma. Ann Intern Med 89(part 1):629–631, 1978.

43. Cassidy DE, Nord HJ, Boyce HW. Management of malignant esophageal strictures: role of esophageal dilation and peroral prosthesis. Am J Gastroenter 75:173, 1981.

44. Lundell L, Leth R, Lind T, Lonroth H, Sjovall M, Olbe L. Palliative endoscopic dilatation in carcinoma of the esophagus and esophagogastric junction. Acta Chir Scand 155:179–184, 1989.

45. Johnson IR, Balfour TW, Bourke JB. Intubation of malignant gastrooesophageal strictures: a modification of the Mousseau-Barbin technique. J R Coll Surg Edinb 21:225–228, 1976.

46. Atkinson M, Ferguson R. Fibreoptic endoscopic palliative intubation of inoperable oesophagogastric neoplasms. BMJ 1:266–267, 1977.

47. Atkinson M, Gerguson R, Parker GC. Tube introducer and modified Celestin tube for use in palliative intubation of oesophagogastric neoplasms at fibreoptic endoscopy. Gut 19:669–671, 1978.

48. Unruh HW, Pagliero KM. Pulsion intubation versus traction intubation for obstructing carcinomas of the esophagus. Ann Thorac Surg 40:337–342, 1985.

49. Pattison CW, Griffin SC, Coker C, Townsend ER, Fountain SW. Palliative intubation of malignant oesophageal strictures. Scand J Thorac Cardiovasc Surg 24:153–155, 1990.

50. Fugger R, Niederle B, Jantsch H, Schiessel R, Schultz F. Endoscopic tube implantation for the palliation of malignant esophageal stenosis. Endoscopy 22:101–104, 1990.

51. Gasparri G, Casalegno PA, Camandona M, et al. Endoscopic insertion of 248 prostheses in inoperable carcinoma of the esophagus and cardia: short-term and long-term results. Gastrointest Endosc 33:354–356, 1987.

52. Ramirez FC, Dennert B, Zierer ST, Sanowski RA. Esophageal self-expandable metallic stents—indications, practice, techniques, and com-

plications: results of a national survey. Gastrointest Endosc 45:360–364, 1997.

53. Knyrim K, Wagner HJ, Bethge N, Keymling M, Vakil N. A controlled trial of an expansile metal stent for palliation of esophageal obstruction due to inoperable cancer. N Engl J Med 329:1302–1307, 1993.

54. De Palma GD, di Matteo E, Romano G, Fimmano A, Rondinone G, Catanzano C. Plastic prosthesis versus expandable metal stents for palliation of inoperable esophageal thoracic carcinoma: a controlled prospective study. Gastrointest Endosc 43:478–482, 1996.

55. Segalin A, Bonavina L, Carazzone A, Ceriani C, Peracchia A. Improving results of esophageal stenting: a study on 160 consecutive unselected patients. Endoscopy 29:701–709, 1997.

56. Shields SJ. Esophageal self-expandable metallic stents. Gastrointest Endosc 45:439–442, 1997.

57. Kinsman KJ, DeGregorio BT, Katon RM, et al. Prior radiation and chemotherapy increase the risk of life-threatening complications after insertion of metallic stents for esophagogastric malignancy [see comments]. Gastrointest Endosc 43:196–203, 1996.

58. Kozarek RA, Raltz S, Brugge WR, et al. Prospective multicenter trial of esophageal Z-stent placement for malignant dysphagia and tracheoesophageal fistula [published erratum appears in Gastrointest Endosc 44:764, 1996]. Gastrointest Endosc 44:562–567, 1996.

59. Song HY, Do YS, Han YM, et al. Covered, expandable esophageal metallic stent tubes: experiences in 119 patients. Radiology 193:689–695, 1994.

60. Kozarek RA, Raltz S, Marcon N, et al. Use of the 25-mm flanged esophageal Z stent for malignant dysphagia: a prospective multicenter trial. Gastrointest Endosc 46:156–160, 1997.

61. Ludwig D, Dehne A, Burmester E, Wiedeman GJ, Strange EF. Treatment of unresectable carcinoma of the esophagus of the gastroesophageal junction by mesh stents with or without radiochemotherapy. Int J Oncol 13:583–588, 1998.

62. Raijman I, Siddique I, Lynch P. Does chemoradiation therapy increase the incidence of complications with self-expanding coated stents in the management of malignant esophageal strictures? Am J Gastroenterol 92:2192–2196, 1997.

63. Fleischer D, Kessler F, Haye O. Endoscopic Nd:YAG laser therapy for carcinoma of the esophagus: a new palliative approach. Am J Surg 143:280–283, 1982.

64. Ell C, Demling L. Laser therapy of tumor stenoses in the upper gastrointestinal tract: an international inquiry. Lasers Surg Med 7:491–494, 1987.

65. Spinelli P, Dal Fante M, Mancini A. Endoscopic palliation of malignancies of the upper gastrointestinal tract using Nd:YAG laser: results and survival in 308 treated patients. Lasers Surg Med 11:550–555, 1991.

66. Hahl J, Salo J, Ovaska J, Haapiainen R, Kalima T, Schroder T. Comparison of endoscopic Nd:YAG laser therapy and oesophageal tube in palliation of oesophagogastric malignancy. Scand J Gastroenterol 26:103–108, 1991.

67. Adam A, Ellul J, Watkinson AF, et al. Palliation of inoperable esophageal carcinoma: a prospective randomized trial of laser therapy and stent placement. Radiology 202:344–348, 1997.

68. Lightdale CJ, Heier SK, Marcon NE, et al. Photodynamic therapy with porfimer sodium versus thermal ablation therapy with Nd:YAG laser for palliation of esophageal cancer: a multicenter randomized trial. Gastrointest Endosc 42:507–512, 1995.

69. Payne-James JJ, Spiller RC, Misiewicz, Silk DBA. Use of ethanol-induced tumor necrosis to palliate dysphagia in patients with esophagogastric cancer. Gastrointest Endosc 36:43–46, 1990.

70. Carazzone A, Bonavina L, Segalin A, Ceriani C, Peracchia A. Endoscopic palliation of oesophageal cancer: results of a prospective comparison of Nd:YAG laser and ethanol injection. Eur J Surg 165:351–356, 1999.

# Chapter 18

# Clinical Aspects and Management of Metastatic Carcinoma of the Esophagus and Gastroesophageal Junction

JAFFER A. AJANI AND GEORGE R. BLUMENSCHEIN

Esophageal and gastroesophageal junction carcinomas are rare in Western countries. Because screening is not feasible or cost-effective, most patients are diagnosed in an advanced stage. Nearly 50% of patients diagnosed with carcinoma of the esophagus or gastroesophageal junction have technically unresectable cancers, often manifesting as metastatic carcinoma. Patients who have metastatic carcinoma of the esophagus or gastroesophageal junction have a life expectancy ranging from 6 to 9 months, and it would be rare for any patient to survive 5 years.

The therapeutic approach to patients with metastatic or locally advanced, unresectable esophageal or gastroesophageal carcinoma is palliative. In addition to supportive care, which may include pain control and other comfort measures, patients may be offered a variety of palliative procedures directed at specific symptoms. These include chemotherapy, chemoradiotherapy, radiotherapy alone, or an endoscopy-directed palliative procedure. The value of chemoradiotherapeutic and endoscopic palliative approaches has been described in Chapter 17.

## Chemotherapy

Proper selection of patients for palliation by chemotherapy is of paramount importance. The likelihood of achieving a response and a positive palliative effect is higher among patients with a better performance status (2 or less) than among those with a poor performance status. Patients with a performance status of 3 or more should not be considered for chemotherapy, as it often results in severe and occasionally fatal toxic effects. In addition, before instituting even a moderately toxic chemotherapy, adequate nutritional support and pain control should be established. The patient's general condition should be improved as much as possible, although such interventions may not be effective in some patients. The degree of weight loss appears to be correlated with performance status. Patients with excessive weight loss (greater than 10% loss of body mass) have a much worse outcome than do those with slight or no weight loss.

When chemotherapy is deemed appropriate, the available options should be discussed thoroughly with the patient and the immediate family members or caretakers.

## Single Agents

In the past, investigations into chemotherapeutic agents that might be effective against squamous cell carcinoma and adenocarcinoma of the esophagus and gastroesophageal junction were largely ignored. As a result, the number of established chemotherapeutic drugs documented to be active against esophageal carcinoma is small. Until 1993, only 16 cytotoxic agents had been investigated systematically against metastatic esophageal carcinoma.[1] Because squamous cell carcinoma was the most commonly encountered histologic type approximately 15 years ago, nearly all conventional chemotherapeutic agents' activity was established against squamous cell cancers. Research into chemotherapy for adenocarcinoma of the esophagus is quite limited.

Among the older group of chemotherapeutic agents, cisplatin is considered to be one of the most active, with a single-agent response rate consistently greater than or equal to 20%.[2,3] Other older chemotherapeutic agents, such as 5 fluorouracil (5-FU), mitomycin, bleomycin, methotrexate, mitoguazone, doxorubicin, and vindesine, are also considered to be active.[4] Cisplatin, 5-FU, and mitomycin are still being used with some degree of frequency against squamous cell carcinoma and adenocarcinoma of the esophagus or gastroesophageal junction. These agents are often used in combination, particularly with newer agents.

Among the newer agents, paclitaxel (Taxol), docetaxel (Taxotere), vinorelbine (Navelbine), lobaplatin, and carboplatin (Para-

**Table 18–1** Results of single-agent chemotherapy in patients with squamous cell carcinoma and adenocarcinoma of the esophagus

| Drug | Total Patients (n) | Responses n (%) |
|---|---|---|
| Bleomycin[9–15] | 81 | 24 (30) |
| CCNU[16] | 19 | 3 (16) |
| Carboplatin[8] | 30 | 2 (7) |
| Cisplatin[1,17–19] | 231 | 56 (24) |
| Dichloromethotrexate[20] | 27 | 0 (0) |
| Doxorubicin[21,22] | 38 | 7 (18) |
| Etoposide[23] | 20 | 0 (0) |
| 5-FU[21,24] | 39 | 15 (38) |
| Ifosfamide[25] | 32 | 2 (6) |
| Methyl-GAG[26–28] | 64 | 15 (23) |
| Mitomycin[18,29] | 33 | 11 (33) |
| Methotrexate[21,30] | 70 | 25 (36) |
| Paclitaxel[5] | 53 | 16 (30) |
| Trimetrexate[31] | 24 | 3 (13) |
| Vindesine[32–34] | 84 | 19 (23) |
| Vinorelbine[35] | 30 | 6 (20) |
| CPT-11[36] | 13 | 1 (8) |

platin) have shown activity.[5–8] Information on the single-agent activity of CPT-11 (irinotecan) is limited. However, this agent also would be expected to have a moderate degree of single-agent activity against squamous cell carcinoma and adenocarcinoma of the esophagus.

Among the taxanes, paclitaxel has been investigated more extensively than docetaxel. However, the overall response rate would be expected to be similar for both agents. Thus, both agents may be considered to be active against carcinoma of the esophagus, producing a response rate of approximately 25%. More importantly, in one study,[5] paclitaxel was found to be active against both squamous cell carcinoma and adenocarcinoma. This finding is important because adenocarcinoma of the esophagus and gastroesophageal junction has become more common than squamous cell carcinoma. CPT-11 has also demonstrated activity against adenocarcinoma of the esophagus. Vinorelbine, carboplatin, and lobaplatin have shown varying levels of activity against squamous cell carcinoma of the esophagus. Results of single-agent trials are summarized in Table 18–1. In summary, single-agent therapy results in a low response rate, short duration of response, and limited palliation. Therefore, the quest for new chemotherapeutic agents that are active against these cancers must continue.

## Combination Chemotherapy

Combination chemotherapy is used frequently for metastatic carcinoma of the esophagus and new approaches continue to evolve. Compared with adenocarcinoma, Therapy of Advanced Carcinoma of squamous cell carcinoma is more sensitive to chemotherapy, chemoradiation, or radiotherapy alone, but the long-term outcome of patients is similar irrespective of histologic type.[37]

Many combination regimens have evolved from older agents, but 5-FU plus cisplatin is considered to be the standard combination of chemotherapy for patients with carcinoma of the esophagus or gastroesophageal junction.[38] It is the most thoroughly investigated and most commonly used regimen. Reported response rates to this combination range from 20% to 50%.[29]

In a randomized phase II study, 92 patients with advanced squamous cell carcinoma were assigned to either 5-FU plus cisplatin or cisplatin alone.[39] Among 88 evaluable patients eligible, the response rate to the combination was 35%, compared with 19% for cisplatin alone. The duration of response was also longer with the combination chemotherapy, but the survival times were similar. It should be noted, however, that this study was not designed to detect a difference in survival time. The combination chemotherapy was more toxic than single-agent therapy. Thus, combination of 5-FU and cisplatin results in a higher response rate and longer response duration compared with 5-FU alone.

Combinations of older and newer drugs are producing some encouraging results. Among these are combinations including paclitaxel or CPT-11. A study evaluating the effects of paclitaxel, 5-FU, and cisplatin in 61 previously untreated patients with advanced adenocarcinoma or squamous cell carcinoma achieved a 48% response rate among 60 evaluable patients. Fourteen of the 30 patients with adenocarcinoma responded, compared with 15 of the 30 patients with squamous cell carcinoma. However, the rate of complete response was much higher in patients with squamous cell carcinoma than in those with adenocarcinoma.[40]

A combination of CPT-11 and cisplatin has also demonstrated activity against squamous cell carcinoma and adenocarcinoma of the esophagus.[41] Table 18–2 summarizes the results of numerous trials of combination chemotherapy. More investigations of these classes of combinations are necessary.

## Conclusion

In summary, chemotherapy for carcinoma of the esophagus has come a long way, but in contrast to clinical investigations for gastric carcinoma, randomized phase III studies are distinctly lacking. Many active combinations have been identified, and a concerted effort could be made to perform systematic phase III studies. Moreover, future investigations should integrate a variety of new classes of agents including antigrowth and antimetastatic agents.

**Table 18–2** Results of combination chemotherapy of advanced squamous cell carcinoma and adenocarcinoma of the esophagus

| Drug Combination | Total Patients (n) | Responses n (%) |
|---|---|---|
| Ara-C + cisplatin + 5-FU[42] | 32 | 13 (41) |
| Bleomycin + cisplatin + vindesine[43–46] | 150 | 72 (48) |
| Bleomycin + cisplatin + methotrexate + methyl-GAG[47] | 14 | 9 (64) |
| Bleomycin + cisplatin + methotrexate[48,49] | 44 | 13 (30) |
| Bleomycin + methotrexate[15] | 5 | 3 (60) |
| Cisplatin + methotrexate[30] | 42 | 32 (76) |
| Cisplatin + bleomycin[50] | 70 | 11 (16) |
| Cisplatin + folinic acid + methotrexate + vincristine[51] | 28 | 19 (68) |
| Cisplatin + methyl-GAG + vindesine[52,53] | 73 | 32 (44) |
| Cisplatin + 5-FU[12,54–56] | 142 | 87 (61) |
| Cisplatin + 5-FU + etoposide[57] | 35 | 17 (49) |
| Cisplatin + 5-FU + interferon-α[58] | 25 | 13 (52) |
| 5-FU + interferon-α[59] | 37 | 10 (27) |
| Cisplatin + paclitaxel[60] | 64 | 29 (45) |
| 5-FU + paclitaxel + cisplatin[40] | 60 | 29 (48) |
| CPT-11 + cisplatin[41] | 35 | 20 (57) |
| Doxorubicin + cisplatin + 5-FU[61] | 21 | 7 (33) |
| Doxorubicin + cisplatin + etoposide[62] | 26 | 13 (50) |

## References

1. Wittes RE, Adrianza ME, Parsons R, et al. Compilation of phase II results with single antineoplastic agents. Cancer Treat Rep 4:91–130, 1985.
2. Kelsen D. Treatment of advanced esophageal cancer. Cancer 50:2576–2581, 1982.
3. Leichman L, Berry BT. Experience with cisplatin in treatment regimens for esophageal cancer. Semin Oncol 18:64–72, 1991.
4. Ajani JA. Contribution of chemotherapy in the treatment of carcinoma of the esophagus: results and commentary. Semin Oncol 21:474–482, 1994.
5. Ajani JA, Ilson DH, Daugherty K, et al. Activity of Taxol in patients with squamous cell carcinoma and adenocarcinoma of the esophagus. J Natl Cancer Inst 86:1086–1091,1994.
6. Conroy T, Etienne PL, Adenis A, et al. Phase II trial of vinorelbine in metastatic squamous cell esophageal carcinoma. J Clin Oncol 14:164–170, 1996.
7. Schmoll HJ, Kohne CH, Papageorglou E, et al. Single-agent lobaplatin is active in patients with oesophageal carcinoma: A phase II evaluation [abstract]. Proc Am Soc Clin Oncol 14:201, 1995.
8. Sternberg C, Kelsen D, Dukeman M, et al. Carboplatin: new platinum analog in the treatment of epidermoid carcinoma of the esophagus. Cancer Treat Rep 69:1305–1307,1985.
9. Kolaric K, Maricic Z, Dujmovic I, et al. Therapy of advanced esophageal cancer with bleomycin, irradiation and combination bleomycin and irradiation. Tumori 62:255–262, 1976.
10. Bonadonna G, de Lena M, Monfardini S, et al. Clinical trial with bleomycin in lymphomas and in solid tumors. Eur J Cancer 8:205–215, 1972.
11. Ravry M, Moertel CG, Schutt AJ, et al. Treatment of advanced squamous cell carcinoma of the gastrointestinal tract with bleomycin (NSC 125066). Cancer Chemother Rep 57:493–395, 1973.
12. Stephens F. Bleomycin: a new approach in cancer chemotherapy. Med J Aust 1:1277–1283, 1973.
13. Yagoda A, Mukherji, B, Young C, et al. Bleomycin, an antitumor antibiotic: clinical experience in 274 patients. Ann Intern Med 77:861–870, 1972.
14. Study of the clinical efficacy of bleomycin in human cancer. BMJ 2:643–645, 1970.
15. Tancini G, Bajetta E, Bonadonna G. Bleomycin alone and in combination with methodrexate in the treatment of carcinoma of the esophagus. Tumori 60:65–71, 1974.
16. Moertel CG, Schutt AJ, Reitemeier RJ, et al. Therapy for gastrointestinal cancer with the nitrosourea alone and in drug combination. Cancer Treat Rep 60:729–732, 1976.
17. Murthy SK, Prabhakaran PS, Chandasekar M, et al. Neoadjuvant cis-DDP in esophageal cancers: an experience at a regional cancer centre, India. J Surg Oncol 45:173–176, 1990.
18. Engstrom PF, Lavin PT, Klaassen DJ. Phase II evaluation of mitomycin and cisplatin in advanced esophageal carcinoma. 67:713–715, 1983.
19. Bleiberg H, Jacob J, Bedenne L, et al. Randomized phase II trial of 5-fluorouracil and cisplatin versus cisplatin alone in advanced esophageal cancer [abstract]. Proc Am Soc Clin Oncol 10:145, 1991.
20. Bajorin D, Kelsen D, Heelan R. Phase II trial of dichloromethotrexate in epidermoid carcinoma of the esophagus. Cancer Treat Rep 70:1245–1246, 1986.
21. Edzinli EZ, Gelber R, Desai DV, et al. Chemotherapy of advanced esophageal carcinoma: Eastern Cooperative Oncology Group experience. Cancer 46:2149–2153,1980.
22. Kolaric K, Maricic Z, Roth A, et al. Adriamycin alone and in combination with radiotherapy in the treatment of inoperable esophageal cancer. Tumori 63:485–491,1977.
23. Coonley CJ, Bains M, Heelan R, et al. Phase II study of etoposide in the treatment of esophageal carcinoma. Cancer Treat Rep 67:397–398, 1983.
24. Lokich JJ, Shea M, Chaffey J. Sequential infusional 5-fluorouracil followed by concomitant radiation for tumors of the esophagus and gastroesophageal junction. Cancer 60:275–279, 1987.
25. Nanus DM, Kelsen DP, Lipperman R, et al. Phase II trial of ifosfamide in epidermoid carcinoma of the esophagus: unexpectant severe toxicity. Invest New Drug 6:239–241, 1988.
26. Ravry MJR, Omura GA, Hill GJ, et al. Phase II evaluation of mitoguazone in cancer of the esophagus, stomach, and pancreas: a Southeastern Cancer Study Group trial. Cancer Treat Rep 70:533–534, 1986.
27. Kelsen D, Chapman R, Bains M, et al. Phase II study of methyl-GAG in the treatment of esophageal carcinoma. Cancer Treat Rep 66:1427–1429, 1982.
28. Falkson G. Methyl-GAG (NSC-32946) in the treatment of esophagus cancer. Cancer Chemother Rep 55:209–212,1971.
29. Whittington R, Close H. Clinical experience with mitomycin C. Cancer Chemother Rep 54:195–198, 1970.
30. Advani SH, Saikia TK, Swaroop S, et al. Anterior chemotherapy in esophageal cancer. Cancer 56:1502–1506, 1985.
31. Alberts AS, Falkson G, Badad M, et al. Trimetrexate in advanced carcinoma of the esophagus. Invest New Drugs 6:319–321, 1988.
32. Kelsen DP, Bains M, Cvitkovic E, et al. Vindesine in the treatment of esophageal carcinoma: a phase II study. Cancer Treat Rep 63:2019–2021, 1979.
33. Bedikian AY, Valdivieso M, Bodey GP, et al. Phase II evaluation of vindesine in the treatment of colorectal and esophageal tumors. Cancer Chemother Pharmacol 2:263–266, 1979.
34. Bezwoda WR, Derman DP, Weaving A, et al. Treatment of esophageal cancer with vindesine: an open trial. Cancer Treat Rep 68:783–785, 1984.
35. Conroy T, Etienne PL, Adenis A, et al. Phase II trial of vinorelbine in metastatic squamous cell esophageal carcinoma. J Clin Oncol 14:164–170, 1996.
36. Hecth JR, Parson M, Rosen LS. A phase II trial of irinotecan (CPT-11) in patients with adenocarcinoma of the esophagus and gastric cardia. Proc Am Soc Clin Oncol 18:287a, 1999.
37. Kelsen DP, Ginsberg R, Pajak T, et al. Preoperative chemotherapy followed by operation versus operation alone for patients with localized esophageal cancers: U.S. National Intergroup Study. N Engl J Med 339:1979–1984, 1998.
38. National Comprehensive Cancer Network. Practice guidelines for upper gastrointestinal carcinomas. Oncology 12:179–213, 1998.
39. Bleiberg H, Conroy T, Paillot B, et al. Randomized phase II study of cisplatin and 5-fluorouracil versus cisplatin alone in advanced squamous cell oesophageal cancer. Eur J Cancer 33:1216–1220, 1997.
40. Ilson DH, Ajani JA, Bhalla K, et al. A phase II trial of paclitaxel, fluorouracil, and cisplatin in patients with advanced carcinoma of the esophagus. J Clin Oncol 16:1826–1834, 1998.
41. Ilson DH, Saltz L, Enzinger P, et al. Phase II trial of weekly irinotecan plus cisplatin in advanced esophageal cancer. J Clin Oncol 17:3270–3275, 1999.
42. Ajani JA, Roth JA, Putnam JB, et al. Feasibility of five courses of preoperative chemotherapy in patients with resectable adenocarcinoma of the esophagus or gastroesophageal junction. Eur J Cancer 31:665–670, 1995.
43. Kelsen D, Hilaris B, Coonley C, et al. Cisplatin, vindesine; and bleomycin chemotherapy of local-regional and advanced esophageal carcinoma. Am J Med 75:645–652, 1983.
44. Dinwoodie WR, Bartolucci AA, Lyman GH, et al. Phase II evaluation of cisplatin, bleomycin, and vindesine in advanced squamous cell carcinoma of the esophagus: a Southeastern Cancer Study Group trial. Cancer Treat Rep 70:267–270, 1986.
45. Roth JA, Pass HI, Flanagan MM, et al. Randomized clinical trial of preoperative and postoperative adjuvant chemotherapy with cisplatin, vindesine, and bleomycin for carcinoma of the esophagus. J Thorac Cardiovasc Surg 96:242–248, 1988.
46. Kelsen DP, Minsky B, Smith M, et al. Preoperative therapy for esophageal cancer. A randomized comparison of chemotherapy versus radiation therapy. J Clin Oncol 8:1352–1361, 1990.
47. Vogl SE, Camacho F, Berenzweig M, et al. Chemotherapy for esophageal cancer with mitoguazone, methotrexate, cisplatin, and bleomycin. Cancer Treat Rep 69:21–23, 1985.
48. DeBesi P, Salvagno L, Endrizzi L, et al. Cisplatin, bleomycin, and methotrexate in the treatment of advanced oesophageal cancer. Eur J Cancer Clin Oncol 20:743–747, 1984.
49. Vogl SE, Greenwald E, Kaplan BH. Effective chemotherapy for esophageal cancer with methotrexate, bleomycin, and cis-diamminedichloroplatinum. Cancer 48:2555–2558, 1981.
50. Coonley CJ, Bains M, Hilaris B, et al. Cisplatin and bleomycin in the treatment of esophageal carcinoma. A final report. Cancer 54:2351–2355, 1984.
51. Resbeut M, Prise-Fleury EL, Ben-Hassel M, et al. Squamous cell carcinoma of the esophagus. Treatment by combined vincristine-methotrexate plus folinic acid rescue and cisplatin before radiotherapy. Cancer 56:1246–1250, 1985.
52. Forastiere AA, Gennis M, Orringer MB, et al. Cisplatin, vindesine, and mitoguazone chemotherapy for epidermoid and adenocarcinoma of the esophagus. J Clin Oncol 5:1143–1149, 1987.

53. Kelsen DP, Fein R, Coonley C, et al. Cisplatin, vindesine, and mitogua-zone in the treatment of esophageal cancer. Cancer Treat Rep 70:255–259, 1986.

54. Ajani JA, Ryan B, Rich TA, et al. Prolonged chemotherapy for localized squamous carcinoma of the esophagus. Eur J Cancer 28A:880–884, 1992.

55. Hilgenberg AD, Carey RW, Wilkins EW, et al. Preoperative chemo-therapy, surgical resection, and selective postoperative therapy for squamous cell carcinoma of the esophagus. Ann Thorac Surg 45:357–363, 1988.

56. Mercke C, Albertsson M, Hambraeus G, et al. Cisplatin and 5-FU com-bined with radiotherapy and surgery in the treatment of squamous cell carcinoma of the esophagus. Acta 30:617–622,1991.

57. Ajani JA, Roth JA, Ryan B, et al. Evaluation of pre- and postoperative chemotherapy for resectable adenocarcinoma of the esophagus or gastro-esophageal junction. J Clin Oncol 8:1231–1238, 1990.

58. Ilson DH, Sirott M, Saltz L, et al. A phase II trial of interferon alpha-2A, 5-fluorouracil, and cisplatin in patients with advanced esophageal carcinoma. Cancer 75:2197–2202, 1995.

59. Kelsen D, Lovett D, Wong J, et al. Interferon alfa-2a and fluorouracil in the treatment of patients with advanced esophageal cancer. J Clin Oncol 10:269–274, 1992.

60. Van der Gaast, Kok TC, Kerkhofs L, et al. Phase I study of a biweekly schedule of a fixed dose of cisplatin with increasing doses of paclitaxel in patients with advanced oesophageal cancer. Br J Cancer 80:1052–1057, 1999.

61. Gisselbrecht C, Calvo F, Mignot L, et al. Fluorouracil, Adriamycin, and cisplatin (FAP) combination chemotherapy of advanced esophageal car-cinoma. Cancer 52:974–977, 1983.

62. Ajani JA, Roth JA, Ryan MB, et al. Intensive preoperative chemother-apy with colony-stimulating factor for resectable adenocarcinoma of the esophagus or gastroesophageal junction. J Clin Oncol 11:22–28, 1993.

# Chapter 19

# Barrett's Esophagus: Molecular Biology and Pathobiology

THOMAS G. PAULSON AND BRIAN J. REID

Barrett's esophagus (BE) is a condition that develops as a consequence of chronic gastroesophageal reflux disease (GERD) and predisposes to the development of esophageal adenocarcinoma (EA).[1] The incidence of EA in the United States has risen more than 350% over the past 20 years.[2] Similar rapid increases have also been reported in Western Europe.[3–5] Unfortunately, most patients with EA present when the cancer is advanced, and more than 90% of patients die from their disease within 5 years.[6] Thus, improvements in diagnosis and treatment are needed to improve disease outcome.

Approximately 10% of patients with GERD develop BE, a condition in which the normal squamous lining of the esophagus is replaced by metaplastic columnar epithelium.[7] Barrett's esophagus is a precursor to EA, and GERD has been shown to be a risk factor for developing EA.[8] The results of several studies suggest that endoscopic biopsy surveillance can detect cancers in BE at an early and curable stage.[9–12] However, multiple prospective studies suggest that, in the vast majority of patients, BE does not progress to cancer.[13–23] In those studies, only 39 of 1127 patients (3.5%) developed cancer, with an estimated incidence ranging from 1 in 52 to 1 in 441 patient-years of follow-up. In addition, the cost-effectiveness of surveillance has been examined. A recent study suggested that 5-year surveillance intervals were optimal.[24] However, most patients with BE are followed at 1- to 2-year intervals or less.[25] Identification of subsets of patients at high and low risk of progression to cancer would more effectively use limited health-care resources by permitting high-risk patients to undergo more frequent surveillance and low-risk patients to be reassured, counseled, and biopsied less frequently.

One approach to improving patient outcome and developing more rational surveillance programs for patients with BE is characterization of the somatic (as opposed to inherited) genetic alterations that take place during neoplastic progression. Such analyses provide information on the genes and molecular pathways whose somatic alterations are involved in the pathogenesis or progression of human cancer in vivo. An understanding of these events may permit identification of high- and low-risk patient subsets and provide molecular targets for therapeutic intervention. Determination of the somatic genetic alterations that characterize progression of BE to EA also allows identification of intermediate biomarkers of disease progression that can lead to objective diagnostic tests to improve identification of individuals at increased risk for progression to cancer. Existing means of assessing patient risk, such as those based on histologic assessment of dysplasia, can be subjective and susceptible to significant inter- and intraobserver variation.[26–29] Genomics-based approaches complement histologic staging and are amenable to high-throughput, laboratory-based screening strategies.

The mortality associated with esophagectomy depends upon the surgical volume of the institution, with low-volume institutions having mortality rates three- to fivefold those of high-volume institutions.[30,31] Given the morbidity and mortality associated with esophagectomy, Barrett's epithelium is not removed upon detection, and the current standard of care is periodic endoscopic surveillance with biopsy.[32] Endoscopic biopsy surveillance according to defined protocols permits tissue samples to be obtained serially during neoplastic disease progression, allowing prospective observations of the same patient and minimizing sampling errors. This is in contrast to the standard of care for other human neoplasms, such as colonic adenomas, in which premalignant lesions are usually removed when detected, making analysis of the temporal evolution of these lesions impossible. Thus, the study of BE and EA provides a unique opportunity for studying the evolution of somatic genetic alterations during human neoplastic progression in vivo.

Molecular analyses of human tumors have traditionally faced a number of other barriers that have been overcome in investigations of BE.[33] Biopsy samples from patients with premalignant and malignant conditions are heterogeneous, contaminated by normal stromal cells (cellular heterogeneity), and contain multiple, distinct neoplastic epithelial cell populations (clonal heterogeneity). These heterogeneities can obscure detection of genetic alterations such as gene mutation or loss of heterozygosity (LOH), which occur during neoplastic progression. In addition, clinical biopsy samples such as endoscopic biopsies or needle aspirates are typically small, reducing the number of analyses that can be performed. Further, the large numbers of patients and samples that must be evaluated make standard molecular biological methods impractical for clinical or population-based studies. Finally, as discussed above, premalignant lesions are frequently removed from patients with other conditions; this limits investigations of the order in which different abnormalities occur in individual patients and prevents studies in which an abnormality at one point in time is used as a predictor of subsequent progression.

We have developed a successful approach for the analysis of clinical samples from patients in the Seattle Barrett's Esophagus Cohort, which is made up of more than 850 individuals whose diagnoses range from Barrett's metaplasia negative for dysplasia to cancer. The fundamental elements to this approach include the following:

1. Standardized endoscopic biopsy protocols that minimize sampling error and permit patients to be followed prospectively over time
2. Flow-cytometric sorting to purify neoplastic cell populations for molecular analyses and to relate molecular analyses to cell-cycle abnormalities and aneuploidy in Barrett's epithelium
3. Whole-genome amplification to permit multiple genetic analyses on small, flow-sorted endoscopic biopsies
4. High-throughput methodologies to evaluate large numbers of patient samples
5. Clonal ordering to determine the order in which two events occurred relative to each other during neoplastic progression
6. Longitudinal studies in which an abnormality at one time point is investigated as a predictor of the development of another abnormality at a subsequent time point.

Ki67/DNA content multiparameter flow-cytometric cell sorting is used to purify proliferating diploid or aneuploid epithelial cell populations from nonproliferating diploid stromal cells.[34,35] Ki67 is a proliferation-associated antigen that can distinguish cells in the $G_1$, S, or $G_2$/M stages of the cell cycle from those in $G_0$.[36] By combining Ki67 detection with a DNA stain (4'6-diamidino-2-phenylindole [DAPI]) in a multiparameter flow-cytometric assay, $G_0$, $G_1$, S, 4N ($G_2$/M or tetraploid) and aneuploid populations can be analyzed and purified by flow-cytometric sorting.

We have addressed the problem of small sample size by using primer-extension preamplification (PEP), a polymerase chain reaction (PCR)–based technique for whole-genome amplification[37,38] that increases the amount of DNA from a given sample approximately 60-fold; this allows 30 or more genetic analyses to be performed on the DNA from a thousand cells. Use of fluorescence-based PCR and ABI PRISM automated DNA sequencers substantially increases throughput, allowing the number of samples necessary for large clinical and population-based studies to be processed and analyzed.[33]

Many studies (e.g., those of colorectal neoplasia) have used the prevalence of abnormalities at different histologic stages of progression to infer a temporal order. The results of these studies are typically represented as linear progressions to cancer, but

actual observed orders of events are frequently at variance with those predicted by such linear models.[39,40] However, esophagectomy specimens frequently contain multiple stages of neoplastic progression, which permits an alternative method of ordering genetic events; this ordering can be combined with data obtained prospectively during endoscopic surveillance. This method, called *clonal ordering,* was originally used to determine the order of events in the yeast cell cycle.[41] Basically, any two events (A and B) in a complex biological pathway such as neoplastic progression can be related to each other in one of four ways: *(1)* A can consistently precede B (e.g., A could cause B or create a condition that permits B to occur); *(2)* B can consistently precede A; *(3)* A and B can occur simultaneously (i.e., both A and B are required for a particular step [interdependent events]); or *(4)* A and B have no order relative to each other (independent events). The determined orders can then be used as hypothesis generators to investigate function or as a basis for larger-scale longitudinal studies in which one abnormality (event A) is used as a predictor of a second event (event B), which is the outcome.

While it is likely that the exact somatic genetic and cell-cycle alterations that occur during progression from BE to EA vary among patients, they do have some general characteristics (Fig. 19–1). The quiescent ($G_0$) squamous cells that normally line the esophagus are replaced by a hyperproliferative metaplastic columnar epithelium. Later, increased 4N fractions and aneuploid populations may emerge. Loss of heterozygosity at chromosomes 17p13 and 9p21, corresponding to the locations of the tumor suppressors p53 and p16$^{INK4a}$ (p16), respectively, occur early during disease progression, as does inactivation of wild-type function of

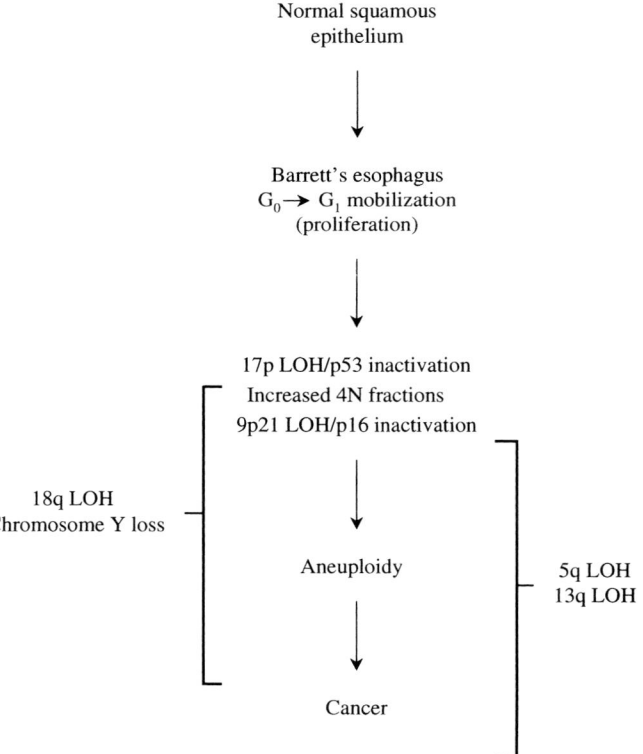

**Figure 19-1** Cell-cycle and somatic genetic alterations observed during progression from Barrett's esophagus (BE) to esophageal adenocarcinoma (EA). This generalized scheme shows the common abnormalities observed in BE and EA; not all events occur in all cases, nor do they always occur in the indicated order (see chapter text and Fig. 19–2).

the remaining allele of *p53* by mutation and the inactivation of the remaining *p16* allele by mutation or promoter hypermethylation. Loss of heterozygosity at chromosome 18q and loss of the Y chromosome frequently occur before the development of EA, but two other frequent LOH events (at chromosomes 5q and 13q) occur as often after the appearance of cancer as before. While it is tempting to view these events as points along a linear pathway, the data discussed below support a more complex view of the interaction between these genetic events during the evolution of neoplastic cell lineages (Fig. 19–2).

## Cell-Cycle and DNA Content Abnormalities

### Mobilization from $G_0$

Increased cell proliferation is a hallmark of Barrett's metaplasia. Exposure of the esophagus to an acidic environment results in

increased cell turnover and an increase in the size of the proliferative zone.[42] Most upper gastrointestinal epithelial cells are in $G_0$ phase, but in Barrett's epithelium the fraction of cells mobilized from this quiescent state into $G_1$ phase is elevated.[35,43] The fraction of Ki67$^+$ cells increases in samples with more advanced histology,[35,44–47] suggesting progressive abrogation of proliferation control during neoplastic progression. Increases in S-phase fractions occur more frequently at later stages, often after the development of aneuploidy. Analysis by Ki67/DNA content multiparameter flow cytometry demonstrated that S-phase fractions greater than 7% were not present in 34 samples of normal fundic or cardiac gland mucosa but were found in 5 out of 31 of metaplastic samples with no dysplasia (16%), 7 of 27 with indefinite/low-grade dysplasia (LGD) (26%), 15 of 20 with high grade dysplasia (HGD) (75%) and 13 of 17 with EA (76%).[35] Only 19 of 73 of diploid specimens (26%) had increased S-phase fractions, in contrast to 21 of 22 aneuploid samples (95%). These findings

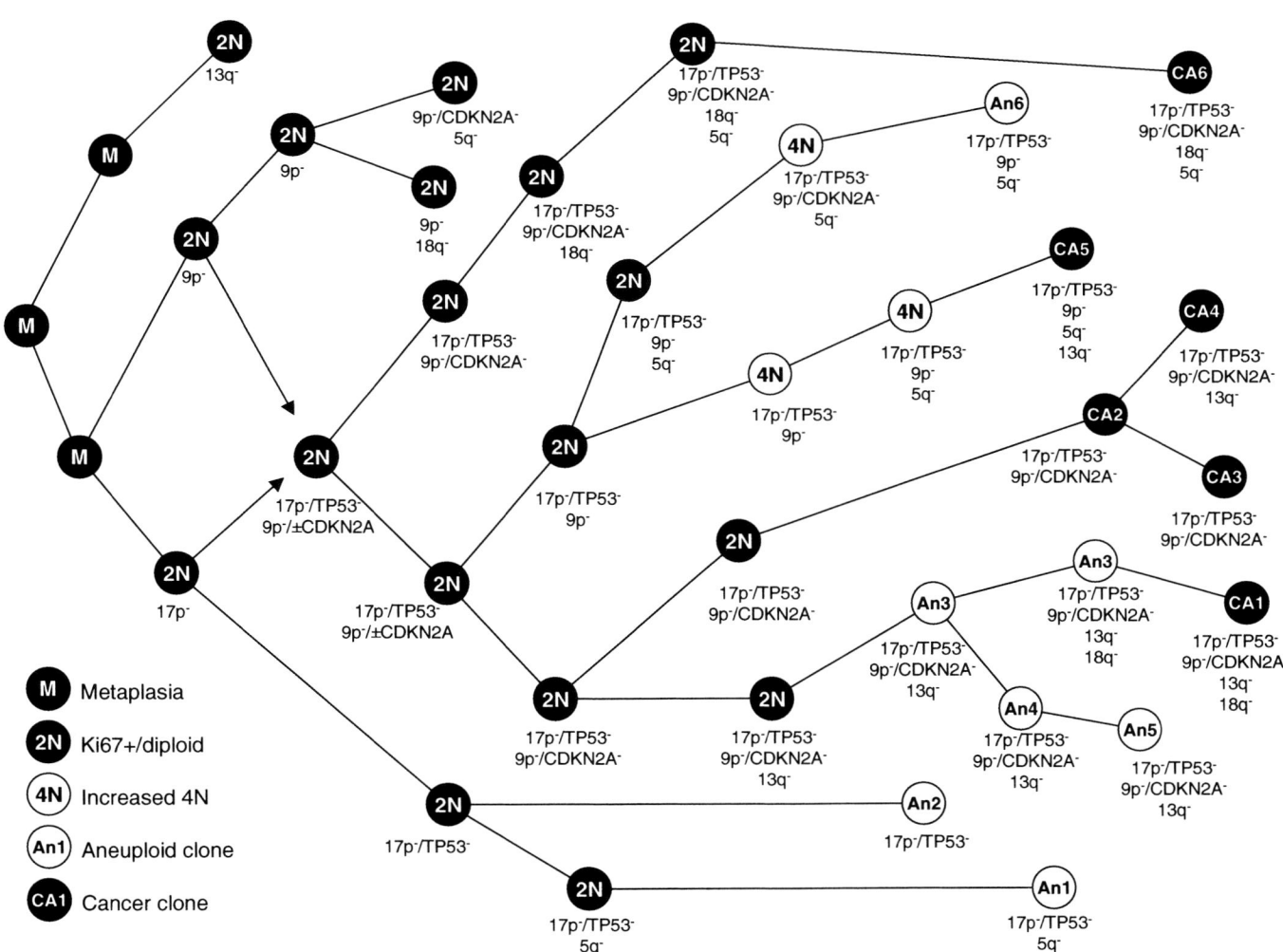

**Figure 19–2** Multiple genetic routes to cancer in Barrett's esophagus (BE). Progression to esophageal adenocarcinoma (EA) is characterized by a general evolution of genetic alterations and increasingly abnormal flow-cytometric abnormalities. Genetic alterations result in frequent bifurcations, leading to the development of a mosaic of clones throughout the esophagus. Some lineages result in cell populations that fail to expand or are eliminated by the growth of other clones. Progression does not stop once cancer develops; alterations and genetic variants continue to arise, resulting in cells with increased metastatic potential. Numbers after the aneuploid and cancer populations indicate these can be characterized by different, distinct genetic alterations. This figure is based on cell populations observed in patients with BE and EA, but is not meant to be exhaustive, nor is it meant to indicate that all alterations must occur in a given patient. (From Barrett MT, Sanchez CA, Prevo LJ, et al. Evolution of neoplastic cell lineages in Barrett oesophagus. Nat Genet 22:106–109, 1999, with permission.)

are consistent with the concept that cells from early-stage BE have intact $G_1/S$ checkpoint controls that are progressively inactivated during neoplastic progression.

### Increased 4N Fractions

Increased 4N fraction is defined as an increase in the percentage of cells (>6%) having a 4N DNA content.[48] Increased 4N fractions can represent diploid cells accumulating in the $G_2/M$, tetraploid, or near-tetraploid aneuploid cell populations. Increased 4N fractions correlate with loss of p53 function; increased 4N fractions are more prevalent in more advanced histologic stages.[35,48–51] For example, increased 4N fractions were not found in any patients with GERD alone (0/44) or with Barrett's metaplasia without dysplasia (0/70) but were found in 22% (7/32) with indefinite/LGD, 88% (7/8) with HGD, and 64% (18/28) with EA.[50] In addition, increased 4N fractions are predictive for development of intermediate events in neoplastic progression. Ninety patients whose biopsies were initially diploid were followed prospectively for an average of 51.4 months to determine if increased 4N fractions were predictive of the subsequent evolution of aneuploid populations.[49] Seventy-five patients had normal 4N fractions over the entire follow-up interval, whereas 15 initially had or developed increased 4N fractions during follow-up. Eleven of the 15 with increased 4N fractions (73%) developed aneuploid populations during follow-up, compared with 8 of the 75 with normal 4N fractions (11%), results strongly suggesting that increased 4N fractions are associated with subsequent progression to aneuploidy ($P < 0.0001$). Coupled with the observation that increased 4N fractions are not detected in all cases of EA,[50] these results suggest that increased 4N populations represent genetically unstable transient intermediates in the progression to EA.

### Aneuploidy

Cell populations with an aneuploid DNA content can arise in premalignant Barrett's epithelium and are found in a majority of patients with EA.[35,48–55] The distribution of aneuploid populations can vary widely by patient. One study reported a patient having a 2.2N population throughout a 10-cm segment of metaplastic epithelium, which suggests a process of clonal expansion;[56] another study found multiple distinct aneuploid populations (range 2–12) that occupied specific, sometimes overlapping regions in 12 of 14 patients with HGD, EA, or both.[51] Microdissection studies have shown that early EA frequently contains only one of multiple aneuploid cell populations present in superficial premalignant epithelium of esophagectomy specimens, but that more advanced cancers can contain multiple aneuploid cell populations.[51,55,57] These findings suggest that cancer develops in Barrett's epithelium through a process of genomic instability that can lead to large changes in DNA content. The aneuploid cell populations that develop as a result of this instability can spread to involve large regions of the esophageal mucosa while continuing to evolve additional variants, eventually leading to an abnormal clone with the capacity for invasion that becomes an early cancer.

The prevalence of aneuploid populations increases with increasing histologic stage.[44,48,53,54,58–60] In one study, aneuploid populations were not detected in any patients with GERD alone (0/44), but were detected in 4% (3/70) with metaplasia without dysplasia, 6% (2/32) with indefinite/LGD, 62% (5/8) with HGD,

and 89% (25/28) with EA.[50] Multiple studies have found aneuploid populations in tissue without HGD or EA, indicating that conventional diagnosis on the basis of histology may be inadequate to detect relatively advanced somatic genetic abnormalities present in the mucosa of some patients. Further studies have demonstrated the utility of aneuploidy as an intermediate marker of disease progression. For example, 62 patients with BE were evaluated prospectively over a mean period of 34 months. Thirteen patients had either aneuploidy or increased 4N fractions at their initial endoscopy; of those, 69% (9/13) progressed to develop HGD or EA during follow-up. None of the 49 patients without these abnormalities progressed to HGD or EA, suggesting that aneuploidy and increased 4N fractions may be used to identify subsets of patients having high or low risks of progression ($P < 0.0001$).[52] In another study, biopsies were obtained from 30 dysplasia-free BE patients every 1–2 years for 13 years. None of the patients whose biopsies remained diploid during that time progressed to dysplasia or EA, whereas 6 of 13 patients who either had aneuploid populations initially or developed them during follow-up developed dysplasia or EA ($P < 0.01$).[61] A recent prospective study of 322 patients reported that baseline diagnoses of increased 4N fractions or aneuploidy were significant predictors of progression to EA, with 5-year cumulative incidences of cancer of 56% (95% confidence interval [CI], 37%–77%) and 43% (95% CI, 28%–62%), respectively. Detection of increased 4N fractions and aneuploid cell populations appears to be especially useful in patients whose biopsy results are negative, indefinite, or LGD, categories difficult to reproducibly distinguish by histology. Among patients whose baseline histologic diagnoses were negative, indefinite, or LGD, those with baseline aneuploidy, increased 4N fractions, or both had a 28% 5-year cumulative incidence of cancer (95% CI, 12%–55%) compared with 0% (95% CI, 0–4.7%) for those whose biopsies were diploid and had normal 4N fractions.[62]

## Somatic Genetic Alterations

### Chromosomal Alterations and Loss of Heterozygosity

A variety of somatic genetic alterations have been observed in BE and EA. These alterations include point mutations, small DNA insertions and deletions, large-scale deletions and amplifications, and whole-chromosome losses. Loss of DNA from one chromosome of a pair (e.g., from the maternally inherited chromosome 17), termed *loss of heterozygosity* (LOH), is observed frequently. In addition, epigenetic alterations, such as methylation, which do not change the coding sequence of the DNA but do affect gene expression, have been observed. Accurate analyses of somatic genetic alterations in BE and EA depend on the purity of the cell populations being analyzed, and it is likely that some of the variability in results from different studies is due to insufficient purification. Microdissection can remove some normal cell contamination; but this technique is operator-dependent, can only separate cells on the basis of morphology, is not possible in some tumors, and is not easily scaleable to high throughput. Flow sorting has the advantage of separation based on objective markers (e.g., proliferation, DNA content, or other measurable characteristics of the population being examined), generates extremely purified cell populations, and is applicable to almost all cell types. For example, multiparameter flow sorting has been used to enrich a 2% fraction of tumor cells in a lymph node from a patient with metastatic breast cancer to greater than 90%.[63]

The progression from BE to EA is characterized by extensive somatic genetic instability. Analyses of this genome wide instability have shown that a number of nonrandom alterations occur in a background of generalized instability. Genomic alterations are often clonal, being observed in both premalignant tissue and EA, and frequently persist over time.[55,56,64] One study using flow-sorted aneuploid populations examined the frequency of LOH by chromosome arm in samples from 20 EAs and 2 HGDs.[38] The background frequency of LOH (the probability that any given chromosome arm would show loss) was 23%, with frequency of losses on chromosomes 5q, 9p, 13q, 17p, and 18q significantly above the background frequency. In this study, fractional allelic loss (the ratio of the number of chromosomal arms with loss to the number of informative chromosomal arms per patient) increased with increasing depth of invasion, from 0.095 in HGD to 0.264 in early adenocarcinoma (intra- and submucosal) to 0.343 in advanced adenocarcinomas (invasion to the muscularis propria or deeper). Other studies have reported frequent losses on chromosomes 1p, 3p, 3q, 4q, 5q, 6q, 9p, 11p, 12q, 13q, 17p, 17q, and 18q.[38,65–74]

The genes associated with some LOH events in EA are known, such as p53 (17p13 LOH) and p16 (9p21 LOH). However, the molecular target or targets, if any, for most of the commonly observed genetic alterations are unknown. Loss of the Y chromosome has been observed in a majority of EAs in a number of studies,[44,64,75–77] similar to findings in studies of other cancers.[78] The pathologic significance of this loss is not known. Gene amplification, increased expression, or both have been reported at some loci in EA, including cathepsin B, cyclin D1, mdm-2, EGRF/erbB-2, and Ki-ras, albeit in a minority of cases.[79–84] Breakage at the chromosomal fragile site Fra3B and concomitant loss of the putative tumor suppressor locus FHIT have been observed in EA.[85] A minority of EAs display sporadic microsatellite instability (replication error phenotype, or RER), suggesting that disruption of mismatch repair does not play a significant role in the pathogenesis or progression of EA.[38,69,86]

### p53 Locus

p53 is the most commonly mutated gene in human cancers,[87] including EA. p53 expression is induced in response to a variety of genotoxic stresses, including exposure to ionizing radiation, antimetabolites, or hypoxia.[88] Through downstream effectors, p53 arrests cells at the $G_1/S$ transition, effectively preventing DNA synthesis under conditions that could lead to chromosome breakage. This function is believed to be a significant part of the tumor suppressor role of p53.

Loss of heterozygosity on chromosome 17p is found in over 90% of EAs[38,55,67,71,72,89] and in 60% of patients with HGD.[90] p53 status has been evaluated in BE and EA either by sequencing or by antibody detection of protein overexpression, which is presumed to be due to p53 mutation. Antibody staining is less labor-intensive and more widely available, whereas sequencing is a more specific method for detecting mutations and may become more available as the technology of the Human Genome Project becomes available for diagnostics. Although many tumors are positive by both techniques, there are numerous exceptions. Approximately 25% of EAs have p53 mutations that lead to protein truncation that might not be detected by protein overexpression.[91,92] By antibody staining and sequencing, cells with p53 mutations are found in more than 70% of EAs.[89,92–100]

The prevalence of p53 mutations increases with increasing histologic stage.[60,101,102] In one study, p53 overexpression was observed in 5% of patients (1 of 21) with BE negative for dysplasia, 15% (2/13) with indefinite/LGD, 45% (5/11) with HGD, and 53% (8/15) with EA.[103] It has been suggested that p53 overexpression may be predictive of progression to HGD or cancer;[104,105] however, large-scale prospective studies of the usefulness of p53 as a predictive marker will be required. p53 mutation, increased 4N fractions, and aneuploidy are all more prevalent in samples having more advanced histologic stage. This is consistent with the role of the p53 pathway in preventing cells that have undergone DNA damage from progressing past the $G_1/S$ checkpoint. Loss of p53 function can result in damaged cells accumulating in $G_2/M$ (i.e., increased 4N fractions) and the eventual development of tetraploid/aneuploid populations.[106–109] The finding that a minority of EAs do not have detectable p53 mutations may be due to technical factors (e.g., insufficient purification) or to the fact that the p53 pathway can be disrupted by means other than p53 mutation (e.g., upstream of p53 via MDM2 or downstream via p21).[110]

Since loss of p53 function is required for the division of cells containing DNA breaks, p53 inactivation should theoretically precede the appearance of other manifestations of genetic instability. Indeed, cells with p53 mutations can appear in premalignant tissue[55] and can occupy large regions of the esophagus.[91] In addition, 17p LOH occurs before most of the other somatic genetic alterations observed in BE. Clonal ordering experiments have demonstrated that 17p LOH occurs before cancer, aneuploidy, and LOH on chromosomes 5q, 13q, and 18q,[34,55,111] simultaneously with the development of increased 4N fractions,[49] and independently of 9p21 LOH,[55] but after the mobilization of cells into $G_1$.[111] Thus, early inactivation of the p53 pathway in BE allows genetically unstable cells to propagate and to generate further manifestations of instability.

### p16 Locus

Loss of heterozygosity at chromosome 9p21, the location of p16, also occurs frequently in EA.[38,67,72,112–114] p16 (also known as CDKN2a) is a cyclin-dependent kinase (CDK) inhibitor that, through its ability to prevent phosphorylation of the retinoblastoma gene (pRb), plays a role in governing the $G_1/S$ transition.[115,116]

In a study of aneuploid cell populations from 32 patients with BE and/or EA, 75% of patients (18 of 24) with EA and 75% (6/8) with only premalignant epithelium were positive for 9p21 LOH.[65] In a recent study of patients having HGD without cancer, 9p21 LOH was found to be more prevalent in diploid cell populations and was present over a larger area of the esophagus than was 17p LOH, suggesting that 9p21 loss plays a role in early clonal expansion.[90] This study also found that 9p21 LOH occurred before or concurrently with 17p LOH in 20 of 21 patients. The concept that p16 inactivation may be a very early event in BE is supported by results of studies demonstrating that p16 inactivation, along with activation of telomerase, is a critical step in allowing cells to bypass normal senescence pathways and extend their life spans.[117] Thus, loss of p16 function may allow the spread of clones with extended proliferation potential over large regions of the esophagus.

In contrast to the situation with p53, mutations in the remaining p16 allele are found in only 23% of EA patients (5 of

22) with 9p21 LOH.[65] This finding is consistent with the high frequency of 9p LOH and low frequency of *p16* mutations found in other cancer types, such as gliomas and lung cancers.[118–120] Homozygous deletion of *p16* has been observed as a mechanism of inactivation in other cancer types,[121,122] but has not been observed in EA.[55,65] An epigenetic mechanism of gene inactivation, the silencing of gene expression through hypermethylation of the promoter region, has been observed at the *p16* locus in a variety of human cancers.[123–125] The methylation status of the p16 promoter can be examined using *(1)* a bisulfite treatment that converts all unmethylated, but not methylated, cytosines to uracil[126] and *(2)* PCR primers that can differentiate between bisulfite-treated methylated and unmethylated p16 promoter sequences.[127] One study using this technique found that methylation of p16 promoter sequences occurred in BE and was more prevalent at higher histologic stages.[128] In another study, 8 of 14 patients with either BE or EA and having 9p21 LOH but no *p16* mutation were found to have methylated p16 promoter sequences, including 3 of 3 patients with BE alone.[129] This study also found that *p16* mutation and promoter hypermethylation were mutually exclusive. Thus, 9p21 LOH, combined with promoter hypermethylation or mutation of the remaining p16 allele, appears to abrogate *p16* expression in BE and EA. Clonal ordering studies have demonstrated that 9p21 LOH precedes aneuploidy, cancer, and LOH at chromosomes 5q and 13q and occurs independently of 17p LOH.[55]

## Clonal Expansion and Pathways to Cancer

Loss of *p16* and *p53* function early during the progression to cancer appears to establish a permissive environment for the evolution of neoplastic cell populations. *p16* inactivation may allow cells to increase in number (i.e., clonal expansion throughout the Barrett's esophageal segment), while *p53* inactivation allows cells with genetic instability to bypass normal checkpoint controls and continue to grow and accumulate genetic alterations (clonal evolution). Thus, a large population of cells with the potential to undergo somatic genetic alterations and evolve into cancer would be established in the esophagus. Indeed, genetic and cell-cycle abnormalities are observed more frequently at later histologic stages, consistent with a predicted evolution of genetic alterations. In addition, the same genetic alterations found in EA are often found in surrounding premalignant epithelium or in biopsies from the same location at earlier time points, indicating expansion of premalignant cell populations and their evolution into cancer. One investigation detailed neoplastic progression in three patients over multiple endoscopies spanning 3 to 6 years.[55] The expansion of clonal populations and the evolution of genetic alterations were clearly demonstrated using ploidy, *p53* and *p16* mutation status, and LOH on chromosomes 5q, 9p, 13q, 17p, and 18q as genetic markers.

The clonal ordering that has been done in BE and EA can differentiate between events occurring in linear (e.g., A before B) or nonlinear (e.g., A occurs independently of B) pathways. The results of these clonal ordering experiments and the observations of somatic genetic alterations in patients who have developed cancer have resulted in a schematic model of cancer progression in BE and EA (Fig. 19–2).[55] The complexity of this model is a function of the ability to follow alterations in patients over time. This model contrasts with that proposed for colorectal cancer, in which a linear pathway has been inferred on the basis of the prevalence of alterations found in lesions of different morpho-

logic stages.[130] A complex model with many pathways to cancer is consistent with that proposed by Nowell, in which malignancies develop as a result of acquired genetic instability and clonal evolution, with cancer as an eventual result.[131] This complex model reconciles the observations that *(1)* EAs frequently have similar genetic alterations but are by no means identical; *(2)* the mosaics of genetic variants that characterize premalignant tissues from different patients are unique, yet each variant may be capable of giving rise to a cancer; and *(3)* clonal populations can arise that are no longer detectable at later time points (generation of variants with limited proliferative potential, or "dead-end" populations).

## Genome and Environment

The growth environment of the esophagus in a patient with GERD likely contributes to the genesis of the genetic alterations that characterize BE and EA.[8] Exposure of esophageal epithelium to low pH and other components of reflux, such as bile salts,[132] puts stress on the normal squamous epithelium of the esophagus. This stress results in cell death, as demonstrated by the corresponding increase in cell proliferation in patients with GERD and BE. Proliferation under inappropriate growth conditions can cause genetic alterations and chromosome breaks.[133–137] Normally, cells that have genetic damage arrest in either G1 or G2/M to repair that damage or are eliminated through apoptotic mechanisms.[115,138,139] However, it has been hypothesized that increased proliferation increases the chance that variants will arise that have lost the normal arrest/apoptosis response, resulting in a growth advantage and expansion of a population of cells at risk for further genomic alterations.[140] It is also possible that the growth of a cell type outside of its normal environment may lead to growth deregulation, genetic alterations, and cancer progression due to the cells' inability to properly respond to environmental growth signals.[141] At the present time, removal of the abnormal environment (acid reflux) through medical or surgical intervention rarely causes reversion to a normal squamous epithelium.[142,143] However, further genetic analysis may lead to identification of the initiating event or events that lead to BE, which could then be targets for intervention.

## Future Directions

The study of neoplastic progression in the BE/EA system, and in other cancer types as well, has benefited significantly from technological advances. The use of flow cytometry has resulted in purification of neoplastic cell samples, allowing less ambiguous analysis of somatic genetic alterations. Advances in sequencing technology and fluorescent detection of PCR products have resulted in greatly increased sample throughput and improved analytic accuracy. This trend is continuing with the development of oligonucleotide-based arrays for detailed analysis of genetic alterations and gene expression.[144] This technology takes advantage of the fact that known oligonucleotides can be either immobilized or synthesized upon substrates in defined positions (e.g., DNA chips) at high density. Two recent examples of this technology are arrays made up of oligonucleotides corresponding to either single-nucleotide polymorphisms (SNPs) from throughout the genome or to sequences corresponding to the coding regions of transcribed genes (expression arrays). The SNP arrays allow genotyping of an entire genome in a single experiment. The high-density LOH maps generated by SNP arrays will greatly facilitate identification of commonly lost tumor suppressor genes and detailed analysis of genome dynamics during neoplastic progression.[145,146]

For expression arrays, a labeled probe derived from the mRNA from a cell population of interest is hybridized to the array. This approach can be used to identify and quantitate the expression of thousands of transcribed genes simultaneously in a given cell population. For example, experiments are currently being performed to compare the gene expression in cells from Barrett's epithelium with those from normal squamous epithelium, in an effort to determine what genes and pathways contribute to the development of premalignant tissue.

A number of questions remain concerning the somatic genetic and cell-cycle alterations that characterize neoplastic progression in BE. Are genetic alterations responsible for the conversion of the normal squamous epithelium to metaplastic columnar epithelium? If so, what are they? Is there a certain genetic background that makes an individual more susceptible to developing BE or EA?[147,148] Certainly the new array of technologies will be useful in addressing these points. Is there a relationship between the types of genetic alterations that occur in BE and the rate at which cancer develops in a given patient? What genetic or expression alterations are responsible for the morphologic changes that lead to histologic diagnoses, and can these alterations be measured more objectively or sensitively using laboratory-based tests? The molecular genetic analyses summarized here have allowed us to determine the important questions concerning disease progression in BE and EA, and future studies (including those utilizing new technologies) may provide the answers needed to improve patient care.

## References

1. Phillips RW, Wong RK. Barrett's esophagus. Natural history, incidence, etiology, and complications. Gastroenterol Clin North Am 20:791–816, 1991.
2. Devesa SS, Blot WJ, Fraumeni JF Jr. Changing patterns in the incidence of esophageal and gastric carcinoma in the United States. Cancer 83:2049–2053, 1998.
3. Hansson LE, Sparen P, Nyren O. Increasing incidence of both major histological types of esophageal carcinomas among men in Sweden. Int J Cancer 54:402–407, 1993.
4. Powell J, McConkey CC. The rising trend in oesophageal adenocarcinoma and gastric cardia. Eur J Cancer Prev 1:265–269, 1992.
5. Bytzer P, Christensen PB, Damkier P, Vinding K, Seersholm N. Adenocarcinoma of the esophagus and Barrett's esophagus: a population-based study. Am J Gastroenterol 94:86–91, 1999.
6. Farrow DC, Vaughan TL. Determinants of survival following the diagnosis of esophageal adenocarcinoma (United States). Cancer Causes Control 7:322–327, 1996.
7. Winters C Jr, Spurling TJ, Chobanian SJ, et al. Barrett's esophagus. A prevalent, occult complication of gastroesophageal reflux disease. Gastroenterology 92:118–124, 1987.
8. Lagergren J, Bergstrom R, Lindgren A, Nyren O. Symptomatic gastroesophageal reflux as a risk factor for esophageal adenocarcinoma. N Engl J Med 340:825–831, 1999.
9. Levine DS, Haggitt RC, Blount PL, et al. An endoscopic biopsy protocol can differentiate high-grade dysplasia from early adenocarcinoma in Barrett's esophagus. Gastroenterology 105:40–50, 1993.
10. van Sandick JW, van Lanschot JJ, Kuiken BW, et al. Impact of endoscopic biopsy surveillance of Barrett's oesophagus on pathological stage and clinical outcome of Barrett's carcinoma. Gut 43:216–222, 1998.
11. Rusch VW, Levine DS, Haggitt R, Reid BJ. The management of high grade dysplasia and early cancer in Barrett's esophagus. A multidisciplinary problem. Cancer 74:1225–1229, 1994.
12. Peters JH, Clark GW, Ireland AP, et al. Outcome of adenocarcinoma arising in Barrett's esophagus in endoscopically surveyed and nonsur-

veyed patients. J Thorac Cardiovasc Surg 108:813–821; discussion 821–812, 1994.
13. O'Connor JB, Falk GW, Richter JE. The incidence of adenocarcinoma and dysplasia in Barrett's esophagus: report on the Cleveland Clinic Barrett's Esophagus Registry. Am J Gastroenterol 94:2037–2042, 1999.
14. van der Burgh A, Dees J, Hop WC, van Blankenstein M. Oesophageal cancer is an uncommon cause of death in patients with Barrett's oesophagus. Gut 39:5–8, 1996.
15. Drewitz DJ, Sampliner RE, Garewal HS. The incidence of adenocarcinoma in Barrett's esophagus: a prospective study of 170 patients followed 4.8 years. Am J Gastroenterol 92:212–215, 1997.
16. Miros M, Kerlin P, Walker N. Only patients with dysplasia progress to adenocarcinoma in Barrett's oesophagus. Gut 32:1441–1446, 1991.
17. Cameron AJ, Ott BJ, Payne WS. The incidence of adenocarcinoma in columnar-lined (Barrett's) esophagus. N Engl J Med 313:857–859, 1985.
18. Spechler SJ, Robbins AH, Rubins HB, et al. Adenocarcinoma and Barrett's esophagus. An overrated risk? Gastroenterology 87:927–933, 1984.
19. Hameeteman W, Tytgat GN, Houthoff HJ, van den Tweel JG. Barrett's esophagus: development of dysplasia and adenocarcinoma. Gastroenterology 96:1249–1256, 1989.
20. Williamson WA, Ellis FH Jr, Gibb SP, et al. Barrett's esophagus. Prevalence and incidence of adenocarcinoma. Arch Intern Med 151:2212–2216, 1991.
21. Robertson CS, Mayberry JF, Nicholson DA, James PD, Atkinson M. Value of endoscopic surveillance in the detection of neoplastic change in Barrett's oesophagus. Br J Surg 75:760–763, 1988.
22. Ovaska J, Miettinen M, Kivilaakso E. Adenocarcinoma arising in Barrett's esophagus. Dig Dis Sci 34:1336–1339, 1989.
23. Achkar E, Carey W. The cost of surveillance for adenocarcinoma complicating Barrett's esophagus. Am J Gastroenterol 83:291–294, 1988.
24. Provenzale D, Schmitt C, Wong JB. Barrett's esophagus: a new look at surveillance based on emerging estimates of cancer risk. Am J Gastroenterol 94:2043–2053, 1999.
25. Falk GW, Ours TM, Richter JE. Practice patterns for surveillance of Barrett's esophagus in the USA [abstract]. Gastrointest Endosc 49:AB50, 1999.
26. Alikhan M, Rex D, Khan A, et al. Variable pathologic interpretation of columnar lined esophagus by general pathologists in community practice. Gastrointest Endosc 50:23–26, 1999.
27. Polkowski W, Baak JP, van Lanschot JJ, et al. Clinical decision making in Barrett's oesophagus can be supported by computerized immuno-quantitation and morphometry of features associated with proliferation and differentiation. J Pathol 184:161–168, 1998.
28. Reid BJ, Haggitt RC, Rubin CE, et al. Observer variation in the diagnosis of dysplasia in Barrett's esophagus. Hum Pathol 19:166–178, 1988.
29. Sagan C, Flejou JF, Diebold MD, Potet F, Le Bodic MF. Reproducibility of histological criteria of dysplasia in Barrett mucosa. Gastroenterol Clin Biol 18:D31–D34, 1994.
30. Begg CB, Cramer LD, Hoskins WJ, Brennan MF. Impact of hospital volume on operative mortality for major cancer surgery. JAMA 280:1747–1751, 1998.
31. Patti MG, Corvera CU, Glasgow RE, Way LW. A hospital's annual rate of esophagectomy influences the operative mortality rate. J Gastrointest Surg 2:186–192, 1998.
32. Sampliner RE. Practice guidelines on the diagnosis, surveillance, and therapy of Barrett's esophagus. The Practice Parameters Committee of the American College of Gastroenterology. Am J Gastroenterol 93:1028–1032, 1998.
33. Paulson TG, Galipeau PC, Reid BJ. Loss of heterozygosity analysis using whole genome amplification, cell sorting, and fluorescence-based PCR. Genome Res 9:482–491, 1999.
34. Blount PL, Galipeau PC, Sanchez CA et al. 17p allelic losses in diploid cells of patients with Barrett's esophagus who develop aneuploidy. Cancer Res 54:2292–2295, 1994.
35. Reid BJ, Sanchez CA, Blount PL, Levine DS. Barrett's esophagus: cell cycle abnormalities in advancing stages of neoplastic progression. Gastroenterology 105:119–129, 1993.
36. Gerdes J, Lemke H, Baisch H, et al. Cell cycle analysis of a cell proliferation-associated human nuclear antigen defined by the monoclonal antibody Ki-67. J Immunol 133:1710–1715, 1984.
37. Zhang L, Cui X, Schmitt K, et al. Whole genome amplification from a single cell: implications for genetic analysis. Proc Natl Acad Sci USA 89:5847–5851, 1992.

38. Barrett MT, Galipeau PC, Sanchez CA, Emond MJ, Reid BJ. Determination of the frequency of loss of heterozygosity in esophageal adenocarcinoma by cell sorting, whole genome amplification and microsatellite polymorphisms. Oncogene 12:1873–1878, 1996.

39. Boland CR. The biology of colorectal cancer. Implications for pretreatment and follow-up management. Cancer 71:4180–4186, 1993.

40. Vogelstein B, Fearon ER, Hamilton SR, et al. Genetic alterations during colorectal-tumor development. N Engl J Med 319:525–532, 1988.

41. Hereford LM, Hartwell LH. Sequential gene function in the initiation of *Saccharomyces cerevisiae* DNA synthesis. J Mol Biol 84:445–461, 1974.

42. Jankowski J. Gene expression in Barrett's mucosa: acute and chronic adaptive responses in the oesophagus. Gut 34:1649–1650, 1993.

43. Pellish LJ, Hermos JA, Eastwood GL. Cell proliferation in three types of Barrett's epithelium. Gut 21:26–31, 1980.

44. Krishnadath KK, Tilanus HW, van Blankenstein M, et al. Accumulation of genetic abnormalities during neoplastic progression in Barrett's esophagus. Cancer Res 55:1971–1976, 1995.

45. Herbst JJ, Berenson MM, McCloskey DW, Wiser WC. Cell proliferation in esophageal columnar epithelium (Barrett's esophagus). Gastroenterology 75:683–687, 1978.

46. Gray MR, Hall PA, Nash J, et al. Epithelial proliferation in Barrett's esophagus by proliferating cell nuclear antigen immunolocalization. Gastroenterology 103:1769–1776, 1992.

47. Hong MK, Laskin WB, Herman BE, et al. Expansion of the Ki-67 proliferative compartment correlates with degree of dysplasia in Barrett's esophagus. Cancer 75:423–429, 1995.

48. Reid BJ, Haggitt RC, Rubin CE, Rabinovitch PS. Barrett's esophagus. Correlation between flow cytometry and histology in detection of patients at risk for adenocarcinoma. Gastroenterology 93:1–11, 1987.

49. Galipeau PC, Cowan DS, Sanchez CA, et al. 17p (p53) allelic losses, 4N (G2/tetraploid) populations, and progression to aneuploidy in Barrett's esophagus. Proc Natl Acad Sci USA 93:7081–7084, 1996.

50. Reid BJ. Barrett's esophagus and esophageal adenocarcinoma. Gastroenterol Clin North Am 20:817–834, 1991.

51. Rabinovitch PS, Reid BJ, Haggitt RC, Norwood TH, Rubin CE. Progression to cancer in Barrett's esophagus is associated with genomic instability. Lab Invest 60:65–71, 1989.

52. Reid BJ, Blount PL, Rubin CE, et al. Flow-cytometric and histological progression to malignancy in Barrett's esophagus: prospective endoscopic surveillance of a cohort. Gastroenterology 102:1212–1219, 1992.

53. McKinley MJ, Budman DR, Grueneberg D, et al. DNA content in Barrett's esophagus and esophageal malignancy. Am J Gastroenterol 82:1012–1015, 1987.

54. Fennerty MB, Sampliner RE, Way D, et al. Discordance between flow cytometric abnormalities and dysplasia in Barrett's esophagus. Gastroenterology 97:815–820, 1989.

55. Barrett MT, Sanchez CA, Prevo LJ, et al. Evolution of neoplastic cell lineages in Barrett oesophagus. Nat Genet 22:106–109, 1999.

56. Raskind WH, Norwood T, Levine DS, et al. Persistent clonal areas and clonal expansion in Barrett's esophagus. Cancer Res 52:2946–2950, 1992.

57. Blount P, rabinovitch PS, Haggitt RC, Reid BJ. Early Barrett's adenocarcinoma arises within a single aneuploid population [abstract]. Gastroenterology 98:A263, 1990.

58. Robaszkiewicz M, Hardy E, Volant A, et al. Flow cytometric analysis of cellular DNA content in Barrett's esophagus. A study of 66 cases. Gastroenterol Clin Biol 15:703–710, 1991.

59. Menke-Pluymers MB, Mulder AH, Hop WC, van Blankenstein M, Tilanus HW. Dysplasia and aneuploidy as markers of malignant degeneration in Barrett's oesophagus. The Rotterdam Oesophageal Tumour Study Group. Gut 35:1348–1351, 1994.

60. Gimenez A, Minguela A, Parrilla P, et al. Flow cytometric DNA analysis and p53 protein expression show a good correlation with histologic findings in patients with Barrett's esophagus. Cancer 83:641–651, 1998.

61. Teodori L, Gohde W, Persiani M, et al. DNA/protein flow cytometry as a predictive marker of malignancy in dysplasia-free Barrett's esophagus: thirteen-year follow-up study on a cohort of patients. Cytometry 34:257–263, 1998.

62. Reid BJ, Levine DS, Longton G, Blount PL, Rabinovitch PS. Predictors of progression to cancer in Barrett's esophagus: baseline histology and flow cytometry identify low- and high-risk patient subsets. Am J Gastroenterol 95:1669–1676, 2000.

63. Glogovac JK, Porter PL, Banker DE, Rabinovitch PS. Cytokeratin labeling of breast cancer cells extracted from paraffin-embedded tissue for bivariate flow cytometric analysis. Cytometry 24:260–267, 1996.

64. Garewal HS, Sampliner R, Liu Y, Trent JM. Chromosomal rearrangements in Barrett's esophagus. A premalignant lesion of esophageal adenocarcinoma. Cancer Genet Cytogenet 42:281–286, 1989.

65. Barrett MT, Sanchez CA, Galipeau PC, et al. Allelic loss of 9p21 and mutation of the *CDKN2/p16* gene develop as early lesions during neoplastic progression in Barrett's esophagus. Oncogene 13:1867–1873, 1996.

66. Barrett MT, Schutte M, Kern SE, Reid BJ. Allelic loss and mutational analysis of the DPC4 gene in esophageal adenocarcinoma. Cancer Res 56:4351–4353, 1996.

67. Dolan K, Garde J, Gosney J, et al. Allelotype analysis of oesophageal adenocarcinoma: loss of heterozygosity occurs at multiple sites. Br J Cancer 78:950–957, 1998.

68. Petty EM, Kalikin LM, Orringer MB, Beer DG. Distal chromosome 17q loss in Barrett's esophageal and gastric cardia adenocarcinomas: implications for tumorigenesis. Mol Carcinog 22:222–228, 1998.

69. Wu TT, Watanabe T, Heitmiller R, et al. Genetic alterations in Barrett esophagus and adenocarcinomas of the esophagus and esophagogastric junction region. Am J Pathol 153:287–294, 1998.

70. Moskaluk CA, Rumpel CA. Allelic deletion in 11p15 is a common occurrence in esophageal and gastric adenocarcinoma. Cancer 83:232–239, 1998.

71. Gleeson CM, Sloan JM, McManus DT, et al. Comparison of p53 and DNA content abnormalities in adenocarcinoma of the oesophagus and gastric cardia. Br J Cancer 77:277–286, 1998.

72. Hammoud ZT, Kaleem Z, Cooper JD, et al. Allelotype analysis of esophageal adenocarcinomas: evidence for the involvement of sequences on the long arm of chromosome 4. Cancer Res 56:4499–4502, 1996.

73. Swift A, Risk JM, Kingsnorth AN, et al. Frequent loss of heterozygosity on chromosome 17 at 17q11.2–q12 in Barrett's adenocarcinoma. Br J Cancer 71:995–998, 1995.

74. Rodriguez E, Rao PH, Ladanyi M, et al. 11p13–15 is a specific region of chromosomal rearrangement in gastric and esophageal adenocarcinomas. Cancer Res 50:6410–6416, 1990.

75. Hunter S, Gramlich T, Abbott K, Varma V. Y chromosome loss in esophageal carcinoma: an in situ hybridization study. Genes Chromosomes Cancer 8:172–177, 1993.

76. Krishnadath KK, Tilanus HW, Alers JC, Mulder AH, van Dekken H. Detection of genetic changes in Barrett's adenocarcinoma and Barrett's esophagus by DNA in situ hybridization and immunohistochemistry. Cytometry 15:176–184, 1994.

77. van Dekken H, Geelen E, Dinjens WN, et al. Comparative genomic hybridization of cancer of the gastroesophageal junction: deletion of 14Q31–32.1 discriminates between esophageal (Barrett's) and gastric cardia adenocarcinomas. Cancer Res 59:748–752, 1999.

78. Heim S, Mitelman F. Numerical chromosome aberrations in human neoplasia. Cancer Genet Cytogenet 22:99–108, 1986.

79. al-Kasspooles M, Moore JH, Orringer MB, Beer DG. Amplification and over-expression of the EGFR and erbB-2 genes in human esophageal adenocarcinomas. Int J Cancer 54:213–219, 1993.

80. Galiana C, Lozano JC, Bancel B, Nakazawa H, Yamasaki H. High frequency of Ki-ras amplification and p53 gene mutations in adenocarcinomas of the human esophagus. Mol Carcinog 14:286–293, 1995.

81. Houldsworth J, Cordon-Cardo C, Ladanyi M, Kelsen DP, Chaganti RS. Gene amplification in gastric and esophageal adenocarcinomas. Cancer Res 50:6417–6422, 1990.

82. Hughes SJ, Glover TW, Zhu XX, et al. A novel amplicon at 8p22–23 results in overexpression of cathepsin B in esophageal adenocarcinoma. Proc Natl Acad Sci USA 95:12410–12415, 1998.

83. Morgan RJ, Newcomb PV, Hardwick RH, Alderson D. Amplification of cyclin D1 and MDM-2 in oesophageal carcinoma. Eur J Surg Oncol 25:364–367, 1999.

84. Soslow RA, Altorki NK, Yang G, Xie D, Yang CS. mdm-2 expression correlates with wild-type p53 status in esophageal adenocarcinoma. Mod Pathol 12:580–586, 1999.

85. Michael D, Beer DG, Wilke CW, Miller DE, Glover TW. Frequent deletions of *FHIT* and *FRA3B* in Barrett's metaplasia and esophageal adenocarcinomas. Oncogene 15:1653–1659, 1997.

86. Muzeau F, Flejou JF, Belghiti J, Thomas G, Hamelin R. Infrequent microsatellite instability in oesophageal cancers. Br J Cancer 75:1336–1339, 1997.

87. Greenblatt MS, Bennett WP, Hollstein M, Harris CC. Mutations in the *p53* tumor suppressor gene: clues to cancer etiology and molecular pathogenesis. Cancer Res 54:4855–4878, 1994.

88. Ko LJ, Prives C. p53: puzzle and paradigm. Genes Dev 10:1054–1072, 1996.

89. Blount PL, Ramel S, Raskind WH, et al. 17p allelic deletions and p53 protein overexpression in Barrett's adenocarcinoma. Cancer Res 51: 5482–5486, 1991.

90. Galipeau PC, Prevo LJ, Sanchez CA, Longton GM, Reid BJ. Clonal expansion and loss of heterozygosity at chromosomes 9p and 17p in premalignant esophageal (Barrett's) tissue. J Natl Cancer Inst 91:2087–2095, 1999.

91. Prevo LJ, Sanchez CA, Galipeau PC, Reid BJ. p53-mutant clones and field effects in Barrett's esophagus. Cancer Res 59:4784–4787, 1999.

92. Hamelin R, Flejou JF, Muzeau F, et al. TP53 gene mutations and p53 protein immunoreactivity in malignant and premalignant Barrett's esophagus. Gastroenterology 107:1012–1018, 1994.

93. Hardwick RH, Shepherd NA, Moorghen M, Newcomb PV, Alderson D. Adenocarcinoma arising in Barrett's oesophagus: evidence for the participation of p53 dysfunction in the dysplasia/carcinoma sequence. Gut 35:764–768, 1994.

94. Sorsdahl K, Casson AG, Troster M, et al. p53 and ras gene expression in human esophageal cancer and Barrett's epithelium: a prospective study. Cancer Detect Prev 18:179–185, 1994.

95. Muzeau F, Flejou JF, Potet F, et al. Profile of p53 mutations and abnormal expression of P53 protein in 2 forms of esophageal cancer. Gastroenterol Clin Biol 20:430–437, 1996.

96. Jankowski J, Coghill G, Hopwood D, Wormsley KG. Oncogenes and onco-suppressor gene in adenocarcinoma of the oesophagus. Gut 33:1033–1038, 1992.

97. Flejou JF, Potet F, Muzeau F, et al. Overexpression of p53 protein in Barrett's syndrome with malignant transformation. J Clin Pathol 46:330–333, 1993.

98. Gleeson CM, Sloan JM, McGuigan JA, Ritchie AJ, Russell SE. Base transitions at CpG dinucleotides in the p53 gene are common in esophageal adenocarcinoma. Cancer Res 55:3406–3411, 1995.

99. Casson AG, Tammemagi M, Eskandarian S, et al. p53 alterations in oesophageal cancer: association with clinicopathological features, risk factors, and survival. Mol Pathol 51:71–79, 1998.

100. Neshat K, Sanchez CA, Galipeau PC, et al. p53 mutations in Barrett's adenocarcinoma and high-grade dysplasia. Gastroenterology 106:1589–1595, 1994.

101. Krishnadath KK, Tilanus HW, van Blankenstein M, Bosman FT, Mulder AH. Accumulation of p53 protein in normal, dysplastic, and neoplastic Barrett's oesophagus. J Pathol 175:175–180, 1995.

102. Younes M, Lebovitz RM, Lechago LV, Lechago J. p53 protein accumulation in Barrett's metaplasia, dysplasia, and carcinoma: a follow-up study. Gastroenterology 105:1637–1642, 1993.

103. Ramel S, Reid BJ, Sanchez CA, et al. Evaluation of p53 protein expression in Barrett's esophagus by two-parameter flow cytometry. Gastroenterology 102:1220–1228, 1992.

104. Weston AP, Banerjee SK, Persons DL, Cherian R, Sharma P. p53 positivity in low-grade dysplasia (LGD) in Barrett's esophagus: marker predictive of progression to cancer or multifocal high-grade dysplasia (mHGD) [abstract]. Am J Gastroenterol 94:2603, 1999.

105. Younes M, Ertan A, Lechago LV, Somoano JR, Lechago J. p53 protein accumulation is a specific marker of malignant potential in Barrett's metaplasia. Dig Dis Sci 42:697–701, 1997.

106. Cross SM, Sanchez CA, Morgan CA, et al. A p53-dependent mouse spindle checkpoint. Science 267:1353–1356, 1995.

107. Fukasawa K, Choi T, Kuriyama R, Rulong S, Vande Woude GF. Abnormal centrosome amplification in the absence of p53. Science 271:1744–1747, 1996.

108. Khan SH, Wahl GM. p53 and pRb prevent rereplication in response to microtubule inhibitors by mediating a reversible G1 arrest. Cancer Res 58:396–401, 1998.

109. Lanni JS, Jacks T. Characterization of the p53-dependent postmitotic checkpoint following spindle disruption. Mol Cell Biol 18:1055–1064, 1998.

110. Prives C. Signaling to p53: breaking the MDM2–p53 circuit. Cell 95:5–8, 1998.

111. Neshat K, Sanchez CA, Galipeau PC, et al. Barrett's esophagus: a model of human neoplastic progression. Cold Spring Harb Symp Quant Biol 59:577–583, 1994.

112. Tarmin L, Yin J, Zhou X, et al. Frequent loss of heterozygosity on chromosome 9 in adenocarcinoma and squamous cell carcinoma of the esophagus. Cancer Res 54:6094–6096, 1994.

113. Suzuki H, Zhou X, Yin J, et al. Intragenic mutations of CDKN2B and CDKN2A in primary human esophageal cancers. Hum Mol Genet 4:1883–1887, 1995.

114. Muzeau F, Flejou JF, Thomas G, Hamelin R. Loss of heterozygosity on chromosome 9 and p16 (MTS1, CDKN2) gene mutations in esophageal cancers. Int J Cancer 72:27–30, 1997.

115. Sherr CJ. Cancer cell cycles. Science 274:1672–1677, 1996.

116. Liggett WH Jr, Sidransky D. Role of the p16 tumor suppressor gene in cancer. J Clin Oncol 16:1197–1206, 1998.

117. Kiyono T, Foster SA, Koop JI, et al. Both Rb/p16INK4a inactivation and telomerase activity are required to immortalize human epithelial cells . Nature 396:84–88, 1998.

118. Okamoto A, Hussain SP, Hagiwara K, et al. Mutations in the p16INK4/MTS1/CDKN2, p15INK4B/MTS2, and p18 genes in primary and metastatic lung cancer. Cancer Res 55:1448–1451, 1995.

119. Rusin MR, Okamoto A, Chorazy M et al. Intragenic mutations of the p16(INK4), p15(INK4B) and p18 genes in primary non-small-cell lung cancers. Int J Cancer 65:734–739, 1996.

120. Li YJ, Hoang-Xuan K, Delattre JY, et al. Frequent loss of heterozygosity on chromosome 9, and low incidence of mutations of cyclin-dependent kinase inhibitors p15 (MTS2) and p16 (MTS1) genes in gliomas. Oncogene 11:597–600, 1995.

121. Okami K, Cairns P, Westra WH, et al. Detailed deletion mapping at chromosome 9p21 in non-small cell lung cancer by microsatellite analysis and fluorescence in situ hybridization. Int J Cancer 74:588–592, 1997.

122. Reed AL, Califano J, Cairns P, et al. High frequency of p16 (CDKN2/MTS-1/INK4A) inactivation in head and neck squamous cell carcinoma. Cancer Res 56:3630–3633, 1996.

123. Herman JG, Merlo A, Mao L, et al. Inactivation of the CDKN2/p16/MTS1 gene is frequently associated with aberrant DNA methylation in all common human cancers. Cancer Res 55:4525–4530, 1995.

124. Gonzalez-Zulueta M, Bender CM, Yang AS, et al. Methylation of the 5' CpG island of the p16/CDKN2 tumor suppressor gene in normal and transformed human tissues correlates with gene silencing. Cancer Res 55:4531–4535, 1995.

125. Merlo A, Herman JG, Mao L, et al. 5' CpG island methylation is associated with transcriptional silencing of the tumour suppressor p16/CDKN2/MTS1 in human cancers. Nat Med 1:686–692, 1995.

126. Clark SJ, Harrison J, Paul CL, Frommer M. High sensitivity mapping of methylated cytosines. Nucl Acids Res 22:2990–2997, 1994.

127. Herman JG, Graff JR, Myohanen S, Nelkin BD, Baylin SB. Methylation-specific PCR: a novel PCR assay for methylation status of CpG islands. Proc Natl Acad Sci USA 93:9821–9826, 1996.

128. Klump B, Hsieh CJ, Holzmann K, Gregor M, Porschen R. Hypermethylation of the CDKN2/p16 promoter during neoplastic progression in Barrett's esophagus. Gastroenterology 115:1381–1386, 1998.

129. Wong DJ, Barrett MT, Stoger R, Emond MJ, Reid BJ. p16INK4a promoter is hypermethylated at a high frequency in esophageal adenocarcinomas. Cancer Res 57:2619–2622, 1997.

130. Fearon ER, Vogelstein B. A genetic model for colorectal tumorigenesis. Cell 61:759–767, 1990.

131. Nowell PC. The clonal evolution of tumor cell populations. Science 194:23–28, 1976.

132. Richter J. Do we know the cause of reflux disease? Eur J Gastroenterol Hepatol 11 (Suppl 1):S3–S9, 1999.

133. Almasan A, Linke SP, Paulson TG, Huang LC, Wahl GM. Genetic instability as a consequence of inappropriate entry into and progression through S-phase. Cancer Metastasis Rev 14:59–73, 1995.

134. Denko NC, Giaccia AJ, Stringer JR, Stambrook PJ. The human Ha-ras oncogene induces genomic instability in murine fibroblasts within one cell cycle. Proc Natl Acad Sci USA 91:5124–5128, 1994.

135. de Vries JE, Kornips FH, Marx P, et al. Transfected c-Ha-ras oncogene enhances karyotypic instability and integrates predominantly in aberrant chromosomes. Cancer Genet Cytogenet 67:35–43, 1993.

136. Fukasawa K, Vande Woude GF. Synergy between the Mos/mitogen-activated protein kinase pathway and loss of p53 function in transformation and chromosome instability. Mol Cell Biol 17:506–518, 1997.

137. Paulson TG, Almasan A, Brody LL, Wahl GM. Gene amplification in a p53-deficient cell line requires cell cycle progression under conditions that generate DNA breakage. Mol Cell Biol 18:3089–3100, 1998.

138. Evan G, Littlewood T. A matter of life and cell death. Science 281:1317–1322, 1998.

139. Elledge SJ. Cell cycle checkpoints: preventing an identity crisis. Science 274:1664–1672, 1996.

140. Ames BN, Gold LS. Mitogenesis, mutagenesis, and animal cancer tests. Prog Clin Biol Res 369:1–20, 1991.

of whom succumbed to other diseases before developing adenocarcinoma in their Barrett's esophagus. The cancer risk and long-term survival for patients with short-segment Barrett's esophagus are not known. Some reports have suggested that such patients may be substantially less likely to develop cancer than patients with long-segment disease,[80-83] but one recent study found no significant difference in the cancer risk for these two groups.[84]

## Dysplasia in Barrett's Esophagus

As discussed in the previous chapter, cancers in Barrett's esophagus develop through a series of genetic alterations that activate proto-oncogenes, disable tumor suppressor genes, or both.[85] These mutations give the cells certain advantages in growth and survival, and the advantaged cells hyperproliferate. During hyperproliferation, the cells acquire more genetic changes that may eventuate in autonomous, clonal growth (neoplasia). Dysplasia becomes cancer when a clone emerges with DNA abnormalities that enable the cells to invade adjacent tissues and to proliferate in unnatural locations. Before the cells acquire enough DNA damage to become cancerous, the earlier genetic alterations often cause histologic changes that can be recognized by the pathologist as dysplasia. The dysplastic changes can be graded as low grade or high grade, depending on the degree of alterations in nuclear morphology and glandular architecture.[86]

High-grade dysplasia is widely regarded as the precursor of invasive cancer in Barrett's esophagus. Endoscopic surveillance is recommended for patients with Barrett's esophagus primarily to seek high-grade dysplasia, with the rationale that removal of this precancerous tissue should prevent the progression to invasive malignancy.[87] Unlike the colon, in which dysplasia and early cancers often take the form of polyps that are easily recognized and removed endoscopically, early neoplasia in Barrett's esophagus is usually flat and inconspicuous. Whereas the dysplastic changes cannot be recognized grossly, endoscopists rely on random biopsy sampling techniques to identify early neoplasms, and this introduces a major problem of biopsy sampling error. Foci of dysplasia can easily be overlooked and, for patients found to have dysplasia, foci of invasive cancer can be missed. Among patients who have esophageal resections performed because endoscopic examination reveals high-grade dysplasia, approximately one-third have been found to have a malignancy in the resected specimen that was missed due to biopsy sampling error.[88]

Extensive biopsy sampling of the Barrett esophagus can reduce, but not eliminate, the problem of biopsy sampling error. One group has reported that they could differentiate high-grade dysplasia from early adenocarcinoma in Barrett's esophagus by adherence to a very rigorous endoscopic biopsy protocol.[89] They obtained four-quadrant biopsy specimens using "jumbo" biopsy forceps at 2-cm intervals throughout the columnar-lined esophagus, and took many additional samples from sites of known dysplasia. After preoperative evaluation by this protocol, none of seven patients who had an esophageal resection for high-grade dysplasia was found to have invasive cancer in the resected esophagus. For each of those seven patients, however, an average of 99 preoperative biopsy specimens were available for review. This extensive sampling undoubtedly minimized the problem of biopsy sampling error. It is not clear that the use of jumbo biopsy forceps contributed to the low rate of sampling error, and another recent study by a different group of investigators suggests that the use of jumbo forceps does not significantly improve the diagnostic yield. In that study, 38 patients with high-grade dysplasia in Barrett's esophagus had preoperative evaluation with four-quadrant biopsy specimens taken at intervals of every 2 cm.[90] In 16 patients in whom the preoperative specimens were obtained with standard biopsy forceps, invasive cancer was found in the resected specimen in 6 (38%). In 12 patients in whom the specimens were taken with jumbo forceps, invasive cancer was found in 4 (33%). This difference was not statistically significant.

Relatively little information is available regarding the natural history of dysplasia in Barrett's esophagus. The speed and frequency with which dysplasia progresses to cancer are not clear, and reports of available studies often describe contradictory results. Hameeteman et al.[91] described eight patients with high-grade dysplasia in Barrett's esophagus, five of whom developed adenocarcinoma within 1 year of the discovery of high-grade dysplasia. In contrast, other investigators have described patients in whom high-grade dysplasia persisted for years with no apparent progression to malignancy.[92] Levine et al.[89] found that 7 of 29 patients (24%) with high-grade dysplasia progressed to invasive cancer during a follow-up period of 2 to 46 months.[89] In a preliminary report from the Hines VA Hospital, only 10 of 69 patients with Barrett's esophagus (14.5%) who had high-grade dysplasia and no evidence of invasive cancer on initial endoscopic evaluation developed adenocarcinoma during a mean follow-up period of 3.8 years.[93] The reasons underlying the disparate results of these studies are not clear. Although high-grade dysplasia may not always progress to cancer, the rate of progression clearly is worrisome.

Another factor that limits the utility of dysplasia as a biomarker for malignancy is the substantial interobserver variation in the grading of this lesion. In one study in which eight expert morphologists were asked to grade dysplastic changes in Barrett's esophagus, interobserver agreement rates were reasonable (85% and 87% agreement for the diagnoses of high-grade dysplasia and intramucosal carcinoma, respectively).[94] When differentiating low-grade dysplasia from reactive epithelial changes caused by reflux esophagitis, however, the interobserver variation was unacceptably low.

Noting the shortcomings of dysplasia as a biomarker for malignancy in Barrett's esophagus, a number of investigators have sought alternative biomarkers. For example, abnormalities in flow cytometry and in the expression of p53 have been found to be earlier and more specific markers for cancer development than the histologic finding of dysplasia[95-98] (see Chapter 19). However, no alternative biomarker has yet been shown to provide sufficient additional information (beyond that provided by histologic examination) to justify its routine application in clinical practice.[97,99] Pending further studies, the finding of dysplasia remains the most appropriate biomarker for the clinical evaluation of patients with Barrett's esophagus.

## Proposed Endoscopic Techniques to Identify Dysplasia

As noted above, dysplastic epithelium in Barrett's esophagus often has no distinguishing endoscopic features. A number of new techniques have been proposed that might highlight dysplastic areas for targeted biopsy sampling during the endoscopic examination. These techniques include chromoendoscopy, endosonography, optical coherence tomography, and fluorescence detection techniques.

In chromoendoscopy, vital dyes (e.g., Lugol's iodine, toluidine blue, methylene blue, indigo carmine) are applied to the esophagus to enhance the endoscopic detection of metaplastic and dysplastic epithelia.[100-104] Available studies on chromoendoscopy in Barrett's esophagus are limited, however, and the results are inconclusive. Presently, this technique cannot be recommended for routine use in clinical practice.

In endosonography, high-frequency ultrasonic waves (e.g., 12 or 20 MHz) are delivered through a transducer that is applied directly to the mucosa of the esophagus to provide detailed images of the esophageal wall and adjacent structures. The technique has been used for the evaluation of tumors and dysplasia in Barrett's esophagus. Preliminary studies have been disappointing, however.[104,105] In one study of nine patients who had esophageal resections for high-grade dysplasia in Barrett's esophagus, preoperative endosonography correctly staged the disease in only four cases.[105] Two patients had early cancers in the resected esophagus even though endosonography revealed no abnormality suggestive of malignancy. Unfortunately, the accuracy of endosonography in staging early neoplasms in Barrett's esophagus appears to be limited. More studies and refinements in technique are needed before endoscopic ultrasonography can be advocated as an adjunct to biopsy sampling for surveillance of Barrett's esophagus.

Optical coherence tomography (OCT) uses infrared light to provide high-resolution cross-sectional imaging of the esophageal mucosa.[106] The technique is similar in principle to endosonography, but image formation in OCT depends on variations in the reflectance of light (rather than ultrasonic waves) from different tissue layers. This method does not require direct contact between the optical fiber and the tissue, and the spatial resolution of the resulting image is up to 10 times higher than that of endosonography. Studies are in progress to determine if OCT will have a role in the management of Barrett's esophagus.

Fluorescence endoscopy is a technique for identifying areas of esophageal dysplasia that can be targeted for biopsy sampling.[107] The technique exploits the fact that cells contain endogenous fluorophores (e.g., NADH, porphyrins) that can absorb laser light and re-emit it as fluorescent light with distinctive spectroscopic characteristics. For some tissues, the fluorescence spectra induced by laser irradiation can distinguish normal from neoplastic epithelia. Panjehpour et al.[108] used laser-induced fluorescence spectroscopy (LIFS) to study 36 patients with Barrett's esophagus, and found an excellent correlation between fluorescence spectral abnormalities and the finding of high-grade dysplasia. A major drawback to the use of LIFS is the time and effort required to sample large areas of mucosa with these pinpoint "optical biopsies." The technique of laser-induced fluorescence endoscopy (LIFE) obviates this problem by using real-time fluorescence imaging to study large areas of the mucosal surface. Preliminary experience with LIFE suggests that it can identify dysplastic lesions in Barrett's esophagus that are not apparent by conventional (white light) endoscopy.[109,110]

The fluorescent signals emitted by endogenous fluorophores are faint, and require expensive, sophisticated instruments for their detection and interpretation. Stronger fluorescence that is far easier to measure can be obtained by administering an exogenous fluorophore that is concentrated selectively by neoplastic tissue.[108-110] Exogenous fluorophores that have been used for this purpose include hematoporphyrin derivatives and 5-aminolevulinic acid (5-ALA), a substance that is metabolized by cells into the potent fluorophore protoporphyrin IX. As for the other techniques mentioned above, more studies are needed before fluorescence endoscopy using either endogenous or exogenous fluorophores can be recommended for widespread clinical application.

## Treatment

The major components of the management of patients with Barrett's esophagus are summarized in Table 20–2.

### Treatment of Gastroesophageal Reflux Disease in Barrett's Esophagus

Modern medical therapy for severe GERD involves aggressive suppression of gastric acid through the administration of proton pump inhibitors (PPIs).[111] This treatment is highly effective in healing the symptoms and endoscopic signs of GERD for patients with Barrett's esophagus.[112,113] However, it is not clear that antireflux therapy can prevent the peptic or neoplastic complications of GERD. Therapy with PPIs clearly improves dysphagia and decreases the need for esophageal dilations in patients who have esophageal strictures,[114,115] but no study has documented that treatment prevents patients with Barrett's esophagus from developing peptic strictures.[116] Gastroesophageal reflux disease is known to be a strong risk factor for esophageal adenocarcinoma and, therefore, effective GERD treatment might be expected to decrease the cancer risk for patients with Barrett's esophagus.[4] However, it is not clear whether GERD predisposes to malignancy by causing Barrett's esophagus to develop in the first place, by promoting the transition from metaplasia to neoplasia in established Barrett's esophagus, or both. The hypothesis that chronic reflux esophagitis might predispose to cancer by increasing proliferation of the metaplastic cells seems reasonable, but no study has established that any form of antireflux therapy reduces the risk of cancer in Barrett's esophagus.

Whereas no study has shown that antireflux therapy decreases the cancer risk in Barrett's esophagus, regression of the metaplastic epithelium with GERD treatment has been proposed as a surrogate marker for decreased cancer risk.[117] Although antireflux therapy rarely, if ever, results in complete regression of the metaplastic lining, partial regression (evidenced by the appearance of islands of squamous epithelium within the metaplastic columnar lining) is observed frequently in patients treated with PPIs or antireflux surgery. Unfortunately, it is not clear that such regression is beneficial.[118] In one recent study, Sharma et al.[119] obtained 39 biopsy specimens from squamous islands in 22 patients with Barrett's esophagus, most of whom had been treated with PPIs. Intestinal metaplasia underlying squamous epithelium was found in 15 of the 39 specimens (39%). Another group found abnormalities in Ki-67 staining and p53 expression frequently in biopsy specimens of squamous islands from patients who had been treated with PPIs.[120] These two observations suggest that the partial regression of metaplasia induced by PPI therapy might have little effect in decreasing cancer risk.

There is some circumstantial evidence to support the notion that control of acid reflux might prevent the progression from metaplasia to malignancy in Barrett's esophagus. For example, biopsy specimens of specialized intestinal metaplasia maintained in organ culture exhibit hyperproliferation when they are exposed

**Table 20-2** Management of patients with Barrett's esophagus

Treat the associated gastroesophageal reflux disease
Advise endoscopic surveillance to detect dysplasia
Treat dysplasia detected
Consider experimental techniques for ablating the metaplastic mucosa

to brief acid pulses (1 hour in duration).[121] This in vitro observation suggests that the episodic acid reflux that occurs frequently in patients with Barrett's esophagus might stimulate cellular hyperproliferation and thereby promote carcinogenesis. Ouatu-Lascar et al.[122] took biopsy specimens from 39 patients with Barrett's esophagus at baseline and after 6 months of therapy with PPIs. The PPIs were given in doses that were sufficient to eliminate symptoms, but not necessarily sufficient to normalize acid reflux. On this regimen, abnormal acid reflux persisted in 15 patients, whereas acid reflux decreased into the normal range in 24 patients. The expression of PCNA (a proliferation marker) decreased and the expression of villin (a differentiation marker) increased significantly only in biopsy specimens from the 24 patients in whom PPI therapy resulted in normalization of esophageal acid exposure.

These studies provide indirect support for the notion that total elimination of acid reflux might be beneficial for patients with Barrett's esophagus. Conventional medical therapy for GERD decreases, but does not eliminate, episodes of acid reflux in most patients. Recent studies have shown that approximately 70% of individuals treated with a PPI twice a day exhibit nocturnal gastric acid breakthrough (defined as a gastric pH <4 for >1 hour at night), and that brief episodes of acid reflux occur frequently during these breakthrough periods in patients with Barrett's esophagus.[123,124] Furthermore, when patients with Barrett's esophagus are treated with PPIs in doses that completely eliminate GERD symptoms and signs, they often exhibit pathological levels of acid reflux nonetheless.[122,125,126]

In some patients, it is ssible to abolish the nocturnal acid breakthrough that occur ing PPI therapy by the addition of a histamine H$_2$-recepto cker at bedtime.[127] Using this combination (a PPI giver e daily and an H$_2$-receptor blocker given at bedtime), it may be possible to eliminate acid reflux in patients with Barrett's esophagus. Some authorities have recommended that this regimen be adopted for widespread clinical use.[128] Others caution against the routine use of this therapy for the following reasons. *(1)* Perfect control of acid reflux clearly is not necessary to effect the healing of reflux esophagitis in most patients. Indeed, the esophageal symptoms and signs of GERD disappear in most patients who are treated simply with a PPI taken in conventional dosage (i.e., only once each day).[129] *(2)* The evidence to support the notion that complete elimination of acid reflux reduces the cancer risk in Barrett's esophagus is indirect and weak at best. It is a large and unsubstantiated leap of faith to assume that effects observed on tissues in organ culture and on proliferation markers in biopsy specimens are useful markers for decreased cancer risk in Barrett's esophagus. *(3)* Some experimental data suggest that elimination of acid reflux may not even be desirable. In an experimental model of esophageal adenocarcinoma involving rats treated with a carcinogen, for example, exposure of the esophagus to acidic gastric juice *protected* against the development of cancer.[130] *(4)* Complete elimination of acid reflux involves considerable inconvenience and expense. This treatment requires the administration of high dosages of expensive medications and the performance of esophageal pH monitoring studies to document the efficacy of therapy in controlling acid reflux. Pending further investigations, it seems reasonable to treat patients with Barrett's esophagus according to the general guidelines established for the medical treatment of patients with GERD.[111] According to these guidelines, medications are used in whatever dosage is necessary to control the symptoms and signs of GERD.

## Endoscopic Surveillance

Two unproved and controversial assumptions underlie the recommendation that regular endoscopic surveillance should be performed for patients with Barrett's esophagus: *(1)* Barrett's esophagus adversely influences survival, and *(2)* endoscopic surveillance can reliably detect early, curable neoplasia in this condition. Regarding the first assumption, two studies have found that the long-term survival of patients with Barrett's esophagus does not differ significantly from that of age- and gender-matched control subjects in the general population.[78,79] However, these studies consisted predominantly of older patients who succumbed to other diseases before they could develop adenocarcinoma in their Barrett's esophagus. Perhaps a study of younger patients would demonstrate an adverse effect on survival, but such a study has not been reported.

Only indirect evidence supports the assumption that surveillance can reliably detect curable neoplasia. One study compared the outcome for 58 patients who first presented to the hospital with symptoms of esophageal cancer (in whom Barrett's esophagus was discovered incidentally during evaluation of the malignancy) with that for 19 patients known to have Barrett's esophagus who had cancers discovered during endoscopic surveillance.[131] The patients whose cancers were discovered during surveillance had tumors in an earlier stage of development and had better long-term survivals than those who presented to the hospital with cancer symptoms. A cost-effectiveness analysis has concluded that the cost of detecting an early cancer by endoscopic surveillance for patients with Barrett's esophagus compares favorably to the cost of mammographic surveillance for women at risk for breast cancer.[75] Some studies have shown that surveillance can detect early esophageal neoplasms in patients with Barrett's esophagus, but no study has proved that endoscopic surveillance reduces the mortality from esophageal cancer.

Provenzale et al.[132,133] have explored the value of different endoscopic surveillance strategies using computer models to construct cohort simulations of patients with Barrett's esophagus. These models are highly sensitive to the value chosen for the incidence of esophageal cancer. As discussed above, reported estimates of cancer incidence in Barrett's esophagus range from 0.2% to 2.9% per year. As shown in Figure 20–5, when the in-

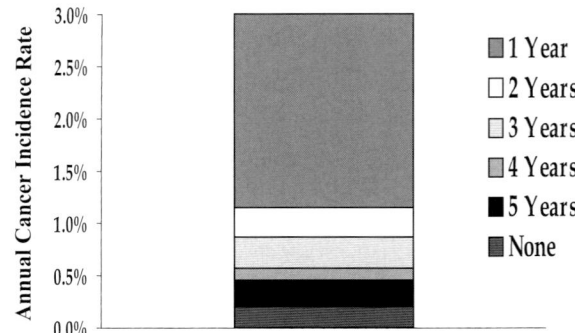

**Figure 20–5** Optimal endoscopic surveillance intervals for quality-adjusted life expectancy in Barrett's esophagus. From a computer model, the graph shows how the optimal endoscopic surveillance intervals vary with the value chosen for the annual rate of cancer incidence in Barrett's esophagus (assuming that the primary goal is to enhance length and quality of life without regard to costs). (Data adapted from Provenzale et al.[133] and reprinted, with permission, from Spechler[71].)

cidence rate falls below 0.2% per year, no endoscopic surveillance at all is the preferred strategy to increase quality-adjusted life expectancy, because this is the point at which procedural risks exceed the benefit of early cancer detection. If one assumes that the annual cancer incidence rate is 1.0%, then endoscopic surveillance every 2 years would be the preferred strategy, whereas surveillance every fourth year would be recommended for a cancer incidence rate of 0.5%. Note that, in this model, the decision whether to recommend yearly surveillance or no surveillance at all hinges on a difference of only 1% in the estimated risk of esophageal cancer.

## Ablative Therapies for Dysplasia and Metaplasia

The only therapy that clearly interrupts the progression from high-grade dysplasia to malignancy in Barrett's esophagus is esophageal resection, a procedure associated with substantial rates of morbidity and morality. The role of this definitive therapy in the management of patients with high-grade dysplasia is disputed.[134] Noting the risks of the procedure, some authorities recommend that patients found to have high-grade dysplasia should be followed with intensive endoscopic surveillance, with esophageal resection performed if and when that surveillance reveals invasive cancer.[134] Others prefer a more aggressive approach, recommending esophageal resection for all fit patients found to have high-grade dysplasia in Barrett's esophagus.[135] Whereas there are no definitive studies on this issue, the controversy will continue.

Endoscopic ablation therapy has been proposed as an alternative to esophageal resection for patients with high-grade dysplasia in Barrett's esophagus.[136,137] Using thermal or photochemical energy delivered endoscopically, it is possible to ablate the metaplastic columnar lining in Barrett's esophagus (Table 20–3).[128] When acid reflux is controlled with PPIs or fundoplication, the ablated columnar epithelium heals with the regeneration of squamous epithelium. The relative merits of the various endoscopic ablation modalities listed in Table 20–3 are disputed, and there appears to be a trade-off between the completeness of mucosal ablation and the frequency of complications. Modalities that cause a deep mucosal injury (e.g., Nd:YAG laser) appear to be effective at eliminating the metaplastic mucosa, but the rate of complications such as esophageal perforation and stricture formation is high. Conversely, modalities that induce relatively superficial mucosal injury (e.g., argon laser) cause few complications, but may leave residual foci of metaplastic tissue behind.

Among the ablative therapies available for Barrett's esophagus, photodynamic therapy (PDT) is perhaps the easiest to administer and the most extensively studied.[136] In PDT, patients are

**Table 20–3** Endoscopic techniques for ablating Barrett's esophagus

*Heat-generating*

Laser (argon, Nd:YAG, KTP)
Multipolar electrocoagulation
Argon beam plasma coagulation

*Freezing*

Cold nitrogen gas

*Photochemical Energy*

Photodynamic therapy

given a systemic dose of a light-activated chemical, usually a porphyrin or porphyrin precursor, that is taken up by the metaplastic columnar cells.[138] The esophagus is then irradiated endoscopically using a low-power laser to activate the chemical. This results in the production of singlet oxygen, a toxic molecule that can destroy epithelial cells and their vasculature. Thus, PDT can be used to ablate metaplastic, dysplastic, and malignant cells in Barrett's esophagus.

Overholt et al.[139] recently described the results of PDT with porfimer sodium for 100 patients who had either superficial cancers or dysplasia in Barrett's esophagus. Patients were followed for a mean duration of 19 months (range 4 to 84 months). For 13 patients with superficial cancers, PDT appeared to eliminate the malignancy in 10 cases (77%). Following PDT for 73 patients with high-grade dysplasia, there was no evidence of dysplasia on follow-up endoscopy in 56 cases (77%). For 14 patients with low-grade dysplasia, PDT resulted in apparent eradication of dysplasia in 13 cases (93%). Unfortunately, the rate of side effects and complications was high. Most patients experienced minor problems with photosensitivity, whereas 4 of the 100 patients experienced substantial problems when they exposed themselves to direct sunlight. Most patients experienced chest pain and dysphagia of mild to moderate severity for 5 to 7 days after the laser treatment, and many required hospitalization to prevent dehydration during that period. Small pleural effusions also developed in most patients, a phenomenon suggesting that PDT often causes transmural injury to the esophagus. Three patients developed atrial fibrillation after PDT, all of whom were treated successfully without sequelae. Perhaps most worrisome was the high rate of esophageal stricture formation: 34% of patients developed esophageal strictures that required one or more sessions of dilation therapy.

Modifications of the PDT procedure have been used in an attempt to reduce the rate of complications. Laukka and Wang[140] tried "low-dose" PDT (porfimer sodium 1.5 mg/kg, 175 J/cm light energy) in five patients who had dysplasia in Barrett's esophagus. The PDT induced partial regression of the columnar metaplasia, but dysplasia persisted in all five cases. Two groups have reported the results of PDT using the alternative photosensitizer 5-ALA in Barrett's esophagus.[141,142] Barr et al.[141] treated five patients with high-grade dysplasia. No evidence of dysplasia was found in any patient on endoscopic examinations performed during follow-up periods ranging from 26 to 44 months, but biopsy specimens taken in treated areas revealed residual foci of columnar metaplasia buried under squamous epithelium in two of the five patients. Gossner et al.[142] used PDT with 5-ALA to treat 22 patients with superficial cancers and 10 patients with high-grade dysplasia in Barrett's esophagus. During a mean follow-up period of 9.9 months, no residual cancer was found in 17 of 22 patients (77%), and high-grade dysplasia appeared to have been eradicated in all 10 cases. Cancers with a thickness of >2 mm were not eliminated by PDT with ALA. The treatment caused only minor side effects, but all patients had residual metaplastic columnar epithelium in the esophagus.

None of the reports showing that metaplastic columnar epithelium in the esophagus can be ablated has established that the procedure is beneficial in any way. When interpreting the studies, furthermore, it is important to consider the substantial problem of biopsy sampling error. As discussed above, esophageal resection for high-grade dysplasia in Barrett's esophagus often reveals invasive cancer that was missed due to biopsy sampling error.[88] Without histologic examination of the resected esophagus or very long periods of follow-up, it is not possible to verify the claims that dysplasia and cancer in Barrett's esophagus are "eliminated" by ablative therapy. The progression from dysplasia to cancer in Barrett's esophagus may be slow,[92] and reports from China have documented that small esophageal cancers can remain asymptomatic for years.[143] Thus, it is inappropriate to conclude on the basis of random biopsy specimens obtained within months of ablation that cancer and dysplasia have been eradicated. Also, ablative therapies usually do not eliminate all of the metaplastic epithelium in the esophagus. Residual foci of metaplasia remain in most patients, and some of these foci may be buried under a superficial layer of squamous epithelium where they are no longer visible. Failure to obliterate all of the metaplastic epithelium might leave patients at high risk for malignancy, and the inability to detect metaplasia hidden by the overgrowth of squamous epithelium might compromise surveillance programs. At least one report has documented the development of intramucosal adenocarcinoma arising under squamous re-epithelialization of Barrett's esophagus.[144] Finally, no study yet has established that ablative therapy has any effect on the risk for cancer development in Barrett's esophagus. Therefore, patients treated with ablation probably require regular endoscopic surveillance. Presently, ablative therapy cannot be recommended for widespread application. However, ablation may be a reasonable choice for patients with high-grade dysplasia or superficial cancers in Barrett's esophagus who are too old, infirm, or unwilling to assume the considerable risks of esophageal resection, provided the procedure is performed as part of an established study protocol.

For patients found to have low-grade dysplasia in Barrett's esophagus, very few data are available to guide the clinician in choosing the appropriate management. It can be difficult to distinguish the changes of low-grade dysplasia from reactive changes in an epithelium that is regenerating in response to inflammatory injury, and the natural history of verified low-grade dysplasia is not well described. Consequently, most authorities are reluctant to recommend a potentially hazardous procedure like esophageal resection for patients with low-grade dysplasia in Barrett's esophagus.

### How the Risk of Cancer Might Affect the Choice of Therapy for Barrett's Esophagus

As mentioned above, no treatment for Barrett's esophagus has been shown to decrease the risk of esophageal cancer. However, antireflux surgery,[145,146] aggressive antisecretory therapy,[128] and endoscopic ablative therapies all have been proposed as potential means to prevent cancer development. One evidence-based tool that can be used to assist clinicians in deciding whether the potential benefits of a treatment outweigh its disadvantages is the calculation of the number needed to treat (NNT).[71,147] This is done using the formula NNT = 1/ARR, where ARR is the absolute risk reduction achieved by the treatment. Assume, for the sake of argument, that there is a highly effective treatment for Barrett's esophagus that will reduce the risk of cancer development by one-half, i.e., from 0.50% to 0.25% per year. This represents an ARR of 0.25%, or 0.0025. In this example, NNT = 1/0.0025 = 400. If this optimistic assessment of risk reduction attributable to therapy is correct, then 400 patients would need to be treated in order to prevent one cancer. Such a large NNT might be acceptable if the treatment were very safe, inexpensive, and convenient. However, none of the proposed treatments for Barrett's esophagus mentioned meet all of these criteria. For an-

tireflux operations, the surgical mortality rate alone (at least 0.2% for laparoscopic Nissen fundoplication[148]) is similar to the proposed ARR for cancer (0.25%). Thus, approximately as many patients would succumb to surgical mortality as would have died from adenocarcinoma if fundoplication were recommended solely for the purpose of cancer prophylaxis in Barrett's esophagus (assuming the operation is highly effective in preventing cancer). Endoscopic ablative therapies also can have serious complications, aggressive antisecretory therapy is inconvenient, and all of these treatments are expensive. Furthermore, the NNT calculation used in this example is based on a reduction of absolute risk that has not been established for any therapy. It is not clear that the treatments mentioned above reduce the risk of cancer development at all, let alone by one-half. A smaller ARR would raise the NNT even higher.

When considering new therapies for GERD and Barrett's esophagus, clinicians must exercise clear, critical thinking. A useful therapy cannot be more dangerous than the disorder it is intended to treat. In their zeal to prevent an uncommon cancer, physicians should not recommend unproved and potentially hazardous therapies for patients with GERD and Barrett's esophagus. The efficacy of such therapies must be verified in controlled trials before they can be recommended for widespread clinical application.

### Management Recommendations

Despite all the controversies discussed above, most authorities continue to recommend regular endoscopic surveillance for patients with Barrett's esophagus.[149] The American College of Gastroenterology recently proposed the following practice guidelines for cancer surveillance in Barrett's esophagus[150]:

- Patients with Barrett's esophagus should undergo surveillance endoscopy and biopsy at an interval determined by the presence and grade of dysplasia. Gastroesophageal reflux disease should be treated aggressively prior to surveillance endoscopy to minimize confusion caused by inflammation in the interpretation of biopsy specimens. The technique of random, four-quadrant biopsies taken every 2 cm in the columnar-lined esophagus for standard histologic evaluation is recommended.
- For patients with no dysplasia, surveillance endoscopy is recommended at an interval of every 2 to 3 years.
- For patients with low-grade dysplasia, surveillance endoscopy every 6 months for the first year is recommended, followed by yearly endoscopy if the dysplasia has not progressed in severity.
- For patients with high-grade dysplasia, two alternatives are proposed after the diagnosis has been confirmed by an expert gastrointestinal pathologist:
  1. One alternative is intensive endoscopic surveillance until intramucosal cancer is detected. The guideline does not recommend a specific interval for such surveillance, but some investigators have studied such patients at an interval of every 3 months.
  2. The other alternative is to recommend esophageal resection.

Although not specifically recommended in the practice guidelines, clinicians can consider the use of experimental ablative therapies such as photodynamic therapy for their patients with high-grade dysplasia in Barrett's esophagus, *provided the therapy is administered as part of an established, approved research protocol.* The use of ablative therapies outside of research protocols cannot be condoned at this time.

### References

1. Spechler SJ, Goyal RK. The columnar lined esophagus, intestinal metaplasia, and Norman Barrett. Gastroenterology 110:614–621, 1996.

2. Antonioli DA, Wang HH. Morphology of Barrett's esophagus and Barrett's-associated dysplasia and adenocarcinoma. Gastroenterol Clin North Am 26:495–506, 1997.

3. Spechler SJ. Laser photoablation of Barrett's epithelium: burning issues about burning tissues. Gastroenterology 104:1855–1858, 1993.

4. Lagergren J, Bergström R, Lindgren A, Nyrén O. Symptomatic gastroesophageal reflux as a risk factor for esophageal adenocarcinoma. N Engl J Med 340:825–831, 1999.

5. Devesa SS, Blot WJ, Fraumeni JF Jr. Changing patterns in the incidence of esophageal and gastric carcinoma in the United States. Cancer 83:2049–2053, 1998.

6. Spechler SJ. Short and ultrashort Barrett's esophagus: what does it mean? Semin Gastrointest Dis 8:59–67, 1997.

7. Tytgat GNJ. Endoscopic features of the columnar-lined esophagus. Gastroenterol Clin North Am 26:507–517, 1997.

8. Kim SL, Waring PJ, Spechler SJ, Sampliner RE, Doos WG, Krol WF, Williford WO, and the Department of Veterans Affairs Gastroesophageal Reflux Study Group. Diagnostic inconsistencies in Barrett's esophagus. Gastroenterology 107:945–949, 1994.

9. Paull A, Trier JS, Dalton MD, Camp RC, Loeb P, Goyal RK. The histologic spectrum of Barrett's esophagus. N Engl J Med 295:476–480, 1976.

10. Weinstein WM, Ippoliti AF. The diagnosis of Barrett's esophagus: goblets, goblets, goblets. Gastrointest Endosc 44:91–95, 1996.

11. Eloubeidi MA, Provenzale D. Does this patient have Barrett's esophagus? The utility of predicting Barrett's esophagus at the index endoscopy. Am J Gastroenterol 94:937–943, 1999.

12. Spechler SJ, Zeroogian JM, Antonioli DA, Wang HH, Goyal RK. Prevalence of metaplasia at the gastro-oesophageal junction. Lancet 344: 1533–1536, 1994.

13. Spechler SJ. The columnar lined oesophagus: a riddle wrapped in a mystery inside an enigma. Gut 41:710–711, 1997.

14. Hirota WK, Loughney TM, Lazas DJ, Maydonovitch CL, Rholl V, Wong RKH. Specialized intestinal metaplasia, dysplasia, and cancer of the esophagus and esophagogastric junction: prevalence and clinical data. Gastroenterology 116:277–285, 1999.

15. Weston AP, Krmpotich P, Makdisi WE, Cherian R, Dixon A, McGregor DH, Banerjee SK. Short-segment Barrett's esophagus: clinical and histological features, associated endoscopic findings, and association with gastric intestinal metaplasia. Am J Gastroenterol 91:981–986, 1996.

16. Sharma P, Morales TG, Sampliner RE. Short-segment Barrett's esophagus—the need for standardization of the definition and of endoscopic criteria. Am J Gastroenterol 93:1033–1036, 1998.

17. Kilgore SP, Ormsby AH, Gramlich TL, Rice TW, Richter JE, Galk GW, Goldblum JR. The gastric cardia: fact or fiction? Am J Gastroenterol 95:921–924, 2000.

18. McClave SA, Boyce HW Jr, Gottfried MR. Early diagnosis of columnar-lined esophagus: a new endoscopic criterion. Gastrointest Endosc 33:413–416, 1987.

19. Spechler SJ. The role of gastric carditis in metaplasia and neoplasia at the gastroesophageal junction. Gastroenterology 117:218–228, 1999.

20. Stemmermann GN. Intestinal metaplasia of the stomach. A status report. Cancer 74:556–564, 1994.

21. Asaka M, Takeda H, Sugiyama T, Kato M. What role does Helicobacter pylori play in gastric cancer? Gastroenterology 113:556–560, 1997.

22. Parsonnet J. Helicobacter pylori in the stomach—a paradox unmasked. N Engl J Med 335:278–280, 1996.

23. Correa P. Helicobacter pylori and gastric carcinogenesis. Am J Surg Pathol 19(Suppl 1):S37–S43, 1995.

24. Watanabe T, Tada M, Nagai H, Sasaki S, Nakao M. Helicobacter pylori infection induces gastric cancer in Mongolian gerbils. Gastroenterology 115:642–648, 1998.

25. Parsonnet J, Friedman GD, Orentreich N, Vogelman H. Risk for gastric cancer in people with CagA-positive or CagA-negative Helicobacter pylori infection. Gut 40:297–301, 1997.

26. O'Connor HJ, Cunnane K. Helicobacter pylori and gastro-oesophageal reflux disease–a prospective study. Ir J Med Sci 163:369–373, 1994.

27. Liston R, Pitt MA, Banerjee AK. Reflux oesophagitis and Helicobacter pylori infection in elderly patients. Postgrad Med J 72:221–223, 1996.

28. Rosioru C, Glassman MS, Halata MS, Schwarz SM. Esophagitis and Helicobacter pylori in children: incidence and therapeutic implications. Am J Gastroenterol 88:510–513, 1993.

29. Talley NJ, Cameron AJ, Shorter RG, Zinsmeister AR, Phillips SF. Campylobacter pylori and Barrett's esophagus. Mayo Clin Proc 63: 1176–1180, 1988.

30. Ursua I, Ramos R, Val-Bernal JF. Helicobacter pylori in Barrett's esophagus. Histol Histopathol 6:403–408, 1991.

31. Loffeld RJLF, Ten Tije BJ, Arends JW. Prevalence and significance of Helicobacter pylori in patients with Barrett's esophagus. Am J Gastroenterol 87:1598–1600, 1992.

32. Abbas Z, Hussainy AS, Ibrahim F, Jafri SM, Shaikh H, Khan AH. Barrett's oesophagus and Helicobacter pylori. J Gastroenterol Hepatol 10: 331–333, 1995.

33. Ricaurte O, Fléjou JF, Vissuzaine C, Goldfain D, Rotenberg A, Cadiot G, Potet F. Helicobacter pylori infection in patients with Barrett's oesophagus: a prospective immunohistochemical study. J Clin Pathol 49:176–177, 1996.

34. Werdmuller BFM, Loffeld RJLF. Helicobacter pylori infection has no role in the pathogenesis of reflux esophagitis. Dig Dis Sci 42:103–105, 1997.

35. Labenz J, Blum AL, Bayerdörffer E, Meining A, Stolte M, Börsch G. Curing Helicobacter pylori infection in patients with duodenal ulcer may provoke reflux esophagitis. Gastroenterology 112:1442–1447, 1997.

36. Weston AP, Badr AS, Topalovski M, Cherian R, Dixon A. Prospective evaluation of the association of gastric H. pylori infection with Barrett's dysplasia and Barrett's adenocarcinoma. Gastroenterology 114: A703, 1998.

37. Chow WH, Blaser MJ, Blot WJ, Gammon MD, Vaughan TL, Risch HA, Perez-Perez GI, Schoenberg JB, Stanford JL, Rotterdam H, West AB, Fraumeni JF Jr. An inverse relation between cagA⁺ strains of Helicobacter pylori infection and risk of esophageal and gastric cardia adenocarcinoma. Cancer Res 58:588–590, 1998.

38. Vicari JJ, Peek RM, Falk GW, Goldblum JR, Easley KA, Schnell J, Perez-Perez GI, Halter SA, Rice TW, Blaser MJ, Richter JE. The seroprevalence of cagA-positive Helicobacter pylori strains in the spectrum of gastroesophageal reflux disease. Gastroenterology 115:50–57, 1998.

39. Graham DY, Yamaoka Y. H. pylori and cagA: relationships with gastric cancer, duodenal ulcer, and reflux esophagitis and its complications. Helicobacter 3:145–150, 1998.

40. Filipe MI, Potet F, Bogomoletz WV, Dawson PA, Fabiani B, Chauveinc P, Fenzy A, Gazzard B, Goldfain D, Zeegen R. Incomplete sulphomucin-secreting intestinal metaplasia for gastric cancer. Preliminary data from a prospective study from three centers. Gut 26:1319–1326, 1985.

41. Craanen ME, Blok P, Dekker W, Ferwerda J, Tytgat GNJ. Subtypes of intestinal metaplasia and Helicobacter pylori. Gut 33:597–600, 1992.

42. Filipe MI, Munoz N, Matko I, Kato I, Pompe-Kirn V, Jutersek A, Teuchmann S, Benz M, Prijon T. Intestinal metaplasia types and the risk of gastric cancer: a cohort study in Slovenia. Int J Cancer 57:324–329, 1994.

43. Tosi P, Filipe MI, Luzi P, Miracco C, Santopietro R, Lio R, Sforza V, Barbini P. Gastric intestinal metaplasia type III cases are classified as low-grade dysplasia on the basis of morphometry. J Pathol 169:73–78, 1993.

44. Zwas F, Shields HM, Doos WG, Antonioli DA, Goldman H, Ransil BJ, Spechler SJ. Scanning electron microscopy of Barrett's epithelium and its correlation with light microscopy and mucin stains. Gastroenterology 90:1932–1941, 1986.

45. Jass JR. Mucin histochemistry of the columnar epithelium of the oesophagus: a retrospective study. J Clin Pathol 34:866–870, 1981.

46. Trier JS. Morphology of the columnar cell-lined (Barrett's) esophagus. In: Spechler SJ, Goyal RK (eds): Barrett's Esophagus: Pathophysiology, Diagnosis, and Management. Elsevier Science, New York, 1985, pp 19–28.

47. Das KM, Prasad I, Garla S, Amenta PS. Detection of a shared colon epithelial epitope on Barrett epithelium by a novel monoclonal antibody. Ann Intern Med 120:753–756, 1994.

48. Griffel LH, Amenta PS, Das KM. Use of a novel monoclonal antibody in diagnosis of Barrett's esophagus. Dig Dis Sci 45:40–48, 2000.

49. Ormsby AH, Goldblum JR, Rice TW, Richter JE, Falk GW, Vaezi MF, Gramlich TL. Cytokeratin subsets can reliably distinguish Barrett's esophagus from intestinal metaplasia of the stomach. Hum Pathol 30: 288–294, 1999.

50. Salo JA, Kivilaakso EO, Kiviluoto TA, Virtanen IO. Cytokeratin profile suggests metaplastic epithelial transformation in Barrett's oesophagus. Ann Med 28:305–309, 1996.

51. Boch JA, Shields HM, Antonioli DA, Zwas F, Sawhney RA, Trier JS. Distribution of cytokeratin markers in Barrett's specialized columnar epithelium. Gastroenterology 112:760–765, 1997.

52. Spechler SJ, Goyal RK. Barrett's esophagus. N Engl J Med 315:362–371, 1986.

53. Hassall E. Columnar-lined esophagus in children. Gastroenterol Clin North Am 26:533–548, 1997.
54. Johnson DA, Winters C, Spurling TJ, Chobanian SJ, Cattau EL Jr. Esophageal acid sensitivity in Barrett's esophagus. J Clin Gastroenterol 9:23–27, 1987.
55. Winter C Jr, Spurling TJ, Chobanian SJ, et al. Barrett's esophagus. A prevalent, occult complication of gastroesophageal reflux disease. Gastroenterology 92:118–124, 1987.
56. Cameron AJ. Management of Barrett's esophagus. Mayo Clin Proc 73:457–461, 1988.
57. Lieberman DA, Oehlke M, Helfand M. Risk factors for Barrett's esophagus in community-based practices. GORGE consortium. Gastroenterology Outcomes Research Group in Endoscopy. Am J Gastroenterol 92:1293–1297, 1997.
58. Cameron AJ, Zinsmeister AR, Ballard DJ, Carney JA. Prevalence of columnar-lined (Barrett's) esophagus. Comparison of population-based clinical and autopsy findings. Gastroenterology 99:918–922, 1990.
59. Collen MJ, Lewis JH, Benjamin SB. Gastric acid hypersecretion in refractory gastroesophageal reflux disease. Gastroenterology 98:654–661, 1990.
60. Mulholland MW, Reid BJ, Levine DS, Rubin CE. Elevated gastric acid secretion in patients with Barrett's metaplastic epithelium. Dig Dis Sci 34:1329–1335, 1989.
61. Gillen P, Keeling P, Byrne PJ, Healy M, O'Moore RR, Hennessy TPJ. Implication of duodenogastric reflux in the pathogenesis of Barrett's oesophagus. Br J Surg 75:540–543, 1988.
62. Iascone C, DeMeester TR, Little AG, Skinner DB. Barrett's esophagus. Functional assessment, proposed pathogenesis, and surgical therapy. Arch Surg 118:543–549, 1983.
63. Zaninotto G, DeMeester TR, Bremner CG, Smyrk TC, Cheng SC. Esophageal function in patients with reflux-induced strictures and its relevance to surgical treatment. Ann Thorac Surg 47:362–370, 1989.
64. Gray MR, Donnelly RJ, Kingsnorth AN. Role of salivary epidermal growth factor in the pathogenesis of Barrett's columnar lined oesophagus. Br J Surg 78:1461–1466, 1991.
65. Hirschowitz BI. Gastric acid and pepsin secretion in patients with Barrett's esophagus and appropriate controls. Dig Dis Sci 41:1384–1391, 1996.
66. Öberg S, DeMeester TR, Peters JH, Hagen JA, Nigro JJ, DeMeester SR, Theisen J, Campos GMR, Crookes PF. The extent of Barrett's esophagus depends on the status of the lower esophageal sphincter and degree of esophageal acid exposure. J Thorac Cardiovasc Surg 117:572–580, 1999.
67. Cameron AJ, Lomboy CT. Barrett's esophagus: age, prevalence, and extent of columnar epithelium. Gastroenterology 103:1241–1245, 1992.
68. Hesketh PJ, Clapp RW, Doos WG, Spechler SJ. The increasing frequency of adenocarcinoma of the esophagus. Cancer 64:526–530, 1989.
69. Blot WJ, Devesa SS, Kneller RW, Fraumeni JF Jr. Rising incidence of adenocarcinoma of the esophagus and gastric cardia. JAMA 265:1287–1289, 1991.
70. Blot WJ, Devesa SS, Fraumeni JF Jr. Continuing climb in rates of esophageal adenocarcinoma: an update. JAMA 270:1320, 1993.
71. Spechler SJ. Barrett's esophagus: an overrated cancer risk factor. Gastroenterology 119:587–589, 2000.
72. Ries LAG, Eisner MP, Kosary CL, Hankey BF, Miller BA, Clegg L, Edwards BK (eds): SEER Cancer Statistics Review, 1973–1997, National Cancer Institute, Bethesda, MD, 2000.
73. Data provided by SEER Program, National Cancer Institute, Bethesda, MD, August 1999.
74. Drewitz DJ, Sampliner RE, Garewal HS. The incidence of adenocarcinoma in Barrett's esophagus: a prospective study of 170 patients followed 4.8 years. Am J Gastroenterol 92:212–215, 1997.
75. Streitz JM Jr, Ellis FH, Tilden RL, Erickson RV. Endoscopic surveillance of Barrett's esophagus: a cost-effectiveness comparison with mammographic surveillance for breast cancer. Am J Gastroenterol 93:911–915, 1998.
76. Shaheen NJ, Crosby MA, Bozymski EM, Sandler RS. Is there publication bias in the reporting of cancer risk in Barrett's esophagus? Gastroenterology 119:333–338, 2000.
77. Van der Burgh A, Dees J, Hop WCJ, van Blankenstein M. Oesophageal cancer is an uncommon cause of death in patients with Barrett's oesophagus. Gut 39:5–8, 1996.
78. Cameron AJ, Ott BJ, Payne WS. The incidence of adenocarcinoma in columnar-lined (Barrett's) esophagus. N Engl J Med 313:857–859, 1985.
79. Van der Veen AH, Dees J, Blankensteijn JD, van Blankenstein M. Adenocarcinoma in Barrett's oesophagus: an overrated risk. Gut 30:14–18, 1989.
80. Spechler SJ. Barrett's esophagus: should we brush off this ballooning problem? Gastroenterology 112:2138–2152, 1997.
81. Spechler SJ. Barrett's esophagus. Semin Oncol 21:431–437, 1994.
82. Ransom JM, Patel GK, Clift SA, Womble NE, Read RC. Extended and limited types of Barrett's esophagus in the adult. Ann Thorac Surg 33:19–27, 1982.
83. Harle IA, Finley RJ, Belsheim M, Bondy DC, Booth M, Lloyd D, McDonald JW, Sullivan S, Valberg LS, Watson WC, Frei JV, Slinger R, Troster M, Meads GE, Duff JH. Management of adenocarcinoma in a columnar-lined esophagus. Ann Thorac Surg 40:330–336, 1985.
84. Rudolph RE, Vaughan TL, Storer BE, Haggitt RC, Rabinovitch PS, Levine DS, Reid BJ. Effect of segment length on risk for neoplastic progression in patients with Barrett's esophagus. Ann Intern Med 132:612–620, 2000.
85. Souza RF, Meltzer SJ. The molecular basis for carcinogenesis in metaplastic columnar-lined esophagus. Gastroenterol Clin North Am 26:583–597, 1997.
86. Schmidt HG, Riddell RH, Walther B, Skinner DB, Riemann JF. Dysplasia in Barrett's esophagus. J Cancer Res Clin Oncol 110:145–152, 1985.
87. Spechler SJ. Endoscopic surveillance for patients with Barrett's esophagus: does the cancer risk justify the practice? Ann Intern Med 106:902–904, 1987.
88. Spechler SJ. Complications of gastroesophageal reflux disease. In: Castell DO (ed): The Esophagus. Little, Brown and Company, Boston, 1992, pp 543–556.
89. Levine DS, Haggitt RC, Blount PL, Rabinovitch PS, Rusch VW, Reid BJ. An endoscopic biopsy protocol can differentiate high-grade dysplasia from early adenocarcinoma in Barrett's esophagus. Gastroenterology 105:40–50, 1993.
90. Falk GW, Rice TW, Goldblum JR, Richter JE. Jumbo biopsy forceps protocol still misses unsuspected cancer in Barrett's esophagus with high-grade dysplasia. Gastrointest Endosc 49:170–176, 1999.
91. Hameeteman W, Tytgat GNJ, Houthoff HJ, van den Tweel JG. Barrett's esophagus: development of dysplasia and adenocarcinoma. Gastroenterology 96:1249–1256, 1989.
92. Lee RG. Dysplasia in Barrett's esophagus. A clinicopathologic study of six patients. Am J Surg Pathol 9:845–852, 1985.
93. Sontag SJ, Schnell TG, Kurucar C, O'Connell S, Levine G, Karpf J, Adelman K, Brand L, Seidel J. Barrett's high-grade dysplasia (HGD): surveillance endoscopy (EGD) once a year is sufficient in most patients. Gastroenterology 116:A304–A305, 1999.
94. Reid BJ, Haggitt RC, Rubin CE, Roth G, Surawicz CM, Van Belle G, Lewin K, Weinstein WM, Antonioli DA, Goldman H, et al. Observer variation in the diagnosis of dysplasia in Barrett's esophagus. Hum Pathol 19:166–178, 1988.
95. Gimenez A, Minguela A, Parrilla P, Bermejo J, Perez D, Molina J, Garcia AM, Ortiz MA, Alvarez R, de Haro LM. Flow cytometric DNA analysis and p53 protein expression show a good correlation with histologic findings in patients with Barrett's esophagus. Cancer 15:83:641–651, 1998.
96. Kim R, Clarke MR, Melhem MF, Young MA, Vanbibber MM, Safatle-Ribeiro AV, Ribeiro U Jr, Reynolds JC. Expression of p53, PCNA, and C-erbB-2 in Barrett's metaplasia and adenocarcinoma. Dig Dis Sci 42:2453–2462, 1997.
97. Ireland AP, Clark GW, DeMeester TR. Barrett's esophagus. The significance of p53 in clinical practice. Ann Surg 225:17–30, 1997.
98. Reid BJ, Blount PL, Rubin CE, Levine DS, Haggitt RC, Rabinovitch PS. Flow-cytometric and histological progression to malignancy in Barrett's esophagus: prospective endoscopic surveillance of a cohort. Gastroenterology 102:1212–1219, 1992.
99. Cameron AJ. Barrett's esophagus and adenocarcinoma: from the family to the gene. Gastroenterology 102:1421–1424, 1992.
100. Woolf GM, Riddell RH, Irvine EJ, Hunt RH. A study to examine agreement between endoscopy and histology for the diagnosis of columnar lined (Barrett's). Gastrointest Endosc 35:541–544, 1989.
101. Chobanian SJ, Cattau EL Jr, Winters C Jr, Johnson DA, Van Ness MM, Miremadi A, Horwitz SL, Colcher H. In vivo staining with toluidine blue as an adjunct to the endoscopic detection of Barrett's esophagus. Gastrointest Endosc 33:99–101, 1987.
102. Canto MIF, Setrakian S, Petras RE, Blades E, Chak A, Sivak MV Jr. Methylene blue selectively stains intestinal metaplasia in Barrett's esophagus. Gastrointest Endosc 44:1–7, 1996.
103. Stevens PD, Lightdale CJ, Green PHR, Siegel LM, Garcia-Carrasquillo RJ, Rotterdam H. Combined magnification endoscopy with chromoendoscopy for the evaluation of Barrett's esophagus. Gastrointest Endosc 40:747–749, 1994.

104. Gangarosa LM, Halter S, Mertz H. Methylene blue staining and endoscopic ultrasound evaluation of Barrett's esophagus with low-grade dysplasia. Dig Dis Sci 45:225–229, 2000.

105. Falk GW, Catalano MF, Sivak MV Jr, Rice TW, Van Dam J. Endosonography in the evaluation of patients with Barrett's esophagus and high-grade dysplasia. Gastrointest Endosc 40:207–212, 1994.

106. Kobayashi K, Izatt JA, Kulkarni MD, Willis J, Sivak MV Jr. High-resolution cross-sectional imaging of the gastrointestinal tract using optical coherence tomography: preliminary results. Gastrointest Endosc 47:515–523, 1998.

107. Stepp H, Stroka R, Baumgartner R. Fluorescence endoscopy of gastrointestinal diseases: basic principles, techniques, and clinical experience. Endoscopy 30:379–386, 1998.

108. Panjehpour M, Overholt BF, Vo-Dinh T, Haggitt RC, Edwards DH, Buckley FP III. Endoscopic fluorescence detection of high-grade dysplasia in Barrett's esophagus. Gastroenterology 111:93–101, 1996.

109. Haringsma J, Tytgat GNJ. The value of fluorescence techniques in gastrointestinal endoscopy: better than the endoscopist's eye? I: The European Experience. Endoscopy 30:416–418, 1998.

110. Marcon NE, Wilson BC. The value of fluorescence techniques in gastrointestinal endoscopy: better than the endoscopist's eye? II: The North American Experience. Endoscopy 30:419–421, 1998.

111. DeVault KR, Castell DO. Updated guidelines for the diagnosis and treatment of gastroesophageal reflux disease. Am J Gastroenterol 94:1434–1442, 1999.

112. Neumann CS, Iqbal TH, Cooper BT. Long-term continuous omeprazole treatment of patients with Barrett's oesophagus. Aliment Pharmacol Ther 9:451–454, 1995.

113. Spechler SJ. Comparison of medical and surgical therapy for complicated gastroesophageal reflux disease in veterans. Department of Veterans Affairs Gastroesophageal Reflux Disease Study Group. N Engl J Med 326:786–792, 1992.

114. Marks RD, Richter JE, Rizzo H, Koehler RE, Spenney JG, Mills TP, Champion G. Omeprazole versus H$_2$-receptor antagonists in treating patients with peptic stricture and esophagitis. Gastroenterology 106:907–915, 1994.

115. Smith PM, Kerr GD, Cockel R, Ross BA, Bate CM, Brown P, Dronfield MW, Green JRB, Hislop WS, Theodossi A, McFarland J, Watts DA, Taylor MD, Richardson PDI, and the Restore Investigator Group. A comparison of omeprazole and ranitidine in the prevention of recurrence of benign esophageal stricture. Gastroenterology 107:1312–1318, 1994.

116. Howden CW, Castell DO, Cohen S, Freston JW, Orlando RC, Robinson M. The rationale for continuous maintenance treatment of reflux esophagitis. Arch Intern Med 155:1465–1471, 1995.

117. Peters FTM, Ganesh S, Kuipers EJ, Sluiter WJ, Klinkenberg-Knol EC, Lamers CBH, Kleibeuker JH. Endoscopic regression of Barrett's oesophagus during omeprazole treamtment: a randomised, double blind study. Gut 45:489–494, 1999.

118. Sampliner RE. New treatments for Barrett's esophagus. Semin Gastrointest Dis 8:68–74, 1997.

119. Sharma P, Morales TG, Bhattacharyya A, Garewal HS, Sampliner RE. Squamous islands in Barrett's esophagus: what lies underneath? Am J Gastroenterol 93:332–335, 1998.

120. Garewal H, Ramsey L, Sharma P, Kraus K, Sampliner R, Fass R. Biomarker studies in reversed Barrett's esophagus. Am J Gastroenterol 94:2829–2833, 1999.

121. Fitzgerald RC, Omary MB, Triadafilopoulos G. Dynamic effects of acid on Barrett's esophagus. An ex vivo proliferation and differentiation model. J Clin Invest 98:2120–2128, 1996.

122. Ouatu-Lascar R, Fitzgerald RC, Triadafilopoulos G. Differentiation and proliferation in Barrett's esophagus and the effects of acid suppression. Gastroenterology 17:327–335, 1999.

123. Peghini PL, Katz PO, Bracy NA, Castell DO. Nocturnal recovery of gastric acid secretion with twice-daily dosing of proton pump inhibitors. Am J Gastroenterol 93:763–767, 1998.

124. Katz PO, Anderson C, Khoury R, Castell DO. Gastro-oesophageal reflux associated with nocturnal gastric acid breakthrough on proton pump inhibitors. Aliment Pharmacol Ther 12:1231–1234, 1998.

125. Katzka DA, Castell DO. Successful elimination of reflux symptoms does not insure adequate control of acid reflux in patients with Barrett's esophagus. Am J Gastroenterol 89:989–991, 1994.

126. Ouatu-Lascar R, Triadafilopoulos G. Complete elimination of reflux symptoms does not guarantee normalization of intraesophageal acid reflux in patients with Barrett's esophagus. Am J Gastroenterol 93:711–716, 1998.

127. Peghini PL, Katz PO, Castell DO. Ranitidine controls nocturnal gastric acid breakthrough on omeprazole: a controlled study in normal subjects. Gastroenterology 115:1335–1339, 1998.

128. Castell DO, Katz PO. Acid control and regression of Barrett's esophagus: is the glass half full or half empty? Am J Gastroenterol 92:2329, 1997.

129. Castell DO, Richter JE, Robinson M, Sontag SJ, Haber MM, and the Lansoprazole Group. Efficacy and safety of lansoprazole in the treatment of erosive reflux esophagitis. Am J Gastroenterol 91:1749–1757, 1996.

130. Ireland AP, Peters JH, Smyrk TC, DeMeester TR, Clark GWB, Mirvish SS, Adrian TE. Gastric juice protects against the development of esophageal adenocarcinoma in the rat. Ann Surg 224:358–371, 1996.

131. Streitz JM Jr, Andrews CW Jr, Ellis FH Jr. Endoscopic surveillance of Barrett's esophagus. Does it help? J Thorac Cardiovasc Surg 105:383–388, 1993.

132. Provenzale D, Kemp JA, Arora S, Wong JB. A guide for surveillance of patients with Barrett's esophagus. Am J Gastroenterol 89:670–680, 1994.

133. Provenzale D, Schmitt C, Wong JB. Barrett's esophagus: a new look at surveillance based on emerging estimates of cancer risk. Am J Gastroenterol 94:2043–2053, 1999.

134. Levine DS. Management of dysplasia in the columnar-lined esophagus. Gastroenterol Clin North Am 26:613–634, 1997.

135. Spechler SJ. Barrett's esophagus. Semin Gastrointestinal Dis 7:51–60, 1996.

136. Van den Boogert J, van Hillegersberg R, Siersema PD, de Bruin RW, Tilanus HW. Endoscopic ablation therapy for Barrett's esophagus with high-grade dysplasia: a review. Am J Gastroenterol 94:1153–1160, 1999.

137. Sampliner RE. Ablative therapies for the columnar-lined esophagus. Gastroenterol Clin North Am 26:685–694, 1997.

138. Nishioka NS. Drug, light, and oxygen: a dynamic combination in the clinic. Gastroenterology 114:604–606, 1998.

139. Overholt BF, Panjehpour M, Haydek JM. Photodynamic therapy for Barrett's esophagus: follow-up in 100 patients. Gastrointest Endosc 49:1–7, 1999.

140. Laukka MA, Wang KK. Initial results using low-dose photodynamic therapy in the treatment of Barrett's esophagus. Gastrointest Endosc 42:59–63, 1995.

141. Barr H, Shepherd NA, Dix A, Roberts DJH, Tan WC, Krasner N. Eradication of high-grade dysplasia in columnar-lined (Barrett's) oesophagus by photodynamic therapy with endogenously generated protoporphyrin IX. Lancet 348:584–585, 1996.

142. Gossner L, Stolte M, Sroka R, Rick K, May A, Hahn EG, Ell C. Photodynamic ablation of high-grade dysplasia and early cancer in Barrett's esophagus by means of 5-aminolevulinic acid. Gastroenterology 114:448–455, 1998.

143. Guanrei Y, Songliang Q, Guizen F. Natural history of early esophageal squamous carcinoma and early adenocarcinoma of the gastric cardia in the People's Republic of China. Endoscopy 20:95–98, 1988.

144. Van Laethem JL. Peny MO, Salmon I, Cremer M, Devière J. Intramucosal adenocarcinoma arising under squamous re-epithelialisation of Barrett's oesophagus. Gut 46:574–577, 2000.

145. Attwood SE, Barlow AP, Norris TL, Watson A. Barrett's oesophagus: effect of antireflux surgery on symptom control and development of complications. Br J Surg 79:1050–1053, 1992.

146. Peters JH. The surgical management of Barrett's esophagus. Gastroenterol Clin North Am 26:647–668, 1997.

147. Schoenfeld P, Cook D, Hamilton F, Laine L, Morgan D, Peterson W. An evidence-based approach to gastroenterology therapy. Gastroenterology 114:1318–1325, 1998.

148. Perdikis G, Hinder RA, Lund RJ, Raiser F, Katada N. Laparoscopic Nissen fundoplication: where do we stand? Surg Laparosc Endosc 7:17–21, 1997.

149. Morales TG, Sampliner RE. Barrett's esophagus. Update on screening, surveillance, and treatment. Arch Intern Med 159:1411–1416, 1999.

150. Sampliner RE and The Practice Parameters Committee of the American College of Gastroenterology. Practice guidelines on the diagnosis, surveillance, and therapy of Barrett's esophagus. Am J Gastroenterol 93:1028–1032, 1998.

# Section 2

## Cancer of the Stomach

# Chapter 21

# Epidemiology and Molecular Epidemiology of Gastric Cancer

STEVEN F. MOSS AND HAIM SHIRIN

Gastric adenocarcinoma is by far the most common malignant gastric neoplasm and worldwide remains the second most common cause of cancer mortality after lung cancer. The much rarer non-Hodgkin's lymphomas and leiomyosarcomas, which account for fewer than 5% of all gastric tumors, are discussed in Chapters 66–70 of this book.

The differentiation of the anatomic site within the stomach and histologic type of gastric adenocarcinoma may be critical in studying the epidemiology and pathogenesis of gastric cancer because cancers of distinct subsites and histology may represent disorders with different etiology and epidemiology. Most gastric cancers arise distally from the antrum and pylorus, but around 20% involve the cardia and fundus and approximately 10% involve the stomach diffusely.[1] The most commonly used histologic distinction is between the intestinal and diffuse subtypes, based on the work of Lauren.[2–4] The intestinal well-differentiated form predominates in high-risk areas, is more common in males, tends to occur in the distal part of the stomach, and is often preceded by a prolonged precancerous phase.[3] The diffuse undifferentiated type occurs more often in young patients, has a more equal male-to-female ratio, and displays a more aggressive clinical course.[4] In recent decades, there has been a decline in the incidence and mortality of gastric cancer in the Western world, due principally to a decrease in the geographically more variable intestinal subtype. The incidence of the diffuse type of cancer may even have gradually increased over this time.[5] The possible reasons for this decline are mainly related to improved environmental and socioeconomic factors including changes in the diet, better preservation and storage of food, and changes in the prevalence of infection with the gastric bacterium *Helicobacter pylori*, as will be discussed later. By contrast, in association with an increase in the incidence of adenocarcinoma of the lower esophagus, there has been a continuing increase in the incidence of adenocarcinoma of the gastric cardia in the U.S. and other Western countries.[6,7]

## Descriptive Epidemiology

According to most recent world estimates, 798,000 new cases of gastric cancer and 628,000 deaths from gastric cancer occur annually.[8] Gastric cancer is responsible for about one-tenth of all deaths from cancer worldwide and is the second most common cancer in men (after lung cancer) and the fourth most frequent cancer in women (after cancer of the breast, colon, and cervix).[8]

A tremendous geographic variation exists in the incidence of carcinoma of the stomach. Age-standardized incidence rates in both genders are very high in Japan (77.9 per 100,000 in men and 33.3 per 100,000 in women) where gastric cancer is the most common malignancy, constituting 31% of all male cancers and 22% of female cancers.[9] High rates are also found in both genders in Korea and China, certain countries in Latin America (particularly Costa Rica and Ecuador), and in Eastern Europe (Fig. 21–1). In contrast, incidence rates are much lower in Eastern and Northern Africa, South and Southeast Asia, Australia, and North America. In the United States, there are estimated to be 21,900 cases annually (13,700 male and 8,200 female) and 13,500 deaths each year—the tenth most common cause of cancer mortality for both males and females.[10] There has been a smooth decline in the incidence of non-cardia gastric cancer in most countries in recent decades, including the United States[6,10] (Fig. 21–2) and a slowing of the rate of increase in the number of cases as the world's population continues to expand.

## Age, Gender, and Ethnic Distribution

Gastric cancer occurs predominantly in older people, and has a peak incidence in those over 60 years of age.[11,12] Gastric cancer at less than 40 years of age comprises 2% to 8% of cases; gastric cancer occurring in patients younger than 30 is very rare.[12,13] According to data from a U.S. national cancer registry, almost

MALES                                             FEMALES

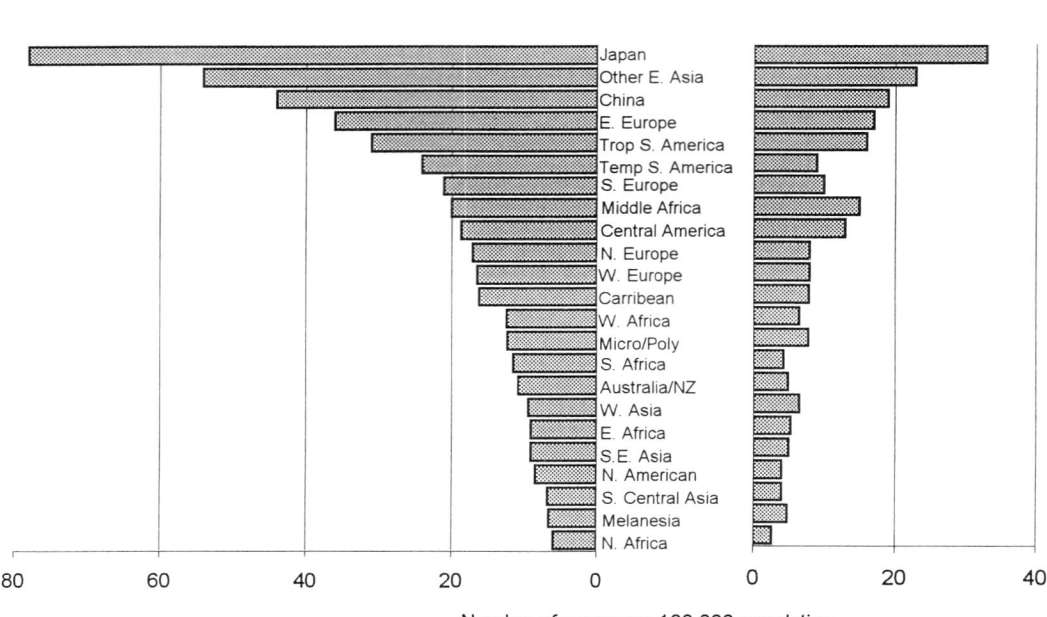

Number of cases per 100.000 population

**Figure 21-1** Incidence of gastric cancer by world region. Micro/Poly, Micronesia/Polynesia; Temp, temperate; Trop, tropical. (Adapted from Parkin DM, Pisani P, Ferlay J. Cancer Statistics, 1999. CA Cancer J Clin 49:32–64, 1999, with publishers' permission.)

50% of gastric carcinoma cases in 1992–93 occurred in patients older than 70 and approximately 20% in patients older than 80 at the time of diagnosis.[14] Although men are more likely to have gastric cancer, the gender ratio varies with age. Below age 40, the male/female ratio is 1:1, and this increases in middle age and beyond to 3.7:1. In the United States, both age and gender distributions have been stable over the last 15 years.[14] The recent ethnic distribution of cases in the United States generally reflects the ethnic mix of the general population, with the exception of a slight excess in patients of Japanese and other Asian ethnicity.[14]

### Early Gastric Cancer

Most Western series report the incidence of early gastric cancer (defined as tumor with invasion limited to the mucosa and submucosa) to be 10% to 20% of resected cases. This fraction falls

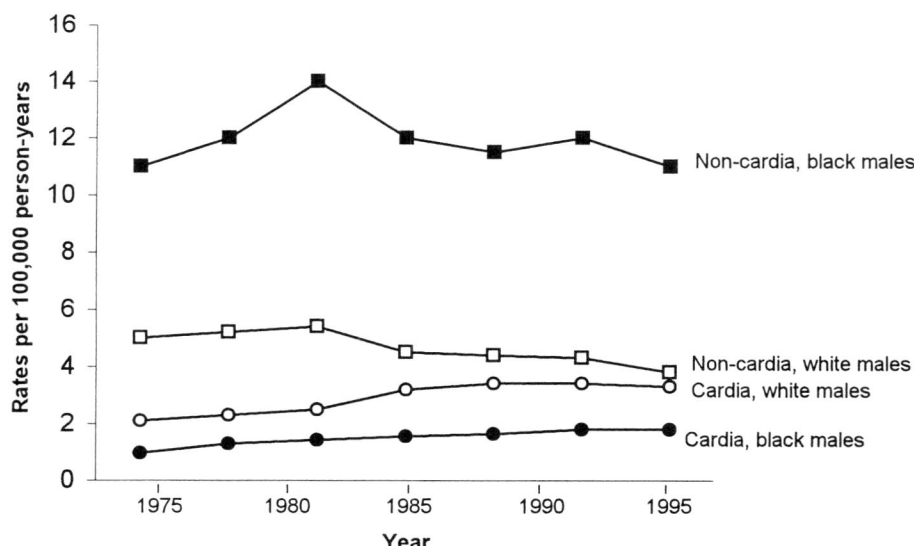

**Figure 21-2** Changes in the age-adjusted incidence rate of gastric cancer by anatomic subsite and race, 1975–1995. (Modified from Devesa SS, Blot WJ, Fraumeni JF. Cancer 83(10):2049–2053, 1998. ©1998 American Cancer Society, with permission of Wiley-Liss, Inc., a subsidiary of John Wiley & Sons, Inc.)

further when the pathology records are examined. In contrast, Japanese national records show that the percentage of early gastric cancers among resected patients was 40% in 1985;[15] in the Cancer Institute of Tokyo, the number of early gastric cancer cases overtook advanced cancers in 1990.[16] Patients with early gastric cancer tend to be younger but show no significant differences in male-to-female ratio when compared with gastric carcinoma patients in general.[17]

## Anatomic Subsite

Examining trends over several decades has revealed a recent increase in the annual incidence of adenocarcinoma of gastric cardia in both white and black males (Fig. 21–2). In white males, the incidence of cancer of the gastric cardia has nearly equaled that of tumors arising in other parts of the stomach.[6,7] Although the incidence has also increased in the young and in females, the upward trend for incidence of gastric cardia carcinoma has been much greater among old men than young men. It has been estimated that gastric cardia cancer and esophageal adenocarcinoma are the most rapidly increasing cancers in the United States.[18]

The possible reasons for these gender and racial differences and the change in incidence observed in the United States and other Western populations are unknown but may relate to an increase in obesity and gastroesophageal reflux in the population. Adenocarcinoma of the gastric cardia shares many epidemiologic features with esophageal adenocarcinoma, and it is often impossible for even experienced pathologists to tell the origin of tumors arising close to the gastroesophageal junction. For these reasons, it has been suggested that some of the apparent increase in the incidence of gastric cardia cancer may be due to misclassification of an esophageal primary tumor.[19–21]

## Histopathologic Precancerous Lesions

Gastric cancer is clearly associated with chronic gastritis and, in the intestinal type of gastric cancer, with a sequence of specific histologic lesions ranging from chronic superficial gastritis through atrophic gastritis and intestinal metaplasia to dysplasia and cancer.[22] Intestinal metaplasia, especially the sulfomucin-rich incomplete type (type IIb or III), and chronic atrophic gastritis can therefore be considered precancerous lesions. The decrease in the risk of gastric cancer observed in migrants from high-risk areas to low-risk areas is accompanied by reductions in the prevalence of intestinal metaplasia,[23–25] suggesting that the etiology of both intestinal metaplasia and gastric cancer is due to environmental exposure, perhaps to *H. pylori* infection. The relationship between other precancerous gastric lesions, including gastric polyps, and gastric cancer will be discussed in Chapter 23.

## Analytical Epidemiology

The many risk factors and associations that have been described for gastric cancer (Table 21–1) likely reflect the multifactorial pathogenesis of gastric cancer. The large variation in the incidence of gastric cancer over time and across geographical regions and the tendency for migrant groups to adopt the incidence rates of their environment after one to two generations support the hypothesis that environmental factors play an important role in the etiology and pathogenesis of gastric cancer.

## Studies of Migrants

Classic epidemiologic studies demonstrated that the second- and third-generation offspring of Japanese immigrants to Hawaii and Eastern European immigrants to the mainland United States adopted rates of gastric cancer similar to those of the native population.[26,27] In a recent study, the incidence of gastric carcinoma in first-generation Japanese males residing in the United States was found to be half that of their counterparts living in Japan, even though the incidence was almost three times higher than in U.S.–born whites.[28] Since most migrant studies of gastric cancer were reported before the *H. pylori* era, the confounding effect of infection with this bacterium needs to be considered in explaining the altered incidence of gastric cancer after migration.

## Occupational Exposure

The observation that environmental factors may have a strong influence on the genesis of gastric cancer has led to several epidemiologic studies investigating the effects of occupational exposures on gastric cancer incidence. Occupations at increased risk include construction workers, quarrymen, carpenters, metal miners, farmers, and those exposed to pesticides and industrial chemicals including petrochemicals and asbestos.[29] In an exhaustive study of the relationship between gastric cancer and occupation or industrial exposure to nearly 300 chemicals in Montreal, Canada, elevated risk was found in excavators and pavers, forestry workers, electrical and electronic workers, motor transport workers, and food industry employees.[30] The substances potentially implicated in the etiology of this increased risk included crystalline silica, leaded gasoline, lead dust, and zinc dust.[30]

A study of occupational exposures specific to cancers of the gastric cardia has revealed that white men employed as financial managers, janitors and cleaners, production inspectors, and truck drivers, and black men employed as railroad workers and carpenters are at increased risk.[31] In the same study of gastric cardia risk factors, industries with elevated risk for white men included pulp and paper milling, newspaper publishing and printing, and water supply and irrigation. With regard to specific exposures, sulfuric acid mists consistently increased risk in white men, but not in black men. Overall, despite some consistent trends of occupational risk in gastric cancer, the effect of specific chemicals has not been well established. Furthermore, it is important to note that some of the studies just mentioned did not stratify for social class and none controlled for infection by *H. pylori*.

## Tobacco, Alcohol, and Socioeconomic Status

A significant dose–response relationship between cigarette smoking and both distal and proximal gastric cancer has been described in several cohort studies.[32–35] In a meta-analysis, the odds ratio for tobacco smoking in gastric carcinogenesis was estimated to be around 1.5 and was higher for men than for women.[36] Habitual smoking may be particularly associated with the differentiated type of gastric cancer, especially in young patients.[37]

Some investigators have reported a positive relationship between alcohol consumption and gastric cancer[38,39] but more recent U.S. studies separating gastric cancer by subsite have not confirmed these findings.[36,40] The positive relationship between low socioeconomic status, defined by parameters of income and education, and gastric cancer risk that has been reported in some studies may be due to confounding variables such as *H. pylori* infection, dietary habits, smoking, and alcohol consumption, as

**Table 21-1** Risk factors and protective factors for gastric cancer

| | Gastric Cancer Type | |
|---|---|---|
| Factor Type | Distal | Proximal |
| *Risk Factors* | | |
| Definite | Male gender | Barrett's esophagus |
| | Age | Intestinal metaplasia |
| | Atrophic gastritis | Body mass index |
| | Intestinal metaplasia | Tobacco use |
| | Dysplasia | Occupational factors |
| | Adenomas | Socioeconomic status |
| | Time post-gastrectomy (>20 years) | |
| | Pernicious anemia | |
| | *Helicobacter pylori* infection | |
| | Hereditary nonpolyposis colorectal cancer | |
| Probable | Family history of gastric cancer | |
| | Familial adenomatous polyposis | |
| | Blood group A | |
| | Salt intake | |
| | Tobacco use | |
| Possible | Low socioeconomic status | |
| | Occupational factors | |
| | Menetrier's disease | |
| | Hamartomas | |
| | Gastric Epstein-Barr virus infection | |
| | Dietary nitrates | |
| | Hetrocyclic amines | |
| *Protective Factors* | | |
| Definite | Refrigeration of food | *CagA*-positive *H. pylori* |
| | Fruits and vegetables | |
| | Prior duodenal ulcer | |
| Probable | Vitamin C | |
| Possible | Carotenoids | |
| | Garlic | |
| | Green tea | |
| | Aspirin and nonsteroidal anti-inflammatory drugs | |
| | Selenium | |

well as occupational factors. None of the studies reported to date have controlled for *H. pylori* infection.[36,40–43]

## Body Mass Index

Increased body weight has been associated with an increased risk for gastric cardia cancer in the United States and China, with an odds ratio of 1.5 to 2.[44–46] Possible explanations for this increased risk include an increasing tendency toward gastroesophageal reflux disease and the development of Barrett's esophagus due to obesity. In contrast, increased body mass index is not a risk factor for adenocarcinoma of the gastric body.

## Helicobacter pylori

*Helicobacter pylori* is found in the stomach of most of the world's population, particularly in the developing world. *H. pylori* is usually acquired in early childhood and is associated with poverty and poor standards of nutrition.[47] In the original description of the culture of this organism from gastric biopsies in 1982, Marshall speculated that *H. pylori* may play a part in the etiology of gastric cancer.[48] Subsequent studies have confirmed the association of *H. pylori* with gastric cancer, and on the strength of the available evidence, *H. pylori* was defined as a definite gastric carcinogen in 1994 by the World Health Organization.[49]

The earliest studies examining the relationship between *H. pylori* and gastric cancer investigated the presence of *H. pylori* in the resected stomachs of patients with gastric cancer. Although some reported *H. pylori* to be more prevalent in gastric cancer patients than controls, others did not, perhaps in part because the detection of *H. pylori* by histology is prone to false-negative results in the presence of coexisting intestinal metaplasia and atrophic gastritis.[50] However, convincing serological evidence of a frequent association of *H. pylori* with a variety of preneoplastic gastric lesions[51] has led to a model of gastric carcinogenesis in which the progressive sequence of histological changes—from chronic gastritis through preneoplastic intermediates such as atrophy, intestinal metaplasia, and dysplasia to gastric cancer—is driven by chronic *H. pylori* infection.[22]

Ecological studies have demonstrated a consistent correlation between geographic areas of high *H. pylori* incidence and high gastric cancer incidence.[52] Exceptions to this rule do exist, however (for example, the relatively low rates of peptic ulcer disease and gastric cancer in sub-Saharan Africa, which are possibly due to dietary confounders). Overall, the strongest evidence for the association between *H. pylori* and gastric cancer has come from prospective seroepidemiologic studies. In three studies reported in 1991, sera were banked from a large number of patients and the cohorts were followed for at least 6 years. Controls were matched for at least one case in each study, and the odds ratio for the development of gastric cancer in these initial studies ranged from 2.8 to 6.0. Subsequently, two other prospective cohort studies from China failed to show such an increased odds ratio. This finding may be due to *H. pylori* infection being almost universal in this population or to the fact that the enzyme-linked immunoadsorbent assay (ELISA) tests used were validated in Western populations and may not reflect true infection rates in the Chinese.[53,54] Indeed, a reanalysis of one of these "negative" studies[54] using antibodies developed against Chinese strains demonstrated that the odds ratio was in fact at least 1.8 and as high as 3.7 with longer follow-up.[55] In a meta-analysis of the available studies to 1996,[56] the combined odds ratio for *H. pylori* in gastric carcinogenesis was calculated at around 2. The odds ratio was much higher in cases where gastric cancer occurred at a younger age because the incidence of *H. pylori* in the controls increased with age. Although only some of the studies specifically defined the location of the cancer within the stomach, no statistically significant association was found between *H. pylori* and tumors of the cardia. This meta-analysis highlighted a particularly strong association between *H. pylori* and early gastric cancer. It also concluded that cancers of the intestinal and diffuse histologic subtypes were equally associated with *H. pylori* infection, even though these two types of cancer are thought to develop through distinct and separate molecular pathways.[57]

Although successful eradication of *H. pylori* in patients with chronic superficial gastritis ultimately leads to a complete histologic normalization of gastric histology, there is considerable doubt whether other intermediate stages of the gastric carcinogenic process can return to normal following the eradication of *H. pylori*. Several studies have reported short-term follow-up on patients with intestinal metaplasia and other preneoplastic histologic conditions associated with *H. pylori* infection. However, most have failed to show regression in the incidence of these lesions after the eradication of *H. pylori*. Large, prospective studies with multiple biopsies (to avoid sampling errors) and long follow-up periods are awaited. Final causal proof implicating *H. pylori* in gastric cancer will require the demonstration of a risk reduction in gastric cancer after the eradication of *H. pylori*. A single study has reported that after the endoscopic removal of early gastric cancer, patients in whom *H. pylori* was eradicated had a reduced incidence of second gastric cancers during short-term follow-up.[58] However, limitations in the blinding and short-term follow-up of the study require that this observation be substantiated in a randomized control study. Prospective intervention studies are currently under way in several areas of the world where gastric cancer incidence is high; they are using as end points either changes in intermediate biomarkers or changes in gastric cancer incidence. It is hoped that these studies will be sufficiently powerful to determine whether the eradication of *H. pylori* will prevent gastric cancer.

## Attributable risk and mechanisms

On the basis of world incidence data from 1990, it has been estimated that *H. pylori* is responsible for about 53% of all gastric cancers in the developing world and 60% of gastric cancers in the developed world.[59] Overall, about 5% of all cancers worldwide are attributable to *H. pylori*.

## Mechanisms of carcinogenesis

*H. pylori* is probably only one of several factors contributing to the development of human gastric cancer; some others are genetic predisposition and environmental factors such as nutrition. Although *H. pylori* is classified as a definite carcinogen,[49] the evidence that it directly promotes neoplasia in the absence of co-

carcinogens was lacking until recently. However, two independent groups in Japan have now demonstrated that in a susceptible animal model (the Mongolian gerbil), chronic infection with *H. pylori* alone can induce gastric adenocarcinoma in a high proportion of animals.[60,61] The relevance of this finding to human gastric cancer still remains uncertain, but this provocative model of *H. pylori* in outbred animals suggests that *H. pylori* may act as a direct carcinogen. For human gastric cancer, Koch's postulates still remain to be proven. However, *H. pylori* does seem to fulfill most, if not all, of the Bradford-Hill guidelines for multifactorial disease determination.[62]

## *H. pylori* CagA

*H. pylori* strains can be subdivided according to certain virulence characteristics. In general, more pathogenic "type I" strains carry the *cag* pathogenicity island, a 40 kilobase DNA fragment encoding a series of virulence-related genes associated with a putative extracellular secretory apparatus.[63] In Western populations, the *cag* island is usually associated with the presence of a vacuolating cytotoxin encoded by the S1a/m1 configuration of the *vacA* gene. Carriage of these more virulent strains is associated with peptic ulcer disease, gastric atrophy, and intestinal metaplasia. Because the *cagA* genotype can be inferred by the presence of antibodies to the immunodominant CagA antigen, two of the large cohorts that demonstrated an association between *H. pylori* and gastric cancer were reanalyzed for CagA serology.[64,65] In both of these cohorts, an increased odds ratio for the intestinal type of gastric cancer was found for *cagA*-positive strains. Furthermore, a retrospective case–control study also demonstrated increased relative risk with the presence of either VacA or CagA antibodies.[66] However, such a relationship does not apply in many parts of the world such as China, Japan, and Korea. In these countries of high gastric cancer incidence, almost all strains are type I and no statistically significant association has been found between carriage of these virulence factors and gastric cancer. Indeed, across countries, the variation in the incidence of CagA seropositivity is not significantly correlated with the incidence of gastric cancer.[67] Putative bacterial factors responsible for associations of *H. pylori* with gastric cancer include sequences in the 3′ region of the *cagA* rather than the presence or absence of the entire *cag* island. Differences in the 3′ region in association with cancer have been reported in Japan, where almost all strains are *cagA* positive.[68] Additional candidate virulence factors include the recently described *iceA* gene, which is independently associated with peptic ulcer disease in Western populations.[69,70]

## *H. pylori* and cancer of the gastric cardia

A recent multicenter case–control study of esophageal and gastric cancers in the United States found *H. pylori* seroprevalence to be inversely related to the presence of esophageal or gastric cardia adenocarcinoma. When subdividing *H. pylori* strains by antibodies to CagA, the investigators found a significant reduction in the odds ratio for esophageal and cardia adenocarcinoma in association with *cagA*-positive *H. pylori* strains, independent of other possible confounding variables.[71] This provocative finding, taken together with a rising incidence of proximal gastric cancer and a spontaneous decline in *H. pylori* infection in the United States,[6,7,18] as well as a possible association between *cagA*-positive *H. pylori* and gastroesophageal reflux disease and Barrett's esophagus,[72] has led to the speculation that *H. pylori* strains carrying the *cag* pathogenicity island may promote distal gastric cancer but protect against proximal gastric cancer.[73] The mechanism responsible for such an association remains unknown, and this provocative hypothesis requires corroboration.

### Epstein-Barr Virus

Increased serum antibody levels to Epstein-Barr virus antigens and the identification of Epstein-Barr viral RNA by in situ hybridization have implicated this virus in the etiology of a minority of gastric cancers.[74,75] The association between Epstein-Barr virus and gastric cancer deserves some reanalysis in light of the strong association between *H. pylori* and gastric lymphoma, especially since the Epstein-Barr virus–associated gastric cancers typically have a very profuse lymphocytic infiltrate.

### Diet

Studies of gastric cancer rates in migrant groups were the first to show that environmental risk factors, particularly those experienced early in life, are important in determining the subsequent risk of gastric cancer. Although much of this early environmental exposure may be due to *H. pylori*, differences in the seroprevalence of *H. pylori* infection cannot explain all of the variability in incidence rates around the world.

There has been a considerable body of work on the relationship between dietary risk factors and gastric cancer, stimulated initially by the demonstration that *N*-nitroso compounds induced gastric cancer in experimental animals.[76] Although many studies in this area are limited by their retrospective nature and the subjective assessment of specific dietary intakes, some consistent trends have emerged.

#### N-nitroso compounds

Nitrates are particularly common in cured foods. Nitrates may be converted into nitrites in the stomach by bacteria and subsequently nitrosated and converted to *N*-nitroso compounds, which are carcinogenic in animals. Concentrations of *N*-nitroso compounds are lowered by the presence of free radical scavengers such as ascorbate or $\alpha$-tocopherol, and the formation of *N*-nitroso compounds is increased by high gastric pH. Despite this possible mechanistic link, the data to support a positive correlation between dietary nitrate intake and gastric cancer are very weak and of marginal statistical significance.[77,78]

#### Salt

The relationship between dietary salt intake and gastric cancer has been extensively studied because early studies implicated preserved (smoked, salted, and pickled) foods in the etiology of gastric cancer. In animal models, salt seems to act synergistically with *N*-nitroso carcinogens to cause gastric cancer and with *Helicobacter* species to cause hyperproliferation.[79] The InterSalt study showed a correlation between urinary sodium excretion and stomach cancer[80] and some case–control studies have found that adding table salt to food is associated with an increase in relative risk for gastric cancer.[77] Although the literature is not entirely consistent, a large number of studies do tend to support a positive association between areas of high gastric cancer incidence and high salt intake. Furthermore, this association has been confirmed in many different regions of the world.

#### Refrigeration

There is consistent evidence that the risk of gastric cancer is decreased by the presence of a home refrigerator.[81] This association is probably due to refrigeration obviating the need to preserve foods by smoking and salting. However, the benefit of home refrigeration may be a surrogate marker for other factors that commonly accompany improved standards of nutrition, such as improved socioeconomic status, affluence, and a low incidence of *H. pylori* infection.

### Fresh vegetables and fruits and micronutrients

Many epidemiologic studies have demonstrated a clear and consistent protective effect of diets high in fresh vegetables and fruits on gastric cancer risk, with a relative risk ratio of 0.1 to 0.9.[81] Recent interest in specific vegetables has focused on allium vegetables such as onions[82] and garlic,[83] perhaps because of a putative negative correlation between garlic and *H. pylori*. Numerous micronutrients are present within fresh fruits and vegetables, any of which may be responsible for the risk reduction. Some examples are described briefly below.

**Vitamin C** A high dietary intake of ascorbate has been associated with a reduced risk of gastric cancer in many studies; the pooled odds ratio is around 0.4.[77] The ability of vitamin C to protect against gastric carcinogenesis may reflect its ability to act as an antioxidant in the stomach, reducing the formation of free oxygen and nitrogen radicals.[84] *H. pylori* infection has been shown to inhibit the secretion of ascorbate from the gastric mucosa into the lumen, thereby potentially reducing the cancer-protective effect of vitamin C.[85]

**Betacarotene and other carotenoids** Betacarotene has antioxidant and other putative cancer-preventive properties.[86] Case–control studies have shown a moderate protective effect of diets rich in betacarotene against gastric cancer,[77] and some studies have found urinary betacarotene levels to be lower in patients with gastric cancer or preneoplastic gastric changes than in patients without them.[81]

**Other micronutrients** At least three studies have shown an inverse relationship between selenium levels and gastric cancer. Alpha-tocopherol has also been investigated in a limited number of studies, but the data are inconsistent and unconvincing.

**Intervention studies of micronutrients and minerals** The potential usefulness of micronutrients and minerals as chemopreventive agents for gastric cancer has been evaluated in a small number of intervention studies. None has shown a significant or consistent benefit from vitamin C, selenium, betacarotene, and vitamin E, either alone or in combination. However, in populations throughout the world that are at high risk for gastric cancer, larger trials of various micronutrients are currently under way, usually in association with *H. pylori* eradication. In these studies, the end points being examined are either precancerous histologic lesions or gastric cancer itself.[81,87]

### Other dietary components

Some, though not all, studies have demonstrated a positive association between gastric cancer and the intake of carbohydrates, particularly starches. Certain heterocyclic amines produced by barbecuing meat and fish have been suggested as risk factors for gastric cancer. In a recent study from Uruguay,[88] the odds ratio for dietary intake of these amines was around 4. Alcohol, coffee, and total tea intake have no relationship with gastric cancer incidence,[89] but green tea specifically may have a protective effect.[81]

### Dietary risk factors and gastric cancer subtypes

Few studies have examined the relationship between dietary risk factors and specific types of gastric cancer. In one recent U.S. study, an attempt was made to examine dietary risk factors with respect to histology. The odds ratios for particular food groups and micronutrients were found to be generally similar for both intestinal and diffuse gastric cancers.[90] Similarly, despite the evidence suggesting different etiologies for distal and proximal gastric cancers in the United States, the relatively few studies that have examined dietary risk factors by subsite within the stomach have found no consistent difference between dietary risk factors for cardia versus noncardia gastric cancers.

## Familial Risk Factors

Cohort and case–control studies have indicated an increased risk for gastric cancer in first-degree relatives of individuals with gastric cancer.[91] This risk may be stronger for the intestinal type of gastric cancer than the diffuse histological type.[92] The available evidence implicates both shared environmental risk factors and specific susceptibility genes in the etiology of familial gastric cancer.

The incidence of gastric cancer is increased in patients with hereditary nonpolyposis colorectal cancer (HNPCC) syndrome. A variety of mutations in genes encoding DNA mismatch-repair enzymes are thought to be responsible for this clinical syndrome, and characteristically tumors in these patients exhibit DNA replication errors. The odds ratio for the development of gastric cancer was 6.9 in patients with HNPPC,[93] and H. pylori infection is rare in these HNPCC-associated gastric tumors.[94] Conversely, a replication error phenotype due to microsatellite instability is very common in gastric cancer, particularly in association with an intestinal morphology, distal location, and H. pylori seropositivity.[95] These findings suggest that H. pylori may in some way predispose to the acquisition of replication errors during gastric carcinogenesis, especially since microsatellite instability may occur in the preneoplastic lesion of intestinal metaplasia.[96]

In familial adenomatous polyposis, gastric polyps are very common, yet gastric cancer is rare. An increased risk of gastric polyps and cancer has also been described in some other rare familial syndromes such as Cowden's syndrome and Peutz-Jeghers syndrome.[91] Recently, germline mutations in the gene encoding E-cadherin have been linked to cases of familial gastric cancer with diffuse-type histology.[97,98]

To investigate the interaction between environmental and familial risk factors, gastric mucosal proliferation rates have been measured as a biomarker of increased risk for cancer in first-degree relatives of gastric cancer patients.[99] Compared with controls, the family members had increased proliferation throughout the stomach, even after excluding H. pylori as a cause of the hyperproliferation. The increased familial risk seems unrelated to dietary factors[100] but may be additive to smoking in increasing the odds ratio for gastric cancer, at all sites within the stomach.[101]

In contrast, two other recent European studies have examined directly the contribution of H. pylori to the familial association of gastric cancer. These reports suggest strongly that much of the previously described familial clustering of noncardia gastric cancer is due to a high prevalence of H. pylori in affected family members.[102,103]

## Associations with Other Medical Conditions and Drug Use

### Pernicious anemia

The standardized incidence rate for gastric cancer is about three times normal in patients with autoimmune pernicious anemia.[104] The recent demonstration that H. pylori may be associated with antigastric autoantibodies suggests that autoimmune pernicious anemia may be part of the spectrum of diseases induced by H. pylori.[105] Since gastric atrophy is a characteristic of pernicious anemia, pernicious anemia may predispose to cancer through decreased acid secretion, bacterial overgrowth, and increased nitrosamine formation. This predisposition to cancer should also occur with hypochlorhydria induced by acid suppression medication, but despite these theoretical concerns, no increased risk of gastric cancer in association with $H_2$ receptor antagonists or protein pump inhibitors has been demonstrated in humans.

### Partial gastrectomy

Prior partial gastrectomy for benign or malignant disease is definitely associated with an increased risk of subsequent gastric cancer in the remaining gastric stump. The odds ratio is at least 2, rising with time since partial gastrectomy after an initial interval of about 10–15 years.[106,107] Persistent H. pylori infection and bile reflux have been implicated in the etiology of this increased risk, but whether prophylactic eradication of H. pylori after partial gastrectomy will be beneficial remains to be determined. The cost-effectiveness of a surveillance program for patients having undergone gastric surgery has not been rigorously evaluated in recent years.

### Duodenal ulcer disease

Analysis of a large Swedish cohort has confirmed the clinical impression that the presence of a duodenal ulcer decreases the risk of subsequent gastric cancer (standardized incidence ratio 0.6). This contrasts with the positive association between gastric ulcers and cancer in this study.[108] There is no simple explanation for this finding, especially since both duodenal ulcers and gastric cancer are associated with H. pylori infection in general, and cagA-positive strains in particular. Differences in the age at acquisition of H. pylori infection or the relative health of the gastric corpus may be important in determining the long-term clinical outcome following infection.

### Aspirin and nonsteroidal anti-inflammatory drugs

In a recent U.S. multicenter study, the use of aspirin and nonsteroidal anti-inflammatory drugs (NSAIDs) was associated with decreased risk for cancer of the distal stomach and esophagus but not the gastric cardia,[109] and this finding was confirmed in a case–control study from Russia.[110] Possible explanations for this seemingly protective effect of aspirin and NSAIDs include their induction of epithelial apoptosis and the inhibition of cyclooxygenase or their precipitation of bleeding which may lead to earlier clinical presentation. In another analysis of this U.S. cohort, none of several drugs with possible effects on the gastroesophageal junction evaluated was associated with an altered risk for gastric adenocarcinoma of the cardia.[111]

### Others

Since the 1950s, an association has been reported between patients with blood group A and gastric cancer.[112] The association is possibly due to differences in the binding of H. pylori to blood group adhesins. Patients with hypogammaglobulinemia may also be at increased risk of gastric cancer; the relationship between Menetrier's disease and gastric cancer is unproven.

## Molecular Epidemiology

Molecular epidemiologic methods aim to identify patients at increased risk for cancer with tissue markers in order to target them with preventive measures. These methods have not been as extensively applied to gastric carcinogenesis as they have been to many other common cancers. This may be due to the relative ease of obtaining gastric biopsies for histologic assessment of intermediate histological steps on the path to gastric cancer or because there are now several simple minimally invasive tests available for *H. pylori*, a major risk factor for gastric cancer. The use of other blood and tissue determinants as biomarkers of increased risk of gastric cancer has been examined in a limited number of studies. Possession of the mutant *ALDH2\*2* allele of acetaldehyde dehydrogenase may be associated with an increased risk of both gastric and esophageal cancer in the Japanese population, thus suggesting a carcinogenic role for alcohol-derived acetaldehyde.[113] A weak association between possession of the null allele of glutathione-*S*-transferase type M1 was reported by one Japanese group[114] but was not confirmed by another.[115] Furthermore, no associations were observed between polymorphisms of cytochrome p450 2E1 and gastric cancer in this same population.[115] A large study in the Portuguese population has implicated polymorphisms of the mucin genes *MUC6* and *MUC1* in the predisposition to gastric cancer.[116,117] Alterations in serum pepsinogen levels and in the ratio of pepsinogen I/II have been described in atrophic gastritis, a precancerous lesion in the pathway to the intestinal form of gastric cancer. However, it is unclear whether the measurement of serum pepsinogens will be superior to routine *H. pylori* serology as a biomarker of risk for gastric cancer.

*H. pylori* infection increases the gastric mucosal concentrations of reactive nitrogen and oxygen species, which may be important mediators of gastric mutagenesis. Increased nitric oxide synthase activity, increased peroxynitrite (a marker of nitrosation), and increased mucosal oxygen radical formation have all been described in association with *H. pylori* infection.[84,118–120] To address whether urinary levels of DNA adducts would serve as useful biomarkers of risk of gastric cancer in molecular epidemiological studies, urinary 8-hydroxyguanine excretion was measured in a large group of healthy volunteers.[121] Unexpectedly, it was found that *H. pylori*–infected individuals had decreased levels. With the ready availability of endoscopy and tests for *H. pylori* in the Western world, it is questionable whether any of the above markers are likely to be useful clinically, although they may contribute to our understanding of pathogenesis.

### p53

Mutations in the *p53* tumor suppressor gene are common in gastrointestinal cancers and are the most frequent mutations in gastric cancer. *p53* mutations have been found in about 50% of histologically advanced gastric cancers and frequently in early gastric cancer of the intestinal histologic subtype, though less often in early diffuse gastric cancer.[122] *p53* mutations and *p53* overexpression (a surrogate marker of *p53* mutation) have also been identified in premalignant gastric lesions, including dysplasia, intestinal metaplasia (particularly type III),[123,124] and possibly even chronic gastritis.[125]

Point mutations affecting the function of *p53* usually affect the evolutionarily conserved middle section of the molecule encoded by exons 4 to 8, with the most common type of mutation being a G:C-to-A:T transition at CpG sites (thought to be secondary to methylation of a cytosine residue, followed by deamination).[126,127] This type of mutation is commonly found in carcinogenesis due to exogenous mutagens and is consistent with an initial DNA nitrosation reaction. Since CpG mutations of *p53*

are more common in gastric cancer cases associated with *H. pylori* infection than those without it,[128] it has been suggested that reactive nitrogen species released by *H. pylori*–associated inflammation are important inducers of this mutation. However, cancers of the gastric cardia also commonly have mutations in *p53*, usually at CpG sites too.[129] Since gastric cardia tumors are not associated with *H. pylori*, this brings into question the concept that CpG *p53* mutations are related to *H. pylori*.

Mutations in *p53* may be associated with circulating serum *p53* antibodies. Serum anti-*p53* antibodies have been found in about one-fifth of gastric cancer cases from Japan. Whether determining the presence of anti-*p53* antibodies will be useful in screening for cancer or as a prognostic marker has not been fully evaluated.[130,131]

### References

1. Lewandrowski KB, Compton CC. The pathology of gastric cancer and conditions predisposing to gastric cancer. In: Rustgi AK (ed): Gastrointestinal Cancers: Biology, Diagnosis, and Therapy. Lippincott-Raven, Philadelphia, 1995, pp 217–242.
2. Jarvi O, Lauren P. On the role of heterotopias of the intestinal epithelium in the pathogenesis of gastric cancer. Acta Pathol Microbiol Scand 29:26–44, 1951.
3. Lauren PA, Nevalainen JT. Epidemiology of intestinal and diffuse types of gastric carcinoma: a time-trend study in Finland with comparison between studies from high and low-risk areas. Cancer 71:2926–2933, 1993.
4. Lauren P. The two histological main types of gastric carcinoma: diffuse and so-called intestinal type carcinoma: an attempt at a histoclinical classification. Acta Pathol Microbiol Scand 64:31–49, 1965.
5. Craanen ME, Dekker W, Blok P, Ferwerda J, Tytgat GNJ. Time trends in gastric carcinoma: changing patterns of type and location. Am J Gastroenterol 87:572–579, 1992.
6. Devesa SS, Blot WJ, Fraumeni JF. Changing patterns in the incidence of esophageal and gastric carcinoma in the United States. Cancer 83:2049–2053, 1998.
7. Powell J, McConkey CC. The rising trend in oesophageal adenocarcinoma and gastric cardia. Eur J Cancer Prev 1:265–269, 1992.
8. Parkin DM, Pisani P, Ferlay J. Global cancer statistics. CA Cancer J Clin 49:33–64, 1999.
9. The Research Group for Population-based Cancer Registration in Japan: Cancer incidence in Japan, 1985–89: re-estimation based on data from eight population-based cancer registries. Jpn J Clin Oncol 28:54–67, 1998.
10. Landis SH, Murray T, Bolden S, Wingo PA. Cancer statistics 1999. CA Cancer J Clin 49:8–31, 1999.
11. Sanchez BF, Garcia MJ, Perez FD, et al. Prognostic factors in a series of 297 patients with gastric adenocarcinoma undergoing surgical resection. Br J Surg 85:255–260, 1998.
12. Mitsudomi T, Matsusaka T, Wakasugi K, et al. A clinicopathological study of gastric cancer with special reference to age of the patients: an analysis of 1,630 cases. World J Surg 13:225–230, 1989.
13. Fujimoto S, Takahashi M, Ohkubo H, et al. Comparative clinicopathologic features of early gastric cancer in young and older patients. Surgery 115:516–520, 1994.
14. Hundahl SA, Menck HR, Mansour EG, Winchester DP. The National Data Base report on gastric carcinoma. Cancer 80:2333–2341, 1997.
15. Shimizu S, Tada M, Kawai K. Early gastric cancer: its surveillance and natural course. Endoscopy 27:27–31, 1995.
16. Nishi M, Ishihara S, Nakajima T, Ohta K, Ohyama S, Ohta H. Chronological changes of characteristics of early gastric cancer and therapy: experience in the Cancer Institute Hospital of Tokyo, 1950–1994. J Cancer Res Clin Oncol 121:535–541, 1995.
17. Everett SM, Axon ATR. Early gastric cancer in Europe. Gut 41:142–150, 1997.
18. Blot WJ, Devesa SS. Rising incidence of adenocarcinoma of esophagus and gastric cardia. JAMA 265:1287–1289, 1991.
19. Locke GR III, Talley NJ, Carpenter HA, Harmsen WS, Zinsmeister AR, Melton LJ III. Changes in the site- and histologic-specific incidence of gastric cancer during a 50-year period. Gastroenterology 109:1750–1756, 1995.
20. Devesa SS, Fraumeni JF Jr. The rising incidence of gastric cardia cancer. J Natl Cancer Inst 91:747–749, 1999.

21. Dolan K, Sutton R, Walker SJ, Morris AI, Campbell F, Williams EMI. New classification of oesophageal and gastric carcinomas derived from changing patterns in epidemiology. Br J Cancer 80:834–842, 1999.

22. Correa P. Human gastric carcinogenesis: a multistep and multifactorial process. First American Cancer Society Award Lecture on Cancer Epidemiology and Prevention. Cancer Res 52:6735–6740, 1992.

23. Correa P, Cuello C, Duque E, et al. Gastric cancer in Columbia. III. Natural history of precursor lesions. J Natl Cancer Inst 57:1027–1035, 1976.

24. Correa P, Cuello C, Duque E. Carcinoma and intestinal metaplasia of the stomach in Colombian migrants. J Natl Cancer Inst 44:297–306, 1970.

25. Stemmerman GN, Ishidate T, Samloff IM, et al. Intestinal metaplasia of the stomach in Hawaii and Japan: a study of its relation to serum pepsinogen I, gastrin and parietal cell antibodies. Am J Dig Dis 23:815–820, 1978.

26. Haenszel W, Kurihara M, Segi S, Lee RKC. Stomach cancer among Japanese in Hawaii. J Natl Cancer Inst 49:969–988, 1972.

27. Staszewski J. Migrant studies in alimentary tract cancer. Recent results. Cancer Res 39:85–97, 1972.

28. Kamineni A, Williams MA, Schwartz SM, Cook LS, Weiss NS. The incidence of gastric carcinoma in Asian immigrants to the United States and their descendants. Cancer Causes Control 10:77–83, 1999.

29. Cocco P, Ward MH, Buiatti E. Occupational risk factors for gastric cancer: an overview. Epidemiol Rev 18:218–234, 1996.

30. Parent ME, Siemiatycki J, Fritschi L. Occupational exposures and gastric cancer. Epidemiology 9:48–55, 1998.

31. Cocco P, Ward MH, Dosemeci M. Occupational risk factors for cancer of the gastric cardia. J Occup Environ Med 40:855–861, 1998.

32. Kneller RW, McLaughlin JK, Bjelke E, et al. A cohort study of stomach cancer in a high-risk American population. Cancer 68:672–678, 1991.

33. Doll R, Peto R, Wheatly K, Gray R, Sutherland I. Mortality in relation to smoking: 40 years' observation on male British doctors. BMJ 309:901–911, 1994.

34. McLaughlin JK, Hrubec Z, Blot WJ, Fraumeni JF Jr. Smoking and cancer mortality among US veterans: a 26-year follow-up. Int J Cancer 60:190–193, 1995.

35. Gammon MD, Schoenberg JB, Ahsan H, et al. Tobacco, alcohol, and socioeconomic status and adenocarcinomas of the esophagus and gastric cardia. J Natl Cancer Inst 89:1277–1284, 1997.

36. Tredaniel J, Boffeta P, Buiatti E, Saracci R, Hirsch A. Tobacco smoking and gastric cancer: review and meta-analysis. Int J Cancer 72:565–573, 1997.

37. Inoue M, Tajima K, Yamamura Y, et al. Influence of habitual smoking on gastric cancer by histologic subtype. Int J Cancer 81:39–43, 1999.

38. Jedrychowski W, Boeing H, Wahrendof J, Popiela T, Tobiasz-Adamczyk B, Kulig J. Vodka consumption, tobacco smoking and risk of gastric cancer in Poland. Int J Cancer 22:606–613, 1993.

39. Wu-Williams AH, Yu MC, Mack TM. Life-style, workplace, and stomach cancer by subsite in young men of Los Angeles County. Cancer Res 50:2569–2576, 1990.

40. Zhang ZF, Kurtz RC, Sun M, et al. Adenocarcinomas of the esophagus and gastric cardia: medical conditions, tobacco, alcohol, and socioeconomic factors. Cancer Epidemiol Biomarkers Prev 5:761–768, 1996.

41. van Loon AJ, Goldbohm RA, van den Brandt PA. Socioeconomic status and stomach cancer incidence in men: results from The Netherlands Cohort Study. J Epidemiol Community Health 52:166–171, 1998.

42. Fontana V, Decensi A, Orengo MA, Parodi S, Torrisi R, Puntoni R. Socioeconomic status and survival of gastric cancer patients. Eur J Cancer 34:537–542, 1998.

43. Hansson LE, Baron J, Nyren O, et al. Early-life risk indicators of gastric cancer. a population-based case–control study in Sweden. Int J Cancer 57:32–37, 1994.

44. Chow WH, Blot WJ, Vaughan TL, et al. Body mass index and risk of adenocarcinomas of the esophagus and gastric cardia. J Natl Cancer Inst 90:150–155, 1998.

45. Vaughan TL, Davis S, Kristal A, Thomas DB. Obesity, alcohol, and tobacco as risk factors for cancers of the esophagus and gastric cardia: adenocarcinoma versus squamous cell carcinoma. Cancer Epidemiol Biomarkers Prev 4:85–92, 1995.

46. Ji BT, Chow WH, Yang G, et al. Body mass index and the risk of cancers of the gastric cardia and distal stomach in Shanghai, China. Cancer Epidemiol Biomarkers Prev 6:481–485, 1997.

47. Dunn BE, Cohen H, Blaser MJ: *Helicobacter pylori*. Clin Microbiol Rev 10:720–741, 1997.

48. Marshall B. Unidentified curved bacilli on gastric epithelium in active chronic gastritis. Lancet i:1273–1275, 1983.

49. Schistosomes, liver flukes and *Helicobacter pylori*. IARC Working Group on the Evaluation of Carcinogenic Risks to Humans, Lyon France, 7–14 June 1994. IARC Monogr Eval Carcinog Risks Hum 61:1–241, 1994.

50. Karnes WE Jr, Samloff IM, Siurala M, et al. Positive serum antibody and negative tissue staining for *Helicobacter pylori* in subjects with atrophic body gastritis. Gastroenterology 101:167–174, 1991.

51. Kuipers EJ. Relationship between *Helicobacter pylori*, atrophic gastritis and gastric cancer. Aliment Pharmacol Ther 12(Suppl 1):25–36, 1998.

52. Eurogast Study Group: An international association between *Helicobacter pylori* and gastric cancer. Lancet 341:1359–1362, 1993.

53. Lin JT, Wang LY, Wang JT, Wang TH, Yang CS, Chen CJ. A nested case–control study on the association between *Helicobacter pylori* infection and gastric cancer risk in a cohort of 9775 men in Taiwan. Anticancer Res 15:603–606, 1995.

54. Webb PM, Yu MC, Forman D, et al. An apparent lack of association between *Helicobacter pylori* infection and risk of gastric cancer in China. Int J Cancer 67:603–607, 1996.

55. Yuan J-M, Yu M, Xu W-W, Cockburn M, Gao Y-T, Ross RK. *Helicobacter pylori* infection and risk of gastric cancer in Shanghai, China: updated results based upon a locally developed and validated assay and further follow-up of the cohort. Cancer Epidemiol Biomarkers Prev 8:621–624, 1999.

56. Huang JQ, Sridhar S, Chen Y, Hunt RH. Meta-analysis of the relationship between *Helicobacter pylori* seropositivity and gastric cancer. Gastroenterology 114:1169–1179, 1998.

57. Solcia E, Fiocca R, Luinetti O, et al. Intestinal and diffuse gastric cancers arise in a different background of *Helicobacter pylori* gastritis through different gene involvement. Am J Surg Pathol 20(Suppl 1):S8–S22, 1996.

58. Uemura N, Mukai T, Okamoto S, et al. Effect of *Helicobacter pylori* eradication on subsequent development of cancer after endoscopic resection of early gastric cancer. Cancer Epidemiol Biomarkers Prev 6:639–642, 1997.

59. Pisani P, Parkin DM, Munoz N, Ferlay J. Cancer and infection: estimates of the attributable fraction in 1990 [review]. Cancer Epidemiol Biomarkers Prev 6:387–400, 1997.

60. Watanabe T, Tada M, Nagai H, Sasaki S, Nakao M. *Helicobacter pylori* infection induces gastric cancer in Mongolian gerbils. Gastroenterology 115:642–648, 1998.

61. Honda S, Fujioka T, Tokieda M, Satoh R, Nishizono A, Nasu M. Development of *Helicobacter pylori*–induced gastric carcinoma in Mongolian gerbils. Cancer Res 58:4255–4259, 1998.

62. Blok P, Craanen ME, Offerhaus GJ, Tytgat GN. Gastric carcinoma: clinical, pathogenic, and molecular aspects. Q J Med 90:735–749, 1997.

63. Covacci A, Telford JL, Del Giudice G, Parsonnet J, Rappuoli R. *Helicobacter pylori* virulence and genetic geography. Science 284:1328–1333, 1999.

64. Blaser MJ, Perez-Perez GI, Kleanthous H, et al. Infection with *Helicobacter pylori* strains possessing *cagA* is associated with an increased risk of developing adenocarcinoma of the stomach. Cancer Res 55:2111–2115, 1995.

65. Parsonnet J, Friedman GD, Orentreich N, Vogelman H. Risk for gastric cancer in people with *cagA* positive or *cagA* negative *Helicobacter pylori* infection. Gut 40:297–301, 1997.

66. Rudi J, Kolb C, Maiwald M, et al. Serum antibodies against *Helicobacter pylori* proteins VacA and CagA are associated with increased risk for gastric adenocarcinoma. Dig Dis Sci 42:1652–1659, 1997.

67. Perez-Perez GI, Bhat N, Gaensbauer J, et al. Country-specific constancy by age in cagA+ proportion of *Helicobacter pylori* infections. Int J Cancer 72:453–456, 1997.

68. Yamaoka Y, Kodama T, Kashima K, Graham DY, Sepulveda AR. Variants of the 3′ region of the *cagA* gene in *Helicobacter pylori* isolates from patients with different *H. pylori*–associated diseases. J Clin Microbiol 36:2258–2263, 1998.

69. Peek RM Jr, Thompson SA, Donahue JP, et al. Adherence to *Helicobacter pylori* gastric epithelial cells induces expression of a gene, *iceA*, that is associated with clinical outcome. Proc Assoc Am Physicians 110:531–544, 1998.

70. van Doorn LJ, Figueiredo C, Sanna R, et al. Clinical relevance of the *cagA*, *vacA*, and *iceA* status of *Helicobacter pylori*. Gastroenterology 115:58–66, 1998.

71. Chow WH, Blaser MJ, Blot WJ, et al. An inverse relation between *cagA*+ strains of *Helicobacter pylori* infection and risk of esophageal and gastric cardia adenocarcinoma. Cancer Res 58:588–590, 1998.

72. Vicari JJ, Peek RM, Falk GW, et al. The seroprevalence of *cagA*-positive *Helicobacter pylori* strains in the spectrum of gastroesophageal reflux disease. Gastroenterology 115:50–57, 1998.

# Chapter 22

# Molecular Biology of Gastric Cancer

EIICHI TAHARA

Striking advances in molecular dissection of precancerous and cancerous lesions of the stomach indicate that genetic and epigenetic alterations in oncogenes, tumor suppressor genes, DNA-repair genes, cell-cycle regulators, telomeres, and telomerase, as well as genetic instability at microsatellite foci, are involved in the multistep process of human stomach carcinogenesis.[1–3] The scenario of these changes found in gastric carcinoma differs depending on the histologic type of gastric cancer, indicating that different carcinogenetic pathways exist for well-differentiated or intestinal-type carcinomas and poorly differentiated or diffuse-type carcinomas. In addition, cancer–stromal interaction through the growth factor/cytokine receptor system, which plays a pivotal role in morphogenesis, cancer progression, and metastasis, is also very different between the two types of gastric carcinoma.[4,5] Moreover, well differentiated–type gastric carcinomas are subdivided into intestinal type and gastric or foveolar type, according to the phenotypic characteristics of cancer cells.[6] More recently, we found that alterations of the *p73* gene, including loss of heterozygosity (LOH) and abnormal expression, may be responsible for the genesis of gastric adenocarcinoma with foveolar epithelial phenotype.[6]

This chapter provides a detailed overview of the molecular machinery that underlies stomach carcinogenesis and describes a system for the molecular–pathologic diagnosis of gastrointestinal cancer. This system may provide a new approach to cancer diagnosis and novel therapeutics for the twenty-first century.[7,8]

## Telomeres and Telomerase

Human telomeres comprise 2 to 20 Kb of tandem repeated sequences (TTAGGG) and telomere-repeat binding proteins (TRF1 and TRF2). Recently, Griffith et al.[9] showed that telomeres in mammalian cells end as large terminal loops. In normal somatic cells without telomerase activity, the telomeres shorten with cell division and increased age, leading to senescence and eventually to crisis. However, in a few types of normal cells, including germ cells and hematopoietic or epithelial stem cells, and in most cancer cells, activation of telomerase allows the telomeres to be regenerated indefinitely, immortalizing these cells.[10,11] Human telomerase consists of several components including human telomerase RNA (hTR), telomerase-associated protein 1 (TEP1), and human telomerase reverse transcriptase (hTERT), which is a catalytic subunit component.[12] The expression of hTERT is closely associated with activation of telomerase in vitro and in vivo.[13,14] Results of a 1998 study on cell immortalization show, however, that activation of telomerase alone is not enough to immortalize certain epithelial cells, and that inactivation of the p16/Rb pathway is needed.[15]

Ninety percent of gastric carcinomas exhibit higher expression of hTERT and higher telomerase activity than does the corresponding non-neoplastic mucosa.[16] Most well-differentiated or intestinal-type carcinomas contain remarkably shortened telomere length, associated with high levels of telomerase activity. More importantly, over 50% of intestinal metaplasias share reduction in telomere length, and 35% of intestinal metaplasias, as well as gastric adenoma, express low levels of telomerase activity equivalent to about one-tenth of the activity in gastric carcinoma.[17] As for mechanisms of telomerase activation, results of a recent study suggest that Akt protein kinase is involved in activation of telomerase through phosphorylation of hTERT.[18] In fact, Akt protein kinase is expressed in gastric cancer tissue at high levels.

Immunohistochemical analysis shows that the hTERT protein is strongly expressed in the nuclei of the tumor cells of all carcinomas but weakly expressed in the nuclei of epithelial cells of intestinal metaplasia and gastric adenoma and in normal fundic mucosa.[16] Thus, hTERT-positive epithelial cells in the above pre-cancerous lesions and normal gastric mucosa may be viewed as epithelial stem cells. Moreover, the prevalence of *Helicobacter pylori* infection in gastric mucosa correlates well with the grade of intestinal metaplasia and the levels of hTR and telomerase activity, the latter of which is frequently associated with hyperplasia of hTERT-positive epithelial cells.[17,19] These observations indicate that *H. pylori* infection may be a strong trigger for hyperplasia of hTERT-positive cells in intestinal metaplasia, followed by increased telomerase activity and telomere reduction. Hyperplasia of hTERT-positive cells caused by *H. pylori* may induce chronic mitogenesis, which can facilitate increased mutagenesis. In fact, DNA hypermethylation at the D17S5 locus, pS2 loss, abnormal CD44 transcripts, CA repeat instability at the D1S19 locus, and *APC* and *p53* mutations, all of which are commonly seen in well-differentiated or intestinal-type gastric cancer, take place in over 30% of incomplete intestinal metaplasias.[20] These data all indicate that telomere reduction and hTERT over-expression due to stem cell hyperplasia are very early events in the multistep carcinogenesis of well-differentiated gastric cancer, followed by the epigenetic and genetic alterations described above. The frequent development of well-differentiated gastric cancer in aged patients with *H. pylori* infection indicates that this type of gastric cancer is a disease of a chronically afflicted genome rather than a genetic disease.

The hTERT gene promoter contains myc protein-binding sites and multiple consensus motifs for transcription factors, including SP1 and AP2.[21] These ubiquitous transcription factors may maintain the expression of hTERT in normal tissues. In fact, normal gastric mucosa expresses SP1, although at a much lower level than does gastric carcinoma.[22] Overexpression of hTERT in gastric carcinoma may be associated with increased levels of regulatory factors such as SP1 and c-myc protein or with low levels or loss of inhibitory factors for hTERT expression.

Recently, a new partner for telomerase, tankyrase, has been identified, a protein with homology to ankyrin and to the catalytic domain of poly (ADP-ribose) polymerase (PARP).[23] Moreover, lack of PARP by gene targeting is associated with severe chromosomal instability.[24] Tankyrase binds to TRF1, a negative regulator of telomere-length maintenance. By ADP ribosylation of TRF1, tankyrase may enable telomerase to replace lost DNA on the chromosome ends. We have found overexpression of TRF1 in most gastric cancer tissues. Of great interest is whether gene alterations or abnormal expression of tankyrase is linked to chromosomal instability implicated in stomach carcinogenesis.

## Genetic Instability

Two types of genetic instability involve microsatellite instability (MSI) and chromosomal instability. Microsatellite instability is caused by altered DNA mismatch repair and has been found in 15% to 39% of sporadic gastric carcinomas worldwide.[25,26] Gastric carcinomas with a high frequency of MSI (MSI-H) can be divided into two subtypes: well-differentiated and poorly differentiated carcinomas, each of which has specific clinicopathologic characteristics. Well differentiated–type gastric cancers with MSI-H are often seen in patients over 73 years of age and often occur in the antrum pylori. They are frequently associated with abundant lymphoid infiltration, a putative favorable prognosis, and cancer multiplicity.[27,28] Hypermethylation of the *hMLH1* gene promoter occurs in over 70% of cases with this type of gastric cancer and is often associated with down-regulation or loss of *hMLH1*.[28,29] This evidence indicates that MSI-H in well-differentiated or intestinal type gastric cancer is mostly due to epigenetic inactivation of the *hMLH1* gene.

Poorly differentiated or diffuse-type gastric cancers with MSI-H occur mostly in patients under 35 years of age, and are often accompanied by scirrhous-type carcinoma with diffusely productive fibrosis.[30] However, poorly differentiated or diffuse-type gastric canceres harbor no germline mutation of *hMLH*1 and *hMSH2* and no alteration at BAT-RII. This type of gastric cancer is frequently associated with LOH on chromosome 17q21, including the *BRCA1* gene, although we have found no mutation of the *BRCA1* gene. There are two possibile explanations for this: *(1)* chromosome 17q12–21, including the *BRCA1* locus, may contain a candidate tumor suppressor gene, and *(2)* allelic loss of the *BRCA1* gene may be linked to frequent genetic instability in young patients with gastric cancer.

Microsatellite instability at the locus D1S191 (chromosome 1q) is found in 46% of well-differentiated or intestinal-type gastric cancers but not in any poorly differentiated–type gastric cancer. Microsatellite alteration at the same locus is also seen in 26% of incomplete-type intestinal metaplasias adjacent to primary gastric cancers. Moreover, an identical pattern of microsatellite alteration at the locus D1S191 is detected in both well-differentiated adenocarcinoma and the adjacent intestinal metaplasia, which suggests the sequential development of well-differentiated adenocarcinoma from incomplete intestinal metaplasia.[31] The results described above indicate that MSI at the D1S191 locus is one of the early events in the multistep process of stomach carcinogenesis.

Chromosomal instability (CIN) leading to DNA aneuploidy also underlies stomach carcinogenesis. Telomere length is necessary for maintaining chromosomal stability as described above. Mutations in the *p53* gene are also linked to CIN.

## Tumor Suppressor Genes

Alterations in the structure and function of tumor suppressor genes, including *p53, p73, APC* and *DCC* and *FHIT,* are involved in stomach carcinogenesis. Among them, inactivation of the *p53* tumor suppressor gene by LOH and mutation is the most frequent genetic event in gastric cancer, occring in over 60% of gastric carcinoma regardless of histologic types.[1,32,33] Alterations in the *p53* gene are also found in 13% to 37% of intestinal metaplasias and 33% to 58% of gastric adenomas or dysplasias,[34–37] indicating that *p53* gene mutation is an early event in stomach carcinigenesis. The mutation spectrum of this gene can serve as a marker of the effect of putative carcinogens.[38] The mutation spectrum of the *p53* gene in gastric cancer patients in Hiroshima displays an intermediate pattern between that of colon cancer and esophagus cancer.[39–41] *p53* mutations at A:T are common in well-differentiated or intestinal-type carcinomas; G:C-to-A:T transitions are predominant in poorly differentiated–type carcinomas.[32] Carcinogenic *N*-nitrosamines, which cause mainly G:C-to-A:T base substitutions, are found in many foods and can also be produced from the amines with nitrates in the acidic environment of the stomach.[42,43]

Loss of heterozygosity of the *p73* gene, a newly discovered *p53*-related tumor suppressor gene, is detected in 38% of gastric cancers, especially well-differentiated adenocarcinomas that exhibit papillary structure–like foveolar epithelium and express the pS2 trefoil factor.[6] This type of gastric cancer with *p73* LOH shows allele-specific expression of *p73* but no gene mutation in the remaining allele. In addition, the incidence of *p53* abnormalities is low (25%). These observations indicate that LOH and abnormal expression of the *p73* gene may play a large role in the genesis of foveolar-type gastric adenocarcinoma, although this is not in line with Knudson's classic two-hit model of carcinogenesis. We have already reported that 25% of well-differentiated gastric cancers show LOH on chromosome 1p by restriction fragment length polymorphism (RFLP) analysis using the MS1 (1p33–p35) probe.[1] However, these loci are rather centromeric when compared with the mapped region of the *p73* gene (1p36.33).

*APC* is a susceptible tumor suppressor gene for familial polyposis coli.[44] Mutations in the *APC* gene also take place in gastric cancers and sporadic colorectal cancers.[45] Interestingly, more than 50% of well-differentiated or intestinal-type gastric cancers harbor *APC* mutations, whereas poorly differentiated gastric cancers harbor no such mutations. Moreover, there is a distinct difference in the nature of *APC* mutations between gastric and colorectal cancers; namely, missense mutation is dominant in gastric cancer while nonsense mutation and frameshift mutation are common in colorectal cancers.[45] Somatic mutations of the *APC* gene are also seen in 20% to 40% of gastric adenomas and 6% of incomplete intestinal metaplsias.[46,47] *APC* alteration is viewed as an early genetic event in the pathogenesis of well-differentiated gastric cancers.[48] Loss of heterozygosity at the *DCC* locus is also one of the characteristics of well-differentiated gastric cancer and is seen in 50% to 60% of primary gastric cancers.[1,49]

The hypothesis that *FHIT* gene alterations are involved in the development of primary gastric cancer remains controversial. Huebner's group reported the rearrangement of the *FHIT* gene, aberrant transcripts, or both in 53% of primary gastric cancers and loss of FHIT protein in 67%.[50,51] Chen and colleagues demonstrated that aberrant transcripts were found not only in 46% of gastric cancers but also in 30% of noncancerous gastric mucosas.[52] Other studies showed that 13% to 16% of primary gastric cancers shared LOH of the *FIHT* gene and no abnormal transcripts,[53,54] although four of seven gastric cancer cell lines exhibited LOH of the *FHIT* gene.[53] *FHIT* gene alterations and loss of FHIT protein should be evaluated in series involving many cases of gastric cancer and precancerous lesions to determine whether environmental factors or putative carcinogens are associated with differences in frequency of FHIT abnormalities between countries.

Several distinct chromosomal loci are deleted in gastric cancers. Loss of heterozygosity at 1q and 7q are frequently associated with well-differentiated gastric cancer, while loss of 1p is relatively common in advanced poorly differentiated gastric cancer.[1] Moreover, LOH at the *bcl-2* gene locus is seen in many well-differentiated gastric cancers and colorectal cancers.[55] Our deletion mapping study on 7q shows that LOH at the D7S95 locus correlates well with peritoneal dissemination.[56] Recently, investigators in a study on allelic loss in xenografted human gastric carcinomas reported a high degree of allelic loss on several chromosomal arms (3p [81%], 4p [64%], 5q [69%], 8p [57%], 13q [59%], 17p [80%], and 18q [61%]) in 18 xenografted gastric adenocarcinomas.[57] From these assigned loci, candidates for the tumor suppressor gene responsible for stomach carcinogenesis may be identified in the future.

pS2, a gastric-specific trefoil factor normally expressed in the gastric feveolar epithelial cells, may function as a gastric-specific tumor suppressor. Recently, we found that the reduction or loss of the *pS2* gene by DNA methylation at the promoter region occurs in intestinal metaplasias and gastric adenomas.[58] Conversely, 32% of gastric cancers display strong expression of the *pS2* gene and 40% of gastric cancers, especially the well-differentiated type, show no expression.[60] Reduced expression or loss of the *pS2* gene due to promoter methylation may play a role in early stages of intestinal-type stomach carcinogenesis. Recent in vivo and in vitro studies suggest that the nuclear retinoid acid receptor β2 (RAR β2) and RUNX3 functions as tumor suppressors and that loss of the RAR β2 and RUNX3 by the promoter CpG hypermethylation is associated with gastric tumorigenesis.[59,60]

## Oncogenes

Several protoncogenes, including c-*met*, K-*sam*, and c-*erbB2*, are frequently activated in gastric carcinomas. The amplification of the c-*met* gene encoding a receptor for hepatocyte growth factor/ scatter factor (HGF/SF) is found in 19% of well-differentiated and 39% of poorly differentiated gastric cancers, frequently accompanied by diffusely productive fibrosis of the scirrhous type.[61] Most gastric carcinomas express two different c-*met* transcripts, one 7.0 kb and the other 6.0 kb. Expression of the 6.0 kb c-*met* transcript, which is expressed preferentially in cancer cells, correlates well with tumor staging, lymphnode metastasis, and depth of tumor invasion.[62] Soman and co-workers[63] reported that the *tpr-met* rearrangement is expressed in gastric carcinomas and gastric precancerous lesions. However, we have not detected *tpr-met* rearrangement in any gastric cancer or intestinal metaplasia.

The K-*sam* (KATO-III cell-derived stomach cancer amplified) gene has at least four transcriptional variants.[64] Type II encodes a receptor for keratinocyte growth factor.[64] Type II transcript is expressed only in carcinoma cells but not in cell lines from sarcomas. K-*sam* is preferentially amplified in 33% of advanced poorly differentiated or scirrhous-type gastric carcinomas but not in well-differentiated gastric carcinomas.[65] Moreover, K-s*am* is never seen in esophageal and colorectal carcinomas. Gastric cancers that overexpress K-sam protein are associated with a less favorable prognosis.

In contrast to K-sam, c-*erb*B2 is preferentially amplified in 20% of well-differentiated gastric cancers but not in poorly differentiated gastric cancer.[66,67] Overexpression of c-*erb*B2 associated with gene amplification is closely correlated with a poor prognosis and liver metastasis.[68,69] The amplification of c-*erb*B1 and c-*erb*B3 is found in 3%[67] and 0%,[70] respectively, of gastric cancers.

K-r*as* mutation is found in gastric intestinal metaplasias, adenomas, and well-differentiated adenocarcinomas,[1,71,72] although its incidence is low (10% to18%). However, K-r*as* mutation is not seen in poorly differentiated gastric cancer. The *hst*-1 gene, isolated from a surgical specimen of human gastric cancer by NIH/3T3 transformation assay, is rarely amplified in gastric cancer (2% of cases).[73]

## Cell-Cycle Regulators

Genetic and epigenetic abnormalities in cell-cycle regulators are involved in the development and progression of gastric cancer by causing unbridled proliferation. Most gastric cancers are commonly associated with overexpression of positive regulators and reduction or loss of negative regulators, both of which cooperate to drive normal cells into malignancy.

The cyclin E gene is amplified in 15% to 20% of gastric carcinomas that are associated with overexpression.[74] The gene amplification, overexpression of cyclin E, or both cause aggressiveness and lymph node metastasis.[74] Cyclin D1 gene amplification, by contrast, is exceptional in gastric carcinomas but frequently occurs in esophageal carcinoma.[75]

CDC25 phosphatases dephosphorylate the threonine and tryosine residues at positions 14 and 15 in the cyclin-dependant kinases (CDKs) and then activate them.[76] Three types of CDC25 have been identified: CDC25A, CDC25B, and CDC25C.[77] CDC25A is expressed early in the $G_1$ phase of the cell cyle, CDC25B is expressed in both the $G_1/S$ and $G_2$ phases.[78] CDC25C is predominantly expressed in the $G_2$ phase. CDC25B is overexpressed in more than 70% of gastric cancers regardless of histologic type and closely correlates with tumor invasion and nodal metastasis.[79] Only 2% of gastric adenomas overexpress CDC25B, however, and no gene amplification of CDC25B has been found in any gastric cancers. In 38% of gastric cancers, CDC25A is overexpressed but CDC25C is at very low or undetectable levels. Thus, the overexpression of CDC25B in tumor cells may stimulate progression of gastric cancer.

In addition to the binding of cyclin/CDK complexes to CDK-inhibitory proteins, CDKs interact with regulatory protein that is the product of the *suc*1 (suppressor of Cdc temperature-sensitive mutations) gene or *Cks1* (Cdc28 kinase subunit) gene in *Saccharomyces*.[80] Cks proteins are necessary for cell-cycle progression in vivo and are physically associated with active forms of CDKs.[80] CKshs1 is a human homolog of the yeast cell-cycle regulatory proteins Cks1 and suc1.[81] We have already found that more than 60% of gastric cancers show higher levels of CKshs1 than do the corresponding normal mucosa.[82] CKshs1 overexpression is less frequent in well-differentiated adenocarcinomas than in poorly differentiated adenocarcinomas. There is no obvious relationship between CKshs1 overexpression and either tumor progression or *p53* mutations. No gene amplification has been found in any gastric cancer cell lines. These findings suggest that overexpression of CKshs1 plays a role in the development of well-differentiated type gastric cancer.

As for negative cell-cycle regulators, the p53-inducible cyclin-dependent kinase inhibitor p21 is associated with the senescence of non-neoplastic gastric epithelial cells.[83] In the neoplastic lesions, the expression of p21 is seen in 78% of gastric adenomas and 76% of gastric adenocarcinomas regardless of *p53* gene mutation. This finding suggests that a *p53*-independent pathway is substantially involved in the induction of p21 in gastric tumors.[84] In fact, the growth inhibition of transforming growth factor β (TGF-β) or retinoic acid is associated with *p53*-independent induction of p21 in a gastric cancer cell line.[85] Moreover, the strong expression of p21 in cancer cells is frequently observed in advanced cancers and nodal metastasis, whereas there is no inverse correlation between p21 expression and proliferative activity measured by Ki-67. These findings overall indicate that the proliferative activity of gastric cancer is not solely dependent on control of the cell cycle by p21.[86] In addition, mutation of the p21 gene is exceptional in gastric cancer[86] and a codon 31 polymorphism does not affect the expression levels of p21.[87]

p27, a member of the cip/kip family of CDK inhibitors, binds to a wide variety of cyclin/CDK complexes and inhibits kinase activity. We have found that growth suppression of interferon-γ is associated with the induction of p27 in a gastric cancer cell TMK-1.[88] More important, reduction in p27 expression is frequently seen in advanced gastric cancers, whereas p27 is well preserved in 90% of gastric adenomas and 85% of early cancers.[89] Gastric adenomas with reduction or loss of p27 are capable of developing into malignacies. Reduced expression of p27 significantly correlates with depth of tumor invasion and nodal metastasis. Moreover, metastatic tumor cells in lymph nodes express p27 at weaker levels than those in primary tumors, which suggests that tumor cells with reduction or loss of p27 may se-lectively metastasize to lymph nodes or distant organs.[90] The expression of p27 in gastric cancer is inversely correlated with the expression of cyclin E.[91] Loss of p27 function and gain of cyclin E evidently stimulate progression and metastasis of gastric carcinomas. Reduction in p27 expression occurs at post-translational levels, resulting from ubiquitin-mediated proteosomal degradation rather than genetic abnormalities.[90]

Deletion or mutations of the *p16* gene are uncommon in primary gastric carcinomas,[91–93] while homozygous deletion of the *p16* gene has been found in two of eight gastric cancer cell lines, and lack of p16 protein expression has been found in five of eight gastric cancer cell lines.[94] Another mechanism of *p16* gene silencing is hypermethylation of the 5 CpG island.[95] In particular, loss of p16 protein is often seen in advanced cancers with nodal metastasis. Loss of p16 and p27 proteins may be associated with the progression of gastric carcinoma. Recently, Chen and co-workers reported that aberrant RNA transcripts of the *p16* gene were noted in 30% to 45% of primary gastric cancers.[96]

Major alterations in the *Rb* gene are also infrequent in primary gastric cancers.[97] All primary tumors and all gastric cancer cell lines express *pRb*.[94]

An important downsteam target of cyclin/Cdks at the $G_1/S$ transition is a family of E2F transcription factors. Gene amplification of *E2F-1* is seen in 4% of gastric cancers and 25% of colorectal cancers.[98] Overexpression of E2F is found in 40% of primary gastric carcinomas.[98] Moreover, E2F and cyclin E tend to be coexpressed in gastric cancer. In contrast, 70% of gastric cancers exhibit lower levels of E2F-3 expression than do corresponding non-neoplastic mucosas. These results suggest that gene amplification and anomalous expression of the *E2F* gene may permit the development of gastric cancer.

## Growth Factors and Cytokines

Gastric cancer cells express a broad spectrum of growth factors, cytokines, or both, including TGF-α, epidermal growth factor (EGF), amphiregulin (AR), cripto, heparin binding (HB)-EGF, platelet-derived growth factor (PDGF), insulin-like growth factor (IGF) II, TGF-$β_1$, basic fibroblast growth factor (bFGF), interleukin (IL)-1α, IL-6, IL-8, and osteopontin (OPN).[2,4,99,100] These growth factors and cytokines function as autocrine, paracrine, and juxtacrine modulators of growth of cancer cells, and they organize the complex interaction between cancer cells and stromal cells that plays a key role in morphogenesis, invasion, neovascularization, and metastasis. Interestingly, the expression of these growth factors, cytokines, or both by cancer cells differs between the two histologic types of gastric carcinoma. The EGF family, including EGF, TGF-α, and cripto, is commonly overexpressed in well-differentiated gastric carcinoma; TGF-β, IGF-II, and bFGF are predominantly overexpressed in poorly differentiated gastric carcinoma.[101] Coexpression of EGF/TGF-α, EGF receptor, and cripto correlates well with the biological malignancy of gastric cancer, because these factors induce metalloproteinases.[102–104] Overexpression of cripto is frequently associated with intestinal metaplasia and gastric adenoma.[105]

In the EGF family, AR, which is overexpressed in more than 60% of gastric carcinomas regardless of histologic type,[106] works as an autocrine growth factor and induces the expression of AR itself, TGF-α, and EGF receptors by gastric cancer cells.[107] Overexpression of the EGF family in gastric cancer usually does not accompany gene amplifications. The relative expression levels of

frequent in patients with gastric carcinoma than in controls, and a significant association has been observed between small *MUC1* genotypes and glandular atrophy due to *H. pylori*.[150] These observations indicate that individuals with small *MUC1* genotypes, especially persons infected with *H. pylori*, are at increased risk for development of gastric carcinoma. It would be interesting to note whether the Japanese population has high frequency of small *MUC1* genotypes, because the highest incidence of gastric cancer is still observed in Japan.

## Genetic Pathway of Two Types of Gastric Cancer

The overall observations on molecular events of gastric cancer may provide supporting evidence for our working hypothesis that there are two distinctive major genetic pathways of stomach carcinogenesis (Fig. 22–1). Genetic and epigenetic alterations found in two types of gastric cancer are summarized in Table 22–1. The scenario of these epigenetic alterations found gastric cancer differs, depending on the two types of gastric cancer, indicating that there are at least two types of CpG island methylator phenotype responsible for the development of intestinal- and diffuse-types gastric cancer. Genetic instability, including microsatellite instability and telomere reduction and immortality (activation of telomerase and expression of *hTERT*), are implicated in an initial step of stomach carcinogenesis. In the multistep process of well differentiated–type or intestinal-type gastric carcinogenesis, infection with *H. pylori* may be a strong trigger for hyperlasia of *hTERT*-positive stem cells in intestinal metaplasia. Genetic instability and hyperplasia of *hTERT*-positive stem cells may pre-

**Table 22–1** Genetic and epigenetic alterations found in two types of gastric cancer of the stomach

| Genetic and Epigenetic Alterations | Incidence of Cases with Indicated Alterations (%) | |
| --- | --- | --- |
| | *Well Differentiated*[a] | *Poorly Differentiated*[a] |
| *Tumor Suppressor Genes* | | |
| p53 LOH, mutation | 60 | 75 |
| p73 LOH | 53[b] | 24 |
| APC LOH, mutation | 40–60 | 0 |
| DCC LOH | 50 | 0 |
| LOH of Chr.1a | 44 | 0 |
| LOH of Chr.7q | 53 | 33 |
| LOH of Chr.17q | 0 | 40[c] |
| Loss of pS2 expression | 49 | 31 |
| Loss of RAR β | 50 | 73 |
| Loss of RUNX3 | 37 | 40 |
| *Cell-Cycle Regulators* | | |
| Cyclin E amplification | 33 | 7 |
| Cyclin E overexpression | 26 | 27 |
| CDC25B overexpression | 33 | 73 |
| Loss of p16 expression | 50 | 10 |
| Loss of p27 expression | 46 | 69 |
| *Oncogenes* | | |
| K-ras mutation | 10 | 0 |
| c-met amplification | 19 | 39 |
| K-sam amplification | 0 | 33 |
| c-erbB2 amplification | 20 | 0 |
| *Adhesion Molecules* | | |
| E-cadherin mutation | 0 | 50 |
| Loss of CDH1 | 55 | 79 |
| CD44 aberrant transcript | 100 | 100 |
| *Growth Factors and Cytokines* | | |
| VEGF overexpression | 46 | 9 |
| IL-8 overexpression | 75 | 85 |
| TGF-β overexpression | 33 | 71 |
| *Microsatellite instability* | 20–40 | 20–70 |
| (h MLH1 methylation) | (5–20) | (0) |
| *Telomere/telomerase* | | |
| Telomere reduction | 62 | 53 |
| Telomerase activity | 100 | 90 |
| TERT expression | 100 | 86 |

IL-8, interleukin-8; TERT, telomerase reverse transcriptase; TGF-β, transforming growth factor β; VEGF, vascular endothelial growth factor.

[a]According to the criteria of the Japanese Classification of Gastric Carcinoma.

[b]Preferentially found in foveolar-type adenocarcinoma.

[c]Preferentially found in patients younger than 35 years of age.

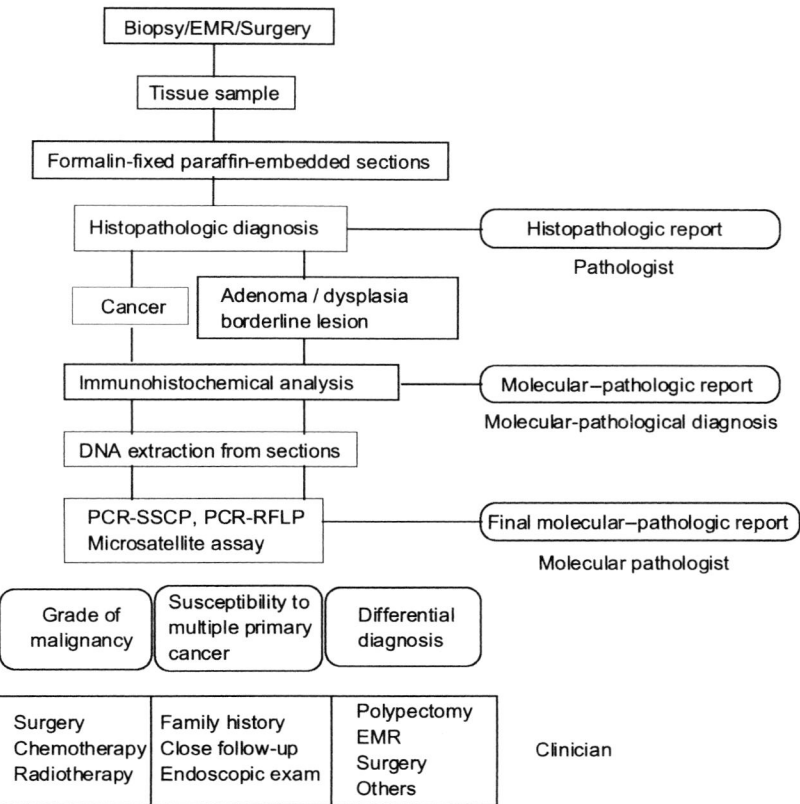

**Figure 22-2** Strategy of molecular–pathological diagnosis of gasterointestinal lesions. EMR, electromagnetic radiation; PCR-RFLP, polymerase chain reaction–restriction fragment length polymorphism; PCR-SSCP, PCR–single-strand conformation polymorphism.

cede replication error at the D1S191 locus, DNA hypermethylation at the D17S5 locus, pS2 loss, p16 loss, CD44 abnormal transcripts, and *p53* mutation, all of which accumulate in at least 30% of in complete intestinal metaplasias. All of these epigentic and genetic alterations are common events in intestinal-type gastric cancer. Incomplete intestinal metaplasia that contains an accumulation of the above multiple molecular events, i.e., metaplastic dysplasia, may be viewed as a bud of intestinal-type gastric cancer at genetic and epigenetic levels. An adenoma–carcinoma sequence is found in about 20% of gastric adenomas with *APC* mutations. In addition to these events, RUNX3 loss, *p53* mutation, and LOH, reduced *p27* expression, cyclin E expression, and presence of c-*met* 6.0 kb transcripts allow malignant transformation from the above precancerous lesions to intestinal-type gastric cancer. *DCC* loss, *APC* mutations, 1q LOH, *p27* loss, reduced TGF-β type I receptor expression, reduced nm23 expression, and c-*erb*B gene amplification, as well as RUNX3 loss, are implicated in the progression and metastasis of intestinal-type gastric cancer. Another pathway for carcinogenesis of well-differentiated gastric cancer involves LOH and abnormal expression of the *p73* gene, which may be responsible for the development of foveolar-type gastric cancers with *pS2* expression.

Loss of heterozygosity at chromosome 17p, mutation or LOH of *p53*, RAR β 2 loss, and mutation or loss of E-cadherin, however, are preferentially involved in the development of poorly differentiated gastric cancers. Interestingly, hypermethylation of the RAR β 2 and CDH1 promoters occurs concordantly. In addition to these changes, gene amplification of K-s*am* and c-*met, p27* loss, and RUNX3 loss as well as reduced

*nm23* obviously confer progression, metastasis, and diffusely productive fibrosis. One point should be added here: mixed gastric carcinomas composed of well-differentiated and poorly differentiated components exhibit some, but not all, of the molecular events described so far for each of the two constituent types of gastric cancer.

Besides these genetic and epigenetic events, well-differentiated and poorly differentiated gastric cancer can also develop different interplay between cancer cells and stromal cells through the growth factor/cytokine receptor system, which plays an important role in cell growth, apoptosis, morphogenesis, angiogenesis, progression, and metastasis.

## Molecular-Pathologic Diagnosis

By analyzing genetic and epigenetic alterations in pathology specimens, we can facilitate and improve cancer diagnosis, predict the grade of malignancy or patient prognosis, identify patients at high risk for developing multiple primary cancers, and discover novel therapeutic approaches. Since 1993, a system of molecular–pathologic diagnosis of gastrointestinal cancer based on the findings discussed in this chapter has been routinely provided by the First Department of Pathology, Hiroshima University School of Medicine, in colllaboration with the Hiroshima City Medical Association Clinical Laboratory.[7,8,150]

The strategy of molecular–pathological diagnosis of gastrointestinal lesions is illustrated in Fig. 22–2. The cases of cancer, adenoma (dysplasia), and borderline lesion are selected for immunohistochemical analysis by using a set of biomarkers

**Table 22-2** Biological markers used for molecular–pathologic diagnosis of gastrointestinal cancer

| Tumor | Biological Marker | Purpose |
|---|---|---|
| Esophagus | p53 | Diagnose disease |
| Esophagus | EGF, TGF-α, EGFR, Ki-67 | Determine malignancy grade |
| Esophagus | Cyclin D1 | Predict metastasis |
| Stomach | p53, APC | Diagnose disease |
| Stomach | TGF-α, EGFR, cripto, c-met, c-erbB2, CyclinE, CDC25B, p27, Ki-67 | Determine malignancy grade Predict metastasis |
| Stomach | nm23, CD44 | Predict susceptibility to multiple cancers |
| Colon | p53, APC, CD44 | Diagnose disease |
| Colon | EGF, TGF-α, cripto, EGFR, Cyclin E, p27, p21, Ki-67 | Determine malignancy grade |
| Colon | nm23, SLX | Predict metastasis |
| Colon | Replication error/mismatch repair genes | Predict NHPCC |

NHPCC, hereditary nonpolyposis colon cancer.

(Table 22–2). Genetic analyses are performed using several primers for detecting p53 and APC mutations, LOH, and microsatellite instabilility at five loci of two CA repeats (D1S191, D17S855, BRCA1) and two polyA tracts (BATRII, BAT40).

As reported recently,[150] 10,419 lesions (from 9241 cases) were examined from August 1993 to November 1998. These consisted of 221 esophageal lesions (216 cases), 4647 gastric lesions (4435 cases), and 5551 lesions colorectal lesions (4590). Their histologic diagnoses were adenoma, dysplasia, borderline lesion, carcinoma, and suspicious lesion for carcinoma. The results of molecular–pathologic diagnosis on gastric lesions are summarized in Table 22–3. Of 1154 adenomas, 10% were diagnosed as adenoma with malignant potential, and 2% were suspected of being adenocarcinoma on the basis of an abnormal accumulation of p53 and mutation or LOH of the p53 gene as well as of the APC gene. Of the borderline lesions, 22% were judged to be carcinomas. Of 2969 adenocarcinomas, more than 80% of which were early cancers, 12% were regarded as high-grade malignancies,

based on overexpression of c-erbB2, EGF receptor, and cyclin E and loss of p27. By microsatellite analysis of about 700 gastric cancer cases, MSI-H was found in approximately 4% of gastric cancers, 50% of which were confirmed as having multiple primary cancers. Follow-up study is necessary to prove the priority of the molecular–pathologic diagnosis. The 2-year survival rates of the patients after surgical removal of gastric and colorectal carcinomas show that the patients with high-grade malignancies had poorer prognoses.

Although the evaluation of our strategy requires continuous assessment and follow-up studies, the evidence cited above indicates that it provides new opportunities for early cancer diagnosis and more accurate evaluation of prognosis. Although DNA-, RNA-, and protein-chip technology will greatly promote new directions in cancer diagnosis and therapeutics in the future, pathologic analysis of precancerous and cancerous lesions remains the first step in DNA, RNA, and protein analyses.

**Table 22-3** Molecular–Pathologic Diagnosis of Gastric Lesions

| Histologic Diagnosis | Lesions | Molecular Diagnosis[a] | n (%) |
|---|---|---|---|
| Adenoma | 1154 | Adenoma with malignant potential | 119 (10) |
|  |  | Suspected adenocarcinoma | 19 (2) |
| Borderline | 469 | Adenoma with malignant potential | 6 (1) |
|  |  | Suspected adenocarcinoma | 45 (10) |
|  |  | Adenocarcinoma | 53 (11) |
| Suspected adenocarcinoma | 250 | Adenocarcinoma | 63 (25) |
|  |  | High-grade malignancy | 3 (1) |
| Adenocarcinoma | 2969 | High-grade malignancy | 357 (12) |

[a]Molecular diagnosis is made according to both molecular and histologic findings.

Definitions of molecular diagnosis are as follows. *Adenoma with malignant potential* is an adenoma with a high probability of becoming carcinoma. Tumors contain some molecular and genetic abnormalities, including abnormality of the p53 gene, but morphologic aberration is within the range for benign tumor. Suspected adenocarcinoma is a tumor that exhibits genetic abnormalities of p53 and/or APC as well as abnormal expression of many cancer-related molecules such as c-erbB2, cyclin E, EGFR, c-met, and so on. Biological atypia is not severe enough to be regarded as carcinoma. Adenocarcinoma is a tumor whose genetic and molecular abnormalities are the same degree as for suspected adenocarcinoma and that can be regarded as malignant histologically if such molecular finding are available.

## References

1. Sano T, Tsujino T, Yoshida K, et al. Frequent loss of heterozygosity on chromosomes 1q, 5q, and 17p in human gastric carcinomas. Cancer Res 51:2926–2931, 1991.
2. Tahara E. Molecular mechanism of stomach carcinogenesis. J Cancer Res Clin Oncol 119:265–272, 1993.
3. Tahara E, Semba S, Tahara H. Molecular biological observations in gastric cancer, Semin Oncol 23:307–315, 1996.
4. Tahara E, Kuniyasu H, Yasui W, Yokozaki H. Abnormal expression of growth factors and their receptors in stomach cancer. In: Nakamura T, Matsumoto K (eds): Gann Monograph on Cancer Research Growth Factors: Cell Growth, Morphogenesis and Transformation. Japan Scientific Society Press, Tokyo, 1994, pp 163–173.
5. Tahara E, Yokozaki H, Yasui W. Growth factors in gastric cancer. In: Nishi M, Ichikawa H, Nakajima T, Maruyama K, Tahara E (eds): Gastric Cancer. Springer-Verlag, Berlin, 1993, pp 209–217.
6. Yokozaki H, Shitara Y, Fujimoto J, Hiyama T, Yasui W, Tahara E. Alterations of *p73* preferentially occur in gastric adenocarcinomas with foveolar epithelial phenotype. Int J Cancer 83:192–196, 1999.
7. Tahara E. Genetic alterations in human gastrointestinal cancer: the application to molecular diagnosis. Cancer Suppl 75:1410–1417, 1995.
8. Yasui W, Yokozaki H, Shimamoto F, Tahara H, Tahara E. Molecular–pathological diagnosis of gastrointestinal tissues and its contribution to cancer histopathology. Pathol Int 49:763–774, 1999.
9. Griffith JD, Comeau L, Rosenfield S, et al. Mammalian telomeres end in a large duplex loop. Cell 97:503–514, 1999.
10. Harley CB, Futcher AB, Greider CW. Telomeres shorten during aging. Nature 345:458–460, 1990.
11. Kim NW, Piatyszek MA, Prowse KR, et al. Specific association of human telomerase activity with immortal cells and cancer. Science 266:2011–2015, 1994.
12. Nakayama J, Tahara H, Tahara E, et al. Telomerase activation by hTRT in human normal fibroblasts and hepatocellular carcinomas, Nat Genet 18:65–68, 1999.
13. Tahara H, Kuniyasu H, Yokozaki H, et al. Telomerase activity in preneoplastic and neoplastic gastric and colorectal lesions. Clin Cancer Res 1:1245–1251, 1995.
14. Tahara H, Tahara E, Tahara E, Ide T. Telomere and telomerase in gastrointestinal cancer. In: Tahara E (ed): Molecular Pathology of Gastroenterological Cancer: Application to Clinical Practice. Springer-Verlag, Berlin, 1997, pp 245–259.
15. Weinberg RA. Bumps on the road to immortality. Nature 396:23–24, 1998.
16. Yasui W, Tahara H, Tahara E, et al. Expression of telomerase catalytic component, telomerase reverse transcriptase, in human gastric carcinomas. Jpn J Cancer Res 89:1099–1103, 1998.
17. Yasui W, Tahara E, Tahara H, et al. Immunohistochemical detection of human telomerase reverse transcriptase in normal mucosa and precancerous lesions of the stomach. Jpn J Cancer Res 90:589–595, 1999.
18. Kang SS, Kwon T, Kown DY, Do SI. Akt protein kinase enhances human telomerase activity through phosphorylation of telomerase reverse transcriptase subunit. J Biol Chem 19:13085–13090, 1999.
19. Kuniyasu H, Domen T, Hamamoto T, et al. Expression of human telomerase RNA is an early event of stomach carcinogenesis. Jpn J Cancer Res 88:103–107, 1997.
20. Tahara E. Molecular mechanism of human stomach carcinogenesis implicated in *Helicobacter pylori* infection. Exp Toxicol Pathol 50:375–378, 1998.
21. Takakura M, Kyo S, Kanaya T, et al. Cloning of human telomerase catalytic subunit (*hTERT*) gene promoter and identification of proximal core promoter sequences essential for transcriptional activation in immortalized and cancer cells. Cancer Res 59:551–557, 1999.
22. Yasui W, Tahara E, Tahara H, et al. Immunohistochemical detection of human telomerase reverse transcriptase in normal mucosa and precancerous lesions of the stomach. Jpn J Cancer Res 90:589–595, 1999.
23. Smith S, Giriat I, Schmitt A, de Lange T. Tankyrase, a poly (ADP-ribose) polymerase at human telomeres. Science 282:1484–1487, 1998.
24. di Fagagna Fd'A, Hande MP, Tong WM, et al. Functions of poly(ADP-ribose) polymerase in controlling telomere length and chromosomal stability. Nat Genet 23:76–80, 1999.
25. Semba S, Yokozaki H, Yamamoto S, Yasui W, Tahara E. Microsatellite instability in precancerous lesions and adenocarcinomas of the stomach. Cancer Suppl 77:1620–1627, 1996.
26. Yokozaki H, Semba S, Fujimoto J, Tahara E. Microsatellite instabilities in gastric cancer patients with multiple primary cancers. Int J Oncol 14:151–155, 1999.
27. Wu MS, Lee CW, Shun CT, et al. Clinicopathological significance of altered loci of replication error and microsatellite instability-associated mutations in gastric cancer. Cancer Res 58:1494–1497, 1998.
28. Leung SY, Yuen ST, Chung LP, et al. hMLH1 promoter methylation and lack of hMLH1 expression in sporadic gastric carcinomas with high-frequency microsatellite instability. Cancer Res 59:159–164, 1999.
29. Fleisher AS, Esteller M, Wang SG, et al. Hypermethylation of the *hMLH1* gene promoter in human gastric cancers with microsatellite instability. Cancer Res 59:1090–1095, 1999.
30. Semba S, Yokozaki H, Yasui W, Tahara E. Frequent microsatellite instability and loss of heterozygosity in the region including BRCA1 (17q21) in young patients with gastric cancer. Int J Oncol 12:1245–1251, 1998.
31. Hamamoto T, Yokozaki H, Semba S, et al. Altered microsatellites in incomplete-type intestinal metaplasia adjacent to primary gastric cancers. J Clin Pathol 50:841–846, 1997.
32. Yokozaki H, Kuniyasu H, Kitadai Y, et al. *p53* point mutations in primary human gastric carcinomas. J Cancer Res Clin Oncol 119:67–70, 1992.
33. Tamura G, Kihana T, Nomura K, et al. Detection of frequent *p53* gene mutations in primary gastric cancer by cell sorting and polymerase chain reaction single-strand conformation polymorphism analysis. Cancer Res 51:2056–3058, 1991.
34. Tohdo H, Yokozaki H, Haruma K, Kajiyama G, Tahara E. *p53* gene mutations in gastric adenomas. Virchows Arch B Cell Pathol Incl Mol Pathol 63:191–195, 1993.
35. Sakurai S, Sano T, Nakajima T. Clinicopathological and molecular biological studies of gastric adenomas with special reference to *p53* abnormality. Pathol. Int 45:51–57, 1995.
36. Ochiai A, Yamauchi Y, Hirohashi S. *p53* mutations in the non-neoplastic mucosa of the human stomach showing intestinal metaplasia. Int J Cancer 69:28–33, 1996.
37. Sakurai S, Sano T, Nakajima T. Clinicopathological and molecular biological studies of gastric adenomas with special reference to *p53* abnormality. Pathol Int 45:51–57, 1995.
38. Harris CC. Chemical and physical carcinogenesis: advances and perspectives for the 1990s. Cancer Res 51:5023–5044, 1991.
39. Maesawa C, Tamura G, Suzuki Y, et al. The sequential accumulation of genetic alterations characteristic of the colorectal adenoma–carcinoma sequence does not occur between gastric adenoma and adenocarcinoma. J Pathol 176:249–258, 1995.
40. Uchino S, Noguchi M, Ochiai A, et al. *p53* mutation in gastric cancer: a genetic model for carcinogenesis is common to gastric and colorectal cancer. Int J Cancer 54:759–764, 1993.
41. Poremba C, Yandell DW, Huang Q, et al. Frequency and spectrum of *p53* mutations in gastric cancer a molecular genetic and immunohistochemical study. Virchows Arch 426:447–455, 1995.
42. Sugimura T, Fujimura S, Baba T. Tumor production in the glandular stomach and alimentary tract of the rat by N-methyl-N'-nitro-N-nitrosoguanidine. Cancer Res 30:455–465, 1970.
43. Mirvish S. Kinetics of nitrosamine formation from alkylureas, N-alkylurethans, and alkylguanidines: possible implications for the etiology of human gastric cancer. J Natl Cancer Inst 46:1183–1193, 1971.
44. Kinzler KW, Nilbert MC, Su LK, et al. Identification of FAP locus genes from chromosome 5q21. Science 253:661–665, 1991.
45. Nakatsuru S, Yanagisawa A, Ichii S, et al. Somatic mutation of the *APC* gene in gastric cancer: frequent mutations in very well differentiated adenocarcinoma and signet-ring cell carcinoma. Hum Mol Genet 1:559–563, 1992.
46. Nishimura K, Yokozaki H, Haruma K, Kajiyama G, Tahara E. Alterations of the APC gene in carcinoma cell lines and precancerous lesions of the stomach. Int J Oncol 7:587–592, 1995.
47. Nakatsuru S, Yanagisawa A, Furukawa Y, et al. Somatic mutations of the *APC* gene in precancerous lesion of the stomach. Hum Mol Genet 2:1463–1465, 1993.
48. Yokozaki H, Kuniyasu H, Semba S, Yasui W, Tahara E. Molecular bases of human stomach carcinogenesis. In: Tahara E (ed): Molecular Pathology of Gastroenterological Cancer: Application to Clinical Practice. Springer-Verlag, Tokyo, 1997, pp 55–70.
49. Uchino S, Tsuda H, Noguchi M, et al. Frequent loss of heterozygosity at the DCC locus in gastric cancer. Cancer Res 52:3099–3102, 1992.

50. Ohta M, Inoue H, Cotticelli MG, et al. The *FHIT* gene, spanning the chromosome 3p14.2 fragile site and renal carcinoma-associated t(3;8) breakpoint, is abnormal in digestive tract cancers. Cell 84:587–597, 1996.

51. Baffa R, Veronese ML, Santoro R, et al. Loss of FHIT expression in gastric carcinoma, Cancer Res 58:4708–4714, 1998.

52. Chen YJ, Chen PH, Lee MD, Chang JG. Aberrant FHIT transcripts in cancerous and corresponding non-cancerous lesions of the digestive tract. Int J Cancer 17:955–958, 1997.

53. Tamura G, Sakata K, Nishizuka S, et al. Analysis of the fragile histidine triad gene in primary gastric carcinomas and gastric carcinoma cell lines. Genes Chromosomes Cancer 20:98–102, 1997.

54. Noguchi T, Muller W, Wirtz HC, Willers R, Gabbert HE. *FHIT* gene in gastric cancer: association with tumor progression and prognosis. J Pathol 188:378–381, 1999.

55. Ayhan A, Yasui W, Yokozaki H, et al. Loss of heterozygosity at the *bcl-2* gene locus and expression of *bcl-2* in human gastric and colorectal carcinomas. Jpn J Cancer Res 85:584–591, 1994.

56. Kuniyasu H, Yasui W, Yokozaki H, et al. Frequent loss of heterozygosity of the long arm of chromosome 7 is closely associated with progression of human gastric carcinomas. Int J Cancer 59:597–600, 1994.

57. Yustein AS, Harper JC, Petroni GR, et al. Allelotype of gastric adenocarcinoma. Cancer Res 59:1437–1441, 1999.

58. Fujimoto J, Yasui W, Tahara H, et al. DNA hypermethylation at the pS2 promoter region is associated with early stage of stomach carcinogenesis. Cancer Lett 149:125–134, 2000.

59. Oue N, Motoshita J, Yokozaki H, et al. Distinct promoter hypermethylation of p16INK4a, CDHI, and RAR-beta in intestinal, diffuse-adherent, and diffuse-scattered type gastric carcinoma. J Pathol 198:55–59, 2002.

60. Li QL, Ito K, Sakakura C, et al. Causal relationship between the loss of RUNX3 expression and gastric cancer. Cell 109:113–124, 2002.

61. Kuniyasu H, Yasui W, Kitadai Y, et al. Frequent amplification of the c-*met* gene in scirrhous-type stomach cancer. Biochem Biophys Res Commun 189:227–232, 1992.

62. Kuniyasu H, Yasui W, Yokozaki H, Kitadai Y, Tahara E. Aberrant expression of c-met mRNA in human gastric carcinomas. Int J Cancer 55:72–75, 1993.

63. Soman NR, Correa P, Ruiz BA, Wogan GN. The TPK-MET oncogenic rearrangement is present and expressed in human gastric carcinoma and precursor lesions. Proc Natl Acad Sci USA 88:4892–4896, 1991.

64. Katoh M, Hattori Y, Sasaki H, et al. K-*sam* gene encodes secreted as well as transmembrane receptor tyrosine kinase. Proc Natl Acad Sci USA 89:2960–2964, 1992.

65. Hattori Y, Odagiri H, Nakatani H, et al. K-*sam*, an amplified gene in stomach cancer, is a member of the heparin-binding growth factor receptor genes. Proc Natl Acad Sci USA 87:5983–5987, 1990.

66. Yokota J, Yamamoto T, Miyajima N, et al. Genetic alterations of the c-*erbB*-2 oncogene occur frequently in tubular adenocarcinoma of the stomach and are often accompanied by amplification of the v-erbA homologue. Oncogene 2:283–287, 1998.

67. Kameda T, Yasui W, Yoshida K, et al. Expression of ERBB2 in human gastric carcinomas: relationship between p185 ERBB2 expression and the gene amplification. Cancer Res 50:8002–8009, 1990.

68. Yonemura Y, Ninomiya I, Ohoyama S, et al. Expression of c-erbB-2 oncoprotein in gastric carcinoma: immunoreactivity for c-erbB-2 protein is an independent indicator of poor short-term prognosis in patients with gastric carcinoma. Cancer 67:2914–2918, 1991.

69. Oda N, Tsujino T, Tsuda T, et al. DNA ploidy pattern and amplification of ERBB and ERBB2 genes in human gastric carcinomas. Virchows Arch B Cell Pathol Incl Mol Pathol 58:273–277, 1990.

70. Katoh M, Terada M. Oncogenes and tumor suppressor genes. In: Nishi M, Ichikawa H, Nakajima T, Maruyama K, Tahara E (eds): Gastric Cancer. Springer-Verlag, Tokyo, 1993, pp 196–208.

71. Lee KH, Lee JS, Suh C, et al. Clinicopathologic significance of the K-*ras* gene codon 12 point mutation in stomach cancer: an analysis of 140 cases. Cancer 75:2794–2801, 1995.

72. Isogaki J, Shinmura K, Yin W, et al. Microsatellite instability and K-*ras* mutations in gastric adenomas, with reference to associated gastric cancers. Cancer Detect Prev 23:204–214, 1999.

73. Yoshida MC, Wada M, Satoh H, et al. Human HST1 (*HSTF1*) gene maps to chromosome band 11q13 and coamplifies with the *INT2* gene in human cancer. Proc Natl Acad Sci USA 85:4861–4864, 1988.

74. Akama Y, Yasui W, Yokozaki H, et al. Frequent amplification of the cyclin E gene in human gastric carcinomas. Jpn J Cancer Res 86:617–621, 1995.

75. Yoshida K, Yasui W, Kagawa Y, Tahara E. Multiple genetic alterations and abnormal growth factor network in human esophageal carcinomas. In Tahara E (eds): Molecular Pathology of Gastroenterological Cancer. Application to Clinical Practice. Springer-Verlag, Tokyo, 1996, pp 31–41.

76. Honda R, Ohba Y, Nagata A, Okayama H, Yasuda H. Dephosphorylation of human p34cdc2 kinase on both Thr-14 and Tyr-15 by human cdc25B phosphatase. FEBS Lett 318:331–334, 1993.

77. Nagata A, Igarashi M, Jinno S, Suto K, Okayama H. An additional homolog of the fission yeast cdc25+ gene occurs in human and is highly expressed in some cancer cells. New Biol 3:959–968, 1991.

78. Jinno S, Suto K, Nagata A, et al. Cdc25A is a novel phosphatase functioning early in the cell cycle. EMBO J 13:1549–1556, 1994.

79. Kudo Y, Yasui W, Ue T, et al. Overexpression of cyclin-dependent kinase-activating CDC25B phosphatase in human gastric carcinomas. Jpn J Cancer Res 88:947–952, 1997.

80. Hadwiger JA, Wittenberg C, Mendenhall MD, Reed SI. The *Saccharomyces cerevisiae CKS1* gene, a homolog of the *Schizosaccharomyces pombe SUC1*+ gene, encodes a subunit of the Cdc28 protein kinase complex. Mol Cell Biol 9:2034–2041, 1989.

81. Richardson HE, Stueland CS, Thomas J, Russell P, Reed SI. Human cDNAs encoding homologs of the small p34cdc28/cdc2-associated protein of *Saccharomyces cerevisiae* and *Schizosaccharomyces pombe*. Genes Dev 4:1332–1334, 1990.

82. Kudo Y, Yasui W, Akama Y, et al. Expression of a cell cycle regulator CKshs1 in human gastrointestinal carcinomas. In: Tahara E, Sugimachi K, Oohara T (eds): Recent Advances in Gastroenterological Carcinogenesis I. Monduzzi Editore, Bologna, 1996, pp 755–759.

83. Harper JW, Adami GR, Wei N, Keyomarsi K, Elledge SJ. The p21 Cdk-interacting protein Cip1 is a potent inhibitor of G1 cyclin-dependent kinases. Cell 75:805–816, 1993.

84. Yasui W, Akama Y, Kuniyasu H, et al. Expression of cyclin-dependent kinase inhibitor p21WAF1/CIP1 in non-neoplastic mucosa and neoplasia of the stomach: relation with p53 status and proliferative activity. J Pathol 180:122–128, 1996.

85. Akagi M, Yasui W, Akama Y, et al. Inhibition of cell growth by transforming growth factor beta1 is associated with p53-independent induction of p21 in gastric cells. Jpn J Cancer Res 87:377–384, 1996.

86. Akama Y, Yasui W, Kuniyasu H, et al. Genetic status and expression of the cyclin-dependent kinase inhibitors in human gastric carcinoma cell lines. Jpn J Cancer Res 87:824–830, 1996.

87. Akama Y, Yasui W, Kuniyasu H, et al. No point mutations but a codon 31 polymorphism and decreased expression of the *p21 SDI1/WAF1/CIP1/MDA6* gene in human gastric carcinomas. Mol Cell Differ 4:187–198, 1996.

88. Kuniyasu H, Yasui W, Kitahara K, et al. Growth inhibitory effect of interferon-β is associated with the induction of cyclin-dependent kinase inhibitor p27 Kip1 in a human gastric carcinoma cell line. Cell Growth Differ 8:47–52, 1997.

89. Yasui W, Kudo Y, Semba S, Yokozaki H, Tahara E: Reduced expression of cyclin-dependent kinase inhibitor p27Kip1 is associated with advanced stage and invasiveness of gastric carcinomas. Jpn J Cancer Res 88:625–629, 1997.

90. Yasui W, Naka K, Suzuki T, et al. Expression of p27Kip1, cyclin E, and E2F-1 in primary and metastatic tumors of gastric carcinoma. Oncol Rep 6:983–987, 1999.

91. Igaki H, Sasaki H, Tachimori Y, et al. Mutation frequency of the *p16/CDKN2* gene in primary cancers in the upper digestive tract. Cancer Res 55:3421–3423, 1995.

92. Gunther T, Schneider-Stock R, et al. Alterations of the *p16/MTS1*-tumor suppressor gene in gastric cancer. Pathol Res Pract 194:809–813, 1998.

93. Lee YY, Kang SH, Seo JY, et al. Alterations of *p16INK4A* and *p15INK4B* genes in gastric carcinomas. Cancer 80:1889–1896, 1997.

94. Akama Y, Yasui W, Kuniyasu H, et al. Genetic status and expression of the cyclin-dependent kinase inhibitors in human gastric carcinoma cell lines. Jpn J Cancer Res 87:824–830, 1996.

95. Merlo A, Herman JG, Lee DJ, et al. 5′CpG island methylation is associated with transcriptional silencing of the tumor suppressor *p16/CDKN2/MTS1* in human cancers. Nat Med 1:686–692, 1995.

96. Chen YJ, Chang G, Shih LS, et al. Frequent detection of aberrant RNA transcripts of the *CDKN2* gene in human gastric adenocarcinoma. Int J Cancer 71:350–354, 1997.

97. Constancia M, Seruca R, Carneiro F, Silva F, Castedo S. Retinoblastoma gene structure and product expression in human gastric carcinomas. Br J Cancer 71:1122, 1995.

98. Suzuki T, Yasui W, Yokozaki H, et al. Expression of the E2F family in human gastrointestinal carcinomas. Int J Cancer 81:535–538, 1999.

99. Tahara E, Yasui W, Yokozaki H: Abnormal growth factor networks in neoplasia. In: Pusztai L, Lewis CE, Yap E (eds): Cell Proliferation in Cancer. Oxford University Press, Oxford, 1996, pp 131–153.

100. Tahara E. Cell growth regulation and cancer: stromal interaction. In: Sugimura T, Sasako M (eds): Gastric Cancer. Oxford University Press, New York. 1997, pp 100–108.

101. Tahara E, Yokozaki H, Yasui W. Stomach–genetic and epigenetic alterations of preneoplastic and neoplastic lesions. In: Srivastava S, Henson DE, Gazdar A (eds): Molecular Pathology of Early Cancer. IOS Press, Amsterdam, 1999, pp 341–361.

102. Yoshida K, Tsujino T, Yasui W, et al. Induction of growth factor-receptor and metalloproteinase genes by epidermal growth factor and/or transforming growth factor-β in human gastric carcinoma cell lines MKN-28. Jpn J Cancer Res 81:793–798, 1990.

103. Yasui W, Hata J, Yokozaki H, et al. Interaction between epidermal growth factor and its receptor in progression of human gastric carcinoma. Int J Cancer 41:211–217, 1988.

104. Kuniyasu H, Yasui W, Akama Y, et al. Expression of cripto in human gastric carcinomas: an association with tumor stage and prognosis. J Exp Clin Cancer Res 13:151–157, 1994.

105. Kuniyasu H, Yoshida K, Yokozaki H, et al. Expression of cripto, a novel gene of the epidermal growth factor family, in human gastrointestinal carcinomas. Jpn J Cancer Res 82:969–973, 1991.

106. Kitadai Y, Yasui W, Yokozaki H, et al. Expression of amphiregulin, a novel gene of the epidermal growth factor family, in human gastric carcinomas. Jpn J Cancer Res 84:879–884, 1993.

107. Akagi M, Yokozaki H, Kitadai Y, et al. Expression of amphiregulin in human gastric cancer cell lines. Cancer 75:1460–1466, 1995.

108. Kitadai Y, Yamazaki H, Yasui W, et al. GC factor represses transcription of several growth factor/receptor genes and causes growth inhibition of human gastric carcinoma cell lines. Cell Growth Differ 4: 291–296, 1993.

109. Dinarello CA: Biology of interleukin 1. FASEB J 2:108–115, 1988.

110. Ito R, Kitadai Y, Kyo E, et al. Interleukin 1α acts as autocrine growth stimulator for human gastric carcinoma cells. Cancer Res 53:4102–4106, 1993.

111. Ito R, Yasui W, Kuniyasu H, Yokozaki H, Tahara E: Expression of interleukin-6 and its effect on the cell growth of gastric carcinoma cell lines. Jpn J Cancer Res 88:953–958, 1997.

112. Yoshida K, Yokozaki H, Niimoto M, et al. Expression of TGF-beta and procollagen type I and type III in human gastric carcinomas. Int J Cancer 44:394–398, 1989.

113. Ito M, Yasui W, Kyo E, et al. Growth inhibition of transforming growth factor-beta on human gastric carcinoma cells: receptor and postreceptor signaling. Cancer Res 52:295–300, 1992.

114. Akagi M, Yasui W, Akama Y, et al. Inhibition of cell growth by transforming growth factor beta1 is associated with p53-independent induction of p21 in gastric carcinoma cells. Jpn J Cancer Res 87:377–384, 1996.

115. Markowitz S, Wang J, Myeroff L, et al. Inactivation of the type II TGF-β receptor in colon cancer cells with microsatellite instability. Science 268:1336–1338, 1995.

116. Yang HK, Kang SH, Kim YS, et al. Truncation of the TGF-beta type II receptor gene results in insensitivity to TGF-beta in human gastric cancer cells. Oncogene 18:2213–2219, 1999.

117. Kim SJ, Yang HK, Im YH, Bang YJ, Yang HK. Mechanisms of TGF-β receptor inactivation and development of resistance to TGF-beta in human gastric cancer. In: Proceedings of the Third International Gastric Cancer Congress, Seoul. Monduzzi Editore, Bologna, 1999, pp 81–90.

118. Ito M, Yasui W, Nakayama H, et al. Reduced levels of transforming growth factor-beta type I receptor in human gastric carcinomas. Jpn J Cancer Res 83:86–92, 1992.

119. Ito Y, Ito K, Bae SC, et al. Hyperplasia of stomach epithelial cells of mice lacking PEBP2αC: possible relation of the gene to human stomach cancer. Proceedings of the 58th Annual Meeting of the Japanese Cancer Association, Hiroshima. Jpn J Cancer Res 90 (Suppl):64, 1999.

120. Shitara Y, Yokozaki H, Yasui W, et al. No mutations of the Smad2 gene in human sporadic gastric carcinomas. Jpn J Clin Oncol 29:3–7, 1999.

121. Yamamoto S, Yasui W, Kitadai Y, et al. Expression of vascular endothelial growth factor in human gastric carcinomas. Pathol Int 48:499–506, 1998.

122. Takahashi Y, Cleary KR, Mai M, Kitadai Y, Bucana CD, Ellis LM. Significance of vessel count and vascular endothelial growth factor and its receptor (KDR) in intestinal-type gastric cancer. Clin Cancer Res 2: 1679–1684, 1996.

123. Tanimoto H, Yoshida K, Yokozaki H, et al. Expression of basic fibroblast growth factor in human gastric carcinomas. Virchows Arch B Cell Pathol Incl Mol Pathol 61:263–267, 1991.

124. Kitadai Y, Haruma K, Sumii K, et al. Expression of interleukin-8 correlates with vascularity in human gastric carcinomas. Am J Pathol 152: 93–100, 1998.

125. Kitadai Y, Haruma K, Mukaida N, et al. Regulation of disease-progression genes in human gastric carcinoma cells by endogenous interleukin-8. Clin Cancer Res 6:2735–2740, 2000.

126. Becker KF, Atkinson MJ, Reich U, et al. E-cadherin gene mutations provide clues to diffuse type gastric carcinomas. Cancer Res 54:3845–3852, 1994.

127. Machado JC, Soares P, Carneiro F, et al. E-cadherin gene mutations provide a genetic basis for the phenotypic divergence of mixed gastric carcinomas. Lab Invest 79:459–465, 1999.

128. Handschuh G, Candidus S, Luber B, et al. Tumour-associated E-cadherin mutations alter cellular morphology, decrease cellular adhesion and increase cellular motility. Oncogene 18:4301–4312, 1999.

129. Muta H, Noguchi M, Kanai Y, et al. E-cadherin gene mutations in signet ring cell carcinoma of the stomach. Jpn J Cancer Res 87: 843–848, 1996.

130. Keller G, Vogelsang H, Becker I, et al. Diffuse type gastric and lobular breast carcinoma in a familial gastric cancer patient with an E-cadherin germline mutation. Am J Pathol 155:337–342, 1999.

131. Guilford P, Hopkins J, Harraway J, et al. E-cadherin germline mutations in familial gastric cancer. Nature 392:402–405, 1998.

132. Iida S, Akiyama Y, Ichikawa W, et al. Infrequent germ-line mutation of the E-cadherin gene in Japanese familial gastric cancer kindreds. Clin Cancer Res 5:1445–1447, 1999.

133. Yoon KA, Ku JL, Yang HK, et al. Germline mutations of E-cadherin gene in Korean familial gastric cancer patients. J Hum Genet 44:177–180, 1999.

134. Kawanishi J, Kato J, Sasaki K, et al. Loss of E-cadherin–dependent cell–cell adhesion due to mutation of the beta-catenin gene in a human cancer cell line, HSC-39. Mol Cell Biol 15:1175–1181, 1995.

135. Caca K, Kolligs FT, Ji X, et al. Beta- and gamma-catenin mutations, but not E-cadherin inactivation, underlie T-cell factor/lymphoid enhancer factor transcriptional deregulation in gastric and pancreatic cancer. Cell Growth Differ 10:369–376, 1999.

136. Ochiai A, Akimoto S, Kanai Y, et al. c-erbB-2 gene product associates with catenins in human cancer cells. Biochem Biophys Res Commun 205:73–78, 1994.

137. Shibata T, Ochiai A, Kanai Y, et al. Dominant negative inhibition of the association between beta-catein and c-erbB-2 by N-terminally deleted beta-catenin suppresses the invasion and metastasis of cancer cells. Oncogene 13:883–889, 1996.

138. Cooper DL, Dougherty G, Harn HJ, et al. The complex CD44 transcriptional unit; alternative splicing of three internal exons generates the epithelial form of CD44. Biochem Biophys Res Commun 182: 569–578, 1992.

139. Matsumura Y, Tarin D. Significance of CD44 gene products for cancer diagnosis and disease evaluation. Lancet 340:1053–1058, 1992.

140. Yokozaki H, Ito R, Nakayama H, Kuniyasu H, Taniyama K, Tahara E. Expression of CD44 abnormal transcripts in human gastric carcinomas. Cancer Lett 83:229–234, 1994.

141. Higashikawa K, Yokozaki H, Ue T, et al. Evaluation of CD44 transcription variants in human digestive tract carcinomas and normal tissues. Int J Cancer 66:11–17, 1996.

142. Yoshida K, Bolodeoku J, Sugino T, et al. Abnormal retention of intron 9 in CD44 gene transcripts in human gastrointestinal tumors. Cancer Res 55:4273–4277, 1995.

143. Weber GF, Ashkar S, Glimcher MJ, Cantor H. Receptor–ligand interaction between CD44 and osteopontin (Eta-1). Science 271:509–512, 1996.

144. Une T, Yokozaki H, Kitadai Y, et al. Co-expression of osteopontin and CD44v9 in gastric cancer. Int J Cancer 79:127–132, 1998.

145. Nakayama H, Yasui W, Yokozaki H, Tahara E. Reduced expression of nm23 is associated with metastasis of human gastric carcinomas. Jpn J Cancer Res 84:184–190, 1993.

146. Lotan R, Ito H, Yasui W, et al. Expression of a 31-kDa lactoside-binding lectin in normal human gastric mucosa and in primary and metastatic gastric carcinomas. Int J Cancer 56:474–480, 1994.

147. Kuniyasu H, Yasui W, Yokozaki H, et al. Frequent loss of heterozygosity of the long arm of chromosome 7 is closely associated with progression of human gastric carcinomas. Int J Cancer 59:597–600, 1994.

148. Reis CA, David L, Correa P, et al. Intestinal metaplasia of human stomach displays distinct patterns of mucin (*MUC1, MUC2, MUC5AC,* and *MUC6*) expression. Cancer Res 59:1003–1007, 1999.

149. Reis CA, David L, Seixas M, Burchell J, Simoes MS. Expression of fully and under-glycosylated forms of *MUC1* mucin in gastric carcinoma. Int J Cancer 79:402–410, 1998.

150. Carvalho F, Seruca R, David L, et al. *MUC1* gene polymorphism and gastric cancer: an epidemiological study. Glycoconj J 14:107–111, 1997.

# Chapter 23

# Pathology and Natural History of Gastric Cancer

## CECILIA FENOGLIO-PREISER, AMY NOFFSINGER, AND GRANT STEMMERMANN

Gastric carcinoma is one of the most common cancers. Annually there are approximately 800,000 new cases of gastric carcinoma and an estimated 650,000 deaths worldwide from this disease. More than 50% of these cancers arise in individuals living in developing countries. The disease is less common in the United States than in other parts of the world. The majority of cancers that develop in the stomach are carcinomas. Their pathologic features will be covered in this chapter. Other primary cancers arising in the stomach include lymphomas, neuroendocrine tumors, and stromal tumors. Other tumors can involve the stomach secondarily, either through direct extension or by metastasis. Metastatic tumors will be covered briefly at the end of this chapter.

The pathologic features of gastric carcinoma are complex, and the natural history varies considerably, depending on the country of origin and the association with specific risk factors. Gastric carcinoma is not a single disease. It can be divided into several types based on either its site of origin in the stomach or its predominant histologic patterns. By site of origin in the stomach, gastric carcinomas are divisible into cardiac (or those involving the gastroesophageal junction) and corporal or antral tumors. Differentiated by their histological features, these carcinomas often are divided into intestinal or diffuse tumors. (The histological features are discussed extensively below.) The intestinal type of gastric carcinoma is predominant in countries with a high risk of developing the disease, whereas the diffuse type is relatively more common in low-risk areas.[1] Intestinal-type tumors account for almost two-thirds of the gastric carcinomas developing in the high-risk areas of northeast Asia, Central America, and Eastern Europe.

## Precursor Lesions and Conditions

As with carcinomas arising elsewhere in the body, gastric carcinomas do not simply emerge from a normal mucosa. Instead, they evolve slowly over a period of time. The antecedent lesions of gastric carcinoma are best understood in intestinal-type carcinomas. Precursor lesions of diffuse gastric cancers are less well understood.

### Precursors of Intestinal-type Gastric Carcinomas

Strong epidemiological evidence links the development of gastric cancer to two environmental influences: diet, and infection with *Helicobacter pylori* (*H. pylori*) (see Chapter 21). Both of these influences lead to the development of chronic gastritis with intestinal metaplasia.

### Multifocal, Environmental Chronic Gastritis

The sequential, multifactorial steps involved in the development of intestinal-type carcinomas have been well studied, largely because of the pioneering work of Correa and colleagues.[2–4] He and others have shown that chronic gastritis results from the combined effects of *H. pylori* infection and a diet high in salt and nitrate and low in antioxidant-containing fresh fruits and vegetables. *H. pylori* infection is the most common cause of chronic gastritis. The bacteria populate the superficial mucosa, adhering to surface foveolar cells and lying in the mucus layer on top of the epithelium. Strains of *H. pylori* are not equally pathogenic. Bacteria containing *cagA* genes cause more epithelial damage than do bacteria lacking these genes. Some *H. pylori* strains also produce a vacuolating cytotoxin named Vac A that causes epithelial damage. An association exists between infection with *cagA*- and Vac A–positive *H. pylori* strains and the development of gastric carcinoma.[5,6]

The pathogenic bacteria damage the gastric epithelium, not on the surface of the mucosa where the bacteria are located, but in the area of the mucous neck and in the gastric glands. *H. pylori* generate a brisk inflammatory response as the replicating cells are invaded by neutrophils and monocytes that generate oxygen free-radicals and the toxic molecule nitric oxide (NO).[7] These free radicals and reactive nitrogen molecules can damage cellular DNA and generate point mutations in genes critical to cell replication and cell death.

Histologically, chronic active gastritis can be diagnosed when both the neutrophils and the mononuclear cells infiltrate the mucosa. The features of chronic antral gastritis consist of an infiltration of the glands by neutrophils, epithelial cell loss, and a compensatory expansion of the replication zone. The surrounding lamina propria contains numerous plasma cells and lymphocytes. The expansion of the replication zone is evident histologically by the presence of an increased number of mitotic figures in the mucous neck region, and it can be highlighted by the increased expression of the proliferation marker Ki-67.

The local production of toxic molecules in the vicinity of the replicating epithelium increases the vulnerability of the latter to DNA damage that may become fixed in the replicating cell populations. With increasing injury, the mucosa becomes atrophic. Simultaneously, the gastric mucosa undergoes a metaplastic process, characterized by replacement of the gastric epithelium with cells that histologically resemble intestinal epithelial cells. The sequential steps in the development of intestinal-type gastric carcinomas are as follows: chronic gastritis, multifocal atrophy, intestinal metaplasia, dysplasia, and carcinoma (Fig. 23–1). In high-risk populations, the process begins in the second and third decades of life. Over time, mucosal atrophy extends from the antral region into the fundus. By the sixth and seventh decades of life, the resulting loss of the acid-secreting cells in the stomach causes an increase in intraluminal gastric pH, thereby allowing anaerobic bacteria that can produce carcinogenic *N*-nitroso compounds to grow.[8,9] This contributes further to the gastric injury, facilitating gastric carcinoma development and progression.

## Autoimmune Gastritis

Autoimmune gastritis also is a precursor to both benign and malignant gastric neoplasias. Less common than multifocal gastritis, autoimmune gastritis develops when patients generate antibodies against their own parietal cells. The major target of the antibodies is the $Na^+$, $K^+$-ATPase pump present in the membranes of the parietal cells.[10] The antibodies destroy cells present in the oxyntic mucosa. Concomitantly, chronic inflammatory cells infiltrate the lamina propria. Because the primary immunological attack is on the oxyntic mucosa, parietal cells are lost early in the disease, allowing hypochlorhydria to develop earlier than in multifocal chronic gastritis. As in multifocal gastritis, the loss of gastric epithelial cells leads to an expansion of the gastric replication zone. Cell loss occurs at a faster pace than does cellular replication, causing the mucosa to atrophy. Also, as in multifocal chronic gastritis, the reacting inflammatory cells can generate endogenous mutagens, causing further damage. The hypochlorhydria predisposes the stomach to an altered bacterial flora, which can generate potential carcinogens from dietary amines. The hypochlorhydria also results in hypergastrinemia with a secondary stimulation of gastric mucosal growth. The increased gastric cancer risk results from the combined effects of several concomitant events. *(1)* The hypochlorhydria allows the emergence of a bacterial flora that can generate potentially carcinogenic compounds from dietary amines. *(2)* The inflammation that develops generates additional potentially carcinogenic compounds. *(3)* Increased cell proliferation increases the number of cells susceptible to accumulating DNA damage. *(4)* The hypergastrinemia stimulates mucosal growth.

## Intestinal Metaplasia

Intestinal metaplasia commonly precedes or accompanies intestinal-type gastric carcinoma, particularly in high-incidence areas. The metaplasia develops against a background of both multifocal chronic gastritis and autoimmune gastritis. The intestinal metaplasia begins to develop concomitantly with the gastric mucosal atrophy. Intestinal metaplasia can be divided into two main types: complete (also designated small intestinal type or type I) and incomplete (also designated colonic intestinal metaplasia or types II and III).[11] Complete intestinal metaplasia resembles small intestinal epithelium. The glands of complete intestinal metaplasia are lined by absorptive cells with well-formed micro-

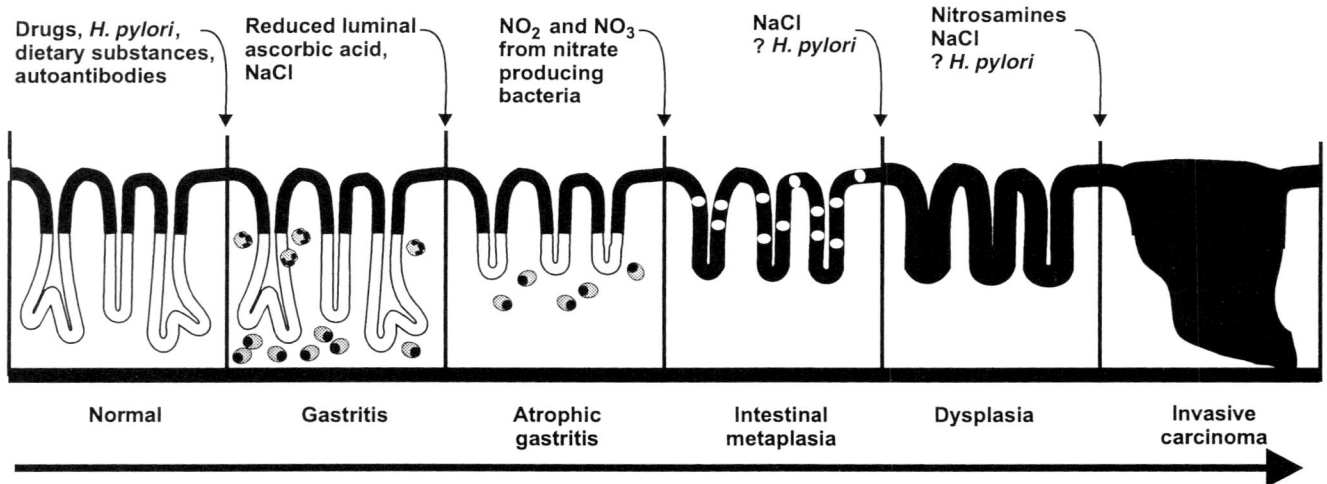

Normal | Gastritis | Atrophic gastritis | Intestinal metaplasia | Dysplasia | Invasive carcinoma

**Figure 23–1** Diagrammatic representation of progressive steps that eventually culminate in development of intestinal-type gastric cancer.

villi, goblet cells, and sometimes Paneth's cells. The Paneth cells and brush border enzymes found in the microvillous border of complete intestinal metaplasia are absent in incomplete metaplasia. The glands in incomplete metaplasia are lined by goblet cells with intervening immature mucous cells that have short, blunted microvilli. Additionally, the mucin expression patterns differ between the two types of metaplasia. Goblet cells in complete intestinal metaplasia produce sialomucins and show decreased expression of "gastric" (MUC1, MUC5AC, and MUC6) mucins and expression of MUC2, an intestinal mucin. The goblet cells in incomplete intestinal metaplasia predominantly produce sulfomucins, and the cells coexpress gastric mucins, with MUC2 mucin reflecting an aberrant differentiation program that does not reproduce any normal adult gastrointestinal epithelial phenotype.[12] More important than the type of metaplasia present is its extent for subsequent cancer risk. Most gastric carcinomas arise in areas of incomplete intestinal metaplasia.

## Dysplasia

*Dysplasia* can be defined as neoplastic epithelium that is not invasive but combines an abnormal architecture, abnormal differentiation, and cytological atypia. Dysplasias arise in either the native gastric epithelium or in areas of intestinal metaplasia. The phenotype of dysplasias arising in intestinalized mucosa is extensively described; the morphology of dysplasia originating in the native (non-intestinalized) stomach is less well established. In the multistage theory of gastric oncogenesis, dysplasia lies between atrophic metaplastic lesions and invasive cancer (Fig. 23–1).

Dysplasia has been graded as mild, moderate, and severe. Currently, consistent with dysplasia arising in other gastrointestinal locations, a three-tier scale (indefinite for dysplasia, low-grade dysplasia, and high-grade dysplasia) is being proposed for gastric lesions (Table 23–1).[13]

Problems associated with diagnosing gastric epithelial dysplasia include *(1)* the distinction between true dysplasia and the reactive or regenerative changes associated with active inflammation of the gastric mucosa, and *(2)* the distinction between dysplasia and truly invasive cancer.[14,15]

### Indefinite for dysplasia

Sometimes doubts arise as to whether a lesion is neoplastic (dysplasia) or non-neoplastic (reactive or regenerative), particularly in small biopsies. Occasionally, reactive regenerating epithelium can be extremely alarming in appearance because of the prominent nuclei and the loss of mucin. In such instances, the diagnostic dilemma is usually resolved by cutting deeper levels of the block, performing Ki-67 immunostains, or obtaining additional biopsies after possible sources of cellular hyperproliferation have been removed. Cases lacking all the attributes required for a definitive diagnosis of dysplasia may be placed into the category "indefinite for dysplasia." In areas of intestinal metaplasia, cells diagnosable as indefinite for dysplasia appear hyperproliferative. The glands may appear closely packed and lined by cells with large,

hyperchromatic, rounded, or especially elongated, basally located nuclei. Nucleoli may be present. It is important to note that the nuclei maintain their normal polarity. Mucin secretions typically are decreased in these areas. The cytological alterations tend to decrease from the base of the glands to their superficial portion. This "maturation gradient" helps distinguish areas of true dysplasia from areas indefinite for dysplasia.

### Low-grade dysplasia

This type of dysplasia has flat, polypoid, and slightly depressed growth patterns. The flat pattern may lack any visible endoscopic or gross changes unless special dyes are used to highlight their presence. This approach is used regularly in Japan during a procedure called dye endoscopy. With this technique, lesions that were previously invisible appear as mucosal irregularities. The term *adenoma* is applied when the proliferation produces a macroscopic, discrete, often protruding lesion. Adenomas also may be flat (Fig. 23–2) or depressed, and they tend to arise in the antrum or mid-stomach in areas of intestinal metaplasia. Overall, adenomas account for approximately 10% of gastric polyps.[16] They are divided into three histological subtypes: tubular, villous, and tubulovillous.

Low-grade dysplasia shows a slightly modified mucosal architecture. Architectural abnormalities include the presence of tubules with budding and branching, papillary infolding, crypt lengthening with serration, and cystic changes (Fig. 23–3). Dysplastic glands are lined by enlarged columnar cells with minimal or no mucin. The homogeneously blue vesicular, rounded, or ovoid nuclei are usually pseudostratified. Cellular atypia and mitoses are confined to the proliferative zone.[17]

### High-grade dysplasia

In contrast to low-grade dysplasia, the high-grade form shows increasing architectural distortion with glandular crowding; cellular atypia is prominent (Fig. 23–4). Tubules are irregular in shape, with frequent branching and folding; no stromal invasion is found. No secretions, or only occasional secretions, are present. The pleomorphic, hyperchromatic, usually pseudostratified nuclei have a typical cigar-shaped appearance. Prominent amphophilic nucleoli are common. Increased proliferative activity is present throughout the dysplasia.[17]

**Table 23–1** Classification of dysplasia

Negative for dysplasia
Indefinite for dysplasia
Dysplasia
    Low-grade
    High-grade

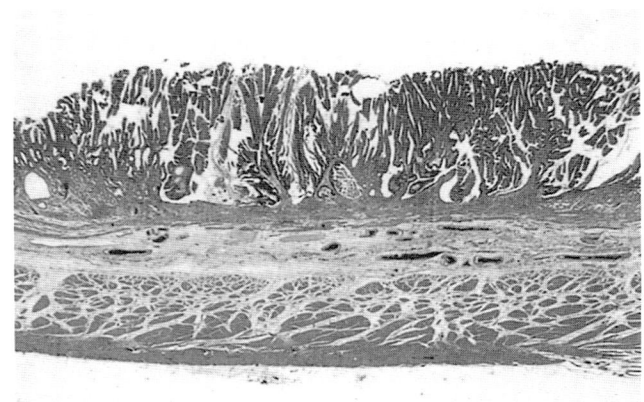

**Figure 23–2** Flat adenoma. The surface of the stomach is replaced by a large patch of adenomatous epithelium that has a tubulovillous configuration. A small amount of residual normal nonadenomatous mucosa is seen at the very left edge of the photograph. The adenoma is slightly elevated above the normal mucosal height.

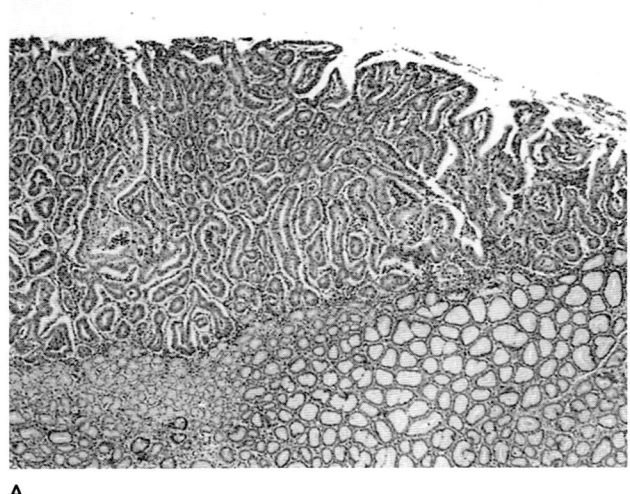

A

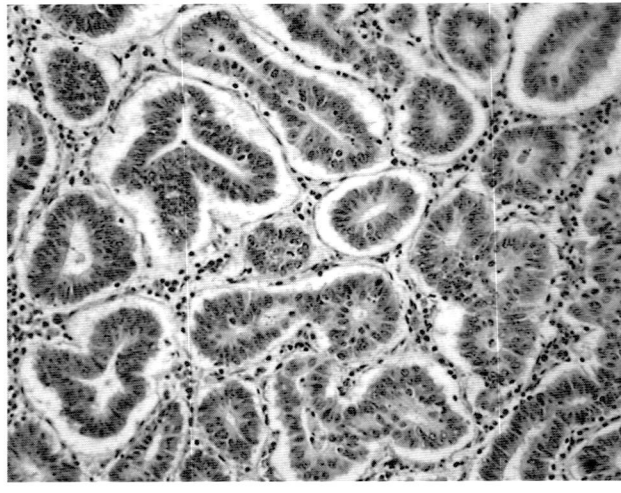

B

**Figure 23–3** Low-grade dysplasia. *A:* Low magnification showing the presence of a large area of dysplastic tubules. *B:* Higher magnification showing the irregular branching of the glands. Individual glands are lined by columnar cells that are mucin depleted and have an increased nuclear/cytoplasmic ratio.

## Invasive carcinoma

Invasive carcinoma is diagnosed when the tumor invades through the basement membrane and into the surrounding lamina propria. Some gastric biopsies contain areas suggestive of true invasion (such as isolated cells or gland-like structures or papillary projections). The diagnosis "suspicious for invasive cancer" is appropriate when the histological picture does not quite fulfill the criteria for an invasive malignancy.[17]

Areas of dysplasia may progress to invasive carcinoma. The extent of the intestinal metaplasia surrounding the dysplastic foci and a sulfomucin phenotype of the epithelium correlate with an increased risk of carcinoma development. In adenomas, the frequency of malignant transformation depends on lesion size and dysplasia grade. Invasive cancer develops in approximately 2% of lesions measuring less than 2 cm and in 40%–50% of lesions greater than 2 cm. Flat adenomas have a greater tendency to contain high-grade dysplasia and to evolve into invasive cancers than do pedunculated adenomas, especially when they are small.[17]

### Hyperplastic polyps

These are one of the most common gastric polyps. They are small (usually less than 2 cm), sessile, or pedunculated lesions arising against a background of *H. pylori*–associated gastritis. Hyperplastic polyps contain a proliferation of surface foveolar cells lining elongated, distorted pits extending deep into the stroma. The surface often erodes. Cancer develops in a minority of hyperplastic polyps, arising in areas of intestinal metaplasia and dysplasia.

### Fundic gland polyps

These may occur sporadically, or they develop in patients with familial adenomatous polyposis coli (APC). These generally are thought to be innocuous lesions, but recently dysplasia and carcinoma have been described in such lesions in a patient with APC.[18]

### Gastric peptic ulcer disease

This disease is related to the subsequent development of gastric neoplasia in two ways. The first is that gastric ulcers typically arise against a background of chronic gastritis, which in itself increases the risk of neoplastic transformation. Moreover, in the past, gastric peptic ulcer disease was treated with antrectomy and vagotomy with anastomosis of the remaining stomach to the small bowel. This procedure predisposed the patient to the development of reflux gastritis, a condition resembling the chronic gastritis associated with *H. pylori* infection and autoimmune gastritis. The gastric cancer risk begins to rise approximately two decades after the gastric surgery. The younger the patient at the time of the gastric surgery, the greater the risk of ultimately developing gastric carcinoma.

### Radiation

Sometimes the stomach is included in the radiation field of patients with abdominal cancers or in young people with lymphomas.

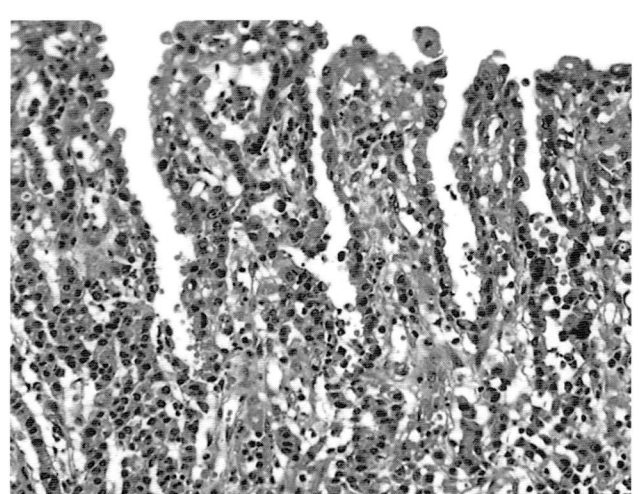

**Figure 23–4** High-grade dysplasia. The glands are irregular in shape and are lined by poorly differentiated cells with high nuclear/cytoplasmic ratios. The cells show loss of polarity and, in some places, glandular crowding.

Some of these patients develop gastric carcinomas decades later, usually as the result of radiation-induced DNA mutations in the gastric mucosa.

## Precursors of Diffuse-type Gastric Carcinomas

Diffuse gastric carcinomas have no well-defined precursor lesion. These tumors usually arise against a background of *H. pylori*–associated chronic superficial gastritis, usually without any evidence of intestinal metaplasia or gastritis. Some diffuse gastric carcinomas have no antecedent histological abnormalities. Some are related to alterations in the foveolar epithelium. The foveolar changes are sometimes referred to as foveolar or "globoid" dysplasia, although the reproducibility of this diagnosis is poor and not all individuals accept this as a diagnostic entity.

## Early Gastric Cancer

Early gastric carcinoma is a carcinoma that remains limited to the mucosa or to the mucosa and submucosa regardless of whether the lymph nodes contain metastatic tumor.[19] Most histological subtypes of gastric carcinoma occur in early gastric carcinoma, in either pure or mixed forms. Elevated cancers with papillary, granular, or nodular-like patterns and a red color are more often moderately to well-differentiated, tubular or papillary tumors with intestinal features; sometimes a preexisting adenoma

is recognizable. Flat early gastric carcinomas surrounded by flat non-neoplastic mucosal islands tend to be poorly differentiated or signet ring carcinomas of the diffuse type. Ulcerated lesions are either intestinal or diffuse cancers.

## Gross Appearance of Gastric Neoplasia

The gross appearances of early gastric cancers are shown in Figure 23–5. The gross features of early gastric cancer are classified into type I, type II (IIa, IIb, Iic), type III, and a combination of IIa+IIc+III,[20] based on the height of the lesion. Elevated, type I early cancers are most likely to occur in the antrum of older male patients with diffuse intestinal metaplasia of the stomach. Flat or ulcerated types II and III early tumors are more likely to occur in younger patients and may arise in the mucosa at the junction of the antrum and corpus of a stomach showing minimal or no intestinal metaplasia.

Advanced gastric carcinomas can develop anywhere in the stomach. In countries without screening programs for this cancer, these tumors are often quite large when diagnosed. The majority arise in the antrum. Advanced gastric cancers may exhibit an exophytic or infiltrative growth pattern that can be modified by surface ulceration.[21] Figure 23–6 shows a Borrmann type I gastric carcinoma. Ulcerating types II or III (Fig. 23–7) are common. Diffuse (infiltrative) tumors (type IV) spread superficially in the mucosa and submucosa, producing flat, plaque-like lesions,

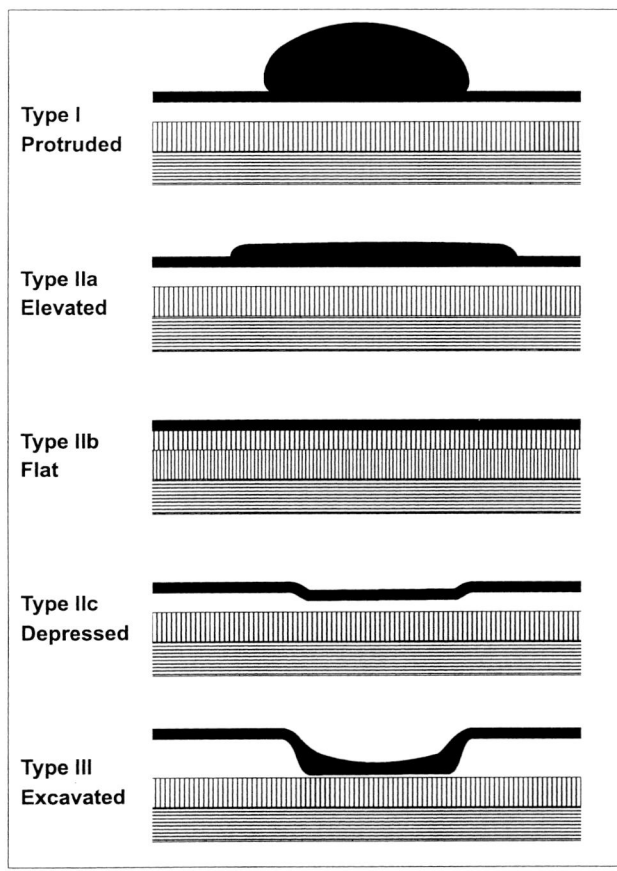

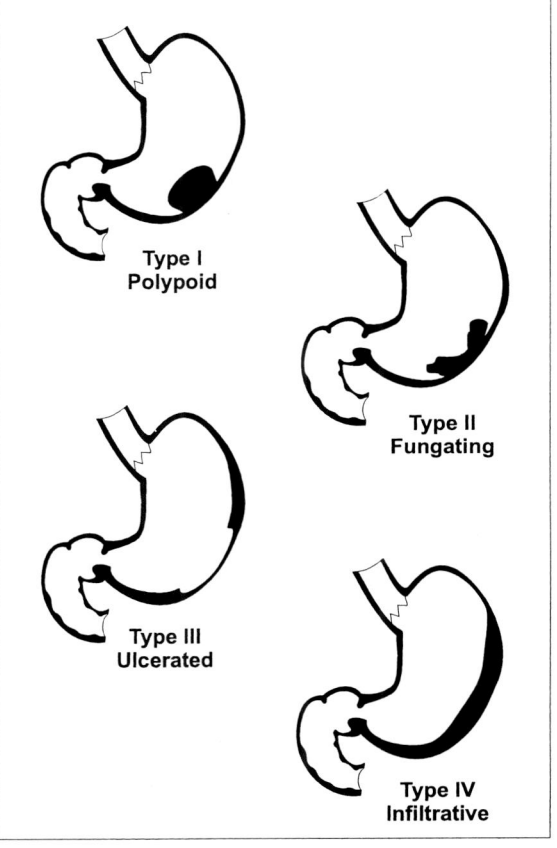

A

B

**Figure 23–5** Diagrammatic representation of the gross appearance of both early and advanced gastric cancers. *A:* Classification according to height of lesion. *B:* Location and shape of types I–IV gastric tumors.

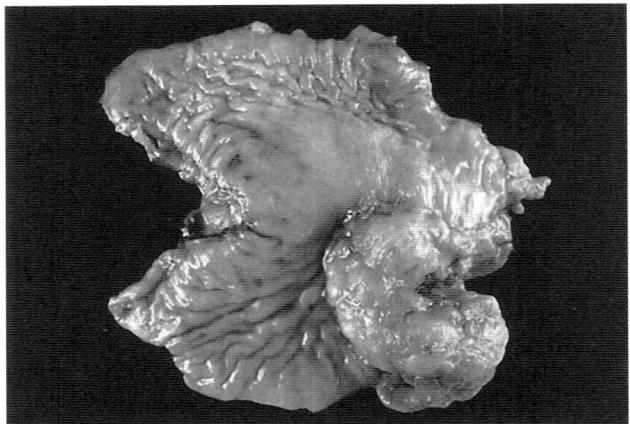

**Figure 23–6** Borrmann type I gastric cancer (polypoid type).

cer. Intestinal-type cancers preferentially arise in older patients in the antrum, usually in association with intestinal metaplasia. These cancers are believed to be related to environmental factors, especially *H. pylori* infection. Most stomach cancers arising in high-risk areas are intestinal. In contrast, diffuse cancers tend to occur in younger individuals, more commonly in the gastric body and not in association with intestinal metaplasia. Some patients with diffuse gastric cancer may have an underlying genetic predisposition to the tumor.[23]

Histologically, the Laurén classification system is based on the observation that many stomach cancers form rudimentary glands that superficially resemble intestinal glands; these tumors are termed *intestinal* in type.

Intestinal carcinomas form recognizable glands and range from well-differentiated (Fig. 23–9) to moderately differentiated tumors, sometimes with poorly differentiated tumor at the advancing margin. These cancers typically arise against a background of intestinal metaplasia. Diffuse cancers contain discohesive cells that fail to form distinct structures and that stimulate an overgrowth of the supporting connective tissues (Fig. 23–10). In diffuse cancers, individual tumor cells may be so widely separated from one another that they are difficult to identify. The cells usually appear round and small, and they are either arranged as single cells or are clustered in abortive, lacy, gland-like, or reticular formations. These tumors resemble those classified as signet ring cell tumors in the World Health Organization (WHO) classification. The mitotic rate is lower in diffuse carcinomas than in intestinal tumors. Small amounts of interstitial mucin may be present. Desmoplasia is more pronounced, and associated inflammation is less evident in diffuse cancers than in the intestinal carcinomas.

*Mixed carcinomas* are gastric cancers that contain approximately equal quantities of intestinal and diffuse tumor cell components. Indeterminate carcinomas are gastric cancers that are too undifferentiated to fit neatly into either category.

with or without shallow ulcerations. With extensive infiltration, a linitis plastica, or "leather-bottle" stomach results (Fig. 23–8). Mucinous gastric carcinomas appear gelatinous with a glistening cut surface. Cancers that arise in the corpus usually are type IV tumors, as are most cancers that occur in women less than 50 years old. All other growth patterns preferentially affect antral tumors, and they are most common in older men from high-risk populations.

## Histological Types of Gastric Carcinoma

Gastric carcinomas are morphologically heterogeneous, resulting in various classifications based on histological appearance, degree of differentiation, growth pattern, and histogenesis. Many gastric carcinomas display two or more distinct histological components. Several of the classification schemes are presented below.

### Laurén Classification

In 1951, Laurén,[22] a Finnish pathologist, devised a simplified classification of gastric carcinomas that subsequently proved helpful to epidemiologists studying the origins of stomach can-

### World Health Organization Classification

A committee of WHO pathologists devised another classification scheme, which identifies many of the histological variants of stomach cancer (Table 23–2).[24]

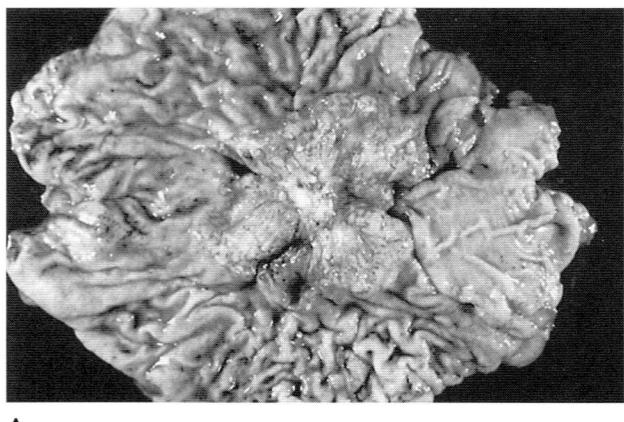

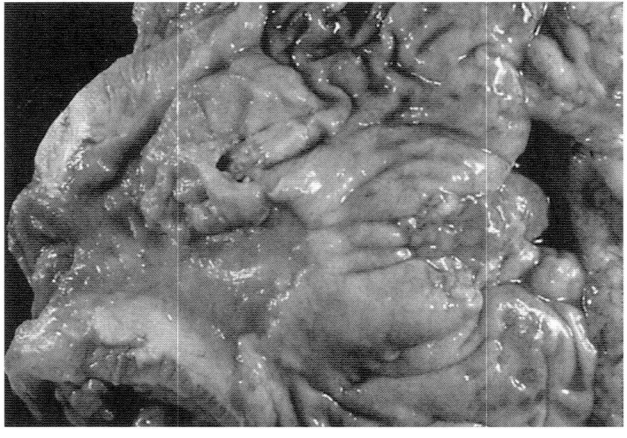

A                                                              B

**Figure 23–7** Gross appearance of gastric cancer. *A:* Borrmann type II cancer—ulcerating and infiltrating. *B:* Borrmann type III gastric cancer (ulcerating type).

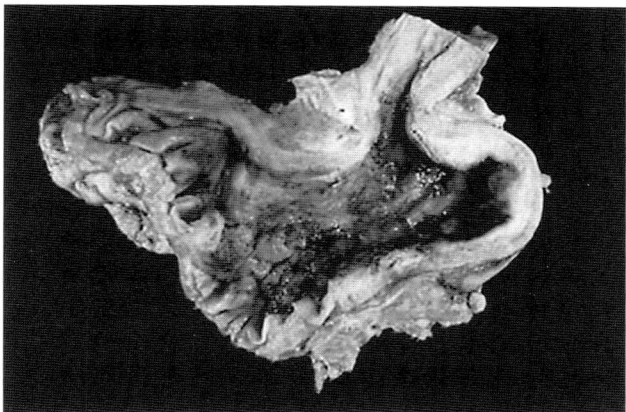

**Figure 23–8** Linitis plastica form of gastric cancer. Note the classical leather bottle–like appearance. The wall is diffusely thickened.

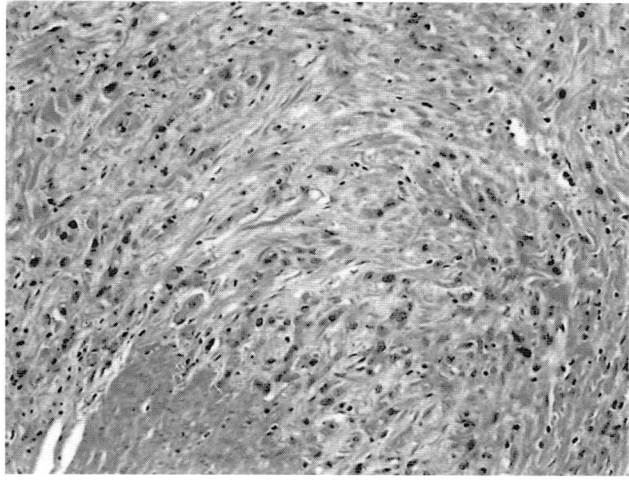

**Figure 23–10** Diffuse carcinoma. The individual tumor cells are widely spaced and supported by a dense desmoplastic stroma.

## Common tumor types

*Tubular adenocarcinomas* contain prominent dilated or slit-like and branching neoplastic tubules varying in diameter; acinar structures may be present (Fig. 23–11). Individual tumor cells may be columnar or cuboidal, or they become flattened by intraluminal mucin. The cells superficially resemble those found in colonic adenocarcinomas. Clear cells also may be present. The degree of cytological atypia varies from low to high grade.[25,26] Poorly differentiated variants are sometimes called *solid carcinomas*. Tumors with a prominent lymphoid stroma sometimes are called *medullary carcinomas* or gastric carcinomas *with lymphoid stroma* (Fig. 23–12).[27] The degree of desmoplasia varies and may be conspicuous in these neoplasms.

*Papillary adenocarcinomas* are well-differentiated exophytic carcinomas with elongated finger-like processes lined by cylindrical or cuboidal cells supported by fibrovascular connective tissue cores. Goblet cells may be present. The cells tend to maintain their polarity. Some tumors show tubular differentiation. Rarely, a micropapillary architecture is present. The degree of cellular atypia and the mitotic index vary, and severe nuclear

atypia may be present. Usually the invading tumor edge is sharply demarcated from surrounding structures. The tumor may be infiltrated by acute and chronic inflammatory cells.

*Mucinous adenocarcinomas* are tumors composed of more than 50% extracellular mucinous pools. The two major growth patterns are *(1)* glands lined by a columnar mucus-secreting epithelium together with interstitial mucin (well-differentiated type) and *(2)* chains or irregular cell clusters floating freely in mucinous lakes (Fig. 23–13). The latter pattern results from glandular rupture. Mucin also may be present in the interglandular stroma. Scattered signet ring cells, when present, do not dominate the histological picture.

*Signet ring cell carcinomas* are adenocarcinomas in which more than 50% of the tumor consists of isolated or small groups of malignant cells containing intracytoplasmic mucin (Fig. 23–14). Superficially, cells lie scattered in the lamina propria, often widening the distances between the pits and glands. The tumor cells can also be quite subtle and can be easily missed when they are few in number. The tumor cells have five morphologies: *(1)* nuclei that push against cell membranes, creating a classical signet ring cell appearance because of an expanded, globoid, optically clear cytoplasm; these contain acid mucin and stain with Alcian blue at pH 2.5; *(2)* bland-appearing cells with central nuclei that are easily mistaken for histiocytes because they show little or no mitotic activity; *(3)* small, deeply eosinophilic cells with prominent, but minute, cytoplasmic granules containing neutral mucin; *(4)* small cells without any mucin; and *(5)* anaplastic cells with little or no mucin. These cell types intermingle and constitute varying tumor proportions. Signet ring cell tumors may also form lacy or delicate trabecular glandular patterns, and they may display a zonal or solid arrangement.[17]

Signet ring cell carcinomas are infiltrative. The number of malignant cells is comparatively small, and desmoplasia may be prominent. Special stains, including mucin stains (periodic acid–Schiff, mucicarmine, or Alcian blue) or immunohistochemical staining with antibodies to cytokeratin, help detect sparsely dispersed tumor cells in the stroma. Cytokeratin immunostains detect a greater percentage of neoplastic cells than do mucin stains. Several conditions mimic signet ring cell carcinoma, including signet ring lymphoma, lamina propria muciphages, xanthomas, and detached or dying cells associated with gastritis.[17]

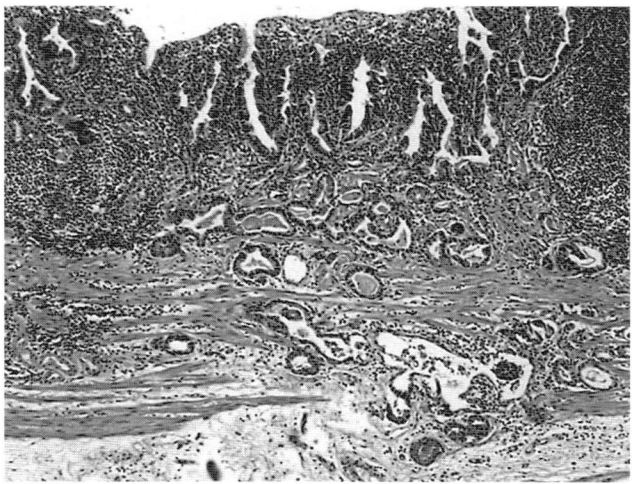

**Figure 23–9** Well-differentiated intestinal-type carcinoma. The cancer arises from an antral mucosa that shows intense gastritis and penetrates through the muscularis mucosae into the underlying submucosa.

**Table 23-2** Histological classification of gastric tumours[a]

| | |
|---|---|
| *Epithelial Tumours* | |
| Dysplasia-adenoma | 8140/0 |
|    Low-grade | |
|    High-grade | |
| *Carcinoma* | |
| Adenocarcinoma | 8140/3 |
|    Intestinal-type | 8144/3 |
|    Diffuse-type | 8145/3 |
| Papillary adenocarcinoma | 8260/3 |
| Tubular adenocarcinoma | 8211/3 |
| Mucinous adenocarcinoma | 8480/3 |
| Signet ring cell carcinoma | 8490/3 |
| Squamous cell carcinoma | 8560/3 |
| Small cell carcinoma | 8070/3 |
| Undifferentiated carcinoma | 8041/3 |
| Others | 8020/3 |
| Carcinoid–well-differentiated endocrine neoplasm | 8240/3 |
| *Nonepithelial Tumors* | |
| Leiomyoma | 8890/0 |
| Schwannoma | 9560/0 |
| Granular cell tumour | 9580/0 |
| Glomus tumour | 8911/0 |
| Leiomyosarcoma | 8890/3 |
| Gastrointestinal stromal tumor | 8936/1 |
|    Benign | 8936/0 |
|    Uncertain malignant potential | 8936/1 |
|    Malignant | 8936/3 |
| Kaposi's sarcoma | 9140/3 |
| Others | |
| *Malignant Lymphomas* | |
| Marginal zone B-cell lymphoma of MALT type | 9699/3 |
| Mantle cell lymphoma | 9673/3 |
| Diffuse large B-cell lymphoma | 9680/3 |
| Others | |
| *Secondary Tumors* | |
| Polyps | |
| Hyperplastic; fundic gland; Peutz-Jeghers | |

[a]Morphology code of the International Classification of Diseases for Oncology (ICD-O) and the Systematized Nomenclature of Medicine (SNOMED). Behavior is coded /0 for benign tumors, /3 for malignant tumours, and /1 for unspecified, borderline, or uncertain behavior.

## Less common tumor types

*Adenosquamous and squamous cell carcinomas* are rare tumors, constituting less than 1% of all gastric carcinomas.[28] Adenosquamous carcinomas combine an adenocarcinoma and squamous cell carcinoma; neither quantitatively prevails. Transitions exist between both components. These tumors grossly resemble other gastric carcinomas.[28] Some appear to be pure squamous cell carcinomas, but on careful examination, some element of glandular differentiation is usually apparent. Recognizing adenosquamous carcinomas is important because these tumors have a worse prognosis than that of ordinary gastric cancers because of their propensity for early invasion of the gastric wall, lymphatics, and blood vessels.[29]

*Small cell carcinomas* (endocrine cell carcinomas) resemble small cell cancers arising elsewhere.

*Undifferentiated carcinomas* lack any differentiated features and fall into the unclassified group in Laurén's scheme. Further

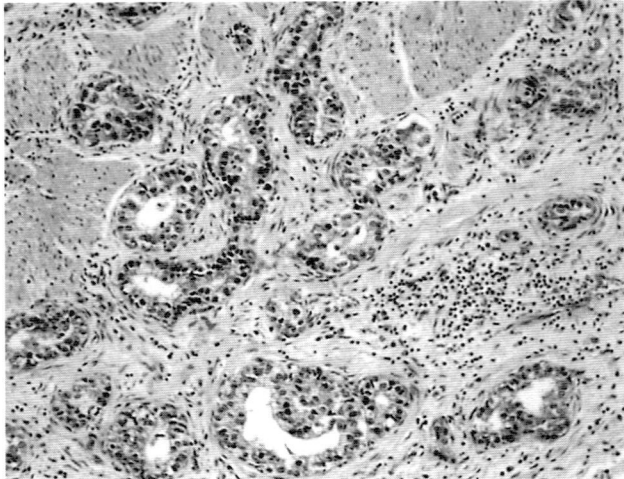

**Figure 23-11** Adenocarcinoma. The carcinoma consists of irregular glands lined by poorly differentiated epithelium.

analysis of this heterogeneous group with ultrastructural and histochemical methods may allow them to be separated into three groups: *(1)* poorly differentiated adenocarcinomas, *(2)* neuroendocrine tumors, and *(3)* composite tumors and cytokeratin-positive B-cell lymphomas and pure undifferentiated carcinoma.

Other rare tumors include parietal cell carcinoma, choriocarcinoma, endodermal sinus tumor, embryonal carcinoma, Paneth cell rich adenocarcinoma, and hepatoid adenocarcinoma.

## Ming Classification

The Ming classification distinguishes gastric carcinomas by their pattern of infiltration into the gastric wall. Tumors are designated *expanding* or *infiltrative* carcinomas (Fig. 23–15).[30] These two patterns tend to correlate with Laurén's intestinal and diffuse-type cancers, respectively. Patients with expanding, well-circumscribed tumors tend to survive twice as long as patients with infiltrative tumors.[31]

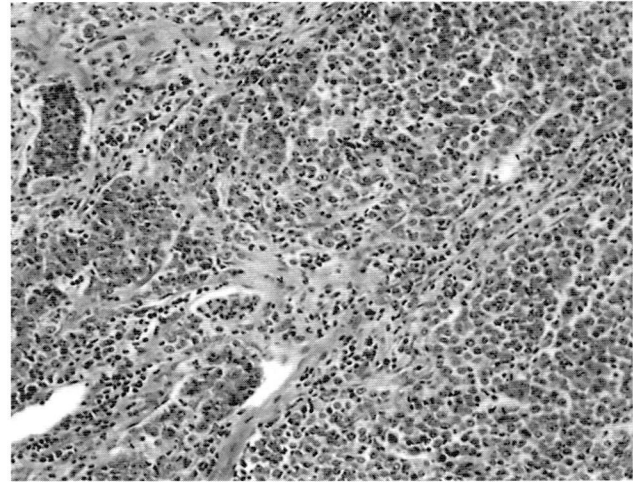

**Figure 23-12** Medullary carcinoma. The cancer consists of darkly stained cells that do not form glandular structures. Stromal desmoplasia is absent. The stroma is infiltrated by numerous lymphocytes.

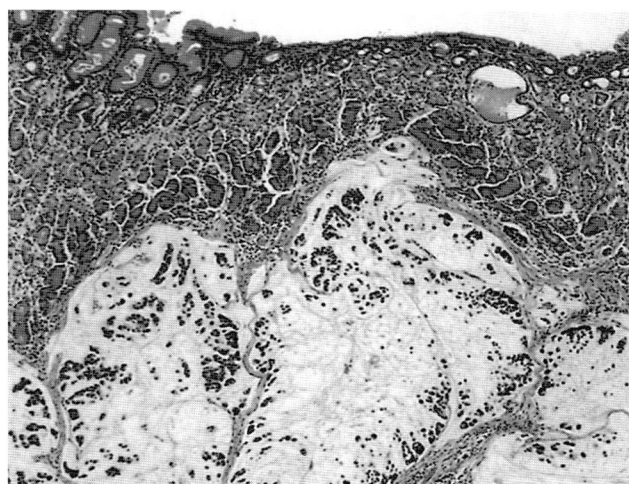

**Figure 23-13** Mucinous carcinoma arising in the gastric corpus. The tumor cells float in lakes of secreted mucus. The supporting stroma shows little or no desmoplasia.

## Goseki Classification

The Goseki classification scheme divides gastric carcinomas into four types. In group I tubular differentiation is good and mucus in cytoplasm is poor. In group II tubular differentiation is good and mucus in cytoplasm is rich. Group III tubular differentiation is poor and mucus in cytoplasm is poor. Group IV tubular differentiation is poor and mucus in cytoplasm is rich. This classification scheme may have prognostic significance.[32]

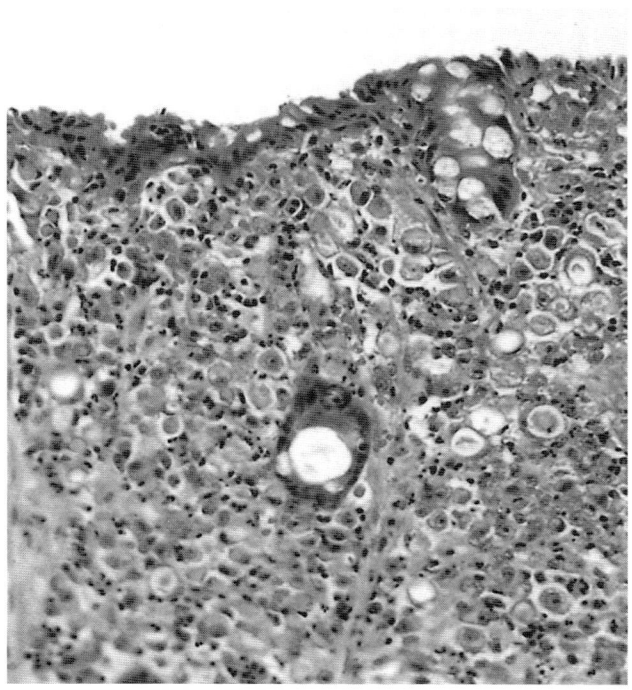

**Figure 23-14** Signet ring cell cancer. Typically, the signet ring cell component of such tumors is best seen in the superficial aspects of the neoplasm.

## Tumor Grading

Some, but not all, gastric carcinomas can be graded. The most easily graded tumors are those that fit into the intestinal type (in the Laurén classification) or the tubular type (in the WHO classification). By definition, all diffuse or signet ring cell gastric carcinomas are poorly differentiated.

*Well-differentiated* tumors are adenocarcinomas with well-formed glands, often resembling metaplastic intestinal epithelium. *Moderately differentiated* tumors are adenocarcinomas that are intermediate between well differentiated and poorly differentiated. *Poorly differentiated* tumors are adenocarcinomas composed of highly irregular glands that are difficult to recognize or of single cells that remain isolated or are arranged in clusters with mucin secretions or acinar structures. These tumors also may be graded as low grade (well and moderately differentiated) or high grade (poorly differentiated).

## Stromal Reactions

Gastric carcinomas may induce a number of stromal reactions to invasive tumor. The most common is desmoplasia. In fact, the presence of desmoplasia is often used to aid in the diagnosis of invasive disease. In some tumors, especially diffuse gastric carcinomas, the desmoplasia can be quite marked. Other stromal reactions include the presence of peritumoral lymphocytic infiltrates, stromal eosinophilia, or a granulomatous response. The lymphoid response is associated with improved survival. The granulomatous reaction is characterized by the presence of single and confluent small sarcoid-like granulomas, often accompanied by a moderately intense mononuclear cell infiltrate.

## Tumors Arising at the Esophagogastric Junction

When a tumor straddles the esophagogastric junction, it can be difficult to determine whether the neoplasm arose from cells in the distal esophagus or in the proximal stomach (the gastric cardia).[33] No universally accepted anatomic landmarks have been established to distinguish *(1)* the distal esophagus from the proximal stomach and *(2)* the extent of the gastric cardia. The term *gastric cardia* is used to refer to the most proximal portion of the stomach and to the presence of a histologically distinct area containing cardiac mucosa.

The esophagogastric junction is an imaginary anatomic line where the esophagus ends and the stomach begins. It is defined endoscopically as the level of the most proximal extent of the gastric folds.[34] In normal individuals, the proximal extent of the gastric folds generally corresponds to the point where the esophagus flares to become the stomach in the region of the lower esophageal sphincter. In patients with hiatal hernias with weak esophageal sphincters, there may be no clear-cut flare at the esophagogastric junction.[35] When the squamocolumnar junction lies proximal to the esophagogastric junction, the esophagus has a distal columnar-lined segment.[36,37] When the squamocolumnar and esophagogastric junctions coincide, the entire esophagus is lined by squamous epithelium. Adenocarcinomas that cross the esophagogastric junction are called *adenocarcinomas of the esophagogastric junction*, regardless of where the bulk of the tumor lies.[37]

The vast majority of cancers arising at the cardia are adenocarcinomas.[38] Histologically, four types are distinguished: papillary, tubular, mucinous, and signet ring cell adenocarcinoma;

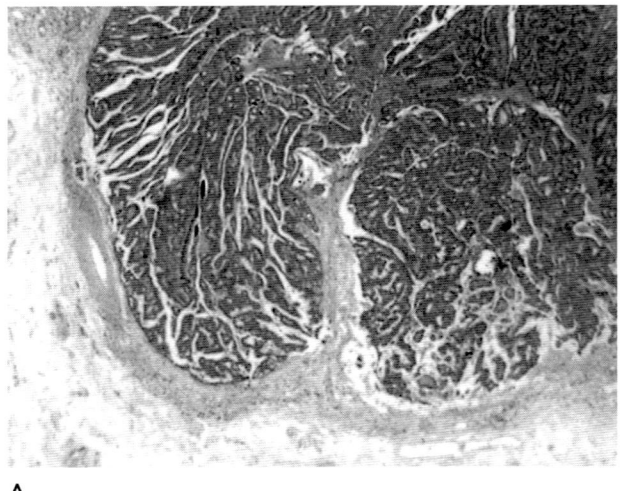

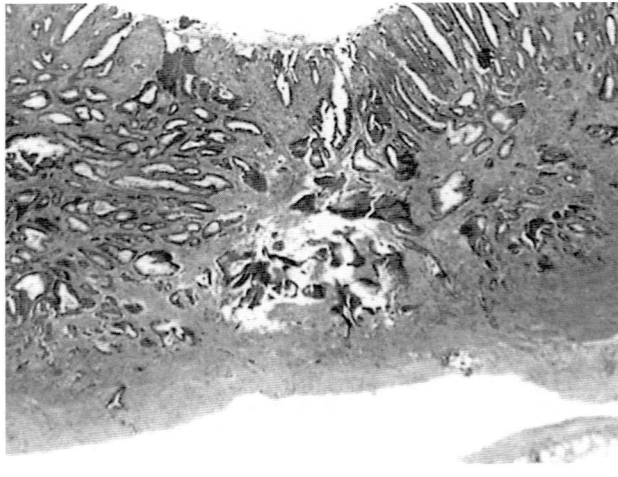

**Figure 23–15** *A:* Expanding gastric carcinoma. The tumor pushes through the gastric wall with nicely rounded edges in the advancing front. *B:* The infiltating tumor sends individual tumor tongues through the gastric wall.

however, the latter two types are uncommon. Signet ring cell cancer is much less common in the proximal stomach than in the distal stomach, and cancers of the proximal stomach generally are not accompanied by atrophic gastritis.[39] Among the less common forms of cancer in the esophagogastric junction region, adenosquamous carcinoma is the one most likely to be encountered. The diagnosis rests on the finding of a mixture of glandular and squamous elements, and not merely on the presence of small squamoid foci in an otherwise typical adenocarcinoma.

### Spread of Gastric Cancer

Gastric carcinomas spread by direct extension, metastasis, or peritoneal dissemination. Early in their development they invade locally in the gastric wall, sometimes extending into adjacent organs. Intestinal and diffuse cancers tend to grow and disseminate differently. Because of their differing growth patterns, the two types of tumors may be treated differently. Intestinal tumors generally grow in a localized, expansile fashion. Diffuse tumors, in contrast, spread widely throughout the stomach. Tumors that invade the duodenum are most often of the diffuse type, and serosal, lymphatic, and vascular invasion and lymph node metastases are common in these lesions. Duodenal invasion occurs through the submucosa or subserosa or via the submucosal lymphatics. The extent of duodenal invasion is often greater than would be expected from gross examination. Therefore, resection margins should be monitored through intraoperative consultation based on frozen sections. Lymph node metastases occur in up to 30% of lesions.[40]

Gastric carcinomas often demonstrate venous and lymphatic invasion. Tubular or intestinal carcinomas tend to show venous invasion, and they preferentially metastasize hematogenously to the liver, lungs, and bone. In contrast, diffuse carcinomas preferentially invade lymphatics, and metastases commonly involve lymph nodes and peritoneal surfaces.[41,42] Mixed tumors exhibit the metastatic patterns of both intestinal and diffuse gastric carcinomas. When cancer penetrates the serosa, peritoneal implants flourish. Bilateral massive ovarian involvement (Krukenberg's tumor) results from transperitoneal or hematogenous spread. These are most commonly encountered among premenopausal women and may be associated with metastasis to the uterus as well.

Adenocarcinomas at the esophagogastric junction exhibit a great propensity for upward lymphatic spread, mainly in the submucosa of the esophagus. For this reason, intraoperative frozen-section examination of the proximal esophageal resection margin is recommended. Upward spread also can involve lower mediastinal nodes. Lymphatic spread from the cardia often extends downward to nodes in the esophagogastric angles and around the left gastric artery and may involve paraceliac and paraaortic lymph nodes.

Lymph node metastases occur in up to 90% of advanced gastric cancers.[43,44] The incidence of metastasis depends on the size of the tumor, the depth of tumor invasion, the presence of lymphatic involvement, and the tumor differentiation.[45,46] Lymph node metastases tend to involve the regional lymph nodes in an orderly fashion, metastasizing to those lymph nodes closest to the tumor first and then metastasizing to more distal lymph nodes later. Occasionally, however, the metastases skip the lymph nodes closest to the tumor, sparing the perigastric nodes.[43]

### Staging

The TNM classification scheme is used worldwide to provide prognostic information about tumors.[47] It classifies gastric carcinomas according to the extent of the primary tumor (T), the presence or absence of nodal metastases (N), and the presence or absence of distant metastases (M). Gastric cancers are classified into four degrees of T, four degrees of N, and two degrees of M, providing 19 categories that are then condensed down to four pathological stages (Table 23–3). The accuracy of pathologic staging is proportional to the number of lymph nodes examined. When only nodes close to the tumor are assessed, 10%–20% of cancers are classified incorrectly.

### Prognosis

The prognosis of patients with gastric cancers varies considerably from country to country. The Japanese have the best prog-

**Table 23–3** TNM classification of gastric cancers

*1. Primary Tumor (T)*

The principal factor is the degree of penetration of the stomach wall.

TX   Primary tumor cannot be assessed
T0   No evidence of primary tumor
Tis   Carcinoma in situ: intraepithelial tumor without invasion of the lamina propria
T1   Tumor invades lamina propria or submucosa
T2   Tumor invades the muscularis propria or subserosa
T2a   Tumor invades muscularis propria
T2b   Tumor invades subserosa
T3   Tumor penetrates the serosa (visceral peritoneum) without invasion of adjacent structures
T4   Tumor invades adjacent structures (spleen, transverse colon, liver, diaphragm, pancreas, abdominal wall, adrenal gland, kidney, small intestine, and retroperitoneum)

*2. Nodal Involvement (N)*

The regional nodes include the perigastric nodes along the lesser and greater curvatures and the nodes along the left gastric, common hepatic, splenic, and celiac arteries. Involvement of other intraabdominal nodes represents distant metastasis.

NX   Regional lymph nodes cannot be assessed
N0   No regional lymph node metastasis
N1   Metastasis in one to six regional lymph nodes
N2   Metastasis in seven to 15 lymph nodes
N3   Metastasis in more than 15 regional lymph nodes

*3. Distant Metastasis (M)*

MX   Presence of distant metastasis cannot be assessed
M0   No distant metastasis
M1   Distant metastasis

nosis because of their earlier-stage diagnosis and the more aggressive extended surgery used in Japan.[48] Patients with early gastric cancers have the best prognosis overall, with 5-year survivals as high as 97% for those with only mucosal disease. The best survivals occur among patients with only superficial mucosal disease. Deep mucosal or submucosal disease may be associated with nodal metastases. Poorly differentiated tumors are more likely to metastasize than are better-differentiated ones. However, well-differentiated tumors with vascular invasion have an unexpectedly poor prognosis because of their tendency to disseminate widely.

Advanced gastric cancer is associated with a much lower survival than early gastric carcinoma. Worldwide the 5-year survival for advanced gastric cancer is only 10%.[49,51] Factors affecting prognosis are listed in Table 23–4. Some are established prognostic factors, whereas others are less clear. Many of the factors are interrelated. As gastric carcinomas grow in the stomach wall, they increase in size and in depth of invasion. The increase in overall tumor mass and depth of invasion correlate with the incidence of nodal metastases.[40,52,53] Poorly differentiated or diffuse gastric tumors tend to widely infiltrate the gastric wall, making adequate tumor resection difficult. These tumors often extend into the duodenum or the peritoneum. At the latter site, they tend to disseminate throughout the abdominal cavity, again making complete removal of the tumor difficult. In some instances, subtle infiltration of the extragastric tissues, or even duodenal or esophageal invasion, can be determined only by using cytokeratin immunostains.

## Secondary Tumors in the Stomach

In postmortem series, 1% to 4% of patients with malignancies reveal metastases to the gastrointestinal tract. The most common primary tumors that spread to the stomach are bronchogenic carcinoma, malignant melanoma, and carcinoma of the breast.[54] Carcinoma of the esophagus also may metastasize to the stomach,[55] in addition to directly invading the cardia. Breast carcinoma may give a diffusely infiltrative appearance, with or without ulceration. Metastatic lobular carcinoma closely mimics primary diffuse gastric carcinoma.

## Handling of Gastric Resection Specimens

The gastrectomy specimen should be sent to the pathology department as soon as possible after its removal. The stomach should be opened along the greater curvature and pinned to a cork board or paraffin plate and floated upside down in 10% neutral buffered formalin for at least 12 hours. The gross limits of the tumor are more easily assessed if the specimen is well fixed, and small, unsuspected multicentric tumors may be identified more easily.

The gross description of the fixed specimen should include the type of resection (proximal subtotal, distal subtotal, or total), the lengths of the greater and lesser curvatures, the length of attached esophagus and/or duodenum, the axial and transverse diameters of the tumor, and the location of the tumor within the stomach. The gross configuration of the tumor should also be noted (i.e., fungating, ulcerated, diffuse). All lesions should be described and sampled, including areas of ulceration, and polypoid or elevated lesions. The location of such lesions should be described accurately in relation to the main tumor mass. In many cases, an explanatory diagram or photograph is useful for documenting the distance of the tumor from resection margins and its relationship to other lesions present in the stomach.

The cut edges of the specimen should be marked with India ink before sectioning. Circumferential blocks are obtained from

**Table 23-4** Factors affecting prognosis

| Factor | Description |
| --- | --- |
| *Established Prognostic Factors* | |
| Tumor size | The larger the tumor, the worse the prognosis. The larger the tumor, the deeper it is likely to extend into the gastric wall. |
| Depth of tumor invasion | The depth of invasion increases with increasing tumor size; the deeper the tumor, the worse the prognosis. |
| Tumor histology | Intestinal tumors have a better prognosis than diffuse tumors. (Intestinal tumors tend to have an expansile growth pattern and are more easily completely resected.) |
| Lymphatic or vascular invasion | Tumors with either of these features are more likely to develop metastases than are tumors without them. |
| Tumor growth pattern | Expansile tumors have a better prognosis than infiltrative ones. |
| Presence of nodal metastases | The presence of regional nodal metastases (and the number of positive nodes) worsens patient prognosis. |
| Status of tumor resection margins | Patients with positive resection margins are more likely to have recurrent disease than are those with negative margins. Diffuse, infiltrative tumors are more likely to have involved resection margins. |
| *Possible Prognostic Factors* | |
| Prominent lymphoid stroma | Tumors with a prominent lymphoid stroma tend to behave less aggressively than tumors without this feature. (Some of the tumors with this feature have microsatellite instability.) |
| Epidermal growth factor receptor (EGFR) expression | Tumors overexpressing EGFR may have a worse prognosis than tumors lacking EGFR overexpression. |
| HER2/neu expression | Tumors overexpressing Her2/neu may have a worse prognosis than tumors lacking Her2/neu overexpression. |
| *Ras* overexpression | Tumors overexpressing *ras* may have a worse prognosis than tumors lacking *ras* overexpression. |
| Carcinoembryonic antigen (CEA) expression | Tumors overexpressing CEA may have a worse prognosis than tumors lacking CEA overexpression. |
| Ploidy status | Aneuploid tumors may have a worse prognosis than diploid tumors. However, signet ring cell tumors tend to have lower proliferative rates and less aneuploidy than tubular carcinomas. As a result, ploidy studies may be prognostic only in intestinal-type tumors. |
| Microsatellite instability (MSI) | MSI-positive tumors tend to have a better prognosis than microsatellite-stable tumors. (This is similar to the situation with colon cancers.) |
| C-*myc* amplification | Tumors with amplified c-*myc* may have a worse prognosis than tumors lacking c-*myc* amplification. |
| E-cadherin mutations | E-cadherin mutations may predispose the patient to the development of diffuse gastric cancers—tumors associated with a poor prognosis. |

the margins of resection to rule out grossly inapparent intramural spread to the surgical margin. Two to four sections should be taken from the tumor, depending on its size. At least one of these sections should include the full thickness of the gastric wall so that the maximum depth of penetration can be determined. A generous sample of the intact non-neoplastic mucosa on the proximal and distal sides of the tumor should be included with the neoplasm to enable precursor lesions, including intestinal metaplasia, atrophic gastritis, or areas of dysplasia to be identified. The pathologist should harvest as many nodes as possible from the lesser curvature and the distal and proximal greater curvature.

Histologic examination should include the following: *(1)* the TNM status of the tumor; *(2)* the histologic type of the cancer, using the Laurén or WHO classification, and its degree of differentiation; *(3)* the presence and extent of vascular and perineural invasion; *(4)* the histologic findings in the non-neoplastic gastric mucosa; and *(5)* the presence or absence of lymph node metastasis. Each report should contain, as a minimum, the information needed to assign an accurate TNM stage, the gastric subsite location of the tumor, a histologic classification of the tumor, and an estimate of its degree of differentiation.

Neoadjuvant treatment with X-ray and chemotherapy is now encountered with increasing frequency, especially for tumors involving the gastroesophageal junction. In such cases, the pathology report should attempt to compare the pretreatment histology with that found in the resected stomach. The TNM staging should indicate that pretreatment has occurred by adding the letter *y* to create a pyTNM stage. A comment may be made concerning tumor viability.

## Conclusion

Cancer of the stomach is a heterogeneous disorder with various histological types of tumors that have been classified in multiple ways. It appears that carcinomas of the cardia, which are increasing in incidence, are a different disease biologically than cancers of the more distal stomach. It also appears that there are multiple subtypes of gastric carcinoma, even at these distinct subsites. Many of the gland-producing carcinomas arise from areas of intestinal metaplasia. Even these areas are not the same throughout the stomach. Those areas that we call intestinal metaplasia actually contain cell populations that are unique with phenotypes shared between both intestinal and gastric mucosa. Eventually, we will learn more about the biology of gastric cancer and whether the histological type is more important than the location in the stomach. If different molecular pathways are involved in the genesis of these cancers, then perhaps more targeted therapies can be designed.

## References

1. Muñoz N. Descriptive epidemiology of stomach cancer. In: Reed PI, Hill MJ (eds): Gastric Carcinogenesis. Excerpta Medica, Amsterdam, 1988, pp 51–69.
2. Correa P. Human gastric carcinogenesis: a multi-step and multi-factorial process. Cancer Res 52:6735–6740, 1992.
3. Brenes F, Ruiz B, Correa P, et al. *Helicobacter pylori* causes hyperproliferation of the gastric epithelium. Pre- and post-eradication indices of proliferating cell nuclear antigen (PCNA). Am J Gastroenterol 88:1870–1875, 1993.
4. Correa P, Miller MJS. Carcinogenesis, apoptosis and cell proliferation. Br Med Bull 54:151–162, 1998.
5. Peek RM, Moss SF, Tham KT, et al. *Helicobacter pylori cagA+* strains and dissociation of gastric epithelial cell proliferation from apoptosis. J Natl Cancer Inst 89:863–868, 1997.
6. Censini S, Lange C, Xiang Z, et al. cag, a pathogenicity island of *Helicobacter pylori*, encodes type I–specific and disease-associated virulence factors. Proc Natl Acad Sci USA 93:14648–14653, 1996.
7. Mannick, EE, Bravo LEB, Zarama G, et al. Inducible nitric oxide synthase, nitrotyrosine and apoptosis in *Helicobacter pylori* gastritis. Cancer Res 56:3238–3243, 1996.
8. Watanabe T, Tada M, Nagai H, Sakasi S, Nakao M. *Helicobacter pylori* infection induces gastric cancer in Mongolian gerbils. Gastroenterology 115:642–648, 1998.
9. Yang D, Tannenbaum SR, Buch C, Lee GCM. 4-Chloro-6-methoxyindole is the precursor of a potent mutagen (4-chloro-6-methoxy-2-hydroxy-1-nitroso-indolin-3-one oxime) that forms during nitrosation of fava beans (Vicia faba). Carcinogenesis 5:1219–1224, 1984
10. Ma JY, Borch K, Sjostrand SE, et al. Positive correlation between H⁺, K⁺-adenosine triphosphatase autoantibodies and *Helicobacter pylori* antibodies in patients with pernicious anemia. Scand J Gastroenterol 29:961–965, 1994.
11. Jass JR, Filipe MI. Sulphomucins and precancerous lesions of the human stomach. Histopathology 4:271–279 1980.
12. Reis C, David L, Correa P, et al. Intestinal metaplasia of stomach displays distinct patterns of mucin (MUC1, MUC2, MUC5AC, and MUC6) expression. Cancer Res 59:1003–1007, 1999.
13. Rugge M, Correa P, Dixon MF, et al. Gastric dysplasia: the *Padova* international classification. Am J Surg Pathol 24:167–176, 2000.
14. Carneiro F. The distinction between dysplasia and truly invasive cancer. Classification of gastric carcinomas. Curr Diagn Pathol 4:51–59, 1997.
15. Schlemper RJ, Itabashi M, Kato Y, et al. Differences in the diagnostic criteria for gastric carcinoma between Japanese and Western pathologists. Lancet 349:1725–1729, 1997.
16. Stolte M, Sticht T, Eidt S, Ebert D, Finkenzeller G. Frequency, location, and age and sex distribution of various types of gastric polyp. Endoscopy 26:659–665, 1994.
17. Hamilton SR, Aaltonen LA. Pathology and Genetics of the Tumours of the Digestive System. World Health Organization Classification of Tumours. International Agency for Research on Cancer, IARC Press, Lyon, 2000.
18. Zwick A, Munir M, Ryan CK, et al. Gastric adenocarcinoma and dysplasia in fundic gland polyps of a patient with attenuated adenomatous polyposis coli. Gastroenterology 113:659–663, 1997.
19. Green PH, O'Toole KM, Weinberg LM, Goldfarb JP. Early gastric cancer. Gastroenterology 81:247–256, 1981.
20. Japanese Research Society for Gastric Cancer. Japanese Classification of Gastric Carcinoma, Kanehara, Tokyo, 1995.
21. Borrmann R. Geschwülste des Magens und Duodenums. In: Henke F, Lubarsch O (eds): Handbuch der Speziellen Pathologischen Anatomie und Histologie, Vol 4. Springer-Verlag, Berlin, 1926, pp 812–865.
22. Laurén T. The two histologic main types of gastric carcinoma. Acta Pathol Microbiol Scand 64:31–49, 1965.
23. Grabiec J, Owen DA. Carcinoma of the stomach in young persons. Cancer 56:388–396, 1985.
24. Watanabe H, Jass JR, Sobin LH. Histological typing of oesophageal and gastric tumours. In: WHO International Histological Classification of Tumours, 2nd ed. Springer-Verlag, Berlin, 1990, pp 5–9.
25. Nishikura K, Watanabe H. Gastric microcarcinoma. Its histopathological characteristics. In: Siewert JR, Roder JD (eds): Progress in Gastric Cancer Research 1997. Monduzzi Editore, Bologna, 1997, pp 251–256.
26. Endoh Y, Motoyama T, Ajioka Y, Watanabe H. Well-differentiated adenocarcinoma mimicking complete-type intestinal metaplasia in the stomach. Hum Pathol 30:826–832, 1999.
27. Watanabe H, Enjoji M, Imai T. Gastric carcinoma with lymphoid stroma—its morphological characteristics and prognostic correlations. Cancer 38:232–243, 1976.
28. Aoki Y, Tabuse K, Wada M, Katsumi M, Uda H. Primary adenosquamous carcinoma of the stomach: experience of 11 cases and its clinical analysis. Gastroenterol Jpn 13:140–145, 1978.
29. Mori H, Iwashita A, Enjoji M. Adenosquamous carcinoma of the stomach. A clinicopathologic analysis of 28 cases. Cancer 57:333–339, 1986.
30. Ming SC. Gastric carcinoma. A pathobiological classification. Cancer 39:2475–2485, 1977.
31. Pagnini CA, Rugge M. Advanced gastric carcinoma and prognosis. Virchows Arch A Pathol Anat Histopathol 406:213–221, 1985.
32. Goseki N, Takizawa T, Koike M. Differences in the mode of the extension of gastric cancer classified by histological type: new histological classification of gastric carcinoma. Gut 33:606–612, 1992.
33. Spechler SJ. The role of gastric carditis in metaplasia and neoplasia at the gastroesophageal junction. Gastroenterology 117:218–228, 1999.
34. McClave SA, Boyce HW Jr, Gottfried MR. Early diagnosis of columnar-lined esophagus: a new endoscopic criterion. Gastrointest Endosc 33:413–416, 1987.
35. Sharma P, Morales TG, Sampliner RE. Short-segment Barrett's esophagus—the need for standardization of the definition and of endoscopic criteria. Am J Gastroenterol 93:1033–1036, 1998.
36. Chandrasoma P. Pathophysiology of Barrett's esophagus. Semin Thorac Cardiovasc Surg 9:270–278, 1997.
37. Öberg S, Peters JH, DeMeester TR, et al. Inflammation and specialized intestinal metaplasia of cardiac mucosa is a manifestation of gastroesophageal reflux disease. Ann Surg 226:522–532, 1997.
38. Sons HU, Borchard F. Cancer of the distal esophagus and cardia. Incidence, tumorous infiltration, and metastatic spread. Ann Surg 203:188–195, 1986.
39. Wang HH, Antonioli DA, Goldman H. Comparative features of esophageal and gastric adenocarcinomas: recent changes in type and frequency. Hum Pathol 17:482–487, 1986.
40. Fukutomi H, Sakita T. Analysis of early gastric cancer collected from major hospitals and institutes in Japan. Jpn J Clin Oncol 11:219–225, 1984.
41. Carneiro F, Sobrinho-Simões M. Metastatic pattern of gastric carcinoma. Hum Pathol 27:213–214, 1996.
42. Mori M, Sakaguchi H, Akazawa K, Tsuneyoshi M, Sueishi K, Sugimachi K. Correlation between metastatic site, histological type, and serum tumor markers of gastric carcinoma. Hum Pathol 26:504–508, 1995.
43. Maruyama B, Gunven P, Okabayashi K, Sasako M, Kinoshita T. Lymph node metastases of gastric cancer: growth pattern in 1931 patients. Ann Surg 210:596–602, 1989.
44. Ringertz N. The pathology of gastric cancer. Natl Cancer Inst Mongr 25:275–285, 1967.
45. Yamao T, Shirao K, Ono H, et al. Risk factors for lymph node metastasis from intramucosal gastric carcinoma. Cancer 77:602–606, 1996.
46. Hirota T, Ochiai A, Itabashi M, Kitaoka H. Significance of histological type of gastric carcinoma as a prognostic factor. Stom Intest 26:1149–58, 1991.
47. Greene FL, Page DL, Fleming ID, Fritz AG, Balch CM, Haller DG, Morrow M, eds. AJCC Cancer Staging Manual, 6th ed. Springer-Verlag, New York, 2002.
48. Hermanek P, Maruyama K, Sobin LH. Stomach carcinoma. In: Hermanek P, Gospodarowicz MK, Hensen DE, Hutter RV, Sobin LH (eds): Prognostic Factors in Cancer. UICC, International Union Against Cancer. Springer-Verlag, Berlin, 1995, pp 47–63.
49. Bizer LS. Adenocarcinoma of the stomach: current results of treatment. Cancer 51:743–745, 1983.
50. Dupont BJ, Cohn Jr I. Gastric adenocarcinoma. Curr Prob Cancer 4:1–46, 1980.
51. Wanebo HJ, Kennedy BJ, Chmiel J, Steele G Jr, Winchester D, Osteen R. Cancer of the stomach. A patient care study by the American College of Surgeons. Ann Surg 218:583–592, 1992.
52. Hirota T, Ming SC. Early gastric carcinoma. In: Ming SC, Goldman H (eds): Pathology of the Gastrointestinal Tract. W.B. Saunders, Philadelphia, 1992, pp 570–583.
53. Johansen AA. Early gastric cancer. Curr Top Pathol 63:1–47, 1976.
54. Telerman A, Gerard B, Van den Heule B, et al. Gastrointestinal metastases from extra-abdominal tumors. Endoscopy 17:99–101, 1985.
55. Saito T, Iizuka T, Kato H, et al. Esophageal carcinoma metastatic to the stomach. A clinicopathologic study of 35 cases. Cancer 56:2235–2241, 1985.

# Clinical Aspects and Management of Gastric Carcinoma: Diagnostic and Staging Procedures

IRVING WAXMAN AND KIRANPREET S. PARMAR

The incidence of gastric carcinoma has decreased dramatically over the past 50 years; the reasons for this decrease are unclear. The prognosis, however, remains poor, with an overall 5-year survival rate of 17%.[1] The mainstay of treatment is surgery, and the prognosis for early gastric carcinoma (50%, 5-year survival) is substantially better than that for late gastric carcinoma (3%, 5-year survival).[2] Hence, optimal treatment for gastric carcinoma requires early diagnosis and staging. Multiple modalities are currently available for diagnosing and staging gastric carcinoma. Initially, a diagnosis can be made by using contrast upper gastrointestinal (UGI) studies, or endoscopy (EGD) with or without vital staining (chromoscopy). Once identified, the tumor can be staged using one of the following modalities: endoscopic ultrasound (EUS), computed tomography (CT) scan, magnetic resonance imaging (MRI), laparoscopy, or laparoscopic ultrasound (LUS).

The outcome of survival is highly dependent upon the stage of gastric carcinoma at the time of detection. Because the symptoms of gastric carcinoma are nonspecific, physicians should have a high index of suspicion for this diagnosis. These symptoms include weight loss, abdominal pain, nausea, anorexia, dysphagia, melena, new-onset dyspepsia, and early satiety. Patients with these symptoms and who are in various high-risk groups, such as those with chronic atrophic gastritis, pernicious anemia, gastric polyps, or prior gastric surgery, should undergo early diagnostic tests to rule out gastric carcinoma.[3]

Gastric carcinoma is initially detected by evaluating the mucosa of the stomach. This evaluation can be done using either a UGI series or an endoscopy. In a blinded, prospective study that compared endoscopy with double-contrast UGI examination in 214 patients, Dekker and co-workers[4] reported that seven malignant lesions were diagnosed by both techniques. The sensitivity and specificity were 100% for both methods. Hamada and

colleagues[5] found that the diagnosis of gastric cancer was made by a radiologist in 79% of the cases in which an abnormality or suspicion for cancer was found, leading to an endoscopy in 94% of the cases. The results of these studies show that the techniques are equally accurate in diagnosing gastric cancer. If performed by a highly skilled radiologist, barium study may be worthwhile in a low-risk patient with symptoms of gastric carcinoma. This imaging study can then be used as a road map by the endoscopist, and any suspicious lesions can be subjected to biopsy using endoscopy.

## Endoscopy

Endoscopy of the upper gastrointestinal tract is a safe and accurate method for detecting gastric cancer. This technique takes about 7 to 10 minutes to perform, is well tolerated by patients, and has multiple advantages over imaging techniques. Through endoscopy, biopsy of suspicious lesions can be performed for a histological diagnosis and the endoscopist can classify morphologically advanced cancers as polypoid, ulcerative, fungating, or infiltrative, in accordance with Bormann's criteria (types I–IV, respectively). Early gastric cancer, in which invasion is limited to the mucosa and submucosa, can also be classified according to the criteria of the Japanese Society for Gastroenterological Endoscopy.[6] Japanese workers have divided this cancer into three basic types: type I lesions protrude more than 5 mm into the lumen and may resemble benign polyps. Lesions found to be malignant upon endoscopic evaluation are defined by irregular borders, friability, and ulceration. Type II lesions are superficial and can be subdivided into type IIa (elevated lesions that protrude less than 5 mm into the lumen), type 2b (flat lesions that may appear as discoloration of the mucosa), and type IIc (depressed lesions with areas of exudate and intact mucous that do not ex-

**Table 24-1** Japanese classification of early gastric cancer

| Type | Configuration |
|---|---|
| Type I (>5 mm elevation) | |
| Type II | |
|    IIa (<5 mm elevation) | |
|    IIb (flat/discoloration) | |
|    IIc (depressed) | |
| Type III (excavated) | |

tend the muscularis mucosa). Type III lesions are large, excavated lesions that penetrate the muscularis mucosa but not the muscularis propria (Table 24–1).

Several studies have evaluated the accuracy of endoscopy, biopsy, and cytology in the diagnosis of gastric carcinoma.[7,8] Cusso and co-workers[9] performed both biopsy and cytological study in 4772 patients. Among the 3810 examinations of patients without malignancy (specificity, 99.8%), 7 were false positive. Cytology yielded positive results in 785 of 903 carcinomas (sensitivity, 86.9%), while biopsies were positive in 826 of the 895 patients with gastric cancer (sensitivity 92.3%).[9] Combining both techniques resulted in a positive diagnosis in 886 of the 903 malignancies (sensitivity, 98.1%).

Once a lesion is identified by endoscopy, multiple biopsies should be taken. Graham and colleagues,[10] recommend that a total of seven biopsies be taken at the site of the lesion, which gives a diagnostic accuracy rate of 98%. If cytology of the gastric aspirate is also performed, the accuracy rate is 100%.[10] If an ulcer is present, biopsies should be taken at the base as well as at the rim of the ulcer. Other methods to increase the accuracy rate are brush cytology, gastric lavage, and endoscopic mucosal resection (EMR). The latter (EMR) should be used in patients in whom gastric carcinoma is suspected, but for whom multiple biopsies have been negative in the past (as in the case of infiltrating carcinoma, in which deep biopsy is helpful).[11]

If a gastric ulcer is found, the current standard of practice dictates that endoscopy be repeated 6 to 8 weeks later. However, in a study by Pruitt and Truss,[7] 148 patients with gastric ulcers were monitored with serial endoscopy for 5 years, and in no case was an unsuspected carcinoma found. Among the 67 cases of gastric carcinoma, 62 were suspected to be malignant by the endoscopist (accuracy 92%), and the accuracy rate of biopsy and/or brush cytology to confirm the diagnosis was 94%. The combined accuracy rate of serial endoscopy with or without brush cytology was 99%, and only one case of gastric carcinoma was diagnosed.[7] Thus, follow-up of lesions initially thought to be benign may not be indicated, but more studies are required.

Another modality used to diagnose gastric carcinoma, especially early carcinomas, is chromoscopy, a method in which a conventional endoscope is used to introduce dyes into the stomach. The dyes bind to either the tumor tissue or normal tissue, forming a contrast between two tissues types and thus improving the ability to detect localized lesions. This method also improves the qualitative diagnosis of localized lesions (by distinguishing between benign and malignant lesions and by enabling the extent of gastric cancer to be assessed) and allows biopsies to be taken with great precision.[12] Indigo carmine is the dye most frequently used to detect gastric cancer, but other dyes, such as methylene blue, Evans blue, or the combination of methylene blue and Congo red, which can be sprayed directly during endoscopy or taken in pill form before endoscopy, are also used. In a study by Tatsutu and co-workers,[13] a combination of Congo red and methylene blue was sprayed on 94 lesions in 85 patients. Seventy-one (76%) of the lesions became white on the surface, in sharp contrast to the surrounding normal mucosa.[13] This method can greatly increase the ability to detect gastric cancer, especially early gastric cancer, and should be used by the gastroenterologist during endoscopic procedures (Color Fig. 24–1, in separate color insert).

## Radiology

The radiographic examination of the stomach consists of four techniques: full-column or barium-filled views, double-contrast or barium-coated and gas-distended views, mucosal relief or barium-coated views of a collapsed stomach, and compression views of the stomach.[14] Advanced gastric carcinoma is easier to identify using barium studies. Findings typically show either a polypoid, lobulated, or fungating mass or a filling defect. The infiltrative type (scirrhous gastric carcinoma) is characterized by loss of rugosity and narrowing of the distal part of the stomach. Double-contrast barium studies typically show a loss of distensibility of the stomach, giving it a "leather-bottle" appearance. In the ulcerative type, benign ulcers must be distinguished from malignant ulcers. The features of a benign ulcer are a round or oval crater surrounded by a smooth rim of edema and/or regular symmetrical folds that radiate to the edge of the ulcer. The mucosa surrounding the ulcer is smooth, with no evidence of nodularity, mass effect, or tumor infiltration that would cause irregularity. The perpendicular view of the ulcer features what is known as the Hampton line, a projection of the ulcer crater into the gastric lumen with overhanging edges. Malignant ulcers can be distinguished from benign ulcers by an irregular/asymmetrical ulcer crater surrounded by distorted areae gastricae. Nodularity and mass effect may be present, leading to clubbing, fusion, and/or obliteration of the radiating folds. If radiography is inconclusive, an endoscopy should be performed to establish a definite diagnosis.

Compared with advanced disease, early gastric carcinoma is more difficult to diagnose with barium studies. Type I lesions appear as elevated masses or as polyps. Type II lesions appear as shallow ulcers, plaque-like growths, or nodules, depending on the stage. Type III lesions appear as irregular ulcerative nodularities with clubbing, fusion, and/or obliteration of the radiating folds. It is recommended that all lesions be studied using endoscopy and that biopsy be performed for a definitive diagnosis (Fig. 24–2).

## Screening

No mass screening program is currently available in the United States. In Japan, the incidence of gastric carcinoma is higher (65 per 100,000 population, accounting for 25% of total cancers) and hence the need for screening programs is greater than in the United States.[15] These programs were started in the 1960s and were used to screen individuals aged 40 years and older. Double-contrast barium studies were performed twice a year. Lambert[15] reported that, because of these screening programs, more cases of early gastric cancer are being detected (currently about 40% of all gastric cancers in Japan), and that the 5-year survival rates in Japan increased from 20% in 1965 to over 40%

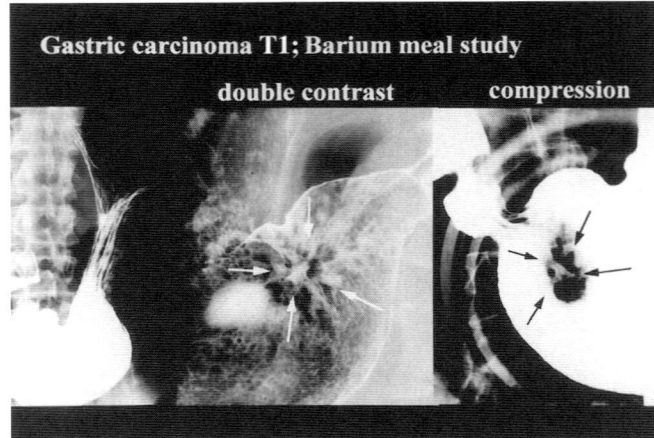

**Figure 24-2** Endoscopy and chromography of gastric cancer. Arrows highlight the gastric cancer.

in 1992. In the United States, the 5-year survival rate has remained around 20%,[16] because gastric carcinomas, when diagnosed, are usually in an advanced stage. In the United States, screening programs for the general population would not be cost-effective, as stomach cancer has only a 2% to 3% mortality rate.[16] However, all patients with symptoms should undergo a diagnostic endoscopy or at least a barium study.

## Staging

Suggested staging classifications for gastric cancer include the Japanese Society for Gastroenterological Endoscopy macroscopic classification of early gastric cancer (Table 24–1),[6] Borrmann's classification of advanced gastric cancer, which is based on the morphological appearance of the tumor; the Lauren classification, which divides stomach cancers into histological types (diffuse and intestinal types). The Mulligan classification divides gastric carcinoma into a mucous cell type, a pylorocardiac gland cell type, and an intestinal type, and the World Health Organization (WHO) system classifies gastric carcinoma according to the grades of dysplasia (well, moderate, and poorly differentiated) as well as the histologic patterns (such as papillary, tubular, mucinous, and signet ring) (Table 24–2).[17] The Ming classification distinguishes an invasive type (which infiltrates freely into the surrounding tissue and usually consists of single cells or glands) from an expanding type (which forms nodules and masses

**Table 24-2** World Health Organization classification

*Dysplasia*

Well differentiated
Moderately differentiated
Poorly differentiated
Undifferentiated

*Histologic Pattern*

Papillary
Tubular
Mucinous
Signet ring
Adenosquamous
Squamous

**Table 24-3** American Joint Committee of Cancer TNM classification

| Stage | Grouping | | |
|---|---|---|---|
| | T | N | M |
| 0 | Tis | N0 | M0 |
| IA | T1 | N0 | M0 |
| IB | T1 | N1 | M0 |
| | T2 | N0 | M0 |
| II | T1 | N2 | M0 |
| | T2 | N1 | M0 |
| | T3 | N0 | M0 |
| IIIA | T2 | N2 | M0 |
| | T3 | N1 | M0 |
| | T4 | N0 | M0 |
| IIIB | T3 | N2 | M0 |
| IV | T4 | N2 | M0 |
| | Any T | Any M | M1 |

*Primary Tumor (T stage)*

TX   Primary tumor cannot be assesed
T0   No evidence of primary tumor
Tis   Carcinoma in situ
T1   Tumor invades the lamina propria or submucosa
T2   Tumor invades muscularis propria or subserosa
T3   Tumor penetrates serosa without invasion of adjacent organs
T4   Tumor invades adjacent structures

*Regional Lymph Nodes (N)*

Nx   Regional nodes cannot be assessed
N0   No regional node metastasis
N1   Nodal metastasis <3 cm from tumor edge
N2   Nodal metastasis >3 cm from tumor edge

*Distance Metastasis (M)*

MX   Distant metastasis cannot be assessed
M0   No distant metastasis
M1   Distant metastasis

usually composed of glandular structures but which may be poorly differentiated or undifferentiated, and the American Joint Committee of Cancer (AJCC) TNM pathological classification of gastric cancer is important in determining the extent of tumor (Table 24–3).[18] Under the latter system, *T* designates the depth of penetration of tumor, *N* indicates the involvement of lymph nodes, and *M* indicates the degree of metastasis to sites other than the lymph nodes. This classification system for gastric cancer is currently the most popular. The system was revised in 1988: the nodal stage was changed and the N3 category was eliminated so that positive lymph nodes found in the periaortic, hepatoduodenal ligament, the posterior aspect of pancreas, or the root of mesentery are now considered stage M1. The prognosis is highly dependent on the stage of the tumor; the prognosis for stage 1 is obviously better than that for stage 4. Other factors that determine the prognosis are tumor site (middle third, distal third of the stomach, or proximal third),[19] tumor size, and histological pattern.

The tools used for staging are CT scan, MRI, EUS, laparoscopy, and laparoscopic ultrasound. The relative merits and limitations of these techniques are described below.

## Computed Tomography Scan

Computed tomography has become one of the most commonly ordered tests for gastric cancer staging. It is used to detect distant metastasis, (i.e., to the liver), direct invasion of surrounding structures, and spread of tumor to the lymph nodes. Performing a good CT scan requires that patients fast overnight. To adequately opacify the bowel, the patient should receive oral contrast 30 minutes to 1 hour before the CT scan. Positive-contrast agents, such as 1-25 barium or water-soluble iodinated contrast media, or negative contrast, such as water, can be used.[20] To obtain accurate images of the mass as well as the thickness of the gastric wall, the patient's stomach should be distended just before the CT scan is performed. Distention can be obtained by giving an additional 300 to 500 cc of oral contrast material, air, carbon dioxide, effervescent powder, or tablets. An intravenous contrast agent should be given to enhance density differences between the lesion and the surrounding parenchyma, to characterize the lesion, and to determine its vascular architecture. The intravenous administration of the contrast should be perfectly timed to get the best views of the lesion and its extent, especially when trying to detect liver metastasis. After the contrast has been given, 5-mm tomographic cuts should be taken throughout the stomach. For proximal gastric lesions, right lateral decubitus positioning, and for antral lesions, left decubitus positioning, may increase the distention in these areas. The prone position is best for reviewing gastroesophageal junction lesions.[21] This area of the stomach should be read carefully by the radiologist because it is difficult to interrupt, as the appearance of a mass may be present in this area in normal subjects. The thickness of the gastric wall is another important feature in the evaluation for gastric carcinoma. Normally, a well-distended gastric wall is about 5 mm thick, and the maximum thickness should not exceed 10 mm in any case. Through CT three layers of the gastric wall can be distinguished: *(1)* the first inner layer, the mucosa, which appears as a markedly enhanced layer; *(2)* the second layer, the submucosa, which is represented by an area of low attenuation; and *(3)* the third outer layer, the muscular–serosal layer, which is represented by an area of high attenution.[22] Disruption of these layers by gastric carcinoma, which appears as an enhanced area, is used to determine the T stage. The loss of the fat plane between the gastric wall and the adjacent organ is used to determine direct infiltration of adjacent organs.[23] Tumor metastasis to the lymph nodes is determined by size greater than 10 mm.[24] It was once thought that CT scanning would replace laparoscopy as a staging tool for gastric carcinoma. This, however, remains an area of great controversy between radiologists and surgeons, with vast amounts of literature supporting both sides. Early studies done by Moss and colleagues[25] showed that CT scans were highly accurate in distinguishing resectable from nonresectable lesions. Multiple studies have since provided the efficacy and limitations of CT scans. In a study of 25 patients with gastric cancer who had preoperative CT scans, Zompetta and co-workers[26] reported that CT was able to detect extension into the serosal layer with 72% accuracy, demonstrate adjacent organ involvement with 84% accuracy, and detect lymph node involvement with 68% accuracy. However, in a report on 75 patients with gastric carcinoma

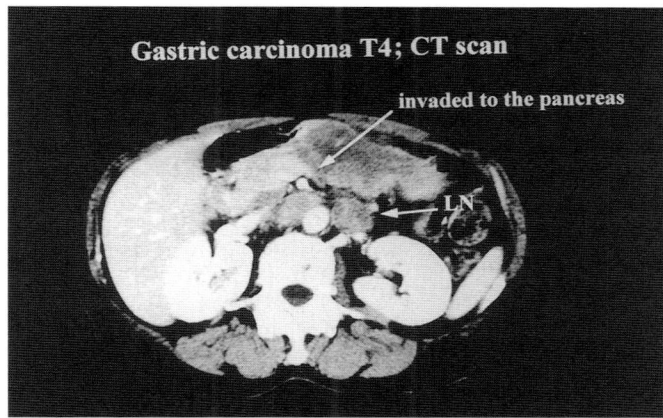

**Figure 24–3** Computed tomography scan of stage T4 gastric carcinoma. LN, lymph nodes.

who underwent preoperative staging with CT scans, Sussman et al.[27] found that CT failed to demonstrate lymphadenopathy in 14 patients, despite the presence of metastasis. In 13 patients, CT scans demonstrated enlarged lymph nodes, but no metastasis was found at surgery. The CT scans predicted spread to the pancreas in 13 patients because of loss of the fat plane between the tumor and the pancreas; of these, 5 lacked a fat plane but had no spread and 8 had a fat plane but had invasion. Computed tomography resulted in incorrect staging in 47% of the patients: 31% were understaged and 16% were overstaged.[27] Although the role of CT scanning in the staging of gastric carcinoma is debated, we believe that it is useful in gastric cancer because it can easily detect liver metastasis. Because of limited resolution, however, CT scans cannot detect the degree of penetration of the gastric wall with great accuracy. In addition, spread to lymph nodes can be determined only by measuring the size of the lymph nodes (>10 mm), which may be enlarged from inflammation rather than metastasis (see Table 24–4).[23,26,28,29] Lastly, in CT scans, loss of fat planes is used to determine the spread of cancer to adjacent organs, but these planes may be lost because of inflammation or cachexia. Hence CT scans should be used in combination with another modality, such as EUS, to increase staging accuracy (Fig. 24–3).

## Magnetic Resonance Imaging

Magnetic resonance imaging is based on the principle that protons in the body absorb and emit radio waves at different rates when placed in a strong magnetic field. These rates can be detected and characterized to produce images. The technique is used to analyze various characteristics of tissue such as hydrogen proton density, T1 and T2 relaxation time in the tissue, and blood flow within the tissue. Hydrogen proton density varies among tissues. T1 measures the time it takes tissue to become magnetized and T2 measures the time it takes for the tissue to become demagnetized. The MRIs taken at T1 usually provide good anatomic detail and are also effective in identifying fat. Those at T2 usually provide better details of pathological processes because of increases in the water content of tissues. Blood flow varies among tissues, thus causing an increase or decrease in signal intensity.

Magnetic resonance imaging of the stomach requires distension of the stomach, which can be accompanied by using either a positive-contrast agent, such as ferric ammonium citrate, mag-

**Table 24–4** Staging accuracy rates of computed tomography scan

| References | T stage (%) | N stage (%) |
|---|---|---|
| Perng et al.[23] | 42 | 49 |
| Zompetta et al.[26] | 84 | 68 |
| Natterman and Dancygier[28] | 24 | 42 |
| Boudiaf et al.[29] | 40 | 60 |

nese chloride, or gadopentetate dimeglumine, to increase the intraluminal signal or a negative-contrast agent, such as perflubron or barium sulfate, to decrease the intraluminal signal. Imaging should be started after the patient has received gadolinium-labeled diethylenetriamine penta-acetic acid (Gd-DTPA), an intravenous contrast agent that shortens T1 and T2 relaxation times. The extent of T1 relaxation is shorter than that of T2 relaxation, resulting in greater signal intensity on T1 images.

Although MRI is not routinely used for staging of gastric carcinoma, technical advances in this field may result in increased use of MRI. The main drawback of MRI is motion artifact caused by breathing. In a study by Matsushita and colleagues,[39] MRI findings in 48 patients with advanced gastric carcinoma were correlated with histopathologic findings. The patients fasted and were given 600 to 1000 ml of water before the procedure to distend the stomach. Coronal, axial, sagittal, and oblique images perpendicular to the stomach wall were taken with a 5- to 7-mm thickness using spoiled gradient recalled acquisition in the steady state. Three or four images were obtained using a single breath hold. Initially, unenhanced images were taken, followed by images taken after intravenous injection of gadopentetate dimeglumine. A band of low signal intensity was found outside the gastric wall during this study and was used to define the presence of invasion. The degree of serosal invasion was classified as MRT1 (no abnormal findings), MRT2 (presence of a band surrounding the lesion), MRT3 (presence of an irregular or interrupted band around the lesion), or MRT4 (absence of a band of low signal intensity and presence of high signal intensity compared with that of adjacent organs. The MRI and histopathologic finding correlated in 11 (79%) of 14 patients in the MRT1 group, 23 (96%) of 24 in the MRT3 group, and 8 (88%) of 10 patients in the MRT4 group. The overall staging accuracy rate of MRI for the T factor was 88%. This study considered the gastric wall as consisting of two layers.

In another study reported by Dux and co-workers[31] resected gastric specimens were compared with MRI findings. This study used T1, T2, and opposed-phase imaging, and three to five layers of the gastric wall were visible, depending on the image. Tumor diagnosis and lymph node detection were best achieved by opposed-phase imaging. Nineteen (95%) of 20 carcinomas were localized by MRI, with the rate of T-stage accuracy being 65% (13 of 20). Five T2 tumors were overstaged as T3 tumors, and one infiltrating T4 carcinoma was understaged as T3. The sensitivity of MRI in detecting lymph node infiltration was 87% (13 of 15) and specificity was 60% (9 of 15). N-staging accuracy of MRI was 80% (16 of 20). Enlarged lymph nodes were classified as being metastatic. As in the study by Costanzi and colleagues,[32] MRI sensitivity in detecting hepatic metastasis was high, but peritoneal carcinomatosis was difficult to demonstrate. Magnetic resonance imaging had a 40.6% sensitivity rate, a 93.87% specificity rate, and 42.08% accuracy in demonstrating lymph node involvement.

In 1995, Inui and colleagues[33] proposed a different MRI technique—the endoscopic MRI, in which the same principle as EUS is used and an MRI coil is attached to the end of an endoscope. This modality had a T-staging accuracy rate of 89% and an N-staging accuracy rate of 56% in nine patients with gastric cancer. Currently, MRI is not routinely used in the diagnosis and staging of gastric carcinoma because of the presence of artifacts (resulting from respiration and peristalsis), the time required to perform MRI, and the overall cost of the procedure. The encouraging results from the above studies and the development of new technologies, such as ultrafast imaging, may make MRI the standard of care in the near future.

## Endoscopic Ultrasound

Endoscopic ultrasound has become the method of choice for locoregional staging of gastric carcinoma. By dividing the gastric wall into five sonographic layers, which correspond to the histological layers,[34] not only the depth of invasion but also the involvement of regional lymph nodes can be determined. The first layer (inner hyperechoic) represents the acoustic interface between the lumen and the gastric epithelium. The second layer (hypoechoic) corresponds to the deep mucosa, lamina propria, and muscularis mucosa. The third layer (hyperechoic) corresponds to the submucosal layer. The fourth layer is the muscularis propria (hypoechoic). The fifth layer (hyperechoic) corresponds to the serosa, or interface, between the gastrointestinal wall and the surrounding tissue.

Endoscopic ultrasound may use a variety of ultrasound frequencies. A 7.5 MHz transducer provides visualization of the organs and lesions extrinsic to the gastrointestinal wall. A 12 MHz probe provides a high-resolution image of the gastrointestinal wall; a 20 MHz provides the highest resolution of the gastrointestinal wall, but the depth of penetration is limited to 15 mm. Whereas conventional EUS shows a five-layered gastrointestinal wall structure, high-frequency ultrasound can delineate the gastric wall as a seven- to nine-layered structure. In 70% of patients the muscularis mucosae are visualized in two layers, and muscularis propria appears as a three-layered structure, (circular, interface, and longitudinal layer).[35] Hence, a decrease in frequency decreases the resolution but increases the depth of visualization, and an increase in frequency increases the resolution at the expense of depth of penetration.[36] Three types of ultrasound systems are available. The first two are radial and used for imaging only: one has a transducer at the end of the ultrasound scope, an ECHO-endoscope, while the other is catheter based and can be passed through the biopsy channel of the endoscope. The third type is a curvilinear array ultrasound scope and is used to obtain biopsies.

The EUS is operator-dependent and requires a highly skilled and experienced gastroenterologist. A standard endoscopic examination must be performed before the EUS is performed to localize the lesion. The examination is usually done under conscious sedation. The scope is passed to the stomach, and the transducer is placed perpendicular to the gastric wall. The balloon is inflated, and air is removed from the stomach, which is then filled with deaerated water. The radial EUS image is oriented like a CT scan, with anterior structures at 12 o'clock, posterior structures at 6 o'clock, left structures at 3 o'clock, and right structure at 9 o'clock The scope is moved back and forth to determine the extent of the lesion, the layer of origin, and the involvement of lymph nodes, and to visualize the normal layers of the gastric wall. The depth of penetration is determined by the disruption of various layers in the gastric wall.

Early gastric carcinomas are limited to the mucosa and the submucosa. Types IIa, IIb, and IIc can be identified as irregularities in the mucosal layer without involvement of the submucosoa, whereas type III has involvement of the submucosa and appears as irregularities in that layer of the bowel wall. It is usually difficult to distinguish between T2 and T3 lesions because the serosa is a very thin layer or absent on some areas of the stomach,[37] making it hard to determine whether the tumor lies in the subserosa or actually penetrates the serosa. As with other imaging modalities, it is also difficult for EUS to differentiate between inflammatory changes and tumor infiltration.[38] This difficulty can lead to overstaging of stage I and II tumors. However, even with this overstaging, the accuracy rate for T stage remains high.

An advanced gastric carcinoma appears as a hypoechoic and inhomogeneous mass arising from the mucosal layer and extending through all the layers of the gastric wall, with destruction of these layers. Scirrhous carcinoma appears as diffuse thickening of the third and fourth layers of the gastric wall, with destruction of the submucosal propria and muscularis propria without the presence of discrete ulceration. Endoscopic ultrasound is also the most accurate method for assessing perigastric lymphadenopathy, and these lymph nodes should be differentiated from blood vessels, which are anechoic and have linear continuity. Limitations of EUS include the short range of ultrasound, which is about 5 to 7 cm. Hence, any lymph nodes beyond that depth cannot be assessed, and the right lobe of the liver also cannot be assessed. Lymph node involvement is determined not only by size but also by morphological characteristics of the nodes. Rounded, sharply demarcated, homogenous, and hypoechoic lymph nodes indicate metastasis. Inflamed lymph nodes usually are triangular or ellipsoid, have poorly defined margins, and are inhomogeneous and hyperechoic. Lymph nodes less than 5 mm and with micrometastasis are difficult to detect. With the advent of the curvilinear ultrasound scope, any suspicious lymph node can easily be biopsied, thereby increasing the accuracy of this modality in staging gastric cancer.

Multiple studies of EUS staging of gastric carcinoma show that the method is about 80% accurate in determining the extent of tumors (T stage) and accurate in assessing lymph node involvement is about 70% (Table 24–5).[39–66] Endoscopic ultrasound plays an important role in preoperative staging of gastric carcinoma and can prevent unnecessary laparotomy. After distal metastasis is ruled out to the liver and lungs, an EUS can be performed to evaluate local extent. Surgical resection of tumors identified by EUS as stage T1–T3 will likely be attempted; endo-

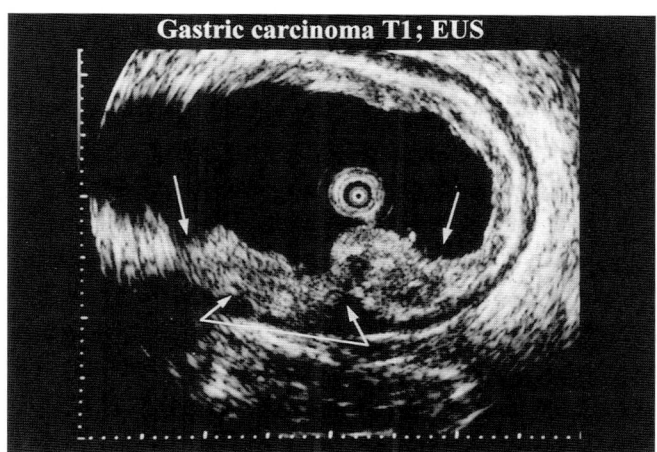

**Figure 24–4** Endoscopic ultrasound of stage T1 gastric carcinoma. Arrows indicate the extent of the gastric lesion.

scopic management may be sufficient for tumors limited to the mucosa (Fig. 24–4).

## Laparoscopy

Most patients presenting with gastric carcinoma in the United States have advanced disease. These patients are usually not candidates for curative resection and would not benefit from exploratory laparotomy. However, these candidates might benefit from more restricted palliative surgery, which does not improve survival but does decrease morbidity. Laparoscopy has been shown to reduce the preoperative stage of gastric carcinoma and thus prevent unnecessary exploratory laparotomy. In addition, laparoscopy is the only modality that allows direct visualization of the peritoneal cavity to detect peritoneal carcinomatosis and occult metastasis to the surface of the liver. Using LUS, the liver and lymph nodes can also be assessed.

Laparoscopy is an easy procedure that takes about 30 to 45 minutes to perform. It is done under general anesthesia with the patient in a supine position. A small incision is made at the umbilicus, through which a 10- to 12-mm port for the camera is passed and a 10- to 12-mm port is passed to the right quadrant. An additional port is placed at the left upper quadrant for biopsies. Surgical staging starts with an examination of the peritoneal cavity, and normal saline is then instilled into the peritoneal cavity, which is then aspirated for cytology. The liver is examined, followed by evaluation of the regional lymph nodes. The size and extent of the primary tumor are then determined.

By identifying inoperable tumors, laparoscopy will help to reduce the morbidity and cost of exploratory laparotomy. Feussner and others[67] reported that in 40% of patients who underwent laparoscopy, management was changed, despite earlier extensive work-up. In their group of 111 patients, 107 had a successful diagnostic laparoscopy. In 56 patients (50.5%) no additional findings were obtained. In 5.4% of cases laparoscopy yielded additional information unrelated to the tumor and changed the method of management. Tumors were downgraded in 17 patients (15.3%) and upgraded in 28 cases (25.2%). Peritoneal implants were found in 26 patients. Laparoscopic ultrasound changed preoperative diagnosis in 8 cases (7.2%) of the whole group. Overall findings of laparoscopy or LUS changed the preoperative diagnosis of 51 patients (46%), leading to a change in management for 45 patients (40.5%).

**Table 24–5** Staging accuracy rates of endoscopic ultrasound

| Reference | T stage | N stage |
| --- | --- | --- |
| Kimura et al.[39] | 85 | — |
| Murata et al.[40] | 79 | — |
| Yasuda et al.[41] | 79 | — |
| Ohashi et al.[42] | 67 | — |
| Tio et al.[43] | 84 | 68 |
| Aibe et al.[44] | 73 | 69 |
| Yoshimi et al.[45] | — | 73 |
| Heintz and Junginger[46] | 79 | 72 |
| Kida et al.[47] | 82 | — |
| Botet et al.[48] | 92 | 78 |
| Saito et al.[49] | 81 | — |
| Akahoshi et al.[50] | 81 | 50 |
| Yasuda et al.[51] | 79 | — |
| Cerizzi et al.[52] | 90 | 55 |
| Rosch et al.[53] | 71 | 75 |
| Ito et al.[54] | 74 | — |
| Dittler and Siewart[55] | 83 | — |
| Grimm et al.[56] | 78 | 87 |
| Ziegler et al.[57] | 86 | 74 |
| Froment et al.[58] | 79 | 70 |
| Natterman et al.[59] | 82 | 78 |
| Caletti et al.[60] | 91 | 61 |
| De Angelis et al.[61] | 80 | 75 |
| Yoshikawa et al.[62] | 72 | — |
| Massari et al.[63] | 89 | 68 |
| Perng et al.[64] | 71 | 65 |
| Hunerbein et al.[65] | 82 | 80 |
| Wang et al.[66] | 70 | 65 |

Kriplani and Kapur[68] noted a 92% diagnostic accuracy rate for laparoscopy. Laparoscopy revealed distant metastasis in 13% of cases and an unresectable tumor in 28% of cases, thus sparing these patients from futile laparotomy. Laparoscopy also accurately predicted resectability in 87% of patients. Possik and colleagues[69] reported that laparoscopy had diagnostic accuracy rates of 89% for detecting peritoneal dissemination and 97% for detecting hepatic metastasis in a cohort of 360 patients. Asencio and colleagues[70] reported that the diagnostic accuracy rate of laparoscopy for determining resectability of gastric tumor was 99%. Consequently, over 40% of patients were spared unnecessary laparotomy in their group of 71 patients.

## Summary

Several modalities for the diagnosis and staging of gastric cancer are available. The main diagnostic modalities used for detecting gastric cancer are barium contrast study and endoscopy. For staging, CT scanning is the most widely used technique, followed by EUS. The CT scan is effective in detecting metastasis (i.e., hepatic involvement) but is somewhat limited in staging locoregional cancer. Endoscopic ultrasound is excellent for locoregional staging but is not effective in detecting distant metastasis. Also, the presence of stenosis is a hindrance to EUS. Magnetic resonance imaging is still a new technology and must be further refined for use in staging of gastric cancer. Laparoscopy with ultrasound is excellent for detection of occult malignancy but is an invasive procedure.

The choice of technique depends on the therapeutic strategy. Patients who will receive multimodal therapy or who are involved in protocols must have the best preoperative assessment possible. This can be provided by using the techniques discussed above to their greatest potential. Presently, combining EUS for locoregional staging and CT scanning to rule out distal metastasis are the techniques of choice and should be viewed as complimentary modalities.

We are indebted to Jiro Watari, M.D., and Yusuke Saitoh, M.D., Ph.D., of the Third Department of Internal Medicine at Asahikawa Medical College in Asahikawa, Hokkaido, Japan for their contribution of Figures 24–1 through 24–4.

## References

1. Wanebo HJ, Kennedy BJ, Chimiel J, et al. Cancer of the stomach: a patient care study by the American College of Surgeons. Ann Surg 218:583–589, 1993.
2. Madden ML, Price SK, Learmanth GM, et al. Surgical staging of gastric carcinoma: sources and consequences of error. Br J Surg 74:119–121, 1987.
3. Stemmerman GN. Intestinal metaplasia of the stomach. Cancer 74:556–562, 1994.
4. Dekker W, Op Den Orth J. Biphasic radiologic examination and endoscope of the gastrointestinal tract: a comparative study. J Clin Gastroenterol 10:461–465, 1988.
5. Hamada T, Kaji F, Shirakabe H, et al. Detectability of gastric cancer by radiology as compared to endoscopy. In: Maruyama M, Kimura K, (eds): Review of Clinical Reasearch in Gastroenterology. Igaku-Shoin, Tokyo, 1988, p 36.
6. Kobayashi S, Prolla JC, Yagi M, et al. Gastroscopic diagnosis of early gastric carcinoma based on Japanese classification. Gastrointest Endosc 16:92–97, 1969.
7. Pruitt RE, Truss CD. Endoscopy, gastric ulcer, and gastric cancer. Follow-up endoscopy for all gastric ulcers? Dig Dis Sci 38:284–288, 1993.
8. Hecker R, Fitch R, Rowland R. The value of endoscopy and biopsy in the diagnosis of gastric carcinoma. Med J Aust 2:472–474, 1975.
9. Cusso X, Mones J, Ocana J, et al. Is endoscopic gastric cytology worthwhile? An evaluation of 903 cases of carcinoma. J Clin Gastroenterol 16:336–339, 1993.
10. Graham DY, Schwartz JT, Cain GD, et al. Prospective evaluation of biopsy number in the diagnosis of esophageal and gastric carcinoma. Gastroenterology 82:228, 1982.
11. Ghosh S, Papachrysostomou M, Welsh M, et al. Diagnostic use of endoscopic mucosal resection. Eur J Gastroenterol Hepatol 9:539–541, 1997.
12. Hiki Y. Endoscopic diagnosis of mucosal cancer. Semin Surg Oncol 17:91–95, 1999.
13. Tatsuta M, Okuda S, Tamura H, et al. Endoscopic diagnosis of early gastric cancer by the endoscopic congo red–methylene blue test. Cancer 50:2956–2960, 1982.
14. Halvorsen RA, Yee J, McCormick VD. Diagnosis and staging of gastric cancer. Semin Oncol 23:3225–3235, 1996.
15. Lambert R. Mass screening programs in Japan: what can we learn in the West? Endoscopy 30:721–723, 1998.
16. Landis SH, Murray T, Bolden S, et al. Cancer statistics, 1999. CA Cancer J Clin 49:8–31, 1999.
17. Arsian Pagnini C, Rugge M. Gastric cancer: problems in histological diagnosis. Histopathology 6:391–398, 1982.
18. The American Joint Committee on Cancer. Manual for Staging, 4th ed. J.B. Lippincott, Philadelphia, 1993.
19. Nakamura K, Veyama T, Yao T, et al. Pathology and prognosis of gastric carcinoma. Cancer 70:1030–1037, 1992.
20. Winter TC, Ager JD, Nghiem HV, et al. Upper gastrointestinal tract and abdomen: water as an orally administered contrast agent for helical CT. Radiology 201:365–370, 1996.
21. Miller FH, Kochman ML, Talamonti MS, et al. Gastric cancer: radiologic staging. Radiol Clin North Am 35:311–329, 1997.
22. Minami M, Kawauchi N, Itai Y, et al. Gastric tumors: radiologic–pathologic correlation and accuracy of T staging with dynamic CT. Radiology 185:173–178, 1992.
23. Perng DS, Jan CM, Chen LT, et al. Computed tomography, endosonography and intraoperative assessment in TN staging of gastric carcinoma. J Formos Med Assoc 95:378–385, 1996.
24. Dehn TCB, Reznek RH, Nockler JB, et al. The preoperative assessment of advanced gastric cancer by computed tomography. Br J Surgery 71:413–417, 1984.
25. Moss AA, Schnyder P, Marks W, et al. Gastric adenocarcinoma: a comparison of the accuracy and economics of staging by computed tomography and surgery. Gastroenterology 80:45–50, 1981.
26. Zompetta C, Catarci M, Polettini E, et al. Diagnostic accuracy of computerized tomography. Preoperative staging of gastric cancer. Clin Ther 146:825–841, 1995.
27. Sussman SK, Halvorsen RA Jr, Illescas FF, et al. Gastric adenocarcinoma: CT versus surgical staging. Radiology 167:335–340, 1988.
28. Nattermann C, Dancygier H. Endosonography in diagnosis and staging of malignant tumors of the stomach. A prospective comparative study between endosonography, computerized tomography and convential ultrsonography. Z Gastroenterol 31:719–726, 1993.
29. Boudiaf M, Bedda S, Soyer P, et al. Preoperative evaluation of gastric adenocarcinomas: comparison of CT results with surgical and pathological results. Ann Chir 53:115–122, 1999.
30. Matsushita M, Oi H, Murakami T, et al. Extraserosal invasion in advanced gastric cancer: evaluation with MRI imaging. Radiology 192:87–91, 1994.
31. Dux M, Roeren T, Kuntz C, et al. MRI for staging of gastric carcionoma: first results of experimental prospective study. J Comput Assist Tomogr 21:66–72, 1997.
32. Costanzi A, Di CesareE, Guadagni S, et al. Gastric adenocarcinoma: magnetic resonance versus surgical staging. Radiol Med (Torino) 92:726–730, 1996.
33. Inui K, Nakazawa S, Yoshino J, et al. Endoscopic MRI: preliminary results of a new technique for visualization and staging of gastrointestinal tumors. Endoscopy 27:480–485, 1995.
34. Kimmey MB, Martin RW, Haggitt RC, et al. Histologic correlates of gastrointestinal ultrasound images. Gastroenterology 96:433–441, 1989.
35. Yanai H, Fujimura H, Suzumi M, et al. Delineation of the gastric muscularis mucosae and assessment of depth of invasion of early gastric cancer using a 20 megahertz endoscopic ultrasound probe. Gastrointest Endosc 39:505–512, 1993.
36. Stolk RUV. Subepithelial lesions. In: Van Dam J, Sivak MV Jr. (eds): Gastrointestinal Endosonography. W.B. Saunders, Philadelphia, 1999, pp 153–165.
37. Ziegler K, Sanft C, Zimmer T, et al. Comparison of computed tomography, endosonography and intraoperative assessment in TN staging of gastric carcinoma. Gut 34:604–610, 1993.
38. Dittler HJ, Siewert JR. Role of endosopic ultrasonography in gastric carcinoma. Endoscopy 25:162–166, 1993.

39. Kimura K, Yamanaka Y, Sakaguchi T, et al. Endoscopic ultrasonography in the assessment of depth of infiltration of gastric cancer. In: Takemoto T, Kaxai K (eds): Recent Topics of Digestive Endoscopy. Experta Medica, Amsterdam 1982, pp 20–26.

40. Murata Y, Suzuki S, Hashimoto H. Endoscopic ultrasonography of the upper gastrointestinal tract. Surg Endosc 2:180–183, 1988.

41. Yasuda K, Nakajima M, Cho E, et al. Benign versus malignant gastric ulcers: a role for endoscopic ultrasonography? In: Dancygier H, Classen M (eds): 5th International Symposium on Endoscopic Ultrasonography. Demeter Verlag (Z Gastrenterol Suppl), Munich, 1989, pp 50–56.

42. Ohashi S, Nakazawa M, Yoshino J, et al. Endoscopic ultrasonography in the assessment of invasive gastric cancer. Scand J Gastroenterol 24: 1039–1048, 1989.

43. Tio TL, Schouwink MH, Cikot RJ, et al. Preoperative TNM classification of gastric carcinoma by endosonography in comparison with the pathological TNM system: a prospective study of 72 cases. Hepatogastroenterology 36:51–56, 1989.

44. Aibe T, Fujimura H, Nogouchi T, et al. Endosonographic detection and staging of early gastric cancer. In: Dancygier H, Classen M (eds): 5th International Symposium on Endoscopic Ultrasonography. Demeter Verlag (Z Gastrenterol Suppl), Munich, 1989, pp 71–78.

45. Yoshimi M, Kusuyama A, Tashiro H, et al. EUS approach to the regional lymph nodes in early gastric cancer. In: Abstracts of the World Congresses of Gastroenterology, Sydney, 1990. The Medicine Group (UK), Abingdon, 1990, no. FP 325.

46. Heintz A, Junginger T. Endosonographisches Staging von Karzinomen in Speiserohre und Magen. Bildgebung 58:4–8, 1991.

47. Kida M, Yamada Y, Sakaguchi T, et al. The diagnosis of gastric cancr by endoscopic ultrasonography. Stomach Intest 26:61–70, 1991.

48. Botet JF, Lightdale CJ, Zauber AG, et al. Preoperative staging of gastric cancer: comparison of endoscopic US and dynamic CT. Radiology 181: 426–432, 1991.

49. Saito N, Takeshita K, Habu H, et al. The use of endoscopic ultrasound in determining the depth of cancer invasion in patients with gastric cancer. Surg Endosc 5:14–19, 1991.

50. Akahoshi H, Misawa T, Fujishima H, et al. Preoperative evaluation of gastric cancer by endoscopic ultrasound. Gut 34:604–610, 1993.

51. Yasuda K, Mukai H, Cho E, et al. Evaluation of the degree of gastric cancer invasion by endscopic ultrasonography (EUS) for endoscopic treatment of early gastric cancer. Stomach Intest 221:1167–1176, 1992.

52. Cerizzi A, Botti F, Carrara A, et al. EUS in preoperative staging of gastric cancer. Endoscopy 24(Suppl I):380(A), 1992.

53. Rosch T, Lorenz R, Zenker K, et al. Local staging and assessmant of resectability in carcinoma of esophagus, stomach and duodenum byendoscopic ultrasonography. Gastrointest Endosc 38:460–467,1992.

54. Ito M, Takasu S, Ikegama F, et al. Endoscopic ultrasonography in gastric cancer. Endoscopy 24:653(A), 1992.

55. Dittler HJ, Siewert JR. Role of endoscopic ultrasonography in gastic carcinoma. Endoscopy 25:162–166, 1993.

56. Grimm H, Binmoeller K, Hamper K, et al. Endosonography for preoperative locoregional staging of esophageal and gastric cancer. Endoscopy 25:224–230, 1993.

57. Ziegler K, Sanft C, Zimmer T, et al. Comparison of computed tomography, endosonography, and intraoperative assessment in TN staging of gastric carcinoma. Gut 5:14–19, 1993.

58. Froment S, Pujol B, Napoleon B, et al. Endoscopic ultrasound (EUS) and adenocarcinoma of the cardia: results and practical usefulness. Gastrointest Endosc 39:305(A), 1993.

59. Nattermann C, Galbenu-Grunwald R, Nier H, et al. Endoskopischer Ultraschall im TN-Staging des Magenkarzinoms. Ein Vergleich mit der Computertomographie und der konventionellen Sonographie. Z Gesamte Inn Med 48:60–64, 1993.

60. Caletti GC, Ferrari A, Brocchi E, et al. Accuracy of endoscopic ultrasonography in the diagnosis and staging of gastric cancer and lymphoma. Surgery 113:14–27, 1993.

61. De Angelis C, Gindro T, Recchia S, et al. Value and limitations of preoperative endoscoped ultrasonography in prediction stage and resectability of gastric cancer. Gastroenterology 106:380(A), 1994.

62. Yoshikawa J, Matsumoto J, Saisho A, et al. Depth of gastric cancer invasion determined by endoscopic ultrasonography. Gastrointest Endosc 40:(A), 1996.

63. Massari M, Cioffi U, De Semone M, et al. Endoscopic ultrasonography for preoperative staging of gastric carcinoma. Hepatogastroenterology 43:542–546,1996.

64. Perng DS, Jan CM, Wang WM, et al. Computed tomography, endoscopic ultrasonography and intraoperative assessment in TN staging of gastric carcinoma. J Formos Med Assoc 95:378–385, 1996.

65. Hunerbein M, Ghadimi BM, Haensch W, et al. Transendoscopic ultrasound of esophageal and gastric cancer using miniaturized ultrasound catheter probes. Gastrointest Endosc 48:371–375, 1998.

66. Wang JY, Hsieh JS, Huang YS, et al. Endoscopic ultrasonography for preoperative locoregional staging and assessment of resectability in gastric cancer. Clin Imaging 22:355–359, 1998.

67. Feussner H, Omote K, Fink U, et al. Pretherapeutic laparoscopic staging in advanced gastric carcinoma. Endoscopy 31:342–347, 1999.

68. Kriplani AK, Kapur BM. Laparoscopy for preoperative staging and asessment of operavility in gastric carcinoma. Gastroentest Endosc 37:441–443, 1991.

69. Possik RA, Franco EL, Pries DR, et al. Sensitivity, specificity, and predictive value laparoscopy for the staging of gastric cancer and for the detection of liver metastases. Cancer 58:1–6, 1986.

70. Ascencio F, Aguilo J, Salvador, et al. Video-laparoscopic staging of gastric cancer. A prospective multicenter comparison with noninvasive technique. Surg Endosc 11:1153–1158, 1997.

# Chapter 25

## Clinical Aspects and Management of Gastric Carcinoma
### Management Options: Potentially Resectable Gastric Cancer

PAUL F. MANSFIELD

Since the 1930s, when gastric cancer was the most common type of cancer in the United States, the incidence of this type of cancer has declined dramatically.[1] Although it is now not even one of the 10 most common cancers, it is the eighth leading cause of cancer death. In 2001, approximately 21,700 patients were diagnosed in the United States, of whom more than half are expected to die from the disease.[1] The prognosis of gastric cancer has improved only marginally over the last two decades despite significant improvements in surgical therapy and perioperative care of patients; the impact of recent advances in adjuvant therapy are yet to be realized. The 5-year survival rate for all stages was only 21% between 1989 and 1996, but this is an improvement over the 15% rate seen between 1974 and 1976.[1] The high mortality rate of this disease is a reflection of the relatively aggressive biology of this cancer as well as the advanced stage of disease present when most gastric cancers are diagnosed. Early lesions are usually asymptomatic, incidental findings in patients undergoing endoscopy for another reason and comprise between 8% and 30% of gastric cancers seen in the United States, depending on the population studied and whether single or multiple institutions were studied.[2–5] In large populations, the incidence of early lesions is quite low, which may be due to a combination of both truly advanced disease at presentation and accurate pathologic assessment.

This chapter will discuss the evaluation and management of patients with potentially resectable gastric cancer, the specifics of operative therapy at M. D. Anderson Cancer Center, and the role of adjuvant and neoadjuvant therapy.

### Preoperative Assessment

The evaluation of the patient with gastric cancer includes the following tests and procedures: physical examination, laboratory studies, computerized tomography (CT), endoscopic ultrasound (EUS), and laparoscopy. On physical examination, special attention should be given to palpating for adenopathy in the supraclavicular fossa (Virchow's node), periumbilical area (Sister Joseph's node), and the left axilla (Irish's node).[6] In addition, the abdomen should be palpated for any masses and percussed for ascites. Digital rectal exam should be performed to assess for any masses or a Blummer's shelf. Laboratory studies include CBC, electrolytes, BUN and creatinine, and liver function tests, and tumor markers (CEA, CA125, CA19-9, etc.) may be considered. Computerized tomography of the abdomen and pelvis should be performed to evaluate for liver metastases, ascites, peritoneal nodules, and nodal metastases outside the anticipated field of resection. For lesions of the proximal stomach, CT of the chest is also performed. Endoscopic ultrasound is used in our institution because of our strong emphasis on neoadjuvant therapy to evaluate the T stage of tumors, so that patients with T1 lesions can be offered immediate resection. It also provides a baseline to aid in the assessment of tumor response.[7]

The role of surgery in gastric cancer begins even before the planned resection. The use of laparoscopy for the staging of gastric cancer is a vital component of the complete staging of the patient. Multiple studies have indicated that laparoscopy for patients who have otherwise potentially resectable gastric cancer results in upstaging of one-fifth to one-fourth of patients.[7–11] This occurs principally through the detection of peritoneal disease, which is not otherwise seen on a CT scan. The detection by laparoscopy of liver metastases not seen on a high-quality CT scan should be less than 5%.[8] Another benefit of laparoscopy is that a feeding jejunostomy tube can be placed for nutritional support during neoadjuvant therapy, with minimal morbidity at the time of staging; however, if ascites is identified, the potential benefits of placing a feeding jejunostomy tube should be carefully weighed against the potential risks. Laparoscopy has also been shown to be cost-effective in patient management.[9] When contemplating surgical resection, several factors must be considered, including organ system function (including pulmonary, cardiac, hepatic, and renal) and general performance status. There are some patients who are so frail from other causes that surgical resection cannot be entertained. One must be aware of the increased risk of surgical morbidity and mortality in patients who have evidence of cirrhosis, although there are a few reports of small numbers of patients who have undergone resection with even Child Class C cirrhosis.[12,13] In the study by Isozaki et al.,[13] there was a 10% mortality rate for cirrhotic patients who underwent gastrectomy and a 16% mortality rate in patients who underwent a D2 dissection, which, in the Japanese experience, is extremely high compared to a typical operative mortality rate.[13] The indication for resection must also be carefully determined, whether for potential cure or as a palliative intervention. When considering palliative resection, the degree of symptoms that a patient has must be clearly understood. Most patients who are able to eat but have diminished intake will improve on chemotherapy;[14] thus this is a relative, rather than an absolute, indication. Those patients who are completely obstructed or bleeding significantly obviously should at least be considered for palliative resection. One must have these considerations clearly in mind prior to taking the patient to the operating room, as intraoperative findings may change the intent of a planned operation. A full discussion of palliative care for these patients is beyond the scope of this chapter but we will briefly mention some of the surgical considerations. While some surgeons advocate resection for palliation, the operative mortality rates can be quite significant in this population.[15–17] In addition, a palliative bypass also carries a very high mortality rate and frequently fails to achieve the desired benefit.[16,18]

Additional preparation of the patient for gastrectomy includes consideration of the method of reconstruction with a particular consideration of any previous operations and the extent of luminal resection that may be required. It is generally recommended that a patient who is obstructed and has a dilated stomach be brought into the hospital 2 to 3 days prior to resection for nasogastric (NG) tube suctioning to decompress the stomach.[19] This maneuver will frequently avoid or minimize delayed gastric emptying in the postoperative course for those patients who undergo a subtotal gastrectomy. We routinely use a bowel prep to empty the colon prior to resection. This can almost always be accomplished on an outpatient basis.

## Surgical Considerations

There are a few issues regarding the surgical management of gastric cancer that have been studied extensively (but not always to a satisfactory conclusion) and merit discussion. The major surgical issues include (1) the extent of luminal resection and (2) lymph node dissection. The choice of operation for gastric cancer is dependent upon the location of the tumor, its histologic type, and the stage of disease. Gastrectomy is the most widely used approach for the treatment of invasive gastric cancer, although very early (in situ) tumors can be treated by endoscopic mucosal resection or laparoscopic wedge excision. Particularly in Japan, this technique has gained widespread acceptance for the earliest tumors with a low histologic grade.[20,21] The specimen is carefully analyzed and, if penetration into the submucosa is identified, the patient is then taken for gastrectomy. Given the rarity of these early tumors in the United States and the degree of experience needed to do this well, gastrectomy should be considered only in the most specialized of centers. The choices for gastric resection include total, distal subtotal, and proximal subtotal gastrectomy. The type of node dissection may be limited or quite extensive.

## Luminal Resection

While some authors have recommended total gastrectomy for tumors of the distal stomach, prospective and randomized studies have indicated no survival advantage of a total gastrectomy over a distal subtotal gastrectomy.[22–24] As reported by Gouzi et al.[24] in a prospective randomized trial of 169 patients with antral adenocarcinomas who were resected with curative intent, patients were assigned to total or subtotal gastrectomy and had postoperative mortality rates of 1.3% for total gastrectomy and 3.2% for subtotal gastrectomy. Complication rates and 5-year survival rates were similar for each group. A second prospective trial, by the Italian Gastrointestinal Tumor Study Group, demonstrated 5-year survival rates of 65% and 62% in the subtotal and total gastrectomy groups, respectively.[23] In most series, the quality of life after a subtotal gastrectomy is superior to that after a total gastrectomy, and therefore subtotal gastrectomy should be performed when an adequate margin can be obtained while maintaining a reasonable-sized gastric remnant.[25,26] One should always be mindful of maintaining an adequate blood supply to the remaining stomach such that subtotal gastrectomy with splenectomy can only truly be safely performed with maintenance of the left gastric artery.

For tumors of the proximal stomach and gastroesophageal (GE) junction, the issues become somewhat more difficult. Three types of GE junction tumors (Siewert classification) have been described by Professor Siewert from Munich:[27,28] type I, in which cancer is associated with Barrett's esophagus or there is true esophageal carcinoma growing down to the GE junction; type II, in which tumor is at the true junction (within 2 cm of the squamocolumnar junction); and type III, which denotes tumors of the subcardial region.

The site of origin of a cancer may be unclear in patients who present with adenocarcinoma involving the GE junction, particularly if the tumor is very advanced. Patients with type I tumors should not be considered for a purely transabdominal approach. These patients are best treated by either a gastric pull up to the neck or an Ivor-Lewis procedure. For patients with type II or III tumors, a total gastrectomy with resection of a portion of the lower esophagus may provide a sufficient margin on the esophagus in patients with well- or moderately differentiated histology.

Type II or III tumors can be approached by either a total gastrectomy or a proximal subtotal gastrectomy (either transabdominally or as an Ivor-Lewis procedure), depending on the local extent of the tumor.[29] For lesions that do not invade a significant portion of the esophagus, a total gastrectomy may be the more appropriate operation. There are two main reasons for this: (1) reflux esophagitis is extremely rare after a Roux-en-Y reconstruction, whereas after proximal subtotal resection roughly one-third of patients will have significant reflux;[26,30,31] and (2) proximal subtotal gastrectomy may fail to fully remove the lymph nodes along the lesser curvature, and thus the most common site of nodal metastases may not be fully treated surgically. However, not all authors would agree that total gastrectomy offers fewer quality-of-life problems.[25] For patients whose carcinoma is associated with Barrett's esophagus, the appropriate operation removes more of the esophagus than can be removed from the abdomen. The relative merits of an Ivor-Lewis procedure vs. a pull up to the neck are beyond the scope of this chapter, although it is clear that the morbidity of an anastomotic leak is far greater with the former. For poorly differentiated tumors, removal of a larger segment of the esophagus is generally recommended. Some surgeons have advocated total esophagogastrectomy with colonic interposition for advanced tumors of the GE junction.[32,33] This operation can carry significant morbidity and mortality rates and should be considered in only the most extenuating circumstances, such as previous surgery or other conditions rendering the stomach not suitable for reconstruction. In some circumstances, the jejunum can be brought up as high as the carina or to the neck with supercharging from the carotid and jugular vessels. Again, it is in relatively rare circumstances that such a maneuver would be needed.

## Node Dissection

One of the areas of greatest controversy in the management of stomach cancer revolves around the issue of lymph node dissection. The Japanese, among others, have strongly advocated the use of radical lymph node dissection, including removal of periaortic lymph nodes. The Japanese Research Society for Gastric Cancer has divided the draining lymph basins into 16 stations, including 6 perigastric stations as well as 10 additional stations along the adjacent major vessels, behind the pancreas, and along the aorta. Retrospective studies from Japan suggest that extended lymphadenectomy can improve survival, with perioperative mortality rates of 1%.[34,35] Similar results have been seen in the prospective study by the German Gastric Cancer Study Group.[36] This therapeutic benefit appears greatest for patients with stages II or IIIA. The extent of lymph node dissection is defined by the designation *D*. A D1 dissection includes just the perigastric lymph nodes. A classic D2 dissection also includes nodes along the hepatic, left gastric, celiac, and splenic arteries as well as those in the splenic hilum. Dissections including nodes along the porta hepatis and periaortic regions are classified as D3. A study by Robertson et al.[37] from Hong Kong found no benefit to performing a D3 dissection over performing a D1. Most Western surgeons would agree that lymph node metastases to the periaortic and porta hepatis regions constitute distant disease and thus routine removal of nodes in these areas is not recommended.

Two large prospective randomized trials comparing results from D1 dissection with those from D2 dissection have been conducted in Western patients.[38,39] The Dutch trial relied heavily on input from a Japanese surgeon, Professor Mitsuro Sasako, from the National Cancer Center in Tokyo.[38] He trained the Dutch surgeons in the technique of radical lymph node dissection, and surgical quality control was carefully scrutinized in this study. The Dutch trial failed to show any benefit for extended lymph node dissection; however, it did demonstrate marked increases in the morbidity and mortality rates with radical lymph node dissection. Careful review of the data from this study, however, reveals that the principal increase in mortality rate was associated with either the male gender undergoing a more extensive dissection or those patients undergoing splenectomy and distal pancreatectomy to effect a complete node dissection. The British also found a similar increase in morbidity associated with splenectomy and distal pancreatectomy in the Medical Research Council trial.[39] The Japanese have routinely employed the use of splenectomy to achieve complete node dissection and have not demonstrated increased morbidity with this maneuver. A large prospective randomized trial in Japan attempting to address this issue is scheduled to begin later this year.

The Dutch trial also compared the risk of recurrence in patients who underwent the more extensive lymph node dissection and survived the operation with that for those who had a D1 dissection. The risk of recurrence was significantly less in the radical dissection group. This has not, however, translated into a survival advantage. In its design, the Dutch trial was based on the assumption that the lymph node dissection would increase the survival rate from 20% to 32%. Surprisingly, 40% of the patients in this study presented with early gastric cancer. In addition, the investigators may have overestimated the potential benefit of extended lymph node dissection. The anticipated benefit of extended lymph node dissection can be calculated by multiplying the frequency of lymph node metastases at a certain site in patients with gastric cancer by the survival of patients with known metastases at those sites. Such a study was undertaken by Sasako et al.[40] and indicated that the incidence of splenic hilar lymph node metastasis is roughly 10% and the survival rate is 10% for patients with positive nodes in that site, therefore, the potential survival benefit of removing those nodes is only 1%. For lymph nodes along the common hepatic, celiac, and left gastric sites, these numbers are slightly higher. Thus, the overall survival benefit to an extended lymph node dissection may be more on the order of 5%–8%, which is less than the added mortality rates seen with this procedure in both the Dutch and MRC trials. Therefore, we believe that aggressive lymph node dissection should only be performed by surgeons who have extremely low operative morbidity and mortality rates for this procedure. The group from Memorial, with a 1.8% mortality rate, has demonstrated such results.[5] Data from the American College of Surgeons would indicate that the risk of mortality, however, is significantly higher across the United States.[41]

Brief mention should be made here of linitis plastica. This extremely virulent form of gastric cancer is considered incurable by many clinicians and some feel these patients should never be subjected to a gastrectomy.[42] At best, 5-year survival rates are in the single-digit range.

The American College of Surgeons has conducted several large studies of patterns of care across the United States.[2,43] Data from these studies have demonstrated the need for careful evaluation of the resected specimen for proper staging. In one American College of Surgeons study, one-third of the patients failed to have any lymph nodes reported in the resected specimen. A similar finding was seen in the Intergroup 0116 trial of adjuvant therapy.[44] This is likely a combination of a less aggressive operation and a reflection of lack of thoroughness (perhaps reflecting a nihilistic perspective) on the part of the pathologist.

The most recent revision of the American Joint Committee on Cancer/International Union (AJCC/UICC) staging systems was published in 1997 (Table 25–1). T stage for the primary tumor

**Table 25–1** AJCC/UICC gastric cancer stage groupings

| T Stage | N Stage | | | |
|---------|---------|------|------|-----|
|         | 0       | 1    | 2    | 3   |
| 1       | IA      | IB   | II   | IV  |
| 2       | IB      | II   | IIIA | IV  |
| 3       | II      | IIIA | IIIB | IV  |
| 4       | IIIA    | IIIB | IV   | IV  |

is defined as follows: T1 disease is confined to the mucosa or submucosa; T2 extends into the muscularis propria; T3 penetrates the serosa; and T4 tumors directly invade adjacent organs. The most significant change was with respect to the delineation of nodal stage. The most recent AJCC staging system reflects the importance of the number of lymph nodes retrieved in a specimen. It is imperative that at least 15 lymph nodes be examined in the specimen. The nodal staging is now divided into four groups: N0, no positive nodes; N1, 1–6 lymph nodes with tumor; N2, 7–15 lymph nodes with tumor; and N3, more than 15 lymph nodes with tumor. It should be noted that N3 disease is considered stage IV disease in the current staging system.

## Technique of Resection

This section will deal only with patients undergoing a subtotal or total gastrectomy and will not discuss the Ivor-Lewis procedure or pull-up procedures for lesions invading the esophagus.

Once a patient is taken to the operating room for a gastrectomy, the patient is placed in the supine position. A mid-line incision is created from the ziphiod to the umbilicus. The falciform ligament is resected, including the associated fat pad. We prefer a Buchwalter retractor system, which provides excellent exposure. While many surgeons have used a bilateral subcostal or chevron incision for total gastrectomy, these are associated with a greater degree of postoperative pain than is a mid-line incision and provide no better access to the upper abdomen. Exploration is again performed to confirm the absence of metastatic disease. The omentum is then dissected off the transverse colon. Some surgeons prefer to perform what is termed an *omental bursectomy* (resecting the anterior leaf off of the transverse mesocolon and the peritoneum off of the pancreas). The stated reason for this is to effect the resection of microscopic peritoneal metastases that might be present there. This, however, is difficult to justify, since any subtotal gastrectomy leaves a portion of the lesser sac, regardless of what type of resection has been performed, and there is no evidence that total gastrectomy (which would be required to remove the entire omental bursa) is a better oncologic procedure. Also, it is extremely optimistic to believe that a resection of microscopic carcinomatosis in and of itself provides any survival advantage. The omentum is resected with the specimen, primarily since the blood supply to the omentum is severely compromised with a gastrectomy.

With the omentum completely reflected superiorly, dissection commences in the left side of the abdomen with identification of the left gastroepiploic vessels and ligation of these. The spleen is pulled down into the operative site with moist packs placed behind it to minimize the risk of injury to the spleen and provide better visualization. The patient is placed in a slight reverse Trendelenberg position to allow gravity to help with exposure. Dissection continues over to the greater curvature of the stomach if a subtotal gastrectomy is planned, or continues cephalad, dividing the short gastric vessels, if a total gastrectomy is to be performed. Once the left side of the stomach has been fully mobilized, dissection of the omentum continues over to the right, and at a point near the hepatic flexure of the colon the omentum is divided up to the duodenum. The right gastroepiploic vein is then identified entering into the middle colic vein and is divided; at this point, there is a packet of lymph nodes adjacent to the right gastric epiploic artery as it arises off the gastroduodenal artery. These nodes are dissected up with the specimen and the artery is ligated. The right gastric vessels are divided near the hepatic

artery and the duodenum is then fully mobilized. With the duodenum elevated, the fatty attachments along the inferior border are ligated with 3-0 silks. Cautery should not be used here, as these vessels are fragile and tend to bleed.

The duodenum is then transected, typically using a stapler. Usually we do not invert the staple line, even though some surgeons may advocate this; however, good blood supply to the duodenum is perhaps the most important factor for adequate healing of the stump. The gastrohepatic ligament is divided with electrocautery, using great care to watch for the presence of an accessory or replaced left hepatic artery. These can almost always be taken with impunity; however, if the vessel is extremely large, a test clamping should be performed.

The stomach is retracted superiorly and dissection then commences across the superior border of the pancreas, reflecting a nodal bearing tissue in a cephalad direction. The left gastric vein is identified, ligated, and divided. This vein may be either in front of or behind the hepatic artery and is quite fragile, so great care should be taken in its dissection.

The dissection continues toward the gastroduodenal artery. The nodal-bearing tissue is reflected cephalad across the hepatic artery. Dissection continues out the splenic artery to the posterior gastric artery, arising from the splenic artery and providing blood supply to the upper posterior-medial wall of the stomach. The left gastric artery is identified at its origin and divided. The nodal-bearing tissue around the celiac axis is dissected back to the crux of the diaphragm. Dissection continues to the right border of the esophagus.

For a subtotal gastrectomy, the nodal-bearing tissue along the right cardia is dissected off the GE junction and upper stomach. All the right cardia nodes are resected even with a subtotal gastrectomy. At this point, for a subtotal resection, a point at least 5 cm proximal to the upper border of the tumor is then selected and the stomach is transected using a stapler, thus concluding a subtotal gastrectomy.

For a total gastrectomy, dissection continues up to the esophagus and, again, a proximal margin of at least 5 cm is performed. If greater exposure of the esophagus is needed, the diaphragm is divided with electrocautery. If still more exposure is needed, the left phrenic vein is suture ligated and divided, providing ample exposure of much of the distal esophagus. Stay sutures of 2-0 silk are placed in the esophagus prior to the transection of the esophagus. It is important to remember to obtain frozen-section analyses of the margins of resection.

## Reconstruction

Two types of reconstruction will be considered here: one for subtotal gastrectomy, and another for total gastrectomy. The principal options for reconstruction after subtotal gastrectomy include a loop (Bilroth II) reconstruction and a Roux-en-Y reconstruction, the latter being our preferred method. Additional loops, pouches, and various reconstructions have been previously described; however, the first two mentioned above are the most common. A loop reconstruction can be performed either at the staple line or by removing the staple line and creating an end of stomach–to–side of small bowel anastomosis. This is typically closed with a two-layer anastomosis (although classic descriptions discuss a three-layer closure). In such situations, we use an inner layer of running 3-0 PDS suture and an outer layer of 3-0 silk Lembert sutures. Frequently, however, we employ a Roux-en-Y reconstruction; roughly 25 cm distal to the ligament of

Treitz, the small bowel is divided and a vascularized pedicle of small bowel is then brought up to the posterior wall of the stomach. This is aligned in such a fashion that a stapled side-to-side anastomosis is created with the tip of the small bowel directed toward the left shoulder. For either anastomosis, it is important to make sure that the anastomosis is at least 6 cm in length to provide optimal emptying of the gastric remnant.[45] To avoid delayed gastric emptying, it is also important to make sure that the gastric remnant left in place is not too large. With Roux-en-Y reconstruction the difficult problem of bile reflux is avoided, which can occur with a Bilroth II reconstruction. The enteroenterostomy is created roughly 45 cm downstream from the gastrojejunostomy. This is performed in a side-to-side fashion with a short defunctionalized side limb, through which a feeding jejunostomy tube may be placed.

The reconstruction of a total gastrectomy can be (but does not need to be) a bit more elaborate than that for a subtotal gastrectomy. The most common reconstruction is the Roux-en-Y reconstruction. This is usually accomplished in an end of esophagus–to–side of jejunum fashion. This anastomosis can be performed with a circular stapler or by sewing in either two layers or one layer, as is our preferred approach. The principal reason for using sewing is a lower rate of anastomotic stricture than with stapling. Leak rates from either sewn or stapled anastomoses are generally equivalent.[46] One other important consideration is that even surgeons who routinely staple an anastomosis will need to perform a sewn anastomosis in roughly 10% of cases. Additional reconstruction options include a Roux-en-Y with a pouch or a jejunal interposition. Unfortunately, the loop reconstructions do not always bypass bile from the esophagojejunostomy and thus a significant incidence of reflux esophagitis can result. For this reason, we do not recommend this reconstruction.

For many years there has been controversy regarding the optimal nutritional reconstructions and the benefits of pouches over a standard Roux-en-Y reconstruction, with results both for and against pouch reconstructions.[30,47–49] One reconstruction, which does make intuitive sense, is a jejunal interposition; however, studies of this technique have not been conclusive.[50] In this technique, a 45-cm segment of small bowel is used, which is interposed between the esophagus and the duodenum, thus creating three anastomoses in series (esophagojejunostomy, duodenojejunostomy, and jejunojejunostomy), the greatest disadvantage of this form of reconstruction. However, patients tend to lose less body weight and certainly have a lower incidence of cholelithiasis and perhaps a better functional result. We consider this reconstruction in patients with extremely early gastric cancers or in patients who otherwise would run into nutritional problems, such as those with a previous bowel resection, since this reconstruction maintains the normal path of food.

The most common reconstruction performed for total gastrectomy is a Roux-en-Y. This is done in a similar fashion to that described above for subtotal gastrectomy, with the exception that the anastomosis is performed to the esophagus in a single layer with 3-0 GI silk sutures. The NG tube is passed across the anastomosis and used to test the anastomosis with air under water prior to completion of the procedure. Postoperatively, we do not routinely obtain a contrast study, but if the patient has unexplained tachycardia or fever or is slow to regain intestinal function, one will be obtained. Typically, the NG tube is removed when there is evidence of bowel function and low output from the NG tube. Otherwise, it is left in for 5–7 days. At this point, the NG tube is removed and the patient is begun on clear liquids and advanced to a post-gastrectomy diet. The nuances of dietary

management of the post-gastrectomy patient in the resumption of oral intake are beyond the scope of this chapter. However, suffice it to say that management of dumping and overcoming the transient loss of appetite are not trivial difficulties to overcome. Many patients may experience fatty food intolerance and increased gas. The feeding jejunostomy tube is removed when the patient no longer requires it for the maintenance of nutrition. This usually takes anywhere from 6–12 weeks. In addition, the feeding jejunostomy tube is an excellent insurance policy for those times when the patient develops a leak and prolonged nothing-by-mouth (NPO) status is required.

## Combined Modality Therapies

### Adjuvant Therapy

*Adjuvant therapy* is treatment given after a potentially curative resection to reduce or eliminate the possibility of recurrence of the cancer at any site. Treatments may include chemotherapy, immunotherapy, radiotherapy, or any combination of these.

### Chemotherapy

The sites of failure after a potentially curative resection can be divided into locoregional (nodal or gastric bed) and distant (liver, peritoneum, nodes, bone, lung, or brain). While many patients fail with peritoneal and/or liver metastases, locoregional recurrence is a significant site of failure. In a reoperative series by Gunderson and Sosin,[51] locoregional recurrence was a component of failure in 88% of patients and was the only site of failure in 45% of patients. Locoregional failure includes any recurrence in the gastric remnant or anastomosis, the bed of resection, or regional nodal basins. In an effort to improve survival from gastric cancer, researchers have sought for many years to develop reliable adjuvant therapy. Initial studies seemed to hold some promise but confirmatory trials failed to confirm the marginal benefits seen. There have been at least 20 prospective randomized trials of adjuvant chemotherapy (or immunochemotherapy) with a surgery-alone control arm in Western or Asian countries. A meta-analysis performed by Hermans et al.[52] in 1993 evaluated 11 prospective randomized trials with over 2000 patients and, after discounting a highly positive single agent trial from the Barcelona group, concluded there was no benefit to adjuvant therapy.[52–54] This study, however, had failed to consider a few other published studies and was heavily criticized. A reanalysis[53] published the following spring suggested a statistically significant benefit to adjuvant therapy, although no specific regimen could be recommended (the odds ratio decreased from 0.88 to 0.67). Obviously, it could be concluded that any benefits of adjuvant chemotherapy are modest at best.

### Chemoradiotherapy

The results of Intergroup Study INT-0116, the most exciting news in the field of gastric cancer, were initially reported by MacDonald at the 2000 American Society of Clinical Oncology (ASCO) meeting and were recently published.[44] This study demonstrated a highly significant survival advantage to the adjuvant therapy used. Patients were randomized after a potentially curative operation to receive either observation or chemoradiation (5-fluorouracil [5-FU]/leucovorin before, during, and after 45 Gy external beam radiation therapy). Over 600 patients were entered into the study, and the patients randomized to the treatment arm had a median survival of 31 months vs. 19 months for the surgery-alone arm ($P < 0.001$) with a median follow-up of 3.3 years. The 3-year disease-free survival rate and overall survival rate were both significantly better with combined therapy than with surgery alone (67% vs. 53%, $P = 0.001$, and 60% vs. 50%, $P = 0.03$, respectively). While treatment-related toxicity was acceptable and treatment-related mortality was 1%, only 65% of patients randomized to the treatment arm completed the therapy as prescribed. Many of the clinicians in the United States who are caring for patients with gastric cancer have accepted this regimen as the new standard of care; however, not everyone shares this sentiment. The argument is offered that this treatment is simply making up for inadequate surgery, as evidenced by the disturbingly high number of patients in this study without any nodes reported in the pathologic report of the resected specimen.

## Neoadjuvant Therapy

*Neoadjuvant therapy* is treatment given before an anticipated definitive surgery. This may be any of the previously mentioned types of therapy, but is frequently a combination of modalities. There are several theoretical reasons for introducing systemic therapy as the first phase of treatment. If the tumor stage is such that there is a high probability that occult metastatic disease is present, initial introduction of chemotherapy may expose micrometastatic disease to the drug when cell growth fraction is high. There is also less tumor cell heterogeneity (i.e., fewer drug-resistant cells), and oxygenation is optimal. Major surgery may delay the introduction of systemic treatment by at least 4 to 6 weeks or, if complications occur, may preclude the ability to treat the patient. In addition, the doses of drug that can be tolerated may be less in patients (especially elderly patients) who are trying to recover from major surgery.

Because of a prolonged postoperative course after gastrectomy, approximately 25% to 35% of patients would never be able to receive adjuvant therapy in a meaningful time frame. The ability to monitor the primary tumor response to neoadjuvant therapy provides very useful information regarding the potential benefits of additional treatment after surgical resection or whether any such treatment should be continued. A significant response in the primary tumor may provide greater insurance of microscopically negative margins at the time of resection by downstaging the tumor.

In rectal cancer, induction chemotherapy and radiation appear to have resulted in increased sphincter preservation, and what was initially intended as neoadjuvant therapy has become the definitive therapy for squamous cell carcinoma of the anal canal. The use of neoadjuvant therapy also appears to be widespread in the treatment of locally advanced breast cancer. An additional benefit of neoadjuvant therapy is that patients who rapidly progress with metastatic disease during induction therapy avoid an unnecessary gastric resection, as these patients almost certainly would not benefit from radical surgery.

## Chemotherapy

Since Wilke, et al.[55] initially reported 34 patients who underwent surgical exploration and were found to have locally advanced unresectable disease, then underwent chemotherapy, and subsequently were re-explored for resection, this combined-modality approach has slowly gained favor. The authors used a combination of etoposide, doxorubicin, and cisplatin (EAP) and found a pathologic complete response (CR) of 15%. This study demonstrated the feasibility of using neoadjuvant chemotherapy in advanced gastric adenocarcinoma. Nakajima et al.[56] found improved survival in patients who were felt to have incurable gastric cancer but responded to treatment with a combination of intravenous 5-FU and leucovorin followed by intraarterial cisplatin and etoposide. There were some long-term survivors among the patients treated by curative surgery after neoadjuvant chemotherapy, thus again demonstrating the importance of downstaging to permit surgical resection in this group of patients.

At M. D. Anderson Cancer Center, we have studied neoadjuvant approaches to the management of gastric cancer for roughly 15 years.[14,57] Our experience with neoadjuvant therapy (using combined etoposide, leucovorin and 5-FU) has progressed from an initial (and admittedly tentative) two cycles of preoperative chemotherapy with three cycles of postoperative therapy for patients whose tumors responded. Surgeons were initially very concerned over the potential risk for increased complications, but as both the surgeons and medical oncologists gained comfort with the neoadjuvant approach, the courses of neoadjuvant therapy were increased to three and ultimately up to five cycles of chemotherapy for patients responding to therapy. The last completed protocol of neoadjuvant chemotherapy alone consisted of 5-FU, interferon, and cisplatin (FIP). Only those patients whose tumor demonstrated a response to therapy continued therapy up to a total of five courses. An evaluation was performed of the 83 patients with pathologically confirmed gastric adenocarcinoma who were treated with these three consecutive phase II neoadjuvant chemotherapy protocols.[58] Upper gastrointestinal series, endoscopy, CT, and pathologic examination were used to assess response. Only in the last group (FIP) was the complete response level of 10% reached. On univariate analysis, T stage, number of positive lymph nodes, and response to chemotherapy were significant predictors of survival, while on multivariate analysis, only response to chemotherapy was found to be an independent predictor of survival. At Memorial Sloan Kettering Cancer Center, Kelsen[59] has combined neoadjuvant systemic chemotherapy with intraperitoneal postoperative therapy. Lenz and Metzger et al.[60,61] have examined the use of neoadjuvant therapy as well as the utility of predictors of response to therapy. They found that elevated levels of thymidilate synthase (TS) and elevated levels of ERCC-1 predicted a poor outcome in response to 5-FU and cisplatin therapies, respectively. The only reported prospective randomized trial of neoadjuvant chemotherapy was a small study from the Dutch Gastric Cancer Group.[62] This study, which started with fewer than 30 patients in each arm (and after exclusion of patients with metastatic disease had fewer than 20 patients in each arm), was grossly underpowered and, not surprisingly, was a negative study. In addition, what is currently considered an ineffective therapy, FAMTX (5-FU, Adriamycin, and methotrexate), was used. There are a few prospective randomized trials of neoadjuvant therapy currently accruing patients, including the EORTC-40954 study, which is comparing results from surgery alone with those from neoadjuvant chemotherapy plus resection for locally advanced gastric cancer. Patients in this study must be considered to be resectable and have at least clinical stage II disease. Patients are randomized to undergo immediate resection or receive two courses of bolus cisplatin every 2 weeks for 6 weeks and bolus 5-FU plus leucovorin weekly for 5 weeks, followed by surgery.

## Radiotherapy

Radiotherapy has been used extensively in the management of cancers of the rectum, esophagus, and head and neck, among other sites. The Intergroup 0116 study was the first to use chemo-radiotherapy in a large study in the adjuvant treatment of gastric cancer. There have been several studies of the use of intraoperative radiotherapy for gastric cancer, most notably the work by Abe et al.[63] and Sindelar et al.[64] Both investigators demonstrated decreased local recurrence rates and Abe suggested a survival advantage.

The earliest studies of radiation with or without chemotherapy were in the 1960s in patients who were not considered curable. In 1998, Zhang et al.,[65] from Beijing, reported the results of a large prospective randomized trial (370 patients) of neoadjuvant radiotherapy in patients with resectable cancer of the gastric cardia. One hundred seventy-one patients were randomized to receive radiotherapy plus surgery and 199 patients were randomized to receive surgery alone. Radiation at 40 Gy was delivered to the cardia, lower segment of the esophagus, fundus, lesser curvature, and hepatogastric ligament, and surgery was conducted 2 to 4 weeks later. The 5-year survival rates were 30.1% for the radiotherapy-plus-surgery group and 19.8% for the surgery-alone group. The survival difference was significant by Kaplan-Meier analysis, with $P = 0.0094$. Interestingly the operative mortality rate was lower in the group undergoing radiation than in the surgery-alone group (0.6% vs. 2.5%). Local failure rates were lower in the radiotherapy group. The authors concluded that there was a survival advantage to using preoperative radiotherapy.

## Chemoradiation

Numerous studies have demonstrated a significant improvement in the effectiveness of radiotherapy when combined with chemotherapy for tumors of the rectum as well as other sites. Moertel et al.[66] reported a randomized trial in 48 patients with locally advanced unresectable gastric cancer, comparing treatment with 35 to 40 Gy external beam radiation with 5-FU to treatment with radiotherapy alone. Median survival was significantly greater in the combined-modality arm. Another study by the Gastrointestinal Tumor Study Group (GITSG) supported this finding.[67] Split-course radiation (50 Gy) given with 5-FU followed by maintenance 5-FU, methotrexate, and Lomustine resulted in a 4-year survival rate of 18%, compared with 6% for the radiation-alone arm. During the mid-1990s we began a pilot study of neoadjuvant chemoradiation for patients with potentially resectable disease.[68] Patients were confirmed to be potentially resectable by CT scan, EUS, and staging laparoscopy. This treatment combined a low dose (300 mg/m²/day) of continuous infusion 5-FU with 45 Gy of external beam radiotherapy given in 25 fractions. Twenty-four patients with potentially resectable but poor-prognosis tumors (at least T2 tumors by EUS) were treated, and all but 1 patient were able to complete therapy, although a few patients required a dose reduction because of toxicity. Nearly 90% of the patients completed the full therapy as prescribed. The feasibility of this treatment was established and a larger phase II study was begun. The preliminary survival data from the two studies were reported at the ASCO in 2000. Of the 44 patients enrolled, 39 had EUS successfully completed, and all of the tumors were stage T2 or greater (82% were T3 or T4). Radiation fields included the entire stomach (including the primary tumor) and regional lymph nodes. Patients were restaged with CT 4 to 6 weeks following treatment and prior to planned resection. All resected patients underwent a spleen-preserving D2 gastrectomy and received 10 Gy of intraoperative radiation. Forty-three patients (97%) completed chemoradiation. Upon

restaging, nine patients (20%) were found to have distant disease and did not require any palliative surgical procedure. Thirty-two patients (73%) underwent resection; 2 patients refused resection. Five patients (11%) had pathologic complete responses, while 18 patients (41%) had partial responses with evidence of downstaging as compared to preoperative EUS. There was one postoperative death (3%) from aspiration and four patients required reoperation. There were four symptomatic leaks, two from esophageal anastomoses and two duodenal stump leaks. With a minimum follow-up of 9 months, overall median survival was 34 months, with disease-specific survival being >60% at 4 years in resected patients.

## Chemotherapy and Chemoradiation

After the feasibility of neoadjuvant chemoradiation (CTX/XRT) was demonstrated in the pilot study and the encouraging pathologic complete responses were seen, an additional neoadjuvant study combining two courses of systemic doses of chemotherapy followed by CTX/XRT was begun. This study, which combined two cycles of 5-FU, cisplatin, and leucovorin, was followed by CTX/XRT as described above. This study has completed accrual and is maturing prior to analysis.

## Conclusions

We have found that response to therapy is the single most important prognostic factor for patients with potentially resectable gastric cancer undergoing neoadjuvant chemotherapy. Whether this is also true for patients receiving chemoradiation or chemotherapy plus chemoradiation is yet to be determined. Well-conceived and conducted randomized trials are clearly needed. The reasons to utilize neoadjuvant therapy are several:

1. Despite an excellent cancer operation, a subset of patients (roughly 10%) will develop aggressive disease that will recur very quickly after gastrectomy and will thus never really benefit from surgical resection.
2. The magnitude of gastric resection is significant enough that up to one-third of patients may not recover from the operation quickly enough to receive any potential adjuvant therapy.
3. Patients with gastric cancer do not typically die of local disease, but rather from disseminated disease. Therefore, treatment of disseminated disease as early as possible would make the most sense. Waiting until after resection could delay such treatment by several months.
4. A neoadjuvant approach allows one to monitor the patient's response to treatment and can be useful in determining if treatment should continue.
5. Treatment is generally better tolerated in patients who have not yet undergone a gastric resection. After gastrectomy, the patient's ability to tolerate the stress of therapy is markedly diminished. In our series, the completion rate for therapy is in excess of 90%, compared to rates of 60%–70% in the adjuvant setting.

While there have been many important advances in the management of gastric cancer, it remains a difficult disease to manage well. Better systemic therapy agents are needed both for patients presenting with unresectable disease and for those with resectable disease who are likely to fail. The surgical management, like other complex upper abdominal procedures, can be performed with low operative morbidity and mortality rates at specialized centers. One must carefully consider the disease being treated before embarking on the specific treatment plan (and considering any available clinical protocols) for the patient with gastric cancer.

## References

1. Greenlee RT, et al. Cancer statistics 2001. CA Cancer J Clin 51:15, 2001.
2. Wanebo H, et al. Cancer of the stomach: a patient care study by the American College of Surgeons. Ann Surg 218:583–592, 1993.
3. Lawrence W Jr, et al. The National Cancer Data Base report on gastric cancer. Cancer 75:1734–1744, 1995.
4. Hundahl SA, Phillips JL, Menck HR. The National Cancer Data Base. Report on poor survival of U.S. gastric carcinoma patients treated with gastrectomy: fifth edition American Joint Committee on Cancer staging, proximal disease, and the "different disease" hypothesis. Cancer 88:921–932, 2000.
5. Karpeh MS, et al. Lymph node staging in gastric cancer: is location more important than number? An analysis of 1,038 patients. Ann Surg 232:362–371, 2000.
6. Davis GR. Neoplasms of the stomach. In: Sleisenger MH, Fordtran JS (eds): Gastrointestinal Disease: Pathophysiology Diagnosis Management. W.B. Saunders, Philadelphia, 1989, p 754.
7. Feussner H, et al. Pretherapeutic laparoscopic staging in advanced gastric carcinoma. Endoscopy 31:342–347, 1999.
8. Lowy A, et al. Staging laparoscopy in potentially resectable gastric cancer. Surgery 119:611–614, 1996.
9. Burke EC, et al. Laparoscopy in the management of gastric adenocarcinoma. Ann Surg 225:262–267, 1997.
10. Possik R, et al. Sensitivity, specificity, and predictive value of laparoscopy for the staging of gastric cancer and for the detection of liver metastases. Cancer 58:1–6, 1986.
11. Stell D, et al. Prospective comparison of laparascopy, ultrasonography and computed tomography in the staging of gastric cancer. Br J Surg 83:1260–1262, 1996.
12. Lorusso D, et al. Complications after elective gastric resection for duodenal ulcer: multivariate analysis of risk factors. Acta Chir Belg 956:247–250, 1995.
13. Isozaki H, et al. Surgery for gastric cancer in patients with chirrhosis. Jpn J Surg 27:17–21, 1997.
14. Ajani JA, et al. Resectable gastric carcinoma, an evaluation of preoperative and postoperative chemotherapy. Cancer 68:1501–1506, 1991.
15. Ellis FH Jr, Gibb SP, Watkins E Jr. Esophagogastrectomy. A safe, widely applicable, and expeditious form of palliation for patients with carcinoma of the esophagus and cardia. Ann Surg 198:531–540, 1983.
16. Meijer S, De Bakker OJ, Hoitsma HF. Palliative resection in gastric cancer. J Surg Oncol, 232:77–80, 1983.
17. Ekbom GA, Gleysteen JJ. Gastric malignancy: resection for palliation. Surgery 884:476–481, 1980.
18. Kikuchi S, et al. Does gastrojejunostomy for unresectable cancer of the gastric antrum offer satisfactory palliation? Hepatogastroenterology 46(25):584–587, 1999.
19. Hocking MP. Postoperative delayed gastric emptying. In: Wickland E (ed): Postgastrectomy Syndromes. W.B. Saunders, Philadelphia, 1991, pp 63–77.
20. Nishi M, et al. Chronological changes of characteristics of early gastric cancer and therapy: experience in the Cancer Institute Hospital of Tokyo, 1950–1994. J Cancer Res Clin Oncol 121(9–10):535–541, 1995.
21. Maruyama K, et al. Surgical treatment for gastric cancer: the Japanese approach. Semin Oncol 233:360–368, 1996.
22. Meyer H, et al. Surgical treatment of gastric cancer: retrospective survey of 1704 operated cases with special reference to total gastrectomy as the operation of choice. Semin Surg Oncol 7:356–364, 1991.
23. Bozzetti F, et al. Subtotal versus total gastrectomy for gastric cancer. Five-year survival rates in a multienter randomized Italian trial. Ann Surg 230:170–178, 1999.
24. Gouzi JL, et al. Total versus subtotal gastrectomy for adenocarcinoma of the gastric antrum. Ann Surg 209:162–166, 1989.
25. Anderson ID, MacIntyre IM. Symptomatic outcome following resection of gastric cancer. Surg Oncol 41:35–40, 1995.
26. Bozzetti F. Total versus subtotal gastrectomy in cancer of the distal stomach: facts and fantasy. Eur J Surg Oncol 186:572–579, 1992.
27. Siewert JR, et al. Surgical resection for cancer of the cardia. Semin Surg Oncol 172:125–131, 1999.
28. Siewert JR, et al. Problem of proximal third gastric carcinoma. World J Surg 19:523–531, 1995.
29. Harrison LE, Karpeh MS, Brennan MF. Total gastrectomy is not necessary for proximal gastric cancer. Surgery 1232:127–130, 1998.
30. Buhl K, Schlag P, Herfarth C. Quality of life and functional results following different types of resection for gastric carcinoma. Eur J Surg Oncol 16:404–409, 1990.
31. Jentschura D, et al. Quality of life after curative surgery for gastric cancer: A comparison between total gastrectomy and subtotal gastric resection. Hepatogastroenterology 44:1137–1142, 1997.
32. Saidi FA, et al. A new approach to the palliation of advanced proximal gastric cancer. J Am Coll Surg 1893:259–268, 1999.
33. Stipa S, Di Giorgio A, Ferri M. Surgical treatment of adenocarcinoma of the cardia. Surgery 1114:386–393, 1992.
34. Noguchi Y, et al. Radical surgery for gastric cancer. A review of the Japanese experience. Cancer 64:2053–2062, 1989.
35. Maruyama K, Okabayashi K, Kinoshita T. Progress in gastric cancer surgery in Japan and its limits of radicality. World J Surg 114:418–425, 1987.
36. Roder JD, et al. Prognostic factors in gastric carcinoma: results of the German Gastric Carcinoma Study 1992. Cancer 727:2089–2097, 1993.
37. Robertson CS, et al. A prospective randomized trial comparing $r_1$ subtotal gastrectomy with $r_3$ total gastrectomy for antral cancer. Ann Surg 220:76–182, 1994.
38. Bonenkamp JJ, et al. Extended lymph-node dissection for gastric cancer. Dutch Gastric Cancer Group. N Engl J Med 340:908–914, 1999.
39. Cuschieri A, et al. Patient survival after D1 and D2 resections for gastric cancer: long-term results of the MRC randomized surgical trial. Br J Cancer 79:1522–1530, 1999.
40. Sasako M, et al. New method to evaluate the therapeutic value of lymph node dissection for gastric cancer. Br J Surg 82:346–351, 1995.
41. Wanebo HJ, et al. Role of splenectomy in gastric cancer surgery: adverse effect of elective splenectomy on longterm survival. J Am Coll Surg 185:177–184, 1997.
42. Cady B, et al. Gastric adenocarcinoma: a disease in transition. Arch Surg 124:303–308, 1989.
43. Wanebo HJ, et al.: Gastric carcinoma: does lymph node dissection alter survival. J Am Coll Surg 183:616–624, 1996.
44. Macdonald JS, et al.: Chemoradiotherapy after surgery compared with surgery alone for adenocarcinoma of the stomach or gastroesophageal junction. N Engl J Med 345:725–730, 2001.
45. Doberneck RC, Berndt GA. Delayed gastric emptying after palliative gastrojejunostomy for carcinoma of the pancreas. Arch Surg 122:827–829, 1987.
46. Fujimoto S, et al. Stapled or manual suturing in esophagojejunostomy after total gastrectomy: a comparison of outcome in 379 patients. Am J Surg 162:256–259, 1991.
47. Kalmar K, et al. Comparison of quality of life and nutritional parameters after total gastrectomy and a new type of pouch construction with simple Roux-en-Y reconstruction: preliminary results of a prospective, randomized, controlled study. Dig Dis Sci 46:1791–1796, 2001.
48. Svedlund J, et al. Quality of life after gastrectomy for gastric carcinoma: controlled study of reconstructive procedures. World J Surg 21:422–433, 1997.
49. Bozzetti F, et al. Comparing reconstruction with Roux-en-Y to a pouch following total gastrectomy. J Am Coll Surg 183:243–248, 1996.
50. Nakane Y, et al. A randomized clinical trial of pouch reconstruction after total gastrectomy for cancer: which is the better technique, Roux-en-Y or interposition? Hepatogastroenterology 48(39):903–907, 2001.
51. Gunderson L, Sosin H. Adenocarcinoma of the stomach: areas of failure in a re-operation series (second or symptomatic look) clinicopathologic correlation and implications for adjuvant therapy. Int J Radiat Oncol Biol Phys 8:1–11, 1982.
52. Hermans J, et al. Adjuvant therapy after curative resection for gastric cancer: meta-analysis of randomized trials. J Clin Oncol 11:1441–1447, 1993.
53. Hermans J, Bonenkamp H. Meta-analysis and gastric cancer [corres]. J Clin Oncol 12:879–880, 1994.
54. Estape J, et al. Mitomycin C as an adjuvant treatment to resected gastric cancer. A 10-year follow-up. Ann Surg 213:219–221, 1991.
55. Wilke H, et al. Preoperative chemotherapy in locally advanced and non-resectable gastric cancer: a phase II study with etoposide, doxorubicin, and cisplatin. J Clin Oncol 7:1318–1326, 1989.
56. Nakajima T, et al. Combined intensive chemotherapy and radical surgery for incurable gastric cancer. Ann Surg Oncol 4:203–208, 1997.
57. Ajani JA, et al. Enhanced staging and all chemotherapy preoperatively in patients with potentially resectable gastric carcinoma. J Clin Oncol 17:2403–2411, 1999.
58. Lowy AM, et al. Response to neoadjuvant chemotherapy best predicts survival after curative resection of gastric cancer. Ann Surg 229:303–308, 1999.
59. Kelsen D, et al. Neoadjuvant therapy of high-risk gastric cancer: a phase II trial of preoperative FAMTX and postoperative Intraperitoneal fluo-

rouracil-cisplatin plus intravenous fluorouracil. J Clin Oncol 14:1818–1828, 1996.

60. Lenz HJ, et al. Thymidylate synthase mRNA level in adenocarcinoma of the stomach: a predictor for primary tumor response and overall survival. J Clin Oncol 14:176–182, 1996.

61. Metzger R, et al. ERCC1 mRNA levels complement thymidylate synthase mRNA levels in predicting response and survival for gastric cancer patients receiving combination cisplatin and fluorouracil chemotherapy. J Clin Oncol 16:309–316, 1998.

62. Songun I, et al. Chemotherapy for operable gastric cancer: results of the Dutch randomised FAMTX trial. The Dutch Gastric Cancer Group (DGCG). Eur J Cancer 35:558–562, 1999.

63. Abe M, et al. Intraoperative radiotherapy in carcinoma of the stomach and pancreas. World J Surg 11:459–464, 1987.

64. Sindelar WF, et al. Randomized trial of intraoperative radiotherapy in carcinoma of the stomach. Am J Surg 165:178–187, 1993.

65. Zhang ZX, et al. Randomized clinical trial on the combination of preoperative irradiation and surgery in the treatment of adenocarcinoma of gastric cardia (AGC)—report on 370 patients. Int J Radiat Oncol Biol Phys 42:929–934, 1998.

66. Moertel CG, et al. Combined 5-fluorouracil and supervoltage radiation therapy of locally unresectable gastrointestinal cancer. Lancet 2(7626):865–867, 1969.

67. A comparison of combination chemotherapy and combined modality therapy for locally advanced gastric carcinoma. Gastrointestinal Tumor Study Group. Cancer 49:1771–1777, 1982.

68. Lowy AM, et al. A pilot study of preoperative chemoradiotherapy for resectable gastric cancer. Ann Surg Oncol 8:519–524, 2001.

# Chapter 26

# Locally Advanced Unresectable Gastric Cancer

JEFFREY W. CLARK

Attempted curative resection is the treatment of choice for gastric adenocarcinoma. However, it is not always possible. In Western countries, less than 50% of patients can have potentially curative resections at the time of initial presentation. In Asian countries where the higher incidence of gastric cancer has led to earlier screening and detection of gastric cancer in high-risk individuals and in those with early symptoms, a greater percentage of patients have their disease diagnosed earlier and thus can have potentially curative resections. For patients whose disease cannot be totally resected but is confined to the perigastric region, additional therapeutic options include radiation therapy, chemotherapy, immunotherapy, and supportive care, each of which can be used alone or in combination. For the most part, these approaches are palliative, although a small percentage of patients will have long-term survival. Most patients will have local and systemic disease progression, so therapeutic approaches need to address both of these issues.

Although locally advanced gastric cancer has been defined in a number of ways, in this chapter it is defined as disease that is either locally unresectable or has been resected but gross residual local disease remains, without evident metastatic disease.

## Surgery

Surgical resection remains the major means of palliation in patients with gastric cancer accompanied by significant bleeding, obstruction, pain, or perforation. This is true even in cases of locally advanced disease in which it is not possible to resect all gross disease. Subtotal or total gastrectomies, when feasible, usually provide better palliation and appear to have no greater morbidity or mortality than less extensive surgical procedures such as gastroenteric anastomosis or intubation of the alimentary tract.[1-8] An exception may be patients with extensive hepatic metastases who do not do as well after palliative gastrectomy. The extent of resection for palliation of local symptoms in this setting needs to be carefully considered. If all gross disease can be resected, then resection of adjacent tissues or organs to accomplish this would appear to be reasonable, given the suggestion that patients whose disease can be completely resected may do better after combined modality treatment (see discussion below under Radiation Therapy). However, if there is unresectable metastatic disease or if the disease cannot be totally resected, then resection of adjacent organs would not be indicated unless necessary to palliate symptoms. It is more difficult to provide relief for patients with diffuse involvement of the stomach (e.g., linitus plastica) via resection, although again, when feasible, surgical resection still appears to offer the best palliation for these patients.

Findings at the time of surgery can significantly aid in design of the radiation therapy fields. In addition, clips can be placed to help better define fields for radiation therapy. Given the relatively high incidence of peritoneal metastases not detected by preoperative radiological studies, staging laparoscopy and analysis of peritoneal washings for cytology may help to better define disease status before deciding on the optimal approach for each patient.[6,8]

For patients in whom comorbid factors make palliative resections too great a risk, there are a number of local therapeutic approaches that can provide palliation. These include direct ethanol injection, laser treatment, phototherapy, endoluminal stents, or gastrostomy tubes.[9-14] Although each of these approaches can offer some palliation, the relief is usually temporary. There is no clear-cut evidence that one of these approaches is superior to the others in all cases, and the decision as to which one to pursue depends on the patient and the available local expertise. There are ongoing efforts attempting to improve each of these approaches.

## Radiation Therapy

Radiation therapy has been evaluated both alone and in combination with chemotherapy, usually 5-fluorouracil (5-FU)–based regimens, as treatment for patients with gastric cancers that cannot be completely resected. Radiation therapy can also help palliate symptoms of bleeding, obstruction, or pain in patients who are not surgical candidates. 5-FU has the benefit of being both a reasonable radiation sensitizer and an active agent against gastric adenocarcinoma. There is some evidence that a combination of chemotherapy and radiation therapy may be better at prolonging survival than either radiation therapy or chemotherapy alone in this setting.[15–23] However, the difference in survival is relatively small, measured in months. The use of radiation in this setting is affected by the amount of tumor present and by the limited tolerance of the stomach and surrounding tissues for irradiation. For this reason, it is usually preferable to use radiation in conjunction with palliative gastric resections whenever feasible.

Reports of nonrandomized series from several institutions have suggested that a small subset of patients who undergo gastric resections but have residual disease (either gross or microscopic) may achieve longer survival after combined chemotherapy and radiation than those who cannot be resected.[16,19–21] Retrospective analysis suggests that survival is better for those patients who have only microscopic residual disease after surgery and are subsequently treated with radiation therapy and chemotherapy.[20,21]

Studies have attempted to identify what role radiation and chemotherapy each play in the benefits of combined-modality therapy. Several randomized studies have shown that a combination of 5-FU–based regimens and radiation therapy provide a survival advantage over radiation alone in treating patients with residual or unresectable gastric cancers. For example, a randomized Mayo Clinic study showed an improvement in both mean and overall survival for patients who received combined-modality therapy.[15] The median survival was approximately 5 months and the 5-year survival rate was 0% for patients who received radiation alone. For those who received combined therapy, the median survival was approximately 7 months and the 5-year survival rate was 12%.

Studies have also addressed the question of whether combined radiation therapy and chemotherapy provides an advantage over chemotherapy alone. An initial Gastrointestinal Tumor Study Group (GITSG) study showed that combined radiation therapy and chemotherapy provided better results than chemotherapy alone.[16] In that study, the median survival was 9 months in the chemotherapy-alone arm and 17 months in the combined modality arm. Eighteen percent of patients were alive 2 to 4 years after treatment in the combined modality arm compared to 7% in the chemotherapy-alone arm. However, a subsequent GITSG study did not show any additional benefit for combined therapy over chemotherapy alone.[24] The relatively small size of studies done to date, as well as the evolution of chemotherapy regimens over time, leaves the question open of whether the addition of radiation therapy to chemotherapy offers a survival advantage over chemotherapy alone.

At the present time, combined-modality therapy (5-FU–based chemotherapy and radiation therapy) for patients with residual local disease remains one of the standard therapeutic approaches when it is feasible in light of comorbid factors. Given the need for better therapy for these patients, further clinical trials evaluating chemotherapy alone and combined-modality therapy in this setting are warranted. Chemotherapeutic agents other than 5-FU that have radiosensitizing properties and are active against gastric cancer (e.g., platinum compounds, taxanes, and irinotecan) need to be further evaluated in combination with radiation therapy (see discussion below under Future Directions).[25,26] In addition, various combinations of agents need to be evaluated as part of combined-modality approaches to determine which of these provides the greatest benefit in terms of palliating symptoms and prolonging survival.

The role of other radiation therapy approaches, such as intraoperative radiation therapy (IORT) alone or in combination with chemotherapy, in this setting is still being defined. Small nonrandomized studies have suggested that a small percentage of patients treated with IORT at the time of incomplete surgical resection survive 5 years.[27–29] However, there are no data from randomized trials showing a survival benefit for the addition of IORT in this setting. Therefore, continued evaluation of IORT in this setting is necessary before it can be considered a component of standard treatment.

## Chemotherapy

A number of chemotherapeutic agents have antitumor activity against gastric cancer. These include 5-FU (and related compounds), anthracyclines (e.g., doxorubicin and epirubicin), platinum compounds (cisplatin and oxaliplatin), mitomycin C, taxanes (e.g., docetaxel and paclitaxel), etoposide, irinotecan, and methotrexate (Table 26–1).[30–40] Various combinations of these have been explored and are continuing to be investigated. The combination of epirubicin, cisplatin, and infusional 5-FU (with or without leucovorin) (ECF) is one of the most active regimens against gastric cancer, with response rates in the 30% to 70% range.[41–44] This combination conferred a small but statistically significant survival benefit when compared with a regimen containing 5-FU, doxorubicin, and methotrexate (FAMTX) (median survival of 8.9 months vs. 5.7 months) in patients with inoperable or metastatic gastric cancer.[44] Since previous studies have shown no such advantage for other combinations over FAMTX, the ECF regimen is the most active one defined to date. However, even though combination chemotherapy regimens provide significant antitumor activity (in terms of response rates), so far the impact of this treatment on long-term survival remains limited.

There clearly remains significant room for improvement in chemotherapy for locally advanced gastric cancers, and this remains an active area of investigation. Given reasonable levels of antitumor activity of the other agents listed in Table 26–1, various combinations of these agents are currently being explored to determine whether improvements in survival can be achieved. The combination of cisplatin and irinotecan (given on a variety of schedules) clearly also has significant activity against gastric cancer.[40,45] Both this combination and ECF are being explored in conjunction with radiation therapy. The results from these and

**Table 26–1** Chemotherapeutic agents with activity against gastric cancer

Thymidylate synthase inhibitors (5-FU and related analogs)
Anthracyclines (doxorubicin, epirubidin)
Platinum compounds (cisplatin, oxaliplatin)
Taxanes (paclitaxel, docetaxel)
Camptothecins (irinotecan)
Topoisomerase II inhibitors (etoposide)
Antifolates (methotrexate)

other studies should be helpful in deciding on future directions for the use of chemotherapy in locally advanced gastric cancers.

The use of intraperitoneal (IP) chemotherapy (with 5-FU, mitomycin C, cisplatin, and other agents) has been evaluated for treating patients with gastric cancer. To date, randomized studies have not shown a clear benefit for this approach in patients with locally advanced disease who have undergone resections.[46,47] Additional studies are continuing to evaluate other IP agents, but at the present time, this remains a potentially interesting but still investigational approach.[47]

A significant recent effort has been made to evaluate preoperative chemotherapy for patients with gastric adenocarcinomas. Although this effort is addressed in greater detail in the previous chapter on potentially resectable patients (Chapter 25), it also has implications for the treatment of patients with locally advanced disease. The ability to directly assess the tumor response pathologically (histologically and evaluating changes in expression of specific genes or proteins) in patients treated in the preoperative setting can provide significant information on what directions to pursue in the future. Neoadjuvant chemotherapy clearly can produce tumor responses in a significant percentage of patients, although pathologic complete responses are uncommon.[48–54] A significant percentage of patients whose disease is deemed unresectable before chemotherapy may be candidates for resection post-treatment, and a small percentage of patients may have the potential for long-term survival.[44,53,54] However, until data from randomized trials are available, the exact role for neoadjuvant therapy in this setting will remain undefined. As is true for patients with metastatic disease, pilot studies of a number of combinations of agents are ongoing in the preoperative setting and may provide new regimens for treating patients with locally advanced disease.

## Immunotherapy

Nonspecific immunotherapy approaches (e.g., the use of OK-432 [a streptococcal preparation] or PSK [a protein-bound polysaccharide derived from *Basidiomycetes*]) have been evaluated for their potential role in treating patients with gastric cancer. Most of these studies have used these agents in conjunction with chemotherapy. The immunostimulants are delivered locally, intraperitoneally, or systemically. Although a number of studies, including several prospective randomized ones, have suggested that the use of immunotherapy combined with chemotherapy prolongs survival, the role of immunotherapy in achieving this result remains undefined.[55–57] Additional prospectively randomized studies are necessary before any role for immunotherapy in treating gastric cancer can be defined.

With the identification of growth factor receptors and other proteins that might be targeted in treating patients with gastric cancer, there is potential for using more specific immunotherapeutic approaches against these gastric cancer cells. A number of early trials evaluating the potential utility of monoclonal antibodies and vaccines are ongoing.[58–60]

## Future Directions

In addition to the continued efforts mentioned to improve treatment for gastric cancer patients, a number of new approaches to treating these patients need to be considered (Table 26–2). The discovery or synthesis of new agents with significant activity against gastric cancer clearly remains a priority. It is hoped that

**Table 26–2** New approaches to treating locally advanced gastric cancer

Improvements in radiation therapy (e.g., external beam and IORT)
New chemotherapy combinations (especially various combinations involving taxanes, cisplatin or oxaliplatin, irinotecan, 5-FU, and related analogs, including oral agents)
Immunotherapy approaches (e.g., monoclonal antibodies, vaccines)
Targeting specific proteins or their functions that are important for the biology of gastric cancer (e.g., growth factor receptors, proteins involved in apoptosis, angiogenic factors)

IORT, intraoperative radiation therapy.

oral analogs of 5-FU, such as capecitabine, will provide a more convenient means of delivering 5-FU on a continuous basis.[61–63] In turn, this should make it easier to deliver 5-FU as part of combined-modality therapy with radiation and as part of combination chemotherapy regimens. Initial trials combining oral 5-FU analogs with other chemotherapeutic agents for gastric cancer have established the feasibility of this approach.[64,65] However, the optimal approach for combining 5-FU analogs with other agents still needs to be evaluated and the exact roles of the camptothecins, taxanes, and other new agents with potential activity in this setting still need to be defined. As discussed above under Radiation Therapy, in addition to 5-FU, other agents (e.g., the taxanes or irinotecan) are being evaluated for use in combination with radiation therapy.[66]

Significant advances have been made in our knowledge of the biology of gastric adenocarcinoma.[67–75] Development and evaluation of new treatment approaches based on this knowledge are a major priority. There are a number of new antitumor approaches evaluating compounds that target specific aspects of gastric cancer biology. Factors such as P-glycoprotein status, growth factor receptor overexpression, mutant *p53* status, thymidylate synthase levels, involvement of specific proteins in the apoptotic pathway, cell-adhesion molecules, and angiogenic factors are all being evaluated as potential targets for modulation in treating patients with gastric cancer. Trials are evaluating the antitumor efficacy of new approaches in settings of both adjuvant and metastatic disease. In addition, efforts continue in the attempt to integrate these approaches with surgery and radiation therapy. New knowledge should also provide clues for earlier diagnosis and prevention.

## Summary

Locally advanced gastric cancer continues to provide a number of challenges to determining the best approach for each patient. When resection of disease is feasible, it offers the best chance for palliation. A number of studies have suggested that radiation therapy, chemotherapy, or a combination of the two provides additional benefit for these patients. In a subset of patients, the additional therapy also prolongs survival. For patients in whom gastric resection is not a viable option because of comorbid factors, a number of other approaches to palliation (mentioned under Surgery above), radiation therapy, and/or chemotherapy may be used. Ongoing studies are attempting to define how best to combine therapeutic approaches and are developing new agents and approaches to improve the treatment of patients with locally advanced gastric cancer.

## References

1. Haugstvedt T, Viste A, Eide GE, Soreide O. The survival benefit of resection in patients with advanced stomach cancer: the Norwegian multicenter experience. Norwegian Stomach Cancer Trial. World 13:617–622, 1989.

2. Monson JR, Sonohue JH, McIlrath DC, Farnell MB, Ilstrup DM. Total gastrectomy for advanced cancer. A worthwhile palliative procedure. Cancer 68:1863–1868, 1991.

3. Kikuchi S, Arai Y, Morise M. Gastric cancer with metastases to the distant peritoneum: a 20-year surgical experience. Hepatogastroenterology 45:1183–1188, 1998.

4. Doglietto GB, Pacelli F, Caprino P. Palliative surgery for far-advanced gastric cancer: a retrospective study on 305 consecutive patients. Am Surg 65:352–355, 1999.

5. Branicki FJ, Chu KM. Gastric cancer in Asia: progress and controversies in surgical management. Aust N Z Journal 68:172–179, 1998.

6. Goh PM, So JB. Role of laparoscopy in the management of stomach cancer. Semin Surg Oncol 16:321–326, 1999.

7. Monson JR, Donohue JH, McIlrath DC, Ilstrup DM. Total gastrectomy for advanced cancer. A worthwhile palliative procedure. Cancer 68:1863–1868, 1991.

8. D'Ugo DM, Persiani R, Carracciolo F, Ronconi P, Coco C, Picciocchi A. Selection of locally advanced gastric carcinoma by preoperative staging laparoscopy. Surg Endosc 11:1159–1162, 1997.

9. Payne-James JJ, Spiller RC, Misiewicz JJ, Silk DB. Use of ethanol-induced tumor necrosis to palliate dysphagia in patients with esophagogastric cancer. Gastrointest Endosc 36:43–46, 1990.

10. Venu RP, Pastika BJ, Kini M, et al. Self-expandable metal stents for malignant gastric outlet obstruction: a modified technique. Endoscopy 30:553–558, 1998.

11. Mason RC, Bright N, McColl I. Palliation of malignant dysphagia with laser therapy: predictability of results. Br J Surg 78:1346–1347, 1991.

12. Topazian M, Ring E, Grendell J. Palliation of obstructing gastric cancer with steel mesh, self-expanding endoprostheses. Gastrointest Endosc 38:58–60, 1992.

13. Loizou LA, Grigg D, Atkinson M, Robertson C, Bown SG. A prospective comparison of laser therapy and intubation in endoscopic palliation for malignant dysphagia. Gastroenterology 100(5 Pt 1):1303–1310, 1991.

14. Brennan FN, McCarthy JH, Laurence BH. Endoscopic Nd-YAG laser therapy for palliation of upper gastrointestinal malignancy. Med J Aust 153:27–31, 1990.

15. Moertel CG, Childs DS Jr, Reitemeir RJ, Colby MY Jr, Holbrook MA. Combined 5-fluorouracil and supervoltage radiation therapy of locally unresectable gastrointestinal cancer. Lancet 2(7626):865–867, 1969.

16. Schein PS, Novak J. Combined modality therapy (XRT-chemo) versus chemotherapy alone for locally unresectable gastric cancer. Cancer 49:1771, 1982.

17. Bleiberg H, Goffin JC, Dalesio O, et al. Adjuvant radiotherapy and chemotherapy in resectable gastric cancer. A randomized trial of the gastrointestinal tract cancer cooperative group of the EORTC. Eur Surg Oncol 15:535–543, 1989.

18. Whittington R, Coia LR, Haller DG, Rubenstein JH, Rosato EF. Adenocarcinoma of the esophagus and esophago-gastric junction: the effects of single and combined modalities on the survival and patterns of failure following treatment. Int J Radiat Oncol Biol Phys 19:593–603, 1990.

19. O'Connell MJ, Gunderson LL, Moertel CG, Kuols LK. A pilot study to determine clinical tolerability of intensive combined modality therapy for locally unresectable gastric cancer. Int J Radiat Oncol Biol Phys 11:1827–1831, 1985.

20. Gunderson LL, Burch PA, Donohue JH. The role of irradiation as a component of combined modality treatment for gastric cancer. J Infus Chemother 5:117–124, 1995.

21. Gunderson LL, Hoskins RB, Cohen AC, Kaufman S, Wood WC, Carey RW. Combined modality treatment of gastric cancer. Int J Radiat Oncol Biol Phys 9:965–975, 1983.

22. Minsky BD. The role of radiation therapy in gastric cancer. Semin Oncol 23:390–396, 1996.

23. Budach VG. The role of radiation therapy in the management of gastric cancer. Ann Oncol 5(Suppl 3):37–48, 1994.

24. The Gastrointestinal Tumor Study Group. The concept of locally advanced gastric cancer. Effective of treatment on outcome. Cancer 66:2324–2330, 1990.

25. Colin PH. Concomitant chemotherapy and radiotherapy: theoretical basis and clinical experience. Anticancer Res 14:2357–2361, 1994.

26. Creane M, Seymour CB, Colucci S, Mothersill C. Radiobiological effects of docetaxel (Taxotere): a potential radiation sensitizer. Int J Radiat Biol 75:731–737, 1999.

27. Takahashi M, Abe M. Intra-operative radiotherapy for carcinoma of the stomach. Eur J Surg Oncol 12:247–250, 1986.

28. Ogata T, Araki K, Matsura K, et al. A 10-year experience of intraoperative radiotherapy for gastric carcinoma and a new surgical method of creating a wider irradiation field for cases of total gastrectomy patients. Int J Radiat Oncol Biol Phys 32:341–347, 1995.

29. Calvo FA, Arista JJ, Azinovic I, et al. Intraoperative and external radiotherapy in resected gastric cancer: updated report of a phase II trial. Int J Radiat Oncol Biol Phys 24:729–736, 1992.

30. Ajani JA. Chemotherapy for gastric carcinoma: new and old options. Oncology 12(10 Suppl 7):44–47, 1998.

31. Wils J. The treatment of advanced gastric cancer. Semin Oncol 23:397–406, 1996.

32. Royce ME, Pazdur R. Novel chemotherapeutic agents for gastrointestinal cancers. Curr Opin Oncol 11:299–304, 1999.

33. Macdonald JS, Havlin KA. Etoposide in gastric cancer. Semin Oncol 19(6 Suppl 13):59–62, 1992.

34. Wils J. Treatment of gastric cancer. Curr Opin Oncol 10:357–361, 1998.

35. Bokemeyer C, Hartmann JJ, Lampe CS, et al. Paclitaxel and weekly 24-hour infusion of 5-fluorouracil/folinic acid in advanced gastric cancer. Semin Oncol 24(6 Suppl 19):S19-96–S19-100, 1997.

36. Philip PA, Azlnpski MM, Gadseed S, Hassain M, Shields S. A phase II study of carboplatin and paclitaxel in the treatment of patients with advanced esophageal and gastric cancer. Semin Oncol 24(6 Suppl 19):S19-86–S19-88, 1997.

37. Schipper DL, Wagener DJ. Chemotherapy of gastric cancer. Anticancer Drugs 7:137–149, 1996.

38. Perez JE, Lacava JA, Dominguez ME. Biochemical modulation of 5-fluorouracil by methotrexate in patients with advanced gastric carcinoma. Am J Clin Oncol 21:452–457, 1998.

39. Einzig AI. Nemberg D, Remick SC, et al. Phase II trial of docetaxel (Taxotere) in patients with adenocarcinoma of the upper gastrointestinal tract previously untreated with cytotoxic chemotherapy: the Eastern Cooperative Oncology Group (ECOG) results of protocol E1293. Med Oncol 13:87–93, 1996.

40. Boku N, Ohtsu A, Shimada Y, et al. Phase II study of a combination of irinotecan and cisplatin against metastatic gastric cancer. J Clin Oncol 17:319–323, 1999

41. Webb A, Cunningham D, Scarffe JH, et al. Randomized trial comparing epirubicin, cisplatin, and fluorouracil versus fluorouracil, doxorubicin, and methotrexate in advanced esophagogastric cancer. J Clin Oncol 15:261–267, 1997.

42. Cascinu S, Labianca R, Nessandroni P, et al. Intensive weekly chemotherapy for advanced gastric cancer using fluorouracil, cisplatin, epidoxorubicin, 6S-leucovorin, glutathione, and filgrastim: a report from the Italian Group for the Study of Digestive Tract Cancer. J Clin Oncol 15:3313–3319, 1997.

43. Wilke H, Korn M, Vanhofer U, et al. Weekly infusional 5-fluorouracil plus/minus other drugs for the treatment of advanced gastric cancer. J Infus Chemother 6:123–126, 1996.

44. Waters JS, Norman A, Cunningham D, et al. Long-term survival after epirubicin, cisplatin and fluorouracil for gastric cancer: results of a randomized trial. Br J Cancer 80:269–272, 1999.

45. Ajani JA, Baker J, Pisters PW, et al. CPT-11 plus cisplatin in patients with advanced, untreated gastric or gastroesophageal junction carcinoma: results of a phase II study. Cancer 94:641–646, 2002.

46. Ogawa M, Taguchi T. Upper gastrointestinal tumors. Cancer Chemother Biol Response Modif 17:464–475, 1997.

47. Bozzetti F, Vaglini M, Deraco M. Intraperitoneal hyperthermic chemotherapy in gastric cancer: rationale for a new approach. Tumori 84:483–488, 1998.

48. Wilke H, Premsser P, Fink N, et al. Preoperative chemotherapy in locally advanced and nonresectable gastric cancer: a phase II study with etoposide, doxorubicin, and cisplatin. J Clin Oncol 7:1318–1326, 1989.

49. Karpeh MS, Kelsen DP. Combined modality therapy of gastric cancer. Surg Oncol Clin North Am 6:741–747, 1997.

50. Kelsen D. Neoadjuvant therapy for upper gastrointestinal tract cancers. Curr Opin Oncol 8:321–328, 1996.

51. Ajani JA, Ota DM, et al. Resectable gastric carcinoma. An evaluation of preoperative and postoperative chemotherapy. Cancer 68:1501–1506, 1991.

52. Ajani JA, Mayer RJ, Ota DM, et al. Preoperative and postoperative combination chemotherapy for potentially resectable gastric carcinoma. J Natl Cancer Inst 85:1839–1844, 1993.

53. Wilke H, Meyer HJ, Fink U. Preoperative chemotherapy in gastric cancer. Recent Results Cancer Res 142:237–248, 1996.

54. Melcher AA, Mort D, Maughan TS. Epirubicin, cisplatin and continuous infusion 5-fluorouracil (ECF) as neoadjuvant chemotherapy in gastro-oesophageal cancer. Br J Cancer 74:1651–1654, 1996.

55. Kim R, Yoshida K, Toge T. Current status and future perspectives of postoperative adjuvant therapy for gastric carcinoma. Anticancer Res 22:283–289, 2002.

56. Kim SY, Park HC, Yoon HJ, Choi YM, Cho KS. OK-432 and 5-fluorouracil, doxorubicin, and mitomycin C (FAM-P) versus FAM chemotherapy in patients with curatively resected gastric carcinoma: a randomized phase III trial. Cancer 83:2054–2059, 1999.

57. Toge T. Effectiveness of immunochemotherapy for gastric cancer: a review of the current status. Semin Surg Oncol 17:139–143, 1999.

58. Tsunoda T, et al. Tumor-specific CTL therapy for advanced cancer and development for cancer vaccine. Hepatoastroenterology 46:Suppl 1: 1287–1292, 1999.

59. Waters JS, et al. New approaches to the treatment of gastrointestinal cancer. Digestion 58:508–519, 1997.

60. Yu B, et al. Phase I trial of iodine 131–labeled COL-1 in patients with gastrointestinal malignancies: influence of serum carcinoembryonic antigen and tumor bulk on pharmacokinetics. J Clin Oncol 14:798–809, 1996.

61. Ravaud A, et al. UFT and oral calcium folinate as first-line chemotherapy for metastatic gastric cancer. Oncology (Huntingt) 13(7 Suppl 3):61–63, 1999.

62. Kim YH, Shin SW, Kim, BS, Park YT, Kim JG, Kim JS. A phase II trial. Oral UFT and leucovorin in patients with advanced gastric carcinoma. Oncology (Huntingt) 11(9 Suppl 10):119–123, 1997.

63. Takiuchi H, Ajani JA. Uracil-tegafur in gastric carcinoma: a comprehensive review. J Clin Oncol 16:2877–2885, 1998.

64. Kim YH, Kim BS, Seo JH, et al. Epirubicin, cisplatin, oral UFT, and calcium folinate in advanced gastric carcinoma. Oncology (Huntingt) 13(7 Suppl 3):64–68, 1999.

65. Grau JJ, Estape J, Fuster J, et al. Randomized trial of adjuvant chemotherapy with mitomycin plus ftorafur versus mitomycin alone in resected locally advanced gastric cancer. J Clin Oncol 16:1036–1039, 1998.

66. Safran H, Akerman O, Cioffi W, et al. Paclitaxel and concurrent radiation therapy for locally advanced adenocarcinomas of the pancreas, stomach, and gastroesophageal junction. Semin Radiat Oncol 9(2 Suppl 1): 53–57, 1999.

67. Cascinu S, et al. P-glycoprotein as an intermediate end point of drug resistance to neoadjuvant chemotherapy in locally advanced gastric cancer. Yonsei Med J 37:397–404, 1996.

68. Chung HC, Gong SJ, Yoo NC, et al. P-glycoprotein as an intermediate end point of drug resistance to neoadjuvant chemotherapy in locally advanced gastric cancer. Yonsei Med J 37:397–404, 1996.

69. Lee HR, Kin JH, Mum HD, et al. Overexpression of c-ErbB-2 protein in gastric cancer by immunohistochemical stain. Oncology 53:192–197, 1996.

70. Cascinu S, Graziano F, Del Ferro E, et al. Expression of p53 protein and resistance to preoperative chemotherapy in locally advanced gastric carcinoma. Cancer 83:1917–1922, 1998.

71. Boku N, Chin K, Hosokawa K, et al. Biological markers as a predictor for response and prognosis of unresectable gastric cancer patients treated with 5-fluorouracil and cisplatinum. Clin Cancer Res 4:1469–1474, 1998.

72. Inada T, Kikuyama S, Ichikawa A, Igarashi S, Ogata Y: Bcl-2 expression as a prognostic factor of survival of gastric carcinoma. Anticancer Res 18:2003–2010, 1998.

73. Velikova G, Banks RE, Gearing A. Circulating soluble adhesion molecules E-cadherin, E-selectin, intercellular adhesion molecule-1 (ICAM-1) and vascular cell adhesion molecule-1 (VCAM-1) in patients with gastric cancer. Br J Cancer 76:1398–1404, 1999.

74. Jang SJ, Park YW, Park MH, et al. Expression of cell-cycle regulators, cyclin E and p21WAF1/CIP1, potential prognostic markers for gastric cancer. Eur J Surg Oncol 25:157–163, 1999.

75. Matturri L, Biodi B, Cazzullo A, et al. Prognostic significance of different biological markers (DNA index, PCNA index, apoptosis, p53, karyotype) in 126 adenocarcinoma gastric biopsies. Anticancer Res 18: 2819–2825, 1998.

# Chapter 27

# Management Options: Metastatic Gastric Carcinoma

MATTHEW H. KULKE AND ROBERT J. MAYER

Approximately 50% of patients with gastric adenocarcinoma have metastatic disease at the time of their initial presentation. Metastatic disease also develops in most patients who undergo potentially curative resection. Systemic cytotoxic chemotherapy remains the most effective treatment modality for patients with metastatic gastric cancer. Studies in the past 30 years have demonstrated that several chemotherapeutic agents are active in this disease, including 5-fluorouracil (5-FU), doxorubicin, cisplatin, and mitomycin C. More recent studies have shown that oral analogues of 5-FU, as well as the taxanes and irinotecan, also have activity. Most of the reports comparing the efficacy of these compounds, given either as single agents or in combination regimens, have generally focused on tumor shrinkage (i.e., the response rate). Recent prospectively randomized trials, in which various drug combinations were compared with either single-agent treatment or with other drug combinations, measured not only response rates but also times to tumor progression and overall survival times. By including these additional end points, these randomized trials have allowed a more precise assessment of the value of systemic chemotherapy. Additional therapies, such as palliative gastrectomy or the administration of intraperitoneal chemotherapy, have also been studied, but their role in the treatment of patients with advanced gastric cancer is less well established. This chapter will review the roles of systemic chemotherapy, intraperitoneal chemotherapy, and palliative resection in patients with metastatic gastric cancer.

## Single Agent Chemotherapy

Numerous agents have been studied in the treatment of advanced gastric cancer (Table 27–1). Many of the trials have been small and uncontrolled, making it difficult to draw firm conclusions on the efficacy of these agents. In general, single-agent chemother-

apy in patients with metastatic gastric cancer has resulted in only modest response rates. Complete responses are rare, and partial responses are brief, lasting only 3 to 6 months. No randomized studies have compared the results of single-agent therapy with those of best supportive care. Whether single-agent therapy confers a survival benefit in patients with metastatic gastric cancer therefore remains unknown.

Among the chemotherapeutic agents used to treat gastric adenocarcinoma, 5-FU, with or without leucovorin, has been studied the most extensively. A retrospective review of 392 patients with gastric cancer treated with 5-FU before 1974 demonstrated an overall response rate of 21%.[1] More recent randomized trials of 5-FU used as a single agent have demonstrated a nearly identical response rate of 20%.[2–5]

In an attempt to improve response rates with 5-FU, Machover and colleagues[6] combined 5-FU (340–400 mg/m$^2$/day) with folinic acid (200 mg/m$^2$/day) using a 5-day treatment schedule followed by a 21-day treatment-free interval. Among 27 patients with gastric cancer, 48% responded to therapy. However, a subsequent trial by the Southwest Oncology Group using Machover's regimen in 40 patients demonstrated a response rate of only 20%.[7] The toxicity of this regimen, while deemed acceptable by the authors, included stomatitis, myelosuppression, and diarrhea.

Studies in metastatic colon cancer showed that a weekly schedule of 5-FU and high-dose leucovorin was as effective as but less toxic than the monthly schedule. These results prompted an evaluation of a similar regimen in gastric cancer. A phase II trial of a weekly schedule of 5-FU (600 mg/m$^2$) and high-dose folinic acid (500 mg/m$^2$) in 28 patients demonstrated a response rate of 11%.[8] Since many patients had been previously treated with combination regimens containing 5-FU, this study may have underestimated the activity of this regimen. Like the weekly bo-

**Table 27-1** Single-agent chemotherapy in advanced gastric cancer

| Agent | Evaluable Patients (n) | Response Rate (%) |
|---|---|---|
| *Antimetabolites* | | |
| 5-Fluorouracil | 392 | 21 |
| Tegafur | 19 | 27 |
| S-1 | 101 | 45 |
| UFT | 286 | 28 |
| Triazinate | 26 | 15 |
| Trimetrexate | 49 | 12 |
| Methotrexate | 28 | 11 |
| Cytarabine | 11 | 27 |
| Gemcitabine | 15 | 0 |
| *Antibiotics* | | |
| Mitomycin C | 211 | 30 |
| *Anthracyclines* | | |
| Doxorubicin | 141 | 17 |
| Epirubicin | 49 | 18 |
| *Heavy Metals* | | |
| Cisplatin | 95 | 21 |
| Carboplatin | 35 | 9 |
| *Alkylating Agents* | | |
| Methyl-CCNU | 37 | 8 |
| BCNU | 23 | 17 |
| Chlorambucil | 18 | 17 |
| *Topoisomerase Inhibitors* | | |
| Etoposide | 29 | 8 |
| Irinotecan | 94 | 21 |
| *Taxanes* | | |
| Paclitaxel | 67 | 13 |
| Docetaxel | 163 | 21 |

lus 5-FU and leucovorin regimen, continuous intravenous infusion of 5-FU is commonly used in advanced colon cancer and is considered by some investigators to be more effective than bolus 5-FU.[9] Infusional 5-FU has not been extensively tested as a single-treatment modality in gastric cancer. In one study, 4 (31%) of 14 patients, responded.[10] This regimen was not associated with myelosuppression and was therefore considered promising for use in combination with other agents.

The activity of oral analogues of 5-FU appears to be similar to that of intravenously administered 5-FU. Oral tegafur, a prodrug of 5-FU, was as effective as intravenous 5-FU in a comparative study in 45 patients with metastatic gastric or colorectal cancer. UFT, a second-generation 5-FU analogue, combines tegafur with uracil, a competitive inhibitor of the catabolic enzyme dihydropyrimidine dehydrogenase (DPD). In review of 286 Japanese patients with gastric cancer, treatment with UFT resulted in an overall response rate of 27.7%.[11] S-1, another oral analogue of 5-FU, combines tegafur with the DPD inhibitor 5-chloro-2,4-dihydropyrimidine. Although preliminary studies of S-1 in patients with gastric cancer have demonstrated response rates of 40% to 51%, larger studies must be performed to confirm activity of this drug.[12,13]

Doxorubicin has also been shown to be active in gastric cancer. Three large multi-institutional studies of doxorubicin demonstrated response rates between 13% and 24%.[14–16] One of the dose-limiting toxicities of doxorubicin is cardiomyopathy.

4-Epidoxorubicin (epirubicin) is a doxorubicin analogue with with antitumor activity similar to that of the parent drug but with less cardiotoxicity.[17] In advanced gastric cancer, the use of epirubicin has yielded response rates of 11% to 21%.[18–20]

Other active drugs in gastric cancer include the platinum analogs, cisplatin and carboplatin. Eight phase II studies[21–28] of cisplatin in a total of 95 patients with advanced gastric cancer demonstrated an overall response rate of 21%. Carboplatin appears to be less active than cisplatin in treating advanced gastric cancer, with a response rate of only 9% in one phase II trial of 35 evaluable patients.[29] A cumulative analysis of clinical trials involving 211 patients with gastric cancer treated with the antitumor antibiotic mitomycin C revealed an overall objective response rate of 30%. When retrospective studies were eliminated from this analysis, however, the response rate was only 24%.

Among the newer chemotherapeutic agents, both the taxanes (e.g., paclitaxel and docetaxel) and the topoisomerase I inhibitor irinotecan are active in gastric cancer. Three studies[30–32] involving a total of 67 evaluable patients treated with paclitaxel showed an overall response rate of 13%. In four phase II studies[33–36] involving a total of 163 patients, docetaxel demonstrated an overall response rate of 21%. A multi-institutional phase II study[37] in 60 evaluable Japanese patients with advanced gastric cancer treated with irinotecan resulted in an overall response rate of 23.3%. The reported probability of disease regression was 16.1% in the 45 patients who had received prior therapy. A subsequent French trial confirmed the activity of irinotecan, demonstrating a response rate of 17.6% in 34 previously untreated patients.[38]

Other drugs with modest activity in gastric cancer include methotrexate (11%), trimetrexate (12%),[39,40] triazinate (15%),[41] the nitrosoureas,[5] and chlorambucil (17%).[42] Gemcitabine does not appear to have activity in gastric cancer.[43]

## Combination Chemotherapy

### 5-Fluorouracil- and Doxorubicin-Containing Regimens

Various combinations of chemotherapeutic agents have resulted in improved response rates among patients with advanced gastric cancer. One of the most widely used combination regimens has been a combination of 5-FU, doxorubicin (Adriamycin), and mitomycin C (FAM). Investigators from Georgetown University introduced the FAM regimen in a trial involving 62 patients. Patients had a response rate of 42%, a median duration of response of 9 months, and a median survival of 5.5 months. The regimen was well tolerated; the most common toxic effects were leukopenia and thrombocytopenia.[44] The original FAM combination was subsequently examined in numerous trials involving a total of 346 patients and found to have an overall response rate of 33% (Table 27–2).[45]

Modifications of the original FAM regimen, including changes in the dosing schedule and intensification of the doxorubicin dose, did not significantly improve the response rate, median duration of response, or survival the.[45] The addition of triazinate, methyl-CCNU, BCNU, and leucovorin to the FAM regimen also did not significantly improve outcomes.[4,46–51] Although these regimens have not been formally compared with the original FAM regimen in randomized trials, response rates in phase II studies of these alternative regimens do not appear to be significantly better than those achieved with FAM alone.

Mitomycin C is associated with delayed myelosuppression, especially leukopenia and thrombocytopenia, and has also been

**Table 27-2** 5-Fluorouracil, doxorubicin, and mitomycin-C (FAM) and FAM variants in treatment of advanced gastric cancer

| Regimen | Evaluable Patients (n) | Response Rate (%) |
|---|---|---|
| FAM (original) | 346 | 33 |
| FAM (dosage intensified) | 122 | 32 |
| FAM (dosage schedule variants) | 188 | 26 |
| FAM + triazinate | 31 | 13 |
| FAM + methyl-CCNU | 49 | 29 |
| FAM + BCNU | 75 | 31 |
| FAM + leucovorin | 26 | 38 |
| FAB | 177 | 43 |
| FAT | 31 | 19 |
| FAP | 217 | 34 |
| FAMe | 147 | 24 |

FAB, 5-fluorouracil, doxorubicin, and BCNU; FAMe, 5-fluorouracil, doxorubicin, and methyl-CCNU; FAP, 5-fluorouracil, doxorubicin, and cisplatin; FAT, 5-fluorouracil, doxorubicin, and triazinate.

associated with microangiopathic hemolytic anemia due to renal damage. These toxicities led several investigators to substitute other agents for mitomycin C in the FAM regimen. The combination of 5-FU, doxorubicin, and methyl-CCNU (FAMe) in a total of 147 patients resulted in an overall response rate of 24%.[16,52-56] Studies of 5-FU, doxorubicin, and BCNU (FAB) in 177 patients demonstrated an overall response rate of 43%.[14,57-59] The combination of 5-FU, doxorubicin, and cisplatin using a variety of dosing schedules yielded response rates ranging from 17% to 53%.[45,56]

## 5-Fluorouracil, Doxorubin, and Methotrexate (FAMTX) Combination Therapy

The regimen consisting of methotrexate administered in high doses followed by 5-FU, given in combination with doxorubicin (FAMTX) was originally reported by Klein and colleagues.[60]. This schedule exploits the reportedly favorable pharmacodynamic properties of the sequential administration of 5-FU and methotrexate and requires that patients undergo leucovorin "rescue" therapy following the administration of high-dose methotrexate. In 116 patients treated according to the original FAMTX schedule, the overall response rate was 58%, and the rate of complete responses was 12%.[61] The median survival time was 9

months, and 6% of patients in this original trial lived longer than 6 years. Subsequent trials of the FAMTX regimen in a total of 472 patients demonstrated an overall response rate of 36% (Table 27-3).[62-67] The regimen was associated with moderate toxicity: neutropenia and mucositis occurred in 10% to 20% of patients and toxic deaths were occurred in 4%.

## Etoposide, Doxorubicin, and Cisplatin (EAP) and Etoposide, Leucovorin, and 5-Fluorouracil (ELF) Combination Therapy

A potential synergistic effect between etoposide and cisplatin led investigators to pursue combination therapy with these agents in gastric cancer, despite the finding that etoposide had minimal activity as a single agent in this disease.[68] An initial phase II trial of etoposide and cisplatin in adenocarcinomas of the upper gastrointestinal tract demonstrated only 1 response among 33 evaluable patients.[68] However, a second study[69] in 48 patients demonstrated a response rate of 28%. Preusser and co-workers[70] reported that a combination of etoposide, doxorubicin, and cisplatin (EAP) in 67 patients yielded responses in 43 patients (64%), including 14 complete responses (21%).[70] The toxicity of this regimen was substantial, however, and grade 3-4 myelosuppression was noted in 64% of patients. Three other trials of EAP showed encouraging response rates of 72%, 70%, and 45% (Table 27-4).[71-73] However, subsequent phase II studies of the EAP regimen resulted in significantly lower response rates and a high incidence of deaths due to toxicity.[74-76]

In response to the significant toxicity observed with EAP, a more tolerable regimen combining etoposide, leucovorin and 5-FU (ELF) was developed for patients over the age of 65 years and for patients with cardiac disease. An initial report on this combination in 51 patients documented an overall response rate of 53% and a complete response rate of 12% (Table 27-5).[77] Toxicity was mild, with only 20% of patients experiencing grade 3 or 4 myelosuppression. However, a second trial involving 41 evaluable patients demonstrated an overall response rate of only 32% and a complete response rate of only 7%.[78] The median duration of response in this trial was 7 months In a trial conducted by another group of investigators,[79] using the ELF regimen in combination with granulocyte-macrophage colony stimulating factor, only 14% of patients achieved a partial response. These more recent studies have called into question the value of the ELF regimen, even in elderly patients and patients with comorbid disease.

**Table 27-3** 5-Fluorouracil, doxorubicin, and methotrexate (FAMTX) in treatment of advanced gastric cancer

| Study | Patients (n) | Responses n (%) | Median Survival (Months) | Rate of Deaths Due to Toxicity (%) |
|---|---|---|---|---|
| Hermann et al. (1984)[63] | 20 | 0 (0) | 3.5 | 10 |
| Wils et al. (1986)[64] | 67 | 22 (33) | 6 | 6 |
| Weh et al. (1989)[62] | 50 | 17 (34) | 7 | 0 |
| Klein (1989)[61] | 116 | 67 (58) | 9 | 3 |
| Wils et al. (1991)[65,a] | 81 | 33 (41) | 10.5 | 4 |
| Kelsen et al. (1992)[66,a] | 30 | 10 (33) | 7 | 0 |
| Wilke et al. (1995)[82,a] | 45 | 9 (20) | 7 | N/A |
| Webb et al. (1997)[67,a] | 108 | 23 (21) | 5.7 | 2 |

N/A, not available.

[a]Data from randomized trial.

**Table 27-4** Etoposide, doxorubicin, and ciplatin (EAP) in treatment of advanced gastric cancer

| Study | Patients (n) | Responses n (%) | Median Survival (Months) | Rate of Deaths Due to Toxicity (%) |
|---|---|---|---|---|
| Preusser et al. (1989)[70] | 67 | 43 (64) | 8 | 0 |
| Wilke et al. (1989)[73] | 33 | 23 (70) | 18 | 0 |
| Katz et al. (1989)[71] | 29 | 21 (72) | 6 | 7 |
| Taguchi (1989)[72] | 31 | 14 (45) | 8 | 6 |
| Taal et al. (1990)[74] | 26 | 4 (15) | N/A | 12 |
| Sparano et al. (1990)[75] | 10 | 1 (13) | N/A | 20 |
| Kelsen et al. (1992)[66,a] | 30 | 6 (20) | 6.1 | 13 |
| Lerner et al. (1992)[76] | 36 | 12 (33) | 7.5 | 11 |

N/A, not available.

[a]Data from a randomized trial

## Cisplatin and 5-Fluorouracil (FP)-Based Combinations

Five studies[80–84] have examined the combination of cisplatin with 5-FU (FP) in treating advanced gastric cancer (Table 27–6). These trials included a total of 260 evaluable patients and demonstrated an overall response rate of 41%. In one study,[83] the addition of the anthracycline epirubicin to FP did not improve the response rates or survival times. However, in a phase II trial,[85] the combination of epirubicin, cisplatin, and 5-FU given as a prolonged continuous intravenous infusion (ECF) to 128 patients with advanced gastroesophageal cancer resulted in an objective tumor response rate of 71%.

Several investigators have attempted to enhance the ECF combination by adding other agents. In one nonrandomized study of 105 patients with advanced gastric cancer, weekly administration of a combination of cisplatin, epirubicin, leucovorin, and 5-FU (PELF) resulted in a response rate of 62% and a median survival of 11 months.[86] A second study[87] evaluated the effects of weekly administration of a combination of etoposide, epirubicin, cisplatin, 5-FU, and leucovorin (EEPFL). Among 42 patients, 71% responded and the overall median survival was 10 months. The efficacy of these regimens has not yet been examined in randomized studies.

## Randomized Trials of Systemic Chemotherapy

### Chemotherapy vs. Best Supportive Care

While numerous trials have demonstrated that cytotoxic chemotherapy shrinks tumors, far fewer studies have sought to determine whether such treatment confers a survival benefit over supportive care alone in patients with metastatic gastric cancer.

Several small, prospectively randomized trials have assessed the benefit of chemotherapy in such patients (Table 27–7). In the first of these studies, patients were randomized to receive either a modified FAMTX regimen or best supportive care. Randomization to this study was stopped prematurely because of evidence of improved survival in the group receiving chemotherapy. At the completion of the study, 30 patients who received chemotherapy had a median survival duration of 10 months, whereas 10 patients who received best supportive care alone had a median survival of only 3 months ($P = 0.001$).[88] In a second study,[89] 41 patients were randomized to receive either combination therapy with 5-FU, epirubicin, and methotrexate (FEMTX) or best supportive care. Accrual to this study was also halted when the group receiving combination chemotherapy showed a survival advantage (12.3 months vs. 3.1 months, $P = 0.0006$). In a third study, 61 patients were randomized to receive either the ELF regimen or best supportive care.[90] Forty percent of the patients in the best supportive care arm of this study did in fact receive chemotherapy at a later time for palliation of symptoms. Despite the use of chemotherapy in a subset of the control group, the quality of life was better and the median survival longer (8 months vs. 5 months, $P = 0.003$) in the group that received immediate chemotherapy than in the control group. Although each of these trials was small, the consistent survival benefit associated with the use of systemic chemotherapy in all three studies provides strong evidence for its efficacy in patients with metastatic gastric cancer.

### Combination Therapy vs. Single-Agent Therapy

While the survival times associated with combination chemotherapy have been longer than those associated with best supportive care, no randomized trials have demonstrated that com-

**Table 27-5** Etoposide, leucovorin, and 5-fluorouracil (ELF) in treatment of advanced gastric cancer

| Study | Patients (n) | Responses n (%) | Median Survival (Months) | Rate of Deaths Due to Toxicity (%) |
|---|---|---|---|---|
| Wilke et al. (1990)[77] | 51 | 27 (53) | 11 | 0 |
| DiBartolomeo et al. (1995)[78] | 41 | 13 (32) | 10 | 0 |
| Wilke et al. (1995)[82,a] | 42 | 9 (21) | 7 | 0 |
| Partyaka et al. (1999)[79] | 29 | 4 (14) | 6.5 | 0 |

[a]Data from a randomized trial.

**Table 27-6** Platinum and 5-fluorouracil (FP) in treatment of gastric cancer

| Study | Patients (n) | Responses n (%) | Median Survival (Months) | Rate of Deaths Due to Toxicity (%) |
|---|---|---|---|---|
| Lacave et al. (1991)[81] | 56 | 22 (41) | 10.6 | 0 |
| Ohtsu et al. (1991)[80] | 20 | 9 (45) | N/A | 0 |
| KRGCGC et al. (1992)[83] | 21 | 5 (24) | N/A | 0 |
| Wilke et al. (1995)[82,a] | 44 | 12 (27) | 8 | 5 |
| Cervantes et al. (1999)[84] | 119 | 59 (50) | 9.3 | 0 |

N/A, not available.

[a]Data from a randomized trial.

bination chemotherapy confers a clear survival advantage over single-agent chemotherapy (Table 27–8). Three trials have compared combination therapy with single-agent doxorubicin. A randomized trial of 139 patients with advanced gastric cancer compared the following three regimens: doxorubicin, 5-FU plus mitomycin C, and 5-fluorouracil plus methyl-CCNU. A comparison of the three arms did not show any significant differences in either the response rates or the median survival times. In the second trial, performed by the Sydney Cooperative Oncology Group, 203 patients were randomized to receive either doxorubicin or FAB.[14] The response rate (40%) was significantly higher in the FAB group than in the doxorubicin group (13%). Interestingly, among the 145 patients with measurable disease, a survival advantage was noted in the FAB group. However, an analysis of the entire group, which included patients with both measurable and unmeasurable disease, showed no statistically significant survival advantage. In the third trial, the Gastrointestinal Tumor Study Group randomized 141 patients to receive either single-agent doxorubicin, FAMe, or a combination of 5-FU mitomycin C, and cytosine arabinoside (FMC).[16] Although the response rates for the three arms were similar, the median survival of patients receiving FAMe (12.9 months) was longer than that of patients receiving doxorubicin (8.2 months, $P < 0.03$).

Five randomized trials have compared combination chemotherapy with therapy with single-agent 5-FU (Table 27–8). In the first of these studies, 167 patients were randomized to receive 5-FU or BCNU, or a combination of these two drugs. Compared with 5-FU alone the combination regimen conferred no significant advantage in either response rates or overall survival times.[5] In 1976, the Southwest Oncology Group reported the results of

a randomized trial in which 5-FU was compared with 5-FU plus methyl-CCNU in 299 patients with advanced gastrointestinal cancers. Only 39 patients in this trial had gastric cancer. Analysis of this small subgroup demonstrated no differences in either response or survival between the arms, although the limited number of patients makes a definitive analysis difficult.[3] A third trial of 82 patients with advanced gastric carcinoma compared 5-FU alone with the combination of BCNU, doxorubicin, 5-FU, and mitomycin C (BAFMi). Despite the larger number of patients, this trial also failed to demonstrate that the combination regimen conferred a benefit over single-agent 5-FU.[4]

In a 1985 trial by the North Central Cancer Treatment Group, single-agent 5-FU treatment was compared with 5-FU and doxorubicin (FA) was compared with FAM in 305 patients with advanced pancreatic or gastric carcinoma.[2] Among the 151 patients with gastric cancer, the three arms showed no significant differences in either response rates or overall survival times. One weakness of this trial was that only 35 patients with gastric cancer had measurable disease, making comparisons of response rates difficult. Nevertheless, this trial casts significant doubt on the use of the FAM combination regimen as standard therapy for advanced gastric cancer.

In a second study performed by the North Central Cancer Treatement Group, 252 patients were randomized to receive either single-agent 5-FU, FAMe, FAP, or a regimen of FAMe alternating with triazinate.[91] Most patients had unmeasurable disease. None of the combination regimens showed survival times longer than those obtained with 5-FU alone, and the toxicity associated with each of the combinations was greater than that with 5-FU alone. The investigators concluded that single-agent 5-FU should remain the standard treatment for advanced gastric cancer.

**Table 27-7** Randomized trials of combination chemotherapy vs. best supportive care for advanced gastric cancer

| Study | Regimen | Evaluable Patients | Median Survival (Months) | P-value |
|---|---|---|---|---|
| Murad et al. (1993)[88] | FAMTX | 30 | 10 | |
| | BSC | 10 | 3 | 0.001 |
| Pyrhonen et al. (1995)[89] | FEMTX | 21 | 12.3 | 0.0006 |
| | BSC | 20 | 3.1 | |
| Glimelius et al. (1997)[90] | ELF | 31 | 8 | 0.003 |
| | BSC | 30[a] | 5 | |

BSC, best supportive care; ELF, etoposide, leucovorin, and 5-fluorouracil; FAMTX, 5-fluorouracil, doxorubicin, and methotrexate; FEMTX, 5-fluorouracil, epirubicin, and methotrexate.

[a]Twelve of 30 patients received chemotherapy.

## 5-Fluorouracil, Doxorubicin, and Mitomycin C (FAM) and Variant Regimens

Despite the lack of data demonstrating longer survival times with combination therapy than with single-agent 5-FU, the higher response rates reported with combination therapy in phase II trials prompted several randomized trials comparing various combination regimens (Table 27–9). Several of these trials did in fact support the use of either FAM or FAMe in the treatment of metastatic gastric cancer. A study performed by the Gastrointestinal Tumor Study Group in 1982 provided the first indirect evidence that combination chemotherapy improves survival in patients with metastatic gastric cancer.[55] In this study, 205 patients were randomized to receive either FAM; FAMe; 5-FU (ICRF-159) and methyl-CCNU (FIMe); or 5-FU and methyl-CCNU (FMe). Because only 59 patients in this trial had measurable disease, it was

**Table 27-8** Single-agent vs. combination chemotherapy in treatment of advanced gastric cancer

| Study | Regimen | Evaluable Patients | Response Rate | Median Survival |
|---|---|---|---|---|
| Kovach et al. (1974)[5] | 5-FU | 59 | 8/28 (28.6%) | 7.4 months |
| | BCNU | 44 | 4/23 (17.4 %) | 3.5 months |
| | 5-FU/BCNU | 64 | 14/34 (41.3%) | 7.7 months |
| Baker et al. (1976)[3] | 5-FU | 9 | 2/9 (22.2%) | 18 weeks[a] |
| | 5-FU/methyl-CCNU | 29 | 6/29 (20.7%) | 18 weeks[a] |
| Cullinan et al. (1985)[2] | 5-FU | 51 | 2/11 (18%) | 29 weeks |
| | FA | 49 | 3/11 (27%) | 29 weeks |
| | FAM | 51 | 5/13 (38%) | 29 weeks |
| DeLisi et al. (1986)[4] | 5-FU | 41 | 6/41 (15%) | 28 weeks |
| | BAFMi | 41 | 9/41 (22%) | 24 weeks |
| Cullinan et al. (1994)[91] | 5-FU | 69 | N/A | 6–8.3 months |
| | FAMe | 53 | N/A | 6–8.3 months |
| | FAP | 51 | N/A | 6–8.3 months |
| | FAMe/triazinate | 79 | N/A | 6–8.3 months |

BAFMi, BCNU, doxorubicin, 5-fluorouracil, and mitomycin C; FA, 5-fluorouracil and doxorubicin; FAM, 5-fluorouracil, doxorubicin, and mitomycin C; FAMe, 5-fluorouracil, doxorubicin, and methyl-CCNU; FAP, 5-fluorouracil, doxorubicin, and cisplatin.
[a]Median survival is for all upper gastrointestinal malignancies.

impossible to compare the objective response rates among the four arms. However, there were clear differences in the median survival times among the four arms. Patients receiving either FAM or FAMe had median survival times of 29.6 and 34.4 weeks, respectively, whereas patients receiving FIMe or FMe had median survivals times of only 22.9 and 17.4 weeks, respectively.

On the basis of these results, the Gastrointestinal Tumor Study Group sought to determine the relative contributions of mitomycin C and methyl-CCNU to 5-FU and doxorubicin (FA) by randomizing 241 patients to receive either FA, FAM, or FAMe.[53] Comparisons of objective response rates were again difficult to make, since only 53 patients had measurable disease. The authors noted a survival benefit in patients receiving FAMe (67

weeks) compared with those receiving FA (43 weeks), but median survival times of the FAMe and FAM groups were not significantly different. Using FAMe as the standard comparison arm, the Gastrointestinal Tumor Study Group subsequently compared FAMe, FAP, and a third regimen combining 5-FU, doxorubicin, and triazinate (FAT).[56] The FAP and FAT regimens resulted in slightly superior survival times compared with FAMe, but there were no significant differences in the response rates between the three regimens.

The FAM regimen was again compared with FAMe in a trial performed by the Eastern Cooperative Oncology Group in 1984.[54] In this trial, 183 previously untreated patients were randomized to receive FAM, FAMe, FMe, or a combination of doxo-

**Table 27-9** Randomized trials of 5-fluorouracil, doxorubicin, and mitomycin C (FAM) and FAM variants

| Study | Regimen | Evaluable Patients | Response Rate | Medial Survival (weeks) |
|---|---|---|---|---|
| GITSG (1982)[55] | FAM | 43 | 3/12 (25%) | 30 |
| | FAMe | 34 | 3/10 (30%) | 34 |
| | FIMe | 46 | 4/19 (21%) | 23 |
| | FMe | 58 | 1/18 (6%) | 17 |
| GITSG (1984)[53] | FA | 78 | 1/19 (5%) | 43 |
| | FAM | 62 | 3/18 (17%) | 33 |
| | FAMe | 62 | 4/16 (25%) | 67 |
| Douglass et al. (1984)[54] | FAM | 46 | 18/46 (39%) | 30 |
| | FAMe | 39 | 11/39 (29%) | 22 |
| | FMe | 44 | 6/44 (14%) | 13 |
| | AM | 46 | 13/46 (29%) | 18 |
| Panettiere et al. (1984)[92] | FAM (original) | 120 | 25/83 (30%) | 23 |
| | FAM (sequential) | 119 | 19/81 (23%) | 22 |
| Schnitzler et al. (1986)[57] | FB | 18 | 2/18 (35%) | 16 |
| | FAB | 17 | 4/17 (24%) | 22 |
| Lacave et al. (1987)[52] | FA | 88 | 3/29 (10%) | 21 |
| | FAMe | 85 | 5/28 (18%) | 32 |
| GITSG (1988)[56] | FAMe | 81 | 5/33 (15%) | 24 |
| | FAP | 85 | 6/30 (20%) | 31 |
| | FAT | 81 | 6/31 (19%) | 30 |

AM, doxorubicin and mitomycin C; FAB< 5-fluorouracil, doxorubicin, and BCNU; FAM, 5-fluorouracil, doxorubicin, and mitomycin C; FAMe, 5-fluorouracil, doxorubicin, and methyl-CCNU; FAP, 5-fluorouracil, doxorubicin, and cisplatin; FAT, 5-fluorouracil, doxorubicin, and triazinate; FB, 5-fluorouracil and BCNU; FIMe, 5-fluorouracil (ICRF-159) and methyl-CCNU; FMe, 5-fluorouracil and methyl-CCNU; GITSG, Gastrointestinal Tumor Study Group.

rubicin and mitomycin C (AM). The response rates for FAM (39%) were higher than those for FAMe (29%), AM (29%), or FMe (14%). The median survival times were also better for the patients receiving FAM (30 weeks) than for those receiving FAMe (22 weeks), AM (18 weeks), or FMe (13 weeks). This Eastern Cooperative Oncology Group trial differed from the Gastrointestinal Tumor Study Group trials in that FAM was given on a weekly rather than on a monthly schedule, a change which appeared to improve the toxicity profile of the regimen. On the basis of these results, the Eastern Cooperative Oncology Group concluded that FAM should be the standard against which future regimens should be compared.

The effect of the dosing schedule in the FAM regimen was formally evaluated by the Southwest Oncology Group in a trial that compared the original FAM regimen, in which all three drugs were given simultaneously, with sequential administration of doxorubicin, mitomycin C, and 5-FU.[92] A total of 239 patients were randomized to receive one of the two combination therapies. The response rates of the two arms were equivalent and the median survival times were nearly identical.

## 5-Fluorouracil, Doxorubicin, and Methotrexate (FAMTX)

In 1991, the European Organization for Research and Treatment of Cancer (EORTC) Gastrointestinal Cooperative Group performed a prospective randomized trial that directly compared the FAMTX regimen with FAM, which many investigators considered the standard of care (Table 27–10).[65] In this trial, 213 patients with advanced gastric cancer received either FAMTX or FAM. Objective response rates among the 160 patients with measurable disease were significantly better in the FAMTX group (41%) than in the FAM group (9%, $P < 0.001$). The median survival time for patients receiving FAMTX (42 weeks) was also longer than that for patients receiving FAM (29 weeks, $P = 0.004$). The toxicities of the two regimens differed, with mucositis being more common in the FAMTX arm and cumulative myelosuppression being more common in the FAM group. One surprising aspect of this trial was the extremely low response rate for FAM, which had consistently yielded response rates of over 30% in previous trials. This finding may have been due in part to differences in techniques for measuring response rates. Whereas physical examination was an accepted technique for measuring response in previous trials, the responses of most pa-

tients in this trial were measured by computed tomography (CT) scan. Despite the low response rates for FAM in this trial, FAMTX became the standard comparison arm in future trials.

A randomized trial involving 60 patients compared EAP chemotherapy with FAMTX.[66] The two groups showed similar response rates and median survival times. However, EAP caused significantly more myelosuppression, and four patients in the EAP arm experienced deaths due to toxicity. The increased risk of death in the EAP arm of this trial led to its early closure and to the subsequent abandonment of the EAP regimen. A more recent trial compared FAMTX with ELF and with cisplatin plus bolus 5-FU.[82] A preliminary analysis of the data revealed no significant differences in the overall survival times or in response rates among the three regimens; however, interpretation of the study was limited by the fact that only 80% of the patients received more than one cycle of chemotherapy.

The encouraging response rates observed with ECF prompted a randomized phase III study that compared ECF with FAMTX in 274 patients.[67] The response rate for ECF (45%) was higher than that for FAMTX (21%, $P = 0.0002$). The median survival time of patients receiving ECF (8.9 months) was also longer than that of patients receiving FAMTX (5.7 months, $P = 0.0009$). The toxicity profiles of the two regimens differed, with ECF causing more alopecia and nausea and FAMTX causing more hematologic toxicity and infections. The two groups had similar quality of life and hospital-based costs. Long-term follow-up results of this trial were reported in 1999, at which time 10 patients in the ECF arm had undergone surgical resection and three pathologic complete responses to chemotherapy had been noted.[93] Three patients in the FAMTX arm had undergone surgery, with no complete responses noted. The 2-year survival rates were 14% for the ECF arm and 5% for the FAMTX arm ($P = 0.03$). Although ECF was relatively well tolerated, one drawback of this regimen is the requirement for a central venous line. In the trial, central venous line complications occurred in 15% of patients. The potential for such complications, as well the inconvenience of using portable home infusion pumps, has prevented the widespread acceptance of ECF as a new standard of care.

Several newer agents, including the taxanes and irinotecan, have activity in advanced gastric cancer and have yet to be evaluated as part of combination regimens in the randomized setting. The continued evaluation of new systemic agents is likely to further increase treatment options and improve outcomes in patients with advanced gastric cancer.

**Table 27–10** Randomized trials of combination chemotherapy regimens in gastric cancer

| Study | Regimen | Evaluable Patients | Response Rate | Median Survival |
|---|---|---|---|---|
| Wils et al. (1991)[65] | FAM | 103 | 7/79 (9%) | 29 weeks |
| | FAMTX | 105 | 33/81 (41%) | 42 weeks |
| Kelsen et al. (1992)[66] | FAMTX | 30 | 10/30 (33%) | 7.3 months |
| | EAP | 30 | 6/30 (20%) | 6.1 months |
| Wilke et al. (1995)[82] | FAMTX | 274[a] | 9/45 (20%) | 7 months |
| | ELF | | 9/42 (21%) | 7 months |
| | FP | | 12/44 (27%) | 8 months |
| Webb et al. (1997)[67] | FAMTX | 130 | 23/108 (21%) | 5.7 months |
| | ECF | 126 | 50/111 (45%) | 8.9 months |

EAP, etoposide, doxorubicin, and cisplatin; ECF, epirubicin, cisplatin, and 5-fluorouracil; ELF, etoposide, leucovorin, and 5-fluorouracil; FAM, 5-fluorouracil, doxorubicin, and mitomycin C; FAMTX, 5-fluorouracil, doxorubicin, and methotrexate; FP, 5-fluorouracil and cisplatin.
[a]Number of patients in all three arms.

## Palliative Resection in Advanced Gastric Cancer

Symptoms of pain, nausea, hemorrhage, and obstruction, which do not reliably respond to chemotherapy, have prompted investigators to consider palliative resection for patients with advanced gastric cancer. In one early retrospective series of 75 patients, 88% of patients who received palliative resection experienced relief of symptoms, compared with 80% of patients who received gastrojejunostomy. The operative mortality rate in this series was greater than 20%.[94] In a more recent series that involved 51 patients,[95] operative mortality for both procedures was low, and the mean survival time after surgery was 9.5 months among patients who had undergone resection, compared with 4.2 months among patients who had undergone bypass. Palliation of symptoms also was significantly better in the group of patients treated with bypass.

A significant problem in these analyses is selection bias: patients who are considered candidates for complete resection are likely to have a better prognosis than those selected to receive only a bypass procedure. Two subsequent studies attempted to stratify patients according to the extent of disease preoperatively. An Italian retrospective analysis compared the outcomes of 105 patients who underwent exploratory laparotomy only, 80 patients who underwent bypass, and 61 patients who underwent palliative resection.[96] The median survival time for patients who had resection was 8.0 months, compared with only 3.5 months for those patients who received bypass procedures and 2.4 months for patients who received laparotomy alone. A benefit of palliative resection was noted among patients with both local disease and distant metastases. In a second series, the outcomes of 45 patients who received palliative resection were compared with those of 21 patients who received laparotomy alone. The two groups had similar extents of disease and the patients who received resection had better overall survival times.[97]

Not all patients with metastatic gastric cancer benefit from palliative resection. In a series of 26 patients with gastric linitis plastica, resection was associated with longer survival times only among patients whose disease was limited to the stomach or lymph nodes.[98] In patients with widespread disease, the median survival was only 4 months. No series to date has assessed the relative contribution of palliative resection in patients undergoing combination therapy. While palliative surgical resection may benefit certain patients, the criteria for selecting such patients have not been firmly established.

## Intraperitoneal Chemotherapy in Advanced Gastric Cancer

The high frequency with which gastric cancer spreads to the peritoneum has led several investigators to examine the utility of intraperitoneal chemotherapy in the prevention and treatment of peritoneal carcinomatosis. Phase II trials of postoperative intraperitoneal cisplatin monotherapy or cisplatin given together with 5-FU or floxuridine have demonstrated that this approach is both feasible and well tolerated by most patients.[99–101] However, a study in which 67 patients with stage III or IV gastric cancer were randomized to receive either intraperitoneal therapy with cisplatin or observation alone failed to demonstrate a survival advantage in the treated group.[102] One small randomized study demonstrated an improved survival rate in patients receiving intraperitoneal mitomycin C bound to carbon particles (M-CH) following surgical resection of gastric cancer.[103] How-

ever, a subsequent randomized study of 91 patients undergoing this procedure failed to show any beneficial effect.[104] Similarly, a randomized study investigating hyperthermic peritoneal perfusion of mitomycin C in patients following resection of gastric cancer failed to demonstrate a survival benefit.[105] Future trials may help to establish the role of intraperitoneal therapy in patients following surgical resection for gastric cancer and in those with peritoneal carcinomatosis from this disease.

## References

1. Comis R, Carter S. Integration of chemotherapy into combined modality treatment of solid tumors. Cancer Treat Rev 1:221–238, 1974.
2. Cullinan S, Moertel C, Fleming T, et al. A comparison of three chemotherapeutic regimens in the treatment of advanced pancreatic and gastric carcinoma. JAMA 253:2061–2067, 1985.
3. Baker L, Vaitkevicius V, Gehan E. Randomized prospective trial comparing 5-fluorouracil to 5-fluorouracil and methyl-CCNU. Cancer Treat Rep 60:733–737, 1976.
4. DeLisi V, Cocconi G, Tonato M, et al. Randomized comparison of 5-FU alone or in combination with carmustine, doxorubicin, and mitomycin (BAFMi) in the treatment of advanced gastric cancer. Cancer Treat Rep 4:481–485, 1986.
5. Kovach J, Moertel C, Schutt A, et al. A controlled study of combined 1,3-bis(2-chloroethyl)-1-nitrosurea and 5-fluorouracil therapy for advanced gastric and pancreatic cancer. Cancer 33:563–567, 1974.
6. Machover D, Goldschmidt E, Chollet P, et al. Treatment of advanced colorectal and gastric adenocarcinomas with 5-fluorouracil and high-dose folinic acid. J Clin Oncol 4:685–696, 1986.
7. Berenberg J, Tangen C, Macdonald J, et al. Phase II study of 5-fluorouracil and folinic acid in the treatment of patients with advanced gastric cancer: a Southwest Oncology Group Study. Cancer 76:715–719, 1995.
8. Arbuck S, Douglass H, Trave F, et al. A phase II study of 5-fluorouracil and high-dose folinic acid in gastric carcinoma. J Clin Oncol 5:1150–1156, 1987.
9. Lokich J, Ahlgren J, Gullo J, et al. A prospective randomized comparison of continuous infusion fluorouracil with a conventional bolus schedule in metastatic colorectal carcinoma: a Mid-Atlantic Oncology Program Study. J Clin Oncol 7:425–732, 1989.
10. Moynihan T, Hansen R, Anderson T, et al. Continuous 5-fluorouracil infusion in advanced gastric carcinoma. Am J Clin Oncol 11:461–464, 1988.
11. Takiuchi T, Ajani J. UFT in gastric cancer: a comprehensive review. J Clin Oncol 16:2877–2885, 1998.
12. Kurihara M, Koizumi W, Hasegawa K, et al. Late phase II study of S-1, a novel oral fluoro-pyrimidine derivative, in patients with advanced gastric cancer. Proc Am Soc Clin Oncol 17:262A, 1998.
13. Ohtsu A, Sakata M, Horikoshi N, et al. A phase II study of S-1 in patients with advanced gastric cancer. Proc Am Soc Clin Oncol 17:262A, 1998.
14. Levi J, Fox R, Tattersall M, et al. Analysis of prospectively randomized comparison of doxorubicin versus 5-fluorouracil, doxorubicin, and BCNU in advanced gastric cancer: implications for future studies. J Clin Oncol 4:1348–1355, 1986.
15. Moertel C, Lavin P. Phase II–III studies in advanced gastric cancer. Cancer Treat Rep 63:1863–1869, 1979.
16. The GITSG. Phase II–III chemotherapy studies in advanced gastric cancer. Cancer Treat Rep 63:1871–1876, 1979.
17. Ganzina F. 4-Epirubicin, a new analog of doxorubicin: a preliminary overview of preclinical and clinical data. Cancer Treat Rev 10:1–22, 1983.
18. Devries E, Nanninga A, Greidanus J, et al. A phase II study of a 21-day continuous infusion schedule with epirubicin in advanced gastric cancer. Eur J Cancer Clin Oncol 25:1509–1510, 1989.
19. Figer A, Loven D, Vigler N. Epirubicin in the treatment of advanced carcinoma of the stomach. Proc Am Soc Clin Oncol 8:112, 1989.
20. Cazap E, Estevez R, Bruno M, et al. Phase II trial of 4′-epi-doxorubicin in locally advanced or metastatic gastric cancer. Tumori 74:313–315, 1988.
21. Lacave A, Izarzugaza I, Aparicio I, et al. Phase II clinical trial of cis-dichloro-diammineplatinum in gastric cancer. Am J Clin Oncol 6:35–38, 1983.
22. Aabo K, Pederson H, Rorth M. Cisplatin in the treatment of advanced gastric carcinoma: a phase II study. Cancer Treat Rep 69:449–450, 1985.

23. Lacave A, Wils J, Diaz-Rubio E. Cisplatinum as second-line chemotherapy in advanced gastric adenocarcinomas: a phase II study of the EORTC gastrointestinal tract cancer cooperative group. Eur J Cancer Clin Oncol 21:1321–1329, 1985.

24. Perry M, Green M, Mick R, et al. Cisplatin in patients with gastric cancer: a cancer and leukeumia group B phase II study. Cancer Treat Rep 70:415–416, 1986.

25. Kantarjian H, Ajani J, Karlin D. Cis-diaminodichloroplatinum chemotherapy for advanced adenocarcinoma of the upper gastrointestinal tract. Oncology 42:69–71, 1985.

26. Leichman L, McDonald B, Dindogru A, et al. Cisplatin: an active drug in the treatment of disseminated gastric cancer. Cancer 53:18–22, 1984.

27. Vogl S, Camacho F, Engstrom P, et al. Phase II trial of cisplatin in advanced gastric cancer. Cancer Treat Rep 68:1497–1498, 1984.

28. Beer M, Cocconi G, Ceci G, et al. A phase II study of cisplatin in advanced gastric cancer. Eur J Cancer Clin Oncol 19:717–720, 1983.

29. Beer M, Cavalli F, Kaye S, et al. A phase II study of carboplatin in advanced or metastatic stomach cancer. Eur J Cancer Clin Oncol 23:1565–1567, 1987.

30. Einzig A, Lipsitz S, Wiernick P, et al. Phase II trial of Taxol in patients with adenocarcinoma of the upper gastrointestinal tract: the Eastern Cooperative Oncology Group (ECOG) results. Invest New Drugs 13:223–227, 1995.

31. Ohtsu A, Boku N, Tamura F, et al. An early phase II study of a 3-hour infusion of paclitaxel for advanced gastric cancer. Am J Clin Oncol 21:416–419, 1998.

32. Ajani J, Fairweather J, Dumas P, et al. Phase II study of Taxol in patients with advanced gastric carcinoma. Cancer J Sci Am 4:269–274, 1998.

33. Sulkes A, Smyth J, Sessa C, et al. Docetaxel in advanced gastric cancer: results of a phase II clinical trial. Br J Cancer 70:380–383, 1994.

34. Mai M, Sakata Y, Kanamura R, et al. A late phase II clinical study of RP56976 (docetaxel) in patients with advanced or recurrent gastric cancer: a cooperative group trial. Gan To Kagaku Ryoho 26:487–496, 1999.

35. Einzig A, Newberg D, Remick S, et al. Phase II trial of docetaxel (Taxotere) in patients with adenocarcinoma of the upper gastrointestinal tract previously treated with cytotoxic chemotherapy: the Eastern Cooperative Oncology Group (ECOG) results of protocol E1293. Med Oncol 13:87–93, 1996.

36. Mavroudis D, Kakolyris S, Kouroussis N, et al. First line treatment of advanced gastric cancer with docetaxel monotherapy and granulocyte colony-stimulating factor (G-CSF). Proc Am Soc Clin Oncol 18:A977, 1999.

37. Futatsuki K, Wakui A, Nakao I, et al. Late phase II study of irinotecan hydrochloride (CPT-11) in advanced gastric cancer. CPT-11 Gastrointestinal Cancer Study Group. Gan To Kagaku Ryoho 21:1033–1038, 1994.

38. Kohne C, Thus-Patience P, Catane R, et al. Final results of a phase II trial of CPT-11 in patients with advanced gastric cancer. Proc Am Soc Clin Oncol 18:258a, 1999.

39. Hantel A, Tangen C, Macdonald J, et al. Phase II trial of trimetrexate in untreated advanced gastric carcinoma. A Southwest Oncology Group Study. Invest New Drugs 12:155–157, 1994.

40. Asbury R, Cnaan A, Haller D. Eastern Cooperative Oncology Group (ECOG) phase II study of trimetrexate in metastatic gastric cancer. Proc Am Soc Clin Oncol 9:A489, 1990.

41. Bruckner H, Lokich J, Stablein D. Studies of Baker's antifol, methotrexate, and razoxane in advanced gastric cancer: a Gastrointestinal Study Group report. Cancer Treat Rep 66:1713–1717, 1982.

42. Moore G, Bross I, Ausman R. Effects of chlorambucil in 374 patients with advanced cancer. Cancer Chemother Rep 52:661–666, 1968.

43. Christman K, Kelsen D, Saltz L, et al. Phase II trial of gemcitabine in patients with advanced gastric cancer. Cancer 73:5–7, 1994.

44. Macdonald J, Schein P, Woolley P, et al. 5-Fluorouracil, doxorubicin, and mitomycin (FAM) combination chemotherapy for advanced gastric cancer. Ann Intern Med 93:533–536, 1980.

45. Preusser P, Achterrath W, Wilke H, et al. Chemotherapy of gastric cancer. Cancer Treat Rev 15:257–277, 1988.

46. Ahlgren J, Smith F, Cazap E, et al. FAM (5-FU, doxorubicin, mitomycin-C) plus triazinate (FAM-T) in gastric carcinoma: a combined phase II trial of the Mid-Atlantic Oncology Progran and the Pan-American Health Organization. Cancer Treat Rep 71:419–420, 1987.

47. Bunn P, Nugent J, Ihde D. 5-Fluorouracil, methyl-CCNU, adriamycin, and mitomycin C in the treatment of advanced gastric cancer. Cancer Treat Rep 62:1287–1293, 1978.

48. Karlin D, Stroehlein J, Bennetts R. Phase I–II Study of the combination of 5-FU, doxorubicin, mitomycin, and semustine (FAMMe) in the

treatment of adenocarcinoma of the stomach. Cancer Treat Rep 66:1613–1617, 1982.

49. Arbuck S, Silk Y, Douglass H, et al. A Phase II trial of 5-fluorouracil, doxorubicin, mitomycin C and leucovorin in advanced gastric cancer. Cancer 65:2442–2445, 1990.

50. Beretta G, Fraschini P, Ravaioli A, et al. FAM/FAMB polychemotherapy for advanced carcinoma of the stomach. Proc Am Soc Clin Oncol 2:C–514, 1983.

51. Bernath A, Thornward C. Treatment of advanced gastric carcinoma with BCNU, adriamycin, 5-FU and mitomycin C (BAFMi). Proc Am Soc Clin Oncol 20:C–87, 1979.

52. Lacave A, Wils J, Bleiberg H, et al. An EORTC Gastrointestinal Group phase III evaluation of combinations of methyl-CCNU, 5-fluorouracil, and Adriamycin in advanced gastric cancer. J Clin Oncol 5:1387–1393, 1987.

53. The GITSG. Randomized study of combination chemotherapy in unresectable gastric cancer. Cancer 53:13–17, 1984.

54. Douglass H, Lavin P, Goudsmit A, et al. An Eastern Cooperative Oncology Group evaluation of combinations of methyl-CCNU, mitomycin-C, Adriamycin, and 5-fluorouracil in advanced measurable gastric cancer (Est 2277). J Clin Oncol 2:1372–1381, 1984.

55. The GITSG. A comparitive clinical assessment of combination chemotherapy in the management of advanced gastric carcinoma. Cancer 49:1362–1366, 1982.

56. The GITSG. Triazinate and platinum efficacy in combination with 5-fluorouracil and doxorubicin: results of a three-arm randomized trial in metastatic gastric cancer. J Natl Cancer Inst 80:1011–1015, 1988.

57. Schnitzler G, Quiesser W, Heim M, et al. Phase III study of 5-FU and carmustine versus 5-FU, carmustine, and doxorubicin in advanced gastric cancer. Cancer Treat Rep 70:477–479, 1986.

58. Levi J, Dalley D, Aroney R. Improved combination therapy in advanced gastric cancer. BMJ 2:1471–1473, 1979.

59. Lopez M, DiLauro L, Papaldo P, et al. Treatment of advanced measurable gastric carcinoma with 5-fluorouracil, adriamycin, and BCNU. Oncology 43:288–291, 1986.

60. Klein H, Wickramanayake P, Dieterle F. Chemotherapie-protokoll zur Behandlung des metastasierenden Magenkarzinoms. Methotrexat, Adriamycin und 5-Fluorouracil. Dtsch Med Wochenschr 45:1708–1712, 1982.

61. Klein H. Long-term results with FAMTX (5-fluorouracil, adriamycin, methotrexate) in advanced gastric cancer. Anticancer Res 9:1025–1026, 1989.

62. Weh H, Platz D, Garbrecht M. Ergebnis eines modifzerten FAMeth Chemotherapie Protokolls beim metastasierten Magenkarzinom. Dtsch Med Wochenschr 114:1391–1396, 1989.

63. Hermann R, Fritz D, Queizer W. Chemotherapie des Magenkarzinom. Dtsch Med Wochenschr 109:1463, 1984.

64. Wils J, Bleiberg H, Dalesio O, et al. An EORTC Gastrointestinal Group evaluation of the combination of sequential methotrexate and 5-fluorouracil combined with Adriamycin in advanced measurable gastric cancer. J Clin Oncol 4:1799–1803, 1986.

65. Wils J, Klein H, Wagener D, et al. Sequential high-dose methotrexate and fluorouracil combined with doxorubicin: a step ahead in the treatment of advanced gastric cancer: a trial of the EORTC Gastrointestinal Tract Cooperative Group. J Clin Oncol 9:827–831, 1991.

66. Kelsen D, Atiq O, Saltz L, et al. FAMTX versus etoposide, doxorubicin, and cisplatin: a random assignment trial in gastric cancer. J Clin Oncol 10:541–548, 1992.

67. Webb A, Cunningham D, Scarffe J, et al. Randomized trial comparing epirubicin, cisplatin, and fluorouracil versus fluorouracil, doxorubicin, and methotrexate in advanced esophagogastric cancer. J Clin Oncol 15:261–267, 1997.

68. Kelsen D, Buckner J, Einzig A, et al. Phase II trial of cisplatin and etoposide in adenocarcinomas of the upper GI tract. Cancer Treat Rep 71:329–330, 1987.

69. Elliot T, Moertel C, Wieand H, et al. A phase II study of the combination of etoposide and cisplatin in the therapy of advanced gastric cancer. Cancer 65:1491–1494, 1990.

70. Preusser P, Wilke H, Achtermath W, et al. Phase II study with the combination etoposide, doxorubicin, and cisplatin in advanced measurable gastric cancer. J Clin Oncol 7:1310–1317, 1989.

71. Katz A, Gansi R, Simon S. Phase II trial of VP-16, Adriamycin, and cisplatin in patients with advanced gastric cancer. Proc Am Soc Clin Oncol 8:98, 1991.

72. Taguchi T. Combination therapy with etoposide, Adriamycin, and cisplatin (EAP) for advanced gastric cancer. Proc Am Soc Clin Oncol 8:108, 1989.

73. Wilke H, Preusser P, Fink U, et al. Preoperative therapy in locally advanced and nonresectable gastric cancer: a phase II study with etoposide, doxorubicin and cisplatin. J Clin Oncol 7:1318–1326, 1989.

74. Taal B, Huinink W, Franklin H. EAP in gastric cancer. J Clin Oncol 8:939–940, 1990.

75. Sparano J, Schwartz E, Salva K. Phase II trial of etoposide, doxorubicin, and cisplatin (EAP regimen) in advanced gastric cancer. Am J Clin Oncol 13:374–378, 1990.

76. Lerner A, Gonin R, Steele G, et al. Etoposide, doxorubicin, and cisplatin (EAP) chemotherapy for advanced gastric carcinoma: results of a phase II trial. J Clin Oncol 10:536–540, 1992.

77. Wilke H, Preusser P, Fink U. New developments in the treatment of gastric cancer. Semin Oncol 17(Suppl 2):61–70, 1990.

78. DiBartolomeo M, Bajetta E, deBraud F, et al. Phase II study of the etoposide, leucovorin and fluorouracil combination for patients with advanced gastric cancer unsuitable for aggressive chemotherapy. Oncology 52:41–44, 1995.

79. Partyka S, Dumas P, Ajani J. Combination chemotherapy with granulocyte-macrophage–colony stimulating factor in patients with locoregional and metastatic gastric adenocarcinoma. Cancer 85:2336–2339, 1999.

80. Ohtsu A, Yoshida S, Saito D, et al. An early phase II study of 5-fluorouracil combined with cisplatinum as a second-line chemotherapy against metastatic gastric cancer. Jpn J Clin Oncol 21:120–124, 1991.

81. Lacave A, Baron F, Anton L, et al. Combination chemotherapy with cisplatin and fluorouracil 5-day infusion in the therapy of advanced gastric cancer: a phase II trial. Ann Oncol 2:751–754, 1991.

82. Wilke H, Wils J, Rougier P, et al. Preliminary analysis of a randomized phase III trial of FAMTX versus ELF versus cisplatin/FU in advanced gastric cancer. A trial of the EORTC Gastrointestinal Tract Cancer Cooperative Group and the AIO. Proc Am Soc Clin Oncol 14:A500, 1995.

83. The Kyoto Research Group for Chemotherapy of Gastric Cancer (KRGCGC). A randomized, comparative study of combination chemotherapies in advanced gastric cancer: 5-fluorouracil and cisplatin (FP) versus 5-fluorouracil, cisplatin and 4′epirubicin. Anticancer Res 12: 1983–1988, 1992.

84. Cervantes A, Navarro M, Carrato A, et al. The addition of cisplatin to continuous infusion 5-fluorouracil for the treatment of advanced gastric cancer. Results of two consecutive phase II trials of the Spanish Group for Tumor Therapy (TTD). Proc Am Soc Clin Oncol 18:A980, 1999.

85. Findlay M, Cunningham D, Norman A, et al. A phase II study in advanced gastro-esophageal cancer using epirubicin and cisplatin in combination with continuous infusion 5-fluorouracil (ECF). Ann Oncol 5: 609–616, 1994.

86. Cascinu S, Labianca R, Allesandroni P, et al. Intensive weekly chemotherapy for advanced gastric cancer using fluorouracil, cisplatin, epidoxorubicin, 6S-leucovorin, glutathione, and filgrastim: a report from the Italian Group for the Study of Digestive Tract Cancer. J Clin Oncol 15:3313–3319, 1997.

87. Chi K, Chao Y, Chan W, et al. Weekly etoposide, epirubicin, cisplatin, 5-fluorouracil and leucovorin: an effective chemotherapy in advanced gastric cancer. Br J Cancer 77:1984–1988, 1998.

88. Murad A, Santiago F, Petroianu A, et al. Modified therapy with 5-fluorouracil, doxorubicin, and methotrexate in advanced gastric cancer. Cancer 72:37–41, 1993.

89. Pyrhonen S, Kuitunen T, Nyandoto P, et al. Randomised comparison of fluorouracil, epidoxorubicin, and methotrexate (FEMTX) plus supportive care with supportive care alone in patients with non-resectable gastric cancer. Br J Cancer 71:587–591, 1995.

90. Glimelius B, Ekstrom K, Hoffman K, et al. Randomised comparison between chemotherapy plus best supportive care with best supportive care in advanced gastric cancer. Ann Oncol 8:163–168, 1997.

91. Cullinan S, Moertel C, Wieand H, et al. Controlled evaluation of three drug combination regimens versus fluorouracil alone for the therapy of advanced gastric cancer. J Clin Oncol 12:412–416, 1994.

92. Panettiere F, Haas C, McDonald B, et al. Drug combinations in the treatment of gastric adenocarcinoma: a randomized Southwest Oncology Group study. J Clin Oncol 2:420–424, 1984.

93. Waters J, Norman A, Cunningham D, et al. Long-term survival after epirubicin, cisplatin, and fluorouracil for gastric cancer: results of a randomized trial. Br J Cancer 80:269–272, 1999.

94. Ekbom G, Gleysteen J. Gastric malignancy: resection for palliation. Surgery 88:476–481, 1980.

95. Meijer S, DeBakker O, Hoitsma H. Palliative resection in gastric cancer. J Surg Oncol 23:77–80, 1983.

96. Bozzetti F, Bonfanti G, Audisio R. Prognosis of patients after palliative surgical procedures for carcinoma of the stomach. Surg Gynecol Obstet 164:151–154, 1987.

97. Boddie A, McMurtrey M, Diacco G, et al. Palliative total gastrectomy and esophagectomy. Cancer 51:1195–1200, 1983.

98. Aranha G, Georgen R. Gastric linitis plastica is not a surgical disease. Surgery 106:758–763, 1989.

99. Jones A, Trott P, Cunningham D, et al. A pilot study of intraperitoneal cisplatin in the management of gastric cancer. Ann Oncol 5:123–126, 1994.

100. Kelsen D, Karpeh M, Schwartz G, et al. Neoadjuvant therapy of high-risk gastric cancer: a phase II trial of preoperative FAMTX and postoperative intraperitoneal fluorouracil-cisplatin plus intravenous fluorouracil. J Clin Oncol 14:1818–1828, 1996.

101. Leichman L, Silberman H, Leichman C, et al. Preoperative systemic chemotherapy followed by adjuvant postoperative intraperitoneal therapy for gastric cancer: a University of Southern California pilot program. J Clin Oncol 10:1933–1942, 1992.

102. Sautner T, Hofbauer F, Depisch D, et al. Adjuvant intraperitoneal cisplatin chemotherapy does not improve long-term survival after surgery for advanced gastric cancer. J Clin Oncol 12:970–974, 1994.

103. Hagiwara A, Takahashi T, Kojima O. Prophylaxis with carbon-adsorbed mitomycin against peritoneal recurrence of gastric cancer. Lancet 339: 629–631, 1992.

104. Rosen H, Jatzko G, Repse S, et al. Adjuvant intraperitoneal chemotherapy with carbon-adsorbed mitomycin in patients with gastric cancer: results of a randomized multicenter trial of the Austrian working group for surgical oncology. J Clin Oncol 16:2733–2738, 1998.

105. Hamazoe R, Maeta M, Kaibara N. Intraperitoneal thermo-chemotherapy for prevention of peritoneal recurrence of gastric cancer. Cancer 73:2048–2052, 1994.

# Section 3

# Cancer of the Pancreas

# Chapter 28

# Epidemiology and Molecular Epidemiology of Pancreatic Cancer

## DONGHUI LI

Pancreatic cancer is a leading cause of cancer-related deaths in developed countries. However, the etiology of this cancer has been poorly understood for several reasons. First, difficulties in early detection and diagnosis have led to most pancreatic cancers being detected only at advanced stages. The prognosis at such stages is poor; many patients with this cancer die before they can be interviewed. Furthermore, clinical means of diagnosing pancreatic cancer have traditionally been unreliable, especially before the advent of advanced imaging techniques. In 1985, approximately 185,000 new cases of pancreatic carcinoma were reported worldwide,[1] with a death/incidence ratio of 0.99, which places pancreatic cancer 13th in incidence but eighth as a cause of cancer death worldwide.[2] In the United States, pancreatic cancer is the fifth leading cause of cancer death in both men and women.[3] Every year, 28,000 Americans die of pancreatic cancer, which accounts for 22% of gastrointestinal cancer deaths and 5% of all cancer deaths.[4]

### Geographic and Demographic Patterns

#### Geographic Variation

The mortality and incidence patterns of pancreatic carcinoma vary worldwide. The mortality rate for pancreatic cancer is high in Denmark, Sweden, Finland, Ireland, Austria, Czechoslovakia, Hungary, and other European countries, and among nonwhite populations in the United States.[5] The mortality rate is low in Hong Kong, Spain, Greece, Portugal, Yugoslavia, India, Kuwait, and Singapore.[5] The mortality rates vary from 12.5 per 100,000 in high-risk countries to less than 2.2 per 100,000 in low-risk countries.[6] In the United States, the incidence of pancreatic cancer has increased since the 1930s until 1973, after which it stabilized at 9 per 100,000 (as measured in 1988).[5] The overall incidence rates also increased in 25 European countries between the 1950s and the 1970s.[5] Part of this increase may have been due to misclassification of pancreatic cancer, but several analyses indicate that some of the rise in incidence was real.[5] Comparisons of the age-adjusted death rates for pancreatic cancer from 1983 to 1987 in 31 countries revealed a decline in the mortality of pancreatic cancer in most countries except for Czechoslovakia, Germany, Japan, Italy, France, and Spain,[5] with the decline more marked for men than for women. The reason for the decline is thought to be related to a reduction in smoking among men.[5]

### Age, Gender, and Race

The most reliable and important predictor of pancreatic cancer incidence is age.[6] The age-specific incidence of pancreatic cancer in white American women and men increases continuously throughout life even after age of 85. About 80% of pancreatic cancer cases occur in people aged 60 to 80 years. Cases in people less than 40 years old are extremely rare; people in the eighth decade of life have approximately 40 times the risk of pancreatic cancer as do those in the fourth decade.[6]

In humans as well as in animal models, pancreatic cancer is more common in males than in females.[6] In the United States, blacks are more frequently affected than whites, with an incidence of 15.2 per 100,000 black men.[7] Mortality rates among African Americans are also higher than those among African blacks, which suggests that environmental factors are involved.[7]

### Host Etiologic Factors

#### Hereditary Factors

Hereditary genetic factors account for less than 10% of pancreatic cancer cases.[8–11] An excess risk of pancreatic cancer has been

### Mixed ductal–endocrine carcinoma

Mixed ductal–endocrine carcinoma, also known as an exocrine-endocrine tumor, is characterized by an intimate admixture of ductal and endocrine cells in the primary tumor as well as in the metastases. Biologically, however, this tumor behaves like a typical ductal adenocarcinoma.[6] By definition, the endocrine cells should comprise at least one-third to one-half of the tumor tissue. The ductal differentiation is defined by mucin production and the presence of a duct-type marker such as CEA. The endocrine cells are characterized by the presence of neuroendocrine markers such as synaptophysin. These neoplasms are exceptionally rare.

## Prognosis and Predictive Factors Associated with Ductal Adenocarcinoma

Ductal adenocarcinoma usually is fatal, with a mean untreated survival time of 3 months and a survival of 10–20 months following radical resection.[44,45] The overall 5-year survival after resection is 3%–4%.[46] Unresectable carcinomas are treated with palliative bypass operations.

### Site, size, stage

Patients with a carcinoma confined to the pancreas and measuring <3 cm in size have a longer survival period than patients with larger tumors or with retroperitoneal invasion. Carcinomas of the body and tail tend to present at a more advanced stage than those located in the head; therefore, patient survival is particularly bad.[44,47]

### Residual tumor tissue

Patients with no residual tumor after resection have the most favorable prognosis. Therefore, the retroperitoneal resection margin is of utmost prognostic importance.[48]

### Recurrence

Local recurrence, especially in the tissues surrounding the large mesenteric vessels, is a major adverse factor in determining survival after resection.[48] Another common site of recurrence is in the regional lymph nodes or in liver metastases that were too small to be detected at the time of surgery.

### Tumor grade

The mean postoperative survival is correlated significantly with the histologic tumor grade (degree of glandular differentiation), mitotic index, and severity of cellular atypia.[49]

### Surgical pathology report

All prognostic and predictive factors should be mentioned in the pathology report in order to alert the clinician to the possible outcome. The report should clearly state the type of pancreatic cancer, its histologic grade, and size and the primary site. The presence or absence of extrapancreatic direct tumor extension (including involvement of surgical resection margins), both vascular and perineural invasion, should be outlined, as these are major predictors of disease recurrence.

## Acinar Cell Carcinoma

Acinar cell carcinomas are rare tumors, constituting 1%–2% of exocrine pancreatic neoplasms. These tumors are recognizable

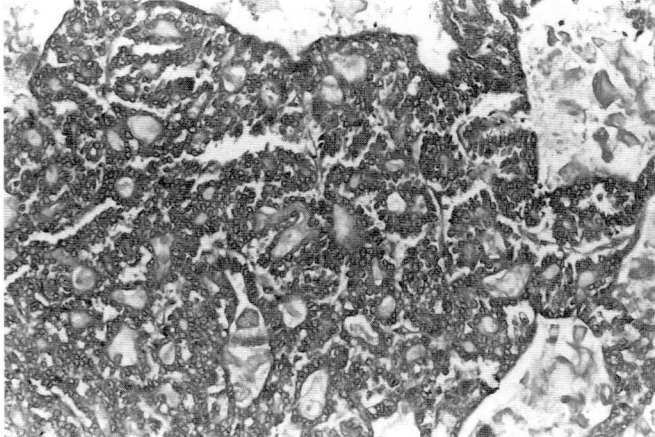

**Figure 30-9** Acinar cell carcinoma. Note the pure acinar growth, reminiscent of normal pancreatic acinar tissue.

by their production of pancreatic enzymes.[6] Most patients are adults (with a mean age of 62 years); these carcinoma can rarely occur in children.[50] Patients usually present with symptoms related to either local spread or metastases. A syndrome of lipase hypersecretion is present in 10%–15% of patients, especially in those with hepatic metastases. This is characterized by excessive secretion of lipase into the serum, with clinical symptoms including subcutaneous fat necrosis and polyarthralgia.[51] The majority of tumors are solid, although cystic changes secondary to the accumulation of secretions in the lumina of neoplastic acini may be seen. Histologically, most tumors are lobulated, with acinar areas alternating with trabeculated and solid forms. A few tumors have a purely acinar growth, reminiscent of normal pancreatic acinar tissue (Fig. 30–9). The predominantly trabecular and solid acinar cell tumors may be confused with pancreatoblastoma and pancreatic endocrine tumors. The key diagnostic feature of acinar cell carcinoma is the abundant stippled eosinophilic cytoplasm of the neoplastic cells, with granules that are PAS positive and diastase resistant. The granules are small and uniform, differing from the granules occasionally seen in solid-pseudopapillary tumors and pancreatoblastoma.

Immunohistochemical studies usually are positive for lipase, trypsin, amylase, chymotrypsin, and $\alpha_1$-antitrypsin.[51,52] All tumors are positive for low-molecular-weight cytokeratin (CAM 5.2). Scattered synaptophysin- and chromogranin-positive endocrine cells are seen in up to 25% of cases.[53] Electron microscopic examination confirms the presence of zymogen granules in the cytoplasm.

Acinar cell carcinomas have an aggressive biologic behavior, and patients have a relatively poor prognosis. Patients younger than 60 years have been reported to have a better prognosis than those over 60 years (25.6 months vs. 13.4 months).[51]

## Pancreatoblastoma

Pancreatoblastoma is a rare pancreatic carcinoma that occurs almost exclusively in infants and childhood; however, it has been reported in adults.[54] This is a primitive tumor that may demonstrate both epithelial and mesenchymal elements. Most of these tumors arise in the head or body of the pancreas as a soft, solid mass, usually surrounded by a fibrous capsule.

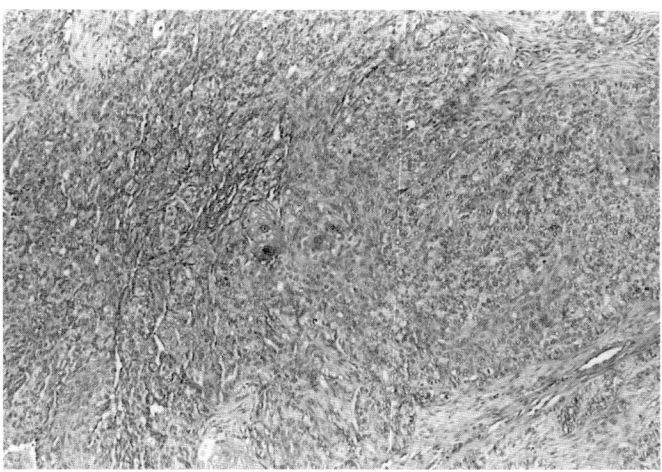

**Figure 30-10** Pancreatoblastoma. A vaguely lobulated tumor shows a mixture of epithelial and mesenchymal elements. Note the presence of squamoid cell nests (arrow).

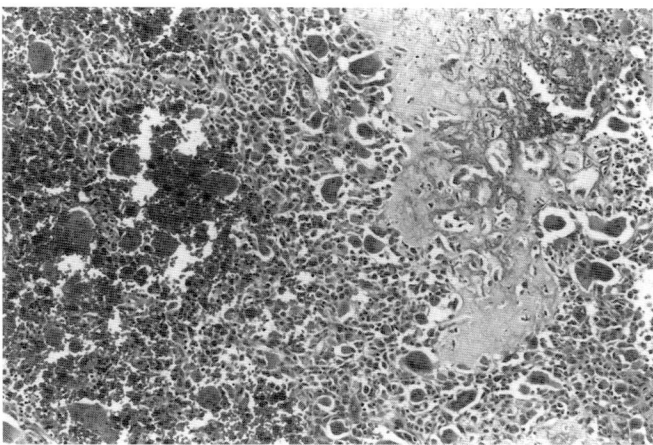

**Figure 30-11** Osteoclast-like giant cell tumor. Osteoclast-like giant cells (uniformly multinucleated) and bizarre tumor giant cells are mixed with a few spindle and small pleomorphic cells. Note the presence of osteoid formation (right) in this neoplasm.

Microscopically, the lobulated neoplasm shows a mixture of epithelial and mesenchymal elements (Fig. 30–10). The epithelial cells are monomorphic, growing in acinar, glandular, or solid patterns. The mitotic activity is usually high. Mesenchymal elements, if present, are in the form of spindle cells and rarely have foci of chondroid or osseous metaplasia. A distinct feature of most pancreatoblastomas is the presence of squamoid cell nests (squamoid corpuscles) that blend with the epithelial component. Immunohistochemically, the epithelial cells are positive for cytokeratin (CAM 5.2), lipase, trypsin, chymotrypsin, and $\alpha_1$-antitrypsin.[52] The squamoid nests are unexpectedly negative for cytokeratin. A few tumors are positive for α-fetoprotein. This immunoprofile reflects the primitive nature of this neoplasm.

The prognosis for patients with pancreatoblastoma is fairly good in the absence of metastases. One-year and 5-year survival rates in these patients are 60% and 25%, respectively. With metastatic disease, or in adult patients with pancreatoblastomas, the outcome is usually fatal, with a mean survival of 1.5 years.[54]

## Osteoclast-like Giant Cell Tumors

Osteoclast-like giant cell tumor of the pancreas is a rare tumor composed of undifferentiated epithelial and/or mesenchymal cells admixed with non-neoplastic osteoclast-like giant cells.[6] Usually the tumor is part of a ductal adenocarcinoma or a mucinous cystic tumor.[55] Although these tumors originally were believed to be epithelial in origin, most fail to demonstrate epithelial markers. Osteoclast-like giant cell tumors can occur at any adult age (with a mean of 60 years). Most occur in the pancreatic head as large, lobulated masses with a rubbery, often hemorrhagic cut surface. Histologically, this tumor resembles the giant cell tumor of bone. It is composed of neoplastic spindle cells with hyperchromatic nuclei, intermixed with non-neoplastic multinucleated (20–40 small bland nuclei) osteoclast-like giant cells (Fig. 30–11). Foci of cartilagenous matrix and osteoid formation are common. The osteoclast-like giant cells have a distinct immunoprofile, which is characterized by cytoplasmic pos-

itivity for histiocytic markers (CD68) and membranous staining for leukocyte common antigen (LCA). The LCA positivity is a unique feature and is not seen in giant cell tumors at other body sites. The prognosis for osteoclast-like giant cell tumor of the pancreas is more favorable than that of ductal adenocarcinoma. Thus, it is important to differentiate this tumor from the sarcomatous components commonly seen in anaplastic ductal adenocarcinoma.

## Miscellaneous Carcinomas

### Oncocytic Carcinoma

Oncocytic carcinomas are rare neoplasms characterized by large cells with granular eosinophilic cytoplasm and large nuclei with well-differentiated nucleoli. Ultrastructurally, the cells show abundant mitochondria and a lack of zymogen and neuroendocrine granules. The differential diagnosis includes endocrine tumor and solid pseudopapillary tumor.

### Choriocarcinoma

Choriocarcinoma is an aggressive tumor associated with elevated levels of human chorionic gonadotropin (hCG). This tumor is composed of cytotrophoblastic cells intermingled with syncytiotrophoblastic cells that are immunoreactive for hCG. Choriocarcinoma can be pure or associated with mucinous cystadenocarcinoma.

### Clear Cell Carcinoma

Clear cell carcinomas are rare tumors composed of clear cells that are rich in glycogen and poor in mucin, and that are morphologically similar to renal cell carcinoma.

### Microglandular Carcinoma

Microglandular carcinoma, also known as *microadenocarcinoma*, is characterized by a cribriform and microglandular pattern of growth and is best regarded as a pattern of growth rather than as a distinct entity.

## Spread of Pancreatic Cancer

Pancreatic carcinoma within the pancreatic head spreads by invading the peripancreatic tissue, often via perineural sheaths (Fig. 30–12). It preferentially involves the retroperitoneal fatty tissues. Subsequently, retroperitoneal veins and nerves are invaded. In advanced cases, direct extension into neighboring organs is seen. Nodal spread involves the retroduodenal (posterior pancreatic or duodenal) and superior pancreatic head groups; the inferior head and superior body groups; and the anterior pancreatic or duodenal and inferior body groups, in descending order of frequency. These lymph node compartments are usually resected along with the pancreatic head in a standard Whipple procedure. More distal nodal metastases may occur in the ligamentum hepatoduodenale, at the celiac trunk, and at the root of the superior mesenteric artery. These lymph node compartments are removed only if an extended Whipple procedure is performed.

Pancreatic cancers within the body and tail are usually detected at a later stage than tumors arising in the head. Thus, they typically show a greater degree of local invasion into the spleen, stomach, left adrenal gland, colon, and retroperitoneum. Nodal metastases involve the superior and inferior body and tail groups and the splenic hilus lymph nodes. The tumor also may spread via lymphatic channels to involve the pleura and lung.

Hematogenous metastases affect the liver, lungs, adrenals, kidneys, bones, brain, and skin, in descending order of frequency.

## Staging of Pancreatic Cancer

The TNM classification scheme is used worldwide to provide prognostic information about tumors. The system classifies pancreatic carcinomas according to the extent of the primary tumor (T), the presence or absence of nodal metastases (N), and the presence or absence of distant metastases (M). The classification of tumors into four degrees of T, two degrees of N, and two degrees of M provides categories that are then condensed into four pathological stages (Table 30–3).

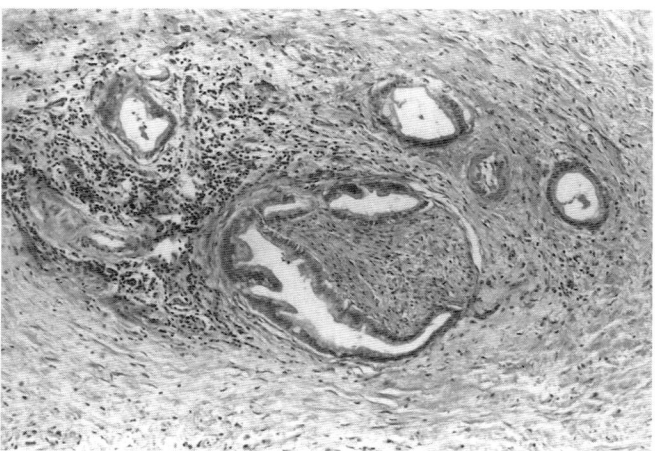

**Figure 30–12** Ductal adenocarcinoma. Note the spread of neoplastic glands along the perineural sheaths (center).

**Table 30–3** TNM classification of tumors of the exocrine pancreas[56]

*Primary Tumor (T)*

| | |
|---|---|
| TX | Primary tumor cannot be assessed |
| T0 | No evidence of primary tumor |
| Tis | Carcinoma in situ |
| T1 | Tumor limited to the pancreas, 2 cm or less in greatest dimension |
| T2 | Tumor limited to the pancreas, >2 cm in greatest dimension |
| T3 | Tumor extends directly into any of the following: duodenum, bile duct, peripancreatic tissues |
| T4 | Tumor extends directly into any of the following: stomach, spleen, colon, adjacent large vessels |

*Regional Lymph Nodes (N)*

| | |
|---|---|
| NX | Regional lymph nodes cannot be assessed |
| N0 | No regional lymph node metastasis |
| N1 | Regional lymph node metastasis |
| N1a | Metastasis in a single regional lymph node |
| N1b | Metastasis in multiple regional lymph nodes |

*Distant Metastasis (M)*

| | |
|---|---|
| MX | Distant metastasis cannot be assessed |
| M0 | No distant metastasis |
| M1 | Distant metastasis |

| Stage | Stage grouping | | |
|---|---|---|---|
| | T | N | M |
| Stage 0 | Tis | N0 | M0 |
| Stage I | T1 | N0 | M0 |
| | T2 | N0 | M0 |
| Stage II | T3 | N0 | M0 |
| Stage III | T1 | N1 | M0 |
| | T2 | N1 | M0 |
| | T3 | N1 | M0 |
| Stage IVA | T4 | Any N | M0 |
| Stage IVB | Any T | Any N | M1 |

## Secondary Tumors of the Pancreas

Secondary tumors of the pancreas are a component of advanced metastatic disease. These tumors account for 3%–16% of pancreatic malignancies and affect men and women equally. Any anatomic region of the pancreas may be involved, with no site predilection. The metastatic lesions can be solitary, multiple, or diffuse. The pancreas may be involved through direct spread (e.g., from stomach, duodenum, liver, bile ducts, or adrenals) or through lymphatic or hematogenous spread from distant sites. The main diagnostic challenge is to distinguish a metastasis from a primary pancreatic neoplasm. Clinical and radiologic findings of multiple tumor nodules and showing an abrupt transition from normal pancreatic tissue to neoplastic tissue without surrounding features of chronic pancreatitis favor a metastatic origin. The absence of pancreatic intraductal carcinoma in situ or dysplasia also suggests a metastatic tumor because most pancreatic adenocarcinomas arise against a background of widespread ductal dysplasia. Immunohistochemical studies of certain primary tumors may be helpful. The most problematic tumors are metastases from the gastrointestinal tract, renal cell carcinoma, and small-cell carcinoma of the lung. The prognosis is generally poor, as most pancreatic metastases indicate an advanced stage of disease.

## References

1. Fritz A, Percy C, Jack A, et al. International Classification of Diseases for Oncology (ICD-O), 3rd ed. World Health Organization, Geneva, 2000.
2. Hamilton SR, Aaltonen LA (eds). WHO Classification of Tumours: Pathology and Genetics of Tumours of the Digestive System. IARC Press, Lyon, 2000.
3. Compagno J, Oertel JE. Microcystic adenomas of the pancreas (glycogen-rich cystadenomas). A clinicopathologic study of 34 cases. Am J Clin Pathol 6:289–298, 1978.
4. Vortmeyer AO, Lubensky IA, Fogt F, Linehan WM, Khettry U, Zhuang Z. Allelic deletion and mutation of the von Hippel–Lindau (VHL) tumor suppressor gene in pancreatic microcystic adenomas. Am J Pathol 151: 951–956, 1997.
5. Egawa N, Maillet B, Schroder S, Foulis A, Mukai K, Klöppel G. Serous oligocystic and ill-demarcated adenoma of the pancreas: a variant of serous cystic adenoma. Virchows Arch 424:13–17, 1994.
6. Solcia E, Capella C, Klöppel G. Tumors of the Pancreas. Armed Forces Institute of Pathology, Washington, DC, 1997.
7. Zamboni G, Scarpa A, Bogina G, et al. Mucinous cystic tumors of the pancreas: clinicopathological features, prognosis, and relationship to other mucinous cystic tumors. Am J Surg Pathol 23:410–422, 1999.
8. Klöppel G, Solcia E, Longnecker DS, Capella C, Sobin LK. WHO: Histological Typing of Tumours of the Exocrine Pancreas, 2nd ed. Springer-Verlag, Berlin, 1996.
9. Parienty R, Ducellier R, Lubrano J, Piccard J, Pradel J, Solarski N. Cystadenomas of the pancreas: diagnosis by computed tomography. J Comput Assist Tomogr 4:364–367, 1980.
10. Yamaguchi K, Enjoi M. Cystic neoplasms of the pancreas. Gastroenterology 92:1934–1943, 1987.
11. Ridder GJ, Maschek H, Flemming P, et al. Ovarian-like stroma in an invasive mucinous cystadenocarcinoma of the pancreas positive for inhibin. A hint concerning its possible pathogenesis. Virchows Arch 432:451–454, 1998.
12. Compagno J, Oertel JE. Mucinous cystic neoplasms of the pancreas with overt and latent malignancy (cystadenocarcinoma and cystadenoma). A clinicopathologic study of 41 cases. Am J Clin Pathol 69:573–580, 1978.
13. Wilentz RE, Albores-Saavedra J, Zahurak M, et al. Pathologic examination accurately predicts prognosis in mucinous cystic neoplasms of the pancreas. Am J Surg Pathol 23:1320–1327, 1999.
14. Yamaguchi K, Tanaka M. Mucin-hypersecreting tumor of the pancreas with mucin extrusion through an enlarged papilla. Am J Gastroenterol 86:835–839, 1991.
15. Klöppel G. Clinicopathologic view of intraductal papillary-mucinous tumor of the pancreas. Hepatogastroenterology 45:1981–1985, 1998.
16. Yamada M, Kozuka S, Yamano K, Nakazawa S, Naitoh Y, Tsukamoto Y. Mucin-producing tumor of the pancreas. Cancer 68:159–168, 1991.
17. Klöppel G, Solcia E, Longnecker DS, et al. (eds). World Health Organization, International Histologic Classification of Tumors. Histologic Typing of Tumors of the Exocrine Pancreas, Vol. 2. Springer-Verlag, Geneva, 1996.
18. Nishihara K, Nagoshi M, Tsuneyoshi M, Yamaguchi K, Hayashi Y. Papillary cystic tumors of the pancreas. Assessment of their malignant potential. Cancer 71:82–92, 1993.
19. Miettinen M, Partanen S, Fraki O, Kivilaakso E. Papillary cystic tumor of the pancreas. An analysis of cellular differentiation by electron microscopy and immunohistochemistry. Am J Surg Pathol 11:855–865, 1987.
20. Adair CF, Wenig BM, Heffess CS. Solid and papillary cystic carcinoma of the pancreas: a tumor of low malignant potential [abstract]. Int J Surg Pathol 2:326, 1995.
21. Jeng LB, Chen MF, Tang RP. Solid and papillary neoplasms of the pancreas. Emphasis on surgical treatment. Arch Surg 128:433–436, 1998.
22. Hruban RH, Adsay NV, Albores-Saavedra J, et al. Pancreatic intraepithelial neoplasia: a new nomenclature and classification system for pancreatic duct lesions. Am J Surg Pathol 25:579–586, 2001.
23. Goggins M, Hruban RH, Kern SE. BRCA2 is inactivated late in the development of pancreatic intraepithelial neoplasia: evidence and implications. Am J Pathol 156:1767–1771, 2000.
24. Heinmoller E, Dietmaier W, Zirngibl H, et al. Molecular analysis of microdissected tumors and preneoplastic intraductal lesions in pancreatic carcinoma. Am J Pathol 157:83–92, 2000.
25. Yamano M, Fujii H, Takagaki T, et al. Genetic progression and divergence in pancreatic carcinoma. Am J Pathol 156:2123–2133, 2000.
26. Klöppel G. Pancreatic, non-endocrine tumours. In: Klöppel G, Heitz PU (eds): Pancreatic Pathology. Churchill Livingstone, Edinburgh, 1994, pp 79–113.
27. Gold EB, Goldin SB. Epidemiology of and risk factors for pancreatic cancer. Surg Oncol Clin North Am 7:67–91, 1998.
28. Greenberg RE, Bank S, Stark B. Adenocarcinoma of the pancreas producing pancreatitis and pancreatic abscess. Pancreas 5:108–113, 1990.
29. Monno S, Nagata A, Homma T, et al. Exocrine pancreatic cancer with humoral hypercalcemia. Am J Gastroenterol 79:128–132, 1984.
30. Warshaw AL, Fernandez-Del CC. Pancreatic carcinoma. N Engl J Med 326:455–465, 1992.
31. Yonezawa S, Sueyoshi K, Nomoto M, et al. Gene expression is found in noninvasive tumors but not in invasive tumors of the pancreas and liver: its close relationship with prognosis of the patients. Hum Pathol 28:344–352, 1997.
32. Takeda S, Nakao A, Ichihara T, et al. Serum concentration and immunohistochemical localization of Span-1 antigen in pancreatic cancer. A comparison with CA19-9 antigen. Hepatogastroenterology 38:143–148, 1991.
33. Batge B, Bosslet K, Sedlacek HH, Kern HF, Klöppel G. Monoclonal antibodies against CEA-related components discriminate between pancreatic duct type carcinomas and nonneoplastic duct lesions as well as nonduct type neoplasias. Virchows Arch A Pathol Anat Histopathol 408: 361–374, 1986.
34. Schussler MH, Skoudy A, Ramaekers F, Real FX. Intermediate filaments as differentiation markers of normal pancreas and pancreas cancer. Am J Pathol 140:559–568, 1992.
35. Yamanaka Y, Friess H, Kobrin MS, et al. Overexpression of *HER2/neu* oncogene in human pancreatic carcinoma. Hum Pathol 24:1127–1134, 1993.
36. Imamura M. Immunohistochemical study of metallothionein in pancreatic carcinomas. J Cancer Res Clin Oncol 122:351–355, 1996.
37. Takada M, Yamamoto M, Saitoh Y. The significance of CD44 in human pancreatic cancer: II. The role of CD44 in human pancreatic adenocarcinoma invasion. Pancreas 9:753–757, 1994.
38. Pignatelli M, Ansari TW, Gunter P, et al. Loss of membranous E-cadherin expression in pancreatic cancer: correlation with lymph node metastasis, high grade, and advanced stage. J Pathol 174:243–248, 1994.
39. Nakaizumi A, Tatsuta M, Uehara H, et al. Cytologic examination of pure pancreatic juice in the diagnosis of pancreatic carcinoma. The endoscopic retrograde intraductal catheter aspiration cytologic technique. Cancer 70: 610–614, 1992.
40. Smith EH, Bartrum RJ Jr, Chang YC, et al. Percutaneous aspiration biopsy of the pancreas under ultrasonic guidance. N Engl J Med 292:825–828, 1975.
41. Ishikawa O, Matsui Y, Aoki I, Iwanaga T, Terasawa T, Wada A. Adenosquamous carcinoma of the pancreas: a clinicopathologic study and report of three cases. Cancer 46:1192–1196, 1980.
42. Tschang TP, Garza GR, Kissane JM. Pleomorphic carcinoma of the pancreas: an analysis of 15 cases. Cancr 39:2114–2126, 1977.
43. Tracey KJ, O'Brien MJ, Williams LF, et al. Signet ring carcinoma of the pancreas, a rare variant with very high CEA values. Immunohistologic comparison with adenocarcinoma. Dig Dis Sci 29:573–576, 1984.
44. Trede M, Schwall G, Saeger HS. Survival after pancreatoduodenectomy. 118 consecutive resections without an operative mortality. Ann Surg 211: 447–458, 1990.
45. Henne BD, Vogel I, Luttges J, Klöppel G, Kremer B. Ductal adenocarcinoma of the pancreas head: survival after regional versus extended lymphadenectomy. Hepatogastroenterology 45:855–866, 1998.
46. Gudjonsson B: Cancer of the pancreas. 50 years of surgery. Cancer 60:2284–2303, 1987.
47. Yeo CJ, Cameron JL, Lillemoe KD, et al. Pancreaticoduodenectomy for cancer of the head of the pancreas. 201 patients. Ann Surg 221:721–731, 1995.
48. Luttges J, Vogel I, Menke M, Henne BD, Kremer B, Klöppel G. The retroperitoneal resection margin and vessel involvement are important factors determining survival after pancreaticoduodenectomy for ductal adenocarcinoma of the head of the pancreas. Virchows Arch 433:237–242, 1998.
49. Klöppel G, Lingenthal G, von-Bulow K, Kern HF. Histological and fine structural features of pancreatic ductal adenocarcinomas in relation to growth and prognosis: studies in xenografted tumours and clinicohistopathological correlation in a series of 75 cases. Histopathology 9: 841–856, 1985.

50. Kuopio T, Ekfors TO, Nikkanen V, Nevelainen TJ. Acinar cell carcinoma of the pancreas. Report of three cases. APMIS 103:69–78, 1995.

51. Klimstra DS, Heffess CS, Oertel JE, Rosai J. Acinar cell carcinoma of the pancreas: a clinicopathologic study of 28 cases. Am J Surg Pathol 16:815–837, 1992.

52. Morohoshi T, Kanda M, Horie A, et al. Immunocytochemical markers of uncommon pancreatic tumors. Acinar cell carcinoma, pancreatoblastoma, and solid cystic (papillary-cystic) tumor. Cancer 59:739–747, 1987.

53. Hoorens A, Lemoine NR, McLellan E, et al. Pancreatic acinar cell carcinoma. An analysis of cell lineage markers, *p53* expression, and Ki-*ras* mutation. Am J Pathol 143:685–698, 1993.

54. Klimstra DS, Wenig BM, Adair CF, Heffess CS. Pancreatoblastoma. A clinicopathologic study and review of the literature. Am J Surg Pathol 19:1371–1389, 1995.

55. Cubilla AL, Fitzgerald PJ. Tumours of the Exocrine Pancreas. Armed Forces Institute of Pathology, Washington, DC, 1984.

56. American Joint Committee On Cancer Staging Manual, 5th ed. J.B. Lippincott, Williams & Wilkins, Philadelphia, 1997.

# Chapter 31

# Clinical Aspects and Management of Pancreatic Adenocarcinoma: Diagnostic and Staging Procedures

CHUSILP CHARNSANGAVEJ AND SANDEEP LAHOTI

Pancreatic cancer ranks twelfth among new cases of cancer diagnosed each year in the United States but is the fifth-leading cause of cancer-related death. In the United States, approximately 27,000 patients receive a diagnosis of pancreatic cancer annually; ductal adenocarcinoma is the most common type, accounting for about 75%–90% of the cases.[1,2] The incidence of pancreatic cancer is highest in patients who are 65 to 80 years old, and the male-to-female ratio of patients is about 1.3:1.0. The incidence of pancreatic cancer has declined among white men since its peak in the early 1970s but has not declined among white women and in the black population.[3] The incidence in Japan has increased over the past 30 years.

Patients with ductal adenocarcinoma have a poor prognosis because of late clinical presentation and the lack of effective treatment. The mortality and incidence rates are identical, suggesting that most patients die within 1 year of diagnosis. This trend has not changed over the past two or three decades. Sixty percent of patients with ductal adenocarcinoma have hepatic metastases, peritoneal carcinomatosis, or both at presentation; only 40% have localized tumors and may be considered surgical candidates. The median survival duration of patients having untreated pancreatic ductal adenocarcinoma is only 3 to 6 months; 2-year survival durations are rare. Surgery offers the only chance for a cure, but only resection with negative margins can provide a survival benefit. Currently, the 5-year survival rate in patients after pancreatoduodenectomy (the Whipple operation) is 18%–21%.[4–6] Of patients who undergo a pancreatoduodenectomy, those who have tumors larger than 2 cm in diameter with vascular invasion and lymph node metastases have a worse prognosis than those who have tumors larger than 2 cm without vascular invasion or nodal metastasis.

The poor prognosis in patients who have pancreatic ductal adenocarcinoma makes imaging studies crucial in the management of this disease, not only for early diagnosis of the tumors but also for proper treatment planning. This chapter addresses the role of imaging studies in the diagnosis and staging of pancreatic cancer.

## Imaging Strategies for Pancreatic Tumors

The goals of imaging studies in patients who have pancreatic masses or suspected pancreatic carcinoma are to accurately diagnose the masses and stage the disease for surgical planning. Imaging of the pancreas should be designed to help determine whether there is a mass in the pancreas, what the diagnosis is, and whether the lesion is resectable.

Currently, there is no screening program for pancreatic cancer because there is no simple screening technique, and only a small group of patients, such as those with hereditary pancreatitis or pancreatic cancer, are known to be at high risk for developing cancer.[3] Common clinical presentations of patients with pancreatic cancer include painless obstructive jaundice, abdominal and back pain, palpable abdominal masses, and weight loss. Transabdominal ultrasonography (US) and computed tomography (CT) are used primarily to screen patients who have clinical evidence of advanced or metastatic disease and are suspected to have a primary tumor in the pancreas. These techniques are effective for the diagnosis of advanced pancreatic carcinoma, particularly when hepatic metastases, peritoneal carcinomatosis, and pancreatic masses are found. Percutaneous fine-needle aspiration biopsy analysis of the pancreatic mass or hepatic metastases under CT or US guidance is usually performed to establish and confirm the diagnosis.

Transabdominal US is frequently used in screening for the cause of obstructive jaundice. If choledocholithiasis can be excluded, CT is frequently used in the evaluation of pancreatic

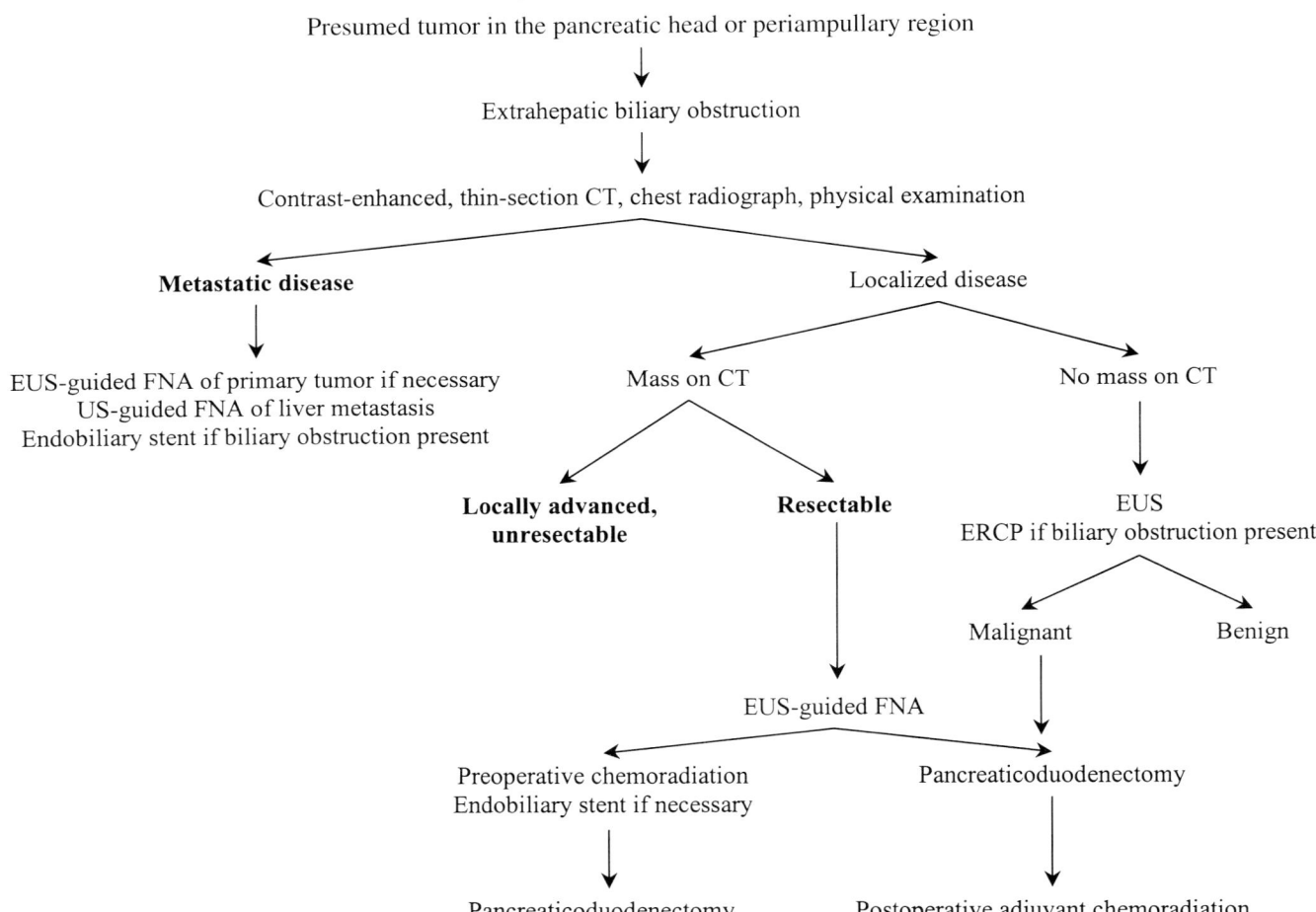

**Figure 32–4** Management algorithm employed at The University of Texas M. D. Anderson Cancer Center for patients with suspected or biopsy-proven adenocarcinoma of the pancreatic head or periampullary region. Patients without a histologic or cytologic diagnosis of adenocarcinoma who have a low-attenuation mass in the pancreatic head (on contrast-enhanced computed tomography ) undergo endoscopic ultrasonography (EUS)–guided fine-needle aspiration (FNA) biopsy. The development of EUS-guided FNA has greatly simplified tissue acquisition in patients with localized, nonmetastatic pancreatic cancer. Laparoscopy should be considered prior to opening the abdomen in patients with potentially resectable disease. In the absence of a mass on CT, diagnostic EUS and endoscopic retrograde cholangiopancreatography (ERCP) are usually performed. When there is no obvious mass to biopsy, or if pretreatment biopsies are nondiagnostic, patients who have clinical and radiologic findings suggesting a pancreatic or periampullary neoplasm undergo pancreaticoduodenectomy.

## Pancreatic Biopsy

Currently, the most common method of pancreatic tumor biopsy is EUS-guided FNA. However, an FNA should be performed only in patients who require cytological confirmation of malignancy prior to the initiation of neoadjuvant chemotherapy or chemoradiation. The routine use of EUS-FNA for resectable tumors may not appear justified. However, most pancreatic resections are not performed in regional referral centers or tertiary cancer centers. Indeed, a recent review of 24,926 patients undergoing pancreaticoduodenectomy nationwide revealed that 58% of patients underwent surgery at rural or urban nonteaching hospitals, where the operative mortality ranged from 10.6% (urban non-teaching) to 19.0% (rural).[29] Because the majority of patients undergo pancreaticoduodenectomy in settings with a high operative mortality, many physicians (including some surgeons) are not willing to proceed with pancreaticoduodenectomy in the absence of a tissue diagnosis of malignancy. Despite improvements in radiographic imaging, such diagnostic uncertainty often results in therapeutic indecision, which in turn often leads to exploratory surgery and surgeons attempting intraoperative biopsy (leading to unnecessary complications) or incorrectly judging a primary pancreatic tumor to be resectable or unresectable. In contrast to the diagnostic and staging evaluation of all other solid tumors, in which the diagnostic phase appears distinct from the treatment phase, with pancreatic and periampullary malignancies, diagnosis and treatment are often a continuum. Patients rapidly transition from excellent health to painless jaundice to the operating room; their first opportunity to seek a second opinion or to explore options for protocol-based therapy is after they have already undergone an unsuccessful attempt at surgical resection or when they are recovering from the complications of an ill-advised intraoperative pancreatic biopsy. The advent of EUS-FNA (combined with high-quality CT and endobiliary stent placement) allows this disease to be treated like all other solid tumors; the diagnostic phase is separated from the treatment phase. Patients with suspected pancreatic or periampullary cancer can be accurately staged with contemporary CT imaging, biliary obstruction can be relieved with endobiliary decompression, and the diagnosis can be established endoscopically with EUS-

FNA. Patients can then be counseled as to available treatment options and the established short- and long-term benefits of referral to a regional center with expertise in pancreatic surgery.

## Preoperative Biliary Drainage

Controversy also exists regarding the use of preoperative biliary drainage (which is necessary if surgery is to be delayed because of, for example, the use of preoperative chemoradiation) and the potential for increased pancreaticoduodenectomy-associated morbidity and mortality. Recent reports suggest increased morbidity and mortality after pancreaticoduodenectomy in patients who have undergone preoperative biliary drainage.[30,31] However, the largest study examining the risk for postoperative morbidity and mortality showed an increase only in the risk of postoperative wound infection in patients who underwent preoperative biliary stent placement.[32] We recently completed a retrospective analysis of 300 consecutive patients who underwent pancreaticoduodenectomy.[6] Multivariate analysis demonstrated no increase in the risk of major postoperative complications or death associated with preoperative stent placement. Others have confirmed this finding.[33] Even the subset of patients who undergo neoadjuvant chemoradiation with stents in place do not suffer clinically significant biliary stent–related complications.[34] Thus, endobiliary decompression as a part of an organized staging evaluation does not increase the risk associated with subsequent therapies, including chemoradiation and surgery.

## Pancreaticoduodenectomy

Pancreaticoduodenectomy involves removal of the pancreatic head, duodenum, gallbladder, and bile duct, with or without removal of the gastric antrum. It represents the standard surgical procedure for neoplasms of the pancreatic head and periampullary region. At the time of surgical exploration for a pancreatic head cancer, the relationship of the tumor to the SMA determines whether a complete resection can be performed. We strongly believe that this critical tumor–vessel relationship should be accurately evaluated prior to taking the patient to the operating room and that it cannot be accurately assessed intraoperatively following a Kocher maneuver. Historically, however, surgeons are taught to perform a Kocher maneuver in an effort to palpate a plane of normal tissue between the firm tumor and the posterior pulsation of the SMA (Fig. 32–5). With larger tumors, or those containing significant peritumoral fibrosis or in reoperative cases (following a previously unsuccessful attempt at pancreaticoduodenectomy), palpation of the relationship of the primary tumor to the SMA (after mobilization of the duodenum) with any reasonable degree of accuracy is impossible. Similarly, attempting to develop a plane of dissection between the anterior surface of the SMPV confluence and the posterior surface of the neck of the pancreas early in the operation to exclude tumor involvement of the SMV or SMPV confluence is unnecessary because tumor involvement of the SMV should not preclude resectability (Fig. 32–6). Furthermore, this maneuver can lead to bleeding at a point in the procedure when neither the SMV inferior to the pancreas nor the portal vein superior to the pancreas have been mobilized. For tumors of the pancreatic head and uncinate process, the anterior wall of the SMV or SMPV confluence is rarely involved in the absence of encasement of the celiac axis or SMA origin (as seen with locally advanced tumors of the pancreatic neck or body). The relationship of a pancreatic head tumor to the lateral and posterior walls of the SMPV confluence

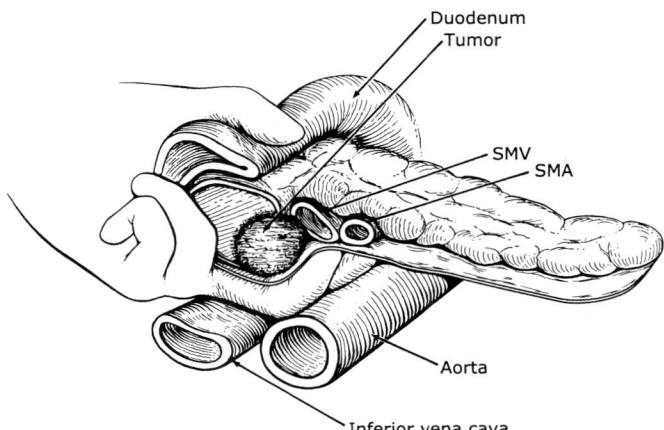

**Figure 32–5** Illustration demonstrating intraoperative palpation to determine the relationship of the tumor to the mesenteric vessels at the time of the Kocher maneuver; this maneuver was commonly taught to surgeons in the past. However, it is difficult or impossible to accurately assess the relationship of the tumor to the posterior pulsation of the superior mesenteric artery (SMA) by palpation. Preoperative assessment of this critical tumor–vessel relationship is the goal of preoperative CT imaging. SMV, superior mesenteric vein.

can be directly inspected only after gastric and pancreatic transection, by which point the surgeon has already committed to resection. Therein lies the rationale for detailed preoperative imaging using high-quality, contrast-enhanced CT, with laparotomy undertaken only in patients who fulfill objective CT criteria for resectability. Both the early Kocher maneuver and dissection of the anterior wall of the SMV–portal vein are founded in surgi-

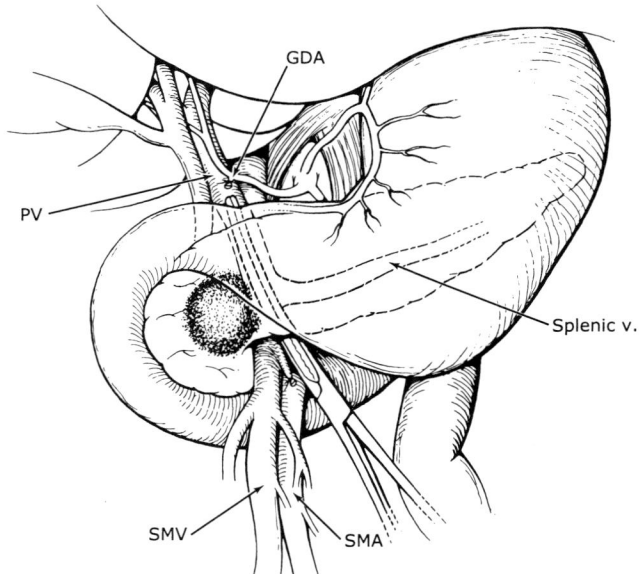

**Figure 32–6** Illustration demonstrating a maneuver commonly performed early in the operation to detect tumor invasion of the anterior wall of the superior mesenteric vein (SMV) or superior mesenteric–portal vein confluence. We do not perform this maneuver because a tumor-free plane often can be developed despite fixation of the tumor to the lateral wall of the SMV. This maneuver may incorrectly suggest that tumor adherence to the SMV does not exist. GDA, gastroduodenal artery; PV, portal vein; SMA, superior mesenteric artery.

cal tradition rather than in surgical anatomy. They are not accurate techniques to assess the resectability of a primary carcinoma of the pancreatic head.

In our recommended technique for pancreaticoduodenectomy, a bilateral subcostal or midline incision is used. The abdomen is carefully explored to exclude extrapancreatic metastatic disease. We do not proceed with tumor resection in the presence of biopsy-proven liver or peritoneal metastases. The issue of lymph node biopsy for frozen-section analysis remains controversial. Positive lymph nodes are a prognostic factor (along with factors such as poorly differentiated histology and microscopically positive resection margins) predictive of decreased survival duration.[4,35,36] However, the majority of resected specimens (60%–90%) contain microscopic metastases in regional lymph nodes. In a good-risk patient with localized, resectable pancreatic cancer, we do not (at this time) view lymph node metastases as an absolute contraindication to pancreaticoduodenectomy when performed as part of a multimodality approach. Therefore, in general, we do not perform random lymph node sampling for frozen-section analysis at the time of pancreaticoduodenectomy. However, each case should be considered individually; for example, in a high-risk patient (with medical comorbidities or oncologic concerns) with suspicious adenopathy, a positive regional lymph node (especially if second echelon) may be viewed as a contraindication to pancreaticoduodenectomy.

The surgical resection is divided into the following six clearly defined steps (Fig. 32–7).

1. The purpose of step 1 is to isolate the infrapancreatic SMV and separate the colon (and its mesentery) from the duodenum and pancreatic head. The lesser sac is entered by taking the greater omentum off the transverse colon. The hepatic flexure of the colon is mobilized from its retroperitoneal attachments, and the right colon is mobilized in the fashion of Cattell and Braasch.[37] The visceral peritoneum is incised to the ligament of Treitz, thereby mobilizing the small bowel mesentery. When complete, this maneuver allows cephalad retraction of the right colon and small bowel, exposing the third and fourth portions of the duodenum. The middle colic vein is divided prior to its junction with the SMV; routine division of the middle colic vein allows greater exposure of the infrapancreatic SMV and prevents iatrogenic traction injury to the SMV during dissection of the middle colic vein–SMV junction.

2. The Kocher maneuver is performed by elevating all fibrofatty and lymphatic tissue medial to the right ureter and anterior to the inferior vena cava with the pancreatic head and duodenum. The Kocher maneuver is continued to the left lateral edge of the aorta, with careful identification of the left renal vein. An incomplete Kocher maneuver makes step 6 difficult; it is important at this time in the operation to fully mobilize the pancreatic head and duodenum to the cephalad aspect of the left renal vein as it crosses the aorta.

3. The portal dissection is initiated by exposing the common hepatic artery proximal and distal to the gastroduodenal artery (GDA). The GDA is then ligated and divided. If the tumor extends to within a few millimeters of the GDA one should obtain proximal and distal control of the hepatic artery and divide the GDA flush at its origin. Dissection of the hepatic artery should be performed with gentle, sharp dissection, especially in patients who have received prior chemotherapy or chemoradiation and in those with extensive peritumoral inflammation. Overly aggressive dissection at the GDA origin can result in intimal dissection of the hepatic artery. The gallbladder is dissected out of the gallbladder fossa, and the common hepatic duct is transected at its junction with the cystic duct. When possible, we place a gentle bulldog clamp on the transected bile duct (step 3 of pancreaticoduodenectomy) to prevent bile spillage until the time of bile duct reconstruction. Because a low-lying right hepatic artery may be injured when the bile duct is divided in an inflamed porta hepatis, its anatomy should be carefully delineated. An accessory or replaced right hepatic artery may course posterolateral to the portal vein, and, rarely, the entire common hepatic artery may arise from the SMA (type IX hepatic arterial anatomy). Fatal hepatic necrosis can result if this is unrecognized and the vessel is sacrificed. The anterior wall of the portal vein is easily exposed following division of the common hepatic duct and medial retraction of the common hepatic artery. The portal vein should be identified but not extensively mobilized until step 6, at which time the stomach and pancreas have been divided.

4. The stomach is transected at the level of the third or fourth transverse vein on the lesser curvature and at the confluence of the gastroepiploic veins on the greater curvature. Care should be taken to ligate and divide the terminal branches of the left gastric artery along the lesser curvature of the stomach prior to gastric transection. The omentum is divided at the level of the greater curvature transection.

5. The jejunum is transected approximately 10 cm distal to the ligament of Treitz, and its mesentery is sequentially ligated and divided. The duodenal mesentery is similarly divided to the level of the aorta, allowing the devascularized segment of duodenum and jejunum to be reflected beneath the mesenteric vessels.

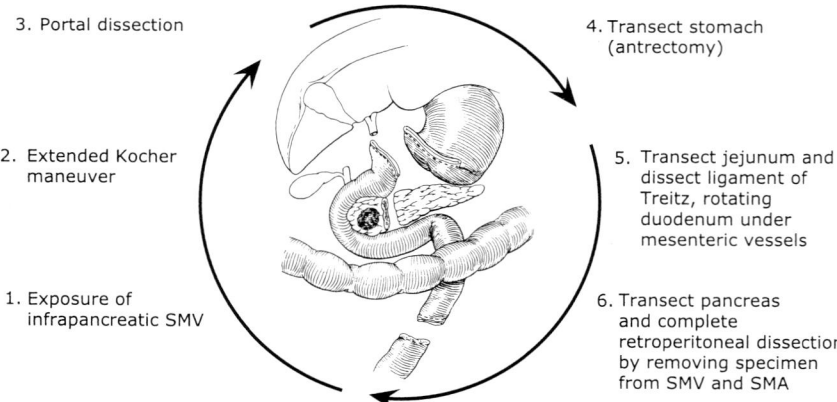

3. Portal dissection

2. Extended Kocher maneuver

1. Exposure of infrapancreatic SMV

4. Transect stomach (antrectomy)

5. Transect jejunum and dissect ligament of Treitz, rotating duodenum under mesenteric vessels

6. Transect pancreas and complete retroperitoneal dissection by removing specimen from SMV and SMA

**Figure 32–7** Six surgical steps of pancreaticoduodenectomy as performed at M. D. Anderson Cancer Center. The operation is performed in a clockwise direction, leading to the final step in tumor resection when the specimen is removed from the right lateral wall of the superior mesenteric artery (SMA). SMV, superior mesenteric vein.

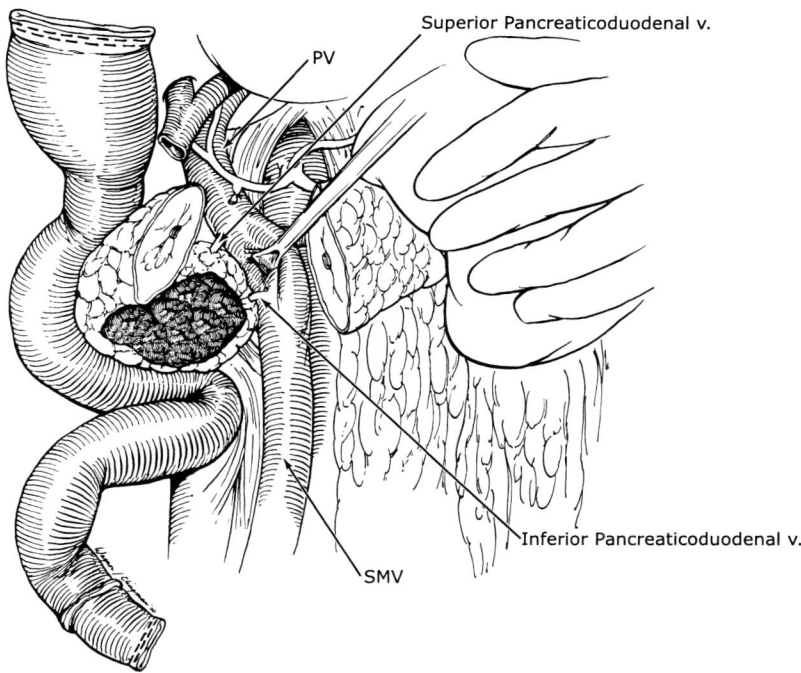

**Figure 32–8** Illustration of step 6 in of pancreaticoduodenectomy. The pancreatic head and uncinate process are separated from the superior mesenteric–portal vein confluence. As illustrated here, the pancreas has been transected at the level of the portal vein (PV) and reflected laterally, allowing identification of small venous tributaries to the PV and superior mesenteric vein (SMV). These tributaries are ligated and divided.

6. The most oncologically important and difficult part of the operation is step 6. After traction sutures are placed on the superior and inferior borders of the pancreas, the pancreas is transected with electrocautery at the level of the portal vein. If there is evidence of tumor adherence to the portal vein or SMV, the pancreas can be divided at a more distal location in preparation for segmental venous resection. The pancreas is separated from the SMV by ligation and division of the small venous tributaries to the uncinate process and pancreatic head (Fig. 32–8). The uncinate process must be completely removed from the SMV to ensure full mobilization of the SMPV confluence and subsequent identification of the SMA. Failure to fully mobilize the SMPV confluence risks injury to the SMA and usually results in a positive margin of resection due to incomplete removal of the uncinate process and the mesenteric soft tissue adjacent to the SMA (Fig. 32–9).

The specimen is then separated from the right lateral wall of the SMA, which is dissected to its origin at the aorta (Fig. 32–2). As mentioned previously, the soft tissue adjacent to the proximal 3–4 cm of the SMA represents the retroperitoneal margin. A grossly positive retroperitoneal margin should not be found if high-quality preoperative imaging is performed. A microscopically positive retroperitoneal margin will occur in 10%–20% of cases.[19] Margin positivity can result from tumor spread along perineural sheaths and does not always result from direct extension of the primary tumor.

Frozen-section evaluation of the pancreaticoduodenectomy specimen is limited to analysis of the pancreatic and common hepatic duct transection margins. Positive resection margins on the biliary or pancreatic duct mandate further resection until clear margins are achieved. However, changes due to pancreatitis should not be confused with margin positivity. Pancreatitis is distal to the tumor and may result in dysplastic cells at the pancreatic transection margin on frozen-section evaluation. Further resection of the pancreas should be performed only if there is histologic evidence on frozen-section analysis of invasive carcinoma at the margin. Dysplasia in the absence of carcinoma is not an indication for further pancreatic resection. Invasive carcinoma extending along the main pancreatic duct is uncommon. Because we remove all tissue to the right of the SMA, further resection at the retroperitoneal margin is not possible. However, this mar-

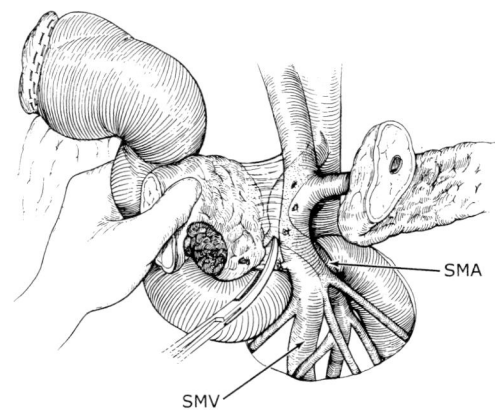

**Figure 32–9** Illustration of attempted removal of the pancreaticoduodenectomy specimen from the mesenteric vessels without mobilization of the superior mesenteric–portal vein confluence and direct identification of the superior mesenteric artery (SMA). This is associated with two potential complications: iatrogenic injury to the SMA and inadequate control of the inferior pancreaticoduodenal arteries because of their mass ligation with adjacent soft tissue. Failure to directly identify and individually ligate the inferior pancreaticoduodenal arteries is the major cause of postoperative hemorrhage. SMA injury and postoperative retroperitoneal hemorrhage are avoidable complications. The maneuver shown in this illustration should be avoided. SMV, superior mesenteric vein.

gin must be identified and inked with the pathologist. It cannot be assessed retrospectively.

## Vascular Resection

It is important to emphasize the distinction between regional pancreatectomy and pancreaticoduodenectomy with segmental resection of the SMV or SMPV confluence. We do not consider venous resection an attempt to improve en bloc lymphatic and soft tissue clearance, as is performed in regional pancreatectomy. It is unlikely that larger local-regional resections (to the left of the SMA and celiac axis) in poorly selected patients with advanced disease will affect survival. Venous resection should be performed only in carefully selected patients who have tumor adherence to the SMV or SMPV confluence but no evidence of tumor extension to the SMA or celiac axis.[38,39] Because the need for venous resection is unexpected in many patients and is discovered only after gastric and pancreatic transection, when non-resectional procedures are no longer an option, surgeons who perform pancreaticoduodenectomies should be familiar with standard vascular techniques for resection and reconstruction of the SMPV confluence.

Tumor adherence to the lateral wall of the SMPV confluence prevents dissection of the SMV and portal vein off the pancreatic head and uncinate process, thereby inhibiting medial retraction of the SMPV confluence and lateral retraction of the specimen. Therefore, the original technique for segmental venous resection involved transection of the splenic vein. Division of the splenic vein allows complete exposure of the SMA medial to the SMV and provides increased SMV and portal vein length (as they are no longer tethered by the splenic vein) for a primary venous anastomosis following segmental vein resection. A generous 2- to 3-cm segment of SMPV confluence can be resected without interposition grafting if the splenic vein is divided. In contrast, we currently preserve the splenic vein–portal vein junction whenever possible (Fig. 32–10). Splenic vein preservation is possible only when tumor invasion of the SMV or portal vein does not involve the splenic vein confluence. Preservation of the splenic vein–SMV–portal vein confluence significantly limits the mobilization of the portal vein and prevents primary anastomo-

sis of the SMV following segmental SMV resection unless segmental resection is limited to 2 cm or less. Therefore, an interposition graft is required in most patients who undergo SMV resection with splenic vein preservation. Our preferred conduit for interposition grafting is the internal jugular vein. Preservation of the splenic vein adds significant complexity to venous resection because it prevents direct access to the most proximal 3–4 cm of the SMA (medial to the SMV). We recently analyzed the effect of SMV–portal vein resection on R0 resection rate and survival during potentially curative pancreaticoduodenectomy for adenocarcinoma of the pancreatic head or uncinate process. No difference was found in R0 resection rate, disease-free survival, or overall 5-year survival regardless of the need for venous resection and reconstruction.

## Pancreatic, Biliary, and Gastrointestinal Reconstruction

Reconstruction after pancreaticoduodenectomy involves three anastomoses performed in a counterclockwise direction (Fig. 32–11). To facilitate construction of a pancreaticojejunostomy, the pancreatic remnant is mobilized from the retroperitoneum and splenic vein for a distance of 2–3 cm. Failure to adequately mobilize the pancreatic remnant results in poor suture placement at the pancreaticojejunal anastomosis. The transected jejunum is brought through a generous incision in the transverse mesocolon to the left of the middle colic vessels. We prefer to bring the jejunum retrocolic rather than retroperitoneal (posterior to the mesenteric vessels in the bed of the resected duodenum). A two-layer, end-to-side, duct-to-mucosa pancreaticojejunostomy is performed over a small Silastic stent if the pancreatic duct is not dilated (Fig. 32–12). A single-layer biliary anastomosis is performed using interrupted 4-0 absorbable monofilament sutures. It is important to align the jejunum with the bile duct to avoid tension on the pancreatic and biliary anastomoses. A stent is rarely used in the construction of the hepaticojejunostomy. Lastly, antecolic, end-to-side gastrojejunostomy is constructed in two layers. The distance between the biliary and gastric anastomoses is at least 50 cm, and the jejunal limb should be aligned so that the efferent limb is adjacent to the greater curvature of the stomach.

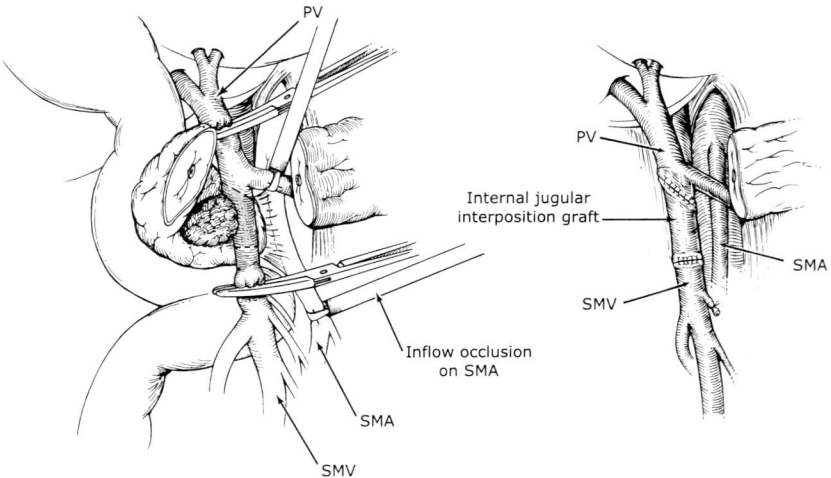

**Figure 32–10** Illustration of segmental resection of the superior mesenteric vein (SMV) with preservation of the splenic vein confluence. The intact splenic vein tethers the portal vein (PV), making a primary anastomosis impossible in most cases. Our preferred method of SMV reconstruction is to use an internal jugular vein interposition graft. Segmental resection of the SMV with splenic vein preservation adds significant complexity to this operation. SMA, superior mesenteric artery.

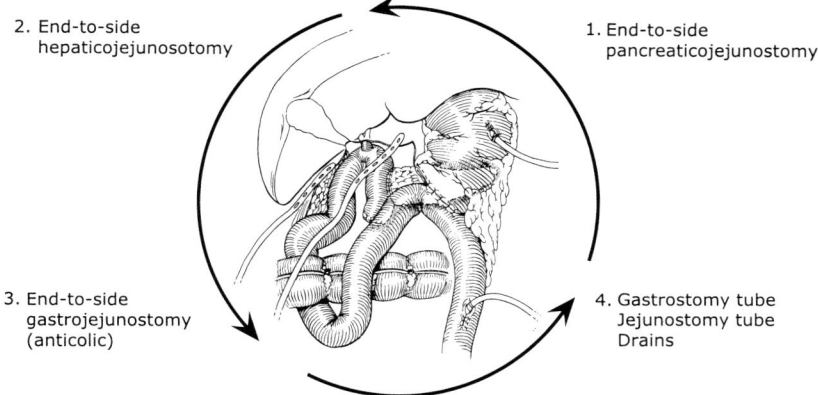

2. End-to-side
hepaticojejunosotomy

1. End-to-side
pancreaticojejunostomy

3. End-to-side
gastrojejunostomy
(anticolic)

4. Gastrostomy tube
Jejunostomy tube
Drains

**Figure 32–11** Illustration demonstrating the steps involved in pancreatic, biliary, and gastrointestinal reconstruction after pancreaticoduodenectomy. A gastrostomy tube and a feeding jejunostomy tube are commonly placed to assist in postoperative management.

Gastrostomy and feeding jejunostomy tubes are placed using the Witzel technique. Delayed gastric emptying is common after pancreaticoduodenectomy; a gastrostomy tube prevents prolonged nasogastric tube placement and facilitates independent patient care. Enteral feeding via a jejunostomy tube avoids a delay in hospital discharge due to poor oral intake. In addition, enteral feeding prevents the expense and potential complications associated with hyperalimentation in patients who require prolonged hospitalization because of perioperative or postoperative complications. Finally, we place the mobilized falciform ligament (carefully preserved when the abdomen was opened) between the hepatic artery and the afferent jejunal limb at the level of the GDA stump, to prevent pseudoaneurysm formation at the site of the GDA stump.

## Pylorus Preservation

Preservation of the antropyloroduodenal segment in combination with pancreaticoduodenectomy was first described by Traverso

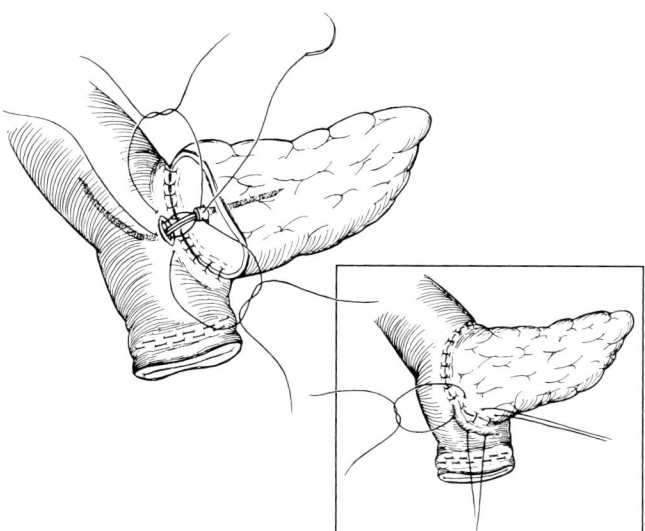

**Figure 32–12** Illustration of a two-layer, end-to-side, duct-to-mucosa pancreaticojejunostomy. When used, the stent (4–5 cm long) is sewn to the pancreatic duct with absorbable suture.

and Longmire in 1978.[40] Since then, increasing numbers of pancreatic surgeons have employed this modification of the procedure, particularly for patients with benign disease or small periampullary lesions. Proponents of the technique argue that preservation of the antropyloric pump mechanism results in improved long-term upper gastrointestinal tract function with enhanced weight gain and few nutritional sequelae.[41–43] Detractors of pylorus preservation counter that the reported improvements in gastrointestinal and nutritional functions are small, if any, and that they come at the expense of an increased incidence of early postoperative delayed gastric emptying.[44,45] Further, leaving the distal stomach and duodenum may compromise margins of excision and prevent adequate peripyloric lymphadenectomy. Published data to date involve retrospective comparisons that have yielded mixed results. Despite the controversy, most pancreatic surgeons would agree that pylorus preservation should not be performed for patients with bulky tumors of the pancreatic head, duodenal tumors involving the first or second portions of the duodenum, or lesions associated with grossly positive pyloric or peripyloric lymph nodes.

The steps in pylorus-preserving pancreaticoduodenectomy are identical to those in standard pancreaticoduodenectomy except in the approach to the antrum, pylorus, and duodenum (steps 3 and 4). Pylorus preservation involves preservation of sufficient blood supply to the proximal duodenum and preservation of vagal innervation to the antrum and pylorus. Therefore, appropriate caution must be exercised during the portal dissection to avoid unnecessary injury to the nerves of Laterjet. This is the fundamental technical difference in the pylorus-preserving procedure and is essential to avoiding postoperative gastroparesis.

## Total Pancreatectomy

Total pancreatectomy is performed by adding dissection of the left upper quadrant of the abdomen following step 1 in our six-step pancreaticoduodenectomy. Following completion of the Cattell-Braasch maneuver and identification of the infrapancreatic SMV, the greater omentum is separated from the left side of the transverse colon, and the splenic flexure is mobilized. The peritoneum lateral to the spleen is then incised in a cephalad direction to the gastroesophageal junction. The short gastric vessels are ligated and divided, allowing medial and cephalad re-

gators to initiate studies in which patients with potentially resectable adenocarcinoma of the pancreas received chemoradiation before pancreaticoduodenectomy.[61] The preoperative use of chemoradiation is supported by several considerations.[24] First, positive gross or microscopic margins of resection along the right lateral border of the SMA are common after pancreaticoduodenectomy, suggesting that surgery alone may be inadequate for local tumor control.[62] Second, because chemoradiation is given first, delayed postoperative recovery does not affect the delivery of multimodality therapy. Third, patients with disseminated disease evident on restaging studies after chemoradiation are not subjected to laparotomy. Fourth, recent data suggest that preoperative chemoradiation may decrease the incidence of pancreaticojejunal anastomotic fistula, the most common complication following pancreaticoduodenectomy.[63]

A recent report from our institution of 132 consecutive patients who received preoperative chemoradiation and pancreaticoduodenectomy for adenocarcinoma of the pancreas supports the use of preoperative chemoradiation.[19] The overall median survival in these 132 patients from the time of tissue diagnosis was 21 months. The dose of preoperative EBRT, the chemotherapy agent used, and the delivery of intraoperative radiation therapy did not influence survival duration. Univariate and multivariate analyses revealed superior survival times among patients who had no evidence of lymph node metastasis ($P = 0.03$). The data suggest that short-course chemoradiation (30 Gy in 2 weeks) combined with pancreaticoduodenectomy performed on accurately staged patients may be equivalent to standard-fractionation chemoradiation (45–50 Gy in 5–6 weeks).

Among patients who receive chemoradiation prior to planned pancreaticoduodenectomy, repeat-staging CT after chemoradiation reveals liver metastases in approximately 25%.[24,64] If these patients had undergone pancreaticoduodenectomy at the time of diagnosis, it is probable that the liver metastases would have been subclinical; therefore, these patients would have undergone a major surgical procedure only to have liver metastases found soon after surgery. In the trials reported from our institution, patients who were found to have disease progression at the time of restaging had a median survival of only 7 months.[61] The avoidance of a lengthy recovery period and the potential morbidity of pancreaticoduodenectomy in patients with such short expected survival duration represent distinct advantages of preoperative over postoperative chemoradiation. When delivering multimodality therapy for any disease, it is beneficial, when possible, to deliver the most toxic therapy last, thereby avoiding morbidity in patients who experience rapid disease progression not amenable to currently available therapies.

More effective radiation sensitization may result in a greater cytotoxic effect at the local tumor site. Gemcitabine (2′,2′-difluorodeoxycytidine, Gemzar) is a deoxycytidine analogue capable of inhibiting DNA replication and repair. Gemcitabine is also a potent radiation sensitizer of human pancreatic cancer cells, and laboratory studies suggest that gemcitabine's inhibitory effect on DNA synthesis when combined with irradiation is prolonged in tumors compared with in normal tissues.[65] We recently reported the results of a phase I study of rapid-fractionation EBRT and concomitant weekly gemcitabine in patients with locally advanced adenocarcinoma of the pancreatic head.[66] Our data suggest that when gemcitabine is given weekly with concomitant radiation therapy to a dose of 30 Gy in 10 fractions, the maximum tolerated dose of gemcitabine is between 350 mg/m²/week and 400 mg/m²/week for 7 weeks. This is approximately one-third the recommended dose of gemcitabine when adminis-

tered as a single agent for the treatment of advanced pancreatic cancer. Seventeen patients were evaluated for response, and eight patients (47%) had evidence of a local anticancer effect. Four of these eight patients had a partial response to therapy. The median survival for the entire group was 6 months. The 1-year survival rate for patients with an objective response to therapy was 66%. The clinical responses observed in this group of patients suggest that gemcitabine is a clinically relevant radiosensitizer in patients with pancreatic adenocarcinoma. However, the toxic effects are significant, thus until dose and scheduling issues are explored further, concomitant administration of gemcitabine and radiation therapy should still be considered investigational.

Because of encouraging results in patients with locally advanced disease, gemcitabine-based chemoradiation is being studied in patients with potentially resectable pancreatic cancer (as defined by CT). The current phase II protocol available at our institution is based on the results of the phase I study discussed above.[66] Patients receive gemcitabine-based chemoradiation followed by a complete restaging evaluation. Patients with no evidence of disease progression are then taken to surgery for pancreaticoduodenectomy. To date, more than 80 patients have been entered on this treatment program, and the histologic response to induction therapy (in the resected specimen) appears superior to that associated with previous regimens; follow-up is immature, preventing survival analysis at this time (Evans, unpublished).

At our institution, current and future treatments for patients with potentially resectable adenocarcinoma of the pancreas emphasize the use of new, more potent radiation-sensitizing agents and the preoperative delivery of systemic therapy. Among patients who undergo a potentially curative pancreaticoduodenectomy, liver metastases are now the dominant form of tumor recurrence. This has caused some investigators to question the need for EBRT in adjuvant and neoadjuvant treatment schemas. The recent interim report from the European Study Group of Pancreatic Cancer (ESPAC)-1 is the largest study to suggest that EBRT may be of no value.[67] The ESPAC-1 trial is a four-arm study with a $2 \times 2$ factorial design that compares the effects of adjuvant chemoradiation (40 Gy in a split course and 5-FU), adjuvant chemotherapy (5-FU and folinic acid), chemoradiation followed by chemotherapy, and observation alone following pancreaticoduodenectomy for pancreatic or periampullary carcinomas. Accrual for this study began in 1994, and medical centers in 11 countries have randomized 530 patients. The majority of patients have been entered into the randomized $2 \times 2$ factorial design. However, because of lack of access to EBRT or specific institutional bias, 188 patients were randomized to receive only chemotherapy or no chemotherapy, and 68 patients were randomized to receive either chemoradiation or no chemoradiation. In the latter two nonfactorial groups, patients could receive nonstandardized therapy at the discretion of their treating physicians. For example, patients who were randomized in the nonfactorial design to chemotherapy or no chemotherapy could receive EBRT. Importantly, nonrandomized treatments were not standardized. Preliminary results suggest no benefit of postoperative chemoradiation.[67] Although we are not ready to remove EBRT from the study of protocol-based treatment for localized pancreatic cancer, the availability of more potent radiation-sensitizing agents and techniques to ensure complete surgical resection makes the study of shorter-course, less toxic EBRT attractive in contemporary clinical trial design.

In the absence of more effective systemic therapies for pancreatic cancer, the length and quality of life of patients with localized pancreatic cancer will be maximized by accurate preoperative assessment of resectability, a standardized technique of tumor resection, and the routine use of protocol-based adjuvant or neoadjuvant therapy. Pancreaticoduodenectomy should always be performed as part of a multimodality approach involving chemotherapy or chemoradiation. Whenever possible, all patients with pancreatic cancers should be offered protocol-based therapy.

## References

1. Whipple AO, Parsons WW, Mullin CR. Treatment of carcinoma of the ampulla of Vater. Ann Surg 225:621–633, 1935.
2. Whipple AO. The rationale of radical surgery for cancer of the pancreas and ampullary region. Ann Surg 114:612, 1941.
3. Waugh JM, Claggett OT. Resection of the duodenum and head of the pancreas for carcinoma. Surgery 20:224, 1946.
4. Yeo CJ, Cameron JL, Sohn TA, et al. Six hundred fifty consecutive pancreaticoduodenectomies in the 1990s: pathology, complications, and outcomes. Ann Surg 226:248–257, 1997.
5. Balcom JH IV, Rattner DW, Warshaw AL, Chang Y, Fernandez-del Castillo C. Ten-year experience with 733 pancreatic resections: changing indications, older patients, and decreasing length of hospitalization. Arch Surg 136:391–398, 2001.
6. Pisters PW, Hudec WA, Hess KR, et al. Effect of preoperative biliary decompression on pancreaticoduodenectomy-associated morbidity in 300 consecutive patients. Ann Surg 234:47–55, 2001.
7. Doerr RJ, Yildiz I, Flint LM. Pancreaticoduodenectomy. University experience and resident education. Arch Surg 125:463–465, 1990.
8. Edge SB, Schmieg RE Jr, Rosenlof LK, Wilhelm MC. Pancreas cancer resection outcome in American University centers in 1989–1990. Cancer 71:3502–3508, 1993.
9. Wade TP, Kraybill WG, Virgo KS, Johnson FE. Pancreatic cancer treatment in the U.S. veteran from 1987 to 1991: effect of tumor stage on survival. J Surg Oncol 58:104–111, 1995.
10. Wade TP, Radford DM, Virgo KS, Johnson FE. Complications and outcomes in the treatment of pancreatic adenocarcinoma in the United States veteran. J Am Coll Surg 179:38–48, 1994.
11. Lieberman MD, Kilburn H, Lindsey M, Brennan MF. Relation of perioperative deaths to hospital volume among patients undergoing pancreatic resection for malignancy. Ann Surg 222:638–645, 1995.
12. Gordon TA, Bowman HM, Tielsch JM, et al. Statewide regionalization of pancreaticoduodenectomy and its effect on in-hospital mortality. Ann Surg 228:71–78, 1998.
13. Simunovic M, To T, Theriault M, Langer B. Relation between hospital surgical volume and outcome for pancreatic resection for neoplasm in a publicly funded health care system. CMAJ 160:643–648, 1999.
14. Sosa JA, Bowman HM, Gordon TA, et al. Importance of hospital volume in the overall management of pancreatic cancer. Ann Surg 228:429–438, 1998.
15. Birkmeyer JD, Finlayson SR, Tosteson AN, et al. Effect of hospital volume on in-hospital mortality with pancreaticoduodenectomy. Surgery 125:250–256, 1999.
16. Birkmeyer JD, Warshaw AL, Finlayson SR, Grove MR, Tosteson AN. Relationship between hospital volume and late survival after pancreaticoduodenectomy. Surgery 126:178–183, 1999.
17. Hillner BE, Smith TJ, Desch CE. Hospital and physician volume or specialization and outcomes in cancer treatment: importance in quality of cancer care. J Clin Oncol 18:2327–2340, 2000.
18. Evans DB, Abbruzzese JL, Willett CG. Cancer of the pancreas. In: DeVita VT, Hellman S, Rosenberg SA (eds): Cancer, Principles and Practice of Oncology, 6th ed. Lippincott Williams and Wilkins, Philadelphia, 2001, pp 1126–1161.
19. Breslin TM, Hess KR, Harbison DB, et al. Neoadjuvant chemoradiotherapy for adenocarcinoma of the pancreas: treatment variables and survival duration. Ann Surg Oncol 8:123–132, 2001.
20. Nitecki SS, Sarr MG, Colby TV, van Heerden JA. Long-term survival after resection for ductal adenocarcinoma of the pancreas. Is it really improving? Ann Surg 221:59–66, 1995.
21. Sohn TA, Yeo CJ, Cameron JL, et al. Resected adenocarcinoma of the pancreas—616 patients: results, outcomes, and prognostic indicators. J Gastrointest Surg 4:567–579, 2000.
22. Geer RJ, Brennan MF. Prognostic indicators for survival after resection of pancreatic adenocarcinoma. Am J Surg 165:68–72, 1993.
23. Fuhrman GM, Charnsangavej C, Abbruzzese JL, et al. Thin-section contrast-enhanced computed tomography accurately predicts the resectability of malignant pancreatic neoplasms. Am J Surg 167:104–111, 1994.
24. Spitz FR, Abbruzzese JL, Lee JE, et al. Preoperative and postoperative chemoradiation strategies in patients treated with pancreaticoduodenectomy for adenocarcinoma of the pancreas. J Clin Oncol 15:928–937, 1997.
25. Jimenez RE, Warshaw AL, Rattner DW, et al. Impact of laparoscopic staging in the treatment of pancreatic cancer. Arch Surg 135:409–414, 2000.
26. Conlon KC, Dougherty E, Klimstra DS, et al. The value of minimal access surgery in the staging of patients with potentially resectable peripancreatic malignancy. Ann Surg 223:134–140, 1996.
27. Merchant NB, Conlon KC. Laparoscopic evaluation in pancreatic cancer. Semin Surg Oncol 15:155–165, 1998.
28. Pisters PW, Lee JE, Vauthey JN, Charnsangavej C, Evans DB. Laparoscopy in the staging of pancreatic cancer. Br J Surg 88:325–337, 2001.
29. Kotwall C, Maxwell JG, Brinker CC, Covington DL, Jones S, Schoepel K. National estimates of mortality rates for radical pancreaticoduodenectomy in 25,000 patients. Presented at the Society of Surgical Oncology 54th Annual Cancer Symposium, Washington DC, 2001.
30. Povoski SP, Karpeh MS Jr, Conlon KC, Blumgart LH, Brennan MF. Preoperative biliary drainage: impact on intraoperative bile cultures and infectious morbidity and mortality after pancreaticoduodenectomy. J Gastrointest Surg 3:496–505, 1999.
31. Povoski SP, Karpeh MS Jr, Conlon KC, Blumgart LH, Brennan MF. Association of preoperative biliary drainage with postoperative outcome following pancreaticoduodenectomy. Ann Surg 230:131–142, 1999.
32. Sohn TA, Yeo CJ, Cameron JL, Pitt HA, Lillemoe KD. Do preoperative biliary stents increase postpancreaticoduodenectomy complications? J Gastrointest Surg 4:258–267, 2000.
33. Martignoni ME, Wagner M, Krahenbuhl L, et al. Effect of preoperative biliary drainage on surgical outcome after pancreatoduodenectomy. Am J Surg 181:52–59, 2001.
34. Pisters PW, Hudec WA, Lee JE, et al. Preoperative chemoradiation for patients with pancreatic cancer: toxicity of endobiliary stents. J Clin Oncol 18:860–867, 2000.
35. Yeo CJ, Abrams RA, Grochow LB, et al. Pancreaticoduodenectomy for pancreatic adenocarcinoma: postoperative adjuvant chemoradiation improves survival. A prospective, single-institution experience. Ann Surg 225:621–633, 1997.
36. Cameron JL, Crist DW, Sitzmann JV, et al. Factors influencing survival after pancreaticoduodenectomy for pancreatic cancer. Am J Surg 161:120–124, 1991.
37. Cattell RB, Braasch JW. A technique for the exposure of the third and fourth portions of the duodenum. Surg Gynecol Obstet 111:378–381, 1960.
38. Bold RJ, Charnsangavej C, Cleary KR, et al. Major vascular resection as part of pancreaticoduodenectomy for cancer: radiologic, intraoperative, and pathologic analysis. J Gastrointest Surg 3:233–243, 1999.
39. Leach SD, Lee JE, Charnsangavej C, et al. Survival following pancreaticoduodenectomy with resection of the superior mesenteric–portal vein confluence for adenocarcinoma of the pancreatic head. Br J Surg 85:611–617, 1998.
40. Traverso LW, Longmire WP Jr. Preservation of the pylorus in pancreaticoduodenectomy. Surg Gynecol Obstet 146:959–962, 1978.
41. Tsao JI, Rossi RL, Lowell JA. Pylorus-preserving pancreatoduodenectomy. Is it an adequate cancer operation? Arch Surg 129:405–412, 1994.
42. Yeo CJ, Cameron JL, Lillemoe KD, et al. Pancreaticoduodenectomy for cancer of the head of the pancreas. 201 patients. Ann Surg 221:721–731, 1995.
43. Crucitti F, Doglietto G, Bellantone R, et al. Digestive and nutritional consequences of pancreatic resections. The classical vs. the pylorus-sparing procedure. Int J Pancreatol 17:37–45, 1995.
44. Patel AG, Toyama MT, Kusske AM, et al. Pylorus-preserving Whipple resection for pancreatic cancer. Is it any better? Arch Surg 130:838–842, 1995.
45. Lin PW, Lin YJ. Prospective randomized comparison between pylorus-preserving and standard pancreaticoduodenectomy. Br J Surg 86:603–607, 1999.
46. Reber HA. Partial subtotal pancreatectomy. In: Nyhus LM, Baker RJ, Fischer J (eds): Mastery of Surgery. Little Brown, Boston, MA, 1996, pp 1029–1049.
47. Ohwada S, Ogawa T, Tanahashi Y, et al. Fibrin glue sandwich prevents pancreatic fistula following distal pancreatectomy. World J Surg 22:494–498, 1998.
48. Konishi T, Hiraishi M, Kubota K, et al. Segmental occlusion of the pancreatic duct with prolamine to prevent fistula formation after distal pancreatectomy. Ann Surg 221:165–170, 1995.
49. Shankar S, Theis B, Russell RC. Management of the stump of the pancreas after distal pancreatic resection. Br J Surg 77:541–544, 1990.

50. Frey CF. Distal pancreatectomy in chronic pancreatitis. In: Trede M, Carter DC (eds): Surgery of the Pancreas. Churchill Livingstone, New York, 1993, pp 321–334.

51. Kajiyama Y, Tsurumaru M, Udagawa H, et al. Quick and simple distal pancreatectomy using the GIA stapler: report of 35 cases. Br J Surg 83: 1711, 1996.

52. Suzuki Y, Kuroda Y, Morita A, et al. Fibrin glue sealing for the prevention of pancreatic fistulas following distal pancreatectomy. Arch Surg 130:952–955, 1995.

53. Suzuki Y, Fujino Y, Tanioka Y, et al. Randomized clinical trial of ultrasonic dissector or conventional division in distal pancreatectomy for nonfibrotic pancreas. Br J Surg 86:608–611, 1999.

54. Bilimoria MM, Cormier JN, Mun Y, Lee JE, Evans DB, Pisters PWT. Pancreatic leak after left pancreatectomy is reduced following main pancreatic duct ligation. Br J Surg 90:190–196, 2003.

55. Staley CA, Cleary KR, Abbruzzese JL, et al. The need for standardized pathologic staging of pancreaticoduodenectomy specimens. Pancreas 12: 373–380, 1996.

56. Evans DB, Rich TA, Byrd DR, et al. Preoperative chemoradiation and pancreaticoduodenectomy for adenocarcinoma of the pancreas. Arch Surg 127:1335–1339, 1992.

57. Porter GA, Pisters PW, Mansyur C, et al. Cost and utilization impact of a clinical pathway for patients undergoing pancreaticoduodenectomy. Ann Surg Oncol 7:484–489, 2000.

58. [No authors listed]. Further evidence of effective adjuvant combined radiation and chemotherapy following curative resection of pancreatic cancer. Gastrointestinal Tumor Study Group. Cancer 59:2006–2010, 1987.

59. Kalser MH, Ellenberg SS. Pancreatic cancer. Adjuvant combined radiation and chemotherapy following curative resection. Arch Surg 120:899–903, 1985.

60. Klinkenbijl JH, Jeekel J, Sahmoud T, et al. Adjuvant radiotherapy and 5-fluorouracil after curative resection of cancer of the pancreas and periampullary region: phase III trial of the EORTC Gastrointestinal Tract Cancer Cooperative Group. Ann Surg 230:776–782, 1999.

61. Evans DB, Pisters PW, Lee JE, et al. Preoperative chemoradiation strategies for localized adenocarcinoma of the pancreas. J Hepatobiliary Pancreat Surg 5:242–250, 1998.

62. Willett CG, Lewandrowski K, Warshaw AL, Efird J, Compton CC. Resection margins in carcinoma of the head of the pancreas. Implications for radiation therapy. Ann Surg 217:144–148, 1993.

63. Lowy AM, Lee JE, Pisters PW, et al. Prospective, randomized trial of octreotide to prevent pancreatic fistula after pancreaticoduodenectomy for malignant disease. Ann Surg 226:632–641, 1997.

64. Pisters PW, Abbruzzese JL, Janjan NA, et al. Rapid-fractionation preoperative chemoradiation, pancreaticoduodenectomy, and intraoperative radiation therapy for resectable pancreatic adenocarcinoma. J Clin Oncol 16:3843–3850, 1998.

65. Epelbaum R, Rosenblatt E, Nasrallah S. A phase II study of gemcitabine (GEM) combined with radiation therapy (RT) in patients with localized, unresectable pancreatic cancer [abstract]. Proc Am Soc Clin Oncol 19: 1029, 2000.

66. Wolff RA, Evans DB, Gravel DM, et al. Phase I trial of gemcitabine combined with radiation for the treatment of locally advanced pancreatic adenocarcinoma. Clin Cancer Res 7:2246–2253, 2001.

67. Neoptolemos JP, Dunn JA, Stocken DD, et al. Adjuvant chemoradiotherapy and chemotherapy in resectable pancreatic cancer: a randomised controlled trial. Lancet 358:1576–1585, 2001.

68. Sewnath ME, Birjmohun RS, Rauws EA, et al. The effect of preoperative biliary drainage on postoperative complications after pancreaticoduodenectomy. J Am Coll Surg 192:726–734, 2001.

# Chapter 33

# Clinical Aspects and Management of Pancreatic Adenocarcinoma

## Management Options: Locally Advanced Unresectable Pancreatic Cancer

MARGARET A. TEMPERO, PAULA TERMUHLEN, RANDALL E. BRAND, AND CORNELIUS McGINN

Current multimodality therapy for patients with pancreatic adenocarcinoma consists of surgery, chemotherapy, and radiation therapy. Unfortunately, more than one-half of patients present with distant metastatic disease and more than two-fifths of patients have locally advanced but unresectable disease.[1] The management of patients with pancreatic adenocarcinoma must include palliation of the symptoms associated with the disease, such as gastric outlet obstruction, biliary obstruction and pain. These patients are often malnourished from tumor cachexia, anorexia, mechanical obstruction, and pancreatic insufficiency, thus further compromising their ability to undergo invasive procedures to control and relieve their symptoms. Furthermore, cancer therapy (chemotherapy or chemoradiation therapy) can cause toxic effects that aggravate the symptom complex. Thus management of patients with pancreatic adenocarcinoma presents many therapeutic challenges. This chapter describes the current options for the palliative management and treatment of patients with locally unresectable pancreatic cancer.

## Determining Resectability

The determination of which patients should receive curative resections is a critical issue in pancreatic cancer. Although some physicians propose that pancreaticoduodenectomy can be used for palliation even for patients with gross residual disease, this belief is not widely held.[2–4] In one study, the morbidity and mortality rates and the period of postoperative recovery among patients who underwent pancreaticoduodenectomy with residual postoperative disease (microscopic or gross) were similar to those of patients who underwent traditional biliary and gastric bypass operations, but the actuarial survival rate was significantly higher in the pancreaticoduodenectomy group.[2] However, the data showing that pancreaticoduodenectomy offers effective palliation with the same risks of morbidity and mortality as those associated with traditional surgical bypass came primarily from patients with positive margins after the procedure had been performed with the intent of a curative resection.[3] Thus the extent of disease was likely greater in the patients who received bypass initially and were not considered for curative resection. This finding suggests, then, that the role of pancreaticoduodenectomy as a palliative treatment remains uncertain. In fact, many practioners hold the opposite opinion, asserting that in cases of locally unresectable or metastatic disease, the median survival of 6–7 months does not justify even operative biliary or gastric bypass unless endoscopic palliation has failed.[5,6] Further support for a nonoperative approach is the finding that patients with a positive margin at the time of resection have survival rates similar to those of patients undergoing palliative chemoradiation therapy.[2,7] The role of traditional surgical biliary and gastric bypass has also been strongly debated.[8–10] Endoprostheses can effectively palliate obstructive jaundice and may help relieve duodenal obstruction in patients with unresectable disease. However, because of the late morbidity associated with endoprostheses, their use may be limited to beyond 6 months.[10]

The experience and philosophy of the surgical team involved in the care of pancreatic cancer patients often determine the definition of resectability. Locally advanced unresectable pancreatic cancer is most commonly distinguished by tumor extension into or around structures that cannot be excised en bloc and by the absence of visceral or peritoneal metastases. Fortunately, in most cases, the resectability of tumors can be determined preoperatively with a minimum of invasive procedures, thus sparing patients unnecessary explorations. At some centers, the determination of whether a tumor is resectable is based on thin-cut contrast-enhanced computed tomography (CT) scanning alone. Curative resection is planned only if no extrapancreatic disease

5-FU plus 40 Gy and 5-FU plus 60 Gy, respectively. The survival advantage associated with the addition of 5-FU was statistically significant ($P < 0.01$). Although the median survival was longer among patients who received a higher dose of radiation (60 Gy) with 5-FU, the difference was not statistically significant. Toxicity included mild to moderate vomiting in approximately one-third of patients and severe vomiting in fewer than 5% of patients. There was no significant hematologic toxicity. This experience serves as a baseline against which other treatment regimens are often compared, with a median survival ranging from 9 months to 1 year for patients with locally advanced, nonmetastatic adenocarcinoma of the pancreas.

A subsequent GITSG trial[80] randomized patients to radiation (40 Gy) with concurrent doxorubicin followed by maintenance doxorubicin to radiation (60 Gy) with 5-FU, as in the trial described above. The rate of hematologic toxicity was significantly greater among patients receiving doxorubicin, and this toxicity generally occurred during the maintenance portion of the regimen. No difference in outcomes was noted, with a median survival time of approximately 9 months in each group. The use of streptozotocin, mitomycin C, and 5-FU (SMF) as maintenance therapy following radiation (50.4 Gy) and concurrent 5-FU, was then tested on the basis of evidence that this chemotherapy regimen resulted in a 15% response rates among patients with advanced disease.[81] However, as in previous studies, the toxicity of the regimen appeared greater than that observed with 5-FU alone and did not increase the median survival time.[82] In the final GITSG trial for patients with unresectable pancreatic cancer, the value of radiotherapy was investigated on the basis of evidence from the Eastern Cooperative Oncology Group (ECOG) which suggested that 5-FU alone was as equally effective as radiotherapy plus 5-FU.[83] In this GITSG trial, patients were randomized to receive either a regimen of streptozotocin, mitomycin C, and 5-FU (SMF) alone or radiotherapy with 5-FU followed by SMF.[84] Despite closure of the trial for lack of funding after only one-third of the projected accrual was achieved, a statistically significant result was obtained: overall survival following combined-modality treatment was 41% at 1 year, compared with 19% in the SMF-alone group ($P < 0.02$).

In each of these trials, the chemotherapy regimen was not effective in the 70%–90% of patients with hepatic metastases. The role of prophylactic hepatic irradiation has been investigated as a means to remedy this pattern of failure and to improve survival. A pilot study suggested that radiation therapy to the liver could be safely delivered during a course of pancreatic irradiation with concurrent 5-FU, prompting a phase I/II RTOG trial.[85] In this trial, 81 patients with unresectable, recurrent, or residual primary tumors and no evidence of liver metastases received 61.2 Gy to the primary tumor with concurrent 5-FU.[86] In the fourth week of treatment, a prophylactic course of whole-liver irradiation (23.4 Gy) was initiated. Most of patients (76%) were able to complete the course of therapy according to protocol. However, severe hepatic toxicity occurred in four patients, one of whom died. Overall, 32% of patients developed hepatic metastases, which suggests that the frequency of hepatic metastases was reduced. Unfortunately, the median survival was only 8.4 months.

Prolonged infusion schedules of 5-FU administered concurrently with radiation have been investigated for their potential to improve outcome.[87,88] By potentially increasing the radiosensitization provided by 5-FU, these schedules may improve local control. Improved control of systemic disease may also occur secondary to increased dosage intensity of 5-FU delivered by prolonged infusion. This approach is particularly appealing given

data from randomized trials of adjuvant treatment for rectal cancer, in which patients receiving protracted venous infusion (PVI) 5-FU with radiotherapy had significantly improved survival times compared to those receiving bolus 5-FU. Indeed, the use of PVI 5-FU during radiotherapy for patients with pancreatic cancer has been accepted as the standard of care, but has not been proved to provide an advantage over bolus injections of 5-FU.

The use of gemcitabine, a novel nucleoside analogue, with concurrent radiotherapy may represent an opportunity to substantially improve the outcome of patients with pancreatic cancer. This agent (discussed in detail below) has been shown to provide a survival advantage over treatment with 5-FU in patients with locally advanced (unresectable) or metastatic pancreatic cancer.[89] Gemcitabine has also been shown to provide symptomatic relief to patients with metastatic pancreatic cancer that did not respond to prior treatment with 5-FU.[90] Thus use of this drug with radiation in a combined modality regimen warrants investigation. Laboratory studies by Lawrence et al.[91] have demonstrated that exposure to noncytotoxic concentrations of gemcitabine produced radiation enhancement ratios of 1.7–1.8 in human cancer cell lines, including pancreatic cancer cell lines. In addition, radiosensitization persisted for 24–48 hours following a brief (2-hour) exposure to gemcitabine. Interestingly, sensitization was not associated with levels of deoxycitadine triphosphate, the cytotoxic metabolite of gemcitabine, but was correlated with depletion of deoxynucleotide pools. In an attempt to maximize radiosensitization, investigators have delivered gemcitabine twice weekly at doses of 10–60 mg/m$^2$ during a course of conventional radiotherapy.[92] This approach attempts to maximize radiosensitization. Thrombocytopenia, neutropenia, and nausea and vomiting were the dose-limiting toxicities at 60 mg/m$^2$. The recommended dose of 40 mg/m$^2$ will be studied further in a cooperative group setting.

Another phase I trial is investigating the maximum tolerated dose (MTD) of gemcitabine when delivered once weekly for 6 weeks during a conventional course of radiotherapy in patients with unresectable pancreatic cancer.[93] Radiation is delivered in 1.8 Gy fractions once daily for a total dose of 50.4 Gy. A margin of 3 cm around the gross target volume is required for the initial field (39.6 Gy). This margin is reduced to 2 cm for the final boost (10.8 Gy). The starting dose of gemcitabine was 300 mg/m$^2$ and was subsequently escalated to 700 mg/m$^2$.

In a trial of an alternative strategy being investigated at the University of Michigan,[94] gemcitabine is delivered at the current recommended dosage (1000 mg/m$^2$/week for 3 weeks every 28 days), with a 3-week course of radiation (15 fractions) delivered concurrently. The regimen aims to maximize systemic drug effect while providing local control through sensitization of a modest radiation dose. Escalation of the radiation dose is achieved by increasing the fraction size, thus keeping the duration of radiation therapy at 3 weeks. A margin of only 1 cm is required around the gross target volume. Doses in the range of 24 to 30 Gy have been investigated.

A comparison of the levels of local toxicity (both acute and late) in gemcitabine dose escalation and "full-dose" gemcitabine with radiation dose escalation may be informative, particularly in terms of the volumes of normal tissue irradiated (as indicated by the margins of expansion). This issue needs to be critically addressed in all chemoradiation studies using gemcitabine, since this agent is a potent radiosensitizer of normal tissues. Once these trials are completed, phase II trials may be conducted to evaluate response and survival as primary end points. Radiation dose escalation is being considered as a neoadjuvant regimen, as patients would receive full-dose systemic therapy as soon as the diagnosis is confirmed and would also receive a local modality that may improve the rate of surgical resection. This approach may also lend itself to integration with alternative systemic approaches using gemcitabine at a fixed dose rate or using gemcitabine in combination with other systemic agents.

## Chemotherapy Alone

To date, the role of chemotherapy without concomitant radiation in the management of locally unresectable pancreatic cancer is poorly understood. As noted above, two studies have compared chemoradiation with either 5-FU alone[79] or with SMF.[80] The conclusions of these trials disagreed: one report suggested that results of 5-FU therapy were comparable to those of chemoradiation, whereas the other report found that SMF obtained results inferior to those of chemoradiation.

As noted above, compared with 5-FU, gemcitabine treatment results in a survival advantage in patients with unresectable and/or metastatic pancreatic cancer.[89] An analysis of more than 3000 patients treated with gemcitabine on an expanded-use protocol included 472 patients with apparent localized disease.[95] The median survival for this group was approximately 7 months, which is within the range (albeit at the lower end) of survival times reported in chemoradiation series.

Currently, researchers are seeking to optimize the effectiveness of gemcitabine through use of infusion schedules that favor the formation of gemcitabine triphosphate (an active metabolite)[96] or that take advantage of synergistic drug combinations, such as gemcitabine with cisplatin.[97] Once this systemic treatment is determined, it should be compared with the most effective chemoradiation regimen.

## Summary

When considering invasive palliative procedures and selecting a treatment plan, the treatment team and the patient should review the potential complications and the expected benefits. Patients must be told that even a minimally invasive procedure may be prolonged because of the debilitating effects of pancreatic cancer. In patients with terminal illness, sustaining quality of life is the goal of treatment, and even successful therapeutic strategies sometimes adversely affect quality of life. An honest discussion with the patient and their loved ones about their specific desires for the time before or after treatment can aid in choosing a procedure or treatment. Equally important is practical discussion of end-of-life issues that respects each patient's desire for a good result. Satisfaction with treatment decisions is highest for patients and their loved ones when the treatment reasonably meets their expectations.

## References

1. Niederhuber JE, Brennan MF, Menck HR. The National Cancer Data Base report on pancreatic cancer. Cancer 76:1671–1677, 1995.
2. Lillemoe KD, Cameron JL, Yeo CJ, et al. Pancreaticoduodenectomy—does it have a role in the palliation of pancreatic cancer? Ann Surg 223:718–728, 1996.
3. Soybel DI. Pancreaticoduodenectomy and palliation in pancreatic carcinoma. Lett Gastroenterol 112:1046–1047, 1996.
4. Klinkenbijl JHG, Jeekel J, Schmitz PIM, et al. Carcinoma of the pancreas and periampullary region: palliation versus cure. Br J Surg 80:1575–1578, 1993.
5. Pretre R, Huber O, Robert J, et al. Results of surgical palliation for cancer of the head of the pancreas and periampullary region. Br J Surg 79:795–798, 1992.
6. Espat NJ, Brennan MF, Conlon KC. Patients with laparoscopically staged unresectable pancreatic adenocarcinoma do not require subsequent surgical biliary or gastric bypass. J Am Coll Surg 188:649–657, 1998.
7. Gastrointestinal Tumor Study Group. Treatment of locally unresectable carcinoma of the pancreas: comparison of combined-modality therapy (chemotherapy plus radiotherapy) to chemotherapy alone. J Natl Cancer Inst 80:751–755, 1988.
8. Wade TP, Neuberger TJ, Swope TJ, et al. Pancreatic cancer palliation: using tumor stage to select appropriate operation. Am J Surg 167:208–213, 1994.
9. Lillemoe KD, Cameron JL, Hardacre JM, et al. Is prophylactic gastrojejunostomy indicated for unresectable periampullary cancer? A prospective randomized trial. Ann Surg 230:322–330, 1999.
10. van den Bosch RP, van der Schelling GP, Klinkenbijl JHG, et al. Guidelines for the application of surgery and endoprostheses in the palliation of obstructive jaundice in advanced cancer of the pancreas. Ann Surg 219:18–24, 1994.
11. Fuhrman GM, Leach SD, Staley CA, et al. Rationale for en bloc vein resection in the treatment of pancreatic adenocarcinoma adherent to the superior mesenteric–portal vein confluence. Ann Surg 223:154–162, 1996.
12. Fuhrman GM, Charnsangavej C, Abbruzzese JL, et al. Thin-section contrast-enhanced computed tomography accurately predicts the resectability of malignant pancreatic neoplasms. Am J Surg 167:104–113, 1994.
13. Rosch T. Diagnosis and staging of pancreatic cancer by EUS: critical analysis. 10th International Symposium on Endoscopic Ultrasonography, Mosby, Cleveland, 1996, pp 153–162.
14. Brand RE, Matamoros A. Imaging techniques in the evaluation of adenocarcinoma of the pancreas. Dig Dis 16:242–252, 1998.
15. Legman P, Vignaus O, Dousser B, et al. Pancreatic tumors: comparison of dual-phase helical CT and endoscopic sonography. Am J Radiol 170:1315–1322, 1998.
16. Rosch T, Lightdale CJ, Botet GA, et al. Localization of pancreatic endocrine tumors by endoscopic ultrasonography. N Engl J Med 326:1721–1726, 1992.
17. Gress F, Savides T, Cummings O, et al. Radial scanning and linear array endosonography for staging pancreatic cancer: a prospective randomized comparison. Gastrointest Endosc 45:138–142, 1997.
18. Lu DA, Reber HA, Krasny RM, et al. Local staging of pancreatic cancer: criteria for unresectability of major vessels as revealed by pancreatic-phase, thin-section helical CT. Am J Radiol 168:1439–1443, 1997.
19. Tierney WM, Carpenter SL, Bansal R, et al. Accuracy and economic impact of helical CT and endoscopic ultrasound in the staging of ampullopancreatic tumors. Gastrointest Endosc 45:183, 1995.
20. Tierney WM, Hirth RA, Fendrick AM, et al. The clinical and economic impact of endoscopic ultrasound, MRA, and helical CT in the staging of pancreatic cancer. Gastrointest Endosc 45:183, 1997.
21. Andren-Sandberg A, Lindberg, CG, Lundstedt C, Ihse I. Computed tomography and laparoscopy in the assessment of the patient with pancreatic cancer. J Am Coll Surg 186:35–40, 1998.
22. Merchant NB, Conlon KC. Laparoscopic evaluation in pancreatic cancer. Semin Surg Oncol 15:155–165, 1998.
23. Singh SM, Longmire WP, Reber HA. Surgical palliation for pancreatic cancer, the UCLA experience. Ann Surg 212:132–139, 1990.
24. Speer AG, Cotton, PB, Russell RCG, et al. Randomised trial of endoscopic versus percutaneous stent insertion in malignant obstructive jaundice. Lancet 2: 57–62, 1987.
25. O'Brien S, Hatfield ARW, Craig PI, Williams SP. A three year follow up of self-expanding metal stents in the endoscopic palliation of long-term survivors with malignant biliary obstruction. Gut 36:618–621, 1995.
26. Schmassmann A, von Gunten, E, Knuchel J, et al. Wallstents versus plastic stents in malignant biliary obstruction: effects of stent patency of the first and second stent on patient compliance and survival. Am J Gastroenterol 91:654–659, 1996.
27. Prat F, Chapat O, Ducot B, et al. A randomized trial of endoscopic drainage methods for inoperable malignant strictures of the common bile duct. Gastrointest Endosc 47:1–7, 1998.
28. Wong RCK, Carr-Locke DL. Endoscopic stents for palliation in patients with pancreatic cancer. In: Reber HA (ed): Pancreatic Cancer—Pathogenesis, Diagnosis, and Treatment. Humana Press, Totowa, NJ, 1998, pp 235–252.
29. Ballinger AB, McHugh M, Catnach SM, et al. Symptom relief and quality of life after stenting for malignant bile duct obstruction. Gut 35:467–470, 1994.
30. Luman W, Cull A, Palmer KR. Quality of life in patients stented for malignant biliary obstruction. Eur J Gastroenterol Hepatol 9:481–484, 1997.

31. Lillemoe KD, Pitt HA. Palliation—surgical and otherwise. CA Suppl 78:605–614, 1996.
32. Lillemoe KD, Barnes SA. Surgical palliation of unresectable pancreatic carcinoma. Surg Clin North Am 5:953–958, 1995.
33. Potts III JR, Broughan TA, Hermann RE. Palliative operations for pancreatic carcinoma. Am J Surg 159:72–78, 1990.
34. DiFronzo LA, Egrari S, O'Connell TX. Choledochoduodenostomy for palliation in unresectable pancreatic cancer. Arch Surg 133:820–825, 1998.
35. Raj PK, Mahoney P, Linderman C. Laparoscopic cholecystojejunostomy: a technical application in unresectable biliary obstruction. J Laparoendosc Adv Surg Tech A 7:47–52, 1997.
36. Shimi S, Banting S, Cuschieri A. Laparoscopy in the management of pancreatic cancer: endoscopic cholecystojejunostomy for advanced disease. Br J Surg 79:317–319, 1992.
37. Scudamore CH, Chow Y, Shackleton CR, Forward AD. Choledochocholecystojejunostomy: a quick, effective method of biliary decompression for carcinoma of the pancreas. Can J Surg 34:543–546, 1991.
38. Chekan EG, Clark L, Wu J, et al. Laparoscopic biliary and enteric bypass. Semin Surg Oncol 16:313–320, 1999.
39. Sarfeh IJ, Rypin EB, Jakowatz JG, et al. A prospective, randomized clinical investigation of cholecystoenterostomy and choledochoenterostomy. Am J Surg 155:411–414, 1988.
40. Sarr MG, Cameron JL. Surgical management of unresectable carcinoma of the pancreas. Surgery 91:122–133, 1982.
41. Shumate CR, Baron TH. Palliative procedures for pancreatic cancer. South Med J 89:27–32, 1996.
42. Tarnasky PR, England RE, Lail LM, et al. Cystic duct patency in malignant obstructive jaundice. An ERCP-based study relevant to the role of laparoscopic cholecystojejunostomy. Ann Surg 221:265–271, 1995.
43. Park A, Schwartz R, Tandan V, Anvari M. Laparoscopic pancreatic surgery. Am J Surg 177:158–163, 1999.
44. Watanapa P, Williamson RCN. Single-loop biliary and gastric bypass for irresectable pancreatic carcinoma. Br J Surg 80:237–239, 1993.
45. Singh SM, Reber HA. Surgical palliation for pancreatic cancer. Surg Clin of North Am 69:599–611, 1989.
46. Egrari S, O'Connell TX. Role of prophylactic gastroenterostomy for unresectable pancreatic carcinoma. Am J Surg 61:862–864, 1989.
47. Zamboni WA, Fisher KS, Ross DS. Surgical palliation for pancreatic carcinoma. Postgrad Med J 67:362–365, 1991.
48. van Wagensveld BA, Coene PPLO, van Gulik TM, et al. Outcome of palliative biliary and gastric bypass surgery for pancreatic head carcinoma in 126 patients. Br J Surg 84:1402–1406, 1997.
49. Watanapa P, Williamson RCN. Surgical palliation for pancreatic cancer: developments during the past two decades. Br J Surg 79:8–20, 1992.
50. Lillemoe KD, Sauter PK, Pitt HA, et al. Current status of surgical palliation of periampullary carcinoma. Surg Gynecol Obstet 176:1–10, 1992.
51. Bergamaschi R, Marvik R, Thoresen JE. Open versus laparoscopic gastrojejunostomy for palliation in advanced pancreatic cancer. Surg Laparosc Endosc 8:92–96, 1998.
52. Ripamonti C, DeConno F, Ventafridda V, et al. Management of bowel obstruction in advanced and terminal cancer patients. Ann Oncol 4:15–21, 1993.
53. Feretis C, Benakes P, Dimopoulos C, et al. Duodenal obstruction caused by pancreatic head carcinoma: palliation with expendable endoprostheses. Gastrointest Endosc 46:161–165, 1997.
54. Sharp KW, Stevens EJ. Improving palliation in pancreatic cancer: intraoperative celiac plexus block for pain relief. South Med J 84:469–471, 1991.
55. Sakorafas GH, Tsiotou AG, Sarr MG. Intraoperative celiac plexus block in the surgical palliation for unresectable pancreatic cancer. Eur J Surg Oncol 25:427–431, 1999.
56. Russell RCG. Review, palliation of pain and jaundice: an overview. Ann Oncol 100 (Suppl 4):165–169, 1999.
57. Wiersama MJ, Wiersema LM. Endosonography-guided celiac plexus neurolysis. Gastrointest Endosc 44:656–662, 1996.
58. Perez MM, Newcomer AD, Moertel CG, et al. Assessment of weight loss, food intake, fat metabolism, malabsorption, and treatment of pancreatic insufficiency in pancreatic cancer. Cancer 52:346–352, 1983.
59. Bruno MJ, Haverkort EB, Tjissen GP, et al. Placebo-controlled trial of enteric-coated pancreatin microsphere treatment in patients with unresectable cancer of the pancreatic head region. Gut 42:92–96, 1998.
60. DiMagno EP, Malagelada JR, Go VLW. The relationships between pancreatic ductal obstruction and pancreatic secretion in man. Mayo Clin Proc 54:157–162, 1979.
61. DiMagno EP, Reber HA, Tempero MA. Epidemiology, diagnosis, and treatment of pancreatic ductal adenocarcinoma. American Gastroenterological Association. Gastroenterology 117:1464–1484, 1999.
62. Haslam JB, Cavanaugh PJ, Stroup SL. Radiation therapy in the treatment of irresectable adenocarcinoma of the pancreas. Cancer 32:1341–1345, 1973.
63. Moertel CG, Frytak S, Hahn RG, et al. Therapy of locally unresectable pancreatic carcinoma: a randomized comparison of high-dose (6000 rads) radiation alone, moderate-dose radiation (4000 rads) + 5-fluorouracil, and high-dose radiation + 5-fluorouracil. Cancer 48:1075–1010, 1981.
64. Flickinger, JC, Jawalekar K, Deutsch M, Webster J. Split-course radiation therapy for adenocarcinoma of the pancreas. Int J Radiat Oncol Biol Phys 15:359–364, 1988.
65. Dobelbower RR, Borgelt BB, Strubler KA, el al: Precision radiotherapy for cancer of the pancreas: technique and results. Int J Radiat Oncol Biol Phys 6:1127–1133, 1980.
66. Kinsella TK, Sindelar WF. Intraloperative radiotherapy for pancreatic cancer. Cancer 78:598–604, 1996.
67. Roldan, GE, Gunderson LL, Nagorney DM, et al. External beam versus intraoperative and external beam irradiation for locally advanced pancreatic cancer. Cancer 61:1110–1116, 1988.
68. Tepper JE, Noyes D, Krall JM, et al. Intraoperative radiation therapy of pancreatic carcinoma: a report of RTOG-8505. Radiation Therapy Oncology Group. Int J Radiat Oncol Biol Phys 21:1145–1149, 1991.
69. Garton GR, Gunderson LL, Nagorney DM, et al. High-dose preoperative external beam and intraoperative irradiation for locally advanced pancreatic cancer. Int J Radiat Ocol Biol Phys 27:1153–1157, 1993.
70. Gunderson, LL, Willett CG, Harrison LB, et al. Intraoperative irradiation: current and future status. Semin Oncol 24:715–731, 1997.
71. Mohiuddin M, Rosato, F, Barbot D, et al. Long-term results of combined modality treatment with I-125 implantation for carcinoma of the pancreas. Int J Radiat Oncol Biol Phys 23:305–311, 1992.
72. Peretz T, Nori D, Hilaris B, et al. Treatment of primary unresectable carcinoma of the pancreas with I-125 implantation. Int J Radiat Oncol Biol Phys 17:931–935, 1989.
73. Raben A, Mychalczak B, Brennan MF, et al. Feasibility study of the treatment of primary unresectable carcinoma of the pancreas with [103]Pd brachytherapy. Int J Radiat Oncol Biol Phys 35:351–356, 1996.
74. DeNittis AS, Stambaugh MD, Lang P, et al. Complete remission of non-resectable pancreatic cancer after infusional colloidal phosphorus-32 brachytherapy, external beam radiation therapy, and 5-fluorouracil: a preliminary report. Am J Clin Oncol 22:355–360, 1999.
75. Gunderson LL, Martin JK, Kvols LK, et al. Intraoperative and external beam irradiation +/− 5-FU for locally advanced pancreatic cancer. Int J Radiat Oncol Biol Phys 13:319–329, 1987.
76. Robertson, JM, Marsh L, TenHaken RK, Lawrence TS. The clinical application of a non-axial treatment plan for pancreatic and biliary malignancies. Radiother Oncol 24:198–200, 1992.
77. Higgins D, Sohn JW, Fine RM, Schell MC. Three-demensional conformal pancreas treatment: comparison of four to six field techniques. Int J Radiat Oncol Biol Phys 31:605–609, 1995.
78. Lichter AS, Lawrence TS. Recent advances in radiation oncology. N Engl J Med 32:371–379, 1995.
79. Moertel CG, Childs DS, Reitemeier RJ, et al. Combined 5-fluorouracil and supervoltage radiation therapy of locally unresectable gastrointestinal cancer. Lancet 2:865–867, 1969.
80. Gastrointestinal Tumor Study Group. Radiation therapy combined with adriamycin or 5-fluorouracil for the treatment of locally unresectable pancreatic carcinoma. Cancer 56:2563–2568, 1985.
81. Gastrointestinal Tumor Study Group. Phase II studies of drug combinations in advanced pancreatic carcinoma: fluorouracil plus doxorubicin plus mitomycin-C and two regimens of streprozoticin plus mitomycin-C plus fluorouracil. J Clin Oncol 4:1774–1798, 1986.
82. Seydel HG, Stablein DM, Leichman LP, et al. Hyperfractionated radiation and chemotherapy for unresectable localized adenocarcinoma of the pancreas. Cancer 65:1478–1482, 1990.
83. Klaasen DJ, MacIntyre JM, Catton GE, et al. Treatment of locally unresectable cancer of the stomach and pancreas: a randomized comparison of 5-fluorouracil alone with radiation plus concurrent and maintenance 5-fluorouracil. J Clin Oncol. 3:373–378, 1985.
84. Gastrointestinal Tumor Study Group. Treatment of locally unresectable carcinoma of the pancreas: comparison of combined-modality therapy (chemotherapy plus radiotherapy) to chemotherapy alone. J Natl Cancer Inst 80:751–755, 1988.
85. Komaki R, Hansen R, Cox, JD, et al. Phase I–II study of prophylactic hepatic irradiation with local irradiation and systemic chemotherapy for

adenocarcinoma of the pancreas. Int J Radiat Oncol Biol Phys 15:1447–1452, 1988.

86. Komaki R, Wadler S, Peters T, et al. High-dose local irradiation plus prophylactic hepatic irradiation and chemotherapy for inoperable adenocarcinoma of the pancreas. A preliminary report of a mult-institutional trial (Radiation Therapy Oncology Group Protocol 8801). Cancer 69:2807–2812, 1992.

87. Poen JC, Collins HL, Niederhuber JE, et al. Chemo-radiotherapy for localized pancreatic cancer: increased dose intensity and reduced acute toxicity with concomitant radiotherapy and protracted venous infusion 5-fluorouracil. Int J Radiat Oncol Biol Phys 40:93–99, 1998.

88. Whittington R, Neuberg D, Tester WJ, et al. Protracted intravenous fluorouracil infusion with radiation therapy in the management of localized pancreaticobiliary carcinoma: a phase I Eastern Cooperative Oncology Group Trial. J Clin Oncol 13:227–232, 1995.

89. Burris HA, Moore MJ, Andersen J, et al. Improvements in survival and clinical benefit with gemcitabine as first-line therapy for patients with advanced pancreas cancer: a randomized trial. J Clin Oncol 15:2405–2413, 1997.

90. Rothenberg ML, Moore MJ, Cripps MC, et al. A phase II trial of gemcitabine in patients with 5-FU-refractory pancreas cancer. Ann Oncol 7:347–353, 1996.

91. Lawrence TS, Chang EY, Hahn TM, et al. Radiosensitization of pancreatic cancer cells by 2',2'-difluoro-2'-deoxycytidine. Int J Radiat Oncol Biol Phys 34:867–872, 1996.

92. Blackstock AW, Bernard SA, Richards F, et al. Phase I trial of twice-weekly gemcitabine and concurrent radiation in patients with advanced pancreatic cancer. J Clin Oncol 17:2208–2212, 1999.

93. McGinn C, Smith D, Szark C, et al. A phase I study of gemcitabine in combination with radiation therapy in patients with localized, unresectable pancreatic cancer [abstract]. Proc Am Soc Clin Oncol 17:1014, 1998.

94. McGinn CJ, Zalupski MM, Shureiqi I, et al. Phase I trial of radiation dose escalation with concurrent weekly full-dose gemcitabine in patients with advanced pancreatic cancer. J Clin Oncol 19:4202–4208, 2001.

95. Storniolo AM, Enas NH, Brown C, et al. An investigational new drug treatment program for patients with gemcitabine. Cancer 85: 1262–1268, 1999.

96. Tempero MA, Plunket W, Ruiz van Haperen V, et al. Randomized phase II trial of dose intense gemcitabine by standard infusion vs. fixed dose rate in metastatic pancreatic adenocarcinoma. Proc Am Soc Clin Oncol 18:273, 1999.

97. Yang LY, Li L, Jian H, et al. Expression of ERCC1 antisense RNA abrogates gemcitabine-mediated cytotoxic synergism with cisplatin in human colon tumor cells defective in mismatch repair but proficient in nucleotide excision repair. Clin Cancer Res 6:773–781, 2000.

# Chapter 34

# Clinical Aspects and Management of Metastatic Pancreatic Cancer

## MACE L. ROTHENBERG AND JORDAN D. BERLIN

Of all malignancies tracked by the National Cancer Institute's (NCI) Surveillance, Epidemiology, and End Results (SEER) program, pancreatic cancer has the lowest 5-year survival rate; 4.1%.[1] The prognosis of this malignancy is poor because of the following factors: *(1)* the limited effectiveness of currently available therapies; *(2)* the lack of effective genetic screening tests that could identify individuals at increased risk of developing pancreatic cancer; *(3)* lack of specific early warning signs and symptoms directly attributable to the disease; *(4)* the inability to detect patients with premalignant lesions or asymptomatic, early-stage pancreatic cancer; and *(5)* the debilitated medical condition of the patient at the time of initiation of treatment that leads to decreased tolerance and increased toxicity from chemotherapy. No other cancer challenges us more to develop novel and innovative therapeutic approaches than does pancreatic cancer. Fortunately, insights gained over the past 15 years into the molecular and genetic processes involved in pancreatic carcinogenesis, angiogenesis, invasion, and metastasis have begun to yield rational targets for therapeutic intervention. This chapter addresses the therapeutic management of patients with metastatic pancreatic cancer.

## Presenting Signs and Symptoms

Pain, the most common symptom associated with advanced pancreatic cancer, is present in up to 89% of patients at the time of diagnosis and is the first symptom of pancreatic cancer in 64% of patients.[2] Other common presenting symptoms include weight loss, anorexia, nausea, jaundice, depression, epigastric bloating, weakness, fatigue, diarrhea, and dark urine (Table 34–1). Except for jaundice and dark urine, these symptoms are nonspecific, thus contributing to an average delay of up to 4.5 months between the onset of symptoms and the diagnosis of pancreatic cancer.[2] De-

pression is underrecognized and undertreated in this group of patients. Upon formal psychological testing, 38% to 71% of patients with pancreatic cancer meet the criteria for clinical depression.[3,4] Furthermore, depression *precedes* the diagnosis of pancreatic cancer in 33% to 50% of patients with this cancer.[4,5]

## Intrinsic Drug Resistance

Despite the fact that adenocarcinoma of the pancreas is one of the most drug-resistant cancers, there are surprisingly few data on the etiology of this drug resistance. One of the reasons for this is that pancreatic tissue is difficult to manipulate in an experimental system because of a heterogeneous cell population (e.g., endocrine, exocrine, ductal, and acinar) and the presence of a substantial amount of proteolytic enzymes making extraction of cellular proteins and nucleic acids difficult.[6] Another reason for the scarcity of data is that pancreatic cancer is characteristically drug-resistant from the outset of therapy. If a pancreatic cancer cell line were available, we could compare this chemosensitive "parental" cell line with a chemoresistant "daughter" cell line to determine specific cellular and genetic differences responsible for the observed resistance.[6] Until these problems are overcome, our efforts to develop more effective therapeutic agents must be based on the extrapolation of observations of other, more chemosensitive tumors and cell lines.

## Single-Agent Chemotherapy

The standard approach to the treatment of patients with advanced pancreatic cancer, as with most cancers, is cytotoxic chemotherapy. Over the past several decades, dozens of agents have been evaluated in phase II trials in metastatic pancreatic cancer, with

**Table 34-1** Frequency of physical signs and symptoms at the time of diagnosis of pancreatic cancer[2-5]

| Symptom | Patients with Symptom at Diagnosis (%) |
|---|---|
| Pain (any site) | 63–89 |
| Abdominal pain | 67–80 |
| Back pain | 58–65 |
| Weight loss | 67–82 |
| Anorexia, nausea, or both | 62 |
| Jaundice | 42–80 |
| Depression | 38–71 |
| Epigastric bloating | 34 |
| Weakness, fatigue, or both | 31 |
| Diarrhea | 25 |
| Dark urine | 25 |
| Hepatomegaly | 19 |
| Palpable gallbladder | 12 |
| Fever | 9 |
| Thrombophlebitis | 3 |
| Splenomegaly | 2 |
| Ascites | 2 |

only limited success.[7] Response rates of 13% to 27% have been reported for single agents such as mitomycin C, doxorubicin, and epirubicin. However, these trials were limited by the small numbers of patients. Furthermore, many of the phase II trials performed before 1980 relied on clinical criteria of response (e.g., decrease in liver span by at least 30% or reduction in the size of a palpable abdominal mass by at least 50%) rather than more sensitive measures, such as computed tomography (CT) scans.[8]

## 5-Fluorouracil

Probably the most studied single agent is 5-fluorouracil (5-FU), which for decades was the cornerstone of therapy for pancreatic cancer. This agent exerts its cytotoxic effect by at least two mechanisms: (1) incorporation of an anabolite, FUTP, into RNA and (2) inhibition of thymidylate synthase, a folate-dependent enzyme essential for the synthesis of nucleic acid precursors, by FdUMP. A third mechanism, DNA chain termination through the incorporation of FdUTP, has also been described. Used as a sin-

gle agent, 5-FU has produced response rates varying from 0% to greater than 20% in patients with advanced pancreatic cancer.[8] However, the response rates reported may be overestimates since many of the studies reporting the highest response rates were performed before 1980 and used the clinical response criteria described above.

One method of possibly enhancing the antitumor activity of single-agent 5-FU has been to combine it with a variety of biochemical modulators that are not cytotoxic by themselves. These agents include leucovorin, N-phosphonacetyl-L-aspartate (PALA), and interferon α (IFN-α) (Table 34–2). The results of phase II trials of these agents have varied widely, with response rates ranging from 0% to 14%, median survival times from 3.7 to 10 months, and 1-year survival rates from less than 10% to approximately 30%.[9-16] In addition, patient selection may have influenced the outcome of these trials. Median and 1-year survival rates have tended to be longer in studies that included patients with locally advanced disease, restricted entry to those patients with a World Health Organization (WHO)/Eastern Cooperative Oncology Group (ECOG) performance status of 0 to 1, and/or included a large proportion of patients who had undergone exploratory laparotomy before chemotherapy. These findings underscore the need for phase III trials in the evaluation of new therapies for advanced pancreatic cancer.

Another method of enhancing the therapeutic efficacy of 5-FU has been to alter the method of administration. Prolonging the infusion of 5-FU may increase the ability of the drug to inhibit thymidylate synthase. In addition, this method allows higher total doses of 5-FU to be administered in a more dose-intense fashion. Phase II trials of infusional 5-FU have produced results similar to those obtained in other trials involving 5-FU (Table 34–2). Oral formulations of 5-FU prodrugs, such as tegafur plus uracil (UFT) and capecitabine, have been developed that promote uptake and retention of 5-FU within the cell and provide a convenient route for chronic drug dosing. Available data on the use of oral 5-FU or 5-FU prodrugs in pancreatic cancer are limited and inconsistent. While some phase II trials of oral 5-FU prodrugs have reported response rates as high as 25%, others have failed to observe any objective responses.[17,18] With the emergence of other, more active agents, the role of single-agent 5-FU in the treatment of patients with metastatic pancreatic cancer has begun to diminish.

**Table 34-2** Phase II trials of biochemically modulated 5-fluorouracil in advanced pancreatic cancer

| Regimen | Patients (n) | Response Rate (%) | Median Survival (Months) | 1-Year Survival (%) |
|---|---|---|---|---|
| LV 500 mg/m² + 5-FU 600 mg/m² every week × 6 of 8 weeks[122] | 42 | 7 | 6.2 | 17 |
| LV 200 mg/m² + 5-FU 370 mg/m² daily × 5 every 4 weeks[123] | 30 | 13 (n = 23) | 3.7 | ~10 |
| LV 20 mg/m² + 5-FU 425 mg/m² daily × 5 every 4 weeks[124] | 31 | 0 | 5.7 | |
| LV 200 mg/m² + 5-FU 400 mg/m² bolus followed by 22-hour infusion of 5-FU 600 mg/m² daily × 2 every 2 weeks[125] | 20 | 10.5 | 6 | 20 |
| LV 500 mg/m² + 5-FU 500 mg/m² + IFN-α 6 million U every week[126,a] | 57 | 14 | 10 | ~30 |
| 5-FU 250 mg/m²/day as CI × 28 days + IFN-α 5 million units 3 × week[108] | 24 | 8 | 4.6 | N/A |
| 5-FU 250 mg/m²/day as CI × 28 days + IFN-α 3 million units 3 × week[107] | 13 | 7.7 | 8.3 | N/A |
| PALA 250 mg/m² on day 1 + 5-FU 2600 mg/m² as CI × 24 hours[127] | 41 | 14 (n = 35) | 5.1 | <10 |

CI, continuous infusion; 5-FU, 5-fluorouracil; IFN, interferon; LV, leucovorin; N/A, not available; PALA, N-phosphonacetyl-L-aspartate.
aIncluded patients with locally advanced disease.

and twenty-six patients with disease-related pain were enrolled in this study. The CBR rate was higher among patients treated with gemcitabine than among those treated with 5-FU (23.8% vs. 4.8%, respectively, P = 0.0022). In addition, survival was significantly longer among gemcitabine-treated patients (median survival 5.65 months vs. 4.41 months, respectively; 1-year survival rates 18% vs. 2%, respectively; P = 0.0025) than among 5-FU-treated patients. In a larger study, both symptomatic and asymptomatic patients received single-agent gemcitabine under an investigational new drug (IND) treatment program.[44] The median survival for these patients was 4.8 months, with a 1-year survival of 15%. The subset of patients not previously treated with chemotherapy had a median survival of 5.1 months (Table 34–3). On the basis of these results, gemcitabine has become the standard therapy for patients with advanced-stage pancreatic cancer and serves as the control arm in most current phase III trials.

## New Combination Chemotherapy Regimens

As noted previously, 5-FU-based combinations, such as FAM or SMF, have no established benefit over treatment with single-agent 5-FU (Table 34–4). Recent efforts have focused on the development of gemcitabine-based combinations and the integration of other active agents into the front-line treatment of advanced pancreatic cancer.

Preclinical data suggest a beneficial interaction when gemcitabine is combined with either cisplatin or 5-FU. Treatment of HT-29 colon cancer cell lines with gemcitabine before 5-fluoro-2'-deoxyuridine (FdUrD) yielded at least additive (and possibly synergistic) effects.[45,46] Compared with the use of either drug alone, this sequence significantly depleted deoxythymidine-5'-triphosphate (dTTP) pools, disturbed the cell cycle, and damaged the DNA. Compared with controls, HT-29 cells preincubated with 5-FU were more sensitive to the cytotoxic effects of gemcitabine.

Clinically, gemcitabine has been combined with 5-FU in several phase I/II and phase II trials (Table 34–5).[47–50] A phase III trial of the combination of gemcitabine plus bolus weekly 5-FU vs. single-agent gemcitabine reported a significant improvement in progression-free survival (3.4 vs. 2.2 months, P = .022), but no improvement in overall survival (5.4 vs. 6.7 months, P = 0.09).[51] It is possible that imbalances in known prognostic factors between the treatment arms and/or the decision to use bolus rather than infusional 5-FU could have contributed to this outcome and, as a result, other gemcitabine plus 5-FU regimens are undergoing expanded evaluation. However, similar results were reported in a small, randomized trial using the gemcitabine–capecitabine combination vs. gemcitabine alone.[52] Other methods for combining these agents may warrant further investigation.

Preclinical pancreatic cancer models have demonstrated synergy between gemcitabine and cisplatin.[53] Clinical evaluation of this combination has generated promising results in early clinical trials, with response rates ranging from 11.5% to 36.4% (Table 34–5).[49,54–56] Preliminary results of a randomized trial underway in Italy comparing this combination to single-agent gemcitabine failed to demonstrate any significant differences in therapeutic outcome.[55] However, these were interim results and subject to change with increased accrual and longer follow-up. Oxaliplatin is a novel platinum derivative with a diaminocyclohexane carrier ligand. Two phase II trials of gemcitabine plus oxaliplatin have generated somewhat inconsistent results, with one trial reporting an objective response rate of 28% and a median survival of 9.2 months while another reported a 13% objective

**Table 34–5** New combination chemotherapy regimens in pancreatic cancer

| Regimen | Patients (n) | Response Rate (%) | Median Survival (Months) | 1-Year Survival (%) |
|---|---|---|---|---|
| Gemcitabine 1000 mg/m$^2$ + 5-FU 600 mg/m$^2$ every week × 3 every 4 weeks[15] | 36 | 14 | 4.4 | >10 |
| Gemcitabine 1000 mg/m$^2$ + 5-FU 600 mg/m$^2$ every week × 3 every 4 weeks[47] | 54 | 4 (19% MR) | 7 | 22 |
| Gemcitabine 1000 mg/m$^2$ + leucovorin 25 mg/m$^2$ + 5-FU 500 mg/m$^2$ [48] | 18 | 22 | 11 | N/A |
| Gemcitabine 1000 mg/m$^2$ + 5-FU 200 mg/m$^2$/day PVI[75] | 26 | 19.2 | 10.3 | 39.5 |
| Leucovorin 400 mg/m$^2$, 5-FU 400 mg/m$^2$ IV bolus followed by 5-FU 3000 mg/m$^2$ CIV over 24 hours + gemcitabine 1250 mg/m$^2$ on day 3[125] | 48 | 19.1 | 8 | 38 |
| Gemcitabine 1000 mg/m$^2$ + leucovorin 200 mg/m$^2$ + 5-FU 750 mg/m$^2$ CIV over 24 hours[16] | 17 | N/A | 7.5+ | N/A |
| Gemcitabine 1500 mg/m$^2$ on days 1 and 14 + leucovorin 250 mg/m$^2$ on day 1, then 7.5 mg po bid × 14 days + UFT 390 mg/m$^2$ on days 1–14[131] | 22 | 13.6 | 8 | N/A |
| Gemcitabine 1000 mg/m$^2$ every week × 3, cisplatin 50 mg/m$^2$ every 2 weeks[49] | 25 evalated | 36.4 (2 CR) (18% SD) | 7.4 | N/A |
| Gemcitabine 1000 mg/m$^2$ every week × 3, cisplatin 50 mg/m$^2$ every 2 weeks[54] | 35 evalated | 11.5 (57.1% SD) | 8.3 | 28 |
| Gemcitabine 1000 mg/m$^2$ every week × 3, cisplatin 25 mg/m$^2$ every week × 3[55] | 32 evalated | 31 | N/A | N/A |
| Docetaxel 100 mg/m$^2$ on day 1 + gemcitabine 1000 mg/m$^2$ every week × 2 every 3 weeks[59] | 56 | 11.6% (n = 43) | 8 | 32 |
| Docetaxel 75 mg/m$^2$ on day 1 + gemcitabine 800 mg/m$^2$ every week × 3 every 4 weeks[60] | 9 | 33.3 | 22% | N/A |
| Gemcitabine 1000 mg/m$^2$/week × 3, every 4 weeks vs. | 160 | N/A | 5.4 | N/A |
| Gemcitabine 1000 mg/m$^2$ followed by 5-FU 600 mg/m$^2$ weekly × 3, every 4 weeks[51] | 158 | N/A | 6.7 P = 0.09 | N/A |

bid, twice a day; CIV, continuous intravenous infusion; CR, complete response; MR, minor response; N/A, not available; po, by mouth; PVI, protracted venous infusion; SD, standard deviation; UFT, tegafur plus uracil.

did not improve outcome: median survival was 6.3 and 6.0 months, respectively ($P = 0.75$).[97] Despite the lack of clinical activity, it does appear that the doses of R115777 blocked farnesyltransferase activity in peripheral blood mononuclear cells.[95]

The strategy of targeting the farnesyltransferase enzyme in pancreatic cancer has been criticized following the observation that the inhibitory effect of FTIs on cellular proliferation in vitro and in vivo is not limited to cells with mutated *Ras*. Ironically, the inhibitory effect of FTIs appears to be even more pronounced in cells with wild-type *Ras*.[98] In addition, farnesylation is not the only mechanism for post-translational modification of Ras proteins, which can be activated by geranylgeranytransferase as well.

The monoterpenes comprise another class of agents thought initially to target Ras mutations. Like the farnesyltransferase inhibitors, they have been shown to inhibit post-translational farnesylation of proteins.[99] Additionally, they inhibit geranylgeranylation, an alternative pathway of post-translational protein modification of Ras. However, subsequent studies have shown that these agents have other mechanisms of action as well. It appears that these agents are capable of inducing apoptosis through induction of receptors related to the TGF-β pathways.[100] This apoptosis appears to be independent of p53, a commonly mutated protein in pancreatic cancer that plays a significant role in apoptosis. One of the earliest monoterpenes to undergo Phase I study, perillyl alcohol, was studied by the ECOG, but did not display activity in patients with advanced pancreatic cancer.[100a]

## Epidermal Growth Factor Receptor Antagonists

Another potent stimulator of cell growth is the epidermal growth factor receptor (EGFR). This receptor, also called HER-1, is part of the HER family of tyrosine kinase receptors. When bound by one of its ligands, which include TGF-α, amphiregulin, and betacellulin as well as epidermal growth factor, the EGFR homodimerizes or heterodimerizes with another member of the HER family. This activates a tyrosine kinase on the intracellular domain, which leads to a phosphorylation cascade resulting in cancer cell growth and proliferation. Two classes of agents have been developed to target the EGFR: monoclonal antibodies directed at blocking ligand binding to the receptor and small molecule tyrosine kinase inhibitors that prevent the signaling cascade of a bound, activated receptor. C225 (cetuximab) is a human-mouse chimeric antibody that was evaluated in combination with gemcitabine in a phase II trial in patients with advanced pancreatic cancer whose tumors overexpressed EGFR.[101] After two cycles of therapy, 12% of patients had achieved a partial response. Median survival with this combination was 6.8 months. A phase III trial comparing this combination to single-agent gemcitabine in patients with advanced pancreatic cancer is scheduled to open in the Southwest Oncology Group in 2003. Small molecules that inhibit the tyrosine kinase (intracellular) domain of the EGFR constitute the second method for targeting EGFR. Agents such as ZD 1839 (Iressa) and OSI 774 (Tarceva) are being evaluated as single agents in ongoing phase II trials.

## Angiogenesis Inhibitors

Tumor-stimulated vasculogenesis is required for cancers to grow beyond 1 to 2 mm in diameter and appears to be essential for both the local growth and the metastasis of malignancies. Expression of certain angiogenic factors has been correlated with a more advanced stage of pancreatic cancer at diagnosis and a worse prognosis for patients with pancreatic cancer.[102] While

several angiogenesis inhibitors have entered clinical trials, no clinical data are available on their activity in pancreatic cancer. In preclinical models, TNP-470 in combination with cisplatin was better than either agent alone in preventing the development of liver metastases in nude mice injected with the liver-metastasizing pancreatic cancer cell line HPC-3H4.[103] It is anticipated that several angiogenesis inhibitors will proceed to phase II evaluation in the advanced pancreatic cancer setting within the next year or two.

## Immunologically Based Therapy

Approaches to the immunotherapy of pancreatic cancer include the use of biologic agents that stimulate one or several components of the immune system, monoclonal antibodies directed against tumor-specific antigens, and tumor vaccines. Interferon and interleukins stimulate many components of the immune system in a relatively nonspecific fashion. These agents act, in part, by enhancing the expression of major histocompatibility complexes I and II on cancer cells and by stimulating effectors of the immune response. Although treatment with interferon and interleukin-2 has been evaluated in a variety of malignancies, only limited trials have been conducted in patients with pancreatic carcinoma. Because many of these phase II trials have been small and have combined interferon with one or more cytotoxic drugs, it is difficult to draw conclusions about the effectiveness of this approach.[104–109] Response rates have ranged from 0% to 35% and median survival times as long as 11 months have been reported. However, more than 50% of patients treated with this therapy experience constitutional, gastrointestinal, or hematologic toxicity. Thus, interferon and interleukin-2 do not have established roles in the treatment of patients with advanced pancreatic cancer.

A more specific form of immunotherapy utilizes monoclonal antibodies designed to target known tumor antigens. The most extensively studied monoclonal antibody (mAb) has been 17-1A. This antibody, created by immunizing mice with the SW1038 colorectal cancer cell line, acts through antibody-dependent cellular cytotoxicity (ADCC).[110] When it was admixed with autologous mononuclear cells, mAb 17-1A was ineffective in the first 18 patients treated and 81% of the patients developed human antimouse antibodies (HAMA). In a later trial that combined mAb 17-1A with interferon to enhance ADCC,[111] limited antitumor effects were seen, with only 1 response among 30 patients and a median survival of only 5 months. Such therapies may become more effective if problems such as the development of HAMA can be overcome through the use of humanized monoclonal antibodies.

A second potential target of monoclonal antibody therapy is the HER-2/neu protein, a glycoprotein with intrinsic tyrosine kinase activity.[112] HER-2/neu appears to be overexpressed in as many as 45% to 58% of pancreatic cancers.[112,113] Trastuzumab (Herceptin), a monoclonal antibody directed against HER-2/neu, has demonstrated activity in patients with HER-2/neu–overexpressing breast cancers.[114] Clinical trials of this agent alone and in combination with cytotoxic drugs have been in initiated in patients with advanced pancreatic cancer.

Three cancer-associated T-cell antigens are shared by 50% to 90% of human pancreatic adenocarcinomas: carcinoembryonic antigen (CEA), MUC-1, and K-ras.[115] Once stimulated, host antigen-presenting cells can prime CD4[+] and CD8[+] cells to generate systemic antitumor immunity. A phase I trial was performed in which 14 patients who had undergone pancreaticoduodenectomy received four vaccinations with allogeneic tumor vaccine.[116] The vaccine was prepared from two cell lines that had been developed from human pancreatic adenocarcinoma specimens and genetically modified to express human GM-CSF. Approximately half of the patients treated at the two highest dose levels had a significant enhancement of delayed-type hypersensitivity reactions to irradiated, autologous tumor. Interestingly, it is this subset of patients who has enjoyed the longest disease-free survival. A follow-up phase II trial of allogeneic tumor vaccine is currently underway.

The k-Ras protein discussed above is an excellent target for immunotherapy. Approaches to vaccination against mutant Ras peptides are being evaluated in clinical trials. Mutations in *Ras* at codons 12 and/or 13 inhibit lymphocyte binding to HLA-A2.1 and extracellular antigen processing.[9] These results have served as the rationale for the use of mutated Ras proteins to create vaccines using pulsed dendritic cells.[10,117] Using another approach, McCarty and colleagues[118] have used p53-specific cytotoxic T lymphocytes (CTLs) to lyse HLA A2.1 restricted panc-1 cells in vitro. These lymphocytes spared AsPC-1 cells that did not express HLA A2.1. The p53-specific CTLs were also effective in delaying growth and prolonging survival of SCID mice inoculated with a human pancreas tumor xenograft, as shown by a comparison with mice inoculated with nonspecific CTLs.

An alternative approach for stimulating an immune response that avoids the need for HLA specificity is the use of "superantigens," which do not require internalization and presentation by antigen-presenting cells to induce a T-lymphocyte response. One study has been conducted using PNU-214565, a fusion protein created by combining the Fab-fragment of the C242 monoclonal antibody and staphylococcal enterotoxin A.[119] In early clinical evaluation, several cytokines, including interleukin-2 and tumor necrosis factor, could be induced in human subjects following a single injection. Multiple injection trials have been initiated.

The newest arena into which immune therapy has crossed is that of gene therapy. Preclinical trials have been conducted in which in vivo injection of pancreas cancer cells transfected with interleukins-2 or -4, or with interleukin-2 and interferon gamma, resulted in measurable antitumor effects.[120,121] These and other similar trials hold promise for future clinical trials in pancreas cancer.

## Conclusions

There is reason for cautious optimism regarding the treatment of patients with metastatic pancreatic cancer. The improvement in survival and relief of tumor-related symptoms with gemcitabine was the first of what is hoped to be many additional advances in this disease. Encouraging results from preclinical and early-phase clinical trials have given rise to a number of phase III trials in which doublets consisting of gemcitabine plus cisplatin, oxaliplatin, 5-FU, irinotecan, rubitecan, or pemetrexed are being compared with single-agent gemcitabine in patients with advanced-stage pancreatic cancer. The results of these trials are expected over the next 3 years and will help to clarify whether any of these combination regimens can further improve survival or control cancer-related symptoms for patients with metastatic pancreatic cancer. At the same time, infusional administration of gemcitabine, which enhances the incorporation of gemcitabine-triphosphate into DNA, will undergo more extensive evaluation as a single agent and in combination with other drugs.

Insights into the processes of angiogenesis, invasion, and metastasis have rapidly been translated into therapeutic opportunities with the development of MMP and angiogenesis inhibitors.

Unfortunately, the results from phase III clinical trials have been disappointing and have failed to demonstrate any therapeutic advantage for this approach. The failure of these to have an impact on the clinical course of this disease underscores the need to develop more accurate preclinical models of *advanced* pancreatic cancer. Therapeutic advances using these molecularly targeted therapies may still be several years off.

Pancreatic cancer appears to be associated with the acquisition of a specific array and sequence of genetic mutations. Here, too, agents specifically targeted to inhibition of EGFR or Ras are undergoing clinical evaluation, often in combination with cytotoxic chemotherapy. Immunologically based therapies are encouraging, but are also at a similar early point in their clinical development.

Over the past few years, there has been a significant shift in our approach to treating patients with metastatic pancreatic cancer. Skepticism has given way to cautious optimism as new agents, drawn from a myriad of classes, become available for clinical evaluation. As a result, we have unprecedented opportunities to improve the outcome for patients with metastatic pancreatic cancer.

## References

1. Ries LAG, Kosary CAL, Hankey BF, Miller BA, Clegg L, Edwards BK (eds). SEER Cancer Statistics Review, 1973–1996. National Cancer Institute, Bethesda, MD, 1999.
2. Gambill EE. Pancreatic and ampullary carcinoma: diagnosis and prognosis in relationship to symptoms, physical findings, and elapse of time as observed in 255 patients. South Med J 63:1119–1122, 1970.
3. Kelsen DP, Portenoy RK, Thaler HT, et al. Pain and depression in patients with newly diagnosed pancreas cancer. J Clin Oncol 13:748–755, 1995.
4. Green AI, Austin CP. Psychopathology of pancreatic cancer. A psychobiologic probe. Psychosomatics 34:208–221, 1993.
5. Joffe RT, Rubinow DR, Denicoff KD, Maher M, Sindelar WF. Depression and carcinoma of the pancreas. Gen Hosp Psychiatry 8:241–245, 1986.
6. Borst P. Multidrug resistance: a solvable problem? Ann Oncol 10(Suppl 4):S162–S164, 1999.
7. Rothenberg ML, Abbruzzese JL, Moore M, Portenoy RK, Robertson JM, Wanebo HJ. A rationale for expanding the endpoints for clinical trials in advanced pancreatic cancer. Cancer 78:627–632, 1996.
8. Ahlgren JD. Chemotherapy for pancreatic carcinoma. Cancer 78:654–663, 1996.
9. Smith MC, Pendleton CD, Maher VE, Kelley MJ, Carbone DP, Berzofsky JA. Oncogenic mutations in *ras* create HLA-A2.1 binding peptides but affect their extracellular antigen processing. Int Immunol 9:1085–1093, 1997.
10. Gjertsen MK, Bakka A, Breivik J, et al. Ex vivo ras peptide vaccination in patients with advanced pancreatic cancer: results of a phase I/II study. Int J Cancer 65:450–453, 1996.
11. Wagener DJ, Verdonk HE, Dirix LY, et al. Phase II trial of CPT-11 in patients with advanced pancreatic cancer, an EORTC early clincial trials group study. Ann Oncol 6:129–132, 1995.
12. Sakata Y, Waklui A, Nakao I, et al. A late phase II study of irinotecan (CPT-11) in advanced pancreatic cancer [abstract]. Proc Am Soc Clin Oncol 12:211a, 1993.
13. Stevenson JP, Scher RM, Kosierowski R, et al. Phase II trial of topotecan as a 21-day continuous infusion in patients with advanced or metastatic adenocarcinoma of the pancreas. Eur J Cancer 34:1358–1362, 1998.
14. Ducreux M, Douillard JY, Pignon JP, et al. Efficacy of 5FU + cisplatin (FUP) compared to bolus 5FU (FU) in advanced pancreatic carcinoma (APC) [abstract]. Eur J Cancer 35:S137, 1999.
15. Berlin JD, Alberti DB, Arzoomanian RZ, et al. A phase I study of gemcitabine, 5-fluorouracil and leucovorin in patients with advanced, recurrent, and/or metastatic solid tumors. Invest New Drugs 16:325–330, 1998.
16. Oettle H, Pelzer U, Hochmuth K, et al. Phase II trial of gemcitabine (GEM) with 24-hour infusion of 5-fluorouracil (FU) and folinic acid (FA) in patients with advanced pancreatic cancer [abstract]. Proc Am Soc Clin Oncol 18:295a, 1999.

17. Ota K, Taguchi T, Kimura K. Report on nationwide pooled data and cohort investigation in UFT phase II study. Cancer Chemother Pharmacol 22:333–338, 1988.

18. Mani S, Kugler JW, Sciortino DF, et al. Phase II trial of uracil/tegafur (UFT) plus leucovorin in patients with advanced pancreatic carcinoma: a University of Chicago phase II consortium study. Ann Oncol 9:1035–1037, 1998.

19. Plunkett W, Huang P, Xu Y-Z, Heinemann V, Grunewald R, Gandhi V. Gemcitabine: metabolism, mechanism of action, and self-potentiation. Semin Oncol 22 (Suppl 11):3–10, 1995.

20. Casper ES, Green MR, Kelsen DP, Heelan RT, Brown TD, Flombaum CD, et al. Phase II trial of gemcitabine (2′2′-difluorodeoxycytidine) in patients with adenocarcinoma of the pancreas. Invest New Drugs 12:1229–1234, 1994.

21. Carmichael J, Fink U, Russell RCG, et al. Phase II study of gemcitabine in patients with advanced pancreatic cancer. Br J Cancer 73:101–105, 1996.

22. Rothenberg ML, Moore MJ, Cripps MC, et al. A phase II trial of gemcitabine in patients with 5-FU refractory pancreas cancer. Ann Oncol 7:347–353, 1996.

23. Touroutoglou N, Gravel D, Raber MN, Plunkett W, Abbruzzese JL. Clinical results of a pharmacodynamically based strategy for higher dosing of gemcitabine in patients with solid tumors. Ann Oncol 9:1003–1008, 1998.

24. Tempero M, Plunkett W, Ruiz van Haperen V, et al. Randomized phase II trial of dose intense gemcitabine by standard infusion vs. fixed dose rate in metastatic pancreatic adenocarcinoma [abstract]. Proc Am Soc Clin Oncol 18:273a, 1999.

25. Wils JA, Kok T, Wagener DJT, Selleslags J, Duez N. Activity of cisplatin in adenocarcinoma of the pancreas. Eur J Cancer 29A:203–204, 1993.

26. Tajiri H, Yoshimori M, Hijikata A, Nakamura K, Ohkura H, Okazaki N. Cis-diamminedichloroplatinum(II) chemotherapy in advanced pancreatic carcinoma. Gan to Kagaku Ryoho 14:3101–3104, 1987.

27. Bergman AM, Ruiz van Haperen VWT, Veerman G, et al. Synergistic interaction between cisplatin and gemcitabine in vitro. Clin Cancer Res 2:521–530, 1996.

28. Fukuda M, Nishio K, Kanzawa F, et al. Synergism between cisplatin and topoisomerase I inhibitors, NB-506 and SN-38, in human small cell lung cancer cells. Cancer 56:789–793, 1996.

29. Abbruzzese JL, Evans D, Gravel D, et al. Docetaxel, a potentially active agent for patients with pancreatic adenocarcinomas [abstract]. Proc Am Soc Clin Oncol 14:221a, 1995.

30. De Forni M, Rougier P, Adenis A, et al. Phase II study of Taxotere® (RP 56976, doxetaxel) in locally advanced and/or metastatic pancreatic cancer [abstract]. Ann Oncol 5 (Suppl 5):202, 1994.

31. Gebbia N, Gebbia V. Single-agent paclitaxel in the treatment of unresectable and/or metastatic pancreatic adenocarcinoma. Eur J Cancer 32A:1822–1823, 1996.

32. Whitehead RP, Jacobson J, Brown TD, et al. Phase II trial of paclitaxel and granulocyte colony–stimulating factor in patients with pancreatic carcinoma: a Southwest Oncology Group study. J Clin Oncol 15:2414–2419, 1997.

33. Stehlin JS, Giovanella BC, Natelson EA, et al. A study of 9-nitro-camptothecin (RFS-2000) in patients with advanced pancreatic cancer. Int J Oncol 14:821–831, 1999.

34. Smith FP, Hoth DF, Levin B, Smythe T, Ueno W, Schein PS. 5-fluorouracil, adriamycin, and mitomycin-C (FAM) chemotherapy for advanced adenocarcinoma of the pancreas. Cancer 46:2014–2018, 1980.

35. Wiggans RG, Woolley PV, Macdonald JS, et al. Phase II trial of streptozocin, mitomycin-C and 5-fluorouracil (SMF) in the treatment of advanced pancreas cancer. Cancer 41:387–391, 1978.

36. Mallinson CN, Rake MO, Cocking JB, et al. Chemotherapy in pancreatic cancer: results of a controlled, prospective, randomised, multicentre trial. BMJ 281:1589–1591, 1980.

37. Cullinan SA, Moertel CG, Fleming TR, et al. A comparison of three chemotherapeutic regimens in the treatment of advanced pancreatic and gastric carcinoma. JAMA 253:2061–2067, 1985.

38. Takada T, Kato H, Matsushiro T, Nimura Y, Nagakawa T, Nakayama T. Comparison of 5-fluorouracil, doxorubicin and mitomycin C with 5-fluorouracil alone in the treatment of pancreatic-biliary carcinomas. Oncology 51:396–400, 1994.

39. Cullinan S, Moertel CG, Wieand HS, et al. A phase III trial of the therapy of advanced pancreatic carcinoma: evaluations of the Mallinson regimen and combined 5-fluorouracil, doxorubicin and cisplatin. Cancer 65:2207–2212, 1990.

40. Oster MW, Gray R, Panasci L, Perry MC. Chemotherapy for advanced pancreatic cancer: a comparison of 5-fluorouracil, adriamycin and mitomycin (FAM) with 5-fluorouracil, streptozocin, and mitomycin (FSM). Cancer 57:29–33, 1986.

41. Palmer KR, Kerr M, Knowles G, Cull A, Carter DC, Leonard RC. Chemotherapy prolongs survival in inoperable pancreatic carcinoma. Br J Surg 81:882–885, 1994.

42. Glimelius B, Hoffman K, Sjoden PO, et al. Chemotherapy improves survival and quality of life in advanced pancreatic and biliary cancer. Ann Oncol 7:593–600, 1996.

43. Burris HA 3rd, Moore MJ, Andersen J, et al. Improvements in survival and clinical benefit with gemcitabine as first-line therapy for patients with advanced pancreas cancer: a randomized trial. J Clin Oncol 15:2403–2413, 1997.

44. Storniolo AM, Enas NH, Brown CA, Voi M, Rothenberg ML, Schilsky R. An investigational new drug treatment program for patients with gemcitabine: results for over 3000 patients with pancreatic carcinoma. Cancer 85:1261–1268, 1999.

45. Ren Q, Kao V, Grem JL. Cytotoxicity and DNA fragmentation associated with sequential gemcitabine and 5-fluoro-2′-deoxyuridine in HT-29 colon cancer cells. Clin Cancer Res 4(11):2811–2818, 1998.

46. Schulz L, Schalhorn A, Wilmanns W, Heinemann V. Synergistic interaction of gemcitabine and 5-fluorouracil in colon cancer cells [abstract]. Proc Am Soc Clin Oncol 17:251a, 1998.

47. Cascinu S, Silva RR, Barni S, et al. A combination of gemcitabine and 5-fluorouracil in advanced pancreatic cancer: a report from the Italian Group for the Study of Digestive Tract Cancer (GISCAD). Br J Cancer 80:1595–1598, 1999.

48. Jovtis S, Marantz A, Almira E, et al. Phase II trial of gemcitabine (GEM), 5-fluorouracil (5-FU) and leucovorin (LV) in advanced pancreatic cancer [abstract]. Eur J Cancer 35:S157, 1999.

49. Philip PA, Zalupski M, Vaitkevicius VK, et al. Phase II study of gemcitabine and cisplatin in advanced or metastatic pancreatic cancer [abstract]. Proc Am Soc Clin Oncol 18:274a, 1999.

50. Berlin JD, Adak S, Vaughn DJ, et al. A phase II study of gemcitabine and 5-fluorouracil in metastatic pancreatic cancer: an Eastern Cooperative Oncology Group study (E3296). Oncology 58:215–218, 2000.

51. Berlin J, Catalano, Thomas J, et al. A phase III study of gemcitabine in combination with 5-FU vs. gemcitabine alone in patients with advanced pancreatic carcinoma (E2297): an Eastern Cooperative Oncology Group trial [abstract]. Proc Am Soc Clin Oncol 20:127a, 2001.

52. Scheithauer W, Schüll, Ulrich-Pur H, et al. Gemcitabine alone or in combination with capecitabine in patients with advanced pancreatic adenocarcinoma [abstract]. Proc Am Soc Clin Oncol 21:126a, 2002.

53. Peters GJ, Bergman AM, Ruiz van Haperen VWT, Veerman G, Kuiper CM, Braakhuis BJM: Interaction between cisplatin and gemcitabine in vitro and in vivo. Semin Oncol 22 (Suppl 11):72–79, 1995.

54. Heinemann V, Wilke H, Possinger K, et al. Gemcitabine and cisplatin in the treatment of advanced and metastatic pancreatic cancer: the final results of a phase II study [abstract]. Proc Am Soc Clin Oncol 18:274a, 1999.

55. Colucci G, Riccardi F, Giuliani F, et al. Randomized trial of gemcitabine alone or with cisplatin in the treatment of advanced pancreatic cancer: a phase II multicenter study of the Southern Italian Oncology Group [abstract]. Proc Am Soc Clin Oncol 18:250a, 1999.

56. Klapdor R, Martin-Svendsen J, Seutter R, Fenner C. Combination therapy with oxaliplatin + gemcitabine in advanced pancreatic cancer [abstract]. Eur J Cancer 35:S146, 1999.

57. Louvet C, André T, Lledo G, et al. Gemcitabine–oxaliplatin combination in advanced pancreatic carcinoma: a GERCOR multicenter phase II study [abstract]. Proc Am Soc Clin Oncol 20:127a, 2001.

58. Alberts S, Townley P, Cha SS, et al. Oxaliplatin and gemcitabine for patients with pancreatic adenocarcinoma: a North Central Cancer Treatment Group phase II study [abstract]. Proc Am Soc Clin Oncol 21:126a, 2002.

59. Androulakis N, Stathopoulos G, Tsavaris N, et al. First-line treatment with docetaxel and gemcitabine in patients with inoperable pancreatic cancer: a multicenter phase II study [abstract]. Eur J Cancer 35:S142–S143, 1999.

60. Jacobs AD, Otero H, Picozzi V, et al. Gemcitabine and Taxotere in patients with unresectable pancreatic carcinoma [abstract]. Proc Am Soc Clin Oncol 18:288a, 1999.

61. Rocha Lima CMS, Savarese D, Bruckner H, et al. Irinotecan plus gemcitabine induces both radiographic and CA 19-9 tumor marker responses in patients with previously untreated advanced pancreatic cancer. J Clin Oncol 20:1182–1191, 2002.

62. Kindler HL, Dugan W, Hochster H, et al. Clinical outcome in patients with advanced pancreatic cancer treated with pemetrexed/gemcitabine [abstract]. Proc Am Soc Clin Oncol 21;125a, 2002.

63. Greenway B, Iqbal MJ, Johnson PJ, Williams R. Oestrogen receptor proteins in malignant and fetal pancreas. BMJ 283:751–753, 1981.

64. Andrén-Sandberg A, Hoem D, Bäckman P. Other risk factors for pancreatic cancer: hormonal aspects. Ann Oncol 10 (Suppl 4):S131–S135, 1999.

65. Iqbal MJ, Greenway B, Wilkinson ML, Johnson PJ, Williams R. Sex-steroid enzymes aromatase and 5-alpha-reductase in the pancreas: a comparison of normal adult, foetal and malignant tissue. Clin Sci 65: 71–75, 1983.

66. Theve NO, Pousette A, Carlstrom K. Adenocarcinoma of the pancreas—a hormone sensitive tumor? A preliminary report on Nolvadex treatment. Clin Oncol 9:193–198, 1983.

67. Tønnenson K, Kamp-Jensen M. Antiestrogen therapy in pancreatic carcinoma: a preliminary report. Eur J Surg Oncol 12:69–70, 1981.

68. Wong A, Chan A. Survival benefit of tamoxifen therapy in adenocarcinoma of pancreas: a case–control study. Cancer 71:2200–2203, 1993.

69. Keating JJ, Johnson PJ, Cochrane AM, et al. A prospective randomised controlled trial of tamoxifen and cyproterone acetate in pancreatic carcinoma. Br J Cancer 60:798–792, 1989.

70. Bakkevold KE, Pettersen A, Arnesjø B, Espehaug B. Tamoxifen therapy in unresectable adenocarcinoma of the pancreas and the papilla of Vater. Br J Surg 77:725–730, 1990.

71. Taylor OM, Benson E, McMahon MJ, Yorkshire Gastrointestinal Group: clinical trial with tamoxifen in patients with irresectable pancreatic adenocarcinoma. Br J Surg 80:384–386, 1993.

72. Corbishley TP, Iqbal MJ, Wilkinson ML, Williams R. Androgen receptors in human normal and malignant pancreatic tissue and cell lines. Cancer 57:1992–1995, 1986.

73. Sharma JJ, Razvillas B, Stephens CD, Hilsenbeck SG, Sharma A, Rothenberg ML. Phase II study of flutamide as second-line chemotherapy in patients with advanced pancreatic cancer. Invest New Drugs 15:361–364, 1997.

74. Greenway BA. Effect of flutamide on survival in patients with pancreatic cancer: results of a prospective, randomised, double-blind, placebo-controlled trial. BMJ 16:1935–1938, 1998.

75. Hidalgo M, Castellano D, Paz-Ares L, et al. Phase I–II study of gemcitabine and fluorouracil as continuous infusion in patients with pancreatic cancer. J Clin Oncol 17:585–592, 1999.

76. Reubi JC, Horisberger U, Essed CE, Jeekel J, Klijn JG, Lamberts SW. Absence of somatostatin receptors in human exocrine pancreatic adenocarcinomas. Gastroenterology 95:760–763, 1988.

77. Buscail L, Saint-Laurent N, Chastre E, et al. Loss of SST2 somatostatin receptor gene expression in human pancreatic and colorectal cancer. Cancer Res 56:1823–1827, 1996.

78. Raderer M, Hamilton G, Kurtaran A, et al. Treatment of advanced pancreatic cancer with the long-acting somatostatin analogue lanreotide: in vitro and in vivo results. Br J Cancer 79:535–537, 1999.

79. Weckbecker G, Tolcsvai L, Liu R, Bruns C. Preclinical studies on the antitumor activity of the somatostatin analogue octreotide (SMS 201-995). Metabolism 41 (Suppl 2):99–103, 1992.

80. Friess H, Büchler M, Beglinger C, et al. Low-dose octreotide is not effective in patients with advanced pancreatic cancer. Pancreas 8:540–545, 1993.

81. Klijn JGM, Hoff AM, Planting AST, et al. Treatment of patients with metastatic pancreatic and gastrointestinal tumors with the somatostatin analogue Sandostatin: a phase II study including endocrine effects. Br J Cancer 62:627–630, 1990.

82. Burch PA, Block M, Schroeder G, et al. Phase III evaluation of octreotide versus chemotherapy with 5-fluorouracil or 5-fluorouracil plus leucovorin in advanced exocrine pancreatic cancer: a North Central Cancer Treatment Group study. Clin Cancer Res 6:3486–3492, 2000.

83. Ebert M, Friess H, Berger HG, Büchler MW. Role of octreotide in the treatment of pancreatic cancer. Digestion 55 (Suppl 1):48–51, 1994.

84. Nelson AR, Fingleton B, Rothenberg ML, Matrisian LM. Matrix metalloproteinases: biologic activity and clinical implications. J Clin Oncol 18:1135–1149, 2000.

85. Rosemurgy A, Harris J, Langleben A, Casper E, Goode S, Rasmussen H. Marimastat in patients with advanced pancreatic cancer: a dose-finding study. Am J Clin Oncol 22:247–252, 1999.

86. Bramhall SR, Rosemurgy A, Brown PD, et al. Marimastat as first-line therapy for patients with unresectable pancreatic cancer: a randomized trial. J Clin Oncol 15:3447–3455, 2001.

87. Carmichael J, Ledermann JA, Woll PJ, et al. Phase IB study of concurrent administration of Marimastat and gemcitabine in non-resectable pancreatic cancer [abstract]. Proc Am Soc Clin Oncol 17:232a, 1998.

88. Moore MJ, Hamm J, Eisenberg P, et al. A comparison between gemcitabine and the matrix metalloproteinase inhibitor BAY 12-9566 in patients with advanced pancreatic cancer [abstract]. Proc Am Soc Clin Oncol 19:240a, 2000.

89. Patterson BC, Sang QXA. Angiostatin-converting enzyme activities of human matrilysin (MMP-7) and gelatinase B/Type IV collagenase (MMP-9). J Biol Chem 272:28823–28825, 1997.

90. O'Reilly MS, Wiederschain D, Stetler-Stevenson, WG, et al. Regulation of angiostatin production by matrix metalloproteinase-2 in a model of concomitant resistance. J Biol Chem 274:29568–29571, 1999.

91. Wen W, Moses MA, Wiederschain D, et al. The generation of Endostatin is mediated by elastase. Cancer Res 59:6052–6056, 1999.

92. Campbell SL, Khosravi-Far R, Rossman KL, Clark CJ, Der CJ. Increasing complexity of Ras signaling. Oncogene 17:1395–1413, 1998.

93. Hudes GR, Schol J, Baab J, et al. Phase I clinical and pharmacokinetic trial of the farnesyltransferase inhibitor R115777 on a 21-day dosing schedule [abstract]. Proc Am Soc Clin Oncol 18:156a, 1999.

94. Eskens F, Awada , Verweij J, et al. Phase I and pharmacologic study of continuous daily oral SCH 66336, a novel farnesyl transferase inhibitor, in patients with solid tumors. Proc Am Soc Clin Oncol 18:156a, 1999.

95. Cohen SJ, Ho L, Ranganathan S, et al. Phase II and pharmacodynamic trial of the farnesyltransferase inhibitor R115777 as initial therapy in patients with metastatic pancreatic adenocarcinoma. Proc Am Soc Clin Oncol 21:137a, 2002.

96. Macdonald JS, Chansky K, Whitehead R, et al. A phase II study of farnesyl trasferase inhibitor R115777 in pancreatic cancer: a Southwest Oncology Group (SWOG) study [abstract]. Proc Am Soc Clin Oncol 21:138a, 2002.

97. van Cutsem E, Karasek P, Oettle H, et al. Phase III trial comparing gemcitabine + R115777 (Zarnestra) versus gemcitabine + placebo in advanced pancreatic cancer (PC) [abstract]. Proc Am Soc Clin Oncol 21:130a, 2002.

98. Lebowitz PF, Prendergast GC. Non-Ras targets of farnesyltransferase inhibitors: focus on Rho. Oncogene 17:1439–1445, 1998.

99. Crowell PL, Chang RR, Ren Z, Elson CE, Gould MN. Selective inhibition of isoprenylation of 21–26 kDa proteins by the anticarcinogen d-limonene and its metabolites. J Biol Chem 266:17679–17685, 1991.

100. Ariazi EZ, Gould MN. Identifying differential gene expression in monoterpene-treated mammary carcinomas using subtractive display. J Biol Chem 271:29286–29294, 1996.

100a. Bailey HH, Levy D, Harris LS, et al. A phase II trial of daily perillyl alcohol in patients with advanced ovarian cancer: Eastern Cooperative Oncology Group Study E2E96. Gynecol Oncol 85:464–468, 2002.

101. Abbruzzese JL, Rosenberg A, Xiong Q, et al. Phase II study of anti-epidermal growth factor receptor antibody cetuximab in combination with gemcitabine in patients with advanced pancreatic cancer [abstract]. Proc Am Soc Clin Oncol 20:130a, 2001.

102. Shimoyama S, Gansauge F, Gansauge S, Oohara T, Kaminishi M, Beger HG. Increased angiogenin expression in pancreatic cancer is related to cancer aggressiveness. Cancer Res 56:2703–2706, 1996.

103. Shishido T, Yasoshima T, Denno R, Mukaiya M, Sato N, Hirata K. Inhibition of liver metastasis of human pancreatic carcinoma by angiogenesis inhibitor TNP-470 in combination with cisplatin. Jpn J Cancer Res 89:963–969, 1998.

104. Toma S, Monteghirfo S, Tasso P, et al. Antiproliferative and synergistic effect of interferon alpha-2a retinoids and their association in established human cancer cell lines. Cancer Lett 82:209–216, 1994.

105. Moore DF Jr, Pazdur R, Sugarman S, et al. Pilot phase II trial of 13-cis-retinoic acid and interferon-α combination therapy for advanced pancreatic adenocarcinoma. Am J Clin Oncol 18:525–527, 1995.

106. Recchia F, Sica G, Casucci D, Rea S, Gulino A, Frati L. Advanced carcinoma of the pancreas: phase II study of combined chemotherapy, β-interferon, and retinoids. Am J Clin Oncol 21:275–278, 1998.

107. John WJ, Flett MQ. Continuous infusion of 5-fluorouracil and interferon-α in pancreatic carcinoma. Am J Clin Oncol 21:147–150, 1998.

108. Sparano JA, Lipsitz S, Wadler S, et al. Phase II trial of prolonged continuous infusion of 5-fluorouracil and interferon-α in patients with advanced pancreatic cancer: Eastern Cooperative Oncology Group protocol 3292. Am J Clin Oncol 19:546–551, 1996.

109. Sparano JA, Fisher RI, Weiss GR, et al. Phase II trials of high-dose interleukin-2 and lymphokine-activated killer cells in advanced breast

carcinoma and carcinoma of the lung, ovary, pancreas and other tumors. J Immunother 16:216–223, 1994.

110. Tempero MA, Haga Y, Sivinski C, Steplewski Z, Kay HD, Pour P. Immunotherapy with monoclonal antibody (Mab) in pancreatic adenocarcinoma. Int J Pancreatol 9:125–134, 1991.

111. Tempero MA, Sivinski C, Steplewski Z, Harvey E, Klassen L, Kay HD. Phase II trial of interferon gamma and monoclonal antibody 17-1A in pancreatic cancer: biologic and clinical effects. J Clin Oncol 8:2019–2026, 1990.

112. Dugan MC, Dergham ST, Kucway R, et al. HER-2/neu expression in pancreatic adenocarcinoma: relation to tumor differential and survival. Pancreas 14:229–236, 1997.

113. Yamanaka Y, Friess H, Kobrin MS, et al. Overexpression of *HER2/neu* oncogene in human pancreatic carcinoma. Hum Pathol 24:1127–1134, 1993.

114. Shak S. Overview of the trastuzumab (Herceptin) anti-HER2 monoclonal antibody clinical program in HER2-overexpressing metastatic breast cancer. Semin Oncol 26 (Suppl 12):71–77, 1999.

115. Laheru DA, Jaffee EM. Potential role of tumor vaccines in GI malignancies. Oncology 14:245–255, 2000.

116. Jaffee EM, Hruban RH, Biedrzycki B, et al. Novel allogeneic granulocyte-macrophage colony-stimulating factor-secreting tumor vaccine for pancreatic cancer: a phase I trial of safety and immune activation. J Clin Oncol 19:145–156, 2001.

117. Gjertsen MK, Saeterdal I, Thorsby E, Gaudernack G. Characterisation of immune responses in pancreatic carcinoma patients after mutant p21 ras peptide vaccination. Br J Cancer 74:1828–1833, 1998.

118. McCarty TM, Liu X, Sun J-Y, Peralta EA, Diamond DJ, Ellenhorn JD. Targeting p53 for adoptive T-cell immunotherapy. Cancer Res 58:2601–2605, 1998.

119. Giantonio BJ, Alpaugh RK, Schultz J, et al. Superantigen-based immunotherapy: a phase I trial of PNU-214565, a monoclonal antibody–staphylococcal enterotoxin A recombinant fusion protein, in advanced pancreatic and colorectal cancer. J Clin Oncol 15:1994–2007, 1997.

120. Kimura M, Yoshida Y, Narita M, et al. Acquired immunity in nude mice induced by expression of the IL-2 or IL-4 gene in human pancreatic cells and antitumor effect generated by in vivo gene transfer using retrovirus. Int J Cancer 82:549–555, 1999.

121. Clary BM, Coveney EC, Blazer DG III, Philip R, Lyerly HK. Active immunotherapy of pancreatic cancer with tumor cells genetically engineered to secrete multiple cytokines. Surgery 120:174–181, 1996.

122. DeCaprio JA, Mayer RJ, Gonin R, Arbuck SG. Fluorouracil and high-dose leucovorin in previously untreated with advanced adenocarcinoma of the pancreas: results of a phase II trial. J Clin Oncol 9:2128–2133, 1991.

123. Weinerman BH, MacCormick RE. A phase II survival comparison of patients with adenocarcinoma of the pancreas treated with 5-fluorouracil and calcium leucovorin versus a matched tumor registry control population. Am J Clin Oncol 17:467–469, 1994.

124. Rubin J, Gallagher JG, Schroeder G, et al. Phase II trials of 5-fluorouracil and leucovorin in patients with metastatic gastric or pancreatic carcinoma. Cancer 78:1888–1891, 1996.

125. Louvet C, Hammel P, Andre T, et al. Multicenter phase II study in advanced pancreatic adenocarcinoma patients with a combination of leucovorin, 5FU bolus and infusion, and gemcitabine (FOLFUGEM Regimen) [abstract]. Proc Am Soc Clin Oncol 18:275a, 1999.

126. Bernhard H, Jager-Arand E, Bernhard G, et al. Treatment of advanced pancreatic cancer with 5-fluorouracil, folinic acid and interferon alpha-2A: the results of a phase II trial. Br J Cancer 71:102–105, 1995.

127. Rosvold E, Schilder R, Walczak J, et al. Phase II trial of PALA in combination with 5-fluorouracil in advanced pancreatic cancer. Cancer Chemother Pharmacol 29:305–308, 1992.

128. Okada S, Sakata Y, Matsuno S, et al. Phase II study of docetaxel in patients with metastatic pancreatic cancer: a Japanese cooperative study. Br J Cancer 80:438–443, 1999.

129. Pederzoli P, Maurer U, Vollmer K, et al. Phase III trial of SMS 201-995 in stage II, III, and IV pancreatic cancer [abstract]. Proc Am Soc Clin Oncol 17:257a, 1998.

130. D'Adamo D, Hammond L, Donehower R, et al. Final results of a phase II study of DX-8951f in advanced pancreatic cancer. Proc Am Soc Clin Oncol 20:134a, 2001.

131. Feliu J, Vincent M, Dorta J, et al. Phase II trial of gemcitabine-UFT-leucovorin (ILV) in advanced carcinoma of the pancreas: preliminary results [abstract]. Eur J Cancer 35:S156–S157, 1999.

132. Roy A, Jacobs A, Bukowski R, et al. Phase III trial of SMS 201–995 pa LAR and continuous infusion 5FU in unresectable stage II, III, and IV pancreatic cancer [abstract]. Proc Am Soc Clin Oncol 17:257a, 1998.

133. Canobbio L, Boccardo F, Cannata D, et al. Treatment of advanced pancreatic carcinoma with the somatostatin analogue BIM 23014. Preliminary results of a pilot study. Cancer 69:648–650, 1992.

# Section 4

# Cancer of the Bile Ducts
# and Gallbladder

# Chapter 35

# Epidemiology, Molecular Epidemiology, and Biomarkers of Biliary Tract Cancers

ROGER D. SOLOWAY AND RAYBURN REGO

Malignant tumors of the biliary tract are rare, accounting for less than 2% of all malignant neoplasms in the United States. Knowledge concerning the etiology of these cancers has come from clinical observations, animal experiments, autopsy series, and descriptive epidemiologic studies. The exact pathogenesis of these tumors, however, still needs to be established, and more sensitive and specific markers need to be developed to screen for these uncommon tumors.

## Demographics

### Gallbladder Cancer

#### United States

In the United States, gallbladder cancer is the sixth most common gastrointestinal malignancy.[1] Women are affected approximately three times more often than men. Gallstones are present in 70% to 90% of patients with gallbladder cancer. The risk of developing gallbladder cancer rises sharply for both men and women after the sixth decade (Fig. 35–1).[1] The outlook for the vast majority of patients with gallbladder cancer is grim. Most large studies of gallbladder cancer have demonstrated overall 5-year survival rates of only 5% to 10%. About 40% of the cancers are diagnosed at stages III and IV,[2] and 90% of these are adenocarcinomas (see Table 35–1 for staging of gallbladder cancer). In the United States, mortality data have revealed higher rates of gallbladder cancer in the Southwest, the Appalachian region, the Midwest, and the upper North Central states and lower rates in the Southeast.[3] The reason for this pattern is not clear, although the higher rates in the Southwest may reflect the higher concentration of American Indians. In the United States, the risk of developing gallbladder cancer is high among American Indians,

Hispanics with an admixture of American Indian genes, and Japanese who have emigrated to the United States, and low among blacks and whites (Fig. 35–2).[3] In the United States, the incidence and mortality rates have been falling steadily since 1970. The downward trends appear related, at least in part, to increasing numbers of cholecystectomies performed annually for gallbladder disease in the United States.[4]

#### Worldwide

The rates for gallbladder cancer are highest in Poland, Hungary, and Czechoslovakia in Eastern Europe; in Chile, Peru, Equador, Colombia, and Costa Rica in Latin American; and in Japan in Asia. Rates are low in the United Kingdom, Spain, France, East Africa, India, New Zealand, Australia, Cuba, and Puerto Rico (Fig. 35–3). Gallbladder cancer is the fourth leading cause of all cancer deaths in Chile; the mortality from gallbladder cancer there (5.2%) is the highest in the world.[5,6] Although most of the Chilean population is Caucasoid, there is an important mixture with Areucanian Indians who inhabited central and southern Chile when the Spaniards arrived there four centuries ago.

Despite the decreasing incidence of gallbladder cancer in countries such as the United States, Czechoslavakia, and Sweden, a rise in both gallbladder and bile duct cancer incidence was noted in Shanghai, China, from 1972 to 1994.[7] The reasons for this trend are unclear but may reflect improvements in disease diagnosis and classification.

### Bile Duct Cancers

In the United States, the incidence of gallbladder cancer has interesting geographic and racial variations; in contrast, there is no significant regional difference in the incidence of extrahepatic bile duct cancers. In a review by Sako in 1957,[8] 570 extra-

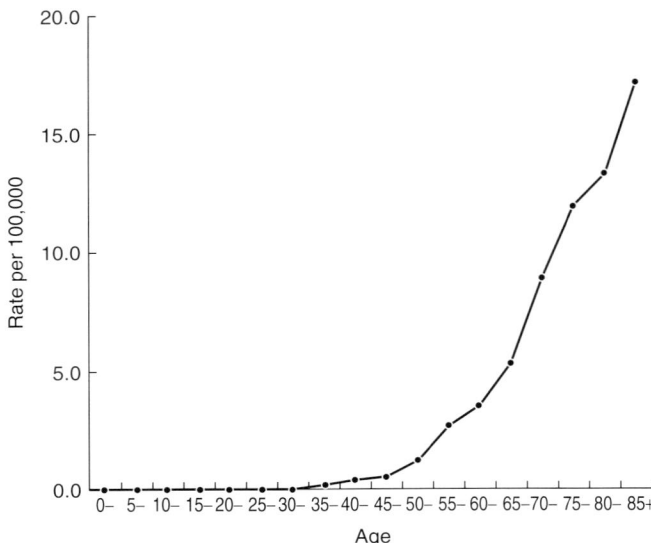

**Figure 35-1** Age-related incidence of gallbladder cancer in women. Note the steep rise in the incidence of gallbladder cancer among women after the age of 60. (From Parkin DM, Whelan SL, Ferlay U, Raymond L, Young J (eds). Cancer Incidence in the Five Continents, Vol. VII [IARC Scientific Publications No. 143]. IARC, Lyon, 1997.)

hepatic cholangiocarcinomas were found in 12 autopsy series (129,571 autopsies) performed in North America, South America, Europe, and Japan during the first half of the twentieth century. The incidence varied from 0.012% to 0.458% among those series. Patient ages ranged from 20 to 89 years, with an average of 59.3 years for men and 56.7 years for women. This retrospective study did not include series from Africa, where the incidence of cholangiocarcinomas is low or from China, where the incidence is high. Unlike gallbladder cancer, which is more common in women, extrahepatic duct cancers are slightly more common in men and occur a median of 10 years earlier than in women. Intrahepatic bile duct cancers are rare in the United States and Europe but are more common in China and Southeast Asia, where the incidence of liver fluke infection and hepatolithiasis is high.

In Taiwan, the incidence of hepatolithiasis during the 1970s and early 1980s ranged from 31% to 52% in all patients undergoing surgery for gallstones.[9-12] More recent reports have shown a decrease in the incidence to about 20%.[13] In Japan, the incidence of hepatolithiasis varies considerably depending on the area surveyed, with the highest incidence of 8.9% found in the Kyushu area.[14] In general, the incidence of hepatolithiasis in Japan varies from 3% to 6%.[15] The incidence of hepatolithiasis in the People's Republic of China also varies according to region.[16] The disease is prevalent in the Pearl River Delta.[17] In Chungking, the incidence is 38%; in Beijing it is 45%.[18] The reported incidence of cholangiocarcinoma in patients with intra-

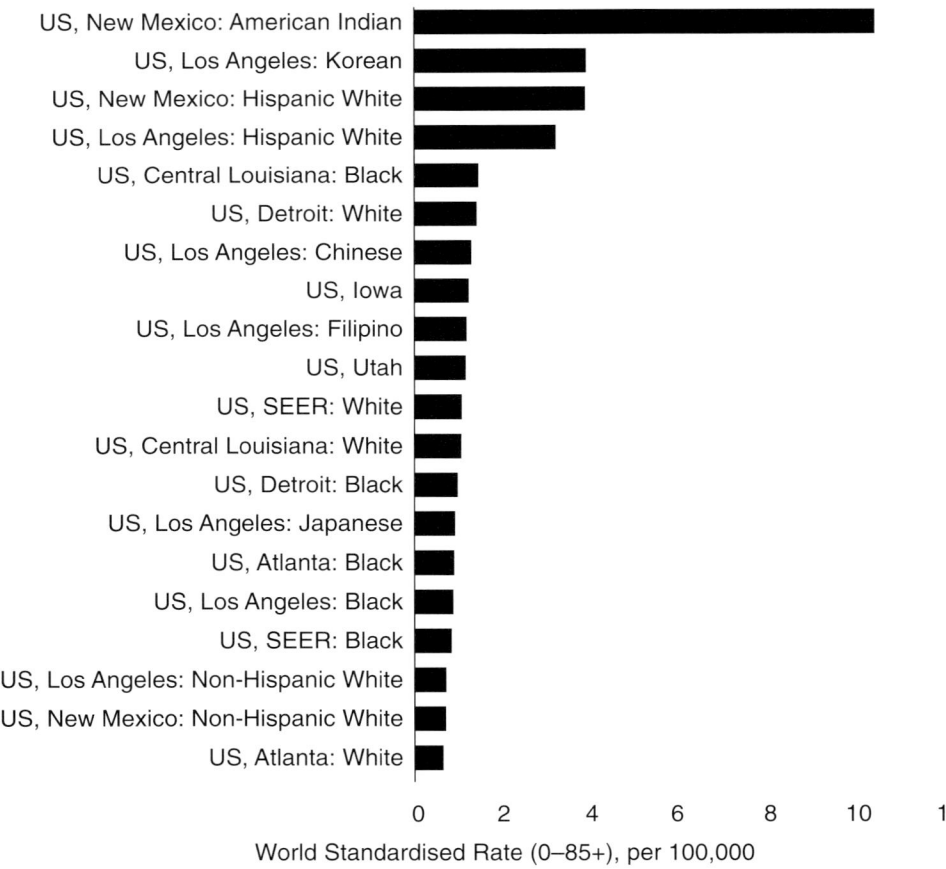

**Figure 35-2** World standardized rates of gallbladder cancer among different ethnic groups in different regions of the United States. Note the highest incidence among American Indians in New Mexico and the low incidences in white and black populations of the United States. (From Parkin DM, Whelan SL, Ferlay U, Raymond L, Young J (eds). Cancer Incidence in the Five Continents, Vol. VII [IARC Scientific Publications No. 143]. IARC, Lyon, 1997.)

**Table 35-1** Staging of gallbladder carcinoma (Nevin's Criteria)

| Stage | Description |
| --- | --- |
| Stage I | Mucosal involvement only |
| Stage II | Extension to muscularis |
| Stage III | Extension to serosa |
| Stage IV | Involvement of regional nodes |
| Stage V | Involvement of liver or other organs |

From Nevin JE, Moran TJ, Kay S, King R, Carcinoma of the gallbadder: staging, treatment, and prognosis. Cancer 37:141–148, 1976.

hepatic duct stones is 1.5% to 9.4% in Japan[19] and 2.4% to 5% in Taiwan.[20-24] Aside from East Asia, increased incidence of intrahepatic duct stones has been reported in Malaysia (10%)[25] and in Colombia (7%).[26]

In the Far East, liver fluke infection due to *Opisthorchis viverrini* or *Clonarchis sinensis* is the most frequently cited cause of cholangiocarcinoma. In Thailand, the proportional incidence rate of cholangiocarcinoma is highest in the Northeast region, where the prevalence of infection with *O. viverrini* is also the highest (Figs. 35–4, 35–5, 35–6). Approximately 34% of the rural Northeast Thai population, or roughly 7 million people, are infected with *O. viverrini*. A formal analysis across five regions of the country showed a strong correlation between the proportional incidence of choangiocarcinoma and the estimated average titers

of antibodies to *O. viverrini* and, to a less degree, fecal egg count.[27-29]

Liver cancer mortality in Korea is the highest in the world.[30] Cholangiocarcinoma accounts for more than 20% of liver cancers in the Pusan area. Two case–control studies of the relationship between *C. sinensis* infection and cholangiocarcinoma have been carried out in the Republic of Korea. Both have shown increased estimated relative risks (6.5 and 6.0).[30] In another case–control study in Hong Kong, the estimated relative risk was 3.1.[30] The incidence of liver cancer was observed to be correlated with the prevalence of infection with *O. felineus* across four areas in the T'umen region of Northwest Siberia.[30] Cases of both cholangiocarcinoma and hepatocellular carcinoma have been reported in people infected with *O. felineus*.

## Risk Factors

### Cholelithiasis

Cholelithiasis is found in about 10% of men and 20% of women in the United States.[31] Many clinical studies have documented a strong association between gallstones and gallbladder cancer, with gallstones being present in 70% to 98% of cancer cases.[32-37] The association with extrahepatic biliary carcinoma is much weaker, on the order of about 30%.[8,38,39] The incidence of gallbladder cancer and gallstones shares demographic characteristics, including female preponderance, racial and ethnic suscepti-

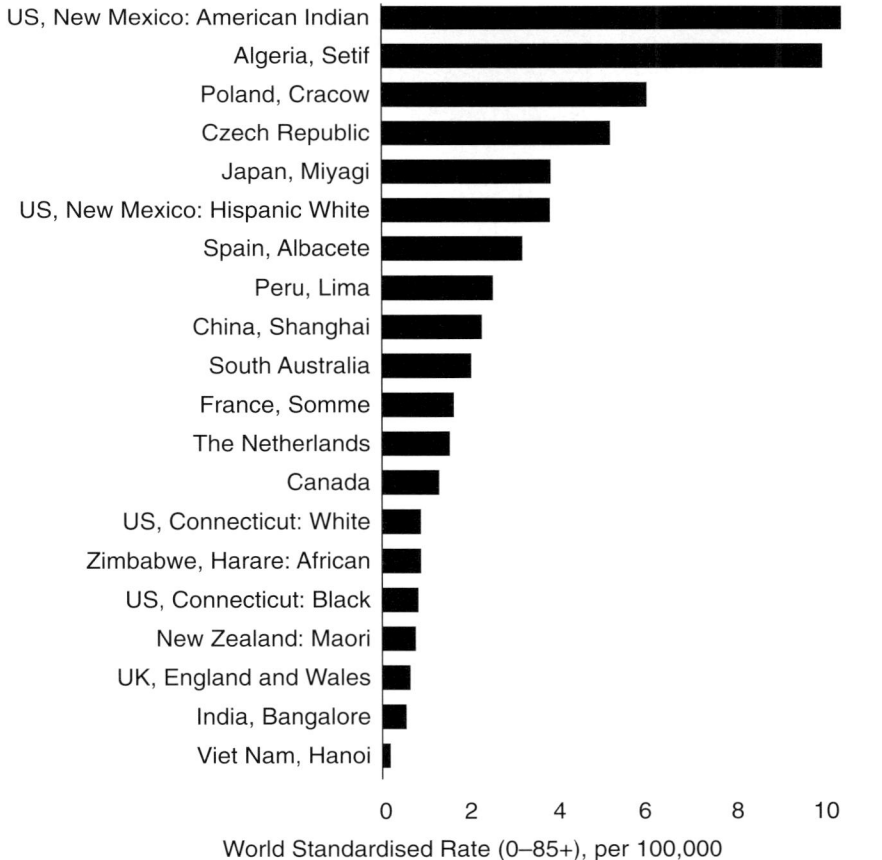

**Figure 35–3** World standardized rates of gallbladder cancer in females. Note the high incidence in New Mexico among American Indians and in Poland, Japan and Lima, Peru. High incidence is also noted in Chile but not shown in this graph. (From Parkin DM, Whelan SL, Ferlay U, Raymond L, Young J (eds). Cancer Incidence in the Five Continents, Vol. VII [IARC Scientific Publications No. 143]. IARC, Lyon, 1997.)

bility, and geographic variation even in the United States. High mortality rates are noted in parts of the Southwest, Midwest, and Appalachia.[4]

The risk for developing gallbladder cancer is increased three-fold in patients with cholelithiasis.[40,41] However, because the actual incidence of gallbladder cancer in patients with asymptomatic cholelithiasis is low, prophylactic gallbladder removal or gallstone dissolution is neither recommended nor cost-effective.[42–44] Older studies reported that cancer was found incidentally in 1% to 2% of cholecystectomies performed for cholelithiasis.[45,46] Autopsy series, by contrast, have shown an incidence of gallbladder cancer of 0.5%.[47–49] Gallstone size is another risk factor for gallbladder cancer. Two studies have revealed a 9- to 10-fold greater risk in subjects with large stones (>3 cm) than that in subjects with small stones (<1 cm). The high risk of gallbladder cancer associated with large stones may be explained by the longer exposure to stones in these patients.[49,50] Identification of a cause of gallstones being associated with gallbladder cancer is more difficult. Chronic trauma and inflammation of the gallbladder mucosa caused by stones might result in epithelial dysplasia and progression to cancer. However, only a small fraction of patients with cholelithiasis later develop cancer, and approximately 20% of patients with gallbladder cancer have no history or evidence of gallstones.

### Liver Flukes

The liver flukes *O. viverrini*, *O. filineus*, and *C. sinensis* are biologically similar foodborne trematodes that chronically infect the bile ducts. Nine million people throughout the world are infected with *O. viverrini*. The fluke is common in Northeast Thailand, where at least one-third of the population is infected. Infection is acquired by eating raw or undercooked freshwater fish containing the metacercaria of flukes. Immature flukes migrate up through the ampulla of Vater into the biliary tree, mature in the small intrahepatic ducts, and produce eggs that are passed in the feces. It has long been recognized that infection with liver flukes is closely associated with cholangiocarcinoma. Studies in experimental animals clearly show that prolonged infection produces a series of epithelial changes in the bile ducts. Epithelial desquamation is followed by regeneration, adenomatous epithelial hyperplasia, ductal fibrosis, and adenomatous hyperplasia which progresses to bile duct cancer in a small proportion of animals.[51] A fermented fish product called *Pla ra* (popular among Northeastern Thais) and other preserved foodstuffs such as dried fish, shrimp, sausage, and cured pork contain high levels of nitrosamines. In several studies, hamsters infected with *O. viverrini* or *C. sinensis* and treated with dimethylnitrosamine developed cholangiocarcinomas, although the hamsters that received either the fluke or the nitrosamine did not develop cancer.[52] It is postulated that the carcinomas arose in these animals because the dimetheylnitrosamine exerted a carcinogenic effect on the altered proliferating epithelial cells of the bile ducts that had been stimulated by the parasite. Therefore, factors other than infection, i.e., nutrition (e.g., nitrosamines, low-protein diet), genetics, environment, and immunology play important roles in the development of cholangiocarcinoma.

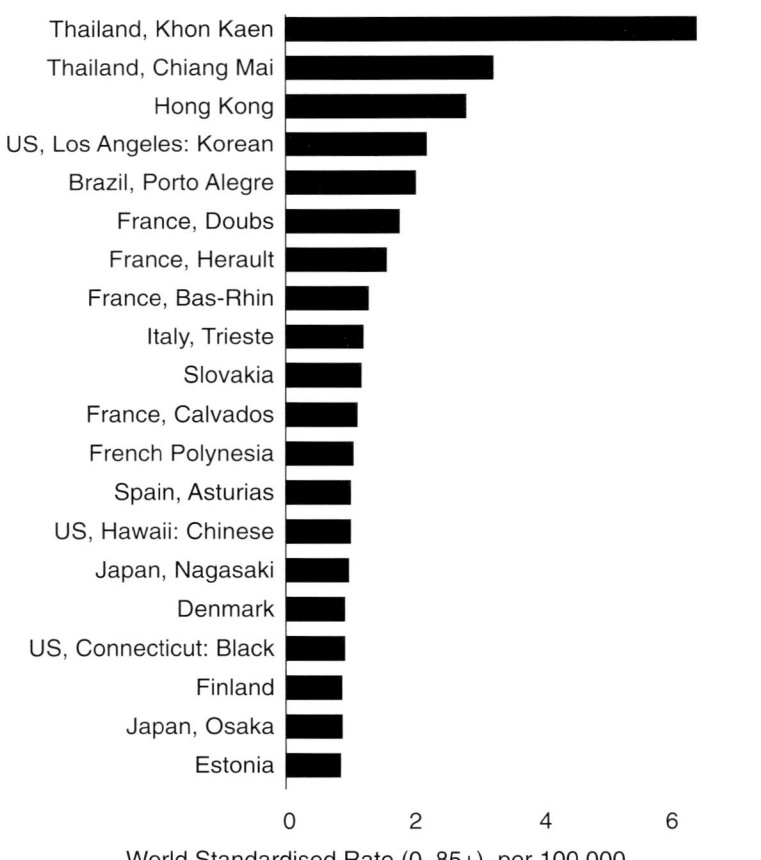

**Figure 35–4** World standardized rates of cholangiocarcinoma in males. The highest incidence is noted in the Far Eastern countries, where there is a high prevalence of liver fluke infestation and hepatolithiasis. (From Parkin DM, Whelan SL, Ferlay U, Raymond L, Young J (eds). Cancer Incidence in the Five Continents, Vol. VII [IARC Scientific Publications No. 143]. IARC, Lyon, 1997.)

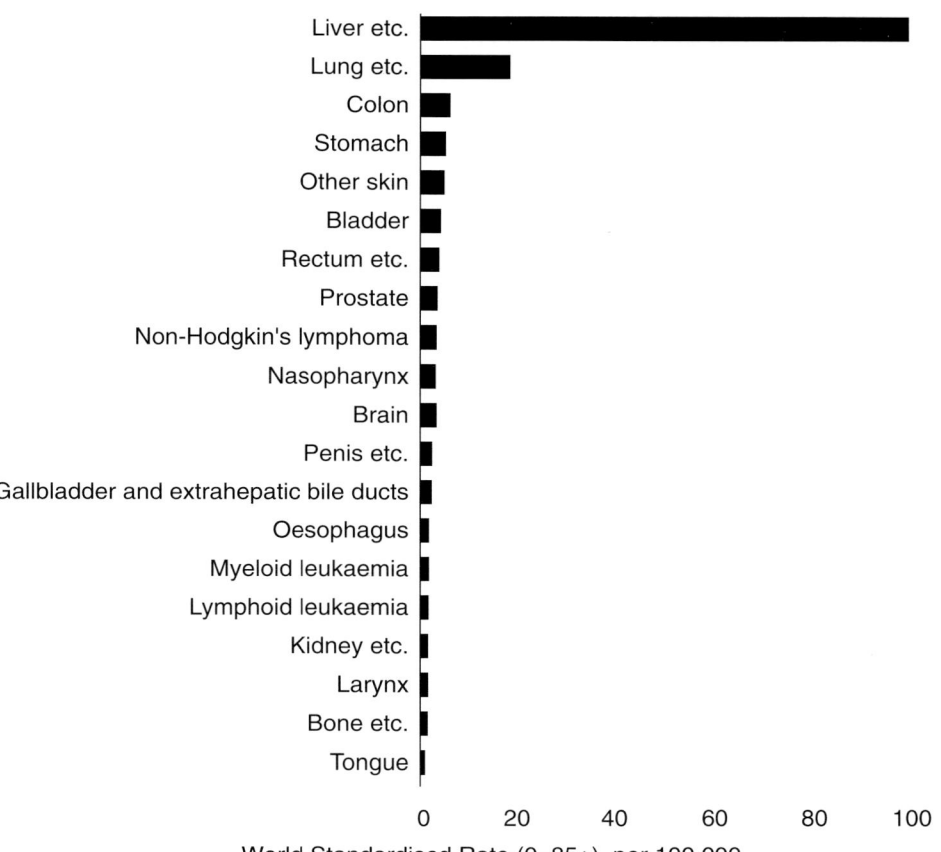

**Figure 35-5** World standardized incidence rates of various cancers in males of Khon Kaen, a northeastern province of Thailand. Note that liver cancer has the highest incidence. (From Parkin DM, Whelan SL, Ferlay J, Raymond L, Young J (eds). Cancer Incidence in Five Continents, Vol. VII [IARC Scientific Publications No. 143]. IARC, Lyon, 1997).

## Typhoid Carriers

There is a strong association between the typhoid carrier state and biliary tract cancer. In a Norwegian study on the epidemiology of typhoid carriers, the overall cancer mortality rate was 17%, and hepatobiliary neoplasms caused 8.5% of total cancer deaths.[53] In a California series, the hepatobiliary cancer death rate for typhoid carriers was 6.1%.[54] In a case–control study of deceased typhoid carriers registered by the New York Health Department between 1922 and 1975, the risk of dying from hepatobiliary cancer was six times more frequent for typhoid carriers than for age-matched controls.[55] It has been suggested that the combination of bile stasis and bacterial infection of the biliary system alters bile salts so that they act as carcinogens in the gallbladder and bile duct. Therefore, all patients who are typhoid carriers should be treated with antibiotics or cholecystectomy.

## Thorotrast

Thorotrast, once a popular radiographic contrast medium, is associated with cholangiocarcinoma about 10 to 30 years after administration.[56–59] About 50,000 to 100,000 patients received thorotrast

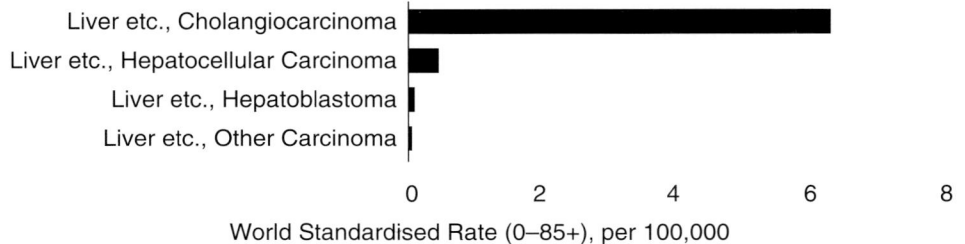

**Figure 35-6** World standardized rates of cholangiocarcinoma, hepatocellular carcinoma, hepatoblastoma, and other cancers of the liver in males of Khon Kaen, Thailand. Note the much higher incidence of cholangiocarcinomas compared with that of hepatocellular carcinoma. This is due to the high prevalence of *O. viverrini* infestation in this northeastern area of Thailand. (From Parkin DM, Whelan SL, Ferlay J, Raymond L, Young J (eds). Cancer Incidence in Five Continents, Vol. VII [IARC Scientific Publications No. 143]. IARC, Lyon, 1997.)

during the 25 years it was used until the mid-1950s.[60] Thorotrast accumulates in the reticuloendothelial system of the liver and cannot be excreted. A relationship between thorotrast administration and the development of hepatic neoplasms has been confirmed by epidemiologic studies.[56–59] Thorotrast is carcinogenic because of its observed fibrogenic activity and radioactivity.[61]

## Occupational Factors

Occupational exposures have been associated with biliary tract cancers. Vinyl chloride was associated with biliary tract cancer in a cohort of male employees of a large Michigan chemical production facility.[62] Statistically significant increased risks for cancer of the gallbladder were observed for men employed in the petroleum refining, paper mill, chemical processing, shoe-making and repair, and textile industries after an analysis of 1960 census data on industry and occupation for all employed individuals in Sweden.[63] A significant increase in the incidence of bile duct cancers was found among asbestos-related workers and among insulation workers.[63] Case reports have linked chlorinated hydrocarbon solvents, widely used as industrial solvents, with cholangiocarcioma.[64] The increased risk of biliary tract cancers among textile workers is further substantiated by another study that looked at cancers of the biliary tract diagnosed between 1980 and 1984 in Shanghai.[65] Although these occupations and occupational agents have been strongly associated with biliary tract cancer, there is no definite proof that these agents are directly responsible for the development of these neoplasms.

## Contraceptives

Use of oral contraceptives may be related to biliary tract cancers. Some studies have shown that gallbladder bile is more saturated with cholesterol during oral contraceptive (OC) use and that there is a significant increase in the lithogenic index.[66,67] In a hospital-based case–control study in 11 large hospitals in New England between 1975 and 1979, the odds ratio for ever-use of OCs as a risk factor for extrahepatic bile duct cancer was 7.8.[68] However, problems with this study included small sample numbers, controls including patients who might have had high (or low) exposures to OCs, lack of adjustment for confounding variables (including age and obesity), and use of the hospital as source of both cases and controls. In contrast, in the World Health Organization (WHO) Collaborative Study of Neoplasia and Steroid Contraceptives, in which history of OC use was compared among 58 hospitals' cases of gallbladder cancer and 355 hospital controls, and data were collected between 1979 and 1986 from participating centers in six countries, no significant association was found between gallbladder cancer and OC used. Also, no clear patterns of increasing or decreasing risk were found with duration of use or with intervals since first or last use.[69]

Results from a large collaborative study did not show an increased risk of biliary tract cancers with use of OCs.[69] There is physiological evidence to show that OCs affect bile composition and promote cholelithiasis.[66,67] Epidemiologic evidence of the impact of OCs on benign gallbladder disease is inconclusive but largely consistent with the hypothesis that OC use accelerates the disease in women who are predisposed to it.[70,71] Benign gallbladder disease is a risk factor for cancers of both the gallbladder and the extrahepatic ducts, but there is little evidence to show that OC use is directly associated with an increased risk of either cancer.

## Primary Sclerosing Cholangitis

Primary sclerosing cholangitis (PSC) is a chronic inflammatory disease characterized by progressive destruction of extrahepatic and intrahepatic bile ducts. About 70% of patients with PSC have inflammatory bowel disease.[72,73] The etiology of PSC is unknown, although both a bacterial origin and manifestation of an autoimmune disorder have been proposed as possible underlying causes. About 10% to 20% of all patients with PSC develop cholangiocarcinoma. The reason for this remains unknown, but chronic inflammation seems to be involved in the pathogenesis. It is extremely difficult to diagnose cholangiocarcinoma in the presence of PSC, despite extensive work-ups prior to liver transplantation. The frequency of undiagnosed cholangiocarcinoma is significant in explanted livers: 9% went undiagnosed in one series[74] and 4 of 11 cases were not diagnosed at another center.[75] In a recent Swedish population-based study of 125 patients with PSC the mean duration between diagnosis of PSC and development of cholangiocarcinoma was 2.3 years, with a cumulative survival of 68.8% 10 years after the diagnosis of PSC.[76]

## Congenital Abnormalities

Anomalous arrangment of the pancreaticobiliary duct (AAPBD) is a rare malformation in which the junction between the major pancreatic duct and the common bile duct is anatomically outside the duodenal wall and beyond the influence of the sphincter of Oddi. This condition is more frequently reported in the Orient, especially in Japan. The incidence rate of gallbladder cancer in people with AAPBD is about 25%.[77] The pathophysiology underlying the development of cancer is thought to be the reflux of pancreatic juice into the gallbladder, resulting in chronic cholecystitis and mucosal metaplasia. The metaplastic change may be a premalignant condition leading to carcinogenesis.

Another congenital anomaly associated with biliary tract cancer is choledochal cyst (Fig. 35–7). Its occurrence is four times more common in women than in men, and has a higher incidence among Japanese and other Asians.[78] The overall incidence of biliary tract cancer is 2.5% among patients with choledochal cyst, about 20 times greater than that in the general population.[79,80] Type IV and V cysts and Caroli's disease are also associated with a higher incidence of carcinoma. Overall, 7% of patients with Caroli's disease are found to have a cholangiocarcinoma, with no female preponderance.[81,82]

## Hepatolithiasis

The prevalence of intrahepatic stones in Western countries is low, ranging from 0.6% to 2.4% of all cases of biliary lithiasis; they are rarely primary.[83–85] This contrasts with the prevalence in Southeast Asia, which ranges from 3% in Hong Kong to 53% in Taiwan.[86] The relationship of parasites to this syndrome is disputed. About 25% of patients with hepatolithiasis have *C. sinensis* ova in stool, but in Taiwan, where the incidence of hepatolithiasis is high, *C. sinensis* infestation is rare. Recurrent bouts of cholangitis predispose patients with hepatolithiasis to biliary

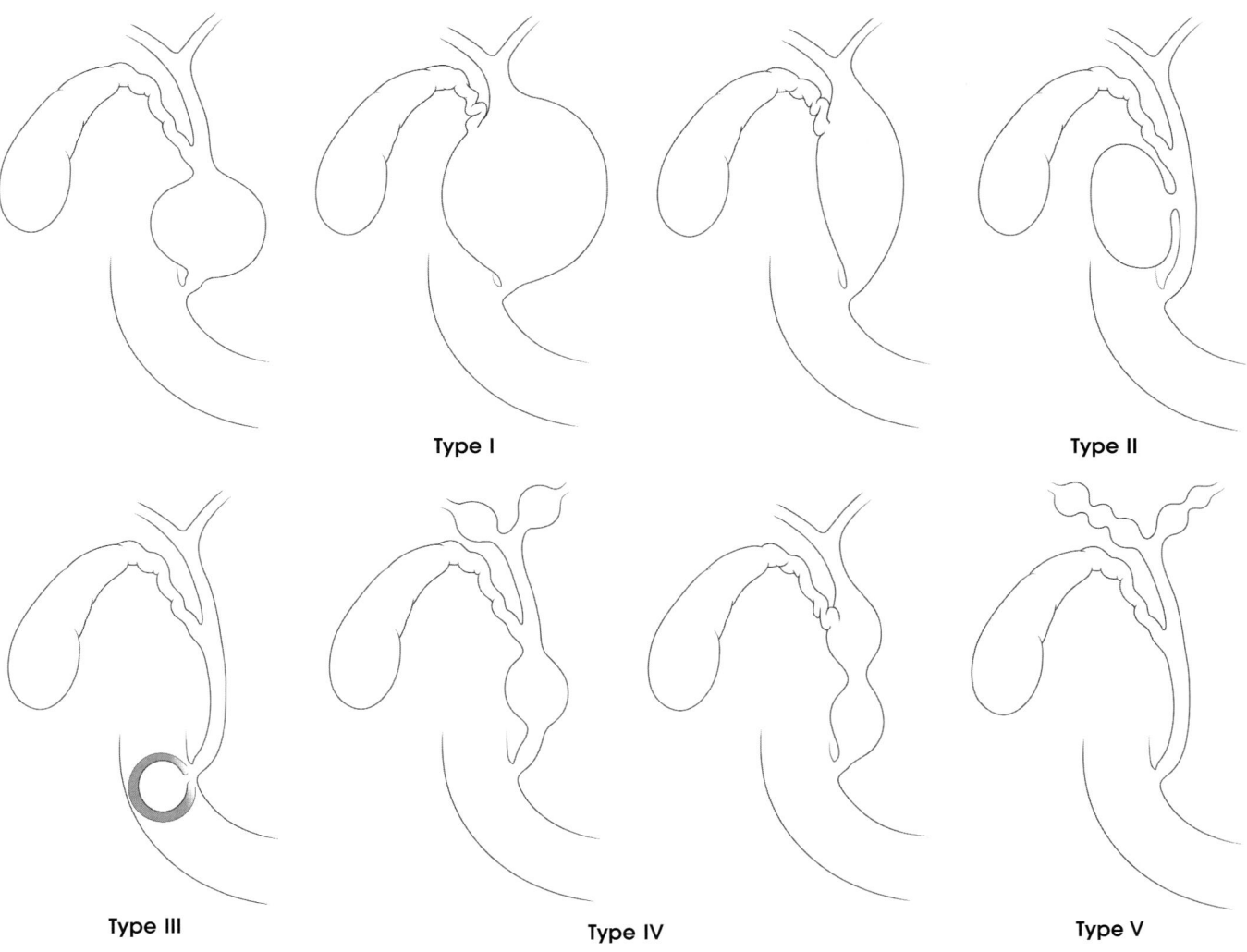

**Figure 35–7** Classification of choledochal cysts.

tract cancer, especially of the intrahepatic type. The development of cholangiocarcinoma is probably multifactorial. One hypothesis is that chronic irritation of the bile duct by bile stasis, bacterial infection, parasitic infestation, or the presence of stones could result in adenomatous hyperplasia of the bile duct epithelium and subsequent development of cholangiocarcinoma.[39,87] The diagnosis of cholangiocarcinoma in patients with hepatolithiasis is notoriously difficult. Positive preoperative diagnosis of cholangiocarcinoma was not made in up to 80% of cases in a recent study from Taiwan.[88] It is difficult to differentiate malignant from benign strictures, even with endoscopic retrograde cholangiopancreatography (ERCP) or percutaneous transhepatic cholangiogram.[20] A space-occupying lesion visible by ultrasonography or CT may be diagnosed as a liver abscess.[89] There is still no established tumor marker for cholangiocarcinoma. A high index of suspicion is therefore necessary in managing patients with hepatolithiasis. In particular, cholangiocarcinoma should be suspected in patients who have weight loss, anemia, hepatomegaly, and intractable abdominal pain.

## Molecular Epidemiology of Biliary Tract Cancers

Genes involved in cancer development include oncogenes and tumor suppressor genes.

### Oncogenes

The *ras* genes are members of a family of oncogenes that is frequently expressed in cancer cells; more than 80% of cancers harbor *ras* mutants. The normal ras protein acts in the cell as a signal-transducing device operating in a complex signaling cascade within the cytoplasm. The normal ras protein growth-stimulatory signals, often released by mitogen receptors at the cell surface, passes them along a pathway to a downstream target that stimulates cell proliferation. Once it has received a growth-stimulatory signal, the normal ras protein binds the nucleotide guanosine triphosphate (GTP) and briefly enters into an active conformation; having released a pulse of growth-stimulatory signals, it then rapidly returns to a resting state by hydrolyzing the bound GTP into guanosine diphosphage (GDP). It is the final hydrolyzing step that is defective in the oncogenic ras proteins found in human tumors. As a result, the ras protein becomes trapped in its excited, signal-emitting mode and thus floods the cell unrelentingly with growth-stimulatory signals.[90] Mutations in *ras* have been identified by techniques involving the polymerase chain reaction (PCR; see below).

In most reported cases, *ras* activation is induced by point mutation. This has been reported in approximately 40% of colon cancers,[91–96] 50% of lung adenocarcinomas,[97,98] 30% of acute myeloid leukemias,[99–102] and up to 90% of pancreatic carcinomas.[103–107] In the case of biliary tract tumors, there are conflicting data about the presence or incidence of this mutation. Almoguera et al.[103] reported finding no mutation in gallbladder cancer using the ribonuclease A mismatch cleavage technique. Tada et al.[107] reported finding *ras* mutations at a low incidence in extrahepatic bile duct carcinoma and not at all in gallbladder carcinoma by using direct sequencing subsequent to PCR. Tada et al.[107] found a high incidence of *ras* gene mutation in hilar type of cholangiocarcinoma—about 67%, especially when these tumors were large. However, Levi et al.[108] found mutations in all cases of carcinoma assessed using a modified two-step PCR method. Also using a modified two-step PCR, Watanabe et al.[109] found that some gallbladder cancers and all extrahepatic bile duct cancers showed point mutations in the K-*ras* codon 12 and that guanosine-to-adenine transitions were most frequent. Petmitr[110] found that the rates of *ras* mutations varied among ethnic groups, with a high frequency of *ras* mutations occurring in cholangiocarcinomas from English patients (l00%) and Japanese patients (60%) and a low frequency occurring in those from Thai patients (4%). These findings may reflect a different etiology of this cancer in the three groups or differences in the development of the mutation, based on ethnicity. The English and Japanese patients in these reports were not infected with liver fluke nor had they been exposed to thorotrast.

Hanada et al.[111] found a higher incidence of K-*ras* mutation in gallbladder cancer patients with AAPBD than in gallbladder cancer patients without it. The significance of this finding is unclear but could be related to chronic bile duct injury by pancreatic enzymes and the formation of surface-active lysolecithin by pancreatic phospholipases. Tada et al.[107] found that the incidence and spectrum of *ras* mutations in gallbladder cancer were similar to those in colon cancer. It is therefore tempting to speculate that the same etiologic agent plays a role in carcinogenesis in both cancers because *ras* gene mutation is known from animal experiments to be induced by specific chemical substances. Dehydroxylated bile acids have been implicated as carcinogens in both colon and biliary tract cancer. However, since the incidence of *ras* gene mutation is low in biliary tract cancer, this mutation is probably not the first carcinogenic event in the biliary tract cancers.

### Tumor Suppressor Genes

In contrast to proto-oncogenes, which induce cancer when they are converted into hyperactive alleles, tumor suppressosr genes trigger cancer when they are inactive (or null) alleles. In normal cells, these genes act to constrain or suppress proliferation. Mutation causes unrestrained growth and leads to malignancy. The tumor suppressor gene associated with biliary tract cancer is *p53*. One mutant *p53* allele often affects cell phenotype even in the presence of the wild-type allele. This effect is attributable to the biochemistry of the p53 protein, which resembles a tetramer. Cells that carry both mutant and wild-type *p53* alleles form mixed tetramers whose functioning is compromised by the defective subunits encoded by the mutant *p53* allele; the mutant allele inhibits its wild-type counterpart. This inhibition is incomplete, however, and most tumor cells gain a further growth advantage by eventually discarding the surviving wild type.[90]

The incidence of *p53* mutation in gallbladder cancer is about 50%.[112–114] However, the spectrum of mutations differs in different regions of the world. A study of *p53* mutations in cholangiocarcinomas from Japanese and Thai patients showed that mutations in both ethnic groups are distributed among exons 5 to 8. The most common change is glycine-to-aspartic acid transition, found in about 50% of the cases.[114] Itoi and colleagues[115] demonstrated that the incidence of p53 overexpression is similar regardless of tumor size or depth of invasion and, thus, that this change is an early event in the development of gallbladder carcinoma. p53 is not overexpressed in non-neoplastic lesions.[113] In a later study, Itoi and his group concluded that p53 protein overexpression correlates well with gene mutation. They also found that the frequency of *p53* mutation and protein overexpression was increased in high-grade compared with low-grade carcinomas, though the difference was not statistically significant.

The incidence of *p53* mutations in cholangiocarcinomas varies in different studies. A study of Thai and Japanese patients with cholangiocarcinoma showed *p53* mutations in about 50% of tumors.[116] A study by Petmitre and co-workers[117] showed this mutation in only 1 of 20 Thai patients with cholangiocarcinoma. Unlike in colon cancer, where there is an adenoma-to-carcinoma sequence and K-*ras* mutation and *p53* gene mutations occur at different points in the sequence, there is no clear progression sequence of mutation pattern in gallbladder cancer.

Resistance to apoptosis, especially via altered expression of B-cell lymphoma/leukemia 2 (Bcl-2) family members, has been implicated in malignant transformation. Gores and associates[118] compared the apoptotic threshold and the expression of the Bcl-2 protein family members Bcl-2, Bcl-xl, and Bax in human nonmalignant cholangiocytes and in a human malignant cholangiocarcinoma cell line. These authors noted a 15-fold increase in Bcl-2 in the malignant cell line over that in the nonmalignant cell line. Moreover, malignant cholangiocytes were resistant to beauvericin-induced apoptosis. They thus concluded that resistance to apoptosis by overexpression of Bcl-2 may be a feature of cholangiocarcinoma. They also speculated that installation of an antisense Bcl-2 construct into bile ducts of patients with cholangiocarcinoma may be a reasonable therapeutic strategy for rendering the tumors more sensitive to apoptosis by anticancer treatments such as radiation or chemotherapy and thereby enhancing the treatment response rates.

### Biomarkers of Biliary Tract Cancers

In epidemiology, a *biomarker* is any substance, structure, or process that can be measured in the human body or its products and that may influence or predict the incidence or outcome of disease. Biomarkers can be used to screen for malignancy. Prostate-specific antigen (PSA), for example, is used to screen for prostatic carcinoma. However, PSA is not specific to prostatic carcinoma. Similarly, biomarkers for biliary tract cancers are not necessarily specific to biliary tract cancers. The two most commonly used and investigated markers for biliary tract cancers are carcinoembryonic antigen (CEA) and carbohydrate antigen 19-9 (CA 19-9).

Carcinoembryonic antigen is a glycoprotein with a molecular weight of 200,000 that has been shown by immunohistochemical methods to be present in malignancies of the colon, pancreas, and the biliary tract. Carbohydrate antigen 19-9 is a mucin-type glycoprotein whose immunodeterminant is present on the carbohydrate moiety of the molecule. This antigen has been found in malignancies of the gastrointestinal tract and is elevated in benign cholestasis and cirrhosis.

Many investigators have tried to use CEA and CA 19-9 to screen patients for cholangiocarcinomas, especially in the setting of PSC. As noted earlier in this chapter, the prevalence of this neoplasm in PSC has been estimated to range between 5% and 15%.[73,119] Adult patients with symptomatic choledochal cysts have a 14% chance of developing cholangiocarcinoma,[120] and between 5% and 10% of patients with hepatolithiasis will develop bile duct malignancy.[20] The differentiation of cholangiocarcinoma from PSC remains challenging. Ultrasonography, CT scanning, and ERCP can establish the diagnosis of cholangiocarcinoma in only a minority of patients. Duplex ultrasonography (86%) and bolus-enhanced CT scanning (59%) have increased the detection rate of intrahepatic and hilar cholangiocarcinomas.[121,122] However, none of these techniques is very sensitive in detecting early extrahepatic tumors in nonjaundiced patients. Brush cytology and biopsy yield a diagnosis in only 30% to 40% of patients.[123] Up to 9% of explant livers from patients also have cholangiocarcinoma despite extensive work-up.[124] In most series, the overall post-transplant prognosis in patients with PSC who have cholangiocarcinoma is very poor.

The utility of CEA and CA 19-9 in the surveillance of patients with PSC for cholangiocarcinoma has been explored in many studies. Both markers have good sensitivities of 70% to 80% but low specificities of 50% to 60%. Nonmalignant hepatobiliary diseases such as cholestasis and bacterial cholangitis also exhibit small increases in serum CA 19-9 levels. However, in one study, the sensitivity and specificity of CA 19-9 values >100 U/ml for cholangiocarcinoma in PSC were found to be 89% and 86%, respectively.[127] Williams and colleagues[125] have come up with an index for the two serum tumor markers (i.e., CA 19-9 + [CEA × 40]) that has an accuracy of 86% in the diagnosis of cholangiocarcinoma in patients with PSC when the index value is over 400. These investigators are using this index in all their PSC patients prior to liver transplantation; when it is positive, it indicates further diagnostic testing.[126]

Soloway and colleagues have shown that CA 19-9 and CEA are useful for discriminating patients with gallbladder cancer from patients with gallstones.[127] In a case–control study of gallbladder cancer in high-risk populations of Mexico City and La Paz, Bolivia, the results suggest that CA 19-9 could be a useful screening test for sufficiently high-risk subpopulations such as Bolivians and Mexican Indians in the United States.[127]

Another biomarker being examined is fibrinonectin (FN). Fibrinonectins are high-molecular-weight extracellular glycoproteins abundant in blood plasma and other body fluids. They are involved in various biological activities such as cell adhesion, motility, and differentiation, hemostasis, and wound healing. The plasma form of FN, which is produced by hepatocytes, differs from the so-called cellular fibrinonectins (cFn), which are produced by other cell types. In several studies, FN concentrations in body fluids such as ascites, urine, and blood have proved to

be useful as a biochemical marker of malignancy. Korner and associates[128] found significantly higher concentrations of both total FN and cFN in bile of patients with carcinoma than in patients without carcinoma. They thus concluded that FN in bile fluid is a sensitive, specific, and easily determined marker for the differential diagnosis of malignant and benign diseases of the biliary tract.[128]

Another potential biomarker is p53 protein overexpression, which has been shown in patients with cholangiocarcinoma. Williams and co-workers[129] detected it in liver tissues in 80% of patients with PSC and cholangiocarcinoma (11/14), in contrast to 0% of patients with PSC but no cholangiocarcinoma (0/15). This finding suggests that immunohistochemical detection of p53 protein could represent an additional criterion for establishing a diagnosis of cholangiocarcinoma in PSC.

## Conclusion

The epidemiology of gallbladder cancer is extremely varied in the different parts of the world and among different races. Like its most common etiological agent, the gallstone, gallbladder cancer is multifaceted. As the different facets of its epidemiology keep expanding, we will be able to better understand its natural history. Epidemiological scientists are continuing in their efforts to uncork the secrets of its origin so that it can be detected in its early stage or even prevented. Of particular interest is the establishment of biomarkers for detection of this cancer in its early stage. Epidemiologists are also looking at factors that lead to the development of cancer, such as race, diet, medications, and bile constituents.

The epidemiology of cholangiocarcioma is also fascinating. Here too, epidemiologists and researchers are trying to come up with early detection methods. Etiological agents differ in the Eastern and Western worlds, with fluke infestation being the primary cause in the East and sclerosing cholangitis or anomalies of the biliary tract being the primary etiology in the West. Meanwhile, the search continues for an ideal biomarker to screen for biliary tract cancer. Until one is found, we will have to rely on the less sensitive and less specific biomarkers discussed here.

## References

1. Donohue J, Stewart K, Menck H. The National Cancer Data Base report on carcinoma of the gallbladder, 1989–1995. Cancer 83:2618–2628, 1998.
2. Henson D. Albores J, Corle D. Carcinoma of the gallbladder: histological types, stage of disease and survival rates. Cancer 70:1493–1497, 1992.
3. Parkin D, Whelan S, Ferlay J, Raymond L, Young J (eds). Cancer Incidence in Five Continents, Vol. VII (IARC Scientific Publications No. 143). IARC, Lyon, France, 1997.
4. Fraumeni JF Jr, Devasa S, McLaughlin, J, Stanford J. Biliary tract cancer. In Schottenfeld D, Fraumeni JF Jr (eds): Cancer Epidemiology and Prevention, 2nd ed. Oxford University Press, New York, 1996, pp 794–803.
5. Armijo R. The epidemiology of cancer in Chile. Natl Cancer Inst Monogr 53:115–118, 1978.
6. Strom BL. Epidemiological and biochemical aspects of an important sequel to to cholelithiasis: gallbladder cancer. In Capocaccia G, Ricci F, Angelico F (eds): Epidemiology and Prevention of Gallstone Disease. MTP Press, Lancaster, 1984, pp. 64–70.
7. Hsing AW, Gao Y, Devasa SS, Jin F, Fraumeni JR. Rising incidence of biliary tract cancers in Shanghai, China. Int J Cancer 75:368–370, 1998.
8. Sako K, Seitzinger GL, Garside E. Carcinoma of the extrahepatic bile ducts: review of literature and report of six cases. Surgery 41:416–437, 1957.

9. Wen CC, Lee HC. Intrahepatic stones: a clinical study. Ann Surg 175:166–177, 1972.

10. Shen PC, Ker CG. Intrahepatic stones. II. Clinical study [in Chinese]. J Formosa Med Assoc 80:1217–1226, 1981.

11. Huang MJ, Liaw YF, Wu CS. Comparison of intravenous radionuclide cholescintigraphy and endoscopic retrograde cholangiography in the diagnosis of intrahepatic gallstones. Br J Radiol 54:302–306, 1981.

12. Chen MF, Wang CS, Chou FF, et al. Surgical treatment of intrahepatic gallstone [in Chinese]. Chang Gung Med J 5:75–78, 1982.

13. Su CH, Lui WY, P'eng FK. Relative prevalence of gallstone disease in Taiwan: a nationwide cooperative study. Dig Dis Sci 37:764–768, 1992.

14. Nagase MN, Hikasa Y, Soloway RD, Tanimura H, Setoyama M, Kato H. Gallstones in Western Japan: factors affecting the prevalance of intrahepatic gallstones. Gastroenterology 78:684–690, 1980.

15. Nakayama F, Furusawa T, Nakama T. Hepatolithiasis in Japan: present status. Am J Surg 216:220, 1980.

16. Nakayama F. Hepatolithiasis and cholangiohepatitis. In: Cohen S, Soloway RD (eds): Gallstones. Churchill Livingstone, New York, 1985, pp 237–246.

17. Stock FE, Fung JHY. Oriental cholagiohepatitis. Arch Surg 84:409–412, 1962.

18. Chen HH, Zhang WH, Wang SS. Twenty-two year experience with the diagnosis and treatment of intrahepatic calculi. Surg Gynecol Obstet 159:519–524, 1984.

19. Tsunoda U. Intrahepatic stones associated with cholangiocarcinoma. Jpn J Gastroenterol Surg 23:118–121, 1990.

20. Sheen-Chen SM, Chou FF, Eng HL. Intrahepatic cholangiocarcinoma in hepato-lithiasis; a frequently overlooked disease. J Surg Oncol 47:131–135, 1991.

21. Chen PH, Lo HW, Wang CS, et al. Cholangiocarcinoma in hepato-lithiasis. J Clin Gastroenterol 6:539–547, 1984.

22. Chen MF, Jan YY, Wang CS, Jeng LBB, Hwang TL, Chen SC. Intrahepatic stones associated with cholangiocarcinoma. Am J Gastroenterol 84:391–395, 1989.

23. Chen MF, Jan YY, Wang CS, et al. A reappraisal of cholangiocarcinoma in patient with hepatolithiasis. Cancer 71:2461–2465, 1993.

24. Ker CG, Sheen PC, Arcillia CE Jr. Choledocoscopic heat probe therapy: an adjunctive palliative treatment for intrahepatic cholangiocarcinoma with hepatolithiasis. Kao Hsiung I Hsueh Ko Hsueh Tsa Chih 7:345–3450, 1991.

25. King MS. Biliary tract disease in Malaya. Br J Surg 58:829–832, 1971.

26. Cobo A, Hall RC, Torres E, Cuello CJ. Intrahepatic calculi. Arch Surg 89:936–941, 1964.

27. Haswell-Elkins MR, Mairiang E, Mairiang P, et al. Cross-sectional study of Opisthorchis viverrini infection and cholangiocarcinoma in communities within a high-risk area in northeast Thailand. Int J Cancer 59:505–509, 1994.

28. Elkins DB, Elkins H, Mairiang E, et al. A high frequency of hepatobiliary disease and cholangiocarcinoma associated with heavy Opisthorchis viverrini infection in a small community in northeast Thailand. Trans R Soc Trop Med Hyg 84:715–719, 1990.

29. Parkin DM, Srivatanakul P, Khlat M, et al. Liver cancer in Thailand: a case–control study of cholangiocarcinoma. Int J Cancer 48:323–328, 1991.

30. Moller H, Heseltine E, Vainio H. Working group report on schistosomes, liver flukes and Helicobacter pylori. Int J Cancer 60:587–589, 1995.

31. Kalser MH. Cholelithiasis: clinical aspects. In Bockus HL, Berk JE, Haubrich WS, et al. (eds): Gastroenterology, 4th ed. W.B. Saunders, Phildelphia, 1985, pp. 3619–3642.

32. Perpetua MM, Valdivieso M, Jeilbrun LK, Nelson RS, Connor T, Bodey GP. Natural history study of gallbladder cancer. Cancer 42:330–335, 1978.

33. Hart J, Shani M, Modan B. Epidemiological aspects of gallbladder and biliary tract neoplasm. Am J Publ Health 62:36–39, 1972.

34. Maram ES, Ludwig J, Kurland LT, Brian DD. Carcinoma of the gallbladder and extrahepatic bile ducts in Rochester, Minnesota, 1935–71. Am J Epidemiol 109:769–772, 1972.

35. Klein JB, Finck FM. Primary carcinoma of the gallbladder. Arch Surg 104:769–772, 1972.

36. Andrews EC, Bennett DE, Arhelger RB. Carcinoma of the gallbladder: report of 45 cases. South Med J 62:573–578, 1969.

37. Black WC, Key CR, Carmany TB, Herman D. Carcinoma of the gallbladder in a population of Southwestern American Indians. Cancer 39:1267–1279, 1977.

38. Longmire WP, McArthur MS, Bastounis EA, Hiatt J. Carcinoma of the extrahepatic biliary tract. Ann Surg 178:333–345, 1973.

39. Koga A, Ichimiya H, Yamaguchi K, Miyazaka K, Nakayama F. Hepatolithiasis associated with cholangiocarcinoma: possible etiological significance. Cancer 55:2826–2829, 1985.

40. Chow WH, Johansen C, Grindley G, Mellemkjaar L, Olsen JH, Fraumeni JF. Gallstones, cholecystectomy and risk of cancers of the liver, biliary tract and pancreas. Br J Cancer 79:640–644, 1999.

41. Maringhini A, Moreau JA, Melton LJ, et al. Gallstones, gallbladder cancer and other gastrointestinal malignancies: an epidemiological study in Rochester, Minnesota. Ann Intern Med 107:30–35, 1987.

42. Comfort MW, Gray HK, Wilson JW. The silent gallstone: a ten- to twenty-year follow-up of 112 cases. Ann Surg 128:931–937, 1948.

43. Lund J. Surgical indications in cholelithiasis: prophylactic cholecystectomy elucidated on the basis of long-term follow-up on 526 non-operated cases. Ann Surg 151:151–162, 1960.

44. Wenckert A, Robertson B. The natural course of gallbladder disease: eleven-year review of 781 non-operated cases. Gastroenterology 50:376–381, 1966.

45. Diehl AK. Epidemiology of gallbladder cancer: a synthesis of recent data. J Natl Cancer Inst 65:1209–1214, 1980.

46. Shukla VK, Khandelwal C, Roy SK, Vaidya MP. Primary carcinoma of the gall-bladder: a review of a 16-year period at the University Hospital. J Surg Oncol 28:32–35, 1985.

47. Lowenfels AB. Gallstones and the risk of cancer. Gut 21:1090–1092, 1980.

48. Crump C. Incidence of gallstones and gallbladder disease. Surg Gynecol Obstet 53:447–455, 1931.

49. Diehl AK. Gallstone size and the risk of gallbladder cancer. JAMA 250:2323–2326, 1983.

50. Lowenfels AB, Walker AM, Althaus DP, Townsen G, Domellof L. Gallstone growth, size and risk of gallbladder cancer: an interracial study. Int J Epidemiol 18:50–54, 1989.

51. Hou PC. Pathological changes in the intrahepatic ducts of cats (Felis catus) infested with Clonorchis sinesis. J Pathol Bacteriol 89:357–364, 1965.

52. Thamavit W, Bhamarapravati N, Sahaphong S, Vajrasthira S, Subhkij A. Effects of dimethylnitrosamine on induction of cholangiocarcinoma in Opisthorchis viverrini–infected Syrin golden hamsters. Cancer Res 38:4634–4639, 1978.

53. Vogelsang TM. Typhoid and paratyphoid B carriers and their treatment. Universitetet I Bergen Arbok 1950, Medisinskrekke Nr I, A.S. John Greigs Biktrykkeri, Bergen, Norway, Nov 1950.

54. Berk MD, Hollister AC. Typhoid Fever Cases and Carriers: An Analysis of Records of the California State Department of Public Health, 1910–1959. State of California Department of Public Health, Berkeley, 1962.

55. Welton JC, Marr JS, Freidman SM. Association between hepatobiliary cancer and typhoid carrier state. Lancet 14:791–794, 1979.

56. Mori T, Maruyama T, Kato Y, et al. Epidemiological follow-up study of Japanese thorotrast cases. Environ Res 18:44–54, 1979.

57. Mori T, Kato Y, Shimamine T, et al. Statistical analysis of Japanese thorotrast-administered autopsy cases. Environ Res 18:231–244, 1979.

58. Van Kaick G, Lorenz D. Malignancies in German thorotrast patients and estimated tissue dose. Health Phys 35:127–136, 1978.

59. Faber M. Twenty-eight years of continuous follow-up of patients injected with thorotrast for cerebral angiography. Environ Res 18:37–43, 1979.

60. Selinger M, Koff RS. Thorotrast and the liver: a reminder. Gastroenterology 68:799–803, 1975.

61. Rubel LR, Ishak K. Thorotrast-associated cholangiocarcinoma: an epidemiological and clinicopathologic study. Cancer 50:1408–1415, 1982.

62. Bond G, McLaren E, Sabel F, et al. Liver and biliary tract cancer among chemical workers. Am J Ind Med 18:19–24, 1990.

63. Maler HSR, McLaughlin JK, Malker BK, et al. Biliary tract cancer and occupation in Sweden. Br J Ind Med 43:257–262, 1986.

64. Zarchy T. Chlorinated hydrocarbon solvents and biliary pancreatic cancer: report of three cases. Am J Ind Med 30:341–342, 1996.

65. Chow W, Ji BT, Dosemeci M, McLaughlin JK, Gao YT, Fraumeni JF Jr. Biliary tract cancer among textile and other workers in Shanghai, China. Am J Ind Med 30:36–40, 1996.

66. Bennion LJ, Ginsberg RL, Garnick MB, Bennett PH. Effects of oral contraceptives on gallbladder bile of normal women. N Engl J Med 294:189–192, 1976.

67. Kern F Jr, Everson GT, De Mark B, et al. Biliary lipids, bile acids and gallbladder function in the human female: effects of contraceptive steroids. J Lab Clin Med 99:798–805, 1982.

68. Yen S, Hsieh CC, MacMahon B. Extrahepatic bile duct cancer and smoking, beverage consumption, past medical history, and oral contraceptive use. Cancer 59:2112–2116, 1987.
69. The WHO Collaborative Study of Neoplasia and Steroid Contraceptives. Combined oral contraceptives and gallbladder cancer. Int J Epidemiol 18:309–314, 1989.
70. Boston Collaborative Drug Surveillance Programme. Oral contraceptives and venous thromboembolic disease, surgically confirmed gallbladder diseases, and breast tumors. Lancet I:1399–1404, 1973.
71. Scragg RKR, McMichael AJ, Seamark RF. Oral contraceptives, pregnancy and endogenous estrogen in gallstone disease: a case–control study. BMJ 288:1795–1799, 1984.
72. Wiesner RH, Grambsch PM, Dickson R, et al. Primary sclerosing cholangitis: natural history, prognostic factors, and survival analysis. Hepatology 10:430–436, 1989.
73. Farrant JM, Hayllar KM, Wilkinson ML, et al. Natural history and prognostic variables in primary sclerosing cholangitis. Gastroenterology 100:1710–1717, 1991.
74. Stieber AC, Marino IR, Iwatsuki S, Starzl TE. Cholangiocarcinoma in sclerosing cholangitis: the role of liver transplantation. Int Surg 74:1–3, 1989.
75. Miros M, Kerlin P, Walker N, Harper J, Lynch S, Strong R. Predicting cholangiocarcinoma in patients with primary sclerosing cholangitis. Ann Surg 207:373–379, 1988.
76. Kornfield D, Ekbom A, Ihre T. Survival and risk of cholangiocarcinoma in patients with primary sclerosing cholangitis: a population-based study. Scand J Gastroenterol 32(10):1041–1045, 1997.
77. Kimura K, Ohto M, Saisho H, et al. Association of gallbladder carcinoma and anomalous pancreaticobiliary ductal union. Gastroenterology 89:1258–1265, 1985.
78. Yamaguchi M. Congenital choledochal cyst: analysis of 1,433 patients in the Japanese literature. Am J Surg 140:653–657, 1980.
79. Ryckman FC, Noseworthy J. Neonatal cholestatic conditions requiring surgical reconstruction. Semin Liver Dis 7:134–154, 1987.
80. Flanigan DP. Biliary carcinoma associated with biliary cysts. Cancer 40:880–883, 1977.
81. Dayton MT, Longmire WP, Tompkins RK. Caroli's disease: a premalignant condition? Am J Surg 145:41–48, 1983.
82. Nagasue N. Successful treatment of Caroli's diaease by hepatic resection: report of six cases. Ann Surg 200:718–723, 1984.
83. Lindstrom CG. Frequency of gallstone disease in a well-defined Swedish population: a prospective necropsy in Malmo. Scand J Gastroentrol 12:341–346, 1977.
84. Simi M, Loriga P, Basoli A, et al. Intrahepatic lithiasis: study of thirty-six cases and review of the literature. Am J Surg 137:317–322, 1979.
85. Grassi G. La litiasi intrepatica. Atti Accad Lancisiana 17:276, 1973.
86. Nakayama F, Soloway RD, Nakama T, et al. Hepatolithiasis in East Asia: retrospective study. Dig Dis Sci 31:21–26,1986.
87. Nakanuma Y, Terada T, Tanaka Y, Ohta G. Are hepatolithiasis and cholangiogram etiologically related? A morphological study of 12 cases of hepatolithiasis associated with cholangiocarcinoma. Virchows Arch A Pathol Anat Histopathol 406:45–58, 1985.
88. Jan YY, Chen MF. Surgical treatment of peripheral cholangiocarcinoma. Asian J Surg 19:105–111, 1996.
89. Kubo S, Kinoshita H, Hirohashi K, Hamba H. Hepatolithiasis associated with cholangiocarcinoma. World J Surg 19:637–641, 1995.
90. Weinberg RA. Molecular mechanisms of carcinogens. In: Leder P, Clayton D, Rubenstine E, (eds): Scientific American Introduction to Molecular Medicine. Scientific American, New York, 1994, pp. 253–276.
91. Bos, JL, Fearson ER, Hamilton SR, et al. Prevalence of ras gene mutations in human colorectal cancers. Nature 327:293–297, 1987.
92. Forrester K, Almoguera C, Han K, Grizzle WE, Perucho M. Detection of high incidence of K-ras oncogenes during human colon tumerogenesis. Nature 327:298–303, 1987.
93. Vogelstine B, Fearson ER, Hamilton SR, et al. Genetic alterations during colorectal tumor development. N Engl J Med 319:525–532, 1988.
94. Sahlab N, Jones DJ, Bos JL, Kinsella A, Schofield PF. Detection of K-ras gene alterations and ras protein in colorectal cancer. Dis Colon Rectum 32:659–664, 1989.
95. Hayakumo T, Azuma T, Nakajima M, et al. Prevalence of K-ras gene mutation in colorectal cancers. Gastroenterol Jpn 88:1539–1544, 1991.
96. Soh K, Yanagisawa A, Hiratsuka H, Sugano H, Kato Y. Variation in K-ras codon 12 point mutation rate with histological atypia within individual colorectal tumors. Jpn J Cancer Res 84:388–393, 1993.
97. Rodenhuis S, Slebos RJ, Boot AJ, et al. Incidence and possible clinical significance of K-ras oncogene activation in adenocarcinoma of the human lung. Cancer Res 48:5738–5741, 1988.
98. Kobayashi T, Tsuda H, Noguchi M, et al. Association of point mutation in C-Ki-ras oncogene in lung adenocarcinoma with particular reference to cytologic subtype. Cancer 66:289–294, 1990.
99. Bos JL. Ras oncogenes in human cancer: a review. Cancer Res 49:4682–4689, 1989.
100. Farr CJ, Saiki RK, Erlich HA, McCormick F, Marshall CJ. Analysis of ras gene mutations in acute myeloid leukemia by polymerase chain reaction and oligonucleotide probes. Proc Natl Acad Sci USA 85:1629–1633, 1988.
101. Barteam CR, Ludwig WD, Hiddeman W, et al. Acute myeloid leukemia: analysis of ras gene mutations and clonality defined by polymorphic X-linked loci. Leukemia 3:247–256, 1989.
102. Radich JP, Kopecky KJ, Willman CL, et al. N-ras mutations in adult de novo myelogenous leukemia: prevalence and clinical significance. Blood 76:801–807, 1990.
103. Almoguera C, Shibata D, Forrester K, Martin J, Arnheim N, Perucho M. Most human carcinomas of exocrine pancreas contain mutant c-K-ras genes. Cell 53:549–554, 1988.
104. Mariyama M, Kishi K, Nakamura K, Obata H, Nishimura S. Frequency and types of point mutation at the 12th codon of the c-K-ras gene found in pancreatic cancers from Japanese patients. Jpn J Cancer Res 80:622–626, 1989.
105. Nagata Y, Abe M, Motoshima K, Nakayama E, Shiku H. Frequent glycine to aspartic acid mutations at codon 12 of c-K-ras gene found in pancreatic cancer in Japanese. Jpn J Cancer Res 81:135–140, 1990.
106. Lemoine NR, Jain S, Hughes CM, et al. Ki-ras oncogene activation in preinvasive pancreatic cancer. Gastroenterology 102:230–236, 1992.
107. Tada M, Yokosuka O, Amata M, Ohto M, Isono K. Analysis of ras gene mutations in biliary and pancreatic tumors by polymerase chain reaction and direct sequencing. Cancer 66:930–935, 1990.
108. Levi S, Urbano-Ispizua A, Gill R, et al. Multiple K-ras codon 12 mutations in cholangiocarcinomas demonstrated with a sensitive polymerase chain reaction technique. Cancer Res 51:3497–3502, 1991.
109. Watanabe M, Masahiro A, Junji T, Mitsutoshi K, Masaharu K, Miyazaki T. Point mutation of K-ras gene codon 12 in biliary tract tumors. Gastroenterology 107:1147–1153, 1994.
110. Petmitr S. Cancer genes and cholangiocarcinoma. Southeast Asian J Trop Med Public Health 28 (Suppl):80–84, 1997.
111. Hanada K, Itoh M, Fuji K, Tsuchida A, Hideo O, Goro K. K-ras and p53 mutations in stage l gallbladder carcinoma with an anomalous junction of the pancreaticobiliary duct. Cancer 77:452–458, 1996.
112. Wistuba I, Gazdar A, Sugio K, Roa I, Albores-Saavedra J. p53 protein overexpression in gallbladder carcinoma and its precursor lesions. Hum Pathol 27:360–365, 1996.
113. Oohashi Y, Watanabe H, Ajoioka Y, Hatakeyama K. p53 immunostaining distinguishes malignant from benign lesions of the gallbladder. Pathol Int 45:58–65, 1995.
114. Yokoyama N, Hitomi J, Watanebe H, et al. Mutations of p53 in gallbladder carcinomas in high incidence areas of Japan and Chile. Cancer Epidemiol Biomarkers Prev 7:297–301, 1998.
115. Itoi T, Watanabe H, Mitsuhiro Y, Ajioka Y, Nishikura K, Saito T. Correlation of p53 protein expression with gene mutation in gallbladder carcinomas. Pathol Int 47:525–530, 1997.
116. Kiba T, Tsuda H, Pairojkul C, Inoue S, Sugimura T, Hiroshashi S. Mutations of the p53 tumor suppressor gene and the ras gene family in intrahepatic cholangiocellular carcinomas in Japan and Thailand. Mol Carcinog 8:312–318, 1993.
117. Petmitr S, Pinloar S, Thousungnoen A, Karalak A, Panata M. K-ras oncogene and p53 gene mutations in cholangiocarcinoma from Thai patients. Southeast Asian J Trop Med Public Health 29:71–75, 1998.
118. Harnois D, Que F, Celli A, LaRusso N, and Gores G: Bcl-2 is overexpressed and alters the threshold for apoptosis in a cholangiocarcinoma cell line. Hepatology 26:884–889,1997.
119. Rosen CB, Nagorney DM, Weisner RH, et al. Cholangiocarcinoma complicating primary sclerosing cholangitis. Ann Surg 213:21–25, 1991.
120. Todani T, Tabuchi K, Watanabe Y, et al. Carcinoma arising in the wall of the congenital bile duct cysts. Cancer 44:1134–1139, 1979.
121. Looser C, Stain SC, Baer HU, et al. Staging of hilar cholangiocarcinoma by ultrasound and duplex sonography: a comparison with angiography and preoperative findings. Br J Radiol 65:871–877, 1992.

122. Yamashita Y, Takahahi M, Kanazawa S, et al. Parenchymal changes of the liver in cholangiocarcinoma: CT evaluation. Gastrointest Radiol 17:161–166, 1992.

123. Desa LA, Akosa AB, Lazzara S, et al. Cytodiagnosis in management of extrahepatic biliary stricture. Gut 32:1118–1191, 1991.

124. Marsh JW, Iwatsuki S, Makowka L, et al. Orthotopic liver transplantation for primary sclerosing cholangitis. Ann Surg 207:21–25, 1988.

125. Nichols JC, Gores GJ, LaRusso NF, Weisner RH, Nagorney DM, Ritts RE. Diagnostic role of serum CA 19-9 for cholangiocarcinoma in patients with primary sclerosing cholangitis. Mayo Clinic Proc 68:874–879, 1992.

126. Ramage J, Donaghy A, Farrant M, Iorns R, Williams R. Serum tumor markers for the diagnosis of cholangiocarcinoma in primary sclerosing cholangitis. Gastroenterology 108:865–869, 1995.

127. Strom B, Maislin G, West S, et al. Serum CEA and CA 19-9: potential future diagnostic or screening tests for gallbladder cancer? Int J Cancer 45:821–824, 1990.

128. Korner T, Kropf J, Hackler R, Brenzel A, Gressner AM. Fibronectin in human bile fluid for diagnosis of malignant biliary diseases. Hepatology 23:423–428, 1996.

129. Rizzi PM, Ryder SD, Portman B, Ramage JK, Naomov NV, Williams R. p53 protein overexpression in cholangiocarcinoma in primary sclerosing cholangitis. Gut 38:265–268, 1996.

# Chapter 36

# Molecular Biology of Cholangiocarcinoma and Gallbladder Carcinoma

## MICHAEL GOGGINS

Neoplasia arises in a cell as a result of damage to multiple cancer-predisposing genes, each providing selection of progressively more autonomous clone(s) until characteristic features of cancer such as invasion and metastasis have been achieved. Many classes of cancer-causing genes are involved in cancer formation. Furthermore, in addition to defects in growth regulatory genes, increasingly, cancers are characterized by defects in genome maintenance.

Cholangiocarcinomas harbor a poor prognosis without optimal surgical treatment. Many patients present with inoperable disease, and even with radical surgery, 5-year survival is typically less than 25%. The prognosis after curative resection for gallbladder carcinoma is similarly poor (10%–30%).[1] A better understanding of the etiology of biliary tract carcinomas is needed to facilitate the development of preventative and treatment strategies.

### Risk Factors for Biliary Tract Carcinoma

The epidemiology of bile duct and gallbladder carcinoma is discussed in greater detail Chapter 35. Most known risk factors for biliary tract carcinomas are those that result in either chronic inflammation (such as primary sclerosing cholangitis, gallbladder or biliary tract stones, infection by parasites or typhoid carriage or, more rarely, Epstein-Barr virus) or carcinogen exposure.[1–6] Congenital anomalies of the biliary tract (maljunction of the biliopancreatic ducts, or cysts) are risk factors for subsequent cancer development acting through as yet unknown mechanisms. The nature of the molecular abnormalities caused by these risk factors remains unknown.

### Natural History of Biliary Tract Carcinomas

Dysplasia is identifiable in liver resection specimens and biopsies from patients with risk factors for biliary tract carcinoma such as primary sclerosing cholangitis.[7] As is probably true for all types of carcinoma, this observation suggests that biliary tract carcinoma evolves through a series of neoplastic precursors best exemplified by the natural history of colorectal carcinoma. The identification of clinically useful markers of biliary tract dysplasia would benefit patients with risk factors for this disease.

Although there is a familial tendency of primary sclerosing cholangitis and Caroli's syndrome,[8–10] there is no recognized inherited syndrome of isolated bile duct or gallbladder carcinoma. Several generalized cancer syndromes, however, target the biliary tract, as outlined below.

Although carcinomas of the biliary tract have not been as extensively studied as those of other more common cancers, a pattern is emerging which suggests that these cancers display genetic features similar, but not identical to, carcinoma of the pancreas and, to a lesser extent, carcinoma of the colon.

### Cancer-Causing Genes: Gatekeepers, Caretakers, and Guardsmen

Several eponyms are now used to describe cancer-causing genes. A *gatekeeper* is a gene whose sole function is to prevent neoplasia, and whose sole biallelic inactivation is sufficient to cause neoplastic transformation. A gatekeeper gene is so vital to the prevention of neoplasia in a given tissue that germline disruption of a gatekeeper typically leads to a recognizable inherited cancer syndrome. Examples of gatekeepers include the *Rb* gene responsible for retinoblastoma, and the *APC* gene mutated in the majority of colorectal cancers.[11] Vogelstein and Kinzler[11] have coined the term *caretaker* for a gene involved in genome maintenance whose inactivation facilitates the development of additional DNA damage, thereby accelerating the evolution to cancer. Examples of caretakers include the *BRCA2* and the mismatch repair genes. A broad class of cancer-causing genes is emerging

that have the common property of DNA or chromosome maintenance. From the many genes involved in recognizing DNA strand breaks (*p53*, *BRCA1*, *BRCA2*, *XRCC1*, and related; *Rad51* and related Rads; *PARP*, *ATM*, *DNA-PK*, *Ku*, and many others) and in recognizing mistakes during cell division (such as spindle cell checkpoint genes, *BUB1*, and others), it is clear that the caretaker group will encompass a large and diverse group of genes. Kern has extended the classification of cancer-related genes with the "guardsmen" concept.[12] *Guardsman* is used to describe the function of most tumor suppressor genes not directly involved in genome maintenance that function to suppress neoplasia, but whose sole inactivation is not sufficient to cause cancer.

## Tumor Suppressor Genes and Their Pathways

Tumor suppressor genes have been demonstrated to suppress oncogenesis by multiple mechanisms. Their functions may include maintaining cell cycle control, transcription regulation, apoptosis control, cytoskeletal function, and growth suppression mediated by several signal transduction pathways. Typically, tumor suppressor genes function within the context of a growth control pathway in which tumor promoting effects may occur when any one gene within a suppressive pathway is inactivated.

Carcinomas of the common bile duct may inactivate the p53, TGF-β, p16, STK11, MKK4, and, possibly, APC pathways. The patterns of tumor suppressor gene inactivation in gallbladder carcinoma have not been extensively studied.

### The TGF-β/*DPC4* pathway

Resistance to TGF-β–mediated growth suppression is a common property of cancer. Up to 80% of cancer cell lines studied lack the property of TGF-β–mediated growth suppression.[13] Many components of this pathway are altered in cancer. *DPC4* (*SMAD4*),[14,15] *TGFBR1* (*ALK-5*),[16] *TGFBR2*,[17,18] and *SMAD2*[19,20] have been identified as targets of inactivation by mutation, homozygous deletion, or loss of expression (in the case of *TGFBR2* and *ALK-5*) in several cancers. TGF-β normally suppresses oncogenesis by binding to TGFBR2, enabling the latter to heterodimerize with ALK-5. ALK-5 signals through SMAD2, SMAD3, and SMAD4,[21] driving DPC4 to the nucleus where it binds DNA and transactivates multiple downstream genes.[22] The introduction of DPC4 into cancer cells that lack DPC4 results in their growth arrest.[23] *ALK-5* activates other SMADs besides *DPC4*, which suggests the existence of some non–DPC4-mediated TGF-β signaling pathways.[21]

*DPC4* is genetically inactivated in ~20% of all bile duct cancers,[24] in 50% of pancreatic cancers and 20% of colorectal cancers,[14,25] and is occasionally targeted in other cancers such as breast and head and neck cancer.[15] Homozygous deletions of the *ALK-5* (*TGFBR1*) gene have also been identified in biliary and pancreatic cancer.[16] Loss of the expression of both the TGF-β type I and type II receptors has been described with moderate frequency in many cancers.[11] Genetic alterations of *TGFBR2* have not been described in bile duct or gallbladder carcinoma.

Inactivation of the TGF-β pathway in cancer has been associated with increased extracellular levels of TGF-β.[13] This gives rise to the apparently paradoxical situation in which a ligand from a tumor suppressor pathway may itself be elevated, and such elevations have been implicated in promoting cancer growth. These data are not in conflict with the tumor-suppressive function of the intracellular TGF-β pathway. Abrogation of the TGF-β pathway by downstream mutations may result in elevated TGF-β secretion into the surrounding matrix. Extracellular TGF-β may promote tumor growth by effects outside the neoplastic cell by promoting immunosuppression, changes in the extracellular matrix, and angiogenesis.[13]

### The *p16/Rb* pathway

The p16 pathway may be the most commonly inactivated tumor-suppressive pathway in human cancer. p16Ink4/CDKN2 is a cyclin-dependent kinase inhibitor that prevents the cooperative action of the cyclin-dependent kinase (CDK) CDK4 and cyclin D1 from phosphorylating Rb, binding to E2F and thereby moving the cell cycle out of late $G_1$ phase.[26,27] Several cancer types, such as small-cell and non–small-cell lung cancer, melanoma, and pancreatic cancer, show inactivation of this pathway in virtually 100% of cancers studied.[28–31] For small-cell lung cancer, *Rb* loss is almost universal, while for pancreatic cancer and non–small-cell lung cancer, *p16* loss by mutation, deletion, or methylation is the mechanism of pathway inactivation. Patients with germline *p16* mutations are at increased risk of melanoma[29] and pancreatic cancer.[30] Yoshida et al.[32] studied *p16* inactivation in biliary tract carcinomas and found that 16 of 25 (64%) biliary tract cancers had point mutations in the *p16* gene. The frequency of *p16* mutations in gallbladder cancer and hilar bile duct cancer was 80% (8 of 10) and 63% (5 of 8), respectively.[30] These figures probably underestimate the rate of genetic inactivation of *p16*, as homozygous deletions of this gene are common but can only rarely be identified when studying primary cancers. *p16* is also occasionally methylated in common bile duct carcinomas.[33] Overall, these data suggest that most biliary tract carcinomas, like many other cancers, have evolved through inactivation of the p16/Rb pathway.

### The *p53* pathway

The *p53* tumor suppressor gene is mutated in close to half of all human cancers.[34] Recent studies have helped refine our understanding of *p53* function, identified new upstream and downstream genes involved in *p53* responses, and characterized *p53* analogues. p53 is a transcription factor induced in response to DNA damage (reviewed in Levine[35]). Proteins known to induce p53 include p14[ARF], a gene that resides in the *p16* locus.[36–39] The viral oncoproteins SV40, adenovirus E1B, and HPVE6 all target p53.[34] Hypoxia induces p53 and this induction can be mediated by HIF-1α (hypoxia-inducible factor 1 alpha),[40–53] which suggests that the hypoxia present in a cancer nodule selects for cells that have lost p53-mediated hypoxia-induced apoptosis. p53 causes cell cycle arrest during $G_1$ through p21 induction and apoptosis mediated by *Bax* and several *PIG* genes.[35,44] p53 also contributes to radiation-induced $G_2$ arrest;[45,46] this function requires the cooperation of the ATM gene product.[47] Experimentally, wild-type *p53* suppresses angiogenesis through inhibition of vascular endothelial growth factor (VEGF),[36] a property that may explain the bystander effect observed when *p53* is delivered in viral vectors in human gene therapy trials for cancer. Additional genes transcriptionally activated by *p53* include *MDM-2*, *GADD45*, *IGF-BP3*,[35] and *p33ING1*.[48] A detailed analysis of genes that are induced by *p53* was carried out by Polyak et al.,[44] using the powerful molecular tool, serial analysis of gene expression (SAGE).[44] The authors identified a large number of p53-induced redox-related genes (PIG genes), leading them to hypothesize that these gene products induce apoptosis by stimulation of oxygen radicals culminating in mitochondrial de-

struction. The recent identification of mitochondrial DNA muta-tions in colorectal cancer raises the possibility that cancers may evade apoptosis and cell death by selecting mitochondria more resistant to apoptosis.[49]

p53 mutations frequently occur in gallbladder carcinoma (in roughly two-thirds of cases in one small series[50]). In cholangio-carcinomas arising in the context of primary sclerosing cholan-gitis, p53 overexpression, a surrogate marker of p53 mutation, is also common.[51]

## BRCA2

The BRCA2 gene product is thought to function as a mitosis maintenance gene. Working with the recombination repair pro-tein Rad51, BRCA2 prevents DNA strand breaks that can occur during normal cell division.[52,53] Patients deficient in functional BRCA2 may be prone to DNA stresses. A potentially significant therapeutic consequence of BRCA2 function is the associated in-creased radiosensitivity of BRCA2-deficient cells that has been observed in vitro and in animal models.[52,53] Investigations are currently underway to determine whether cancers from patients with germline BRCA2 mutations are more sensitive to radio-therapy. Such patients could also be sensitive to other types of radiation, such as X-rays. Although breast, ovarian, and pancre-atic carcinoma are the cancers most known for BRCA2 carri-ers,[54–57] recent data from the Breast Cancer Consortium suggest that BRCA2 mutation carriers also have a fivefold increased risk of carcinomas of the bile duct and gallbladder.[58] This study also suggests that patients with germline BRCA2 mutations may have increased lifetime risks of prostate, stomach, and melanoma skin cancer.[58] BRCA2 mutation carriers have a reduced penetrance of cancer and often a late age of onset, making it difficult to iden-tify gene carriers by clinical features alone.

## The Peutz-Jeghers (STK11) gene

STK11 is somatically mutated in a small proportion of pancreatic and biliary cancers.[59] Polyps in the common bile duct have been rarely described among patients with Peutz-Jeghers syndrome.[60]

## Other tumor suppressor genes

MKK4 is an occasional target of mutation in biliary cancer.[61] Cur-rently, the selective advantage provided by MKK4 inactivation in cancers is not known. A mutation profile of several recently iden-tified tumor suppressor genes such as PTEN, SNF5, and ptch have not been reported in carcinomas of the biliary tract.

## The APC (adenomatous polyposis coli) pathway

APC normally prevents tumorigenesis by sequestering β-catenin in the cytoplasm. The central portion of APC has a phosphory-lation domain that binds β-catenin. The absence of APC func-tion allows β-catenin to reach the nucleus and stimulate the ex-pression of the HMG box transcription factor, TCF4.[62] TCF4 stimulates c-myc (and probably other oncogenic pathways), ac-counting for the frequent overexpression, yet lack of amplifica-tion, of c-myc in colorectal carcinomas.[63] Over 80% of colorectal carcinomas exhibit mutation of the APC gene. In colorectal car-cinomas that do not target APC, β-catenin and, more recently, TCF4 mutations have been identified.[64,65] It is not certain whether patients with familial adenomatous polyposis (FAP) have an in-creased risk of cholangiocarcinoma, as not one case was observed in a large cohort of FAP kindreds.[66] While APC mutations have not been reported among patients with biliary tract carcinomas, patients with FAP occasionally develop cholangiocarcinoma.[67]

## Oncogenes

### K-ras

K-ras is commonly mutated in bile duct and gallbladder cancers (~75%).[68,69] The function of the K-ras pathway remains in-completely understood. Mutant K-ras induces transformation of cells in culture, and several downstream signals are induced by mutant K-ras in this setting. A more modest level of activation of the K-ras pathway results from mutation of K-ras in vivo, whereas in vitro studies create much higher levels of activation of the K-ras pathway.[70] For this reason, the important down-stream components of the K-ras pathway remain uncertain.

The K-ras protein requires farnesylation and methylation for binding the cell membrane and function. The ability of farnesyl transferase inhibitors to inhibit K-ras signal transduction has led to clinical trials of their use in cancer.[71]

Other oncogenes that may be important in biliary tract carci-noma include Her2 neu (Her2 or erbB2). Approximately two-thirds of cholangiocarcinomas display evidence of over-expression of Her2 on immunohistochemical analysis.[72,73] The identification of Her2 overexpression and subsequent elucidation of Her2 function have led to therapeutic targeting of this recep-tor. In clinical trials, Herceptin treatment improves survival of patients with breast cancers that overexpress the Her2 receptor.[74] Currently, trials are underway to study the effects of herceptin on other Her2-overexpressing carcinomas.

## Mismatch Repair Genes

Mismatch repair genes function to correct mistakes made in DNA synthesis during DNA replication. The identification of kindreds with the hereditary nonpolyposis colon cancer (HNPCC) syn-drome[75,76] and the discovery that tumors from patients with HNPCC typically have microsatellite instability (RER$^+$) sug-gestive of a mismatch repair defect ultimately led to the identi-fication of the human mismatch repair genes.[77] Six human DNA mismatch repair genes have been identified to date: hMSH2, hMLH1, hPMS1, hPMS2, hMSH6/GTBP, and hMSH3. Micro-satellite instability has been demonstrated in a wide variety of cancers.[78] Once both copies of a mismatch repair gene are inac-tivated, de novo mutations are not repaired appropriately and car-cinomas evolve relatively rapidly. This altered pathway of tumori-genesis may account for the clinicopathological differences between RER$^+$ and RER$^-$ cancers.[79–81]

There are no published reports of analysis of cholangiocarci-nomas or gallbladder carcinomas for evidence of microsatellite instability. Lynch et al. have reported several cases of cholan-giocarcinoma in HNPCC syndrome kindreds.[81,82]

## Chromosome Instability and Mitotic Checkpoint Genes

Genetic instability is an inherent feature of cancer, but investi-gators are only beginning to identify the molecular mechanisms underlying this instability. On the basis of studies in colorectal carcinoma, Lengauer et al.[83] have proposed that cancers can be classified as having one of two forms of genetic instability: mi-crosatellite instability (MIN) or chromosomal instability (CIN).[83] Cahill et al.[84] found that CIN cancers have a defect in mitotic spindle checkpoint function. In response to a mitotic spindle toxin, MIN cells with an intact checkpoint stop undergoing mi-tosis, but CIN cells do not. Two genes that regulate the mitotic

diated by the alternative reading frame product p19ARF. Cell 91:649–659, 1997.

39. Graeber TG, Peterson JF, Tsai M, Monica K, Fornace AJ Jr, Giaccia AJ. Hypoxia induces accumulation of p53 protein, but activation of a G1-phase checkpoint by low-oxygen conditions is independent of p53 status. Mol Cell Biol 14:6264–6277, 1994.

40. Graeber TG, Osmanian C, Jacks T, Housman DE, Koch CJ, Lowe SW, Giaccia AJ. Hypoxia-mediated selection of cells with diminished apoptotic potential in solid tumours. Nature 379:88–91, 1996.

41. An WG, Kanekal M, Simon MC, Maltepe E, Blagosklonny MV, Neckers LM. Stabilization of wild-type p53 by hypoxia-inducible factor 1alpha. Nature 392:405–408, 1998.

42. Carmeliet P, Dor Y, Herbert JM, Fukumura D, Brusselmans K, Dewerchin M, Neeman M, Bono F, Abramovitch R, Maxwell P, Koch CJ, Ratcliffe P, Moons L, Jain RK, Collen D, Keshet E. Role of HIF-1alpha in hypoxia-mediated apoptosis, cell proliferation and tumour angiogenesis. Nature 394:485–490, 1998.

43. Polyak K, Xia Y, Zweier JL, Kinzler KW, Vogelstein B. A model for p53-induced apoptosis. Nature 389:300–305, 1997.

44. Hermeking H, Lengauer C, Polyak K, He TC, Zhang L, Thiagalingam S, Kinzler KW, Vogelstein B. 14-3-3 sigma is a p53-regulated inhibitor of G2/M progression. Mol Cell 1:3–11, 1997.

45. Bunz F, Dutriaux A, Lengauer C, Waldman T, Zhou S, Brown JP, Sedivy JM, Kinzler KW, Vogelstein B. Requirement for p53 and p21 to sustain G2 arrest after DNA damage. Science 282:1497–501, 1998.

46. Waterman MJ, Stavridi ES, Waterman JL, Halazonetis TD. ATM-dependent activation of p53 involves dephosphorylation and association with 14-3-3 proteins. Nat Genet 19:175–178, 1998.

47. Bouvet M, Ellis LM, Nishizaki M, Fujiwara T, Liu W, Bucana CD, Fang B, Lee JJ, Roth JA. Adenovirus-mediated wild-type p53 gene transfer down-regulates vascular endothelial growth factor expression and inhibits angiogenesis in human colon cancer. Cancer Res 58:2288–2292, 1998.

48. Garkavtsev I, Grigorian IA, Ossovskaya VS, Chernov MV, Chumakov PM, Gudkov AV. The candidate tumour suppressor p33ING1 cooperates with p53 in cell growth control. Nature 391:295–298, 1998.

49. Polyak K, Li Y, Zhu H, Lengauer C, Willson JK, Markowitz SD, Trush MA, Kinzler KW, Vogelstein B. Somatic mutations of the mitochondrial genome in human colorectal tumours. Nat Genet 20:291–293, 1998.

50. Hanada K, Itoh M, Fujii K, Tsuchida A, Ooishi H, Kajiyama G. K-ras and p53 mutations in stage I gallbladder carcinoma with an anomalous junction of the pancreaticobiliary duct. Cancer 77:452–458, 1996.

51. Rizzi PM, Ryder SD, Portmann B, Ramage JK, Naoumov NV, Williams R. p53 protein overexpression in cholangiocarcinoma arising in primary sclerosing cholangitis. Gut 38:265–268, 1996.

52. Sharan SK, Morimatsu M, Albrecht U, Lim DS, Regel E, Dinh C, Sands A, Eichele G, Hasty P, Bradley A. Embryonic lethality and radiation hypersensitivity mediated by Rad51 in mice lacking BRCA2. Nature 386:804–810, 1997.

53. Abbott DW, Freeman ML, Holt JT. Double-strand break repair deficiency and radiation sensitivity in BRCA2 mutant cancer cells. J Natl Cancer Inst 90:978–985, 1998.

54. Struewing JP, Hartge P, Wacholder S, Baker SM, Berlin M, McAdams M, Timmerman MM, Brody LC, Tucker MA. The risk of cancer associated with specific mutations of BRCA1 and BRCA2 among Ashkenazi Jews. N Engl J Med 336:1401–1408, 1997.

55. Goggins M, Schutte M, Lu J, Moskaluk CA, Weinstein CL, Petersen GM, Yeo CJ, Jackson CE, Lynch HT, Hruban RH, Kern SE. Germline BRCA2 gene mutations in patients with apparently sporadic pancreatic carcinomas. Cancer Res 56:5360–5364, 1996.

56. Ozcelik H, Schmocker B, Di Nicola N, Shi XH, Langer B, Moore M, Taylor BR, Narod SA, Darlington G, Andrulis IL, Gallinger S, Redston M. Germline BRCA2 6174delT mutations in Ashkenazi Jewish pancreatic cancer patients. Nat Genet 16:17–18, 1997.

57. Tonin P, Weber B, Offit K, Couch F, Rebbeck TR, Neuhausen S, Godwin AK, Daly M, Wagner-Costalos J, Berman D, Grana G, Fox E, Kane MF, Kolodner RD, Krainer M, Haber DA, Struewing JP, Warner E, Rosen B, Lerman C, Peshkin B, Norton L, Serova O, Foulkes WD, Garber JE, et al. Frequency of recurrent BRCA1 and BRCA2 mutations in Ashkenazi Jewish breast cancer families. Nat Med 2:1179–1183, 1996.

58. Cancer risks in BRCA2 mutation carriers. J Natl Cancer Inst 91:1310–1316, 1999.

59. Su GH, Hruban RH, Bansal RK, Bova GS, Tang DJ, Shekher MC, Westerman AM, Entius MM, Goggins M, Yeo CJ, Kern SE. Germline and somatic mutations of the STK11/LKB1 Peutz-Jeghers gene in pancreatic and biliary cancers. Am J Pathol 154:1835–1840, 1999.

60. Nichols PH, Armstrong CP. Obstructed common bile duct from a Peutz-Jeghers polyp. Br J Surg 84:232, 1997.

61. Su GH, Hilgers W, Shekher MC, Tang DJ, Yeo CJ, Hruban RH, Kern SE. Alterations in pancreatic, biliary, and breast carcinomas support MKK4 as a genetically targeted tumor suppressor gene. Cancer Res 58:2339–2342, 1998.

62. He TC, Sparks AB, Rago C, Hermeking H, Zawel L, da Costa LT, Morin PJ, Vogelstein B, Kinzler KW. Identification of c-MYC as a target of the APC pathway. Science 281:1509–1512, 1998.

63. Morin PJ, Sparks AB, Korinek V, Barker N, Clevers H, Vogelstein B, Kinzler KW. Activation of beta-catenin-Tcf signaling in colon cancer by mutations in beta-catenin or APC. Science 275:1787–1790, 1997.

64. Sparks AB, Morin PJ, Vogelstein B, Kinzler KW. Mutational analysis of the APC/beta-catenin/Tcf pathway in colorectal cancer. Cancer Res 58:1130–1134, 1998.

65. Duval A, Gayet J, Zhou X-P, Iacopetta B, Thomas G, Hamelin R. Frequent frameshift mutations of the tcf-4 gene in colorectal cancers with microsatellite instability. Cancer Res 59:4213–4215, 1999.

66. Giardiello FM, Offerhaus GJ, Lee DH, Krush AJ, Tersmette AC, Booker SV, Kelley NC, Hamilton SR. Increased risk of thyroid and pancreatic carcinoma in familial adenomatous polyposis. Gut 34:1394–1396, 1993.

67. Smith MD, Robbins PD, Cullingford GL, Levitt MD. Cholangiocarcinoma and familial adenomatous polyposis. Aust N Z J Surg 63:324–327, 1993.

68. Watanabe M, Asaka M, Tanaka J, Kurosawa M, Kasai M, Miyazaki T. Point mutation of K-ras gene codon 12 in biliary tract tumors. Gastroenterology 107:1147–1153, 1994.

69. Matsubara T, Sakurai Y, Sasayama Y, Hori H, Ochiai M, Funabiki T, Matsumoto K, Hirono I. K-ras point mutations in cancerous and noncancerous biliary epithelium in patients with pancreaticobiliary maljunction. Cancer 77:1752–1757, 1996.

70. Hua VY, Wang WK, Duesberg PH. Dominant transformation by mutated human ras genes in vitro requires more than 100 times higher expression than is observed in cancers. Proc Natl Acad Sci USA 94:9614–9619, 1997.

71. Liu M, Bryant MS, Chen J, Lee S, Yaremko B, Lipari P, Malkowski M, Ferrari E, Nielsen L, Prioli N, Dell J, Sinha D, Syed J, Korfmacher WA, Nomeir AA, Lin CC, Wang L, Taveras AG, Doll RJ, Njoroge FG, Mallams AK, Remiszewski S, Catino JJ, Girijavallabhan VM, Bishop WR, et al. Antitumor activity of SCH 66336, an orally bioavailable tricyclic inhibitor of farnesyl protein transferase, in human tumor xenograft models and wap-ras transgenic mice. Cancer Res 58:4947–4956, 1998.

72. Chow NH, Huang SM, Chan SH, Mo LR, Hwang MH, Su WC. Significance of c-erbB-2 expression in normal and neoplastic epithelium of biliary tract. Anticancer Res 15:1055–1059, 1995.

73. Terada T, Ashida K, Endo K, Horie S, Maeta H, Matsunaga Y, Takashima K, Ohta T, Kitamura Y. c-erbB-2 protein is expressed in hepatolithiasis and cholangiocarcinoma. Histopathology 33:325–331, 1998.

74. Pegram MD, Lipton A, Hayes DF, Weber BL, Baselga JM, Tripathy D, Baly D, Baughman SA, Twaddell T, Glaspy JA, Slamon DJ. Phase II study of receptor-enhanced chemosensitivity using recombinant humanized anti-p185HER2/neu monoclonal antibody plus cisplatin in patients with HER2/neu-overexpressing metastatic breast cancer refractory to chemotherapy treatment. J Clin Oncol 16:2659–2671, 1998.

75. Vasen HF, Mecklin JP, Khan PM, Lynch HT. The International Collaborative Group on Hereditary Non-Polyposis Colorectal Cancer (ICG-HNPCC). Dis Colon Rectum 34:424–425, 1991.

76. Lynch HT, Smyrk TC, Lynch JF. Overview of natural history, pathology, molecular genetics and management of HNPCC (Lynch syndrome). Int J Cancer 69:38–43, 1996.

77. Boland CR. Hereditary non-polyposis colorectal cancer. In: Vogelstein B, Kinzler K (eds): The Genetic Basis of Human Cancer. MacGraw Hill, New York, 1998, pp 333–346.

78. Jass JR, Smyrk TC, Stewart SM, Lane MR, Lanspa SJ, Lynch HT. Pathology of hereditary non-polyposis colorectal cancer. Anticancer Res 14:1631–1634, 1994.

79. Kim H, Jen J, Vogelstein B, Hamilton SR. Clinical and pathological characteristics of sporadic colorectal carcinomas with DNA replication errors in microsatellite sequences. Am J Pathol 145:148–156, 1994.

80. Mecklin JP, Jarvinen HJ, Virolainen M. The association between cholangiocarcinoma and hereditary nonpolyposis colorectal carcinoma. Cancer 69:1112–1114, 1992.

81. Lynch HT, Richardson JD, Amin M, Lynch JF, Cavalieri RJ, Bronson E, Fusaro RM. Variable gastrointestinal and urologic cancers in a Lynch syndrome II kindred. Dis Colon Rectum 34:891–895, 1991.

82. Aarnio M, Mecklin JP, Aaltonen LA, Nystrom-Lahti M, Jarvinen HJ. Life-time risk of different cancers in hereditary non-polyposis colorectal cancer (HNPCC) syndrome. Int J Cancer 64:430–433, 1995.

83. Lengauer C, Kinzler KW, Vogelstein B. Genetic instability in colorectal cancers. Nature 386:623–627, 1997.

84. Cahill DP, Lengauer C, Yu J, Riggins GJ, Willson JK, Markowitz SD, Kinzler KW, Vogelstein B. Mutations of mitotic checkpoint genes in human cancers. Nature 392:300–303, 1998.

85. Goelz SE, Vogelstein B, Hamilton SR, Feinberg AP. Hypomethylation of DNA from benign and malignant human colon neoplasms. Science 228:187–190, 1985.

86. Feinberg AP, Vogelstein B. Hypomethylation distinguishes genes of some human cancers from their normal counterparts. Nature 301:89–92, 1983.

87. Lengauer C, Kinzler KW, Vogelstein B. DNA methylation and genetic instability in colorectal cancer cells. Proc Natl Acad Sci USA 94:2545–2550, 1997.

88. Chen RZ, Pettersson U, Beard C, Jackson-Grusby L, Jaenisch R. DNA hypomethylation leads to elevated mutation rates. Nature 395:89–93, 1998.

89. Nan X, Ng HH, Johnson CA, Laherty CD, Turner BM, Eisenman RN, Bird A. Transcriptional repression by the methyl-CpG-binding protein MeCP2 involves a histone deacetylase complex. Nature 393:386–389, 1998.

90. Baylin SB, Herman JG, Graff JR, Vertino PM, Issa JP. Alterations in DNA methylation: a fundamental aspect of neoplasia. Adv Cancer Res 72:141–196, 1998.

91. Toyota M, Ahuja N, Ohe-Toyota M, Herman JG, Baylin SB, Issa JP. CpG island methylator phenotype in colorectal cancer. Proc Natl Acad Sci USA 96:8681–8686, 1999.

92. Feinberg AP. Genomic imprinting and cancer. In: Vogelstein B, Kinzler K (eds): The Genetic Basis of Human Cancer. MacGraw Hill, New York, 1998, pp. 95–108.

93. Cui H, Horon IL, Ohlsson R, Hamilton SR, Feinberg AP. Loss of imprinting in normal tissue of colorectal cancer patients with microsatellite instability. Nat Med 4:1276–1280, 1998.

94. Kim NW, Piatyszek MA, Prowse KR, Harley CB, West MD, Ho PL, Coviello GM, Wright WE, Weinrich SL, Shay JW. Specific association of human telomerase activity with immortal cells and cancer. Science 266:2011–2015, 1994.

95. Niiyama H, Mizumoto K, Kusumoto M, Ogawa T, Suehara N, Shimura H, Tanaka M. Activation of telomerase and its diagnostic application in biopsy specimens from biliary tract neoplasms. Cancer 85:2138–2143, 1999.

96. Kolquist KA, Ellisen LW, Counter CM, Meyerson M, Tan LK, Weinberg RA, Haber DA, Gerald WL. Expression of TERT in early premalignant lesions and a subset of cells in normal tissues. Nat Genet 19:182–186, 1998.

97. Snijders PJ, van Duin M, Walboomers JM, Steenbergen RD, Risse EK, Helmerhorst TJ, Verheijen RH, Meijer CJ. Telomerase activity exclusively in cervical carcinomas and a subset of cervical intraepithelial neoplasia grade III lesions: strong association with elevated messenger RNA levels of its catalytic subunit and high-risk human papillomavirus DNA. Cancer Res 58:3812–3818, 1998.

98. Ozaki S, Harada K, Sanzen T, Watanabe K, Tsui W, Nakanuma Y. In situ nucleic acid detection of human telomerase in intrahepatic cholangiocarcinoma and its preneoplastic lesion. Hepatology 30:914–919, 1999.

# Chapter 37

# Pathology and Natural History of Cholangiocarcinoma and Gallbladder Carcinoma

ASIF RASHID AND STEVEN A. AHRENDT

Malignant tumors of the bile ducts and gallbladder are uncommon neoplasms. The bile ducts and gallbladder give rise to a wide variety of histopathological types of cancers, with adenocarcinoma being the most common type.[1,2] Bile duct cancers and gallbladder cancers differ in incidence, gender distribution, clinical features, association with lithiasis and other risk factors, frequency of histological types, and treatment. For example, gallbladder cancers are two to three times more common in women than in men, but no gender difference is present for bile duct cancer. Cholelithiasis is present in up to 90% of patients with gallbladder cancer but is no more common in patients who develop bile duct cancers than in the general population. Cancer of the extrahepatic bile ducts is associated with primary sclerosing cholangitis, choledochal cysts, or parasitic infections.

Malignancies of the bile ducts and gallbladder can be classified histopathologically into epithelial, endocrine, mesenchymal, and miscellaneous tumors (Table 37–1). Epithelial tumors can be further classified into adenocarcinomas, squamous cell carcinomas, adenosquamous carcinomas, and small cell carcinomas. Adenocarcinomas can be further subclassified as gland-forming adenocarcinomas (adenocarcinomas, not otherwise specified) or papillary, intestinal, pleomorphic giant cell, signet ring cell, mucinous (colloid), and clear cell types.

## Pathology and Natural History of Cholangiocarcinoma

Extrahepatic bile duct cancer arises in the common bile duct, cystic duct, common hepatic duct, the hepatic duct bifurcation, and the extrahepatic portions of the right and left hepatic ducts. These cancers present clinically with biliary obstruction and jaundice and are distinct from intrahepatic bile duct cancer, which presents with pain and/or a mass on imaging studies. The incidence of cholangiocarcinoma is approximately 1.0 case per 100,000 population per year in the United States.[3] The peak incidence of extrahepatic bile duct cancer occurs between ages 70 and 74 years. The median age of patients with bile duct cancer is 69 years, in contrast to 73 years for patients with gallbladder cancer.[3] Bile duct carcinomas are associated with choledochal cyst,[4,5] Caroli's disease–congenital hepatic fibrosis with intrahepatic biliary cysts,[6,7] primary sclerosing cholangitis,[8–13] liver fluke infestations,[14] and typhoid carrier state.[15]

Several anatomic classifications have been proposed for cholangiocarcinoma. Nakeeb and colleagues,[16] divided these tumors into intrahepatic, perihilar, and distal cholangiocarinomas. This scheme is particularly useful because it stratifies patients both by their clinical presentation and by the appropriate resection. Perihilar cholangiocarcinomas, or Klatskin tumors,[17] are the most common (67% of cases). They present with jaundice, and, when respectable, are managed through resection of the extrahepatic bile duct with or without a partial hepatectomy.[18–20] Distal cholangiocarcinomas, which are the second most common type (27% of cases), also present with jaundice. If possible, these tumors are managed by pancreaticoduodenectomy, similar to pancreatic and other periampullary neoplasms.[21–24] Intrahepatic cholangiocarcinomas are the least common (6% of cases) and are managed by hepatic resection, similar to hepatocellular carcinoma. Occasionally, cholangiocarcinomas may be multiple or diffuse and may require more extended resections.

Bismuth and colleagues[25] have classified cancers of the hepatic duct bifurcation according to their anatomic location. In this system, type I tumors are confined to the common hepatic duct; and type II tumors involve the bifurcation without involving secondary intrahepatic ducts. Type IIIa and IIIb tumors extend into either the right or left secondary intrahepatic ducts, respectively, and type IV tumors involve the secondary intrahepatic ducts on both sides.

**Table 37-1** Histopathological classification of malignant neoplasms of the bile duct, ampulla of vater, and gallbladder

*Malignant Epithelial Tumors*

Adenocarcinoma
    Not otherwise specified
    Papillary adenocarcinoma
    Mucinous adenocarcinoma
    Intestinal-type adenocarcinoma
    Clear cell adenocarcinoma
    Signet ring cell carcinoma
Adenosquamous carcinoma
Squamous cell carcinoma
Small cell (oat cell) carcinoma
Undifferentiated carcinoma

*Endocrine Tumors*

Carcinoid tumor
Mixed carcinoid–adenocarcinoma
Paraganglioma

*Malignant Mesenchymal Tumors*

Rhabdomyosarcoma
Leiomyosarcoma
Malignant fibrous histiocytoma
Kaposi's sarcoma
Angiosarcoma

*Miscellaneous Malignant Tumors*

Carcinosarcoma
Lymphoma
Melanoma

Bile duct carcinoma has several morphological variants: papillary (polypoid) or nodular, stricturing or sclerosing, and diffusely infiltrating. Papillary (16% of cases) and nodular (11% of cases) tumors are less common than the infiltrating or sclerosing types. Papillary and nodular tumors are most likely to extend superficially through the mucosa distant from the main tumor mass.[26] In contrast, the diffusely infiltrating type commonly extends through the submucosa or outside the bile duct via direct, vascular, lymphatic, or perineural invasion. Characteristically, extensive fibrosis and an inflammatory cell infiltrate accompany submucosal extension in diffusely infiltrating tumors. The proximal extension of a cancer usually is the critical factor in determining resectability in patients with perihilar cholangiocarcinoma. Sakamoto and colleagues[26] carefully analyzed the proximal extent of tumor in 62 patients with perihilar cholangiocarcinoma. Among patients with mucosal extension, usually nodular or papillary tumors, the mean proximal extension from the main tumor mass was 11 ± 11 mm, although extension up to 31 mm was observed. Among patients with submucosal extension, the mean proximal extension from the main tumor mass was 6 ± 4 mm, with the maximal proximal extent reaching 19 mm from the primary cancer. No anastomotic recurrences were observed in 32 patients in whom a tumor-free proximal margin of at least 5 mm was achieved.

The histological classification of adenocarcinomas of the bile duct includes well-differentiated, pleomorphic giant cell, adenosquamous, oat cell, and colloid types (Table 37–1).[1–3] Ninety-nine percent of extrahepatic bile duct cancers are carcinomas, and the vast majority of these (92%) are adenocarcinomas.[3] In this series of more than 3400 cases of extrahepatic bile duct cancer compiled from the Surveillance, Epidemiology, and End Results (SEER) Program of the National Cancer Institute, adeno-

carcinoma, not otherwise specified, was the most common subtype observed, accounting for 72% of the total cases.[3,27] Less common types included papillary adenocarcinomas and mucinous adenocarcinomas, accounting for 9% and 5%, respectively, of all carcinomas. In the series reported by Albores-Saavedera and colleagues,[2,28] 76% of carcinomas of the extrahepatic bile ducts were adenocarcinomas, 5.5% were adenosquamous carcinomas, 4.1% were papillary adenocarcinomas, and 4.1% were undifferentiated carcinomas.

Benign bile duct tumors can undergo malignant transformation.[29] Malignant transformation of both intrahepatic and extrahepatic cystadenomas, and biliary cystadenocarcinoma also have been recognized.[30–33] Similarly, biliary papillomatosis is characterized by multifocal papillary lesions involving the intrahepatic bile ducts, extrahepatic bile ducts, or both and can undergo malignant transformation.[34,35] Most adenocarcinomas of the extrahepatic bile duct express carcinoembryonic antigen (CEA), carbohydrate antigen 19.9 (CA 19.9), p21, and pS2.[36,37]

The sequence of dysplasia–carcinoma in situ–invasive carcinoma has been described in the bile duct but is observed less often than in the gallbladder.[38–41] Dysplasia was present in 10% of the bile duct carcinomas reported by Albores-Saavadera and Henson.[42] However, fewer than 1% of bile duct carcinomas were reported to develop within a preexisting adenoma in a review of the larger SEER database.[3]

Histologically, cholangiocarcinomas range from well-differentiated adenocarcinomas to undifferentiated carcinomas.[1–3,27,28] Often, nests of malignant cells are surrounded by an extensive desmoplastic reaction. The low neoplastic cellularity of these tumors contributes to the low sensitivity of diagnostic biliary cytology. In addition, the reactive epithelial cells due to presence of the inflammatory cell infiltrate associated with cholangitis or the presence of a biliary stent further adds to the difficulty in distinguishing between reactive and malignant cells. Brush cytology during endoscopic retrograde cholangiopanceatography (ERCP) plays an important role in distinguishing between benign stricture and malignancy and in confirming diagnosis before definitive treatment.[43]

Bile duct cancers usually spread by direct extension to adjacent organs and blood vessels. Proximal cancers may directly invade the liver. Extrahepatic bile duct cancers may also invade adjacent blood vessels, including the main, right, or left hepatic arteries or the main, right, or left portal veins. Approximately one-fourth of bile duct cancers are confined to the bile duct or show local vascular involvement at the time of diagnosis. However, 15%–30% of patients initially believed to have localized disease are found to have liver or peritoneal metastases during operative exploration.[44] Regional lymph node metastases or adjacent organ involvement (liver, gallbladder, duodenum) are common and are found in up to 50% of patients.[3] Distant metastases are found in 26% of patients at the time of diagnosis.[3]

Tumor stage at the time of diagnosis is the most important factor in determining prognosis.[45–52] The current staging system of extrahepatic bile duct cancer, based on the extent of tumor (T) at the primary site, presence or absence of regional lymph node involvement (N), and presence or absence of distant metastases (M), is shown in Table 37–2.[45] The 5-year survival rates for patients with localized (stages I and II) bile duct cancer is 26%.[3] The 5-year survival rates for patients with regional disease (stage III) at the time of diagnosis is 12%.[3] Median survival for patients with distant disease at diagnosis is 6 months. Left untreated, most patients with bile duct cancer will develop progressive hepatic failure. With appropriate palliative treatment, most patients die of tumor progression.

**Table 37-2** Primary tumor (T), lymph node (N), and metastasis (M) staging definitions for biliary tract cancers

| Category | Gallbladder | Extrahepatic Bile Ducts | Ampulla of Vater |
|---|---|---|---|
| **Primary Tumor (T)** | | | |
| TX | Primary tumor cannot be assessed | Primary tumor cannot be assessed | Primary tumor cannot be assessed |
| T0 | No evidence of primary tumor | No evidence of primary tumor | No evidence of primary tumor |
| Tis | Carcinoma in situ | Carcinoma in situ | Carcinoma in situ |
| T1 | Tumor invades lamina propria or muscle layer | Tumor confined to the bile duct histologically | Tumor limited to ampulla of Vater or spincter of Oddi |
| T1a | Tumor invades lamina propria | | |
| T1b | Tumor invades muscle layer | | |
| T2 | Tumor invades perimuscular connective tissue; no extension beyond serosa or into liver | Tumor invades beyond the wall of the bile duct | Tumor invades duodenal wall |
| T3 | Tumor perforates the serosa (visceral peritoneum), and/or directly invades one adjacent organ | Tumor invades the liver, pancreas, gallbladder, and/or unilateral branches of the portal view or hepatic artery | Tumor invades pancreas |
| T4 | Tumor invades main portal vein or hepatic artery or invades multiple extrahepatic organs | Tumor invades main portal vein or its branches bilaterally, or common hepatic artery or other adjacent structures such as colon, stomach, duodenum, or abdominal wall | Tumor invades peripancreatic soft tissues and/or into other adjacent organs |
| **Lymph Node (N)** | | | |
| NX | Regional lymph nodes cannot be assessed | Regional lymph nodes cannot be assessed | Regional lymph nodes cannot be assessed |
| N0 | No regional lymph node metastasis | No regional lymph node metastasis | No regional lymph node metastasis |
| N1 | Regional lymph mode metastasis | Regional lymph mode metastasis | Regional lymph node metastasis |
| **Distant Metastasis (M)** | | | |
| MX | Presence of distant metastasis cannot be assessed | Presence of distant metastasis cannot be assessed | Presence of distant metastasis cannot be assessed |
| M0 | No distant metastasis | No distant metastasis | No distant metastasis |
| M1 | Distant metastasis | Distant metastasis | Distant metastasis |
| **Stage Groupings** | | | |
| Stage 0 | Tis N0 M0 | Tis N0 M0 | Tis N0 M0 |
| Stage IA | T1 N0 M0 | T1 N0 M0 | T1 N0 M0 |
| Stage IB | T2 N0 M0 | T2 N0 M0 | T2 N0 M0 |
| Stage IIA | T3 N0 M0 | T3 N0 M0 | T3 N0 M0 |
| Stage IIB | T1 N1 M0 | T1 N1 M0 | T1 N1 M0 |
| | T2 N1 M0 | T2 N1 M0 | T2 N1 M0 |
| | T3 N1 M0 | T3 N1 M0 | T3 N1 M0 |
| Stage III | T4 Any N M0 | T4 Any N M0 | T4 Any N M0 |
| Stage IV | Any T Any N M1 | Any T Any N M1 | Any T Any N M1[a] |

Table modified from the American Joint Committee on Cancer Staging Manual.[45]

Several additional factors influence the natural history of patients with cholangiocarcinoma. The histological subtype may influence prognosis. Patients with papillary adenocarcinoma have an overall 5-year survival rate of 34%. In contrast, patients with adenocarcinoma not otherwise specified have an 11% 5-year survival.[3] Tumor differentiation also influences outcome in distal cholangiocarcinoma, with shorter survival times occurring among patients with poorly differentiated tumors.[16]

## Ampullary Cancers

Most ampullary carcinomas occur between the ages of 50 and 60 years. It is difficult to differentiate clinically tumors arising in the head of the pancreas, second part of the duodenum, ampulla, or terminal portion of the common duct. This distinction is important, however, as management and prognosis depend on whether the cancer arises in the ampulla, pancreas, common bile duct, or duodenal mucosa. An adenoma at the ampulla of Vater may be indistinguishable in presentation from the malignant lesion. Ampullary cancers are mostly adenocarcinomas, but a variety of other histological types can be seen.[1,2] Most ampullary carcinomas arise from adenomas, in contrast to gallbladder and bile duct carcinomas.[53] Yamaguchi and Enjoji[54] found 20 cases of unequivocal adenoma at the margins of 109 resected ampullary carcinomas. In addition, they detected carcinoma in situ in five adenomas of the ampulla of Vater.

The prognosis of ampullary carcinoma is associated with tumor differentiation and stage.[45,55–64] Akwari et al.[56] reported survival rates for 87 patients with ampullary carcinomas. Five-year survival rates for well-differentiated, moderately differentiated, and poorly differentiated tumors were 60%, 24%, and 0%, respectively. Two-year survival rates in moderately differentiated and poorly differentiated tumors were 58% and 30%, respectively. A similar trend has been reported in a smaller series.[55]

## Pathology of Gallbladder Cancer

Carcinoma of the gallbladder is the fifth most common malignancy of the gastrointestinal tract, with an incidence of 1.2–1.4 cases per 100,000 population per year in the United States, and is present in 1% of cholecystectomies performed in the United States.[2,3,41,65–68] Gallbladder carcinoma was present in 0.08% of all patients admitted at the M. D. Anderson Cancer Center.[69] The peak incidence of gallbladder cancer occurs between ages 70 to 75 years, and the female-to-male predominance is 3:1.[3,41,70] Carcinoma of the gallbladder is associated with gallstones in 70%–90% of cases,[42,71,72] and it is more likely to occur in association with gallstones among women. In two reported series of gallbladder carcinomas, cholelithiasis was present in 91% and 85% of women, but in only 59% and 68% of men, respectively.[42,72] Other conditions associated with an increased incidence of gallbladder carcinoma include an anomalous pancreatobiliary duct junction,[73–75] choledochal cyst,[76] 'porcelain' (calcified) gallbladder,[77,78] and *Salmonella typhi* carrier state.[79] In addition, gallbladder cancer has been diagnosed in up to 7% of elderly patients presenting with acute cholecystitis.[80]

A metaplasia–dysplasia–carcinoma sequence appears to be the major pathway to invasive gallbladder cancer.[81–85] Dysplasia and carcinoma in situ of the gallbladder are preinvasive forms of neoplasia. Dysplasia is histologically characterized by loss of uniform alignment of the epithelial cells, and pseudostratification and hyperchromasia of nuclei. Carcinoma in situ is histologically characterized by large nuclei and coarse chromatin granules. Carcinoma in situ may extend into Rokitansky-Aschoff sinuses and mucous glands in the mucosa.[86] In two reported series, dysplasia was present in 3.5% and 16% of gallbladders removed for cholelithiasis,[81,87] and carcinoma in situ was present in 2.5% of gallbladders removed for cholelithiasis.[87] Recent molecular genetics studies have shown that the genetic abnormalities found in dysplasia are the same as those of invasive carcinoma, providing additional support to the concept that dysplasia is precursor of invasive gallbladder cancer.[88] Rarely, invasive carcinoma arises from tubular or papillary adenomas of the gallbladder.[1,85,89]

According to the Surveillance, Epidemiology, and End Results (SEER) Program of the National Cancer Institute,[3] approximately 99% of all gallbladder cancers are carcinomas. Of these, 90% are adenocarcinomas. Well- or moderately differentiated adenocarcinoma is the most common histological subtype of gallbladder adenocarcinoma, accounting for 74% of invasive carcinoma. Papillary adenocarcinoma, mucinous adenocarcinoma, and squamous cell carcinomas, with or without glandular differentiation, are uncommon; each of these subtypes accounts for about 5% of cases.

Adenocarcinoma can arise in the body (30%), fundus (60%), or neck (10%) of the gallbladder.[42] These malignancies may appear as a raised mucosal plaque, a polypoid or papillary tumor, a large fungating mass, or as a focal or diffuse induration and thickening of the wall of the gallbladder. Tumors in the neck of the gallbladder or cystic duct can lead to collapse and contraction or to hydrops of the gallbladder. Those arising in the body of the gallbladder may cause an hourglass deformity. The infiltrating carcinomas are grayish-white and may be glistening if they are producing abundance of mucin.

Adenocarcinomas are characterized by glandular differentiation. The glands may be small and tubular, branching, or cystically dilated. In poorly differentiated adenocarcinomas, the neoplastic cells may grow in sheets or ribbons, in addition to forming glands. The cytoplasm is lightly eosinophilic. Nuclei are round to oval, hyperchromatic, and often vesicular; nucleoli are inconspicuous. The number of mitoses varies considerably from one tumor to another. The neoplastic cells have cytoplasmic and luminal mucin. The tumor cells typically express cytokeratin, CEA, and epithelial membrane antigen. α-Fetoprotein production is extremely rare.[90]

Papillary adenocarcinomas form branching, papillary fronds consisting of a fibrovascular stalk covered by columnar or cuboidal cells. The cells have basally located, hyperchromatic nuclei with variable atypia and mitotic activity. Mucin production is common. Tumors with many goblet cells have been subclassified as intestinal-type adenocarcinomas.[1,2,91]

Mucinous carcinomas produce a large quantity of mucus. The neoplastic cells are floating in a mucin pool. The in situ component may be gland-forming or papillary. Mucinous adenocarcinomas have a propensity to spread to the peritoneum and grow along the bile ducts more often than other histological types of adenocarcinomas.[1,2] Signet ring cell carcinoma is a variant of mucinous carcinoma.[1,2]

Clear cell carcinoma is an unusual but distinctive primary gallbladder cancer.[92] Because of the clear cell component, these tumors can be confused with metastatic renal cell carcinoma. However, clear cell carcinomas have shown foci of conventional adenocarcinoma that contain mucin and often are CEA positive. Cytokeratin 7 and CEA are useful immunohistochemical markers for distinguishing clear cell carcinoma of the gallbladder from metastatic renal cell carcinoma.

Squamous carcinomas have pure squamous cell differentiation, and adenosquamous carcinomas have an admixture of squamous and glandular differentiation.[1,2] Transition from dysplasia and squamous metaplasia of the gallbladder epithelium to squamous carcinoma has been noted.[2]

Small cell (oat cell) carcinoma of the gallbladder, which is comparable to small cell carcinoma of the lung, is a histologically distinct type of carcinoma with small round cells, usually mixed with a spindle cell component.[1–3,93–95] The carcinoma may show glandular or squamous component. Most patients with these tumors are women in the sixth or seventh decade of life who have coexisting gallstone disease. The tumor is highly lethal, with early metastases and death shortly after diagnosis. Cushing's syndrome due to adrenocorticotrophic hormone-secreting small cell carcinomas of the gallbladder has been reported.[95] Because of its characteristic morphological features, highly aggressive clinical behavior, occasional association with endocrine manifestations, and sensitivity to chemotherapy, small cell carcinoma should be distinguished from undifferentiated carcinoma.

Undifferentiated carcinoma is composed of variable proportions of spindle and giant cells and resembles a sarcoma.[96,97] Foci of well- to moderately differentiated adenocarcinoma or severe dysplasia are present in two-thirds of cases. The sarcomatoid component stains with cytokeratin and with vimentin in two-thirds of cases. Carcinoembryonic antigen staining is present in one-fifth of cases. This variant of carcinoma has an extremely poor prognosis. In one study, only 3 of 37 patients survived for more than 1 year.[97]

Carcinoid tumors of the gallbladder represent fewer than 1% of all digestive tract carcinoid tumors.[98,99] Composite tumors of the gallbladders consisting of a carcinoid tumor and an adenocarcinoma have been reported.[100,101]

All primary sarcomas of the gallbladder are rare.[1–3] These include rhabdomyosarcoma,[102] leiomyosarcoma, malignant fibrous histiocytoma, and angiosarcoma.

Carcinosarcomas are malignant tumors consisting of carcinomatous and sarcomatous elements.[2,103–106] These tumors are large and polypoid and often fill the gallbladder lumen. The carcinomatous component is either glandular or squamous, whereas the sarcomatous component may be fibrosarcoma, chondrosarcoma, or osteosarcoma. Malignant melanoma is rarely primary in the gallbladder.[2,107–110]

Fine-needle aspiration (FNA) biopsy of the gallbladder has a role in confirming the diagnosis of malignancy in patients with advanced carcinoma. In one study of 88 patients with a gallbladder mass, FNA had a sensitivity and specificity for diagnosing carcinoma of 88.5% and 100%, respectively.[111]

Nevin et al.,[112] developed the first clinically useful staging system for gallbladder cancer. The TNM system, described by the American Joint Committee on Cancer, is the preferred staging system (Table 37–2).[45] Patients with gallbladder cancer typically have tumor extending into the liver or distant metastases. Regional lymph node metastases are present in 50%–80% of patients at the time of diagnosis. Lymph node metastasis is an early event and is present in 15% of T1 lesions.[113,114] Local spread to the stomach, duodenum, colon, peritoneal surface, and cystic duct is common, as are hematogenous metastases to the liver and lung.

Lymphatic drainage from the gallbladder occurs in a reproducible and predictable fashion and correlates with the pattern of lymph node metastases seen in gallbladder cancer.[115,116] Lymph flow from the gallbladder initially drains to the cystic duct node and then descends along the common bile duct to the pericholedochal lymph nodes. Flow then proceeds to nodes posterior to the head of the pancreas and then to the interaortocaval lymph nodes. Secondary routes of lymphatic drainage include the retroportal and right celiac lymph nodes.[116]

Hepatic involvement can occur by direct invasion through the gallbladder bed, angiolymphatic portal tract invasion, or distant hematogenous spread.[117] Spread via the angiolymphatic portal tracts is the predominant mode of hepatic metastasis. Such spread may extend more than 1 cm from the main tumor mass, and it correlates well with the depth of direct invasion of the liver. Distant spread beyond the region of the gallbladder is associated with hematogenous metastases elsewhere.

## Natural History of Gallbladder Cancer

The prognosis of patients with gallbladder carcinoma is dismal. Overall, 60%–80% are dead within 1 year of diagnosis, and the 5-year survival is only 12%.[3,65,118] Although histological type and histological grade correlate with outcome, disease stage at the time of diagnosis is the most important predictor of outcome.[3,45,65–67,118] In one study, the 5-year survival for patients with localized disease was 42%, compared with only 4% for patients with regional stage disease and less than 1% for those with distant stage disease.[1] Stage T1a gallbladder carcinoma has the most favorable prognosis. In one series, 35 patients with incidentally discovered T1a gallbladder cancer had an overall 5-year survival of 100%.[119] Invasion into the muscular wall of the gallbladder increases the risk of recurrent cancer after curative resection. In a survey of 172 major hospitals in Japan, the 5-year survival for patients with T1b tumors was 72%.[120] Invasion into either the muscularis or into the subserosa increases the risk of regional lymph node metastases to 15% and 50%, respectively.[114] Five-year survival in patients with either lymph node or distant metastases is 5% or less.[3,121]

Compared with other major histological subtypes of carcinomas, papillary adenocarcinomas have a better stage at presentation and a better outcome.[3] Carriaga and Henson[3] reported that the relatively high survival rate of patients with papillary adenocarcinoma was related to the stage of disease: 64% of patients with papillary adenocarcinomas had localized disease at diagnosis. In contrast, 11% of patients with nondistinctive adenocarcinomas and 19% of those with mucinous adenocarcinomas had localized disease at diagnosis. The 5-year survival rate of papillary adenocarcinomas was 41%, whereas it was 11% for patients with nondistinctive adenocarcinomas and 8% for those with mucinous adenocarcinomas. The undifferentiated and small cell variants of carcinomas are associated with a uniformly poor prognosis; most patients die within a few months of diagnosis.[2]

## References

1. Albores-Saavedra J, Henson DE, Sobin LH. In: Albores-Saavedra J, Henson DE, Sobin LH (eds): WHO Histological Classification of Tumors of the Gallbladder and Extrahepatic Bile Ducts. Springer-Verlag, Berlin, 1991, pp 1–75.
2. Albores-Saavedra J, Henson DE, Klimstra DS. Histological typing of tumours of the gallbladder and extrahepatic bile ducts. In: Rosai J (ed): Tumors of the Gallbladder and Extrahepatic Bile Ducts, Series 3, Fascicle 27. Armed Forces Institute of Pathology, Washington, DC, 2000, pp 1–265.
3. Carriaga MT, Henson DE. Liver, gallbladder, extrahepatic bile ducts, and pancreas. Cancer 75:171–190, 1995.
4. Kagawa Y, Kashihara S, Kuramoto S, Maetani S. Carcinoma arising in a congenitally dilated biliary tract: report of a case and review of the literature. Gastroenterology 74:1286–1294, 1978.
5. Voyles CR, Smadja C, Shands WC, Blumgart LH. Carcinoma in choledochal cysts: age-related incidence. Arch Surg 118:986–988, 1983.

6. Bismuth H, Corlette MB. Intrahepatic cholangioenteric anastomosis in carcinoma of the hilus of the liver. Surg Gynecol Obstet 140:170–178, 1975.

7. Dayton MT, Longmire WP Jr, Tompkins RK. Caroli's disease: a premalignant condition? Am J Surg 145:41–48, 1983.

8. Wee A, Ludwig J, Coffey RJ Jr, LaRusso NF, Wiesner RH. Hepatobiliary carcinoma associated with primary sclerosing cholangitis and chronic ulcerative colitis. Hum Pathol 16:719–726, 1985.

9. Mir-Madjlessi SH, Farmer RG, Sivak MV Jr. Bile duct carcinoma in patients with ulcerative colitis. Relationship to sclerosing cholangitis: report of six cases and review of the literature. Dig Dis Sci 32:145–154, 1987.

10. Cullingford GL, Carr-Locke DL. Sclerosing cholangitis: variations in its clinical course. Eur J Gastroenterol Hepatol 3:329–335, 1991.

11. Rosen CB, Nagorney DM. Cholangiocarcinoma complicating primary sclerosing cholangitis. Semin Liver Dis 11:26–30, 1991.

12. Bergquist A, Glaumann H, Persson B, Broome U. Risk factors and clinical presentation of hepatobiliary carcinoma in patients with primary sclerosing cholangitis: a case–control study. Hepatology 27:311–316, 1998.

13. Ahrendt SA, Pitt HA, Nakeeb A, et al. Diagnosis and management of cholangiocarcinoma in primary sclerosing cholangitis. J Gastrointest Surg 3:357–368, 1999.

14. Kurathong S, Lerdverasirikul P, Wongpaitoon V, et al. *Opisthorchis viverrini* infection and cholangiocarcinoma. Gastroenterology 89:151–156, 1985.

15. Welton JC, Marr JS, Friedman SM. Association between hepatobiliary cancer and typhoid carrier state. Lancet 1:791–794, 1979.

16. Nakeeb A, Pitt HA, Sohn TA, et al. Cholangiocarcinoma: a spectrum of intrahepatic, perihilar, and distal tumors. Ann Surg 224:463–475, 1996.

17. Klatskin G. Adenocarcinoma of the hepatic duct at its bifurcation within the porta hepatis: an unusual tumor with distinctive clinical and pathological features. Am J Med 38:241–256, 1965.

18. Bengmark S, Ekberg H, Evander A, Klofver-Stahl B, Tranberg KG. Major liver resection for hilar cholangiocarcinoma. Ann Surg 207:120–125, 1988.

19. Burke EC, Jarnagin WR, Hochwald SN, Pisters PW, Fong Y, Blumgart LH. Hilar cholangiocarcinomas: patterns of spread, the importance of hepatic resection for curative operation, and a presurgical staging system. Ann Surg 228:385–394, 1998.

20. Iwasaki Y, Okamura T, Ozaki A, et al. Surgical treatment for carcinoma at the confluence of the major hepatic ducts. Surg Gynecol Obstet 162:457–464, 1986.

21. Langer JC, Langer B, Taylor BR, Zeldin R, Cummings B. Carcinoma of the extrahepatic bile ducts: results of an aggressive surgical approach. Surgery 98:752–759, 1985.

22. Madariaga JR, Iwatsuki S, Todo S, Lee RG, Irish W, Starzl TE. Liver resection for hilar and peripheral cholangiocarcinomas: a study of 62 patients. Ann Surg 227:70–79, 1998.

23. Pichlmayr R, Weimann A, Klempnauer J, et al. Surgical treatment in proximal bile duct cancer: a single-center experience. Ann Surg 224:628–638, 1996.

24. Pinson CW, Rossi RL. Extended right hepatic lobectomy, left hepatic lobectomy, and skeletonization resection for proximal bile duct cancer. World J Surg 12:52–59, 1988.

25. Bismuth H, Nakache R, Diamond T. Management strategies in resection for hilar cholangiocarcinoma. Ann Surg 215:31–38, 1992.

26. Sakamoto E, Nimura Y, Hayakawa N, et al. The pattern of infiltration at the proximal border of hilar bile duct carcinoma: a histological analysis of 62 resected cases. Ann Surg 227:405–411, 1998.

27. Nakajima T, Kondo Y. Well-differentiated cholangiocarcinoma: diagnostic significance of morphologic and immunohistochemical parameters. Am J Surg Pathol 13:569–573, 1989.

28. Albores-Saavedra J, Delgado R, Henson DE. Well-differentiated adenocarcinoma, gastric foveolar type, of the extrahepatic bile ducts: a previously unrecognized and distinctive morphological variant of bile duct carcinoma. Ann Diagn Pathol 3:75–80, 1999.

29. Ishak KG, Willis GW, Cummins SD, Bullock AA. Biliary cystadenoma and cystadenocarcinoma: report of 14 cases and review of the literature. Cancer 39:322–338, 1977.

30. Wheeler DA, Edmondson HA. Cystadenoma with mesenchymal stroma (CMS) of the liver and bile ducts: a clinicopathologic study of 17 cases, 4 with malignant change. Cancer 56:1434–1445, 1985.

31. O'Shea JS, Shah D, Cooperman AM. Biliary cystadenocarcinoma of extrahepatic duct origin arising in previously benign cystadenoma. Am J Gastroenterol 82:1306–1310, 1987.

32. Akwari OE, Tucker A, Seigler HF, Itani KMF. Hepatobiliary cystadenoma with mesenchymal stroma. Ann Surg 211:18–27, 1990.

33. Sielezneff I, Ferrero A, Chapel F, Le Treut Y-P. Le cystadenomes des voies bilares extra hepatiques: une cause rare d'ictere cholestatique. Gastroenterol Clin Biol 16:708–713, 1992.

34. Neumann RD, LiVolsi VA, Rosenthal NS, et al. Adenocarcinoma in biliary papillomatosis. Gastroenterology 70:779–782, 1976.

35. Gouma DJ, Mutum SS, Benjamin IS, Blumgart LH. Intrahepatic biliary papillomatosis. Br J Surg 71:72–74, 1984.

36. Yamaguchi K, Enjoji M, Nakayama F. Cancer of the extrahepatic bile duct: a clinicopathologic study of immunohistochemistry for CEA, CA 19-9, and p21. World J Surg 12:11–17, 1988.

37. Seitz G, Thelsinger B, Tomasetto G, et al. Breast cancer–associated protein pS2 expression in tumors of the biliary tract. Am J Gastroenterol 86:1491–1494, 1991.

38. Laitio M. Histogenesis of epithelial neoplasms of human gallbladder I: dysplasia. Pathol Res Pract 178:51–56, 1983.

39. Kurashina M, Kozuka S, Nakasima N, Hirabayasi N, Ito M. Relationship of intrahepatic bile duct hyperplasia to chonangiocellular carcinoma. Cancer 61:2469–2474, 1988.

40. Haworth AC, Manley PN, Groll A, Pace R. Bile duct carcinoma and biliary tract dysplasia in chronic ulcerative colitis. Arch Pathol Lab Med 113:434–436, 1989.

41. Henson DE, Albores-Saavedra J, Corle D. Carcinoma of the gallbladder: histologic types, stage of disease, grade, and survival rate. Cancer 70:1493–1497, 1992.

42. Albores-Saavedra J, Henson DE. Precursor lesions. In: Hartmann WH (ed): Tumors of the Gallbladder and Extrahepatic Bile Ducts, Series 2, Fascicle 22. Armed Forces Institute of Pathology, Washington, DC, 1986, pp 44–53.

43. Ferrari AP Jr, Lichtenstein DR, Slivka A, Chang C, Carr-Locke DL. Brush cytology during ERCP for the diagnosis of biliary and pancreatic malignancies. Gastrointest Endosc 40:140–145, 1994.

44. Cameron JL, Pitt HA, Zinner MJ, Kaufman SL. Management of proximal cholangiocarcinoma by surgical resection and radiotherapy. Am J Surg 159:91–97, 1990.

45. American Joint Committee on Cancer. Gallbladder, extrahepatic bile ducts, and ampulla of Vater. In: Green FL, Page DL, Fleming ID, et al. (eds): AJCC Cancer Staging Manual, 6th ed. Springer-Verlag New York, Inc., New York, 2002, pp 139–156.

46. Tompkins RK, Thomas D, Wile A, Longmire WP Jr. Prognostic factors in bile duct carcinoma. Ann Surg 194:447–457, 1981.

47. Alexander F, Rossi RL, O'Bryan M, Khettry U, Braasch JW, Watkins E Jr. Biliary carcinoma: a review of 109 cases. Am J Surg 147:503–509, 1984.

48. Saunders K, Tompkins R, Longmire W Jr, Roslyn J. Bile duct carcinoma in the elderly: a rationale for surgical management. Arch Surg 126:1186–1190, 1991.

49. Henson DE, Albores-Saavedra J, Corle D. Carcinoma of the extrahepatic bile ducts: histological types, stage of disease, grade, and survival rate. Cancer 70:1498–1501, 1992.

50. Schoenthaler R, Phillips TL, Castro J, Efird JT, Better A, Way LW. Carcinoma of the extrahepatic bile ducts: the University of California at San Francisco experience. Ann Surg 219:267–274, 1994.

51. Su C-H, Tsay S-H, Wu C-C, et al. Factors influencing postoperative morbidity, mortality, and survival after resection for hilar cholangiocarcinoma. Ann Surg 223:384–394, 1996.

52. Klempnauer J, Ridder GJ, von Wasielewski R, Werner M, Weimann A, Pichlmayr R. Resectional surgery of hilar cholangiocarcinomas: a multivariate analysis of prognostic factors. J Clin Oncol 15:947–954, 1997.

53. Baczako K, Buchler M, Berger HG, Kirkpatrick CJ, Haferkamp O. Morphogenesis and possible precursor lesions of invasive carcinoma of the papilla of Vater: epithelial dysplasia and adenoma. Hum Pathol 16:305–310, 1985.

54. Yamaguchi K, Enjoli M. Carcinoma of the ampulla of Vater: a clinicopathologic study and pathologic staging of 109 cases of carcinoma and 5 cases of adenoma. Cancer 59:506–515, 1987.

55. Blumgart LH, Kennedy A. Carcinoma of the ampulla of Vater and duodenum. Br J Surg 60:33–40, 1973.

56. Akwari OE, van Heerden JA, Adson MA, Baggenstoss AH. Radical pancreatoduodenectomy for cancer of the papilla of Vater. Arch Surg 112:451–456, 1977.

57. Delcore R Jr, Connor CS, Thomas JH, Friesen SR, Hermreck AS. Significance of tumor spread in adenocarcinoma of the ampulla of Vater. Am J Surg 158:593–596, 1989.

58. Allema JH, Reinders ME, van Gulik TM, et al. Prognostic factors for survival after pancreaticoduodenectomy for patients with carcinoma of the pancreatic head region. Cancer 75:2069–2076, 1995.

59. Allema JH, Reinders ME, van Gulik TM, et al. Results of pancreati-coduodenectomy for ampullary carcinoma and analysis of prognostic factors for survival. Surgery 117:247–253, 1995.

60. Bakkevold KE, Kambestad B. Staging of carcinoma of the pancreas and ampulla of Vater. Tumor (T), lymph node (N), and distant metastasis (M) as prognostic factors. Int J Pancreatol 17:249–259, 1995.

61. El-Ghazzawy AG, Wade TP, Virgo KS, Johnson FE. Recent experience with cancer of the ampulla of Vater in a national hospital group. Am Surg 61:607–611, 1995.

62. Bottger TC, Boddin J, Heintz A, Junginger T. Clinicopathologic study for the assessment of resection for ampullary carcinoma. World J Surg 21:379–383, 1997.

63. Howe JR, Klimstra DS, Moccia RD, Conlon KC, Brennam MF. Factors predictive of survival in ampullary carcinoma. Ann Surg 228:87–94, 1998.

64. Klempnauer J, Ridder GJ, Pichlmayr R. Prognostic factors after resection of ampullary carcinoma: multivariate survival analysis in comparison with ductal cancer of the pancreatic head. Br J Surg 82:1686–1691, 1995.

65. Piehler JM, Cricklow RW. Primary carcinoma of the gallbladder. Surg Gynecol Obstet 147:929–942, 1978.

66. Jones RS. Carcinoma of the gallbladder. Surg Clin North Am 70:1419–1428, 1990.

67. Pitt HA, Dooley WC, Yeo CJ, Cameron JL. Malignancies of the biliary tree. Curr Probl Surg 32:1–90, 1995.

68. Silverberg E, Lubera JA. Cancer statistics, 1989. CA Cancer J Clin 39:3–20, 1989.

69. Perpetuo MD, Valdivieso M, Heilbrun LK, Nelsen RS, Connor T, Bodey GP. Natural history study of gallbladder cancer. A review of 36 years, experience at M. D. Anderson Hospital and Tumor Institute. Cancer 42:330–335, 1978.

70. Solan MJ, Jackson BT. Carcinoma of the gallbladder: a clinical appraisal and review of 57 cases. Br J Surg 58:593–597, 1971.

71. Ohlsson EG, Aronsen KF. Carcinoma of the gallbladder: a study of 181 cases. Acta Chir Scand 140:475–480, 1974.

72. Thorbjarnarson B, Glenn F. Carcinoma of the gallbladder. Cancer 12:1009–1014, 1959.

73. Kinoshita H, Nagata E, Hirohashi K, Sakai K, Kobayashi Y. Carcinoma of the gallbladder with an anomalous connection between the choledochus and the pancreatic duct: report of 10 cases and review of the literature in Japan. Cancer 54:762–769, 1984.

74. Tanaka K, Nishimura A, Yamada K, et al. Cancer of the gallbladder associated with anomalous junction of the pancreatobiliary duct system without bile duct dilatation. Br J Surg 80:622–624, 1993.

75. Tanno S, Obara T, Maguchi H, et al. Association between anomalous pancreaticobiliary ductal union and adenomyomatosis of the gallbladder. J Gastroenterol Hepatol 13:175–180, 1998.

76. Komi M, Tamura T, Miyoshi Y, Kunitomo K, Udaka H, Takehara H. Nationwide survey of cases of choledochal cyst: analysis of coexistent anomalies, complications and surgical treatment in 64 cases. Surg Gastroenterol 3:69–73, 1984.

77. Ashur H, Siegal B, Oland Y, Adam YG. Calcified gallbladder (porcelain gallbladder). Arch Surg 113:594–596, 1978.

78. Polk HC Jr. Carcinoma and the calcified gallbladder. Gastroenterology 50:582–585, 1966.

79. Caygill CP, Hill MJ, Braddick M, Sharp JC. Cancer mortality in chronic typhoid and paratyphoid carriers. Lancet 343:83–84, 1994.

80. Liu KJ, Richter HM, Cho MJ, Jarad J, Nadimpalli V, Donahue PE. Carcinoma involving the gallbladder in elderly patients presenting with acute cholecystitis. Surgery 122:748–756, 1997.

81. Albores-Saavedra J, Alcantara-Vazquez A, Cruz-Ortiz H, Herrera-Goepfert R. The precursor lesions of invasive gallbladder cancer: hyperplasia, atypical hyperplasia and carcinoma in situ. Cancer 45:919–927, 1980.

82. Albores-Saavedra J, de Jesus Manrique J, Angeles-Angeles A, Henson DE. Carcinoma in situ of the gallbladder. Am J Surg Pathol 8:323–333, 1984.

83. Yamaguchi K, Enjoji M. Carcinoma of the gallbladder: a clinicopathology of 103 patients and a newly proposed staging. Cancer 62:1425–1432, 1988.

84. Yamamoto M, Nakajo S, Tahara E. Dysplasia of the gallbladder: its histogenesis and correlation to gallbladder adenocarcinoma. Pathol Res Pract 185:454–460, 1989.

85. Kijima H, Watanabe H, Iwafuchi M, Isihara N. Histogenesis of gallbladder carcinoma from investigation of early carcinoma and microcarcinoma. Acta Pathol Jpn 39:235–244, 1989.

86. Born MW, Ramey WG, Ryan SF, Gordon PE. Carcinosarcoma and carcinoma of the gallbladder. Cancer 53:2171–2177, 1984.

87. Duarte I, Llanos O, Domke H, Harz C, Valdivieso V. Metaplasia and precursor lesions of gallbladder carcinoma. Cancer: frequency, distribution, and probability of detection in routine histological samples. Cancer 72:1878–1884, 1993.

88. Wistuba I, Miquel AF, Gazdar AF, Albores-Saavedra J. Gallbladder adenomas have molecular abnormalities different from those present in gallbladder carcinomas. Hum Pathol 30:21–25, 1999.

89. Kozuka S, Tsubone M, Yasui A, Hachisuka K. Relation of adenoma to carcinoma in the gallbladder. Cancer 50:2226–2234, 1982.

90. Watanabe M, Hori Y, Nojima T, et al. Alpha-fetoprotein producing carcinoma of the gallbladder. Dig Dis Sci 38:561–564, 1993.

91. Albores-Saavedra J, Cruz-Ortiz H, Alcantara-Vazquez A, Henson DE. Unusual types of gallbladder cancer: a report of 16 cases. Arch Pathol Lab Med 105:287–293, 1981.

92. Vardaman C, Albores-Saavedra J. Clear cell carcinoma of the gallbladder and extrahepatic bile ducts. Am J Surg Pathol 19:91–99, 1995.

93. Albores-Saavedra J, Soriano J, Larraza-Hernandez O, Aguirre J, Henson DE. Oat cell carcinoma of the gallbladder. Hum Pathol 15:639–646, 1984.

94. Iida Y, Tsutsumi Y. Small cell (endocrine cell) carcinoma of the gallbladder with squamous and adenocarcinomatous components. Acta Pathol Jpn 42:119–125, 1992.

95. Spence RW, Burns-Cox CJ. ACTA-secreting 'apudoma' of gallbladder. Gut 16:473–476, 1975.

96. Appelman HD, Coopersmith N. Pleomorphic spindle cell carcinoma of the gallbladder: relation to sarcoma of the gallbladder. Cancer 25:535–541, 1970.

97. Albores-Saavedra J, Molberg K, Henson DE. Unusual malignant epithelial tumors of the gallbladder. Semin Diagn Pathol 13:326–338, 1996.

98. Bosl GJ, Yagoda A, Camara-Lopes LH. Malignant carcinoid of the gallbladder: third reported case and review of the literature. J Surg Oncol 13:215–222, 1980.

99. Goodman ZD, Albores-Saavedra J, Lundblad DM. Somatostatinoma of the cystic duct. Cancer 53:498–502, 1984.

100. Wisniewski M, Token C. Composite tumor of the gallbladder exhibiting both carcinomatous and carcinoidal patterns. Am J Gastroenterol 58:633–637, 1972.

101. Muto Y, Okamoto K, Urhimura M. Composite tumor (ordinary adenocarcinoma) typical carcinoid, and goblet cell adenocarcinoma of the gallbladder: a variety of composite tumor. Am J Gastroenterol 79:647–649, 1984.

102. Mihara S, Matsumoto H, Tokunaga F, Yano H, Ota M, Yamashita S. Botryoid rhabdomyosarcoma of the gallbladder in a child. Cancer 49:412–418, 1982.

103. Mehrotra TN, Gupta SC, Naithani YP. Carcinosarcoma of the gallbladder. J Pathol 104:145–148, 1971.

104. Higgs WR, Mocega EE, Jordan PH Jr. Malignant mixed tumour of the gallbladder. Cancer 32:471–475, 1973.

105. Mansori KS, Cho SY. Malignant mixed tumor of the gallbladder. Am J Clin Pathol 73:709–711, 1980.

106. von Kuster LC, Cohen C. Malignant mixed tumors of the gallbladder: report of two cases and a review of the literature. Cancer 50:1166–1182, 1982.

107. Sierra-Callejas JL, Warecka K. Primary malignant melanoma of the gallbladder. Virchows Arch A Pathol Anat Histol 370:233–238, 1976.

108. Peison B, Rabin L. Malignant melanoma of the gallbladder: report of three cases and review of the literature. Cancer 37:2448–2454, 1976.

109. Hatae Y, Kikuchi M, Segawa M, Yonemitsu K. Malignant melanoma of the gallbladder. Pathol Res Pract 163:281–287, 1978.

110. Anderson JB, Hughes RG, Williamson RCN. Malignant melanoma of the gallbladder. Postgrad Med J 59:390–391, 1983.

111. Zargar SA, Khuroo MS, Mahajan R, Jan GM, Shah P. US-guided fine needle aspiration biopsy of gallbladder masses. Radiology 179:275–278, 1991.

112. Nevin JE, Moran TJ, Kay S, King R. Carcinoma of the gallbladder: staging, treatment, and prognosis. Cancer 37:141–148, 1976.

113. Wilkinson DS. Carcinoma of the gallbladder: an experience and review of the literature. Aust N Z J Surg 65:724–727, 1995.

114. Tsukada K, Hatakeyama K, Kurosaki I, et al. Outcome of radical surgery for carcinoma of the gallbladder according to the TNM stage. Surgery 120:816–822, 1996.

115. Fahim RB, McDonald JR, Richards JC, et al. Carcinoma of the gallbladder: a study of its modes of spread. Ann Surg 156:114–123, 1962.

116. Shirai Y, Yoshida K, Tsukada K, Ohtani T, Muto T. Identification of the regional lymphatic system of the gallbladder by vital staining. Br J Surg 79:659–662, 1992.

117. Shirai Y, Tsukada K, Ohtani T, Watanabe H, Hatakeyama K. Hepatic metastases from carcinoma of the gallbladder. Cancer 75:2063–2068, 1995.

118. Bartlett DL, Fong Y, Fortner JG, Brennan MF, Blumgart LH. Long-term results after resection for gallbladder cancer: implications for staging and management. Ann Surg 224:639–646, 1996.

119. Shirai Y, Yoshida K, Tsukada K, Muto T. Inapparent carcinoma of the gallbladder: an appraisal of a radical second operation after simple cholecystectomy. Ann Surg 215:326–331, 1992.

120. Ogura Y, Mizumoto R, Isaji S, Kusuda T, Matsuda S, Tabata. Radical operations for carcinoma of the gallbladder: present status in Japan. World J Surg 15:337–343, 1991.

121. Donohoe JH, Stewart AK, Menck HR. The National Cancer Data Base report on carcinoma of the gallbladder, 1989–1995. Cancer 83:2618–2628, 1998.

# Chapter 38

# Clinical Aspects and Management of Cholangiocarcinoma and Gallbladder Carcinoma: Diagnostic and Staging Procedures

ISAAC RAIJMAN

Bile duct and gallbladder cancers are diagnosed primarily by combining the clinical presentation with laboratory work and cross-imaging studies of the abdomen. These studies determine the likely diagnosis, which can be then confirmed by direct cholangiography or choledochoscopy. Thereafter, the diagnosis is confirmed by cytopathologic assessment with or without associated molecular biologic techniques and immunochemistry. However, even with all the technological advances now available, tissue confirmation sometimes fails to detect disease even when the diagnosis is strongly suspected. This chapter describes the current practical techniques and technologies that can be used in the diagnosis and staging of bile duct and gallbladder cancers.

## Diagnosis

### Tumor Markers

Serologic testing for the diagnosis of cholangiocarcinoma or gallbladder cancer has proved to be of limited value. Patients with benign tumors, without or with jaundice, may have an elevated carbohydrate antigen (CA) 19-9 concentration.[1] The detection of serum tumor markers has been used primarily in patients with primary sclerosing cholangitis (PSC) and suspected cholangiocarcinoma. In a recent study involving 37 patients with PSC, a serum CA 19-9 concentration above 100 U/ml was 89% sensitive and 86% specific to detect disease.[2] The concentration of serum and bile carcinoembryonic antigen (CEA) in patients with PSC and cholangiocarcinoma is approximately five times that of patients with benign strictures.[3] The combination of serum CA 19-9 and CEA identified 66% of patients with cholangiocarcinoma, including those with occult disease. In another study, combined CEA and CA 19-9 testing in patients with PSC was 86% accurate in detecting cholangiocarcinoma.[4] There are no data on

the use of tumor markers in gallbladder cancer, and this testing has been used as a final diagnosis in patients who present with obstructive jaundice.

### Endoscopy

#### Endoscopic Retrograde Cholangiography

Endoscopic retrograde cholangiography (ERCP) is the gold standard for the detection of biliary strictures regardless of their location or etiology (Fig. 38–1). This technique provides needed information to not only determine the location and extent of the stricture or tumor but also collect adequate tissue samples and ensure optimum therapy. Cholangiography can be used to classify cholangiocarcinomas according to the Bismuth classification on the basis of the tumor location in the extrahepatic bile duct. Once a stricture is identified, cytology, histology, or both must be performed to confirm the diagnosis. Brush cytology alone is associated with low sensitivity values ranging from 35% to 70%, compared with 43% to 88% for forceps biopsy of malignant strictures.[5–9] Biliary brushings were assessed in 86 patients with biliary strictures of unknown etiology.[5] A final diagnosis was achieved in 78 patients on the basis of intraoperative findings and histological investigation, autopsy, or prolonged follow-up. Strictures were malignant in 57 patients and benign in 21 patients. The sensitivity for brush cytology was 56%, the specificity was 90%, the positive predictive value was 94%, the negative predictive value was 43.2 %, and the accuracy was 65%. The sensitivity was significantly higher in cholangiocarcinoma, 80%, compared with pancreatic carcinoma, 35%.

Cholangiocarcinoma may develop in approximately 10% of patients with PSC, and distinguishing it from benign strictures can be difficult. In a recent study, the results of 47 brush cytol-

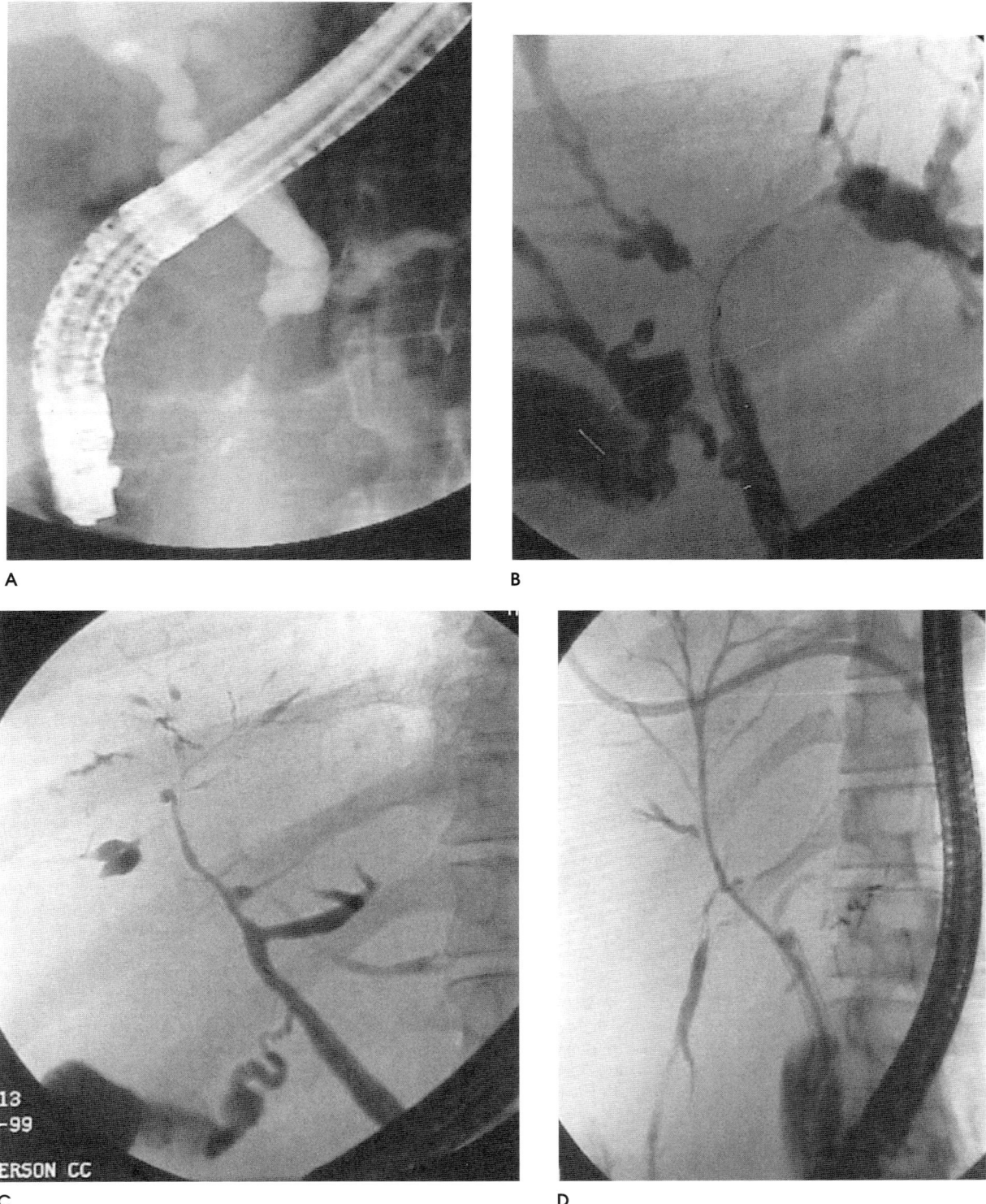

**Figure 38-1** Series of cholangiographic images showing various types of bile duct strictures secondary to cholangiocarcinoma. All pictures were obtained using endoscopic retrograde cholangiography. *A:* Distal chol- angiocarcinoma; *B:* hilar cholangiocarcinoma; *C:* intrahepatic cholangiocarcinoma; *D:* intrahepatic cholangiocarcinoma.

ogy specimens obtained from dominant strictures from 43 patients with PSC were compared with the histological diagnosis or clinical status of the patients at least 2 years later.[6] In 27 specimens, p53 immunocytochemical examination was done and K-ras mutation analysis was performed in 25 patients. For the

detection of malignancy, brush cytology showed a sensitivity of 60%, a specificity of 89%, a positive predictive value of 59%, and negative predictive value of 89%. Adding the results of p53 and K-ras analysis did not improve the results. Similar conclusions were reached in another study assessing the diagnostic value of p53 immunoreactivity in 143 brush cytology specimens from patients with various pancreatobiliary strictures.[7] Sixty-three of 89 (71%) malignant strictures were identified cytologically while 45 cases (51%) were p53 immunoreactive. Atypical cytology was found cytologically in 19 specimens (13.3%), of which p53 expression was positive in 12 cases. Of these 12 cases, 4 were carcinomas and 8 were benign. Thus, adding p53 immunostaining did not increase diagnostic accuracy. During a recent retrospective study of 31 patients, 34 endoscopic biliary brushings were obtained from bile duct strictures.[8] Cytology showed cholangiocarcinoma in 15%, results suspicious for cholangiocarcinoma in 6%, atypical hyperplasia in 18%, and results negative for malignancy in 62%. All positive diagnoses were histologically confirmed. The cases that were suspicious for cholangiocarcinoma and the five atypical hyperplasia cases were also subsequently diagnosed by histology as cholangiocarcinoma. Of the 21 patients with negative cytology, negative biopsies were obtained in 15 and clinical follow-up inconsistent with carcinoma was found in 6. Overall, endoscopic bile duct brushing was diagnostically accurate in 48% for malignancy. Importantly, atypical hyperplasia may represent carcinoma and follow-up is necessary.

Other authors have assessed the sensitivity of brush cytology by measuring DNA and proliferation.[9] Analysis included morphometry, DNA quantification, and characterization of nuclear chromatin distribution and condensation. Brush cytology samples were obtained during ERCP from various diseases, including 22 cases of chronic pancreatitis, 11 pancreatic adenocarcinomas, 13 PSC, and 11 cholangiocarcinomas, and were compared to 25 normal epithelia specimens. The sensitivity for distinguishing chronic pancreatitis from pancreatic adenocarcinoma was 82% and the specificity was 82%. The sensitivity in distinguishing PSC from cholangiocarcinoma was 82% and the specificity was 85%. It thus appears that cytometry may add to cytology alone in the diagnosis of malignant bile duct strictures. A new scraping brush consisting of a 10 Fr tapered dilator with a semi-rigid 1-cm pad of Velcro was designed, and in all 15 patients in whom this brush was tested, a positive diagnosis of malignancy was obtained.[10] This device is not yet widely available.

The combination of brush cytology, forceps biopsy, and needle aspiration provides a sensitivity of 80%, which is greater than the sensitivity of any of these methods alone.[11] Transpapillary biopsy performed with forceps had a reported sensitivity of 88% in 18 patients with cholangiocarcinoma.[12] The use of CEA staining of obtained tissue has improved cytopathologic recognition of cancer and the differentiation of benign and malignant lesions.[13,14] In situ hybridization for telomerase RNA in routine cytologic brushings has been used in the diagnosis of various malignancy-related biliary strictures.[15] This technique was used in 18 patients with benign and malignant biliary strictures, 3 of whom had cholangiocarcinoma and 1 who had gallbladder cancer. Among the eight malignant strictures, routine cytology was positive in five and telomerase RNA in six, for a sensitivity of 75%. Interestingly, both techniques were positive in only three patients. The role of telomerase RNA as an adjunct to routine cytology remains to be determined.

With the advent of smaller, more durable miniendoscopes with improved optical resolution, choledochoscopy is being reintroduced as an important part of the diagnostic and therapeutic armamentarium for biliary diseases (Fig. 38–2). In our initial experience using a 9 Fr miniendoscope (Pentax, Orange, NY), choledochoscopy was useful in providing information to recognize undetected disease and provide directed therapy.[16,17] Chole-

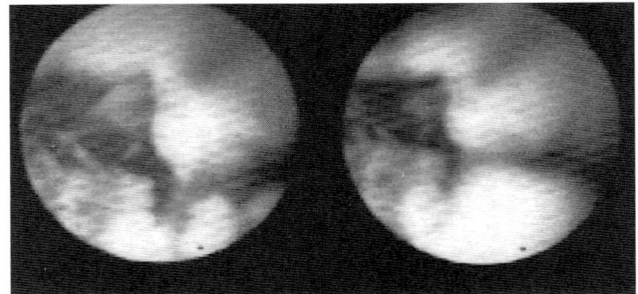

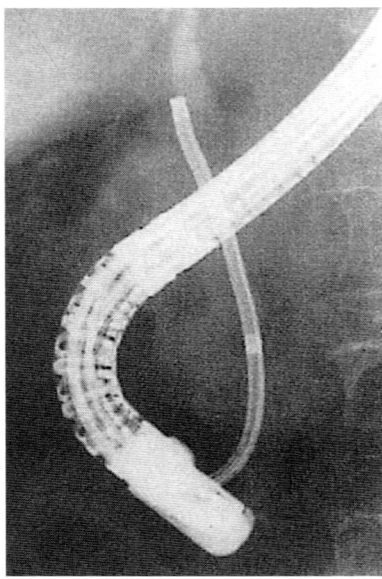

**Figure 38–2** *A:* choledochoscopic evidence of cholangiocarcinoma. *B:* Fluoroscopic view of the choledochoscope.

dochoscopy confirmed the diagnosis in 44 (51%) and provided additional diagnostic information in 43 (49%) patients, including undiagnosed viral and fungal infections, ischemic injury, ductal ulceration, bleeding angiodysplasia, and localized and diffuse cancers. Choledochoscopy was helpful in providing targeted treatment in 82% of patients in whom it was used with therapeutic purposes. In our experience with 61 patients, 11 of whom had malignant biliary disease, choledochoscopy confirmed the anticipated diagnosis in 59%, provided additional diagnostic information in 30%, and allowed targeted treatment in 44% of the patients. Thus far, our current experience of 132 patients (unpublished results) corroborates our initial findings. See et al.[18] reported their results in 111 patients with benign or malignant bile duct tumors who underwent cholangioscopy. The appearance of adenocarcinoma as well as other malignant and benign conditions showed characteristic cholangioscopic findings that helped in establishing the diagnosis. Cholangioscopy can be very useful in determining the local extent of the disease, even when the result of cholangiography is negative (Fig. 38–3).

The role of ERCP in the diagnosis of gallbladder cancer per se is extremely limited. The combination of a proximal duodenal stricture or luminal narrowing, a mid-choledochal stricture, and cystic duct obstruction is highly suggestive of gallbladder cancer. Otherwise, the role of ERCP in gallbladder cancer is useful in diagnosing those patients presenting with obstructive jaundice. In a few cases ERCP may identify, if the cystic duct is patent, intraluminal gallbladder masses.

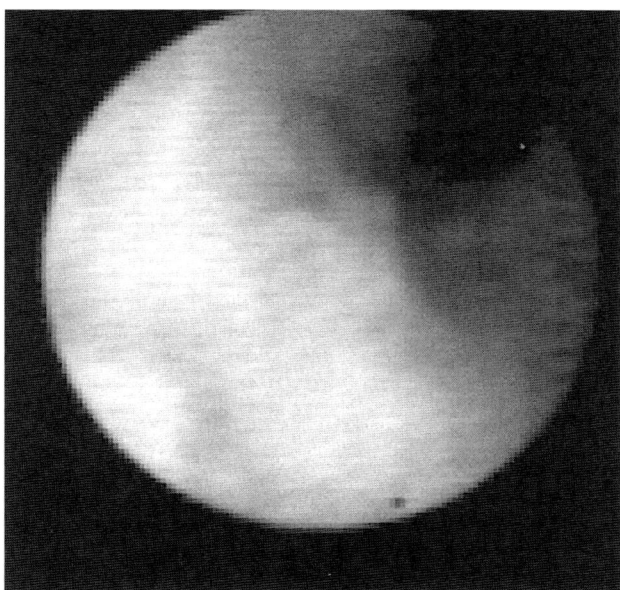

**Figure 38-3** Choledochoscopic image showing local extension of cholangiocarcinoma not detected by cholangiography.

## Endoscopic Ultrasound and Intraductal Probes

Unlike endosonography in other areas of the gastrointestinal tract or in the pancreas, endosonography of the biliary tree and gallbladder has not proved as useful. The technique has only limited ability to characterize the inner layer of the bile duct, detect invasion of peripheral structures, and assess the luminal contents of the gallbladder. Dedicated radial and linear echoendoscopes or intraductal ultrasonographic probes do not accurately measure the depth of invasion of bile duct tumors.[19,20] In addition, extensive experience is required in the performance of echoendoscopy of the bile duct. In the presence of a biliary stricture that precludes passage of the echoprobe, it is not possible to determine the depth of invasion of the lesion.[21]

To establish the diagnostic ability and the criteria for depth invasion of gallbladder cancer of endoscopic ultrasonography, Kim and colleagues compared the ultrasonographic and pathologic findings for 12 patients.[22] The endoscopic ultrasonography findings were classified according to four types: type A, findings were characterized by a smooth, pedunculated mass without changes of the outer hyperechoic layer; type B, an elevated lesion with thickened, heterogeneous, low echoic wall but no change in the outer hyperechoic layer; type C, the same characteristics of type B but with irregularity of the outer hyperechoic wall; and type D, definite destruction of the outer hyperechoic wall. The positive predictive value for type A was 75%; for type B, 77%; for type C, 75%; and for type D, 100%. The sensitivity for subserosal invasion was 77% and 82% for serosal involvement.

Endoscopic ultrasonography has also been used to differentiate neoplastic from non-neoplastic gallbladder polyps. In a study of 132 patients undergoing endoscopic ultrasonography and cholecystectomy, multivariate analysis showed that the most important predictor for the finding of a neoplasm was polyp size. All polyps less than 5 mm in greatest dimension were non-neoplastic and the risk for neoplasm was greater in patients with polyps greater than 15 mm.[23]

Intraductal endosonography with high-frequency transducers has been used to characterize biliary strictures and to distinguish between benign and malignant disease. Intraductal endosonography has shown 68% sensitivity in accurately predicting disease stages I–IV according to the TNM classification.[24] Limitations of this technique include its inability to detect mild invasion to the perimuscular loose connective tissue and its inability to detect lymph node or distal metastases. In a recent study, a thin-caliber ultrasonic probe with a 2-mm diameter and a 20 mHz frequency was inserted into the bile duct in 42 patients with bile duct strictures or filling defects, and the resultant findings were compared with those obtained with percutaneous choledochoscopy and biopsy. The sensitivity of intraductal endosonography for diagnosing bile duct cancer was 89% and the specificity was 50%.[25] In the same study, the sensitivity values of bile duct cytology and percutaneous cholangioscopic biopsy improved when these tests were performed in combination with intraductal endosonography. Intraductal endosonography has been useful in determining tumor invasion to the pancreas,[26] right hepatic artery,[27] and portal vein.[28]

Three-dimensional intraductal ultrasonography has been used in conjunction with intraductal ultrasonography to determine the depth of invasion of bile duct tumors.[19] In a study involving 146 patients with various cancers, including 33 cases of bile duct cancer and 8 cases of gallbladder cancer, three different probes with frequencies of 7.5 mHz, 12 mHz, and 20 mHz were used via percutaneous and peroral approaches. Intraductal ultrasonography had an accuracy rate of 85% for diagnosing the depth of tumor in 13 patients with bile duct cancer, 89% for determining when the tumor invaded the pancreas, 92% for determining when the tumor invaded the portal vein, and 85% for determining the presence of intraductal spread. The diagnostic accuracy of three-dimensional intraductal ultrasonography was not better than the diagnostic accuracy of intraductal ultrasonography alone.

In a recent study involving eight patients with extrahepatic bile duct cancer and three patients with intrahepatic bile duct cancer, the accuracy rates for determining the extent of tumor (T stage) using intraductal endosonography was 88% for extrahepatic cancer and 100% for intrahepatic cancer. For determining the regional lymph node involvement (N stage) of extrahepatic cancer, the sensitivity and specificity were each 75%, compared with a 75% sensitivity and 50% specificity using endoscopic ultrasonography.[29] The use of endosonography-guided fine-needle aspiration in 10 patients with brush cytology–negative, potentially operable hilar cholangiocarcinoma was studied.[30] Adequate material was obtained in nine patients, seven of whom demonstrated cholangiocarcinoma and hepatocellular carcinoma in one. One benign inflammatory lesion identified on cytology proved to be a false-negative finding by frozen section. Metastatic locoregional hilar lymph nodes were detected in two patients, and in one patient the celiac and paraaortic lymph nodes revealed metastatic disease. Thus, adding fine-needle aspiration in this difficult area is helpful in establishing a definitive diagnosis and avoiding unnecessary surgery when metastatic disease is demonstrated.

## Radiology

### Ultrasonography

Ultrasonography of the right upper quadrant of the abdomen is the initial test of choice when cancer of the bile duct and gallbladder is suspected. Ultrasonography of patients with this disease typically reveals dilation of the intrahepatic ducts in proximal lesions and dilation of both the intrahepatic and the extrahepatic ducts in more distal lesions. Ductal papillary and nodular type cholangiocarcinoma show polypoid intraluminal masses, whereas ductal nodular cholangiocarcinoma manifests as a discrete smooth mass with associated mural thickening. The nodular form predominates and appears as a solitary mass with a distinct right lobe predilection, whereas the infiltrative form is rare and manifests as a diffusely abnormal liver echotexture.[31] However, the ducts may not be dilated in patients with PSC or in those with underlying cirrhosis. While useful as an initial test to assess the initial presentation, ultrasonography is inadequate in providing detail sufficient to determine the extent of disease and appropriate therapy.

Percutaneous ultrasonography, by contrast, is useful in the diagnosis of gallbladder cancer. Thickening of the gallbladder wall and the presence of an intraluminal mass and a mass in the gallbladder fossa are findings highly suggestive of the diagnosis.[32,33] Limitations of ultrasonography include its inability to detect very small lesions or to distinguish benign polyps from cancer, and the need to rely on findings that are sometimes present in benign disorders.

## Computed Tomography

Computed tomography (CT), especially when performed using the helical technique, can provide information important in determining the extent of the disease (Fig. 38–4). However, this technology has limited ability to detect lesions localized in the periphery, where minimal contrast enhancement may occur. In some instances, particularly for tumors localized in the hilum, it is crucial to obtain delayed images, as fibrotic tissue tends to retain contrast longer than the surrounding tissue. Most cholangiocarcinomas manifest focal or diffuse ductal dilation.

In a study of 24 patients with 25 peripheral cholangiocarcinomas, incremental dynamic nonhelical CT was performed in 4 cases and helical CT in 21 cases.[34] Bile duct dilatation was present in 52%, regional lymph node enlargement was in 24%, retraction of the liver capsule was in 36%, and satellite nodules were in 32%. During the portal phase, all tumors were hypo-

dense, whereas during delayed images, 70% of tumors showed hyperattenuation. Portal venous encasement was seen in 40%. The CT features of intraductal intrahepatic cholangiocarcinoma include segmental or lobar dilatation of the intrahepatic bile ducts associated with or without intraductal polypoid mass, amorphous structures, or both with slight hyperattenuation.[35] Using quadruple-phase helical CT, 45 patients with newly diagnosed bile duct cancer and hepatoma were studied.[36] In cholangiocarcinoma, tumor attenuation increased during the delayed phase. In the majority of lesions, the greatest tumor conspicuity was seen during the portal venous phase. As shown in other studies, the delayed phase is particularly important in diagnosing these cancer.

Dynamic CT scanning (D-CT) was compared with dynamic magnetic resonance imaging (D-MRI) for the diagnosis of peripheral cholangiocarcinoma in 20 patients,[37] with results showing that D-CT and D-MRI exhibited a similar tumoral enhancement pattern. Both showed a wedge-like enhancement area peripheral to the tumor in about 50% of the patients, and both techniques showed ductal dilatation in 65% of the patients. Vascular involvement and extrahepatic invasion were seen in 45% of the patients by D-CT but in only 10% by D-MRI.

The role of CT in staging gallbladder cancer is limited, as CT is effective in identifying only tumors that are usually large. As many as 56% of patients with gallbladder cancer do not show any abnormalities on CT.[38] In addition, CT does not reveal existing lymphatic involvement in up to 48% of patients and in only 60% of patients can metastasis be fully delineated.[39]

## Magnetic Resonance Imaging

The role of magnetic resonance imaging (MRI) in the diagnosis of cholangiocarcinoma and gallbladder cancer is unclear. The technique has sensitivity and specificity similar to those of CT but is more expensive (Fig. 38–5). With the administration of gadolinium, MRI may help distinguish between inflammatory changes and tumor and should help in assessing the extent of the cancer.[40] Magnetic resonance cholangiopancreatography (MRCP) is a relatively new modality that uses magnetic resonance technology to create a three-dimensional image of the biliary tree (Fig. 38–6). Recently, MRCP was compared with ERCP for diagnosis in 20 patients with malignant hilar ob-

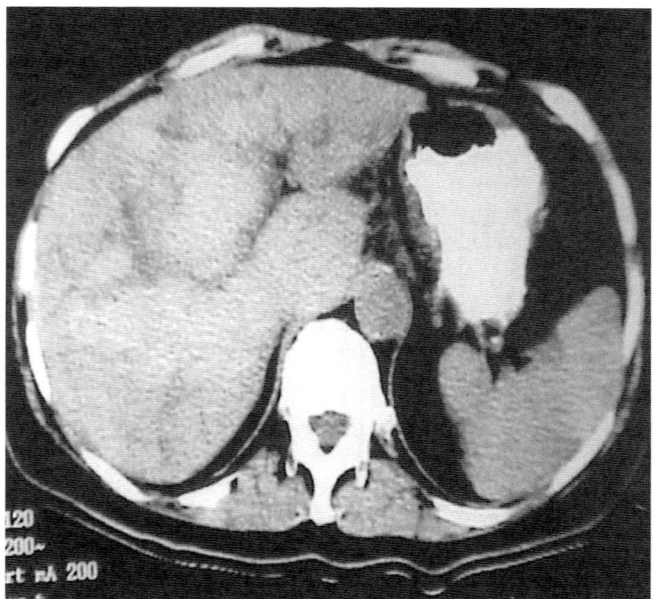

**Figure 38–4** Computed tomography showing an advanced cholangiocarcinoma.

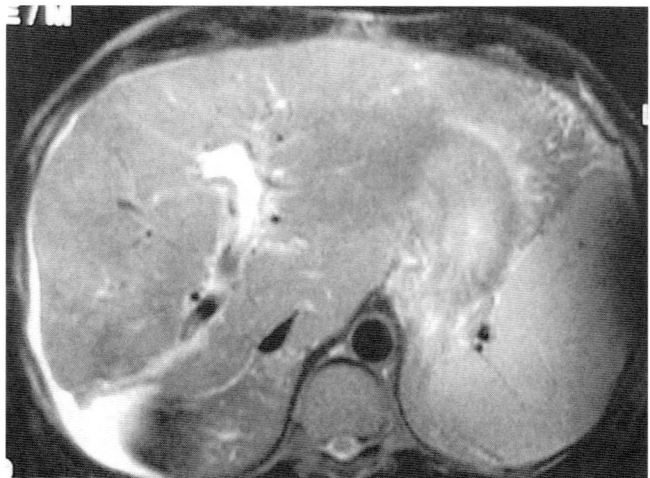

**Figure 38–5** Magnetic resonance imaging showing a cholangiocarcinoma.

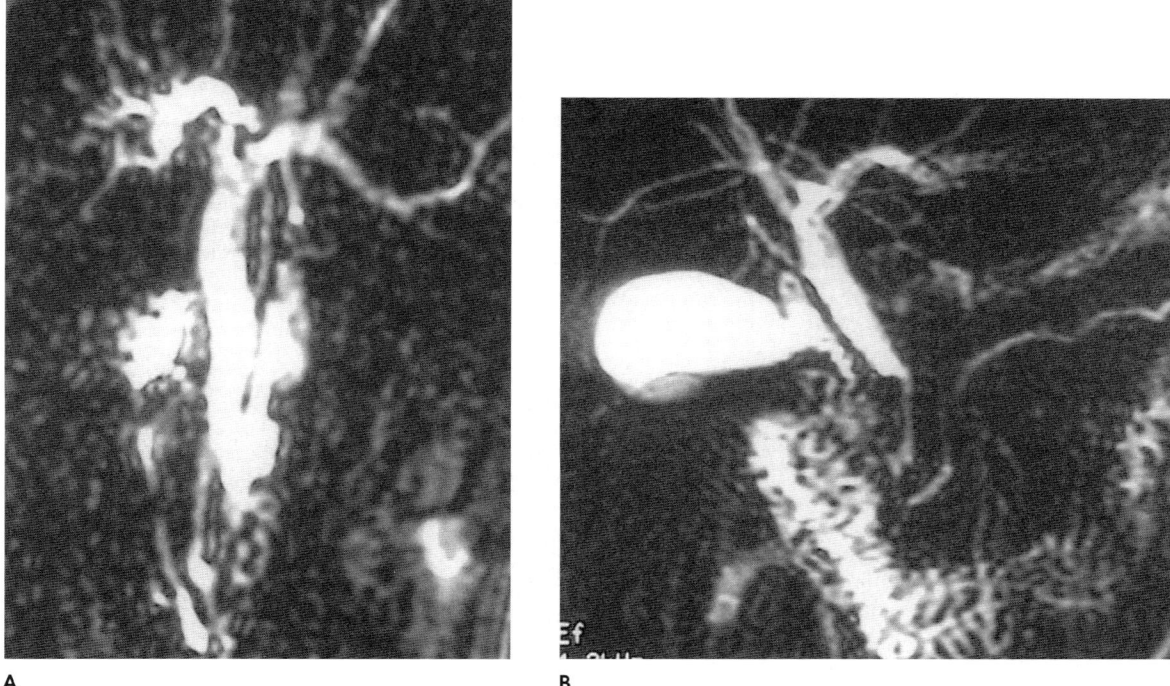

A                                                    B

**Figure 38-6** Magnetic resonance cholangiography showing a distal bile duct stricture in a patient with cholangiocarcinoma. *A:* Lateral view; *B:* anteroposterior view.

struction, 15 of which were cholangiocarcinomas. Using the Bismuth's classification, ERCP diagnosed type I in 20%, type II in 35%, type III in 35%, and type IV in 10%. MRCP correctly classified 78% of the patients and underestimated tumor extension in 22%.[41] Other authors have suggested that the combination of MRI and MRCP as an "all-in-one" approach may provide the identification, characterization, and staging of the lesion, giving the clinician all the information necessary for the planning of adequate treatment.[42] In another series, MRCP was compared with ERCP in 78 patients: MRCP showed 71% sensitivity for the recognition of normal bile ducts, 83% sensitivity for recognition of ductal dilation, 85% sensitivity for the recognition of strictures, and 77% sensitivity for the correct stricture location.[43] In addition, MRCP had a 50% sensitivity for identifying benign strictures and an 80% sensitivity for identifying malignant strictures. The limitation of MRCP is that it relies on the presence of associated biliary dilation to diagnose a stricture; that is, benign or malignant strictures not associated with biliary dilation, such as those encountered in PSC or scirrhous cancers, may not be detected.

### Positron Emission Tomography

In a small study in which the role of positron emission tomography (PET) for the diagnosis of cholangiocarcinoma was examined,[44] PET scanning of the liver was performed in nine patients with PSC, in six patients with PSC and known cholangiocarcinoma, and in five control patients. The PET scanning correctly revealed hot spots in all six patients with cholangiocarcinoma but not in the other patients. The specialized equipment needed for PET scanning limits the utility of this imaging modality. The role of PET in gallbladder cancer has not been evaluated.

### Other Techniques

Radiolabeling techniques may be used for detecting cholangiocarcinomas expressing specific receptors. Tissue from seven surgically resected human cholangiocarcinomas was studied for binding and growth-active properties of somatostatin and its analogues. All specimens expressed SSTR2 messenger RNA. In one patient, a cholangiocarcinoma could be localized using gamma camera imaging with an 111In-SS analogue.[45] The future widespread application of these techniques is unknown.

## Staging

### Cholangiocarcinoma

Staging of the disease is relevant only if the patient is a candidate for surgical resection. However, staging may also be used in patients with unresectable disease if specific therapy, such as radiation of bone metastasis, is a possibility. Bile duct cancer can be classified on the basis of clinical or cholangiographic findings. The T (tumor at primary site), N (regional lymph node involvement), M (distant metastases) classification system is used for clinical staging, while the Bismuth classification is the standard system used with cholangiography.

### Cholangiographic Classification

Intrahepatic bile duct cancer is usually classified according to the Bismuth classification, in which malignancies are classified according to the location of the tumor around the hilum (Table 38–1). This classification is not applicable to distal or mid-common bile duct cancers. Type I tumors are those located within

**Table 38–1** Bismuth classification of cholangiocarcinoma (hilar tumors)

| | |
|---|---|
| Type I | Within the common hepatic duct |
| Type II | Right and left hepatic duct involvement |
| Type III a | Right secondary intrahepatic involement |
| Type III b | Left secondary intrahepatic involvement |
| Type IV | Bilateral secondary intrahepatic involvement |

the common hepatic duct; type II tumors involve the right and left hepatic ducts; type IIIa and IIIb tumors involve the right and left secondary intrahepatics ducts, respectively; and type IV tumors involve bilateral intrahepatic ducts.[46] Extrahepatic bile duct cancer is classified according to its anatomic location: the upper third involves the common hepatic duct from the cystic duct to the bifurcation; middle third involves the area from the cystic duct to the upper border of the duodenum; and lower third characterizes tumor localized between the suprapapillary portion of the bile duct and the upper border of the duodenum.[47] Location is a reliable indicator of the histologic type of the tumor. Sclerosing tumors tend to involve the upper third and the hilum; nodular cancers, the middle third; and papillary tumors, the lower third. In addition, tumors can be characterized as central or as peripheral as described above, when localized away from the choledochus and bifurcation.

## Clinical Classification

Clinical staging is defined in four stages under the TNM classification as delineated in Table 38–2. Stage I tumors are limited to the bile duct mucosa or the muscular layer, stage II tumors extend up to the periductal area but do not involve the lymph nodes, stage III tumors involve regional lymph nodes, and stage IV tumors invade adjacent structures or have distal metastases.

A tumor is deemed unresectable when there is extensive involvement of the bile duct, involvement of the main portal vein, hepatic artery, or portal venous branches bilaterally, involvement of the hepatic arterial branches and the contralateral ductal system, or local or distant metastases.

## Gallbladder Cancer

The staging of gallbladder cancer is based primarily on surgical findings. Clinical staging of gallbladder cancer is inadequate because of the limitations of cross-imaging studies as described above. This limitation applies particularly to early-stage tumors. When cross-imaging studies do correctly identify the stage, the disease is in an advanced stage and thus the prognosis is extremely poor.

**Table 38–2** TNM classification of cholangiocarcinoma

| Stage | Classification | Description |
|---|---|---|
| Stage I | T1, N0, M0 | Disease limited to the mucosa or muscular layer |
| Stage II | T2, N0, M0 | Invasion of periductal tissue without local or distant metastases |
| Stage III | T1–2, N1, M0 | Metastases to regional lymph nodes |
| Stage IVa | T3, any N, M0 | Invasion of adjacent structures |
| Stage IVb | Any T, any N, M1 | Distant metastases |

**Table 38–3** TNM staging for gallbladder cancer

| Stage | Classification | Description |
|---|---|---|
| Stage I | T1, N0, M0 | Disease limited to the mucosa or muscular layer |
| Stage II | T2, N0, M0 | Invasion of periductal tissue without local or distant metastases |
| Stage III | T1–3, N1, M0 | Metastases to cystic duct, pericholedochal or hilar nodes or extends <2 cms |
| Stage IVa | T4, N1, M0 | Local invasion > 2 cms, regional metastases but no distant metastases |
| Stage IVb | T1–4, N1–0, M1 | Distant metastases |

As with cholangiocarcinoma, gallbladder cancer is classified according to the TNM staging system.[48] Stage I tumors invade the mucosa or muscle layer; stage II tumors involve the perimuscular connective tissue but not the serosa; stage III tumors extend into one adjacent organ, the cystic duct, or the pericholedochal and/or hilar nodes; and stage IV tumors invade the adjacent organs and more distant regional nodes or involve distal metastases (see Table 38–3).

## Conclusion

While significant advances have been made in the diagnosis and staging of bile duct cancer and gallbladder cancer, detection of either cholangiocarcinoma and gallbladder cancer at an early stage remains elusive. Despite these advances, the mortality of both diseases remains high. The ongoing improvement and advances in technology, in addition to being less invasive, will enable clinicians to make an earlier diagnosis and determine accurate staging of the disease. This will translate into better treatments, including less unnecessary surgeries and, perhaps, a true potential for cure of the disease in a larger number of patients.

## References

1. Paganuzzii M, Onetto M, Marroni P, et al. CA 19-9 and CA 50 in benign and malignant pancreatic and biliary diseases. Cancer 61:2100–2108, 1987.
2. Nichols JC, Gores GJ, LaRusso NF, et al. Diagnostic role of serum CA 19-9 for cholangiocarcinoma in patients with primary sclerosing cholangitis. Mayo Clin Proc 68:874, 1993.
3. Nakeeb A, Lipsett PA, Lillemoe KD, et al. Biliary carcinoembryonic antigen levels are a marker for cholangiocarcinoma. Am J Surg 171:147, 1996.
4. Ramage JK, Donaghy A, Farrant JM, et al. Serum tumor markers for the diagnosis of cholangiocarcinoma in primary sclerosing cholangitis. Gastroenterology 108:865, 1995.
5. Glasbrenner B, Ardan M, Boeck W, et al. Prospective evaluation of brush cytology of biliary strictures during endoscopic retrograde cholangiopancreatography. Endoscopy 31:712–717, 1999.
6. Ponsioen CY, Vrouenraets SM, van Milligen de Wit AW, et al. Value of brush cytology for dominant strictures in primary sclerosing cholangitis. Endoscopy 31:305–309, 1999.
7. Stewart CJ, Burke GM. Value of p53 immunostaining in pancreaticobiliary brush cytology specimens. Diagn Cytopathol 23:308–313, 2000.
8. Trent V, Khurana KK, Pisharodi LR. Diagnostic accuracy and clinical utility of endoscopic bile duct brushing in the evaluation of biliary strictures. Arch Pathol Lab Med 123:712–715, 1999.
9. Sears RJ, Duckworth CW, Decaestecker C, et al. Image cytometry as a discriminatory tool for cytologic specimens obtained by endoscopic retrograde cholangiopancreatography. Cancer 84:119–126, 1998.
10. Parasher VK, Huibregtse K. Endoscopic retrograde wire-guided cytology of malignant biliary strictures using a novel scraping brush. Gastrointest Endosc 48:288–290, 1998.

11. Wiersema MJ, Lehman GA, Sherman S, et al. Endoscopic brush cytology, fine needle aspiration and forceps biopsy in the evaluation of malignant biliary strictures. Gastrointest Endosc 39:336A, 1993.

12. Kubota Y, Takaoka M, Tani K, et al. Endoscopic transpapillary biopsy for diagnosis of patients with pancreatobiliary ductal strictures. Am J Gastroenterol 88:1700–1704, 1993.

13. Maxwell P, Davis RI, Sloan JM. Carcinoembryonic antigen in benign and malignant epithelium of the gallbladder, extrahepatic bile ducts and ampulla of Vater. J Pathol 170:73–76, 1993.

14. Wolber RA, Greene CA, Dupuis BA. Polyclonal carcinoembryonic antigen staining in the cytologic differential diagnosis of primary and metastatic hepatic malignancies. Acta Cytol 35:215–220, 1991.

15. Morales CP, Burdick JS, Saboorian MH, et al. In situ hybridization for telomerase RNA in routine cytologic brushings for the diagnosis of pancreatobiliary malignancies. Gastrointest Endosc 48:402–405, 1998.

16. Siddique I, Galati J, Ankoma-Sey V, et al. The role of choledochoscopy in the diagnosis and management of biliary tract disease. Gastrointest Endosc 50:67–73, 1999.

17. Raijman, V Ankoma-Sey, H Monsour, et al. The role of choledochoscopy in the diagnosis and management of non-transplant biliary tract disease. Hepatology 26:1829A, 1997.

18. Seo DW, Lee SK, Yoo KS, et al. Cholangioscopic findings in bile duct tumors. Gastrointest Endosc 52:630–634, 2000.

19. Inui K, Nakazawa S, Yoshino J, et al. Ultrasound probes for biliary lesions. Endoscopy 30(Suppl 1):A120–A123, 1998.

20. Tamada K, Ido K, Ueno N, et al. Preoperative staging of extrahepatic bile duct cancer with intraductal ultrasonography. Am J Gastroenterol 90:239–246, 1994.

21. Fujita N, Noda Y, Kobayashi G, et al. Staging of bile duct carcinoma by EUS and IDUS. Endoscopy 30(Suppl 1);A132–A134, 1998.

22. Kim J, Ciaccia D, Kiel J, Shermann S. Endoscopic ultrasonography for evaluating the depth of invasion of gallbladder cancer. Gastrointest Endosc 49:164A, 1999.

23. Choi WB, SK Lee, Kim MH, et al. A new strategy to predict the neoplastic polyps of the gallbladder based on a scoring system using endoscopic ultrasonography. Gastrointest Endosc 49:168A, 1999.

24. Tamada K, Ido K, Ueno N, et al. Preoperative staging of extrahepatic bile duct cancer with intraductal ultrasonography (IDUS). Am J Gastroenterol 89:239–246, 1994.

25. Tamada K, Ueno N, Tomiyama T, et al. Characterization of biliary strictures using intraductal ultrasonography: comparison with percutaneous cholangioscopic biopsy. Gastrointest Endosc 47:341–349, 1998.

26. Tamada K, Ueno N, Ichiyama M, et al. Assessment of pancreatic parenchymal invasion by bile duct cancer using intraductal ultrasonography. Gastrointest Endosc 28:492–496, 1996.

27. Tamada K, Ueno N, Ichiyama M, et al. Assessment of hepatic artery invasion using intraductal ultrasonography. Gastrointest Endosc 27:579–583, 1995.

28. Tamada K, Ueno N, Ichiyama M, et al. Assessment of portal vein invasion by bile duct cancer using intraductal ultrasonography. Gastrointest Endosc 27:573–578, 1995.

29. Sechopoulos P, Leach S, Mertz H. Evaluation of intraductal ultrasonography (IDUS) in the diagnosis and staging of pancreatico-biliary tumors. Gastrointest Endosc 49:187A, 1999.

30. Fritscher-Ravens A, Broering DC, Sriram PV, et al. EUS-guided fine-needle aspiration cytodiagnosis of hilar cholangiocarcinoma: a case series. Gastrointest Endosc 52:534–540, 2000.

31. Bloom CM, Langer B, Wilson SR. Role of US in the detection, characterization, and staging of cholangiocarcinoma. Radiographics 19:1199–1218, 1999.

32. Oikarinen H, Paivansalo M, Lahde S, et al. Imaging in gallbladder carcinoma. Eur J Radiol 17:179–183, 1993.

33. Kersting-Sommerhoff B, Helmberger H, Bautz W. Radiologic diagnosis and staging of gallbladder and bile duct tumors. Endoscopy 17:179–183, 1993.

34. Valls C, Guma A, Puig I, et al. Intrahepatic peripheral cholangiocarcinoma: CT evaluation. Abdom Imaging 25:490–496, 2000.

35. Lee JW, Han JK, Kim TK, et al. CT features of intraductal intrahepatic cholangiocarcinoma. AJR Am J Roentgenol 175:721–725, 2000.

36. Loyer EM, Chin H, DuBrow RA, et al. Hepatocellular carcinoma and intrahepatic peripheral cholangiocarcinoma: enhancement patterns with quadruple phase helical CT—a comparative study. Radiology 212:866–875, 1999.

37. Zhang Y, Uchida M, Abe T, et al. Intrahepatic peripheral cholangiocarcinoma: comparison of dynamic CT and dynamic MRI. J Comput Assist Tomogr 23:670–677, 1999.

38. Ohtani T, Shirai Y, Tsukada K, et al. Carcinoma of the gallbladder: CT evaluation of lymphatic spread. Radiology 189:875–880, 1993.

39. Oikarinen H, Paivansalo M, Lahde S, et al. Imaging in gallbladder carcinoma. Eur J Radiol 17:179–183, 1993.

40. Fan ZM, Yamashita Y, Harada M, et al. Intrahepatic cholangiocarcinoma: spin-echo and contrast-enhanced dynamic MR imaging. AJR Am J Roentgenol 161:313–317, 1993.

41. Zidi SH, Prat F, Le Guen O, Rondeau Y, Pelletier G. Performance characteristics of magnetic resonance cholangiography in the staging of malignant hilar strictures. Gut 46:103–106, 2000.

42. Pavone P, Laghi A, Passariello R. MR cholangiopancreatography in malignant biliary obstruction. Semin Ultrasound CT MR 20:317–323, 1999.

43. Hintze RE, Adler A, Velzke W, et al. Clinical significance of magnetic resonance cholangiopancreatography (MRCP) compared to endoscopic retrograde cholangiopancreatography (ERCP). Endoscopy 29:182–187, 1997.

44. Keiding S, Hansen SB, Ramsussen H, et al. Detection of cholangiocarcinoma in primary sclerosing cholangitis by positron emission tomography. Hepatology 28:701, 1998.

45. Tan CK, Podila PV, Taylor JE, et al. Human cholangiocarcinomas express somatostatin receptors and respond to somatostatin with growth inhibition. Gastroenterology 108:1908–1916, 1995.

46. Bismuth H, Nakache R, Diamond T. Management strategies in resection for hilar cholangiocarcinoma. Ann Surg 215:31–38, 1992.

47. Adam A, Benjamin IS. The staging of cholangiocarcinoma. Clin Radiol 46:299–303, 1992.

48. Beahrs OH. Gallbladder. In: Beahrs OH (ed): Manual for Staging of Cancer. Philadelphia, Lippincott, 1992, pp 93–98.

or noncontiguous metastases as well as enlarged periportal lymph nodes suggesting nodal metastases.[14,15] Even intraoperative ultrasonography is suboptimal for detecting intraductal spread by hilar cholangiocarcinoma; it can correctly demonstrate the extent of tumor spread away from the primary biliary tumor in only 18% of cases.[16] Intraoperative ultrasonography can be used to screen for noncontiguous liver metastases from the primary biliary cancer and can accurately detect direct tumor invasion of the portal vein or hepatic artery in 83.3% and 60% of cases, respectively.[16] Recently, endoscopic ultrasonography and intraductal sonography findings have been described in patients with hilar bile duct cancer, but the small number of patients studied precludes determination of the staging accuracy of these techniques.[17]

Like the intrahepatic variety, hilar cholangiocarcinoma is usually hypointense on T1- and hyperintense on T2-weighted MRI. Dilated intrahepatic bile ducts are evident in patients with obstructing tumors, and lobar atrophy is seen in cases of portal venous occlusion. Fast low-angle shot (FLASH) MR with contrast-enhanced coronal imaging has been used to demonstrate intraluminal extension of tumor and to distinguish between blood vessels and bile ducts.[18,19] Magnetic resonance cholangiopancreatography (MRCP) and MR virtual endoscopy can demonstrate hilar bile duct obstruction by tumor with dilated intrahepatic ducts.[18,20] The advantages of MRCP over direct cholangiography include its noninvasiveness and ability to visualize isolated bile ducts. Relative to direct cholangiography, however, MRCP evaluation of tumor extent is limited by spatial resolution.[20]

Cholangiography can definitively demonstrate a lesion obstructing the left and right hepatic duct at the hilar confluence (Fig. 39–5), and percutaneous transhepatic cholangiography (PTC) and endoscopic retrograde cholangiopancreatography (ERCP) are both useful in assessing patients with extrahepatic biliary obstruction. A prospective, randomized comparison of PTC and ERCP in jaundiced patients concluded that both techniques had similar diagnostic accuracy.[21] Percutaneous transhepatic cholangiography was 100% accurate at demonstrating obstruction at the confluence of the left and right hepatic ducts, while ERCP had an accuracy of 92% in demonstrating these lesions. Endoscopic retrograde cholangiopancreatography has the additional benefit of providing a pancreatogram. A normal pancreatogram helps to exclude a small carcinoma of the head of the pancreas as a cause of biliary obstruction. Some investigators have recommended combining PTC and ERCP to establish the extent of a lesion in the bile ducts; however, such concomitant studies are helpful only in selected patients with complete obstruction of the biliary tree.[22] Cytologic specimens can be obtained at the time of PTC and ERCP. The presence of malignant cells in bile or bile duct brushings is confirmed in approximately 50% of patients undergoing PTC or ERCP.[21,22]

Drainage of the obstructed biliary tree with partial or complete relief of jaundice and associated symptoms can be achieved with PTC. Improvements in catheter technology have led to the development of endoprostheses that can be placed across the malignant obstruction into the duodenum to allow internal drainage.[23] It must be emphasized that providing symptomatic relief for patients by decompressing the biliary tract should not be the primary reason for placing these catheters. Prospective, randomized studies have failed to demonstrate a benefit in terms of a decrease in hospital morbidity or mortality by preoperative decompression of biliary obstruction.[24,25] However, the catheters are useful in identifying and dissecting the hepatic duct bifurcation at the time of operation and in reconstructing the biliary tract following extirpation of the tumor.[26,27] Although ERCP can be employed to place an internal stent across a malignant hilar obstruction, the success rate with this procedure is much lower than with PTC.[28]

Positron emission tomography (PET) is being evaluated as a diagnostic tool in patients with all types of malignant tumors. In this method, in vivo metabolism of positron-emitting radiolabeled tracers is assessed, such as [[18]F]fluoro-2-deoxy-D-glucose (FDG), a glucose analogue that accumulates in various malignant tumors because of their high glucose metabolic rates. FDG-PET does not provide anatomic detail to assess resectability of hilar cholangiocarcinomas or intrahepatic malignancies, but it may prove useful in detecting distant metastatic disease that would preclude a curative resection. In patients with primary sclerosing cholangitis, FDG-PET studies may be able to detect small hilar and intrahepatic cholangiocarcinomas and thus may be useful in therapeutic and transplant decision making in these patients.[29]

The final radiologic study to consider is celiac and superior mesenteric arteriography with late-phase portography. Arteriography in patients with hilar cholangiocarcinoma is important because extensive encasement of the hepatic arteries or portal vein precludes curative resection. Combining the findings on cholangiography with vascular involvement by tumor on arteriography has been found to have a greater than 80% accuracy in predicting unresectability.[30] However, occasionally a patient will have compression or displacement of vascular structures rather than true malignant invasion or encasement. A high-resolution, thin-section CT scan with intravenous bolus contrast administration can demonstrate hepatic artery and portal vein involvement by a hilar tumor and obviate the need for more invasive angiographic studies. We obtain an arteriogram in less than 5% of our patients with hilar cholangiocarcinoma.

The role of laparoscopy as part of the diagnostic and staging evaluation of patients with hilar cholangiocarcinoma is being evaluated at our institution. Several patients with seemingly re-

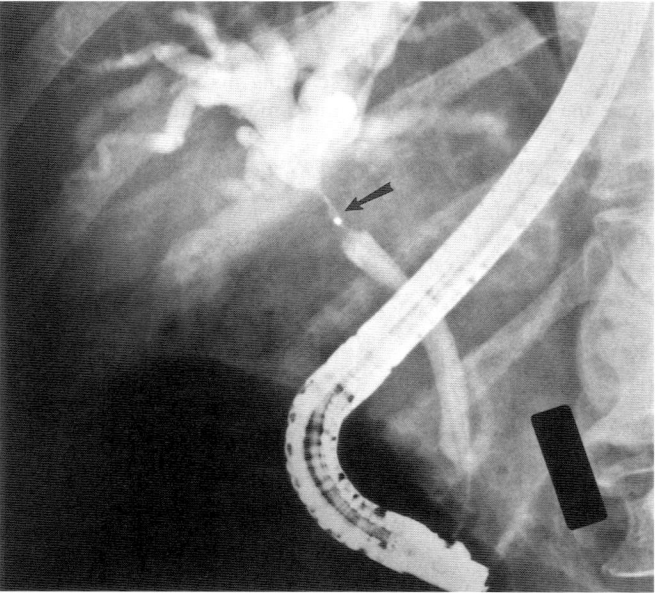

**Figure 39–5** Endoscopic retrograde cholangiopancreatography (ERCP) showing a focal stricture of the proper hepatic bile duct (arrow) and marked dilatation of the intrahepatic bile ducts. This hilar cholangiocarcinoma was completely resected with Roux Y hepaticojejunostomy reconstruction of biliary–enteric continuity.

sectable tumors avoided an exploratory laparotomy when peritoneal tumor implants were found by laparoscopy. Patients at high risk of developing peritoneal carcinomatosis may be identified by positive cytologic specimens obtained from laparoscopic washings. Laparoscopic ultrasonography can be used to exclude the presence of noncontiguous liver metastases or extensive hilar tumor infiltration in patients with extrahepatic bile duct cancers (Fig. 39–6).[31]

## Treatment of Intrahepatic Cholangiocarcinoma

Most patients with intrahepatic cholangiocarcinoma present with large tumors and usually have evidence of regional lymph node, pulmonary, and/or bone metastases at the time of diagnosis. Patients who present with jaundice due to large intrahepatic cholangiocarcinomas usually die within a year of diagnosis. Patients with an elevated serum bilirubin level associated with an intrahepatic cholangiocarcinoma are rarely candidates for curative resection because of coexistent hepatic artery and portal vein invasion, extensive lymph node metastases, bilobar liver involvement by tumor, and/or distant metastases.[32] Intrahepatic cholangiocarcinomas may be detected before they metastasize or cause jaundice in 30%–45% of patients.[32,33] These patients should be considered for operation because long-term survival has been reported in a proportion of the patients undergoing curative liver resection for intrahepatic cholangiocarcinoma.[32–40] In a study of 19 patients who underwent resection of intrahepatic cholangiocarcinoma, patients with no porta hepatis lymph node metastases had a 3-year survival rate of 64% compared with 0% for patients with nodal metastases.[37] A larger cohort of 32 patients who underwent resection of intrahepatic cholangiocarcinomas confirmed the negative prognostic impact of regional lymph node metastases and large primary tumor size (>5 cm diameter).[38] The

5-year overall survival rates reported for patients who underwent a margin-negative liver resection for intrahepatic cholangiocarcinoma range from 20% to 48%, with regional lymph node metastases, presence of satellite tumor nodules, portal vein invasion by tumor, and large primary tumors identified as poor prognostic indicators.[32–38] Large primary tumor size is a poor prognostic indicator because of the increased frequency of vascular and lymphatic invasion by the tumor as well as its growth along neighboring bile duct walls.[39]

Orthotopic liver transplantation has been described in patients with intrahepatic cholangiocarcinoma.[38,41–43] In series prior to 1990, the 1-year survival was 29.4%, and only two of the patients who underwent liver transplantation were alive 5 years following the transplant.[43] Almost 90% of the patients who survived at least 90 days after the liver transplant died of recurrent cholangiocarcinoma, frequently at extrahepatic sites. Recent small series of patients describe 5-year post-transplantation survival rates of up to 53%.[41,42] The improved survival is based on careful selection of cholangiocarcinoma patients for liver transplantation, specifically by not transplanting patients with lymph node metastases or invasion of major intrahepatic or extrahepatic blood vessels.

## Surgical Treatment of Hilar Bile Duct Cholangiocarcinoma

In 1922, Fardel first reported a primary malignancy of the extrahepatic biliary tract.[44] A report in 1957 described three patients with small adenocarcinomas involving the confluence of the left and right hepatic ducts.[45] Such primary cholangiocarcinomas arising at the bifurcation of the extrahepatic biliary tree are known commonly as Klatskin's tumors, following his report in 1965 of a larger series of patients with these lesions.[46]

Cholangiocarcinomas arising in the hilar bile ducts are relatively rare. Extrahepatic biliary cancer has an incidence of 0.01%–0.46% in autopsy series.[47] Of the 17,500 projected new cases of primary hepatobiliary cancers that occur annually in the United States, approximately 2000 are Klatskin's tumors.[48]

### Prognostic factors

In contrast to reports from two or three decades ago, most patients with hilar cholangiocarcinoma are now diagnosed before death. The most important factor affecting prognosis is resectability of the tumor. Patients who undergo curative (margin-negative) resection have 3-year survival rates from 40% to 87% and 5-year survival rates between 10% and 73%.[49–52] The wide range of survival rates is explained by variations in the incidence of poor prognostic factors in the various series. Significant determinants of improved prognosis in patients undergoing curative resection include well-differentiated tumors, absence of lymph node metastases, absence of direct tumor extension into the liver, papillary (vs. nodular or sclerotic) histology, serum bilirubin at presentation of less than 9 mg/dl, and near-normal or normal performance status.[49] Palliative resection, surgical bypass procedures, and various types of intubation and drainage procedures are associated with 3-year survival rates of 0%–4%.[50] Hilar cholangiocarcinomas have a poorer prognosis than carcinomas arising in the middle or distal third of the extrahepatic bile duct, which is related directly to presentation of hilar tumors at a more locally advanced stage with bilobar liver involvement by tumor and resultant lower rates of curative resection.[53,54] However, like hilar cholangiocarcinoma, the presence of regional lymph node metastases reduces the 5-year overall survival rate following resection

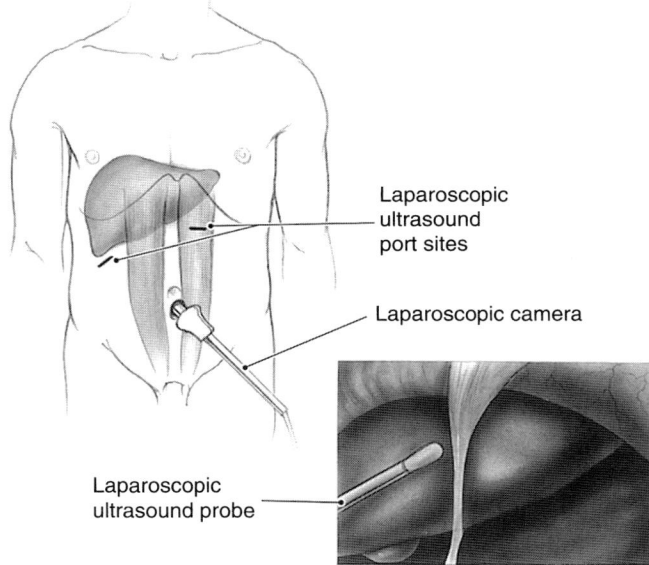

Laparoscopic ultrasound port sites

Laparoscopic camera

Laparoscopic ultrasound probe

**Figure 39–6** Schematic showing periumbilical placement of a laparoscopic camera and location of port sites for introduction of a laparoscopic ultrasound probe. Parietal and visceral peritoneal surfaces are inspected to exclude the presence of carcinomatosis in patients with cholangiocarcinoma. Laparoscopic ultrasonography is used to detect noncontiguous liver metastases.

of middle or distal third bile duct cancer to 21%, compared with 65% in patients with node-negative disease.[54]

Pathologic features of bile duct cancer are predictors of outcome. Prognosis is affected adversely if the tumor infiltrates through the serosa of the bile duct, invades directly into the liver, invades blood vessels, or has metastasized to regional lymph nodes.[55] Histologic type and grade also are important factors. Patients with the relatively unusual papillary bile duct adenocarcinoma have the most favorable prognosis, with 3-year survival rates of up to 75%.[50,55,56] Patients with the more common nodular or sclerotic types of hilar cholangiocarcinoma have 3-year survival rates of less than 30%. A pathologic study that correlated gross tumor type with patterns of spread provides evidence that may explain these observed differences in survival outcomes. Papillary and superficial nodular tumors spread predominantly by mucosal extension, rarely invading deeper layers of the bile duct wall or lymphatic channels, whereas nodular infiltrating or diffuse infiltrating tumors spread by direct or lymphatic extension in the submucosa.[57] The distance of mucosal or submucosal spread away from the gross tumor can be as great as 30 mm, but there were no local or anastomotic recurrences if at least a 5-mm tumor-free margin was attained. Patients with well- or moderately differentiated carcinomas have a 3-year survival rate of up to 51%, whereas no patient with a poorly differentiated carcinoma survived longer than 2 years.[55]

### Resection

Resection of a hilar cholangiocarcinoma affords the patient the best chance for significant survival; however, 5-year survival rates after resection of hilar cancers are 40% in the most hopeful reports and 10% or less in others. Long-term survival rates after resection of middle or distal common bile duct cholangiocarcinomas (the latter requiring pancreaticoduodenectomy) are generally higher than after resection of hilar tumors.[3] This is most likely related to higher rates of margin-negative resection of middle or distal extrahepatic bile duct tumors and the absence of direct tumor extension into the liver.

The patterns of failure after curative extrahepatic bile duct resection for hilar cholangiocarcinoma have been described in a few series of patients (Table 39–1).[58] Locoregional tumor recurrence developed in a high percentage of patients, with failure in the liver in 62%, the tumor bed in 42%, and regional lymph nodes in 20%. The caudate lobe is the most frequent site of liver recurrence. Regional lymph nodes include porta hepatis, retroduodenal, and perigastric node groups along the gastrohepatic ligament. Distant metastasis develops in most patients who suffer a locoregional recurrence but is the site of first failure in only 24%.

Detailed anatomic studies have offered an explanation for the high incidence of liver and local recurrence following resection of only the extrahepatic biliary tree for a hilar cholangiocarci-

noma. In a series of 25 patients undergoing surgery for hilar cholangiocarcinoma, direct invasion of hepatic parenchyma at the hilum was noted in 12 patients (46.2%), with 11 patients (42.3%) also having carcinoma extending into the bile ducts draining the caudate lobe or directly invading the caudate lobe parenchyma.[59] In a study of 106 adult human cadavers, 97.2% had bile ducts draining the caudate lobe that entered directly into the main left hepatic duct, right hepatic duct, or both.[60] These caudate lobe bile ducts frequently enter the main left or right hepatic ducts within 1 cm of the proper hepatic duct. Thus, a carcinoma arising at the confluence of the right and left hepatic ducts need not be large to extend into the bile ducts draining the caudate lobe.

Because cholangiocarcinoma is known to spread along the walls of the bile ducts and because the caudate lobe and hepatic hilum are frequent sites of tumor recurrence following extrahepatic duct resection, a number of authors now recommend more aggressive resections that include the caudate lobe and hepatic hilar parenchyma.[60–66] An understanding of the Bismuth-Corlette classification of hilar cholangiocarcinoma is useful in planning the extent and site of liver resection (Fig. 39–7).[67] The improved equipment and understanding of techniques requisite for a safe liver resection allow more aggressive extended resections with little or no increase in operative morbidity and mortality (Figs. 39–8 to 39–16). The median survival associated with a more radical surgical approach has ranged from 10 to 37 months, with 5-year survival rates of 20%–44% and 10-year survival rates as high as 14%.[60–66] These studies clearly show that liver resection is worthwhile only if completely tumor-negative resection margins can be attained because there were no 5-year survivors when resection margins were involved by tumor.

While aggressive surgical resection of hilar cholangiocarcinomas, including hepatic resection, provides the best chance for long-term patient survival, these operative procedures are associated with significant risk. The operative mortality rate in modern series ranges from 5% to 12%, with postoperative liver failure following extensive liver resection being the most common cause of death.[60–66] Surgical complications occur in 25%–45% of surviving patients. Infectious complications are the most common postoperative problem, and preoperative placement of biliary stents with resultant contamination of the obstructed biliary tree increases the incidence of infection.[68] Very extensive operations that include major hepatectomy, resection of the extrahepatic bile ducts, and en bloc pancreaticoduodenectomy have been used in patients with hilar cholangiocarcinoma.[69] Given an operative mortality rate of at least 30%, a 100% complication

**Table 39-1** Sites of tumor recurrence after curative resection of proximal hilar cholangiocarcinoma

| Site | Frequency (%) |
| --- | --- |
| Liver | 62 |
| Tumor bed | 42 |
| Regional lymph nodes | 20 |
| Peritoneum | 16 |
| Lungs | 71 |
| Bone | 31 |
| Skin | 7 |

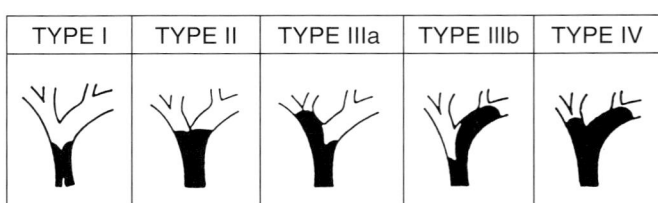

| TYPE I | TYPE II | TYPE IIIa | TYPE IIIb | TYPE IV |
| --- | --- | --- | --- | --- |

**Figure 39-7** Bismuth-Corlette classification of hilar cholangiocarcinoma. Types 1 and 2 can be resected with excision of the extrahepatic bile duct with or without the hilar plate and caudate lobe. Types 3A and 3B can be resected with the addition of an en bloc right or left hepatic lobectomy, respectively. Type 4 is unresectable because of bilobar liver involvement with resultant inability to achieve tumor-free resection margins. (From Bismuth H, Corlette MB. Intrahepatic cholangioenteric anatomosis in carcinoma of the hilus of the liver. Surg Gynecol Obstet 140:170-178, 1975, with permission.)

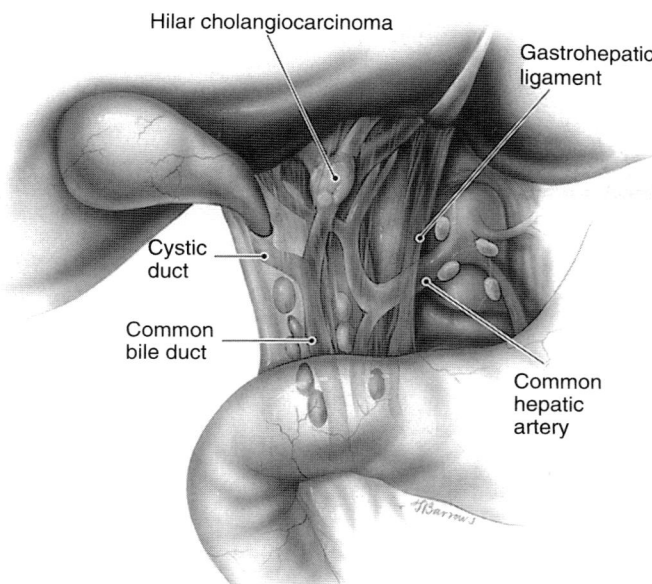

**Figure 39-8** Location of a hilar cholangiocarcinoma arising at the base of the liver at the confluence of the left and right hepatic ducts. The association of the extrahepatic bile duct with the hepatic arteries and portal vein is evident. Lymph nodes in the gastrohepatic ligament, retroduodenal, and celiac region are included to indicate possible pathways of lymphatic spread.

rate, and rare survival of patients for more than 2 years after operation, such ultraradical procedures are of dubious value.

## Multidisciplinary treatment

A multimodality approach to reduce locoregional recurrence rates and improve survival after resection of hilar cholangiocarcinoma has been reported.[70] Of 53 patients who underwent resection of a hilar cholangiocarcinoma, 38 received postoperative external beam radiotherapy to the resection bed at a dose of 50–60 Gy. In addition, 27 of these 38 patients received brachytherapy with iridium-192 seeds temporarily loaded into their transhepatic biliary stents in the area of the hepaticojejunostomies. These 27 patients received 20 Gy of internal radiation after completion of external-beam radiotherapy. There was no significant difference in the 1-, 2-, and 3-year survival rates for patients who underwent resection with or without radiotherapy, but there were no survivors after 3 years in the group that did not receive radiotherapy. The 5- and 10-year survival rates in the group receiving radiotherapy were 11% and 5%, respectively. Stented hepaticojejunostomies allow access to the remaining biliary tree following resection of hilar cholangiocarcinomas and can be used for diagnostic and therapeutic purposes.[71] Because hilar cholangiocarcinomas are rare tumors, no large-scale randomized studies have evaluated the role of adjuvant chemotherapy and/or radiotherapy following resection. Thus, there is no definitive proof that adjuvant treatment improves survival when compared with surgery alone.

We recently reviewed our experience in patients with extrahepatic cholangiocarcinoma treated at The University of Texas M. D. Anderson Cancer Center.[72] Of 91 patients evaluated between 1983 and 1996, 51 (56%) presented with unresectable disease and 40 (44%) underwent resection. The median survival for the resectable vs. unresectable patients was 22.2 months vs. 10.7 months ($P < 0.0001$). Nine patients, five with hilar and four with

distal common duct cholangiocarcinoma, were treated with preoperative chemoradiation therapy (continuous intravenous infusion of 5-fluorouracil at 300 mg/m²/day combined with external beam irradiation). Three of these nine patients had a pathologic complete response to chemoradiation treatment; the remaining six patients had varying degrees of histologic response to treatment. The rate of margin-negative resection was 100% for the preoperative chemoradiation group, compared with 54% for the group not receiving preoperative treatment ($P < 0.01$). The patients treated with preoperative chemoradiation had no operative or postoperative complications related to treatment, thus it appears that neoadjuvant chemoradiation for extrahepatic bile duct cancer can be performed safely, produces significant antitumor response, and may improve the ability to achieve tumor-free resection margins.

## Palliation

In general, curative surgical resection is possible in less than 30% of patients with hilar cholangiocarcinoma.[49–52,73] In patients deemed unresectable on the basis of diagnostic studies, laparotomy can be avoided by placing external drains percutaneously or endoprostheses endoscopically.[74,75] Conventional 10- or 12-French polyethylene endoprostheses have a high rate of occlusion and cholangitis.[76] However, new expandable metal wall

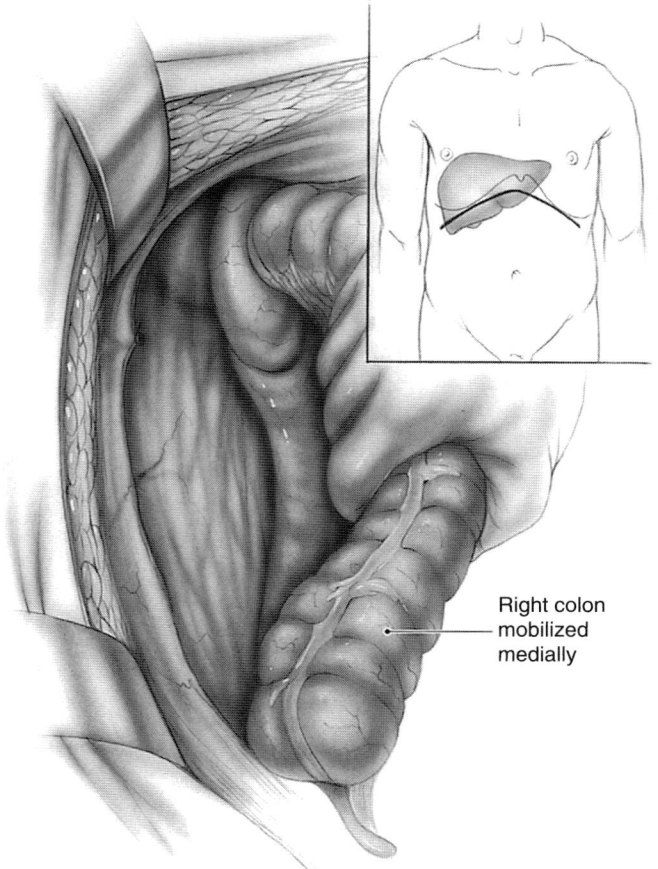

**Figure 39-9** Bilateral subcostal skin incision used for hepatobiliary resection. After exploration of the peritoneal cavity and liver to exclude the presence of distant or noncontiguous liver metastases, the entire right colon is rotated lateral to medial to gain access to the retroperitoneum for complete regional lymphadenectomy.

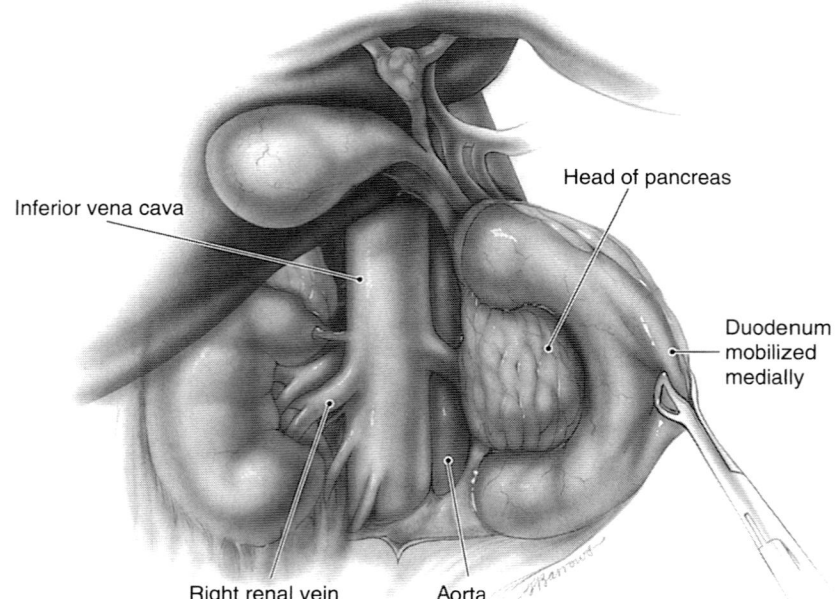

Inferior vena cava

Head of pancreas

Duodenum mobilized medially

Right renal vein          Aorta

**Figure 39-10** Complete regional lymphadectomy for a primary hilar cholangiocarcinoma deemed resectable. After mobilizing the right colon, all of the retroperitoneal tissue anterior to the capsule of the kidney, right renal vein, and inferior vena cava and posterior to the duodenum and pancreatic head is resected. This lymphadenectomy leaves the structures shown here in the field of dissection.

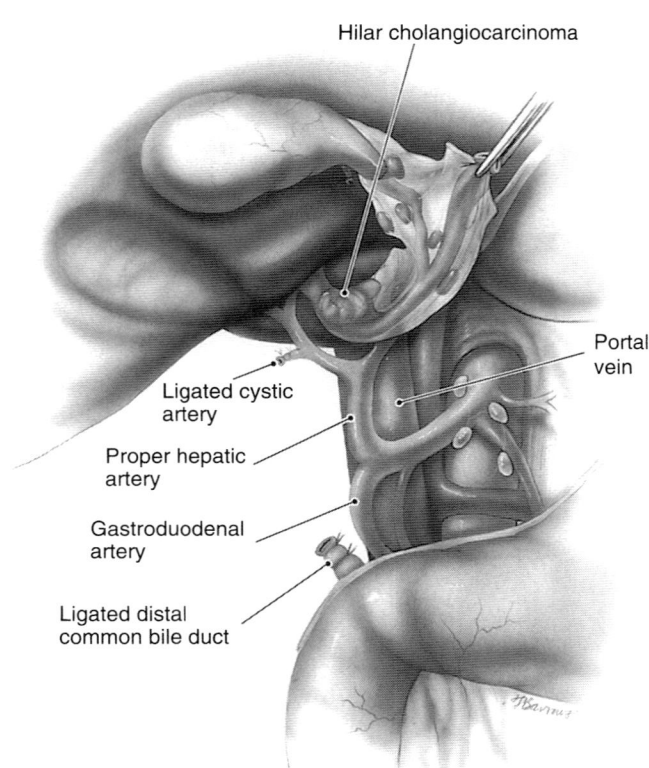

Hilar cholangiocarcinoma

Portal vein

Ligated cystic artery

Proper hepatic artery

Gastroduodenal artery

Ligated distal common bile duct

**Figure 39-11** Porta hepatis dissection in a patient with hilar cholangiocarcinoma. The common bile duct is ligated and divided at the cephalad aspect of the duodenum. The common bile duct is then reflected anteriorly and superiorly as the bile duct, including the gallbladder and cystic duct. Lymphatics in the porta hepatis and gastrohepatic ligament are dissected away from the gastroduodenal artery, hepatic arteries, and portal vein.

stents appear to stay patent longer and may be used to deliver palliative high-dose rate endoluminal brachytherapy.[77,78] When a patient is deemed unresectable at the time of laparotomy, a decision must be made between surgical bypass and operative intubation to drain the obstructed biliary tree. It is clear that techniques for surgical bypass, operative intubation, and percutaneous external drainage are equivalent in providing partial or complete relief of jaundice in 70%–100% of patients.[49] The only apparent advantage to the patient who undergoes surgical bypass

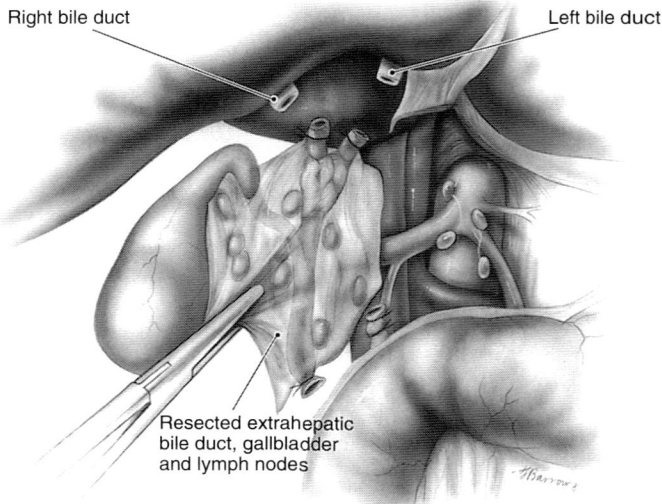

Right bile duct                                    Left bile duct

Resected extrahepatic bile duct, gallbladder and lymph nodes

**Figure 39-12** Dissection of a hilar cholangiocarcinoma off of the hepatic arteries and portal vein, followed by dissection of the left and right bile ducts proximal to the tumor. The right and left bile ducts are divided at points at least 1 cm away from palpable tumor, thus completing the resection of the hilar bile duct cancer and associated lymphatics.

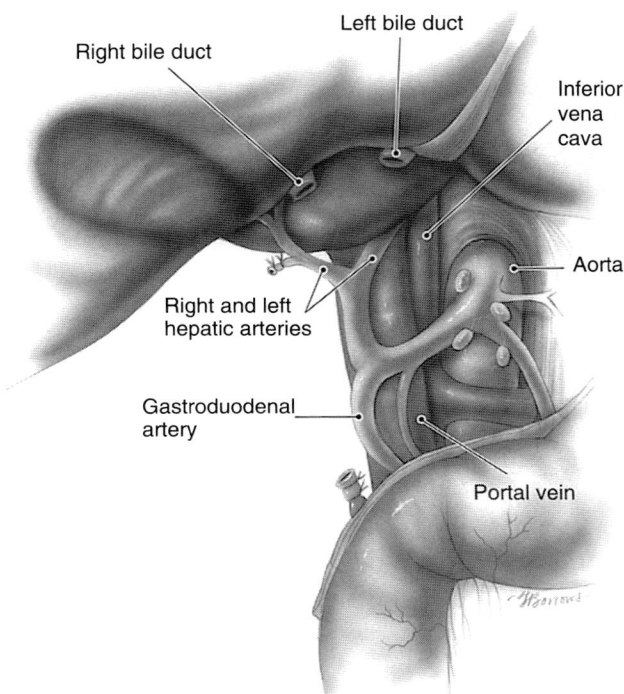

**Figure 39-13** Field of dissection in the porta hepatis following resection of a hilar cholangiocarcinoma. The bile duct and all lymphatic-bearing tissue have been completely removed, leaving only the hepatic arteries and portal vein in the porta hepatis. The resection is completed by removing the caudate lobe of the liver prior to biliary reconstruction.

instead of operative intubation is the absence of an external drainage catheter.

The advantage of not having an external biliary drainage catheter or an internal endoscopically placed biliary endoprosthesis should not be underestimated because it is known that the incidence of cholangitis, occlusion, or displacement of the catheter or endoprosthesis ranges from 28% to almost 100%.[74–76,79] Assessments of quality of life in patients with hilar cholangiocarcinoma who undergo surgical bypass, operative intubation, or percutaneous drainage have shown no distinct advantage for any one of these palliative treatments.[49,80] However, some studies suggest that the duration of well-being is longest in patients who undergo a surgical bypass.[80–83] There is no significant difference in survival related to the type of palliative procedure used to relieve biliary obstruction; the median survival in patients undergoing palliative drainage is 8 months or less. However, effective palliation of biliary obstruction in patients with unresectable hilar cholangiocarcinomas is important because 50% will survive for at least 1 year, 20% for 2 years, and 10% for 3 or more years.[84]

## Gallbladder Carcinoma

Adenocarcinoma of the gallbladder is the fifth most common gastrointestinal malignancy. When compared with the worldwide incidence of hepatocellular carcinoma, the incidence of gallbladder carcinoma is low (less than 10% of the annual cases of primary hepatobiliary cancer). In Western countries such as the United States, however, where the incidence of hepatocellular carcinoma is low, gallbladder cancer is relatively more frequent (4000 new cases in 1993 compared with 10,000 cases of hepatocellular carcinoma in the same year).[85] Autopsy and biliary tract operation data from 112,713 patients revealed an average inci-

dence of gallbladder carcinoma ranging from 0.55% to 1.91%.[86] Over the past three decades, there appears to have been a slight increase in the incidence of gallbladder carcinoma in Western countries, but this may be ascribed to more thorough reporting rather than a true increase in incidence.[86] Gallbladder carcinoma is diagnosed most frequently in the sixth and seventh decades of life. Unlike hepatocellular carcinoma (HCC) and cholangiocarcinoma, gallbladder carcinoma has a higher incidence in females than males, with a ratio of approximately 3:1.[86] This preponderance is even greater in patients less than 40 years old, with a female-to-male ratio of 20:1.[87]

Gallbladder carcinoma is more prevalent in Southwest American Indians. The incidence in this group is six times that in non-Indian populations.[88] Gallbladder carcinoma has been found in 6% of Southwest American Indians undergoing biliary tract surgery.[88] Gallbladder carcinoma is the second most common gastrointestinal malignancy in this population, and the youngest reported case of gallbladder carcinoma occurred in an 11-year-old Navajo girl.[89]

Other human populations also have an increased incidence of gallbladder cancer. In Chile, the incidence of gallbladder cancer is rising, and gallbladder cancer is the number one cause of cancer mortality in Chilean women.[90] The geographic and population-based variations in the incidence of gallbladder cancer suggest that environmental risk factors, including carcinogens, infectious agents such as *Salmonella typhi* and *Helicobacter pylori*, and diet, likely play a role in gallbladder tumorigenesis.

### Clinical Presentation

The most common symptoms and signs in patients with gallbladder carcinoma are nonspecific. Right upper-quadrant abdominal pain, which may or may not be exacerbated by eating a fatty meal, is the predominant presenting complaint in 75%–97% of patients.[86,91,92] Right upper-quadrant abdominal tenderness is present in a slightly smaller percentage of patients. These symptoms and signs usually are ascribed to cholelithiasis or cholecystitis. Nausea, vomiting, and anorexia are present in 40%–64% of patients; clinically evident jaundice, in 45%; and loss of greater than 10% of normal body weight, in 37%–77%.

Although 45% of patients are obviously jaundiced at presentation, 70% of patients present with serum bilirubin levels at least two times greater than normal.[92] Serum alkaline phosphatase levels are elevated in two-thirds of patients with gallbladder carcinoma. Alanine aminotransferase and aspartate aminotransferase levels are elevated in one-third of patients and are consistent with advanced hepatic invasion and metastases. Serum CEA levels generally are obtained only in patients diagnosed preoperatively with advanced (TNM stage III or IV) disease, and are elevated in over 80% of these patients.[92] The incidence of elevated serum CEA levels in early-stage disease is not known.

### Diagnostic Studies

Before ultrasonography and CT became widely available, the preoperative diagnosis rate for gallbladder carcinoma was only 8.6%–16.3%.[86,93] Ultrasonography is the primary imaging study for symptomatic patients with presumed cholelithiasis or choledocholithiasis. A high-resolution ultrasound is able to detect early and locally advanced gallbladder carcinoma.[94] Early tumors as small as 5 mm can be recognized as a polypoid mass projecting into the gallbladder lumen or as a focal thickening of the gallbladder wall.[95,96] In patients with locally advanced gallbladder

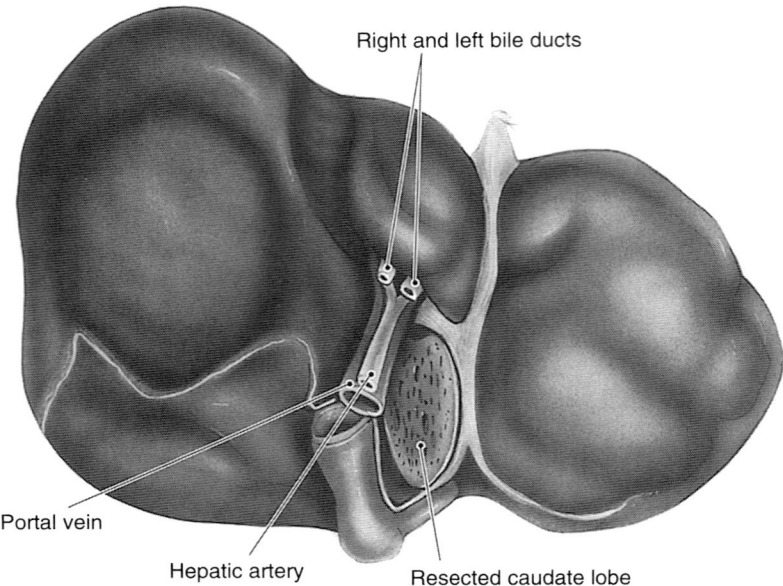

**Figure 39–14** Inferior aspect of the liver following resection of the extrahepatic bile duct and caudate lobe of the liver for a hilar cholangiocarcinoma.

carcinoma, ultrasound can demonstrate extrahepatic and intrahepatic bile duct obstruction, porta hepatis lymphadenopathy, direct hepatic extension of tumor, and hepatic metastases. Preoperative ultrasonography may suggest the correct diagnosis in up to 75% of patients with gallbladder carcinoma.[95,97,98] However, ultrasonography does not accurately detect celiac or paraortic lymphadenopathy or peritoneal dissemination of tumor.[99] Blood flow studies with color Doppler ultrasonography are also useful

because 90% of gallbladder cancers have high-velocity arterial flow, while benign lesions have minimal flow.[100] Recent advances in endoscopic ultrasonography, including the use of contrast-enhancing agents, may improve the diagnostic accuracy in assessing gallbladder cancer stage.[101]

Computed tomography scans are performed less frequently in patients with presumed benign biliary tract disease. However, if gallbladder carcinoma is suspected, CT findings can predict cor-

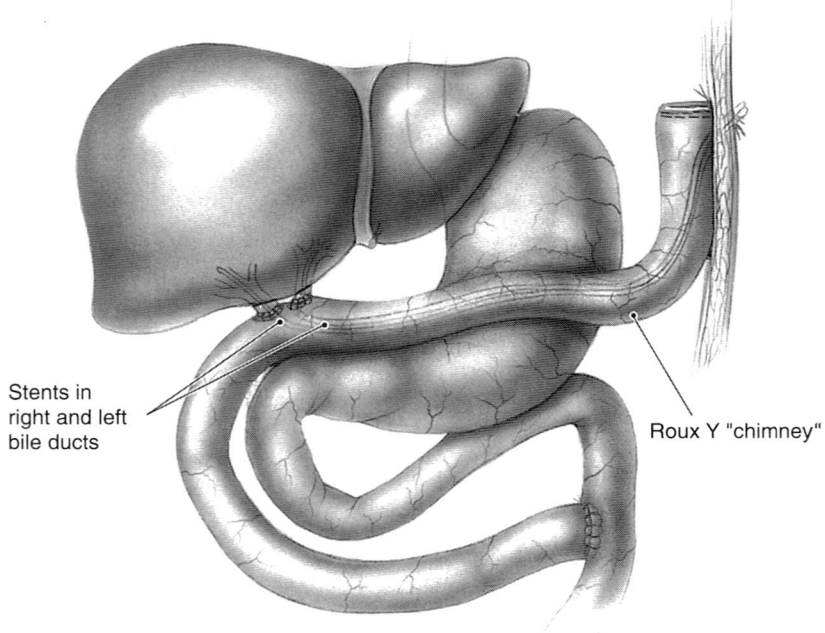

**Figure 39–15** Following resection of the extrahepatic bile ducts for a hilar cholangiocarcinoma, biliary–enteric continuity is restored with a Roux Y hepaticojejunostomy. A "chimney" of bowel can be sutured to the parietal peritoneum, thus allowing stents placed across the biliary–enteric anastomoses to be directed through the lumen of the "chimney" and then out through the abdominal wall and skin.

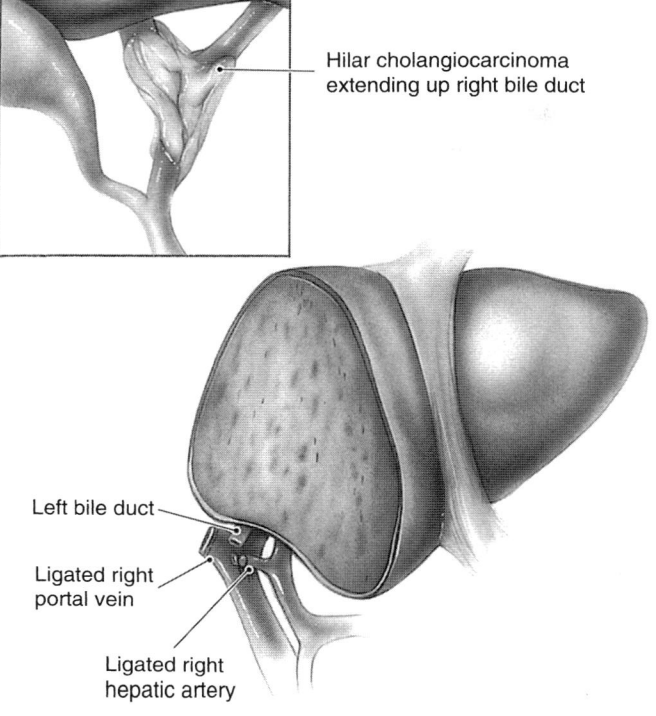

Hilar cholangiocarcinoma
extending up right bile duct

Left bile duct

Ligated right
portal vein

Ligated right
hepatic artery

**Figure 39-16** Inset diagram showing a hilar cholangiocarcinoma extending proximally into the intrahepatic portion of the right bile duct (Bismuth-Corlette type IIIa). In this situation, in addition to resection of the extrahepatic bile ducts and complete porta hepatis and retroduodenal lymphadenectomy, an en bloc resection of the right hepatic lobe and caudate lobe is performed. Biliary–enteric construction is completed with a single hepaticojejunostomy to the left bile duct using a Roux Y limb.

rectly the diagnosis in 88%–95% of patients.[102–105] The CT characteristics of gallbladder carcinoma include diffuse or focal gallbladder wall thickness of greater than 0.5 mm (95% of patients), gallbladder wall contrast enhancement (95%), intraluminal mass (90%), direct liver invasion by tumor (85%, Fig. 39–17), regional lymphadenopathy (65%), concomitant cholelithiasis (52%), dilated intrahepatic or extrahepatic bile ducts (50%), noncontiguous liver metastases (12%), invasion of contiguous gastrointestinal tract organs (8%), and intraluminal gallbladder gas (4%).[104] Computed tomography can also demonstrate calcification of the gallbladder wall (Fig. 39–18).

## Prognostic Factors

Advanced local and regional disease usually is present at the time of diagnosis of gallbladder carcinoma. Only 10% of patients with this disease have cancer confined to the gallbladder wall.[91] Direct extension of the carcinoma into the gallbladder fossa of the liver is found in 69%–83% of patients (Fig. 39–19).[106–108] Direct invasion of the liver usually indicates the presence of other regional disease because less than 12% of patients with liver involvement have no other sites of regional disease. Direct invasion of the extrahepatic biliary tract occurs in 57% of cases; the duodenum, stomach, or transverse colon, in 40%; and the pancreas, in 23% (Fig. 39–19).[86] The hepatic artery or portal vein is encased by tumor in 15% of patients. Regional lymph node metastases in the cystic, choledochal, or pancreaticoduodenal

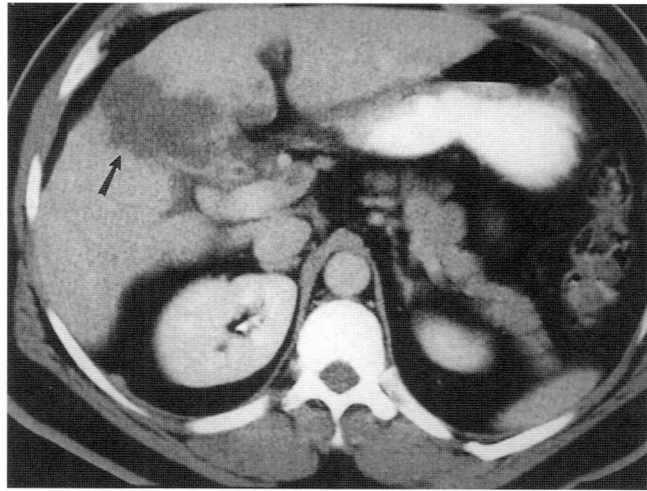

**Figure 39-17** High-resolution, helical CT scan in a patient with gallbladder carcinoma. Direct tumor invasion into the hepatic parenchyma is evident (arrow).

lymphatic drainage basins are present in 42%–70% of patients.[106] Regional lymph node metastases and/or direct tumor invasion of the hepatic parenchyma are indicators of poor prognosis and associated with significant reductions in 5-year overall survival rates.[109–111] Somewhat more distant lymph node metastases occur along the aorta or inferior vena cava in approximately 25% of patients. Importantly, lymph node metastases can occur even in the absence of liver or other contiguous organ involvement by the gallbladder carcinoma.

The pattern of lymph node metastasis from gallbladder carcinoma is predictable on the basis of anatomical studies that have identified three pathways (cholecystoretropancreatic, cholecystoceliac, and cholecystomesenteric) of lymphatic drainage of the gallbladder (Fig. 39–20).[112] The primary pathway is the cholecystoretropancreatic pathway, in which lymphatic vessels on the anterior and posterior surface of the gallbladder converge at a

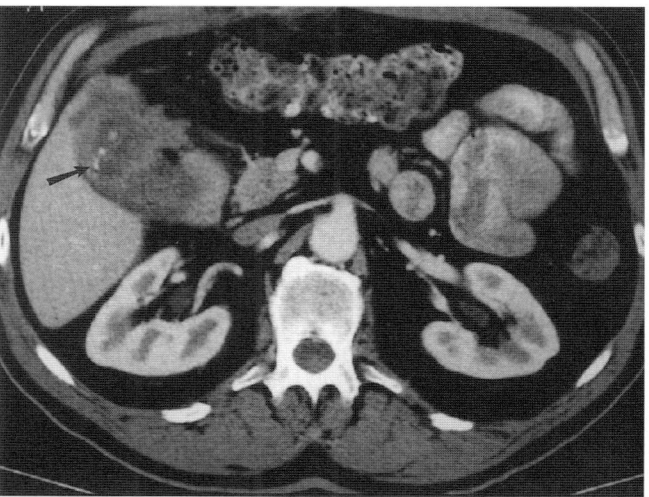

**Figure 39-18** High–resolution, helical CT scan in another patient with gallbladder cancer. A locally invasive tumor is again noted, with areas of calcification (arrow) noted in the thickened gallbladder wall.

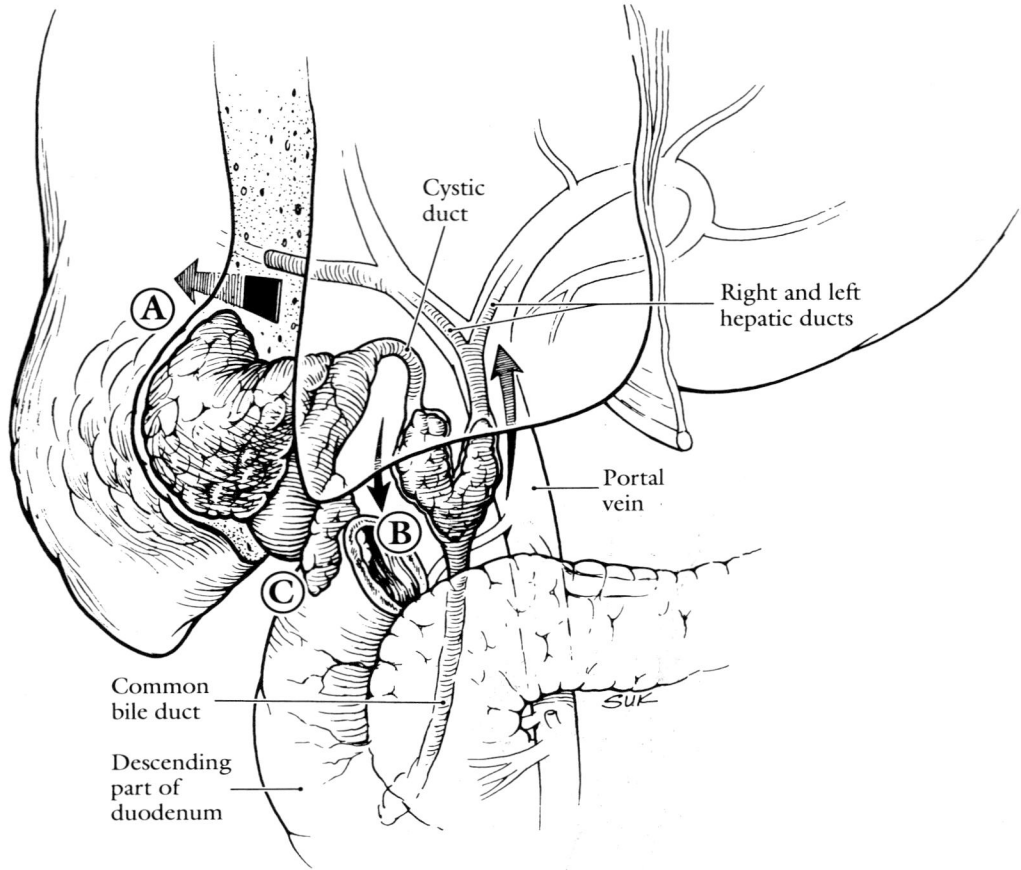

Cystic duct

Right and left hepatic ducts

Portal vein

Common bile duct

Descending part of duodenum

**Figure 39–19** Direct tumor extension from gallbladder carcinoma can lead to invasion of hepatic parenchyma adjacent to the gallbladder (A); the extrahepatic biliary tree (B); or the duodenum, stomach, or transverse colon (C).

large retroportal lymph node. This principal retroportal lymph node communicates with the choledochal and pancreaticoduodenal lymph nodes. The cholecystoceliac pathway consists of lymphatics from the anterior and posterior wall of the gallbladder that run to the left in front of the portal vein and then communicate with groups of pancreaticoduodenal lymph nodes. The cholecystomesenteric pathway drains from the gallbladder to aortocaval lymph nodes lying near the left renal vein. The final pattern of spread of gallbladder carcinoma is related to vascular invasion. Noncontiguous liver, pulmonary, and bone metastases have been found in 66%, 24%, and 12% of gallbladder carcinoma patients, respectively.[106] Pathologic evidence of vascular or lymphatic invasion indicates more aggressive disease and an increased risk for disease recurrence following resection.

The staging systems used for gallbladder carcinoma are based on the pathologic characteristics of local invasion by the tumor and lymph node metastases (Table 39–2). Before the American Joint Cancer Committee (AJCC) developed a tumor–node–metastasis (TNM) staging schema for gallbladder carcinoma, the Nevin staging system was frequently used.[113] Studies of gallbladder carcinoma in Japan generally apply the staging system of the Japanese Society of Biliary Surgery.[114] However, most recent studies have staged patients according to the TNM criteria. Carcinoma in situ corresponds to T1a, N0, M0 in the AJCC staging system.

## Surgical Treatment

### Resection

The curative resection rates for gallbladder carcinoma range from 10% to 30%.[115–117] Most patients are not candidates for curative resection because they have extensive locoregional disease, noncontiguous liver metastases, and/or distant metastases. While it is clear that long-term survival can be achieved in some patients with resectable lesions, the extent of resection remains a controversial issue.

Most surgeons consider simple cholecystectomy to be adequate treatment for gallbladder carcinoma confined to the mucosa (T1a, N0, M0). The 5-year survival rate for patients undergoing simple cholecystectomy for disease confined to the mucosa ranges from 57% to 100%.[118–121] There is no universal agreement on simple cholecystectomy as the sole treatment for patients with T1a, N0, M0 tumors; some authors recommend extended cholecystectomy (cholecystectomy; wedge resection of the gallbladder fossa including a 3- to 5-cm margin of normal liver; and a cystic, pericholedochal, gastrohepatic, pancreaticoduodenal, and paraaortic lymphadenectomy) for patients with these very early–stage lesions.[122,123] These same authors recommend that all gallbladders be opened at the time of cholecystectomy to obtain samples for frozen-section evaluation of any suspicious areas in the mucosa. If an unsuspected gallbladder

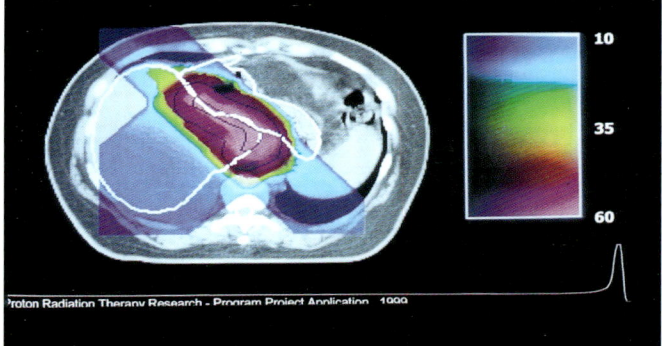

**Color Figure 7-1** A 4-field proton plan of a patient who has undergone a resection of a bile duct cancer with microscopic residual tumor along the liver transection margin. The color scheme indicates the dose distribution with 60 Gy (pink) covering the tumor volume. The uninvolved liver receives substantially less irradiation (<20 Gy).

**Color Figure 7-2** A 5-field intensity modulated radiation treatment (IMXT) plan of the same patient with a resected bile duct cancer with microscopic residual tumor at the liver transection margin. In comparison to the proton plan, substantially higher doses of radiation go to the uninvolved liver (40% to 80% of prescription dose, 60 Gy).

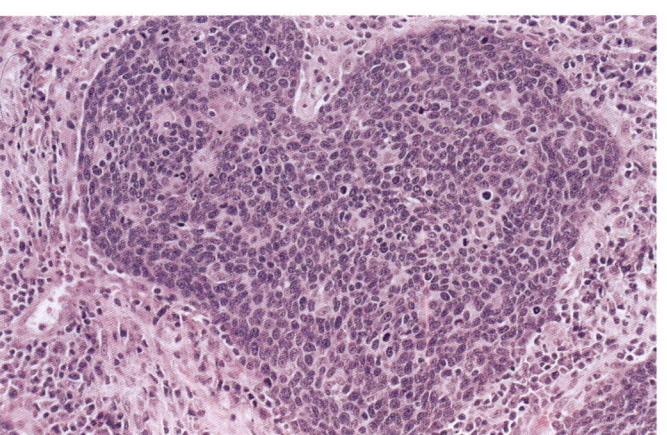

**Color Figure 14-2** High-power view of a basaloid carcinoma showing a large aggregate of cells containing irregular pleomorphic, somewhat pale nuclei with numerous mitotic figures and intervening hyalin-like material in the intercellular space. Focal palisading of tumor cells is noted at the edge of this lobule. In other areas, the tumor showed dysplastic changes in the overlying squamous mucosa.

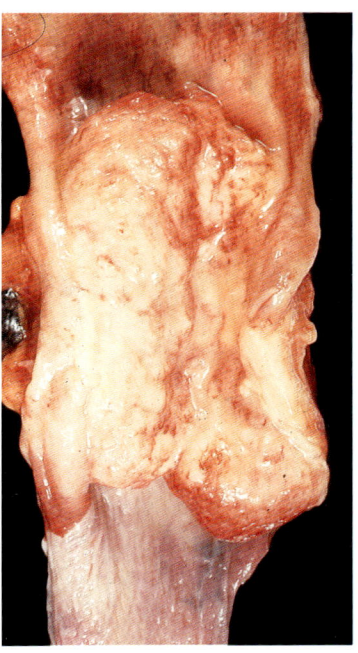

**Color Figure 14-6** Resection specimen from a patient with adenocarcinoma arising in Barrett's esophagus. In the center of the field, there is an exophytic irregular tumor mass arising a few centimeters above the original gastroesophageal junction (bottom of photo). The mucosa surrounding and above the tumor mass shows a nodular pattern and is similar in appearance to the columnar mucosa in the distal gastroesophageal and proximal stomach region. The neosquamocolumnar junction (top of photo) is present 5–6 cm above the gastroesophageal junction.

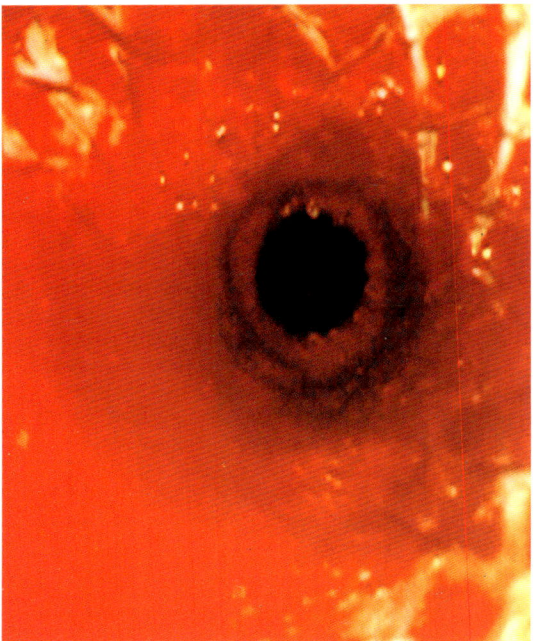

**Color Figure 17-3** Endoscopic view of a deployed esophageal stent.

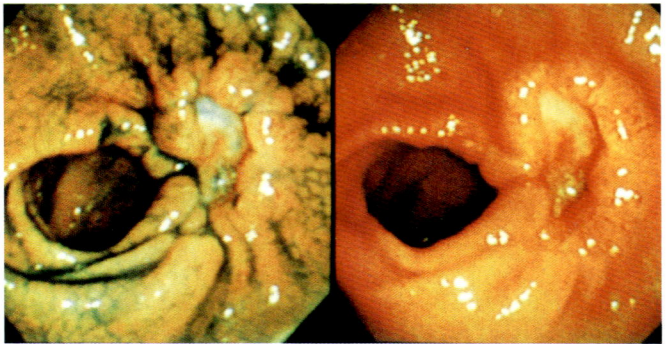

**Color Figure 24–1** Endoscopic identification of gastric cancer.

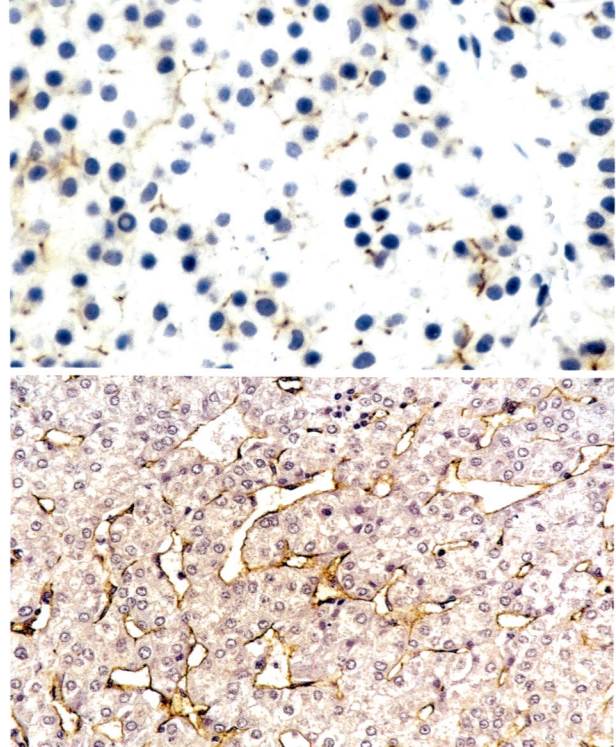

**Color Figure 43–10** Immunohistochemistry in hepatocellular carcinoma. Carcinoembryonic antigen (CEA) polyclonal antibodies cross-react with biliary glycoprotein 1, producing a specific staining pattern (top). Capillarization of sinusoids occurs with expression of CD34 (bottom).

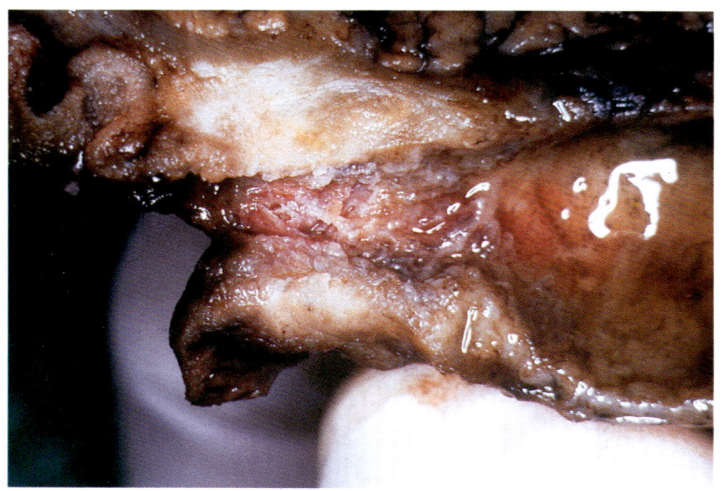

**Color Figure 48–1** Ampulla of Vater. Adenocarcinoma. Longitudinal section through the ampulla and distal common bile duct. Carcinoma thickens wall of ampulla, causing partial obstruction and dilatation of bile duct.

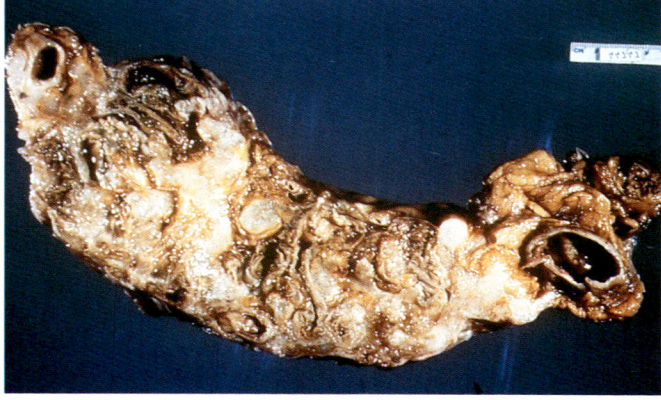

A

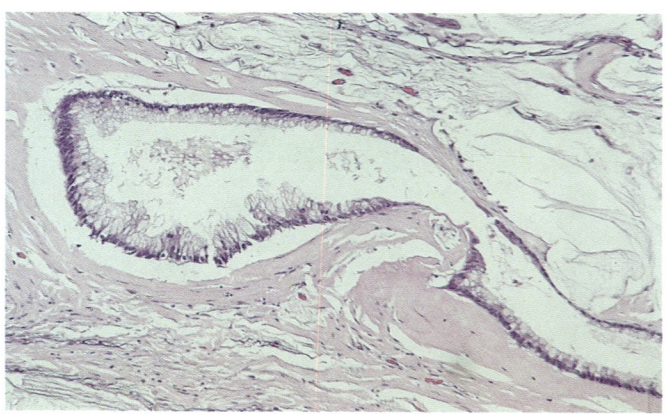

B

**Color Figure 48–8** Peritoneum. Metastatic mucinous adenocarcinoma (pseudomyxoma peritonei). *A:* Several loops of small intestine are encased in a mass of loculated mucus and fibrous tissue. *B:* Well- differentiated mucus-producing epithelium embedded in a fibrous matrix. Mucus is within the lumen and is extravasated in the stroma.

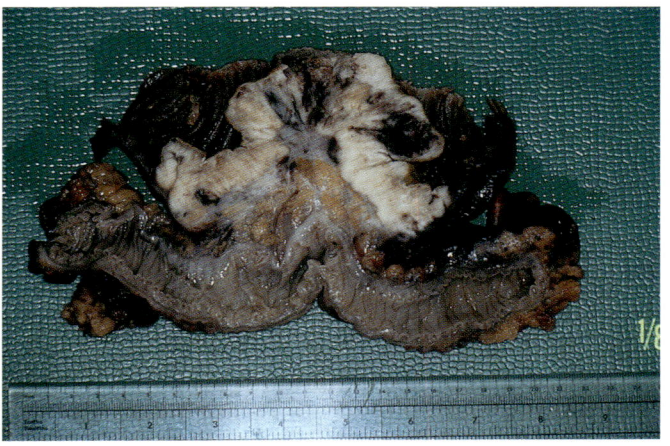

**A**

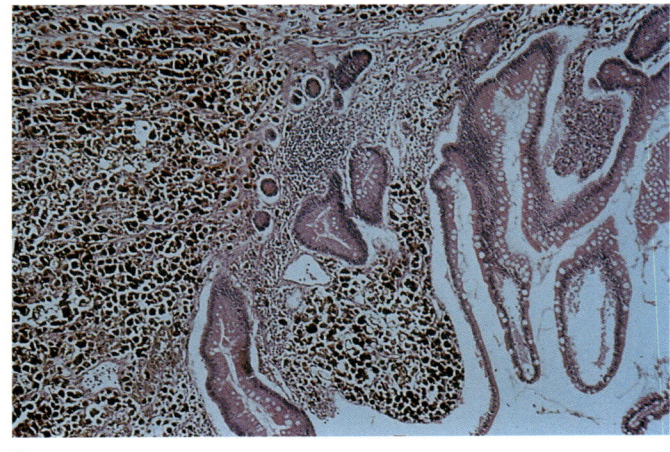

**B**

**Color Figure 48–16** Small intestine. Metastatic malignant melanoma. *A:* A large tumor fusing the small and large intestine. *B:* Heavily pigmented melanoma cells diffusely infiltrating the mucosa.

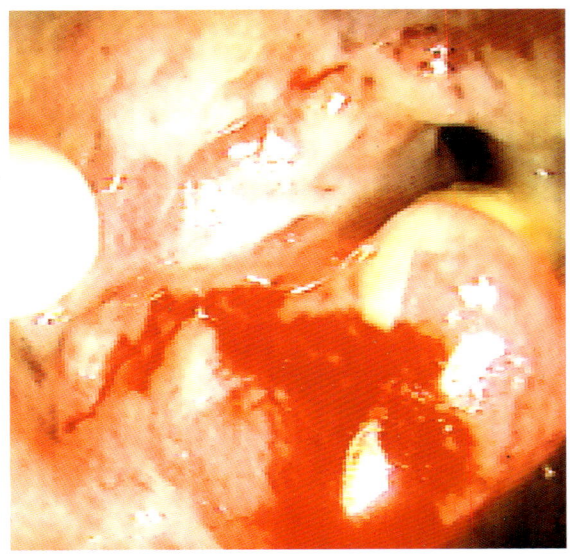

**Color Figure 58–1** Colonoscopic image of a nearly obstructing rectal cancer.

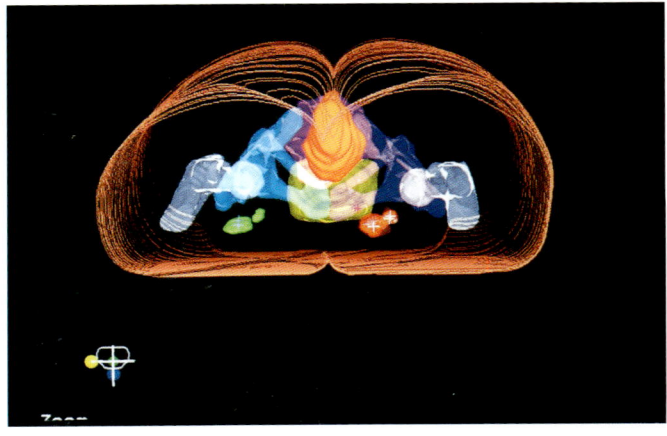

**A**

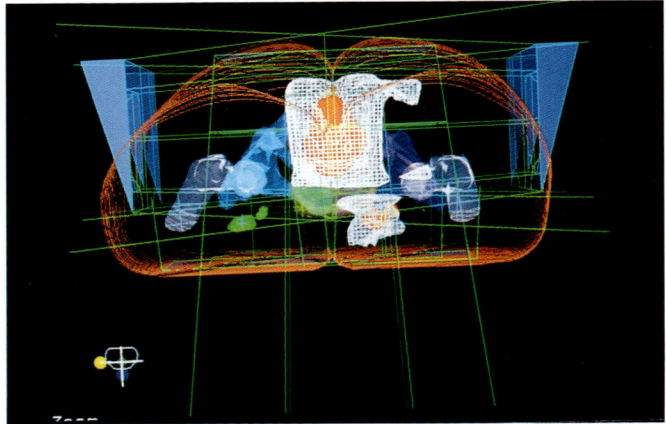

**B**

**Color Figure 63–3** Three-dimensional conformal boost plan for a patient with a T3 N1 M0 squamous cell carcinoma of the anal canal treated with a total dose of 55.8 Gy with concurrent cisplatin and 5-fluorouracil. This patient was treated in the prone position. *A:* Computed tomography images of the patient's primary cancer with the target volume delineated in orange. Normal tissues, such as the bladder, are also contoured. *B:* In the same patient, the 98% isodose curve encompasses the target volume. Also shown is the 98% isodose curve surrounding the lymph node in the patient's right groin that was positive for metastases upon biopsy and was treated with electron boost.

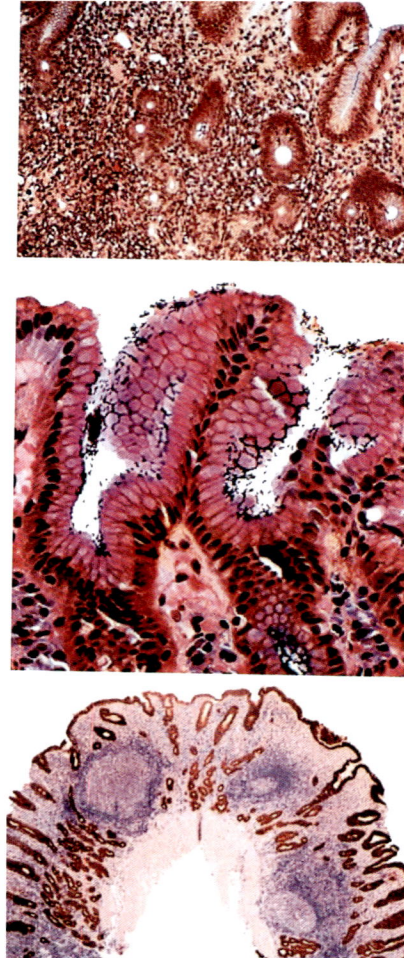

**Color Figure 66–2** *H. pylori* gastritis and mucosa-associated lymphoid tissue (MALT) in the stomach. The *upper* panel shows chronic active gastritis, with mononuclear and polymorphonuclear cell infiltration in the gastric mucosa. The *middle* panel shows large numbers of *H. pylori* organisms, stained brown with a Genta stain, attached to the gastric surface epithelium. In the *lower* panel, a cytokeratin (AE1/AE3) stain highlights prominent lymphoid follicles pushing the normal glandular epithelium.

**Color Figure 66–3** Low-grade mucosa-associated lymphoid tissue (MALT) lymphoma. The *left* panel shows diffuse infiltration of the gastric mucosa by centrocyte-like cells. The *middle* panel shows a higher-power magnification of the area, demonstrating an effaced lymphoid follicle that resulted from follicular colonization by the lymphoma cells. The follicle center can still be recognized by the presence of tingible-body macrophages, which contain abundant, pale cytoplasm. The *right* panel shows an example of the epithelial destruction caused by lymphoepithelial invasion. Isolated gastric epithelial cells with abundant eosinophilic cytoplasm are surrounded by the lymphoid infiltrate (hematoxylin and eosin stain).

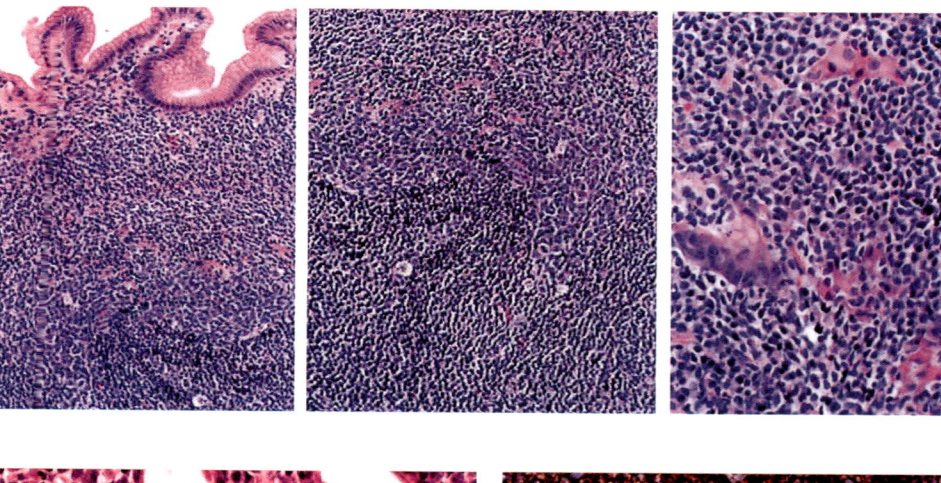

**Color Figure 66–5** Diffuse infiltrate in high-grade large B-cell lymphoma. The tumor lymphocytes are uniformly stained with the CD20 marker on immunohistochemical stains, confirming the B-cell lineage of the lymphoma.

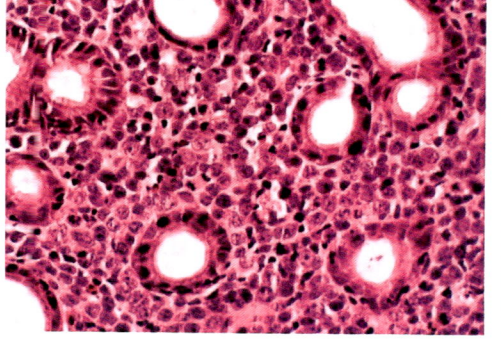

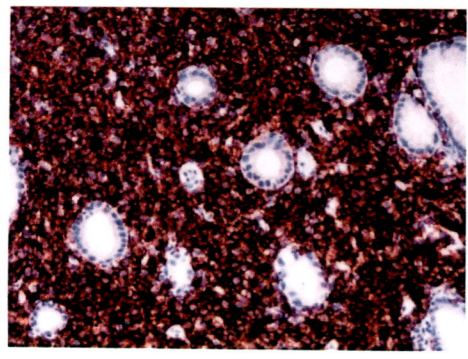

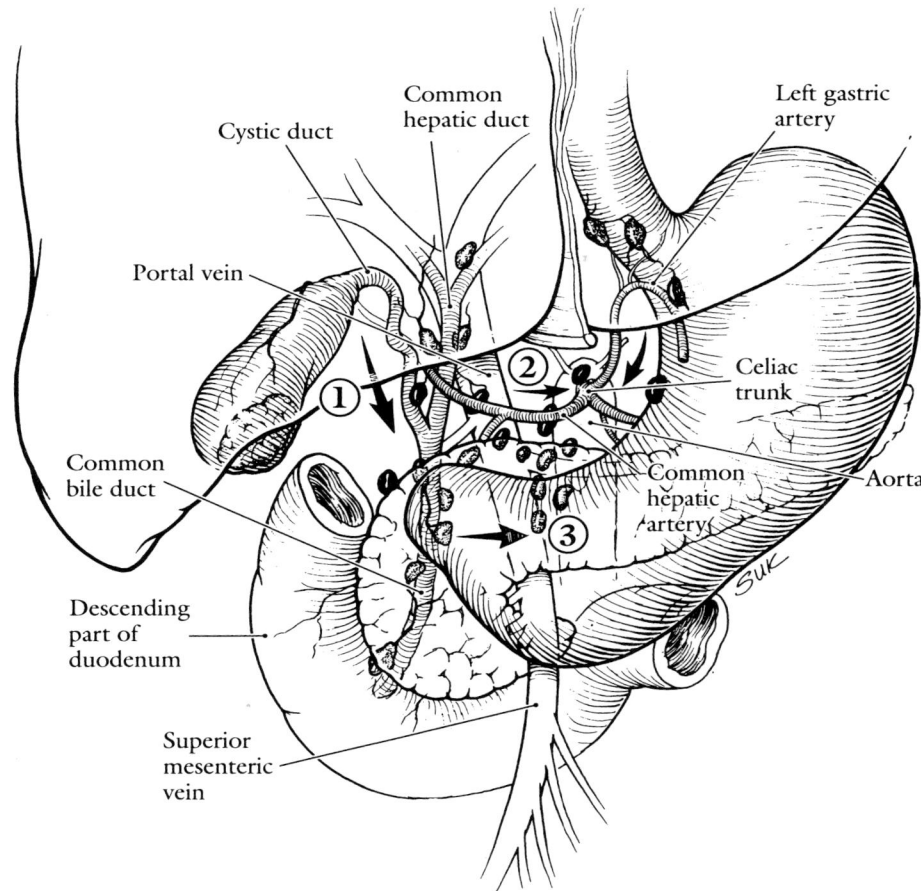

**Figure 39-20** Patterns of lymphatic drainage from the gallbladder. The main pathway of lymphatic drainage and, thus, lymph node metastasis from gallbladder cancer is to the cholecystoretropancreatic nodes (1). This pathway drains from the gallbladder to nodes along the cystic duct and common bile duct and then to nodes posterior to the duodenum and pancreatic head. The cholecystoceliac pathway (2) courses from the gallbladder through the gastrohepatic ligament to celiac nodes. A third lymphatic drainage route, the cholecystomesenteric pathway (3), courses from the gallbladder posterior to the pancreas to the aortocaval lymph nodes.

carcinoma is diagnosed by frozen-section biopsy or if a T1a, N0, M0 gallbladder carcinoma is diagnosed on final pathological review, these authors advocate that an extended cholecystectomy be performed. The rationale for this aggressive surgical treatment of T1a, N0, M0 gallbladder carcinoma is based on the small number of cases of regional lymph node recurrence in patients treated with simple cholecystectomy alone. No rationale is provided for liver resection in these early-stage patients; the small number of patients who did fail after simple cholecystectomy developed metastases in pericholedochal or cystic lymph nodes and not in the liver. Furthermore, the incidence of subsequent lymph node metastases in T1a, N0, M0 patients was less than 10% in two small groups of 32 and 36 patients, respectively.[122,123] In a study of patients who underwent cholecystectomy and regional lymphadenectomy, the incidence of lymph node metastases in 201 patients with gallbladder carcinoma confined to the mucosa was only 2.5%.[119] The mortality rate for extended resection ranges from 2% to 5%, and the rates of major postoperative morbidity range from 13% to 40%.[118–120,124] Therefore, the morbidity and mortality associated with extended cholecystectomy is excessive compared with the potential survival benefit to less than 5% of patients with T1a, N0, M0 lesions.

There is a rationale for performing extended cholecystectomy in patients with T1b tumors or AJCC TNM stage II and III gallbladder carcinomas (Fig. 39–21). In 165 patients with T1b gallbladder carcinomas, there was a 15.6% incidence of regional lymph node metastasis.[119] Of 867 patients with T2 primaries, 56.1% had regional lymph node metastases.[119] The 453 patients with T3 tumors had a 74.4% incidence of regional lymph node metastases.[119] The 5-year survival rates following extended cholecystectomy for AJCC stage II and III gallbladder carcinoma range from 7.5% to 37%.[118–120,122,124,125] Patients with AJCC stage II or III gallbladder carcinoma treated with simple cholecystectomy alone had a 0% 5-year survival rate, compared with a 29% 5-year survival rate in those patients treated with extended cholecystectomy.[124] Microscopically positive liver resection margins have a negative impact on survival; patients with these margins had a median survival of 8.9 months, compared to 67.2 months for patients with tumor-free margins.[109] Preoperative helical CT scans and intraoperative ultrasonography are used to assess the extent of direct invasion into the hepatic parenchyma. If adequate tumor-negative resection margins are attained, the radicality of liver resection does not have an impact on survival, as attested to by similar long-term survival rates following right

**Table 39-2** Comparison of the most commonly used staging systems for gallbladder carcinoma

| Stage | Nevin | JSBS | AJCC TNM |
|---|---|---|---|
| I | Cancer confined to the mucosa | Cancer confined to subserosal layers | T1a, N0, M0<br>T1b, N0, M0 |
| II | Cancer involves the mucosa and muscularis | Direct invasion of the liver and/or bile duct, porta hepatis lymph node metastases | T2, N0, M0 |
| III | Cancer extends through the serosa (all three layers of the gallbladder wall involved) | More extensive liver invasion by cancer, more extensive regional lymph node metastases (gastrohepatic, retropancreatic) | T1, N1, M0<br>T2, N1, M0<br>T3, Any N, M0 |
| IV | Tumor through all three layers of the gallbladder wall with cystic lymph node metastasis | Liver, peritoneal, and/or distant organ metastases | T4, Any N, M0<br>Any T, Any N, M1 |
| V | Tumor invades the liver by direct extension and/or metastasis to any distant organ | No stage V | No stage V |

AJCC, American Joint Committee on Cancer; JSBS, Japanese Society of Biliary Surgery; TNM, primary Tumor, regional lymph Node, distant Metastasis; T1, tumor invades mucosa or muscle layer; T1a, tumor invades mucosa; T1b, tumor invades muscle; T2, tumor invades perimuscular connective tissue, no extension beyond serosa or into liver; T3, tumor invades beyond serosa or into one adjacent organ or both (extension <2 cm into liver); T4, tumor extends >2 cm into liver and/or into two or more adjacent organs (stomach, duodenum, colon, pancreas, omentum, extrahepatic bile ducts). N0, no regional lymph node metastasis; N1, regional lymph node metastasis; N1a, metastasis in cystic duct, pericholedochal, and/or gastrohepatic lymph nodes; N1b, metastasis in peripancreatic, periduodenal, periportal, celiac, and/or superior mesenteric artery lymph nodes. M0, no distant metastasis; M1, distant metastasis.

lobectomy, extended right lobectomy, right trisegmentectomy, and central bisegmentectomy for gallbladder cancer.[118–120,126–128] T1b patients are classified as stage I in the AJCC system but, arguably, with a 15.6% incidence of regional lymph node metastases, long-term survival benefit may occur in a significant number of these patients who undergo an extended cholecystectomy (see Fig. 39–21).

En bloc resection of the extrahepatic bile duct is not always done as part of an extended cholecystectomy. An en bloc resection of the proper hepatic and common bile duct with Roux Y hepaticojejunostomy should be included in an extended cholecystectomy of transmurally invasive tumors because tumor invades the extrahepatic bile duct in 57% of cases (Fig. 39–22). This includes those cases in which a clinically unsuspected gallbladder carcinoma is diagnosed pathologically following a simple cholecystectomy with a positive margin at the cystic duct. Gallbladder cancer involving the cystic duct and gallbladder neck frequently grows along the proper hepatic and right bile ducts, necessitating a right or extended right hepatic lobectomy and excision of the extrahepatic ducts to remove all disease.[129]

Extremely radical operations have been proposed for patients with extensive T3, N1, M0 or T4, N0–1, M0 tumors. This includes hepatopancreaticoduodenectomy and abdominal organ cluster transplantation for locally advanced gallbladder carcinoma.[119,130,131] The operative mortality rate for these radical procedures is at least 15% with a greater than 90% incidence of major morbidity. Resection of the portal vein and/or hepatic artery with vascular reconstruction is frequently necessary to resect all malignant disease completely. The largest report of patients undergoing hepatopancreaticoduodenectomy for gallbladder carcinoma is 150 cases from Japan, with a 5-year survival rate of 14%.[119] The patients who did not die from intraoperative or postoperative complications all succumbed to recurrent and/or metastatic carcinoma.

## Impact of laparoscopic cholecystectomy

It is estimated that 70,000 laparoscopic cholecystectomies are performed each year in the United States.[132] On average, gall-

bladder carcinoma is diagnosed in 2% of patients undergoing cholecystectomy for presumed benign biliary tract disease.[86] Thus, approximately 1400 patients annually who undergo laparoscopic cholecystectomy could suffer inadvertent dissemination of gallbladder carcinoma.[132–138] The spillage of tumor cells at the time of laparoscopic cholecystectomy has caused seeding of peritoneal surfaces and laparoscopic port tracts in several patients.[139,140] This dissemination of tumor cells is an unfortunate occurrence because it may preclude a potentially curative open resection and limit the patient's long-term survival. However, the potential laparoscopic dissemination of tumor cells may not significantly alter the natural history of gallbladder cancer in most patients. At The University of Texas M. D. Anderson Cancer Center, a review of our experience with diagnostic and therapeutic laparoscopy in patients with gastrointestinal malignancies indicated that port site recurrence is a harbinger of widespread metastasis in greater than 95% of patients.[141] Thus, a laparoscopic port site is rarely an isolated site of recurrent malignant disease.[141] Furthermore, a report drawn from the National Cancer Data Base on gallbladder carcinoma in the United States between 1989 and 1995 revealed no change in incidence or survival from gallbladder cancer during the time laparoscopic cholecystectomy supplanted open cholecystectomy as the procedure of choice for presumed benign gallbladder disease.[142] Nonetheless, because of the large number of cholecystectomies being performed laparoscopically and the small but measurable risk of dissemination of tumor cells, it has been recommended that (1) unless the surgeon feels capable of performing a definitive extended cholecystectomy for gallbladder carcinoma, cases in which gallbladder carcinoma is suspected preoperatively by clinical or radiologic criteria should be referred without laparoscopy, laparotomy, or percutaneous biopsy; and (2) if gallbladder carcinoma is suspected on visual inspection during an attempted laparoscopic cholecystectomy, either an open definitive operation should be performed or the operation should be terminated without biopsy and the patient referred for appropriate surgical therapy.[133] Patients who undergo laparoscopic cholecystectomy and are then found on pathologic analysis to have gallbladder cancer should

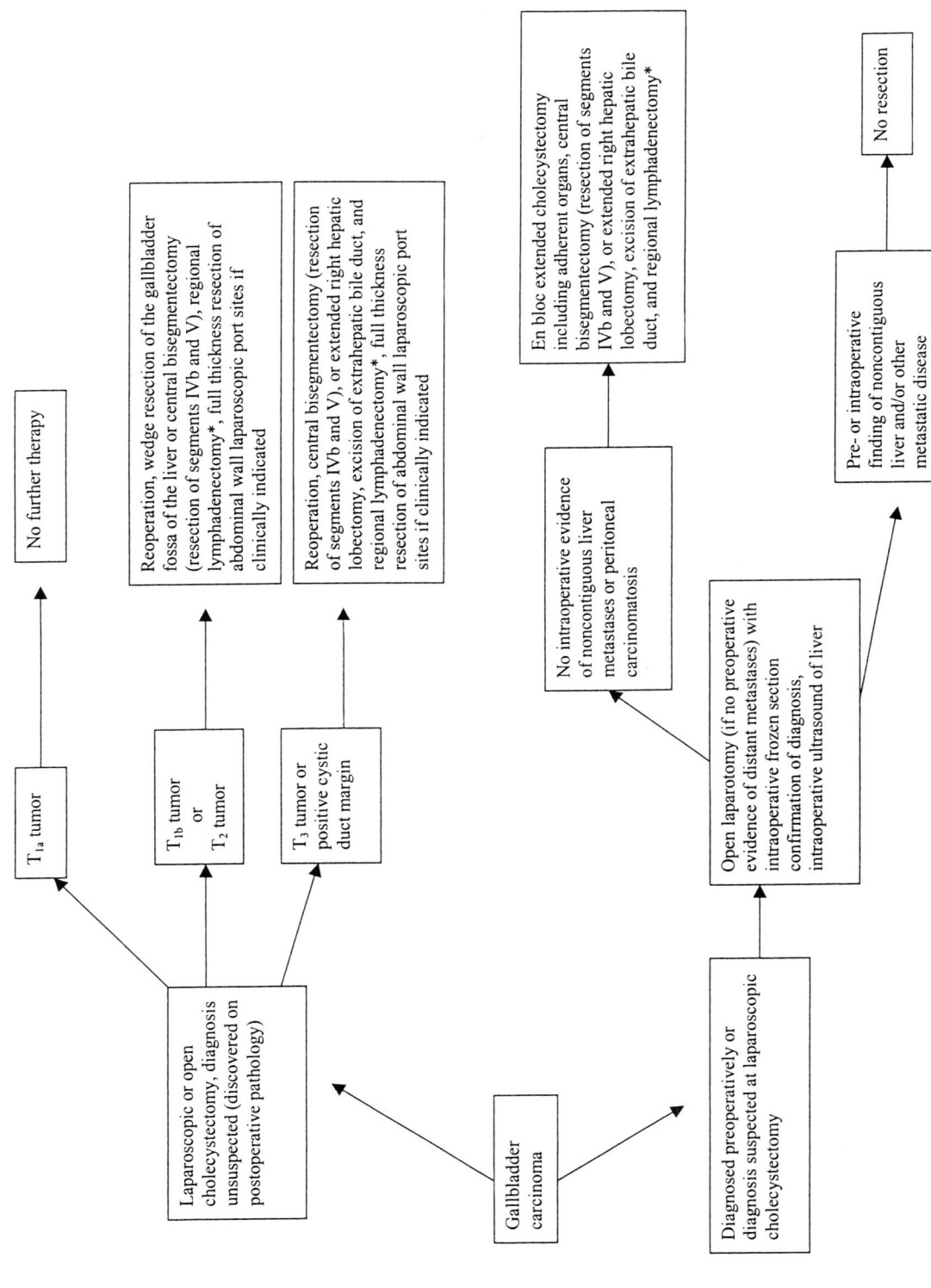

**Figure 39-21** Algorithm for guiding surgical decision making in patients with gallbladder cancer. *Regional lymphadenectomy includes complete dissection and removal of the cystic, pericholedochal, pancreaticoduodenal, gastrohepatic, and paraaortic lymph nodes.

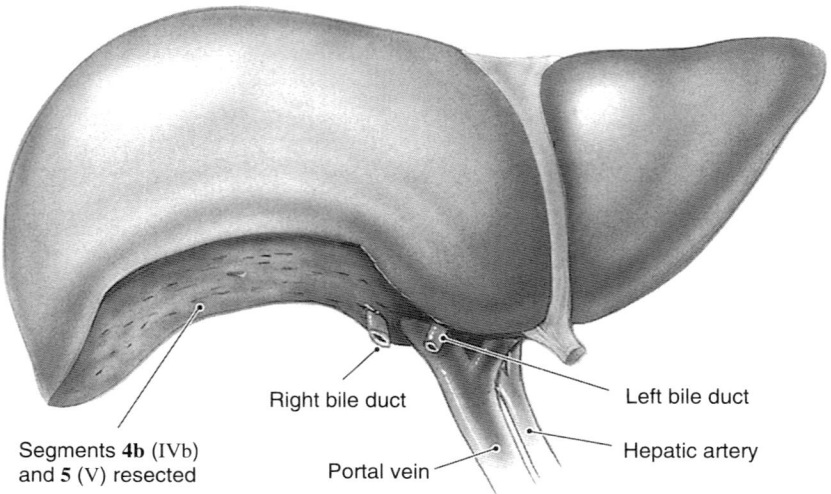

Figure 39-22 Stage II or III gallbladder cancer with minimal hepatic invasion can be treated by regional lymphadenectomy and resection of segments IVb and V of the liver. The extrahepatic bile duct is also resected when tumor extends down the cystic duct or directly invades the proper hepatic duct. Biliary–enteric continuity in this instance is established with a Roux Y hepaticojejunostomy. For more extensive hepatic invasion by gallbladder cancer, right hepatic trisegmentectomy may be required.

still be considered for aggressive surgical treatment because long-term disease-free survival will occur in a subset of these patients (Fig. 39–21).[143]

Palliation

Most patients with gallbladder carcinoma are diagnosed at an advanced, unresectable stage of disease. As in patients with hilar bile duct cancer, relief of symptomatic jaundice is an important consideration that can affect quality of life. Patients with unresectable gallbladder carcinoma often have extensive involvement of the extrahepatic bile duct and may have bulky porta hepatis lymphadenopathy, making endoscopic placement of an internal stent difficult. When unresectable gallbladder carcinoma is diagnosed at the time of laparotomy, a surgical biliary bypass, such as an intrahepatic cholangioenteric anastomosis, can be performed, resulting in significant symptomatic relief in greater than 90% of patients.[49] When the diagnosis is made on the basis of radiographic and percutaneous biopsy findings, jaundice can be relieved by placing transhepatic biliary catheters percutaneously.

In contrast to patients with hilar bile duct carcinoma in which gastroduodenal obstruction is a relatively rare event, 30%–50% of patients with advanced gallbladder carcinoma will develop a clinically significant element of gastroduodenal obstruction.[144] This can be treated surgically with a bypass procedure, such as gastrojejunostomy, or by placing decompressing gastrostomy and feeding jejunostomy tubes. A percutaneous endoscopic gastrostomy tube can also be used to decompress the obstructed stomach in patients with advanced disease and limited life expectancy.

Multidisciplinary treatment

Most patients who undergo an extended cholecystectomy or more radical resection for AJCC stage II, II, or IV gallbladder carcinoma develop tumor recurrence and die as a result of their disease. Nonrandomized studies and case reports have suggested that overall survival can be improved by administering adjuvant radiation therapy and/or chemotherapy after resection of stage II, III, or IV tumors.[145,146] Unfortunately, the number of patients who have received postsurgical adjuvant treatment is small, and

a variety of treatment regimens have been used. In a nonrandomized study, 9 patients with stage IV gallbladder carcinoma were treated with complete surgical resection alone, while 17 patients were treated with complete resection combined with 20–30 Gy of intraoperative radiation therapy.[147] Ten of these 17 patients also received 36.4 Gy of postoperative external-beam radiation therapy. The surgical procedures performed in both groups of patients included extended cholecystectomy and a variety of more radical procedures, including hepatopancreaticoduodenectomy. There were no 3-year survivors in the 9 patients treated with resection alone, but there was a 10.1% 3-year survival in the 17 patients treated with resection and radiation therapy. There is a single report of 18 patients treated with preoperative chemoradiation therapy (4500 cGy, 180 cGy/fraction, 5 days/week, continuous intravenous infusion of 5-fluorouracil (5-FU) 350 mg/m$^2$/day on days 1–5 and 21–25) prior to a planned resection of known gallbladder cancer.[148] Thirteen of the 18 patients underwent resection; one patient refused operation, one patient did not complete preoperative chemoradiation, one patient progressed after chemoradiation, and two patients had unresectable disease found at laparotomy. The 5-year actuarial survival rate in the 13 resected patients was 57%. Unfortunately, there are no randomized trials of patients with stage II and III gallbladder carcinoma treated with a coherent program of adjuvant or neoadjuvant therapy. Such trials will be necessary to demonstrate an improvement in survival in patients who receive pre- or postoperative therapies combined with a curative resection for gallbladder carcinoma.

## References

1. Anthony PP: Tumours and tumour-like lesions of the liver and biliary tract. In: MacSween RNM, Anthony PP, Scheuer PJ (eds): Pathology of the Liver, 2nd ed. Churchill Livingstone, Edinburgh, 1987, p 574.
2. Thuluvath PJ, Rai R, Venbrux AC, Yeo CJ. Cholangiocarcinoma: a review. Gastroenterologist 5:306–315, 1997.
3. Nakeeb A, Pitt HA, Sohn TA, et al. Cholangiocarcinoma: a spectrum of intrahepatic, perihilar, and distal tumors. Ann Surg 224:463–475, 1996.
4. Pitt H, Dooley W, Yeo C, Cameron J. Malignancies of the biliary tree. Curr Probl Surg 32:1–90, 1995.

**Table 40-1** TNM staging of gallbladder cancer

| Stage | Tumor | Description | Nodes | Description | Metastases | Description |
|---|---|---|---|---|---|---|
| Stage 0 | Tis | Carcinoma in situ | N0 | No nodal involvement | M0 | No distant metastases |
| Stage I | T1 | Tumor limited to mucosa or muscularis | N0 | | M0 | |
| Stage II | T2 | Tumor invades serosa | N0 | | M0 | |
| Stage III | T1–2 | | N1 | Metastasis in cystic duct, bile duct, or hilar lymph nodes | M0 | |
| | T3 | Tumor invades liver (<2 cm) or one adjacent organ | N0–1 | | M0 | |
| Stage IVa | T4 | Tumor extends >2 cm into liver or two or more adjacent organs | N0–1 | | M0 | |
| Stage IVb | T1–4 | | N2 | Metastasis in other lymph nodes | M0 | |
| | T1–4 | | N0–2 | | M1 | Distant metastases |

bar peripheral hepatic metastases, extrahepatic disease, or occlusion of the common hepatic artery or main portal vein generally are considered to be contraindications to resection. Nonsurgical palliative therapy to relieve obstructive jaundice is accomplished through percutaneous transhepatic cholangiographic catheters or endoscopically placed stents to decompress the biliary tree. Surgical palliative procedures for proximal lesions can include a Roux-en-Y hepaticojejunostomy with transhepatic stent placement or a segment III bypass to the left intrahepatic duct.[14,15] For distal tumors, a Whipple procedure, a choledochojejunostomy, hepaticojejunostomy, or cholecystojejunostomy to decompress the biliary tree and a prophylactic gastrojejunostomy to avoid possible late gastroduodenal obstructions can be performed.[9,14,15]

## Treatment of Unresectable Gallbladder Carcinoma and Cholangiocarcinoma

### Radiation Therapy

External-beam radiation therapy has traditionally been thought of as a palliative form of therapy in gallbladder cancer and cholangiocarcinomas.[16–30] Surrounding tissues limit the dose of radiation that can be effectively delivered to the cancer cells. In 1997, Todokori et al. extensively reviewed the role of radiotherapy in the treatment of primary gallbladder cancer in 113 patients.[18] Detailed descriptions of radiotherapy were provided for 82 patients: 67 patients underwent external-beam therapy (mean total dose, 42.3 Gy), 8 patients had intraoperative radiotherapy (range, 12.5 to 30 Gy, with some receiving external-beam therapy as well), 4 patients were given 131-iodine Rose Bengal injections, and 3 patients underwent brachytherapy with 192-iridium wires. Overall survival time following radiotherapy was 6.3 months. When examined by type of radiotherapy, mean survival time for external beam therapy was 4.2 months compared with a mean survival time for intraoperative therapy of 11 months.

In 1988, Meyers and Jones[23] reported on the effectiveness of 192-iridium brachytherapy among 27 patients with cholangiocarcinoma (24 whom had tumors deemed unresectable). Two patients also had received chemotherapy, and all but five were receiving external-beam radiotherapy as well. The specific treatment regimen was not described. Average survival after brachytherapy was 11.5 months. Hayes and colleagues[21] reported the results of radiation therapy on 24 patients with cholangiocarcinoma. Ten patients received no radiation or only palliative radiation, and 14 patients received so-called definitive radiation therapy. The second group of patients consisted of four patients who received external-beam therapy only (51.3 to 58.8 Gy total dose), two patients who received brachytherapy only (58.8 to 63.5 Gy total dose), and eight patients who received a combination of therapy (combined dosage of 63.5 to 108.2 Gy) of external-beam

**Table 40-2** TNM staging of bile duct cancer

| Stage | Tumor | Description | Nodes | Description | Metastases | Description |
|---|---|---|---|---|---|---|
| I | T1 | Tumor limited to mucosa or muscularis | N0 | No nodal involvement | M0 | No distant metastases |
| II | T2 | Tumor invades periductal tissue | N0 | | M0 | |
| III | T1–2 | | N1 | Metastases in regional lymph nodes | M0 | |
| IVA | T3 | Tumor invades adjacent structures | N0–1 | | M0 | |
| IVB | T1–3 | | N0–1 | | M1 | Distant metastases |

therapy (41.0 to 60.2 Gy) and brachytherapy (13.1 to 58 Gy). Median survival of the two groups was 2.0 and 12.8 months, respectively. Houry and colleagues[16] described the results of a retrospective review of the effectiveness of radiotherapy in patients with unresectable gallbladder carcinoma. Sixteen patients (4 of whom underwent palliative surgery) received a mean total dose of 4200 rad of external-beam therapy. Mean survival was 9.2 months for patients with Nevin stage IV carcinomas and 7.2 months for those with Nevin stage V carcinomas. In 1991, Todoroki and colleagues[20] studied the effects of resection combined with intraoperative radiotherapy in 26 patients with TNM stage IV gallbladder carcinoma. The first group (17 patients) received a single intraoperative dose of 20 to 30 Gy; in addition, 10 of these patients also received postoperative external-beam radiotherapy (mean dose, 36.4 Gy). The second group of nine patients underwent resection alone. Resection plus intraoperative radiotherapy (with or without external radiation therapy) achieved 2-year and 3-year survival rates of 20.2% and 10.1%, respectively, compared to no 2-year survival rate in the group undergoing resection alone. Leung and colleagues[22] studied the effectiveness of intraluminal brachytherapy in patients with cholangiocarcinomas. Sixteen patients underwent one to three treatments of intraluminal brachytherapy consisting of iridium-192 strands passed through biliary stents. The median dose of the first treatment was 60 Gy, the median dose of the second was 38 Gy, and the median dose of the third was 60 Gy. Median survival duration was 23 months, with 1- and 2-year survival rates of 61% and 42%, respectively.

In 1996, Kamada and colleagues[24] studied the role of radiation therapy in 145 patients with cholangiocarcinoma. The patients fell into one of four groups. The first group consisted of 54 patients with unresectable disease who were given so-called radical radiotherapy, consisting of external-beam radiotherapy combined with intraluminal radiotherapy, to a mean total radiation dosage of 83.1 Gy. The second group, which consisted of 23 patients with unresectable disease, received palliative radiotherapy. The third group, with 59 patients, received postoperative radiotherapy, and the last group received preoperative radiotherapy. Patients who received radical radiotherapy had 1-, 3-, and 5-year survival rates of 56%, 13%, and 8%, respectively. Furthermore, the use of expandable metallic biliary stents in these patients seemed to prolong median survival time from 9.3 months to 14.9 months. Foo and colleagues[25] evaluated external-beam radiotherapy with a brachytherapy boost in 24 patients with cholangiocarcinoma. The median dose of external-beam therapy was 50.4 Gy, and the median dose of brachytherapy was 20 Gy. Nine patients received concurrent chemotherapy with 5-FU, and two patients underwent surgery. Median survival was 12.8 months, and 2- and 5-year survival rates were 18.8% and 14.1%, respectively.

Mcmasters and colleagues[31] reported on the ability of preoperative chemoradiation to downstage previously unresectable disease in six patients with cholangiocarcinoma (as part of a larger study assessing the utility of neoadjuvant therapy in the treatment of cholangiocarcinoma). The treatment consisted of 5-FU (300 mg/m$^2$/day, Monday through Friday) administered with external-beam radiation therapy (delivered to a total dose of 45 to 50.4 Gy). All six patients received further radiotherapy boosts of 10 Gy dosages either intraoperatively or via brachytherapy postoperatively. All six patients had negative resection margins. During follow-up, two deaths occurred, one from disease recurrence and one from comorbid disease.

Robertson and colleagues[32] described the long-term results of hepatic artery infusion of fluorodeoxyuridine (0.2 mg/kg/day) and concurrent conformal radiation therapy (1.5–1.65 Gy, twice a day to a total dose of 48 or 66 Gy) in 22 patients (11 with hepatocellular carcinoma and 11 with cholangiocarcinomas). The median survival for the group was 16 months, with a 4-year survival rate of nearly 20%. Freedom from hepatic progression at 2 years was approximately 50% (slightly better in the cholangiocarcinoma group). In 1996, Huse and colleagues[33] examined the use of radiation therapy with 5-FU and low-dose folinic acid in 8 patients with advanced biliary or gallbladder carcinoma. Radiation was given as a split course of 40 Gy. Toxicity was substantial with some patients unable to complete the planned therapy. In 1999, de Aretxabala and colleagues[34] studied the role of preoperative chemoradiotherapy in the treatment of gallbladder carcinoma. Eighteen patients were given concurrent 5-FU (350 mg/m$^2$/day on days 1–5 and days 21–25) and external-beam radiation (4500 cGy delivered in fractions of 180 cGy/day for 5 days per week). Fifteen patients went on to reexploration, and 13 underwent resection. Seven patients were alive at 24 months. Median survival times were not given.

## Chemotherapy

Chemotherapy has not shown promising results.[35–45] The overall response rate is usually reported as less than 20%. In 1983 Morrow and colleagues[35] showed that adjuvant systemic chemotherapy (5-fluorouracil [5-FU] and methyl-CCNU) or hepatic arterial 5-FU therapy when combined with radiation therapy to the liver improved survival by 4.5 months (the specifics of this therapy and the overall response rate were not given). Smith and colleagues[39] later looked at combined 5-FU and mitomycin C in the treatment of 11 patients with hepatobiliary carcinomas. In this study, hepatic artery infusion of 5-FU (1200 mg/m$^2$/day for 4 days) and mitomycin C (6 mg/m$^2$ on days 1 and 4) repeated every 4 weeks produced a complete response in 9% and a partial response in 55% of patients. This effect was more pronounced in the patients with gallbladder carcinoma. Falkson and colleagues[36] studied the efficacy of three regimens in 87 patients with hepatobiliary carcinoma (53 with gallbladder carcinoma and 34 with cholangiocarcinoma): group 1 received oral 5-FU (600 mg/m$^2$/day, days 1 through 5, every 5 weeks); group 2 received oral 5-FU (as above) plus streptozotocin (500 mg/m$^2$/day intravenously for 5 days, alternating courses with the 5-FU), and group 3 received oral 5-FU (as above) and methyl-CCNU (a single oral dose of 150 g/m$^2$ on day 1). Five of the patients with gallbladder carcinoma (two each in groups 1 and 2, and one in group 3) had objective responses to treatment. Three of the patients with cholangiocarcinoma (one in group 1 and two in group 3) had objective responses to the treatment.

In 1996, Gebbia and colleagues[45] studied the effects of 5-FU, high-dose levofolinic acid, and oral hydroxyurea on advanced gallbladder adenocarcinomas. Patients were given levofolinic acid (100 mg/m$^2$ intravenously over 2 hours) followed by 5-FU (600 mg/m$^2$ intravenous bolus) and oral hydroxyurea (1000 mg/m$^2$) 1 day a week for 6 weeks, followed by 15 days of rest. Thirty percent of patients achieved a partial response rate and the mean duration of survival was 8 months.

Also in 1996, Jones and colleagues[44] studied the effect of paclitaxel on unresectable biliary tree carcinomas. Fifteen patients (4 with gallbladder carcinoma and 11 with cholangiocarcinoma) were treated with 170–200 mg/m$^2$ over 3 hours every 21 days.

No complete or partial responses were noted. Patt and colleagues[43] looked at the efficacy of intravenous 5-FU and subcutaneous interferon (IFN) $\alpha_{2b}$ (IGN-$\alpha_{2b}$) in treating hepatobiliary cancers. Thirty-five patients (10 with gallbladder carcinoma and 25 with cholangiocarcinoma) were treated every 14 days with a regimen consisting of 5-FU (750 mg/m$^2$/day) on days 1 through 5 and rIFN-$\alpha_{2b}$ (5 MU/m$^2$/day) on days 1, 3, and 5. A partial response was seen in 34% of the patients (gallbladder, 25%; biliary, 37.5%). Median time to disease progression was 9.5 months, and median survival duration was 12 months.

In 1998, Takada and colleagues[42] reported on a multicenter, randomized trial of 5-FU, doxorubicin, and mitomycin C in the treatment of nonresectable pancreatic and hepatobiliary carcinoma. Ten patients with gallbladder carcinoma and four with cholangiocarcinoma were given 5-FU (200 mg/m$^2$), doxorubicin (15 mg/m$^2$), and mitomycin C (5 mg/m$^2$) 1 day per week for the first 4 weeks, then were off the regimen for 1 week. Although the regimen showed no benefit in either response or survival among patients with cholangiocarcinoma, those with gallbladder carcinoma experienced a 50% inhibition of tumor progression compared with controls, and survival duration was 207 days. Also in 1998, Sanz-Altamira and colleagues[41] studied patients with unresectable biliary tree carcinoma treated with 5-FU, leucovorin, and carboplatin. On days 1 through 4, 5-FU (400 mg/m$^2$) and leucovorin (25 mg/m$^2$) were given, and on day 1, carboplatin (300 mg/m$^2$) was given. No response was achieved in the patients with gallbladder carcinoma. Among the 10 patients with cholangiocarcinoma, 2 patients achieved a partial response and 1 patient achieved a complete response.

Finally, in 1999, Pazdur and colleagues[40] studied the efficacy of docetaxel in the treatment of cholangiocarcinoma. Seventeen patients underwent 1-hour infusions of docetaxel (100 mg/m$^2$) once every 21 days. No complete or partial responses were achieved. It should be stressed that these studies were handicapped by small numbers, most were nonrandomized, and control groups, when present, were often not completely matched.

## Other Treatments for Unresectable Gallbladder Carcinoma and Cholangiocarcinoma

Although surgery, chemotherapy, and radiotherapy have been the usual modalities employed against gallbladder carcinoma and cholangiocarcinoma, other therapeutic strategies offer promise as alternative treatments, especially when dealing with unresectable or metastatic disease. Cryosurgery, ethanol injection, matrix gel/cisplatin injection, radiofrequency ablation, photodynamic therapy, and gene therapy have been used to treat various neoplasms, and they have the potential to be useful in treating gallbladder and bile duct carcinoma as well.

Cryosurgery has been used extensively to treat primary hepatocelullar carcinoma and colorectal disease metastatic to the liver, and it has been applied to many other primary and secondary hepatic lesions as well.[46–50] Under ultrasound guidance, a liquid nitrogen probe is inserted into the center of an unresectable tumor, and a surrounding 1-cm margin is frozen, thawed, and then refrozen. Cryosurgery may also be used to freeze positive margins when further resection cannot be performed. No prospective, randomized studies have compared cryosurgery to other treatment modalities, and long-term survival data are lacking, but most series report median survival durations of more than 2 years.[47] Whether this experience primarily with colorectal

metastases can be extrapolated to unresectable gallbladder carcinoma or cholangiocarcinoma remains to be seen.

Percutaneous ethanol injection has been used as an ablative technique to treat hepatocellular carcinomas for more than 10 years. Solitary tumors between 3 and 5 cm or as many as three tumors less than 4 cm in diameter can be effectively treated with ultrasound-directed injections. The ethanol is delivered in small amounts in multiple sessions or as the so-called one-shot technique. Five-year survival rates approach 60% in properly selected patients.[51,52] Again, this technique has been used only for primary hepatocellular carcinomas and there are no data regarding its use with other hepatobiliary tumors.

Developed at The University of Texas M. D. Anderson Cancer Center,[53] direct intratumoral injection of a collagen matrix gel impregnated with cisplatin has been used in several types of unresectable liver tumors, including gallbladder carcinoma and cholangiocarcinoma. No long-term data are available yet, but initial tumor response has been between 50% and 90%, and the technique has the potential to treat tumors up to 10 cm in diameter.

Radiofrequency ablation is a technique in which an electrode produces an alternating electric current operating in the range of radiofrequency waves (460 kHz) that agitates the ions in the surrounding tissue. The agitation induces a coagulative necrosis in a zone of up to 3.5 cm around the electrode.[54–59] The electrode can be introduced percutaneously or surgically. Several lesions can be treated in one sitting and larger lesions can be treated with overlapping ablations. In a recent large, prospective, nonrandomized trial, the local recurrence rate was 1.8%. However, metastatic disease developed in new sites in 27.6% of patients, a result that emphasizes the importance of regional and systemic therapy.[56] Long-term data are not unavailable in this study, but other studies with fewer patients have shown 1- and 5-year survival rates of 94% and 40%, respectively, for patients with hepatocellular carcinoma; less impressive results were obtained for those with metastatic lesions.[55] Nagata and colleagues[59] did show that in treating metastatic lesions, radiofrequency ablation, combined with chemoembolization, resulted in long-term recurrence rates comparable to those with radiofrequency ablation alone in the treatment of hepatocellular carcinoma. The addition of chemoembolization to radiofrequency ablation of hepatocellular carcinoma did not improve recurrence rates.[59] This study further supports the need for regional and systemic therapy, especially for metastatic disease.

Photodynamic therapy is a local cancer therapy already used to treat various types of cancers. As described by Ortner and colleagues,[60] tissue death is achieved first by injecting a photosensitizer intravenously and then activating this compound with nonthermal light at the appropriate wavelength. It is believed that an energy transfer from light to oxygen results in the formation of cytotoxic oxygen derivatives. Because tumor microvasculature has a selective sensitivity to photodynamic therapy, cell death occurs through ischemic necrosis as well as by direct tumor cytotoxicity. In the above study, 13 patients with unresectable cholangiocarcinoma were initially treated with biliary drainage via stents, and those who did not improve went on to photodynamic therapy. End points measured included median survival time, 30-day mortality, serum bilirubin levels, and quality-of-life indices. No deaths occurred in the first 30 days, and median survival time was 439 days. Both end points were significant improvements over reported results for biliary drainage alone among patients with matched stage of tumor. Serum bilirubin levels declined from 318 ± 72 to 103 ± 35 µmol/L. Quality of life, as measured by the Karnofsky index, World Health Organization (WHO) index, and performance-rating scale, improved significantly and remained stable. Although this was a small, nonrandomized study, the results do suggest a role for photodynamic therapy in the therapy of unresectable cholangiocarcinoma.

Gene therapy has been explored in many diseases, including cancers of the gallbladder and biliary tract. Mutations of the Ki-*ras* proto-oncogene and the *p53* tumor suppressor gene have been observed in intrahepatic cholangiocarcinomas.[61–63] In experimental protocols, gene vectors are being used to insert the *p53* gene into patients with hepatic tumors in an effort to arrest neoplastic growth. Ideally, this work could be applied to other neoplastic processes, including cholangiocarcinoma and gallbladder cancer. Another novel approach is to use gene therapy to augment more traditional treatments. Pederson and colleagues[64] described an approach in which an adenovirus vector is used to insert an enzyme into a human cholangiocarcinoma cell line, rendering it more susceptible to traditional chemoradiotherapy. These methods, while experimental, provide hope that additional clinical choices will be available to patients with unresectable disease.

## Conclusion

Unresectable gallbladder carcinoma and cholangiocarcinoma are devastating diagnoses for thousands of patients annually. While early diagnosis and surgery still provide the best hope for patients with these cancers, there continues to be a role for aggressive treatment of select patients with advanced disease, using the therapies discussed above. Further investigative protocols are needed to clarify the exact place for each of these tools in the clinician's armamentarium.

## References

1. Piehler JM, Crichlow RW. Primary carcinoma of the gallbladder. Surg Gynecol Obstet 147:929–992, 1978.
2. Donohue JH, Stewart AK, Menck HR. The National Cancer Data Base report on carcinoma of the gallbladder, 1989–1995. Cancer 83:2618–2628, 1998.
3. Jemal A, Murray T, Samuels A, et al: Cancer statistics, 2003. CA Cancer J Clin 53:5–26, 2003.
4. Nevin JE, Moran TJ, Kay S, King R. Carcinoma of the gallbladder: staging, treatment, and prognosis. Cancer 37:141–148, 1976.
5. Frezza EE, Mezghebe H. Gallbladder carcinoma: a 28-year experience. Int Surg 82:295–300, 1997.
6. de Aretxabala X, Roa I, Burgos L, et al: Gallbladder cancer in Chile: a report on 54 potentially resectable tumors. Cancer 69:60–65, 1992.
7. Wanebo HJ, Vezeridis MP. Treatment of galbladder cancer: In: Sugarbaker P (ed): Hepatobiliary Cancer. Kluwer Academic Publishers, Amsterdam, 1994, pp. 97–110.
8. Maibenco DC, Smith JL, Nava HR, Petrelli NJ, Douglass HO. Carcinoma of the gallbladder. Cancer Invest 16:33–39, 1998.
9. Pearlstone DB, Curley SA, Feig BW. The Management of gallbladder cancer: before, during and after laparasopic cholecystectomy. Semin Laparosc Surg 5:121–128, 1998.
10. Kimura K, Ohto M, Saisho H, et al. Association of gallbladder carcinoma and anomalous pancreaticobliary ductal union. Gastroenterology 89:1258–1265, 1985.
11. Yoshida T, Shibata K, Matsumoto T, et al. Carcinoma of the gallbladder associated with anomalous junction of the pancreaticobiliary duct in adults. J Am Coll Surg 189:57–62, 1999.
12. Suda K, Miyano T, Konuma I, Matsumoto M. An abnormal pancreaticocholedcho-ductal junction in cases of biliary tract carcinoma. Cancer 52:2086–2088, 1983.
13. Tompkins RK, Saunders K, Roslyn JJ, Longmire WP. Changing patterns in diagnosis and management of bile duct cancer. Ann Surg 211:614–622, 1990.
14. Yeo CJ, Cameron JL. Tumors of the gallbladder and bile ducts. In: Zinner MJ, et al. (eds): Maingot's Abdominal Operations. Appleton and Lang, Stamford, CT, 1997, pp 1835–1854.
15. Bartlett DL, Fung Y. Tumors of the galbladder. In: Blumgart LH, Fung Y (eds): Surgery of the Liver and Biliary Tract. W.B. Saunders, Philadelphia, 2000, pp 993–1015.
16. Houry S, Schlienger M, Huguier M, Lacaine F, Penne F, et al. Gallbladder carcinoma: role of radiation therapy. Br J Surg 76:448–450, 1989.
17. Bosset J-F, Mantion G, Gillet M, Pelissier E, Boulenger M, et al. Primary carcinoma of the gallbladder: adjuvant postoperative external irradiation. Cancer 64:1843–1847, 1989.
18. Todoroki T. Radiation therapy for primary gallbladder cancer. Hepatogastroenterology 44:1229–1239, 1997.
19. Busse PM, Cady B, Bothe A, Jenkins R, McDermott WV, et al. Intraoperative radiation therapy for carcinoma of the gallbladder. World J Surg 15:352–356, 1991.
20. Todoroki T, Iwasaki Y, Orii K, Otsuka M, Ohara K, et al. Resection combined with intraoperative radiation therapy (IORT) for stage IV (TNM) gallbladder carcinoma. World J Surg 15:357–366, 1991.
21. Hayes JK, Sapoznik MD, Miller FJ. Definitive radiation therapy in bile duct carcinoma. Int J Radiat Oncol Biol Phys 15:735–744, 1988.
22. Leung J, Guiney M, Das R. Intraluminal brachytherapy in bile duct cancer. Aust N Z J Surg 66:74–77, 1996.
23. Myers W, Jones RS. Internal radiation for bile duct cancer. World J Surg 12:99–104, 1988.
24. Kamada T, Saitou H, Takamura A, Nojima T, Okushiba S-I. The role of radiotherapy in the management of extrahepatic bile duct cancer: an analysis of 145 consecutive patients treated with intraluminal and/or external beam radiotherapy. Int J Radiat Oncol Biol Phys 34:767–774, 1996.
25. Foo ML, Gunderson LL, Bender CE, Buskirk SJ. External radiation therapy and transcatheter iridium in the treatment of extrahepatic bile duct carcinoma. Int J Radiat Oncol Biol Phys 39:929–935, 1997.
26. Kubota Y, Takaoka M, Kin H, Ogura M, Yamamoto S, et al. Endoscopic irradiation and parallel arrangement of Wallstents for hilar cholangiocarcinoma. Hepatogastroenterology 45:415–419, 1998.
27. Hishinuma S, Ogata Y, Matsui J, Ozawa I, Imura J. Preoperative radiotherapy for cancer of the extrahepatic bile duct. Am J Clin Oncol 21:203–208, 1998.
28. Kuvshinoff BW, Armstrong JG, Fong Y, Schupak K, Gertradjman G, Heffernan N, et al. Palliation of irresectable hilar cholangiocarcinoma with biliary drainage and radiotherapy. Br J Surg 82:1522–1525, 1995.
29. Milella M, Salvetti M, Cerotta A, Cozzi G, Uslenghi E, et al. Interventional radiology and radiotherapy for inoperable cholangiocarcinoma of the extrahepatic bile ducts. Tumori 84:467–471, 1998.
30. Urego M, Flickenger JC, Carr BI. Radiotherapy and multimodality management of cholangocarcinoma. Int J Radiat Oncol Biol Phys 44:121–126, 1999.
31. McMasters KM, Tuttle TM, Leach SD, Rich T, Cleary KR, et al. Neoadjuvant chemoradiation for extrahepatic cholangioarcinoma. Am J Surg 174:605–609, 1997.
32. Robertson JM, Lawrence TS, Andrews JC, et al. Long-term results of hepatic artery fluorodeoxyuridine and conformal radiation therapy for primary hepatobiliary cancers. Int J Radiat Oncol Biol Phys 37:325–330, 1997.
33. Hsue V, Wong CS, Moore M, et al. A phase I study of combined radiation therapy with 5-fluorouracil and low-dose folinic acid in patiets with locally advanced pancreatic or biliary carcinoma. Int J Radiat Oncol Biol Phys 34:445–450, 1996.
34. de Aretxabala X, Roa I, Burgos L, et al. Preoperative chemoradiotherapy in the treatment of gallbladder cancer. Am Surg 65:241–246, 1999.
35. Morrow CE, Sutherland DE, Florack G, Eisenberg M, Grage TB. Primary gallbladder carcinoma: significance of subserosal lesions and results of aggressive surgical treatment and adjuvant chemotherapy. Surgery 94:709–714, 1983.
36. Falkson G, MacIntyre JM, Moertel CG. Eastern Cooperative Oncology Group experience with chemotherapy for inoperable gallbladder and bile duct cancer. Cancer 54:965–969, 1984.
37. Gallardo J, Fodor M, Gamargo C, Orlandi L. Efficacy of gemcitabine in the treatment of patients with gallbladder carcinoma: a case report. Cancer 83:2419–2421, 1998.
38. Robertson JM, McGinn CJ, Walker S, et al. A phase I trial of hepatic arterial bromodeoxyuridine and conformal radiation therapy for patients with hepatobiliary cancers or colorectal liver metastases. Int J Radiat Oncol Biol Phys 39:187–1092, 1997.
39. Smith GW, Bukowski RM, Hewlett JS, Groppe CW. Hepatic artery infusion of 5-fluorouracil and mitomycin C in cholangiocarcinoma and gallbladder carcinoma.
40. Pazdur R, Royce ME, Rodriguez GI, et al. Phase II trial of docetaxel for cholangiocarcinoma. Am J Clin Oncol 22:78–81, 1999.

41. Sanz-Altamira PM, Ferrante K, Jenkins RL, Lewis WD, Huberman MS. A phase II trial of 5-fluorououracil, leucovorin, and carboplatin in patients with unresectable biliary tree carcinoma. Cancer 82:2321–2325, 1998.

42. Takada T, Nimura Y, Katoh H, et al. Prospective randomized trial of 5-fluorouracil, doxorubicin, and mitomycin C or nonresectable pancreatic and biliary carcinoma: multicenter randomized trial. Hepatogastroenterology 45:2020–2026, 1998.

43. Patt YZ, Jones DV, Hoque A, et al. Phase II trial of intravenous fluorouracil and subcutaneous interferon α-2b for biliary tract cancer. J Clin Oncol 14:2311–2315, 1996.

44. Jones DV, Lozano R, Hoque A, Markowitz A, Patt YZ. Phase II study of paclitaxel therapy for unresectable biliary tree carcinomas. J Clin Oncol 14:2306–2310, 1996.

45. Gebbia V, Majello E, Testa A, et al. Treatment of advanced adenocarcinomas of the exocrine pancreas and the gallbladder with 5-fluorouracil, high-dose levofolinic acid and oral hydroxyurea on a weekly schedule: results of a multicenter study of the Southern Italy Oncology Group. Cancer 78:1300–1307, 1996.

46. Weaver ML, Atkinson D, Zemel R. Hepatic cryosurgery in treating colorectal metastases. Cancer 76:210–214, 1995.

47. Seifert JK, Junginger T, Morris DL. A collective review of the world literature on hepatic cryotherpay. J R Coll Surg Edinb 43:141–154, 1998.

48. Haddad FF, Chapman WC, Wright K, Blair TK, Pinson CW. Cliical experience with cryosurgery for advanced hepatobiliary tumors. J Surg Res 75:103–108, 1998.

49. Adam R, Akpinar E, Johann M, et al. Place of cryosurgery in the treatment of malignant liver tumors. Ann Surg 225:39–59, 1997.

50. Shafir M, Shapiro R, Sung M, et al. Cryoablation of unresectable malignant liver tumors. Am J Surg 171:27–31, 1996.

51. Livraghi T, Benedini V, Lazzaroni S, Meloni F, Torzilli G. Long-term results of single session percutaneous ethanol injection in patients with large hepatoceluluar carcinoma. Cancer 83:48–57, 1998.

52. Livraghi T, Bolondi L, Lazzaroni S, et al. Percutaneous ethanol injection in the treatment of hepatocellular carcinoma in cirrhosis: a study of 207 patients. Cancer 69:925–929, 1992.

53. Davidson BS, Izzo F, Cromeens DM, et al. Collagen matrix cisplatin prevents local tumor growth after margin-positive resection. J Surg Res 58:618–624, 1995.

54. Nagata Y, Hiraoka M, Nishimura Y, et al. Clinical results of radiofrequency hyperthermia for malignant liver tumors. Int J Radiat Oncol Biol Phys 38:359–365, 1997.

55. Rhim H, Dodd G. Radiofrequncy thermal ablation of liver tumors. J Clin Ultrasound 27:221–229, 1999.

56. Curley SA, Izzo F, Delrio P, et al. Radiofrequency ablation of unresectable primary and metastatic hepatic malignancies: results in 123 patients. Ann Surg 230:1–8, 1999.

57. Jiao LR, Hansen PD, Havlik R, et al. Clinical short-term results of radiofrequency ablation in primary and secondary liver tumors. Am J Surg 177:303–306, 1999.

58. Scudamore CH, Lee SI, Patterson EJ, et al. Radiofrequency ablation followed by resection of malignant liver tumors. Am J Surg 177:411–417, 1999.

59. Nagata Y, Hiraoka M, Akuta K, et al. Radiofrequency thermotherapy for malignant liver tumors. Cancer 65:1730–1736, 1990.

60. Ortner MJ, Liebertruth J, Schreiber S, et al. Photodynamic therapy of nonresectable cholangiocarcinoma. Gastroenterology 114:536–542, 1998.

61. Kang YK, Kim WH, Lee HW, Lee HK, Kim YI. Mutation of *p53* and *K-ras*, and loss of heterozygosity of *APC* in intrahepatic cholagiocarcinoma. Lab Invest 79:477–483, 1999.

62. Ahrendt SA, Eisenberger CF, Yip L, et al. Chromosome 9p21 loss and p16 inactivation in primary sclerosing cholangitis-associated cholangiocarcinoma. J Surg Res 84:88–93, 1999.

63. Ohashi K, Nakajima Y, Kanehiro H, et al. Ki-*ras* mutations and p53 protein expressions in intrahepatic cholangiocarcinoma: relation to gross tumor morphology. Gastroenterology 109:1612–1617, 1995.

64. Pederson LC, Buchsbaun DJ, Vickers SM, et al. Molecular chemotherapy combined with radiation therapy enhances killing of cholangiocarcinoma cells in vitro and in vivo. Cancer Research 57:4325–4332, 1997.

# Section 5

# Hepatocellular Cancer

# Chapter 41

# Epidemiology and Molecular Epidemiology of Hepatocellular Cancer

MANAL M. HASSAN AND YEHUDA Z. PATT

Hepatocellular carcinoma (HCC), a common cancer worldwide, causes more than 250,000 deaths annually,[1] including more than 5000 deaths per year in the United States.[2] A recently published study reported a statistically significant increase in the incidence of HCC in the United States over the past two decades.[3] The incidence rose from 1.4 per 100,000 from 1976 to 1980 to 2.4 per 100,000 from 1991 to 1995. With respect to gender and race, the same report showed that in the United States, HCC occurs three times more often in men than in women and twice as often in African Americans than in whites. The peculiar pattern of HCC— the rise in incidence among young persons and its varied incidence among different populations and races—suggests that this tumor is caused by several factors and that interactions among these factors may significantly increase the risk for HCC. Most patients with HCC have associated chronic liver disease, including chronic hepatitis and liver cirrhosis.[4]

Many environmental and genetic factors have been identified as increasing the risk of developing HCC. Furthermore, synergy between these factors has been shown to be significant in hepatocarcinogenesis. This chapter reviews the available data on these risk factors and generally discusses their molecular effect on HCC development.

## Environmental Risk Factors for Hepatocellular Carcinoma

### Hepatitis B Virus

The hepatitis B virus (HBV) genome is a partially double-stranded, circular DNA molecule. The structure of the virus has been described in detail by Tiollais and Buendia.[5] It is composed of a lipid envelope and nucleocapsid structure. The first consists of hepatitis B surface antigen (HBsAg), and the second is com-posed of core protein and the viral DNA genome. Since the identification of HBsAg and recognition of its importance as a marker of chronic HBV infection,[6] several seroepidemiologic, cohort, and case–control studies have established the significant hepato-carcinogenicity of chronic infection with HBV in humans.[7–14] The magnitude of this association is extremely high in some populations, and the relative risk has exceeded 100 in Asian studies.[11]

The molecular biology of HBV in relation to the development of HCC has been reviewed extensively,[15,16] and the mechanism by which HBV may induce HCC has been investigated through different approaches. Several studies have suggested direct involvement of the HBV genome in causing the genetic changes of hepatocarcinogenesis.[17–19] Evidence for the direct role of HBV on HCC development is supported by the integration of HBV DNA in the infected hepatocyte. An estimated 83% of HBsAg-positive patients with HCC have integrated HBV DNA in their tumor DNA.[20] Such integration of the virus may be associated with microdeletion in the DNA at the integration site,[21] secondary chromosomal rearrangement,[22,23] chromosomal translocation,[22,24] or large chromosomal deletion.[25] HBV integration is likely to be a random process, however, a recently documented exception to this is that HBV DNA is found at a gene locus that encodes the thyroid hormone–retinoic acid receptor[26] and at a gene locus that encodes cyclin A.[27] Another direct mechanism for HBV involvement is the transactivator activity attributed to the X gene[28,29] as well as the preS/S antigen gene[30] of HBV. This transactivating function of HBV could activate the promoters of several cellular genes related to cell growth.[31] Other studies have postulated that HBV carcinogenesis also is indirectly related to the underlying infection by making the infected hepatocyte more susceptible to genetic changes caused by other risk factors. In other words, HBV may act as an initiator of hepatocarcinogenesis and other environmental risk factors, such as ethanol consumption[32] or aflatoxin ingestion,[33] or another viral infection may accelerate the carcinogenesis in the liver.[34] As HBV continues to replicate, causing persistent hepatitis, the liver responds with continuous regeneration and fibrosis, an outcome that eventually results in cirrhosis. Experimental studies have shown that mice develop cirrhosis after months of inflammation, fibrosis, and hepatocyte regeneration.[19] Moreover, cirrhosis is clearly associated with a high risk for HCC. About 70% of the time, HCC develops on top of cirrhosis,[35] and clinical follow-up of patients with large regenerative nodules has revealed the development of liver cancer in some of these patients.[36] These findings support the concept that HBV not only is a direct causative factor for HCC but also has an indirect role in hepatocarcinogenesis.

## Hepatitis C Virus

Hepatitis C virus (HCV) is a small, single-stranded RNA virus, 30–238 nm in diameter, with a lipid envelope.[37] At the 5′ end of the virus, there is a terminal region composed of 329–341 nucleotides. This region apparently has a role in the translation of the viral genome, and its highly conserved character renders it suitable for diagnostic detection of viral nucleic acid by polymerase chain reaction (PCR) of HCV-cDNA.[38] The prevalence of HCV infection varies widely by geographic areas. The highest prevalence has been reported among healthy Egyptian blood donors (10.9% to 15%),[39,40] whereas the prevalence in northern Europe and the United States is much lower (0.5% to 1.8%).[41,42] Epidemiologic studies show that the most efficient transmission of HCV is through transfusion of blood and blood products or the sharing of contaminated needles by drug users.[43,44] Antischistosomiasis injection treatment was reported as an independent risk factor for the high prevalence of HCV in rural Egypt.[40] Several studies have demonstrated the significant role of HCV in the development of HCC in different countries.[45–48] In the United States, the odds ratio (OR) for HCV infection has ranged from 4.8 to 7.3. In a case–control study at The University of Texas M. D. Anderson Cancer Center in Houston, we observed a 15-fold increase in HCC risk among HCV-positive patients compared with HCV-negative patients and an estimated population-attributable risk of 23% related to HCV alone. In addition to being the major risk factor for HCC, HCV is a major factor contributing to the increase in HCC incidence in the United States. Our data from M. D. Anderson showed that 26 patients (18%) and 66 patients (31%) with anti-HCV antibodies were diagnosed with HCC from 1993 to 1995 and from 1996 to 1998, respectively ($P = 0.01$). Although the age distribution of these patients did not differ significantly during the periods 1993–1995 and 1996–1998, the increase in HCV-associated HCC was greatest among patients 40 to 49 years old. Hepatitis B surface antigen or anti-HBc was found in 37 patients (26%) with HCC from 1993 to 1995 and in 37 patients (17%) with HCC from 1996 to 1998 ($P = 0.06$). Moreover, a significant decrease in the prevalence of HBsAg from 1996 to 1998 (21 patients, 10%) compared with that in 1993 to 1995 (25 patients, 18%) was observed ($P = 0.03$) (M. Hassan, unpublished data, 2000).

Hepatitis C virus, a nonintegrating RNA virus, is widely assumed to cause HCC through a pathogenic mechanism that induces chronic liver disease and cirrhosis. About 60% to 80% of anti–HCV-positive HCC patients were found to have liver cirrhosis. Progression toward cirrhosis in individuals infected with HCV seems to be significantly different from that associated with HBV-induced cirrhosis. More than 20% of anti–HCV-positive cases developed advanced cirrhosis compared with 8.7% in HBsAg-positive cases.[49,50]

Like other RNA viruses, HCV displays a high genetic variability. On the basis of nucleotide sequence homology, whole-sequenced HCV isolates are classified in type I (1a), type II (1b), type III (2a), and type IV (2b). Provisionally, type V (3a) and type VI (3b) isolates were reported on the basis of data on partially sequenced genomes.[51] The geographic distribution of these genotypes demonstrated that types I, II, and III are predominant in Western countries and the Far East, whereas type IV is predominant in the Middle East.[52]

Some evidence suggests that the HCV genotype 1b is more aggressive and more closely associated with advanced chronic liver diseases such as liver cirrhosis and HCC,[53,54] although a high prevalence of HCV type 1b has been reported among patients with HCC and no cirrhosis.[55] This information may indicate that in some instances, the neoplastic transformation in type 1b infection may not require transition through the stage of cirrhosis. The observation that many HCCs can develop in patients with HCV but no cirrhosis and the fact that many of the HCV structural and nonstructural proteins have not been investigated entirely indicate that the molecular mechanism of HCV in hepatocarcinogenesis is not well established. Interestingly, a recent study has reported that HCV encodes a selenium (Se)-dependent antioxidant enzyme, glutathione peroxidase (GPx), and GPx may have a regulatory role in HCV replication.[56] The virus-induced overexpression of GPx may lead to a decreased level of Se in the host due to the competition of HCV for Se. In fact, patients with HCV have been shown to have a significant decline in their serum Se.[57] This information may suggest the implication of oxidative stress in HCV hepatocarcinogenicity.

## Alcohol Consumption

Numerous studies, including a review by the International Agency for Research on Cancer (IARC), have indicated that heavy alcohol consumption and alcoholic cirrhosis are important risk factors for HCC, primarily in countries with a low incidence of HBV infection.[58–60] Others have suggested that the carcinogenic effects of alcohol are not directly mediated but rather evolve with the development of liver cirrhosis.[61] Moreover, it has been reported that once cirrhosis develops, cessation of alcohol use does not prevent the development of HCC.[62] This findings suggests that among people with alcoholic cirrhosis, the risk for HCC development is closely related to the cirrhosis.

In the United States, the risk for HCC was found to increase with consumption of more than 80 g of ethanol per day.[58] In Italy, a history of alcohol consumption (more than 80 g of ethanol daily for at least 5 years) was found in 58.1% of patients with HCC and in 36.4% of the controls (OR, 4.6; 95% confidence interval [CI], 2.7–7.8).[63] Indeed, in previous case–control studies, heavy alcohol intake seems to be the single most relevant cause of HCC.[63,64] In separate studies, the estimated population-attributable risk for HCC related to heavy alcohol consumption was 40% in the United States (M. Hassan, unpublished data, 2000) and 45% in Italy.[63] Both studies suggested a positive interaction between hepatitis viral infection and heavy alcohol consumption, especially among patients with genotype 1b. The estimated OR reached 126 (95% CI, 42–373) among individuals who consumed more than 80 g of ethanol a day.[64] Despite this close relationship between HCV and alcohol consumption in HCC development, there is little understanding of how HCV and alcohol might interact. In most studies, anti-HCV in alcoholics was found to be closely associated with the presence of HCV RNA in serum (a marker of HCV replication).[65] This suggests that the immunosuppression associated with chronic alcohol consumption may enhance HCV replication.[66] Another possibility is that the interaction between hepatitis virus infection and alcohol consumption could be related to oxidative stress. Patients infected with the human immunodeficiency virus (HIV) experienced a significant drop in serum Se level when they were co-infected with HCV compared to those without concurrent infection with HCV.[57] Moreover, the hepatotoxicity of ethanol and its associated malnutrition will further reduce the cellular Se level. This additive decline in the Se level makes the cell more susceptible to reactive oxygen species and may be associated with enhanced viral replication and higher viral load.

## Aflatoxin Exposure

Aflatoxins (AFs) are toxic secondary fungal metabolites (mycotoxins) produced by *Aspergillus flavus* and *Aspergillus parasiticus*. These types of molds are very common; however, their production of toxins requires high temperature and humidity. In general, there are four AF compounds: $B_1$, $B_2$, $G_1$, and $G_2$.[67,68] The most common and most toxic AF is $AFB_1$, and the most important target organ is the liver, where the toxicity can lead to liver necrosis and bile duct proliferation.[68] Experimental data from animal studies have provided ample evidence of a positive correlation between AF and HCC.[67] Geographic studies indicate that areas with a high incidence of liver cancer such as China and Africa experience higher rates of exposure to AF. Moreover, epidemiologic research has documented a significant risk for HCC development among individuals who consume high amounts of AF,[69-71] as well as a positive linear relationship between HCC mortality and estimated $AFB_1$ level.[72] The estimated OR was 13.9 and 17 for moderate and heavy dietary AF loads, respectively. However, measurement of human AF exposure through dietary studies and analysis of food samples is a relatively crude method of assessing AF exposure. It does not provide data on the biologically effective dose of AF at the individual level. Molecular dosimetry and techniques to identify markers that indicate past exposure to AF, by contrast are very useful in determining the population at risk.

The toxic and carcinogenic effects of $AFB_1$ are manifested only after the compound is metabolized by endogenous cytochrome P-450 (CYP). In other words, $AFB_1$ must be converted to its highly reactive 8,9 epoxide metabolite by the action of the mixed function (CYP-dependent) mono-oxygenase enzyme systems in the liver.[73,74] Therefore, development of AF biomarkers is based on detection of the $AFB_1$ active metabolites, which can interact covalently with cellular molecules, including DNA, RNA, and protein. The two major macromolecular adducts that have been identified are the AF-$N^7$-guanine adduct in the DNA adduct found in urine[75] and a lysine adduct found in serum albumin.[76] Monitoring levels of AF-albumin and AF-$N^7$-guanine adducts revealed a highly significant association between the adduct level and AF intake.[77-79] However, the biologic half-lives of AF-$N^7$-guanine adducts (8 hours)[80,81] and of AF-albumin adduct (2 to 3 weeks)[82,83] are short. Therefore, both urinary DNA adducts and serum albumin adducts may reflect recent dietary exposure to AF and are not appropriate markers of long-term or chronic exposure to AF; they can nonetheless be useful tools in studies that monitor humans for genetic instability caused by AF exposure.

A detoxification process carried out through two enzymatic pathway oposes the activation process of AF. Epoxide hydrolase catalyzes hydrolysis of epoxide to $AFP_1$-diol, and glutathione-S-transferase (GST) catalyzes reaction of the 8,9-epoxide to glutathione and subsequent biliary excretion of this conjugated product.[84] Any deficiency in the activity of these enzymes can enhance the carcinogenecity of AF. Therefore, detection of the mutant alleles of either of these enzymes in an individual may indicate elevated susceptibility to HCC because of the diminished capacity for AF detoxification. Mutant alleles of both enzymes have been correlated with the presence of an AF-albumin adduct, and individuals with an adduct level greater than 5 pg/mg albumin have been found to be more likely to have mutant alleles of either enzyme than are individuals with no detectable level of AF-albumin adduct.[85] Moreover, in China the frequency of mutant alleles in the two AF-detoxifying enzymes was significantly higher in patients with HCC than in controls ($P = 0.04$).[85] This information suggests that the combination of dietary exposure, biological markers for AF, and genetic variation in AF-detoxifying enzymes is more important than any single factor in the epidemiologic assessment of the role of AF in HCC.

## Genetic Risk Factors for Hepatocellular Carcinoma

### Familial Aggregation

Only limited attention has been given to the role of primary genetic factors in HCC development. Early reports described the observation of HCC occurrence in siblings who had no hepatitis infection or other risk factors for HCC.[86-88] Later, a complex segregation analysis of 490 extended families in China was undertaken to examine the effects of HBV infection and genetic susceptibility.[89] The study found that the lifetime risk of developing HCC in the presence of HBV infection and genetic susceptibility was 0.84 for males and 0.46 for females. However, these lifetime risks dropped to 0.09 for males and 0.01 for females in the presence of HBV infection only. Similar findings were demonstrated in a case series of 14 Alaska natives with familial clustering of HCC, early onset for HCC development (79% were less than 24 years old), and no evidence of *p53* mutation.[90] Therefore, it appears that among families with a clustering of HBV, there are differences in the risk of developing HCC; some families have multiple occurrences of HCC, whereas others have none. This may suggest that some genetic predisposition to chronic liver disease, including HCC, does exist and that more studies are needed to clarify this association.

### Inherited Diseases

#### Hereditary hemochromatosis

Hereditary hemochromatosis (HHC) is an autosomal recessive genetic disorder of iron metabolism that causes excessive intestinal absorption of dietary iron and deposition of iron in organs, including the liver.[91] Elevated transferrin saturation (TS) and serum ferritin have been suggested as sensitive and specific tools for diagnosing HHC in healthy asymptomatic individuals.[92] However, elevated TS and serum ferritin may also be secondary to chronic liver diseases such as HCV infection, liver cirrhosis, or HCC. Recently, a major histocompatibility complex (MHC) class I gene named *HLA-H* or *HFE* was cloned. Two mutations have been described: Cys282Tyr (*C282Y*) and His63Asp

(*H63D*).[93] The *C282Y* mutation is more common in HHC. Whereas the prevalence of the homozygous gene mutation is 0.3% to 0.5% in the white population,[94] the estimated prevalence of the heterozygous *C282Y* mutation is 10% to 16% among white Americans and 3% among African Americans.[95] It has been recommended that when TS levels exceed 50%, *HFE* gene mutation tests of *C282Y* should be performed to distinguish HHC from secondary liver iron overload.[92] In the United States, the *C282Y* mutation can be detected in 82.3% of homozygous HHC and in 6.8% of heterozygous HHC.[96]

Growing evidence suggests that even mildly increased amounts of iron in the liver can be damaging, especially when combined with other hepatotoxic factors such as alcohol consumption and chronic viral hepatitis. Recently, Smith and co-workers[97] demonstrated that individuals who carry only one allele of the *C282Y* gene had minor increases in iron stores; however, these heterozygous individuals appear to develop more fibrosis of the liver in association with chronic HCV infection.

Iron enhances the pathogenicity of microorganisms, adversely affects the function of macrophages and lymphocytes, and enhances fibrogenic pathways,[98,99] all of which can increase hepatic injury caused by iron alone or by iron and other factors such as chronic HCV infection. Indeed, a synergistic relationship between HCV and iron overload from hemochromatosis has been suggested.[100] In a study by Hayashi and co-workers,[101] iron depletion improved liver function tests in HCV-infected individuals. In a study by Mazzella and associates,[102] response of chronic HCV to interferon was shown to be related to hepatic iron concentration. Possible factors contributing to the actions of iron in chronic viral hepatitis include enhancement of oxidative stress, enhancement of lipid peroxidation, exacerbation of immune-mediated tissue inflammation, and possible enhancement of the rate of viral replication or viral mutation.[103]

Because the prevalence of heterozygous *C282Y* mutation is as high as 10% in the general population,[95] the likelihood of an interaction of the gene mutation with HCV infection may be quite significant. However, well-designed epidemiological studies are recommended to establish this association.

### α₁-Antitrypsin Deficiency

$\alpha_1$-Antitrypsin deficiency (AATD) is an autosomal dominant genetic disorder characterized by a deficiency in a major serum protease inhibitor (PI).[104] This order is caused by a mutation in the 12.2 kb $\alpha_1$-antitrypsin gene on chromosome 14.[104] More than 75 different PI alleles have been identified, most of which are not associated with disease.[105] A relationship exists between PI phenotypes and serum concentrations of $\alpha_1$-antitrypsin. Thus, the MM phenotype (normal) is associated with a serum concentration of 100%; MZ, 60%; SS, 60%; FZ, 60%; M, 50%; PS, 40%; SZ, 42.5%; ZZ, 15%; and Z, 0 to 10%.

The most common deficiency variant, PIZ, in its homozygote state often is associated with liver cirrhosis and liver cancer.[106] The role of heterozygous PIZ in the development of primary liver cancer is controversial. Several studies have suggested a significant association between heterozygous PIZ and liver cirrhosis, liver fibrosis, and primary liver cancer.[107–109] Despite these reports, increasing evidence suggests that chronic liver disease develops only when another factor, such as HCV infection, is present and acts as a promoter for the liver damage. In a recent study, chronic liver disease was found in 40% of PIZ-positive patients, whereas 62% to 75% were positive for anti-HCV.[110] In a case report of a 39-year-old man with chronic HCV infection whose liver disease progressed over 4 years from mild hepatitis to se-

vere cirrhosis despite interferon treatment, the patient was found to be heterozygous for AATD (PIMZ). This case suggests a synergistic effect between HCV and AATD in the development of liver cirrhosis or liver cancer.[111]

$\alpha_1$-Antitrypsin is an acute-phase reactant whose major role is to inhibit the actions of neutrophil elastase, proteases, and cathepsin G.[112] Any condition that triggers the acute-phase response would be expected to stimulate the production of $\alpha_1$-antitrypsin by the liver. Therefore, it is suggested that chronic HCV infection could stimulate the hepatocytes to produce the mutant $\alpha_1$-antitrypsin continuously leading to more liver damage.[111]

Other less common inherited disorders, such as glycogen storage disease type I (von Gierke's disease),[113] porphyria cutanea tarda,[114] and Wilson's disease,[115] have been found to be associated with HCC. However, the interactions between these diseases and other established risk factors, such as HCV or HBV, have not be studied.

### p53 Mutation

Genetic susceptibility to HCC is recognized in experimental animals as well as in humans. The most interesting genetic alteration reported in HCC is mutation of the *p53* gene. This mutation has been observed in both HBsAg-positive and -negative patients and in areas of both high and low AF exposure.[116–120] Recent evidence indicates that p53 alterations in patients with HCC appear to be unique, with a high frequency of GC → TA mutations in codon 249 of the *p53* gene with the substitution of arginine for serine. This particular mutation has been observed more often in areas with high AF exposure, such as China and Africa,[121,122] than in areas with low AF exposure, such as the United States and Australia.[123,124] In addition, a positive association was found between the prevalence of this specific mutation and the levels of AF-albumin adducts.[85] Because geographic areas that are endemic for HBV are also highly exposed to AF contamination, it is not clear whether HBV or AF is the cause of this *p53* mutation in HCC. However, the occurrence of this mutation in patients infected with HBV and exposed to AF, but not in patients infected with HBV and not exposed to AF, suggests that it is more likely that AF and not HBV is the cause of this *p53* mutation.[125]

Another tumor suppressor gene involved in hepatocarcinogenesis is the retinoblastoma gene (*Rb*). Loss of heterozygosity (LOH) of the *Rb* gene was found in 43% of human HCC.[126] A previous study showed that polymorphism of the *Rb* gene was present in 12.9% of advanced HCC with no evidence of HBV or HCV.[127] Moreover, 86% of patients with HCC with a *p53* mutation had LOH at the *Rb* gene, compared with none of the HCC patients with no *p53* mutation.[128]

### Metabolic Polymorphism

Genetic differences in the enzymes responsible for activation and detoxification of environmental carcinogens are likely to be important sources for interindividual variability in cancer susceptibility. Cytochrome P-450s are involved in phase I metabolism and detoxification of carcinogens.[129] This metabolic process may create highly reactive intermediates that can be carcinogenic or mutagenic.

#### Cytochrome P-450A1

Cytochrome P-450A1 (CYPA1) is associated with cigarette smoking and has been involved in the biotransformation of tobacco-derived polycyclic aromatic hydrocarbons into carcinogenic metabolites.[130] Two closely related polymorphisms at the *CYPA1* gene locus have been identified. One is a restriction fragment length polymorphism (RFLP), Msp1. The second is located in exon 7 and is responsible for an isoleucine-for-valine (Ile–Val) substitution in the protein catalytic region that affects the protein's function.[131,132] A more recent study reported that both alleles, the Ile–Val and the Msp1, increased HCC risk among smokers but not among nonsmokers. The study suggests that the two alleles may have different mechanisms for increasing the susceptibility to smoking-related HCC.[133]

### Cytochrome P-450E1

Cytochrome P-450E1 (CYP2E1) is induced by ethanol[134] and is critically important in the metabolic activation of many low-molecular-weight carcinogens, including *N*-nitrosamines, benzene, and aniline[135,136] Induction of CYP2E1 by ethanol has been shown to increase the occurrence of HCC in animals exposed to *N*-nitrosodimethylamine (NDMA). Rats exposed to low doses of NDMA developed HCC only when they were simultaneously treated with ethanol.[137] The RFLPs of the *CYP2E1* gene have been identified: the RFLPs detected by *Pst*I and *Rsa*I digestion were associated with transcriptional regulation of gene expression; the rare *c2* gene has a higher transcriptional activity than its *c1* counterpart.[138] Several studies have suggested that CYP2E1 may play a role in hepatocarcinogenesis in individuals exposed to hepatotoxic compounds, such as ethanol and vinyl chloride monomer.[139–141] Yu and co-workers[139] showed that the *c1/c1* genotype of *CYP2E1*, detected by *Pst*I or *Rsa*I digestion, was found in 83.3% of patients with HCC and in 63.3% of controls ($P = 0.034$). The study concluded that habitual alcohol drinking modified the HCC risk of cigarette smoking among those with the *c1/c1* genotype. Another study demonstrated that the *c2* allele frequency was 0.108 in 37 patients who habitually had drunk more than 50 g of ethanol per day ($P = 0.0035$) and the OR was 4.67 (95% CI, 1.57–13.81).[140] Furthermore, the study results suggested that carrying one copy of the *c2 CYP2E1* gene increases the risk of HCC in previous ethanol users.

### Cytochrome P-4502D6

Cytochrome P-4502D6 (CYP2D6) is involved in activation of some mutagens such as AF.[142,143] One study found that individuals who were homozygous for the *CYP2D6* gene appeared to have a sixfold higher risk for HCC.[144] Moreover, Agundez and associates[145] reported that the OR for developing HCC among patients without hepatitis who had two active *CYP2D6* genes was 5.6 (95% CI, 1.4–33.3).

### Arylamine *N*-acetyltransferase

Arylamine *N*-acetyltransferase (NAT2) is another polymorphic enzyme that is involved in the activation and inactivation of carcinogens through *N*-acetylation. One study found that the genetic polymorphism of *NAT2* is associated with hepatocarcinogenesis, and that the relationship between the slow acetylator *NAT2* genotype and HCC is more pronounced in patients without any HBV or HCV markers.[145]

### Glutathione-*S*-transferase

Glutathione-*S*-transferases are phase II detoxification enzymes that catalyze the conjugation of a wide variety of endogenous and exogenous toxins. There are four different mammalian classes of soluble enzymes: α, μ, π, and θ.[146] In humans, polymorphisms have been demonstrated in the μ class (GSTM1) and the θ class (GSTT1). Polymorphisms rarely occur in other classes.[147] Zhou and associates[148] reported that total GST activity was significantly higher in normal tissues than in tumor tissues from 32 HCC patients. Moreover, the study found that patients positive for HBV DNA had significantly lower GST activity than those who were HBV negative. A similar finding was reported in another matched case–control study, which compared 32 patients with HCC to 73 age-matched controls and found a significant OR of 12.4 and 10.2 for HBsAg carriers with high-level serum AFB$_1$-albumin adduct in the null *GSTM1* and the null *GSTT1* genotypes, respectively.[149]

By contrast, two recent case–control studies[139,150] found no independent effect of GSTM1 deficiency on smoking-related HCC risk. However, the latest study suggested that the *GSTM1* genotype modified the association between HCC and cigarette smoking as well as that between alcohol use and HCC among subjects with low levels of plasma β-carotene. The study found a threefold increase in the risk of HCC among *GSTM1*-null subjects after adjustment for smoking and an eightfold increase in the risk after adjustment for alcohol drinking.[150]

### Epoxide hydrolase

Epoxide hydrolase (EH) is also a phase II enzyme that catalyzes the conjugation of polycyclic aromatic hydrocarbons, including benzo-[a]-pyrene, to highly electrophilic metabolites. McGlynn and co-workers,[151] examined the associations of genetic variations in two AFB$_1$ detoxification genes, *EH* and *GSTM1*, with the presence of serum AFB$_1$-albumin adducts, HCC, and *p53* codon 249 mutations. Mutant alleles at both loci were significantly overexpressed in individuals with serum AFB$_1$ adducts. Mutant alleles of *EH* were significantly overexpressed in patients with HCC. The relationship of EH to HCCs varied by HBsAg and was indicative of the synergistic effect.

### Codon 72 *p53* polymorphism

An association between HCC and the codon 72 *p53* polymorphism was assessed in a recent study.[152] The study found that the pro/pro genotype of the *p53* polymorphism was a predictor of HCC risk among HBV carriers who smoked and were homozygous for the *GSTM1*-null allele. This association was not found among nonsmoking carriers or those who had at least one intact *GSTM1* allele. The study suggests that both cigarette smoking and *GSTM1* genotype modified the HCC risk associated with the *p53* polymorphism.

### Summary

Sufficient evidence suggests that HCC is a multifactorial cancer that involves environmental and genetic components. The etiologic roles of many of these risk factors, in terms of their molecular impact on hepatocarcinogenesis, have not been elucidated entirely. Moreover, the interaction among these risk factors is evident and can be highly determined in high-risk populations by using more specific markers and by applying the appropriate epidemiologic designs. It is well established that HCC is a difficult-to-treat cancer with a poor prognosis. Therefore, strategies for preventing liver cancer should be the main objective for future studies. Such strategies include prevention of HCV and possibly chemoprevention in patients with advanced chronic liver diseases caused by viral hepatitis.

### References

1. Bosch FX, Munoz N. Hepatocellular carcinoma in the world: epidemiologic questions. In: Tabor E, Di Bisceglie AM, Purcell RH (eds): Etiology, Pathology, and Treatment of Hepatocellular Carcinoma in North America, Vol 13. Portfolio Publishing Company and Gulf Publishing Company, Houston, TX, 1991, pp 35–54.

2. Surveillance, Epidemiology, and End Results (SEER) Program. National Cancer Institute, Bethesda, MD, August, 1998.
3. El-Serag HB, Mason AC. Rising incidence of hepatocellular carcinoma in the United States. N Engl J Med 340:745–750, 1999.
4. Okuda K. Early recognition of hepatocellular carcinoma. Hepatology 6:729–738, 1986.
5. Tiollais P, Buendia MA. Hepatitis B virus. Sci Am 264:116–123, 1991.
6. Blumberg BS, Alter HJ, Visnich S. A 'new' antigen in leukemia sera. JAMA 191:101–106, 1956.
7. Sherlock S, Fox RA, Niazi SP, Scheuer PJ. Chronic liver disease and primary liver-cell cancer with hepatitis-associated (Australia) antigen in serum. Lancet 1:1243–1247, 1970.
8. Tong MJ, Weiner JM, Ashcavai MW, et al. Evidence for clustering of hepatitis B virus infection in families of patients with primary hepatocellular carcinoma. Cancer 44:2338–2344, 1979.
9. Szmuness W. Hepatocellular carcinoma and the hepatitis B virus: evidence for a causal association. Prog Med Virol 24:40–69, 1978.
10. Maupas P, Melnick JL. Hepatitis B infection and primary liver cancer. Prog Med Virol 27:1–5, 1981.
11. Beasley RP, Hwang LY, Lin CC, et al. Hepatocellular carcinoma and hepatitis B virus: a prospective study of 22, 707 men in Taiwan. Lancet 2:1129–1133, 1981.
12. Tu JT, Gao RN, Zhang DH, et al. Hepatitis B virus and primary liver cancer on Chongming Island: People's Republic of China. Natl Cancer Inst Monogr 69:213–215, 1985.
13. Prince AM, Szmuness W, Michon J, et al. A case–control study of the association between primary liver cancer and hepatitis B infection in Senegal. Int J Cancer 16:376–383, 1975.
14. Yu MC, Tong MJ, Coursaget P, et al. Prevalence of hepatitis B and C viral markers in black and white patients with hepatocellular carcinoma in the United States. J Natl Cancer Inst 82:1038–1041, 1990.
15. Rogler CE. Cellular and molecular mechanisms of hepatocarcinogenesis associated with Hepadnavirus infection. Curr Top Microbiol Immunol 168:103–140, 1991.
16. Buendia MA. Hepatitis B viruses and hepatocellular carcinoma. Adv Cancer Res 59:167–226, 1992.
17. Brechot C, Pourcel C, Louise A, et al. Presence of integrated hepatitis B virus DNA sequences in cellular DNA of human hepatocellular carcinoma. Nature 286:533–535, 1980.
18. Ganem D, Varmus HE. The molecular biology of the hepatitis B viruses. Annu Rev Biochem 56:651–693, 1987.
19. Chisari FV, Klopchin K, Moriyama T, et al. Molecular pathogenesis of hepatocellular carcinoma in hepatitis B virus transgenic mice. Cell 59:1145–1156, 1989.
20. Hino O, Kitagawa T, Sugano H. Relationship between serum and histochemical markers for hepatitis B virus and rate of viral integration in hepatocellular carcinomas in Japan. Int J Cancer 35:5–10, 1985.
21. Nakamura T, Tokino T, Nagaya T, et al. Microdeletion associated with the integration process of hepatitis B virus DNA. Nucl Acids Res 16:4865–4873, 1988.
22. Tokino T, Matsubara K. Chromosomal sites for hepatitis B virus integration in human hepatocellular carcinoma. J Virol 65:6761–6764, 1999.
23. Ogata N, Tokino T, Kamimura T, et al. A comparison of the molecular structure of integrated hepatitis B virus genomes in hepatocellular carcinoma cells and hepatocytes derived from the same patient. Hepatology 11:1017–1023, 1990.
24. Hino O, Shows TB, Rogler CE. Hepatitis B virus integration site in hepatocellular carcinoma at chromosome 17;18 translocation. Proc Natl Acad Sci USA 83:8338–8342, 1986.
25. Rogler CE, Sherman M, Su CY, et al. Deletion in chromosome 11p associated with a hepatitis B integration site in hepatocellular carcinoma. Science 230:319–322, 1985.
26. Dejean A, Bougueleret L, Grzeschik KH, et al. Hepatitis B virus DNA integration in a sequence homologous to v-erb-A and steroid receptor genes in a hepatocellular carcinoma. Nature 322:70–72, 1986.
27. Wang J, Zindy F, Chenivesse X, et al. Modification of cyclin A expression by hepatitis B virus DNA integration in a hepatocellular carcinoma. Oncogene 7:1653–1656, 1992.
28. Wollersheim M, Debelka U, Hofschneider PH. A transactivating function encoded in the hepatitis B virus X gene is conserved in the integrated state. Oncogene 3:545–552, 1988.
29. Takada S, Kido H, Fukutomi A, et al. Interaction of hepatitis B virus X protein with a serine protease, tryptase TL2 as an inhibitor. Oncogene 9:341–348, 1994.
30. Kekule AS, Lauer U, Meyer M, et al. The preS2/S region of integrated hepatitis B virus DNA encodes a transcriptional transactivator. Nature 343:457–461, 1990.
31. Natoli G, Avantaggiati ML, Chirillo P, et al. Induction of the DNA-binding activity of c-jun/c-fos heterodimers by the hepatitis B virus transactivator pX. Mol Cell Biol 14:989–998, 1994.
32. Okuda K, Ohnishi K. The role of viral infections in alcoholic liver disease. In: Hall P (ed): Alcoholic Liver Disease: Pathology and Pathogenesis, 2nd ed. Edward Arnold, London, 1995, pp. 147–159.
33. Wogan GN. Aflatoxins as risk factors for hepatocellular carcinoma in humans. Cancer Res 7:2114s–2118s, 1992.
34. Donato F, Boffetta P, Puoti M. A meta-analysis of epidemiological studies on the combined effect of hepatitis B and C virus infections in causing hepatocellular carcinoma. Int J Cancer 75:347–354, 1998.
35. Okuda K, Nakashima T, Sakamoto K, et al. Hepatocellular carcinoma arising in noncirrhotic and highly cirrhotic livers: a comparative study of histopathology and frequency of hepatitis B markers. Cancer 49:450–455, 1982.
36. Arakawa M, Kage M, Sugihara S, et al. Emergence of malignant lesions within an adenomatous hyperplastic nodule in a cirrhotic liver: observations in five cases. Gastroenterology 91:198–208, 1986.
37. Choo QL, Kuo G, Weiner AJ, et al. Isolation of a cDNA clone derived from a blood-borne non-A, non-B viral hepatitis genome. Science 244:359–362, 1989.
38. Choo QL, Richman KH, Han JH, et al. Genetic organization and diversity of the hepatitis C virus. Proc Natl Acad Sci USA 88:2451–2455, 1991.
39. Darwish NM, Abbas MO, Abdelfattah FM, Darwish MA. Hepatitis C virus infection in blood donors in Egypt. Egypt Public Health Assoc 67:223–236, 1992.
40. Kamel MA, Ghaffar YA, Wasef MA, et al. High HCV prevalence in Egyptian blood donors. Lancet 340:427, 1992.
41. Aceti A, Taliani G, Bruni R, et al. Hepatitis C virus antibody in Swaziland. Acta Trop 51:159–161, 1992.
42. Murphy EL, Bryzman S, Williams AE, et al. Demographic determinants of hepatitis C virus seroprevalence among blood donors. JAMA 275:995–1000, 1996.
43. Alter MJ, Hadler SC, Judson FN, et al. Risk factors for acute non-A, non-B hepatitis in the United States and association with hepatitis C virus infection. JAMA 264:2231–2235, 1990.
44. van der Poel C, Cuypers H, Reesink H, et al. Risk factors in hepatitis C virus–infected blood donors. Transfusion 31:777–779, 1991.
45. Yu MC, Tong MJ, Coursaget P, Ross RK, Govindarajan S, Henderson BE. Prevalence of hepatitis B and C viral markers in black and white patients with hepatocellular carcinoma in the United States [see comments]. J Natl Cancer Inst 82:1038–1041, 1990.
46. Yu MC, Yuan JM, Ross RK, et al. Presence of antibodies to the hepatitis B surface antigen is associated with an excess risk for hepatocellular carcinoma among non-Asians in Los Angeles County, California. Hepatology 25:226–228, 1997.
47. Di Bisceglie AM, Order SE, Klein JL, et al. The role of chronic viral hepatitis in hepatocellular carcinoma in the United States. Am J Gastroenterol 86:335–338, 1991.
48. Tanaka K, Hirohata T, Koga S, et al. Hepatitis C and hepatitis B in the etiology of hepatocellular carcinoma in the Japanese population. Cancer Res 51:2842–2847, 1991.
49. Mendenhall CL, Seeff L, Diehl AM, et al. Antibodies to hepatitis B virus and hepatitis C virus in alcoholic hepatitis and cirrhosis: their prevalence and clinical relevance. Hepatology 14:581–589, 1991
50. Shiratori Y, Shiina S, Imamura M, et al. Characteristic difference of hepatocellular carcinoma between hepatitis B and C viral infection in Japan. Hepatology 22:1027–1033, 1995.
51. Simmonds P. Variability of hepatitis C virus. Hepatology 21:570–583, 1995.
52. Dusheiko G, Schmilovitz-Weiss H, Brown D, et al. Hepatitis C virus genotypes: an investigation of type-specific differences in geographic origin and disease. Hepatology 19:13–28, 1994.
53. Nousbaum JB, Pol S, Nalpas B, et al. Hepatitis C virus type 1b (II) infection in France and Italy: Collaborative Study Group. Ann Intern Med 122:161–168, 1995.
54. Silini E, Bono F, Cividini A, et al. Differential distribution of hepatitis C virus genotypes in patients with and without liver function abnormalities. Hepatology 21:285–290, 1995.
55. De Mitri MS, Poussin K, Baccarini P, et al. HCV-associated liver cancer without cirrhosis. Lancet 345:413–415, 1995.
56. Zhang W, Cox AG, Taylor EW. Hepatitis C virus encodes a selenium-dependent glutathione peroxidase gene. Implications for oxidative stress as a risk factor in progression to hepatocellular carcinoma. Med Klin Suppl 3:2–6, 1999.
57. Look MP, Rockstroh JK, Rao GS, et al. Serum selenium, plasma glutathione (GSH) and erythrocyte glutathione peroxidase (GSH-Px) lev-

els in asymptomatic versus symptomatic human immunodeficiency virus-1 (HIV-1) infection. Eur J Clin Nutr 51:266–272, 1997.

58. Yu MC, Mack T, Hanisch R, Peters RL, Henderson BE, Pike MC. Hepatitis, alcohol consumption, cigarette smoking, and hepatocellular carcinoma in Los Angeles. Cancer Res 43:6077–6079, 1983.

59. Austin H, Delzell E, Grufferman S, et al. A case–control study of hepatocellular carcinoma and the hepatitis B virus, cigarette smoking, and alcohol consumption. Cancer Res 46:962–966, 1986.

60. Tanaka K, Hirohata T, Takeshita S. Blood transfusion, alcohol consumption, and cigarette smoking in causation of hepatocellular carcinoma: a case–control study in Fukuoka, Japan. Jpn J Cancer Res 79:1075–1082, 1988.

61. Ohnishi K, Shinji S, Nobuaki G. The effect of habitual alcohol intake on the development of liver cirrhosis and hepatocellular carcinoma. Cancer 49:672–677, 1981.

62. Lee FI. Cirrhosis and hepatoma in alcoholics. Gut 7:77–85, 1966.

63. Donato F, Tagger A, Chiesa R, et al. Hepatitis B and C virus infection, alcohol drinking, and hepatocellular carcinoma: a case–control study in Italy. Brescia HCC Study. Hepatology 26:579–584, 1997.

64. Tagger A, Donato F, Ribero ML, et al. Case–control study on hepatitis C virus (HCV) as a risk factor for hepatocellular carcinoma: the role of HCV genotypes and the synergism with hepatitis B virus and alcohol. Brescia HCC Study. Int J Cancer 81:695–699, 1999.

65. Oshita M, Hayashi N, Kasahara A, et al. Increased serum hepatitis C virus RNA levels among alcoholic patients with chronic hepatitis C. Hepatology 20:1115–1120, 1994.

66. Paronetto F. Immunologic reactions in alcoholic liver disease. Semin Liver Dis 13:183–195, 1993.

67. Busby WF, Wogan GN Jr. Aflatoxins. Am Cancer Soc Monogr 182:945–1136, 1984.

68. Ueno Y. The toxicology of mycotoxins. Crit Rev Toxicol 14:99–132, 1985.

69. Van Rensburg SJ, Cook-Mozaffari P, Van Schalkwyk DJ, et al. Hepatocellular carcinoma and dietary aflatoxin in Mozambique and Transkei. Br J Cancer 51:713–726, 1985.

70. Peers F, Bosch X, Kaldor J, et al. Aflatoxin exposure, hepatitis B virus infection and liver cancer in Swaziland. Int J Cancer 39:545–553, 1987.

71. Yeh FS, Yu MC, Mo CC, et al. Hepatitis B virus, aflatoxins, and hepatocellular carcinoma in southern Guangxi, China. Cancer Res 49:2506–2509, 1989.

72. Bulatao-Jayme J, Almero EM, Castro MC, et al. A case–control dietary study of primary liver cancer risk from aflatoxin exposure. Int J Epidemiol 11:112–119, 1982.

73. Guengerich FP, Shimada T. Oxidation of toxic and carcinogenic chemicals by human cytochrome P-450 enzymes. Chem Res Toxicol 4:391–407, 1991.

74. Shimada T, Guengerich F. Evidence for cytochrome P450NF's, being the principal enzyme involved in the bioactivation of aflatoxins in human liver. Proc Natl Acad Sci USA 87:8306–3810, 1990.

75. Essigmann JM, Croy RG, Nadzan AM, et al. Structural identification of the major DNA adduct formed by aflatoxin B1 in vitro. Proc Natl Acad Sci USA 74:1870–1874, 1977.

76. Sabbioni G, Skipper PL, Buchi G, et al. Isolation and characterization of the major serum albumin adduct formed by aflatoxin B1 in vivo in rats. Carcinogenesis 8:819–824, 1987.

77. Groopman JD, Roebuck BD, Kensler TW. Molecular dosimetry of aflatoxin DNA adducts in humans and experimental rat models. Prog Clin Biol Res 374:139–155, 1992.

78. Zarba J, Shabar F, Wogan G, Montesano R, Wild C. Molecular dosimetry of aflatoxin B1 exposures in a human population with high hepatitis B virus infection. Proc Am Assoc Cancer Res 31:230, 1990.

79. Autrup H, Seremet T, Wakhisi J, et al. Aflatoxin exposure measured by urinary excretion of aflatoxin B1-guanine adduct and hepatitis B virus infection in areas with different liver cancer incidence in Kenya. Cancer Res 47:3430–3433, 1987.

80. Wild CP, Jiang YZ, Allen SJ, et al. Aflatoxin-albumin adducts in human sera from different regions of the world. Carcinogenesis 11:2271–2274, 1990.

81. Qian GS, Ross RK, Yu MC, et al. A follow-up study of urinary markers of aflatoxin exposure and liver cancer risk in Shanghai, People's Republic of China. Cancer Epidemiol Biomarkers Prev 3:3–10, 1994.

82. Wild CP, Garner RC, Montesano R, et al. Aflatoxin B1 binding to plasma albumin and liver DNA upon chronic administration to rats. Carcinogenesis 7:853–858, 1986.

83. Wild CP, Jiang YZ, Sabbioni G, et al. Evaluation of methods for quantitation of aflatoxin-albumin adducts and their application to human exposure assessment. Cancer Res 50:245–251, 1990.

84. Liu YH, Taylor J, Linko P, et al. Glutathione S-transferase μ in human lymphocyte and liver: role in modulating formation of carcinogen-derived DNA adducts. Carcinogenesis 12:2269–2275, 1991.

85. McGlynn KA, Rosvold EA, Lustbader ED, et al. Susceptibility to hepatocellular carcinoma is associated with genetic variation in the enzymatic detoxification of aflatoxin B1. Proc Natl Acad Sci USA 92:2384–2387, 1995.

86. Kaplan L, Cole S. Faternal primary hepatocellular carcinoma in three male, adult siblings. Am J Med 39:305–311, 1968.

87. Hagstrom RM, Baker TD. Primary hepatocellular carcinoma in three male siblings. Cancer 22:142–150, 1968.

88. Lynch HT, Srivatanskul P, Phornthutkul K, et al. Familial hepatocellular carcinoma in an endemic area of Thailand. Cancer Genet Cytogenet 11:11–18, 1984.

89. Shen FM, Lee MK, Gong HM, et al. Complex segregation analysis of primary hepatocellular carcinoma in Chinese families: interaction of inherited susceptibility and hepatitis B viral infection. Am J Hum Genet 49:88–93, 1991.

90. Alberts SR, Lanier AP, McMahon BJ, et al. Clustering of hepatocellular carcinoma in Alaska Native families. Genet Epidemiol 8:127–139, 1991.

91. Fairbanks V, Baldus W. Disorders of iron metabolism. In: Wiliams WJ, Beutler E, Erslev A, Lichtman M (eds): Hematology, 4th ed. McGraw-Hill, New York, 1990, pp 752–758.

92. Piperno A. Classification and diagnosis of iron overload. Haematologica. 83:447–455, 1998.

93. Feder JN, Gnirke A, Thomas W, et al. A novel MHC class I–like gene is mutated in patients with hereditary haemochromatosis. Nat Genet 13:399–408, 1996.

94. Bothwell TH, MacPhail AP. Hereditary hemochromatosis: etiologic, pathologic, and clinical aspects. Semin Hematol 35:55–71, 1998.

95. Monaghan KG, Rybicki BA, Shurafa M, et al. Mutation analysis of the HFE gene associated with hereditary hemochromatosis in African Americans. Am J Hematol 58:213–217, 1998.

96. Beutler E, Gelbart T, West C, et al. Mutation analysis in hereditary hemochromatosis. Blood Cells Mol Dis 22:187–194, 1996.

97. Smith BC, Gorve J, Guzail MA, et al. Heterozygosity for hereditary hemochromatosis is associated with more fibrosis in chronic hepatitis C. Hepatology 27:1695–1699, 1998.

98. Bullen JJ, Rogers HJ, Griffiths E, et al. Role of iron in bacterial infection. Curr Top Microbiol Immunol 80:1–35, 1978.

99. Bullen JJ, Ward CG, Rogers HJ. The critical role of iron in some clinical infections. Eur J Clin Microbiol Infect Dis 10:613–617, 1991.

100. Miller M, Crippin JS, Klintmalm G, et al. End-stage liver disease in a 13-year-old secondary to hepatitis C and hemochromatosis. Am J Gastroenterol 91:1427–1429, 1996.

101. Hayashi H, Takikawa T, Nishimura N, et al. Serum aminotransferase levels as an indicator of the effectiveness of venesection for chronic hepatitis C. J Hepatol 22:268–271, 1995.

102. Mazzella G, Accogli E, Sottili S, et al. Alpha interferon treatment may prevent hepatocellular carcinoma in HCV-related liver cirrhosis. J Hepatol 24:141–147, 1996.

103. Bonkovsky HL, Banner BF, Rothman AL. Iron and chronic viral hepatitis. Hepatology 25:759–768, 1997.

104. Sifers RN, Finegold MJ, Woo SL. Molecular biology and genetics of alpha 1-antitrypsin deficiency. Semin Liver Dis 12:301–310, 1992.

105. Fabbretti G, Sergi C, Consales C, Faa G, Brisigotti M, Romeo G, Callea F. Genetic variants of alpha-1-antitrypsin (AAT) [review]. Liver 12:296–301, 1992.

106. Eriksson S, Carlson J, Velez R. Risk of cirrhosis and primary liver cancer in alpha 1-antitrypsin deficiency. N Engl J Med 314:736–739, 1986.

107. Blenkinsopp WK, Haffenden GP. Alpha-1-antitrypsin bodies in the liver. J Clin Pathol 30:132–137, 1977.

108. Carlson J, Eriksson S. Chronic 'cryptogenic' liver disease and malignant hepatoma in intermediate alpha 1-antitrypsin deficiency identified by a Pi Z-specific monoclonal antibody. Scand J Gastroenterol 20:835–842, 1985.

109. Zhou H, Fischer HP. Liver carcinoma in PiZ alpha-1-antitrypsin deficiency. Am J Surg Pathol 22:742–748, 1998.

110. Vogel W, Propst T, Propst A, et al. Causes of liver disease in an adult population with heterozygous and homozygous alpha 1-antitrypsin deficiency. Acta Paediatr Suppl 393:24–26, 1994.

111. Banner BF, Karamitsios N, Smith L, et al. Enhanced phenotypic expression of alpha-1-antitrypsin deficiency in an MZ heterozygote with chronic hepatitis C. Am J Gastroenterol 93:1541–1545, 1998.

112. Teckman JH, Qu D, Perlmutter DH. Molecular pathogenesis of liver disease in alpha₁-antitrypsin deficiency. Hepatology 24:1504–1516, 1996.

113. Bianchi L. Glycogen storage disease, and hepatocellular tumors. Eur J Pediatr 152 (Suppl 1):S63–S70, 1993.

114. Siersema PD, ten Kate FJ, Mulder PG, et al. Hepatocellular carcinoma in porphyria cutanea tarda: frequency and factors related to its occurrence. Liver 12:56–61, 1992.

115. Cheng WS, Govindarajan S, Redeker AG. Hepatocellular carcinoma in a case of Wilson's disease. Liver 12:42–45, 1992.

116. Nishida N, Fukuda Y, Kokuryu H, et al. Role and mutational heterogeneity of the *p53* gene in hepatocellular carcinoma. Cancer Res 53: 368–372, 1993.

117. Sheu JC, Huang GT, Lee PH, et al. Mutation of *p53* gene in hepatocellular carcinoma in Taiwan. Cancer Res 52:6098–6100, 1992.

118. Kazachkov Y, Khaoustov V, Yoffe B et al. p53 abnormalities in hepatocellular carcinoma from United States patients: analysis of all 11 exons. Carcinogenesis 17:2207–2212, 1996.

119. Hsia CC, Kleiner DE Jr, Axiotis CA, et al. Mutations of *p53* gene in hepatocellular carcinoma: roles of hepatitis B virus and aflatoxin contamination in the diet. J Natl Cancer Inst 84:1638–1641, 1992.

120. Scorsone KA, Zhou YZ, Butel JS, et al. *p53* mutations cluster at codon 249 in hepatitis B virus–positive hepatocellular carcinomas from China. Cancer Res 52:1635–1638, 1992.

121. Hsu IC, Metcalf RA, Sun T, et al. Mutational hotspot in the *p53* gene in human hepatocellular carcinomas. Nature 350:427–428, 1991.

122. Bressac B, Kew M, Wands J, et al. Selective G to T mutations of *p53* gene in hepatocellular carcinoma from southern Africa. Nature 35:429–431, 1991.

123. Patel P, Stephenson J, Scheuer PJ, et al. *p53* codon 249ser mutations in hepatocellular carcinoma patients with low aflatoxin exposure. Lancet 339:881, 1992.

124. Hayward NK, Walker GJ, Graham W, et al. Hepatocellular carcinoma mutation. Nature 352:764, 1991.

125. Kirby GM, Batist G, Fotouhi-Ardakani N, et al. Allele-specific PCR analysis of p53 codon 249 AGT transversion in liver tissues from patients with viral hepatitis. Int J Cancer 68:21–25, 1996.

126. Zhang X, Xu HJ, Murakami Y, et al. Deletions of chromosome 13q, mutations in retinoblastoma 1, and retinoblastoma protein state in human hepatocellular carcinoma. Cancer Res 54:4177–4182, 1994.

127. Yumoto Y, Hanafusa T, Hada H, et al. Loss of heterozygosity and analysis of mutation of *p53* in hepatocellular carcinoma. J Gastroenterol Hepatol 10:179–185, 1995.

128. Murakami Y, Hayashi K, Hirohashi S, et al. Aberrations of the tumor suppressor *p53* and retinoblastoma genes in human hepatocellular carcinomas. Cancer Res 51:5520–5525, 1991.

129. Guengerich FP. Roles of cytochrome P-450 enzymes in chemical carcinogenesis and cancer chemotherapy. Cancer Res 48:2946–2954, 1988.

130. Shimada T, Yun CH, Yamazaki H, et al. Characterization of human lung microsomal cytochrome P-450 1A1 and its role in the oxidation of chemical carcinogens. Mol Pharmacol 41:856–864, 1992.

131. Nakachi K, Imai K, Hayashi S, et al. Polymorphisms of the CYP1A1 and glutathione *S*-transferase genes associated with susceptibility to lung cancer in relation to cigarette dose in a Japanese population. Cancer Res 53:2994–2999, 1993.

132. Sivaraman L, Leatham MP, Yee J, et al. *CYP1A1* genetic polymorphisms and in situ colorectal cancer. Cancer Res 54:3692–3695, 1994.

133. Yu MW, Chiu YH, Yang SY, et al. Cytochrome P450 1A1 genetic polymorphisms and risk of hepatocellular carcinoma among chronic hepatitis B carriers. Br J Cancer 80:598–603, 1999.

134. Takahashi T, Lasker JM, Rosman AS, et al. Induction of cytochrome P-4502E1 in the human liver by ethanol is caused by a corresponding increase in encoding messenger RNA. Hepatology 17:236–245, 1993.

135. Guengerich FP, Kim DH, Iwasaki M. Role of human cytochrome P-450 IIE1 in the oxidation of many low molecular weight cancer suspects. Chem Res Toxicol 4:68–79, 1991.

136. Yang CS, Yoo JS, Ishizaki H, et al. Cytochrome P450IIE1: roles in nitrosamine metabolism and mechanisms of regulation. Drug Metab Rev 22:147–159, 1990.

137. Tsutsumi M, Matsuda Y, Takada A. Role of ethanol-inducible cytochrome P-450 2E1 in the development of hepatocellular carcinoma by the chemical carcinogen, *N*-nitrosodimethylamine. Hepatology 18: 1483–1489, 1993.

138. Hayashi S, Watanabe J, Kawajiri K. Genetic polymorphisms in the 5'-flanking region change transcriptional regulation of the human cytochrome P450IIE1 gene. J Biochem 110:559–565, 1991.

139. Yu MW, Gladek-Yarborough A, Chiamprasert S, et al. Cytochrome P450 2E1 and glutathione *S*-transferase M1 polymorphisms and susceptibility to hepatocellular carcinoma. Gastroenterology 109:266–273, 1995.

140. Ladero JM, Agundez JA, Rodriguez-Lescure A, et al. *RsaI* polymorphism at the cytochrome P4502E1 locus and risk of hepatocellular carcinoma. Gut 39:330–333, 1996.

141. Huang CY, Huang KL, Cheng TJ, et al. The GST T1 and CYP2E1 genotypes are possible factors causing vinyl chloride induced abnormal liver function. Arch Toxicol 71:482–488, 1997.

142. Crespi CL, Penman BW, Gelboin HV, et al. A tobacco smoke–derived nitrosamine, 4-(methylnitrosamino)-1-(3-pyridyl)-1-butanone, is activated by multiple human cytochrome P450s including the polymorphic human cytochrome P4502D6. Carcinogenesis 12:1197–1201, 1991.

143. Aoyama T, Yamano S, Guzelian PS, et al. Five of 12 forms of vaccinia virus–expressed human hepatic cytochrome P450 metabolically activate aflatoxin B1. Proc Natl Acad Sci USA 87:4790–4793, 1990.

144. Agundez JA, Ledesma MC, Benitez J, et al. *CYP2D6* genes and risk of liver cancer. Lancet 345:830–831, 1995.

145. Agundez JA, Olivera M, Ladero JM, et al. Increased risk for hepatocellular carcinoma in NAT2-slow acetylators and CYP2D6-rapid metabolizers. Pharmacogenetics 6:501–512, 1996.

146. Ketterer B, Harris JM, Talaska G, et al. The human glutathione *S*-transferase supergene family, its polymorphism, and its effects on susceptibility to lung cancer. Environ Health Perspect 98:87–94, 1992.

147. Seidegard J, Pero RW, Markowitz MM, et al. Isoenzyme(s) of glutathione transferase (class Mu) as a marker for the susceptibility to lung cancer: a follow-up study. Carcinogenesis 11:33–36, 1990.

148. Zhou T, Evans AA, London WT, et al. Glutathione *S*-transferase expression in hepatitis B virus–associated human hepatocellular carcinogenesis. Cancer Res 57:2749–2753, 1997.

149. Chen CJ, Yu MW, Liaw YF, et al. Chronic hepatitis B carriers with null genotypes of glutathione *S*-transferase M1 and T1 polymorphisms who are exposed to aflatoxin are at increased risk of hepatocellular carcinoma. Am J Hum Genet 59:128–134, 1996.

150. Yu MW, Chiu YH, Chiang YC, et al. Plasma carotenoids, glutathione *S*-transferase M1 and T1 genetic polymorphisms, and risk of hepatocellular carcinoma: independent and interactive effects. Am J Epidemiol 149:621–629, 1999.

151. McGlynn KA, Rosvold EA, Lustbader ED, et al. Susceptibility to hepatocellular carcinoma is associated with genetic variation in the enzymatic detoxification of aflatoxin B1. Proc Natl Acad Sci USA 92: 2384–2387, 1995.

152. Yu MW, Yang SY, Chiu YH, et al. A *p53* genetic polymorphism as a modulator of hepatocellular carcinoma risk in relation to chronic liver disease, familial tendency, and cigarette smoking in hepatitis B carriers. Hepatology 29:697–702, 1999.

# Chapter 42

# Molecular Biology of Hepatocellular Cancer

## JOE W. GRISHAM

Hepatocellular carcinoma (HCC) is one of the most common visceral neoplasms; more than 430,000 new cases occur worldwide each year.[1] Detection of HCC is difficult in its early stages, and current treatment modalities are ineffective in late-stage cancers.[2] Consequently, the number of deaths from HCC each year approximates the number of new cases identified. Despite this unsatisfactory situation, the major risk factors for HCC are better known than those for perhaps any other human cancer. Worldwide approximately 80% of the attributable risk for HCC is due to chronic infections with hepatitis B virus (HBV) or/and hepatitis C virus (HCV).[1,3] Most of the remaining risk for HCC results from the consumption of foods contaminated with the fungal toxin aflatoxin B1 and from excessive consumption of ethanol-containing beverages.[1,4] Exposure to a few chemicals and drugs and to external and internal irradiation, affliction with certain congenital metabolic diseases, and, possibly, tobacco smoking are other risk factors for HCC.[1,4] The etiology of HCC is multifactorial, and various combinations of these causal factors appear to be able to amplify risk.[4] Exposure to specific risk factors varies in different geographic areas around the world,[3] leading to large variations in the incidence of HCC in different regions.[1,4]

Identification of the most important causal factors for HCC has provided the basis for prevention and treatment strategies.[2,3] This knowledge also has led to the identification of behavioral modifications that avoid or reduce risky personal practices; to the development of grain production and storage methods that reduce fungal growth; to the screening of blood donors for hepatitis B and C antigens to reduce viral contamination of the blood supply; and to the elaboration of specific therapies to prevent viral infection (hepatitis B vaccination),[5] reduce viral burden in patients with chronic hepatitis (interferon treatment of patients with hepatitis B and C)[6] and increase the breakdown of promu-

tagenic metabolites of aflatoxin in hepatocytes (treatment with oltipraz).[7]

This chapter reviews the molecular pathogenesis of HCC—that is, the aberrations in the molecular control of hepatocyte proliferation, differentiation, death, and maintenance of genomic integrity that are associated with and are presumably responsible for development and progression of HCC in humans.[8] When relevant information is available, these molecular abnormalities are related to the metabolic actions of some of the major etiologic agents for HCC. Insight into the molecular mechanisms by which the known risk factors transform hepatocytes and produce malignant tumors will expand the bases for new strategies to prevent HCC and, possibly, to eradicate newly detected tumors.[9]

## Molecular Genetic Alterations in Hepatocellular Carcinoma

In this section we review the molecular aberrations that have been detected in fully malignant HCC. The data on molecular genetic aberrations available today are derived from tissue specimens that have included HCC at all stages of malignant progression, including tumors that range in size from a few millimeters to several centimeters in diameter and that represent various grades of differentiation and clinical stages. As might be expected, given the different sizes, grades, and stages of the HCCs that have been analyzed, the molecular aberrations that have been identified yield a somewhat heterogeneous pattern. The variability in molecular aberrations identified in different HCCs can be reduced somewhat by relating molecular alterations to tumor grade and stage, which can also provide information on the molecular changes that accompany tumor progression. However, molecular heterogeneity remains even when the data are segregated by tumor grade or stage, suggesting that aberrations in many different genes and molecules, which involve several regulatory pathways, can lead to HCC.

Multiple molecular changes have been detected in HCC, even though the data are not yet complete. Thus far, most studies have analyzed only one, or occasionally two, genes or gene products in each tumor studied, preventing a full understanding of the variety of regulatory molecules that may be involved and of the patterns of regulatory pathways that are affected in individual HCC. The data reviewed here are grouped around the involvement of molecules in specific signal transduction and cellular regulatory pathways that participate in the control of hepatocyte proliferation, differentiation, death, and genomic integrity. In future studies, it will be desirable to assess the simultaneous expression of multiple genes in each HCC.

Molecular alterations occur in tumor cell populations that initially are often monoclonal, proliferate rapidly, and undergo frequent clonal divergence. The populations of tumor cells were monoclonal in 105 (96%) of 109 small HCCs, based on the pattern of integration of HBV DNA into the tumor cell genome, the random silencing of a polymorphic X-linked gene in females, and/or DNA fingerprint patterns obtained by polymerase chain reaction (PCR) amplification of multilocus minisatellite probes or random primers.[10–23] Tumor cells of HCC proliferate much more rapidly than hepatocytes in either healthy livers or livers that are the sites of chronic hepatitis or cirrhosis in which HCC usually develops, and tumor cell proliferation increases as HCC progresses.[8] Hepatocellular carciomas undergo clonal divergence as they enlarge,[24] and molecular alterations that increase cell formation or reduce cell death are selected and rapidly permeate the tumor cell populations.

## Growth Factors and Receptors

Various growth factor/receptor combinations are up-regulated or newly expressed in HCC. These growth factor/receptor combinations include several that strongly activate mitogenic pathways, such as transforming growth factor (TGF)-α/epidermal growth factor receptor (EGFR), insulin-like growth factor (IGF)-II/IGF-I receptor (IGF-IR), and hepatocyte growth factor (HGF)/HGF receptor (c-met), as well as some growth factor/receptor combinations that are so-called comitogens for hepatocytes, such as adrenergic compounds/adrenergic receptor (AdR) and fibroblast growth factor (FGF)/fibroblast growth factor receptors (FGFRs). In addition, the inflammatory cytokines tumor necrosis factor (TNF)-α and interleukin (IL)-6 are hepatocyte comitogens, and they are strongly expressed in the pathologic livers in which HCC tumors arise. Vascular endothelial growth factor (VEGF)/VEGF receptor and platelet-derived endothelial cell growth factor (PD-ECGF)/PD-ECGF receptor combinations are primarily mitogenic for endothelial cells. (All of the hepatocyte mitogens and comitogens also function as vascular growth factors.) These various mitogenic/comitogenic growth factor/receptor combinations send signals through multiple transduction pathways (discussed in Components of Intracellular Signaling Pathways, below) to the hepatocyte nucleus to regulate the expression of specific gene sets. The major growth factor/receptor combination that is strongly antimitogenic for hepatocytes is TGF-β/TGF-β RI, RII. TGF-β expression is up-regulated in HCC, but its signaling pathway is impaired.

### Transforming growth factor-α, epidermal growth factor, epidermal growth factor receptor, HER2/erbB2

Transforming growth factor α and epidermal growth factor (EGF) are ligands that bind to and activate the receptors of the epidermal growth factor group, which include HER2/erbB2, HER3, and HER4, in addition to EGFR (HER1). Multimolecular receptors composed of different heteromeric combinations of these EGFR-related molecules appear to be able to activate different signal transduction pathways.

Transforming growth factor α is not expressed in unaltered hepatocytes,[25] but it has been detected (by immunohistochemistry) in 238 (67%) of 354 HCCs.[26–34] Serum levels of TGF-α were 2- to 20-fold higher in 135 patients with HCC (median level 45 to 100 pg/ml) than in 173 healthy controls (median level, 6 to 21 pg/ml).[35,36] Urinary excretion also was increased about sixfold in 31 patients with HCC (21.5 ± 20.3 μg/g creatinine) compared to that in 33 individuals without liver disease (4.9 ± 2.8 μg/g creatinine).[37] Expression of TGF-α was most intense in the more highly differentiated HCCs[27,29–31] and, in most studies, correlated positively with elevated cell proliferation.[36,38] The mechanism by which TGF-α expression is up-regulated in HCC is not known, but it may partly involve gene transactivation by proteins expressed by HBV and HCV.

Epidermal growth factor was detected by immunohistochemistry in 14 (25%) of 56 HCCs.[39] Urinary excretion of EGF was not increased in HCC patients,[37] but several EGF-like proteins were identified in the urine of HCC patients.[40] Much of the urinary EGF-like protein was of low molecular weight and may have represented breakdown products of TGF-α/EGF. In keeping with this possibility, expression of EGF in HCC did not correlate with any diagnostic or prognostic characteristics of the tumor.[32]

Epidermal growth factor receptor, which is a component of the heteromeric receptor for both TGF-α and EGF, continues to be expressed at functional levels by neoplastic hepatocytes, providing the molecular basis for an autocrine pathway that stimulates the proliferation of neoplastic hepatocytes.[32] In 25 HCCs, EGFR was quantified at a concentration of 8.9 ± 14.6 fmol/mg protein, compared with 11.4 ± 9.2 fmol/mg protein in 18 normal livers.[41] EGFR was expressed at about the same level in both HCC and adjacent nontumorous liver tissues in 18 cases in which both tissues were compared.[33,34] HER2/erbB2 can form heteromeric complexes with EGFR (along with HER3 and HER4) and thereby modify the effect of ligand binding to receptor in some tissues. HER2/erbB2 (also called Neu) appears to have an important role in the development of mammary cancer, for example. But the potential role of this EGFR-related molecule in HCC is not clear because HER2/erbB2 does not appear to be expressed by normal hepatocytes. HER2 protein was expressed focally (by immunohistochemistry) in only 4 (11%) of 35 HCCs in three studies,[42–44] but in another larger study it was detected in 60 (80%) of 75 HCCs.[34] ErbB2 protein concentrations (by ELISA) in 31 HCCs ranged from 0.02 to 4.5 U/mg protein, with a median level of 0.43 U/mg protein.[45] Hepatocellular carcinomas that expressed HER2 at concentrations greater than the median level for all HCCs in the group were correlated with shorter patient survival times. Furthermore, in keeping with the expression of HER2 by HCC, the level of this peptide (by ELISA) was 40% higher in the sera of 22 patients with HCC than that in 23 control subjects.[45]

### Insulin-like growth factor II, insulin-like growth factor I receptor, mannose 6-phosphate/insulin-like growth factor II receptor

Insulin-like growth fcator II, which is highly expressed in the embryonic liver and is down-regulated in the healthy adult liver, sends metabolic and mitogenic signals through the IGF-IR, as well as through the insulin receptor if the ambient level is sufficiently high. Mannose 6-phosphate (M6P)/IGF-IIR (sometimes called 1the IGF-IIR) is a multifunctional receptor involved in the lysosomal degradation of many mannose-containing molecules and in other functions as well (see TGF-β, below). In the instance of IGF-II, M6P/IGF-IIR shuttles the bound ligand to lysosomes, where it is catabolized, thereby reducing the concentration of IGF-II at the cell membrane and competing with IGF-IIR for available ligand.

Expression of IGF-II was strongly up-regulated in HCC (by as much as ninefold), as measured by quantifying the level in tissue,[46] assessing immunohistochemical staining in tissue,[47] and quantifying mRNA by blot hybridization or RNase-protection assay.[46,48-54] The concentration of IGF-II in 10 HCCs was 369.2 ± 373.5 ng/g, compared with 41.3 ± 18.7 ng/g in healthy liver tissue.[46] Expression of IGF-II was immunohistochemically intense in 182 (79%) of 231 HCCs, but no stained hepatocytes were detected in 29 normal livers.[31,47,48,55,56] Interestingly, the level of IGF-II was not elevated in the sera of patients with HCC, even though hepatic production was greatly increased. The serum concentration of IGF-II was 738 ± 189 μg/L in 23 healthy individuals and 475 ± 205 μg/L in 32 patients with HCC,[57] and these concentration ranges were corroborated in another study.[46] This situation may imply that IGF-II is completely consumed by the same HCC cells that produce it. This possibility is supported by the observation that IGF-II and the cell proliferation marker Ki-67 colocalized predominantly in the same tumor cells in 10 HCCs,[58] another indication that IGF-II expression correlates positively with tumor cell proliferation.

Increased expression of IGF-II in HCC is associated with conjoint alterations in allelic activity and promoter usage by the IGF-II gene, which appears to reflect a partial reversion to fetal patterns of gene expression. The IGF-II gene is expressed only from the P2, P3, and P4 promoters of the paternal allele during embryonic development of the liver,[59,60] whereas the maternal allele is imprinted, similar to the H19 gene.[61] The P3 promoter is responsible for about 80% of the IGF-II transcripts in fetal hepatocytes.[62] Postnatally, maternal imprinting of the IGF-II gene is lost in human liver, in coordination with loss of imprinting and down-regulation of the H19 gene, dominant use of the P1 promoter, and reduced expression of IGF-II.[60,61] The P1 promoter is responsible for more than 50% of the IGF-II transcripts produced in the healthy adult liver from both alleles.[62]

The P1 promoter was partially down-regulated, but not completely silenced, in 49 (93%) of 53 HCCs and the P3 promoter was up-regulated in 19 (51%) of 37 HCCs[54,55,63] in association with renewed imprinting of the H19 gene to the maternal allele.[64,65] Transcription from the IGF-II gene demonstrated marked allelic imbalance, approaching monoallelic transcription in 24 (62%) of 39 HCCs, although allelic heterozygosity was retained in 38 (97%) of 39 HCCs.[54,66] However, the extent of allelic imbalance of the IGF-II gene varied markedly in different HCCs.[66-68] Paternal imprinting and P1 promoter use do not appear to be complete in most instances.[67,69] In a few HCCs, paternal imprinting was detected even when the P1 promoter continued to be active.[68]

Complex alterations in allelic activity and promoter transcriptional usage seem to be responsible for the increased expression of IGF-II in HCC. This appears to represent a partial reversion from the adult status of biallelic transcription to the fetal condition of monoallelic transcription. Therefore, increased IGF-II expression in HCC in adults does not result from the loss of imprinting of this gene.

The signaling receptors for IGF-II, IGF-IR and the insulin receptor (INSR), are ubiquitously expressed by normal liver tissue, but their expression status by HCC apparently has not been assessed. Additionally, the availability of IGF-II can be modulated by IGF-binding proteins (IGFBPs), which also have not received detailed study in HCC. Increased expression of IGFBP-1 was detected in four of five HCCs,[70] but the other binding proteins apparently have not been assessed.

Expression of M6P/IGF-IIR mRNA was markedly reduced in 7 (64%) of 11 HCCs, and this reduction was associated with diminished immunohistochemical staining of receptor protein on HCC tumor cells.[71] Loss of one allele (LOH) of the M6P/IGF-IIR gene on chromosome 6q26–27 was detected in 69 (49%) of 140 HCCs[72-76] and the remaining allele was mutated in 18 (17%) of 109 HCCs that showed LOH.[75-77] In addition, homozygous deletion of the M6P/IGF-IIR alleles was reported in 5 (15%) of 34 HCCs.[73] Combined LOH and mutation of the remaining allele are characteristics of aberrant tumor suppressor genes, thus M6P/IGF-IIR may function as a tumor suppressor in hepatocytes. Loss of function of M6P/IGF-IIR may provide a relative growth advantage for affected HCC cells. Nevertheless, several studies from Japan have failed to detect mutations in the M6P/IGF-IIR gene.[75,78,79] This variation may indicate that the mutation is found only in subsets of HCC.

### Insulin-like growth factor I

Although the liver is the major source of IGF-I in adults, increased production of this growth factor appears to have no direct role in the development of HCC. However, the tissue concentration of IGF-I in HCC apparently has not been studied. Transcription of the gene was down-regulated in seven (100%) of seven HCCs,[51] and the concentration of IGF-I in the serum of 32 patients with HCC was only 26.9 ± 32.6 μg/L, compared with 277.1 ± 101.7 μg/L in 23 control subjects.[57] Reduced hepatic expression of IGF-I may reflect the inhibitory effect of high serum levels of IGF-II on secretion of growth hormone from the pituitary gland,[57] or it may result from the loss of growth hormone receptors on HCC tumor cells (see Hormones and Receptors, below).[80]

### Hepatocyte growth factor and c-met

Hepatocyte growth factor normally is expressed in the liver by mesenchymal, endothelial, and biliary epithelial cells but not by hepatocytes. It is also stored in the liver bound to matrix proteins. However, HGF has been detected by immunohistochemistry in the tumorous hepatocytes of 136 (64%) of 214 HCCs,[33,81-85] but HGF mRNA either was not detected in HCC[86] or was identified in only a small fraction of tumor cells.[87] These findings suggest that the HGF detected immunohistochemically in tumor cells reflects receptor-mediated uptake, an opinion supported by the observation that HGF staining did not correlate with increased cell proliferation[84] or with patient survival.[85] Instead, tumor cell proliferation and patient survival were highly correlated with expression of c-met, the cognate receptor for HGF (see below). Nevertheless, the concentration of HGF in the serum of 39 patients with HCC increased to 1.06 ± 1.05 ng/ml, compared with 0.27 ± 0.08 ng/ml in 200 subjects without liver disease.[88] This may reflect the release of liver matrix-associated HGF as a consequence of matrix destruction.

Receptors c-met and c-ron (a c-met–related receptor for HGF-like protein) were expressed by both healthy hepatocytes and HCC tumor cells.[89] Expression of c-met was detected by immunohistochemistry in 235 (84%) of 281 HCCs,[33,81,82,84,89-94] and c-met was considered to be overexpressed in 137 (56%) of 244 HCCs.[33,82,84,89-94] Quantification of c-met mRNA (by reverse transcriptase–polymerase chain reaction [RT-PCR]) showed that 11 HCCs contained 0.41 ± 0.20 pg/μg total mRNA whereas 4 normal livers contained 0.20 ± 0.15 pg/μg total mRNA.[86] Elevated expression of c-met was correlated with increased tumor cell proliferation and impaired survival of patients with HCC.[85] In some studies,[92,93] but not all,[84,85,92] elevated expression of c-met was also correlated with poor differentiation of tumor cells. The mechanism that leads to increased expression of c-met in HCC is unclear; studies in cultured HCC tumor cells indicate that the c-*met* gene is up-regulated by exposing the cells to either HGF or EGF or to the inflammatory cytokines TNF-$\alpha$, IL-1, or IL-6.[89] Whether these molecules regulate expression of the c-*met* gene in vivo is not known.

### Adrenergic receptors

The adrenergic compounds—epinephrine, norepinephrine, and vasopressin—are ligands for the G protein–coupled AdR. The density of $\alpha_1$AdR on tumor cells was uniformly decreased by more than 50% in 32 HCCs, as compared with the concentration in normal livers ($61.9 \pm 19.7$ fmol/mg protein), whereas it was decreased about twofold in liver tissue adjacent to HCC.[95] The dissociation constant for prazosin-binding was unchanged in these different tissues (normal liver, $210.1 \pm 31.4$ pM). The density of $\alpha_2$AdR was reduced on tumor cells in 19 (70%) of 27 HCCs. In contrast, the density of $\beta_2$AdR was approximately doubled in 22 HCCs, compared with that in either 24 normal livers ($89.7 \pm 17.9$ fmol/mg protein) or 22 liver tissues adjacent to HCC, but the dissociation constant for pindolol-binding was unchanged (normal liver, $112.5 \pm 32.1$ pM).[95] Along with these changes in AdR density, cAMP production (reflecting adenyl cyclase activity) was stimulated by isoproterenol to a significantly greater extent in HCC tissue ($66.6 \pm 4.7$ pmol/min/mg protein) than in either adjacent nontumorous tissue ($29.6 \pm 7.0$ pmol/min/mg of protein) or healthy liver tissue ($32.4 \pm 13.6$ pmol/min/mg of protein).[95]

### Fibroblast growth factors/receptors

Acidic and basic forms of FGF were each expressed focally by tumor cells (detected by immunohistochemistry) in about one-third of 56 HCCs, and both forms were detected concurrently in about 20%. Expression of FGF, however, was found only in endothelial cells and macrophages of nontumorous liver.[39,96] Basic FGF gene transcripts were detected in 20 (43%) of 46 HCCs in other studies.[97–99] Increased expression of FGF by HCC was correlated with the extent of tumor vascularity.[39] The expression of FGF receptors in HCC has not received detailed study, although FGFR-4 was found to be up-regulated in HCC in a parallel hybridization analysis of multiple protein kinase genes.[100]

### Vascular endothelial growth factor

Strong expression of VEGF protein was detected by immunohistochemistry in 131 (72%) of 183 HCCs[101–105] and by immunoblot of protein in 21 (75%) of 28 HCCs;[106] mRNA transcripts were identified in 102 (73%) of 139 HCCs examined by RT-PCR.[99,101,107–109] Three of the VEGF isoforms expressed in normal liver ($VEGF_{121}$, $VEGF_{165}$, and $VEGF_{189}$) were also expressed in HCC,[103,107] but $VEGF_{206}$ was not.[103] The relationship of VEGF expression by HCC to tumor size, differentiation, and vascularity is uncertain because several studies have yielded conflicting results on all of these correlations.[101,103,104,107–109] Despite many VEGF studies, the role of VEGF in the development and growth of HCC is not yet clear. Receptors for VEGF (Flt-1 and Fkt-1) apparently have not been evaluated in HCC.

### Platelet-derived endothelial cell growth factor

The concentration of PD-ECGF (by ELISA) was significantly elevated in the plasma of 34 patients with HCC ($6.0 \pm 2.5$ U/ml), compared with that in 17 healthy individuals ($4.2 \pm 1.1$ U/ml), and the majority of tumor cells stained diffusely for PD-ECGF by immunohistochemistry.[110] Platelet-derived endothelial cell growth factor mRNA was also detected by RNA blot in 19 (68%) of 28 HCCs, correlating with the expression of VEGF.[106] Expression of PD-ECGF transcripts was higher in HCCs that were associated with tumor thrombi in the portal vein. Apparently no data are available on expression of receptors for PD-ECGF in HCC.[106]

### Tumor necrosis factor $\alpha$ and interleukin-6

Although TNF-$\alpha$ and IL-6 are potent mitogenic factors for hepatocytes,[111] expression of these inflammatory cytokines and of their receptors apparently has not been studied in HCC. Nevertheless, both cytokines are copiously expressed in the chronically inflamed livers in which HCC often arises, a finding suggesting that these cytokines are likely to be involved in the development of HCC.

### Transforming growth factor $\beta$ and transforming growth factor $\beta$ receptors I and II

In healthy livers, TGF-$\beta_1$ is expressed by mesenchymal cells but not appreciably by hepatocytes. However, TGF-$\beta_1$ mRNA (as well as mRNAs for TGF-$\beta_2$ and -$\beta_3$) was highly overexpressed in 34 HCCs.[112–114] TGF-$\beta$ protein was localized to tumor cells (by immunohistochemistry) in most HCC,[113–115] and the levels of TGF-$\beta$ mRNA and protein were highly correlated in a few HCCs in which this relationship was directly examined.[113] The expression of TGF-$\beta_1$ protein in HCC correlated inversely with tumor cell proliferation as measured by the proliferating cell nuclear antigen (PCNA) index,[32] indicating that the growth factor retained some degree of negative control of tumor cell growth. The concentration of TGF-$\beta_1$ in the plasma of 26 patients with HCC was sharply increased ($19.3 \pm 19.5$ ng/ml), compared with the plasma concentration in 20 healthy controls ($1.4 \pm 0.8$ ng/ml).[116,117] The plasma level of TGF-$\beta_1$ correlated with tumor vascularity, as assessed angiographically.[118] Urinary excretion of TGF-$\beta_1$ also was higher in 140 patients with HCC ($64.1 \pm 47.3$ $\mu$g/g creatinine) than in 50 healthy controls ($14.9 \pm 10.5$ $\mu$g/g creatinine).[119] Resection or embolization of HCC was followed by a prompt decrease in both serum concentration and urinary excretion of TGF-$\beta$.[117–119]

Transforming growth factor $\beta$ exerts its antimitogenic action by binding to heterodimeric complexes of type I and type II TGF-$\beta$ receptors, which initiate a signal that is passed to the nucleus. Both TGF-$\beta$ RI and TGF-$\beta$ RII are expressed by normal hepatocytes, but expression of the receptors was sharply decreased or extinguished entirely in 18 (72%) of 25 HCCs and reduced in the other 7 tumors.[120] In other studies, TGF-$\beta$ RII was detected by immunohistochemistry in all of 104 HCC, but the receptor was decreased in 25 tumors (24%) compared with levels in adjacent liver tissue.[33,114] The level of TGF-$\beta$ RI mRNA was reduced in 10 of 11 HCCs by an average of 40%, and TGF-$\beta$ RII mRNA was decreased by an average of 51% in 8 of the tumors, and receptor protein was decreased by 30%.[71] The mechanisms by which TGF-$\beta$ receptors are down-regulated in HCC are not entirely clear. In one study, in 32 (44%) of 73 HCCs the RII gene was mutated by the deletion of a single nucleotide in the $A_{10}$ microsatellite tract in exon 3, producing a frameshift that resulted in a downstream stop codon and an inactive truncated receptor protein; the frequency of mutations correlated with poor differentiation of HCC.[121] However, similar mutations were not found in either the polyA or polyG microsatellite tracts of the TGF-$\beta$ gene in a total of 195 HCCs examined in five other studies;[78,79,122–124] the overall frequency of mutational inactivation of the TGF-β RII gene in 268 HCC in the six studies was 8%.[78,79,121–124]

Impaired activation of latent TGF-β also may partly explain the defective antimitogenic function of TGF-β in HCC. In addition to involvement in the degradation of IGF-II, M6P/IGF-IIR participates in the activation of proTGF-β by serving as a scaffold on which the latent molecule is proteolytically cleaved. The marked reduction in expression of M6P/IGF-IIR that results from a combination of LOH and mutation of the remaining allele[72–77] (see above) may reduce the activation of latent TGF-β that is produced in excess by HCC with a malfunctioning M6P/IGF-IIR gene. The ratio of activated-to-latent TGF-β in the liver and serum of patients with HCC apparently has not been examined.

## Hormones and Receptors

Several of the classic hormones, including insulin, thyroid hormone, parathyroid hormone, and the sex steroids, are considered to be comitogens for hepatocytes.[108] Some of these classic hormones and their receptors may be involved in the development of HCC, although the data are still fragmentary.

### Insulin and insulin receptor

Although insulin (INS) and INSR expression apparently has not been examined in HCC, considerable evidence suggests their involvement in the development of this neoplasm. Epidemiologic studies indicate that the risk of HCC is increased in patients with type II diabetes, even when the population studies are controlled for other risk factors, including alcoholism, hemochromatosis, and cirrhosis.[125] Type II diabetes is associated with INS resistance and with compensatory elevation in the concentration of circulating INS. By binding to and activating IGF-IR, elevated INS levels may stimulate hepatocyte proliferation and produce the other cellular effects that result from the overexpression of IGF-II. However, the molecular mechanisms that relate chronically elevated levels of circulating INS and HCC are not known. Type II diabetes in patients with HCC has also been associated with rapid tumor recurrence after surgical resection.[126] Increased signaling through INSR and its related receptors is suggested by the observation that insulin receptor substrate 1 (IRS-1) is overexpressed in HCC.[127]

### Growth hormone and growth hormone receptor

The potential role of growth hormone (GH) and its receptor in HCC has not received much study. That the circulating level of GH is significantly elevated in patients with chronic hepatitis and cirrhosis[128] suggests the possibility that this hormone may play a role in the early stages of hepatocarcinogesis. It is of interest that HCC cells appear to acquire molecular changes that block their ability to respond to GH. Expression of growth hormone receptor (GHR) (detected by radioreceptor assay using radiolabeled recombinant GH) was totally extinguished in six HCCs, although GHR was expressed on hepatocytes in adjacent liver tissue that was the site of chronic hepatitis.[80] In keeping with the loss of GHR on HCC cells, the transcription of the IGF-I gene (which is regulated by GH and produces many of the hepatic metabolic actions formerly attributed to GH) was strongly downregulated in tumor cells, and the level of IGF-I in the serum of patients was markedly diminished in patients with HCC.[57]

### Thyroid hormone and receptors

Elevated plasma levels of thyroxine have been reported in many patients with HCC, in association with increased concentrations of thyroid hormone (TH)–binding protein.[129–133] The functional effect of these changes is not clear, as affected patients showed no evidence of hyperthyroidism. Thyroid hormone nuclear receptor α and β proteins were truncated in 9 (56%) of 16 HCCs.[134] The thyroid hormone receptor (TR)α gene contained point mutations in 10 (63%) of 16 HCCs, and the TRβ gene was mutated in 12 (75%) of 16 HCCs.[134] Mutational hot spots were detected at codons 209 to 228 and 245 to 256.[134] These alterations were correlated with overexpression of the TRβ1 protein and with variably altered expression of TRα protein.[135] Overexpression of TRβ1 was associated with increased invasiveness of HCC.[136] Although TH-binding to TR was not affected by the mutation and truncation of receptors, its ability to bind to DNA was reduced or abolished, leading to the suggestion that mutant TR may have lost the ability to repress gene expression and gained a dominant negative action.

### ErbA

Expression of the erbA oncogene, which has close homology to the TR gene, was markedly enhanced in six HCCs and adjacent liver tissues, as indicated by RNA blotting.[137] The erbA molecule appears to function as a constitutive transcriptional repressor.

### Retinoids and retinoic acid receptors

Retinoids influence several hepatocellular properties, including cellular growth and differentiation, by binding to one of two retinoic acid receptors (RAR) (α or β) that are expressed by hepatocytes. The RARβ gene was first identified near an HBV genomic insertion site in an HCC.[138–141] Two studies of small numbers of HCCs have not agreed on whether RARβ or RARα is overexpressed in this tumor.[139,142]

### Androgens and estrogens

The incidence of HCC is two- to fourfold higher in males than in females regardless of the causative factors involved,[1,4] thus androgenic steroids or the balance between androgens and estrogens may have important roles in the development of this neoplasm. This suggestion is strengthened by observations that therapeutic uses of androgenic steroids are associated with increased risk to development of hepatocellular neoplasms in males, including both benign hepatocellular adenoma (HCA) and HCC.[143,144] Furthermore, use of contraceptive mixtures containing certain formulations of estrogens and progestins has been associated with increased risk of HCC in women.[145] Cirrhosis, which often precedes HCC, is associated with abnormal metabolism of steroid hormones, resulting in males in generally decreased serum levels of testosterone, dihydrotestosterone, and dehydroepiandrosterone, and increased levels of estradiol, estrone, and androstenedione.[146] Although androgen levels are generally diminished in male patients with cirrhosis, those who have the highest testosterone levels also have the greatest risk of developing HCC. This was shown by an epidemiologic study of 9691 Taiwanese men, which found that the eventual development of HCC, which occurred in 35 men during the period of study, was 4.1-fold (95% confidence limits, 1.3- to 13.2-fold) more likely to develop in the men whose plasma testosterone levels (measured up to 4.6 years before HCC was detected) were in the upper tertile for the entire group.[147] Although the men were matched by age and known HCC risk factors (infection with HBV or HCV, alcohol use, diet, etc.), those who had testosterone levels in the lower three tertiles for the group had a much lower risk of developing HCC.[147] These results suggest that androgens may play a role in the development of HCC, even at near-physiological levels.

## Androgen receptors

Androgen receptors (AR) have been detected (by binding/displacement assays) in 197 (64%) of 306 HCCs in concentrations ranging from the normal level (6 to 35 fmol/mg protein) to increases of about 10-fold, with the receptor concentration almost always greater in HCC than in adjacent nontumorous tissue. Binding affinities of AR in HCC approximated those found in normal liver (2 to 30 nM).[148–158] Androgen receptor was preferentially expressed in small (<3 cm) HCC.[158] In females, AR was expressed in only 7 (37%) of 19 HCCs,[154] a result suggesting higher expression in males. The functional competence and heightened activity of AR expressed by HCC was shown by the ability of tumor nodules to concentrate radiolabeled testosterone from incubation medium in vitro more avidly than the surrounding liver tissue.[151] Moreover, surgically resected HCC that expressed AR had a significantly higher rate of recurrence during the subsequent 2 to 5 years than did resected HCC that was AR negative.[151,158]

## Estrogen receptors

Estrogen receptors were detected in 98 (44%) of 225 HCCs at concentrations similar to or slightly higher than in the adjacent nontumorous liver tissue (2 to 6 fmol/mg protein) and with similar binding affinities (1–3 nM).[148,150,153,155,156,159,160] Estrogen receptors also were detected immunohistochemically in up to 68% of the nuclei in six to eight HCCs (75%), as well as in up to 50% of the nuclei of adjacent liver tissue and of nondiseased livers.[160] In one study, ER-negative HCC tumors were slightly larger than ER-positive tumors.[156] Although ER status did not significantly influence 5-year survival following surgical resection of the primary tumors, the difference was suggestive; among 68 patients with HCC who were followed for 5 years, 2 (10%) of 21 patients with ER-positive tumors survived, compared with 11 (23%) of 47 patients with ER-negative tumors.[156]

Truncated ER transcripts that lacked exon 5, including part of the hormone-binding domain, were detected by PCR in seven of seven HCC from males, but not in any of seven HCCs from females.[161] The truncated ER could not bind estradiol, leading to speculation that the mutated transcripts might retain constitutive transcriptional activity without needing to be occupied by bound estrogen.[161] In a larger subsequent study, 9 (36%) of 25 HCCs in males and 3 (20%) of 15 HCCs in females expressed only the mutant transcript.[162] A mixture of both truncated and wild-type ER was expressed by 11 (44%) of 25 HCCs in males and 7 (47%) of 15 HCCs in females, whereas the remaining tumors in both sexes expressed only the wild-type ER.[162]

Androgen receptor and ER appeared to interact weakly in affecting the 5-year survival of 57 patients following surgical resection of primary tumors;[156] 10 (67%) of 15 patients whose HCC expressed neither AR nor ER survived for 5 years. Estrogen receptor expression in the absence of AR expression was associated with 5-year survival of two (50%) of four patients, but none of 38 patients whose HCC expressed AR survived for 5 years, irrespective of whether ER was expressed (13 patients) or not (25 patients).[156]

These results suggest that androgens/AR strongly and estrogens/ER slightly promote the process of hepatocarcinogenesis. Nevertheless, mechanistic understanding of the sex steroids' role in the development of HCC is lacking. Analysis of concentrations of androgens and estrogens and their receptors in both patients and their HCC could provide useful information on the mechanisms involved.

## Neuropeptide receptors

Receptors for somatostatin and vasoactive intestinal polypeptide were detected by binding of radioactive substrates in about 24 (41%) of 59 HCC.[163] With this technique, receptor for substance P was detected in only 5% and cholecystokinin (gastrin) receptor was not found on any HCC. However, another study detected gastrin receptor on 21 (90%) of 23 HCCs by immunohistochemistry.[164] Expression of neuropeptide receptors by HCC probably reflects their neuroendocrine differentiation.

## Components of Intracellular Signaling Pathways

The binding of a growth factor to its cognate receptor energizes the passage of a signal that ultimately activates transcription factors in the nucleus to stimulate expression of a selected set of genes. Multiple signal transduction pathways connect receptors on the cell membrane to the nucleus, and other receptors are located in the cytosol or the nucleus.

### Mitogen-activated protein kinase pathway

Molecular elements of the mitogen-activated protein kinase (MAPK) pathway have been most often analyzed in HCC, but other mitogenic pathways apparently have not been studied. The MAPK cascade contains multiple molecules that participate in the passage of a signal from a ligand-occupied receptor to nuclear transcription factors. Not all of the molecular components of the MAPK cascade have been examined in HCC.

IRS-1 transfers phosphotyrosine signals from ligand-occupied INSR (and possibly some other tyrosine kinase receptors) to downstream molecules. The IRS-1 gene was overexpressed by more than twofold in 9 (41%) of 22 HCCs[127,165] and IRS-1 protein was more highly expressed in five HCCs than in the adjacent nontumorous liver tissue.[127,166]

Expression of ras p21 protein was detected by immunohistochemistry in 130 (49%) of 265 HCCs, and tumor cells appeared to be more intensely stained in most studies than did adjacent nontumorous hepatocytes.[34,167–171] Only a few studies have examined expression of specific ras mRNAs, and most of these used relatively insensitive blotting methods that yielded variable results. However, overexpression of transcripts for H-ras and N-ras was reported in studies that included fewer than 12 HCCs each.[34,172–175]

Activating mutations in codons 12, 13, and 61 of the H-*ras*, K-*ras*, and N-*ras* genes were sought in 24 to 141 HCCs. Codon 12 of the H-*ras* gene was mutated in 3 (2.1%) of 141 HCCs;[176–181] of the K-*ras* gene, in 2 (2.3%) of 86 HCCs;[178,179,181–184] and of the N-*ras* gene, in none of 43 HCCs.[178,179,181] Mutations involving codon 13 were not detected in any *ras* gene (H-, K-, or N-*ras*) in 24 HCCs.[178,181] Codon 61 of the H-*ras* gene contained no mutations in 56 HCCs,[178–181] whereas the K-*ras* gene was mutated at this locus in 1 (2%) of 50 HCCs,[178,179,181,184] and codon 61 of the N-*ras* gene was mutated in 4 (5.4%) of 74 HCCs.[175,176,178,179] These results indicate that *ras* gene mutations do not play a prominent role in activating the MAPK pathway in human HCC. Instead, the available data suggest that upregulation of the MAPK pathway in HCC is mainly driven by the binding of mitogenic growth factors to their cognate receptors.

The mitogen-activated kinases (MEK1, 2) and the extracellular signal-regulated kinases (ERK1, 2) are located farther downstream in the MAPK pathway. As evaluated by immunoblotting of electrophoretically separated proteins, MEK1 located in the particulate fraction was increased by more than fourfold and MEK2 was increased by more than threefold in five HCCs as compared with adjacent nontumor tissue.[185] A MEK kinase (MEKK-3) also was found to be strongly up-regulated in two HCCs in a parallel hybridization analysis of protein kinase genes.[100] In another study, particulate fraction ERK1 was increased by more than fivefold; ERK1 in the soluble fraction, by nearly sevenfold; and soluble ERK2, by threefold in five HCCs.[185] In addition, the ability of ERK2 from particulate and cytosolic fractions of HCC to phosphorylate myelin basic protein was increased by three- to sixfold.[185] These results on ERK2 were confirmed in a larger study, which showed that ERK2 was significantly up-regulated in 15 (58%) of 26 HCCs compared with the activity in adjacent nontumorous tissue, and in 17 (65%) of 26 HCCs compared with healthy liver tissue.[185]

ERK1 and ERK2 were localized by immunohistochemistry to nuclei of tumor cells, and their activities were significantly correlated with the extent of expression of the nuclear transcription factor c-fos and with the cell cycle regulatory molecule, cyclin D1[186] (see below). These findings indicate that the increased activity of the MAPK pathway is directly correlated with the activation of common nuclear transcription factors (c-myc, c-fos, c-jun) and with the molecular changes that allow increased cell cycling.

The tyrosine kinase activity of src p60 protein was augmented by two- to fivefold in 20 HCCs, compared with that in the adjacent liver tissue, further supporting the amplification of activity of the MAPK pathway in HCC.[187] Significantly higher activity of src protein kinase was found in 5 poorly differentiated HCC tumors, compared with 15 moderately differentiated and 5 well-differentiated tumors, a finding suggesting that protein kinase activity continued to increase with the progression of HCC.[187]

### G protein pathway

The heterotrimeric G proteins transmit a signal from adrenergic receptors (for example) to the downstream effectors adenyl cyclase/cyclic adenosine monophosphate. The $G_{\alpha i}$ class of proteins was generally up-regulated in six HCCs as compared with adjacent liver tissue.[188] $G_{\alpha i1}$ was increased by threefold in five of six HCCs and was unchanged in one; $G_{\alpha i1-2}$ was increased by twofold in four of six HCC tumors and was unchanged in two; $G_{\alpha i3}$ was increased in four of six HCCs by less than twofold and decreased in two of six by about 4%.[188] The $G_{\alpha i}$ proteins showed a fourfold increase in functional activity in four of six HCCs, as demonstrated by pertussis toxin–catalyzed ADP-dependent phosphorylation, and the level was not changed in two.[188] The $G_{\alpha s}$ proteins were decreased by 70% in all six HCC tumors, and their functional activity was also decreased, as indicated by threefold impairment in stimulation of adenyl cyclase by forskolin.[188]

### Nuclear transcription factors

Among nuclear transcription factors, c-myc has been investigated the most thoroughly in HCC. Increased expression of myc p62 protein was detected in 61 (56%) of 109 HCCs by immunohistochemistry and immunoblot of extracted protein,[169–171,189–192] in some instances exceeding the level in adjacent liver tissue by 15-fold. Increased expression of myc protein was more common in moderately and poorly differentiated tumors than in well-differentiated tumors.[191,192] Expression of c-myc mRNA was detected in 91 (94%) of 97 HCCs at relative levels of three- to more than fivefold compared with that in adjacent liver tissue.[172–175,191,192]

In addition to increased activity of the MAPK pathway, several other mechanisms are responsible for the up-regulation of the c-myc gene in HCC, including hypomethylation of the c-myc promoter and gene amplification.[193,194] Substantial hypomethylation of the c-myc gene was found in 15 (56%) of 27 HCCs[193,194] involving most heavily the third exon.[194] Amplification of the c-myc gene was detected in 50 (31%) of 163 HCCs[168,195–198] and was associated more frequently with high tumor cell proliferation, p53 overexpression, large tumors, poorly differentiated tumors, and poor prognosis.[197,198]

The N-myc gene was amplified and rearranged in 2 (20%) of 10 HCCs.[175] A polymorphism of the L-myc gene that eliminates the SS genotype was associated with a nearly ninefold increase in susceptibility to HCC.[199]

In a small number of studies, the patterns of expression[186,189] and methylation[200] of the c-fos and c-jun genes in HCC appeared to mirror those of c-myc. Expression of c-fos protein (by immunoblot) was increased in 12 (26%) of 46 HCCs[186] whereas expression of c-jun was increased in 13 (50%) of 26 HCCs.[186]

### Transforming growth factor β signaling pathway

Occupancy of TGF-β RI/RII heterodimers by TGF-β activates a series of signaling molecules termed Smads (mothers against decapentaplegic homolog), to stimulate expression of various genes. No allelic losses of the Smad2 gene were identified in 35 HCCs,[201] and only 1 (1.5%) contained a mutation of the gene among 65 HCCs.[123,201,202] Loss of heterozygosity of the Smad4 gene was detected in 8 (15%) of 54 HCCs,[202,203] and 2 (3%) with mutations were found among 73 HCCs.[123,201,203] These findings suggest the possibility that Smad4 functions as a tumor suppressor in a fraction of HCCs. The Smad6 and Smad7 molecules regulate transcriptional activity of complexes of Smad2/Smad4, possibly by controlling entry of transcriptionally active complexes into nuclei. Smad2 protein was detected in the nuclei of HCC cells (by immunohistochemistry), but was found only in the cytoplasm in hepatocytes of adjacent nontumorous liver tissue.[204] Expression of Smad6 and Smad7 mRNAs was down-regulated in HCC in association with localization of Smad2 protein in HCC nuclei.[204] These results were interpreted to suggest that down-regulation of Smad6 and Smad7 genes in HCC resulted in conversion of TGF-β from a growth inhibitor to a growth stimulator of hepatocytes.[204]

## Cell Cycle Regulatory Molecules

Transit through the cell cycle is regulated by the actions of several proteins—cyclins, cyclin-dependent kinases, and cyclin kinase inhibitors. Cyclin and cyclin-dependent kinases form active complexes that can phosphorylate appropriate substrates, which in the case of the G1 cyclins (cyclins D, E, and A) is the RB protein. The cyclin kinase inhibitors (only p16[INK4A], p21[WAF1/CIP1], p27[KIP1], and p57[KIP2] have been studied in HCC) regulate the phosphorylating activity of cyclin/cyclin-kinase complexes by binding to them. Expression of cyclins is regulated by c-myc, together with other transcription factors and other regulatory molecules. Expression of p21[WAF1/CIP1] is partially regulated by p53, whereas p27[KIP1] responds to TGF-β. The major G1 cyclins and their cyclin-kinase inhibitors have been studied in HCC, but the cyclin kinases have not been examined yet.

### Cyclin D1

Cyclin D1 protein was overexpressed (by immunohistochemistry) in 70 (44%) of 158 HCCs,[186,205,206] and increased expression was significantly associated with early recurrence after resection.[205] The cyclin D1 gene was amplified by 3- to 20-fold (by Southern blot) in 12 (12%) of 100 HCCs.[186,206,207] In HCC containing an amplified cyclin D1 gene, mRNA was up-regulated in each of 5 HCCs examined,[207] and protein was overexpressed in 20 (69%) of 29 HCCs.[206,207] The cyclin D1 gene and the *int-2* gene, which are located nearby on chromosome 11q13, were simultaneously amplified in 7 (8%) of 91 HCCs.[208] Expression of the cyclin D1 gene was not altered in liver tissue adjacent to HCC.[206] Up-regulation of the cyclin D1 gene was detected in only 4 (6%) of 71 HCCs in another study,[209] in coordination with strong up-regulation of the cyclin E gene in the same tumors (see below).

Cyclin D1 antibodies were not found in the sera of any of 100 HCC patients.[210]

## Cyclin E

Expression of the cyclin D1 and E genes in HCC appears to be correlated. In studies in which both cyclins were examined in the same group of HCC, cyclin D1 mRNA (by RT-PCR) was overexpressed in only 4 (6%) of 71 HCCs, whereas cyclin E expression was increased and cyclin D1 expression was simultaneously down-regulated in 29 (41%) of 71 HCCs.[209] This observation may reflect the fact that cyclins D and E are normally expressed sequentially and interact through feedback mechanisms that involve cyclin kinase inhibitors. It seems possible that overexpression of either or both D1 and E cyclins may be a feature of aberrant cell cycle regulation in HCC. However, most studies have not evaluated more than one cyclin in the same group of HCC.

Overexpression of the cyclin E gene was detected in 77 (44%) of 175 HCCs and in adjacent tissue in 5 (7%) of 71 livers.[209] Concordance of mRNA (by RT-PCR) and protein expression (by immunohistochemistry) was over 90%.[209] Up-regulation of the cyclin E gene was significantly associated with mutation of the *p53* gene (detected in 25 [35%] of 71 HCC), as well as with poor differentiation, large size, and local invasion of tumors and poor 4-year survival.[209]

Antibodies to cyclin E were not detected in the sera of any of 100 patients with HCC.[210]

## Cyclin A

Cyclin A mRNA was overexpressed (by slot blot) in 18 (42%) of 43 HCCs,[211] and protein expression was increased (by immunoblot) in 12 (39%) of 31 HCCs.[212] Increased cyclin A protein was associated with gene amplification (by Southern blot) in 6 (50%) of 12 HCCs.[212] The cyclin A–associated protein, Skp2, was overexpressed in 17 (55%) of 31 HCCs and it was increased concurrently with cyclin A in 11 (65%) of 17 tumors.[212] Expression of cyclin A was positively correlated with the fraction of tumor cells in S/G$_2$ phases of the cell cycle and negatively with the length of patient survival.[212]

Hepatitis B virus genomic DNA was integrated into the cyclin A gene in one HCC associated with gene truncation and the production of a cyclin A-HBV fusion protein.[213,214] Truncation of the cyclin A gene by HBV genomic integration led to the deletion of the N-terminus of the cyclin A protein containing the degradation signal, which was replaced by the HBV preS/S promoter and some downstream sequences.[214] The resulting fusion protein was highly expressed and resisted degradation. This HBV genomic insertion into the cyclin A gene appears to have been an uncommon event, rarely found in HCC generally. Loss of heterozygosity of the cyclin A gene on chromosome 4q27 was detected in 1 (5%) of 20 unselected HCCs.[215]

Antibodies to cyclin A protein were detected in the sera of 1 of 100 patients with HCC.[210]

## Cyclin B

Cyclin B1 expression apparently has been evaluated in only one HCC, in which it was not overexpressed.[216] However, aberrant expression of cyclin B1 may be an important feature of HCC because antibodies to the protein were detected in the sera of 15 (15%) of 100 patients with HCC.[210]

## Cyclin kinase inhibitor p16$^{INK4A}$

The p16$^{INK4A}$ protein was reduced or absent (by immunohistochemistry or immunoblot) in 53 (52%) of 101 HCCs.[217,218] Expression of mRNA was detected by RT-PCR in all 22 HCC tumors examined, and mRNA was detected even when protein was not expressed.[217] Reduction and extinction of p16$^{INK4A}$ protein expression were associated with gene hypermethylation in 95 (51%) of 185 HCCs.[219–223] Protein expression was totally suppressed when more than 65% of the available sites were methylated, and lesser degrees of methylation were associated with reduced expression.[219] Reduced or no expression of p16$^{INK4A}$ correlated inversely with tumor grade and was observed most often in poorly differentiated HCC.[217,219] Hypermethylation of the *p16$^{INK4A}$* gene in HCC was associated with the presence of methylated p16$^{INK4A}$ DNA in the sera of 13 (81%) of 16 patients.[223]

Various structural aberrations have also been detected in the *p16$^{INK4A}$* gene in HCC. Intragenic somatic mutations were detected in 15 (5%) of 312 HCCs,[217–222,224–227] and homozygous deletions were found in 32 (10%) of 315 tumors.[217–219,221,222,224–228] Loss of heterozygosity on chromosome 9p21 in the vicinity of the *p16$^{INK4A}$* gene locus was detected in 67 (37%) of 183 HCCs,[218,220,222,224,226,227] and microsatellite instability (MSI) was found in 4 of 17 (24%).[227] Germline mutation of the *p16$^{INK4A}$* gene was identified in 4 (15%) of 26 patients with HCC with somatic loss of the remaining allele in two of the four patients with germline mutation and HCC.[220] Hepatocellular carcinoma associated with germline mutation of the *p16$^{INK4A}$* gene occurred at a relatively early age, and in one situation this mutation was found in a mother and son, suggesting familial susceptibility.[220]

In contrast to the results of the studies discussed above, low levels of p16$^{INK4A}$ were detected by immunohistochemistry in both 104 HCCs and 99 adjacent nontumorous liver tissues.[201] The protein was predominantly localized to nuclei, and HCC contained a larger fraction of stained nuclei than did adjacent liver tissue.[205] It is difficult to interpret these results in relation to those of the other reported studies. The differences may reflect variations in methods and reagents.

The p19$^{ARF}$ transcript, an alternate transcript from the *p16$^{INK4A}$* gene, was not homozygously deleted in 15 HCCs.[228]

## Cyclin kinase inhibitor p21$^{WAF1/CIP1}$

Reduced expression of p21$^{WAF1/CIP1}$ mRNA (by RT-PCR) was found in 23 (58%) of 40 HCCs, compared with that found in adjacent liver tissue.[229,230] Expression of p21$^{WAF1/CIP1}$ protein was detected in the cell nuclei of 151 (75%) of 201 HCCs and in all adjacent liver tissues, but only 3%–6% of nuclei were stained in both settings.[205,231] In a group of 97 HCCs, p21$^{WAF1/CIP1}$ mRNA expression in individual tumors at levels greater than the median level for the group correlated with fewer tumor nodules, but not with tumor size or grade.[231]

Correlation between *p53* mutation and p21$^{WAF1/CIP1}$ expression was not perfect. Coordinate expression of p21$^{WAF1/CIP1}$ and p53 proteins (by immunohistochemistry) was detected in 28

(29%) of 97 HCCs, whereas p53 was expressed in the absence of p21[WAF1/CIP1] in 20 (21%) of 97 HCCs, and p21[WAF1/CIP1] was expressed in the absence of p53 in 35 (36%) of 97 HCCs.[231] The relative level of p21[WAF1/CIP1] mRNA was significantly decreased in 4 (67%) of 6 HCCs that contained a mutated *p53* gene, as compared with 5 (25%) of 20 HCCs with wild-type *p53*. No differences were detected in the expression of p21[WAF1/CIP1] between HCC and adjacent liver tissues that each contained wild-type p53. Low levels of p21[WAF1/CIP1] mRNA were detected in 5 (24%) of 21 HCCs containing a mutated *p53* gene, but 3 (14%) of 21 HCCs with a wild-type *p53* gene also expressed low levels of p21[WAF1/CIP1] mRNA.[230] Reduced expression of p21[WAF1/CIP1] mRNA was detected in 12 (63%) of 19 HCCs, although only one tumor had a mutated *p53* gene. A second HCC in this group contained a mutation in the *p21[WAF1/CIP1]* gene itself, which suggests that mutation is another mechanism by which *p21[WAF1/CIP1]* gene expression is reduced.[229] Supporting this opinion is the finding that among three HCCs in which *p21[WAF1/CIP1]* expression was reduced, one contained a mutated gene and another contained a gene that was rearranged.[232] These results suggest that mutations in both the *p53* gene and the *p21[WAF1/CIP1]* gene may be responsible for decreased expression of p21[WAF1/CIP1] protein, but the relative frequency of each mechanism, or whether other mechanisms exist, is not yet clear.

### Cyclin kinase inhibitor p27[KIP1]

Transcripts of the *p27[KIP1]* gene were significantly reduced (by RT-PCR ratio to β-actin mRNA) in 21 HCCs.[233] Expression of mRNA was significantly reduced in 11 (52%) of 21 HCC, but the level of expression was not correlated with HCC size or differentiation grade.[233] In a study of 104 HCCs and 90 adjacent tissues, p27[KIP1] protein was increased (by immunoblot) in tumors but not in nontumorous liver tissue.[205] The p27[WAF1/CIP1] protein was localized (by immunohistochemistry) to cell nuclei in both tissues.[205] Expression of p27[KIP1] in more than 50% of HCC nuclei was correlated with longer disease-free survival following surgical resection, whereas staining of smaller fractions of tumor cell nuclei was correlated with large size, poor differentiation, and portal vein invasion of HCC.[205] These results suggest that relatively small changes in the expression of p27[KIP1] may affect HCC growth.

The mechanisms that regulate the expression of p27[KIP1] in HCC apparently have not been examined. In particular, studies of the role of TGF-β in the regulation of p27[KIP1] in HCC appear to be lacking at this time.

### Cyclin kinase inhibitor p57[KIP]

The *p57[KIP2]* gene contained neither mutations nor LOH in 17 HCC.[227] Expression of the gene apparently has not been examined in HCC.

## RB and E2F1

RB p110 protein is complexed with E2F1 protein (and other E2F proteins) in nonproliferating cells. Cells pass through the $G_1$ phase of the cell cycle in coordination with the progressive activation of the cyclin/cyclin kinase heteromers, as the regulatory influence of the various cyclin kinase inhibitors is overcome. Each activated cyclin kinase partially phosphorylates the RB protein, culminating with the activated cyclinA/cyclin kinase complex, which completes RB phosphorylation. Full phosphorylation of RB sites disrupts the RB/E2F1 complex, enabling E2F1 (a transcription factor) to enter nuclei and activate the genes required for completion of S phase.

### RB

RB protein was not detected (by immunohistochemistry) in 125 (54%) of 231 HCCs,[205,234–236] whereas overexpression was found in 15 (19%) of 81 HCCs. Loss of RB protein expression correlated closely with LOH of the *RB* gene, which was detected in 10 (48%) of 21 HCCs, all but one of which lacked RB protein expression.[236] Of nine HCCs with both LOH and loss of expression of the *RB* gene, the remaining allele contained small deletions in two (22%).[236] The mechanism for loss of RB protein associated with LOH in the absence of mutation of the residual allele is not clear. Methylation of the promoter region of the *RB* gene was not found in any of 19 HCCs in which RB protein was not expressed.[237]

Overall, LOH of the RB gene has been reported in 55 (34%) of 161 HCCs assessed with locus-specific probes.[203,236,238–244] Multiple microsatellite and restriction fragment length polymorphism (RFLP) probes for loci in the region of chromosome 13q14.3 (the site of the *RB1* gene) detected LOH in 32 (91%) of 35 HCCs.[236,243] In some instances, LOH was coupled with retention of some *RB* gene sequences, which suggests that a breakpoint was located within the *RB* gene.[240] Such interstitial deletions were detected in only 1 (4%) of 25 HCCs,[241] but a combination of homozygous deletion and replication error involved the *RB* gene in 2 (29%) of 7 HCCs.[234]

Lack of expression and/or LOH of the *RB* gene and *p53* mutation often occurred simultaneously in the small number of HCC cases studied. In seven HCCs with a mutated *p53* gene, six (86%) also had LOH of the *RB* gene.[234] Of five HCCs that did not express RB protein, four (80%) also expressed nuclear p53 (by immunohistochemistry),[234] a characteristic of mutated p53 protein.

### E2F1

When released from binding to RB, E2F1 is a nuclear transcription factor. In a study of mutations and deletions of the RB-binding domain of E2F1in 382 cancers, none were found in 24 HCCs.[245] Other E2F proteins apparently have not been examined in HCC.

## p53, mdm2, p73, and p51

Many cellular processes are regulated by p53 protein, including aspects of cell proliferation, apoptosis, and the response of cells to DNA damage. The mdm2 molecule regulates p53 availability by forming inactive complexes of the two molecules. The p73 and p51 molecules bear significant homology with p53 protein and may share common functional properties.

### p53

The overexpression of p53 is indicated by nuclear localization of protein (by immunohistochemistry), which appears to reflect both gene mutation and other causes of p53 protein stabilization (see below). Nuclear localization of p53 protein (by immunohistochemistry) was detected in 343 (31%) of 1109 HCCs.[246–272] The frequency of nuclear staining correlated with the differentiation grade and size of HCC.[257,259,266,270,271]

Sequence analyses of exons 5 to 8 or 9 have detected mutations at various locations in the gene in 541 (27%) of 2034 HCCs.[180,184,209,230,231,238,248–250,299–301,303–308] Mutation of the *p53* gene is significantly associated with poor survival,[264,299] tumor grade,[253,264,276,285,286,295] and size.[295]

Transversion mutation in the third base of codon 249 (G to T) is the most frequent mutation found in the *p53* gene in HCC, having been detected in 192 (8%) of 2324 HCC tumors.[180,184,230,231,238,247–250,253–255,260–265,267–269,273–280,284–288, 290–295,297–299,301–317] The frequency of this specific mutation varies markedly in different geographic regions around the world; for example, four studies, including 90 HCC tumors from patients in North America, Europe, and Australia, detected no mutations at this site,[260,295,310,314] whereas four studies, including 71 HCC tumors from patients in China and southern Africa, detected this specific mutation in 44 (62%).[308,312,316–318] This variation in mutation site appears to reflect varying exposure to dietary aflatoxins.[305] However, it has been difficult to relate *p53* mutations in codon 249 precisely to past exposure to aflatoxins because of the transient nature of many metabolic markers of exposure and the long period between exposure and emergence of HCC.[319] Furthermore, the specific impact of aflatoxin on HCC incidence is difficult to discern because populations in geographic areas with a high dietary burden of aflatoxin also are frequently afflicted by a high incidence of chronic HBV infection of the liver.[319,320] However, application of molecular markers of exposure (including urinary excretion of AFM1 and AFB1-$N^7$-guanine) in cohort studies has produced strong evidence that aflatoxin exposure is an important risk factor for HCC in humans.[321,322] Furthermore, in recent epidemiological studies that have applied the detection and quantification in plasma of DNA containing the codon 249 mutation as a specific molecular marker of aflatoxin exposure, the presence of the mutation has been associated with a greatly increased risk of HCC.[317]

The data on the fraction of HCC that show nuclear staining for p53 protein and the fraction that contain mutations somewhere in the gene indicate that mutation is responsible for many, but not all, of the instances of nuclear staining. Among a group of 84 HCCs containing mutations in exons 5 to 8 or 9, the nuclei in 64 stained for p53 (76%), whereas the nuclei in 20 (24%) did not stain for p53.[259,263,269,298] Nuclei were stained in 14 (27%) of 52 HCCs expressing wild-type p53 and were not stained in 38 (73%).[259,263,269,298] Among 77 HCCs in which nuclei did not stain for p53, the gene was mutated in 12 (16%).[250,259,263,268,269,298] Four (80%) of five HCCs with codon 249 mutations showed nuclear staining.[247,298] Thus the concordance between nuclear staining and *p53* mutation in HCC in separate studies appears to vary between 65% and 85%, indicating that mutation is a major but not sole cause of p53 overexpression and nuclear localization. This conclusion was confirmed by a recent study in which immunohistochemical staining and sequencing of the *p53* gene were performed in the same group of 28 HCCs; 16 (94%) of 17 HCCs in which the *p53* gene was mutated showed intense nuclear staining, but so did 3 (27%) of 11 HCCs that contained wild-type p53.[323] Several other mechanisms may stabilize p53 protein sufficiently to allow it to accumulate in HCC cells. Plausible alternate mechanisms include sequestration of p53 by binding to overexpressed or mutated mdm2, its regulatory partner, and by complexing with viral proteins such as the HBV X protein (see below).

Loss of heterozygosity of the *p53* gene has been detected in 364 (42%) of 871 informative HCC tumors.[180,203,238,240–242,247, 254,267,273,277,283–286,288–290,294,304,308 ,309,316,317,323–332] The frequency of *p53* LOH correlates with increasing HCC grade[286] and size.[327]

Antibodies to p53 protein have been detected in the sera of 73 (15%) of 502 patients with HCC[268,298,333–336] but not in the sera of 107 patients with non-neoplastic liver diseases.[333,336] Presence of serum antibody was a moderately specific but not very sensitive indicator of p53 overexpression in HCC: 10 (53%) of 19 patients whose HCC overexpressed p53 protein had antibody, whereas 4 (21%) of 19 patients with HCC that did not overexpress p53 also had serum antibody.[298,336] The presence of anti-p53 antibody in the serum seemed to reflect the extent of nuclear accumulation of p53 protein,[336] but it did not correlate with patient survival.[335,336]

## mdm2

Mouse double minute (mdm)2 protein binds to and inactivates p53. In a study of the *mdm2* gene in several types of cancer, two HCCs expressed low levels of mdm2 mRNA and protein, and both also weakly expressed p53 protein.[337] In each HCC, the *mdm2* gene contained a mutation that produced a stop codon and resulted in a truncated protein that reacted weakly with antibody.[337] The effect of the mutations on the binding affinity of mdm2 and p53 proteins was apparently not investigated, and the relation of these *mdm2* mutations to p53 expression is not certain.

The level of mdm2 mRNA (byRT-PCR) normalized to β-actin mRNA was significantly higher in 42 HCCs than in the adjacent liver tissues, and the elevated level correlated with the local invasiveness, but not the size, of HCC.[302] In 23 HCCs without *p53* mutation, mdm2 expression was significantly higher than in 18 HCCs that expressed mutated *p53*.[302] Among 10 HCCs that expressed mdm2 mRNA at levels greater than the median level for the entire group, only 1 HCC (10%) contained a mutated *p53* gene, whereas among the 32 HCCs that expressed mdm2 transcripts at levels below the median level for the group, 17 (55%) contained a mutated *p53* gene.[302] Furthermore, the expression of the *mdm2* gene was significantly higher in 13 HCCs that recurred or metastasized within 1 year after surgical resection than in 19 HCCs that did not recur or metastasize within a year.[302] These results suggest that overexpression of mdm2 may be an important mechanism for suppressing *p53* gene function in HCC.

## p73

Loss of heterozygosity of the *p73* gene, located on chromosome 1p36.3, was detected in 5 (20%) of 25 informative HCCs.[338] Nevertheless, p73 mRNA was overexpressed in 25 (34%) of 74 HCCs and p73 protein was overexpressed in 61 (32%) of 193 HCCs.[339] In this study, no correlation was found between the expression of *p73* and *p53* genes in HCC.[339] In a study of 35 HCC, p73 expression was detected in three HCCs (9%) even in the face of LOH on chromosome 1p36.3,[340] a deletion that should have included one allele of the *p73* gene. Loss of heterozygosity of chromosome 1p36 affected 10 (22%) of 45 HCCs, and both α and β p73 transcripts were expressed in 8 (33%) of 24 HCCs, but not in normal liver tissue.[340] Expression of the *p73* gene was detected in 6 (40%) of 15 HCCs that contained LOH of the *p53* locus.[340]

## p51

No mutations were detected in the *p51* gene by PCR–single-strand conformational polymorphism (SSCP) in 54 HCCs,[341] which suggests that this gene is not often involved in HCC. Loss of heterozygosity of this gene apparently has not been studied in HCC.

It seems unlikely that the *p73* gene functions as a conventional tumor suppressor gene. Whether either the *p73* or *p51* genes can partly compensate for *p53* loss in HCC is not clear. One study found no relationship between expression of *p73* and *p53* genes in HCC, whereas another detected a possible association between *p73* expression and *p53* LOH.

## The Wingless Signal Pathway

The Wingless (Wnt) signal cascade includes the frizzled receptor, the adenomatous polyposis coli (APC) protein, axin, β-catenin, and E-cadherin, among other components. Axin, APC, and E-cadherin control the availability of β-catenin, largely by sequestering the latter in protein–protein complexes or by facilitating its breakdown. β-Catenin participates with E-cadherin and other proteins in the formation of intercellular adhesion junctions, and free β-catenin migrates to the cell nucleus where it activates the Tcf1 transcription factor, driving cell proliferation. Molecular components of this important signaling pathway are involved in both the regulation of cell proliferation and the maintenance of cell–cell adhesion and cell differentiation.

### APC

Loss of heterozygosity of the *APC* locus was detected in 8 (6%) of 128 informative HCCs.[203,242,331,342–345] No mutations of the *APC* gene were found in 69 unselected HCCs or in 30 HCCs selected because they lacked mutations of the β-catenin gene.[345] These results suggest that the *APC* gene does not function as a tumor suppressor in HCC.

### Axin

Mutations in the *axin1* gene were detected in 5 (6%) of 87 HCCs that lacked mutations in the β-catenin gene.[346] All of the mutations yielded a truncated protein lacking the β-catenin binding site. Mutations in the axin gene were associated with nuclear accumulation of β-catenin.[346]

### β-Catenin

Expression of β-catenin was increased (by immunohistochemistry) in 85 (57%) of 149 HCCs.[347–349] Overexpression of β-catenin was common in HCC of all grades, but it was highest in the well-differentiated tumors, decreasing in those that were poorly differentiated.[347] Mutations and small deletions in exon 3 (which includes the glycogen synthase kinase-3β phosphorylation site that is responsible for triggering the breakdown of β-catenin), were detected in 85 (21%) of 415 HCCs.[345,346,348–352] Mutations were associated with the nuclear accumulation of β-catenin, which was correlated with elevated cell proliferation,[348,349] but not with HCC grade or size.[345]

### E-Cadherin

E-cadherin is normally expressed by hepatocytes, and expression was detected by immunohistochemistry in 113 (80%) of 142 HCCs.[353–357] Reduced or extinguished expression of E-cadherin occurred in poorly differentiated HCC[346,353–356,358] and was correlated with tumor invasion and rapid recurrence following surgical resection.[357] E-cadherin transcripts were markedly reduced in three HCCs that lacked expression of protein.[357] Reduced or extinguished expression was associated with methylation of the E-cadherin promoter and frequent LOH on chromosome 16q near the site of the gene.[356,359] Loss of heterozygosity near the E-cadherin locus was detected in 18 (64%) of 28 HCC,[360] and the nearby haptoglobin gene also contained LOH in more than 90%.[361]

These results indicate that aberrations in the molecular components of the Wnt signaling pathway play important roles in the pathogenesis of HCC.

## Other Tumor-Associated Genes

Several genes that are involved in neoplasms of other tissues have also been studied in a few HCCs, and some (as well as other genes not yet examined) may have important roles in HCC.

### FHIT

The fragile histidine triad (*FHIT*) gene, located on chromosome 3p14.2, is the most frequently abnormal locus in the human genome, and it is a translocation breakpoint in several neoplasms. Altered *FHIT* gene transcripts often are found in HCC: aberrant transcripts lacking several exons (4–5, 4–6, 5–6, 5–7, 5–8, and/or 8) and producing truncated transcripts were found in 32 (57%) of 56 HCCs,[362–364] and FHIT protein was lacking in 5 (50%) of 10 HCCs.[365] Loss of heterozygosity of the *FHIT* gene was detected in 3 (11%) of 28 HCC[364] and either MSI or LOH was found in 10 (29%) of 34 HCCs.[365]

Whether *FHIT* aberrations are specifically associated with HCC has been debated because of the frequency with which aberrations of the gene are found in nondiseased and non-neoplastic liver tissue.[362–364,366] However, the *FHIT* gene appears to be abnormal more frequently in HCC than in adjacent nontumorous liver tissue; in particular, the extent of exonic deletion and transcript truncation seems to be greater in HCC.[362–365] Furthermore, FHIT protein expression was lacking in 5 (50%) of 10 HCC, whereas the protein was expressed in adjacent nontumorous tissue.[365] These data suggest that aberrations in the *FHIT* gene may play an important role in the development and expression of HCC. The FRA3B locus containing the *FHIT* gene is the site in the human genome most sensitive to the effects of exogenous mutagens. As a result, the frequent presence of aberrations in nontumorous liver tissue may simply reflect the actions of the numerous mutagens/carcinogens to which all humans are exposed. Such alterations in the *FHIT* gene in non-neoplastic liver tissue may represent alterations in the hepatocyte genome that are potentially preneoplastic and that eventuate in HCC in some individuals.

### PTEN/MMAC1

The phosphatase and tensin homolog/mutated in many advanced cancers (*PTEN/MMAC1*) gene, located on chromosome 10q23, showed LOH in 29 (25%) of 115 HCCs and the remaining allele was mutated in 6 (16%) of the 37 HCCs that contained LOH.[367,368] These results suggest that the *PTEN/MMAC1* gene is a tumor suppressor gene in human hepatocytes and that it is involved in a significant fraction of HCC. In another study of 96 HCCs, which were not selected because they contained LOH of the *PTEN/MMAC1* gene, the gene was mutated in only 3 (3%),[369] a finding suggesting that mutation of the gene is of little importance in hepatocarcinogenesis in the absence of associated LOH.

### nm23-H1, H2

Loss of heterozygosity of the nonmetastatic *(nm)23* gene on chromosome 17q21.3 was detected in 4 (18%) of 22 informative HCCs.[203] The protein expressed by the *nm23* gene is homologous to the enzyme nucleoside diphosphate kinase.[370] Among 42 HCCs, this protein was expressed (by immunohistochemistry) less intensively in HCC that had metastasized at the time of study than in tumors that had not metastasized.[370,371] In another study of 25 HCCs, immunohistochemical expression of nm23 protein was detected in 15 (60%) or 17 (68%), depending on the antibody used, and survival was higher in patients whose tumors stained, even though expression of the gene was not correlated with HCC size, grade, or vessel invasion.[372] In this study, 7 (70%) of 10 intrahepatic satellite tumor nodules did not stain,[372] which suggests that lack of expression was associated with the local spread of HCC within the liver. Expression of nm23-H1 mRNA (but not of H2) also correlated inversely with the frequency of intrahepatic metastases, but not with tumor grade.[373] Among 17 patients with single cirrhosis-associated HCC nodules in the liver that were surgically resected, 8 (80%) of 10 patients whose nodules expressed nm23 mRNA at levels three- to fivefold higher than the adjacent liver tissue were recurrence-free after 30 months.[374] In contrast, only one (14%) of seven patients whose HCC expressed nm23 mRNA at or below the level of adjacent nontumorous liver tissue was recurrence-free 30 months after resection.[374]

These results suggest that the expression of nm23-H1 is related to intrahepatic spread and extrahepatic metastasis of HCC. However, the findings of another study of 27 HCCs cast doubt on such a relationship: included in this group of HCC were 13 that occurred as single intrahepatic nodules—seven that had intrahepatic satellite nodules, and seven that were associated with extrahepatic metastasis.[375] Many of the HCC that were located within the liver overexpressed nm23 protein, and no differences were found between the main tumor and satellite nodules. Furthermore, among extrahepatic metastases, only one of seven expressed nm23 weakly, but no more weakly than did the primary tumor.[375]

### KAI1

Reduced expression of the Kangai (KAI)1 gene, which codes an integral membrane glycoprotein of the TM4 family, is associated with metastasis of some tumors. The KAI1 gene was downregulated by 2.6-fold in 39 HCCs as compared with 10 nondiseased livers.[376] Expression of KAI1 mRNA was significantly reduced or lacking entirely in 36 metastatic HCC tumors.[376]

### Tg737

The Tg737 gene is homologous to a gene that regulates proliferation and sporulation in fission yeast. A similar gene was defective in rodent HCC. Tumor-specific deletions in either exons 3, 5, 14, or 22 were detected in 4 (36%) of 11 HCCs.[377] However, another study of 23 HCCs in humans failed to identify deletions or rearrangements of the Tg737 gene in any tumors,[378] casting doubt on its role in human HCC.

### HIP/PAP

Transcription of the Huntingtin interactive protein/pancreatitis associated protein (HIP/PAP) gene, which expresses a protein with significant homology to human pancreatic stone protein/pancreatic thread/regenerating islet-derived proteins, was upregulated in seven (24%) of 29 HCC.[379] The protein, which binds efficiently to collagens I and IV or to heparan sulfate, was expressed (by immunohistochemistry) in 10% to 50% of the cells of five HCCs, and it was expressed most strongly in tumor cells forming pseudoglands.[380]

### MAG

The malignancy-associated gene (MAG) is a largely uncharacterized gene that has a short sequence homologous to a sequence in the c-met gene and a longer sequence homologous to sequences in the ERCC2 gene cluster. MAG was expressed in 8 (80%) of 10 HCC, and in all of 16 cirrhotic livers but in none of 4 normal livers.[381] This gene has not been studied intensively, and the implications of its expression in HCC and cirrhosis are unknown.

### MAGE/GAGE gene family

MAGE genes code for tumor antigens of the melanoma antigen group, and the related GAGE genes code for antigens of the T cell–antigen group. Both MAGE and GAGE proteins are highly immunogenic. The MAGE family contains at least 12 genes, MAGE-1 through MAGE-12. MAGE-1 protein was expressed (by immunohistochemistry) in 43 (66%) of 65 HCCs and in 5 (8%) of 65 adjacent liver tissues.[382,383] MAGE-1 protein was also detected (by immunoblot) in 12 (85%) of 15 HCCs. MAGE-1 mRNA was expressed (by RT-PCR) in 25 (77%) of 33 HCCs.[84] Expression of the MAGE-1 gene correlated with portal vein invasion but not with tumor grade or stage. MAGE-3 protein was expressed in 8 (53%) of 15 HCCs, and MAGE-3 mRNA was expressed in 14 (42%) of 33 HCCs.[384] Neither MAGE-3 nor MAGE-4 protein expression correlated with HCC grade or stage.[384] In a study in which expression of all of the MAGE genes was evaluated by PCR in 22 HCCs, MAGE-1 and MAGE-3 mRNAs were expressed in about 68%; MAGE-8, in 46%; and the other MAGE genes, in about 30% each.[385] MAGE-4 proteins were significantly increased in the sera of patients with HCV-related HCC: sera of 45 patients with HCV-related HCC contained 2.2 ± 2.7 ng/ml, as compared with 0.39 ± 0.33 ng/ml in the sera of 92 controls.[386] These data suggest that HCV-positive patients with HCC may express higher levels of MAGE proteins. GAGE-1 and -2 mRNAs were also detected by PCR in 6 of 10 HCCs, but not in any of 10 nondiseased livers.[363]

### BRCA2

Mutations in the breast cancer (BRCA)2 gene were detected in 3 (5%) of 60 HCCs by sequencing the entire gene.[387]

### Various tumor suppressor genes

Loss of heterozygosity of the BRCA1 gene was detected in 3 (12%) of 26 HCCs, of the extoses (EXT)1 gene, in 5 (20%) of 25 HCCs, of the Von Hippel–Lindau (VHL) gene, in 2 (8%) of 24 HCCs; and of the Wilms tumor (WT)-1 gene, in 1 (5%) of 22 HCCs.[203] Loss of heterozygosity of the deleted in colorectal cancer (DCC) gene was found in 5 (8%) of 66 HCCs.[203,331]

## Apoptotic Pathways

Apoptotic signals, which lead to cell death, are stimulated by several mechanisms, some entirely intrinsic to the cell and others energized by extracellular molecules. Apoptosis can be activated by p53 or c-myc, acting within a cell, and by the binding of extracellular ligands to receptors on cell surfaces. Receptor/ligand combinations that may stimulate apoptosis include TGF-β/TGF-β RI, RII; TNF-α/TNFR-1; and FasL/Fas (also termed CD95 and APO-1). Generation of apoptosis involves complex signaling pathways comprised of multiple interacting molecules. Among the molecules in the death signaling pathways, only those of the Bcl-2 class have been examined in HCC.

### Bcl-2 and Bcl-X

B-cell lymphoma (Bcl)-2 and Bcl-X genes modulate apoptosis. Bcl-2 is not expressed strongly in normal liver, and it was detected focally in only 8 (7%) of 107 HCCs.[105,387–389] Bcl-$X_L$ and Bcl-$X_S$ proteins, which appear to be predominantly expressed in liver, apparently have not been evaluated in HCC.

## Fas and FasL

Fas (or CD95), a member of the tumor necrosis factor receptor (TNFR) super family, is a receptor for Fas ligand (FasL). Normal hepatocytes express Fas only weakly by immunohistochemistry,[390,391] but expression was readily detected on the majority of hepatocytes in five normal livers using a more sensitive in situ hybridization technique.[392] Fas receptor was strongly upregulated in chronic hepatitis and cirrhosis.[390-396] In contrast, Fas was markedly down-regulated in 42 (64%) of 66 HCCs,[393,394] in which expression was limited to about 6% of neoplastic hepatocytes,[395] and it was totally extinguished in 23 (35%) of 66 HCCs.[393,394] These observations were confirmed by RNase protection assay in six HCCs, in which Fas transcripts were reduced compared with adjacent liver tissue.[396]

Acquisition by neoplastic hepatocytes of the ability to express FasL was detected in 26 (39%) of 66 HCCs (by in situ hybridization or immunohistochemistry).[393,394] FasL-expressing tumor cells killed cytotoxic T lymphocytes on contact in vitro.[393] Fas-negative HCC were associated with more frequent intrahepatic spread and shorter disease-free survival after surgical resection.[394] Patients whose HCC were FasL negative also had reduced survival after surgical removal of the primary tumor.[394]

In other studies, expression of both Fas and FasL was detected in 41 HCCs, as well as in adjacent nontumorous liver tissue.[395,396] However, the methods used in these studies could not clearly distinguish expression by normal and neoplastic hepatocytes from that by infiltrating T lymphocytes.

Truncated Fas molecules lacking membrane-anchoring sequences (soluble Fas, or sFas) were detected at higher levels in the sera of patients with HCC or cirrhosis than in healthy patients.[394,397] The serum level of sFas (by ELISA) in 61 patients with HCC ranged from 0.21 to 29.2 ng/ml (mean 4.1) as compared with 0 to 4.9 ng/ml (mean 0.29) in 59 healthy control subjects and 0.24 to 8.4 ng/ml (mean 2.2) in 27 patients with cirrhosis.[397] Significantly higher sFas levels were found in patients who had multiple, as compared with single, intrahepatic nodules of HCC, and surgical removal of single tumor nodules was followed by rapid decreases in serum sFas.[397] Serum sFas clearly was produced from a truncated gene contained in neoplastic hepatocytes (by RT-PCR) and not by lymphocytes.[394]

CD40, a transmembrane glycoprotein that is homologous to TNFR, but lacks death domains, was detected (by immunohistochemistry) in 27 (60%) of 45 HCC, but not in adjacent liver tissues involved with chronic hepatitis or cirrhosis.[398] CD40 can bind TNF-α and thereby sequester it.

In combination, HCC's loss of Fas expression, acquisition of the capacity to express FasL and CD40, and increased expression of sFas may allow many tumors to escape immune surveillance by cytotoxic T lymphocytes. In addition, high serum levels of TGF-β, which typify HCC patients (see above), also inhibit the immune system. Impaired cellular immunity may have an important role in the growth and spread of HCC.

## Differentiation Molecules

Defective regulation of hepatocyte differentiation appears to be an important element in the development and progression of HCC. Regulation of hepatocyte differentiation is a complex function of multiple factors, including several hormones, growth factors, retinoids, matrix molecules, adjacent hepatocytes, and hepatocyte-intrinsic molecules. Among the latter are the hepato-cyte-enriched transcription factors, hepatocyte nuclear factors (HNF)-1, -3, -4, -6, and CAAT sequence enhancer binding protein (C/EBP) isoforms. Few studies have examined molecular abnormalities in the regulation of hepatocyte differentiation in HCC. In two studies that included 65 HCC, the ratio of HNF-1α to HNF-1β or the level of HNF-1 in tumor cells relative to that in adjacent liver tissue correlated with the HCC differentiation grade.[399,400] A nuclear transcription factor termed HTF was upregulated in HCC by two- to threefold compared with that in normal liver.[401]

## Telomeres and Telomerase

The ends of chromosomes, the telomeres, are composed of repeated $TTAGGG_n$ sequences. Telomeric DNA is not replicated by the cell's DNA synthesis proteins but instead requires a molecular complex containing template RNA, telomerase reverse transcriptase (hTERT), and telomerase-associated protein. The hTERT controls the overall activity of the enzyme complex. Because hepatocytes in normal human livers do not express telomerase, the telomeres shorten by a few hundred kilobases with each replicative cycle. Chromosome ends from which telomeres are completely eroded are "sticky," acting like a double-strand break. Thus, telomere erosion can facilitate the development of chromosome aberrations, and many cells with eroded chromosomes lose the capacity to complete replicative cycles unless they regain the ability to express telomerase. Reexpression of telomerase may relieve the limits on repetitive cycling, allowing affected cells to become immortal. Thus, both telomere erosion and reexpression of telomerase are likely to be important molecular elements in hepatocarcinogenesis.

### Telomere shortening

The lengths of chromosomal telomeres in hepatocytes are reduced considerably during the accelerated cell proliferation that accompanies chronic hepatitis, cirrhosis, and HCC; telomeres measured $8.3 \pm 1.5$ kb in 17 normal livers and $5.3 \pm 2.4$ kb in 73 HCCs.[402-408] These relative telomere lengths were confirmed in a study that measured telomere repeat content by blotting DNA with a radiolabeled d(TTAGGG)$_3$ probe normalized to a d(CCT)$_7$ probe.[409] Telomere lengths remained stable in HCC of different grades, possibly reflecting the reexpression of telomerase.

### Telomerase activity

Telomerase activity (by telomeric repeat amplification [TRAP] assay) was strongly expressed in 143 (90%) of 159 HCCs, as compared with weak expression in 30 (23%) of 128 adjacent nontumorous liver tissues.[402-404,410-415] Expression of hTERT correlated with differentiation grade in 117 HCCs.[401,411-414] Semi-quantitative estimation of telomerase levels (normalized to levels measured in cultured tumor cells) showed that in 56 (92%) of 61 HCC tumors, telomerase activity was significantly increased above the level of activity expressed in adjacent liver tissue.[413,416] Relative telomerase levels in HCC correlated with tumor grade and size,[413] and this was confirmed by assessing expression of telomerase mRNA (normalized to β-actin mRNA).[417] In 23 HCCs, telomerase mRNA was expressed at levels 2 logs greater than that expressed in nondiseased liver and 1 log greater than that in chronic hepatitis or cirrhosis.[417] Expression of high levels of telomerase correlated with rapid recurrence of HCC following surgical resection.[418]

## DNA Mismatch Repair Genes and Microsatellite Instability

Defective DNA mismatch repair is associated with the accumulation of small deletions, frameshifts, base substitutions, and small rearrangements in the microsatellite sequences—repetitive sequences of mono, di-, tri-, and tetranucleotides—located in both coding and noncoding regions of many genes. Mismatch repair deficiency and microsatellite instability (MSI) are associated with increased risk of cancer in affected individuals, as exemplified by hereditary nonpolyposis cancer of the colon.[419] Loss of heterozygosity of the mismatch repair gene, mutS homolog2 (*hMSH2*), was detected in 6 (13%) of 46 HCCs, and the *hMLH1* gene showed LOH in 9 (20%) of 46 HCCs; LOH of both mismatch repair genes occurred in 5 (11%) of 46 HCCs.[331] In a separate study, the *hMSH2* gene was mutated in 7 (18%) of 38 HCCs, but both LOH and mutation do not appear to have been assessed in the same group of HCC.[307] The available data suggest that aberrations in mismatch repair genes are associated with MSI in HCC. At least one of 16 MS loci evinced MSI among 16 (36%) of 46 HCCs, and MSI was significantly greater in the HCC that showed LOH of one or both mismatch repair genes studied.[331] The number of unstable microsatellite loci in nine HCCs that had LOH of *hMSH2* and/or *hMLH1* genes ranged from 0.77 to 2.33 band shifts per microdomain, compared with an average of much less than one band shift per microdomain in the 36 HCCs that lacked LOH of either the *hMSH2* or *hMLH1* genes.[331] Mutation of the *hMSH2* gene or of the *p53* gene also was correlated with MSI in at least one of five microsatellite loci in 8 (62%) of 13 HCCs, compared with 5 (20%) of 25 HCCs that lacked these mutations.[307] Microsatellite instability was significantly associated with shortened disease-free survival following surgical resection of primary lesions.[307]

Microsatellite instability has been evaluated in several studies that have included 449 HCCs. In studies that examined 4 to 29 microsatellite loci, MSI of at least one locus was found in 68 HCCs (15%).[78,79,123,124,304,307,331,420–426] In 12 studies that each examined more than 10 HCCs, the fraction of HCC in each study that showed MSI ranged from 0 to 63%.[78,79,123,124,304,307,331,420–422,424–426] This variation may reflect that only a subset of HCCs are affected by MSI. Two comprehensive allelotype studies of 116 HCCs, which each employed more than 230 microsatellite probes for loci located throughout the genome, found that most HCCs exhibited MSI at a small number of loci.[426,427] In one study, the ratio of unstable loci to the total number of loci examined averaged 0.13 and ranged from 0 to 0.14.[427] The other study found that 12 (5%) of 231 microsatellite loci were unstable in some HCCs and that at least one locus was unstable in 9 (26%) of 34 HCCs.[426] No particular microsatellite loci appear to be unstable with an unusually high frequency. Although numerous microsatellite loci have been assessed for instability, few studies have analyzed the same loci, preventing a detailed analysis of instability at specific loci among a large group of HCCs. Microsatellite instability was detected in the *p53* gene in 11 (19%) of 58 HCCs.[121–123] The *p53* gene contained MSI in 2 (6%) of 34 HCCs that formed solitary hepatic nodules and in 4 (29%) of 14 HCCs that formed multiple intrahepatic nodules.[121] However, *p53* gene LOH did not correlate with LOH of the *hMSH2* and *hMLH1* genes.[121]

Minisatellite loci, which are tandemly repeated noncoding sequences of up to about 100 bp located terminally on chromosomes, are also altered in many HCC. Rearrangements in minisatellite sequences were detected in either 17 or 18 (49% or 51%) of 35 HCCs using two multilocus probes (termed 33.15 and 33.6).[21,428] When single-locus probes derived from the multilocus probes were used, rearrangements were located on chromosome 1p33–p35 in 23% of HCC, on chromosome 7q36–qter in 19%, and on chromosome 12q24.3–qter in 15%.[428]

These observations implicate defects in mismatch repair enzymes and MSI in the development and progression of HCC. Most of the MSI detected in HCC falls into the category of low-frequency MSI (MSI-L, as designated by a recent review panel),[419] but the implication of differences in the frequencies of MSI (MSI-H or MSI-L) in for cancer development is not clear.

Direct evidence of increased mutation frequency in erythrocytes[429] and lymphocytes[430] among patients with HCC raises the possibility that poorly understood constitutional factors may affect their susceptibility to gene mutation and HCC.

## Allelic Losses

Loss of function of both alleles by deletion of one allele, coupled with inactivation of the remaining allele by mutation, hypermethylation, and/or other possible mechanisms, is necessary to abolish the function of tumor suppressor genes. The 39 nonacrocentric arms of the autosomes have been allelotyped fairly densely in several hundred HCCs by means of RFLP and/or microsatellite probes. Four studies have allelotyped more than 270 HCCs with multiple microsatellite probes located about every 20 cM throughout the autosomal genome.[426,427,431,432] Several individual chromosome arms have been allotyped with more locus probes than were used in the studies that comprehensively investigated the autosomal genome (for example, 1p,[332,433] 4p,[434] 4q,[435–437] 5q,[344] 8p,[438–441] 9p,[219,222,226] 11p,[442] 13q,[235,241,243] 16p,[443,444] 16q,[304,435,443,445] 17p,[277,284,304,308,325] and 22q[326]). A few chromosome arms have been examined by microsatellite probes located about every 1 to 2 cM along their lengths.[437,441] In addition, many studies have examined fewer loci for LOH, some examining only one or two often anonymous probes for an entire chromosome arm and a few using probes known to be located in specific genes (for a complete survey of allelic losses, see Grisham[8]). The combined results of these studies yield a fairly comprehensive picture of allelic losses in HCC. Among all HCC that have been examined to date, 13 autosome arms (1p, 1q, 4q, 5q, 6q, 8p, 8q, 9p, 13q, 14p, 16p, 16q, and 17p) contain allelic losses in 30% to 60% (Table 42–1), whereas the remaining autosomal arms contain allelic losses in 20% or less. Allelic deletions accumulate in at least nine of these chromosome arms as HCC progresses from small, well-differentiated, and localized tumors to large, poorly differentiated, and metastatic tumors[203,241,281,328,330] (Table 42–1). A larger fraction of poorly differentiated HCC show LOH of these loci than do well-differentiated tumors, and the number of LOH/HCCs also increase in concert.

Some affected chromosome arms contain LOH "hot spots" (Table 42–2). Several well-known tumor suppressor genes (e.g., *p53* [chromosome 17p13.1], *RB1* [chromosome 13q14], *p16^{INK4A}* [chromosome 9p21–p22], E-cadherin [chromosome 16q22.1], and *M6P/IGF-IIR* [chromosome 6q26–q27]) often appear to be included in these common allelic deletions in HCC. Other tumor suppressor genes located on some of the chromosome arms that contain frequent allelic deletions, however, do not show high rates of LOH in HCC (e.g., *p73* [chromosome 1p36.3], *APC* and *MCC* [chromosome 5q22], *BRCA1* [chromosome 17q21], and *nm23* [chromosome 17q21.3]). Despite attempts to identify and isolate

**Table 42-1** Allelic deletions on autosome arms in hepatocellular carcinoma

| Autosome Arms | HCC Unselected by Grade or Size with Deletions in Autosome Arms[a] (%) | HCC of Different Grades with Deletions in Autosome Arms[b] (%) | | | |
| --- | --- | --- | --- | --- | --- |
| | | Early[c] | Well Differentiated | Moderately Differentiated | Poorly Differentiated |
| 1p | 36 ± 17 | 18 | 10 | 30 | 35 |
| 1q | 42 ± 20 | | | | |
| 4q | 52 ± 24 | 0 | 18 | 33 | 54 |
| 5q | 33 ± 19 | — | 20 | 30 | 35 |
| 6q | 30 ± 20 | | | | |
| 8p | 58 ± 18 | — | 20 | 46 | 56 |
| 8q | 38 ± 23 | | | | |
| 9p | 39 ± 15 | | | | |
| 13q | 42 ± 22 | 0 | 7 | 25 | 41 |
| 14q | 36 ± 10 | | | | |
| 16p | 49 ± 18 | | | | |
| 16q | 47 ± 19 | 0 | 4 | 24 | 48 |
| 17q | 53 ± 14 | 0 | 20 | 48 | 59 |

[a]Data derived from Table 42–1 in Grisham.[8] Less than 20% of HCCs contain allelic deletions in other autosome arms.

[b]See Nishida et al.,[241] Konishi et al.,[281] Kuroki et al.,[328] and Tamura et al.[330]

[c]As defined in Oda et al.[276]

new tumor suppressor genes from some of the chromosome regions affected by LOH hot spots,[446,447] the specific genes affected by most allelic losses in HCC are still unknown. It is uncertain whether these deleted loci contain as yet unknown tumor suppressor genes or merely represent random, nonspecific chromatin losses as a consequence of the general genomic instability that characterizes malignant neoplasms. However, the fact that several of these chromosomal deletions recur frequently in HCC suggests that the deletions are not random, but rather have essential pathogenic roles in the development and progression of this tumor.

**Table 42-2** Common losses of chromosome arms and deletions of chromosome segments (hot spots) in hepatocellular carcinoma

| Chromosome Number | Chromosome Arm | | Chromosome Segment | | | |
| --- | --- | --- | --- | --- | --- | --- |
| | KT | CGH | KT | FISH | CGH | ALLELO |
| 1 | 1p | 1p | 1p11 | | | 1p34–36 | 1p13–21 |
| | | | 1p22 | | | 1p31–32 |
| | | | 1p32–33 | | | 1p36–36.2 |
| 3 | | | | 3p14 | | |
| 4 | | 4q | | 4q21 | 4q12–21 | Multiple |
| 5 | | 5q | | | 5q12–21 | 5q21–22 |
| | | | | | | 5q35–qter |
| 6 | 6q | 6q | 6q13–25 | 6q14 | 6q13–16 | 6q26–27 |
| | | | 6q22–25 | | | |
| 8 | 8p | 8p | | 8p12 | 8p21–23 | 8p21–23 |
| | | | | 8p22 | | |
| | | | 8q10 | | | 8q22–24 |
| 9 | | | | 9p21 | | |
| | | | | 9p24 | | |
| 10 | | 10q | | | | |
| 13 | 13p | | | | | |
| | | 13q | | | 13q13–14 | 13q12–13 |
| | | | | | | 13q14–14.3 |
| | | | | | | 13q27 |
| | | | | | | 13q32 |
| 16 | | 16p | | | | 16p13–pter |
| | 16q | 16q | 16q24 | | | 16q22–22.3 |
| | | | | | | 16q24–qter |
| 17 | 17p | 17p | 17p11 | | | 17p11–13 |

Abbreviations: ALLELO, allelotype; CGH, comparative genomic hybridization; FISH, fluorescence in situ hybridization; KT, karyotype.

Karyotype dat are from reference 8, Table 6. Fluorescence in situ hybridization data are from references 449–456. Comparative genomic hybridization data are from references 457–462. Allelotype data are from reference 8, Table 1.

## Aberrations in Chromosome Structure and Number

### Karyotypes

Complete banded karyotypes have been published for only a few hundred tumor cells from 20 HCCs (for reviews Grisham[8] and Parada et al.[448]), reflecting the technical difficulty involved in producing adequately spread mitotic figures from solid tumors. The HCC tumor cells examined were highly aneuploid, and the individual chromosomes showed complex structural aberrations and frequent numerical changes. Chromosome 1 was most frequently involved in structural aberrations that affected both arms, followed in decreasing frequency by abnormalities involving chromosomes 8, 6, 7, 9, 10, and 16. Specific bands involved in breaks and rearrangements clustered at chromosomes 1p11, 1p22, 1p32, 1p34, and 1p36; 1q10, 1q12, and 1q25; 6q13–q15 and 6q22–25; 8q10; 16q24; and 17p11. Entire copies of chromosomes 5, 8, 13, 16, 17, 18, 21, and 22 were lost (or were involved in complex rearrangements) in up to half of the cells examined, along with extra copies of chromosomes 3, 6, 7, and 20. Partial losses often involved chromosome arms 1p, 6q, 8p, 13p, 16q, and 17p, whereas the most frequent partial gains included the 1q, 8q, and 17q arms.

### Fluorescence in situ hybridization

Losses and gains of selected individual chromosomes have been examined by fluorescence in situ hybridization (FISH) with probes for chromosome-specific α-satellite DNA located at the centromeres.[449–456] Chromosome gains were frequent, involving 13 different chromosomes in many HCC (Table 42–2); extra copies of chromosomes 1, 6, 8, 18, and 20 were found in a large fraction of tumor cells in more than half of all the HCC examined. Chromosome losses were less frequent (Table 42–2), most often involving chromosomes 4 and 16 in 22% and 26% of the HCC examined, respectively.

Unique sequence yeast artificial chromosome (YAC) probes were used for FISH examination of eight noncentromeric regions located on five chromosomes in 17 HCCs.[455] Deletions were detected at 4q21 in 13 HCCs (77%), at 8p22 in 10 (59%), at 6q14 in 8 (47%), at 8p12 in 6 (35%), at 9p21 and 9p24 in 4 each (24%), and at 3p14 in 2 (12%). Each of the 17 HCCs showed at least one deleted locus and/or was aneuploid. Examination of the 6p14–p22 region with eight YAC probes and a chromosome 6–specific α-satellite probe disclosed that 16 of 25 HCCs contained more than two copies of chromosome 6, whereas 8 of the remaining 9 HCCs each contained one copy (only 1 of 25 HCCs was euploid for this chromosome).[456] Allelic losses in the 6q14–q22 region were detected in 12 (48%) of 25 HCCs, all but one of which were polysomic for chromosome 6. The minimal common area of loss was a 2-cM region at 6q14, and 6q14 loss was associated with longer patient survival but not with any characteristics of the HCC.[456]

### Comparative genomic hybridization

Losses and gains of specific chromosome arms and regions were determined by comparative genomic hybridization (CGH) in six studies examining 247 HCCs.[457–462] Losses of 4q were detected in 141 (57%) of 247 HCCs; of 8p in 83 (41%) of 203 HCCs; of 17p in 74 (41%) of 180 HCCs; of 16q in 79 (40%) of 196 HCCs; of 13q in 75 (32%) of 237 HCCs; and of 6q in 27 (32%) of 85 HCCs. Losses of 1p in 13 (29%) of 45 HCCs; of 5q in 12 (34%) of 35 HCCs; of 16p in 19 (46%) of 41 HCCs; of 10q in 7 (17%)

of 41 HCCs; and of 19p in 4 (40%) of 10 HCCs also were noted, but only in relatively small numbers (Table 42–2). Gains of 1q were detected in 156 (63%) of 247 HCCs; of 8q in 119 (48%) of 247 HCCs; of 17q in 60 (31%) of 196 HCCs; and of 6p in 33 (26%) of 129 HCCs. Gains of 20q were found in 25 (37%) of 67 HCCs and of 5p in 3 (30%) of 10 HCCs. Losses of 1p, 4q, 8p, 16q, and 17p accumulated in high-grade HCC, and 8p loss was correlated with tumor metastasis in one study. Specific chromosome bands often lost included 1p34–p36, 4q12–q21, 5q13–q21, 6q13–q16, 8p21–p23, and 13q13–q14, whereas bands 1q24–q25 and 8q21–q24 frequently were gained. Amplifications involved 11p12, 12p11, 14q12, and 17p12.

## Other Aberrantly Expressed Genes in Hepatocellular Carcinoma

Many genes are aberrantly expressed in HCC in addition to the so-called oncogenes and tumor suppressor genes that may be directly involved in the initiation and expression of this neoplasm. Every gene may be equally susceptible to the random genomic aberrations that accompany the development of HCC. Many metabolic housekeeping genes are abnormal in HCC, contributing to the overall phenotypic characteristics of tumor cells. The application of techniques for evaluating the expression of multiple genes simultaneously in HCC and in adjacent nontumorous tissue (subtractive hybridization, differential display, serial analysis of gene expression, etc.) has yielded results suggesting that gene expression is globally distorted in HCC tumor cells.[70,463,464] Future studies using gene arrays will ascertain the extent and patterns of gene expression abnormalities in HCC.

Increased expression of some metabolic genes, such as glutamine synthetase (GS) and ornithine decarboxylase (ODC), is required to provide the substrates needed to support the rapid proliferation of HCC tumor cells. GS transcripts were up-regulated significantly (by 3- to 46-fold) in 23 (68%) of 34 HCCs, as compared with adjacent liver tissue, and the activity of the enzyme was increased by 2- to 90-fold in six of eight HCCs selected for study.[465,466] Histochemical and immunoblot analyses showed that GS protein accumulated in 40% to 56% of advanced HCC, and the fraction of GS-positive HCC correlated with tumor grade and with disease-free interval after surgical resection.[467] Expression of ODC, which catalyzes the formation of polyamines necessary for cell proliferation, was strongly up-regulated in 35 HCCs as compared with adjacent liver tissue.[468] ODC enzyme activity was also increased in 13 HCCs, and enzyme activity was highly correlated with increased cell proliferation.[469] The *ODC* gene in HCC contained frequent mutations in the region rich in proline, glutamic acid, serine, and threonine residues (PEST region), which slowed the degradation of the protein and contributed to its accumulation in HCC cells.[469] Mutations in the PEST region of the *ODC* gene increased in frequency along with increasing HCC grade.[469]

The genes involved in methylating DNA have important roles in HCC development, because aberrations in gene methylation are associated with both silencing and overexpression of some genes and, possibly, with the development of allelic deletions at some loci in this tumor.[276,356,470] DNA methyltransferase (DNMT), which catalyzes gene methylation, was up-regulated by more than twofold in chronic hepatitis and cirrhosis prior to the emergence of HCC, and elevated expression was maintained in HCC of all grades.[471] Expression of genes for the enzymes that control the level of *S*-adenosylmethionine (SAM), the substrate for DNMT, also was altered in HCC. The molecular forms of S-adenosylmethionine synthetase (SAMS), which catalyze the formation of SAM, were noted to shift in HCC from the α and β isoforms to the δ isoform.[472] The δ isoform, which normally is expressed in the kidneys but not in the liver, has a higher affinity for methionine than the α and β isoforms, and it is more efficient in utilizing methionine at low ambient levels. Expression of the δ isoform in HCC may give tumor cells a relative advantage in making SAM available for intracellular methylations. A third enzyme involved in controlling the intracellular level of SAM, glycine-N-methyltransferase (GMT), was markedly diminished in HCC cells.[473] GMT reduces the intracellular level of SAM by consuming it to make sarcosine.[473] Reduction of sarcosine production in HCC cells increases the level of SAM available for other methylation reactions.

## Molecular Genetic Alterations That Precede HCC

In this section we review the molecular genetic alterations that develop in livers that are the site of chronic hepatitis and/or cirrhosis before HCC emerge. Of particular interest are molecular changes that occur in nodular aggregates of hepatocytes, especially dysplastic nodules that often are the precursor lesions of HCC. Our goal is to begin to delineate the sequence of molecular alterations that first appear in preneoplastic hepatocytes and then culminate in advanced, metastatic HCC. Information on the molecular genetic alterations that precede HCC is even less complete than that for HCC. Nevertheless, aberrant molecular patterns that may lead to HCC are already discernible.

### Cytokines and Growth Factors

Accelerated hepatocyte proliferation in chronic hepatitis and cirrhosis is driven by cytokines and growth factors that are secreted by inflammatory cells and aberrantly expressed by residual hepatocytes.[474] The cells of the inflammatory infiltrate secrete a variety of cytokines, including several growth factors that are highly mitogenic for hepatocytes, as well as a variety of matrix-degrading enzymes.[111,474] Matrix destruction releases growth factors that are sequestered on matrix molecules, especially high concentrations of HGF.[111,475] In addition to the mitogen-promoting cytokines and mitogenic growth factors secreted by inflammatory cells, the residual hepatocytes are also induced to up-regulate or newly express growth factors, especially TGF-α and IGF-II. These two growth factors are ligands for growth factor receptors that these cells already express, thus creating autocrine mitogenic pathways. Increased expression of the mitogenic growth factors TGF-α and IGF-II is induced in hepatocytes at the earliest stages of chronic hepatitis and cirrhosis, with expression continuing in HCC precursor lesions and in the HCC that ultimately emerges.

#### Transforming growth factor α and epidermal growth factor receptor

Transforming growth factor α expression was detected immunohistochemically in hepatocytes in 12 (60%) of 20 livers involved with chronic hepatitis and in all of 22 cirrhotic livers.[25] TGF-α mRNA was significantly elevated in livers involved with chronic hepatitis and cirrhosis as compared with healthy livers, and expression correlated with increased hepatocyte proliferation.[31,36–38,476] The mechanism by which TGF-α is up-regulated is not known, but expression was most intense in dysplastic hepatocytes infected with HBV.[25–29,477] A role for HBV in trans-

ducing TGF-α expression is supported by studies in which transfection of whole HBV genomic DNA or of the HBV preS1 gene induced expression of the growth factor in cultured cells.[478,479] Expression of the major component of the heteromeric receptor for TGF-α, EGFR, or HER1 was unchanged in chronic hepatitis and cirrhosis.[33,34,36] Expression of HER3 and HER4 has not been assessed in preneoplastic liver tissue, but HER2 (erbB2) was detected focally on hepatocytes in 2 (13%) of 15 cirrhotic livers.[43] HER2 peptide also was significantly elevated in the sera of 12 patients with cirrhosis (1498 ± 701 U/ml) as compared with the concentration in 23 control subjects with healthy livers (911 ± 389 U/ml).[480]

#### Insulin-like growth factor II

Expression of IGF-II is up-regulated in chronic hepatitis and cirrhosis. Immunohistochemical analysis demonstrated the expression of this growth factor in hepatocytes in 58 (53%) of 109 livers with chronic hepatitis[31,47] and in 172 (73%) of 237 cirrhotic livers.[31,47,48] The concentration of IGF-II in cirrhotic livers was more than threefold that in healthy livers, but serum levels usually were not elevated in patients with cirrhosis.[46,57] Induction of IGF-II expression in chronic hepatitis and cirrhosis is associated with complex changes in promoter and allele usage.[66,67] Imbalanced expression of IGF-II alleles was noted in 13 (68%) of 19 cases of chronic hepatitis and 4 (80%) of 5 cases of cirrhosis,[67] and was especially strong in dysplastic nodules, along with a shift in dominance from the P1 to the P3 promoter.[66] These changes in promoter and allele usage from the typical adult pattern are identical to those that occur in HCC.

Insulin-like growth factor II signals the nucleus predominately through the IGF-I receptor. No studies on expression of the IGF-I receptor in chronic hepatitis and cirrhosis have been found. Expression of IGFBP-1 was up-regulated in 35 patients with chronic hepatitis and cirrhosis, whereas IGFBP-3 expression was significantly down-regulated.[128] The effects of changes in binding proteins on the availability of IGF-II to hepatocytes are not known. M6P/IGF-IIR competes with IGF-IR for available IGF-II. The M6P/IGF-II gene located on chromosome 6q26–q27 showed LOH in 8 (57%) of 14 dysplastic nodules,[74–76] and expression presumably was reduced. Cirrhotic nodules located adjacent to HCC had lost the same allele of the M6P/IGF-IIR gene as had the tumors in 9 of 10 instances,[74] which suggests that the LOH occurred first in hepatocytes in cirrhotic nodules from which the HCC developed.

#### Insulin-like growth factor I

Serum levels of IGF-I were reduced by about half in 35 patients with chronic hepatitis and cirrhosis, as compared with 10 healthy control subjects (mean level in controls, 193 ng/ml; range, 151 to 235 ng/ml).[57]

#### Hepatocyte growth factor/c-met

The liver is flooded with HGF in chronic hepatitis and cirrhosis, probably as a result of the destruction of hepatic matrix, which sequesters large amounts of the growth factor.[111] The sera of 27 patients with cirrhosis contained two to five times the concentration of HGF found in the sera of 200 healthy subjects (0.27 ± 0.08 ng/ml), and the serum concentration in 40 patients with chronic hepatitis was increased by an average of 50%;[88] another study, however, detected no change in serum concentration.[82] Hepatocytes in 12 (40%) of 30 livers with chronic hepatitis and in 6 (67%) of 9 livers with cirrhosis stained heavily for HGF by immunohistochemistry,[82] and this was considered to represent

ation and other mechanisms, handicaps the current implementation of strategies to block or reverse them.

None of the potential molecular therapies would appear to be panaceas that apply to all HCC. Much investigation is required to determine the different molecular mechanisms that may lead to HCC and to test the safety and efficacy of possible molecular therapeutic procedures before any molecular therapy will be available for human use. Until that time, the most effective strategies for combating HCC will continue to be the prevention of liver damage by hepatocarcinogenic risk factors, combined with conventional and emerging therapies to prevent formation of toxic AFB1 metabolites in hepatocytes and to eradicate or reduce the multiplicity of infecting hepatitis B and C viruses in chronically infected livers. Overall, prevention of HCC appears to be the most feasible and effective strategy for the foreseeable future.

## Summary

Hepatocarcinogenesis is a slowly developing, molecularly complex process that requires years from the time of initial contact with a liver carcinogen before HCC emerges. Although contemporary knowledge of the complex molecular alterations that drive HCC development is still incomplete, the details are being filled in rapidly. During most of the prolonged preneoplastic phase of HCC, development of molecular genetic aberrations is limited to quantitative (epigenetic) changes in gene expression that are potentially reversible. Available evidence indicates that irreversible structural aberrations in genes develop relatively late in the preneoplastic process, but they accumulate rapidly with the emergence of HCC. The slowly developing sequence of potentially reversible, and then irreversible, molecular genetic changes, coupled with rapidly expanding knowledge of the molecular regulation of hepatocytes and of the mechanisms by which the major hepatocarcinogenic agents perturb hepatocellular regulation, allows reasonable hope that ultimately it will be possible to control the expression of critical aberrant regulatory molecules, thereby preventing or delaying development of HCC.

## Note Added In Proof

For an updated discussion and additional references that have appeared since this review was completed, see S.S. Thorgeirsson and J.W. Grisham. Molecular pathogenesis of human hepatocellular carcinoma. Nature-Genetics 31:339–346, 2003.

This review was written during a Fogarty Scholarship held by the author at the National Cancer Institute. The author is grateful to Dr. Snorri S. Thorgeirsson, Chief of the Laboratory of Experimental Carcinogenesis, for his interest and support. Especially helpful were numerous discussions with Dr. Thorgeirsson on the molecular pathogenesis of HCC. This research was partly supported by United States Public Health Service grant CA 29323 from the National Cancer Institute. Ms. Fumi Wells produced the final text and Ms. Carol Troutner made editorial revisions.

## References

1. Parkin DM, Pisani P, and Ferlay J. Global cancer statistics. CA Cancer J Clin 49:33–64, 1999.
2. Venook AP. Treatment of hepatocellular carcinoma: too many options? J Clin Oncol 12:1323–1334, 1994.
3. Stuver SO. Towards global control of liver cancer? Semin Cancer Biol 8:299–306, 1998.
4. Grisham JW. Interspecies comparison of liver carcinogenesis: implications for cancer risk assessment. Carcinogenesis 18:59–81, 1997.
5. Chang MH, Chen CJ, Lai MS, et al. Universal hepatitis B vaccination in Taiwan and the incidence of hepatocellular carcinoma in children. N Engl J Med 336:1855–1859, 1997.
6. Marques AR, Lau DT, McKenzie R, et al. Combination therapy with famciclovir and interferon-alpha for the treatment of chronic hepatitis B. J Infect Dis 178:1483–1486, 1998.
7. Wang JS, Shen X, He X, et al. Protective alterations in phase 1 and 2 metabolism of aflatoxin B1 by oltipraz in residents of Qidong, People's Republic of China. J Natl Cancer Inst 91:347–354, 1999.
8. Grisham J. Molecular genetic alterations in primary hepatocellular neoplasms: hepatocellular adenoma, hepatocellular carcinoma, and hepatoblastoma. In: Coleman WB, Tsongalis GJ (eds): The Molecular Basis of Cancer. Humana Press, New Jersey, 2002, pp 269–346.
9. Qian C, Drozdzik M, Caselmann WH, Prieto J. The potential of gene therapy in the treatment of hepatocellular carcinoma [review]. J Hepatol 32:344–351, 2000.
10. Shafritz DA, Shouval D, Sherman HI, Hadziyannis SJ, Kew MC. Integration of hepatitis B virus into the genome of liver cells in chronic liver diseases and hepatocellular carcinoma. Studies on percutaneous liver biopsies and post-mortem tissue specimens. N Engl J Med 305:1067–1073, 1981.
11. Esumi M, Aritaka T, Arii M, et al. Clonal origin of human hepatoma determined by integration of hepatitis B virus DNA. Cancer Res 46:5767–5771, 1986.
12. Govindarajan S, Craig JR, Valinluck B. Clonal origin of hepatitis B–associated hepatocellular carcinoma. Hum Pathol 19:403–405, 1988.
13. Tsuda H, Hirohashi S, Shimosato Y, Terada M, Hasegawa H. Clonal origin of atypical adenomatous hyperplasia of the liver and clonal identity with hepatocellular carcinoma. Gastroenterology 95:1664–1666, 1988.
14. Aoki N, Robinson WS. State of the hepatitis B viral genomes in cirrhotic and hepatocellular carcinoma nodules. Mol Biol Med 6:395–408, 1989.
15. Chen PJ, Chen DS, Lai MY, et al. Clonal origin of recurrent hepatocellular carcinomas. Gastroenterology 96:527–529, 1989.
16. Sakamoto M, Hirohashi S, Tsuda H, Shimosato Y, Makuuchi M, Hosoda Y. Multicentric independent development of hepatocellular carcinoma revealed by analysis of hepatitis B virus integration pattern. Am J Surg Pathol 13:1064–1067, 1989.
17. Hsu HC, Chou TJ, Chen JY, Lee CS, Lee PH, Peng SY. Clonality and clonal evolution of hepatocellular carcinoma with multiple nodules. Hepatology 13:923–928, 1991.
18. Sheu JC, Huang GT, Chou H-C, et al. Multiple hepatocellular carcinomas at an early stage have different clonality. Gastroenterology 105:1471–1476, 1993.
19. Aihara T, Noguchi S, Sasaki Y, Nakano H, Imaoka S. Clonal analysis of regenerative nodules in hepatitis C virus–induced cirrhosis. Gastroenterology 107:1805–1811, 1994.
20. Kawai S, Imazeki F, Yokosuka O, et al. Clonality in hepatocellular carcinoma: analysis of methylation pattern of pleomorphic X-chromosome-linked phosphoglycerate kinase gene in females. Hepatology 22:112–117, 1995.
21. Aihara T, Noguchi S, Sasaki Y, Nakano H, Monden M, Imaoka S. Clonal analysis of precancerous lesion of hepatocellular carcinoma. Gastroenterology 111:455–462, 1996.
22. Paradis V, Laurent A, Flejou JF, Vidaud M, Bedossa P. Evidence for the polyclonal nature of focal nodular hyperplasia of the liver by the study of X-chromosome inactivation. Hepatology 26:891–895, 1997.
23. Yamamoto T, Kajino K, Kudo M, Sasaki Y, Arakawa Y, Hino O. Determination of the clonal origin of multiple human hepatocellular carcinomas by cloning and polymerase chain reaction of integrated hepatitis B virus DNA. Hepatology 29:1445–1452, 1999.
24. Sirivatnauksorn Y, Sirivatnauksorn V, Battacharaya S, et al. Evolution of genetic abnormalities in hepatocellular carcinomas demonstrated by DNA fingerprinting. J Pathol 189:344–350, 1999.
25. Castilla A, Prieto J, Fausto N. Transforming growth factors beta 1 and alpha in chronic liver disease: effects of interferon alpha therapy. N Engl J Med 324:933–940, 1991.
26. Hsia CC, Axiotis CA, DiBisceglie AM, Tabor E. Transforming growth factor-α in human hepatocellular carcinoma and coexpression with hepatitis B surface antigen in adjacent liver. Cancer 70:1049–1056, 1992.
27. Collier JD, Guo K, Gullick WJ, Bassendine MF, Burt AD. Expression of transforming growth factor alpha in human hepatocellular carcinoma. Liver 13:151–155, 1993.
28. Schaff Z, Hsia CC, Sarosi I, Tabor E. Overexpression of transforming growth factor-alpha in hepatocellular carcinoma and focal nodular hyperplasia from European patients. Hum Pathol 25:644–651, 1994.
29. Morimitsu Y, Hsia CC, Kojiro M, Tabor E. Nodules of less-differentiated tumor within or adjacent to hepatocellular carcinoma: relative expression of transforming growth factor-alpha and its receptor in different areas of tumor. Hum Pathol 26:1126–1132, 1995.

30. Nalesnik MA, Lee RG, Carr BI. Transforming growth factor alpha (TGF-α) in hepatocellular carcinomas and adjacent parenchyma. Hum Pathol 29:228–234, 1998.

31. Park BC, Huh MH, Seo JH. Differential expression of transforming growth factor alpha and insulin growth factor II in chronic active hepatitis B, cirrhosis and hepatocellular carcinoma. J Hepatol 22:286–294, 1995.

32. Yamaguchi K, Carr BI, Nalesnik MA. Concomitant and isolated expression of TGF-α and EGF-R in human hepatoma cells supports the hypothesis of autocrine, paracrine, and endocrine growth of human hepatoma. J Surg Oncol 58:240–245, 1995.

33. Kiss A, Wang NJ, Xie JP, Thorgeirsson SS. Analysis of transforming growth factor (TGF)-α/epidermal growth factor receptor, hepatocyte growth factor/c-met, TGF-β receptor type II, and p53 expression in human hepatocellular carcinomas. Clin Cancer Res 3:1059–1066, 1997.

34. Tang Z, Qin L, Wang X, et al. Alterations of oncogenes, tumor suppressor genes and growth factors in hepatocellular carcinoma: with relation to tumor size and invasiveness. Chinese Med J 111:313–318, 1998.

35. Tomiya T, Fujiwara K. Serum transforming growth factor alpha as a marker of hepatocellular carcinoma complicating cirrhosis. Cancer 77:1056–1060, 1996.

36. Harada K, Shiota G, Kawasaki H. Transforming growth factor-alpha and epidermal growth factor receptor in chronic liver disease and hepatocellular carcinoma. Liver 19:318–325, 1999.

37. Yeh YC, Tsai JF, Chuang LY, et al. Elevation of transforming growth factor α and its relationship to the epidermal growth factor receptor and α-fetoprotein levels in patients with hepatocellular carcinoma. Cancer Res 47:896–901, 1987.

38. Masuhara M, Yasunaga M, Tanigawa K, et al. Expression of hepatocyte growth factor, transforming growth factor alpha, and transforming growth factor beta 1 messenger RNA in various human liver diseases and correlation with hepatocyte proliferation. Hepatology 24:323–329, 1996.

39. Motoo Y, Sawabu N, Nakanuma Y. Expression of epidermal growth factor and fibroblast growth factor in human hepatocellular carcinoma: an immunohistochemical study. Liver 11:272–277, 1991.

40. Chuang LY, Tsai JH, Yeh YC, et al. Epidermal growth factor-related transforming growth factors in the urine of patients with hepatocellular carcinoma. Hepatology 13:1112–1116, 1991.

41. Hamazaki K, Yunoki Y, Tagashira H, Mimura T, Mori M, Orita K. Epidermal growth factor receptor in human hepatocellular carcinoma. Cancer Detect Prev 21:355–360, 1997.

42. Mori S, Akiyama T, Morishita Y, et al. Light and electron microscopical demonstration of c-erbB-2 gene product–like immunoreactivity in human malignant tumors. Virchows Arch B Cell Pathol Incl Mol Pathol 54:8–15, 1987.

43. Brunt EM, Swanson PE. Immunoreactivity for c-erbB-2 oncopeptide in benign and malignant diseases of the liver. Am J Clin Pathol 97 (Suppl 1):s53–s61, 1992.

44. Collier JD, Guo K, Mathew J, et al. c-erbB-2 oncogene expression in hepatocellular carcinoma and cholangiocarcinoma. J Hepatol 14:377–380, 1992.

45. Heinze T, Jonas S, Kärsten A, Neuhaus P. Determination of the oncogenes p53 and c-erbB2 in the tumor cytosols of advanced hepatocellular carcinoma (HCC) and correlation with survival time. Anticancer Res 19:2501–2504, 1999.

46. Cariani E, Seurin D, Lasserre C, Franco D, Binoux M, Brechot C. Expression of insulin-like growth factor II (IGF-II) in human primary liver cancer: mRNA and protein analysis. J Hepatol 11:226–231, 1990.

47. Su Q, Liu YF, Zhang JF, Zhang SX, Li DF, Yang JJ. Expression of insulin-like growth factor II in hepatitis B cirrhosis and hepatocellular carcinoma: its relationship with hepatitis B virus antigen expression. Hepatology 20:788–799, 1994.

48. Fiorentino M, Grigioni WF, Baccarini P, et al. Different in situ expression of insulin-like growth factor type II in hepatocellular carcinoma: an in situ hybridization and immunohistochemical study. Diagn Mol Pathol 3:59–65, 1994.

49. Cariani E, Lasserre C, Seurin D, et al. Differential expression of insulin-like growth factor II mRNA in human primary liver cancers, benign liver tumors, and liver cirrhosis. Cancer Res 48:6844–6849, 1988.

50. Cariani E, Lasserre C, Kemeny F, Franco D, Brechot C. Expression of insulin-like growth factor II, α-fetoprotein, and hepatitis B virus transcripts in human primary liver cancer. Hepatology 13:644–649, 1991.

51. Su TS, Liu WY, Han SH, et al. Transcripts of insulin-like growth factors I and II in human hepatoma. Cancer Res 49:1773–1777, 1989.

52. D'Arville CN, Nouri-Aria KT, Johnson P, Williams R. Regulation of insulin-like growth factor II gene expression by hepatitis B virus in hepatocellular carcinoma. Hepatology 13:310–315, 1991.

53. Lamas E, LeBail B, Housset C, Boucher O, Brechot C. Localization of insulin-like growth factor-II and hepatitis B virus mRNAs and proteins in human hepatocellular carcinomas. Lab Invest 64:98–104, 1991.

54. Li X, Nong Z, Ekström C, et al. Disrupted IGF2 promoter control by silencing of promoter P1 in human hepatocellular carcinoma. Cancer Res 57:2048–2054, 1997.

55. Sohda T, Yun K, Iwata K, Soejima H, Okumura M. Increased expression of insulin-like growth factor 2 in hepatocellular carcinoma is primarily regulated at the transcriptional level. Lab Invest 75:307–311, 1996.

56. Sohda T, Kamimura S, Iwata K, Shijo H, Okumura M. Immunohistochemical evidence of insulin-like growth factor II in human small hepatocellular carcinoma with hepatitis C virus infection: relationship to fatty change in carcinoma cells. J Gastroenterol Hepatol 12:224–228, 1997.

57. Daughaday WH, Wu J-C, Lee S-D, Kapadia M. Abnormal processing of pro-IGF-II in patients with hepatoma and in some hepatitis B virus antibody-positive asymptomatic individuals. J Lab Clin Med 116:555–562, 1990.

58. Sohda T, Oka Y, Iwata K, et al. Co-localization of insulin-like growth factor II and the proliferation marker M1B1 in hepatocellular carcinoma cells. J Clin Pathol 50:135–137, 1997.

59. Davies SM. Developmental regulation of genomic imprinting of the IGF2 gene in human liver. Cancer Res 54:2560–2562, 1994.

60. Ekström TJ, Cui H, Li X, Ohlsson R. Promoter-specific IGF2 imprinting status and its plasticity during human liver development. Development 121:309–316, 1995.

61. Li X, Cui H, Sandstedt B, Nordliner H, Larsson E, Ekström TJ. Expression levels of the insulin-like growth factor-II gene (IGF-2) in the human liver: developmental relationships of the four promoters. J Endocrinol 149:117–124, 1996.

62. Lustig O, Ariel I, Ilan J, Lev-Lehman E, DeGroot N, Hochberg A. Expression of the imprinted H19 gene in the human fetus. Mol Reprod Dev 38:239–246, 1994.

63. Nardone G, Romano M, Calabro A, et al. Activation of fetal promoters of insulin-like growth factor II gene in hepatitis C virus–related chronic hepatitis, cirrhosis, and hepatocellular carcinoma. Hepatology 23:1304–1312, 1996.

64. Ariel I, Miao HQ, Ji XR, et al. Imprinted H19 oncofetal RNA is a candidate tumor marker for hepatocellular carcinoma. Mol Pathol 51:21–25, 1998.

65. Sohda T, Iwate K, Soejima H, Kamimura S, Shijo H, Yun K. In situ detection of insulin-like growth factor II (IGF2) and H19 gene expression in hepatocellular carcinoma. J Hum Genet 43:49–53, 1998.

66. Aihara T, Noguchi S, Miyoshi Y, et al. Allelic imbalance of insulin-like growth factor gene expression in cancerous and precancerous lesions of the liver. Hepatology 28:86–89, 1998.

67. Takeda S, Kondo M, Kumada T, et al. Allelic-expression imbalance in the insulin-like growth factor 2 gene in hepatocellular carcinoma and underlying disease. Oncogene 12:1589–1592, 1996.

68. Uchida K, Kondo M, Takeda S, et al. Altered transcriptional regulation of the insulin-like growth factor 2 gene in human hepatocellular carcinoma. Mol Carcinog 18:193–198, 1997.

69. Kim KS, Lee YI. Biallelic expression of H19 and IGF2 genes in hepatocellular carcinoma. Cancer Lett 119:143–148, 1997.

70. Kondoh N, Wakatsuki T, Ryo A, et al. Identification and characterization of genes associated with hepatocellular carcinogenesis. Cancer Res 59:4990–4996, 1999.

71. Sue SR, Chari RS, Kong FM, et al. Transforming growth factor beta receptors and mannose 6-phosphate/insulin-like growth factor-II receptor expression in human hepatocellular carcinoma. Ann Surg 222:171–178, 1995.

72. DeSouza AT, Hankins GR, Washington MK, et al. Frequent loss of heterozygosity on 6q at the mannose 6-phosphate/insulin-like growth factor-II receptor locus in human hepatocellular tumors. Oncogene 10:1725–1729, 1995.

73. Piao Z, Choi Y, Park C, Lee WJ, Park J-H, Kim H. Deletion of the M6P/IGF2r gene in primary hepatocellular carcinoma. Cancer Lett 120:39–43, 1997.

74. Yamada T, DeSouza AT, Finkelstein S, Jirtle RL. Loss of the gene encoding mannose 6-phosphate/insulin-like growth factor II receptor is an early event in liver carcinogenesis. Proc Natl Acad Sci USA 94:10351–10355, 1997.

75. Wada I, Kanda H, Nomura K, Kato Y, Machinami R, Kitagawa T. Failure to detect genetic alteration of the mannose-6-phosphate/insulin-like growth factor 2 receptor (M6P/IGF2R) gene in hepatocellular carcinoma in Japan. Hepatology 29:1718–1721, 1999.

76. Oka Y, Killian JK, Jang HS, et al. M6P/IGF2R is mutated in hepato-

cellular carcinomas in Japan [abstract]. Proc Am Assoc Cancer Res 42:61–62, 2001.

77. DeSouza AT, Hankins GR, Washington MK, Orton TC, Jirtle RL. M6P/IGF2R gene is mutated in human hepatocellular carcinomas with loss of heterozygosity. Nat Genet 11:447–449, 1995.

78. Saeki A, Tamura S, Ito N, et al. Lack of frameshift mutations at coding mononucleotide repeats in hepatocellular carcinoma in Japanese patients. Cancer 88:1025–1029, 2000.

79. Yamamoto H, Itoh F, Fukushima H, et al. Infrequent widespread microsatellite instability in hepatocellular carcinoma. Int J Oncol 16:543–547, 2000.

80. Chang TC, Lin JJ, Yu SC, Chang TJ. Absence of growth-hormone receptor in hepatocellular carcinoma and cirrhotic liver. Hepatology 11:123–126, 1990.

81. Ljubimova JY, Petrovic LM, Wilson SE, Geller SA, Demetriou AA. Expression of HGF, its receptor c-met, c-myc, and albumin in cirrhotic and neoplastic human liver tissue. J Histochem Cytochem 45:79–87, 1997.

82. Okano JI, Shiota G, Kawasaki H. Expression of hepatocyte growth factor (HGF) and HGF receptor (c-met) proteins in liver diseases: an immunohistochemical study. Liver 19:151–159, 1999.

83. Yoshinaga Y, Matsuno Y, Fujita S, et al. Immunohistochemical detection of hepatocyte growth factor/scatter factor in human cancerous and inflammatory lesions of various organs. Jpn J Cancer Res 84:1150–1158, 1993.

84. D'Errico A, Fiorentino M, Ponzetto A, et al. Liver hepatocyte growth factor does not always correlate with hepatocellular proliferation in human liver lesions: its specific receptor c-met does. Hepatology 24:60–64, 1996.

85. Ueki T, Fujimoto J, Suzuki T, Yamamoto H, Okamoto E. Expression of hepatocyte growth factor and its receptor c-met proto-oncogene in hepatocellular carcinoma. Hepatology 25:862–866, 1997.

86. Noguchi O, Enomoto N, Ikeda T, Kobayashi F, Marumo F, Sato C. Gene expressions of c-met and hepatocyte growth factor in chronic liver disease and hepatocellular carcinoma. J Hepatol 24:286–292, 1996.

87. Selden C, Farnaud S, Ding SF, Habib N, Foster C, Hodgson HJF. Expression of hepatocyte growth factor mRNA, and c-met mRNA (hepatocyte growth factor receptor) in human liver tumours. J Hepatol 21:227–234, 1994.

88. Shiota G, Okano JI, Kawasaki H, Kawamoto T, Nakamura T. Serum hepatocyte growth factor levels in liver diseases: clinical implications. Hepatology 21:106–112, 1995.

89. Chen Q, Seol DW, Carr B, Zarnegar R. Expression and relation of Met and Ron proto-oncogenes in human hepatocellular carcinoma tissues and cell lines. Hepatology 26:59–66, 1997.

90. DiRenzo MF, Narsimhan RP, Olivero M, et al. Expression of the HGF receptor in normal and neoplastic tissues. Oncogene 6:1997–2004, 1992.

91. Prat M, Narsimhan RP, Crepaldi T, Nicotra MR, Natali PG, Comoglio PM. The receptor encoded by the human c-met oncogene is expressed in hepatocytes, epithelial cells and solid tumors. Int J Cancer 49:323–328, 1991.

92. Boix L, Rosa JL, Ventura F, et al. c-met mRNA overexpression in human hepatocellular carcinoma. Hepatology 19:88–91, 1994.

93. Suzuki K, Hayashi N, Yamada Y, et al. Expression of the c-met proto-oncogene in human hepatocellular carcinoma. Hepatology 20:1231–1236, 1994.

94. Grigioni WF, Fiorentino M, D'Errico A, et al. Overexpression of c-met proto-oncogene product and raised Ki67 index in hepatocellular carcinomas with respect to benign liver conditions. Hepatology 21:1543–1546, 1995.

95. Bevilacqua M, Norbisto G, Chebat E, et al. Changes in α-1 and β-2 adrenoceptor density in human hepatocellular carcinoma. Cancer 67:2543–2551, 1991.

96. Motoo Y, Sawabu N, Yamaguchi Y, Terada T, Nakanuma Y. Sinusoidal capillarization of human hepatocellular carcinoma: possible promotion by fibroblast growth factor. Oncology 50:270–274, 1993.

97. Shimoyama Y, Gotoh M, Ino Y, Sakamoto M, Kato K, Hirohashi S. Characterization of high-molecular-mass forms of basic fibroblast growth factor in hepatocarcinogenesis. Jpn J Cancer Res 82:1263–1270, 1991.

98. Li D, Bell J, Brown A, Berry CL. The observation of angiogenic and basic fibroblast growth factor gene expression in human colonic adenocarcinoma, gastric adenocarcinomas, and hepatocellular carcinomas. J Pathol 172:171–175, 1994.

99. Mise M, Arii S, Higashituj H, et al. Clinical significance of vascular endothelial growth factor and basic fibroblast growth factor gene expression in liver tumor. Hepatology 23:455–464, 1996.

100. Tsou AP, Wu KM, Tsen TY, et al. Parallel hybridization analysis of multiple protein kinase genes: identification of gene expression patterns characteristic of human hepatocellular carcinoma. Genomics 50:331–340, 1998.

101. El-Assal O, Yamanoi A, Soda Y, et al. Clinical evidence of microvessel density and vascular endothelial growth factor expression in hepatocellular carcinoma and surrounding liver: possible involvement of vascular endothelial growth factor in angiogenesis of cirrhotic liver. Hepatology 27:1554–1562, 1998.

102. Chow NH, Hsu PI, Lin X-Z, et al. Expression of vascular endothelial growth factor in normal liver and hepatocellular carcinoma: an histochemical study. Hum Pathol 28:698–703, 1997.

103. Torimura T, Sata M, Ueno T, et al. Increased expression of vascular endothelial growth factor is associated with tumor progression in hepatocellular carcinoma. Hum Pathol 29:986–991, 1998.

104. Yamaguchi R, Yano H, Iemura A, Ogasawara S, Haramaki M, Kojiro M. Expression of vascular endothelial growth factor in human hepatocellular carcinoma. Hepatology 28:68–77, 1998.

105. Kobayashi N, Ishii M, Ueno Y, et al. Co-expression of Bcl-2 protein and vascular endothelial growth factor in hepatocellular carcinomas treated by chemoembolization. Liver 19:25–31, 1999.

106. Zhou J, Tang ZY, Fan J, et al. Expression of platelet-derived endothelial cell growth factor and vascular endothelial growth factor in hepatocellular carcinoma and portal vein thrombus. J Cancer Res Clin Oncol 126:57–61, 2000.

107. Suzuki K, Hayashi N, Miyamoto Y, et al. Expression of vascular permeability factor/vascular endothelial growth factor in human hepatocellular carcinoma. Cancer Res 56:3004–3009, 1996.

108. Li XM, Tang Zy, Zhou G, Lui YK, Ye SL. Significance of vascular endothelial growth factor mRNA expression in invasion and metastasis of hepatocellular carcinoma. J Exp Clin Cancer Res 17:13–17, 1998.

109. Shimoda K, Mori M, Shibuta K, Banner BF, Bernard GF. Vascular endothelial growth factor/vascular permeability factor mRNA expression in patients with chronic hepatitis C and hepatocellular carcinoma. Int J Oncol 14:353–359, 1999.

110. Jin-no K, Tanumizu M, Hyodo I, et al. Circulating platelet-derived endothelial cell growth factor increases in hepatocellular carcinoma patients. Cancer 82:1260–1267, 1998.

111. Michalopoulos GK, DeFrances MC. Liver regeneration. Science 276:60–66, 1997.

112. Ito N, Kawata S, Tamura S, et al. Expression of transforming growth factor-beta 1 mRNA in human hepatocellular carcinoma. Jpn J Cancer Res 81:1202–1205, 1990.

113. Ito N, Kawata S, Tamura S, et al. Elevated levels of transforming growth factor beta messenger RNA and its polypeptide in human hepatocellular carcinoma. Cancer Res 51:4048–4083, 1991.

114. Abou-Shady M, Baer HU, Friess H, et al. Transforming growth factor betas and their signaling receptors in human hepatocellular carcinoma. Am J Surg 177:209–215, 1999.

115. Orsatti G, Hytiroglou P, Thung SN, Ishak KG, Paronetto F. Lamellar fibrosis in the fibrolamellar variant of hepatocellular carcinoma: a role for transforming growth factor beta. Liver 17:152–156, 1997.

116. Shirai Y, Kawata S, Ito N, et al. Elevated levels of transforming growth factor-beta in patients with hepatocellular carcinoma. Jpn J Cancer Res 83:676–679, 1992.

117. Shirai Y, Kawata S, Tamura S, et al. Plasma transforming growth factor-beta 1 levels in patients with hepatocellular carcinoma. Comparison with chronic liver diseases. Cancer 73:2275–2279, 1994.

118. Ito N, Kawata S, Tamura S, et al. Positive correlation of plasma transforming growth factor-beta 1 levels with tumor vascularity in hepatocellular carcinoma. Cancer Lett 89:45–48, 1995.

119. Tsai JF, Chuang LY, Jeng JE, et al. Clinical relevance of transforming growth factor-beta 1 in the urine of patients with hepatocellular carcinoma. Medicine 76:213–226, 1997.

120. Bedossa P, Peltier E, Terris B, Franco D, Poynard T. Transforming growth factor-beta1 (TGF-β1) and TGF-β 1 receptors in normal, cirrhotic and neoplastic human livers. Hepatology 21:760–766, 1995.

121. Furuta K, Misao S, Takahashi K, et al. Gene mutation of transforming growth factor beta 1 type II receptor in hepatocellular carcinoma. Int J Cancer 81:851–899, 1999.

122. Vincent F, Hagiwara K, Ke Y, Stoner GD, Demetrick DJ, Bennett WP. Mutation analysis of the transforming growth factor beta type II receptor in sporadic human cancers of the pancreas, liver, and breast. Biochem Biophys Res Commun 223:561–564, 1996.

123. Kawate S, Takenoshita S, Ohwada S, et al. Mutation analysis of transforming growth factor beta type II receptor, Smad2, and Smad4 in hepatocellular carcinoma. Int J Oncol 14:127–131, 1999.

124. Salvucci M, Lemoine A, Saffroy R, et al. Microsatellite instability in European hepatocellular carcinoma. Oncogene 18:181–187, 1999.

125. Legiou P, Kuper H, Stuver SO, Tzonou A, Trichopoulos D, Adami HO. Role of diabetes in the etiology of hepatocellular carcinoma. J Natl Cancer Inst 92:1096–1099, 2000.

126. Ikeda Y, Shimada M, Hasegawa H, et al. Prognosis of hepatocellular carcinoma with diabetes mellitus after hepatic resection. Hepatology 27:1567–1571, 1998.

127. Nishiyama M, Wands JR. Cloning and increased expression of an insulin receptor substrate-1-like gene in human hepatocellular carcinoma. Biochem Biophys Res Commun 183:280–285, 1992.

128. Donaghy A, Ross R, Gimson A, Hughes SC, Holly J, Williams R. Growth hormone, insulin-like growth factor-I, and insulin-like growth factor binding proteins 1 and 3 in chronic liver disease. Hepatology 21:680–688, 1995.

129. Nelson RB. Thyroid-binding globulin in hepatoma. Arch Intern Med 139:1063, 1979.

130. Kalk WJ, Kew M, Danielwitz MD, Jacks F, Van Der Walt LA, Levin J. Thyroxine-binding globulin and thyroid function tests in patients with hepatocellular carcinoma. Hepatology 2:72–76, 1982.

131. Alexopoulos A, Hutchinson W, Bari A, Keating JJ, Johnson PJ, Williams R. Hyperthyroxinemia in hepatocellular carcinoma: relation to thyroid binding globulin in the clinical and preclinical stages of the disease. Br J Cancer 57:313–316, 1988.

132. Hutchinson WL, Johnson PJ, White YS, Williams R. Differential hormone–binding characteristics of thyroxine-binding globulin in hepatocellular carcinoma and cirrhosis. J Hepatol 9:265–271, 1989.

133. Hutchinson WL, White YS, Fagan EA, Johnson PJ, Williams R. Impaired binding properties of thyroxine-binding globulin in hepatocellular carcinoma and chronic liver disease. Hepatology 14:116–120, 1991.

134. Lin KH, Shieh HY, Chen SL, Hsu HC. Expression of mutant thyroid hormone nuclear receptors in human hepatocellular carcinoma cells. Mol Carcinog 26:53–61, 1999.

135. Lin KH, Zhu XG, Hsu HC, et al. Dominant negative activity of mutant thyroid hormone alpha 1 receptors from patients with hepatocellular carcinoma. Endocrinology 138:5308–5315, 1997.

136. Lin K-H, Lin YW, Lee HF, et al. Increased activity of human hepatocellular carcinoma cells is associated with an overexpression of thyroid hormone beta nuclear receptor and low expression of anti-metastatic nm23 gene. Cancer Lett 98:89–95, 1995.

137. Arbuthnot P, Kew M, Parker I, Fitschen W. Expression of c-erbA in human hepatocellular carcinoma. Anticancer Res 9:885–888, 1989.

138. Dejean A, Bougueleret L, Grzeschik KH, Tiollais P. Hepatitis B virus DNA integration in a sequence homologous to v-erb-A and steroid receptor genes in hepatocellular carcinoma. Nature 322:70–72, 1986.

139. DeThé H, Marchio A, Tiollais P, Dejean A. A novel thyroid hormone receptor-related gene inappropriately expressed in human hepatocellular carcinoma. Nature 330:667–670, 1987.

140. Brand N, Petkovich M, Krust A, et al. Identification of a second human retinoic acid receptor. Nature 332:850–853, 1988.

141. Benbrook D, Lenhardt E, Pfahl M. A new retinoic acid receptor identified from a hepatocellular carcinoma. Nature 333:669–672, 1988.

142. Sever CE, Locker J. Expression of retinoic acid alpha and beta receptor genes in liver and hepatocellular carcinoma. Mol Carcinog 4:138–144, 1991.

143. Sweeney EC, Evans DJ. Hepatic lesions in patients treated with synthetic anabolic steroids. J Clin Pathol 29:626–633, 1976.

144. Boyd PR, Mark GJ. Multiple adenomas and a hepatocellular carcinoma in a man on oral methyl testosterone for eleven years. Cancer 40:1765–1770, 1977.

145. Hsing AW, Hoover RN, McLaughlin JK, et al. Oral contraceptives and primary liver cancer among young women. Cancer Causes Control 3:43–48, 1992.

146. Guéchot J, Piegny N, Ballet F, Vanbourdolle M, Giboudeau J, Poupon R. Sex hormone imbalance in male alcoholic patients with and without hepatocellular carcinoma. Cancer 62:760–762, 1988.

147. Yu MW, Chen CJ. Elevated serum testosterone levels and risk of hepatocellular carcinoma. Cancer Res 53:790–794, 1993.

148. Iqbal MJ, Wilkinsin ML, Johnson PJ, Williams R. Sex steroid receptor proteins in foetal, adult and malignant human liver tissue. Br J Cancer 48:791–796, 1983.

149. Nagasue N, Ito A, Yukaya H, Ogawa Y. Androgen receptors in hepatocellular carcinoma and surrounding parenchyma. Gastroenterology 89:643–647, 1985.

150. Eagon PK, Francavilla A, DiLeo A, et al. Quantitation of estrogen and androgen receptors in hepatocellular carcinoma and adjacent normal human liver. Digest Dis Sci 36:1303–1308, 1991.

151. Nagasue N, Yukaya H, Chang YC, Ogawa Y, Kohno H, Ito A. Active uptake of testosterone by androgen receptors of hepatocellular carcinomas in humans. Cancer 57:2162–2167, 1986.

152. Nagasue N, Yamanoi A, Kohno H, et al. Androgen receptor in cirrhotic liver, adenomatous hyperplastic nodule and hepatocellular carcinoma in the human. Hepatogastroenterology 39:455–460, 1992.

153. Onishi S, Murakami T, Moriyama T, Mitamura K, Imawari M. Androgen and estrogen receptors in hepatocellular carcinomas and the surrounding noncancerous liver tissue. Hepatology 6:440–443, 1989.

154. Nagasue N, Chang YC, Hayashi T, et al. Androgen receptor in hepatocellular carcinoma as a prognostic factor after hepatic resection. Ann Surg 209:424–427, 1989.

155. Nagasue N, Kohno H, Chang YC, et al. Androgen and estrogen receptors in hepatocellular carcinoma and the surrounding liver in women. Cancer 63:112–116, 1989.

156. Nagasue N, Yu L, Yukaya H, Kohno H, Nakamura T. Androgen and estrogen receptors in hepatocellular carcinoma and surrounding liver parenchyma: impact on intrahepatic recurrence after hepatic resection. Br J Surg 82:542–547, 1995.

157. Boix L, Bruix J, Castells A, et al. Sex hormone receptors in hepatocellular carcinoma. Is there a rationale for hormonal treatment? J Hepatol 17:187–191, 1993.

158. Boix L, Castells A, Bruix J, et al. Androgen receptors in hepatocellular carcinoma and surrounding liver: relationship with tumor size and recurrence rate after surgical resection. J Hepatol 22:616–622, 1995.

159. Nagasue N, Ito A, Yukaya H, Ogawa Y. Estrogen receptors in hepatocellular carcinoma. Cancer 57:87–91, 1986.

160. Nagasue N, Kohno H, Chang YC, et al. Clinicopathologic comparisons between estrogen receptor–positive and –negative hepatocellular carcinoma. Ann Surg 212:150–154, 1990.

161. Villa E, Camellini L, Dugani A, et al. Variant estrogen receptor messenger RNA species detected in human primary hepatocellular carcinoma. Cancer Res 55:498–500, 1995.

162. Villa E, Dugani A, Moles A, et al. Variant liver estrogen receptor transcripts already occur in an early stage of chronic liver disease. Hepatology 27:983–988, 1998.

163. Ruebi JC, Zimmermann A, Jonas S, et al. Regulatory peptide receptors in human hepatocellular carcinomas. Gut 45:766–774, 1999.

164. Caplin M, Khan K, Savage K, et al. Expression of gastrin in hepatocellular carcinoma, fibrolamellar carcinoma, and cholangiocarcinoma. J Hepatol 30:519–526, 1999.

165. Tanaka S, Mohr L, Schmidt EV, Sugimachi K, Wands JR. Biological effects of insulin receptor substrate-1 overexpression in hepatocytes. Hepatology 26:598–604, 1997.

166. Furusaka A, Nishiyama M, Ohkawa K, et al. Expression of insulin receptor substrate-1 in hepatocytes: an investigation using monoclonal antibodies. Cancer Lett 84:85–92, 1994.

167. Nonomura A, Ohta G, Hayashi M, et al. Immunohistochemical detection of ras oncogene p21 product in liver cirrhosis and hepatocellular carcinoma. Am J Gastroenterol 82:512–518, 1987.

168. Jagirdar J, Nonomura S, Patil J, Thor A, Paronetto F. ras oncogene p21 expression in hepatocellular carcinoma. J Exp Pathol 4:37–46, 1989.

169. Tiniakos D, Spandidos DA, Kakkanas A, Pintzas A, Pollice L, Tiniakos G. Expression of ras and myc oncogenes in human hepatocellular carcinoma and non-neoplastic liver tissues. Anticancer Res 9:715–722, 1989.

170. Tiniakos D, Spandidos DA, Yiagnisis M, Tiniakos G. Expression of ras and c-myc proteins and hepatitis B surface antigen in human liver disease. Hepatogastroenterology 40:37–40, 1993.

171. Radosevich JA, Gould KA, Koukoulis GK, et al. Immunolocalization of ras oncogene p21 in human liver diseases. Ultrastruct Pathol 17:1–8, 1993.

172. Zhang XK, Huang DP, Chiu DK, Chiu JF. The expression of oncogenes in human developing liver and hepatomas. Biochem Biophys Res Commun 142:932–938, 1987.

173. Himeno Y, Fukuda Y, Hatanaka M, Imura H. Expression of oncogenes in human liver disease. Liver 8:208–212, 1988.

174. Gu JR, Hu LF, Cheng YC, Wan DF. Oncogenes in primary hepatic cancer. J Cell Physiol 4(Suppl.):13–20, 1986.

175. Zhang XK, Huang D, Qiu DK, Chiu J. The expression of c-myc and c-N-ras in human cirrhotic livers, hepatocellular carcinomas and liver tissue surrounding the tumors. Oncogene 5:909–914, 1990.

176. Ogata N, Kamimura T, Asakura H. Point mutation, allelic loss and increased methylation of c-Ha-ras gene in human hepatocellular carcinoma. Hepatology 13:31–37, 1991.

177. Fukuda K, Ogasawara S, Maruiwa M, Yano H, Murakami T, Kojiro M. Structural alterations in c-myc and c-Ha-ras proto-oncogenes in human hepatocellular carcinoma. Kurume Med J 35:77–87, 1988.

178. Tada M, Omata M, Ohto M. Analysis of *ras* gene mutations in human hepatic malignant tumors by polymerase chain reaction and direct sequencing. Cancer Res 50:1121–1124, 1990.

179. Challen C, Guo K, Collier JD, Cavanagh D, Bassendine MF. Infrequent point mutations in codons 12 and 61 of *ras* oncogenes in human hepatocellular carcinoma. J Hepatol 14:342–346, 1992.

180. Kress S, Jahn U-R, Buchmann A, Bannasch P, Schwarz M. *p53* point mutations in hepatocellular carcinomas from Germany. Cancer Res 52:3220–3223, 1992.

181. Leon M, Kew MC. Analysis of *ras* gene mutations in hepatocellular carcinoma in Southern African blacks. Anticancer Res 15:859–862, 1995.

182. Tsuda H, Hirohashi S, Shimosato Y, Ino Y, Yoshida T, Terada M. Low incidence of point mutation of c-Ki-*ras* and N-*ras* oncogenes in human hepatocellular carcinoma. Jpn J Cancer Res 80:196–199, 1989.

183. Stok P, Loda M, Bosari S, Wiley B, Poppenhausen K, Wolfe H. Detection of K-*ras* mutations in pancreatic and hepatic neoplasms by nonisotopic mismatched polymerase chain reaction. Oncogene 6:857–862, 1991.

184. Imai Y, Oda H, Arai M, et al. Mutational analysis of the *p53* and K-*ras* genes and allelotype study of the *Rb-1* gene for investigating the pathogenesis of combined hepatocellular-cholangiocellular carcinomas. Jpn J Cancer Res 87:1056–1062, 1996.

185. Schmidt CM, McKillop IH, Cahill PA, Sitzmann JV. Increased MAPK expression and activity in primary hepatocellular carcinoma. Biochem Biophys Res Commun 236:54–58, 1997.

186. Ito Y, Sasaki Y, Horimoto M, et al. Activation of mitogen-activated protein kinases/extracellular signal-related kinases in human hepatocellular carcinoma. Hepatology 27:951–958, 1998.

187. Masaki T, Okada M, Shiratori Y, et al. pp60c-src activation in hepatocellular carcinoma of humans and LEC rats. Hepatology 27:1257–1264, 1998.

188. Schmidt CM, McKillpo IH, Cahill PA, Sitzman JV. Alterations in guanine nucleotide regulatory protein expression and activity in human hepatocellular carcinoma. Hepatology 26:1189–1194, 1997.

189. Arbuthnot P, Kew M, Fitschen W. c-fos and c-myc oncoprotein expression in human hepatocellular carcinomas. Anticancer Res 11:921–924, 1991.

190. Gan FY, Gesell MS, Alousi M, Luk GD. Analysis of ODC and c-*myc* gene expression in hepatocellular carcinoma by in situ hybridization and immunohistochemistry. J Histochem Cytochem 41:1185–1196, 1993.

191. Saegusa M, Takano Y, Kishimoto H, Wakabayashi G, Nohga K, Okudaira M. Comparative analysis of p53 and c-myc expression and cell proliferation in human hepatocellular carcinomas: an enhanced immunohistochemical approach. J Cancer Res Clin Oncol 119:737–744, 1993.

192. Su TS, Lin LH, Lui WY, et al. Expression of c-*myc* gene in human hepatomas. Biochem Biophys Res Commun 132:264–268, 1985.

193. Kaneko Y, Shibuya M, Nakayama T, et al. Hypomethylation of c-*myc* and epidermal growth factor receptor genes in human hepatocellular carcinoma and fetal liver. Jpn J Cancer Res 76:1136–1140, 1985.

194. Nambu S, Inoue K, Saski H. Site-specific hypomethylation of the c-*myc* oncogene in human hepatocellular carcinoma. Jpn J Cancer Res 78:695–704, 1987.

195. Fujiwara Y, Monden M, Mori T, Nakamura Y, Emi M. Frequent multiplication of the long arm of chromosome 8 in hepatocellular carcinoma. Cancer Res 53:857–860, 1993.

196. Peng SY, Lai PL, Hsu HC. Amplification of the c-*myc* gene in human hepatocellular carcinoma: biologic significance. J Formosan Med Assoc 92:866–870, 1993.

197. Abou-Elella A, Gramlich T, Fritsch C, Gansler T. c-*myc* amplification in hepatocellular carcinoma predicts unfavorable prognosis. Mod Pathol 9:95–98, 1996.

198. Kawate S, Fukusato T, Ohwada S, Watanuki A, Morishita Y. Amplification of c-*myc* in hepatocellular carcinoma: correlation with clinicopathologic features, proliferative activity and p53 overexpression. Oncology 57:157–163, 1999.

199. Taylor JA, Bell A, Nagorney D. L-*myc* proto-oncogene alleles and susceptibility to hepatocellular carcinoma. Int J Cancer 54:927–930, 1993.

200. Choi EK, Uyeno S, Nishida N, et al. Alterations of c-fos methylation in the processes of aging and tumorigenesis in human liver. Mutat Res 354:123–128, 1996.

201. Yakicier MC, Irmak MB, Romano A, Kew M, Ozturk M. *Smad2* and *Smad4* mutations in hepatocellular carcinoma. Oncogene 18:4879–4883, 1999.

202. Schutte M, Hruban RH, Hedrick L, et al. *DPC4* gene in various tumor types. Cancer Res 56:2527–2530, 1996.

203. Piao Z, Kim H, Jeon BK, Le WJ, Park C. Relationship between loss of heterozygosity of tumor suppressor genes and histologic differentiation in hepatocellular carcinoma. Cancer 80:865–872, 1997.

204. Matsuzaki K, Date M, Furukawa F, et al. Autocrine stimulatory mechanism of transforming growth factor beta in human hepatocellular carcinoma. Cancer Res 60:1394–1402, 2000.

205. Ito Y, Matsuura N, Sakon M, et al. Expression and prognostic roles of the G1-S modulators in hepatocellular carcinoma: p27 independently predicts the recurrence. Hepatology 30:90–99, 1999.

206. Zhang YJ, Jiang W, Chen CJ, et al. Amplification and overexpression of cyclin D1 in human hepatocellular carcinoma. Biochem Biophys Res Commun 196:1010–1016, 1993.

207. Nishida N, Fukuda Y, Komeda T, et al. Amplification and overexpression of cyclin D1 gene in aggressive human hepatocellular carcinoma. Cancer Res 54:3107–3110, 1994.

208. Tanigami A, Tokino T, Takita KI, Ueda M, Kasumi F, Nakamura Y. Detailed analysis of an amplified region at chromosome 11q13 in malignant tumors. Genomics 13:21–24, 1992.

209. Peng SY, Chou SP, Hsu HC. Association of down-regulation of cyclin D1 and of overexpression of cyclin E with *p53* mutation, high tumor grade and poor prognosis in hepatocellular carcinoma. J Hepatol 29:281–289, 1998.

210. Covini G, Chan EKL, Nishioka M, Morshed SA, Reed SI, Tan EM. Immune response to cyclin B1 in hepatocellular carcinoma. Hepatology 25:75–80, 1997.

211. Paterlini P, Flejou JF, DeMitri MS, Pisi E, Franco D, Bréchot C. Structure and expression of the cyclin A gene in human primary liver cancer. Correlation with flow cytometric parameters. J Hepatol 23:47–52, 1995.

212. Chao Y, Shih YL, Chiu JH, et al. Overexpression of cyclin A but not Skp2 correlates with the tumor relapse of human hepatocellular carcinoma. Cancer Res 58:985–990, 1998.

213. Wang J, Chenivesse X, Henglein B, Bréchot C. Hepatitis B virus integration in a cyclin A gene in a hepatocellular carcinoma. Nature 343:555–557, 1990.

214. Wang J, Zindy F, Chenivesse X, Lamas E, Henglein B, Bréchot C. Modification of cyclin A expression by hepatitis B virus DNA integration in a hepatocellular carcinoma. Oncogene 7:1653–1656, 1992.

215. DeMitri MS, Pisi E, Brechot C, Paterlini P. Low frequency of allelic loss in the cyclin A gene in human hepatocellular carcinomas: a study based on PCR. Liver 13:259–261, 1993.

216. Gorczyca W, Sarode V, Juan G, Melamed MR, Darzynkiewicz Z. Laser scanning cytometric analysis of cyclin B1 in primary human malignancies. Mod Pathol 10:457–462, 1997.

217. Hui A-M, Sakamoto M, Kanai Y, et al. Inactivation of *p16INK4* in hepatocellular carcinoma. Hepatology 24:575–579, 1996.

218. Piao Z, Park C, Lee JS, Yang CH, Choi KY, Kim H. Homozygous deletions of the *CDKN2* gene and loss of heterozygosity of 9p in primary hepatocellular carcinoma. Cancer Lett 122:201–207, 1998.

219. Matsuda Y, Ichida T, Matsuzawa J, Sugimura K, Asakura H. *p16INK4* is inactivated by extensive CpG methylation in human hepatocellular carcinoma. Gastroenterology 116:394–400, 1999.

220. Chaubert P, Gayer R, Zimmermann A, et al. Germ-line mutations of the *p16INK4* (MTS1) gene occur in a subset of patients with hepatocellular carcinoma. Hepatology 25:1376–1381, 1997.

221. Lin YW, Chen CH, Huang GT, et al. Infrequent mutations and no methylation of CDKN2A (p16/MTS1) and CDKN2B (p15/MTS2) in hepatocellular carcinoma in Taiwan. Eur J Cancer 34:1789–1795, 1998.

222. Liew CT, Li HM, Lo KW, et al. High frequency of *p16INK4A* gene alterations in hepatocellular carcinoma. Oncogene 18:789–795, 1999.

223. Wong IHN, DennisLo YM, Zhang J, et al. Detection of aberrant p16 methylation in the plasma and serum of liver cancer patients. Cancer Res 59:71–73, 1999.

224. Kita R, Nishida N, Fukuda Y, et al. Infrequent alterations in the *p16INK4A* gene in liver cancer. Int J Cancer 67:176–180, 1996.

225. Qin LX, Tang ZY, Liu KD, et al. Alterations of CDKN2(p16/MTS1) exon 2 in human hepatocellular carcinoma. Oncology Rep 3:405–408, 1996.

226. Biden K, Young J, Buttenshaw R, et al. Frequency of mutation and deletion of the tumor suppressor gene *CDKN2A* (*MTS1/p16*) in hepatocellular carcinoma from an Australian population. Hepatology 25:593–597, 1997.

227. Bonilla F, Orlow I, Cordon-Cardo C. Mutational study of *p16CDKN2/MTS1/INK4A* and *p57KIP2* genes in hepatocellular carcinoma. Int J Oncol 12:583–588, 1998.

228. Laes J, Parada LA, Johansson B, Levan G, Szpirer C, Szpirer J. Alterations in P19ARF in rodent hepatoma cell lines but not in human primary liver cancer. Cancer Genet Cytogenet 17:118–124, 2000.

229. Furutani M, Arii S, Tanaka H, et al. Decreased expression and rare somatic mutation of the *CIP1/WAF1* gene in human hepatocellular carcinoma. Cancer Lett 111:191–197, 1997.

230. Hui A-M, Kanai Y, Sakamoto M, Tsuda H, Hirohashi S. Reduced *p21^WAF1/CIP1* expression and *p53* mutation in hepatocellular carcinoma. Hepatology 25:575–579, 1997.

231. Qin LF, Ng IO, Fan ST, Ng M. p21/WAF1, p53 and PCNA expression and *p53* mutation status in hepatocellular carcinoma. Int J Cancer 79:424–428, 1998.

232. Watanabe H, Fukuchi K, Takagi Y, Tomoyasu S, Tsuruoka N, Gomi K. Molecular analysis of *Cip1/Waf1 (p21)* gene in diverse types of human tumors. Biochim Biophys Acta 1263:275–280, 1995.

233. Hui AM, Sun L, Kanai Y, Sakamoto M, Hirohashi S. Reduced p27^Kip1 expression in hepatocellular carcinomas. Cancer Lett 132:67–73, 1998.

234. Hsia CC, DiBisceglie AM, Kleiner DE, Farshid M, Tabor E. *RB* tumor suppressor gene expression in hepatocellular carcinomas from patients infected with the hepatitis B virus. J Med Virol 44:67–73, 1994.

235. Zhang X, Xu HJ, Murakami Y, et al. Deletions of chromosome 13q, mutations in *Retinoblastoma 1*, and retinoblastoma protein state in human hepatocellular carcinoma. Cancer Res 54:4177–4182, 1994.

236. Hui AM, Li X, Makuuchi M, Takayama T, Kubota K. Overexpression and lack of retinoblastoma protein are associated with tumor progression and metastasis in hepatocellular carcinoma. Int J Cancer (Pred Oncol) 84:604–608, 1999.

237. Hada H, Koide N, Morita T, et al. Promoter-independent loss of mRNA and protein of the *Rb* gene in a human hepatocellular carcinoma. Hepatogastroenterology 43:1185–1189, 1996.

238. Murakami Y, Hayashi K, Hirohashi S, Sekiya T. Aberrations of the tumor suppressor *p53* and retinoblastoma genes in human hepatocellular carcinomas. Cancer Res 51:5520–5525, 1991.

239. Nakamura T, Iwamura Y, Kaneko M, et al. Deletions and rearrangements of the retinoblastoma gene in hepatocellular carcinoma, insulinoma and some neurogenic tumors as found in a study of 121 tumors. Jpn J Clin Oncol 21:325–329, 1991.

240. Walker GJ, Hayward NK, Falvey S, Cooksley WGE. Loss of somatic heterozygosity in hepatocellular carcinoma. Cancer Res 51:4367–4370, 1991.

241. Nishida N, Fukada Y, Kokuryu H, et al. Accumulation of allelic loss on arms of chromosomes 13q, 16q and 17p in advanced stages of human hepatocellular carcinoma. Int J Cancer 51:862–868, 1992.

242. Fujimoto Y, Hampton LL, Wirth PJ, Wang NJ, Xie JP, Thorgeirsson SS. Alterations of tumor suppressor genes and allelic losses in human hepatocellular carcinoma in China. Cancer Res 54:281–285, 1994.

243. Kuroki T, Fujiwara Y, Nakamori S, Imaoka S, Kanematsu T, Nakamuri Y. Evidence for the presence of two tumor-suppressor genes for hepatocellular carcinoma on chromosome 13q. Br J Cancer 72:383–385, 1995.

244. Ashida K, Kishimoto Y, Nakamoto K, et al. Loss of heterozygosity of the retinoblastoma gene in liver cirrhosis accompanying hepatocellular carcinoma. J Cancer Res Clin Oncol 123:489–495, 1997.

245. Nakamura T, Monden Y, Kawashima K, Naruke T, Nishimura S. Failure to detect mutations in the retinoblastoma protein-binding domain of the transcription factor E2F-1 in human cancers. Jpn J Cancer Res 87:1204–1209, 1996.

246. Zhao M, Zhang NX, Laissue JA, Zimmermann A. Immunohistochemical analysis of p53 protein overexpression in liver cell dysplasia and hepatocellular carcinoma. Virchows Arch 424:613–621, 1994.

247. Goldblum JR, Bartos RE, Carr KA, Frank TS. Hepatitis B and alterations of the *p53* tumor suppressor gene in hepatocellular carcinoma. Am J Surg Pathol 17:1244–1251, 1993.

248. Ng IO, Chung LP, Tsang SWY, et al. *p53* gene mutation spectrum in hepatocellular carcinomas in Hong Kong Chinese. Oncogene 9:985–990, 1994.

249. Ng IO, Srivastava G, Chung LP, Tsang SW, Ng MM. Overexpression and point mutations of *p53* tumor suppressor gene in hepatocellular carcinomas in Hong Kong Chinese people. Cancer 74:30–37, 1994.

250. Volkmann M, Hofmann WJ, Müller M, et al. p53 overexpression is frequent in European hepatocellular carcinoma and largely independent of codon 249 hot spot mutations. Oncogene 9:195–204, 1994.

251. Livni N, Eid A, Ilan Y, et al. p53 expression in patients with cirrhosis with and without hepatocellular carcinoma. Cancer 75:2420–2426, 1995.

252. Ojanguren I, Ariza A, Castellà EM, Fernández-Vasalo A, Mate JL, Navas-Palacios JJ. p53 immunoreactivity in hepatocellular adenoma, focal nodular hyperplasia, cirrhosis and hepatocellular carcinoma. Histopathology 26:63–68, 1995.

253. Kang YK, Kim CJ, Kim WH, Kim HO, Kang GH, Kim YI. *p53* mutation and overexpression in hepatocellular carcinoma and dysplastic nodules in the liver. Virchows Arch 432:27–32, 1998.

254. Hosono S, Lee CS, Chou MJ, Yang, CS, Shih C. Molecular analysis of the p53 alleles in primary hepatocellular carcinomas and cell lines. Oncogene 6:237–243, 1991.

255. Challen C, Lunec J, Warren W, Collier J, Bassendine MF. Analysis of the *p53* tumor-suppressor gene in hepatocellular carcinomas from Britain. Hepatology 16:1362–1366, 1992.

256. Hsia CC, Kleiner DE, Axiotis CA, et al. Mutations of *p53* gene in hepatocellular carcinoma: roles of hepatitis B virus and aflatoxin contamination in the diet. J Natl Cancer Inst 84:1638–1641, 1992.

257. Laurent-Puig P, Flejou JF, Fabre M, et al. Overexpression of p53: a rare event in a large series of white patients with hepatocellular carcinoma. Hepatology 16:1171–1175, 1992.

258. Choi SW, Hytiroglu P, Geller SA, et al. The expression of p53 antigen in primary malignant epithelial tumors of the liver: an immunohistochemical study. Liver 13:172–176, 1993.

259. Hsu HC, Tseng HJ, Lai PL, Lee PH, Peng SY. Expression of *p53* gene in 184 unifocal hepatocellular carcinomas: association with tumor growth and invasiveness. Cancer Res 53:4691–4694, 1993.

260. Kar S, Jaffe R, Carr BI. Mutation at codon 249 of *p53* gene in a human hepatoblastoma. Hepatology 18:566–569, 1993.

261. Shieh YSC, Nguyen C, Vocal MV, Chu HW. Tumor-suppressor *p53* gene in hepatitis C and B virus–associated hepatocellular carcinoma. Int J Cancer 54:558–562, 1993.

262. Kennedy SM, MacGeogh C, Jaffe R, Spurr NK. Overexpression of the oncoprotein p53 in primary hepatic tumors of childhood does not correlate with gene mutations. Hum Pathol 25:438–442, 1994.

263. Bourdon JC, D'Errico A, Paterlini P, Grigioni W, May E, Debuire B. p53 protein accumulation in European hepatocellular carcinoma is not always dependent on p53 gene mutation. Gastroenterology 108:1176–1182, 1995.

264. Hayashi H, Sugio K, Matsumata T, Adachi E, Takenaka K, Sugimachi K. The clinical significance of *p53* gene mutation in hepatocellular carcinomas from Japan. Hepatology 22:1702–1707, 1995.

265. Kubicka S, Trautwein C, Schrem H, Tillmann H, Manns M. Low incidence of *p53* mutations in European hepatocellular carcinomas with heterogeneous mutation as a rare event. J Hepatol 23:412–419, 1995.

266. Nakopoulou L, Janinis J, Giannopoulou I, Lazaris AC, Koureas A, Zacharoulis D. Immunohistochemical expression of p53 protein and proliferating cell nuclear antigen in hepatocellular carcinoma. Pathol Res Pract 191:1208–1213, 1995.

267. DeBenedetti VMG, Welsh JA, Yu MC, Bennett WP. *p53* mutations in hepatocellular carcinoma related to oral contraceptive use. Carcinogenesis 17:145–149, 1996.

268. Soini Y, Chia SC, Bennett WP, et al. An aflatoxin-associated mutational hotspot at codon 249 in the *p53* tumor suppressor gene occurs in hepatocellular carcinomas from Mexico. Carcinogenesis 17:1007–1012, 1996.

269. Lunn RM, Zhang YJ, Wang LY, et al. *p53* mutations, chronic hepatitis B virus infection and aflatoxin exposure in hepatocellular carcinoma in Taiwan. Cancer Res 57:3471–3477, 1997.

270. Nakashima Y, Hsia CC, Yuwen H, et al. p53 overexpression in small hepatocellular carcinomas containing two different histologic grades. Int J Oncol 12:455–459, 1998.

271. Qin G, Su J, Ning Y, Duan X, Luo D, Lotlikar PD. p53 protein expression in patients with hepatocellular carcinoma from the high incidence area of Guangxi, Southern China. Cancer Lett 121:203–210, 1997.

272. Feitelson MA, Zhu M, Duan LX, London WT. Hepatitis B X antigen and p53 are associated in vitro and in liver tissues from patients with primary hepatocellular carcinoma. Oncogene 8:1109–1117, 1993.

273. Hosono S, Chou MJ, Lee CS, Shih C. Infrequent mutation of *p53* gene in hepatitis B virus positive primary hepatocellular carcinoma. Oncogene 8:491–496, 1993.

274. Bressac B, Kew M, Wands J, Ozturk M. Selective G to T mutations of *p53* gene in hepatocellular carcinoma from southern Africa. Nature 350:429–431, 1991.

275. Buetow KH, Sheffield VC, Zhu M, et al. Low frequency of *p53* mutations observed in a diverse collection of primary hepatocellular carcinomas. Proc Natl Acad Sci USA 89:9622–9626, 1992.

276. Oda T, Tsuda H, Scarpa A, Sakamoto M, Hirohashi S. Mutation pattern of the *p53* gene as a diagnostic marker for multiple hepatocellular carcinoma. Cancer Res 52:3674–3678, 1992.

277. Oda T, Tsuda H, Scarpa A, Sakamoto M, Hirohashi S. *p53* gene mutation spectrum in hepatocellular carcinoma. Cancer Res 52:6358–6364, 1992.

278. Sheu JC, Huang GT, Lee PH, et al. Mutation of *p53* gene in hepatocellular carcinoma in Taiwan. Cancer Res 52:6098–6100, 1992.

380. Christa L, Carnot F, Simon MT, et al. HIP/PAD is an adhesive protein expressed in hepatocarcinoma, normal paneth, and pancreatic cells. Am J Physiol 271:G993–G1002, 1996.

381. Ljubimova JY, Wilson SE, Petrovic LM, et al. Novel human malignancy-associated gene (MAG) expressed in various tumors and in some tumor pre-existing conditions. Cancer Res 58:4475–4479, 1998.

382. Yamashita N, Ishibashi H, Hayashida K, et al. High frequency of the MAGE-1 gene expression in hepatocellular carcinoma. Hepatology 24:1437–1440, 1996.

383. Liu BB, Ye SL, He P, Liu Y-K, Tang Z-Y. MAGE-1 and MAGE gene expression may be associated with hepatocellular carcinoma. J Cancer Res Clin Oncol 125:685–689, 1999.

384. Kariyama K, Higashi T, Kobayashi Y, et al. Expression of MAGE-1 and -3 genes and gene products in human hepatocellular carcinoma. Br J Cancer 81:1080–1087, 1999.

385. Tahara T, Mori M, Sadanaga N, Sakamoto Y, Kitano S, Makuuchi M. Expression of the MAGE gene family in hepatocellular carcinoma. Cancer 85:1234–1240, 1999.

386. Tsuzurahara S, Sata M, Iwamoto O, et al. Detection of MAGE-4 protein in the sera of patients with hepatitis-C virus–associated hepatocellular carcinoma and liver cirrhosis. Jpn J Cancer Res 88:915–918, 1997.

387. Katagiri T, Nakamura Y, Miki Y. Mutations in the BRCA2 gene in hepatocellular carcinoma. Cancer Res 56:4575–4577, 1996.

388. Charlotte F, L'Hermine A, Martin N, et al. Immunohistochemical detection of bcl-2 normal and pathological human liver. Am J Pathol 144:460–465, 1994.

389. Zhao M, Zhang NX, Economou M, Blaha I, Laissue JA, Zimmermann A. Immunohistochemical detection of bcl-2 protein in liver lesions; bcl-2 protein is expressed in hepatocellular carcinomas but not in liver cell dysplasia. Histopathology 25:237–245, 1994.

390. Hiramatsu N, Hayashi N, Katayama K, et al. Immunohistochemical detection of Fas antigen in liver tissue of patients with chronic hepatitis C. Hepatology 19:1354–1359, 1994.

391. Mochizuki K, Hayashi N, Hiramatsu N, et al. Fas antigen expression in liver tissues of patients with chronic hepatitis B. J Hepatology 24:1–7, 1996.

392. Galle PR, Hofmann WJ, Walczak H, et al. Involvement of the CD95 (APO-1/Fas) receptor and ligand in liver damage. J Exp Med 182:1223–1230, 1995.

393. Strand S, Hofmann WJ, Hug H, et al. Lymphocyte apoptosis induced by CD95 (APO-1/Fas) ligand-expressing tumor cells—a mechanism of immune invasion? Nat Med 2:1361–1366, 1996.

394. Nagao M, Nakajima Y, Hisanaga M, et al. The alteration of Fas receptor and ligand system in hepatocellular carcinomas: how do hepatoma cells escape from the host immune surveillance in vivo? Hepatology 30:413–421, 1999.

395. Kubo K, Matsuzaki Y, Okazaki M, Kato A, Kobayashi N, Okita K. The Fas system is not significantly involved in apoptosis in human hepatocellular carcinoma. Liver 18:117–123, 1998.

396. Shin EC, Shin JS, Park JH, Kim JJ, Kim H, Kim SJ. Expression of Fas-related genes in human hepatocellular carcinomas. Cancer Lett 134:155–162, 1998.

397. Jodo S, Kobayashi S, Nakajima Y, et al. Elevated serum levels of soluble Fas/APO-1 (CD95) in patients with hepatocellular carcinoma. Clin Exp Immunol 112:166–171, 1998.

398. Sugimoto K, Shiraki K, Ito T, et al. Expression of functional CD40 in human hepatocellular carcinoma. Hepatology 30:920–926, 1999.

399. Ninomiya T, Hayashi Y, Saijon K, et al. Expression ratio of hepatocyte nuclear factor-1 to variant hepatocyte nuclear factor-1 in differentiation of hepatocellular carcinoma and hepatoblastoma. J Hepatol 25:445–453, 1996.

400. Wang W, Hayashi Y, Ninomiya T, et al. Expression of HNF-1 α and HNF-1 β in various histological differentiations of hepatocellular carcinoma. J Pathol 184:272–278, 1998.

401. Kishimoto T, Kokura K, Ohkawa N, et al. Enhanced expression of a new class of liver-enriched b-Zip transcription factors, hepatocarcinogenesis-related transcription factor, in hepatocellular carcinomas of rats and humans. Cell Growth Differ 9:337–344, 1998.

402. Tahara T, Nakanishi T, Kitamoto M, et al. Telomerase activity in human liver tissue: comparison between chronic liver disease and hepatocellular carcinomas. Cancer Res 55:2734–2736, 1995.

403. Kojima H, Yokosuka O, Imazeki F, Saisho H, Omata M. Telomerase activity and telomere length in hepatocellular carcinoma and chronic liver disease. Gastroenterology 112:493–500, 1997.

404. Miura N, Horikawa I, Nishimoto A, et al. Progressive telomere shortening and telomerase reactivation during hepatocellular carcinogenesis. Cancer Genet Cytogenet 93:56–62, 1997.

405. Kitada T, Seki S, Kawakita N, Kuroki T, Monna T. Telomere shortening in chronic liver diseases. Biochem Biophys Res Commun 211:33–39, 1995.

406. Ohashi K, Tsutsumi M, Kobitsu K, et al. Shortened telomere length in hepatocellular carcinomas and corresponding background liver tissues of patients infected with hepatitis virus. Jpn J Cancer Res 87:419–422, 1996.

407. Ohashi K, Tsutsumi M, Nakajima Y, Kobitsu K, Nakano H, Konishi Y. Telomere changes in human hepatocellular carcinomas and hepatitis virus infected noncancerous livers. Cancer 77(Suppl 8):1747–1751, 1996.

408. Urabe Y, Nouso K, Higashi T, et al. Telomere length in human liver diseases. Liver 16:293–297, 1996.

409. Isokawa O, Suda T, Aoyagi Y, et al. Reduction of telomeric repeats as a possible predictor for development of hepatocellular carcinoma: convenient evaluation by slot-blot analysis. Hepatology 30:408–412, 1999.

410. Nakayama J, Tahara H, Tahara E, et al. Telomerase activation by hTRT in human normal fibroblasts and hepatocellular carcinomas. Nat Genet 18:65–68, 1998.

411. Wada E, Hisatomi H, Moritoyo T, Kanamaru T, Hikiji K. Genetic diagnostic test of hepatocellular carcinoma by telomerase catalytic subunit mRNA. Oncol Rep 5:1407–1412, 1998.

412. Ohta K, Kanamaru T, Yamamoto M, Saitoh Y. Clinical significance of telomerase activity in hepatocellular carcinoma. Kobe J Med Sci 42:207–217, 1996.

413. Nakashio R, Kitamoto M, Tahara H, Nakanishi T, Ide T, Kajiyama G. Significance of telomerase activity in the diagnosis of small differentiated hepatocellular carcinoma. Int J Cancer 74:141–147, 1997.

414. Hisatomi H, Nagao K, Kanamura T, Endo H, Tomimatsu M, Hikiji K. Levels of telomerase catalytic subunit mRNA as a predictor of potential malignancy. Int J Oncol 14:727–732, 1999.

415. Hytiroglou P, Kotoula V, Thung SN, Tsokos M, Fiel MI, Papadimitriou CS. Telomerase activity in precancerous hepatic nodules. Cancer 82:1831–1838, 1998.

416. Kojima H, Yokosuka O, Kato N, et al. Quantitative evaluation of telomerase activity in small liver tumors: analysis of ultrasonography-guided liver biopsy specimens. J Hepatol 31:514–520, 1999.

417. Ogami M, Ikura Y, Nishiguchi S, Kuroki T, Ueda M, Sakurai M. Quantitative analysis and in situ localization of human telomerase RNA in chronic liver disease and hepatocellular carcinoma. Lab Invest 79:15–26, 1999.

418. Suda T, Isokawa O, Aoyagi Y, et al. Quantitation of telomerase activity in hepatocellular carcinoma: a possible aid for a prediction of recurrent disease in the remnant liver. Hepatology 27:402–406, 1998.

419. Boland CR, Thibodeau SN, Hamilton SR, et al. A National Cancer Institute workshop on microsatellite instability for cancer detection and familial predisposition: development of international criteria for the determination of microsatellite instability in colorectal cancer. Cancer Res 58:5248–5257, 1998.

420. Han HJ, Yanagisawa A, Kato Y, Park JG, Nakamura Y. Genetic instability in pancreatic cancer and poorly differentiated type of gastric cancer. Cancer Res 53:5087–5089, 1993.

421. Kazachkov Y, Yoffe B, Khaoustov VI, Solomon H, Klintmalm GB, Tabor E. Microsatellite instability in human hepatocellular carcinoma: relationship to p53 abnormalities. Liver 18:156–161, 1998.

422. Takagi K, Esumi M, Takano S, Iwai S. Replication error frequencies in primary hepatocellular carcinoma: a comparison of solitary primary versus multiple primary cancers. Liver 18:272–276, 1998.

423. Horii A, Han HJ, Shimada M, et al. Frequent replication errors at microsatellite loci in tumors of patients with multiple primary cancers. Cancer Res 54:3373–3375, 1994.

424. Yakushiji H, Sinsuke M, Matsukura S, et al. DNA mismatch repair in curatively resected sextuple primary cancers in different organs: a molecular case report. Cancer Lett 142:17–22, 1999.

425. Kondo Y, Kanai Y, Sakamoto M, Mizokami M, Ueda R, Hirohashi S. Microsatellite instability associated with hepatocarcinogenesis. J Hepatol 31:529–536, 1999.

426. Sheu JC, Lin YW, Chou HC, et al. Loss of heterozygosity and microsatellite instability in hepatocellular carcinoma in Taiwan. Br J Cancer 80:468–476, 1999.

427. Boige V, Laurent-Puig L, Fouchet P, et al. Concerted nonsyntenic allelic losses in hyperploid hepatocellular carcinoma is determined by a high-resolution allelotype. Cancer Res 57:1986–1990, 1997.

428. Kaplanski C, Srivatanakul P, Wild C. Frequent rearrangements at minisatellite loci D1S7 (1p33–35), D7S22 (7q36–ter) and D12S11 (12q24.3–ter) in hepatitis B virus–positive hepatocellular carcinomas from Thai patients. Int J Cancer 72:248–254, 1997.

429. Okada S, Ishii H, Nose H, et al. Evidence for increased somatic cell mutations in patients with hepatocellular carcinoma. Carcinogenesis 18:445–449, 1997.
430. Wu X, Gu J, Patt Y, et al. Mutagen sensitivity as a susceptibility marker for human hepatocellular carcinoma. Cancer Epidemiol Biomarkers Prev 7:567–570, 1998.
431. Nagai H, Pineau P, Tiollais P, Buendia MA, Dejean A. Comprehensive allelotyping of human hepatocellular carcinoma. Oncogene 14:2927–2933, 1997.
432. Piao Z, Park C, Park JH, Kim H. Allelotype analysis of hepatocellular carcinoma. Int J Cancer 75:29–33, 1998.
433. Yeh SH, Chen PJ, Chen HL, Lai MY, Wang CC, Chen DS. Frequent genetic alterations at the distal region of chromosome 1p in human hepatocellular carcinomas. Cancer Res 54:4188–4192, 1994.
434. Buetow KH, Murray JC, Israel JL, et al. Loss of heterozygosity suggests tumor suppressor gene responsible for primary hepatocellular carcinoma. Proc Natl Acad Sci USA 86:8852–8856, 1989.
435. Yeh SH, Chen PJ, Lai MY, Chen S. Allelic loss on chromosomes 4q and 16q in hepatocellular carcinoma: association with elevated alpha-fetoprotein production. Gastroenterology 110:184–192, 1996.
436. Piao Z, Park C, Park JH, Kim H. Deletion mapping of chromosome 4q in hepatocellular carcinoma. Int J Cancer 79:356–360, 1998.
437. Bando K, Nagai H, Matsumoto S, et al. Identification of a 1-cM region of common deletion on 4q35 associated with progression of hepatocellular carcinoma. Genes Chromosomes Cancer 25:284–289, 1999.
438. Emi M, Fujiwara Y, Ohata H, et al. Allelic loss at chromosome band 8p21.3–p22 is associated with progression of hepatocellular carcinoma. Genes Chromosomes Cancer 7:152–157, 1993.
439. Fujiwara Y, Ohata H, Emi M, et al. A 3-Mb physical map of the chromosome region 8p21.3–p22, including a 600-kb region commonly deleted in human hepatocellular carcinoma, colorectal cancer, and non-small cell lung cancer. Genes Chromosomes Cancer 10:7–14, 1994.
440. Piao Z, Kim N-G, Kim H, Park C. Deletion mapping of the short arm of chromosome 8 in hepatocellular carcinoma. Cancer Lett 138:227–232, 1999.
441. Pineau P, Nagai H, Prigent S, et al. Identification of three distinct regions on the short arm of chromosome 8 in hepatocellular carcinoma. Oncogene 18:3127–3134, 1999.
442. Wang HP, Rogler CE. Deletion in human chromosome arms 11p and 13q in primary hepatocellular carcinomas. Cytogenet Cell Genet 48:72–78, 1988.
443. Tsuda H, Zhang W, Shimosato Y, et al. Allele loss on chromosome 16 associated with progression of human hepatocellular carcinoma. Proc Natl Acad Sci USA 87:6791–6794, 1990.
444. Koyama M, Nagai H, Bando K, Ito M, Moriyama Y, Emi M. Localization of a target region of allelic loss to a 1-cM interval on chromosome 16p13.13 in hepatocellular carcinoma. Jpn J Cancer Res 90:951–956, 1999.
445. Piao Z, Park C, Kim JJ, Kim H. Deletion mapping of chromosome 16q in hepatocellular carcinoma. British J Cancer 80:850–854, 1999.
446. Fujiwara Y, Ohata H, Kuroki T, et al. Isolation of a candidate tumor suppressor gene on chromosome 8p21.3–p22 that is homologous to an extracellular domain of the PDGF receptor beta gene. Oncogene 10:891–895, 1995.
447. Yuan B-Z, Miller MJ, Keck CL, Zimonjic DB, Thorgeirsson SS, Popescu NC. Cloning, characterization, and chromosomal localization of a gene frequently deleted in human liver cancer (DLC-1) homologous to rat RhoGAP. Cancer Res 58:2196–2199, 1998.
448. Parada LA, Hallén M, Tranberg KG, et al. Frequent rearrangements of chromosomes 1, 7, and 8 in primary liver cancer. Genes Chromosomes Cancer 23:26–35, 1998.
449. Nasarek A, Werner M, Nolte M, Klempnauer J, Georgii A. Trisomy 1 and 8 occur frequently in hepatocellular carcinoma but not in liver cell adenoma and focal nodular hyperplasia. A fluorescence in situ hybridization study. Virchows Arch 427:373–378, 1995.
450. Hamon-Benais C, Ingster O, Terris B, et al. Interphase cytogenetic studies of human hepatocellular carcinomas by fluorescent in situ hybridization. Hepatology 23:429–435, 1996.
451. Kimura H, Kagawa K, Deguchi T, et al. Cytogenetic analyses of hepatocellular carcinoma by in situ hybridization with a chromosome-specific DNA probe. Cancer 77:271–277, 1996.
452. Ohsawa N, Sakamoto M, Saito T, Kobayashi M, Hirohashi S. Numerical chromosome aberrations in hepatocellular carcinoma detected by fluorescence in situ hybridization. J Hepatol 25:655–662, 1996.
453. Zimmermann U, Feneux D, Mathey G, Gayral F, Franco D, Bedossa P. Chromosomal aberrations in hepatocellular carcinomas: relationship with pathological features. Hepatology 26:1492–1498, 1997.
454. Kato A, Kubo K, Kurokawa F, Okita K, Oga A, Murakami T. Numerical aberrations of chromosomes 16, 17, and 18 in hepatocellular carcinoma: a FISH and FCM analysis of 20 cases. Dig Dis Sci 43:1–7, 1998.
455. Huang SF, Hsu HC, Fletcher JA. Investigation of chromosomal aberrations in hepatocellular carcinomas by fluorescence in situ hybridization. Cancer Genet Cytogenet 111:21–27, 1999.
456. Huang SF, Hsu HC, Cheng YM, Chang TC. Allelic loss at chromosome band 6q14 correlates with favorable prognosis in hepatocellular carcinoma. Cancer Genet Cytogenet 116:23–27, 2000.
457. Marchio A, Meddeb M, Pineau P, et al. Recurrent chromosomal abnormalities in hepatocellular carcinoma detected by comparative genomic hybridization. Genes Chromosomes Cancer 18:59–65, 1997.
458. Kusano N, Shiraishi K, Kubo K, Oga A, Okita K, Sasaki K. Genetic aberrations detected by comparative genomic hybridization in hepatocellular carcinomas: their relationship to clinicopathological features. Hepatology 29:1858–1862, 1999.
459. Lin YW, Sheu JC, Huang GT, et al. Chromosomal abnormality in hepatocellular carcinoma by comparative genomic hybridization in Taiwan. Eur J Cancer 35:652–658, 1999.
460. Qin LX, Tang ZY, Sham JST, et al. The association of chromosome 8p deletion and tumor metastasis in human hepatocellular carcinoma. Cancer Res 59:5662–5665, 1999.
461. Sakakura C, Hagiwara A, Taniguchi H, et al. Chromosomal aberrations associated with hepatitis C virus infection detected by comparative genomic hybridization. Br J Cancer 80:2034–2039, 1999.
462. Wong N, Lai P, Lee SW, et al. Assessment of genetic changes in hepatocellular carcinoma by comparative genomic hybridization analysis. Relationship to disease stage, tumor size, and cirrhosis. Am J Pathol 154:37–43, 1999.
463. Barnard GF, Staniunas RJ, Bao S, et al. Increased expression of human ribosomal phosphoprotein PO messenger RNA in hepatocellular carcinoma and colon cancer. Cancer Res 52:3067–3072, 1992.
464. Huang LR, Hsu HC. Cloning and expression of CD24 gene in human hepatocellular carcinoma: a potential early tumor marker gene correlates with p53 mutation and tumor differentiation. Cancer Res 55:4717–4721, 1995.
465. Christa L, Simon MT, Flinois JP, Gebhardt R, Bréchot C, Lasserre C. Overexpression of glutamine synthetase in human primary liver cancer. Gastroenterology 106:1312–1320, 1994.
466. Osada T, Sakamoto M, Nagawa H, et al. Acquisition of glutamine synthetase expression in human hepatocarcinogenesis. Relation to disease recurrence and possible regulation by ubiquitin-dependent proteolysis. Cancer 85:819–831, 1999.
467. Gan FY, Gesell MS, Moshier JA, Alousi M, Luk GD. Detection of ornithine decarboxylase messenger RNA in human hepatocellular carcinoma by in situ hybridization. Epithel Cell Biol 1:13–17, 1992.
468. Tamori A, Nishiguchi S, Kuroki T, et al. Relationship of ornithine decarboxylase activity and histological findings in human hepatocellular carcinoma. Hepatology 20:1179–1186, 1994.
469. Tamori A, Nishiguchi S, Kuroki T, et al. Point mutation of ornithine decarboxylase gene in human hepatocellular carcinoma. Cancer Res 55:3500–3503, 1995.
470. Kanai Y, Ushijima S, Tsuda H, Sakamoto M, Sugimura T, Hirohashi S. Aberrant DNA methylation on chromosome 16 is an early event in hepatocarcinogenesis. Jpn J Cancer Res 87:1210–1217, 1996.
471. Sun L, Hui AM, Kanai Y, Sakamoto M, Hirohashi S. Increased DNA methyltransferase expression is associated with an early stage of human hepatocarcinogenesis. Jpn J Cancer Res 88:1165–1170, 1997.
472. Cai J, Sun WM, Hwang JJ, Stain SC, Lu SC. Changes in S-adenosylmethionine synthetase in human liver cancer: molecular characterization and significance. Hepatology 24:1090–1097, 1996.
473. Chen YM, Shiu JY, Tzeng SJ, et al. Characterization of glycine-N-methyltransferase-gene expression in human hepatocellular carcinoma. Int J Cancer 75:787–793, 1998.
474. Simpson KJ, Lukas NW, Colletti L, Strieter RM, Kunkel SL. Cytokines and the liver. J Hepatol 27:1120–1132, 1997.
475. Martinez-Hernandez A, Amenta PS. The extracellular matrix in hepatic regeneration. FASEB J 9:1401–1410, 1995.
476. Tanaka S, Takenaka K, Matsumata T, Mori R, Sugimachi K. Hepatitis C–virus replication is associated with expression of transforming growth factor-alpha and insulin-like growth factor-II in cirrhotic livers. Dig Dis Sci 41:208–215, 1996.
477. Hsia CC, Thorgeirsson SS, Tabor E. Expression of hepatitis B surface and core antigens and transforming growth factor-alpha in "oval cells" of the liver in patients with hepatocellular carcinoma. J Med Virol 43:216–221, 1994.

478. Tabor E, Farshid K, Di Bisceglie A, Hsia CC. Increased expression of transforming growth factor alpha after transfection of a human hepatoblastoma cell line with the hepatitis B virus. J Med Virol 37:271–273, 1992.

479. Ono M, Morisawa K, Nie J, et al. Transactivation of transforming growth factor alpha gene by hepatitis B virus preS1. Cancer Res 58: 1813–1816, 1998.

480. Luo JC, Yu MW, Chen CJ, Santella RM, Carney WP, Brandt-Rauf PW. Serum c-erbB-2 oncopeptide in hepatocellular carcinogenesis. Med Sci Res 21:305–307, 1993.

481. Nagy P, Schaff Z, Lapis K. Immunohistochemical detection of transforming growth factor-beta 1 in fibrotic liver diseases. Hepatology 14: 269–273, 1991.

482. Milani S, Herbst H, Schuppan D, Stein H, Surrenti C. Transforming growth factors beta 1 and beta 2 are differentially expressed in fibrotic liver disease. Am J Pathol 139:1221–1229, 1991.

483. Annoni G, Weiner FR, Zern MA. Increased transforming growth factor-beta 1 gene expression in human liver disease. J Hepatol 14:259–264, 1992.

484. Roulot D, Durand H, Coste T, et al. Quantitative analysis of transforming growth factor beta 1 messenger RNA in the liver of patients with chronic hepatitis C: absence of correlation between high levels and severity of disease. Hepatology 21:298–304, 1995.

485. Haritani H, Esumi M, Uchida T, Shikata T. Oncogene expression in the liver tissue of patients with nonneoplastic liver disease. Cancer 67: 2594–2598, 1991.

486. Aguilar F, Harris CC, Sun T, Hollstein M, Cerutti P. Geographic variation of *p53* mutational profile in nonmalignant human liver. Science 264:1317–1319, 1994.

487. Iwamoto KS, Mizuno T, Kurata A, Masuzawa M, Mori T, Seyama T. Multiple, unique, and common *p53* mutations in a thoratrast recipient with four primary cancers. Hum Pathol 29:412–416, 1998.

488. Tsopanomichalou M, Kouroumanlis E, Ergazaki M, Spandidos DA. Loss of heterozygosity and microsatellite instability in human non-neoplastic hepatic lesions. Liver 19:305–311, 1999.

489. Salvucci M, Lemoine A, Azoulay D, et al. Frequent microsatellite instability in post-hepatitis B viral cirrhosis. Oncogene 13:2681–2685, 1996.

490. Kishimoto Y, Shiota G, Wada K, et al. Frequent loss in chromosome 8p loci in liver cirrhosis accompanying hepatocellular carcinoma. J Cancer Res Clin Oncol 122:585–589, 1996.

491. Roncalli M, Bianchi P, Grimaldi GC, et al. Fractional allelic loss in non–end-stage cirrhosis: correlation with hepatocellular carcinoma during follow-up. Hepatology 31:846–850, 2000.

492. Tokino T, Matsubara K. Chromosomal sites for hepatitis B virus integration in human hepatocellular carcinoma. J Virol 65:6761–6764, 1991.

493. Haruna Y, Hayashi N, Katayama K, et al. Expression of X protein and hepatitis B virus replication in chronic hepatitis. Hepatology 13:417–421, 1991.

494. Wang WL, London WI, Feitelson MA. Hepatitis B virus X antigen in hepatitis B virus carrier patients with liver cancer. Cancer Res 51: 4971–4977, 1991.

495. Paterlini P, Poussin K, Kew M, Franco D, Brechot C. Selective accumulation of the X transcript of the hepatitis in patients negative for hepatitis B surface antigen with hepatocellular carcinoma. Hepatology 21: 313–321, 1995.

496. Greenblatt MS, Feitelson MA, Zhu M, et al. Integrity of p53 in hepatitis B X antigen-positive and -negative hepatocellular carcinoma. Cancer Res 57:426–432, 1997.

497. Su Q, Schröder CH, Hoffmann WJ, Otto G, Pichlmayr R, Bannasch P. Expression of hepatitis B virus X protein in HBV-infected livers and hepatocellular carcinoma. Hepatology 27:1109–1120, 1998.

498. Zhang XK, Egan JO, Huang D, Sun ZL, Chien VK, Chiu JF. Hepatitis B virus DNA integration and expression of an erb B–like gene in human hepatocellular carcinoma. Biochem Biophys Res Commun 188: 344–351, 1992.

499. Zhou YZ, Slagle BL, Donehower LA, vanTuinen P, Ledbetter DH, Butel JS. Structural analysis of a hepatitis B virus genome integrated into chromosome 17p of a human hepatocellular carcinoma. J Virol 62: 4224–4231, 1988.

500. Becker SA, Zhou YZ, Slagle BL. Frequent loss of chromosome 8p in hepatitis B virus–positive hepatocellular carcinomas from China. Cancer Res 56:5092–5097, 1996.

501. Hatada I, Tokino T, Ochiya T, Matsubara K. Co-amplification of integrated hepatitis B virus DNA and transforming gene *hst-1* in a hepatocellular carcinoma. Oncogene 3:537–540, 1988.

502. Rogler CE, Sherman M, Su CY, et al. Deletion in chromosome 11p associated with a hepatitis B integration site in hepatocellular carcinoma. Science 230:319–322, 1985.

503. Fisher JH, Scoggin CH, Rogler CE. Sequences which flank an 11p deletion observed in an hepatocellular carcinoma map to 11p13. Hum Genet 75:66–69, 1987.

504. Simon D, Carr BI. Integration of hepatitis B virus and alteration of the 1p36 region found in cancerous tissue of primary hepatocellular carcinoma with viral replication evidenced only in noncancerous, cirrhotic tissue. Hepatology 22:1393–1398, 1995.

505. Pasquinelli C, Garreau F, Bougueleret L, et al. Rearrangement of a common cellular DNA domain on chromosome 4 in human primary liver tumors. J Virol 62:629–632, 1988.

506. Blanquet V, Garreau F, Chenivesse X, et al. Regional mapping to 4q32.1 by in situ hybridization of a DNA domain rearranged in human liver cancer. Hum Genet 80:274–276, 1988.

507. Tokino T, Fukushige S, Nakamura T, et al. Chromosome translocation and inverted duplication associated with integrated hepatitis B virus in hepatocellular carcinomas. J Virol 61:3848–3854, 1987.

508. Meyer M, Wiedorn KH, Hofschneider PH, Koshy R, Caselmann WH. A chromosome 17:7 translocation is associated with a hepatitis B virus DNA integration in human hepatocellular carcinoma DNA. Hepatology 15:665–671, 1992.

509. Hino O, Shows TB, Rogler CE. Hepatitis B virus integration site in hepatocellular carcinoma at chromosome 17;18 translocation. Proc Natl Acad Sci USA 83:8338–8342, 1986.

510. Okabe H, Ikai I, Matsuo K, et al. Comprehensive allelotype study of hepatocellular carcinoma: potential differences between hepatitis B virus–positive and –negative tumors. Hepatology 31:1073–1077, 2000.

511. Kawai H, Suda T, Aoyagi Y, et al. Quantitative evaluation of genomic instability as a possible predictor for development of hepatocellular carcinoma: comparison of loss of heterozygosity and replication error. Hepatology 31:1246–1250, 2000.

512. Schlueter V, Meyer M, Hofschneider PH, Koshy R, Caselmann WH. Integrated hepatitis B virus X and 3′ truncated preS/S sequences derived from human hepatomas encode functionally active transactivators. Oncogene 9:3335–3344, 1994.

513. Maguire HF, Hoeffler JP, Siddiqui A. HBVx protein alters the DNA binding specificity of CREB and ATF-2 by protein–protein interactions. Science 252:842–844, 1991.

514. Cheong JH, Yi M, Lin Y, Murakami S. Human RPB5, a subunit shared by eukaryotic nuclear RNA polymerases, binds human hepatitis B virus X protein and may play a role in X transactivation. EMBO J 14: 143–150, 1995.

515. Williams JS, Andrisani OM. The hepatitis B virus X protein targets the basic region–leucine zipper domain of CREB. Proc Natl Acad Sci USA 92:3819–3823, 1995.

516. Lin Y, Nomura T, Cheong J, Dorjsuren D, Iida K, Murakami S. Hepatitis B virus X protein is a transcriptional modulator that communicates with transcription factor II B and the RNA polymerase II subunit 5. J Biol Chem 272:7132–7139, 1997.

517. Twu JS, Schloemer RH. Transcriptional trans-activation function of hepatitis B virus. J Virol 61:3448–3453, 1987.

518. Zhou DX, Tarablous A, Ou JH, Yen TS. Activation of class 1 major histocompatibility complex gene expression by hepatitis B virus. J Virol 64:4025–4028, 1990.

519. Mahe Y, Mukaida N, Kuno K, et al. Hepatitis B virus X protein transactivates human interleukin-8 gene through acting on nuclear factor B and CCAAT/enhancer-binding protein-like *cis*-elements. J Biol Chem 266:13759–13763, 1991.

520. Aufiero B, Schneider RJ. The hepatitis B virus X-gene product transactivates both RNA polymerase II and III promoters. EMBO J 9: 497–504, 1990.

521. Menzo S, Clementi M, Alfani E, et al. Transactivation of epidermal growth factor receptor gene by the hepatitis B virus X-gene product. Virology 196:878–882, 1993.

522. Cross JC, Wen P, Rutter WJ. Transactivation by hepatitis B virus X protein is promiscuous and dependent on mitogen-activated cellular serine/threonine kinases. Proc Natl Acad Sci USA 90:8078–8082, 1993.

523. Kekule AS, Lauer U, Weiss L, Luber B, Hofschneider PH. Hepatitis B virus transactivator HBx uses a tumour promoter signalling pathway. Nature 361:742–745, 1993.

524. Benn J, Schneider RJ. Hepatitis B virus HBx protein activates Ras-GTP complex formation and establishes a Ras, Raf, MAP kinase signalling cascade. Proc Natl Acad Sci USA 91:10350–10354, 1994.

525. Balsano C, Avantaggiati ML, Natoli G, et al. Full-length and truncated versions of the hepatitis B virus (HBV) X protein (pX) transactivate the c-*myc* protooncogene at the transcriptional level. Biochem Biophys Res Commun 176:985–992, 1991.

526. Avantaggiati ML, Natoli G, Balsano C, et al. The hepatitis B virus (HBV) pX transactivates the c-fos through multiple *cis*-acting elements. Oncogene 8:1567–1574, 1993.

527. Twu JS, Lai MY, Chen DS, Robinson WS. Activation of protooncogene c-*jun* by the X-protein of the hepatitis B virus. Virology 192:346–350, 1993.

528. Natoli G, Avantaggiati ML, Chirillo P, et al. Induction of the DNA-binding activity of c-*jun*/c-*fos* heterodimers by the hepatitis B virus transactivator pX. Mol Cell Biol 14:989–998, 1994.

529. Zhou MX, Watabe M, Watabe K. The X gene of human hepatitis B virus transactivates the c-*jun* and alpha-fetoprotein genes. Arch Virol 134:369–378, 1994.

530. Su F, Schneider RJ. Hepatitis B virus HBx protein sensitizes cells to apoptotic killing by tumor necrosis factor alpha. Proc Natl Acad Sci USA 94:8744–8749, 1997.

531. Kim H, Lee H, Yun Y. X-gene product of hepatitis B virus up-regulates tumor necrosis factor alpha gene expression in hepatocytes. Hepatology 28:1012–1013, 1998.

532. Lara-Pezzi E, Majano PL, Gomez-Gonzalo M, et al. The hepatitis B virus X protein up-regulates tumor necrosis factor alpha gene expression in hepatocytes. Hepatology 28:1013–1021, 1998.

533. Benn J, Schneider RJ. Hepatitis B virus HBx protein deregulates cell cycle checkpoint controls. Proc Natl Acad Sci USA 92:11215–11219, 1995.

534. Doria M, Klein N, Lucito R, Schneider RJ. The hepatitis B virus HBx protein is a dual specificity cytoplasmic activator of Ras and nuclear activator transcription factors. EMBO J 14:4747–4757, 1995.

535. Klein NP, Schneider RJ. Activation of Src family kinases by hepatitis B virus HBx protein and coupled signalling to Ras. Mol Cell Biol 17:6427–6436, 1997.

536. Benn J, Su F, Doria M, Schneider RJ. Hepatitis B virus HBx protein induces transcription factor AP-1 by activation of extracellular signal-regulated and c-jun N-terminal mitogen-activated protein kinases. J Virol 70:4978–4985, 1996.

537. Minami M, Poussin K, Kew M, Okanoue T, Brechot C, Paterlini P. Precore/core mutations of hepatitis B virus in hepatocellular carcinomas developed in noncirrhotic livers. Gastroenterology 111:691–700, 1996.

538. Poussin K, Dienes H, Sirma H, et al. Expression of mutated hepatitis B virus X genes in human hepatocellular carcinomas. Int J Cancer 80:497–505, 1999.

539. Sirma H, Giannini C, Poussin K, Paterlini P, Kremsdorf D, Brechot C. Hepatitis B virus X mutants, present in hepatocellular carcinoma tissue, abrogate both the antiproliferative and transactivation effects of HBx. Oncogene 18:4848–4859, 1999.

540. Wang XW, Forrester K, Yeh H, Feitelson MA, Gu JR, Harris CC. Hepatitis B virus X protein inhibits p53 sequence-specific DNA binding, transcriptional activity, and association with transcription factor ERCC3. Proc Natl Acad Sci USA 91:2230–2234, 1994.

541. Henkler F, Waseam N, Golding MH, Alison MR, Koshy R. Mutant p53 but not hepatitis B virus X protein is present in hepatitis B virus–related human hepatocellular carcinoma. Cancer Res 55:6084–6091, 1995.

542. Puisieux A, Ji J, Guillot C, et al. p53-mediated cellular response to DNA damage in cells with replicative hepatitis B virus. Proc Natl Acad Sci USA 92:1342–1346, 1995.

543. Truant R, Antunovic J, Greenblatt J, Prives C, Cromlish JA. Direct interaction of the hepatitis B virus HBx protein with p53 leads to inhibition by HBx of p53 response element-directed transactivation. J Virol 69:1851–1859, 1995.

544. Jia W, Wang XW, Harris CC. Hepatitis B virus x protein inhibits nucleotide excision repair. Int J Cancer 80:875–879, 1999.

545. Wang XW, Gibson MK, Vermeulen W, et al. Abrogation of p53-induced apoptosis by the hepatitis B virus X gene. Cancer Res 55:6012–6016, 1995.

546. Chirillo P, Pagano S, Natoli G, et al. The hepatitis B virus X gene induces p53-mediated programmed cell death. Proc Natl Acad Sci USA 94:8162–8167, 1997.

547. Elmore LW, Hancock AR, Chang SF, et al. Hepatitis B virus X protein and p53 tumor suppressor interactions in the modulation of apoptosis. Proc Natl Acad Sci USA 94:14707–14712, 1997.

548. Gottlob K, Fulco M, Levrero M, Graessmann A. The hepatitis B virus HBx protein inhibits caspase 3 activity. J Biol Chem 273:33347–33353, 1998.

549. Terradillos O, Pollicino T, Lacoeur H, et al. p53-independent apoptotic effects of the hepatitis B virus HBx protein in vivo and in vitro. Oncogene 17:2115–2123, 1998.

550. Sakamuro D, Furukawa T, Takegami T. Hepatitis C virus nonstructural protein NS3 transforms NIH 3T3 cells. J Virol 69:3893–3896, 1995.

551. Ray RB, Lagging LM, Meyer K, Ray R. Hepatitis C virus core protein cooperates with ras and transforms primary rat embryo fibroblasts to tumorigenic phenotype. J Virol 70:4438–4443, 1996.

552. Sullivan D, Gerber MA. Conservation of hepatitis C virus 5′ untranslated sequences in hepatocellular carcinoma and the surrounding liver. Hepatology 19:551–553, 1994.

553. Kim DW, Suzuki R, Harada T, Saito I, Miyama T. Transsuppression of gene expression by hepatitis C viral core protein. Jpn J Med Sci Biol 47:211–220, 1994.

554. Matsumoto M, Hseih TY, Zhu N, et al. Hepatitis C virus core protein interacts with the cytoplasmic tail of lymphotoxin-beta receptor. J Virol 71:1301–1309, 1997.

555. Zhu N, Khoshnan A, Schneider R, et al. Hepatitis C virus core protein binds to the cytoplasmic domain of tumor necrosis factor (TNF) receptor 1 and enhances TNF-induced apoptosis. J Virol 72:3691–3697, 1998.

556. Hsieh TY, Matsumoto M, Chou HC, et al. Hepatitis C virus core protein interacts with heterogeneous nuclear ribonucleoprotein K. J Biol Chem 273:17651–17659, 1998.

557. Shih C, Chen C, Chen S, Wu C, Lee Y. Modulation of the *trans*-activity of hepatitis C virus core protein by phosphorylation. J Virol 69:1160–1171, 1995.

558. Ray RB, Steele R, Meyer K, Ray R. Transcriptional repression of p53 promoter by hepatitis C virus core protein. J Biol Chem 272:10983–10986, 1997.

559. Ray RB, Steele R, Meyer K, Ray R. Hepatitis C virus core protein represses p21WAF1/Cip1/Sid1 promoter activity. Gene 208:331–336, 1998.

560. Ghosh AK, Steale R, Meyer K, Ray R, Ray RB. Hepatitis C virus NS5A protein modulates cell cycle regulatory genes and promotes cell growth. J Gen Virol 80:1179–1183, 1999.

561. Tsuchihara K, Hijikata M, Fukuda K, Kuroki T, Yamamoto N, Shimotohno K. Hepatitis C virus core protein regulates cell growth and signal transduction pathway transmitting growth stimuli. Virology 258:100–107, 1999.

562. Fujita T, Ishido S, Muramatsu S, Itoh M, Hotta H. Suppression of actinomycin D–induced apoptosis by the NS3 protein of hepatitis C virus. Biochem Biophys Res Commun 229:825–831, 1996.

563. Ray RB, Meyer K, Ray R. Suppression of apoptotic cell death by hepatitis C virus core protein. Virology 226:176–182, 1996.

564. Ray RB, Meyer K, Steele R, Shrivastava A, Aggarwal BB, Ray R. Inhibition of tumor necrosis factor (TNF-α)–mediated apoptosis by hepatitis C virus core protein. J Biol Chem 273:2256–2259, 1998.

565. Ruggieri A, Harada T, Matsuura Y, Miyamura T. Sensitization to Fas-mediated apoptosis by hepatitis C virus core protein. Virology 229:68–76, 1997.

566. Marusawa H, Hijikata M, Chiba T, Shimotohno K. Hepatitis C virus core protein inhibits Fas- and tumor necrosis factor α–mediated apoptosis via NF-κ B activation. J Virol 73:4713–4720, 1999.

567. Hengstler JG, van den Burg B, Steinberg P, Oesch F. Interspecies differences in cancer susceptibility and toxicity. Drug Metab Rev 81:917–970, 1999.

568. Wang JS, Groopman JD. DNA damage by mycotoxins. Mutat Res 421:161–181, 1999.

569. Guengerich FP, Johnson WW, Shimada T, Ueng YF, Yamasaki H, Langouët S. Activation and detoxification of aflatoxin B1. Mutat Res 402:121–128, 1998.

570. McGlynn KA, Rosvold EA, Lustbaden ED, et al. Susceptibility to hepatocellular carcinoma is associated with genetic variation in the enzymatic detoxification of aflatoxin $B_1$. Proc Natl Acad Sci USA 92:2384–2387, 1995.

571. Yu MW, Gladek-Yarborough A, Chiamprasert S, Santella RM, Lian YF, Chen CJ. Cytochrome P450 2E1 and glutathione *S*-transferase M1 polymorphisms and susceptibility to hepatocellular carcinoma. Gastroenterology 109:1266–1273, 1995.

572. Greenblatt MS, Bennett WP, Hollstein M, Harris CC. Mutations of the *p53* tumor suppressor gene, clues to cancer etiology and molecular pathogenesis. Cancer Res 54:4855–4878, 1994.

573. Tarao K, Ohkawa S, Shimizu A, et al. Significance of hepatocellular proliferation in the development of hepatocellular carcinoma from anti-hepatitis C virus–positive cirrhotic patients. Cancer 73:1149–1153, 1994.

574. Borzio M, Trerè D, Borzio F, et al. Hepatocyte proliferation is a powerful parameter for predicting hepatocellular carcinoma development in liver cirrhosis. J Clin Pathol (Mol Pathol) 51:96–101, 1998.

575. Su Q, Benner A, Hofmann WJ, Otto G, Pichlmayr R, Bannasch P. Human hepatic preneoplasia: phenotypes and proliferation kinetics of foci and nodules of altered hepatocytes and their relationship to liver cell dysplasia. Virchows Arch 431:391–406, 1998.

576. Tiniakos DG, Brunt EM. Proliferating cell nuclear antigen and Ki-67 labeling in hepatocellular nodules: a comparative study. Liver 19:58–68, 1999.

577. Matsuno Y, Hirohashi S, Furuya S, Sakamoto M, Mukai K, Shimosato Y. Heterogeneity of proliferative activity in nodule-in-nodule lesions of small hepatocellular carcinoma. Jpn J Cancer Res 81:1137–1140, 1990.

578. LeBail B, Belleannee G, Bernard PH, Saric J, Balabaud C, Bioulac-Sage P. Adenomatous hyperplasia in cirrhotic liver; histological evaluation, cellular density, and proliferative activity of 35 macronodular lesions in cirrhotic explants of 10 adult French patients. Hum Pathol 26: 897–906, 1995.

579. Sugitani S, Sakamoto M, Ichida T, Genda T, Asakura H, Hirohashi S. Hyperplastic foci reflect the risk of multicentric development of human hepatocellular carcinoma. J Hepatol 28:1045–1053, 1998.

580. Terasaki S, Kaneko S, Kobayashi K, Nonomura A, Nakanuma Y. Histological features predicting malignant transformation of nonmalignant hepatocellular nodules: a prospective study. Gastroenterology 115: 1216–1222, 1998.

# Chapter 43

# Pathology and Natural History of Hepatocellular Carcinoma

ULYSSES J. BALIS AND GREGORY Y. LAUWERS

Hepatocellular carcinoma (HCC) is heterogeneous in both its gross and microscopic features. Importantly, an increasing number of its characteristics are being demonstrably associated with tumor progression and outcome. Thus, a broad-based understanding of the pathology of HCC is of particular importance to the clinician charged with the management of patients afflicted with this disease.

As the fifth most prevalent malignancy in the world in overall frequency, with 0.5 to 1 million new cases occurring each year,[1-3] there is an ample body of data characterizing this disease and its etiologies. The world areas with the greatest incidences include China and Southeast Asia, and sub-Saharan Africa, where hepatitis B virus (HBV) is the principal etiologic factor and where the comprehensive hepatitis vaccination programs promise a significant reduction in the overall local incidence of HCC.[4,5] In contrast, in Western nations with traditionally low incidence, such as the United States,[6] Japan,[7,8] and United Kingdom,[9] hepatitis C virus (HCV) has emerged as a major etiologic agent, with suggestions that the increasing incidence of HCC in these populations is indeed tied to the increased incidence of HCV.[10]

In other classes of individuals at risk for developing HCC, the risk is tied to the onset and progression of their cirrhosis; these cases are often (but not uniquely) related to alcohol-related cirrhosis and end-stage hemochromatosis. Several studies suggest that the baseline incidence of HCC in cases of ethanol-induced cirrhosis is between 15% and 20%, with chronicity playing a potentiating role.[11,12]

## Preneoplastic Lesions Associated with Hepatocellular Carcinoma

Since the detection of early HCC in cirrhotic patients is being facilitated by the development of high-resolution noninvasive im-

aging techniques, the attention of hepatopathologists is now more directed toward the premalignant processes. Several studies support the concept of a multistep carcinogenesis of HCC in cirrhotic liver.[13-15] The different steps are constituted by a series of nodular lesions characterized by various histologic features. A recently revised terminology of nodular hepatic lesions, developed by an International Working Party, is gaining acceptance worldwide and will be used here.[16] The chronologically successive lesions are macroregenerative nodules, dysplastic nodules (DNs), and well-differentiated HCC.

Dysplastic nodules, which represent the penultimate step of the hepatocellular carcinogenic sequence, usually measure between 0.8 and 1.5 cm in diameter and rarely more than 2.0 cm (Fig. 43–1). They are tan or greenish, characteristically bulge from the cut surface of the liver, and have a soft consistency. Dysplastic nodules have been subclassified into low- and high-grade lesions. Practically, the diagnosis of a DN on frozen section and on cytologic material is an impossible task, and remains challenging on routinely processed material.[16,17]

### Low-Grade Dysplastic Nodules

Low-grade DNs show a significant overlap with macroregenerative nodules and fail to demonstrate significant architectural or cytologic atypia with the exception of large cell changes. They usually contain many portal tracts and hepatic venules and may be subdivided by fibrous septa. The hepatocytes are normal appearing, arranged in plates that are one to two cells thick, and an orderly growth pattern is maintained. The cellular density is essentially comparable to that of the surrounding tissue.[16] One study[18] has suggested that the increased number of unpaired arteries to bile duct suggest a DN rather than a regenerative nodule. Large cell changes (or dysplasia as it was previously called) can be identified either focally or throughout the nodule. These

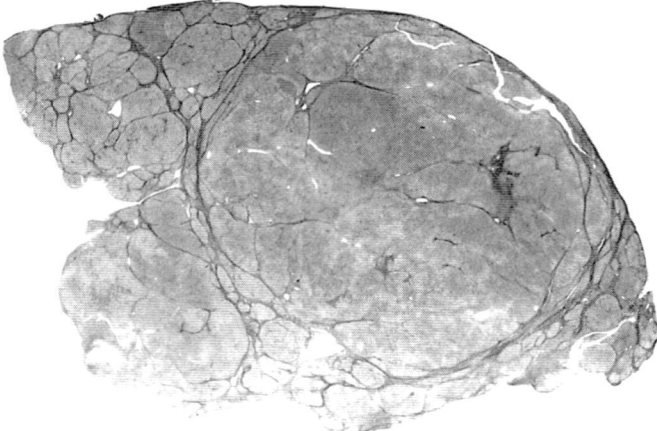

**Figure 43-1** Dysplastic nodule. The expansile lesion is characteristically larger than the surrounding cirrhotic nodules. Residual fibrous septa harboring portal tracts and hepatic venules are identified.

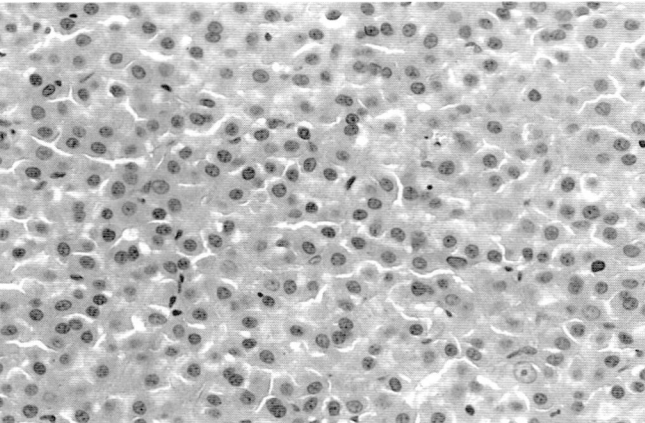

**Figure 43-3** Small cell changes characterized by compact sheets of small, monotonous, atypical hepatocytes exhibiting high nuclear/cytoplasmic ratio.

changes refer to the cellular enlargement of hepatocytes with nuclear pleomorphism and frequent multinucleation (Fig. 43–2). The significance of large changes has been long debated, interpreted as being either a premalignant lesion or a marker of increased risk of HCC. In his 1973 paper that first reported large cell dysplasia, Anthony[19] showed that it was about three times more frequent in cirrhotic liver with HCC than in cirrhotic liver without tumor, in a series of HBV-infected patients from Uganda. These results were later supported by Japanese and European studies.[17,20] However, one well-designed, matched case–control study suggested that large cell dysplasia resulted from hepatocytic polyploidization and thus does not represent a direct premalignant lesion.[21]

## High-Grade Dysplastic Nodules

High-grade DNs can present with a large constellation of cytologic and architectural changes. These include diffuse or focal small cell changes and architectural disarray.[22–24] The latter changes include pseudoacinar formation and thickened liver plates. Histologically, high-grade dysplastic nodules are charac-

terized by small atypical hepatocytes with a high nuclear/cytoplasmic ratio, thickened nuclear membrane, and rare mitoses (Fig. 43–3). Other changes can include clear cell changes, clustering of Mallory bodies, and fatty changes. Iron resistance has also been noted in patients with hemochromatosis. Occasionally, evidence of overt HCC can be seen arising within a high-grade dysplastic nodule (carcinoma in situ).[17,25,26]

To differentiate high-grade DN from well-differentiated HCC is a difficult exercise with diverse criteria advocated by different teams. Also, because of limited experience in the diagnosis of very early lesions, Western pathologists frequently diagnose as DNs lesions that would be diagnosed as well-differentiated HCC in Japan. Features generally accepted as evidence of HCC transformation include the capillarization of sinusoids, development of macrovesicular steatosis with Mallory bodies, clear cell changes, and sinusoidal deviation of nuclei.[26,27] The close relation between high-grade DNs and HCCs is confirmed by the high rate of malignant transformation (50%–78% of cases) arising after a short follow-up period (6–16 months).[27,28]

### Gross Tumor Pattern Classification

The autopsy series-based gross classification of Eggel,[29] now over a century old, divides HCCs into nodular, massive, and diffuse types. The nodular type is composed of tumor nodules scattered within the cirrhotic parenchyma. The massive type consists of a circumscribed, huge tumor nodule occupying most or all of a hepatic lobe (Fig. 43–4). The diffuse type is considerably more rare and characterized by many and indistinct tumor foci, disseminated throughout the cirrhotic liver. To respond to the limitations of Eggel's classification, mostly with regard to small nodular tumors, several proposals modeled after the classification of the Liver Cancer Study Group of Japan have been advanced.[30,31] These proposals have promoted the division of nodular HCC into three subgroups: single nodular (SN, or type 1) (Fig. 43–4), single nodular with extranodular growth (SNEG, or type 2), and confluent multinodular (CMN, or type 3). Patients with type 2 were found to have a worse survival rate. Shimada et al.[31] also reported that among the three subtypes, the SNEG type showed higher rates of portal vein invasion, intrahepatic metastasis, and poorly differentiated histology. Irrespective of the gross appearance, most HCCs are soft neoplasms often display-

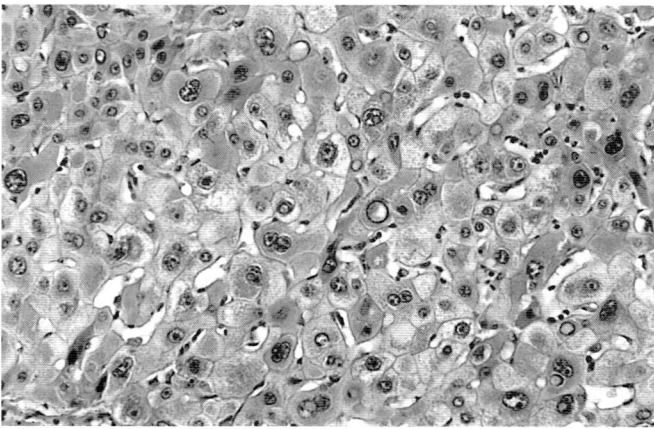

**Figure 43-2** Large cell changes showing enlarged hepatocytes with pleomorphic and multinucleation.

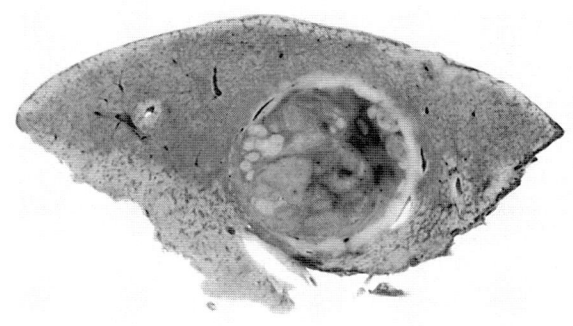

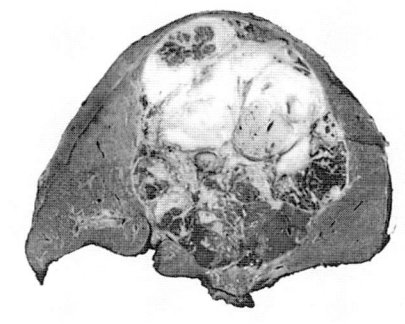

**Figure 43–4** Gross appearance of hepatocellular carcinoma (HCC). Encapsulated, nodular-type HCC is shown in the top image. Massive-type HCC, consisting of a huge tumor occupying most of a hepatic lobe, is shown in the bottom image.

ing necrotic foci of various sizes. Their color ranges from tan–gray to green, depending on the degree of bile production.

## Microscopic Features of Hepatocellular Carcinoma

The microscopic evaluation of HCC is compounded by its variegation in architectural and cytologic features. Cytologically, neoplastic hepatocytes are usually large polygonal and eosinophillic cells with prominent cytoplasmic granularity and well-defined borders.

Hepatocellular carcinomas usually manifest several common architectural arrangements. The World Health Organization has established a five-tier classification of histologic patterns, with only one of these, the fibrolamellar variant, being of prognostic value; the others—trabecular, pseudoglandular, compact, and scirrhous—are not infrequently encountered as any combination of these patterns.[32]

The trabecular pattern, which attempts to recapitulate the normal hepatic architecture, is observed most commonly. In well-differentiated cases of HCC, the hepatic plate architecture is recapitulated, with trabeculae as few as three cells thick (microtrabecular variant), to larger nested sheets, wider than a dozen cells (macrotrabecular variant) (Fig. 43–5).[32,33] A final variant of the trabecular pattern is the solid type, in which the sinusoids are either absent, or collapsed or compressed by broad cords of malignant hepatocytes, giving the tumor a very compact appearance. In large HCCs, it is not unusual to see a spectrum of trabecular morphologies represented across areas of the tumor.

The pseudoglandular (or acinar) pattern is also typically encountered in cases of well-differentiated HCC. It shows hepatocytes forming rosettes with centrally placed or peripherally located bile canaliculi (Fig. 43–5).[34,35] Interestingly, it is this pattern that is most commonly identified with transformed hepatocyte cell lines in vitro, which suggests that this morphology is closely associated with loss of contact inhibition.[36,37]

The scirrhous pattern, which is more often encountered in patients who have received either embolization therapy, radiation, or chemotherapy, exhibits expansive fibrous bands infiltrated by slits or cords of malignant cells. Infrequently, this pattern may arise de novo.[32,38]

A wide spectrum of intracytoplasmic inclusions can be observed in HCCs. These include glycogen, fat, bile, fibrinogen (pale bodies), Mallory's hyaline bodies (Fig. 43–6), α-fetoprotein, giant lysosomes, and $\alpha_1$-antitrypsin.[32]

## Histologic Grading of Hepatocellular Carcinoma

Thorough compendia of current histologic grading of HCC have been reported.[38,39] Briefly, the system of Edmondson and Steiner,[39] first proposed in 1954 and still in widespread use, categorizes tumors into four grades (I to IV) of architectural and cytologic severity, with higher grades putatively predicting worse outcome. Grade I (Fig. 43–7) is composed of well-differentiated

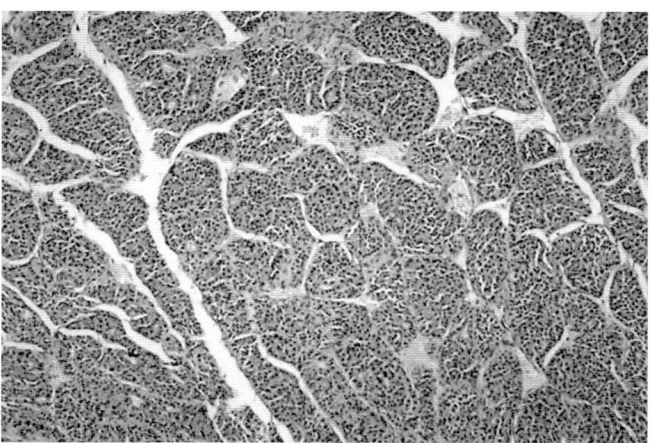

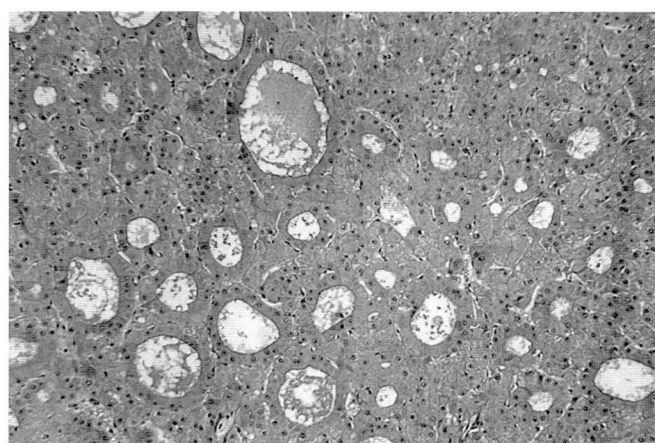

**Figure 43–5** Microscopic architecture of hepatocellular carcinoma. The macrotrabecular variant is composed of wide hepatocytic plates (left) and a pseudoglandular (or acinar) pattern (right).

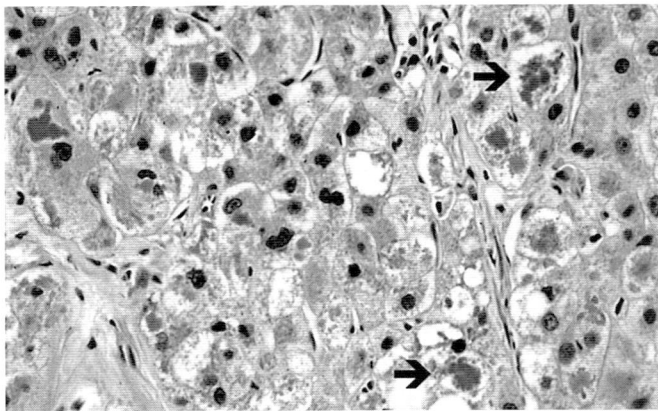

**Figure 43–6** Intracytoplasmic inclusions can be observed in hepatocellular carcinomas. Shown here is an example of Mallory's hyaline bodies (arrows).

neoplastic hepatocytes arranged in thin trabeculae. In grade II, the cells are larger and more atypical, sometimes organized in an acinar pattern. In grade III (Fig. 43–7), architectural and cytologic anaplasia are prominent, but the tumor is still readily identified as hepatocytic in origin. In grade IV, the neoplastic cells are markedly anaplastic and not easily identified as hepatocytic.

As a slight modification of the Edmondson and Steiner system, the Liver Cancer Study Group[38] of Japan classifies HCC into well-, moderately, or poorly differentiated, or undifferentiated forms, based on slightly different architectural and cytologic features. Whether these grading systems are of prognostic utility remains controversial.[40]

## Cytologic and Histologic Subtypes

While of importance in allowing for correct diagnosis, classification of HCC subtypes continues to be controversial with regard to whether tumor subtype plays a role in prognosis. The utility of recognizing these variants remains essentially in the ability to be able to distinguish them from secondary hepatic malignancies.

The clear cell variant of HCC exhibits large, uniform cells with extensive cytoplasmic clearing, occurring as a result of in-

creased intracytoplasmic accumulation of glycogen.[32] It should be distinguished from either metastatic renal cell or adrenocortical carcinoma. Preliminary reports of favorable prognosis associated with this subtype have not been reproduced.[41,42]

The giant cell variant, first described by Kuwano et al. in 1984,[43] contains malignant osteoclast-like giant cells resembling those seen in giant cell tumor of bone. This tumor, also known as pleomorphic variant, typically displays bizarre pleomorphic nuclei and marked anaplasia, seen in combination with more common HCC morphologies. Interestingly, Kojiro et al.[44] and Kyotani et al.[45] provided reasonably compelling evidence that, in some cases, sarcomatous changes may represent, but not exclusively, a specific response to hepatic artery embolization therapy with cisplatin microspheres. However, areas of transition with typical HCC are frequently seen, and in one series cytokeratin staining has been reported in 62% of the cases.[46]

## Prognostically Relevant Variants of Hepatocellular Carcinoma

The recognition of *fibrolamellar carcinoma* (FLC) is of importance, as these tumors typically exhibit a slow growth rate in comparison to the common variants.[47] They are rare, accounting for less than 5% of cases, and typically arise in the second and third decades of life, without gender predilection.[32,48,49] Macroscopically, they can be quite large, ranging from 7 to 20 cm,[48] with the tumor presenting as a sharply demarcated mass without capsule formation. A central fibrous scar is seen in as many as 71% of cases as determined by computerized tomography (CT) imaging.[50] Histologically, they exhibit a characteristic lamellar organized connective tissue with polygonal macrohepatocytes with oncocytic cytoplasm, corresponding ultrastructurally with increased, swollen mitochondria.[32,48] (Fig. 43–8). Additionally, they can show $\alpha_1$-antitrypsin globules and unique pale, ground-glass, cytoplasmic inclusions of fibrinogen known as pale bodies.[32,48] The reduced growth rate and the usual development on non-cirrhotic liver confer an improved prognosis for any given tumor size, with 5-year survival ranging from 35% to 56%.[51,52] However, skeletal metastasis has been reported, with some recurrences manifesting far beyond the 5-year remission interval, illustrating the indolent progression of this variant.[53] At the molecular level, FLCs lack intratumoral genetic heterogeneity or evidence of clonal evolution, in contrast to conventional HCCs.[54,55] However, Wilkens and co-workers[55] reported that there may be

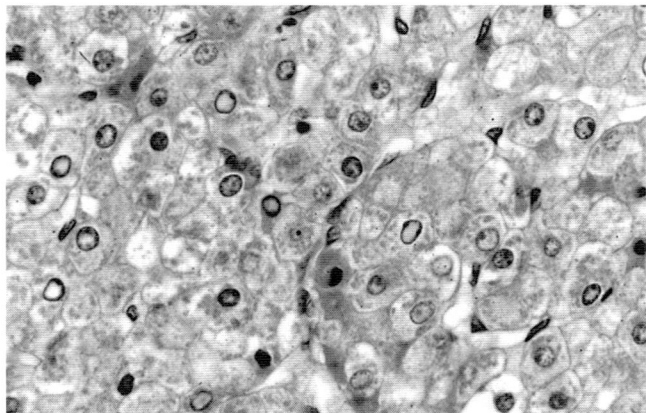 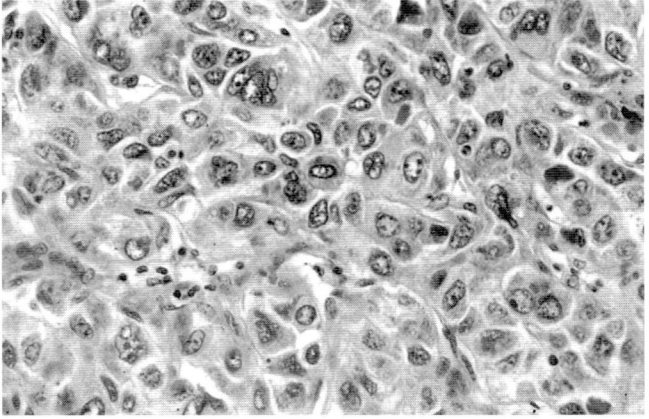

**Figure 43–7** Histologic grading of hepatocellular carcinoma (HCC). Grade I is composed of well-differentiated neoplastic hepatocytes (left). Grade III is characterized by prominent cytologic anaplasia (right).

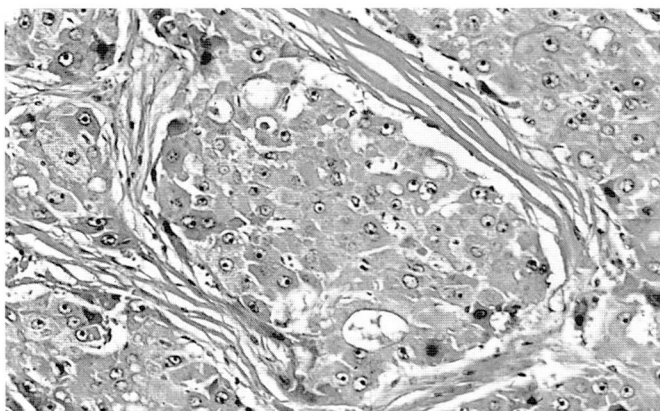

**Figure 43-8** Fibrolamellar carcinoma. This type of hepatocellular carcinoma is characterized by the lamellar organization of connective tissue surrounding polygonal macrohepatocytes with oncocytic cytoplasm.

a large number of genetic aberrations in recurrent lesions, not originally present in the primary tumor, suggesting that clonal evolution is indeed possible in this subtype, albeit slower in manifesting. Recently, a clear cell variant of FLC has been reported.[56] It is important to distinguish this variant from the conventional clear cell HCC, as the former is associated with a favorable prognosis.

Combined hepatocellular and cholangiocarcinoma (HCC/CC) manifests as the juxtaposing and intimate association of HCC and cholangiocarcinoma (CC) elements.[32] Characteristically, α-fetoprotein (AFP) levels are low, while higher concentrations of serum carcinoembryonic antigen (CEA) and CA 19-9 can be detected.[57,58] In cases in which the HCC morphology predominates, cirrhosis is present at least 55% of the time,[57] whereas in cases where the CC component predominates, it is relatively infrequent, occurring in less than 13% of cases. Usually parts of these tumors show bile production, intercellular bile canaliculi, or a trabeculae (characteristics of HCC), while the CC component can be recognized by gland formation by cells resembling biliary epithelium, intracellular mucin production, or positive cytokeratin 7 and 19 immunoreactivity.[57,59,60] There is anecdotal evidence suggesting that these tumors exhibit extremely unfavorable prognosis, with intrahepatic metastasis and regional lymph node spread being likely in addition to a predilection for pulmonary spread.[61] Genetic studies of combined HCC and cholangiocarcinoma have elucidated three separate developmental pathways: (1) collision tumor with two independent neoplastic clones, (2) single clonal tumor with homogenous genetic background in both components, and (3) single clonal tumor where genetic heterogeneity in the process of clonal evolution parallels histologic diversity.[62]

## Prognostically Relevant Pathologic Features of Hepatocellular Carcinoma

### Macroscopic Characteristics

The macroscopic features of HCC reported as having prognostic significance include tumor size, venous invasion, capsule formation, intrabiliary growth, and multiplicity.[63-68] Of these, tumor size remains the more significant factor, with several studies suggesting that 5 cm is a significant threshold: HCCs larger than 5 cm are likely to develop intrahepatic metastasis, portal vein tumor thrombus, or hematogenous metastasis.[68-70] The rate of intrahepatic me-

tastasis rises from 60% to 96% and the rate of portal vein thrombosis almost doubles from 40% to 75% for these larger HCCs.[68,70] Major portal vessel thrombosis also portends a poor prognosis, with recurrence being likely within 1 year and death occurring within 2 years after the resection in most patients.[71,72]

Tumor invasion into the hepatic duct and/or common bile duct is a relatively rare finding associated with a poor prognosis.[73] Patients present with obstructive jaundice and/or hemobilia and are frequently incorrectly diagnosed as having a cholangiocarcinoma or choledocholithiasis.[74]

Capsular formation has become the subject of interest from the perspective of tumorigenesis, with at least one recent study[75] providing evidence that capsule formation (Fig. 43-9) results from an α-smooth muscle actin (α-SMA)–positive mesenchymal cell population proliferating in response to tumor growth. Accordingly, the incidence of capsule formation is a function of tumor size, as mechanical stress on neighboring parenchyma increases with continued tumor growth. In one study,[76] a capsule was found in 46% of HCCs less than 2 cm in diameter, in 84% of tumors between 2 and 5 cm, and in 45% of HCCs greater than 5 cm. Whether the presence of a capsule is associated with lower nuclear grades, improved survival, lower intrahepatic recurrence rate, or reduced incidence of local venous invasion has been debated.[77,78]

Tumor multicentricity, noted in 16% to 74% of resected HCCs,[66-68,76] is an important prognostic feature associated with intrahepatic recurrence following surgery as well as with overall survival. The two mechanisms that account for the multiplicity of HCC are metastasis and multicentric carcinogenesis, with the latter being the spread of intrahepatic metastases via the portal system.[32,79,80] Secondary tumors are considered metastases if (1) they consist of a portal vein tumor thrombus or grow contiguously with a thrombus, (2) multiple small satellite lesions surround a larger main tumor, or (3) a single tumor is present near the main tumor but is significantly smaller in size and exhibits the same histology.[80]

### Microscopic Characteristics

Microscopic vascular invasion has been predictive of not only overall survival but also disease-free survival.[79,81,82] Given the rich vascular stroma of HCC, it is not surprising that in some series, microscopic vascular invasion is found in about half of the total number of cases resected. Poon and colleagues[83] have dem-

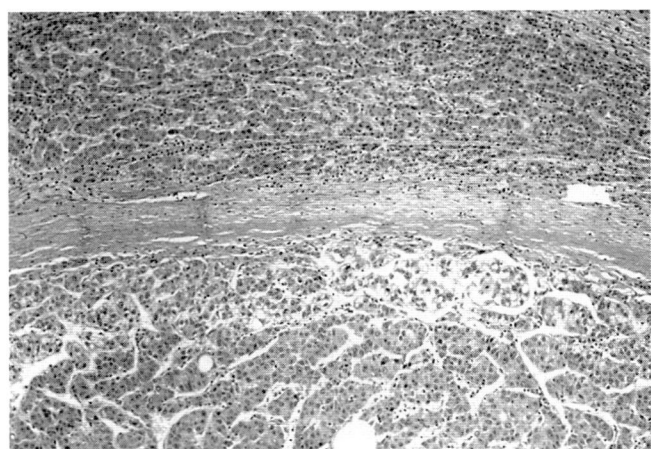

**Figure 43-9** Encapsulated hepatocellular carcinoma. The thick fibrous band at the interface between the tumor and the surrounding parenchyma has been associated with improved survival.

onstrated that increased tumor angiogenesis, as assessed by pre-operative serum vascular endothelial growth factor (VEGF) quantification, may be used as a positive predictor of microscopic venous invasion. Pathologic risk factors for microvascular invasion are tumor size greater than 5 cm, high nuclear grade, and high mitotic rate.[40,63]

Nuclear grade and mitotic activity, which also reflect tumor aggressiveness, are significant predictors of survival for patients with resected HCCs. Mitotic activity has also been reported as a valid prognostic indicator.[40,63,81,84]

### Importance of Surrounding Cirrhotic Parenchyma

Between 50% and 60% of HCCs arise in cirrhotic livers.[78,85] In addition to providing a fertile ground for hepatocellular carcinogenesis, cirrhosis plays a role (beyond issues of operability and hepatic function reserve) in the prognosis of patients with HCC. Differences in the multiplicity of tumors and the incidence of capsule formation and venous invasion have been reported in these tumors. Only 12% of HCCs arising in noncirrhotic liver present with multiple tumors,[86] but these grow faster and are larger than those in cirrhotic livers.[85–87] In contrast, HCCs arising in cirrhotic liver tend to exhibit slower growth and smaller size, presumably because of mechanical tumor growth restriction conferred by surrounding fibrotic parenchyma.[88] Yet, whether tumor encapsulation is more frequent in patients without cirrhosis is a debated issue.[78,89,90]

Controversies also exist as to the influence of cirrhosis and the histologic grade. It has not been determined whether or not venous invasion is more frequent in patients with cirrhosis than in those without it.[63,78] Also, heightened aggressiveness of HCCs arising in cirrhotic liver, as evidenced by mitotic activity, microvascular invasion (MVI), nuclear grade, and architectural pattern, has been advanced by some investigators[40,78] but is contested by others.[63] However, the importance of the surrounding hepatic parenchyma for long-term survival after curative resection[91,92] is well accepted. In that setting, metachronous carcinogenesis and not the recurrence of the original neoplasm has been implicated as the biologic mechanism underlying the long-term prognosis of cirrhotic patients with resected HCCs.[80,93,94]

### Histochemical and Immunohistochemical Studies Facilitating the Diagnostis of Hepatocellular Carcinoma

Although comprehensive compendia of ancillary immunohistochemical studies are available in the standard pathology texts, a general survey of routinely employed antibodies is relevant. It should be stressed, however, that special studies are generally meant to complement routine hematoxylin and eosin evaluation, and are not intended as a substitution for a proper and methodical histologic review.

### Carcinoembryonic Antigen

Biliary glycoprotein 1 exhibits an antigenic structure similar to that of CEA and thus is immunoreactive for polyclonal anti-CEA (Color Fig. 43–10; see separate color insert). Staining will be present in a canalicular or pericanalicular pattern, which is characteristic of HCC and is positively correlated with the degree of tumor differentiation.[95,96] Conversely, cholangiocarcinoma and metastatic adenocarcinoma to the liver will express a diffuse cytoplasmic pattern.[95,97,98]

### α-Fetoprotein

Histologic sections immunostained for AFP may show positivity even when only low serologic levels are detected.[99] Immunopositivity for AFP is mostly seen in HCC cases of intermediate degrees of differentiation, with both very well–differentiated and anaplastic tumors often lacking AFP expression. While it has been putatively touted as a relatively specific marker for HCC, immunoreactivity may be seen with various metastatic adenocarcinomas and germ cell tumors. Finally, AFP immunopositivity has been reported in benign hepatocytes.[100,101]

### Cytokeratins

As a general rule, the cytokeratin (CK) class of antibodies plays an important role in the identification and classification of epithelial tumors. Hepatocellular carcinomas are usually positive for low-molecular-weight keratins such as CAM 5.2, CK 8, and CK 18.[100,102] CK 7 and CK 19 are often positive in transformed biliary epithelial cells of HCC/CC and CC. Since a common epithelial (biliary) progenitor cell is thought to play a role in the oncogenesis of both HCC and CC, use of cytokeratin staining is of limited utility in distinguishing these two primary hepatic lesions, as some reports suggest that as many as 12% of HCCs express CK 19 immunoreactivity.[96,100]

### Albumin

While albumin immunopositivity is highly prevalent in cases of HCC, it also can be seen occasionally in CC and other tumors, thus lowering overall specificity.[103,104] However, the role of albumin mRNA in situ hybridization has recently been highlighted as a more specific technique. This method appears to be of particular value in distinguishing primary and metastatic tumors.[103,105]

### CD34

Absent in the specialized fenestrated hepatic endothelial cells of normal liver, CD34 immunoreactivity can be seen in association with chronic liver diseases and HCCs (Color Fig. 43–10 in separate color insert).[106–108] Of particular utility is the observation that macroregenerative nodules are generally negative for CD34, whereas dysplastic nodules and early HCC may exhibit focal staining. The extent of CD34 immunoreactivity is variable in early stages of HCC progression and, according to some investigators, more positive in advanced tumors.[106,109]

### Hep Par 1

Specific for hepatocytes (benign as well as malignant), Hep Par 1 is one of the more recent antibodies used to differentiate HCCs and tumors with hepatocytic differentiation from other neoplasms. Hep Par 1 exhibits relatively high sensitivity and specificity (82% and 90%, respectively).[101] Typically, the intensity and extent of staining are positively correlated with the degree of tumor differentiation, and the sclerosing variant may be completely devoid of staining.[96,110]

### CD10

CD10 or CALLA (common ALL antigen; Neprilysin), a type 2 cell metalloproteinase, has been recently tested in hepatic tumors. Morphologically, this stain manifests as a canalicular pattern. A recent publication[111] reports sensitivity and specificity values of 68.3% and 100%, respectively, for hepatocytic differentiation. Although CD10 does not distinguish between benign and malignant processes, it can be useful in differentiating between HCC and non-HCC.

In practice, since no single antibody is exclusively expressed by malignant hepatocytes, experience suggests that the use of a panel of immunohistochemical stains (instead of the use of select, individual antibodies) greatly improves sensitivity and specificity for the diagnosis of HCC, with some reports touting near-100% specificity for HCC inclusion.[96,101,111]

## References

1. Okuda K. Hepatocellular carcinoma. J Hepatol 32:225–237, 2000.
2. Parkin D, Whelan S, Ferlay J. Cancer Incidence in Five Continents, Vol. VII, International Agency for Research on Cancer, Lyon, 1997.
3. Bosch FX, Ribes J, Borras J. Epidemiology of primary liver cancer. Semin Liver Dis 19:271–285, 1999.
4. Chang M H, et al. Universal hepatitis B vaccination in Taiwan and the incidence of hepatocellular carcinoma in children. Taiwan Childhood Hepatoma Study Group. N Engl J Med 336:1855–1859, 1997.
5. Lee CL, Ko YC. Hepatitis B vaccination and hepatocellular carcinoma in Taiwan. Pediatrics 99:351–353, 1997.
6. El-Serag HB, Mason AC. Rising incidence of hepatocellular carcinoma in the United States. N Engl J Med 340:745–750, 1999.
7. Makimoto K, Higuchi S. Alcohol consumption as a major risk factor for the rise in liver cancer mortality rates in Japanese men. Int J Epidemiol 28:30–34, 1999.
8. Okuda K, et al. Changing incidence of hepatocellular carcinoma in Japan. Cancer Res 47:4967–4972, 1987.
9. Taylor-Robinson SD, et al. Increase in primary liver cancer in the UK, 1979–94. Lancet 350:1142–1143, 1997.
10. Mori M, et al. Prospective study of hepatitis B and C viral infections, cigarette smoking, alcohol consumption, and other factors associated with hepatocellular carcinoma risk in Japan. Am J Epidemiol 151:131–139, 2000.
11. Seitz HK, Poschl G, Simanowski UA. Alcohol and cancer. Recent Dev Alcohol 14:67–95, 1998.
12. Naccarato R, Farinati F. Hepatocellular carcinoma, alcohol, and cirrhosis: facts and hypotheses. Dig Dis Sci 36:1137–1142, 1991.
13. Wada K, Kondo F, Kondo Y. Large regenerative nodules and dysplastic nodules in cirrhotic livers: a histopathologic study. Hepatology 8:1684–1688, 1988.
14. Arakawa M, et al. Emergence of malignant lesions within an adenomatous hyperplastic nodule in a cirrhotic liver. Observations in five cases. Gastroenterology 91:198–208, 1986.
15. Sakamoto M, Hirohashi S, Shimosato Y. Early stages of multistep hepatocarcinogenesis: adenomatous hyperplasia and early hepatocellular carcinoma. Hum Pathol 22:172–178, 1991.
16. International Working Party. Terminology of nodular hepatocellular lesions. Hepatology 22:983–993, 1995.
17. Kojiro M. Premalignant lesions of hepatocellular carcinoma: pathologic viewpoint. J Hepatobiliary Pancreat Surg 7:535–541, 2000.
18. Hytiroglou P, Theise ND. Differential diagnosis of hepatocellular nodular lesions. Semin Diagn Pathol 15:285–299, 1998.
19. Anthony PP. Primary carcinoma of the liver: a study of 282 cases in Ugandan Africans. J Pathol 110:37–48, 1973.
20. Borzio M, et al. Liver cell dysplasia is a major risk factor for hepatocellular carcinoma in cirrhosis: a prospective study. Gastroenterology 108:812–817, 1995.
21. Lee RG, Tsamandas AC, Demetris AJ. Large cell change (liver cell dysplasia) and hepatocellular carcinoma in cirrhosis: matched case–control study, pathological analysis, and pathogenetic hypothesis. Hepatology 26:1415–1422, 1997.
22. Watanabe S, et al. Morphologic studies of the liver cell dysplasia. Cancer 51:2197–2205, 1983.
23. Ferrell LD, et al. Proposal for standardized criteria for the diagnosis of benign, borderline, and malignant hepatocellular lesions arising in chronic advanced liver disease. Am J Surg Pathol 17:1113–1123, 1993.
24. Nakashima O, et al. Pathomorphologic characteristics of small hepatocellular carcinoma: a special reference to small hepatocellular carcinoma with indistinct margins. Hepatology 22:101–105, 1995.
25. Terada T, Nakanuma Y. Iron-negative foci in siderotic macroregenerative nodules in human cirrhotic liver. A marker of incipient neoplastic lesions. Arch Pathol Lab Med 113:916–920, 1989.
26. Nakanuma Y, et al. Analytical histopathological diagnosis of small hepatocellular nodules in chronic liver disease. Histol Histopathol 13:1077–1087, 1998.
27. Terasaki S, et al. Histological features predicting malignant transformation of nonmalignant hepatocellular nodules: a prospective study. Gastroenterology 115:1216–1222, 1998.
28. Takayama T, et al. Malignant transformation of adenomatous hyperplasia to hepatocellular carcinoma. Lancet 336:1150–1153, 1990.
29. Eggel H: Uber das primare Carcinom der Leber. Beitr Pathol Anat 30:506–604, 1901.
30. Hui AM, et al. Predictive value of gross classification of hepatocellular carcinoma on recurrence and survival after hepatectomy. J Hepatol 33:975–979, 2000.
31. Shimada M, et al. The role of macroscopic classification in nodular-type hepatocellular carcinoma. Am J Surg 182:177–182, 2001.
32. Hirohashi S, et al. Hepatocellular carcinoma. In: Hamilton S, Aaltonen L (eds): World Health Organization Classification of Tumors. Pathology and Genetics of Tumours of the Digestive System, IARC Press, Lyon, 2000, pp 159–172.
33. Nagato Y, et al. Histological and morphometrical indicators for a biopsy diagnosis of well-differentiated hepatocellular carcinoma. Hepatology 14:473–478, 1991.
34. Kondo Y, Wada K. Intrahepatic metastasis of hepatocellular carcinoma: a histopathologic study. Hum Pathol 22:125–130, 1991.
35. Cohen MB, et al. Cytologic criteria to distinguish hepatocellular carcinoma from nonneoplastic liver. Am J Clin Pathol 95:125–130, 1991.
36. Yano H, Kojiro M, Nakashima T. A new human hepatocellular carcinoma cell line (KYN-1) with a transformation to adenocarcinoma. In Vitro Cell Dev Biol 22:637–646, 1986.
37. Vasiliev JM, et al. Contact inhibition of phagocytosis in epithelial sheets: alterations of cell surface properties induced by cell–cell contacts. Proc Natl Acad Sci USA 72:719–722, 1975.
38. Japanese Liver Cancer Study Group. The General Rules for the Clinical and Pathological Study of Primary Liver Cancer, Kanehira & Co., Tokyo, Japan, 1997.
39. Edmondson H, Steiner P. Primary carcinoma of the liver: a study of 100 cases among 48,900 necropsies. Cancer 7:462–503, 1954.
40. Lauwers G, et al. Prognostic histologic indicators of curatively resected hepatocellular carcinomas: a multi-institutional analysis of 425 patients with definition of a histologic prognostic index. Am J Surg Pathol 26:25–34, 2002.
41. Yang SH, et al. Clinicopathologic study on clear cell hepatocellular carcinoma. Pathol Int 46:503–509, 1996.
42. Lai CL, et al. Histologic prognostic indicators in hepatocellular carcinoma. Cancer 44:1677–1683, 1979.
43. Kuwano H, et al. Hepatocellular carcinoma with osteoclast-like giant cells. Cancer 54:837–842, 1984.
44. Kojiro M, et al. Hepatocellular carcinoma with sarcomatous change: a special reference to the relationship with anticancer therapy. Cancer Chemother Pharmacol 23(Suppl):S4–S8, 1989.
45. Kyotani S, et al. A study of embolizing materials for chemo-embolization therapy of hepatocellular carcinoma: antitumor effect of cis-diamminedichloroplatinum(II) albumin microspheres, containing chitin and treated with chitosan on rabbits with VX2 hepatic tumors. Chem Pharm Bull (Tokyo) 40:2814–2816, 1992.
46. Maeda T, et al. Spindle cell hepatocellular carcinoma. A clinicopathologic and immunohistochemical analysis of 15 cases. Cancer 77:51–57, 1996.
47. Scoazec JY, et al. Fibrolamellar carcinoma of the liver: composition of the extracellular matrix and expression of cell-matrix and cell-cell adhesion molecules. Hepatology 24:1128–1136, 1996.
48. Berman MA, Burnham JA, Sheahan DG. Fibrolamellar carcinoma of the liver: an immunohistochemical study of nineteen cases and a review of the literature. Hum Pathol 19:784–794, 1988.
49. Craig JR. Cirrhosis, hepatocellular carcinoma, and survival. Hepatology 26:798–799, 1997.
50. Ichikawa T, et al. Fibrolamellar hepatocellular carcinoma: imaging and pathologic findings in 31 recent cases. Radiology 213:352–361, 1999.
51. Ringe B, et al. Results of hepatic resection and transplantation for fibrolamellar carcinoma. Surg Gynecol Obstet 175:299–305, 1992.
52. Soreide O, et al. Characteristics of fibrolamellar hepatocellular carcinoma. A study of nine cases and a review of the literature. Am J Surg 151:518–523, 1986.
53. Kutluk MT, et al. Fibrolamellar hepatocellular carcinoma with skeletal metastases. Pediatr Hematol Oncol 18:273–278, 2001.
54. Sirivatanauksorn Y, et al. Genomic homogeneity in fibrolamellar carcinomas. Gut 49:82–86, 2001.
55. Wilkens L, et al. Cytogenetic aberrations in primary and recurrent fibrolamellar hepatocellular carcinoma detected by comparative genomic hybridization. Am J Clin Pathol 114:867–874, 2000.
56. Cheuk W, Chan JK. Clear cell variant of fibrolamellar carcinoma of the liver. Arch Pathol Lab Med 125:1235–1238, 2001.

57. Kojiro M. Pathology of Hepatocellular Carcinoma, New York: Churchill Livingstone. 1997, pp 165–187.

58. Nakamura S, et al. Surgical treatment of patients with mixed hepatocellular carcinoma and cholangiocarcinoma. Cancer 78:1671–1676, 1996.

59. Maeda T, et al. Combined hepatocellular and cholangiocarcinoma: proposed criteria according to cytokeratin expression and analysis of clinicopathologic features. Hum Pathol 26:956–964, 1995.

60. Goodman ZD, et al. Combined hepatocellular-cholangiocarcinoma. A histologic and immunohistochemical study. Cancer 55:124–135, 1985.

61. Koskinas J, et al. Combined hepatocellular-cholangiocarcinoma presented with massive pulmonary embolism. Hepatogastroenterology 47:1125–1128, 2000.

62. Fujii H, et al. Genetic classification of combined hepatocellular-cholangiocarcinoma. Hum Pathol 31:1011–1017, 2000.

63. Adachi E, et al. Factors correlated with portal venous invasion by hepatocellular carcinoma: univariate and multivariate analyses of 232 resected cases without preoperative treatments. Cancer 77:2022–2031, 1996.

64. Hanazaki K, et al. Prognostic factors after hepatic resection for hepatocellular carcinoma with hepatitis C viral infection: univariate and multivariate analysis. Am J Gastroenterol 96:1243–1250, 2001.

65. Liver Cancer Study Group of Japan. The general rules for the clinical and pathological study of primary liver cancer. Jpn J Surg 19:98–129, 1989.

66. Lai EC, et al. The pathological basis of resection margin for hepatocellular carcinoma. World J Surg 17:786–790; discussion 791, 1993.

67. Nagao T, et al. Postoperative recurrence of hepatocellular carcinoma. Ann Surg 211:28–33, 1990.

68. Yuki K, et al. Growth and spread of hepatocellular carcinoma. A review of 240 consecutive autopsy cases. Cancer 66:2174–2179, 1990.

69. Liver Cancer Study Group of Japan. Primary liver cancer in Japan: clinicopathologic features and results of surgical treatment. Ann Surg 211: 277–287, 1989.

70. Adachi E, et al. Risk factors for intrahepatic recurrence in human small hepatocellular carcinoma. Gastroenterology 108:768–775, 1995.

71. Izumi R, et al. Prognostic factors of hepatocellular carcinoma in patients undergoing hepatic resection. Gastroenterology 106:720–727, 1994.

72. Ikai I, et al. Surgical intervention for patients with stage IV-A hepatocellular carcinoma without lymph node metastasis: proposal as a standard therapy. Ann Surg 227:433–439, 1998.

73. Nakashima T, Kojiro M. Pathologic characteristics of hepatocellular carcinoma. Semin Liver Dis 6:259–266, 1986.

74. Kojiro M, et al. Hepatocellular carcinoma presenting as intrabile duct tumor growth: a clinicopathologic study of 24 cases. Cancer 49:2144–2147, 1982.

75. Ishizaki M, et al. The formation of capsule and septum in human hepatocellular carcinoma. Virchows Arch 438:574–580, 2001.

76. Nagao T, et al. Hepatic resection for hepatocellular carcinoma. Clinical features and long-term prognosis. Ann Surg 205:33–40, 1987.

77. Arii S, et al. Predictive factors for intrahepatic recurrence of hepatocellular carcinoma after partial hepatectomy. Cancer 69:913–919, 1992.

78. Nzeako UC, Goodman ZD, Ishak KG. Hepatocellular carcinoma in cirrhotic and noncirrhotic livers. A clinico-histopathologic study of 804 North American patients. Am J Clin Pathol 105:65–75, 1996.

79. Toyosaka A, et al. Pathologic and radiographic studies of intrahepatic metastasis in hepatocellular carcinoma; the role of efferent vessels. J Hepatobiliary Pancreat Surg 10:97–103; discussion 103–104, 1996.

80. Sakamoto M, et al. Multicentric independent development of hepatocellular carcinoma revealed by analysis of hepatitis B virus integration pattern. Am J Surg Pathol 13:1064–1067, 1989.

81. Haratake J, et al. Predictable factors for estimating prognosis of patients after resection of hepatocellular carcinoma. Cancer 72:1178–1183, 1993.

82. Vauthey JN, et al. Factors affecting long-term outcome after hepatic resection for hepatocellular carcinoma. Am J Surg 169:28–34; discussion 34–25, 1995.

83. Poon RT, et al. Serum vascular endothelial growth factor predicts venous invasion in hepatocellular carcinoma: a prospective study. Ann Surg 233:227–235, 2001.

84. Ouchi K, et al. Mitotic index is the best predictive factor for survival of patients with resected hepatocellular carcinoma. Dig Surg 17:42–48, 2000.

85. Smalley SR, et al. Hepatoma in the noncirrhotic liver. Cancer 62:1414–1424, 1988.

86. Bismuth H, Chiche L, Castaing D. Surgical treatment of hepatocellular carcinomas in noncirrhotic liver: experience with 68 liver resections. World J Surg 19:35–41, 1995.

87. Kishi K, et al. Hepatocellular carcinoma. A clinical and pathologic analysis of 57 hepatectomy cases. Cancer 51:542–548, 1983.

88. Lunevicius R, et al. Clinicopathological significance of fibrotic capsule formation around liver metastasis from colorectal cancer. J Cancer Res Clin Oncol 127:193–199, 2001.

89. Kemeny F, et al. Morphological and histological features of resected hepatocellular carcinoma in cirrhotic patients in the West. Hepatology 9:253–257, 1989.

90. Ng IO, et al. Tumor encapsulation in hepatocellular carcinoma. A pathologic study of 189 cases. Cancer 70:45–49, 1992.

91. Bilimoria MM, et al. Underlying liver disease, not tumor factors, predicts long-term survival after resection of hepatocellular carcinoma. Arch Surg 136:528–535, 2001.

92. Nagasue N, et al. Lack of intratumoral heterogeneity in DNA ploidy pattern of hepatocellular carcinoma. Gastroenterology 105:1449–1454, 1993.

93. Vauthey J, et al. Importance of field cancerization in clinical oncology. Lancet Oncol 1:15–16, 2000.

94. Sakon M, et al. Clinical significance of hepatic resection in hepatocellular carcinoma: analysis by disease-free survival curves. Arch Surg 135:1456–1459, 2000.

95. Christensen WN, Boitnott JK, Kuhajda FP. Immunoperoxidase staining as a diagnostic aid for hepatocellular carcinoma. Mod Pathol 2:8–12, 1989.

96. Leong AS, et al. Hep Par 1 and selected antibodies in the immunohistological distinction of hepatocellular carcinoma from cholangiocarcinoma, combined tumours and metastatic carcinoma. Histopathology 33:318–324, 1998.

97. Balaton AJ, et al. Distinction between hepatocellular carcinoma, cholangiocarcinoma, and metastatic carcinoma based on immunohistochemical staining for carcinoembryonic antigen and for cytokeratin 19 on paraffin sections. J Pathol 156:305–310, 1988.

98. Ma CK, et al. Comparative immunohistochemical study of primary and metastatic carcinomas of the liver. Am J Clin Pathol 99:551–557, 1993.

99. Kondo Y. Histologic features of hepatocellular carcinoma and allied disorders. Pathol Annu 20 Pt 2:405–430, 1985.

100. Hurlimann J, Gardiol D. Immunohistochemistry in the differential diagnosis of liver carcinomas. Am J Surg Pathol 15:280–288, 1991.

101. Minervini MI, et al. Utilization of hepatocyte-specific antibody in the immunocytochemical evaluation of liver tumors. Mod Pathol 10:686–692, 1997.

102. Johnson DE, et al. The diagnostic utility of the keratin profiles of hepatocellular carcinoma and cholangiocarcinoma. Am J Surg Pathol 12:187–197, 1988.

103. Krishna M, Lloyd RV, Batts KP. Detection of albumin messenger RNA in hepatic and extrahepatic neoplasms. A marker of hepatocellular differentiation. Am J Surg Pathol 21:147–152, 1997.

104. D'Errico A, et al. Histogenesis of primary liver carcinomas: strengths and weaknesses of cytokeratin profile and albumin mRNA detection. Hum Pathol 27:599–604, 1996.

105. Oliveira AM, et al. Differentiation of primary and metastatic clear cell tumors in the liver by in situ hybridization for albumin messenger RNA. Am J Surg Pathol 24:177–182, 2000.

106. Cui S, et al. Enhanced CD34 expression of sinusoid-like vascular endothelial cells in hepatocellular carcinoma. Pathol Int 46:751–756, 1996.

107. Couvelard A, Scoazec JY, Feldmann G. Expression of cell-cell and cell-matrix adhesion proteins by sinusoidal endothelial cells in the normal and cirrhotic human liver. Am J Pathol 143:738–752, 1993.

108. Sakamoto M, et al. Phenotype changes in tumor vessels associated with the progression of hepatocellular carcinoma. Jpn J Clin Oncol 23:98–104, 1993.

109. Tanigawa N, et al. Quantitation of sinusoid-like vessels in hepatocellular carcinoma: its clinical and prognostic significance. Hepatology 26:1216–1223, 1997.

110. Wennerberg AE, Nalesnik MA, Coleman WB. Hepatocyte paraffin 1: a monoclonal antibody that reacts with hepatocytes and can be used for differential diagnosis of hepatic tumors. Am J Pathol 143:1050–1054, 1993.

111. Borscheri N, Roessner A, Rocken C. Canalicular immunostaining of neprilysin (CD10) as a diagnostic marker for hepatocellular carcinomas. Am J Surg Pathol 25:1297–1303, 2001.

# Chapter 44

# Clinical Aspects and Management of Hepatocellular Cancer: Diagnostic and Staging Procedures

MICHAEL A. CHOTI

Hepatocellular carcinoma (HCC) is among the most common malignancies worldwide, accounting for more than 1,000,000 new cases per year.[1,2] Surgical therapy of early-stage disease provides the only hope for curative therapy. Therefore, early diagnosis and appropriate determination of extent of disease and hepatic function are critical in optimizing treatment planning and improving survival rates. Advances in imaging techniques and other tests have improved the ability to carefully evaluate patients with HCC. However, the array of options available to the clinician has also resulted in increased complexity and confusion regarding optimal patient evaluation. This chapter will review the variety of diagnostic and staging procedures, ranging from blood tests and imaging modalities to intraoperative staging. Three important goals should be addressed when patients with HCC are evaluated: *(1)* confirmation of the diagnosis, *(2)* staging of the extent of disease, and *(3)* assessment of hepatic functional reserve.

## Diagnosis and Staging of Hepatocellular Carcinoma

Diagnosis of symptomatic HCC is often made late in the course of the disease, manifested with nonspecific symptoms of advanced disease, including abdominal pain, weakness, and weight loss. More commonly, diagnosis in high risk patients with cirrhosis and/or chronic hepatitis is made through routine use of serum α-fetoprotein (AFP) levels and transabdominal ultrasound. Further staging evaluation is then warranted to determine the extent of disease.

### α-Fetoprotein

Measurement of serum AFP is useful both in screening of high-risk individuals and in determining the diagnosis in a patient with a focal hepatic lesion. The basis of screening for HCC is typically the interval measurements of AFP levels in asymptomatic high-risk patients, often in combination with routine ultrasound or computed tomography (CT) examination.[3–5] Although the true benefit of screening for HCC has not been clearly documented,[6] screening programs have been established in several countries. Individuals at high risk who should be considered candidates for screening include those with cirrhosis or documented viral hepatitis and persons with a family history of HCC.

α-Fetoprotein is a fetal protein that is not normally detectable in healthy adults but is elevated in most persons with HCC.[7] In high-incidence areas, over 90% of HCC patients have elevated serum AFP concentrations (>10 ng/ml); in low-incidence areas, AFP is elevated in only 50% to 70% of cases.[8] It is clear that the sensitivity and specificity of AFP in diagnosing HCC depends on the level chosen as the cut-off value. In one study, when 20 ng/ml was used as the cut-off, the sensitivity for detecting HCC was 87% and the specificity was 31%. When the cut-off value was raised to 530 ng/ml, specificity increased to 95% but sensitivity fell to 56%.[7] In general, an AFP level of greater than 500 ng/ml may indicate HCC and warrants further investigation. In the presence of a space-occupying hepatic lesion and such an elevated AFP level, the diagnosis of HCC is virtually certain.

A variety of benign conditions can be associated with modest elevations in AFP levels (between 10 and 500 ng/ml), including hepatic inflammation, biliary tract obstruction, and cirrhosis.[9,10] Up to 20% of individuals with chronic hepatitis and 40% of those with cirrhosis have an AFP elevation of greater than 10 ng/ml.[11,12] In patients with chronic liver disease, therefore, AFP levels between 10 and 500 ng/ml should be considered inconclusive, and in such cases there are no clear management guidelines.[13] Time trends may be helpful, as steadily increasing levels may be more suggestive of HCC than fluctuating AFP levels. Even in cases where no identifiable lesion is found on imaging studies, elevated and rising serum AFP levels may indicate an early HCC. These patients should be followed carefully. Careful hepatic imaging may identify early lesions in some cases but in many cases also can lead to false-positive findings from regenerating nodules.

Several investigators have attempted to improve the specificity of AFP as a diagnostic test by identifying tumor-specific isoforms. Earlier approaches were based on detecting differences in the affinity to binding of the AFP molecules to various lectins.[14,15] More recently, investigators have used isoelectric focusing to identify isoforms directly.[7,16] These studies have demonstrated that such qualitative assessment of the tumor-specific band can increase the positive predictive value from 41.5% with the conventional assay of total AFP to 73.1% using the specific isoform.[7]

### Ultrasonography

Ultrasonography (US) is the most commonly used imaging modality for detecting HCC. It has the advantage of being widely available, less costly than other methods, and relatively noninvasive. However, it is also the most operator-dependent imaging modality. Perhaps the most common use of US in the evaluation of the HCC patient is in screening. As discussed, routine US is often employed in combination with serum AFP measurements in high-risk populations, and this screening combination can increase the detection rate of HCC in high-risk populations over that found by using AFP alone.[6] Yet, not all cases of HCC can be detected early with US. In one recent study,[17] ultrasonography performed prior to liver transplantation detected only 33% of the HCC, which ranged from 0.6 to 5.0 cm in diameter. In another study, the sensitivity and specificity of screening US were approximately 70% and 93%, respectively.[6]

Ultrasonography can also play a role in the anatomic evaluation and assessment of the extent of disease. Size, lesion number, and location can often be determined, typically detecting tumors as small as 1–2 cm in diameter.[18,19] Ultrasonography can also provide an estimate of the severity of underlying liver disease, and Doppler imaging can provide information regarding blood flow. Duplex or color Doppler displays the velocity and direction of flow relative to the position of the ultrasound transducer.[20,21] More importantly, this information is useful for determining tumor vascular involvement and intravascular thrombi.

More recently, advances in ultrasound technology include the use of contrast enhancement with intravascular microbubble agents. When injected intravenously, these microbubbles are stable enough to pass through pulmonary capillary beds and produce vascular enhancement in hypervascular lesions such as HCC, particularly when harmonic pulse-inversion mode US imaging is used.[22] Early experience with these materials suggests improved imaging compared with conventional Doppler US.[23,24] Further studies are necessary to determine whether these new US methods will play an increasing role in the assessment of patients with HCC.

### Computed Tomography

Computed tomography (CT) is the most commonly used imaging modality for HCC in many Western countries, including the United States.[25] It has the advantage of producing high-resolution cross-sectional images and is less operator-dependent in both acquisition and interpretation of the images.[26] Computed tomography plays an important role in both confirming diagnosis and determining the extent of disease. The size and number of lesions can be assessed, as well as evidence of associated features such as vascular invasion and satellite nodules. Moreover, the extent of cirrhosis and portal hypertension can be determined. The more recent introduction of helical CT has improved the quality significantly.[27] With this technique, the procedure allows continuous tube rotation and data acquisition while the patient simultaneously moves through the gantry. In addition to the ability to image during a single breath-hold, this helical CT allows for imaging during precise time points of maximal arterial and portal opacification. Typical HCC are hypervascular and usually display enhancement on arterial phase.[28] Therefore, it is important to acquire images on both arterial and portal phases when evaluating a patient with a liver tumor.[29,30] Although resolution is improved with the newer techniques, whether these techniques offer an improved ability to detect small tumors compared with other imaging modalities is not clear.

In addition to its use in lesion detection, CT is extremely useful in the assessment of hepatic anatomy, determination of resectability, and surgical planning in the case of resectable disease. Newer imaging rendering, including three-dimensional viewing, has helped to improve the ability to evaluate the liver.[31,32]

### Angiographic Imaging

Because most hepatocellular tumors are hypervascular, hepatic arterial angiographic approaches can detect even small HCC lesions (Fig. 44–1). Although less commonly used today, conventional angiography is still being used in some centers routinely for diagnostic and preoperative evaluation.[33,34] It remains an essential component of assessment of tumor vasculature in patients undergoing planned chemoembolization.

Computed tomographic arteriography or CT portography involves placing a catheter into the hepatic or superior mesenteric artery, respectively, and performing CT scanning during the infusion of contrast agent.[35–37] Hepatocellular cancers will appear as high-attenuation peripheral blushes within the liver on hepatic arterial injection and as diminished lesion conspicuity on portal (mesenteric artery) injection.[35,38–41] As with conventional angiography, CT arteriography has largely been supplanted by mul-

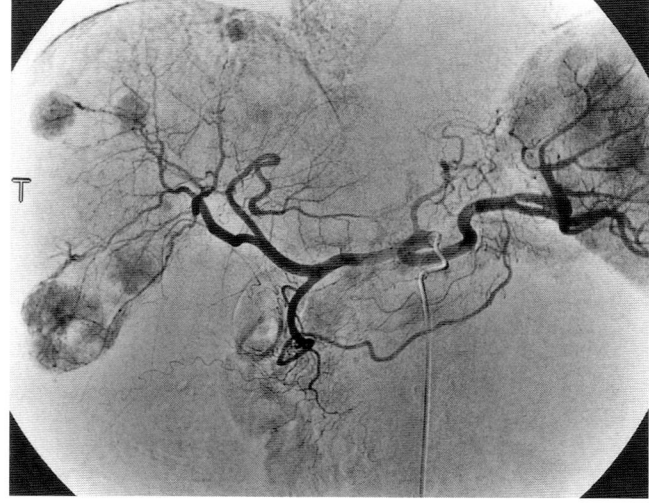

**Figure 44–1** Hepatic arterial angiography demonstrating multiple hypervascular tumors in a patient with multifocal hepatocellular carcinoma.

tiphase, contrast-enhanced helical CT and magnetic resonance imaging (MRI) and is used less commonly in most centers.

Perhaps the most sensitive angiographic imaging modality for HCC is CT-Lipiodol. Lipiodol, an iodized oily agent that is most often used with bland or chemoembolization, was found to be retained in hypervascular tumors such as HCC because of the particle size and composition. When administered angiographically, a subsequent CT scan may reveal areas of increased density due to the high iodine content of the agent (Fig. 44–2). Several comparative imaging studies have demonstrated superior sensitivity of CT-Lipiodol for lesions 1 cm or smaller in diameter (>70% sensitivity), making it the most sensitive preoperative imaging modality.[42–46] In spite of these data, the cost, relative invasiveness, and technical variability in quality have limited enthusiasm for its use in most hospitals, particularly in Western centers.

## Magnetic Resonance Imaging

Magnetic resonance imaging (MRI) is being used with increasing frequency as a diagnostic and staging procedure for HCC. Much as with CT, significant advances have been made in MRI technology. Smaller surface coils, decreased scan times, higher resolution, and single breath-hold images have all resulted in dramatic improvement in image quality. Magnetic resonance imaging may be superior to CT or US at characterization of lesions suspected to be HCC.[43,47,48] T2-weighted images may demonstrate characteristic features of HCC such as mosaic or nodular patterns of signal intensity. More importantly, as with contrast-enhanced CT, HCC typically demonstrates arterial-phase signal enhancement after bolus injection of contrast agents. The most commonly used agent is the intravenous administration of gadolinium, which results in arterial and portal phase images much like those on CT (Fig. 44–3). Contrast-enhanced imaging in the cirrhotic patient is sometimes impaired by the limited arterial blood flow to the liver. As MRI requires less contrast material administration than CT, this imaging modality may be more useful in patients with significant cirrhosis.

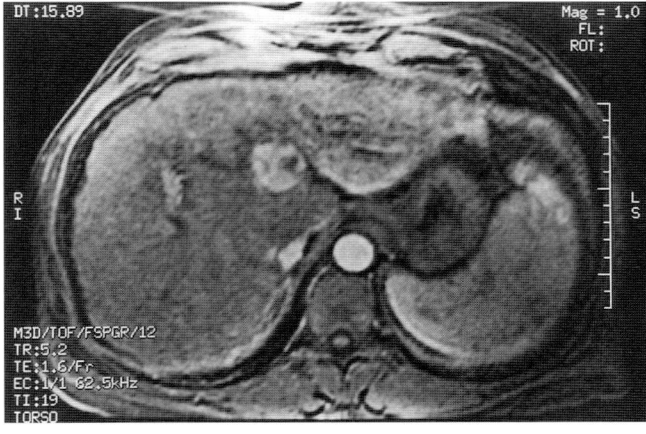

A

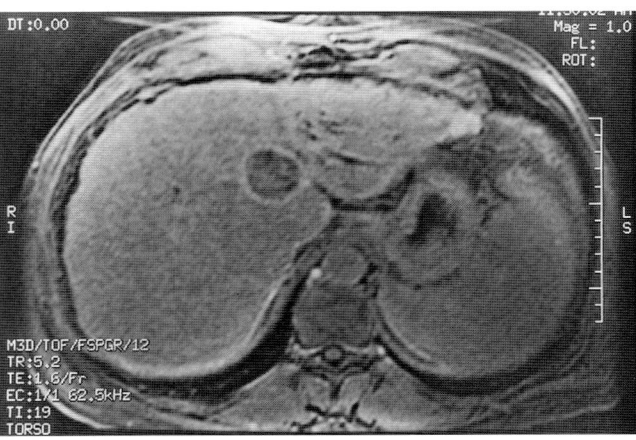

B

**Figure 44-3** Gadolinium contrast–enhanced magnetic resonance image (MRI) in a patient with left lobe hepatocellular carcinoma. *A:* Arterial phase demonstrating a hypervascular tumor. *B:* Reduced enhancement in the same tumor in delayed images.

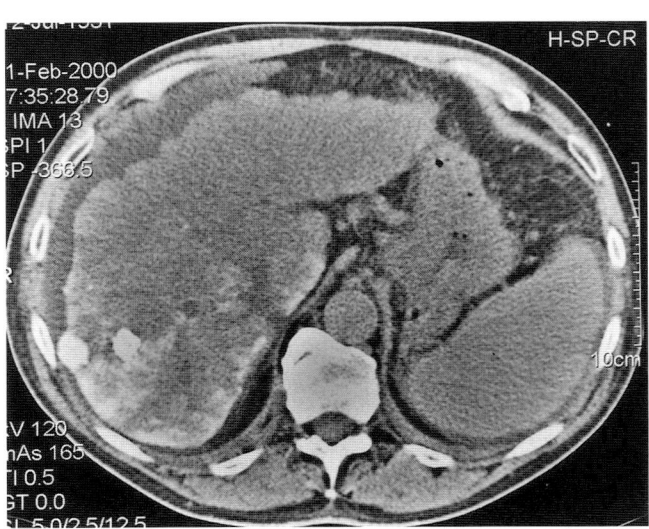

**Figure 44-2** Computed tomography–Lipiodol study demonstrating multifocal disease in the right hepatic lobe in a cirrhotic patient with hepatocellular carcinoma.

More recently, newer contrast agents have been developed to assess differences between tumor and normal liver parenchyma in order to improve lesion detection and identification. Ferumoxide,[49] Mn-DPDP,[50] and Gd-EOB/DTPA,[51–54] among others, have demonstrated various properties of uptake within the reticuloendothelial system and hepatocytes. These novel approaches to enhanced MRI are undergoing extensive research, and early studies suggest they may provide increased sensitivities over those with standard MRI or dual-phase helical CT.[50,55]

## Fluorodeoxyglucose Positron Emission Tomography Imaging

Fluorodeoxyglucose positron emission tomography (FDG-PET) is a functional imaging technique for tumor detection based on the uptake and intercellular accumulation of a radioactively labeled glucose analogue by metabolizing tumors. FDG is labeled with $^{18}F$, the radioactive isotope of fluorine that rapidly decays by positron emission. FDG-PET is now being recognized as one of the most powerful noninvasive methods for tumor staging for a variety of malignancies.

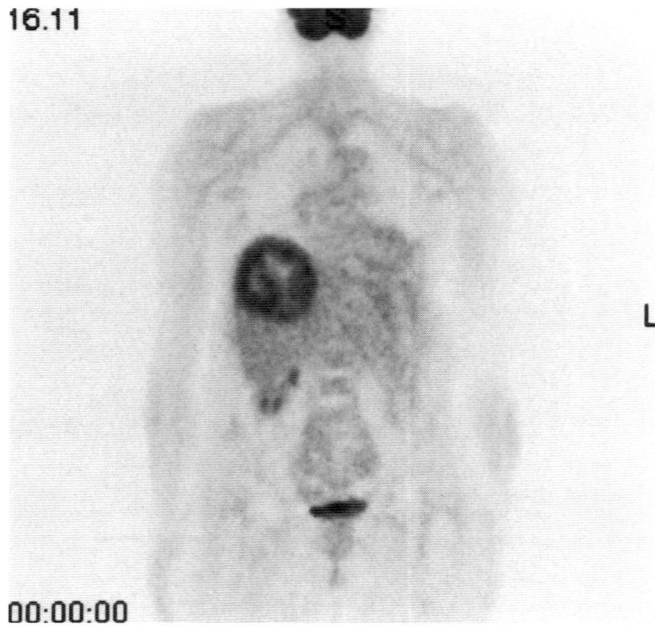

**Figure 44-4** Fluorodeoxyglucose positron emission tomography (FDG-PET) image of large hepatocellular carcinoma. L, left.

A variety of investigators have examined the potential role of FDG-PET in the diagnosis and staging of HCC.[56-59] Theoretically, FDG-PET may serve to stage the extent of disease by identifying metastatic deposits in lymph nodes and other sites. Moreover, PET may prove useful diagnostically in differentiating benign and malignant hepatic nodules or in differentiating high- and low-grade tumors (Fig. 44-4).

Few studies to date, however, have demonstrated any advantage of FDG-PET over other imaging modalities in HCC. While able to detect larger and more poorly differentiated tumors, FDG-PET is least helpful in cases of well-differentiated HCC, small tumors,[58,59] or those associated with low AFP levels. These, of course, are situations in which such functional imaging would be most important. Clearly, further investigative work is necessary to define the role of FDG-PET in the diagnosis and management of HCC.

## Percutaneous Needle Biopsy

Preoperative needle biopsy is rarely necessary in patients with unequivocal diagnosis of HCC and resectable disease (i.e., AFP >500 ng/ml and lesion identified on imaging studies). In most cases, the diagnosis is evident and preoperative biopsy rarely alters management.[60] Percutaneous biopsy is most useful in cases of unresectable disease or in some cases when a patient with compensated liver disease is being considered for liver transplantation.[61] In selected cases in which the diagnosis is unclear or when multifocal disease is being ruled out, needle biopsy should be considered prior to major resection.[62] Other roles for biopsy include evaluating cases in which nonoperative ablative therapy is being contemplated or in evaluating the extent of cirrhosis in the nontumorous liver.

Needle biopsy, when utilized, can result in accurate diagnosis in most cases.[63-67] In one study,[66] the highest diagnostic accuracy was achieved when the combined analysis of both fine needle aspiration plus intranodular core needle biopsy was used (91%), compared with the use of fine needle aspiration alone or needle biopsy alone (48% and 67%, respectively). However, needle biopsy is associated with potential risks, for example, bleeding or tumor rupture in some cases. In addition, there is a potential risk of tumor spillage or dissemination of malignant cells along the needle biopsy tract.[68,69]

## Intraoperative Staging

The most common surgical treatment for HCC is hepatic resection. When such a patient is judged to be an operative candidate and when preoperative staging suggests resectable disease, two additional diagnostic procedures should be considered prior to resection: *(1)* laparoscopy and *(2)* intraoperative ultrasonography.

### Laparoscopy

Because up to 30% of patients are found at operation to have unresectable disease,[70] minimally invasive intraoperative assessment of the liver and abdomen can prove useful in some cases. Laparoscopy can often visualize peritoneal implants and multifocal disease when present. Moreover, laparoscopy can be used to examine the liver and evaluate the extent of cirrhosis and portal hypertension. Laparoscopic ultrasonography can improve assessment by allowing visualization of smaller lesions within the liver. Lo et al.[71,72] reported on 500 patients undergoing surgical exploration for HCC, 198 of whom underwent laparoscopy and laparoscopic ultrasonography. Unresectable disease was found in approximately 20% of patients in each group. The majority of such cases in the laparoscopy group were found prior to laparotomy, reducing the number of unnecessary open explorations. Overall, the resectability rate at laparotomy improved from 80% to 86% with the use of this approach. Another role for laparoscopy may be in the setting of suspected HCC but unknown diagnosis. Some centers, for example, have advocated diagnostic laparoscopy in cases of elevated AFP and no detectable lesion on imaging studies, particularly when transplantation is being considered.[73] Although conceptually appealing, the yield and clinical cost-effectiveness of laparoscopy in this setting remain to be demonstrated.

### Intraoperative Ultrasonography

In addition to laparoscopic ultrasonography, intraoperative ultrasonography at laparotomy is an important component of staging and assessment of the liver prior to resection. Considerably more sensitive than transcorporeal ultrasonography, the intraoperative application can detect lesions as small as 5 mm.[74] There are some limitations to the accuracy of detecting small lesions in patients with cirrhosis compared with those without cirrhosis, however, due to the reduction in image resolution and stiffness from the fibrous liver. Moreover, regenerating nodules within the liver can be mistaken for multifocal tumor. Indeterminate lesions seen only on intraoperative ultrasonography should be biopsied to confirm unresectability. Equally important as assessment of the extent of disease, intraoperative ultrasonography also serves to delineate hepatic anatomy, allowing for a more carefully planned resection. In addition, operative ablative approaches such as radiofrequency ablation, cryotherapy, and others require intraoperative ultrasound for biopsy, probe targeting, and operative ablation monitoring.

## Assessment of Hepatic Function

When evaluating a patient with HCC for treatment planning, perhaps as important as tumor staging is the determination of baseline hepatic function. At least 75% of HCC patients worldwide have associated cirrhosis. The presence of cirrhosis limits the amount of liver that can resected with partial hepatectomy and is associated with significantly higher operative morbidity and mortality.[75-80] Patients with cirrhosis and portal hypertension are coagulopathic and thrombocytopenic, increasing the risk of postoperative hemorrhage. Moreover, the cirrhotic liver has a diminished regenerative capacity, resulting in a higher risk of perioperative complications associated with liver failure. The severity of underlying disease is often the most important factor in determining the choice between partial hepatectomy and liver transplantation.

### Clinical Evaluation and Liver Function Tests

Several formulas and biochemical tests have been proposed to grade cirrhosis and estimate hepatic functional reserve. Perhaps the most commonly used and accepted is the Child-Pugh classification (Table 44–1). This scale utilizes simple laboratory tests such as bilirubin, prothrombin time, and albumin, as well as clinical variables such as ascites and encephalopathy. Because of the prohibitively high operative risk, patients in Child class C and some in class B are considered not to be candidates for liver resection, regardless of tumor size and location. In patients with small tumors and poor hepatic function, orthotopic liver transplantation is perhaps the optimal treatment.

### Dynamic Measurements of Hepatic Function

A variety of other, more specific functional tests have been advocated by some investigators for use in the preoperative patient. One of the first of these dynamic tests was the bromosulfophathlein retention test[81] reported in 1913. The functional test used perhaps most frequently by some groups is the indocyanine green (ICG) clearance test.[82,83] Indocyanine green is a synthetic dye used as a test of liver function by measuring its blood clearance after intravenous administration. More recently, a more rapid dynamic measurement of hepatic function, the monoethylglycinexylidide (MEGX) test, has been used in some centers.[84,85] This test relies on the measurement of rapid clearance of a lidocaine metabolite, therefore estimating both hepatic metabolic capacity and hepatic blood flow. Although these dynamic studies can assess the severity of underlying liver disease, they are not useful in most cases at predicting hepatic function following resection or other therapy. Therefore, most centers do not use these tests preoperatively on a routine basis.

### Measurement of Blood Flow and Portal Pressures

Physiologic test studies measuring portal pressures have also been used by some surgeons to assess operative risk. Wedged hepatic venous pressure and hepatic venous pressure gradient can be measured through introduction of a venous catheter into the hepatic vein, and portal pressure can be estimated. Patients with cirrhosis with increased portal pressure are at higher risk of hepatic decompensation after resection of HCC. Patients with portal pressures >10 mmHg are believed by some not to be candidates for resection.[86]

Preoperative assessment of hepatic function and the determination of whether the patient is a candidate for surgical resection are most often based on the surgeon's impression, which is formed by the clinical Child-Pugh score, the appearance of the liver on preoperative imaging studies, and the overall assessment of the patient's performance status.

## Summary

Accurate diagnosis and staging of HCC are essential when considering the variety of potential treatment options. Diagnosis of early HCC in asymptomatic patients relies on screening strategies in identified high-risk populations. Aggressive screening modalities, including measurement of AFP levels and cross-sectional imaging, may result in earlier detection and improved survival. Because advances in radiologic techniques have allowed the detection of smaller tumors and more accurate characterization of localized disease, a progressively larger number of patients will derive benefit from local treatment approaches. The rapidly changing array of diagnostic and imaging options, particularly MRI, CT, US, and PET imaging, will certainly alter management approaches to this disease in the future.

### References

1. Schafer DF, Sorrell MF. Hepatocellular carcinoma. Lancet 353:1253–1257, 1999.
2. El-Serag HB. Epidemiology of hepatocellular carcinoma. Clin Liver Dis 5:87–107, 2001.
3. Oka H, Tamori A, Kuroki T, Kobayashi K, Yamamoto S. Prospective study of alpha-fetoprotein in cirrhotic patients monitored for development of hepatocellular carcinoma. Hepatology 19:61–66, 1994.
4. Chen DS, Sung JL, Sheu JC, Lai MY, How SW, Hsu HC, Lee CS, Wei TC. Serum alpha-fetoprotein in the early stage of human hepatocellular carcinoma. Gastroenterology 86:1404–1409, 1984.
5. Wong LL, Limm WM, Severino R, Wong LM. Improved survival with screening for hepatocellular carcinoma. Liver Transpl 6:320–325, 2000.
6. Pateron D, Ganne N, Trinchet JC, Aurousseau MH, Mal F, Meicler C, Coderc E, Reboullet P, Beaugrand M. Prospective study of screening for hepatocellular carcinoma in Caucasian patients with cirrhosis. J Hepatol 20:65–71, 1994.
7. Johnson PJ, Williams R. Serum alpha-fetoprotein estimations and doubling time in hepatocellular carcinoma: influence of therapy and possible value in early detection. J Natl Cancer Inst 64:1329–1332, 1980.
8. Kew MC. Hepatic tumors and cysts. In: Feldman M, Scharschmidt M, Sleisenger H (eds): Sleisenger and Fordtran's Gastrointestinal and Liver Disease: Pathophysiology/Diagnosis/Management. W.B. Saunders Company, Philadelphia, pp 1364–1387.
9. Bates SE, Longo DL. Tumor markers: value and limitations in the management of cancer patients. Cancer Treat Rev 12:163–207, 1985.
10. Wu JT. Serum alpha-fetoprotein and its lectin reactivity in liver diseases: a review. Ann Clin Lab Sci 20:98–105, 1990.

**Table 44–1** Child-Pugh classification of cirrhosis[a]

| Test | Points | | |
|------|--------|---|---|
| | 1 | 2 | 3 |
| Bilirubin (mg/dl) | 2.0 | 2.0–2.9 | >2.9 |
| Prothrombin time Prolongation (sec) | 1–3 | 4–6 | >6 |
| Albumin (g/dl) | >3.5 | 2.8–3.4 | <2.8 |
| Ascites | None | Mild | Moderate to severe |
| Encephalopathy | None | Grade 1 or 2 | Grade 3 or 4 |

[a]Child-Pugh classification: A = 5–6 points; B = 7–9 points; C = 10–15 points.

11. Silver HK, Deneault J, Gold P, Thompson WG, Shuster J, Freedman SO. The detection of alpha 1-fetoprotein in patients with viral hepatitis. Cancer Res 34:244–247, 1974.

12. Bloomer JR, Waldmann TA, McIntire KR, Klatskin G. Alpha-fetoprotein in noneoplastic hepatic disorders. JAMA 233:38–41, 1975.

13. Tangkijvanich P, Anukulkarnkusol N, Suwangool P, Lertmaharit S, Hanvivatvong O, Kullavanijaya P, Poovorawan Y. Clinical characteristics and prognosis of hepatocellular carcinoma: analysis based on serum alpha-fetoprotein levels. J Clin Gastroenterol 31:302–308, 2000.

14. Du MQ, Hutchinson WL, Johnson PJ, Williams R. Differential alpha-fetoprotein lectin binding in hepatocellular carcinoma. Diagnostic utility at low serum levels. Cancer 67:476–480, 1991.

15. Taketa K, Endo Y, Sekiya C, Tanikawa K, Koji T, Taga H, Satomura S, Matsuura S, Kawai T, Hirai H. A collaborative study for the evaluation of lectin-reactive alpha-fetoproteins in early detection of hepatocellular carcinoma. Cancer Res 53:5419–5423, 1993.

16. Burditt LJ, Johnson MM, Johnson PJ, Williams R. Detection of hepatocellular carcinoma-specific alpha-fetoprotein by isoelectric focusing. Cancer 74:25–29, 1994.

17. Kim CK, Lim JH, Lee WJ. Detection of hepatocellular carcinomas and dysplastic nodules in cirrhotic liver: accuracy of ultrasonography in transplant patients. J Ultrasound Med 20:99–104, 2001.

18. Sheu JC, Sung JL, Chen DS, Yu JY, Wang TH, Su CT, Tsang YM. Ultrasonography of small hepatic tumors using high-resolution linear-array real-time instruments. Radiology 150:797–802, 1984.

19. Tanaka S, Kitamura T, Imaoka S, Sasaki Y, Taniguchi H, Ishiguro S. Hepatocellular carcinoma: sonographic and histologic correlation. AJR Am J Roentgenol 140:701–707, 1983.

20. Furuse J, Maru Y, Yoshino M, Mera K, Sumi H, Sekiguchi R, Satake M, Hasebe T, Ochiai A. Assessment of arterial tumor vascularity in small hepatocellular carcinoma. Comparison between color doppler ultrasonography and radiographic imagings with contrast medium: dynamic CT, angiography, and CT hepatic arteriography. Eur J Radiol 36:20–27, 2000.

21. Lencioni R, Pinto F, Armillotta N, Bartolozzi C. Assessment of tumor vascularity in hepatocellular carcinoma: comparison of power Doppler US and color Doppler US. Radiology 201:353–358, 1996.

22. Kim TK, Choi BI, Han JK, Hong HS, Park SH, Moon SG. Hepatic tumors: contrast agent-enhancement patterns with pulse-inversion harmonic US. Radiology 216:411–417, 2000.

23. Wilson SR, Burns PN, Muradali D, Wilson JA, Lai X. Harmonic hepatic US with microbubble contrast agent: initial experience showing improved characterization of hemangioma, hepatocellular carcinoma, and metastasis. Radiology 215:153–161, 2000.

24. Bertolotto M, Dalla PL, Quaia E, Locatelli M. Characterization of unifocal liver lesions with pulse inversion harmonic imaging after Levovist injection: preliminary results. Eur Radiol 10:1369–1376, 2000.

25. Peterson MS, Baron RL. Radiologic diagnosis of hepatocellular carcinoma. Clin Liver Dis 5:123–144, 2001.

26. Bluemke DA, Soyer P, Fishman EK. Helical (spiral) CT of the liver. Radiol Clin North Am 33:863–886, 1995.

27. Kuszyk BS, Bluemke DA, Urban BA, Choti MA, Hruban RH, Sitzmann JV, Fishman EK. Portal-phase contrast-enhanced helical CT for the detection of malignant hepatic tumors: sensitivity based on comparison with intraoperative and pathologic findings. AJR Am J Roentgenol 166:91–95, 1996.

28. Murakami T, Kim T, Takamura M, Hori M, Takahashi S, Federle MP, Tsuda K, Osuga K, Kawata S, Nakamura H, Kudo M. Hypervascular hepatocellular carcinoma: detection with double arterial phase multidetector row helical CT. Radiology 218:763–767, 2001.

29. Hann LE, Winston CB, Brown KT, Akhurst T. Diagnostic imaging approaches and relationship to hepatobiliary cancer staging and therapy. Semin Surg Oncol 19:94–115, 2000.

30. Peterson MS, Baron RL, Marsh JW, Oliver JH, Confer SR, Hunt LE. Pretransplantation surveillance for possible hepatocellular carcinoma in patients with cirrhosis: epidemiology and CT-based tumor detection rate in 430 cases with surgical pathologic correlation. Radiology 217:743–749, 2000.

31. Soyer P, Lacheheb D, Levesque M. False-positive CT portography: correlation with pathologic findings. Am J Roentgenol Radium Ther Nucl Med 160:285–289, 1993.

32. Soyer P, Bluemke DA, Choti MA, Fishman EK. Variations in the intrahepatic portions of the hepatic and portal veins: findings on helical CT scans during arterial portography. AJR Am J Roentgenol 164:103–108, 1995.

33. Ishiguchi T, Shimamoto K, Fukatsu H, Yamakawa K, Ishigaki T. Radiologic diagnosis of hepatocellular carcinoma. Semin Surg Oncol 12:164–169, 1996.

34. Bartolozzi C, Lencioni R, Caramella D, Palla A, Bassi AM, Di Candio G. Small hepatocellular carcinoma. Detection with US, CT, MR imaging, DSA, and Lipiodol-CT. Acta Radiol 37:69–74, 1996.

35. Soyer P, Bluemke DA, Fishman EK. CT during arterial portography for the preoperative evaluation of hepatic tumors: how, when, and why? AJR Am J Roentgenol 163:1325–1331, 1994.

36. Heath DG, Soyer PA, Kuszyk BS, Bliss DF, Calhoun PS, Bluemke DA, Choti MA, Fishman EK. Three-dimensional spiral CT during arterial portography: comparison of three rendering techniques. Radiographics 15:1001–1011, 1995.

37. Murakami T, Oi H, Hori M, Kim T, Takahashi S, Tomoda K, Narumi Y, Nakamura H. Helical CT during arterial portography and hepatic arteriography for detecting hypervascular hepatocellular carcinoma. AJR Am J Roentgenol 169:131–135, 1997.

38. Tanaka Y, Sasaki Y, Katayama K, Hiramatsu N, Ito A, Murata H, Enomoto N, Oshita M, Mochizuki K, Tsujii M, Tsuji S, Kasahara A, Tomoda K, Nakamura H, Hayashi N, Hori M. Probability of hepatocellular carcinoma of small hepatocellular nodules undetectable by computed tomography during arterial portography. Hepatology 31:890–898, 2000.

39. Makita O, Yamashita Y, Arakawa A, Nakayama Y, Mitsuzaki K, Ando M, Namimoto T, Takahashi M. Diagnostic accuracy of helical CT arterial portography and CT hepatic arteriography for hypervascular hepatocellular carcinoma in chronic liver damage. An ROC analysis. Acta Radiol 41:464–469, 2000.

40. Takayasu K, Muramatsu Y, Furukawa H, Wakao F, Moriyama N, Takayama T, Yamasaki S, Sakamoto M, Hirohashi S. Early hepatocellular carcinoma: appearance at CT during arterial portography and CT arteriography with pathologic correlation. Radiology 194:101–105, 1995.

41. Bluemke DA, Soyer PA, Chan BW, Bliss DF, Calhoun PS, Fishman EK. Spiral CT during arterial portography: technique and applications. Radiographics, 15:623–637, 1995.

42. Choi BI, Park JH, Kim BH, Kim SH, Han MC, Kim CW. Small hepatocellular carcinoma: detection with sonography, computed tomography (CT), angiography and Lipiodol-CT. Br J Radiol 62:897–903, 1989.

43. De Santis M, Romagnoli R, Cristani A, Cioni G, Casolo A, Vici FF, Ventura E. MRI of small hepatocellular carcinoma: comparison with US, CT, DSA, and Lipiodol-CT. J Comput Assist Tomogr 16:189–197, 1992.

44. Eurvilaichit C. Lipiodol-enhanced CT scanning of malignant hepatic tumors. J Med Assoc Thai 83:398–406, 2000.

45. Lencioni R, Pinto F, Armillotta N, Di Giulio M, Gaeta P, Di Candio G, Marchi S, Bartolozzi C. Intrahepatic metastatic nodules of hepatocellular carcinoma detected at Lipiodol-CT: imaging-pathologic correlation [see comments]. Abdom Imaging 22:253–258, 1997.

46. Valls C, Figueras J. Detection of hepatocellular carcinoma in cirrhotic livers with Lipiodol-CT. Hepatology 28:273–275, 1998.

47. Onaya H, Itai Y. MR imaging of hepatocellular carcinoma. Magn Reson Imaging Clin North Am 8:757–768, 2000.

48. Sharma R, Saini S. Role and limitations of magnetic resonance imaging in the diagnostic work-up of patients with liver cancer. J Comput Assist Tomogr 23(Suppl 1):S39–S44, 1999.

49. Hagspiel KD, Neidl KF, Eichenberger AC, Weder W, Marincek B. Detection of liver mestastases: comparison of superparamagnetic iron oxide–enhanced and unenhanced MR imaging at 1.5 T with dynamic CT, intraoperative US, and percutaneous US. Radiology 196:471–478, 1995.

50. Bartolozzi C, Donati F, Cioni D, Crocetti L, Lencioni R. MnDPDP-enhanced MRI vs dual-phase spiral CT in the detection of hepatocellular carcinoma in cirrhosis. Eur Radiol 10:1697–1702, 2000.

51. Stern W, Schick F, Kopp AF, Reimer P, Shamsi K, Claussen CD, Laniado M. Dynamic MR imaging of liver metastases with Gd-EOB-DTPA. Acta Radiol 41:255–262, 2000.

52. Min JS, Kim NK, Park JK, Yun SH, Noh JK. A prospective randomized trial comparing intravenous 5-fluorouracil and oral doxifluridine as postoperative adjuvant treatment for advanced rectal cancer. Ann Surg Oncol 7:674–679, 2000.

53. Earls JP, Bluemke DA. New MR imaging contrast agents. Magn Reson Imaging Clin North Am 7:255–273, 1999.

54. Clement O, Siauve N, Lewin M, de Kerviler E, Cuenod CA, Frija G. Contrast agents in magnetic resonance imaging of the liver: present and future. Biomed Pharmacother 52:51–58, 1998.

55. Bluemke DA, Paulson EK, Choti MA, DeSena S, Clavien PA. Detection of hepatic lesions in candidates for surgery: comparison of ferumoxides-enhanced MR imaging and dual-phase helical CT. AJR Am J Roentgenol 175:1653–1658, 2000.

56. Iwata Y, Shiomi S, Sasaki N, Jomura H, Nishiguchi S, Seki S, Kawabe J, Ochi H. Clinical usefulness of positron emission tomography with fluorine-18-fluorodeoxyglucose in the diagnosis of liver tumors. Ann Nucl Med 14:121–126, 2000.

57. Delbeke D, Martin WH, Sandler MP, Chapman WC, Wright JK, Pinson CW. Evaluation of benign vs malignant hepatic lesions with positron emission tomography. Arch Surg 133:510–515, 1998.

58. Trojan J, Schroeder O, Raedle J, Baum RP, Herrmann G, Jacobi V, Zeuzem S. Fluorine-18 FDG positron emission tomography for imaging of hepatocellular carcinoma. Am J Gastroenterol 94:3314–3319, 1999.

59. Khan MA, Combs CS, Brunt EM, Lowe VJ, Wolverson MK, Solomon H, Collins BT, Di Bisceglie AM. Positron emission tomography scanning in the evaluation of hepatocellular carcinoma. J Hepatol 32:792–797, 2000.

60. Torzilli G, Minagawa M, Takayama T, Inoue K, Hui AM, Kubota K, Ohtomo K, Makuuchi M. Accurate preoperative evaluation of liver mass lesions without fine-needle biopsy. Hepatology 30:889–893, 1999.

61. Klintmalm GB. Liver transplantation for hepatocellular carcinoma: a registry report of the impact of tumor characteristics on outcome. Ann Surg 228:479–490, 1998.

62. Farges O, Malassagne B, Flejou JF, Balzan S, Sauvanet A, Belghiti J. Risk of major liver resection in patients with underlying chronic liver disease: a reappraisal. Ann Surg 229:210–215, 1999.

63. Koutselini H, Lazaris AC, Kavantzas N, Kiritsi T, Davaris PS. Significance of nuclear morphometry as a diagnostic tool in fine-needle aspirates of the liver. Eur J Gastroenterol Hepatol 12:913–921, 2000.

64. Longchampt E, Patriarche C, Fabre M. Accuracy of cytology vs. microbiopsy for the diagnosis of well-differentiated hepatocellular carcinoma and macroregenerative nodule. Definition of standardized criteria from a study of 100 cases. Acta Cytol 44:515–523, 2000.

65. de Boer WB, Segal A, Frost FA, Sterrett GF. Can CD34 discriminate between benign and malignant hepatocytic lesions in fine-needle aspirates and thin core biopsies? Cancer 90:273–278, 2000.

66. Borzio M, Borzio F, Macchi R, Croce AM, Bruno S, Ferrari A, Servida E. The evaluation of fine-needle procedures for the diagnosis of focal liver lesions in cirrhosis. J Hepatol 20:117–121, 1994.

67. Hertz G, Reddy VB, Green L, Spitz D, Massarani-Wafai R, Selvaggi SM, Kluskens L, Gattuso P. Fine-needle aspiration biopsy of the liver: a multicenter study of 602 radiologically guided FNA. Diagn Cytopathol 23:326–328, 2000.

68. Navarro F, Taourel P, Michel J, Perney P, Fabre JM, Blanc F, Domergue J. Diaphragmatic and subcutaneous seeding of hepatocellular carcinoma following fine-needle aspiration biopsy. Liver 18:251–254, 1998.

69. Kim SH, Lim HK, Lee WJ, Cho JM, Jang HJ. Needle-tract implantation in hepatocellular carcinoma: frequency and CT findings after biopsy with a 19.5-gauge automated biopsy gun. Abdom Imaging 25:246–250, 2000.

70. Babineau TJ, Lewis WD, Jenkins RL, Bleday R, Steele GD, Forse RA. Role of staging laparoscopy in the treatment of hepatic malignancy. Am J Surg 167:151–154, 1994.

71. Lo CM, Lai EC, Liu CL, Fan ST, Wong J. Laparoscopy and laparoscopic ultrasonography avoid exploratory laparotomy in patients with hepatocellular carcinoma. Ann Surg 227:527–532, 1998.

72. Lo CM, Fan ST, Liu CL, Poon RT, Lam CM, Yuen WK, Yeung C, Wong J. Determining resectability for hepatocellular carcinoma: the role of laparoscopy and laparoscopic ultrasonography. J Hepatobiliary Pancreat Surg 7:260–264, 2000.

73. Ido K, Nakazawa Y, Isoda N, Kawamoto C, Nagamine N, Ono K, Hozumi M, Sato Y, Kimura K, Sugano K. The role of laparoscopic US and laparoscopic US-guided aspiration biopsy in the diagnosis of multicentric hepatocellular carcinoma. Gastrointest Endosc 50:523–526, 1999.

74. Ezaki T, Stansby GP, Hobbs KE. Intraoperative ultrasonographic imaging in liver surgery: a review. HPB Surg 3:1–4, 1990.

75. Capussotti L, Polastri R. Operative risks of major hepatic resections. Hepatogastroenterology 45:184–190, 1998.

76. Kim ST, Kim KP. Hepatic resections for primary liver cancer. Cancer Chemother Pharmacol (33 Suppl):S18–S23, 1994.

77. Lai EC, Fan ST, Lo CM, Chu KM, Liu CL, Wong J. Hepatic resection for hepatocellular carcinoma. An audit of 343 patients. Ann Surg 221:291–298, 1995.

78. Shimada M, Takenaka K, Fujiwara Y, Gion T, Shirabe K, Yanaga K, Sugimachi K. Risk factors linked to postoperative morbidity in patients with hepatocellular carcinoma. Br J Surg 85:195–198, 1998.

79. Eguchi H, Umeshita K, Sakon M, Nagano H, Ito Y, Kishimoto SI, Dono K, Nakamori S, Takeda T, Gotoh M, Wakasa K, Matsuura N, Monden M. Presence of active hepatitis associated with liver cirrhosis is a risk factor for mortality caused by posthepatectomy liver failure. Dig Dis Sci 45:1383–1388, 2000.

80. Shimada M, Rikimaru T, Sugimachi K, Hamatsu T, Yamashita Y, Aishima S, Taguchi K, Tanaka S, Shirabe K. The importance of hepatic resection for hepatocellular carcinoma originating from nonfibrotic liver. J Am Coll Surg 191:531–537, 2000.

81. Rowntree L. An experimental and clinical study of the value of phenoltetrachlorphthalein as a test of hepatic function. Bull Johns Hopkins Hosp 24:327. 1913.

82. Merkel C, Gatta A, Zoli M, Bolognesi M, Angeli P, Iervese T, Marchesini G, Ruol A. Prognostic value of galactose elimination capacity, aminopyrine breath test, and ICG clearance in patients with cirrhosis. Comparison with the Pugh score. Dig Dis Sci 36:1197–1203, 1991.

83. Nonami T, Nakao A, Kurokawa T, Inagaki H, Matsushita Y, Sakamoto J, Takagi H. Blood loss and ICG clearance as best prognostic markers of post-hepatectomy liver failure. Hepatogastroenterology 46:1669–1672, 1999.

84. Ercolani G, Grazi GL, Calliva R, Pierangeli F, Cescon M, Cavallari A, Mazziotti A. The lidocaine (MEGX) test as an index of hepatic function: its clinical usefulness in liver surgery. Surgery 127:464–471, 2000.

85. Testa R, Valente U, Risso D, Caglieris S, Giannini E, Fasoli A, Botta F, Dardano G, Lantieri PB, Celle G. Can the MEGX test and serum bile acids improve the prognostic ability of Child-Pugh's score in liver cirrhosis? Eur J Gastroenterol Hepatol 11:559–563, 1999.

86. Bruix J, Castells A, Bosch J, Feu F, Fuster J, Garcia-Pagan JC, Visa J, Bru C, Rodes J. Surgical resection of hepatocellular carcinoma in cirrhotic patients: prognostic value of preoperative portal pressure. Gastroenterology 111:1018–1022, 1996.

# Chapter 45

# Clinical Aspects and Management of Hepatocellular Cancer

## Management Options: Potentially Resectable Hepatocellular Carcinoma

JASON M. ROBKE AND MARK S. ROH

Patients with hepatocellular carcinoma (HCC) have been treated with a number of different modalities over the years, including observation, systemic chemotherapy, surgical resection with and without adjuvant chemotherapy, radiation, and chemoembolization. Surgical resection used to be the only hope of prolonging survival or curing this disease. During the 1980s, resection rates ranged from 15% to 60%, with recurrence rates of 50% to 70%.[1] Survival at this time for cirrhotic patients ranged from 55% to 85% at 1 year, to 26% to 58% at 3 years, to less than 15% at 5 years. Noncirrhotic patients had a higher survival rate. In the 1990s the resection rate increased to greater than 75% with 1-, 3-, and 5-year survival estimated at 89%, 82%, and 50%, respectively, for noncirrhotic patients.[2–7] In recent years, cirrhotic patients have had similar survival statistics.[8] Also in the 1990s, 1-, 3-, and 5-year tumor-free survival rates of 78%, 40%, and 25% were reported.[4,9] Recent advances in technology along with appropriate patient selection can offer potentially curative therapy, possibly without undergoing hepatic resection.[10] Although chemoembolization has not been shown to cure HCC, some physicians think it can prolong survival. Percutaneous ethanol injection (PEI) and cryotherapy in the appropriate patients may show promise as well. Untreated HCC, however, is fatal, and surgical resection remains the most promising option for treatment. Unfortunately, only 30% of patients present with resectable lesions.[11] This chapter will discuss treatment options available for these patients.

## Anatomy of the Liver

An understanding of the anatomy of the liver is required before work-up and resectability can be undertaken. When one listens to people describe the location of tumors in their liver one quickly learns how confusing the anatomy of the liver can be. Often an incorrect description is given. What must be understood first is that there are two ways of dividing up the liver, based on morphologic anatomy or functional anatomy.[12,13]

*Morphologic (lobar) anatomy* examines the liver on the basis of its external appearance and attachments as seen in the abdomen during laparotomy. A *lobe* is defined as a part of parenchyma limited by fissures or grooves. From this view, the falciform ligament and umbilical fissure can be seen dividing the liver into a larger right lobe and a smaller left lobe. Tracing the falciform inferiorly, it wraps toward the hilus and the hilar fissure, which outlines the posterior extent of the right lobe. Lying anterior to the hilar fissure and between the gallbladder fossa and falciform is the quadrate lobe. Lying posterior and wrapping around the inferior vena cava (IVC) is the caudate (Spigel) lobe. This anatomy allows description of classic hemihepatectomies and lobectomies but is not sufficient to describe segmentectomies. This description does not take into account the vascular and metabolic divisions of the parenchyma.

*Functional anatomy* does address these divisions. It is based on the 1957 description by Couinaud[14] which separates the liver parenchyma according to portal venous flow and hepatic vein drainage. The three hepatic veins divide the liver into four sectors. They enter the liver along three portal scissurae and then divide to drain adjacent sectors. The portal vein branches enter the liver via hepatic scissurae and directly enter into the four sectors defined by the hepatic veins. For example, the falciform ligament lies on a hepatic scissura, meaning that a branch of the left portal vein enters the liver there, and hepatic veins enter the parenchyma adjacent to the area. The liver is divided into left and right hemilivers by the main portal scissura (which contains the middle hepatic vein). To the left of this are segments IV, III,

522

and II, which are fed by the left portal vein and drained by the left hepatic vein and branches of the middle hepatic vein. Thus the left liver extends to the right of the falciform. The right liver is fed by the right portal veins and drained by the right hepatic vein and half of the middle hepatic vein.

Location of the portal scissurae is often confusing, because there are no external landmarks for easy identification, such as with the morphologic anatomy. The main portal scissura (Cantle's line), which divides the liver into left and right hemilivers, lies along a line 75° from the horizontal plane opened to the left of the ex vivo liver, beginning at the IVC. This separates the liver into two hemilivers, which have different portal and arterial supplies as well as separate biliary drainage. Thus one can easily appreciate where the confusion arises: the morphological left lobe lies to the left of the falciform only, and the functional left lobe (or left liver/hemiliver) extends to the right of the falciform, encompassing a portion of the morphologic right lobe.

Each of the two hemilivers are further divided by the remaining two portal scissurae into segments as defined by Goldsmith and Woodburne,[15] or sectors defined by Couinaud.[14] The right portal scissura is inclined 40° to the right at the IVC, and divides the right hemiliver into anteromedial and posterolateral sectors. When the liver is in vivo, the right portal scissura lies approximately horizontal, making the anteromedial sector entirely anterior and the posterolateral sector entirely posterior. The right two sectors are further divided into two segments each, which are fed and drained by separate branches of their sector's respective portal and hepatic veins. The anterior sector of the right hemiliver contains segment VIII superiorly and segment V inferiorly. The posterior sector contains segment VII superiorly and segment VI inferiorly. The left liver contains segment IV anterior and to the right of the falciform. This segment extends posteriorly to the umbilical fissure and contains the quadrate lobe. Posterior to the umbilical fissure lies the caudate lobe, which will be addressed separately. Left of the falciform lies segments II superiorly and III inferiorly.

The caudate lobe, Spigel's lobe or segment I, is considered separate from the right and left livers because, from a functional view, its vasculature does not follow any of the above rules. Its veins drain directly into the IVC. Both left and right portal veins and hepatic arteries feed this segment. By some accounts it is considered a third liver, and this difference in vascular supply becomes evident in conditions such as Budd-Chiari syndrome, in which the hepatic veins thrombose but the caudate drainage remains patent and the lobe hypertrophies. This separation leads to difficulty in resecting lesions in this segment.

## Types of Resection

A *hepatectomy* involves removing one of the functional hemilivers, either right or left. This differs from a *lobectomy*, which involves resecting one of the morphologic lobes. Thus in a left hepatectomy, segment IV is resected as well, which is part of the right lobe. Hepatectomies can also be called *hepatic lobectomies,* a procedure that is still distinct from lobectomy. Resection of the left lobe is also known as a *left lateral segmentectomy,* and resection of the right lobe is also called a *right extended lobectomy* or a *trisegmentectomy* (removing the anteromedial and posterolateral segments of the right lobe as well as segment IV of the left liver). *Sectorectomies* involve resection between portal scissurae, and segmentectomies are resections of the individual segments named. The caudate is considered a separate segment from a right or left hepatectomy.

## Preoperative Evaluation

Before operative intervention can be undertaken, an appropriate preoperative work-up must be performed. Failure to adequately evaluate the patient, the liver, and the tumor can result in unnecessary laparotomies, inadequate resections, or patient death. The patient evaluation begins with determination of the patient's desire to undergo the risks of a resection. While surgery can prolong life, or even offer a cure, mortality rates from 0% to 10% have been reported for extensive hepatic resections in noncirrhotic patients.[1,3,16] For cirrhotic patients, morbidity rates of 50% and mortality rates of 10% to 20% are seen with resections.[1,2,3,17–19] Some patients and their families are not willing to accept the risk of a premature death from surgery, even though their disease will lead to their early death anyway.

A careful history and physical examination are then performed. While postoperative liver failure accounts for a number of deaths, other comorbidities increase this number. Cardiac, respiratory, renal, and hematologic conditions can be uncovered and possibly improved prior to operation.

The patient's age will affect recovery and must be taken into consideration before undergoing a resection. Studies with rats suggest that as the patient ages, the liver will tolerate less of a resection,[20] so what might be resectable in a younger population might not be resectable in the elderly. Preclinical studies suggest that the voluminal regenerative properties of the liver are not affected by age, but rather a decline in postoperative protein synthesis in patients.[21] A postoperative hospital death rate due to hepatic failure of greater than 40% has been reported in patients over 70, compared with less than 5% for younger patients undergoing similar resections.[22] Others have reached similar conclusions that patients over 70 have markedly increased morbidity and mortality.[22–25]

Nutritional state can be assessed for cachectic patients or those with malnutrition and lean body mass wasting from loss of appetite. Nutritional supplements or total parenteral nutrition (TPN) should be considered prior to surgery.[26–31]

Preoperative blood work should include serum electrolytes, BUN, creatinine, liver function tests, coagulation panel, complete blood counts, and an albumin level. An electrocardiogram (EKG) and chest X-ray should be reviewed and evaluated by the appropriate specialists. An adequate supply of cross-matched blood and coagulation factors should be readily available.

The liver and tumor can then be evaluated through a variety of methods. The standard screening test of the liver for HCC is ultrasound. The usual advantages of ultrasound use apply, such as low cost, noninvasiveness, and ease on the patient. Ultrasound also has a sensitivity for detection of HCC of greater than 85%,[32] and as the technology improves this sensitivity will only increase. Ultrasound can detect lesions smaller than 1 cm in diameter.[33] There are, however, disadvantages to relying solely on ultrasound. In patients with end-stage cirrhotic livers that were removed for transplant and then examined, the sensitivity was about 50%.[34] Ultrasound has been shown to be better at differentiating HCC from benign lesions in cirrhotic livers,[35] and development of ultrasound contrast media to further improve this is under study.[36] Infiltrative forms of HCC may be undetectable by ultrasound when the lesions are less than 3 cm in diameter.[34] As the size of the tumor increases, the ultrasound characteristics change.

Tumors less than 2 cm tend to be hypoechoic, with less than 10% being hyperechoic. As the tumor grows larger than 2 cm, about 50% remain hypoechoic. The degree of heterogeneity depends on the amount of fat, sinusoidal dilatation, hemorrhage, and necrosis. Ultrasound works well for detecting a capsule, which appears as a hypoechoic halo. Parenchymal changes that occur around many tumors also produce a halo, so this finding on ultrasound alone is of limited use. What ultrasound is very useful for, however, is detecting invasion of the portal veins. Ultrasound is superior to computed tomography (CT) and magnetic resonance imaging (MRI) in this area. Although it is difficult to detect subsegmental invasion major segmental invasion should be seen. Ultrasound is not always reliable in accurately identifying invasion of the hepatic veins, IVC, and bile ducts. Bile duct dilatation can be seen, which should prompt cholangiography.

For many abdominal pathologies, a CT of the abdomen is usually an excellent diagnostic tool. In the case of HCC, CT has limitations. Because of the hypervascularity of HCC, the tumor is best seen when the entire liver can be scanned while the intravenous contrast is enhancing it. Older, slower CT machines fail to sequence the entire liver in this short time span. This failure may lead to underappreciation of the extent of the tumor. The newer, helical CT machines have changed this situation. Another drawback to CT is its decreased sensitivity to venous invasion, compared with ultrasound. Computed tomography scans should be performed with intravenous contrast when possible. Abdominal CT with contrast can delineate lesions less than 1 cm in diameter and has been shown to be better than MRI at detecting such small lesions.[33,37] Hepatocellular carcinoma appears as an enhancing lesion during the arterial phase and becomes hypodense or isodense during the portal venous phase or during unenhanced scans. Capsules, when present, can be seen with CT but may have enhancement delayed by about 5 minutes. Another, more invasive method for detecting small HCCs is through intraarterial injection of Lipiodol.

The radiological study of choice for HCC is MRI. The sensitivity and specificity of MRI surpass those of CT and ultrasound, and ongoing improvements in the technology continue.[38–40] It also detects lesions smaller than 1 cm.[33] Two-thirds of the time, T1-weighted images show the tumor to be hypointense, with hyperintense surrounding liver. A surrounding capsule appears as a hypointense halo. Hepatocellular carcinoma is hyperintense on T2-weighted images, and a capsule shows as a single, hypointense or double-layered halo. Gadolinium-enhanced MRI enhances the tumor best during the arterial phase, and then diminishes to iso- or hypointense in later images. Ultrasound still surpasses MRI at detecting vein and bile duct invasion. Although CT is not as useful as MRI, an MRI need not be ordered if an adequate CT is performed.[41] However, MRI has been reported to be better at detecting tumor pseudocapsule,[42] and it may[43] or may not[35] be better than CT at determining whether a hepatic lesion is benign or malignant.

Another method of observing the liver and identifying possible HCC is through CT or MR arterial portography (AP).[11,19,44–49] This involves performing an angiogram to place an arterial catheter into the mesenteric circulation and then directly injecting contrast material into the liver during the scan. Yu and co-workers[43] found fewer false-positive lesions with MRAP than with CTAP. Magnetic resonance AP required less contrast medium than does CTAP. They concluded that MRAP optimally shows liver parenchyma, even in cirrhosis, and "offers high sensitivity in the early detection of focal lesions with decreased portal flow." Some investigators consider spiral CT to have surpassed AP in imaging accuracy, and spiral CT is probably the study of choice, even over MRI, in imaging HCC.[33]

If the patient remains a surgical candidate, mesenteric angiography is required prior to resection. The vascular supply to the liver should be known to the operative surgeon, specifically the presence of an aberrant arterial supply. The angiogram will also further outline the tumor and its blood supply and may help with situations of questionable vascular invasion. It should not be used as the sole diagnostic tool. Angiography exhibits high sensitivity for HCC but is surpassed by the combination of ultrasound and MRI. An initial examination by ultrasound, complemented by MRI, and finally angiography before surgery are also a recommended strategy.[34]

The previous comments refer to the work-up of a noncirrhotic liver. Cirrhotic livers have scar tissue, fibrosis, regenerating nodules, and necrosis. All of these change the architecture of the liver and affect its appearance on radiologic scans. Not infrequently they mask a tumor on one scan, which can then only be seen with another. A liberal combination of the methods discussed above should be used in this case to ensure the most accurate evaluation of the liver.

Any patient with suspicion of metastases to bone or brain should undergo the appropriate nuclear medicine scan prior to operation. Confirmation of extrahepatic disease is a contraindication to surgery, and percutaneous or intravascular methods of treatment are the only alternatives.

After it has been determined that the patient can tolerate a major surgery and the extent of the hepatic resection is known, the next question to be answered is whether the liver can survive a partial resection. Major resection of noncirrhotic livers has been established to be a safe procedure with less than 10% mortality. Normal liver can tolerate up to 70% resection. This changes with cirrhotic patients, as mortality increases from 12% to 37%. Those patients with elements of liver failure need further evaluation of the liver. Several methods are available to evaluate hepatic function and reserve. The most simple measures of hepatic function are the classification systems of Child and Pugh.[50,51] These systems group patients into three groups, A, B, and C, according to the presence or absence of ascites and encephalopathy and patient nutritional status as determined by serum laboratory values. The Child system measures serum albumin and bilirubin. The Pugh system substitutes prothrombin time for albumin and bilirubin. Variable success has been reported in using these classifications as predictors of outcome. Reports of increased in-hospital and long-term survival in class A over B and C have been seen,[2] as well as reports stating no correlation.[17,52] One limit to these studies is the lack of sufficient numbers in the C class. More recent investigations support higher mortalities for patients in class C and recommend that such patients be evaluated for liver transplant instead of resection. Patients who did not have cirrhosis had better in-hospital and overall survival.[1]

Another popular method of evaluating the liver is based on hepatic blood flow and clearance of indocyanine green (ICG). This medium is used in several different ways as a sensitive indicator of hepatic function.[53] One method measures ICG clearance (ICGC), which involves injecting 0.5 mg/kg of ICG into a peripheral vein and then measuring ICG levels in the contralateral vein at 2, 4, 6, 8, 10, 15, 20, 25, 30, 40, 50, 60, and 90 minutes. A two-compartment model of ICG elimination calculates the mean blood clearance using the following formula:[54]

$$[(\text{Dose} / \text{AUG}) \times (1 - \text{Hct})] \times 100 = \text{Total clearance \%}$$

where AUG is the area under the elimination curve and Hct is the hematocrit.

Using this model, Hemming and co-workers[53] found a 30-day postoperative mortality rate of 18%. The type of resection did not appear to be a factor and no significant difference existed in preoperative laboratory results or age between survivors vs. non-survivors. A significant difference was found in ICGC. Survivors had an ICGC of 7.7 ± 0.7 (SEM) ml/min/kg, and nonsurvivors had an ICGC of 2.5 ± 3.5 ml/min/kg. Analysis yielded a discriminating point of 5.2 ml/min/kg.

Hemming and co-workers concluded that age, cirrhosis, and preoperative liver function tests should not be contraindications to resection, but that an ICGC of less than 5.0 ml/min/kg should be. It should be pointed out that their mortality using this model is markedly greater than that for other reports, and they did not differentiate between extents of resections.

Another model of liver evaluation is the ICG retention rate at 15 minutes (ICG15).[55] Makuuchi and co-workers[56] summarize nicely the experiences of two specialized centers in Japan and provide a simple algorithm for determining the extent of resection a patient can survive. If a patient has uncontrollable ascites, even with diuretics, then they are not candidates for hepatectomy. Patients with controllable ascites should have their serum bilirubin concentration determined; if the value is normal, then they can undergo ICG15 testing. Patients with bilirubin values between 1.1 and 1.5 mg/dl can have limited resections. Patients with bilirubin values between 1.6 and 1.9 mg/dl will tolerate enucleation only. Patients with bilirubin levels greater than 2.0 mg/dl cannot be resected. Patients with normal bilirubin values and normal ICG15 results can tolerate resection of two-thirds of the noncancerous liver, which includes right hepatectomy, extended right hepatectomy, and left hepatectomy. If the volume of noncancerous liver required for an adequate resection exceeds 60% of the total noncancerous liver volume, then portal vein embolization (PVE) is performed.[56] Patients with ICG15 values of 10%–19% tolerated resection of one-third of the noncancerous liver. If greater than one-third of the noncancerous liver needed to be resected, then these patients underwent PVE. If the ICG15 value was 20%–29%, then Couinand's single segmentectomy was performed by cannulating the portal vein feeding the cancerous area, injecting indigocarmine, and resecting the stained area. Patients with ICG15 values of 30%–39% and of greater than 40% tolerated limited resection and enucleation, respectively, at best.

Using these criteria for ICG15, these authors reported in-hospital and surgical mortalities of 0.82% and 0.27%, respectively.[57] One-, 3-, and 5-year survival rates were 92%, 73%, and 47%; tumor-free survival rates were 62%, 32%, and 13%. Sectorectomy, segmentectomy, and subsegmentectomy provided significantly better tumor-free survival ($P < 0.05$). The authors boldly state that if surgeons follow their preoperative guidelines, mortality will be limited to less than 1%, and "if jaundice occurs after hepatic resection, this should be considered a failure to select the most appropriate surgical procedure, even if jaundice resolves." Others have reported similar results.[6,58]

Other methods of estimating liver reserve exist. Use of monoethylglycinexyloiodide (MEGX),[59] and determination of maximum removal rate of ICG[60] and arterial ketone body ratio[61] have been described, but their clinical applications are questioned.[62–64]

## Liver Resection and Related Considerations

Once the location of the lesions and the maximum estimated volume of liver that can be resected have been determined, the ac-tual operation can be planned. First to be considered is whether any preoperative therapies should be given. Preoperative PVE to the resected side is advocated by some practioners.[65] The rationale behind this method is that by diminishing blood flow to the pathological side, the rest of the liver will hypertrophy prior to resection, thus decreasing the incidence of postoperative liver failure. Increases in volume from 44% to 90% have been reported.[66,67] No controlled trials have been undertaken to prove that this technique decreases morbidity and mortality.[33] Preoperative transarterial embolization appears to have no role in treating HCC.[68,69] Neoadjuvant chemotherapy also does not improve survival, nor does it decrease recurrence.[70]

When the extent of resection is planned, several points need to be considered. Decreased recurrence and increased survival occur with anatomic resections, in contrast to local excisions, and with at least a 1-cm margin.[6,8,71–74] Among patients who undergo anatomic resection, mortality rates are higher with hepatic resections than with segmentectomies, with similar long-term survival.[1,73,74] Performance of a segmentectomy allows for repeated resections should recurrence occur. In general, if the liver can tolerate it, the smallest anatomic resection should be performed to ensure at least a 1-cm margin. If the liver cannot tolerate a segmentectomy, then local excision is performed.

Special mention should be made of tumors of the caudate lobe. Because of its location adjacent to the IVC and hepatic veins, exposure and resection are possible but more complicated. Often an isolated resection of the entire caudate lobe is not appropriate. Further investigation into the efficacy of isolated caudate resections needs to be performed.[75,76] Because of the difficulty of caudate lobe exposure and resection, patients with caudate tumors need to be referred to surgeons and hospitals experienced in handling these resections.

Many studies have listed various indications and contraindications for HCC resections. The most important point to remember is that if the surgeon feels the patient and the liver can tolerate a resection, then surgery should be performed. Resections of multicentric tumors have been done, albeit with a higher recurrence and decreased overall survival than for solitary tumors, but with improved survival compared to any other modality of treatment.[77] Of the contraindications to surgery, several are worth mentioning. Diffuse spread of tumor throughout the liver is obviously not curable by surgery. Liver transplantation studies are reporting better survival than resection but are hindered by the lack of available livers. Patients that are definitely not candidates for resection should be evaluated for transplantation.[3,11,78–82] While tumor invasion into the intrahepatic vascular or biliary tree decreases survival, it is not a contraindication to surgery. Tanaka and co-workers[83] noted, however, that evidence of intrahepatic metastases and IVC thrombus resulted in 100% mortality from early recurrence. Tumor thrombus extending into the IVC or hepatic veins can be removed by performing hepatic vascular exclusion and thrombectomy or replacing the IVC with a prosthetic conduit, but no long-term improvement in survival has been proven,[81,84] and subjecting the patient to such a major undertaking must be strongly weighed against a questionable short-term improvement.

Recent technical advances have allowed for extensive hepatic resections with limited intraoperative mortality. The ability to control the pre- and posthepatic vasculature has greatly improved hepatic surgery. Complete mobilization of the liver should be perfomed prior to beginning the resection. The surgeon will then be able to rapidly compress portions of the liver to stop or diminish any bleeding that may occur, while the assistant achieves he-

mostasis. Selective inflow control limits blood loss by ligating or embolizing all inflow to the target area as soon as possible. Total inflow occlusion (Pringle maneuver) can also be performed by clamping all of the inflow vessels in the gastrohepatic ligament. A normal liver should be able to withstand 1 hour of inflow occlusion, but most surgeons interrupt the warm ischemia time by unclamping for 5 or 10 minutes every 15 to 30 minutes. Total vascular isolation of the liver using the Pringle maneuver and atrial-caval shunts enables surgery in and around the hepatic veins and IVC with a great reduction in potential blood loss.[85] For complicated tumors with difficult exposures, ex vivo resections can be performed by surgeons experienced in this technique.

Predictors of positive outcome and prognosis include absence of tumor-related symptoms, early stage, size less than 5 cm, fewer than three tumors, low α-fetoprotein, presence of a capsule, absence of vascular invasion, at least a 1-cm margin, and anatomic resection.[1,73,74,86–90]

Adjuvant therapy has little to offer HCC patients after resection. Chemotherapy, systemic and intraarterial, has not been shown to significantly change recurrence,[70,91–95] but postoperative injection of chemotherapeutic agents suspended in Lipiodol may significantly decrease intrahepatic recurrence of HCC.[91] Another promising therapy that is still in its infancy is use of synthetic retinoids. In experimental animals treated with synthetic retinoids, recurrence of HCC decreased from 49% to 27%.[96]

Should evidence of tumor recurrence occur, the best option is re-resection as long as the work-up of the recurrent tumor leaves this as an option. Results of re-resection are as good as primary resection and offer the best prognosis.[97–102] Chemoembolization for recurrence has not been proven to significantly prolong survival.

Future treatments for hepatocellular carcinoma include further study of retinoids,[96] percutaneous ethanol injection, and microwave tissue coagulation.[21,103–106]

## References

1. MacIntosh IL, Minuk HY. Hepatic resection in patients with cirrhosis and hepatocellular carcinoma. Surg Gynecol Obstet 174:245–254, 1992.
2. Franco D, Capussotti L, Smadja C, et al. Resection of hepatocellular carcinomas: results in 72 European patients with cirrhosis. Gastroenterology 98:733–738, 1990.
3. Philosophe B, Greig P, Hemming A, et al. Surgical management of hepatocellular carcinoma: resection or transplantation? J Gastrointest Surg 2:21–27, 1998.
4. Shuto T, Hirohashi K. Changes and results of surgical strategies for hepatocellular carcinoma: results of a 15-year study on 452 consecutive patients. Jpn J Surg 28:1124–1129, 1998.
5. Nagasue N, Kohno G, Chang Y, et al. Liver resection for hepatocellular carcinoma, results of 229 consecutive patients during 11 years. Ann Surg 217:375–384, 1993.
6. Lai E, Fan S, Lo C, Chu K, Liu C, Wong J. Hepatic resection for hepatocellular carcinoma, an audit of 343 patients. Ann Surg 221:291–298, 1995.
7. Vauthey J, Klinstra D, Franceschi D, et al. Factors affecting long-term outcome after hepatic resection for hepatocellular carcinoma. Am J Surg 169:28–35, 1995.
8. Mazziotti A, Grazi G, Cavallari A. Surgical treatment of hepatocellular carcinoma on cirrhosis: a Western experience. Hepatogastroenterology 45:1281–1287, 1998.
9. Ikeda K, Saitoh S, Tsubota A, et al. Risk factors for tumor recurrence and prognosis after curative resection of hepatocellular carcinoma. Cancer 7:19–25, 1993.
10. Palma D. Diagnostic imaging and interventional therapy of hepatocellular carcinoma. Br J Radiol 71:808–818, 1998.
11. Olthoff K. Surgical options for hepatocellular carcinoma: resection and transplantation. Liver Transplant Surg 4(5, Suppl 1):S98–S104, 1998.
12. Bismuth H, Castaing D, Roccuia J, Nyhus L, Baker R, Fischer J. Surgical anatomy of the liver and bile ducts. In: Bismuth L (ed): Mastery of Surgery, 3rd ed. Little, Brown and Company, Boston, 1997, pp 1003–1015.
13. Blumgart LH, Hann L, Fong Y. Surgical and radiologic anatomy of the liver and biliary tract. In: Blumgart LH and Fong Y (eds): Surgery of the Liver and Biliary Tract, 3rd ed. W.B. Saunders, London, 2000, pp 3–33.
14. Couinaud C. Le Foie. Etudes Anatomiques et Chirurgicales. Masson, Paris, 1957.
15. Goldsmith NA, Woodburne RT. Surgical anatomy pertaining to liver resection. Surg Gynecol Obstet 195:310–318, 1957.
16. Bowman D, Walt A. Current status of resection for hepatic neoplasms. Semin Liv Dis 3:193–202, 1983.
17. Nagao T, Inone S, Goto S, et al. Hepatic resection for hepatocellular carcinoma: clinical features and longterm prognosis. Ann Surg 205:33–40, 1997.
18. Kanematsu T, Takenaka K, Matsumata T, Juruto T, Sugimachi K, Inokuchi K. Limited hepatic resection effective for selected cirrhotic patients with primary liver cancer. Ann Surg 199:51–56, 1984.
19. Lee N, Wong J, Ong G. The surgical management of primary carcinoma of the liver. World J Surg 6:66–75, 1982.
20. Bucher N. Influence of age upon incorporation of thymidine-2-C$_{14}$ into DNA of regenerating rat liver. Cancer Res 24:509–512, 1964.
21. Carrillo MC, Carnovale CE, Favre C, Monti JA, Scapini C. Hepatic protein synthesis and serum amino acid levels during liver regeneration in young and old malnourished rats. Mech Ageing Dev 91:55–64, 1996.
22. Yamamoto K, Takinaka K, Matsumato T, et al. Right hepatic lobectomy in elderly patients with hepatocellular carcinoma. Hepatogastroenterology 44:514–518, 1997.
23. Takenaka K, Shimada M, Higashi H, et al. Liver resection for hepatocellular carcinoma in the elderly. Arch Surg 129:846–850, 1994.
24. Fong Y, Blumgart L, Fortnes J, Brennan M. Pancreatic or liver resection for malignancy is safe and effective for the elderly. Ann Surg 222:426–437, 1995.
25. Karl R, Smith S, Fabri P. Validity of major cancer operations in elderly patients. Ann Surg Oncol 2:107–113, 1995.
26. Muller J, Thul P, Ablassmaier B. Perioperative nutritional therapy and its relevance for postoperative outcome. Chirurg 68:574–582.
27. Heys S, Walker L, Erimin O. The value of perioperative nutrition in the sick patient. Proc Nutr Soc 56(1B):443–457, 1997.
28. Heys S, Gaugh D, Erimin O. Is nutritional support in patients with cancer undergoing surgery beneficial? Eur J Surg Oncol. 22(3):292–297, 1996.
29. Hill A, Daly J. Current indications for intravenous nutritional support in oncology patients. Surg Oncol Clin North Am 4:549–563, 1995.
30. Buzby G. Overview of randomized clinical trials of TPN for malnourished surgical patients. World J Surg 17:173–177, 1993.
31. Daly J, Redmond H, Gallagher H. Perioperative nutrition in cancer patients. JPEN J Parenter Enteral Nutr 16(Suppl):1005–1055, 1992.
32. Kanematsu T, Sonoda T, Takenaka K, et al. The value of ultrasound in the diagnosis and treatment of small hepatocellular carcinoma. Br J Surg 72:23–25, 1985.
33. Hemming M, Greig P, Langer B. Current surgical management of primary hepatocellular carcinoma. Adv Surg 32:169–193, 1999.
34. Yves M. Hepatocellular carcinoma radiological findings. Hepatogastroenterology 45:1232–1235, 1998.
35. Kanematsu M. Small hepatic nodules in cirrhosis: ultrasound, CT and MR imaging findings. Abdomin Imaging 24:47–55, 1999.
36. Tanaka S, Kitmara T, Fujiito M, Yoshioka F. Value of contrast-enhanced color Doppler sonography in diagnosing hepatocellular carcinoma with special attention to the "color-filled pattern." J Clin Ultrasound 26:207–212, 1998.
37. Hori M, Murakami T, Oi H, et al. Sensitivity in detection of hypervascular hepatocellular carcinoma by helical CT with intraarterial injection of contrast medium, and by helical CT and MR imaging with intravenous injection of contrast medium. Acta Radiol 39:144–151, 1998.
38. Earls J, Theise N, Weinreb J, et al. Dysplastic nodules and hepatocellular carcinoma: thin-section MR imaging of explanted cirrhotic livers with pathologic correlation. Radiology 201:207–214, 1996.
39. Peterson M, Baron R, Marukami T. Hepatic malignancies: usefulness of acquisition of multiple arterial and portal venous phase images at dynamic gadolinium-enhanced MR imaging. Radiology 201:337–345, 1996.

40. Yamashita Y, Mitsuzaki K, Yi T, et al. Small hepatocellular carcinoma in patients with chronic liver damage: prospective comparison of detection with dynamic MR imaging, and helical CT of the whole liver. Radiology 200:79–84, 1996.

41. Coffin C, Diche T, Mahfouy A, et al. Benign and malignant hepatocellular tumor: evaluation of tumoral enhancement after mangafodipir trisodium injection of MR imaging. Eur Radiol 9:444–449, 1999.

42. Grazide L, Olivetti L, Fugazzola A, et al. The pseudocapsule in hepatocellular carcinoma: correlation between dynamic MR imaging and pathology. Eur Radiol 9:62–67, 1999.

43. Yu J, Kim K, See J, Yoo H. MR imaging during arterial portography for assessment of hepatocellular carcinoma: comparison with CT during arterial portography. AJR Am J Roentgenol 170:1501–1506, 1998.

44. Matsui O, Kaduya M, Kameyama T, et al. Benign and malignant nodules in cirrhotic livers: distinction based on blood supply. Radiology 178:494–497, 1991.

45. Takayasu K, Muramatsu Y, Furukawa H, et al. Early hepatocellular carcinoma: appearance at CT during arterial portography and CT arteriography with pathologic correlation. Radiology 194:101–105, 1995.

46. Merine K, Takayasu K, Wakao F. Detection of hepatocellular carcinoma: comparison of CT during arterial portography with CT after intraarterial injection of iodized oil. Radiology 175:123–126, 1990.

47. Pavone P, Giuliani A, Cardone G, et al. Intraarterial portography with gadopentetate dimeglumine: improved liver to lesion contrast in MR imaging. Radiology 179:693–697, 1991.

48. Soyer P, Laissy JP, Sibert A, et al. Focal hepatic masses: comparison of detection during arterial portography with MR imaging and CT. Radiology 1990:737–740, 1994.

49. Dravid V, Shapiro M, Mitchell D, et al. MR portography: preliminary comparison with CT portography and conventional MR imaging. J Magn Reson Imaging 4:767–771, 1994.

50. Child C. The Liver and Portal Hypertension. W.B. Saunders, Philadelphia, 1954.

51. Pugh R, Murray-Lyon I, Dawson J, et al. Transection of the esophagus for bleeding esophageal varices. Br J Surg 60:646–649, 1973.

52. Nagasue N, Hukaya H, Ogawa Y, Sasaki Y, Chang Y, Neimi K. Clinical experience with 118 hepatic resections for hepatocellular carcinoma. Surgery 99:694–701, 1986.

53. Gottlieb ME, Stratton H, Newell J, Shah D. Indocyanine green its use as an early indicator of hepatic dysfunction following injury in man. Arch Surg 119:264–268, 1984.

54. Hemming AW, Scudamore CH, Shackleton C, Pudek M, Erb S. Indocyanine green clearance as a predictor of successful hepatic resection in cirrhotic patients. Am J Surg 163:515–518, 1992.

55. Kubota K, Maduuchi M, Kusaka K, et al. Measurement of liver volume and hepatic functional reserve as a guide to decision-making in resectional surgery for hepatic tumors. Hepatology 26:1176–1181, 1997.

56. Makuuchi M, Le Thai B, Takayasu K, et al. Preoperative portal embolization to increase safety of major hepatectomy for hilar bile duct carcinoma: preliminary report. Surgery 107:521–527, 1990.

57. Makuuchi M, Takayama T, Kubota K, et al. Hepatic resection for hepatocellular carcinoma Japanese experience. Hepatogastroenterology 45:1267–1274, 1998.

58. Takenaka K, Kawahara N, Yamamoto K, et al. Results of 280 liver resections for hepatocellular carcinoma. Arch Surg 131:71–76, 1996.

59. Shiffman M, Luketic VA, Sanyal A, et al. Hepatic lidocaine metabolism and liver histology in patients with chronic hepatitis and cirrhosis. Hepatology 19:933–940, 1994.

60. Moody FG, Rillers LF, Aldrete JS. Estimation of the functional reserve of human liver. Ann Surg 180:592–598, 1974.

61. Yamaoka Y, Washida M, Manaka D, et al. Arterial ketone body ratio as a predictor of donor liver viability in human liver transplantation. Transplantation 55:92–95, 1993.

62. Leclercq I, Saliez A, Wallemacq P, Horsmans Y, Lambotti L. The monoethylglycinexylidide test does not correctly evaluate lidocaine metabolism after ischemic liver injury in the rat. Hepatology 26:1182–1118, 1997.

63. Kawasaki S, Sugiyama Y, Iga T, et al. Pharmacokinetic study on hepatic uptake of indocyanine green in cirrhotic patients. Am J Gastroenterol 80:801–806, 1985.

64. Matsushita K, Kawasaki S, Makuuchi M, et al. Arterial ketone body ratio in liver surgery. Hepatology 20:331–335, 1994.

65. Kinoshita H, Sakai K, Hirohashi K, Igawa S, Yamasaki O, Kubo S. Preoperative portal vein embolization for hepatocellular carcinoma. World J Surg 10:803–808, 1986.

66. De Baere T, Roche A, Elias D, Lassa P, Lagrange C, Bousson V. Preoperative portal vein embolization for extension of hepatectomy indications. Hepatology 24:1386–1391, 1996.

67. Shimamura T, Nakajimi Y, Une Y, et al. Efficacy and safety of preoperative percutaneous transhepatic portal embolization with absolute alcohol: a clinical study. Surgery 121:135–141, 1997.

68. Nagasue N, Galizia G, Kohno H, et al. Adverse effects of preoperative hepatic artery chemoembolization for resectable hepatocellular carcinoma: a retrospective comparison of 138 liver resections. Surgery 106:81–86, 1989.

69. Adachi E, Matsumata T, Nishizaki T, Hashimoto H, Tsuneyoshi M, Sugimachi K. Effects of preoperative transcatheter hepatic arterial chemoembolization for hepatocellular carcinoma. The relationship between postoperative course and tumor necrosis. Cancer 72:3593–3598, 1993.

70. Rougier P, Mitry E, Clavero-Fabri M. Chemotherapy and medical treatment of hepatocellular carcinoma. Hepatogastroenterology 45:1264–1266, 1998.

71. Nonami T, Harada A, Kwokawa T, Nakao A, Takagi H. Advances in hepatic resection and results for hepatocellular carcinoma. Semin Surg Oncol 12:183–188, 1996.

72. Miyagawa S, Kawasaki S. Subsegmentectomy or segmentectomy in hepatocellular carcinoma. Hepatogastroenterology 45:2–6, 1998.

73. Kanematsu T, Sugimachi K, Kohno H, Matsumata T, Kobayashi M, Inokuchi K. Minute liver cancer and concomitant esophageal varices: detection and successful surgical treatment. World J Surg 5:707–711, 1981.

74. Wolff H, Winkler H, Lippert H. Liver transplantation for malignant liver disease. Trans Proc 21:2406, 1989.

75. Takayama T, Makuuchi M. Segmental liver resections, present and future caudate lobe resection for liver tumors. Hepatogastroenterology 45:20–23, 1998.

76. Asahara T, Dohi K, Hiroshi H, et al. Isolated caudate lobectomy by anterior approach for hepatocellular carcinoma originating in the paracaval portion of the caudate lobe. J Hepatobiliary Pancreat Surg 5:416–421, 1998.

77. Okusaka T, Okada S, Nose H, et al. The prognosis of patients with hepatocellular carcinoma of multicentric origin. Hepatogastroenterology 43:919–925, 1996.

78. Houben K, McCall J. Liver transplantation for hepatocellular carcinoma in patients without underlying liver disease: a systematic review. Liver Transplant Surg 5:91–95, 1999.

79. Van Thiel D, Colantoni A, De Maria N. Liver transplantation for hepatocellular carcinoma? Hepatogastroenterology 45:1944–1949, 1998.

80. Yokoyama I, Takagi H. Liver transplantation and hepatocellular carcinoma. Semin Surg Oncol 12:212–216, 1996.

81. Otto G, Heuschen U, Hofmann W, Krumm G, Hiny U, Herfarth C. Survival and recurrence after liver transplantation versus liver resection for hepatocellular carcinoma. Ann Surg 227:424–432, 1998.

82. Schwartz M. Primary hepatocellular carcinoma: transplant versus resection. Semin Liver Dis 14:135–139, 1994.

83. Tanaka A, Morimoto T, Oyaki N, et al. Extension of surgical indication for advanced hepatocellular carcinoma: is it possible to prolong life span or improve quality of life? Hepatogastroenterology 43:1172–1181, 1996.

84. Nonami T, Nakao A, Harada A, Kaneko T, Kurokawa T, Takagi H. Hepatic resection for hepatocellular carcinoma with a tumor thrombus extending to inferior vena cava. Hepatogastroenterology 44:798–802, 1997.

85. Mattox K, Pachter H, Liang H, Hofstetter S, Feliciano D, Moore E. Liver and biliary tract trauma. Trauma, 4th ed. McGraw-Hill, New York, 2000, pp 661–662.

86. Bismuth H, Chiche L, Adam R, Castaing D, Diamond T, Dennison A. Liver resection versus transplantation for hepatocellular carcinoma in cirrhotic patients. Ann Surg 218:145–151, 1993.

87. Otto G, Heuschen U, Hofmann W, Krumm H, Hinz U, Herfarth C. Is transplantation really superior to resection in the treatment of small hepatocellular carcinoma? Transplant Proc 29:489–491, 1997.

88. Iwatsuki S, Starzl T, Sheahan D, et al. Hepatic resection versus transplantation for hepatocellular carcinoma. Ann Surg 214:221–229, 1991.

89. Colella G, DeCarlis L, Rondinara G, et al. Is hepatocellular carcinoma in cirrhotics an actual indication for liver transplantation? Transplant Proc 29:492–494, 1997.

90. Mazzaferro V, Regalia E, Doci R, et al. Liver transplantation for the treatment of small hepatocellular carcinoma in patients with cirrhosis. N Engl J Med 334:393–399, 1996.

91. Takenaka K, Yoshida K, Nisfizaki T, et al. Postoperative prophylactic lipiodolization reduces the intrahepatic recurrence of hepatocellular carcinoma. Am J Surg 169:400–405, 1995.

92. Lai E, Lo C, Fan S, Liu C, Wong J. Postoperative adjuvant chemotherapy after curative resection of hepatocellular carcinoma. Arch Surg 133:183–188, 1998.

93. Okada S. Chemotherapy in hepatocellular carcinoma. Hepatogastroenterology 45:1259–1263, 1998.

94. Sasaki Y, Imaoka S, Fujita M, et al. Regional therapy in the management of intrahepatic recurrence after surgery for hepatoma. Ann Surg 206:40–47, 1987.

95. Izumi R, Shimizu K, Miyazaki I. Postoperative adjuvant locoregional chemotherapy in patients with hepatocellular carcinoma. Hepatogastroenterology 43:1415–1420, 1996.

96. Muto Y, Moriwaki H, Ninomiya M, et al. Prevention of second primary tumors by an acyclic retinoid, polyprenoic acid, in patients with hepatocellular carcinoma. N Engl J Med 334:1561–1567, 1996.

97. Hu R, Lee P, Yu S, et al. Surgical resection for recurrent hepatocellular carcinoma: prognosis and analysis of risk factors. Surgery 120:23–29, 1996.

98. Farges O, Regimbeau J, Belghiti J. Aggressive management of recurrence following surgical resection of hepatocellular carcinoma. Hepatogastroenterology 45:1275–1280, 1998.

99. Matsuda Y, Ito T, Oguchi Y, Nakajuma K, Izukura T. Rationale of surgical management for recurrent hepatocellular carcinoma. Ann Surg 217:28–34, 1993.

100. Shimada M, Mastumata T, Taketomi A, Yamamoto K, Itasaka H, Sugimachi K. Repeat hepatectomy for recurrent hepatocellular carcinoma. Surgery 115:703–706, 1994.

101. Jeng K, Yang F, Chiang H, Ohta I. Repeat operation for nodular recurrent hepatocellular carcinoma within the cirrhotic liver remnant: a comparison with transcatheter arterial chemoembolization. World J Surg 16:1188–1192, 1992.

102. Kanematsu T, Matsumata T, Takenaka K, Yoshida Y, Higashi H, Sugimachi K. Clinical management of recurrent hepatocellular carcinoma after primary resection. Br J Surg 75:203–206, 1988.

103. Castellano L, Calandra M, Del Vecchio Blanco C, de Sio I. Predictive factors of survival and intrahepatic recurrence of hepatocellular carcinoma in cirrhosis after percutaneous ethanol injection: analysis of 71 patients. J Hepatology 27:862–870, 1997.

104. Tanikawa K, Majima Y. Percutaneous ethanol injection therapy for recurrent hepatocellular carcinoma. Hepatogastroenterology 40:324–327, 1993.

105. Seki T, Wakabayashi M, Nakagawa T, et al. Ultrasonically guided percutaneous microwave coagulation therapy for small hepatocellular carcinoma. Cancer 74:817–825, 1994.

106. Ryu M, Watanabe K, Yamamoto H. Hepatectomy with microwave tissue coagulation for hepatocellular carcinoma. J Pancreat Surg 5:184–191, 1998.

# Chapter 46

# Clinical Aspects and Management of Hepatocellular Cancer

## Management Options: Metastatic Hepatocellular Carcinoma

YEHUDA Z. PATT AND MANAL M. HASSAN

Hepatocellular carcinoma (HCC) is common worldwide with varying geographic incidence and is frequently encountered in Southeast Asia and sub-Saharan Africa.[1,2] The disease was once rare in the United States, Western Europe, and Australia, but its incidence has been rising in the United States. The incidence of hepatobiliary cancers increased 48% between 1993[3] (15,000 new cases) and 2000[4] (20,200 new cases). In 1999, El-Serag and Mason[5] reported an increase in the incidence of HCC in the United States, mostly in the African American population.

The majority (60%) of patients with HCC have underlying liver cirrhosis,[6] the etiology of which may be related to exposure to the hepatitis C virus (HCV) exposure to the hepatitis B virus (HBV), alcohol intake,[7] or exposure to a combination of these. The latency period between exposure to HCV and the development of liver cirrhosis may be as long as 20 years, and it may take as long as 30 years from exposure to develop HCC.[8] Heavy alcohol abuse may decrease the length of the latency period and accelerate the development of HCC.[9] It is estimated that approximately 1.8% of the U.S. population has been exposed to HCV and is anti-HCV reactive, indicating that approximately 4 million individuals in the United States are infected with the virus.[10] The incidence of HCC among patients with HBV-related cirrhosis increases annually, but reaches a plateau of 30% in approximately 8 to 9 years following the diagnosis of cirrhosis. The incidence of HCC in patients with HCV-related cirrhosis, however, tends to follow a nonrelenting course with an annual risk of 3% to 6%[11,12] It has been estimated that 5% to 10% of individuals infected with HCV may eventually develop HCC.[13] Considering the major etiologic role of HCV and alcohol consumption in the development of HCC, it is not surprising that a large proportion of HCC patients in the United States have clinical, radiologic, or histologic evidence of liver cirrhosis. Indeed, a pathologic analysis of 804 cases of HCC indicated that 60% of the patients had histologic evidence of liver cirrhosis.[6]

## Hepatocellular Carcinoma and Liver Cirrhosis

Liver cirrhosis and the associated portal hypertension, thrombocytopenia, and synthetic dysfunction have a major impact on the management of HCC, and therefore it is extremely important to discuss both the interaction between cirrhosis and HCC and the role of cirrhosis in the staging of HCC.

The most commonly used staging classification for liver cirrhosis has been the one suggested by Child and Pugh.[14] Clinical and biochemical variables are considered and a score is generated on the basis of the severity of each variable. The clinical variables are encephalopathy and the presence of ascites; the biochemical variables are serum albumin and bilirubin levels and prothrombin time. With increasing severity, each of these variables gets a higher score, and with increasing severity of the cirrhosis, the Child-Pugh score becomes higher. The severity of the cirrhosis is classified as class A, class B, or class C.[14]

The traditional TNM staging of liver tumors[15] takes into account only the size of the primary tumor in the liver (T), regional lymph nodes (N), and distant metastasis (M), and the stage is a product of these considerations. Conversely, the staging system proposed by Okuda et al.[16] not only takes into account the tumor size, lymph nodes, and distant metastasis but also, and more importantly, acknowledges the major role played by liver cirrhosis in the management and prognosis of HCC. The Okuda staging system assigns weight to the percentage of liver that is replaced by tumor, to biochemical indicators of the severity of liver cirrhosis (serum albumin and bilirubin levels and prothrombin time), and to the presence or absence of ascites. Thus,

a patient with severe liver cirrhosis with an albumin level of less than 3 g/dl, a serum bilirubin level of greater than 3 m g/dl, and the presence of ascites will be considered to have Okuda stage III disease even if the HCC replaces less than 50% of the liver parenchyma or is only as small as 3 cm in diameter. In view of the major impact that liver cirrhosis has on the treatment options for HCC, the staging system suggested by Okuda et al. is more practical and relevant to the treatment outcome than is TNM staging. A similar approach has been used by the Cancer of the Liver Italian Program (CLIP) and the Barcelona groups.[17,18]

## The Challenge of Treating Hepatocellular Carcinoma

Approximately 50% of patients with primary biliary tree cancers present with obstructive jaundice that requires adequate decompression.[19] In such cases, the underlying liver parenchyma function is not compromised because the disease process affects mostly the biliary tree and is less commonly associated with liver cirrhosis. Following endoscopic retrograde cholangiopancreatography (ERCP) or percutaneous transhepatic cholangiopancratography (PTC), these patients may be treated with single chemotherapeutic agents or combinations administered at conventional doses. Conversely, about 60% of all patients with HCC present with liver cirrhosis that requires management. Thus, portal hypertension and associated ascites may be treated with potassium-sparing diuretics, such as spironolactone, as well as mechanical devices, such as the transjagular intrahepatic portosystemic shunts required at times in patients with refractory ascites. Hematopoietic growth factors such as thromboproietin or Neumega may be used for the management of significant thrombocytopenia. However, when synthetic liver dysfunction becomes apparent and is associated with significant hypoabluminemia and decreased levels of clotting factors, orthotopic liver transplantation (OLT) becomes the only potentially curative approach.[20]

### Management of Small Hepatocellular Carcinoma

The approaches to small HCC are surgical resection, radiofrequency ablation or cryoablation, percutaneous ethanol injection, and OLT. These approaches are limited by the tumor size and location, the number of tumor nodules, and the severity of the underlying liver cirrhosis. Moreover, none of these approaches addresses the possible multifocal liver disease or micrometastatic disease that is likely to be present in sites outside the liver.

The surgical resection of HCC, even though considered the only curative approach to the tumor, does not usually result in greater than a 28% long-term survival rate.[21,22] Various approaches to prevent tumor recurrence following the resection of HCC have been reported, including the use of an acyclic retinoid[23] and the use of I[131] Lipiodol embolization,[24] the latter of which in a randomized trial significantly improved the duration of survival among treated patients. However, recurrence is not the only limiting factor to the resection of HCC. The primary tumor size, location, and proximity to major blood vessels, the number of satellite lesions, the severity of underlying liver cirrhosis, and the quantity of residual functioning tumor-free liver are all crucial factors in determining tumor resectability. Moreover, there are no standard definitions of "resectable" and "nonresectable" disease, and the decision about whether to resect is usually a subjective one that is best left to the surgeon. Occa-

sionally, a right hepatic lobectomy may be contraindicated because the residual left lobe is too small to support the patient postoperatively. Investigators have developed techniques to induce left lobe hypertrophy.[25,26] Embolization of the right portal vein containing the tumor may promote hypertrophy of the tumor-free left liver lobe. Such hypertrophy of the residual unaffected liver may allow the surgeon to resect a tumor-containing right liver lobe and leave the patient with enough functioning left liver lobe to survive.

Orthotopic liver transplantation was recently suggested as a reasonable approach to small HCC because it helps to mange not only the tumor but also liver cirrhosis and portal hypertension.[20,25] Such transplantation is limited by the number and the size of liver metastases.[25] Also, OLT does not address micrometastatic disease, and some researchers have suggested that tumor growth may be accelerated in OLT cases by the use of antirejection drugs.[26] Additionally, the paucity of livers available for transplantation mandates that priority be given to those patients who are likely to benefit the longest from the transplanted liver. Since patients with HCC are likely to develop recurrent disease, the wisdom of using this limited resource of organs in patients who are likely to develop tumor recurrence has to be questioned. However, the likelihood of tumor recurrence could be decreased substantially by preoperative systemic or hepatic arterial chemotherapy, thus supporting an argument in favor of OLT, resection, or ablation following a response to preoperative neoadjuvant treatment.

### Transarterial Approach to Hepatocellular Carcinoma

Regional hepatic artery, chemotherapy, or hepatic artery chemoembolization (HACE) may be appropriate only in patients with HCC that is confined to the liver. These approaches may be precarious in patients with severe liver dysfunction, however, because of further compromise in liver function due to ischemia of nontumor liver parenchyma, chemotherapy-related hepatotoxicity and nephrotoxicity, or fluid-volume shifts related to liver cirrhosis. Indeed, use of HACE in patients with portal vein occlusion may exacerbate portal hypertension and associated ascites and "third spacing." Yet, HACE has been employed at The University of Texas M. D. Anderson Cancer Center in carefully selected patients with painful liver masses that can be selectively chemoembolized for palliative purposes.

When considering the transarterial treatment of HCC in carefully selected patients without cirrhosis; hepatic artery infusion (HAI) of chemotherapy combinations such as the FLAP regimen (floxuridine, leucovorin, doxorubicin, and cisplatin)[27] or HAI of chemobiotherapy regimens, such as the PIAF regimen (cisplatin, interferon [IFN]-$\alpha_{2b}$, doxorubicin, and 5-fluorouracil [5-FU])[28,29] have been preferred. Hepatic artery infusion is feasible even in the presence of portal vein occlusion or hepatofugal blood flow, and it may be accomplished with implantable pumps, thereby improving patients' quality of life.[30]

When implanting infusion devices, we have preferred to use implantable infusion pumps rather than ports so as to increase the likelihood of long-term hepatic artery patency. This patency can be maintained by the constant flow of fluids from a pump into the hepatic artery. Conversely, when using a hepatic artery port, the liquid in the arterial catheter is stagnant, resulting in the back-flow of blood into the catheter and increasing the risk of hepatic arterial catheter occlusion.[30]

## Systemic Chemotherapy

The pyrimidine antimetabolite 5-FU was the first reported chemotherapeutic agent tested in the treatment of HCC. The treatment schedules, dosages, and duration in different studies have varied. However, overall response rates of about 10% and a median survival of 3 to 5 months have discouraged further use of 5-FU as a single agent.[31,32] Therefore, various chemotherapeutic agents have been added to 5-FU in the treatment of HCC, making up such regimens as 5-FU plus leucovorin, or 5-FU plus IFN-α. Other agents have included doxorubicin[31,33,34] alone or in combination with IFN; amsacrine;[31] epirubicin;[35] VP-16;[34] cisplatin;[36–38] 5-epirubicin and IFN; mitoxantrone[39] and IFN-β;[40–42] ifosfamide;[43–45] pyrazoloacridine;[46] cisplatin combined with IFN-γ;[47,48] and 5-FU plus IFN-α.[49,50] Doxorubicin seems to be the single most active agent, with a response rate of 25% and a survival advantage over no treatment.[33] Capizzi and associates[36] have tested the combination of gemcitabine, amifostine, and cisplatin (GAP) and observed an objective response in six (86%) of seven patients with HCC and viral hepatitis, splenomegaly, and esophageal varices. Fuloria and colleagues[37] studied the combination of gemcitabine and cisplatin in cases of advanced-stage HCC and reported that 25% of the patients in that series achieved a partial response and 58% showed stable disease. Patt and colleagues[50] used the PIAF combination systemically and reported an initial impressive response in a patient with liver and extrahepatic disease.[50] The same regimen was tested in Chinese patients in Hong Kong by Leung and colleagues.[51] An objective radiologic partial response was observed in only 26% of the patients in that series. Nine (18%) patients in that series with nonresectable tumors became eligible for surgical resection, and complete histologic remission was documented in four patients (9%). However, this drug combination, which includes cisplatin and doxorubicin, is unlikely to be tolerated in patients with advanced cirrhosis since cisplatin requires intravascular volume expansion to prevent renal toxicity. Such a volume expansion is extremely hard to accomplish in patients with severe liver cirrhosis, portal hypertension, and hypoalbuminemia. Moreover, doxorubicin cannot be given to patients with hyperbilirubinemia.

## Tamoxifen

The presence of estrogen receptors in 33% of HCC[52] has prompted the use of tamoxifen in patients with this disease. However, in a phase II study of tamoxifen in HCC patients there were no responses, the duration of stable disease ranged from 5 to 13 months, and there was a median survival time of 6 months from the initiation of tamoxifen therapy.[52] The patients with cirrhosis and advanced HCC who received tamoxifen did not survive longer than those who received a placebo.[53] A comparison of tamoxifen to best supportive care showed that tamoxifen did not prolong survival of patients with HCC.[54] In another study, tamoxifen combined with VP-16 showed modest activity and acceptable toxicity in patients with far-advanced HCC, and seemed to be a useful palliative treatment in 25% of such patients.[55] Data from studies have suggested that tamoxifen significantly enhanced the cytotoxicity of doxorubicin in an HCC cell line.[56] Thus, high-dose tamoxifen seems to be a biochemical modulator of doxorubicin in the treatment of HCC.[53] Yet, a clinical trial of doxorubicin and oral tamoxifen in vivo failed to prolong survival when compared with tamoxifen alone in patients with advanced HCC.[57] Recently, Javed and colleagues[58] reported a higher partial response rate and improved survival in patients randomly assigned to receive 40 mg/day of tamoxifen orally than in those given the same dose of tamoxifen plus radiotherapy with 180 cGy 5 days a week for a total of 2500 to 3000 cGy in 3 to 3.5 weeks.[58]

## Interferon

Interferon α as a single agent in patients with HCC initially seemed quite appealing because of its antiviral and antitumor activity. The initial phase II trials of IFN-α in patients with HCC failed to demonstrate an antitumor response.[59,60] Subsequently, Lai and colleagues[61] demonstrated that patients who received high-dose single-agent recombinant IFN-α had an improved survival compared to control patients who received no treatment[61] or patients who received doxorubicin as a single agent. More recently, Llovet and associates[62] have reported the results of a randomized controlled trial for patients with advanced HCC who received either recombinant IFN-α$_{2b}$ or a placebo. The survival rates at 1 year and 2 years according to intent to treat among treatment and control arms were 58% and 38% vs. 36% and 12%, respectively ($P = 0.15$). A review of these data and the survival confidence interval in the treated and control groups shows no overlap, indicating that the survival difference may be real. It is possible that the conclusions drawn by Llovet and colleagues were not entirely correct, and IFN may prolong the survival of HCC patients. Moreover, there is disagreement about whether patients with HCV-related cirrhosis who receive recombinant IFN-α treatment have a lower incidence of HCC following long-standing cirrhosis than patients who do not receive IFN. The results of meta-analysis conducted recently suggest that IFN may prevent hepatoma in HCV-infected cirrhotic patients.[47,48,63] Because the decrease in the incidence of hepatoma was independent of a decrease in hepatitis C viral RNA researchers have sought additional mechanisms to explain the prevention of HCC. One such mechanism could be the effect of recombinant IFN-α on angiogenesis. rIFN-α has been shown to enhance thymidine phosphorylase (TP) gene expression.[64] Increased TP expression may have a proangiogenic effect, mostly on larger tumors.[65] However, the effects on early tumor vascularity may be inhibitors.[65]

Interferon α treatment in patients with HBV significantly decreased the rate of HCC development compared with no treatment, especially among patients with a higher serum titer of HBV DNA.[48] In a recent study, patients with HCC received either intraarterial cisplatin infusion plus systemic IFN-α (group I), intraarterial cisplatin infusion alone (group II), or supportive care only (group III). The partial response rate of group I was higher than that of group II (33% vs. 14%, $P = 0.05$). The median survival of group I (19 weeks) was significantly longer than that of group II (11 weeks) or group III (5 weeks) ($P = 0.05$ and $P = 0.01$, respectively). Thus, intraarterial cisplatin infusion plus systemic IFN-α may be useful as a palliative treatment for HCC patients with major vascular involvement or extrahepatic metastasis.[66] Stuart and colleagues[67] treated 10 patients with advanced HCC with 5-FU at 750 mg/m$^2$ and IFN-α at $9 \times 10^6$ units three times weekly. Toxicity, including mucositis and neurologic and hematologic side effects, was encountered in this cirrhotic population without sustained antitumor responses. The median survival of this heavily pretreated group was 10 months.[67]

A phase II clinical trial evaluated the efficacy of 5-FU administered as a continuous intravenous infusion at a total dose of 750 mg/m$^2$/day for 5 consecutive days plus recombinant IFN-α$_{2b}$ administered subcutaneously at a dose of $5 \times 10^6$ μ/m$^2$ once a day on days 1, 3, and 5 of the 5-FU infusion. The treatment

was repeated every 14 days as tolerated. A partial response rate of 18% and a minor response rate of 4% were observed, lasting from 2 to 24 months (median, 11.5 months). The patients experienced mucositis (54%), diarrhea (15%), and dermatitis (17%), but fatigue, thrombocytopenia, granulocytopenia, neurologic toxicity, and nausea and vomiting did not occur frequently. Interestingly, a durable partial response was observed in 5 (31%) of 16 patients with HCC who had low levels of serum $\alpha$-fetoprotein (AFP) and in patients with a tumor burden of <50% liver replacement. Conversely, the treatment was ineffective among patients with a high level of serum AFP or extensive liver disease.[68] A more recent phase II clinical trial extended the duration of 5-FU infusion and IFN administration to 21 days, with a 7-day rest period. The median survival was 18.2 months, with a 1-year survival rate of 64%. The treatment was associated with only mild toxicity,[69] thus this therapy may have a role as neoadjuvant treatment in patients with potentially resectable HCC. In both of these studies, the overall partial response rate among 11 patients with fibromellar HCC was 50%.[49,69]

## Capecitabine

Capecitabine is an oral fluoropyrimidine, a prodrug developed to generate 5-FU. Thymidine phosphorylase (TP) is the rate-limiting enzyme that metabolizes 5′-deoxy-5-fluorouridine (5′-dFUrd, doxifluoridine), an intermediate metabolite of capecitabine, to the active drug 5-FU, whereas dihydropyrimidine dehydrogenase (DPD) catablozies 5-FU to an inactive molecule. Tumor susceptibility to fluoropyrimidines correlates with the levels of these enzymes within the tumor.[70] Because the levels of TP are higher in tumors than in plasma and surrounding nontumor tissues, the tumor-to-plasma 5-FU ratios may be as high as 20. Lozano and colleagues[71] described 55 patients with unresectable hepatobiliary carcinoma treated with capecitabine at 2000 mg/m$^2$ in two divided doses given orally every day for 14 days. Sixteen percent of the patients had a response; the median time to progression was 6.3 months and the 1-year survival rate was 67% for patients with HCC. Hand-foot syndrome was the most common side effect occurring in 37% of patients. The treatment was well tolerated even by patients with cirrhosis.[71] A more recent analysis indicated a 13% response rate (RR) (95% confidence interval [CI], 4% to 23%) among 31 patients with HCC, a 6% RR (95% CI, 0% to 15%) among 16 patients with cholangiocarcinoma, and a 50% RR (95% CI, 21% to 79%) among eight patients with gallbladder cancer. Although the activity of capecitabine is modest, the drug deserves further evaluation, alone or in combination with other drugs, in patients with liver cirrhosis and either HCC or gallbladder carcinoma. rIFN-$\alpha$ has been shown to enhance TP gene expression, thereby modulating 5-FU antitumor activity.[64,65] Additionally, metabolism of capecitabine to 5-FU is enhanced by increased TP expression, therefore a trial of rIFN-$\alpha$ and capecitabine combination seems warranted.

## UFT

UFT is a combination of the 5-FU prodrug (tegafur) and uracil at a 1:4 molar ratio.[72] Tegafur is converted to 5-FU by liver microsomes. Degradation into inactive metabolites is inhibited by uracil, allowing higher tumor levels of the active compound 5-FU. On the basis of the results of phase I trials[73] and recognized activity of UFT in other gastrointestinal malignancies,[74,75] Mani and colleagues[76] studied UFT in 16 patients with advanced, unresectable HCC. UFT was given at a starting dose of 300 mg/m$^2$/

day and leucovorin at 90 mg/day, with both drugs given in three divided doses daily for 28 days, repeated every 35 days. Neither complete nor partial responses were observed,[76] and three patients had stable disease lasting 17 to 22 months.

## Antiangiogenic Agents

Angiogenesis is a process of new blood vessel formation[77,78] controlled by several molecules with positive and negative regulatory properties.[79] Vascular endothelial growth factor (VEGF) and basic fibroblast growth factor (bFGF) are the most specific and potent mitogenic stimulants of the endothelial cells.[79-81] Tumor size usually does not exceed several millimeters unless the tumor formation can be sustained by a vascular net that will provide oxygen and nutrients. Hepatocellular carcinoma is characterized by increased pathologic angiogenesis that can be correlated with increased serum VEGF and bFGF levels. Increased serum bFGF levels have been associated with a poorer prognosis in multiple studies.[59,82-86] Chow and colleagues[87] demonstrated that the expression of bFGF was associated with a higher proliferative index and sonographic evidence of portal vein thrombosis. However, VEGF expression did not correlate with the biochemical liver profile, AFP levels, histologic grading, gender of the patients, or clinical stage of cirrhosis. The authors concluded that VEGF expression may characterize progression toward higher proliferation in hepatocarcinogenesis in vivo.[87] Because the inhibition of angiogenesis induces a dormant state in which tumors do not grow, antiangiogenic therapy has attracted considerable interest. Several studies have attempted to block HCC neovasculature as therapy.[88-92] Kim and associates[92] evaluated the effects of the angiogenesis inhibitor TNP-470 on HCC in rats. Treatment with TNP-470 reduced the incidence of HCC and the size and frequency of HCC in treated animals compared with control animals. As expected, however the agent did not affect either the histology of liver cirrhosis or liver function. Rather, the treatment with TNP-470 significantly reduced tumor vascularity in the treated rats relative to the control animals and the frequency of apoptotic hepatoma cells was higher in the treated rats than in the control rats. Thus, TNP-470 suppressed the progression of HCC in rats by inhibiting angiogenesis, a result suggesting that TNP-470 is therapeutic against HCC.[92]

### Thalidomide

Thalidomide is an antiangiogenic and immunomodulatory agent that inhibits the processing of several mRNA encoding peptide molecules, including tumor necrosis factor (TNF)-$\alpha$ and the angiogenic VEGF.[90] Thalidomide is currently being tested alone or in combination in a number of solid tumors, including HCC.[90,93,94]

Because HCC tumors are known to be highly vascularized, Patt et al., after noticing a dramatic response to thalidomide in a patient compassionately treated with the agent,[93] have conducted a phase II trial of thalidomide in patients with HCC.[94] Preliminary results indicated a 5% partial response rate and a 45% rate of disease stability. Disease stability was associated with a decrease in serum AFP levels. The major toxicity was drowsiness, observed in 87% of the patients, who required dose reduction to no more than 400 mg given at bedtime. Allergic skin reactions were in observed about 30% of the patients. Initial results indicated a median patient survival of 12 months. However, a recent analysis indicated a median survival of only 7.7 months (unpublished results) thus decreasing the interest in pursuing use of the agent in HCC patients.

## Octreotide

Octreotide is a somatostatin analogue that possess antimitotic activity against a variety of nonendocrine tumors.[95] Reubi and colleagues[96] demonstrated that 41% of tissue samples obtained from 59 HCC patients expressed somatostatin receptors and showed a high affinity for both somatostatin and octreotide.[96]

Kouroumalis and associates[95] conducted a randomized trial in 58 patients with advanced HCC randomly assigned to receive either subcutaneous octreotide at 250 μg twice daily or no treatment. The treated patients had longer median survival than that of the untreated patients (13 months vs. 4 months, $P = 0.002$). The cumulative 6- and 12-month survival rates were longer for the treated patients than for the control subjects (75% vs. 37% and 56% vs. 13%, respectively). Decreases in the serum AFP levels were observed following 6 months of octreotide treatment.[95] If these results can be confirmed by additional randomized trials, octreotide could be added to the armamentarium of treatment of HCC in patients with advanced liver cirrhosis.

## Prevention of Hepatocellular Carcinoma

The prognosis of patients with HCC remains dismal. Even in cases in which the HCC is amenable to surgical resection, the 5-year survival rate is less than 25%, and the median survival of patients with more advanced disease is less than 1 year.[97] Therefore, the prevention of HCC has to be explored. The primary prevention of HCC would require the elimination of infection with HBV and HCV viruses and an anti–alcohol consumption campaign to prevent liver cirrhosis. The feasibility of such a primary prevention strategy has been demonstrated in Taiwan. Indeed, the rate of HCC in Taiwanese children aged 6 to 9 years decreased from 5.2 per million before the neonatal vaccination program for HBV began in 1984 to 1.3 per million in the first vaccinated cohort.[98] The secondary prevention of the progression from HCV-related cirrhosis to HCC has been attributed to IFN treatment in patients with cirrhosis.[99,100] Multi-institutional prevention trials in patients with advanced HCV-related cirrhosis using IFN-α analogues are being planned. Agents with the potential for preventing second primary tumors following HCC resection, such as polyprenoic acid and acyclic retinoids, have also been investigated.[23]

## Conclusion

The poor prognosis of HCC and the therapeutic challenge posed by underlying liver cirrhosis mandate that research efforts and resources be directed toward prevention strategies. The investment in prevention trials is likely to result in a greater return than what can be expected from treatment of advanced disease.

### References

1. Parkin DM, Pisani P, Ferlay J. Estimates of the worldwide incidence of eighteen major cancers in 1985. Int J Cancer 54:113, 1993.
2. Parkin DM, Muir CS, Whelan SL, et al. Cancer Incidence of Five Continents, Vol. VI. International Agency for Research on Cancer Scientific Publications, Lyon, No. 12, 1992.
3. Boring CC, Squires TS, Tong T, et al. Cancer statistics, 1994. CA Cancer J Clin 44:7–26, 1994.
4. Greenlee RT, Murray T, Bolden S, Wingo PA. Cancer statistics, 2000. Cancer J Clin 50:27–33, 2000.
5. El-Serag HB, Mason AC. Rising incidence of hepatocellular carcinoma in the United States. N Engl J Med 340:745–750, 1999.
6. Nzeko UC, Goodman ZD, Ishak KG. Hepatocellulr carcinoma in cirrhotic and noncirrhotic livers. A clinicohistopathologic study of 804 North American patients. Am J Clin Pathol 105:65–75, 1996.
7. Conn HO. Cirrhosis. In: Schiff L, Schiffer ER (eds): Diseases of the Liver, 5th ed. 1982, pp 847–977.
8. Kiyosawa K, Sodeyama T, Tanaka E, et al. Interrelationship of blood transfusion, non-A–non-B hepatitis and hepatocellular carcinoma: analysis by detection of antibody to hepatitis C virus. Hepatology 12: 671–675, 1990.
9. Tagger A, Donato F, Ribero ML, et al. Case–control study on heptitis C virus (HCV) as a risk factor for hepatocellular carcinoma: the role of HCV genotypes and the synergism with hepatitis B virus and alcohol. Int J Cancer 81:695–699, 1999.
10. Alter MJ, Kruszon MD, Nainan OV, et al. The prevalence of hepatitis C virus infection in the United States, 1988 through 1994. N Engl J Med 341:556–562, 1999.
11. Gentilini P, Melani L, Riccardi D, Casini Raggi V, Romanelli RG. Hepatocellular carcinoma and viral cirrhosis. Hepatology 20:764–765, 1994.
12. Ikeda K, Saitoh S, Koida I, et al. A multivariate analysis of risk factors for hepatocellular carcinogenesis: a prospective observation of 795 patients with viral and alcoholic cirrhosis. Hepatology 18:47–53, 1993.
13. Hofnagle JH. Hepatitis C: the clinical spectrum of disease. Hepatology 26:15S–20S, 1997.
14. Pugh RNH, Murray-Lyon IM, Dawson JL, Pietroni MC, Williams R. Transection of the oesophagus for bleeding oesophageal varices. Br J Surg 60:646–649, 1973.
15. American Joint Committee on Cancer. AJCC Cancer Staging Manual, 6th ed. 2002, p 131.
16. Okua K, Ohtsuki T, Obata H, et al. Natural history of hepatocellular carcinoma and prognosis in relation to 5-fluorouracil treatments. A study of 850 patients. Cancer 56:918–928, 1985.
17. The Cancer of the Liver Italian Program (CLIP) Investigators. Prospective validation of the CLIP score: a new prognostic system for patients with cirrhosis and hepatocellular carcinoma. Hepatology 31:840–845, 2000.
18. Llovet JM, Bru C, Bruix J. Prognosis of hepatocellular carcinoma. The BCLV staging classification. Semin Liver Dis 19:329–338, 1999.
19. Patt YZ, Jones DV Jr, Hoque A, et al. Phase II trial of intravenous and subcutaneous interferon α-2b for biliary tract cancer. J Clin Oncol 14: 2311–2315, 1996.
20. Mazzaferro V, Regalia E, Doci R, et al. Liver transplantation for the treatment of small hepatocellular carcinomas in patients with cirrhosis. N Engl J Med 14: 728–729, 1996.
21. Vauthey N, Klimstra D, Franceschi D, et al. Factors affecting long-term outcome after hepatic resection for hepatocellular carcinoma. Am J Surg 169:28–35, 1995.
22. Ringe B, Pichlmayr R, Wittekind C, et al. Surgical treatment of hepatocellular carcinoma: experience with liver resection and transplantation in 198 patients. World J Surg 15:270–285, 1991.
23. Muto Y, Moriwaki H, Ninomiya M, et al. Prevention of second primary tumors by an acyclic retinoid, polyprenoic acid, in patients with hepatocellular carcinoma. Hepatoma Prevention Study Group. N Engl J Med 334:1561–1567, 1996.
24. Lau WY, Leung TW, Ho SK, et al. Adjuvant intra-arterial iodine-131 labelled Lipiodol for resectable hepatocellular carcinoma: a prospective randomised trial. Lancet 353:797–801, 1999.
25. Rolles K. Transplantation for liver cancer. In: Okuda K, Tabor E (eds): Liver Cancer. Churchill Livingstone, New York, 1997, pp 531–536.
26. Yokoyama I, Carr B, Saitsu H, et al. Accelerated growth rates of recurrent hepatocellular carcinoma after liver transplantation. Cancer 68: 2095–2100, 1991.
27. Patt YZ, Charnsagavej C, Yoffe B, et al. Hepatic arterial infusion of floxoridine, leucovorin, doxorubicin, and cisplatin for heptocellular carcinoma: effects of hepatitis B and C viral infection on drug toxicity and patient survival. J Clin Onc 12:1204–1211, 1994.
28. Lozano RD, Patt YZ, Ellis L, et al. A phase II trial of a hepatic arterial infusion of platinol (CDDP) recombinant to human interferon alpha-2b (rIFNα) Adrimycin® (DOX) and 5-FU (PIAF) for the treatment of hepatocellular carcinoma (HCC). Proc Am Soc Clin Oncol 20:167a (Abst. No. 666), 2001.
29. Patt YZ, Hoque A, Roh M, et al. Durable clinical and pathologic response of hepatocellular carcinoma to systemic and hepatic arterial administration of platinol, recombinant interferon alpha 2B, doxorubicin, and 5-fluorouracil: a communication. Oncology 22:209–213, 1999.
30. Doci, R, Bignami P, Quagliuolo V. Continuous hepatic arterial infusion with 5-fluorodeoxyuridine for treatment of colorectal metastases. Reg Cancer Treat 3:13–18, 1990.
31. Friedman MA. Primary hepatocellular cancer—present results and future prospects. Int J Radiat Oncol Biol Phys 9:1841–1845, 1983.

32. Lin DY, Lin SM, Liaw YF. Non-surgical treatment of hepatocellular carcinoma. J Gastroenterol Hepatol 12:S319, 1997.

33. Lai CL, Wu PC, Chan GC, et al. Doxorubicin versus no antitumor therapy in inoperable hepatocellular carcinoma. A prospective randomized trial. Cancer 62:479–483, 1988.

34. Melia WM, Johnson PJ, Williams R. Induction of remission in hepatocellular carcinoma. A comparison of VP 16 with Adriamycin. Cancer 51:206–210, 1983.

35. Hochster HS, Green MD, Speyer J, et al. 4′Epidoxorubicin (epirubicin): activity in hepatocellular carcinoma. J Clin Oncol 3:1535–1540, 1985.

36. Capizzi RL, Hann HL, Feeney KJ, et al. Gemcitabine, amifostine, and cisplatin (GAP) treatment for unresectable hepatocellular carcinoma (HCC). Program/Proceedings of the 36th Annual Meeting of the American Society of Clinical Oncology, New Orleans, 2000, p 285a.

37. Fuloria J, Parikh PM, Prabhakaran M, et al. A multicenter, phase II trial of gemcitabine and cisplatin in unresectable hepatocellular carcinoma. Program proceedings of the 36th Annual Meeting of the American Society of Clinical Oncology, New Orleans, 2000, p 292a.

38. Melia WM, Westaby D, Williams R. Diamminodichloride platinum (cisplatinum) in the treatment of hepatocellular carcinoma. Clin Oncol 7: 275–280, 1981.

39. Falkson G, Coetzer BJ. Phase II studies of mitoxantrone in patients with primary liver cancer. Invest New Drugs 3:187–189, 1985.

40. Bernardinello E, Cabaletto L, Chemello L, et al. Long-term clinical outcome after beta-interferon therapy in cirrhotic patients with chronic hepatitis C. TVVH Study Group. Hepatogastroenterology 46:3216–3222, 1999.

41. Ikeda K, Arase Y, Saitoh S, et al. Interferon beta prevents recurrence of hepatocellular carcinoma after complete resection or ablation of the primary tumor. A prospective randomized study of hepatitis C virus–related liver cancer. Hepatology 32:228–232, 2000.

42. Zein NN. Interferons in the management of viral hepatitis. Cytokines Cell Mol Ther 4:229–241, 1998.

43. Lin J, Shiu W, Leung WT, et al. Phase II study of high-dose ifosfamide in hepatocellular carcinoma. Cancer Chemother Pharmacol 31:338–339, 1993.

44. Malik IA, Khan WA, Haq S, et al. A prospective phase II trial to evaluate the efficacy and toxicity of hepatic arterial infusion of ifosfamide in patients with inoperable localized hepatocellular carcinoma. Am J Clin Oncol 20:289–292, 1997.

45. Thongprasert S, Klunklin K, Phornphutkul K, et al. Phase II study of ifosfamide (Holoxan) in hepatoma. Eur J Cancer Clin Oncol 24:1795–1796, 1988.

46. Adjei AA. Current status of pyrazoloacridine as an anticancer agent. Invest New Drugs 17:43–48, 1999.

47. Ikeda K, Saitoh S, Arase Y, et al. Effect of interferon therapy on hepatocellular carcinogenesis in patients with chronic hepatitis type C: a long-term observation study of 1,643 patients using statistical bias correction with proportional hazard analysis. Hepatology 29:1124–1130, 1999.

48. Ikeda K, Saitoh S, Suzuki Y, et al. Interferon decreases hepatocellular carcinogenesis in patients with cirrhosis caused by the hepatitis B virus: a pilot study. Cancer 82:827–835, 1998.

49. Hassan MM, Patt YZ, Lozano RD, et al. Continuous IV infusion of 5-FU and subcutaneous recombinant interferon alpha 2b is an active regimen in fibrolamelar hepatocellular carcinoma. Program/Proceedings of the 36th Annual Meeting of the American Society of Clinical Oncology, New Orleans, 2000, p 383a.

50. Patt YZ, Hogue A, Roh M, et al. Durable clinical and pathologic response of hepatocellular carcinoma to systemic and hepatic arterial administration of platinol, recombinant interferon alpha 25, doxorubicin, and 5-fluorouracil: a communication. Am J Clin Oncol. 22:209–213, 1999.

51. Leung TW, Patt YZ, Lau WY, et al. Complete pathological remission is possible with systemic combination chemotherapy for inoperable hepatocellular carcinoma. Clin Cancer Res 5:1676–1681, 1999.

52. Engstrom PF, Levin B, Moertel CG, et al. A phase II trial of tamoxifen in hepatocellular carcinoma. Cancer 65:2641–2643, 1990.

53. Riestra S, Rodriguez M, Delgado M, et al. Tamoxifen does not improve survival of patients with advanced hepatocellular carcinoma. J Clin Gastroenterol 26:200–203, 1998.

54. Cancer of the Liver Italian Programme Group. Tamoxifen in treatment of hepatocellular carcinoma: a randomized controlled trial. Cancer of the Liver Italian Programme. Lancet 352:17–20, 1998.

55. Cheng AL, Chen YC, Yeh KH, et al. Chronic oral etoposide and tamoxifen in the treatment of far-advanced hepatocellular carcinoma. Cancer 77:872–877, 1996.

56. Cheng AL, Yeh KH, Fine RL, et al. Biochemical modulation of doxorubicin by high-dose tamoxifen in the treatment of advanced hepatocellular carcinoma. Hepatogastroenterology 45:1955–1960, 1998.

57. Schachschal G, Lochs H, Plauth M. Controlled clinical trial of doxorubicin and tamoxifen versus tamoxifen monotherapy in hepatocellular carcinoma. Eur J Gastroenterol Hepatol 12:281–284, 2000.

58. Javed AA, Gurchani SA, Maud AI. Tamoxifen and radiotherapy in advanced unresectable hepatocellular carcinoma. Program/Proceedings of the 36th Annual Meeting of the American Society of Clinical Oncology, New Orleans, 2000, p 286a.

59. Gastrointestinal Tumor Study Group. A prospective trial of the recombinant interferon alpha 2b in previously untreated patients with HCC. Cancer 66:135–139, 1990.

60. Kardinal CG, Moertel CG, Wieand HS, et al. Combined doxorubicin and alpha interferon therapy of advanced hepatocellular carcinoma. Cancer 71:2187–2190, 1993.

61. Lai CL, Lau J, Wu PC, et al. Recombinant interferon alpha in inoperable hepatocellular carcinoma: a randomized control trial. Hepatology 17:3889–394, 1993.

62. Llovet JM, Sala M, Castells L, et al. Randomized controlled trial of interferon treatment for advanced hepatocellular carcinoma. Hepatology 31:54–58, 2000.

63. Baffis V, Shrier I, Sherker AH, Azilagyi A. Use of interferon for prevention of hepatocellular carcinoma in cirrhotic patients with hepatitis B or hepatitis C virus infection. Ann Intern Med 131:696–701, 1999.

64. Morita T, Tokue A. Biomodulation of 5-fluorouracil by interferon-α in human renal carcinoma cells; relationship to the expression of thymidine phosphorylase. Cancer Chemother Pharmacol 44:91–96, 1999.

65. Marchetti S, Chazal M, Dubreuil A, et al. Impact of thymidine phosphorylase surexpression on fluoropyrimidine activity and on tumour angiogenesis. Br J Cancer 85:439–445, 2001.

66. Chung YH, Song IH, Song BC, et al. Combined therapy consisting of intraarterial cisplatin infusion and systemic interferon-alpha for hepatocellular carcinoma patients with major portal vein thrombosis or distant metastasis. Cancer 88:1986–1991, 2000.

67. Stuart K, Tessitore, Huberman M. 5-fluorouracil and alpha-interferon in hepatocellular caracinoma. Am J Clin Oncol 19:136–139, 1996.

68. Patt YZ, Yoffe B, Charnsangavej C, et al. Low serum alpha-fetoprotein level in patients with hepatocellular carcinoma as a predictor of response to 5-FU and interferon-alpha-2b. Cancer 72:2574–2582, 1993.

69. Patt YZ, Lozano R, Hassan MM, et al. Continuous IV infusion of (5-FU) and subcutaneous recombinant interferon alpha 2b (rIFNα2b) is an active regimen in hepatocellular carcinoma. Proc Am Soc Clin Oncol 20:1681 (Abst. 671), p 168a, 2001.

70. Mori K, Hasegawa M, Nishida M, et al. Expression levels of thymidine phosphorylase and dihydropyrimidine dehydrogenase in various human tumor tissues. Int J Oncol 17:33–38, 2000.

71. Lozano RD, Patt YZ, Hassan MM, et al. Oral capecitabine (Xeloda) for the treatment of hepatobiliary cancers (hepatocellular carcinoma, cholangiocarcinoma, and gallbladder cancer). Program/Proceedings of the 36th Annual Meeting of the American Society of Clinical Oncology, New Orleans, 2000, p 264a.

72. Maehara Y, Kakeji Y, Ohno S, et al. Scientific basis for the combination of tegafur with uracil. Oncolgy (Huntingt) 11:14–21, 1997.

73. Pazdur R. Phase I and pharmacokinetic evaluations of UFT plus oral leucovorin. Oncology (Huntingt) 11:35–39, 1997.

74. Pazdur R. Phase II study of UFT plus leucovorin in colorectal cancer. Oncology 54:19–23, 1997.

75. Pazdur R. UFT: East meets West in drug development. Oncology (Huntingt) 11:11–13, 1997.

76. Mani S, Sciortino D, Samuels B, et al. Phase II trial of uracil/tegafur (UFT) plus leucovorin in patients with advanced biliary carcinoma. Invest New Drugs 17:97–101, 1999.

77. Folkman J. Angiogenesis in cancer, vascular, rheumatoid and other disease. Nat Med 1:27–31, 1995.

78. Folkman J, Shing Y. Angiogenesis. J Biol Chem 267:10931–10934, 1992.

79. Bussolino F, Albini A, Camussi G, et al. Role of soluble mediators in angiogenesis. Eur J Cancer 32A:2401–2412, 1996.

80. Leung DW, Cachianes G, Kuang WJ, et al. Vascular endothelial growth is a secreted aniogenic mitogen. Science 246:1306–1309, 1989.

81. Montesano R, Vassalli JD, Baird A, et al. Basic fibroblast growth factor induces angiogenesis in vitro. Proc Natl Acad Sci USA 83:7297–7301, 1986.

82. An FQ, Matsuda M, Fujii H, et al. Expression of vascular endothelial growth factor in surgical specimens of hepatocellular carcinoma. J Cancer Res Clin Oncol 126:153–160, 2000.

83. Chung YS, Maeda K, Sowa M. Prognostic value of angiogenesis in gastrointestinal tumours. Eur J Cancer 32A:2501–2505, 1996.

84. El-Assal ON, Yamanoi A, Soda Y, et al. Clinical significance of microvessel density and vascular endothelial growth factor expression in hepatocellular carcinoma and surrounding liver: possible involvement of vascular endothelial growth factor in the angiogenesis of cirrhotic liver. Hepatology 27:1554–1562, 1998.

85. Hollingsworth HC, Kohn EC, Steinberg SM, et al. Tumor angiogenesis in advanced stage ovarian carcinoma. Am J Pathol 147:33–41, 1995.

86. Honda H, Tajima T, Kajiyama K, et al. Vascular changes in hepatocellular carcinoma: correlation of radiologic and pathologic findings. AJR Am J Roentgenol 173:1213–1217, 1999.

87. Chow NH, Hsu PI, Lin XZ, et al. Expression of vascular endothelial growth factor in normal liver and hepatocellular carcinoma: an immunohistochemical study. Hum Pathol 28:698–703, 1997.

88. Ahmed MH, Konno H, Nahar L, et al. The angiogenesis inhibitor TNP-470 (AGM-1470) improves long-term survival of rats with liver metastasis. J Surg Res 64:35–41, 1996.

89. Diaz-Flores L, Gutierrez R, Varela H. Angiogenesis: an update. Histol Histopathol 9:807–843, 1994.

90. Eisen T, Boshoff C, Mak I, et al. Continuous low-dose thalidomide: a phase II study in advanced melanoma, renal cell, ovarian and breast cancer. Br J Cancer 82:812–817, 2000.

91. Folkman J. Tumor angiogenesis: therapeutic implications. N Engl J Med 285:1182–1186, 1971.

92. Kim M, Torimura T, Ueno T, et al. Angiogenesis inhibitor TNP-470 suppressed the progression of experimentally induced hepatocellular carcinoma in rats. Int J Oncol 16:375–382, 2000.

93. Patt YZ, Hassan MM, Lozano RD, et al. Durable clinical response of refractory hepatocellular carcinoma to orally administered thalidomide. Am J Clin Oncol 23:319–321, 2000.

94. Patt YZ, Hassan MM, Lozano RD, et al. Phase II trial of thalomid (thalidomide) for treatment of non-resectable hepatocellular carcinoma. Proc Am Soc Clin Oncol 19:266a (Abst. 1035), 2000.

95. Kouroumalis E, Skordilis P, Thermos K, et al. Treatment of hepatocellular carcinoma with octreotide: a randomized controlled study. Gut 42:442–447, 1998.

96. Reubi JC, Zimmermann A, Jonas S, et al. Regulatory peptide receptors in human hepatocellular carcinomas. Gut 45;766–774, 1999.

97. Dancey JE, Shepherd FA. Carcinoma of the liver. In: Foley JF, Vose JM, Armitage JO (eds): Current Therapy in Cancer, 2nd ed. W.B. Saunders, Philadephia, 1999, pp 81–89.

98. Chang MH, Chen CJ, Lai MS, et al. Universal hepatitis B vaccination in Taiwan and the incidence of hepatocellular carcinoma in children. Taiwan Childhood Hepatoma Study Group. N Engl J Med 336:1855–1859, 1997.

99. Kasahara A, Hayahsi N, Mochizuki K, et al. Risk factors for hepatocellular carcinoma and its incidence after interferon treatment in patients with chronic hepatitis C. Osaka Liver Disease Study Group. Hepatology 27:1394–1402, 1998.

100. Nishiguchi S, Kuroki T, Nakatani S, et al. Randomised trial of effects of interferon-alpha on incidence of hepatocellular carcinoma in chronic active hepatitis C with cirrhosis. Lancet 346:1051–1055, 1995.

# Section 6

# Cancer of the Small Bowel and Appendix

# Chapter 47

# Epidemiology, Molecular Epidemiology, and Molecular Biology of Small Bowel and Appendiceal Adenocarcinomas

ALFRED I. NEUGUT AND NADIR ARBER

Most articles and studies on a specific cancer site begin by describing how important the particular cancer is in terms of its incidence and mortality rates. For example, two gastrointestinal (GI) tract cancers, gastric cancer and large bowel cancer, are indeed major contributors to the cancer burden of the world overall, and to the cancer burden of the United States in particular. Thus, what is most interesting about the small bowel, located as it is between two high cancer incidence organs and containing 90% of the mucosal surface area of the alimentary tract and 75% of its length, is that it is one of the rarest types of cancer.[1–6] Its significance, therefore, is a direct consequence of its rarity. This is an optimistic message, for if one could elucidate the precise reasons for its low incidence and mortality, perhaps new preventive strategies could be devised for cancers of the stomach, the large bowel, or other major sites.

Given its potential significance, it is therefore disappointing to learn how little has actually been done to study small bowel cancer. Of course, this reflects in large part the disease's uncommonness and the consequent difficulty in obtaining significant numbers of cases for study, as well as some degree of short-sightedness regarding the potential of this organ to provide important information regarding carcinogenesis.

## Descriptive Epidemiology

At present, an estimated 4800 new cases of small bowel cancer and 1200 related deaths occur each year in the United States. This can be contrasted with almost 22,000 cases of gastric cancer and 124,500 cases of colorectal cancer during the same period.[7] Details regarding the pathology of small bowel cancer are covered in Chapter 48. Briefly, small bowel cancer has four major histologic subtypes: adenocarcinoma, carcinoid, sarcoma, and lymphoma. In some parts of the world, lymphoma is the most

common type of small bowel cancer, though in most industrialized countries it is much less common (see Section 10 in this volume).[1,3,8,9] Sarcomas and carcinoid tumors are also covered in other sections of this volume.

In this chapter, the focus is on adenocarcinomas, which represent the most common subtype in North America and Europe, constituting roughly 40%–50% of small bowel cancers.[1,4,5,10–14] The average major medical center can expect to see two to four cases during the course of a year.[3] In fact, much of the descriptive epidemiology and analytic epidemiology that has been published regarding small bowel cancer has not been analyzed or described in terms of specific histologic subgroups and thus combines together a variety of tumors that may or may not share common features. A good example of this variety is the subsite distribution. Small bowel adenocarcinomas tend to arise in the duodenum, particularly in proximity to the ampulla of Vater. Carcinoids and lymphomas are predominantly ileal or jejunal, while sarcomas tend to be relatively evenly distributed throughout the small bowel.

We have previously noted a striking resemblance between the epidemiology of adenocarcinomas of the large bowel and small bowel (see Table 47–1).[1] They tend to share a number of specific risk factors, such as Crohn's disease, familial adenomatous polyposis (FAP), and a prior history of adenomas. They also tend to occur together in the same individuals, with an elevated risk of colorectal cancer in survivors of small bowel adenocarcinoma and vice versa. While small bowel adenocarcinomas occur at 1/50th the rate of large bowel adenocarcinomas, both tend to share the same geographic and international variability, with predominance in Western countries and relatively low occurrence in the Third World.[6] Finally, both tend to arise out of adenomatous polyps, sharing the adenoma–carcinoma sequence,[15] although this is still under study in the small bowel.

**Table 47-1** Risk factors for adenocarcinoma of the small bowel and large bowel

| Risk Factor | Small Bowel | Large Bowel |
|---|---|---|
| Adenomas | + + + | + + + |
| Familial adenomatous polyposis | + + | + + + + |
| Crohn's disease | + + + + | +/+ + |
| Other GI tract cancer | + + + | + + + |
| Animal fat intake | + | + + |
| Smoking | + + | +/+ + |
| Alcohol use | +/+ + | ? |
| Radiation exposure | + | ? |
| Cholecystectomy | + | + |

Number of plus signs refers to strength and/or consistency of association. GI, gastrointestinal. ? = equivocal. Adapted from Neugut AI, Jacobson JS, Suh S, Mukherjee R, Arber N. Epidemiology of cancer of the small intestine. Cancer Epidemiol Biomarkers Prev 7:243–251, 1998.[1]

Given the shared characteristics of small bowel and large bowel cancer, it is particularly surprising that small bowel adenocarcinomas tend to cluster at the gastric end of the small intestine rather than at the more distal end, closer to the large bowel. This tendency has aroused considerable speculation in the literature, particularly by Lowenfels, that bile and/or its metabolites may play a role in small bowel carcinogenesis.[4,16,17]

## Geographic Distribution

As noted previously, the incidence of small bowel cancer varies among different populations. In general, the incidence tends to be higher in the industrialized West than in less industrialized countries. However, it should be borne in mind that most of these figures represent overall statistics for small bowel cancer, without subtyping. Very little population registry information is available for assessing variations in the incidence of small bowel adenocarcinoma and small bowel lymphoma on a population-based scale among different countries. However, numerous hospital-based series from hospitals and cancer centers in different countries indicate a predominance of adenocarcinoma in the West and lymphomas in the Third World.[3]

In 1973, an important paper by Lowenfels[6] showed a strong linear correlation between the international distributions of small bowel and large bowel cancer, but data from the 1990s suggest a much weaker correlation (Jacobson et al., unpublished observations). Most of the detailed population-based data regarding small bowel cancer come from several studies in North America (see Table 47–2). In these studies, spanning from 1965 to the 1990s, the overall incidence of small bowel cancer was approximately 10–14 cases per million people per year. In most of the registries cited, adenocarcinoma is the predominant subtype, with incidence ranging from 3.0 to 6.5 cases per million per year. The concomitant mortality rates have generally been approximately one-fourth of the incidence rates. Stang et al., in describing their experience with the German Cancer Registry,[14] found the age-standardized incidence of small bowel cancer to be 3.3–6.2 cases per million per year.

## Gender Differences

In most studies, males have had higher small bowel cancer incidence rates than females (see Table 47–3).[1,4,5,10–14] Generally, this ratio has held true in international studies as well,[3,18] and for all four of the main histologic subgroups when those subgroups

**Table 47-2** Population-based studies of small bowel cancer histology and incidence

| Cancer Registries | Histology | n (%) | Incidence (per million per year)[a] |
|---|---|---|---|
| Los Angeles County, California, 1972–1985[4] | Adenocarcinoma | 446 (37.5) | N/A |
| | Carcinoid | 503 (42.3) | N/A |
| | Sarcoma | 152 (12.8) | N/A |
| | Lymphoma | 89 (7.5) | N/A |
| | Total[a] | 1190 | N/A |
| SEER Registries, 1973–1982[5] | Adenocarcinoma | 732 (40.0) | 3.9 |
| | Carcinoid | 542 (29.6) | 2.9 |
| | Sarcoma | 232 (12.7) | 1.2 |
| | Lymphoma | 312 (17.0) | 1.6 |
| | Total[a] | 1832 | 9.6 |
| Western Canada, 1966–1990[10] | Adenocarcinoma | 521 (41.9) | N/A |
| | Carcinoid | 334 (26.8) | N/A |
| | Sarcoma | 140 (11.3) | N/A |
| | Lymphoma | 244 (19.6) | N/A |
| | Total[a] | 1244 | 11.0 |
| Utah, 1966–1990[11] | Adenocarcinoma | 80 (24.4) | 3.0 |
| | Carcinoid | 136 (41.5) | 6.5 |
| | Sarcoma | 36 (11.0) | 1.5 |
| | Lymphoma | 72 (22.0) | 2.5 |
| | Total[a] | 328 | 14.0 |
| SEER, 1973–1991[12] | Adenocarcinoma | 1609 | 6.5 |
| | Carcinoid | 1683 | 6.5 |
| | Total[a,b] | 3292 | 13.0 |

N/A, data not available; SEER, Surveillance, Epidemiology, and End Results.

[a] Total includes other histologies.

[b] Excludes lymphomas and sarcomas.

**Table 47–3** Age-adjusted incidence rate of small bowel cancer per 100,000 population by race and gender, SEER, 1973–1993

|                | 1973 | 1983 | 1993 |
|----------------|------|------|------|
| White males    | 0.9  | 1.2  | 1.6  |
| White females  | 0.7  | 0.8  | 1.1  |
| Black males    | 1.8  | 1.8  | 2.4  |
| Black females  | 1.2  | 1.3  | 2.0  |

Adapted in part from Neugut AI, Jacobson JS, Suh S, Mukherjee R, Arber N. Epidemiology of cancer of the small intestine. Cancer Epidemiol Biomarkers Prev 7:243–251, 1998.[1] Also adapted from Ries LAG, Kosary CL, Hankey BF, Harris A, Miller BA, Edwards BK (eds). SEER Cancer Statistics Review, 1973–93. National Cancer Institute, Bethesda, MD, 1996.[19]

were studied. Interestingly, the gender distribution of small bowel cancer is similar to that of colorectal and gastric cancer.[19] Our own study of this phenomenom,[13] utilizing the U.S. National Cancer Institute Surveillance, Epidemiology, and End Results Program (SEER) data, yielded similar results.

### Racial Differences

There has been no extensive study of racial differences in small bowel cancer incidence. Population-based studies in the United States have suggested somewhat higher incidence rates for blacks than whites (see Table 47–3). The Los Angeles County Cancer Surveillance Program in particular found an age-adjusted incidence of 1.5 cases per 100,000 per year for black males vs. 0.9 per 100,000 per year for white males and a similar ratio for black vs. white females (1.0 vs. 0.6 per 100,000 per year). The specific adenocarcinoma rates reflected a similar pattern.[4]

### Time Trends

Three studies have investigated the time trends for small bowel malignancies; all three used SEER data spanning from 1973 to the present.[5,12,13] The first decade, between 1973 and 1982, saw little change in the overall or specific rates of adenocarcinoma. In the second decade, from 1983 to 1993, the incidence of small bowel cancer increased from 1.2 to 1.6 per 100,000 among white males, from 0.8 to 1.1 per 100,000 among white females, from 1.8 to 2.4 per 100,000 among black males, and from 1.3 to 2.0 per 100,000 among black females (see Table 47–3).

### Age Distribution

As for many other cancers, the incidence of small bowel cancer tends to increase with age. In most studies, the mean age at diagnosis has been approximately 60 years.[1–3] Adenocarcinomas tend to be diagnosed in somewhat older people than do the other histologic subtypes.

## Analytic Epidemiology

Some risk factors have been identified for small bowel cancer, particularly small bowel adenocarcinoma (see Table 47–1). We discuss a number of these below.

### Crohn's Disease

Crohn's disease has been recognized as a possible risk factor for small bowel adenocarcinoma since 1956.[20] Since that time, over 100 cases have been reported in the medical literature.[21] Inter-

estingly, while most small bowel adenocarcinomas occur in the duodenum, those associated with Crohn's disease tend to occur in the ileum.[21] Furthermore, there seems to be a latency period of 20 years or so after the onset of the Crohn's disease, similar to the latency period between ulcerative colitis and large bowel adenocarcinoma.

Two cases of small bowel cancer, both in the ileum, were found in a Danish cohort study of 373 patients with Crohn's disease diagnosed between 1962 and 1987 and followed for 10 to 15 years.[22] In this study, 0.04 cases would have been expected, giving a relative risk of small bowel cancer of 50 (95% confidence interval [CI], 37.1–65.9). A similarly conducted retrospective cohort study in Stockholm[23] found a relative risk of 15.6 (95% CI, 4.3–40.1). Another group estimated a 0.3% probability of Crohn's disease and small bowel cancer occurring in the same individual.[24]

We conducted a small case–control study comparing 19 cases of small bowel adenocarcinoma diagnosed at Columbia-Presbyterian Medical Center, New York, from 1980 to 1987 with 52 control cases of patients undergoing benign non-gastrointestinal surgical procedures such as herniorrhaphy and transurethral resection of the prostate.[17] Four of the 19 adenocarcinomas were in the ileum, and three of these were associated with prior Crohn's disease. In another case group, 14 of 17 carcinoid tumors were also found in the ileum but none occurred in the context of prior Crohn's disease. In a different study, Lashner[25] compared 7 patients with Crohn's disease who developed adenocarcinoma with 28 patients with Crohn's disease, matched for age and gender, who did not develop a small bowel malignancy. Several factors were found to enhance the risk of developing small bowel adenocarcinoma, including treatment with 6-mercaptopurine and occupational exposure to aromatic compounds or other potential carcinogens (odds ratio [OR], 20.3; 95% CI, 2.7–150.5).

### Adenomas

Sellner[15] previously described circumstantial evidence linking adenomatous polyps to subsequent small bowel adenocarcinoma, a sequence similar to the adenoma–carcinoma sequence in the large bowel. As in the case of large bowel disease, patients with small bowel carcinoma are, on average, several years older than those with small bowel adenomas; invasive carcinoma is often found in the context of adenomatous tissue; the site, size, and villous histology of small bowel adenomas are associated with the risk of invasive carcinoma; small bowel adenomas and adenocarcinomas have similar male/female ratios; and the international variation in the prevalence of small bowel adenomas and carcinomas is similar to each other. Furthermore, there have been three case reports of small bowel adenomas that were left in place after pathologic diagnosis; one of these adenomas subsequently progressed to adenocarcinoma.[26–28]

In addition, it has been found that one of the malignancies that arises in the context of FAP is small bowel adenocarcinoma.[29–34] Patients with FAP tend to develop multiple adenomas in the small bowel like those in the mucosa of the large bowel; as is typical for adenocarcinoma of the small bowel, these malignancies tend to arise in the duodenum. Indeed, a recent study indicated that periampullary carcinoma was the most common extracolonic malignancy in FAP patients, with 2.9% developing this type of malignancy.[29] Another study of 1262 FAP patients followed at St. Mark's Hospital, London, showed that 47 ultimately developed duodenal cancer and that periampullary carcinoma was the most common cause of death in this population.[30]

Interestingly, one study found that bile from the duodenums of 29 FAP patients was more mutagenic than bile from 24 non-FAP patients.[31] Another group at Johns Hopkins (Baltimore, MD) found 11 cases of duodenal and ampullary adenocarcinoma in FAP patients during 18,679 person-years of follow-up.[32] This gave a relative risk of >300 for duodenal adenocarcinoma and 123.7 for ampullary adenocarcinoma (95% CI, 33.7–316.7). There was no elevation in risk of gastric or nonduodenal small bowel cancer in this population. Some studies have also suggested that patients with Peutz-Jeghers syndrome have an elevated risk of developing small bowel adenocarcinoma.[2]

### Prior Colon Cancer

As stated earlier, patients with FAP have an increased risk of developing small bowel adenocarcinoma. An increased risk has also been observed for patients with hereditary nonpolyposis colorectal cancer (HNPCC).[35,36] As some studies have suggested, the lifetime risk for small bowel adenocarcinoma among HNPCC patients is 1%. Neugut and Santos[37] demonstrated an elevated risk of small bowel adenocarcinoma following prior colorectal cancer in the general population, with a standardized incidence ratio (SIR) of 7.1 (95% CI, 4.7–10.3) in males and 9.0 (95% CI, 6.0–12.9) in females. Interestingly, they also demonstrated an elevated risk of colorectal cancer after small bowel adenocarcinoma, with similar risk ratios. This finding reinforces the notion of similarities in the epidemiology of small bowel and large bowel adenocarcinoma. Small bowel carcinoid tumors were not associated with an elevated risk of colorectal cancer or other malignancies.

### Other Medical Conditions

Some authors have suggested a significant role for bile in the etiology of small bowel adenocarcinoma, particularly its concentration in the periampullary region of the duodenum.[4,16] One small case–control study found that 3 of 19 patients with adenocarcinoma had had a previous cholecystectomy, but none of 52 control subjects had (P = 0.004).[17] Lightdale and co-workers[38] suggested that the alkaline environment of the small bowel accounted for the lower cancer rate there than in the stomach and other portions of the GI tract. In the same small case–control study of 19 adenocarcinoma cases,[17] two patients had a prior history of peptic ulcer disease but none of the 52 controls did (P = 0.02).

Another medical condition associated with small bowel adenocarcinoma is cystic fibrosis. Several case reports have suggested an association between cystic fibrosis and adenocarcinoma in the ileum. A cohort study of 412 cystic fibrosis patients found one case of small bowel adenocarcinoma; an incidence of 0.001 was expected, based on population incidence rates (P = 0.003).[39] In contrast, a larger retrospective cohort study of 28,511 patients with cystic fibrosis, with follow-up to 7 years, found only two small bowel cancers.[40]

Small bowel adenocarcinoma has also been reported to be associated with celiac sprue.[41]

### Radiation Therapy

Radiation therapy to the abdomen and pelvis is used in a number of settings. One large cohort study of almost 50,000 women treated with radiation therapy and 16,713 women treated without radiation therapy for cervical cancer found a relative risk of 1.8 for small bowel cancer (95% CI, 1.1–2.0). The study did not, however, describe the histologic subtypes of small bowel cancer observed.[42]

### Diet

Several groups have studied the association of diet with small bowel cancer. Chow and colleagues[43] examined the association of various dietary risk factors with it. The study utilized data on decedents from the 1986 National Mortality Follow-Back Survey of the National Center for Health Statistics. That survey used a probability sample of 1% of U.S. deaths for 1986. Chow and colleagues identified 430 patients who died of small bowel cancer (all white and aged 25–74 years) and compared them with 921 randomly selected controls of the same age range who died of other causes. Information on risk factors was obtained from next of kin. Unfortunately, this large study of small bowel cancer did not provide information regarding histologic subtypes. The study did, however, find statistically significant odds ratios in the range of 2 to 3 for intake of red meat and salt-cured and smoked foods.

In a population-based case–control study, Wu and colleagues[44] compared 36 small bowel adenocarcinoma cases with 998 population controls. Information on risk factors was obtained by interview. The results suggested an association with intake of fried, smoked, or barbecued meat and fish, although this finding was not statistically significant. An increase in risk was associated with sugar intake in the form of nonalcoholic beverages (OR, 3.3; 95% CI, 1.2–9.4). An ecologic study of small bowel cancer mortality and food data found a correlation coefficient of 0.61 (P ≤ 0.005) for per capita daily consumption of animal fat and 0.75 (P ≤ 0.005) for per capita daily animal consumption of protein.[45]

### Tobacco and Alcohol

The association of tobacco and alcohol with small bowel cancer has been studied too. Chow and colleagues[43] found no association in the context of their study described above, where no histologic subtyping was available. A small case–control study by Chen and co-workers[17] based on medical record review was the first to find an association between small bowel adenocarcinoma and smoking (OR, 6.2; 95% CI, 1.5–26.7) and between small bowel adenocarcinoma and alcohol consumption (OR, 5.5; 95% CI, 1.4–21.4). Similar results were obtained by Wu and colleagues[44] for ethanol intake (OR, 2.9; 95% CI, 1.2–7.1) and for smoking (OR, 2.1; 95% CI, 0.8–5.1), although the association with smoking was not significant.

## Molecular Genetics

One of the major advances in cancer research in the past 10 to15 years has been the elucidation of the molecular genetics of colorectal cancer. Elegant studies by Vogelstein and others have explored the somatic genetic changes that take place in the course of colorectal carcinogenesis.[46–48] We now have a clearer perception of the process of colorectal carcinogenesis on a molecular genetic level than that of any other solid tumor. Clinical benefits have included the identification of germline mutations and predisposing factors. Research efforts are currently under way to take advantage of these new findings in developing new screening tools for colon cancer[49,50] and pharmacologic agents for treating colorectal cancer.[51,52] In contrast, very little research has been carried out on molecular markers in small bowel cancer, and the few studies that have been done have been limited in size. How-

ever, a morphologic adenoma–carcinoma sequence has been described for tumors in the small intestine.[15,53–56]

The few studies that have been done suggest that certain oncogenes are altered in ways and in frequencies that correspond to similar events in large bowel cancer. Given the overall similarities in the epidemiology and the adenoma–carcinoma sequence for both small bowel adenocarcinoma and colorectal adenocarcinoma, it is highly likely that the same molecular genetic changes are involved.[1,57,58] However, further work is needed to confirm this. If true, then a potentially important future research program should be to determine the protective effect in small bowel mucosa, given the similar frequency of these molecular genetic changes in the small and large bowels.

## Cell Culture Studies

Uncontrolled cell proliferation is the hallmark of cancer, and there is increasing evidence that tumors undergo damage to genes that directly regulate their cell cycle.[59–63] Genetic alterations affecting the $G_1$ phase of the cell cycle are so frequent in human cancers that abnormalities in this pathway may actually be necessary for tumor development. Like the tumor suppressor protein p53, other participants in the $G_1$ phase may participate in checkpoint functions that regulate homeostatic tissue renewal throughout life. Oncogenic processes often exert their effects by targeting specific regulators of $G_1$-phase progression.[60,61]

Transfection of normal enterocytes derived from rat jejunum (RIE cells) with the c-H-ras oncogene and transfection of normal enterocytes derived from the rat ileum (IEC 18 cells) with both c-H-ras[64] and the c-K-ras[65] oncogenes resulted in malignant transformation of these cells. These results imply that the ras oncogene plays its major role early in the multistep process of small bowel tumorigenesis. Ras-transformed enterocytes displayed increased expression of both cyclin D1 and Rb genes, thus revealing novel effects of these oncogenes in small bowel carcinogenesis.[64,65] Overexpression of cyclin D1 by IEC 18 cells resulted in their malignant transformation.[66]

## Animal Studies

### The min mouse system

Animal models and cell culture systems have shed some light on potential molecular biomarkers of small bowel tumors. Of particular importance is the min mouse model.[67–71] Min mice carry a dominant mutation in the homologue of the adenomatous polyposis coli (APC) gene on chromosome 18.[69] Mutations in the APC gene appear to be responsible not only for FAP but also for many sporadic cases of GI tract cancer. APC gene modification may be a critical event in the initiation of small bowel tumor formation. Mendelian transmission of the mutated gene causes most homozygous min mice to develop multiple polyps throughout the intestinal tract, mostly in the small bowel. Loss of the wild-type APC allele precedes the formation of adenomas.[67,71] In a recent elegant study, Oshima and associates[71] crossed COX2 knockout mice with APC-mutated min mice and demonstrated a marked reduction in the number of intestinal adenomas in the progeny.

### mom-1

Further analysis of the min mouse model has identified, by quantitative trait loci studies, a locus designated mom-1 that dramatically modifies the min-induced tumor number. This locus is frequently rearranged or mutated in intestinal tumors and maps to the distal region of chromosome 4, in a region syntenic to human chromosome 1p35-36. This region of human chromosome 1 is frequently rearranged or mutated in intestinal tumors. mom-1 is estimated to account for approximately 50% of the genetic variation in adenomas in min mice.[72] Further analysis of the mom-1 gene in tumors produced by min mice should indicate if it is comutated during tumor progression. MacPhee and colleagues[73] have suggested that secretory phospholipase A2 is the protein encoded by mom-1 and that it modifies polyp number by affecting the cellular microenvironment within the intestinal crypt.

### Strain B10.A

Fijneman and Demant[74] reported that a high percentage of B10.A mice treated with the carcinogen N-ethyl-N-nitrosourea developed macroscopic tumors of the small intestine. These tumors were described as adenocarcinomas containing cells of four histologically different types, each resembling one of the four main differentiated cell types in the mouse small intestine: mucosa, enteroendocrine, Paneth, and columnar. Because these four cell types all originate from a common pluripotent stem cell, the crypt-base columnar cell, it is believed that tumors of the small intestine originate from neoplastically affected crypt-base columnar cells.

### Loss of heterozygosity

Loss of heterozygosity (LOH) studies have presented a powerful tool for following the development and progression of cancer. In human tumors, however, LOH can be difficult to interpret because of the small numbers of tumors of a precise type, stage, genetic background, and environmental exposure.[75] Transgenic mice would appear to be ideal for performing genome-wide scans for LOH. However, when the overall genome-wide rate of LOH of carcinoid tumors was tested in transgenic mice expressing the SV40 tumor antigen (Tag), it was found to be quite low. Moreover, chromosomes 9 and 16 showed high rates of allelic loss. The locus in chromosome 9 lies in a region syntenic to human 3q, 6q12, 15q24, and 3p21, whereas the locus on chromosome 16 lies in a region syntenic to human chromosomes 3q and 22q. Since these regions do not encode either pRb or p53, the two tumor suppressor genes known to interact with SV40 Tag, it is possible that novel genes are involved in the loss of function that contributes to multistage tumorigenesis.[75]

SV40 Tag, human K-ras, and a dominant negative mutant of human p53 have been expressed singly, and in all possible combinations, in postmitotic enterocytes of transgenic mice to assess their role in the pathogenesis of gut neoplasia. Transgenic mice producing K-ras and/or p53 had no detectable phenotypic abnormalities. K-ras cooperated with SV40 Tag to generate marked proliferative and dysplastic changes; yet, mice that carried one, two, or three of these transgenes did not form adenomas or adenocarcinomas. A modest increase in tumor number was noted in animals that expressed the min mutation and either SV40 Tag, SV40 Tag with K-ras, or SV40 Tag, K-ras, and p53. These results demonstrate the remarkable protective effect of the continuously and rapidly renewing epithelium in the small bowel.[76]

## Human Studies

### Allelic loss of 5q

In a human study, deletion in the long arm of chromosome 5 was noted in one of seven cases (14%) of Crohn's disease–associated adenocarcinomas, while none were noted in 13 sporadic cases.[77] In a similar study, deletions in chromosome 5q were noted in

17% of sporadic adenocarcinomas of the ampulla.[78] This suggests that the rate of allelic loss at 5q in small bowl cancer is therefore significantly lower than that seen in colorectal cancer, where the rate of allelic loss is around 40%.[79] However, the most common mutations in the *APC* gene are due to truncating mutations, for which allelic loss is not a very sensitive marker.

### c-K-*ras*

Several groups have evaluated the frequency of c-K-*ras* in small bowel adenocarcinoma by using a polymerase chain reaction (PCR)-based assay of restriction fragment length polymorphism (RFLP). The first group to do so observed c-K-*ras* mutations at codon 12 in five of six cases.[80] Subsequent studies evaluating alterations in sporadic and Crohn's disease associated–adenocarcinomas of the small intestine[77] found six c-K-*ras* mutations (at both codon 12 and 13) in 15 of 37 sporadic cases (40%), and 4 of 8 Crohn's disease associated–cases (50%). In a large study of 262 formalin-fixed, paraffin-embedded sections of GI tumors, c-K-*ras* mutations (at codon 12) were detected in 8 of 20 small bowel adenomas (40%) and in 10 of 28 adenocarcinomas (36%) (Arber, unpublished data). Younes and co-workers,[81] by contrast, found codon 12 mutations in only 4 of 28 cases (14.3%).

### DCC

Deletion of the *DCC* gene in the long arm of chromosome 18 has been demonstrated in only one study, where it was found in only 1 of 15 cases (6%).[77]

### p53

Rashid and Hamilton[77] found increased expression of p53 protein in 47% of sporadic adenocarcinomas, 57% of Crohn's-associated adenocarcinomas, and 29% of adenomas. Arber and colleagues[82] evaluated p53 in 20 adenomas and 24 adenocarcinomas using immunohistochemical methods and found increased expression in 47% of adenomas and in 65% of adenocarcinomas ($P \leq 0.05$). This suggested a significant increase in p53 expression with tumor progression. In the same study, increased p53 levels were more prevalent in tumors removed from females than in those from males (71% vs. 37%, $P < 0.05$). Spandidos and co-workers[83] reported similar findings. p53 was seen in 46% of small bowel tumors, including lymphoma, leiomyosarcoma, and adenocarcinoma. Increased expression of p53 was associated with a poorer prognosis in two studies.[82,84]

### Cell cycle proteins

We have looked for the expression of cell cycle proteins p16, p21, p27, cyclin D1, and cyclin E in small bowel adenomas and adenocarcinomas using immunohistochemical methods.[82] All normal-appearing mucosa samples expressed the p27[kip1] protein, but none displayed appreciable nuclear staining for p16[ink4a], p21[cip1], cyclin D1, or cyclin E. Rarely, in approximately 1 cell per 20 crypts, positive nuclear staining for these proteins was noted near the base of the crypt. The abnormalities identified in the tumors are summarized in Table 47–4. The most common alteration involved an increase in the p16[ink4a] protein, which was overexpressed in 92% of the adenomas and 91% of the adenocarcinomas.

There was also increased expression of the cyclin D1, cyclin E, p21[cip1], and p27[kip1] proteins in both adenomas and adenocarcinomas but no evidence that their expression increased with tumor progression (Table 47–5). The p27[kip1] protein was seen in all of the normal mucosa samples but 83% of the adenomas and 77% of the adenocarcinomas.

Increased expression of cyclin D1 in the small bowel neoplasms was associated with advanced patient age ($P < 0.05$) and a decrease in 3-year survival. Of 15 subjects who died within the 3-year period, 7 (47%) showed increased expression of cyclin D1, and 11 had mutated *p53*. Increased expression of cyclin D1 was closely associated with mutated *p53* in adenomas, and increased expression of cyclin E was closely associated with increased p53 in adenocarcinomas ($P < 0.05$). Tumor stage and grade were not significantly associated with any of the above abnormalities.

### erbB-2-neu (HER-2)

erbB-2-neu encodes a transmembrane glycopotein that has tyrosine-specific kinase activity. Cohen and co-workers[85] examined the expression of the p185 neu protein in normal and malignant tumors at several GI sites, including the small intestine, and found a point mutation in the *neu* gene, leading to a single amino acid substitution (valine to glutamine at residue 664), to be responsible for the transforming phenotype. In the normal mucosa, there was prominent neu expression in the villus, with little or no staining in the crypts; immunoreactivity was consistently greater in adenomatous polyps than in normal tissues. These findings suggest that p185 neu may play a role in the transformation of these cells. In another study,[84] neu protein was overexpressed in 9 of 15 adenocarcinomas (60%) from the duodenum and was associated with a poorer prognosis.

### Transforming growth factor α

Transforming growth factor α (TGF-α) expression was evaluated in one study by immunohistochemistry. It was found in 9 of 15 tumors but was not associated with patient survival, tumor stage, or tumor grade.[84]

**Table 47–4** Comparison of small and large bowel tumors

| | Small Bowel Tumors (%) | | Large Bowel Tumors (%) | |
| Abnormality | Polyp | Adenocarcinoma | Polyp | Adenocarcinoma |
| --- | --- | --- | --- | --- |
| Allelic loss of 5q | 0 | 5 | 40 | 40 |
| K-*ras* overexpression | 35 | 40 | 40 | 40–50 |
| Allelic loss of 18q | 10 | 5 | 40 | 60 |
| p53 | 33 | 47 | 30 | 50 |
| Microsatellite instability | — | 13 | — | 15 |

Adapted from Arber N, Hibshoosh H, Yasui W, et al. Abnormalities in the expression of cell-cycle related proteins in tumors of the small bowel. Cancer Epidemiol Biomarkers Prev 8:1101–1105, 1999.[82]

**Table 47–5** Cell cycle–related protein abnormalities in small bowel tumors[a]

| Protein | Tumor Type (%)[a] | |
| --- | --- | --- |
| | Adenoma | Adenocarcinoma |
| Cyclin D1 | 31 | 30 |
| Cyclin E | 31 | 38 |
| p16 | 92 | 91 |
| p21 | 50 | 46 |
| p27 | 83 | 77 |
| p53 | 47 | 65 |

[a]Each percentage indicates percentage of patients with detectable levels of the protein. Adapted from Arber N, Hibshoosh H, Yasui W, et al. Abnormalities in the expression of cell-cycle related proteins in tumors of the small bowel. Cancer Epidemiol Biomarkers Prev 8:1101–1105, 1999.[82]

## Microsatellite instability

Genomic instability and replication errors play an important role in the pathogenesis of tumors, especially intestinal tumors and those of the small bowel.[86] Rashid and Hamilton[77] found replication errors in 3 of 23 cases studied. Hibi and associates[87] observed replication errors in 5 of 11 cases. Keller and colleagues[88] found microsatellite instability in one of five cases.

## Tumor markers

Carcinoembryonic antigen (CEA) expression was evaluated in 15 patients by Zhu and co-workers[84] using an avidin-biotin-peroxidase complex technique and was found in 73%. Tobi and colleagues[89] recently found increased expression of adenoma monoclonal antibodies in 16 of 18 cases of small bowel adenocarcinomas (89%) but only weak staining in normal mucosa.

## Why Are Small Bowel Tumors So Rare?

Like the spleen, the small intestine is remarkably resistant to carcinogenesis. When gastric carcinoma recurs after gastrojejunostomy, the recurrence is five times more likely to be gastric rather than jejunal. However, when peptic ulcers recur after gastrojejunostomy, the recurrence is nearly always jejunal.[90] Likewise, the terminal ileum is highly resistant to tumor invasion from the proximal colon; only 0.7% of colon cancers recur locally after an ileocolic anastamosis compared with 14% after colocolic anastamosis.[90]

Several theories have been offered to explain the low incidence of small bowel cancer:

1. Small intestinal mucosal cells are lost and replaced very rapidly, at an estimated rate of 1 g of intestinal mucosa every 16 minutes.[76,91] Therefore, mutated cells may be shed into the lumen before a tumor can develop.
2. There are relatively few bacteria in the normal small bowel.[92,93]
3. The rapid transit of small bowel contents and the sparseness of bacterial flora there may minimize exposure to potential carcinogenic products.[6,94]
4. Liquified chyme may reduce mechanical trauma to the small bowel and protect it from carcinogens.[6,94]
5. The alkaline pH of small bowel contents prevents formation of nitrosamines that may be carcinogenic in the acidic environment of the stomach.[38,94]
6. The small bowel has a well-developed, protective local immunoglobulin A (IgA)-mediated immune system.[91]
7. In the small bowel, carcinogens induce apoptosis, and cells that contain genetic defects are quickly removed.[91]
8. The small bowel has fewer stem cells (carcinogen target cells) than the colon or the stomach.[94] Moreover, these stem cells lie deep within crypts and are therefore shielded from potential carcinogens by mucosal layers and other efficient mechanisms that maintain the stem cells' genetic integrity.[95]
9. The duodenum contains a water-soluble tumor-inhibiting component.[96]
10. The small bowel contains relatively low levels of enzymes that activate precarcinogens.[97]

None of these hypotheses has been very well investigated. Certainly, little research has been done on these issues in the human small bowel. In particular, although the rapid turnover of small bowel mucosal cells has been suggested as a possible mechanism for the low rate of small bowel cancer in humans (i.e., partially transformed cells are shed before full carcinogenesis can occur), most experts feel that a high proliferation and turnover rate directly correlates with carcinogenesis. On the other hand, the higher proliferation rate in the large bowel has been suggested by Lipkin and others[98] to be an etiologic factor, or at least a marker for cancer risk.

## Appendiceal Cancer

### Epidemiology

Primary adenocarcinoma of the appendix is rare and seldom diagnosed at presentation or even during appendectomy. Pathologic examination still remains the primary method of diagnosis. Primary appendiceal adenocarcinoma was first described in 1882 by Berger, and by 1999 only about 500 cases had been described. It is found during 0.1% of all appendectomies, corresponding to an estimated incidence of 0.2 per 100,000 people per year.[99,100] It accounts for 0.2% to 0.5% of all intestinal malignancies and 4% to 6% of primary appendiceal neoplasms. The mean age at presentation is around 60 years, with males being affected 1.5 times more frequently than females.[101]

### Pathology

There are no macroscopic characteristics that distinguish appendiceal adenocarcinoma from other appendiceal lesions. Seventy percent of appendiceal adenocarcinomas present as a nodule at the base of the appendix. Grossly, these tumors may appear polypoid or ulcerative.[102] The two main types of appendiceal adenocarcinoma are mucinous cystadenocarcinoma, which may develop from a precursor cystadenoma, and colonic adenocarcinoma, which may develop from a tubular or tubulovillous adenoma.[103] Cystadenocarcinoma produces abundant extracellular mucin, tends to be well differentiated, and tends to metastasize to the ovary. Colonic adenocarcinoma lacks mucin and is poorly differentiated. Lymph node metastases are noted in 25% of cases at presentation and are more commonly associated with adenocarcinoma than with cystadenocarcinoma. Cystadenocarcinoma is generally less virulent than adenocarcinoma, despite its ability to produce pseudomyxoma peritonei.[100]

### Clinical Presentation

Appendiceal cancer can present in a variety of forms, depending on the type of tumor (mucinous or colonic) and the stage at presentation. Scott[104] reported that patients with these tumors presented with acute appendicitis with or without abscess formation in 65% of cases, an abdominal mass in 13%, and ileus in 3%; in 7% of cases, tumor was detected incidentally during unrelated elective surgery. The appendix is narrow; therefore, even a small growth can occlude its lumen, resulting in symptoms of acute appendicitis.[102] More unusual presentations have included vaginal bleeding, infiltration of the abdominal wall, melena, bladder infiltration, hydronephrosis,[100] cecal–cecal intussusception, and symptoms of Crohn's disease.[104] There are some rare reports of association with long-standing ulcerative colitis[105] and synchronous development of mucinous tumors of the appendix and ovaries.

Appendiceal malignancies are the most frequently perforating carcinomas of the entire GI tract. Anatomically, there appear to be several reasons for this: (1) an extremely thin subserosal and peritoneal coat, (2) a delicate vascular submucosa supplied by a terminal artery, and (3) the thinnest longitudinal and inner circular muscles in the GI tract.[106] An abscess is often a sequela of perforation. This is most likely due to the desmoplastic reaction created by the cancer and the release, in response to surrounding chronic inflammation, of factors that elicit the omentum to wall off the process.[107]

If a cystadenocarcinoma ruptures, it may shed malignant mucin-producing cells throughout the peritoneal cavity, thereby causing generalized pseudomyxoma peritonei. Patients with this condition present with abdominal distention suggesting ascites but without shifting dullness.[100] Also, they may present with anemia, a mass in the right groin, or even dyspareunia.[106]

## Mucinous Tumors of the Appendix and Ovaries

The simultaneous appearance of pseudomyxoma peritonei and mucinous tumors involving the appendix and ovaries has been noted for many years. Two theories have recently been proposed regarding the origin of pseudomyxoma peritonei: the tumors arise as independent primaries,[99,100] or they represent an appendiceal tumor that has metastasized to ovary.[108] Several lines of evidence support the first theory: (1) the predominance of right-sided ovarian lesions in association with pseudomyxoma peritonei, which might be explained by the proximity of the right ovary to the appendix; (2) the high percentage of bilateral ovarian mucinous tumors; (3) the presence of mucus and atypical mucinous cells on the ovarian surface, suggesting an "implantation lesion"[108]; (4) the different embryologic origins of the ovary and appendix (mesodermal and endodermal, respectively); and (5) the rarity of having both tumors in the absence of pseudomyxoma peritonei.

Chuaqui and colleagues[109] evaluated 12 cases of simultaneous appendiceal and ovarian involvement and found genetic alterations in p53, *MLH1* and *APC* genes in one or both tumors in six cases. In three of those cases, a selective alteration on chromosome 17q (typically ovarian) was found on the ovarian lesion, but not the appendiceal.

Guerrieri and co-workers[108] examined the expression of cytokeratin 7 (CK-7) in appendiceal and ovarian tumors. They noted that ovarian epithelial and mucinous tumors were always CK-7 positive while colonic adenocarcinomas were typically CK-7 negative. They also found that most (60%) of the simultaneous mucinous tumors stained positive for CK-7, which supports an appendiceal origin of these tumors.

## References

1. Neugut AI, Jacobson JS, Suh S, Mukherjee R, Arber N. Epidemiology of cancer of the small intestine. Cancer Epidemiol Biomarkers Prev 7:243–251, 1998.
2. Schottenfeld D, Islam SS. Cancers of the small intestine. In: Schottenfeld D, Fraumeni J Jr (eds): Cancer Epidemiology and Prevention, 2nd ed. Oxford University Press, New York, 1996, pp 806–812.
3. Neugut AI, Marvin M, Rella VA, Chabot JA. An overview of adenocarcinoma of the small intestine. Oncology 11:529–536, 1997.
4. Ross RK, Hartnett NM, Bernstein L, Henderson BE. Epidemiology of adenocarcinomas of the small intestine: is bile a small bowel carcinogen? Br J Cancer 63:143–145, 1991.
5. Weiss NS, Yang C. Incidence of histologic types of cancer of the small intestine. J Natl Cancer Inst 78:653–656, 1987.
6. Lowenfels AB. Why are small bowel tumors so rare? Lancet 1:24–26, 1973.
7. Landis SH, Murray T, Bolden S, Wingo PA. Cancer statistics, 1999. CA Cancer J Clin 49:8–31, 1999.
8. Silberman H, Crichlow RW, Caplan HS. Neoplasms of the small bowel. Ann Surg 180:157–161, 1974.
9. Frand VI, Ramot B. Malignant lymphomata: an epidemiological study. Harefuah 5:83–86, 1963.
10. Gabos S, Berkel J, Band P, Robson D, Whittaker H. Small bowel cancer in western Canada. Int J Epidemiol 22:198–206, 1993.
11. DiSario JA, Burt RW, Vargas H, McWhorter WP. Small bowel cancer: epidemiological and clinical characteristics from a population-based registry. Am J Gastroenterol 89:699–701, 1994.
12. Severson RK, Schenk M, Gurney JG, Weiss LK, Demers RY. Increasing incidence of adenocarcinomas and carcinoid tumors of the small intestine in adults. Cancer Epidemiol Biomarkers Prev 5:81–84, 1996.
13. Chow JS, Chen CC, Ahsan H, Neugut AI. A population-based study of the incidence of malignant small bowel tumors: SEER, 1973–90. Int J Epidemiol 25:722–728, 1996.
14. Stang A, Stegmaier C, Eisinger B, Stabenow R, Metz KA, Jockel KH. Descriptive epidemiology of small intestinal malignancies: the German Cancer Registry experience. Br J Cancer 80:1440–1444, 1999.
15. Sellner F. Investigations on the significance of the adenoma–carcinoma sequence in the small bowel. Cancer 66:702–715, 1990.
16. Lowenfels AB. Does bile promote extra-colonic cancer? Lancet 2:239–241, 1978.
17. Chen CC, Neugut AI, Rotterdam H. Risk factors for adenocarcinomas and malignant carcinoids of the small intestine: preliminary findings. Cancer Epidemiol Biomarkers Prev 3:205–207, 1994.
18. Parkin D, Muir C, Whelan SL, Gao WT, Ferlay J. Cancer Incidence in Five Continents, 6th ed. IARC Scientific Publication #120. Oxford University Press, New York, 1993.
19. Ries LAG, Kosary CL, Hankey BF, Harris A, Miller BA, Edwards BK (eds). SEER Cancer Statistics Review, 1973–93. National Cancer Institute, Bethesda, MD, 1996.
20. Ginsburg L, Schneider KM, Dreizin DH, Levinson C. Carcinoma of the jejunum occurring in a case of regional enteritis. Surgery 39:347–351, 1956.
21. Michelassi F, Testa G, Pomidor WJ, Lashner BA, Block GE. Adenocarcinoma complicating Crohn's disease. Dis Colon Rectum 35:654–661, 1993.
22. Munkholm P, Langholz E, Davidsen M, Binder V. Intestinal cancer risk and mortality in patients with Crohn's disease. Gastroenterology 105:1716–1723, 1993.
23. Persson PG, Karlen P, Burnell O, et al. Crohn's disease and cancer: a population-based cohort study. Gastroenterology 107:1675–1678, 1994.
24. Darke SG, Parks AG, Grogono JL, Pollock J. Adenocarcinoma and Crohn's disease: a report of two cases and analysis of the literature. Br J Surg 60:169–175, 1973.
25. Lashner BA. Risk factors for small bowel cancer in Crohn's disease. Dig Dis Sci 37:1179–1184, 1992.
26. Greenwald E, Parker J, Schultz S, Reed E. Benign papillary adenoma of the ampullary region of the duodenum with intussusception. Gastroenterology 43:344–350, 1962.
27. Uppaputhangkule V, Maas L, Gelzayd E. Endoscopic diagnosis of villous adenoma of the duodenum. Gastrointest Endosc 22:97–98, 1976.
28. Hessler P, Braunstein E. Adenocarcinoma of the duodenum arising in a villous adenoma. Gastrointest Radiol 2:355–357, 1978.
29. Jagelman DG, DeCosse JJ, Bussey HJR, and the Leeds Castle Polyposis Group. Upper gastrointestinal cancer and familial adenomatous polyposis. Lancet 1:1149–1151, 1988.
30. Spigelman AD, Talbot IC, Penna C, et al. Evidence for adenoma–carcinoma sequence in the duodenum of patients with familial adenomatous polyposis. J Clin Pathol 47:709–710, 1994.
31. Spigelman AD, Crofton-Sleigh C, Venitt S, Phillips RKS. Mutagenicity of bile and duodenal adenomas in familial adenomatous polyposis. Br J Surg 77:878–881, 1989.
32. Offerhaus GJ, Giardiello FM, Krush AJ, et al. The risk of upper gastrointestinal cancer in familial adenomatous polyposis. Gastroenterology 102:1980–1982, 1993.

33. Nugent KP, Spigelman AD, Williams CB, Talbot IC, Phillips RK. Surveillance of duodenal polyps in familial adenomatous polyposis: progress report. J R Soc Med 87:704–706, 1994.

34. Spigelman AD, Williams CB, Talbot IC, Domizio P, Phillips RKS. Upper gastrointestinal cancer in patients with familial adenomatous polyposis. Lancet 2:783–785, 1989.

35. Watson P, Lynch HT. Extracolonic cancer in hereditary nonpolyposis colorectal cancer. Cancer 71:677–685, 1993.

36. Aarnio M, Mecklin JP, Aaltonen LA, Nystrom-Lahti M, Jarvinen HJ. Lifetime risk of different cancers in hereditary non-polyposis colorectal cancer (HNPCC) syndrome. Int J Cancer 64:430–433, 1995.

37. Neugut AI, Santos J. The association between cancers of the small and large bowel. Cancer Epidemiol Biomarkers Prev 2:551–553, 1993.

38. Lightdale CJ, Koepsell T, Sherlock P. Small intestine. In: Schottenfeld D, Fraumeni JF Jr (eds): Cancer Epidemiology and Prevention, 1st ed. W.B. Saunders, Philadelphia, 1982, pp 692–702.

39. Sheldon CD, Hodson ME, Carpenter LM, Swerdlow AJ. A cohort study of cystic fibrosis and malignancy. Br J Cancer 68:1025–1028, 1993.

40. Neglia JP, Fitzsimmons SC, Maisonneuve P, et al. The risk of cancer among patients with cystic fibrosis. N Engl J Med 332:494–499, 1995.

41. Begos DG, Kuan S, Dobbins J, Ravikumar TS. Metachronous small-bowel adenocarcinoma in celiac sprue. J Clin Gastroenterol 20:233–236, 1985.

42. Kleinerman RA, Boice JD Jr, Storm HH, et al. Second primary cancer after treatment for cervical cancer: an international cancer registries study. Cancer 76:442–452, 1995.

43. Chow WH, Linet MS, McLaughlin JK, Hsing AW, Chien HT, Blot WJ. Risk factors for small intestine cancer. Cancer Causes Control 4:164–169, 1993.

44. Wu AH, Yu MC, Mack TM. Smoking, alcohol use, dietary factors and risk of small intestinal adenocarcinoma. Int J Cancer 70:512–517, 1997.

45. Lowenfels AB, Sonni A. Distribution of small bowel tumors. Cancer Lett 3:83–86, 1977.

46. Vogelstein B, Kinzler KW. Colorectal cancer and the intersection between basic and clinical research. Cold Spring Harbor Symp Quant Biol 59:517–521, 1994.

47. Real MA, Fearon ER. Gene effects in colorectal tumorigenesis. In: Young GP, Rozen P, Levin B (eds): Prevention and Early Detection of Colorectal Cancer. W.B. Saunders, London, 1996, pp 63–86.

48. Cho RK, Vogelstein B. Genetic alterations in the adenoma–carcinoma sequence. Cancer 70:1727–1731, 1992.

49. Sidransky D, Tokin T, Hamilton SR, et al. Identification of ras oncogene mutations in the stool of patients with curable colorectal tumors. Science 256:102–105, 1992.

50. Wargovich MJ. Precancer markers and prediction of tumorigenesis. In: Young GP, Rozen P, Levin B (eds): Prevention and Early Detection of Colorectal Cancer. W.B. Saunders, London, 1996, pp 89–101.

51. Schulz S, Nyce JW. Inhibition of protein isoprenylation and p21 ras membrane association by dehydroepiandrosterone in human colonic adenocarcinoma cells in vitro. Cancer Res 51:6563–6567, 1991.

52. Dansei R, McLellan CA, Myers CE. Specific labeling of isoprenylated proteins: application to study inhibitors of the post-translational farnesylation and geranylgeranylation. Biochem Biophys Res Commun 206:637–643, 1995.

53. Seifert E, Schulte F, Stolte M. Adenoma and carcinoma of the duodenum and papilla of Vater: a clinicopathologic study. Am J Gastroenterol 87:37–42, 1992.

54. Perzin HK, Bridge M. Adenomas of the small intestine: a clinicopathologic review of 51 cases and a study of their relationship to carcinoma. Cancer 48:799–819, 1981.

55. Kozuka S, Tsubone M, Yamaguchi A, Hachisuka K. Adenomatous residue in cancerous papilla of Vater. Gut 22:1031–1034, 1981.

56. Hermanek P. Adenoma/Dysplasie-Karzinom-Sequence im Dunndarm. Z Gastroenterol 25:166–167, 1987.

57. Arber N, Neugut AI, Weinstein IB, Holt PR. Molecular genetics of small bowel cancer. Cancer Epidemiol Biomarkers Prev 7:243–251, 1998.

58. Arber N: Small bowel adenocarcinoma (commentary). Oncology 11:549, 1997.

59. Pines J. Cyclins: wheels within wheels. Cell Growth Differ 2:305–310, 1991.

60. Hunter T, Pines J. Cyclins and cancer. II. cyclin D and CK inhibitors come of age. Cell 79:573–582, 1994.

61. Hall M, Peters G. Genetic alterations of cyclins, cyclin-dependent kinases, and CDK inhibitors in human cancer. Adv Cancer Res 68:67–108, 1996.

62. Pardee AB. GI events and regulations of cell proliferation. Science 246:603–608, 1989.

63. Sherr CJ. G1 phase progression: cycling on cue. Cell 79:551–555, 1994.

64. Filmus J, Robles AI, Shi W, Wong MJ, Colombo LL, Conti CJ. Induction of cyclin D1 overexpression by activated ras. Oncogene 9:3627–3633, 1994.

65. Arber N, Sutter T, Miyake M, et al. Increased expression of cyclin D1 and the Rb tumor suppressor gene in c-K-ras transformed rat enterocytes. Oncogene 12:1903–1908, 1996.

66. Arber N, Kaznov D, Meltzer E, Brill S, Rattan J, Halpern Z. Overexpression of cyclin D1 in normal enterocytes (IEC18) increases proliferation and inhibits apoptosis [abstract]. Gastroenterology A372, G1630, 1999.

67. Luongo C, Moser A, Gledhill S, Dove WF. Loss of APC in intestinal adenomas from min mice. Cancer Res 54:5947–5952, 1994.

68. Fod R, Edelmann W, Yang K, et al. A targeted chain-termination mutation in the mouse APC gene results in multiple intestinal tumors. Proc Natl Acad Sci USA 91:8969–8973, 1994.

69. Luongo C, Gould KA, Su LK, et al. Mapping of multiple intestinal neoplasia (min) to proximal chromosome 18 of the mouse. Genomics 15:3–8, 1993.

70. Oshima M, Oshima H, Kitagawa K, Kobayashi M, Itakura C, Taketo M. Loss of APC heterozygosity and abnormal tissue building in nascent intestinal polyps in mice carrying a truncated APC gene. Proc Natl Acad Sci USA 92:4482–4486, 1995.

71. Oshima M, Dinchuk JE, Kargman SL, et al. Suppression of intestinal polyposis in APC knockout mice by inhibition of cyclooxygenase 2 (COX-2). Cell 87:803–809, 1996.

72. Dietrich WF, Lander ES, Smith JS, et al. Genetic identification of mom-1, a major modifier locus affecting min-induced intestinal neoplasia in the mouse. Cell 75:631–639, 1993.

73. MacPhee M, Chepenick KP, Liddell RA, Nelson KK, Siracusa LD, Buchberg AM. The secretory phospholipase A2 gene is a candidate for the mom-1 locus, a major modifier of APC min-induced intestinal neoplasia. Cell 81:957–966, 1995.

74. Fijneman RJA, Demant P. A gene for susceptibility to small intestinal cancer, ssicl, maps to the distal part of mouse chromosome 4. Cancer Res 55:3179–3182, 1995.

75. Dietrich WF, Radany EH, Smith JS, Bishop JM, Hanahan D, Lander ES. Genome-wide search for loss of heterozygosity in transgenic mouse tumors reveals candidate tumor suppressor genes on chromosomes 9 and 16. Proc Natl Acad Sci USA 91:9451–9455, 1994.

76. Boyle WJ, Brenner DA. Molecular and cellular biology of the small intestine. Curr Opin Gastroenterol 11:121–127, 1995.

77. Rashid A, Hamilton SR. Genetic alterations in sporadic and Crohn's-associated adenocarcinomas of the small intestine. Gastroenterology 113:127–135, 1997.

78. Achille A, Scupoli MT, Magalini AR, et al. APC gene mutations and allelic losses in sporadic ampullary tumors: evidence of genetic differences from tumors associated with familial adenomatous polyposis. Int J Cancer 68:305–312, 1996.

79. Kern SE, Fearon ER, Tersmette KEF, et al. Allelic loss in colorectal carcinoma. JAMA 261:3099–3103, 1989.

80. Sutter T, Arber N, Moss SF, et al. Frequent c-K-ras mutations in small bowel adenocarcinomas. Dig Dis Sci 41:115–118, 1996.

81. Younes N, Fulton N, Tanaka R, Wayne J, Straus FH, Kaplan EL. The presence of K-12 ras mutations in duodenal adenocarcinomas and the absence of ras mutations in other small bowel adenocarcinomas and carcinoid tumors. Cancer 79:1804–1808, 1997.

82. Arber N, Hibshoosh H, Yasui W, et al. Abnormalities in the expression of cell-cycle related proteins in tumors of the small bowel. Cancer Epidemiol Biomarkers Prev 8:1101–1105, 1999.

83. Spandidos DA, Zoumpourlis V, Gorgoulis V, Gourtsoyiannis NC. p53 expression in human small intestinal tumors. Oncol Rep 1:885–887, 1997.

84. Zhu L, Kim K, Domenico R, Appert HE, Howard JM. Adenocarcinoma of duodenum and ampulla of Vater: clinicopathology study and expression of p53, c-neu, TGF-α, CEA, EMA. J Surg Oncol 61:100–105, 1996.

85. Cohen JA, Weiner B, More KF, et al. Expression pattern of 185neu (NGL) gene encoded growth factor receptor protein (p185neu) in normal and transformed epithelial tissues of the digestive tract. Oncogene 1:81–88, 1989.

86. Lynch HT, Lynch JF. 25 years of HNPCC. Anticancer Res 14:1617–1624, 1994.

87. Hibi K, Kondo K, Akiyama S, Ito K, Takagi H. Frequent genetic instability in small intestine carcinomas. Jpn J Cancer Res 86:357–360, 1995.

88. Keller G, Rotter M, Vogelstein H, et al. Microsatellite instability in adenocarcinoma of the upper gastrointestinal tract. Am J Pathol 14:593–600, 1995.
89. Tobi M, Kaila V, Hassan N, et al. Monoclonal antibody Adnab-9 defines a preneoplastic marker in epithelium at risk for adenocarcinoma of small intestine. Hum Pathol 30:467–473, 1999.
90. Martin RG: Malignant tumors of the small intestine. Surg Clin North Am 66:779–785, 1985.
91. Kim SH, Roth KA, Moser AR, Gordon JI. Transgenic mouse models that explore the multistep hypothesis of intestinal neoplasia. J Cell Biol 123:877–893, 1993.
92. Laqueur GK, McDaniel EG, Matsumoto H. Neoplasms in female Fischer rats following intraperitoneal injection of methylazoxy-methanol. J Natl Cancer Inst 39:55, 1967.
93. Hill MJ, Brasar BD, Hawkswoth G, Aries V, Crother JS, Williams RE. Bacteria and etiology of cancer of large bowel. Lancet 1:95–96, 1977.
94. Potten CS. Clonogenic, stem and carcinogen-target cells in small intestine mucosa. Scand J Gastroenterol 104:3–10, 1984.
95. Potten CS. The significance of spontaneous and induced apoptosis in the gastrointestinal tract of mice. Cancer Metastasis Rev 11:179–195, 1992.
96. Arbuna J, Cruicchi ET. A factor responsible for resistance to cancer. Curr Ther Res 40:745–749, 1996.
97. Wattenberg LW. Carcinogen detoxifying mechanisms in the gastrosintestinal tract. Gastroenterology 51:932–935, 1996.
98. Lipkin M, Higgins P. Biological markers of cell proliferation and differentiation in human gastrointestinal disease. Adv Cancer Res 50:1–24, 1988.
99. Proulx GM, Willett CG, Daley W, Shellito PC. Appendiceal carcinoma: patterns of failure following surgery and implications for adjuvant therapy. J Surg Oncol 66:51–53, 1997.
100. Deans GT, Spence RAJ. Neoplastic lesions of the appendix. Br J Surg 82:299–306, 1995.
101. Connor SJ, Hanna GB, Frizelle FA. Appendiceal tumors: retrospective clinicopathologic analysis of appendiceal tumors from 7,970 appendectomies. Dis Colon Rectum 41:75–80, 1998.
102. Lyss A. Appendiceal malignancies. Semin Oncol 15:129–137, 1998.
103. Rutledge R, Alexander J. Primary appendiceal malignancies: rare but important. Surgery 111;244–249, 1992.
104. Scott MJ. Primary adenocarcinoma of the vermiform appendix masquerading as Crohn's disease: case report. Eur J Surg 157:153–154, 1991.
105. Odze RD, Medline P, Cohen Z. Adenocarcinoma arising in an appendix involved with chronic ulcerative colitis. Am J Gastroenterol 89:1905–1907, 1994.
106. Cortina R, McCormick J, Kolm P, Perry R. Management and prognosis of adenocarcinoma of the appendix. Dis Colon Rectum 38:848–852, 1995.
107. Cerame M. A 25-year review of adenocarcinoma of the appendix—a frequently perforating carcinoma. Dis Colon Rectum 31:145–149, 1988.
108. Guerrieri C, Franlund B, Fristedt S, Gillooley JF, Boeryd B. Mucinous tumors of the vermiform appendix and ovary, and pseudomyxoma peritonei: histogenic implications of cytokeratin 7 expression. Hum Pathol 28:1039–1045, 1997.
109. Chuaqui RF, Zhuang Z, Emmert-Buck MR, et al. Genetic analysis of synchronous mucinous tumors of the ovary and appendix. Hum Pathol 27:165–167, 1996.

# Chapter 48

# Pathology and Natural History of Small Bowel and Appendiceal Cancers

NORMAN J. CARR AND LESLIE H. SOBIN

In this chapter, mesenchymal tumors and lymphomas will be discussed together. However, the differences between other lesions occurring in the appendix and small intestine are such that we have given them separate sections. The classification we use for gastrointestinal neoplasms is that of the World Health Organization.[1] In general, the definitions are the same as for tumors of the large intestine.

Small intestinal malignancies are uncommon. In the United States, the National Cancer Institute's Surveillance, Epidemiology and End Results (SEER) program showed adenocarcinomas and carcinoids to be the most frequent primary malignancies in the small intestine, with an approximately equal age-adjusted incidence of 0.4 per 100,000 each.[2] However, for part of the study period the program recorded only carcinoids designated malignant. For small cell malignant lymphoma, the SEER program[2] found an age-adjusted incidence of 0.3 per 100,000. One study found metastatic malignancies to be more frequent than primary tumors in the small bowel.[3]

The most common primary appendiceal tumor is the carcinoid, but most of these tumors are clinically benign, in contrast to small intestinal carcinoids. Classical carcinoids are covered in Chapter 64, but two distinctive lesions of the appendix with neuroendocrine differentiation, the goblet cell carcinoid and the tubular carcinoid, are included in this chapter.

## Adenocarcinoma of the Small Intestine

Although the small intestine constitutes the largest portion of the gastrointestinal tract, in most industrialized countries it is the site of less than 5% of gastrointestinal malignancies.[4,5] Approximately two-thirds of small bowel tumors are malignant. Adenocarcinomas are the most common histologic type in most Western populations, while in some other parts of the world lymphomas are more common.

According to the SEER data, the age-adjusted incidence of small intestinal carcinoma is 0.4 per 100,000, the median age of patients at diagnosis is 67 years, and the most common disease site is the duodenum.[2] These findings are generally consistent with data from other studies;[4–7] a population-based study from Hawaii found higher rates.[8]

Although carcinomas of the ampulla of Vater are usually classified separately, they show many similarities with duodenal lesions, and a distinction between tumors arising on the duodenal papilla and in the ampulla frequently cannot be made. Tumors in the ampulla are more likely to produce obstructive jaundice than those on the papilla (Color Fig. 48–1; see separate color insert).

The small intestine is more resistant to the development of epithelial malignancies than other gastrointestinal sites, such as the colon. A number of hypotheses have been expounded to account for this observation;[4,5] some of the more reasonable ones are listed in Table 48–1, but there is little direct evidence to favor any in particular.

### Etiology and Pathogenesis

There is good evidence for an adenoma–carcinoma sequence in the small intestine, analogous to that which is generally held to occur in the colon. For example, adenocarcinomas are frequently associated with an adjacent adenoma (Fig. 48–2), and many adenomas contain foci of invasion.[4,6,9] Adenomas with high-grade dysplasia or villous morphology are most likely to be associated with invasive carcinoma.[9]

Patients with familial adenomatous polyposis often have multiple adenomas of the small intestine (Fig. 48–3) and an increased

**Table 48-1** Possible reasons for the relatively low incidence of small intestinal adenocarcinoma

*Factors Limiting Exposure to Intraluminal Carcinogens*

Scarcity of luminal bacteria (particularly anaerobes) and their metabolic products
Rapid transit of small bowel contents, minimizing exposure time
Alkaline environment that reduces production of nitrosamines
High levels of benzopyrene hydrolase

*Immunoprotection*

Well-developed lymphoid tissue
High levels of immunoglobulin A (IgA) expression

*Other Factors*

Reduction in mechanical trauma due to liquified nature of chyme
Possibly lower bcl-2 expression in the small intestine than in the colon
Presence of a water-soluble tumor-inhibiting component in the duodenum

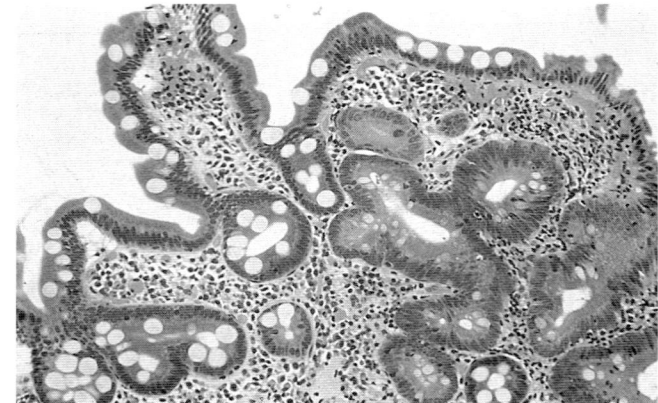

**Figure 48-3** Small intestine. Adenoma in patient with familial adenomatous polyposis. A small focus of adenomatous glands in small bowel mucosa. (From Jass JR, Sobin LH. Histological Typing of Intestinal Tumors, 2nd ed. Springer-Verlag, Berlin, 1989, p 56, with permission.)

risk of small intestinal adenocarcinoma.[10] In a study of patients with familial adenomatous polyposis who had undergone colectomy, random biopsy specimens of ileal mucosa showed foci of abnormal, dysplastic crypts resembling dysplastic aberrant crypt foci of the colon in a proportion of patients.[11] These foci were not associated with inflammation, metaplasia, or lymphoid follicles. The authors suggested that these lesions are microadenomas or oligocryptal adenomas, supporting the concept of the following sequence: normal ileal mucosa, microadenoma, gross adenoma, adenocarcinoma.

The duodenum is the most common site for small intestinal adenocarcinomas, and these tumors tend to occur in the periampullary region.[12] This phenomenon has led to the hypothesis that bile or its metabolites may be involved in oncogenesis at this site.[4,5] However, in patients with Crohn's disease, carcinomas are more likely to occur in the ileum, suggesting the possibility of a role for inflammation in their development.[4,12]

Celiac disease is associated with an increased risk of small intestinal adenocarcinoma. A recent report documents two cases in which the diagnosis of adenocarcinoma preceded that of celiac disease.[13]

There is some epidemiological evidence that cigarette use and alcohol consumption are risk factors for the development of small intestinal adenocarcinoma.[4]

Adenocarcinomas may arise in ileostomies and ileal conduits.[14–16] The interval between ileostomy formation and the development of carcinoma is usually prolonged, typically around 25 years.[14] Histological assessment is required to distinguish these carcinomas from the non-neoplastic inflammatory cap polyps that can occur at these sites as a manifestation of mucosal prolapse phenomenon.

Ileal pouches fashioned as part of the treatment of adenomatous polyposis have a relatively high incidence of adenomas; the cumulative number of patients with ileal pouch adenomas increases with time from surgery. There is an obvious theoretical risk of developing carcinoma under these circumstances, and careful pouch surveillance is indicated[17] A case of pouch carcinoma in a 35-year-old female who had a proctocolectomy for adenocarcinoma in ulcerative colitis has been described.[16]

There has been a well-documented increase in the incidence of other malignancies in patients with small bowel carcinoma.[7,8] For example, a registry-based study found associated carcinomas in 42% of such patients.[7] Most of these other primaries are colonic adenocarcinomas; other primary sites include prostate, female genital tract, lung, urinary tract, skin, and breast.[6–8] It has also been demonstrated that there is an increased risk of small intestinal adenocarcinomas in patients with hereditary nonpolyposis colorectal cancer (HNPCC).[18]

In patients with Peutz-Jeghers syndrome, the lifetime risk of developing small intestinal cancer has been estimated at 2.4%.[4] However, the pathologist must take care to distinguish true invasive carcinoma from the pseudoinvasion, or epithelial misplacement, that is common in Peutz-Jeghers polyps (Fig. 48–4).[19,20]

There is little information concerning the genetic changes in small intestinal adenocarcinoma. K-*ras* mutations at codon 12 are found in a proportion of cases, most commonly in duodenal lesions.[21] Patients with HNPCC and small intestinal carcinomas have been shown to have germline mutations of *hMLH1* or *hMSH2*.[18] In some tumors with high levels of microsatellite instability, mutations of the TGF-β-RII gene have been found.[1]

## Pathologic Features

Although adenocarcinomas can arise anywhere in the small intestine, the duodenum is the most common site.[2,4,12] Grossly, adenocarcinomas of the small intestine may have a polypoid, fun-

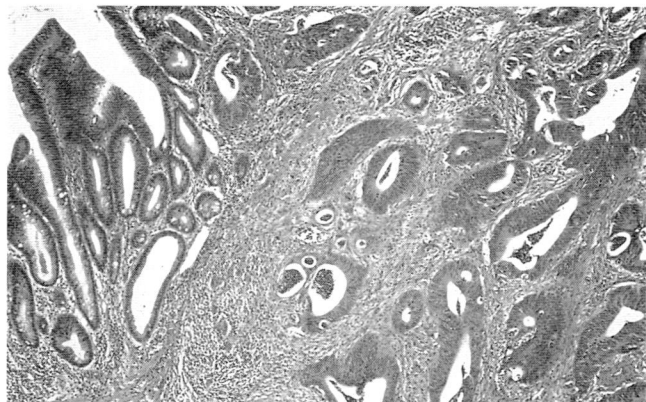

**Figure 48-2** Small intestine. Adenocarcinoma arising in an adenoma. Disorganized glands of carcinoma undermine the adenoma. (From Jass JR, Sobin LH. Histological Typing of Intestinal Tumors, 2nd ed. Springer-Verlag, Berlin, 1989, p 56, with permission.)

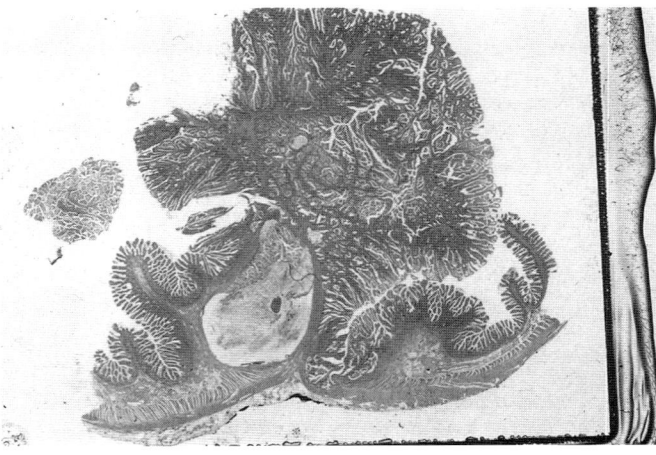

**Figure 48–4** Small intestine. Peutz-Jeghers polyp with pseudoinvasion. An intramural cystic lesion containing mucus and small bowel mucosa beneath the typical arborizing structure of a Peutz-Jeghers polyp.

gating, sessile, ulcerated, or annular appearance.[12] Histologically, they are similar to colonic lesions. As for epithelial neoplasms of the colon, it has been suggested that the definition of malignancy in small intestine epithelial neoplasms is invasion beyond the muscularis mucosae.[9,12] However, an alternative view is found in the TNM classification,[22] where T1 is defined as "tumor invades lamina propria or submucosa." The presence of desmoplasia is a useful feature in making this diagnosis in biopsy material. Adenocarcinomas of the small intestine usually produce mucin and may be well, moderately, or poorly differentiated; some have papillary morphology. Occasionally, Paneth cells are present.[12] Mucinous adenocarcinomas are not uncommon, but signet ring cell carcinoma is rare and should raise the suspicion of disease spread from a gastric primary tumor.

Immunoexpression of epithelial membrane antigen and cytokeratin is the rule, and some tumors express carcinoembryonic antigen (CEA), p53, c-neu, and tranforming growth factor α (TGF-α).[23] Some adenocarcinomas contain scattered endocrine cells, which can be identified histochemically, immunohistochemically, or ultrastructurally. Provided their morphology is that of an adenocarcinoma, such lesions should be classified as adenocarcinomas rather than neuroendocrine carcinomas.[4,12]

## Prognosis

The prognosis for patients with adenocarcinoma of the small bowel is generally held to be poor. According to the SEER data, the overall 5-year survival for adenocarcinoma was 28% and for

**Table 48-2** TNM classification of small intestinal carcinomas (summary)

| Classification | Description |
| --- | --- |
| T1 | Lamina propria, submucosa |
| T2 | Muscularis propria |
| T3 | Subserosa, nonperitonealized perimuscular tissues (mesentery, retroperitoneum) ≤2 cm |
| T4 | Visceral peritoneum, other organs/structures (including mesentery, retroperitoneum) >2 cm |
| N1 | Regional lymph node metastasis |

This classification does not apply to carcinomas of the Ampulla of Vater.

**Table 48-3** Stage grouping of small intestinal carcinomas according to TNM classification

| Stage | T | N | M |
| --- | --- | --- | --- |
| Stage 0 | Tis | N0 | M0 |
| Stage I | T1 | N0 | M0 |
| | T2 | N0 | M0 |
| Stage II | T3 | N0 | M0 |
| | T4 | N0 | M0 |
| Stage III | Any T | N1 | M0 |
| Stage IV | Any T | Any N | M1 |

mucinous adenocarcinoma, 22%.[2] However, a recent population-based study from Sweden showed 5- and 10-year survival rates of 39% and 37% for duodenal tumors and 46% and 41% for jejunoileal tumors.[24] Furthermore, the Swedish study found a temporal trend toward improved survival in recent years.

Survival is related to pathologic stage; nodal involvement in particular confers a poor prognosis.[6] The TNM classification is the recommended approach to staging (see Tables 48–2 and 48–3).[22] Well-differentiated tumors may have a better prognosis than moderately or poorly differentiated ones,[6] although this observation has not been made in every series of cases.[7] One study found a significant negative association between survival and immunoexpression of c-neu in duodenal adenocarcinomas.[23]

As discussed previously, there is a high incidence of other malignancies in patients with small intestinal adenocarcinoma. Thus, the clinician should consider the possibility of other neoplastic lesions in any patient with small intestinal adenocarcinoma.

## Rare Primary Carcinomas of the Small Intestine

Small cell carcinomas have been described as primary tumors in the small intestine.[25] They have neurosecretory granules ultrastructurally, and they resemble their pulmonary counterparts in both their morphology and their aggressive behavior. There is evidence of a spectrum of increasing malignancy, as observed elsewhere in the gastrointestinal tract, from low-grade carcinoids to high-grade small cell carcinomas via neuroendocrine carcinomas of non–small cell type showing intermediate behavior.[26] However, although mixed lesions composed of adenoma or adenocarcinoma and small cell carcinoma do occur (Fig. 48–5), mixed lesions composed of carcinoids and small cell carcinomas do not.

Rarely, small intestinal carcinomas are biphasic and exhibit areas of sarcomatoid morphology along with areas of conventional adenocarcinoma. The sarcomatoid areas show ultrastructural and immunohistochemical evidence of epithelial differentiation. The preferred nomenclature for such lesions is *sarcomatoid carcinoma*. The prognosis is poor.[27]

Adenosquamous carcinomas can occur.[28] Either the glandular or squamous component may predominate.

A few cases of primary small intestinal choriocarcinoma have been reported; presentation may be with melena.[29] Serum human chorionic gonadotrophin levels are raised, as in choriocarcinomas arising in more conventional sites.

## Adenocarcinoma of the Appendix

Primary adenocarcinomas of the appendix are unusual. The age-adjusted incidence of appendiceal adenocarcinoma in the SEER study was 0.2 per 100,000, and there was a slight preponderance in males.[2] By analogy with the rest of the large intestine, it is

## References

1. Hamilton SR, Aaltonen LA. World Heath Organization Classification of Tumours: Pathology and Genetics of Tumours of the Digestive System. IARC Press, Lyon, 2000.

2. Thomas RM, Sobin LH. Histology of cancer. Gastrointestinal cancer: incidence and prognosis by histologic type. SEER population-based data, 1973–1987. Cancer 5(Suppl):154–170, 1995.

3. Minardi AJ, Zibari GB, Aultman DF, McMillan RW, McDonald JC. Small bowel tumors. J Am Coll Surg 186:664–668, 1998.

4. Neugut AI, Jacobson JS, Suh S, Mukherjee R, Arber N. The epidemiology of cancer of the small bowel. Cancer Epidemiol Biomarkers Prev 7:243–251, 1998.

5. O'Riordan BG, Vilor M, Herrera L. Small bowel tumors: an overview. Dig Dis 14:245–257, 1996.

6. Ouriel K, Adams JT. Adenocarcinoma of the small intestine. Am J Surg 147:66–71, 1984.

7. Ripley D, Weinerman BH. Increased incidence of second malignancies associated with small bowel adenocarcinoma. Can J Gastroenterol 11:65–68, 1997.

8. Stemmermann GN, Goodman MT, Nomura AM. Adenocarcinoma of the proximal small intestine: a marker for familial and multicentric cancer? Cancer 70:2766–2771, 1992.

9. Attanoos R, Williams GT. Epithelial and neuroendocrine tumors of the duodenum. Semin Diagn Pathol 8:149–162, 1991.

10. Spigelman AD, Talbot IC, Penna C, et al. Evidence for adenoma–carcinoma sequence in the duodenum of patients with familial adenomatous polyposis. J Clin Pathol 47:709–710, 1994.

11. Bertoni G, Sassatelli R, Nigrisoli E, et al. First observation of microadenomas in the ileal mucosa of patients with familial adenomatous polyposis and colectomies. Gastroenterology 109:374–380, 1995.

12. Fenoglio-Preiser CM, Pascal RR, Perzin KH. Tumors of the Intestines. Atlas of Tumor Pathology, 2nd Series, fascicle 27. Armed Forces Institute of Pathology, Washington, DC, 1990, pp 175–187.

13. MacGowan DJL, Hourihane DO, Tanner WA, O'Morain C. Duodenojejunal adenocarcinoma as a first presentation of coeliac disease. J Clin Pathol 49:602–604, 1996.

14. Attanoos R, Billings PJ, Hughes LE, et al. Ileostomy polyps, adenomas, and adenocarcinomas. Gut 37:840–844, 1995.

15. Sakano S, Yoshihiro S, Joko K, et al. Adenocarcinoma developing in an ileal conduit. J Urol 153:146–148, 1995.

16. Vieth M, Grunewald M, Niemeyer C, Stolte M. Adenocarcinoma in an ileal pouch after prior proctocolectomy for carcinoma in a patient with ulcerative pancolitis. Virchows Arch 433:281–284, 1998.

17. Wu JS, McGannon EA, Church JM. Incidence of neoplastic polyps in the ileal pouch of patients with familial adenomatous polyposis after restorative proctocolectomy. Dis Colon Rectum 41:552–557, 1998.

18. Rodriguez-Bigas MA, Vasen HF, Lynch HT, et al. Characteristics of small bowel carcinoma in hereditary nonpolyposis colorectal carcinoma. Cancer 83:240–244, 1998.

19. Shepherd NA, Bussey H, Jass JR. Epithelial misplacement in Peutz-Jeghers polyps: a diagnostic pitfall. Am J Surg Pathol 11:743–749, 1987.

20. Sobin LH. Pseudoinvasive intestinal polyps. Dig Dis Pathol 2:1–12, 1989.

21. Younes N, Fulton N, Tanaka R, Wayne J, Straus FH, Kaplan EL. The presence of K-12 ras mutations in duodenal adenocarcinomas and the absence of ras mutations in other small bowel adenocarcinomas and carcinoid tumors. Cancer 79:1804–1808, 1997.

22. Sobin LH, Wittekind Ch (eds). TNM Classification of Malignant Tumors, 5th ed John Wiley & Sons, New York, 1997, pp 63–65.

23. Zhu L, Kim K, Domenico DR, Appert H, Howard JM. Adenocarcinoma of duodenum and ampulla of Vater: clinicopathology study and expression of p53, c-neu, TGF-α, CEA, and EMA. J Surg Oncol 61:100–105, 1996.

24. Zar N, Holmberg L, Wilander E, Rastad J. Survival in small intestinal adenocarcinoma. Eur J Cancer 32A:2114–2119, 1996.

25. Zamboni G, Franzin G, Bonetti F, et al. Small cell neuroendocrine carcinoma of the ampullary region. A clinicopathologic, immunohistochemical, and ultrastructural study of three cases. Am J Surg Pathol 14:703–713, 1990.

26. Emory RE, Emory TS, Goellner JR, Grant CS, Nagorney DM. Neuroendocrine ampullary tumors: spectrum of disease including the first report of a neuroendocrine carcinoma of non–small cell type. Surgery 115:762–766, 1994.

27. Lam KY, Leung CY, Ho JWC. Sarcomatoid carcinoma of the small intestine. Aust N Z J Surg 66:636–639, 1996.

28. Griesser GH, Schumacher U, Elfeldt R, Horny H-P. Adenosquamous carcinoma of the ileum: report of a case and review of the literature. Virchows Arch A 406:483–487, 1985.

29. Chan GS, Ng WK, Chua DT, Wu PC. Raised serum hCG in a male patient caused by primary jejunal choriocarcinoma. J Clin Pathol 51:413–415, 1998.

30. Qizilbash AH. Mucoceles of the appendix: their relationship to hyperplastic polyps, mucinous cystadenomas and cystadenocarcinomas. Arch Pathol 99:548–555, 1975.

31. Carr NJ, McCarthy WF, Sobin LH. Epithelial noncarcinoid tumors and tumor-like lesions of the appendix: a clinicopathologic study of 184 patients with a multivariate analysis of prognostic factors. Cancer 75:757–768, 1995.

32. Higa E, Rosai J, Pizzimbono CA, Wise L. Mucosal hyperplasia, mucinous cystadenoma, and mucinous cystadenocarcinoma of the appendix: a reevaluation of the appendiceal "mucocele". Cancer 32:1525–1541, 1973.

33. Williams GR, du Boulay CEH, Roche WR. Benign epithelial neoplasms of the appendix: classification and clinical associations. Histopathology 21:447–451, 1992.

34. Williams RA, Whitehead R. Non-carcinoid epithelial tumours of the appendix—a proposed classification. Pathology 18:50–53, 1986.

35. Deans GT, Spence RAJ. Neoplastic lesions of the appendix. Br J Surg 82:299–306, 1995.

36. Younes M, Katikaneni PR, Lechago J. Association between mucosal hyperplasia of the appendix and adenocarcinoma of the colon. Histopathology 26:33–37, 1995.

37. Carr NJ, Sobin LH. Unusual tumors of the appendix and pseudomyxoma peritonei. Semin Diagn Pathol 13:314–325, 1996.

38. Ronnett BM, Zahn CM, Kurman RJ, Kass KA, Sugarbaker PH, Shmookler BM. Disseminated peritoneal adenomucinosis and peritoneal mucinous carcinomatosis: a clinicopathologic analysis of 109 cases with emphasis on distinguishing pathologic features, site of origin, prognosis, and relationship to "pseudomyxoma peritonei." Am J Surg Pathol 19:1390–1408, 1995.

39. Matsuoka Y, Masumoto T, Suzuki K, et al. Pseudomyxoma retroperitonei. Eur Radiol 9:457–459, 1999.

40. Szych C, Staebler A, Connolly D, Wu R, Cho KR, Ronnett BM. Molecular genetic evidence supporting the clonality and appendiceal origin of pseudomyxoma peritonei in women. Am J Pathol 154:1849–1855, 1999.

41. Young RH, Rosenberg AE, Clement PB. Mucin deposits within inguinal hernia sacs: a presenting finding of low grade mucinous cystic tumours of the appendix. A report of two cases and a review of the literature. Mod Pathol 10:1228–1232, 1997.

42. Hinson FL, Ambrose NS. Pseudomyxoma peritonei. Br J Surg 85:1332–1339, 1998.

43. Sugarbaker PH. Pseudomyxoma peritonei: a cancer whose biology is characterized by a redistribution phenomenon. Ann Surg 219:109–111, 1994.

44. Ronnett BM, Shmookler BM, Diener-West M, Sugarbaker PH, Kurman RJ. Immunohistochemical evidence supporting the appendiceal origin of pseudomyxoma peritonei in women. Int J Gynecol Pathol 16:1–9, 1997.

45. Mortman KD, Sugarbaker PA, Shmookler BM, DeGuzman VC, Soberman MS. Pulmonary metastases in pseudomyxoma peritonei syndrome. Ann Thorac Surg 64:1434–1436, 1997.

46. Costa MJ. Pseudomyxoma peritonei: histologic predictors of patient survival. Arch Pathol Lab Med 118:1215–1219, 1994.

47. McCarthy JH, Aga A. A fallopian tube lesion of borderline malignancy associated with pseudomyxoma peritonei. Histopathology 13:223–225, 1998.

48. Gough DB, Donohue JH, Schutt AJ, et al. Pseudomyxoma peritonei: long-term patient survival with an aggressive regional approach. Ann Surg 219:112–119, 1994.

49. Kurita M, Komatsu H, Hata Y, et al. Pseudomyxoma peritonei due to adenocarcinoma of the lung: case report. J Gastroenterol 29:344–348, 1994.

50. Zanelli M, Casadei R, Santini D, et al. Pseudomyxoma peritonei associated with intraductal papillary-mucinous neoplasm of the pancreas. Pancreas 17:100–102, 1998.

51. Prayson RA, Hart WR, Petras RE. Pseudomyxoma peritonei: a clinicopathologic study of 19 cases with emphasis on site of origin and nature of associated ovarian tumors. Am J Surg Pathol 18:591–603, 1994.

52. Young RH, Gilks CB, Scully RE. Mucinous tumors of the appendix associated with mucinous tumors of the ovary and pseudomyxoma peritonei: a clinicopathologic analysis of 22 cases supporting an origin in the appendix. Am J Surg Pathol 15:415–429, 1991.

53. Cortina R, McCormick J, Kolm P, Perry RR. Management and prognosis of adenocarcinoma of the appendix. Dis Colon Rectum 38:848–852, 1995.

54. Nitecki SS, Wolff BG, Schlinkert R, Sarr MG. The natural history of surgically treated primary adenocarcinoma of the appendix. Ann Surg 219:51–57, 1994.

55. Smith JW, Kemeny N, Caldwell C, Banner P, Sigurdson E, Huvos A. Pseudomyxoma peritonei of appendiceal origin. Cancer 70:396–401, 1992.

56. Subbuswamy SG, Gibbs NM, Ross CF, et al. Goblet cell carcinoid of the appendix. Cancer 34:338–344, 1974.

57. Warkel RL, Cooper PH, Helwig EB. Adenocarcinoid, a mucin-producing carcinoid tumor of the appendix. Cancer 42:2781–2793, 1978.

58. Edmonds P, Merino MJ, Livolsi V, et al. Adenocarcinoid (mucinous carcinoid) of the appendix. Gastroenterology 86:302–309, 1984.

59. Park K, Blessing K, Kerr K, et al. Goblet cell carcinoid of the appendix. Gut 31:322–324, 1990.

60. Butler JA, Houshiar A, Lin F, et al. Goblet cell carcinoid of the appendix. Am J Surg 168:685–687, 1994.

61. Ramnani DM, Wistuba II, Behrens C, et al. K-ras and p53 mutations in the pathogenesis of classical and goblet cell carcinoids of the appendix. Cancer 86:14–21, 1999.

62. Anderson NH, Somerville JE, Johnston CF, Hayes DM, Buchanan KD, Sloan JM. Appendiceal goblet cell carcinoids: a clinicopathological and immunohistochemical study. Histopathology 18:61–65, 1991.

63. Isaacson P. Crypt cell carcinoma of the appendix (so-called adenocarcinoid tumor). Am J Surg Pathol 5:213–224, 1981.

64. Burke AP, Sobin LH, Federspiel BH, et al. Appendiceal carcinoids: correlation of histology and immunohistochemistry. Mod Pathol 2:630–637, 1989.

65. Burke AP, Sobin LH, Federspiel BH, Shekitka KM, Helwig EB. Goblet cell carcinoids and related tumors of the vermiform appendix. Am J Clin Pathol 94:27–35, 1990.

66. Shaw PA, Pringle JH. The demonstration of a subset of carcinoid tumours of the appendix by in situ hybridization using synthetic probes to proglucagon mRNA. J Pathol 167:375–380, 1992.

67. Suster S. Gastrointestinal stromal tumors. Semin Diagn Pathol 13:297–313, 1996.

68. Sarlomo-Rikala M, Kovatich A, Barusevicius A, Miettinen M. CD117: a sensitive marker for gastrointestinal stromal tumors that is more specific than CD34. Mod Pathol 11:728–734 , 1998.

69. Sircar K, Hewlett BR, Huizinga JD, Chorneyko K, Berezin I, Riddell RH. Interstitial cells of Cajal as precursors of gastrointestinal stromal tumors. Am J Surg Pathol 23:377–389, 1999.

70. Kindblom LG, Remotti HE, Aldenborg F, Meis-Kindblom JM. Gastrointestinal pacemaker cell tumor (GIPACT): gastrointestinal stromal tumors show phenotypic characteristics of the interstitial cell of Cajal. Am J Pathol 152:1259–1269, 1998.

71. Hirota S, Isozaki K, Moriyama Y, et al. Gain-of-function mutations of c-kit in human gastrointestinal stromal tumors. Science 279:577–580, 1998.

72. Miettinen M, Monihan JM, Sarlomo-Rikala M, et al. Gastrointestinal stromal tumors/smooth muscle tumors (GISTs) primary in the omentum and mesentery: clinicopathologic and immunohistochemical study of 26 cases. Am J Surg Pathol 23:1109–1118, 1999.

73. Shanks JH, Harris M, Banerjee SS, Eyden BP. Gastrointestinal autonomic nerve tumours: a report of nine cases. Histopathology 29:111–121, 1996.

74. Min K-W. Small intestinal stromal tumors with skeinoid fibers. Am J Surg Pathol 16:145–155, 1992.

75. Emory TS, Sobin KH, Lukes L, Lee DH, O'Leary TJ. Prognosis of gastrointestinal smooth-muscle (stromal) tumors: dependence on anatomic site. Am J Surg Pathol 23:82–87, 1999.

76. Friedman SL, Wright TL, Altman DF. Gastrointestinal Kaposi's sarcoma in patients with acquired immunodeficiency syndrome: endoscopic and autopsy findings. Gastroenterology 89:102–108, 1985.

77. Laine L, Politoske EJ, Gill P. Protein-losing enteropathy in acquired immunodeficiency syndrome due to intestinal Kaposi's sarcoma. Arch Intern Med 147:1174–1175, 1987.

78. Deziel DJ, Saclarides TJ, Marshall JS, Yaremko LM. Appendiceal Kaposi's sarcoma: a cause of right lower quadrant pain in the acquired immunodeficiency syndrome. Am J Gastroenterol 86:901–903, 1991.

79. Zebrowska G, Walsh NM. Human immunodeficiency virus–related Kaposi's sarcoma of the appendix and acute appendicitis: report of a case and review of the literature. Arch Pathol Lab Med 115:1157–1160, 1991.

80. Carr NJ, Sobin LH. Gastrointestinal tract. In: Al-Sam SZ, Lakhani SR, Davies JD (eds): Practical Atlas of Pseudomalignancy. Arnold, London, 1998, pp 204–227.

81. Muller G, Dargent JL, Duwel V, et al. Leukaemia and lymphoma of the appendix presenting as acute appendicitis or acute abdomen: four case reports with a review of the literature. J Cancer Res Clin Oncol 123: 560–564, 1997.

82. Crump M, Gospodarowicz M, Shepherd FA. Lymphoma of the gastrointestinal tract. Semin Oncol 26:324–337, 1999.

83. Isaacson PG. Gastrointestinal lymphoma. Hum Pathol 25:1020–1029, 1994.

84. Chan JKC. Gastrointestinal lymphomas: an overview with emphasis on new findings and diagnostic problems. Semin Diagn Pathol 13:260–296, 1996.

85. Kelly MD, Stuart M, Tschuchnigg M, et al. Primary intestinal Hodgkin's disease complicating ileal Crohn's disease. Aust N Z J Surg 67:485–489, 1997.

86. Ben-Ayed F, Halphen M, Najjar T, et al. Treatment of alpha chain disease: results of a prospective study in 21 Tunisian patients by the Tunisian-French Intestinal Lymphoma Study Group. Cancer 63:1251–1256, 1989.

87. Domizio P, Owen RA, Shepherd NA, et al. Primary lymphoma of the small intestine: a clinicopathological study of 119 cases. Am J Surg Pathol 17:429–442, 1993.

88. Isaacson PG, MacLennan KA, Subbuswamy SG. Multiple lymphomatous polyposis of the gastrointestinal tract. Histopathology 8:641–656, 1983.

89. O'Briain DS, Kennedy MJ, Daly PA, et al. Multiple lymphomatous polyposis of the gastrointestinal tract: a clinicopathologically distinctive form of non-Hodgkin's lymphoma of B-cell centrocytic type. Am J Surg Pathol 13:691–699, 1989.

90. Chott A, Vesely M, Simonitsch I, et al. Classification of intestinal T-cell neoplasms and their differential diagnosis. Am J Clin Pathol 111 (Suppl 1):S68–S74, 1999.

91. Carbonnel F, Grollet-Bioul L, Brouet JC, et al. Are complicated forms of celiac disease cryptic T-cell lymphomas? Blood 92:3879–3886, 1998.

92. Thomas JA, Allday MJ, Crawford DH. Epstein-Barr virus–associated lymphoproliferative disorders in immunocompromised individuals. Adv Cancer Res 57:329–380, 1991.

93. Burke AP, Helwig EB. Gangliocytic paraganglioma. Am J Clin Pathol 92:1–9, 1989.

94. Dookhan DB, Miettinen M, Finkel G, Gibas Z. Recurrent duodenal gangliocytic paraganglioma with lymph node metastases. Histopathology 22:399–401, 1993.

95. Hashimoto S, Kawasaki S, Matsuzawa K, Harada H, Makuuchi M. Gangliocytic paraganglioma of the papilla of Vater with regional lymph node metastasis. Am J Gastroenterol 87:1216–1218, 1992.

96. Inai K, Kobuke T, Yonehara S, Tokuoka S. Duodenal gangliocytic paraganglioma with lymph node metastasis in a 17-year-old boy. Cancer 63:2540–2545, 1989.

97. Washington K, McDonagh D. Secondary tumors of the gastrointestinal tract: surgical pathologic findings and comparison with autopsy survey. Mod Pathol 8:427–433, 1995.

98. Elsayed AM, Albahra M, Nzeako UC, Sobin LH. Malignant melanomas in the small intestine: a study of 103 patients. Am J Gastroenterol 91: 1001–1006, 1996.

# Chapter 49

# Clinical Aspects and Management of Small Bowel and Appendiceal Cancers: Diagnostic and Staging Procedures

### KAREN M. HORTON AND ELLIOT K. FISHMAN

Neoplasms of the small bowel continue to pose a significant diagnostic challenge to both the clinician and the radiologist for several reasons. First, these tumors are uncommon, with an annual incidence of only 0.5 to 1.0 per 100,000 people in the western hemisphere.[1] Thus, small intestinal neoplasms are often overlooked. Second, these tumors typically result in nonspecific symptoms such as abdominal pain, gastrointestinal bleeding, nausea, vomiting, and weight loss.[2] This contributes to a delay in diagnosis. Third, most small bowel neoplasms are small, especially in the early stages.[3] This makes detection by conventional radiologic studies difficult. Although small bowel enteroscopy may come to play a larger role in the diagnosis of small bowel tumors,[4,5] this technology is still evolving and has not yet replaced more traditional radiologic examinations.[6]

Radiologic examination of the small intestine has improved significantly over the past 20 years. Today, contrast examinations (dedicated small bowel series and enteroclysis) and computed tomography (CT) are the major radiologic examinations performed for evaluation of small bowel pathology.[7] In addition, magnetic resonance imaging (MRI) may be utilized in select problem cases.

## Technique

### Contrast Studies

The dedicated small bowel series is the most commonly performed radiologic examination for evaluation of suspected small bowel disease. It is a simple and noninvasive test. After a scout abdominal radiograph is obtained, the patient drinks 400–600 ml of thin barium. Overhead radiographs are obtained at 20-minute intervals to follow the progression of the contrast agent through the entire small bowel and into the right colon. Fluoroscopy is performed intermittently by the radiologist to observe peristalsis. Also, the radiologist uses a compression device to fully evaluate the small intestine by separating overlapping loops. Spot compression films are obtained of the small bowel, with attention paid to areas of suspected abnormalities.

Enteroclysis is a more invasive examination of the small intestine that can be performed in patients in whom there is a high suspicion of small bowel pathology.[8] During enteroclysis, a tube is placed through the patient's nose or mouth and advanced through the esophagus, stomach, and duodenum to the ligament of Treitz. A balloon is inflated to secure the tube. Some radiologists routinely administer mild sedation to relieve patient anxiety.[8] Next, a barium mixture is infused followed by methylcellulose. Often, a mechanical pump is utilized to administer the contrast agent. The goal is to fully distend the small intestine to maximize detection of a mass or obstruction. This technique results in distended small bowel loops that are coated with barium. The appearance is similar to that produced by a barium enema; thus, enteroclysis is referred to as a "small bowel enema."

The exact role of the small bowel series and enteroclysis is controversial. Most radiologists agree that because of the low prevalence of small bowel cancer, the dedicated small bowel series is a good inexpensive screening test. However, in patients for whom there is a high clinical suspicion of small bowel disease, enteroclysis may be performed as the primary examination.[9] Enteroclysis is more sensitive than the dedicated small bowel series and more accurate. However, it is also more invasive and more expensive. In one series comparing the dedicated small bowel series with enteroclysis, enteroclysis demonstrated additional information in 50% of cases.[10] In a series by Maglinte and co-workers,[11] 42 lesions were detected on enteroclysis that were not visualized by the small bowel series. The failure of the small bowel series was due to both technical and perceptual errors.[11] The literature supports the conclusion that enteroclysis is more sensitive than the dedicated small bowel series for detection of small bowel malignancies.[2,6,11–13]

## Computed Tomography

Optimal CT examination of the small intestine requires careful attention to technique. Patients should be examined after an overnight fast or should eat and drink nothing for at least 6 hours before the examination. Adequate opacification of the small intestine is essential, as nondistended segments may mimic or mask disease. We routinely administer 750 ml of flavored Hypaque 30 to 45 minutes before the study and an additional 250 ml immediately before the examination. Although high-attenuation agents such as Hypaque have traditionally been used as CT oral contrast agents, there has been recent interest in low-density agents such as water or milk.[14,15] Unlike high-attenuation oral contrast agents, these low-attenuation agents do not interfere with three-dimensional studies of the abdomen. In addition, low-attenuation contrast agents allow better visualization of the enhancing bowel wall and may improve detection of small bowel disease and neoplasms.

To maximize the detection of small bowel pathology, the small intestine should be adequately distended. To improve small bowel distention, CT enteroclysis can be performed.[16] This technique is a combination of enteroclysis and CT. The CT is performed after the administration of a low-density contrast agent through a duodenal tube using a mechanical pump. This allows maximum distention of the small intestine, which is especially helpful when diagnosing low-grade obstruction or small masses.[17] However, this examination is invasive, and more research is needed to determine if CT enteroclysis will improve the detection or staging of small bowel neoplasms.[16]

Regardless of the type of oral contrast agent administered, the use of an intravenous contrast agent is essential in the detection and staging of small bowel neoplasms. An intravenous contrast agent is necessary to determine the presence and pattern of enhancement of small bowel neoplasms as well as to opacify adjacent vessels to detect encasement. In addition, intravenous contrast is necessary to detect liver metastasis. We routinely administer 120 ml of Omnipaque 350 (Nycomed, Princeton, NJ) at 2 to 3 ml per second. Scanning should be performed 40 seconds after the start of the injection, which allows evaluation of the liver in the portal phase of enhancement. Spiral scanning offers a distinct advantage over conventional CT by allowing rapid scanning during intravenous contrast administration and narrow collimation. For small bowel imaging, spiral or helical CT is optimal with 5 mm collimation and a table speed of 8 mm/second. Reconstruction is typically performed at 5-mm intervals. Additional targeted images or delayed scans can be obtained as needed.

## Appearance of Tumors

### Adenocarcinoma

The appearance of adenocarcinoma on barium studies varies with location. In the duodenum, 75% of adenocarcinomas appear as polypoid masses. Other appearances include infiltrative or stenotic lesions with or without ulceration. The upper gastrointestinal (GI) series has a reported accuracy of 70% to 80% for the detection of duodenal malignancies.[18] If substances such as glucagon are administered during the upper GI series, the accu-

racy can be increased to 85% to 90% by maximizing duodenal distention and decreasing peristalsis.[19–21] In a report of 67 patients with adenocarcinoma of the duodenum, the upper GI series allowed diagnosis in 88% of cases.[18] In that study, endoscopic exam (EGD) allowed diagnosis in 89% of cases.[18] The upper GI series is a useful complementary study when combined with EGD, especially if the entire duodenum is not visualized by endoscopy.

On barium studies, adenocarcinomas of the mesenteric small bowel (jejunum and ileum) classically appear as focal areas of luminal narrowing, fold destruction, and overhanging edges (apple core lesion) (Fig. 49–1).[9] The mass is typically rigid and will not compress. Ulceration may be present. If the lumen is narrowed significantly, small bowel obstruction will occur. However, not all apple core lesions in the small intestine are due to primary adenocarcinoma. Metastasis to the small bowel can have an identical appearance (Fig. 49–2).[22] Also, inflammatory diseases such as Crohn's disease can result in segmental areas of stenosis that may mimic the appearance of adenocarcinoma.[23,24] Usually, however, there are other indications that Crohn's disease may be present, such as involvement of other segments of the GI tract. Overall, lesions smaller than 2 cm in diameter may be difficult to visualize by CT. These are better detected by small bowel series or enteroclysis.[25]

In addition to having the apple core appearance, adenocarcinomas may also appear as polypoid intraluminal or intramural masses, rarely resulting in intussusception. Differentiating these from other polypoid lesions can be difficult. Rarely, adenocarcinomas can appear as subtle, eccentric plaque-like lesions in the small bowel, which can be detected on enteroclysis.[9]

On CT, small bowel adenocarcinomas may demonstrate a variety of appearances (Figs. 49–3 and 49–4). The tumor most frequently appears as an eccentric or circumferential wall thickening (usually greater than 1.5 cm) involving a short segment of the small bowel.[26,27] This may result in an apple core appearance similar to that seen on barium contrast studies. Although inflammatory diseases of the small bowel may also produce diffuse or segmental wall thickening, this usually does not exceed

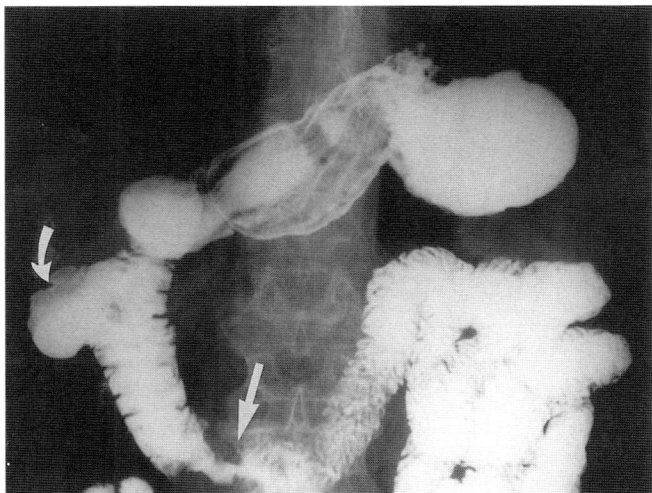

**Figure 49-1** Duodenal adenocarcinoma. Upper gastrointestinal series with small bowel follow-through demonstrates a focal segment of irregular luminal narrowing in the third portion of the duodenum (arrow). This is an example of the "apple core" appearance of adenocarcinoma. Note also a duodenal diverticulum (curved arrow).

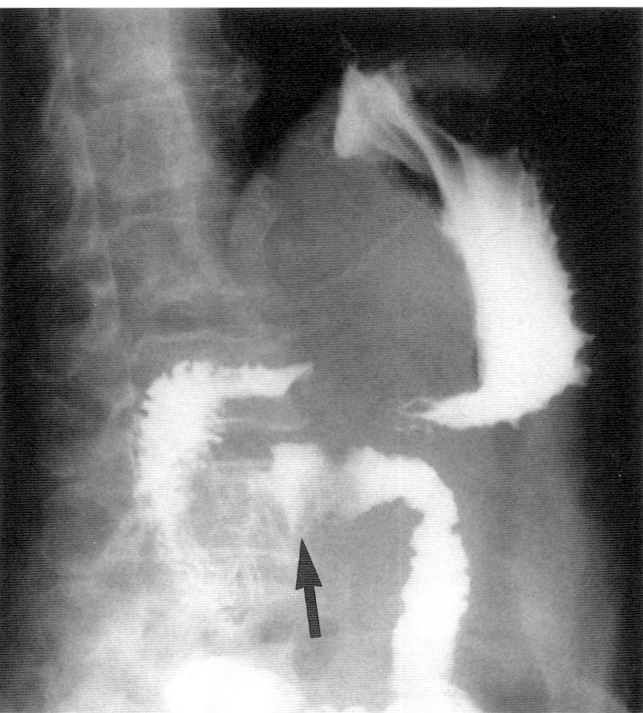

**Figure 49–2** Metastasis to duodenum. Upper gastrointestinal series with small bowel follow-through in a female with breast cancer demonstrates a focal segment of irregularity and fold destruction in the third portion of the duodenum, compatible with metastases (arrow). Note also nodularity of the stomach due to metastatic infiltration.

1.5 cm. Also, inflammatory or ischemic diseases of the small intestine can produce a halo of alternating high and low attenuation within the wall. This is characteristic of a nonneoplastic process.

In cases of adenocarcinoma of the small intestine, which produce significant wall thickening, there may be luminal narrowing and proximal obstruction. Ulceration has been reported to occur in approximately 40% of cases of small bowel adenocarcinoma.[28] However, this is usually not as well demonstrated on CT as on barium studies.[25] Adenocarcinomas can in rare cases present as polypoid masses, which may result in obstruction or

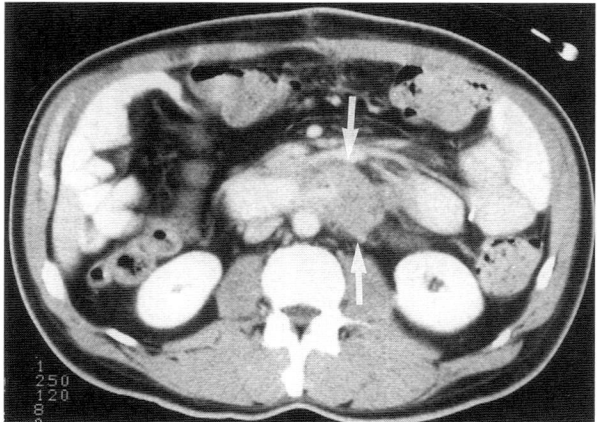

**Figure 49–3** Duodenal adenocarcinoma. Contrast-enhanced spiral CT scan demonstrates a soft tissue mass (arrows) surrounding the third portion of the duodenum and causing luminal narrowing.

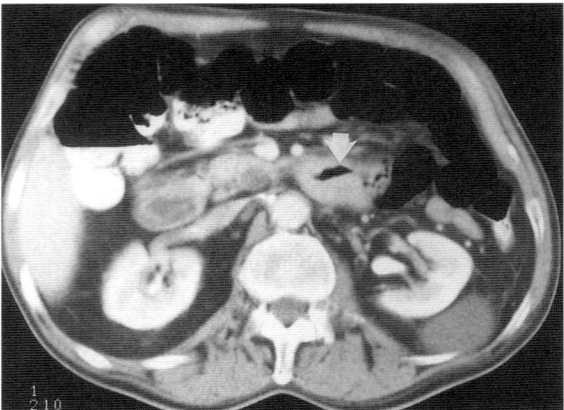

**Figure 49–4** Duodenal adenocarcinoma. Contrast-enhanced spiral CT scan demonstrates a subtle mass at the junction of the third and fourth portion (arrow) of the duodenum consistent with carcinoma.

intussusception. On CT, adenocarcinomas may appear homogeneous in attenuation or, in cases of large tumors with ischemia and necrosis, may appear heterogeneous. Contrast enhancement of the tumor may also be demonstrated.[29]

In addition to detecting primary small bowel adenocarcinoma, CT may aid in tumor staging. Although CT is not able to resolve the individual layers of the bowel wall, it can delineate tumors confined to the muscular wall and distinguish these from tumors that extend into the adjacent mesenteric fat. Irregular tumor margins and stranding in the adjacent mesenteric fat are indications of local tumor invasion.[25,26,28] Also, obliteration of fat planes between bowel loops or between the bowel and adjacent structures is suggestive of local tumor extension. Computed tomography can detect enlarged mesenteric lymph nodes that may be involved with tumor. From the location of the primary tumor, the regional draining lymph nodes can be predicted. For instance, tumors involving the duodenum tend to involve the lymph nodes in the peripancreatic, gastroduodenal, pyloric, and superior mesenteric artery regions.[26] Regional lymph nodes for both the jejunum and the ileum drain along the superior mesenteric vessels, while the terminal ileum may drain into lymph nodes in the cecal and ileocolic regions.[26] Typically, mesenteric nodes greater than 1 cm in short axis diameter are suspicious for neoplastic involvement. However, the sensitivity and specificity of CT are limited because even very small nodes may harbor malignancy and large nodes may simply be reactive.

Computed tomography is currently the imaging modality of choice for the detection of liver metastasis. To maximize the detection of metastasis to the liver, imaging should be performed during the portal venous phase of enhancement.[30] This will maximize the detection of small low-attenuation lesions.

Staging of small bowel adenocarcinoma is based on the TNM system (Tables 49–1 and 49–2).[31] This classification does not apply to lymphoma, sarcoma, or carcinoid tumors.

## Carcinoid Tumors

The radiologic appearance of carcinoid tumors varies depending on their size and location. The ileum is the most common location for small bowel carcinoid, followed by the jejunum. Carcinoid tumors arise from the Kulchitsky cells in the crypts of Lieberkühn. Therefore, they grow as submucosal nodules. At this stage, the small bowel series and enteroclysis are much more sen-

**Table 49-1** TNM system of staging of small bowel adenocarcinoma

| Stage | Description |
|---|---|
| TX | Primary tumor not assessed |
| T0 | No evidence of primary tumor |
| Tis | Carcinoma in situ tumor |
| T1 | Tumor invades the lamina propria or submucosa |
| T2 | Tumors invades the muscularis propria |
| T3 | Tumor extends <2 cm into the serosa or into the mesentery (jejunum and ileum) or retroperitoneum (duodenum) |
| T4 | Tumor perforates the visceral peritoneum or directly invades adjacent structures |
| NX | Regional lymph nodes not assessed |
| N0 | No regional lymph node metastases |
| N1 | Regional lymph node metastases |
| MX | Presence of distant metastases not assessed |
| M0 | No distant metastases |
| M1 | Distant metastases |

Adapted from Beachers ON, Henson DE, Hutter RVP, Kennedy BJ (eds). Handbook for the Staging of Cancer. J.B. Lippincott, Philadelphia, 1993, pp 89–93, with permission.[31]

sitive for detection.[13] The CT scan may be normal when the tumors are small and confined to the submucosa. On small bowel series or enteroclysis, submucosal carcinoid tumors appear as smooth solitary intraluminal defects, most commonly in the distal ileum. This appearance is not specific for carcinoid tumors, however, other submucosal masses such as leiomyoma, lipoma, or submucosal metastasis or lymphoma may have an identical appearance. When the submucosal carcinoid tumor ulcerates, this can produce the appearance of a "target lesion" on the contrast studies. However, this appearance is not specific for carcinoid and can occur in other tumors, such as lymphoma, melanoma, metastatic breast cancer, or Kaposi's sarcoma. Since approximately 30% of carcinoid tumors are multicentric, the contrast study may reveal multiple submucosal nodules. As the small intestinal carcinoid grows, there may be extension and thickening of the muscular layers of the wall. On contrast studies, this appears as thickening of the wall and mucosal folds.[32] If the tumor extends outside the bowel loop, it can infiltrate the mesentery and result in a desmoplastic reaction. On contrast studies, this will appear as angulation and tethering as well as fixation of the involved small bowel loops.[9] Retraction of the loops toward the root of the mesentery can also be seen. If there is an extensive mesenteric component with fibrosis, the mesenteric vessels can be encased, resulting in ischemia of the loops.

Although CT scans typically cannot demonstrate a small primary mass within the wall of the small bowel, CT is an excel-

**Table 49-2** American Joint Commission on Cancer (AJCC) staging of small bowel carcinoma

| Stage | T | N | M |
|---|---|---|---|
| Stage 0 | Tis | N0 | M0 |
| Stage 1 | T1 or T2 | N0 | M0 |
| Stage 2 | T3 or T4 | N0 | M0 |
| Stage 3 | Any T | N1 | M0 |
| Stage 4 | Any T | Any N | M1 |

Adapted from Beachers ON, Henson DE, Hutter RVP, Kennedy BJ (eds). Handbook for the Staging of Cancer. J.B. Lippincott, Philadelphia, 1993, pp 89–93, with permission.[31]

lent modality for demonstrating the mesenteric extension of tumors. Carcinoids that have infiltrated the mesentery demonstrate a characteristic appearance on CT (Figs. 49–5 and 49–6), namely an ill-defined mesenteric mass containing calcification in up to 70% of cases.[33] The mesenteric mass appears spiculated with a stellate pattern.[34] Computed tomographic scans obtained using an intravenous contrast agent nicely demonstrate the encasement or occlusion of mesenteric vessels. Thickening and ischemia of the involved small bowel loops may also be demonstrated as a result of mesenteric vessel encasement. Although the CT appearance of a mesenteric mass with calcification and desmoplastic reaction is suggestive of carcinoid tumor, other conditions such as treated lymphoma or retractile mesenteritis can have a similar CT appearance.[35]

In cases where there is a high clinical suspicion of carcinoid tumor but inconclusive barium studies or CT, angiography can be performed and may demonstrate the submucosal mass on the basis of its vascularity.[32]

Computed tomography is especially useful for evaluation of patients with suspected carcinoid tumor because of the high incidence of metastasis of such tumors. Over 80% of tumors measuring greater than 2 cm in diameter are associated with metastatic disease. The major sites of metastasis from carcinoid tumor include the liver, nodes, bones, and lungs.

Carcinoid metastases to the liver have a characteristic CT appearance due to their vascularity.[36] On early-phase (arterial-phase) imaging after the administration of intravenous contrast, these metastases are brightly enhanced (Fig. 49–6). On delayed imaging, these lesions may become isodense with liver parenchyma. Therefore, if metastatic carcinoid tumor is suspected, arterial-phase imaging should be performed. Computed tomography or ultrasound can be used for guidance if percutaneous biopsy is indicated.

In addition to contrast studies and CT, nuclear scintigraphy is a useful diagnostic tool in patients with carcinoid syndrome. Radionuclide scanning following the injection of radioactive somatostatin analogues such as [111]indium (or [123]I)-labeled octreotide or [123]I-labeled metaiodobenzylguanidine (MIBG) is a sensitive, noninvasive method for diagnosing and localizing carcinoid as well as other neuroendocrine tumors.[37] This technique is especially useful for localizing occult tumors and detecting

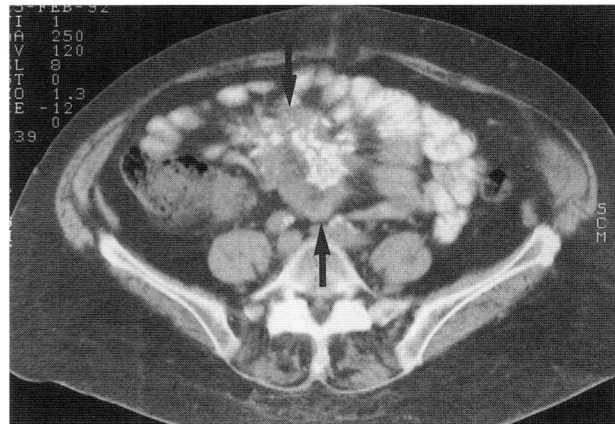

**Figure 49-5** Carcinoid. Oral contrast-enhanced abdominal CT scan demonstrates a 6-cm mesenteric mass (arrows) with focal calcifications as well as signs of tethering of the mesentery due to fibrosis and desmoplastic reaction. This is the classic CT appearance of carcinoid.

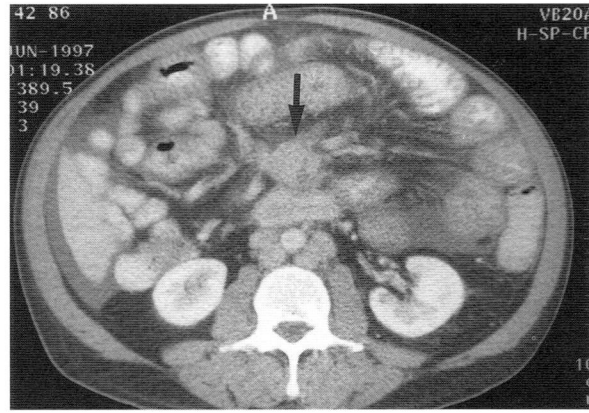

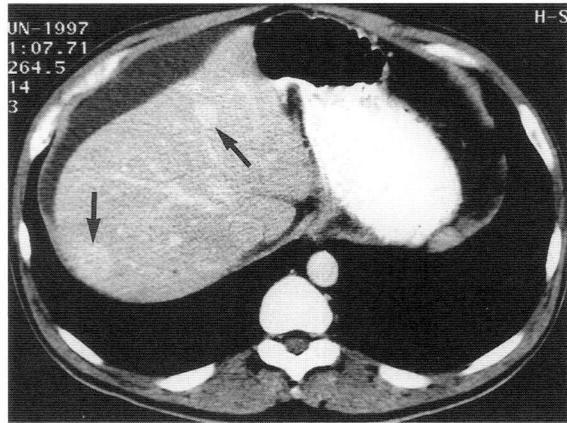

**Figure 49–6** Carcinoid. *A:* Contrast-enhanced spiral CT scan demonstrates a subtle soft tissue mass (arrow) in the root of the mesentery, compatible with known carcinoid. Note thickening of several small bowel loops as well as minimal ascites. *B:* Note also multiple hypervascular liver metastases (arrows).

chemically active metastases. However, scintigraphy does not provided precise anatomic detail.

Usually, contrast studies, CT, and nuclear scintigraphy play complementary roles in the diagnosis and staging of patients with suspected carcinoid metastases.

## Lymphoma

Most small bowel lymphomas are of the non-Hodgkin's cell type involving the mesenteric small bowel and in rare cases the duodenum.[38] The primary tumor can often be detected with small bowel contrast studies and CT. However, CT offers the advantage of simultaneously detecting adenopathy as well as the extraluminal extent of disease.

There are four major patterns of small bowel lymphoma identified on radiographic studies.[26] First, lymphoma can appear as multiple nodules or filling defects within the small bowel. The nodules may coalesce and result in the appearance of asymmetric wall thickening and luminal narrowing. Second, lymphoma may appear as a single polypoid lesion, which may vary in size. If small (1–2 cm), this lesion may not be visible on CT but can be detected on enteroclysis. Polypoid lesions can result in complications such as intussusception, which is nicely demonstrated on CT. Third, lymphoma can be infiltrating. The radiographic appearance will include wall thickening, destruction of the normal small bowel fold pattern, and luminal narrowing. This appear-

ance may simulate adenocarcinoma of the small bowel on contrast studies and CT. However, lymphoma usually involves a relatively longer segment of small bowel than adenocarcinoma and small bowel lymphoma, as opposed to adenocarcinoma, typically does not result in obstruction. This is because the lymphoma usually weakens the muscular wall of the bowel and does not induce the typical fibrosis or desmoplastic reaction that occurs with adenocarcinoma.[39,40] Also, the presence of associated significant retroperitoneal adenopathy favors the diagnosis of lymphoma over adenocarcinoma. In addition to luminal narrowing, aneurysmal dilatation of the effected bowel loops has been described in up to 50% of cases (Figs. 49–7 and 49–8).[25,28] The fourth pattern is that of a large exophytic mass that may ulcerate or fistulize to adjacent bowel loops.

The small bowel can be involved secondarily when lymphoma develops in the adjacent mesenteric lymph nodes and spreads by direct extension into small bowel loops (Fig. 49–9). The small bowel loops can be displaced or completely encased by the enlarged nodes. Bulky mesenteric disease can form a mantle of nodes that envelope mesenteric vessels and small bowel loops, producing the "sandwich sign."[41]

## Leiomyosarcoma

Leiomyosarcoma is a gastrointestinal stromal tumor (GIST) that arises from smooth muscle cells in the muscularis propria. Such tumors are estimated to comprise between 10% and 16% of all intestinal neoplasms.[42] When small, leiomyosarcomas are difficult to distinguish from benign leiomyomas by radiographic or even pathologic appearance. Leiomyosarcomas are characterized pathologically by their differentiation into smooth muscle or neural elements and are then categorized as benign, borderline, of low malignant potential, or malignant.

Leiomyosarcomas are rare in the duodenum but occur with equal incidence in the jejunum and ileum. These tumors typically appear exophytic and bulky (Fig. 49–10).[25] There is often central ulceration or low attenuation compatible with necrosis. These tumors can be so large that it becomes difficult to determine their site of origin. Three-dimensional CT imaging may be helpful in these instances. Leiomyosarcomas typically do not produce significant adenopathy. This can also help distinguish leiomyosarcomas from lymphomas on CT.[43] Com-

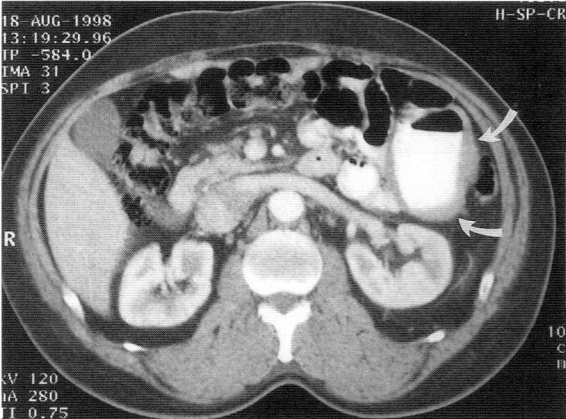

**Figure 49–7** Small bowel lymphoma. Contrast-enhanced spiral CT scan demonstrates moderate circumferential thickening of a small bowel loop in the left upper quadrant and associated dilatation of the lumen (curved arrows). This is an example of a small bowel lymphoma resulting in aneurysmal dilation of the involved bowel loop.

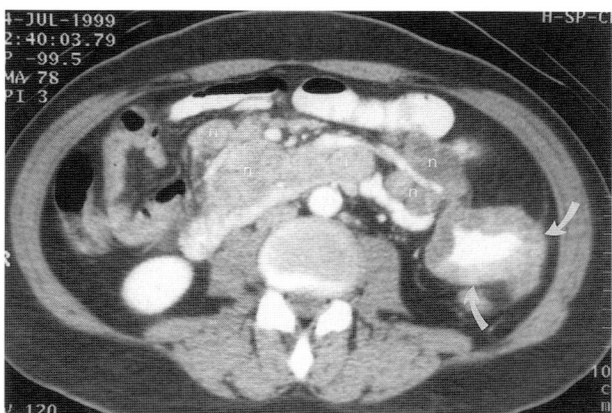

**Figure 49-8** Small bowel lymphoma. Spiral CT scan demonstrates aneurysmal dilatation of a loop of small bowel in the mid left abdomen (arrows) compatible with lymphoma. Note also moderate associated adenopathy (n) in the mesentery.

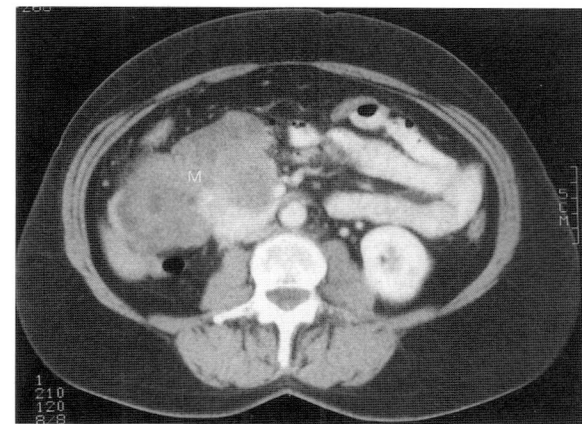

**Figure 49-10** Duodenal leiomyosarcoma. Contrast-enhanced spiral CT scan reveals an 11 × 6 × 5 cm complex mass (M) involving the second and third portions of the duodenum and encasing the superior mesenteric vein. The mass has central low attenuation compatible with necrosis. Leiomyosarcomas are often large and exophytic.

puted tomography can also detect direct invasion of adjacent organs or distant metastasis, which typically involves the liver. Metastatic leiomyosarcoma to the liver classically appears cystic on CT and should not be mistaken for benign hepatic cysts.[43]

## Metastases

Metastases can involve the small intestine by three distinct routes. First, neoplasms in organs such as the pancreas or colon can grow to directly invade nearby small bowel loops (Fig. 49–11). This can be detected on contrast studies as tethering, serosal spiculation, or mass effect indicating extrinsic involvement of the bowel. Computed tomography can demonstrate extension of the primary tumor to encase or invade adjacent bowel loops.

Second, the small intestine may be involved by intraperitoneal seeding by primary tumors such as ovarian cancer or in pseudomyxoma peritonei (Fig. 49–12). Computed tomography can nicely demonstrate the intraperitoneal implants on the small intestine as well as implants on solid organs such as the liver or spleen.

Third, metastases may involve the small intestine by hematogenous spread in patients with cancers such as lung cancer, breast cancer, or melanoma (Fig. 49–13). In such cases, the radiographic appearance may simulate that of primary small bowel tumors. On contrast studies, metastases to the small bowel can appear as target lesions in the submucosa (simulating lymphoma) or as apple core lesions (simulating primary adenocarcinoma). On CT, metastases may appear as a focal mass or focal thickening of the small bowel, similar to the CT appearance of primary small bowel tumors.

## Malignancies of the Appendix

Neoplasms of the appendix are rare, occurring in only 0.5% of appendices.[44] The most common appendiceal malignancy is carcinoid, which accounts for up to 15% of all gastrointestinal carcinoid tumors.[44]

Since 80% of appendiceal carcinoid tumors are less than 1 cm in size, the diagnosis is usually not made preoperatively on radiologic examination.[45–47] Contrast studies are not usually use-

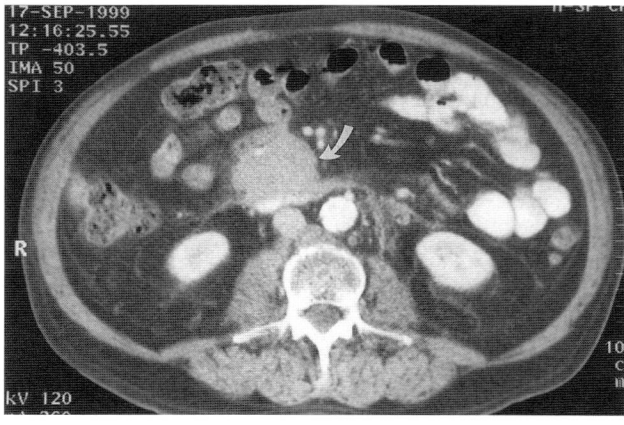

**A**

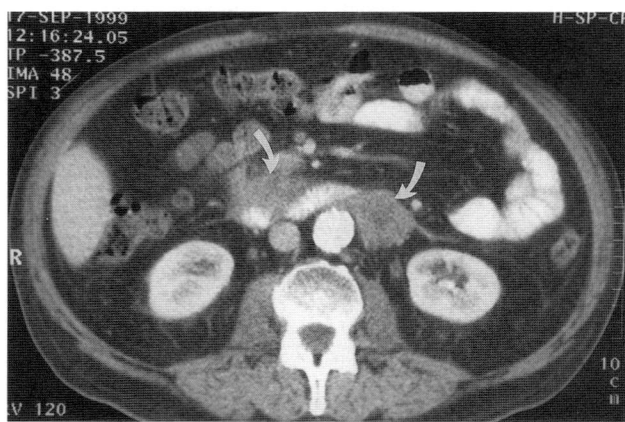

**B**

**Figure 49-9** Lymphoma. *A, B:* Contrast-enhanced spiral CT scan demonstrates a nodal mass (arrows) in the mesentery with secondary involvement and encasement of adjacent small bowel loops. This is an ex-

ample of secondary involvement of the small bowel in a patient with lymphoma.

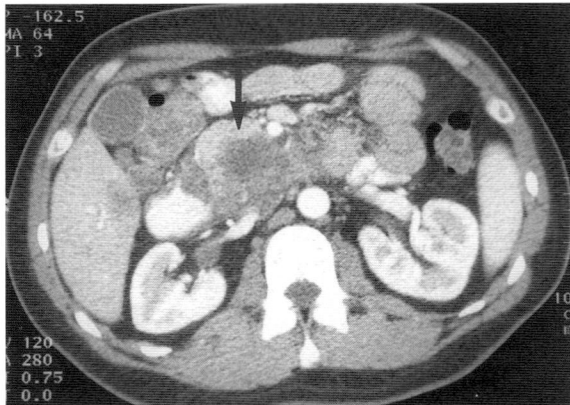

**Figure 49-11** Small bowel metastases. Contrast-enhanced CT scan demonstrates a low density mass in the head and uncinate process of the pancreas (arrow) with local extension and invasion of the third portion of the duodenum.

ful in the diagnosis of primary appendiceal carcinoid, although they may demonstrate nonfilling of the appendix or, in some cases, mass effect of the cecum. Similarly, although CT cannot usually visualize small appendiceal masses, it is useful for evaluation of possible metastasis. The primary site of metastasis is the liver. Carcinoid metastases are hypervascular and are best visualized on scans performed with intravenous contrast agents and imaged in the arterial phase of liver enhancement. As for carcinoid tumors of the small intestine, any extension beyond the appendix into the adjacent mesenteric fat can be detected by CT.

Adenocarcinoma of the appendix occurs in 0.1% of appendices. Most, and possibly all, appendiceal adenocarcinomas are thought to arise from preexisting adenomas.[44] There are two main types of adenocarcinoma of the appendix: cystadenocarcinoma and colorectal adenocarcinoma.

Since almost 70% of patients with adenocarcinoma of the appendix present with signs and symptoms suggesting acute appendicitis, the diagnosis is usually not made until surgery or after examination of the pathologic specimen. In cases of appendiceal adenocarcinoma, the contrast enema is not usually

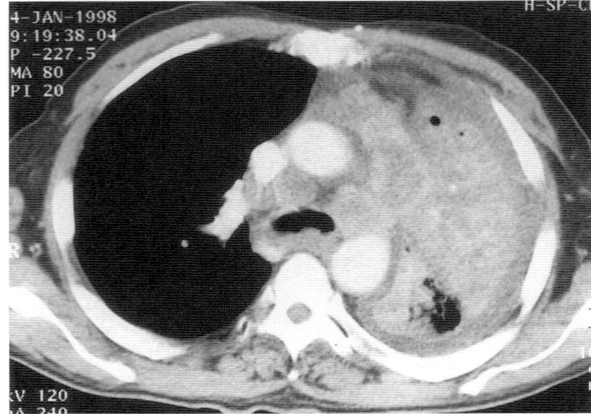

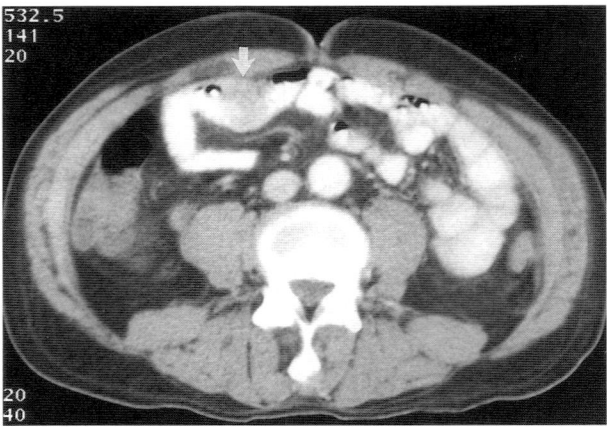

**Figure 49-13** Small bowel metastases. *A:* Contrast-enhanced spiral CT scan reveals a dense soft tissue mass filling almost the entire left hemithorax, compatible with atelectasis and patient's known lung cancer. Note bulky lymph nodes in the precarinal space. Tumor also encases and narrows the left pulmonary artery and left mainstem bronchus (not shown). *B:* Contrast-enhanced spiral CT scan of the abdomen revealing a 2.5-cm soft tissue mass (arrow) in a mid small bowel loop compatible with a metastasis

helpful in making the diagnosis. It typically demonstrates nonfilling of the appendix and possibly mass effect on the cecum. It cannot distinguish between acute appendicitis and adenocarcinoma of the appendix. Likewise, the findings on CT can be identical, consisting of inflammation and soft tissue thickening of appendix and adjacent fat.

Cystadenocarcinomas typically demonstrate abundant extracellular mucin. This can lead to a condition called "mucocele of the appendix" caused by an abnormal accumulation of mucus in the dilated appendix. The reported prevalence of mucocele in appendectomy specimens is 0.2% to 0.3%. Preoperative diagnosis of mucocele of the appendix is crucial in attempting to avoid rupture at surgery.[48] Mucocele of the appendix can arise from hyperplasia, a benign mucinous cystadenoma, or a mucinous cyst adenocarcinoma.[49] The etiology of the mucocele is determined on pathologic examination and cannot typically be determined on radiologic examination.

Barium enemas in patients with mucocele of the appendix classically demonstrate extrinsic compression of the cecum or adjacent small bowel (Fig. 49–14). They can also demonstrate nonfilling of the appendix. However, these findings are very nonspecific.

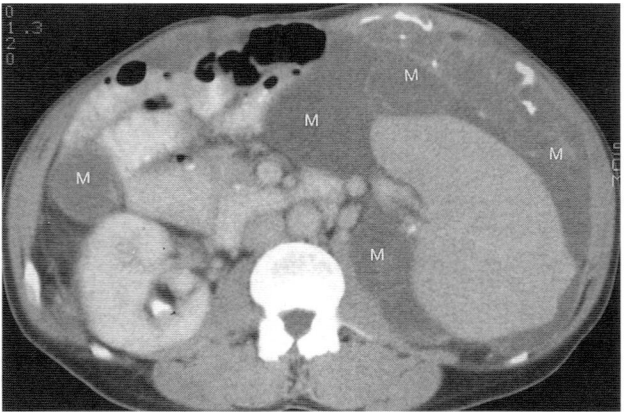

**Figure 49-12** Small bowel metastases. Contrast-enhanced CT scan demonstrates multiple cystic masses (M) throughout the abdomen with a few focal calcifications. These findings are compatible with pseudomyxoma peritonei. Note also the extensive peritoneal metastases involving the small bowel in the right abdomen.

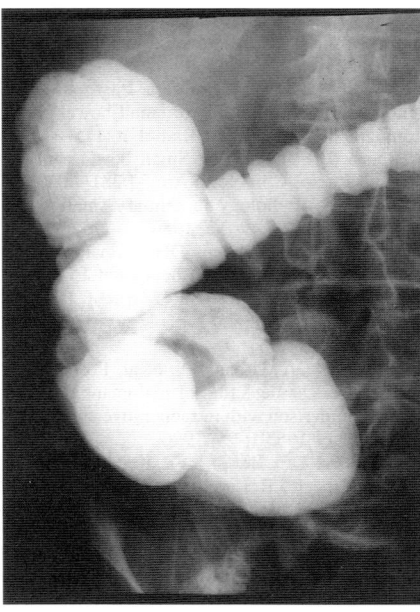

**Figure 49-14** Mucocele. Contrast enema demonstrates a smooth contour defect in the cecum (arrow). At surgery, a mucocele of the appendix was discovered.

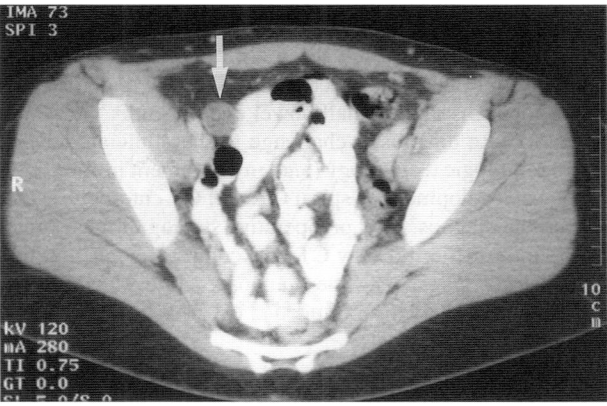

**Figure 49-16** Mucocele. Contrast-enhanced spiral CT scan demonstrates a dilated fluid-filled appendix (arrow) without associated inflammatory changes in the periappendiceal fat. In this case, a mucocele of the appendix was diagnosed at surgery.

On CT, the normal appendix appears as a tubular structure with thin walls and should not measure more than 6 mm in diameter (Fig. 49–15). A mucocele of the appendix appears as a low-attenuation, well-defined mass in the right lower quadrant adjacent to the cecum (Fig. 49–16). Mucoceles are typically retrocecal because 65% of appendixes are retrocecal. The attenuation of the mass is dependent on the amount of mucin. Computed tomography may also demonstrate mass effect. A key differential point is the lack of appendiceal inflammation. This helps distinguish mucocele from acute appendicitis. On CT, there is enhancement of the wall of the mucocele. The wall may either be thick or thin. The thickness of the wall does not help distinguish between neoplastic and non-neoplastic causes of mucocele of the appendix. The presence of an intramural nodule may help suggest the diagnosis of cystadenocarcinoma as the cause of the mucocele.[50]

On ultrasound, a mucocele typically appears as a cystic mass in the right lower quadrant adjacent to the cecum. Ultrasonography usually demonstrates good through-transmission and posterior enhancement.[48] The internal echoes are dependent on the amount and viscosity of the mucin. On ultrasound scans, the mucocele wall is typically thin, which helps distinguish a mucocele from the appendiceal wall thickening seen in appendicitis.[48,50]

Almost 50% of patients with cyst adenocarcinoma of the appendix will develop pseudomyxoma peritonei.[51] This can be well visualized on CT. Pseudomyxoma peritonei appears as multiple foci of gelatinous material throughout the peritoneum (Fig. 49–17).[52,53] This can make the liver and spleen as well as the GI tract appear scalloped. Computed tomography is also helpful in detecting lymph node metastases, which are noted in 25% of cases at presentation. Prognosis of adenocarcinoma of the appendix is determined by Dukes staging and degree of differentiation.

Metastasis to the appendix has been reported for ovarian, breast, stomach, and lung cancers. Other malignant tumors of the appendix have been reported but are extremely rare. These include malignant lymphoma, smooth muscle tumors, nerve sheath tumors, ganglioneuromas, and Kaposi's sarcoma.

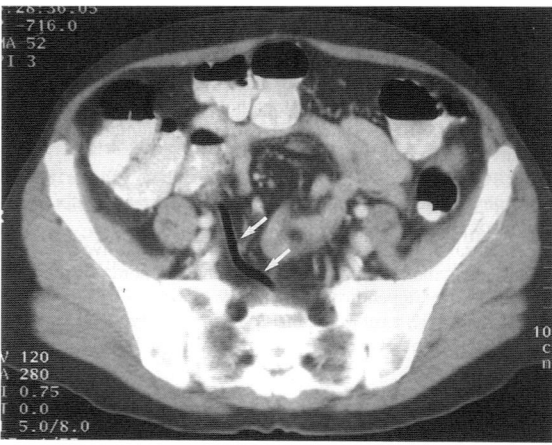

**Figure 49-15** Normal appendix. Contrast-enhanced spiral CT scan demonstrates the CT appearance of a normal air-filled appendix (arrows).

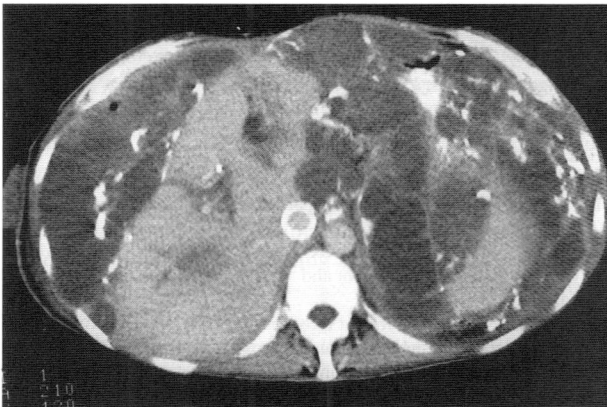

**Figure 49-17** Pseudomyxoma peritonei. Contrast-enhanced spiral CT scan demonstrates multiple cystic masses throughout the abdomen, some of which are calcified. This is the classic CT appearance of pseudomyxoma peritonei.

ovaries. Immunohistochemical and ultrastructural studies and literature review. Arch Pathol Lab Med 109:930–933, 1985.

64. Jones R, McFarlane A. Carcinomas and carcinoid tumors of the appendix in a district general hospital. J Clin Pathol 29:687–692, 1976.

65. Miller R, Sarikaya H, Jenison E. Adenocarcinoid tumor of the appendix presenting as unilateral Krukenberg tumor. J Surg Oncol 37:65–71, 1988.

66. Merino M, Edmonds P, Li V, Olsi L. Appendiceal carcinoma metastatic to the ovaries am mimicking primary ovarian tumors. Int J Gynecol Pathol 4:110–120, 1985.

67. Thomas R, Barnhill D, Worsham F, Hoskins W. Krukenberg tumor of the ovary from an occult appendiceal primary: case report and review of the literature. Obstet Gynecol 65:95S–98S, 1985.

68. Zirkin R, Brown S, Hertz M. Adenocarcinoid of the appendix presenting as bilateral ovarian tumors: a case report with histochemical and ultrastructural studies. Diagn Gynecol Obstet 2:269–274, 1980.

69. Hood I, Jones B, Watt J. Mucinous carcinoid tumor of the appendix presenting as bilateral ovarian tumors. Arch Pathol Lab Med 110:336–340, 1986.

70. Friedland J, Allardice J, Wyatt A. Pseudomyxoma peritonei. J R Soc Med 79:480–482, 1993.

71. Sugarbaker P. Pseudomyxoma peritonei: a cancer whose biology is characterized by a redistribution phenomenon. Ann Surg 219:109–111, 1994.

72. Smith J, Kemeny N, Caldwell C, Banner P, Sigurdson E, Huvos A. Pseudomyxoma of appendiceal origin: the Memorial Sloan-Kettering Cancer Center experience. Cancer 70:396–401, 1992.

73. Fernandez R, Daly J. Pseudomyxoma peritonei. Arch Surg 115:409–414, 1980.

74. Gough D, Donohue J, Schutt A. Pseudomyxoma peritonei. Long-term patient survival with an aggressive regional approach. Ann Surg 219:112–119, 1994.

75. Long R, Spratt J, Dowling E. Pseudomyxoma peritonei: new concepts in management with a report of seventeen patients. Am J Surg 117:162–169, 1969.

76. Cortina R, McCormick J, Kolm P, Perry R. Management and prognosis of adenocarcinoma of the appendix. Dis Colon Rectum 38:848–852, 1995.

77. Lenriot J, Huguier M. Adenocarcinoma of the appendix. Am J Surg 155:470–475, 1988.

78. Lin J, Cogbill C, Athota P, Tsung S, Kwak Y. Superfical spreading adenocarcinoma of appendix, cecum and terminal ileum. Dis Colon Rectum 23:587–589, 1980.

79. Didolkar M, Fanous N. Adenocarcinoma of the appendix: a clinicopathologic study. Dis Colon Rectum 20:130–134, 1977.

80. Flint F, Kahn A, Passaro E. Adenocarcinoma of the appendix. Surgery 120:707–709, 1970.

81. Pugeda F, Hishaw J. Primary adenocarcinoma of the appendix. Dis Colon Rectum 12:457–461, 1969.

82. Reichle F, Brigham M, Fleegler E, Rosemond G. Adenocarcinoma of the vermiform appendix. Am Surg 37:344–350, 1977.

# Section 7

## Cancer of the Colorectum

# Chapter 52

# Epidemiology and Prevention of Colorectal Cancer

ERNEST T. HAWK, JAYE L. VINER, AND PAUL J. LIMBURG

Colorectal cancer (CRC) is the fourth most frequently diagnosed cancer in the United States and has the second highest cancer-related mortality rate after lung cancer.[1] While the incidence of CRC has declined over recent years, the disease remains a major public health burden in the United States. Advanced CRC is largely refractory to conventional therapeutics and is one of the least curable malignancies. Despite continuing advances in cancer therapy, long-term survival has not improved significantly over the last four decades, a situation that mandates improvements in early detection of this surgically curable disease and preventive interventions to reduce the incidence of the disease and its downstream morbidities and mortality. Indeed, given our understanding of the pathogenesis of CRC, current screening technologies, and effective preventive interventions, CRC should be highly preventable. Continued efforts to raise awareness of the merits of CRC screening and prevention and to stimulate adherence to current guidelines are critical in order to realize major progress against CRC. Emerging molecular technologies to improve CRC risk assessment and target interventions are already challenging traditional concepts of "health" and "disease" and will progressively transform our approach to managing colorectal carcinogenesis. This chapter will review the epidemiologic distribution and determinants of CRC, screening technologies used to identify those at greater than average risk, and preventive interventions—both established and emerging.

## Colorectal Carcinogenesis: The Basis of Risk, The Premise for Prevention

While CRC was once considered a clinically catastrophic event, we now understand that it is but one late stage in a long disease process driven by cumulative alterations in DNA structure and function, which are subsequently and sequentially expressed within each and ultimately across all higher levels of biologic organization (e.g., RNA, protein, organelle, cell, tissue, organ, organism). For example, at the molecular level, structural changes in oncogenes (e.g., K-*ras*), tumor suppressor genes (e.g., *APC*, *p53*), or mismatch repair genes (e.g., *hMSH-2*) or changes in gene expression driven by aberrancies in regulatory control signals (e.g., hypermethylation of the estrogen receptor gene) are initiating or contributing influences.[2–5] At the cellular and tissue levels, key derangements of colorectal carcinogenesis include characteristic morphologic changes collectively termed *atypia* or *dysplasia,* an imbalance in cellular population dynamics via increased proliferation, suppressed apoptosis or sloughing, and altered phenotypic features of functional maturity (e.g., loss of the differentiated profile of Lewis blood group antigens).[6]

Progression toward significant clonal anarchy is mitigated by multiple endogenous mechanisms, including carcinogen detoxification, DNA repair, selective apoptosis, and immunologic surveillance. Nevertheless, in progressive colorectal carcinogenesis, a clonal population of cells is eventually identifiable as an aberrant crypt focus (ACF).[7,8] Aberrant crypt foci are large colorectal crypts raised slightly above the surrounding normal mucosa and usually have a slit-like or irregularly shaped lumen. They can be visualized in many ex vivo colorectal specimens with methylene blue or other topical dyes,[9] and recently have been identified in vivo by high-resolution/magnifying endoscopy.[10,11] Only a fraction of ACF harbor significant genetic alterations known to underlie colorectal carcinogenesis (e.g., loss of wild-type APC protein or mutations of K-*ras*) or are histologically dysplastic (5%–54%), but many are believed to be true adenoma precursors.[12,13] The prevalence of colorectal ACF increases with age and appears to correlate with the cross-sectional risk for more advanced neoplastic lesions within a population,[11] just as persons with adenomas are at increased risk for CRC.

The carcinogenic continuum challenges traditional notions of biologic and chronologic boundaries of disease and, consequently, of disease prevention. *Prevention* is defined as an active intervention that reduces the probability of subsequent development of disease. As such, the definition of prevention depends on definitions of both health and disease which, in the case of carcinogenesis, are drawn from a complex biology. Indeed, within the last 20 years, preinvasive colorectal carcinogenesis, represented by the adenomatous polyp, has become widely recognized as a stage of disease worthy of clinical intervention largely on the basis of the risk for progression.[14] Debate persists as to whether earlier pathologies identified at the tissue level (e.g., aberrant crypt foci, dysplasia), the cellular level (e.g., atypia), or even the molecular level (e.g., altered APC protein, overexpression of cyclooxygenase-2 [COX-2] m-RNA, *APC* gene mutation) far in advance of clinical disease should be considered worthy markers of risk,[15] targets for intervention,[16] or end points for clinical prevention trials.[17,18] Technologic advances that enable the detection of progressively earlier stages of carcinogenesis further kindle the debate, ensuring that controversy over the definition of disease and the risks, benefits, and costs of prevention will continue.

Definition of disease informs the language of risk and preventive oncology. For example, when CRC is the "disease" of interest, *primary prevention* is defined as an intervention that reduces the risk of incident CRC in individuals without overt pathology;[19] *secondary prevention* involves discovering cancer through screening before the emergence of signs and symptoms. In this scenario, the effectiveness of secondary CRC prevention depends on the subsequent intervention of cancer resection. *Tertiary prevention* involves interventions to reduce the risk of complications or side effects associated with a therapy or with the natural history of cancer.

As suggested above, in biopsy-accessible target organs such as the colorectum, technologies that increase our sensitivity for detecting asymptomatic, precancerous stages of neoplasia in the colorectum, ACF, and adenomatous polyps at a minimum have allowed us to shift the definition to earlier disease states and thus have blurred the distinction between primary and secondary prevention. For colorectal neoplasia (i.e., ACF, adenomas, and cancer), secondary prevention includes screening to identify lesions, and an individual's risk is subsequently reduced by endoscopic removal of the lesions. Improved understanding of early neoplastic lesions, their relationship to cancer, and the importance of early detection, combined with interventions directed at all stages of neoplasia, may account for the recent declines in CRC incidence and mortality. Further advances in CRC risk identification coupled with broadly implemented behavioral, pharmaceutical, and surgical interventions should continue to reduce the personal and societal burdens of this common malignancy.

## Epidemiology: Evaluating the Evidence

*Epidemiology* is the study of disease distribution and determinants in human populations, typically using observational methods independent of intentional interventions. Just as laboratory-based investigations are critical for elucidating mechanistic pathways involved in colorectal carcinogenesis, observational population-based studies are instrumental for identifying the key host and environmental factors associated with gastrointestinal tumor development. Comparisons of cohorts stratified by age, geography, gender, ethnicity, medical history, dietary practices, and lifestyle have yielded valuable insights into colorectal carcinogenesis. Even so, the full spectrum of risk and protective factors remains to be determined.

Randomized controlled trials are ideal for assessing the cause-and-effect relationships between a given exposure variable (e.g., fiber intake) and a defined clinical outcome (e.g., CRC incidence). However, intervention trials are logistically complex, expensive, and time-consuming, and cannot ethically be used to assess the effect of an agent likely to be harmful. As a result, most host and environmental factors putatively associated with colorectal neoplasia have been identified from observational studies.

Fundamental differences in observational study designs should be considered to appropriately interpret data generated by observational studies. In general, cohort, nested case–cohort, and nested case–control studies provide the strongest epidemiologic evidence for making causative inferences, as the exposure variables are measured before disease onset and outcome variables are documented prospectively. Retrospective studies, such as case–control studies, are prone to methodologic biases that could affect the magnitude and nature of the risk associations. Case series, case reports, and ecologic studies should be used for hypothesis generation only, as these designs do not incorporate individual subject controls. Other key elements to consider when assessing and interpreting observational data are the biologic plausibility of the proposed risk association, the consistency of the risk association across multiple studies, the magnitude of the assumed causative effect, and the generalizability of the results to nonstudy population subgroups.

### Geographic Distribution

Cancer registries are used to monitor the distribution of malignancies within geographically or otherwise defined populations. The International Agency for Research on Cancer (IARC) compiles data such as these to create GLOBOCAN, which serves as a centralized source of information on global cancer incidence and mortality. The IARC provides regularly updated statistics on its Internet site (www.iarc.fr). According to recent incidence data,[20] CRC ranks fourth in incidence among cancers overall (excluding nonmelanoma skin cancer), with an estimated 783,000 new cases diagnosed annually. Age-adjusted incidence rates are 15.3/100,000 for women and 19.4/100,000 for men. Colorectal malignancies also have the fourth highest cancer mortality rate, causing approximately 437,000 deaths worldwide per annum. Age-adjusted mortality rates are 8.6/100,000 for women and 10.7/100,000 for men.

In the United States, the Surveillance, Epidemiology, and End Results (SEER) program tracks the occurrence of colorectal and other malignancies. SEER records contain data from 11 cancer registries, representing a 14% nonrandom sample of the national population.[21] The most current SEER data are available in public use format (cancer incidence only) and can be obtained through the program's Internet site (www.seer.cancer.gov). According to SEER data, colorectal malignancies are the fourth most common cause of cancers and the second most common cause of cancer deaths in the United States; approximately 147,000 new cases and 57,100 disease-related fatalities were estimated for the year 2003.[1] Age-adjusted incidence and mortality rates for women are 36.7/100,000 and 13.0/100,000, respectively. For men, both rates are higher, at 51.8/100,000 and 20.9/100,000, respectively.[22] The incidence figures for the United

States exceed global averages, consistent with an international pattern of increased CRC risk among industrialized societies.[23]

Secular trends in SEER data highlight a recent overall decline in CRC incidence and mortality in the United States; incidence rates peaked in 1985 and have subsequently dropped by an average of 1.8% per year among women (−0.4% since 1992) and 2.0% per year among men (−1.1% since 1992).[22,24] Mortality rates have also decreased, but the temporal pattern differs between men and women. Among women, CRC mortality rates began declining in 1949. Since 1992, the annual change has been −1.7%. Among men, CRC mortality rates did not show a consistent downturn until 1978. Since then, a −1.3% annual change has been observed (−2.1% since 1992). The mechanisms underlying these favorable trends are largely unknown. However, earlier detection of colorectal neoplasms (including precursor adenomas as well as resectable malignancies) through increasingly widespread use of CRC screening may be partially responsible. Improved cancer treatments have also reduced mortality, but the contributions from such advances are unlikely to fully account for the decline of CRC in the population.

## Race and Ethnicity

Colorectal cancer risks differ across racial and ethnic population subgroups within the United States. Early SEER data categorized only whites and blacks, but more recently recorded cancer cases (from 1992 forward) classify patients according to five subgroups: blacks, whites, Asian and Pacific Islanders, Hispanics, and Native Americans/Alaskan Natives. Of these subgroups, blacks have the highest rates of both CRC incidence and mortality (Table 52–1). In addition, the 5-year CRC survival rate of blacks is lower than that of whites. From 1974 to 1996, the gap between the survival rates of blacks and whites increased from a difference of 5% (46% vs. 51%) to a difference of 11% (52% versus 63%) for colon cancer, and from 7% (42% vs. 49%) to 9% (52% vs. 61%) for rectal cancer.[1] Blacks overall present with more advanced disease at the time of the initial detection, a factor that may partially explain survival differences between the two groups.[25] However, when within-stage survival comparisons are made, this discrepancy in prognosis persists. Race-related differences in CRC treatment have also been impugned in some, but not all, reports.[26,27] Additional possibilities for survival differences include as-yet undetected biologic or environmental factors that account for racial dissimilarities in age at diagnosis,[28]

anatomic subsite distribution,[29–31] and histopathologic characteristics[28] of colorectal tumors.

## Anatomic Subsite

Subsegments of the colorectum differ in embryologic origin, physiologic function, and vascular supply. Differences in tumor morphology, histology, and genetics have been observed across anatomic subsites within the large bowel.[32–36] Region-specific CRC incidence rates also differ, and the incidence of adenocarcinomas located in the proximal colon appears to be increasing relative to incidences in the distal colon and rectum (Table 52–2). In 1976, the distribution pattern for large bowel malignancies was 36% in the cecum, ascending colon, hepatic flexure, transverse colon, or splenic flexure; 31% in the descending colon or sigmoid colon; and 31% in the rectum (including the rectosigmoid junction). Twenty years later, these percentages were 42%, 27%, and 28%, respectively. Age-adjusted incidence rates for cecal and ascending colon cancers have increased over the same period, in contrast to stable or decreased rates for all other anatomic subsegments. Whites have experienced recent declines in proximal colon, distal colon, and rectal cancer incidence rates.[37] Conversely, blacks have demonstrated a more mixed pattern, with increasing rates of proximal colon cancer, unchanged rates of distal colon cancer, and decreasing rectal cancer incidence rates among women only. Mechanistic hypotheses to explain these subsite trends remain largely underexplored.

## Migrant Populations

Geographically mobile populations afford unique opportunities to study the potential role of environmental factors in chronic disease. Migrant groups tend to assume risks of CRC similar to those of their adopted country with increasing duration of residence. This finding strongly supports the assumption that adult life exposures are important modulators of large bowel carcinogenesis. However, risk assimilation is seldom complete, emphasizing the importance of multiple, complex interactions between heritable factors (e.g., genetic code) and environmental factors (e.g., diet, physical activity, exposures) in CRC causation. Earlier this century, Japanese and Chinese immigrants experienced increases in CRC upon relocation to the United States, perhaps

**Table 52-1** Colorectal cancer incidence and mortality by race/ethnicity (United States, 1990–1997)

| Demographic Subgroup | Age-Adjusted Rates[a] | |
| --- | --- | --- |
| | Incidence[b] | Mortality[c] |
| Blacks | 50.7 | 23.0 |
| Whites | 43.6 | 17.2 |
| Asian and Pacific Islanders | 38.1 | 10.8 |
| Hispanics | 28.8 | 10.3 |
| American Indians and Alaskan Natives | 16.3 | 10.1 |

[a]Per 100,000 persons, age-adjusted to the 1970 United States standard population.

[b]From SEER 11 Registries public use data, National Cancer Institute, Division of Cancer Control and Population Sciences, 2000.[1]

[c]Derived by SEER from data originating from the National Center for Health Statsitics, Centers for Disease Control and Prevention, 2000.[1]

**Table 52-2** Colorectal cancer incidence by anatomic subsite, 1976 vs. 1996 (United States)

| Anatomic Subsite | 1976 | | 1996 | |
| --- | --- | --- | --- | --- |
| | Rate[a] | % | Rate[a] | % |
| All colorectal subsites[b] | 44.7 | 100 | 40.2 | 100 |
| Cecum | 6.6 | 15 | 6.7 | 17 |
| Ascending | 3.7 | 8 | 4.5 | 12 |
| Transverse[c] | 5.6 | 13 | 5.1 | 13 |
| Descending | 2.7 | 6 | 1.8 | 4 |
| Sigmoid | 11.2 | 25 | 9.6 | 23 |
| Rectosigmoid junction | 4.4 | 10 | 4.0 | 10 |
| Rectum | 9.6 | 21 | 7.6 | 18 |

[a]Per 100,000 persons, age-adjusted to the 1970 U.S. standard population (SEER 9 Registries public use dataset, August 1998 submission, 1973–1996).

[b]Excluding appendix.

[c]Including hepatic flexure and splenic flexure.

owing in part to changes in physical activity, dietary habits, or available food sources.[38,39] Just as resettlement in a high-risk region can increase CRC risk, migration to a low-risk region can decrease risk. Native European immigrants in Australia experienced reductions in CRC mortality rates for up to 30 years post-migration, although a gradient of increasing CRC risk was observed over time among southern Europeans, the subgroup that had the lowest relative risk before migration.[40] This phenomenon is even more apparent among Italian immigrants to South America; CRC rates decreased among Italian migrants to a low-risk area of Sao Paulo, Brazil, whereas they increased among migrants to a high-risk area of Argentina.[41]

## Determinants of Colorectal Carcinogenesis

### Longitudinal Cohorts

Colorectal cancer risk and protective factors have been extensively evaluated within five large prospective cohorts: the Nurses' Health Study (NHS),[42-57] the Cancer Prevention Study II (CPS-II),[58-64] the Health Professionals Follow-up Study (HPFS),[44,57,65-71] the Iowa Women's Health Study (IWHS),[72-77] and the Netherlands Cohort Study (NCS).[78-85] Brief descriptions of these studies, including their subjects' demographics, exposure assessment instruments, and published CRC outcome measures, are outlined for general reference (Table 52–3). Additional prospective, retrospective, and compilation (i.e., meta-analysis) studies that have provided more limited epidemiologic information are included under the following topic headings.

### Host Factors

#### Age

As with most malignancies, CRC risks increase with advancing age. The SEER data suggest that age-specific CRC incidence rates begin to rise more rapidly during the fifth decade of life in the United States (Fig. 52–1). Colorectal cancer subsite distributions may also vary by age. In a study of more than 75,000 Medicare enrollees, Cooper and colleagues[86] observed that proximal colon cancers appear to be disproportionately more common among elderly patients. Comparing persons aged 85 years and above with those aged 65–69 years, these investigators noted relative increases of 333%, 179%, and 192% for the rates of cancer in the proximal colon, distal colon, and rectum, respectively. The incidence of adenomatous polyps, the precursor lesions of most sporadic CRC, also increases with age. Furthermore, multiple adenomas and larger adenomas are more common among older patients.[87] Among residents of developed countries, age-stratified prevalence estimates for adenomas are 30% at 50 years, 40%–50% at 60 years, and 50%–65% at 70 years.[88,89] Several important clinical features of adenomas may be age related as well. In the National Polyp Study (a multicenter clinical trial designed to evaluate surveillance strategies among 1418 patients with one or more colorectal adenomas), the risk of having a polyp with high-grade dysplasia was 80% higher (odds ratio [OR] = 1.8; 95% confidence interval [CI] = 1.2–5.4) among subjects 60 years of age or older than that of younger counterparts.[90]

#### Personal history of colorectal neoplasia

Nearly all CRCs are thought to arise from benign neoplasia through the well-established adenoma–adenocarcinoma sequence.[91,92] However, most colorectal adenomas do not progress to become cancers. In fact, it is estimated that fewer than 10% of adenomatous polyps undergo malignant transformation.[93] Nonetheless, individuals with a personal history of colorectal neoplasia are at increased risk for developing metachronous (recurrent) tumors. Neither hyperplastic polyps nor small, solitary tubular adenomas are strong risk factors for subsequent colorectal neoplasms.[94,95] However, important predictors of CRC risk include adenoma size (typically defined as 1 cm or larger in diameter), villous histology, or multiplicity. Several retrospective and prospective studies have shown that these characteristics are positively associated with future tumor development.[95-100] In a cohort of 842 patients who had at least one tubulovillous, villous, or large distal colorectal adenoma at baseline, the standardized incidence ratio for colon cancer after an average follow-up period of 13.8 years per patient (in the absence of routine surveillance) was 3.6 (95% CI = 2.4–5.0).[95] More strikingly, this risk measure increased to 6.6 (95% CI = 3.3–11.8) among patients with more than one rectosigmoid adenoma at baseline. Persons who have undergone surgical resection for CRC represent another high-risk group for metachronous neoplasia. These patients are prone to recurrent primary cancers, second primary cancers, and adenomatous polyps.[101-103] The distinction between recurrent and second primary colorectal neoplasias (adenomas and carcinomas) can be difficult to distinguish without detailed serial endoscopic mapping. Nevertheless, persons with prior CRC resections tend to develop "recurrent" adenomas relatively soon, with the median time to detection ranging from 19 to 32 months.[103-105]

#### Family history of colorectal neoplasia

Genetic syndromes, such as familial adenomatous polyposis (FAP) and hereditary nonpolyposis colorectal cancer (HNPCC), account for fewer than 5% of all CRCs.[106] Yet, despite the absence of a well-defined inherited predisposition in most cases, familial clustering among CRC patients is common. Burt and others have postulated that inheritance establishes an underlying susceptibility to tumor formation, while gene–environment interactions determine the eventual expression of colorectal neoplasia.[106,107] Large epidemiologic investigations have reported remarkably consistent risk estimates for large bowel cancer among first-degree relatives of patients with sporadic neoplasia. Analysis of combined data from the Nurses' Health Study and the Health Professionals Follow-up Study yielded a multivariate relative risk (RR) of 1.72 (95% CI = 1.33–2.20) for subjects with vs. those without family histories of CRC.[57] The risk was even higher among subjects younger than 45 years who had more than one first-degree relative with CRC. In the Iowa Women's Health study,[75] the age-adjusted RR for colon cancer was 1.8 (95% CI = 1.3–2.4) among postmenopausal women with a father, mother, sister, or brother who had the same disease. Similarly, Winawer and others[108] observed a RR for CRC of 1.78 (95% CI = 1.18–2.67) among parents and siblings of patients with adenoma (referent to spouse controls) in the National Polyp Study. Family history was less strongly associated with CRC in the Cancer Prevention Study II, but this study assessed only fatal cases and could thus have been influenced by a nondifferential misclassification bias related to earlier neoplasms, which might have attenuated the true relative risk.[60] Although less thoroughly investigated, CRC in a second- or third-degree relative also appears to be associated with a modest increase in risk.[109]

**Table 52-3** Large epidemiologic prospective studies of colorectal neoplasia

| | Nurses' Health Study[42-57] | Cancer Prevention Study II[58-64] | Health Professionals Follow-up Study[44,57,65-71] | Netherlands Cohort Study[78-85] | Iowa Women's Health Study[72-77] |
|---|---|---|---|---|---|
| Year initiated | 1976 | 1982 | 1986 | 1986 | 1986 |
| No. of subjects | 121,700 | 1,185,124 | 51,529 | 120,852 | 41,837 |
| Age at enrollment | 30–55 years | ≥30 years | 40–75 years | 55–69 years | 55–69 years |
| Sex | Women | Women and men | Men | Women and men | Women |
| Cohort characteristics | Registered nurses from 11 U.S. states | Recruited from all 50 U.S. states, District of Columbia, and Puerto Rico | Dentists, optometrists, osteopaths, podiatrists, pharmacists, and veterinarians | Recruited from 204 municipal population registries throughout the country | Assembled from Iowa Department of Transportation driver's license list |
| Exposure assessments | Baseline and follow-up questionnaires | Baseline questionnaire | Baseline and follow-up questionnaires | Baseline questionnaire | Baseline and follow-up questionnaires |
| Observed neoplastic outcomes | Adenoma incidence and cancer incidence | Cancer mortality | Adenoma incidence and cancer incidence | Cancer incidence | Cancer incidence |

**Table 52-5** Colorectal neoplasia prevention trials evaluating calcium (*Continued*)

| Study | Sample Size[a] | Design/Cohort[b] | Intervention[c] | Primary Results[d] |
|---|---|---|---|---|
| Hofstad et al.[202,544] | 116 | DBRCT in patients with current adenomas (those <1 cm were retained) | 1.6 g/day + β-carotene 15 mg + vitamin C 150 mg + vitamin E 75 mg + selenium 101 μg/day × 36 months | Growth of small adenomas, no effect Adenoma incidence/recurrence, increased* Fecal bile acids, no effect |
| Baron et al.[203] | 930 | DBRCT in patients with prior adenoma | 3.0 g/day × 48 months | Patients with adenoma recurrence, 19% reduction* Adenoma number, 24% reduction* |
| Faivre et al.[176,177] | 655 | RDBCT in patients with prior adenoma; 35–75 years old | 2.0 g/day (vs 3.8 g/day ispaghula husk) vs. placebo × 36 months | Adenoma incidence/recurrence, 34% reduction (NS) |
| Women's Health Initiative[147] | 45,000– 48,000 | Complex factorial, DBRCT in post-menopausal women 50–79 years old | Calcium + vitamin D; hormone replacement therapy; low-fat diet × approximately 9 years | Colorectal cancer incidence (among many others), ongoing |

BrdU, bromodeoxyuridine; CCPR, crypt cell proliferation; CRC, colorectal cancer; FAP, familial adenomatous polyposis; NS, nonsignificant; PCNA, proliferative cell nuclear antigen; TID, three times a day.

*Statistically significant result ($P < 0.05$).

[a]Number randomized.

[b]Trial designs: SBRCT, single-blind, randomized, controlled trial; DBRCT, double-blind, randomized, controlled trial; DBRCXT, double-blind, randomized, controlled crossover trial; RCXT, unblinded, randomized, controlled crossover trial.

[c]Calcium carbonate unless noted otherwise.

[d]Proliferation assessed via random biopsies of normal-appearing mucosa.

**Table 52-6** Colorectal neoplasia prevention trials of antioxidant micronutrients

| Study | Sample Size[a] | Design/Cohort[b] | Intervention | Primary Results |
|---|---|---|---|---|
| Bussey et al.[225] | 49 | DBRCT in familial adenomatous polyposis | Vitamin C 3 g/days × 9–24 months | Rectal adenoma number, reduced (NS) |
| DeCosse et al.[169] | 58 | DBRCT in familial adenomatous polyposis | Placebo + wheat bran fiber 2.2 g/day vs. vitamin C 4 g/day + vitamin E 400 mg/day + wheat bran fiber 2.2 gm/day vs. vitamins C + E + wheat bran fiber increased to 22.5 g/day vs. placebo × 48 months | Rectal adenoma number, reduced in the fiber + vitamin group (NS) |
| Paganelli et al.[226] | 41 | DBRCT in patients with prior adenoma | Vitamin A, vitamin C, vitamin E × 6 months | Proliferation, no effect; Proliferative pattern, normalized (thymidine)* |
| Cahill et al.[217] | 60 | Case series in patients with past adenoma = 40; and volunteers = 20 | Vitamin E 160 mg/day vs. vitamin C 750 mg vs. β-carotene 9 mg/day × 1 month | Proliferation, reduced with vitamin C (BrdU)* or β-carotene*; Proliferation pattern, normalized with vitamin C (BrdU)*; vitamin E, no effect |
| McKeown-Eyssen et al.[227] | 185 | DBRCT in patients with prior adenoma | Vitamin C 400 mg/day + vitamin E 400 mg/day × 24 months | Adenoma recurrence, 14% reduction (NS) |
| Roncucci et al.[228] | 255 | PBRCT in patients with prior adenoma | Vitamin A 30,000 IU/day.+ vitamin E 70 mg/day + vitamin C 1 g/day vs. lactulose 20 g/day vs. no treatment × 12–36 months (average of 18 months) | Adenoma recurrence, 84% reduction with vitamins*; 59% reduction with lactulose* |
| Greenberg et al.[218] | 864 | DBRCT in patients with prior adenoma | β-carotene 25 mg/day vs. vitamin C 1 g/day + vitamin E 400 mg/day vs. both vs. neither, 2 × 2 factorial × 48 months | Adenoma recurrence, no effect with β-carotene (1.01) or vitamins C + E (NS) |
| Hofstad et al.[202] | 116 | DBRCT in patients with prior adenoma | β-carotene 15 mg/day + vitamin E 75 mg/day + vitamin C 150 mg/day + selenium 101 μg/day + calcium 1.6 g/day × 36 months | Adenoma recurrence or growth, no effect (NS) |
| MacLennan et al.[145] | 378 | PBRCT in patients with prior adenoma | β-carotene 20 mg/day vs. wheat bran 11 g/day vs. fat <25% calories/day × 48 months | Adenoma recurrence, no effect |
| Clark et al.[234,545] | 1,312 | DBRCT in patients with a history of basal or squamous cell skin cancer | 200 selenium μg/d (as high-selenium brewer's yeast) × mean of 54 months | Cancer incidence, 58% reduction (secondary end point on 27 cases)* |
| ATBC[221,222] | 15,538 | DBRCT in male smokers 50–69 years old | β-carotene 20 mg/day vs. vitamin E 50 mg/day vs. both vs. neither × mean of 76 months | Adenoma incidence, 66% increase with vitamin E*; no effect with β-carotene; Cancer incidence, no effect with vitamin E or β-carotene on cancer |
| Hennekens et al.[219] | 22,071 | DBRCT in male physicians | β-carotene 50 mg QOD × 60 months | β-carotene, no effect on adenoma or cancer incidence; Cancer incidence, no effect |
| Women's Health Study[220,232] | 39,876 | 2 × 2 factorial DBRCT in female health professionals ≥45 years old | β-carotene 50 mg QOD × 27 months with median of 24 months follow-up; vitamin E ± aspirin × years | Cancer incidence, no effect from β-carotene (stopped early); aspirin and vitamin E components ongoing |
| SUVIMAX[229,230] | 15,000 | DBRCT in volunteers | β-carotene 6000 μg/day + vitamin C 120 mg/day + vitamin E 15 mg/day + selenium 101 μg/d + zinc 20 mg/day × 96 months | Cancer incidence; cardiovascular disease, ongoing |
| Moertel et al.[233] | 100 | DBRCT in patients with advanced colorectal cancer, chemotherapy-naive | Vitamin C 10 g/day × weeks | Cancer progression, no effect; Overall survival, no effect |

BrdU, bromodeoxyuridine; NS, nonsignificant; QOD, every other day.

*Statistically significant result (P < 0.05).

[a]Number randomized.

[b]Trial design: DBRCT, double-blind, randomized, controlled trial; PBRCT, partially-blind, randomized, controlled trial.

studied the effects of other retinoids. One small study evaluating a mixture of antioxidants including β-carotene reduced proliferation marginally,[217] whereas larger studies with more definitive end points have shown no substantial benefit.[145,209,218–222] These disappointing results, coupled with the findings from two studies (i.e., the Alpha-Tocopherol Beta Carotene Trial and the Beta Carotene and Retinol Efficacy Trial) in which β-carotene supplementation increased the incidence of lung cancer among smokers, has dampened the enthusiasm for additional research with β-carotene for CRC prevention.[223,224] Nevertheless, the promising mechanistic hypotheses and significant animal data with other retinoids suggest that further research is warranted.

Several prevention trials investigating antioxidants have used vitamin C or vitamin E or both, most often in combination with other micronutrients.[169,202,217,218,221–223,225–232] While two studies noted beneficial effects against proliferation or adenoma recurrence,[217,228] several larger trials conducted over longer periods failed to demonstrate significant effects against adenoma recurrence and CRC incidence.[202,218,231] In addition, one of the largest trials, involving 15,538 male smokers given α-tocopherol, reported a statistically significant (66%) increase in colorectal adenomas[221] but a discordant, nonsignificant (16%) reduction in CRC incidence.[222] Explanations for these findings include a slightly higher rate of gastrointestinal symptoms (e.g., gastrointestinal bleeding), which may have led to more endoscopies in those on vitamin E, although this explanation is quite speculative. Long-term follow-up will be essential to determine the importance of the higher rates of adenomas in the persons receiving vitamin E. Another large trial, evaluating the incidence of cancer in 15,000 persons taking a combination of antioxidant agents, is ongoing.[229,230] An early therapeutic trial of vitamin C used a very high dose of 10 g/day, yet failed to show an effect against CRC progression or overall survival in 100 patients with therapy-naive advanced CRC.[233]

Selenium's effect against CRC has been tested (albeit as a secondary endpoint) in a placebo-controlled, randomized trial involving 1312 persons with a history of skin cancer given selenium for several years.[234] At an average follow-up of 6.4 years, Clark et al.[234] reported a significant (58%) reduction in CRC incidence, based on 27 total cases. While far from definitive, this result suggests that further investigation is warranted.

### Folate and methionine

Fresh fruits and leafy green vegetables are rich in folate, whereas red meat, chicken, and fish have relatively high concentrations of methionine. Both folate and methionine supply the methyl groups necessary for critical cellular functions, such as nucleotide synthesis and gene regulation. Diets deficient in methyl donor compounds might contribute to colorectal carcinogenesis by altering the capacity for DNA synthesis, repair, or transcriptional control. Retrospective and prospective studies generally support an inverse association between folate or methionine intake and the risk of colorectal neoplasia.[44,53,70,235–239] Among participants in the Health Professionals Follow-up Study and the Nurses' Health Study, subjects in the highest folate and methionine quintiles had 35% and 25% lower risks, respectively, for distal colorectal adenomas.[44] Additionally, women who reported long-term (≥15 years) use of multivitamins containing folic acid were up to 85% less likely to develop colon cancer. In several studies, the occurrence of colon neoplasms has been shown to be significantly lower among patients with ulcerative colitis who took supplemental folate than among those who did not.[240,241] Finally, alcohol consumption and methylenetetrahydrofolate re-

ductase (MTHFR) gene polymorphisms affect methyl group availability and each of these factors appears to modify the proposed cancer protection benefits obtained from folate and methionine.[44,70,242,243] At least two trials are currently evaluating the efficacy of folate supplements in preventing the development of colorectal adenomas.[244]

### Sucrose

Refined sugars (including sucrose) can affect intestinal transit, fecal bile acid levels, and serum insulin concentration, all of which may play a role in colorectal tumorigenesis.[164,245] Some, but not all, case–control studies have found a positive association between sugar consumption and large bowel cancer risk.[246] In the Iowa Women's Health Study, subjects in the highest vs. the lowest total sucrose intake categories were more likely to develop incident colon cancer (RR = 1.74; 95 CI = 1.06–2.87).[72] Nondairy sucrose-containing foods conferred the largest type-specific RR (RR = 2.00; 95% CI = 1.21–3.30). Despite the latter findings, the evidence of sucrose as a potentially modifiable risk factor for CRC remains inconclusive.

### Coffee and tea

Both coffee and tea have been proposed as preventive agents for colorectal neoplasia. Coffee is a complex mixture of substances that, at least individually, have potentially mutagenic as well as antimutagenic properties.[247] A meta-analysis of coffee consumption and CRC risk showed that frequent drinkers had a 24% lower risk for CRC relative to infrequent drinkers or nondrinkers (OR = 0.76; 95% CI = 0.66–0.89).[248] However, this inverse risk association was heavily influenced by retrospective data. When cohort studies were considered separately, the inverse association disappeared (RR = 0.97; 95% CI = 0.73–1.29). Coffee intake was also found to have no association with recurrent colorectal adenomas in nested analyses from a vitamin supplementation trial.[249]

Tea contains catechins, such as (-)-epigallocatechin-3-gallate, which are powerful antioxidants. The chemopreventive potential of green tea appears to be greater than that of black tea, because catechins are less oxidized in green tea. Case–control studies from China and Japan support a beneficial effect from green tea, but no cohort studies have been reported to date.[250] Prospective evaluations of the possible relationship between black tea consumption and colorectal neoplasia risk have been inconclusive.[84,249,251]

## Lifestyle Factors

### Alcohol

Alcoholic beverages may stimulate colorectal neoplasia growth and development through a combination of direct and indirect mechanisms.[252,253] Ethanol (or its metabolites) can induce cellular proliferation, block methyl group donation, and inhibit DNA repair. The hepatotoxic effects of alcohol might additionally cause altered activation or clearance of colorectal carcinogens. A meta-analysis based on 27 cohort and case–control studies published through March 1989 predicted that 24 g of alcohol (about 2 drinks) per day had only a modest promotional effect on both colon and rectal cancer risks.[254] Subsequent prospective data suggest that these risk associations may be more substantial, particularly among select subgroups of alcohol users. Among male health professionals, the RR for colon cancer with moderate to heavy alcohol consumption (>2 vs. ≤0.25 drinks per day) was 2.07 (95% CI = 1.29–3.32), which rose dramatically to 3.30

(95% CI = 1.58–6.88) when low folate and methionine intakes were also considered.[70] Frequent beer consumption ($\geq$5 vs. <1.1 glasses per week) was significantly associated with rectal cancer risk (RR = 1.8; 95% CI = 1.0–3.5) in the Netherlands Cohort Study, although neither this factor nor other alcohol consumption variables were associated with colon cancer risk in the same population.[85] The most curious finding from the major cohort studies was a 38% risk reduction for distal colon cancer among wine drinkers ($\geq$4 g/day vs. 0 g/day) in the Iowa Women's Health Study, despite the absence of an overall correlation between alcohol use and CRC risk.[77] This unusual observation could be due to undefined hormonal factors that may differentially affect subsite-specific colorectal carcinogenesis in postmenopausal women.

## Tobacco

Tobacco smoke contains a number of putative carcinogens, including polycyclic aromatic hydrocarbons (PAHs), nitrosamines, and aromatic amines.[45] At least 23 prospective studies have investigated the association between tobacco use and CRC risk and report qualitatively and quantitatively different results.[45,160,255,256] One plausible explanation for the discrepancy in risk estimates is that smoking may be an initiator of carcinogenesis in the large bowel and that a prolonged latency period may therefore be required before adverse effects are detectable.[46,66,257] Most of the earlier cohort studies included relatively short follow-up periods and consequently may have underestimated the true risk association. Giovannucci et al.[45] reviewed 17 observational studies and noted that the risk for the development of colorectal adenomas was 2–3 times higher among long-term smokers than among non-smokers. These studies further suggest a dose–response relationship between pack-years of tobacco use and adenomatous polyps. In contrast, Baron and colleagues[258] found no increase in the risk of recurrent adenomas among smokers enrolled in a polyp prevention trial. In total, the epidemiologic data on the association between tobacco use and CRC risk are compelling, though somewhat inconsistent. The inconsistencies may be due in part to the durations of exposure and observation, and longer studies may provide more relevant data.

## Physical activity

The effects of physical activity on colorectal neoplasia risk are difficult to assess from observational data, primarily because of the diversity of metrics and the large number of potentially confounding variables (e.g., dietary habits, other coexisting behaviors, body mass index, and abdominal adiposity). Nevertheless, an inverse association has been observed in multiple studies. Three major hypotheses have been proposed to explain how an active lifestyle might reduce CRC risk. First, increased exertion appears to stimulate intestinal transit, which could diminish the duration of contact between the colorectal epithelium and intraluminal toxins.[259] Second, physical activity may prevent hyperinsulinemia, a putative promoter of colorectal tumorigenesis.[260] Third, energy expenditure has been negatively correlated with the concentration of prostaglandin $E_2$, a procarcinogen, in the rectal mucosa.[261]

Colditz and colleagues[262] recently summarized the existing literature addressing physical activity and CRC risk. Among 23 case–control studies and 18 cohort studies, the risk of CRC is consistently 40%–50% lower among subjects reporting high activity levels than among subjects reporting low levels. The beneficial effects derived from exercise seem to be more pronounced in the colon (particularly the distal colon) than in the rectum. Relatively few studies have investigated the relationship between physical activity and the risk for colorectal adenoma, but the available data suggest an inverse association and a site-specific pattern similar to those reported for CRC.[47,69]

## Chemoprevention

### Elements of Chemoprevention Research

#### Agents

*Cancer chemoprevention* is defined as the use of specific chemical compounds to prevent, inhibit, or reverse carcinogenesis prior to the development of clinical cancer.[263,264] Chemopreventive interventions may be applied throughout carcinogenesis—from the inception of the process before the first relevant genetic aberration, through the cumulative molecular, cellular, and histopathologic alterations (such as the formation of ACF or adenomatous polyps), to the invasion of the neoplastic clone across the basement membrane, which characterizes invasive cancer. Chemopreventive agents are typically used at specific doses and frequencies by defined routes of administration to specific risk cohorts. Persons with germline abnormalities in cancer-promoting genes, such as those with familial adenomatous polyposis (FAP) or hereditary nonpolyposis colorectal cancer (HNPCC), are most likely to benefit from chemopreventive interventions that complement established preventive measures such as screening, surveillance, polypectomy, and prophylactic surgery. In addition, because chemopreventive agents are often administered systemically, they have the potential to reduce the risk of cancer in more than one organ system affected by a given germline condition. Typically, prolonged exposure is anticipated, but at least one study suggests that some chemopreventive agents may not require lifelong administration to be of long-term benefit.[265]

In contrast, as reviewed above, dietary approaches to cancer prevention employ dietary modifications (e.g., higher fiber and lower fat) or isolated dietary substituents (e.g., wheat bran or cruciferous vegetables) to interrupt the carcinogenic process. These approaches are attractive because they may benefit a broad segment of the population rather than only those at greater than average risk. Obviously, there are many areas of overlap between dietary and chemopreventive approaches (e.g., vitamins or calcium). An important difference is that chemopreventive drugs may be useful in high-risk subjects for whom dietary modifications may be inadequate.[146,175]

Antineoplastic phamacologic agents (i.e., chemotherapeutic agents) are traditionally characterized as cytotoxic or cytostatic based on in vitro activity against cancer cell lines. This distinction is primarily qualitative; indeed many cytotoxic agents are cytostatic to different (e.g., more resistant) cell lines, or when given at lower concentrations or for shorter durations. It is likely that agents developed for cancer therapy also have activity against preinvasive neoplasia. Provided that the therapeutic index (i.e., risk vs. benefit) is acceptable for a specific risk cohort, such agents could be developed as chemopreventive drugs as well. Several cytostatic agents—angiogenesis inhibitors, COX inhibitors, farnsyltransferase inhibitors, epithelial growth factor receptor (EGFR) inhibitors—are currently under investigation as both cancer preventive and therapeutic agents.

A preventive agent's therapeutic index depends on the agent's mechanisms of action; pharmacokinetic properties (absorption, distribution, metabolism, and excretion); the intended route, frequency, and duration of use; and the clinical risks and options of the intended cohorts. Each of these factors potentially has enormous impact on the utility of an agent for cancer prevention. Nonsteroidal antiinflammatory drugs (NSAIDs), for example, are associated with a number of unacceptable toxicities, such as gastrointestinal irritation or ulceration, platelet dysfunction, and renal insufficiency. The therapeutic index of this class of drugs might be enhanced through several approaches such as antineoplastic mechanistic specificity (e.g., COX-2 inhibitors); targeted distribution (e.g., topical administration to limit systemic exposure); optimization of dose, frequency, or duration of use; and synergistic combinations with other chemopreventive agents or dietary manipulations (without greater toxicity) (Table 52–7).[266]

## Cohorts

Cohorts appropriate for chemopreventive interventions range from the general population to subsets of the population at greater than average risk owing to germline defects or environmental conditions. Specific examples are outlined (Table 52–8). Environmental risk cohorts include individuals exposed to tobacco smoke or consuming unhealthy diets. Persons at germline risk include those with FAP, HNPCC, Peutz-Jaeger syndrome, and juvenile polyposis syndrome. Additional high-risk cohorts, likely defined by a mix of environmental and germline factors, include persons with inflammatory bowel disease or with first- or second-degree relatives with colorectal neoplasia (i.e., adenomas or carcinomas).

## End points or efficacy biomarkers

Within the colorectum, chemopreventive efficacy is routinely assessed via one or more study end points: cellular or subcellular biomarker modulation in the at-risk mucosa or neoplastic epithelium, regression of prevalent adenomas, suppression of recurrent adenomas following resection, or prevention of incident adenomas in individuals without prior neoplasia. The United States Food and Drug Administration (FDA) has recently re-

**Table 52–7** Methods for improving the therapeutic index of candidate agents (e.g., NSAIDs) for chemoprevention of colorectal neoplasia

*Regimen Optimization*

Dose
Frequency
Duration

*Regional/Topical Administration*

Enema
Suppository
Targeted oral delivery system

*Mechanistic Targeting*

COX-2 selective inhibitors
Sulindac sulfone
*R*-flurbiprofen

*Combination Regimens with*

Calcium
Matrix metalloproteinases inhibitor
Selenium
Ursodiol
Difluoromethylornithine
9-*cis* retinoic acid
HMG-CoA reductase inhibitor
EGFR inhibitor

COX-2, cyclooxygenase-2; EGFR, epidermal growth factor receptor.

**Table 52–8** Cohorts at risk for colorectal cancer

*Environmental Risk*

Age >55 years
Tobacco use
Obesity
Unhealthy diets (low in fruits/vegetables and high in fats)
Personal history of colorectal neoplasia (e.g., aberrant crypt foci [ACF], adenomas, or carcinomas)

*Germline Risk*

Familial adenomatous polyposis (FAP)
Hereditary nonpolyposis colorectal cancer (HNPCC)
Peutz-Jaeger syndrome
Juvenile polyposis syndrome

*Mix of Germline and Environmental Risk Factors*

Inflammatory bowel disease (IBD)
Family history of adenomas or carcinomas

viewed and approved celecoxib on the basis of its ability in conjunction with standard care to reduce the number of colorectal adenomas in persons with FAP (http://www.fda.gov/cder/approval/index.htm). This approval represents an important advance for the field of cancer chemoprevention.

Biomarker studies typically evaluate cellular or tissue morphology, proliferation, apoptosis, and biochemical or molecular effects within the normal-appearing flat mucosa or preinvasive neoplastic lesions to judge the bioavailability and mechanistic pharmacodynamics of a chemopreventive agent. These trials are usually small, quick, and relatively easy to conduct, although estimates of the ultimate benefits (e.g., cancer risk reduction) associated with the use of agents effective in these studies are not necessarily conclusive. Nevertheless, biomarker studies provide an important opportunity to investigate the natural history of molecular and cellular oncogenesis within target tissues, to identify mechanisms of potential chemopreventive agents, and to assess preliminary efficacy.[266] For these reasons, biomarkers are commonly employed as primary end points in early clinical trials or as secondary end points nested within definitive trials.

In adenoma regression studies, subjects with existing adenomas are given chemopreventive agents and evaluated for changes in the size, area, or histopathology of prevalent adenomas. These trials are relatively short and efficient, but the relevance of a positive result is again somewhat uncertain because, by definition, the measured outcome (i.e., regression of prevalent neoplasia) deals with neoplastic lesions that are more advanced than those targeted in incidence reduction trials. Biomarker assessments within the neoplastic lesions are often performed in tandem with the clinical and histopathologic end points to obtain complementary mechanistic data. Adenoma regression trials are particularly sensitive to agents that affect cellular population dynamics—increasing apoptosis or cellular shedding and/or reducing proliferation—within prevalent neoplastic tissues.

Trials of adenoma suppression begin with complete polyp removal by surgical polypectomy, endoscopic ablation, or laser fulguration, followed by adjuvant administration of a potential chemopreventive agent. Subjects are monitored with serial endoscopies, focusing on recurrent adenoma number, size, area, or histopathology. Finally, in adenoma prevention trials, persons harboring germline or somatic mutations but who do not yet manifest the neoplastic phenotype (e.g., ACF or adenomas) are administered chemopreventive agents. Subsequent examinations are performed to gauge the investigational agent's effects on incident polyp number, area, size, and histopathology. Adenoma suppression and adenoma prevention trials may afford the best opportunities to predict whether the incidence of cancer can be reduced. Of course, these trial designs also require the largest sample sizes, longest study durations, and greatest resource expenditures. Each of the four study designs has intrinsic merit, and how they should be integrated to develop optimal chemopreventive compounds in the most efficient and reliable manner is a matter of considerable importance and debate.

The potential direct benefits to personal health from successful CRC chemoprevention for average-risk individuals seem obvious—reducing the frequency of invasive endoscopy; preserving colorectal anatomy; complementing the effectiveness of screening, surveillance, and polypectomy; and treating the chronic disease of neoplasia in a mechanistically targeted manner. Even more likely to benefit are patients with hereditary CRC syndromes, such as FAP or HNPCC, for whom CRC chemoprevention might reduce the need for diagnostic or therapeutic procedures, eliminate the physical disfigurement associated with prophylactic surgery, or reduce the mortality of these diseases, and thereby reduce parental concerns over the passage of a potentially lethal genetic trait.[267] On a public health level, substantial declines in health-care resource utilization may be appreciated through effective CRC chemoprevention. Consequently, strategies that complement (or more optimistically, delay or replace) current management options should be enthusiastically received by patients, physicians, and third-party payers alike.

## Agents in Development

### Nonsteroidal anti-inflammatory drugs

As a class, NSAIDs are structurally diverse, yet seem to share several common activities, namely, to reduce cellular proliferation, to slow cell cycle progression, and to stimulate apoptosis. These antineoplastic effects appear to be significantly, though perhaps not exclusively, linked to the inhibition of COX activity, which facilitates the conversion of arachidonic acid into biologically active prostanoids (e.g., prostaglandins, thromboxanes, and prostacyclins) that are believed to be important promoters of carcinogenesis.[268,269] COX activity is derived from two isozymes: COX-1 and COX-2. COX-1 is constitutively expressed and is believed to play a homeostatic and physiologic role, whereas COX-2 is induced by growth factors, cytokines, and tumor promoters and contributes to both inflammation and neoplasia. Traditional NSAIDs, such as aspirin or sulindac, suppress the activities of both isozymes, resulting in profound anticancer effects as well as unintended toxic effects such as gastric ulceration, renal insufficiency, and bleeding.[270] COX-2 is commonly overexpressed in colorectal carcinogenesis; studies demonstrate its presence in more than 50% of adenomas and in 80%–85% of adenocarcinomas, whereas it is rarely expressed in normal colorectal epithelium.[271] This overexpression appears to be functionally important for neoplastic progression, as evidenced by the lower incidence of intestinal polyps in mice without a functional COX-2 gene.[272] These and other data suggest that selective inhibition of the COX-2 isoenzyme offers a more refined target for CRC prevention with fewer side effects, compared with nonselective COX inhibitors.[273] Finally, there is some evidence that NSAIDs and NSAID derivatives such as *R*-flurbiprofen and sulindac sulfone may also regulate cell growth via COX-independent pathways.[274,275]

More than 90 studies in rodent models of both genetic and carcinogen-induced colon carcinogenesis have been conducted with NSAIDs or NSAID derivatives (data not shown). With few exceptions,[276–282] these studies have demonstrated the profound activity of NSAIDs against most stages of colorectal carcinogenesis including aberrant crypt formation; adenoma and adenocarcinoma multiplicity, incidence, and size; metastasis; and survival. The NSAIDs prevent the development of neoplastic lesions and in some cases are effective in regressing established adenomas. The remarkable consistency of data across animal models, investigators, time, specific agents within this class, and end points inspires considerable confidence in the validity of the observations. In addition, several animal studies suggest that combinations of NSAIDs with other effective chemopreventives, including difluoromethylornithine,[283–287] epidermal growth factor inhibitors,[288] or lovastatin,[289] may be even more effective.

Among 30 studies (21 retrospective[290–310] and 9 prospective[59,68,311–318]), all studies but two[311–313] reported statistically significant inverse associations between NSAID use and colorectal neoplasia risk (Figs. 52–2 to 52–4), with reductions ranging from 16% to 92% (averaging approximately 40%–50%) for adenomas, incident cancers, or fatal cancers among demographically diverse populations. The first negative study, which prospectively evaluated 12,180 residents of a large retirement community with a median age of 73 years,[311,312] reported an association between daily aspirin use and increased CRC risks for both men (RR = 1.38) and women (RR = 1.10) after 8.5 years of follow-up. Subsequently, an observational follow-up of the Physicians' Health Study reported no effect of aspirin against incident CRC.[313] These atypical results may be related in part to misclassification of the exposure variable measured at baseline or to cohort idiosyncrasies. A recent positive study is noteworthy as well. Garcia-Rodriguez and Huerta-Alvarez[318] conducted a population-based cohort study with a secondary case–control analysis of more than 940,000 individuals in the United Kingdom. They noted a significant 40% reduction in colorectal cancer risk among long-term aspirin users taking 300 mg daily, but no significant benefit in persons taking 75 or 150 mg aspirin daily. In sum, the observational data are compelling in their strength and consistency, clearly suggesting the preventive effectiveness of COX inhibitors against all stages of sporadic colorectal neoplasia.

In the setting of germline risk, more than 15 case series and reports have described the effects of NSAIDs, primarily sulindac, against prevalent adenomas in persons with FAP (Table 52–9).[267] The first report described almost complete regression of colorectal adenomas in four patients treated with sulindac over 4–12 months.[319] Subsequent studies have reported significant reductions in adenoma size and number associated with sulindac or indomethacin treatment. Furthermore, four controlled trials have shown significant reductions in colorectal adenoma size or number or both with sulindac (Table 52–10).[320–323] Responses to NSAIDs are generally evident within a few months; however, complete regression of all tumors is rare, and the long-term implications of NSAID administration have yet to be established. To date, four cases of CRC diagnosed in FAP patients while taking sulindac have been reported.[324–328] However, these cases are difficult to interpret, given that the total number of treated individuals is unknown and some of these cancers may have predated treatment with sulindac and only became visible after reduction of the general polyp burden. Moreover, the clonal burden of subjects with FAP may be too great to be controlled by any single chemopreventive agent.

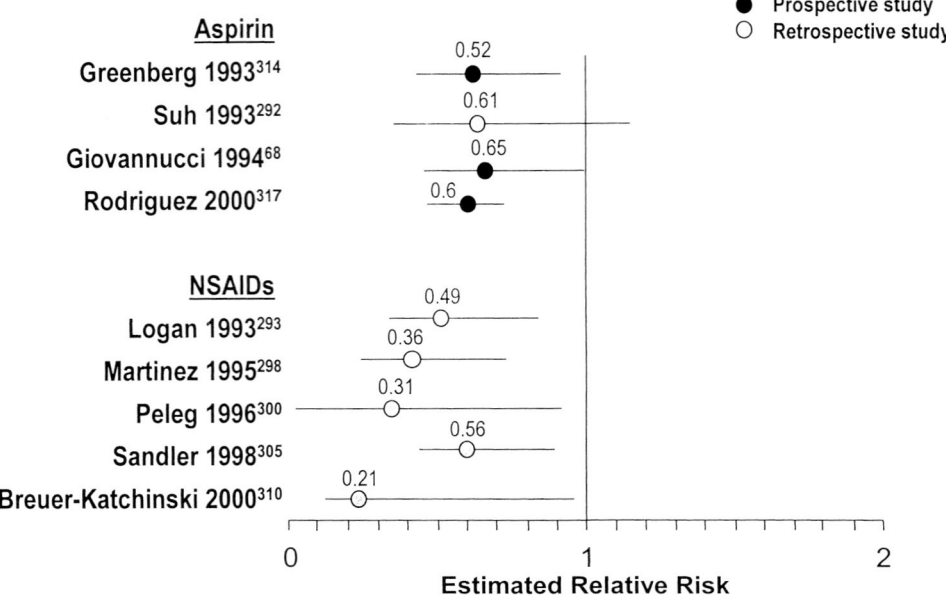

**Figure 52–2** Nonsteroidal anti-inflammatory drug (NSAID) use and colorectal polyp/adenoma incidence.

Chemoprevention of sporadic colorectal neoplasia with NSAIDs has been reported experimentally in three small studies measuring polyp regression[329–331] and in one large, controlled trial evaluating cancer occurrence.[332] Mixed results were obtained in the regression studies after 4–6 months of sulindac or piroxicam therapy, although a trial by Disario (reported only in abstract form) observed significant regressions when sulindac was administered over 12 months. The most definitive NSAID chemoprevention trial reported thus far is the Physicians' Health Study (PHS), in which 22,071 subjects were randomized to re-

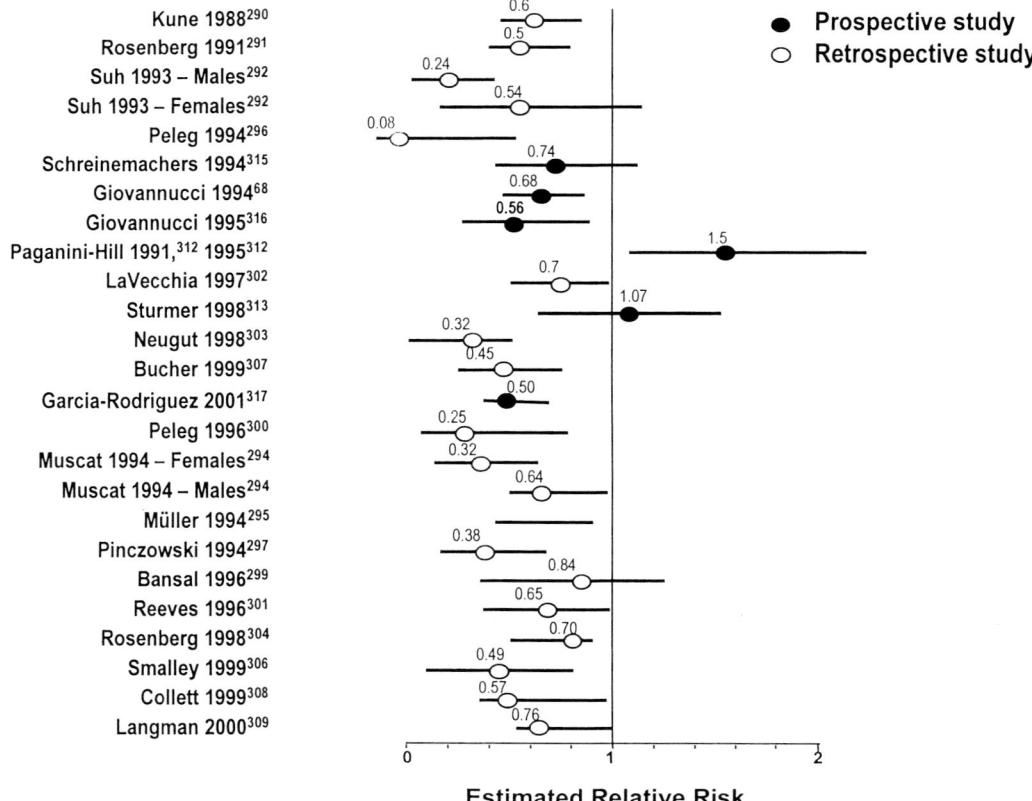

**Figure 52–3** Nonsteroidal anti-inflammatory drug use and colorectal cancer incidence.

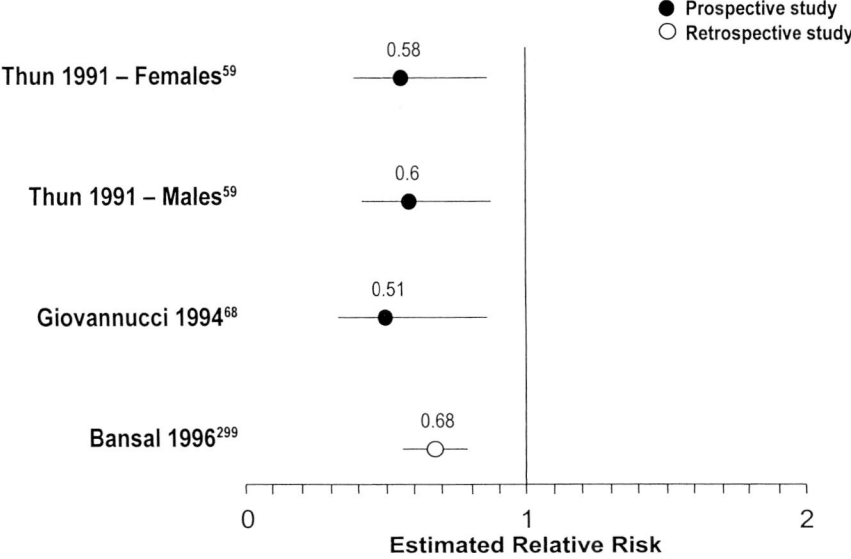

**Figure 52–4** Nonsteroidal anti-inflammatory drug use and colorectal cancer mortality.

ceive aspirin 325 mg every other day or placebo for an average of 5 years.[332] At the end of the initial follow-up period, no significant difference was seen between intervention groups in the self-reported frequency of new large bowel malignancies (RR = 1.15; 95% CI = 0.80–1.65). Extension of the follow-up period to 12 years did not significantly alter the incidence rate ratio

(RR = 1.07; 95% CI = 0.67–1.70), though presumably many of the participants randomized to receive placebo would have taken cardioprotective doses of aspirin following the demonstration of cardiovascular preventive effects.[313] Design limitations of the PHS must be considered, particularly the highly selective nature of the cohort (in contrast to the diverse at-risk population in

**Table 52–9** Nonsteroidal anti-inflammatory drugs and prevention of colorectal neoplasia in familial adenomatous polyposis patients, uncontrolled studies

| Study | Sample Size[a] | Intervention[b] | Primary Result(s) |
|---|---|---|---|
| Waddell and Loughry[319] | 4 | Sulindac 75–150 mg po bid × 4–12 months | Adenoma number, reduced |
| Gonzaga et al.[546] | 1 | Sulindac (not specified) × 12 months | Adenoma number, reduced |
| Waddell et al.[547] | 10 | Sulindac 75–200 mg po bid × 21–92 months | Adenoma number, reduced |
| Charneau et al.[548] | 8 | Sulindac 200–300 mg po qd × 1–8 months | Microadenoma number, reduced |
| Friend[549] | 3 | Sulindac 150 mg po qd–bid × 1.5–3 months | Adenoma number, reduced |
| Iwama et al.[550] | 10 | Sulindac 150 mg po qd × 3 months | Adenoma number and size, no overall effect<br>Mild reduction in selected subjects |
| Rigau et al.[551] | 4 | Sulindac 200 mg po bid × 6 months | Adenoma number and size, reduced<br>Prostanoids reduced* |
| Tonelli et al.[324,552] | 13 | Sulindac 100 mg po bid × 6 months | Adenoma number and size, reduced[c] |
| Muller et al.[553] | 10 | Sulindac 100 mg po tid × 4 months | Adenoma number and size, reduced |
| Niv and Fraser[325] | 1 | Sulindac 150 mg po tid × 16 months | Adenoma burden, no overall effect[c] |
| Spagnesi et al.[554] | 20 | Sulindac 100 mg po bid × 2 months | Adenoma number or size, reduced*<br>Proliferative index, no effect |
| Thorson et al.[326] | 1 | Sulindac 150 mg po bid × 3 months | Adenoma number, reduced[c] |
| Giardiello et al.[555] | 22 | Sulindac 150 mg po bid × 3 months | Adenoma number and size, reduced* |
| Hirata et al.[556] | 2 | Indomethacin 50 mg ir qd–bid × 1–3 months | Adenoma number, reduced |
| Hirota et al.[557] | 7 | Indomethacin 50 mg qd–bid × 1–2 months | Adenoma number, reduced*<br>Proliferative index, increased |
| van Stolk et al.[336] | 18 | Sulindac sulfone 200–400 mg po bid × 6 months | Adenoma number and size, stable<br>Apoptosis within lesions, increased |
| Dolara et al.[348] | 7 | Nimesulide 2 mg/kg qd po × 2.5 months | Endoscopic effect, none<br>Proliferative index, unchanged |

bid, twice a day; po, orally; qd, every day; tid, three times a day.

*Statistically significant result ($P < 0.05$).

[a]Number of subjects evaluated at study completion.

[b]Duration of agent administration until described effect.

[c]One subject with adenocarcinoma on extended follow-up.

**Table 52-10** Nonsteroidal anti-inflammatory drugs and prevention of colorectal neoplasia in familial adenomatous polyposis patients, controlled trials

| Study | Sample Size[a] | Design[b] | Intervention[c] | Primary Result(s) |
|---|---|---|---|---|
| Labayle[320] | 9 | DBRXT | Sulindac 100 mg po tid × 4 months | Adenoma number and size, reduced* |
| Giardiello[321,328] | 22 | DBRCT | Sulindac 150 mg po bid × 9 months | Adenoma number and size, reduced* Mucosal prostanoids, reduced*[d] |
| Nugent[322] | 14 | DBRCT | Sulindac 200 mg po bid × 6 months | Adenoma burden, reduced* Proliferative index, reduced* |
| Winde[323] | 38 | CCTRL | Sulindac 25–150 mg ir bid × 3–48 months | Adenoma number and size, reduced* Proliferative index, reduced* Prostanoids, reduced |
| Steinbach[349] | 77 | DBRCT | Celecoxib 100, 400 mg po bid × 6 months | Focal and global adenoma number and burden, reduced* (400 mg bid dose vs. placebo) |

bid, twice a day; ir, intrarenal; po, orally; tid, three times a day.

*Statistically significant result ($P < 0.05$).

[a]Number of subjects evaluated.

[b]DBRCT, double-blind, randomized, controlled trial; DBRXT, double-blind, randomized, crossover trial; CCTRL, case–control study.

[c]Duration of agent administration until described effect.

[d]One subject with adenocarcinoma on extended follow-up.

the United States, all subjects in the PHS were male physicians), the lack of uniform colorectal surveillance guidelines, and the limited aspirin dose and treatment duration. Three ongoing phase III trials of aspirin in colorectal adenoma and CRC prevention are using the same or higher doses in diverse cohorts and will therefore provide additional data on aspirin's effectiveness as a chemopreventive agent.[244]

### Nonsteroidal anti-inflammatory derivatives and selective COX-2 inhibitors

Nonselective COX inhibitors (i.e., traditional NSAIDs) cause significant side effects in approximately 3% of chronic users, creating considerable incentive to develop related compounds with improved safety profiles that retain chemopreventive efficacy. The sulfone metabolite of sulindac, sulindac sulfone, reportedly does not produce appreciable COX inhibition or anti-inflammatory activities in animal models, but significantly reduces tumor incidence, multiplicity, and burden in azoxymethane (AOM)-treated rats when administered early.[333,334] However, the effects in *Min* mice have been less striking.[275,335] A phase I/II trial in 18 FAP patients over 6 months suggests that sulindac sulfone, unlike sulindac, does not induce polyp regression but, compared with historical controls, may stabilize polyp numbers.[336] Additional clinical trials have been undertaken but are not yet published.

*R*-flurbiprofen is an enantiomer believed to lack the ulcerogenic tendency of racemic mixtures of the parent molecule.[337] Two studies in *Min* mice have shown substantial reductions in tumor multiplicity and prolonged survival, although species-specific racemization may explain part of the observed efficacy.[275,338] To date, no human trials have been reported.

Selective COX-2 inhibitors recently approved for treatment of arthritis and pain provide yet another avenue for improving the therapeutic index of NSAIDs to allow their use in cancer prevention settings.[269,339] Compared with normal mucosa, COX-2 is overexpressed in 50% of adenomas and 80%–85% of adenocarcinomas in the colorectum, providing a specific target for antineoplastic interventions. Nine studies of COX-2 selective inhibitors—two with NS-398, one with MF tricyclic, two with nimesulide, one with rofecoxib, and three with celecoxib—have

proven the efficacy of this class of agents in reducing ACF and colorectal tumors in carcinogen- and genetically driven rodent models at nontoxic doses.[272,340–347] The first study by Oshima et al.[272] was particularly noteworthy for three reasons. First, it showed that COX-2 is overexpressed at a very early stage of adenoma formation. Second, it demonstrated that a selective COX-2 inhibitor (MF tricyclic) was at least as effective as a nonselective COX inhibitor, sulindac. Third, the study provided direct evidence of the mechanistic importance and specificity of COX-2 inhibition, since a knockout mutation of the *COX-2* gene resulted in significant reductions in adenomas, with the percentage of inhibition being proportional to the degree of genetic impairment (i.e., *COX-2* null mice had fewer adenomas than did *COX-2* heterozygous mice, which in turn had fewer adenomas than *COX-2* wild-type mice).

On the basis of these preclinical data, COX-2 selective inhibitors have now advanced to human trials in cancer prevention. Although a small case series reported that nimesulide administered over 10 weeks did not reduce the rectal adenoma burden in seven persons with FAP,[348] a randomized, placebo-controlled trial of celecoxib administered over 6 months to 83 subjects with FAP showed significant regression and reductions in colorectal adenoma number and size, with a frequency and profile of side effects comparable to those of placebo (Table 52–10).[349] In addition, celecoxib improved the endoscopic appearance of both the colorectum and the duodenum of these patients, which suggests that it may reduce neoplastic risk in both organs. These data served as the premise for a landmark FDA approval of celecoxib to complement the standard care (i.e., surveillance and prophylactic surgery) of patients with FAP. Whether celecoxib, or any single drug, can reduce the extraordinarily high cancer risk of this cohort needs to be established in long-term trials. On the basis of positive results in FAP adenoma regression, celecoxib is now under study in additional clinical trials involving persons at elevated risk for CRC due to germline mutations or prior sporadic neoplasia.

The long-term benefit of chemopreventive agents can only be definitively established through rigorous trials. Certainly, NSAIDs and COX-2 selective inhibitors are among the most promising agents under investigation and may confer benefits that extend well beyond CRC prevention, such as risk reduction for cardiovascular events, Alzheimer's disease, and other cancers (e.g., esophageal, gastric, bladder, and skin cancers).[64,350–353]

Exogenous estrogens

Estrogenic compounds decrease bile acid flow,[354] thereby lowering the concentration of potentially harmful secondary bile acids within the colorectum. Estrogens may also affect tumor development through cell receptor–mediated mechanisms[5] or by reducing serum insulin-like growth factors,[355] which appear to stimulate epithelial proliferation. More than 35 epidemiologic studies have evaluated the association between exogenous estrogens (alone or in combination with progestins) and the risk of colorectal neoplasia. In a recent meta-analysis (including 10 prospective studies) reported by Grodstein and others,[356] the composite relative risk for women who had ever used postmenopausal hormone therapy relative to those who had never used such therapy was 0.80 (95% CI = 0.74–0.86) for colon cancer and 0.81 (95% CI = 0.72–0.92) for rectal cancer. Current use was associated with an even greater risk reduction (34%), although the total duration of use was not an important effect modifier. Substantially fewer studies have examined the risk association between estrogen-containing compounds and colorectal adenomas, but the existing data appear to support a protective effect.[49,357–360] Because of the strength of these associations and the number of women who are presently exposed to these compounds, exogenous estrogens might contribute substantially to CRC prevention. The Women's Health Initiative Trial will help to confirm or refute the observational data.[147]

Difluoromethylornithine (DFMO or eflornithine)

Difluoromethylornithine is an enzyme-activated, irreversible inhibitor of ornithine decarboxylase (ODC), the enzyme that catalyzes the conversion of ornithine to putrescine.[361] This conversion is the first critical step in the synthesis of polyamines, which are ubiquitous and strongly implicated in cell proliferation. The role of ODC and polyamines in neoplasia are evident from several lines of research. NIH 3T3 cells are induced to a transformed phenotype via experimental overexpression of ODC. In addition, several types of tumor promoters have been shown to increase ODC activity. In human and animal tissues treated with carcinogens, ODC activity and polyamine content of colorectal adenomas and cancers are markedly higher than those of adjacent normal or healthy control tissues.[362,363] Meyskens and Gerner[364] have hypothesized that the loss of functional APC, common in human and animal colorectal carcinogenesis, may result in overexpression of c-myc, which in turn would lead to overexpression of ODC mRNA, excess polyamines, and supraphysiologic epithelial proliferation. Some recent data suggest that ODC activity is indeed linked to the APC signaling pathway.[365] Finally, DFMO consistently and profoundly suppresses polyamine concentrations and tumorigenesis in carcinogen-driven, genetic, and xenograft-based preclinical models of colorectal carcinogenesis.[283–286,366–375] More specifically, DFMO exerts its most profound effect on the post-initiation phase of tumorigenesis,[371] reducing the incidence, multiplicity, and growth rate and/or volume of aberrant crypt foci, adenomas, and carcinomas.[286,372,375,376]

There are several mechanistic explanations for DFMO's preventive efficacy. At the cellular level, DFMO results in the depletion of cellular polyamines, which reduces proliferation in neoplastic cells but leaves normal colorectal epithelium unaffected in at least some models.[286,368,376] A proapoptotic effect of DFMO has been described in a carcinogen-induced animal

model.[286] At the molecular level, a variety of other DFMO effects have been described—reductions in AOM-induced tyrosine phosphokinase activity,[377] accumulation of decarboxylated adenosyl methionine with attendant terminal differentiation and genome-wide loss of DNA methylation,[378] reductions in cellular prostanoid levels,[376] and reductions in AOM-induced cells with mutated ras genes.[379]

Difluoromethylornithine was first tested as a chemotherapeutic in the late 1980s. Despite promising in vitro and in vivo testing, phase II treatment trials at doses of 2–8 g/m²/day were associated with significant thrombocytopenia, nausea, vomiting, abdominal pain, diarrhea, and reversible hearing loss.[380,381] In the early 1990s, DFMO's potential as a chemopreventive agent was recognized, and DFMO was retested in several trials at doses several times lower than those used in the earlier therapeutic trials.[382–384] Initial trials demonstrated that ODC activity and polyamine concentrations could be suppressed in relevant target tissues, including the colorectum, at doses of 0.2–1.0 g/m²/day, with a dose-limiting toxicity of reversible hearing loss. Subsequent trials have confirmed that DFMO at doses of 0.2–0.4 g/m²/day over 12 months significantly suppress rectal polyamine levels in patients with personal or familial histories of colorectal neoplasia and is reasonably tolerated, with rare reports of ototoxicity.[385,386]

Exciting data on DFMO suggest that the drug shows synergistic efficacy in combination with other chemopreventive agents.[283–287,373,374,387] Five studies show that the combination of DFMO with a COX inhibitor (e.g., piroxicam or aspirin) acts synergistically to reduce intestinal neoplasia compared with placebo, even when doses are reduced by 50%.[283–287] Two NCI-contracted clinical trials are currently testing DFMO combined with NSAIDs in subjects with prior sporadic adenomas and in persons with FAP. The synergistic efficacy of DFMO has been demonstrated not only with COX inhibitors but also in vitro and in vivo with mitomycin C,[373] cyclosporine,[387] and selenium.[374] Finally, in animal models, DFMO appears to be active against carcinogenesis in a wide variety of target organs, which suggests that this agent may be particularly promising for cancer risk reduction at multiple sites (e.g., inheritable cancer syndromes).

Ursodeoxycholic acid

Unconjugated fecal bile acids are mutagenic and cytotoxic to the colorectal epithelium, possibly promoting the transformation of adenomatous lesions to invasive carcinoma.[388,389] Deoxycholic acid, a secondary bile acid, stimulates colorectal epithelial proliferation in animal models.[390] In humans, serum levels of deoxycholic acid have been shown to correlate with rectal mucosal proliferation rates.[390]

Ursodeoxycholic acid (UDCA), a noncytotoxic, hydrophilic epimer of chenodeoxycholate, has shown promising chemopreventive efficacy in two rat models of colorectal carcinogenesis.[391,392] Specifically, Earnest et al.[391] described a significant reduction in the incidence of both AOM-induced colorectal adenomas and carcinomas after exposure to UDCA.[391] More recently, Narisawa and colleagues[392] reported significant reductions in colorectal ACF, tumors, and telomerase levels in response to UDCA treatment. The mechanisms underlying these effects are not yet completely defined. UDCA stimulates expression of major histocompatibility complex antigens on premalignant tissues, modulates carcinogen-induced changes in protein kinase C, and stabilizes cellular membranes.[393–397] More intriguing, however, are recent reports that UDCA reduces the mucosal concentrations of phospholipase A2 at the mRNA and protein levels, the concentrations of mucosal PGE2 and 6-keto PGF 1-α, and the incidence of aberrant crypt foci in azoxymethane-exposed rats.[398] In the only clinical chemoprevention data published thus far, UDCA administered at 10 mg/kg/day over an average of 9.2 months did not change rectal mucosal proliferation in 19 patients,[399] however a recent cross-sectional study reported a significantly lower prevalence of colonic dysplasia in patients with ulcerative colitis and sclerosing cholangitis who were treated with UDCA.[400] Given that UDCA therapy among patients with primary biliary cirrhosis (the only current FDA-approved indication for usage) is virtually free of serious side effects,[401] further research is certainly warranted. Clinical data regarding UDCA effectiveness in colorectal adenoma chemoprevention are expected from two ongoing phase III trials in postpolypectomy patients.[402]

### 3-Hydroxy-3-methylglutaryl coenzyme A (HMG-CoA) reductase inhibitors

In addition to their known cholesterol-lowering effects, HMG-CoA reductase inhibitors suppress cell growth in several model systems.[403–405] Data show that this class of agents may be active against two conditions that account for most mortalities in the United States, namely, cardiovascular and malignant diseases. Lovastatin, pravastatin, and simvastatin have been found to inhibit carcinogen-induced colon tumors in mice,[289,406,407] but relevant human data are sparse. Hebert and colleagues[408] conducted a meta-analysis of 29,000 subjects treated with HMG-CoA reductase inhibitors for an average of 3.3 years and observed no significant effects on cancer incidence overall (RR = 1.03, 95% CI = 0.90–1.17).[408] To our knowledge, no clinical intervention studies specifically focused on HMG-CoA reductase inhibitors and colorectal tumorigenesis are under way.

### Perillyl alcohol/limonene

Perillyl alcohol is a hydroxylated derivative of *d*-limonene. Both substances are reported to selectively inhibit post-translational isoprenylation of small guanine nucleotide-binding (G) proteins, including the *ras* oncogene product.[409,410] Additional chemopreventive activities attributed to perillyl alcohol include inhibition of tumor cell proliferation, induction of apoptosis, and induction of carcinogen-metabolizing phase II enzymes. Preclinical evidence indicates that *d*-limonene and perillyl alcohol inhibit carcinogen-induced ACF, as well as the incidence and multiplicity of colorectal tumors, probably through the induction of apoptosis.[411,412]

### Protease inhibitors

Bowman-Birk inhibitor (BBI), a protease inhibitor derived from soybeans, suppresses carcinogen-induced transformation in vitro and carcinogenic progression in vivo. In 1985, Weed and colleagues[413] reported a significant reduction in adenomas in dimethylhydrazine (DMH)-treated mice given nontoxic doses of a soybean extract. Subsequently, BBI was isolated and found to inhibit adenomas in a similar manner to that of the soybean extract, with the key functional activity being a trypsin inhibitory domain.[414] In *Min* mice, BBI caused approximately a 50% reduction in the number of tumors in both the small intestine and colon and a 40% reduction in colon tumor incidence.[415] One preclinical study suggests that BBI is useful in treating inflammatory bowel disease and reduces the attendant neoplastic risk.[416] Bowman-Birk inhibitor also demonstrates substantial preclinical activity in several other target organs and seems to be well tolerated; investigations in humans are ongoing.[417]

Matrix metalloproteinases (MMPs) have traditionally been implicated in later steps of carcinogenesis, such as basement membrane invasion and metastasis. Recently, however, Matrisian and colleagues[418] have demonstrated that one MMP family member, matrilysin, is frequently expressed in adenomas in *Min* mice and humans, and that it can, surprisingly, be immunolocalized to the lumenal surface of dysplastic crypts.[419] A strain of *Min* mice genetically engineered to be deficient in matrilysin exhibited a 60% reduction in tumor multiplicity and reduced tumor size.[419] Subsequently, a study of the synthetic MMP inhibitor batimastat in *Min* mice resulted in a 48% reduction in intestinal tumor multiplicity, suggesting that MMP inhibitors targeting matrilysin may be useful in CRC prevention.[420,421]

### Future Directions in Chemopreventive Agent Development for Colorectal Cancer

Optimizing the therapeutic index of an agent for a given patient cohort is the fundamental goal of all drug development efforts. In cancer prevention, achieving this acceptable balance is particularly challenging because the targeted populations may be heterogeneous, ranging from those at a marginally elevated risk for cancer (e.g., person's with a history of a remote, small adenoma) to those at an extremely high risk (e.g., persons with a highly penetrant, dominant germline predisposition such as familial adenomatous polyposis) compared with the general population. The potential for side effects may be unacceptable in the former, relatively healthy cohort, but completely acceptable to persons who are at extreme risk for incident cancer or who must consider less palatable preventive options such as surgical extirpation of organs at risk. Given the expansion of our understanding of the molecular basis of colorectal carcinogenesis and thus potential targets for biophamacologic interventions in prevention and treatment, we anticipate that colorectal chemoprevention will soon involve a much broader range of agents, as well as agents of greater specificity and activity (Table 52–11).

Most studies to date have examined the chemopreventive effects of traditional pharmacologics. However, recent advances in our understanding of nutrition and the availability of genetically enhanced seeds have created a broad range of food products, engineered foods, and nutriceutical derivatives for prevention testing and development. Vaccines, biologic agents, gene-based agents, and traditional chemotherapeutics are likely to offer additional areas for investigation. Indeed, as chemotherapeutic drugs move away from targeting cytotoxicity a priori to include a wider scope of biologic modulations, the distinctions between therapeutic and preventive agents may be progressively blurred, although the targeted cohorts and ultimate goals of each approach are likely to remain distinct. As new agents are tested in traditional therapeutic settings, there may be opportunities for concomitant efficacy assessments against target organ-based preventive endpoints. This approach may improve the efficiency of agent evaluations (e.g., by obviating the need for phase IIa trials) and create an alternate pathway for the identification of promising preventive agents.

Another major goal of chemoprevention research is to improve the predictiveness and efficiency of clinical trials. Fortunately, the number of promising agents for colorectal cancer chemoprevention is rapidly outgrowing our ability to test each agent in definitive clinical trials. To address this need, a hierarchy of cancer prevention trial designs—phases I–IV—have been promulgated.[422] As in other disciplines, this developmental strategy builds the scientific premise for an agent in an incremental manner, and allows one to prioritize across agents, thus reserving only the most compelling agents for definitive (phase III) tri-

**Table 52–11** Mechanism-driven prevention of colorectal carcinogenesis—proposed molecular targets and interventions

| Proposed Molecular Target | Potential Preventive Agent |
|---|---|
| APC mutation[558] | APC gene or protein replacement[559–561] |
| DCC mutation[562] | DCC gene or protein replacement[563,564] |
| Ras mutation[565] | Farnysltransferase inhibitors,[566] folate[567] |
| COX-2 overexpression[269] | COX-2 inhibitors[272,273] |
| Growth factor overexpression[568-570] | EGFR inhibitors[288,571,572] |
| p53 mutation/hypofunction[3,573] | p53 gene or protein replacement,[574,575] p53-sensitive adenovirus[576–578] |
| Matrilysin overexpression[418,421] | Matrix metalloproteinases inhibitors,[419,420] Bowman-Birk inhibitor[415] |
| Neoangiogenesis[579,580] | Antiangiogenic agents[269,581] |
| IGF overexpression[52,127,582] | IGF inhibitors[583] |
| Aberrant methylation[584–586] | 5-aza-cytidine,[587] folate[588,589] |
| Mismatch repair defects[590] | Gene or protein replacement |
| Telomerase[434,591] | Telomerase inhibitors[592] |

EGFR, epidermal growth factor receptor; IGF, insulin-like growth factor.

als. In this schema, phase I and phase II investigations are necessarily performed using intermediate biomarkers to rapidly provide measures of preliminary efficacy and mechanistic insights. Inherent in this strategy is the need to validate the applied biomarkers for their accuracy, reliability, and predictiveness for later events of ultimate interest. Because of the complex nature of colorectal carcinogenesis, the use of several surrogate end points in tandem may be better than a single measurement performed in isolation. This goal may be facilitated by the recent advent of such technologies as gene expression arrays, which have the capacity to simultaneously evaluate thousands of potentially relevant targets.[423]

Another area in need of further research involves serial measures of drug effects. Adenoma regression has provided some of the most convincing preliminary data on efficacy, but it is problematic to employ in the sporadic setting because of current practice standards. In addition, adenoma regression may be an inappropriate measure of efficacy for some agents. Subclinical neoplastic pathologies such as ACF may be more amenable to serial monitoring since they are not routinely resected at the time of initial identification and can now be quantitatively assessed using high-resolution endoscopy.[11]

The identification of risk cohorts will improve through our progressive understanding of the molecular determinants of carcinogenic progression and the application of that knowledge to improve familial and genetic screening. The identification of important, highly penetrant germline aberrations (e.g., HNPCC-related mutations) that predispose gene carriers to cancer at several sites is increasing the need for chemoprevention. Recently, technologies designed to evaluate personal risk via multiple genetic polypmorphisms of carcinogen-metabolizing enzymes have become available.[424] These technologies offer another approach to improve cohort selection for chemopreventive testing.

Progress in colorectal chemopreventive research depends on the rational application of emerging technologies designed to improve the selection of agents, end points, and cohorts for clinical chemoprevention trials. In the NCI's Chemoprevention Program, a series of trials are conceptualized to move an agent efficiently and effectively along a developmental path from phase I through phase III trials.[422] Recently, NCI's early phase II clinical trials have been conducted using the most promising chemopreventive agents in high-risk genetic cohorts (e.g., FAP) because of the extreme unmet medical need[425,426] and the biologic rele-

vance of APC-driven colorectal carcinogenesis to both the FAP and sporadic settings.[336,349] Because most FAP patients have prevalent neoplastic lesions that progress relatively rapidly, agents can be tested for regressive or preventive effects within a short period. Agents that are effective can then be moved forward into definitive phase III trials in persons with FAP (and in those at elevated risk in the sporadic setting) with greater confidence in the pharmacodynamic relevance of the agent, dose, frequency, and duration of administration (Fig. 52–5).

The most effective means of chemoprevention may involve gene-based interventions that specifically target relevant mutations or their downstream effects. With several phase III trials of promising agents in progress and clear paths to the next generation of definitive trials, we have every reason to anticipate success in bringing effective chemopreventive agents into the standard care of persons at risk for CRC in the near future.

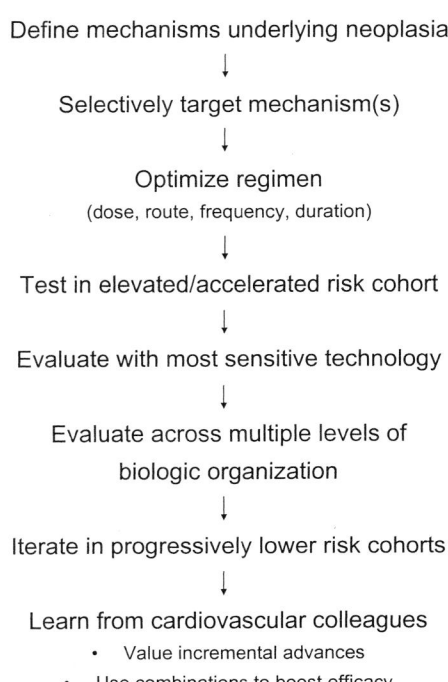

**Figure 52–5** Colorectal cancer prevention–drug development paradigm.

## Colorectal Neoplasia Screening

### Rationale

As outlined earlier, the genesis of colorectal carcinoma is becoming increasingly better understood. Alterations in the structure or function of genes are induced, selectively retained, and expressed cumulatively and sequentially across progressively higher levels of biologic organization and may result in ACF, adenomas, and carcinoma. The evidence for molecular progression underlying this process is compelling, with many genes and signaling pathways apparently involved.[2,92] Similarly, evidence of adenomas as carcinoma precursors (i.e., at the cellular or histopathologic level of progression) is compelling, though necessarily somewhat indirect, because adenomas are usually excised upon discovery to ensure the removal of occult cancer and reduce the risk of cancerous progression. Certainly, most cancers arise from adenomas, although most adenomas do not progress to cancer.[427,428] Nevertheless, ACF, adenomas, and carcinomas are visible with endoscopy and, in the case of larger lesions ($\geq$1.0 cm in diameter), by barium enema as well. Neoplasia evolves over years and is essentially asymptomatic until the later stages. This extended time frame provides enormous opportunities—and responsibilities—for detecting evidence of early neoplasia via colorectal screening long before the onset of symptoms.[429,430]

Screening provides several potential benefits. First, cancers identified at an early stage (stage I or II) have a better prognosis than those detected at later stages.[431] Among persons without cancer, screening serves to identify those who are at greater than average risk owing to prevalent adenomas. Removal of these adenomas reduces the risk of CRC by as much as 70%–90%.[432] In addition, persons with adenomas may benefit from nonsurgical preventive interventions, such as chemoprevention. Therefore, optimal preventive or curative interventions are founded on the early detection of precursors or cancers via endoscopic screening of the colorectum or via detection of neoplastic precursors (i.e., biomarkers) in stool, colonic washings, or, perhaps in the future, in blood.[433,434] Indeed, a reasonable literature now supports the theory that CRC screening, by any of several methods, reduces cancer mortality.[433,435–437] However, to be effective, CRC screening must be recommended by health-care professionals and acceptable to the general population. Assimilation of widely accepted CRC screening recommendations for the U.S. population continues to be slow.[438–440]

## Screening Methods

### Fecal Occult Blood Testing

Stool testing is simple, inexpensive, noninvasive, and theoretically representative of the entire colorectum. For these reasons, and because it is widely available, fecal occult blood testing (FOBT) is currently the most frequently employed method of screening for colorectal neoplasia. Because most small and medium-sized adenomas are associated with negligible blood loss, FOBT primarily detects advanced adenomas and cancer.[430] A positive FOBT requires follow-up diagnostic testing with a complete structural evaluation of the colorectum.

Estimates of FOBT sensitivity and specificity vary because of differences in sample rehydration and the specific tests employed, but have been reported to be as high as 92% and 98%, respectively.[441–445] However, sensitivity may be routinely overestimated owing to failure to confirm negative results, thus prompting certain authors to argue that the true sensitivity of a single fecal occult blood stool test could be as low as 30%.[446,447] Nevertheless, the effectiveness of FOBT to reduce CRC mortality, presumably through the identification of large adenomas or early-stage cancers with subsequent endoscopic or surgical removal, has been documented in two case–control studies;[448,449] one nonrandomized, controlled trial;[445] and three of four randomized, controlled trials (Table 52–12).[442,450–460] Although screening reduced CRC mortality in these trials, CRC incidence in the screened and unscreened arms was generally comparable,[453,456] with one notable exception. Mandel et al.[451] recently reported an approximate 20% reduction in incident CRC after 18 years of follow-up in persons screened annually or biennially compared to controls. The difference in CRC incidence between the American, British, and Danish studies may be a function of the longer duration of follow-up available in the study by Mandel et al. Thus, reductions in CRC mortality may arise from the detection and treatment of cancers at earlier stages over the short term (beneficial stage shift),[442,453,456] and from the identification and removal of adenomas, which reduces CRC incidence, over the longer term.[451] Therefore, despite a variety of valid theoretical concerns related to potential biases (i.e., selection bias, lead time bias, length bias, overdiagnosis bias) in the generation and interpretation of data from screening studies,[461,462] the cumulative evidence derived from well-designed trials involving more than 350,000 participants undergoing a variety of FOBT tests administered annually or biennially suggests that FOBT screening affords a modest though significant reduction in CRC mortality (16%)[463] and incidence (20%).[451]

Despite the favorable reduction in CRC mortality, FOBT screening has important limitations that warrant further study. Proper FOBT technique involves collecting two samples from three consecutive stools for analysis. If any of the six samples is positive, a focused evaluation of the colon should be performed. Because blood is an indirect biomarker for colorectal neoplasia, intermittent bleeding from tumors or other non-neoplastic gastrointestinal lesions may compromise FOBT's sensitivity and specificity. In addition, interpretation of a FOBT is somewhat subjective and may be influenced by dietary factors and recently ingested medications. The low positive predictive value of FOBT further results in frequent follow-up diagnostic evaluations, which add time, expense, complexity, and procedure-related risks to the overall screening program.

Compliance with FOBT screening in the reported trials has been remarkably good—up to 94% in a Danish trial.[456] However, the compliance in community-based screening programs has been far less impressive, reportedly as low as 15%–30% in one study.[464] In addition, because FOBT is a screening test without diagnostic capabilities, a patient's lack of compliance with subsequent diagnostic tests, and the quality of those tests, may undermine a patient's benefit from screening. Indeed, recent reports have noted that up to 25% of subjects with positive FOBTs fail to seek appropriate follow-up care, and as many as 50% of those seeing a physician in follow-up fail to receive an adequate colorectal evaluation.[465]

### Flexible sigmoidoscopy

Approximately 50%–60% of colonic neoplasms are located in the distal 60 cm of the colorectum and are therefore amenable to identification by flexible sigmoidoscopy. The sensitivity of this technique is a function of the adequacy of the bowel preparation, the training and experience of the endoscopist, and the size of

**Table 52-12** Fecal occult blood testing and colorectal cancer

| Study | Period of Conduct | Design/Cohort | Sample Size | Test Employed | Dukes A Cancer (%) Screen | Dukes A Cancer (%) Control | Reduction in CRC Mortality (and Secondary End Points) |
|---|---|---|---|---|---|---|---|
| Wahrendorf et al.[448] | 1983–1986 | Case–control study; population-based in Saarland, Germany; matched by birth year, short period of observation | 1912: 372 cases, 1540 controls | At least one asymptomatic FOBT in prior 6–36 months | — | — | 57% (95% CI = 0.27–0.68) in females*; 8% in males |
| Selby et al.[449] | 1981–1988 | Case–control study; Kaiser Permanente Medical Care Program; matched by age and gender | 1212: 485 cases, 727 controls | At least one screening FOBT in prior 5 years | — | — | 31% (95% CI = 0.52–0.91)* |
| Winawer et al.[445] | 1975–1979 | Nonrandomized controlled trial; New York; persons ≥40 years old | 21,756 | Annual FOBT (primarily nonrehydrated) + rigid sigmoidoscopy vs. annual rigid sigmoidoscopy alone | 43 | 22 | 43% at 10 years follow-up ($P = 0.05$)* |
| Mandel et al.[442,450,451] | 1975–1992 (= period of screening) | Randomized, controlled trial; volunteers Minnesota; 50–80 years old | 46,551 | Rehydrated Hemoccult II – annually vs. biennially vs. control × 10 years | 33 | 25 | 33%* annual, 6% biennial at 13-year follow-up 33%* annual, 21%* biennial at 18 years follow-up PPV = 31% for adenoma and carcinoma; survival advantage* CRC incidence = 20% reduction,* annual 17% reduction biennial* at 18 years follow-up |
| Hardcastle et al.[452,453] | 1981–1995 | Randomized, controlled trial; population-based in Nottingham, U.K.; 45–74 years old | 152,850 | Biennial nonrehydrated Hemoccult × up to 12 years | 20 | 11 | 15%* at 7.8 years PPV = 53% for adenoma and carcinoma; survival advantage* |
| Kronborg et al.[454–456] | 1985–1995 | Randomized, controlled trial; population-based in Funen, Denmark; 45–75 years old | 61,938 | Biennial, nonrehydrated Hemoccult II × 10 years | 22 | 11 | 18%* at 10 years follow-up ($P = 0.03$) PPV = 58% for adenoma and carcinoma; survival advantage* |
| Kewenter et al.[457–460] | 1982– | Randomized, controlled trial; population-based in Gotheburg, Sweden; 60–64 years old | 68,308 | Biennial, nonrehydrated Hemoccult II only screened twice with follow-up of 2–7 years after last rescreening | 34 | 15 | Preliminarily 12% at 16 years follow-up; still ongoing |
| Towler et al.[463] | | Meta-analysis of four randomized, controlled trials | | | | | 16%* |

CRC, colorectal cancer; FOBT, fecal occult blood testing; PPV, positive predictive value. *Statistically significant result.

the neoplasm. Tandem colonoscopic studies have shown that endoscopy can detect lesions less than 5 mm in diameter in approximately 75%–85% of cases and larger lesions in 85%–90% of cases.[466–468] The sensitivity of flexible sigmoidoscopy for lesions in the distal colorectum should be similar. Sigmoidoscopy cannot detect neoplasia in the proximal colon. However, approximately 20% of patients with proximal cancers have synchronous distal adenomas; thus, adenomas found by sigmoidoscopy are often considered an indication for complete colonoscopy, especially if the distal adenoma is large.[469]

Most sigmoidoscopic screening studies have shown that cancers are detected at an earlier stage and that survival rates are higher among those screened than among those not screened (Table 52–13). However, many of these studies lack optimal controls or are subject to a variety of biases. Case–control studies have demonstrated that flexible sigmoidoscopy reduces the risk of distal CRC incidence by 45%–50%[470] and mortality by up to 60%–80%.[471–473] Three large, nonrandomized case series involving sigmoidoscopy (with adenoma removal) have also found an improved survival, favorable stage shifts, or reductions in cancer incidence between those screened and those in various control groups.[474–476] Conversely, Atkin and colleagues did not find a lower CRC incidence rate (standardized incidence rate [SIR] = 1.2, 95% CI = 0.7–2.1) after a mean of 14 years of follow-up in over 1600 subjects receiving one-time screening with rigid sigmoidoscopy plus polypectomy.[95] Two large multicenter randomized trials of flexible sigmoidoscopic screening are under way and should give definitive evidence of the risks and benefits associated with this screening method (and the attendant preventive intervention, polypectomy).[477–479] Nevertheless, in view of the strength and consistency of data already available, many professionals would prefer to screen by colonoscopy rather than flexible sigmoidoscopy.[480]

Endoscopic examination of the distal colorectum by flexible sigmoidoscopy is typically quick, well tolerated, and performed without sedation. Nonetheless, estimates of compliance with flexible sigmoidoscopic screening vary widely, ranging from less than 10% to 100%.[438] A strong family history of CRC is the most common denominator among populations with high compliance rates. In general, the rate of compliance with sigmoidoscopy is considered to be lower than that with FOBT because of patients' fear of procedure-related discomfort and expense.[481]

Disadvantages of endoscopic examination include enema bowel preparation and a 1–2/10,000 perforation rate, which, although quite low, is a potential obstacle to population-based screening.[433,470] Additionally, adenomatous polyps identified by flexible sigmoidoscopy cannot be removed unless the bowel is first cleansed thoroughly. Another obvious limitation of flexible sigmoidoscopic screening is that colorectal tumors originating in the proximal colon (up to 50% of all colorectal neoplasms) will not be detected using this technique alone.[480,482,483]

### Barium enema

Double-contrast barium enema (DCBE) examination represents another CRC screening option. In contrast to flexible sigmoidoscopy, DCBE allows the entire large bowel to be examined for neoplasms. However, as with endoscopic evaluations, adequate bowel purgation is necessary, and the procedure is not entirely risk-free, with the reported risk of perforation or death approximating 1 in 25,000 and 1 in 56,000, respectively.[484] In addition, the quality of an exam and its interpretation is highly operator-dependent—a function of the training, skill, and experience of the radiologist.[485,486] Mass lesions identified radiologically also

require endoscopic or surgical biopsy to establish a tissue diagnosis, since DCBE does not incorporate any therapeutic capabilities. Based on retrospective studies, the sensitivity of barium enema for CRC ranges from 70% to 95%, and its sensitivity for colorectal adenomas <1 cm in diameter is approximately 50%–80%.[487–493] Prospective data are somewhat less impressive, with tumor detection rates ranging from 50% to 75% among patients with signs or symptoms of colorectal disease.[494–496] The false-positive rates of DCBE, which are largely due to retained stool or mucosal irregularities, may be substantial for small polyps (up to 50%), but are less problematic for large polyps (5%–10%) or cancers (<1%).[488,497,498] Two studies have reported that DCBE misses up to 25% of neoplasms in patients with positive FOBTs.[445,496] A recent trial to evaluate the relative merits of colonoscopy vs. DCBE for surveillance found that DCBE had limited sensitivity, detecting only 32%, 53%, or 48% of polyps with a diameter less than 0.6 cm, between 0.6 cm and 1.0 cm, or greater than 1.0 cm, respectively.[499]

No randomized trials of DCBE-based screening have been reported to date; however, one randomized trial compared diagnostic DCBE with flexible sigmoidoscopy in persons with low-grade gastrointestinal bleeding.[500] This 380-patient study demonstrated that colonoscopy was more sensitive than DCBE in detecting polyps less than 0.9 cm in diameter, though the technologies were comparable for lesions ≥0.9 cm.

### Colonoscopy

Colonoscopy is the most sensitive and specific tool currently available for identifying polyps and cancers located anywhere in the large intestine. Experienced endoscopists can perform pancolonic evaluations in greater than 95% of cases.[501] Furthermore, preventive interventions such as polypectomy can be implemented during the initial examination, curtailing discomfort and costs associated with multiple screening and preventive procedures. Tandem colonoscopy studies have shown that approximately 15%–27% of adenomas <1 cm in diameter may be missed by experienced endoscopists.[466–468] In the study by Rex and colleagues,[468] 6% of clinically important neoplastic lesions (i.e., polyps ≥1 cm in size or CRCs) were missed on same-day, back-to-back colonoscopies. A follow-up report by Rex[502] notes that the rate of missed adenomas may be related to the withdrawal technique of the colonoscopist.

Evidence of the effectiveness of colonoscopy as a screening tool derives from one case–control study,[503] several uncontrolled prospective case series,[501,504,505] one controlled prospective case series,[506] and indirect evidence of CRC risk reduction associated with proper management after positive FOBT. Muller and colleagues demonstrated that endoscopy (either proctosigmoidoscopy or colonoscopy) with polypectomy reduces CRC incidence by 40%–50%,[470] and diagnostic endoscopy with appropriate polypectomy significantly reduces CRC mortality (OR = 0.41, 95% CI = 0.33–0.50), with beneficial effects lasting up to 5 years.[473] Rex and others[501] performed colonoscopies in 210 asymptomatic FOBT-negative, average-risk subjects and reported adenomas in 25% of the subjects, along with two Dukes' A cancers. Approximately half the persons with neoplasia did not have distal lesions identifiable by flexible sigmoidoscopy. DiSario et al.[504] performed colonoscopy in 119 asymptomatic, FOBT-negative, average-risk men, 41% of whom had adenomas and 2% of whom had cancer. In another study involving 639 average-risk subjects, Rogge and others[505] reported prevalent adenomas in 34%, with half the lesions located proximal to the sigmoid colon. Thiis-Evensen and colleagues[506] offered flexible sigmoidoscopy with follow-up

**Table 52–13** Sigmoidoscopic screening and colorectal cancer

| Study | Period of Conduct | Design/Cohort | Sample Size | Test Employed | Rate of Sigmoidoscopy | Impact on Incidence, Survival, and Mortality |
|---|---|---|---|---|---|---|
| Hertz[474] | — | Uncontrolled case series; Memorial-Strang Clinic | 26,124 | Rigid sigmoidoscopy | — | Survival rate in 58 persons with cancers = 90% after 15 year follow-up, but no controls or adjustment for biases |
| Gilbertsen[475] | 1948–1976 | Case series compared to Minnesota cancer incidence rates | 21,150 | Annual rigid sigmoidoscopy with polypectomy | Average of 5.4 exams per patient | 85% reduction in rectal cancer incidence; favorable stage shift; 5-year survival was twice the average |
| Friedman[476] | 1964–1980 | Randomized, controlled trial; Kaiser-Permanente, Oakland; 35–54 years old | 10,713: 5156 study; 5557 control | Annual urging for Multiphasic Health Check-up (including sigmoidoscopy ≥40 years old) over 16 years; mean exams in study period = 6:1 | Sigmoidoscopy performed in 8.1% and 5.2% of person-years in study and control groups, respectively | 56%* reduction in colorectal mortality between study and control groups; favorable stage shift (NS); survival rate (NS); difference in those with cancers within reach of the sigmoidoscope not significant |
| Atkin[95] | — | Case series of patients with rectosigmoid adenomas; compared to age, gender, year-specific population rates | 1618 | One-time rigid sigmoidoscopy and polypectomy with 22,482 person years of follow-up (mean = 14 years per patient) | — | SIR = 1.2 (NS); subgroups at high risk were those with large adenomas or those with a villous component or those incompletely excised; small, isolated adenomas caused no increased risk |
| Muller[470, 461] | 1981–dx | Case–control; U.S. veterans; matched by age, race, gender, time of discharge | 32,702: 16,351 cases, 16,351 controls | Any endoscopic procedure (with polypectomy as appropriate) since 1981 | — | 49%* and 45%* reductions in colon and rectal cancer incidence, respectively; protective influence lasting approx. 6 years; 59%* reduction in CRC-associated mortality |
| Newcomb[471] | 1979–1988 | Case–control; Greater Marshfield Community Health Plan; matched by age, gender, enrollment duration | 262: 66 cases, 196 controls | Any screening sigmoidoscopy over 9 years | 10% cases vs. 30% controls | 79%* reduction in CRC death; benefit limited to rectal and distal colon tumors; FOBT and DRE not associated with a reduction |
| Selby[472] | 1971–1988 | Case–control; Kaiser-Permanente Medical Care Program; matched by age, gender, enrollment duration | 1129: 261 cases, 868 controls | Any screening rigid sigmoidoscopy to 30 cm over prior 10 years | 8.8% cases vs. 24.2% controls | 59%* reduction in rectosigmoid cancer mortality; benefit continued for 10 years; adjusted OR = 0.96 for more proximal colon cancers |
| Atkin[477,478] | — | Randomized, controlled multi-center pilot trial; residents of Welwyn Garden City and Leicester; 55–54 years old | 23,246 | Flexible sigmoidoscopy ± colonoscopy vs. passive follow-up | — | Ongoing at 12 centers |
| PLCO[479] | 1994– | Randomized, controlled, multi-center trial; 60–74 years old | 148,000 persons | Sigmoidoscopy at baseline and year 5; up to 16 years | — | Ongoing at 10 centers |

CRC, colorectal cancer; DRE, digital rectal examination; FOBT, fecal occult blood test; NS, nonsignificant; OR, odds ratio; SIR, standardized incidence rate. *Statistically significant result.

colonoscopy to 400 men and women drawn from a population registry in Telemark, Norway. Those who were screened had a reduced risk of CRC (RR = 0.20; 95% CI = 0.03–0.95) but a higher risk of overall mortality (RR = 1.57; 95% CI = 1.03–2.4). In the National Polyp Study, indirect evidence for the effectiveness of colonoscopy with polypectomy was demonstrated by the 75%–90% lower CRC incidence rates observed, as compared with three external reference populations.[432] Finally, the reductions in CRC incidence[451] and mortality[442,450,452–460] from FOBT screening provide indirect though compelling evidence of colonoscopy's effectiveness in reducing colorectal cancer mortality.

Despite these encouraging data, population-based colonoscopy screening programs face substantial challenges. Colonoscopic exams require bowel preparation and conscious sedation. In addition, the rates of complications are higher than with other screening modalities, approximating 1 perforation per 1000 exams, 3 episodes of major bleeding per 1000 exams, and procedure-related mortality in 1–3 per 10,000 exams.[433] In addition, the test is quite costly and is not currently reimbursed by most third-party payers as a screening test for persons at average risk, although this situation may be changing.

Nevertheless, two recent studies demonstrate the potential merits of colonoscopic screening. Mutually confirmatory studies by Lieberman and others[482] and Imperiale and others[483] reported high rates of isolated, advanced proximal neoplasms (approximately 62% in each study) that were inaccessible by flexible sigmoidoscopy, a widely accepted method of screening. Despite all of the suggestions that colonoscopy may be an optimal screening method for CRC, randomized controlled trials have not yet been conducted to fastidiously document its effectiveness in reducing CRC mortality, establish its relative effectiveness over other forms of CRC screening, or determine the risks associated with its use for screening, rather than diagnostic or therapeutic, purposes. A large multi-institutional randomized, controlled trial of colonoscopic screening is being considered to investigate whether a single, screening colonoscopy effectively reduces the incidence and mortality of CRC.[429] Despite gaps in knowledge, some authorities have already questioned the prudence of promoting flexible sigmoidoscopy rather than colonoscopy as the primary endoscopic screening technology,[480] and beginning in July 2001, colonoscopic screening every 10 years will be a covered option in the U.S. Medicare program (http://www.medicare.gov/publications/pubs/pdf/prevent.pdf).

## Current Screening Guidelines

As reviewed in the preceding sections, a large body of data supports the theory that screening, by any of several methods, can effectively reduce CRC mortality. Within the last 5 years, at least four groups—the Agency for Health Care Policy and Research (AHCPR),[433] the United States Preventive Services Task Force,[507] the American Cancer Society,[435,436] and the American College of Gastroenterology (ACG)[437] have promulgated recommendations for CRC screening. Most practitioners accept the AHCPR recommendations regarding the type and frequency of screening as reasonable standard-of-care guidelines because they were developed by a multidisciplinary consortium and endorsed by several scientific/professional bodies, including the American Cancer Society.[433] Coupled with an intensive public awareness campaign stressing the need for CRC screening, these algorithms define the standard of practice as recognized by most patients, physicians, and third-party payers.

Physicians and other health professionals, especially those in the fields of primary care, oncology, gastroenterology, and ge-

netics, should be familiar with the characteristics associated with an increased risk for CRC, as well as the strengths and limitations of available screening approaches. For CRC screening to be worthwhile, the applied technology must be accessible, affordable, and accurate. Unfortunately, none of the existing options is ideal. Patient compliance with the requisite tests, follow-up diagnostic studies, preventive interventions (i.e., polypectomy and perhaps chemoprevention in the future), and long-term surveillance examinations are essential for screening and early detection strategies to be maximally effective. If these stipulations are not met, the program becomes less effective, regardless of the screening modality.

The AHCPR guidelines are presented as an algorithm for CRC screening and surveillance procedures and require sequential symptom assessment, risk assessment, screening, diagnosis, and surveillance (Fig. 52–6). Entry into the screening component is premised on an asymptomatic individual's risk status (i.e., average vs. increased risk for cancer) as determined by personal and family history of colorectal neoplasia and by age.

### Average risk population

Asymptomatic persons aged 50 years or older without a personal history of colorectal neoplasia, significant family history of colorectal neoplasia, or medical conditions associated with increased risk for colorectal neoplasia (such as inflammatory bowel disease) are considered to be at average risk for CRC. This group effectively represents the population well served by generalized screening using current screening options: annual FOBT, flexible sigmoidoscopy every 5 years, annual FOBT with flexible sigmoidoscopy every 5 years, DCBE every 5 years, or colonoscopy every 10 years.[433,436] If any of these tests are positive, complete colonic diagnostic evaluation via colonoscopy or DCBE with flexible sigmoidoscopy is indicated (Fig. 52–6). While this approach is generally regarded as the standard of care, recent guidelines published by the ACG are of interest because for the first time, they suggest that colonoscopy every 10 years should now be considered the "preferred" screening strategy, with flexible sigmoidoscopy every 5 years plus annual FOBT being a reasonable alternative.[437]

### Personal history of colorectal neoplasia

Because persons with a personal history of colorectal adenomas or carcinoma are at increased risk for CRC, periodic colonoscopies are performed following removal of a neoplasm. The frequency of colonoscopic surveillance required post-polypectomy depends on factors such as the number, size, and histology of the baseline neoplasms. Atkin and colleagues[95] demonstrated that persons with adenomas of tubulovillous or villous histology or adenomas larger than 1 cm in diameter were approximately three times more likely to develop CRC than individuals in the general population. In general, to ensure the absence of residual adenomas, a second examination is advised within 1 year. After technically adequate clearing, testing is repeated 3 years later.[96] If the study in the third year is also negative, repeat colonoscopy in 5 years may be appropriate. However, if recurrent adenomas are present at the year 3 study, colonoscopy should be performed again in 3 years. Exceptions to this schema may be considered. For example, the risk of developing CRC among patients with a single, small (<1 cm in diameter), benign adenoma is controversial, and therefore formal surveillance may not be required.[508] However, large polyps (>2 cm in diameter) are typically reassessed after 3–6 months to document complete resection. Cancerous polyps with favorable histology (low-grade) can be managed by endoscopic treatment alone, but follow-up colonoscopy in 3 months may be warranted.[509]

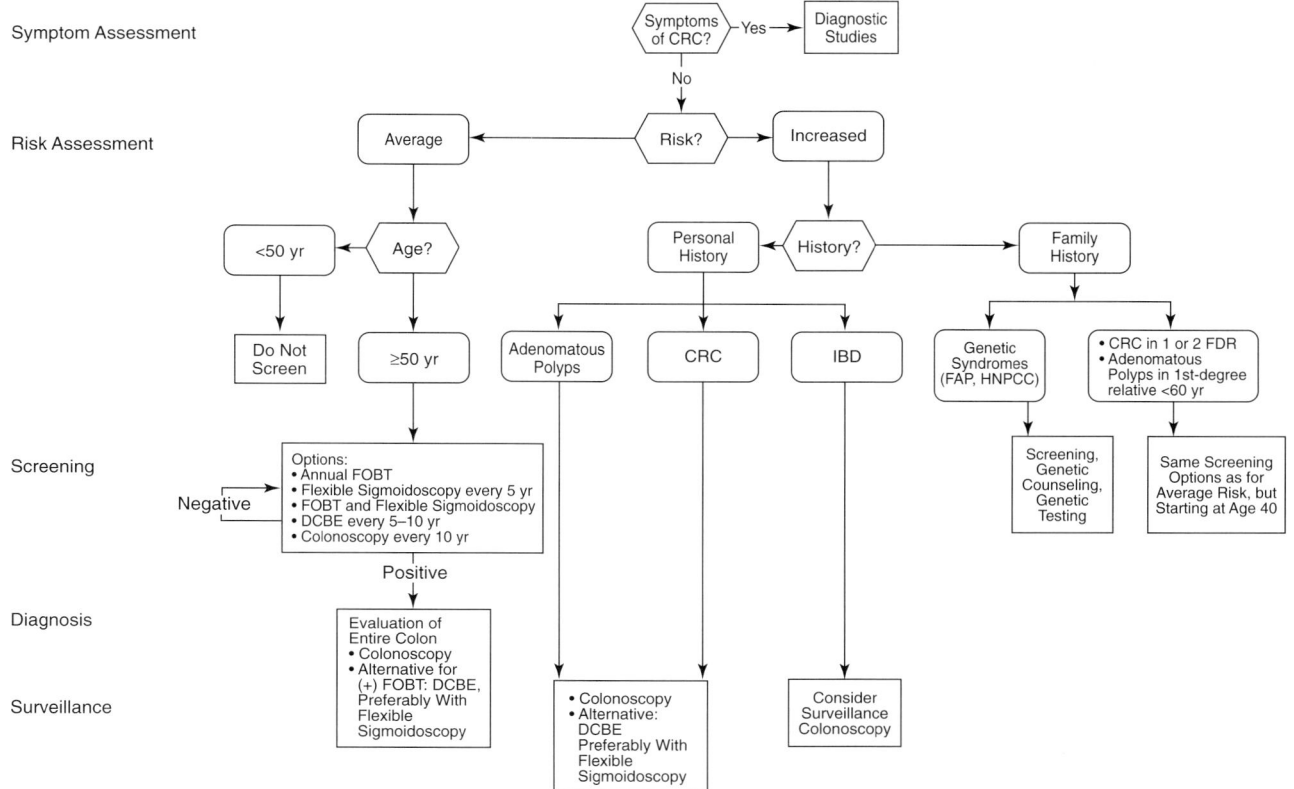

**Figure 52–6** Colorectal cancer screening and surveillance algorithm promulgated by the Agency for Health Care Policy and Research (AHCPR), 1997. (From Winawer SJ, Fletcher RH, Miller L, et al. Colo- rectal cancer screening: clinical guidelines and rationale. Gastroenterology 112:594–642, 1997, with permission.)

Surveillance after curative resection for CRC is essentially identical to that described for patients with prior resected adenomas. An initial perioperative colonoscopy is needed to rule out synchronous lesions. Subsequent evaluations are then performed at intervals of 3–5 years (Fig. 52–6).

## Family history of colorectal neoplasia

Two familial forms of CRC—FAP and hereditary nonpolyposis CRC (HNPCC or Lynch syndrome)—are associated with well-recognized clinical and genetic abnormalities, as described elsewhere. Patients with FAP typically develop polyps after the onset of puberty, which is the time screening colonoscopies should be initiated (Fig. 52–6). Annual examinations are advised until subjects manifest phenotypic expression of the genetic syndrome (i.e., multiple polyps distributed throughout the colorectum), at which point total colectomy is strongly encouraged. The inherited chromosomal abnormality in FAP is likely uniform within kindreds; therefore relatives of individuals with the disease may seek genetic counseling to assess the need for aggressive screening or chemopreventive interventions.

Patients with HNPCC, however, are identified clinically using the Amsterdam criteria: three or more family members with CRC, one of whom is a first-degree relative of the other two, affecting at least two successive generations, with a minimum of one case of CRC diagnosed before the age of 50 years.[510] Persons with HNPCC should undergo colonoscopy at least every 2 years, beginning 10 years prior to the age at which the youngest family member was diagnosed with colorectal cancer. After age 40 years, annual colonoscopy is recommended. Indeed, both colorectal screening[511,512] and surveillance[513] have been shown to reduce CRC mortality (as well as CRC stage and incidence) in persons with HNPCC.

Blood-based testing for germline alterations that predispose to hereditary CRC is available for several known mutations (e.g., *APC* in FAP; *hMLH1* and *hMSH2* in HNPCC).[514] These tests are particularly useful to identify a germline mutation in phenotypically negative individuals from a known FAP or HNPCC family. The most commonly employed test for mutations of *APC* is based on identification of a truncated in vitro protein product,[515] although this test has a clinical sensitivity of only 80% due to mutations outside of the coding region. For HNPCC, commercial testing is available for *hMLH1* and *hMSH2*, two of the six known predisposing genetic alterations.[516,517] Again, this testing is done by an in vitro synthesized protein assay or by gene sequencing in selected individuals who may be at higher than average risk. Assuming that the familial genetic defect is known, these tests can be clinically useful to distinguish between a prephenotypic gene carrier who is likely to benefit from aggressive CRC screening and preventive measures and an individual who does not carry the mutation and who can therefore adopt the CRC screening recommendations for an individual at average risk. While it is possible that subtle germline polymorphisms of carcinogen-metabolizing enzymes, or combinations of them, predispose individuals to CRC, this issue remains experimental.[141]

In the absence of a clear genetic syndrome, persons with a first- (e.g., parent, sibling, or child) or second-degree (e.g., grandparent, aunt/uncle, cousin) relative with CRC before age 55 years or a first-degree relative under age 60 years when an adenomatous polyp is detected should be screened by any of the methods approved for persons at average risk; however, screening should be initiated 10 years earlier (i.e., at age 40 years).

### Inflammatory bowel disease

While data endorsing surveillance colonoscopy in Crohn's disease are currently lacking, two studies have found a screening benefit in patients with chronic ulcerative colitis.[518,519] Monitoring routinely begins after 8 years of disease for those with pancolitis and after 15 years of disease for those with left-sided colitis only. Dysplastic mass lesions arising from areas of inflammation require surgical resection. The optimal management strategy for patients with low-grade dysplasia identified from random biopsies obtained at surveillance colonoscopy remains controversial (Fig. 52–6).

## Screening Utilization and Implementation

Education and adherence by both patients and practitioners to CRC screening recommendations are fundamental to their effectiveness.[520] Screening identifies individuals at greater than average risk, i.e., those most likely to assume risks of side effects and a postdiagnostic surveillance regimen and comply with and benefit from preventive interventions for personal, familial, and public motives. Nevertheless, compliance with any of the available CRC screening modalities is generally suboptimal,[438,521] despite coverage by Medicare and many private insurers. State-mandated insurance coverage for CRC screening is rare, in contrast to mandated coverage for breast, prostate, and cervical cancer.[522]

Participation in FOBT screening varies widely and depends somewhat on the population studied (i.e., patient vs. community based). Overall, median participation is approximately 40%–50% with somewhat greater participation in the context of specific programs and media campaigns as opposed to isolated surveys. Noncompliance with FOBT recommendations is largely attributable to inconvenience, disinterest, cost, embarrassment, noxiousness, lack of symptoms, denial of risk, and technical challenges associated with the test.[438] Despite such limitations, FOBT is a potent tool for which colonoscopy is the effector of screening efficacy.

Adherence to sigmoidoscopic recommendations is highest among those with a family history of CRC (45%–70%), intermediate in those offered worksite-based programs, and lowest in studies of the general population. The most recent U.S. survey conducted by the Centers for Disease Control demonstrated that only 28% of persons aged 50 years or older reported having undergone sigmoidoscopy within the past 5 years.[523] Reasons for nonadherence are similar to those for FOBT—lack of symptoms, inconvenience, disinterest, and cost—but also include concerns about procedure-related pain, discomfort, or injury.[524–526] Despite these obstacles, it appears that having experienced an invasive screening once before may partially alleviate a patient's concerns, because several studies have noted an increased willingness of subjects to undergo the procedure again, as necessary.[527,528] Little is known about subjects' acceptance of colonoscopic screening because the procedure is still not widely practiced. In a recent trial, Rex and colleagues[529] reported that less than 15% of medical personnel responded to an offer to participate in a free colonoscopic screening study.

Strategies to improve participation in CRC screening have included programs targeting the public or at-risk individuals. However, few such programs have included valid and reliable evaluations of effectiveness. This area is an important one for future research; public education programs employed in cardiovascular prevention (e.g., cholesterol education programs, hypertension education programs) may serve as useful models. Women and persons at higher socioeconomic levels typically are more receptive to offers of screening. Ethnic differences are also evident, with minorities being underrepresented in most programs, for multiple reasons. Efforts to promote screening may be advanced by offering multiple screening techniques, embedding testing in the context of routine medical care, and offering incentives such as employer-sponsored programs.[438] The age at which to stop CRC screening, if ever, is a matter of considerable complexity and controversy.

Based on models of cost-effectiveness, CRC screening appears to be an economically sound investment, although effectiveness is contingent upon several key factors, including subject compliance and test sensitivity.[530–533] One recent study determined that CRC costs approximately $15,000–$25,000 per year of life saved, which is on par with many other commonly employed medical procedures.[530] However, it is difficult to rely on modeling for specific recommendations because several different models have been developed, each relies on myriad assumptions, and none have been completely validated.

## Future Considerations

Existing screening methods are effective in reducing CRC mortality, and emerging technologies may prove less invasive, more sensitive, and more specific. For example, computed tomographic (CT) or magnetic resonance (MR) colography, also known as virtual colography, uses sophisticated imaging software to reconstruct complex two- and three-dimensional images of the colon from volumetric CT or MR data. These studies are performed after patients have undergone traditional bowel preparation followed by air-insufflation. Colography detects polyps $\geq 1$ cm in diameter with 75% sensitivity and 90% specificity,[534] although lower sensitivity (38%) and specificity (63%) have been reported.[535] Challenges associated with these approaches include image artifacts from retained colonic fluid or stool and suboptimal colonic distention, as well as long interpretation times.[536] Further research and software development are likely to address many of these flaws. Even so, cost analysis suggests that, if it is to supplant or complement current methods of CRC screening, virtual colography must be inexpensive or improve compliance rates significantly over those obtained with colonoscopy.[537]

Stool-based screening has several advantages over structural screening by endoscopy or CT colography. Fecal screening is noninvasive, requires no cathartic preparations, and can be performed remotely from the medical practitioner's office. Moreover, because these screening methods can target one or, optimally, a cluster of common genetic alterations that underlie colorectal neoplasia, they are likely to be more sensitive and specific than current stool tests. DNA is a particularly appealing target for CRC screening assays because it is released continuously into the fecal stream and in relatively greater quantities than DNA from normal mucosa.[538] Neoplastic DNA has a unique molecular signature that provides multiple targets for screening assays and can be obtained from stool without adjusting dietary or medical regimens. In addition, the DNA is quite stable, allowing for ease of specimen transport and storage. Early investigations targeting single mutations of K-*ras* or *p53* have confirmed that mutations from colorectal neoplasms are detectable in stool.[539–541] Multitargeted detection systems that assess signature genetic alterations are likely to prove even more sensitive and specific, and several proprietary studies utilizing this approach are under way. Preliminary data from one of these studies suggest that stool-based DNA assays may even detect neoplastic lesions high in the aerodigestive tract (e.g., in the esophagus or stomach).[542]

## Conclusion

Colorectal cancer, the second-leading cause of cancer death in the United States, is a preventable disease. However, available screening technologies, although effective, are not consistently applied. This conveys a sobering message: efficient development of new screening tools and chemopreventives is meaningless without professional and public implementation. Results of clinical trials are the critical threshold in discerning useful tools from ingenious concepts. Ironically, new technologies are now prospectively validated in clinical trials against the best available screening tools, which remain vastly underutilized.

Early technologies have limitations (e.g., costs, inconvenience, invasiveness) that typically decrease over time. By foregoing implementation of available CRC screening methods, we not only deprive ostensibly healthy patients the benefits of early detection but also reduce the pace of future developments. Aversion to the existing technology should not dampen enthusiasm for its promise. The efficacy of CRC screening is indisputable, whereas the best techniques, schedules, and cohorts have yet to be defined.

## Note Added in Proof

Since the submission of this chapter, several important developments in colorectal cancer, epidemiology, and prevention have been published. With regard to colorectal cancer screening, workshops convened by the National Cancer Institute[593] and American Association for Cancer Research[594] highlighted the importance of the adenoma as a meaningful endpoint for CRC risk reduction trials. In addition, long-term updates from the FOBT screening studies in Nottingham[595] and Funen[596] show continued reductions in CRC mortality of 13%–27% at 11 years, and 18%–30% at 13 years, respectively, Finally, another summary of the evidence in support of CRC screening have been promulgated by the American Preventive Services Task Force.[597]

In CRC prevention, data supporting the preventive effect of NSAIDs continue to accrue. Most recently, two randomized controlled trials of aspirin in persons at moderate risk for cancer demonstrated significant reductions in recurrent colorectal neoplasia (primarily, adenomas).[598,599] The first trial by Sandler et al. evaluated the efficacy of 325 mg of aspirin per day vs. placebo in 635 patients with prior early stage CRC and reported a significant 35% reduction in recurrent adenomas, with a significant delay in the time to detect a first adenoma.[6] Baron et al. randomized 1121 patients with a prior sporadic adenoma to aspirin at 81 or 325 mg/day vs. placebo and reported a significant 19% reduction (with 81 mg), or nonsignificant 4% reduction (with 325 mg) in patients with recurrent adenomas.[7] While this reverse dose-response is unexplained, both groups experienced a reduced risk of advanced neoplasia (41% and 17% reductions in advanced adenomas/cancer with each dose, respectively). In both trials, aspirin was relatively well tolerated. These trials suggest that patients with a moderate risk of colorectal neoplasia may wish to consider aspirin as a complement to traditional colonoscopic surveillance and polypectomy. Finally, the Women's Health Initiative reported that the use of conjugated equine estrogen with medroxyprogesterone acetate vs. placebo in 16,608 postmenopausal women resulted in a significant 37% reduction in colorectal cancer incidence, although other health risks associated with hormone replacement tempered enthusiasm for this approach to CRC risk reduction.[600]

## References

1. Jemal A, Murray T, Samuels A, et al. Cancer statistics, 2003. CA Cancer J Clin 53:5–26, 2003.
2. Vogelstein B, Fearon ER, Hamilton SR, et al. Genetic alterations during colorectal tumor development. N Engl J Med 319:525–532, 1988.
3. Fujiwara T, Stolker JM, Watanabe T, et al. Accumulated clonal genetic alterations in familial and sporadic colorectal carcinomas with widespread instability in microsatellite sequences. Am J Pathol 153:1063–1078, 1998.
4. Kinzler KW, Vogelstein B. Cancer-susceptibility genes. Gatekeepers and caretakers. Nature 386:761, 763, 1997.
5. Issa JP, Ottaviano YL, Celano P, et al. Methylation of the oestrogen receptor CpG island links ageing and neoplasia in human colon. Nat Genet 7:536–540, 1994.
6. Boone CW, Bacus JW, Bacus JV, et al. Properties of intraepithelial neoplasia relevant to cancer chemoprevention and to the development of surrogate end points for clinical trials. Proc Soc Exp Biol Med 216: 151–165, 1997.
7. McLellan EA, Medline A, Bird RP. Dose response and proliferative characteristics of aberrant crypt foci: putative preneoplastic lesions in rat colon. Carcinogenesis 12:2093–2098, 1991.
8. Bird RP, Good CK. The significance of aberrant crypt foci in understanding the pathogenesis of colon cancer [review]. Toxicol Lett 112–113:395–402, 2000.
9. Shpitz B, Bomstein Y, Mekori Y, et al. Aberrant crypt foci in human colons: distribution and histomorphologic characteristics. Hum Pathol 29:469–475, 1998.
10. Axelrad AM, Fleischer DE, Geller AJ, et al. High-resolution chromoendoscopy for the diagnosis of diminutive colon polyps: implications for colon cancer screening. Gastroenterology 110:1253–1258, 1996.
11. Takayama T, Katsuki S, Takahashi Y, et al. Aberrant crypt foci of the colon as precursors of adenoma and cancer. N Engl J Med 339:1277–1284, 1998.
12. Nucci MR, Robinson CR, Longo P, et al. Phenotypic and genotypic characteristics of aberrant crypt foci in human colorectal mucosa. Hum Pathol 28:1396–1407, 1997.
13. Shpitz B, Bomstein Y, Shalev M, et al. Oncoprotein coexpression in human aberrant crypt foci and minute polypoid lesions of the large bowel. Anticancer Res 19:3361–3366, 1999.
14. Kronborg O, Fenger C. Clinical evidence for the adenoma–carcinoma sequence. Eur J Cancer Prev 9(Suppl 1):S73–86, 1999.
15. McKerrow JH, Bhargava V, Hansell E, et al. A functional proteomics screen of proteases in colorectal carcinoma. Mol Med 6:450–460, 2000.
16. Roche K. The 1st AACR-NCI-EORTC International Conference on Molecular Targets and Cancer Therapeutics. Washington DC, 16–19 November, 1999. American Association for Cancer Research. European Organisation for Research and Treatment of Cancer. Eur J Cancer 36: 286–287, 2000.
17. Schatzkin A, Freedman LS, Dorgan J, et al. Using and interpreting surrogate endpoints in cancer research. IARC Sci Publ 142:265–271, 1997.
18. Temple R. Are surrogate markers adequate to assess cardiovascular disease drugs? JAMA 282:790–795, 1999.
19. U.S. Preventive Services Task Force. Methodology. Guide to Clinical Preventive Services: Report of the U.S. Preventive Services Task Force. Williams & Wilkins, Baltimore: 1996. p. xl–xli.
20. Parkin DM, Pisani P, Ferlay J. Estimates of the worldwide incidence of 25 major cancers in 1990. Int J Cancer 80:827–841, 1999.
21. Hankey BF, Ries LA, Edwards BK. The surveillance, epidemiology, and end results program: a national resource. Cancer Epidemiol Biomarkers Prev 8:1117–1121, 1999.
22. Howe HL, Wingo PA, Thun MJ, et al. Annual report to the nation on the status of cancer (1973 through 1998), featuring cancers with recent increasing trends. J Natl Cancer Inst 93:824–842, 2001.
23. Pisani P, Parkin DM, Bray F, Ferlay J. Estimates of the worldwide mortality from 25 cancers in 1990 [published erratum appears in Int J Cancer 1999;83(6):870–873]. Int J Cancer 83:18–29, 1999.
24. Wingo PA, Ries LA, Giovino GA, et al. Annual report to the nation on the status of cancer, 1973–1996, with a special section on lung cancer and tobacco smoking. J Natl Cancer Inst 91:675–690, 1999.
25. Mayberry RM, Coates RJ, Hill HA, et al. Determinants of black/white differences in colon cancer survival. J Natl Cancer Inst 87:1686–1693, 1995.
26. Ball JK, Elixhauser A. Treatment differences between blacks and whites with colorectal cancer. Med Care 34:970–984, 1996.

27. Cooper GS, Yuan Z, Landefeld CS, Rimm AA. Surgery for colorectal cancer: race-related differences in rates and survival among Medicare beneficiaries. Am J Public Health 86:582–586, 1996.

28. Chen VW, Fenoglio-Preiser CM, Wu XC, et al. Aggressiveness of colon carcinoma in blacks and whites. National Cancer Institute Black/White Cancer Survival Study Group. Cancer Epidemiol Biomarkers Prev 6:1087–1093, 1997.

29. Thomas CRJ, Jarosz R, Evans N. Racial differences in the anatomical distribution of colon cancer. Arch Surg 127:1241–1245, 1992.

30. Johnson HJ, Carstens R. Anatomical distribution of colonic carcinomas. Interracial differences in a community hospital population. Cancer 58:997–1000, 1986.

31. Demers RY, Severson RK, Schottenfeld D, Lazar L. Incidence of colorectal adenocarcinoma by anatomic subsite. An epidemiologic study of time trends and racial differences in the Detroit, Michigan area. Cancer 79:441–447, 1997.

32. Delattre O, Olschwang S, Law DJ, et al. Multiple genetic alterations in distal and proximal colorectal cancer. Lancet 2:353–356, 1989.

33. Thibodeau SN, Bren G, Schaid D. Microsatellite instability in cancer of the proximal colon. Science 260:816–819, 1993.

34. Breivik J, Lothe RA, Meling GI, et al. Different genetic pathways to proximal and distal colorectal cancer influenced by sex-related factors. Int J Cancer 74:664–669, 1997.

35. Zhang H, Evertsson S, Sun X. Clinicopathological and genetic characteristics of mucinous carcinomas in the colorectum. Int J Oncol 14:1057–1061, 1999.

36. Jernvall P, Makinen MJ, Karttunen TJ, et al. Microsatellite instability: impact on cancer progression in proximal and distal colorectal cancers. Eur J Cancer 35:197–201, 1999.

37. Troisi RJ, Freedman AN, Devesa SS. Incidence of colorectal carcinoma in the U.S.: an update of trends by gender, race, age, subsite, and stage, 1975–1994. Cancer 85:1670–1676, 1999.

38. Locke FB, King H. Cancer mortality risk among Japanese in the United States. J Natl Cancer Inst 65:1149–1156, 1980.

39. Whittemore AS, Wu-Williams AH, Lee M, et al. Diet, physical activity, and colorectal cancer among Chinese in North America and China. J Natl Cancer Inst 82:915–926, 1990.

40. McCredie M, Williams S, Coates M. Cancer mortality in migrants from the British Isles and continental Europe to New South Wales, Australia, 1975–1995. Int J Cancer 83:179–185, 1999.

41. Bouchardy C, Khlat M, Mirra AP, Parkin DM. Cancer risks among European migrants in Sao Paulo, Brazil. Eur J Cancer 10:1418–1423, 1993.

42. Colditz GA. The nurses' health study: a cohort of US women followed since 1976. J Am Med Womens Assoc 50:40–44, 1995.

43. Colditz GA, Manson JE, Hankinson SE. The Nurses' Health Study: 20-year contribution to the understanding of health among women. J Womens Health 6:49–62, 1997.

44. Giovannucci E, Stampfer MJ, Colditz GA, et al. Folate, methionine, and alcohol intake and risk of colorectal adenoma. J Natl Cancer Inst 85:875–884, 1993.

45. Giovannucci E, Martinez ME. Tobacco, colorectal cancer, and adenomas: a review of the evidence. J Natl Cancer Inst 88:1717–1730, 1996.

46. Giovannucci E, Colditz GA, Stampfer MJ, et al. A prospective study of cigarette smoking and risk of colorectal adenoma and colorectal cancer in U.S. women. J Natl Cancer Inst 86:192–199, 1994.

47. Giovannucci E, Colditz GA, Stampfer MJ, Willett WC. Physical activity, obesity, and risk of colorectal adenoma in women (United States). Cancer Causes Control 7:253–263, 1996.

48. Platz EA, Martinez ME, Grodstein F, et al. Parity and other reproductive factors and risk of adenomatous polyps of the distal colorectum (United States). Cancer Causes Control 8:894–903, 1997.

49. Grodstein F, Martinez ME, Platz EA, et al. Postmenopausal hormone use and risk for colorectal cancer and adenoma. Ann Intern Med 128:705–712, 1998.

50. Fuchs CS, Giovannucci EL, Colditz GA, et al. Dietary fiber and the risk of colorectal cancer and adenoma in women. N Engl J Med 340:169–176, 1999.

51. Platz EA, Hankinson SE, Rifai N, et al. Glycosylated hemoglobin and risk of colorectal cancer and adenoma (United States). Cancer Causes Control 10:379–386, 1999.

52. Giovannucci E, Pollak MN, Platz EA, et al. A prospective study of plasma insulin-like growth factor-1 and binding protein-3 and risk of colorectal neoplasia in women. Cancer Epidemiol Biomarkers Prev 9:345–349, 2000.

53. Giovannucci E, Stampfer MJ, Colditz GA, et al. Multivitamin use, folate, and colon cancer in women in the Nurses' Health Study. Ann Intern Med 129:517–524, 1998.

54. Martinez ME, Giovannucci E, Spiegelman D, et al. Leisure-time physical activity, body size, and colon cancer in women. Nurses' Health Study Research Group. J Natl Cancer Inst 89:948–955, 1997.

55. Hu FB, Manson JE, Liu S, et al. Prospective study of adult onset diabetes mellitus (type 2) and risk of colorectal cancer in women. J Natl Cancer Inst 91:542–547, 1999.

56. Willett WC, Stampfer MJ, Colditz GA, et al. Relation of meat, fat, and fiber intake to the risk of colon cancer in a prospective study among women. N Engl J Med 323:1664–1672, 1990.

57. Fuchs CS, Giovannucci EL, Colditz GA, et al. A prospective study of family history and the risk of colorectal cancer. N Engl J Med 331:1669–1674, 1994.

58. No authors listed. Cancer Prevention Study II. The American Cancer Society Prospective Study. Stat Bull Metrop Insur Co 73:21–29, 1992.

59. Thun MJ, Namboodiri MM, Heath CWJ. Aspirin use and reduced risk of fatal colon cancer. N Engl J Med 325:1593–1596, 1991.

60. Thun MJ, Calle EE, Namboodiri MM, et al. Risk factors for fatal colon cancer in a large prospective study. J Natl Cancer Inst 84:1491–1500, 1992.

61. Calle EE, Miracle-McMahill HL, Thun MJ, Heath CWJ. Estrogen replacement therapy and risk of fatal colon cancer in a prospective cohort of postmenopausal women. J Natl Cancer Inst 87:517–523, 1995.

62. Stellman SD, Demers PA, Colin D, Boffetta P. Cancer mortality and wood dust exposure among participants in the American Cancer Society Cancer Prevention Study-II (CPS-II). Am J Ind Med 34:229–237, 1998.

63. Kahn HS, Tatham LM, Thun MJ, Heath CWJ. Risk factors for self-reported colon polyps. J Gen Intern Med 13:303–310, 1998.

64. Thun MJ, Namboodiri MM, Calle EE, et al. Aspirin use and risk of fatal cancer. Cancer Res 53:1322–1327, 1993.

65. Giovannucci E, Stampfer MJ, Colditz G, et al. Relationship of diet to risk of colorectal adenoma in men. J Natl Cancer Inst 84:91–98, 1992.

66. Giovannucci E, Rimm EB, Stampfer MJ, et al. A prospective study of cigarette smoking and risk of colorectal adenoma and colorectal cancer in U.S. men. J Natl Cancer Inst 86:183–191, 1994.

67. Giovannucci E, Rimm EB, Stampfer MJ, et al. Intake of fat, meat, and fiber in relation to risk of colon cancer in men. Cancer Res 54:2390–2397, 1994.

68. Giovannucci E, Rimm EB, Stampfer MJ, et al. Aspirin use and the risk for colorectal cancer and adenoma in male health professionals. Ann Intern Med 121:241–246, 1994.

69. Giovannucci E, Ascherio A, Rimm EB, et al. Physical activity, obesity, and risk for colon cancer and adenoma in men. Ann Intern Med 122:327–334, 1995.

70. Giovannucci E, Rimm EB, Ascherio A, et al. Alcohol, low-methionine, low-folate diets, and risk of colon cancer in men. J Natl Cancer Inst 87:265–273, 1995.

71. Platz EA, Giovannucci E, Rimm EB, et al. Dietary fiber and distal colorectal adenoma in men. Cancer Epidemiol Biomarkers Prev 6:661–670, 1997.

72. Bostick RM, Potter JD, Kushi LH, et al. Sugar, meat, and fat intake, and non-dietary risk factors for colon cancer incidence in Iowa women (United States). Cancer Causes Control 5:38–52, 1994.

73. Steinmetz KA, Kushi LH, Bostick RM, et al. Vegetables, fruit, and colon cancer in the Iowa Women's Health Study. Am J Epidemiol 139:1–15, 1994.

74. Doyle TJ, Zheng W, Cerhan JR, et al. The association of drinking water source and chlorination by-products with cancer incidence among postmenopausal women in Iowa: a prospective cohort study. Am J Public Health 87:1168–1176, 1997.

75. Sellers TA, Bazyk AE, Bostick RM, et al. Diet and risk of colon cancer in a large prospective study of older women: an analysis stratified on family history (Iowa, United States). Cancer Causes Control 9:357–367, 1998.

76. Zheng W, Anderson KE, Kushi LH, et al. A prospective cohort study of intake of calcium, vitamin D, and other micronutrients in relation to incidence of rectal cancer among postmenopausal women. Cancer Epidemiol Biomarkers Prev 7:221–225, 1998.

77. Gapstur SM, Potter JD, Folsom AR. Alcohol consumption and colon and rectal cancer in postmenopausal women. Int J Epidemiol 23:50–57, 1994.

78. van den Brandt PA, Goldbohm RA, van 't Veer P, et al. A large-scale prospective cohort study on diet and cancer in The Netherlands. J Clin Epidemiol 43:285–295, 1990.

79. van den Brandt PA, Goldbohm RA, van 't Veer P, et al. A prospective

cohort study on toenail selenium levels and risk of gastrointestinal cancer. J Natl Cancer Inst 85:224–229, 1993.

80. Kampman E, Goldbohm RA, van den Brandt PA, van 't Veer P. Fermented dairy products, calcium, and colorectal cancer in The Netherlands Cohort Study. Cancer Res 54:3186–3190, 1994.

81. Dorant E, van den Brandt PA, Goldbohm RA. A prospective cohort study on the relationship between onion and leek consumption, garlic supplement use and the risk of colorectal carcinoma in The Netherlands. Carcinogenesis 17:477–484, 1996.

82. Goldbohm RA, van den Brandt PA, van 't Veer P, et al. Cholecystectomy and colorectal cancer: evidence from a cohort study on diet and cancer. Int J Cancer 53:735–739, 1993.

83. Goldbohm RA, van den Brandt PA, van 't Veer P, et al. A prospective cohort study on the relation between meat consumption and the risk of colon cancer. Cancer Res 54:718–723, 1994.

84. Goldbohm RA, Hertog MG, Brants HA, et al. Consumption of black tea and cancer risk: a prospective cohort study. J Natl Cancer Inst 88:93–100, 1996.

85. Goldbohm RA, Van den Brandt PA, Van 't Veer P, et al. Prospective study on alcohol consumption and the risk of cancer of the colon and rectum in The Netherlands. Cancer Causes Control 5:95–104, 1994.

86. Cooper GS, Yuan Z, Landefeld CS, et al. A national population-based study of incidence of colorectal cancer and age. Implications for screening in older Americans. Cancer 75:775–781, 1995.

87. Itzkowitz SH. Gastrointestinal adenomatous polyps. Semin Gastrointest Dis 7:105–116, 1996.

88. Vatn MH, Stalsberg H. The prevalence of polyps of the large intestine in Oslo: an autopsy study. Cancer 49:819–825, 1982.

89. Eide TJ. The age-, sex-, and site-specific occurrence of adenomas and carcinomas of the large intestine within a defined population. Scand J Gastroenterol 21:1083–1088, 1986.

90. O'Brien MJ, Winawer SJ, Zauber AG, et al. The National Polyp Study. Patient and polyp characteristics associated with high-grade dysplasia in colorectal adenomas. Gastroenterology 98:371–379, 1990.

91. Morson BC. Evolution of cancer of the colon and rectum. Cancer 34:845–849, 1974.

92. Fearon ER, Vogelstein B. A genetic model for colorectal tumorigenesis. Cell 61:759–767, 1990.

93. Kim EC, Lance P. Colorectal polyps and their relationship to cancer. Gastroenterol Clin North Am 26:1–17, 1997.

94. Rex DK, Cummings OW, Helper DJ, et al. 5-year incidence of adenomas after negative colonoscopy in asymptomatic average-risk persons. Gastroenterology 111:1178–1181, 1996.

95. Atkin WS, Morson BC, Cuzick J. Long-term risk of colorectal cancer after excision of rectosigmoid adenomas. N Engl J Med 326:658–662, 1992.

96. Winawer SJ, Zauber AG, O'Brien MJ, et al. Randomized comparison of surveillance intervals after colonoscopic removal of newly diagnosed adenomatous polyps. The National Polyp Study Workgroup. N Engl J Med 328:901–906, 1993.

97. Jorgensen OD, Kronborg O, Fenger C. A randomized surveillance study of patients with pedunculated and small sessile tubular and tubulovillous adenomas. The Funen Adenoma Follow-up Study. Scand J Gastroenterol 30:686–692, 1995.

98. Otchy DP, Ransohoff DF, Wolff BG, et al. Metachronous colon cancer in persons who have had a large adenomatous polyp. Am J Gastroenterol 91:448–454, 1996.

99. Fornasarig M, Valentini M, Poletti M, et al. Evaluation of the risk for metachronous colorectal neoplasms following intestinal polypectomy: a clinical, endoscopic and pathological study. Hepatogastroenterology 45:1565–1572, 1998.

100. Yang G, Zheng W, Sun QR, et al. Pathologic features of initial adenomas as predictors for metachronous adenomas of the rectum. J Natl Cancer Inst 90:1661–1665, 1998.

101. Cali RL, Pitsch RM, Thorson AG, et al. Cumulative incidence of metachronous colorectal cancer. Dis Colon Rectum 36:388–393, 1993.

102. Rex DK. Colonoscopy: a review of its yield for cancers and adenomas by indication. Am J Gastroenterol 90:353–365, 1995.

103. Neugut AI, Lautenbach E, Abi-Rached B, Forde KA. Incidence of adenomas after curative resection for colorectal cancer. Am J Gastroenterol 91:2096–2098, 1996.

104. Carlsson G, Petrelli NJ, Nava H, et al. The value of colonoscopic surveillance after curative resection for colorectal cancer or synchronous adenomatous polyps. Arch Surg 122:1261–1263, 1987.

105. Chen F, Stuart M. Colonoscopic follow-up of colorectal carcinoma. Dis Colon Rectum 37:568–572, 1994.

106. Burt RW. Screening of patients with a positive family history of colorectal cancer. Gastrointest Endosc Clin N Am 7:65–79, 1997.

107. Easton D, Peto J. The contribution of inherited predisposition to cancer incidence. Cancer Surv 9:395–416, 1990.

108. Winawer SJ, Zauber AG, Gerdes H, et al. Risk of colorectal cancer in the families of patients with adenomatous polyps. National Polyp Study Workgroup. N Engl J Med 334:82–87, 1996.

109. Slattery ML, Kerber RA. Family history of cancer and colon cancer risk: the Utah Population Database [published erratum appears in J Natl Cancer Inst 1994;86(23):1802]. J Natl Cancer Inst 86:1618–1626, 1994.

110. Andres PG, Friedman LS. Epidemiology and the natural course of inflammatory bowel disease. Gastroenterol Clin North Am 28:255–281, 1999.

111. Hendriksen C, Kreiner S, Binder V. Long-term prognosis in ulcerative colitis—based on results from a regional patient group from the county of Copenhagen. Gut 26:158–163, 1985.

112. Devroede GJ, Taylor WF, Sauer WG, et al. Cancer risk and life expectancy of children with ulcerative colitis. N Engl J Med 285:17–21, 1971.

113. Karlen P, Lofberg R, Brostrom O, et al. Increased risk of cancer in ulcerative colitis: a population-based cohort study. Am J Gastroenterol 94:1047–1052, 1999.

114. Lewis JD, Deren JJ, Lichtenstein GR. Cancer risk in patients with inflammatory bowel disease. Gastroenterol Clin North Am 28:459–477, 1999.

115. Nuako KW, Ahlquist DA, Sandborn WJ, et al. Primary sclerosing cholangitis and colorectal carcinoma in patients with chronic ulcerative colitis: a case–control study. Cancer 82:822–826, 1998.

116. Shetty K, Rybicki L, Brzezinski A, et al. The risk for cancer or dysplasia in ulcerative colitis patients with primary sclerosing cholangitis. Am J Gastroenterol 94:1643–1649, 1999.

117. Gillen CD, Andrews HA, Prior P, Allan RN. Crohn's disease and colorectal cancer. Gut 35:651–655, 1994.

118. Ribeiro MB, Greenstein AJ, Sachar DB, et al. Colorectal adenocarcinoma in Crohn's disease. Ann Surg 223:186–193, 1996.

119. Walsh SV, Loda M, Torres CM, et al. P53 and beta-catenin expression in chronic ulcerative colitis–associated polypoid dysplasia and sporadic adenomas: an immunohistochemical study. Am J Surg Pathol 23:963–969, 1999.

120. Slattery ML, Benson J, Berry TD, et al. Dietary sugar and colon cancer. Cancer Epidemiol Biomarkers Prev 6:677–685, 1997.

121. Bennion LJ, Grundy SM. Effects of diabetes mellitus on cholesterol metabolism in man. N Engl J Med 296:1365–1371, 1977.

122. Andersen E, Hellstrom P, Hellstrom K. Cholesterol biosynthesis in non-ketotic diabetics before and during insulin therapy. Diabetes Res Clin Pract 3:207–214, 1987.

123. Will JC, Galuska DA, Vinicor F, Calle EE. Colorectal cancer: another complication of diabetes mellitus? Am J Epidemiol 147:816–825, 1998.

124. Kono S, Honjo S, Todoroki I, et al. Glucose intolerance and adenomas of the sigmoid colon in Japanese men (Japan). Cancer Causes Control 9:441–446, 1998.

125. Durrant LG, Watson SA, Hall A, Morris DL. Co-stimulation of gastrointestinal tumour cell growth by gastrin, transforming growth factor alpha and insulin like growth factor-I. Br J Cancer 63:67–70, 1991.

126. Jenkins PJ, Besser GM, Fairclough PD. Colorectal neoplasia in acromegaly. Gut 44:585–587, 1999.

127. Ma J, Pollak MN, Giovannucci E, et al. Prospective study of colorectal cancer risk in men and plasma levels of insulin-like growth factor (IGF)-I and IGF-binding protein-3. J Natl Cancer Inst 91:620–625, 1999.

128. Giovannucci E, Colditz GA, Stampfer MJ. A meta-analysis of cholecystectomy and risk of colorectal cancer. Gastroenterology 105:130–141, 1993.

129. Reid FD, Mercer PM, Harrison M, Bates T. Cholecystectomy as a risk factor for colorectal cancer: a meta-analysis. Scand J Gastroenterol 31:160–169, 1996.

130. Todoroki I, Friedman GD, Slattery ML, et al. Cholecystectomy and the risk of colon cancer. Am J Gastroenterol 94:41–46, 1999.

131. Schatzkin A, Kelloff G. Chemo- and dietary prevention of colorectal cancer. Eur J Cancer 31A:1198–1204, 1995.

132. Haenszel W, Correa P. Cancer of the large intestine: epidemiologic findings. Dis Colon Rectum 16:371–377, 1973.

133. Willett W. The search for the causes of breast and colon cancer. Nature 338:389–394, 1989.

134. Haenszel W, Berg JW, Segi M, et al. Large-bowel cancer in Hawaiian Japanese. J Natl Cancer Inst 51:1765–1779, 1973.

135. Giovannucci E, Goldin B. The role of fat, fatty acids, and total energy intake in the etiology of human colon cancer. Am J Clin Nutr 66:1564S–1571S, 1997.

136. Howe GR, Aronson KJ, Benito E, et al. The relationship between dietary fat intake and risk of colorectal cancer: evidence from the com-

bined analysis of 13 case–control studies. Cancer Causes Control 8: 215–228, 1997.

137. Gaard M, Tretli S, Loken EB. Dietary factors and risk of colon cancer: a prospective study of 50,535 young Norwegian men and women. Eur J Cancer Prev 5:445–454, 1996.

138. Kato I, Akhmedkhanov A, Koenig K, et al. Prospective study of diet and female colorectal cancer: the New York University Women's Health Study. Nutr Cancer 28:276–281, 1997.

139. Probst-Hensch NM, Sinha R, Longnecker MP, et al. Meat preparation and colorectal adenomas in a large sigmoidoscopy-based case–control study in California (United States). Cancer Causes Control 8:175–183, 1997.

140. Sinha R, Rothman N. Role of well-done, grilled red meat, heterocyclic amines (HCAs) in the etiology of human cancer. Cancer Lett 143: 189–194, 1999.

141. Lang NP, Butler MA, Massengill J, et al. Rapid metabolic phenotypes for acetyltransferase and cytochrome P4501A2 and putative exposure to food-borne heterocyclic amines increase the risk for colorectal cancer or polyps. Cancer Epidemiol Biomarkers Prev 3:675–682, 1994.

142. Chen J, Stampfer MJ, Hough HL, et al. A prospective study of N-acetyl-transferase genotype, red meat intake, and risk of colorectal cancer. Cancer Res 58:3307–3311, 1998.

143. Roberts-Thomson IC, Butler WJ, Ryan P. Meat, metabolic genotypes and risk for colorectal cancer. Eur J Cancer Prev 8:207–211, 1999.

144. McKeown-Eyssen GE, Bright-See E, Bruce WR, et al. A randomized trial of a low fat high fibre diet in the recurrence of colorectal polyps. Toronto Polyp Prevention Group [published erratum appears in J Clin Epidemiol 1995;48(2):i]. J Clin Epidemiol 47:525–536, 1994.

145. MacLennan R, Macrae F, Bain C, et al. Randomized trial of intake of fat, fiber, and beta carotene to prevent colorectal adenomas. The Australian Polyp Prevention Project. J Natl Cancer Inst 87:1760–1766, 1995.

146. Schatzkin A, Lanza E, Corle D, et al. Lack of effect of a low-fat, high-fiber diet on the recurrence of colorectal adenomas. Polyp Prevention Trial Study Group. N Engl J Med 342:1149–1155, 2000.

147. No authors listed. Design of the Women's Health Initiative clinical trial and observational study. The Women's Health Initiative Study Group. Control Clin Trials 19:61–109, 1998.

148. Anti M, Armelao F, Marra G, et al. Effects of different doses of fish oil on rectal cell proliferation in patients with sporadic colonic adenomas. Gastroenterology 107:1709–1718, 1994.

149. Anti M, Marra G, Armelao F, et al. Modulating effect of omega-3 fatty acids on the proliferative pattern of human colorectal mucosa. Adv Exp Med Biol:605–610, 1997.

150. Steinmetz KA, Potter JD. Vegetables, fruit, and cancer. II. Mechanisms. Cancer Causes Control 2:427–442, 1991.

151. Potter JD. Colorectal cancer: molecules and populations. J Natl Cancer Inst 91:916–932, 1999.

152. Potter JD, Slattery ML, Bostick RM, Gapstur SM. Colon cancer: a review of the epidemiology. Epidemiol Rev 15:499–545, 1993.

153. Steinmetz KA, Potter JD. Food-group consumption and colon cancer in the Adelaide Case–Control Study. I. Vegetables and fruit. Int J Cancer 53:711–719, 1993.

154. Haenszel W, Locke FB, Segi M. A case–control study of large bowel cancer in Japan. J Natl Cancer Inst 64:17–22, 1980.

155. Graham S, Dayal H, Swanson M, et al. Diet in the epidemiology of cancer of the colon and rectum. J Natl Cancer Inst 61:709–714, 1978.

156. Tuyns AJ, Kaaks R, Haelterman M. Colorectal cancer and the consumption of foods: a case–control study in Belgium. Nutr Cancer 11: 189–204, 1988.

157. Manousos O, Day NE, Trichopoulos D, et al. Diet and colorectal cancer: a case–control study in Greece. Int J Cancer 32:1–5, 1983.

158. Tajima K, Tominaga S. Dietary habits and gastro-intestinal cancers: a comparative case–control study of stomach and large intestinal cancers in Nagoya, Japan. Jpn J Cancer Res 76:705–716, 1985.

159. Hu JF, Liu YY, Yu YK, et al. Diet and cancer of the colon and rectum: a case–control study in China. Int J Epidemiol 20:362–367, 1991.

160. Le Marchand L, Wilkens LR, Kolonel LN, et al. Associations of sedentary lifestyle, obesity, smoking, alcohol use, and diabetes with the risk of colorectal cancer. Cancer Res 57:4787–4794, 1997.

161. Lin HJ, Probst-Hensch NM, Louie AD, et al. Glutathione transferase null genotype, broccoli, and lower prevalence of colorectal adenomas. Cancer Epidemiol Biomarkers Prev 7:647–652, 1998.

162. Kritchevsky D. Dietary fibre and cancer. Eur J Cancer Prev 6:435–441, 1997.

163. Chaplin MF. Bile acids, fibre and colon cancer: the story unfolds. J R Soc Health 118:53–61, 1998.

164. Giovannucci E. Insulin and colon cancer. Cancer Causes Control 6: 164–179, 1995.

165. Howe GR, Benito E, Castelleto R, et al. Dietary intake of fiber and decreased risk of cancers of the colon and rectum: evidence from the combined analysis of 13 case–control studies. J Natl Cancer Inst 84: 1887–1896, 1992.

166. Pietinen P, Malila N, Virtanen M, et al. Diet and risk of colorectal cancer in a cohort of Finnish men. Cancer Causes Control 10:387–396, 1999.

167. Harris PJ, Ferguson LR. Dietary fibres may protect or enhance carcinogenesis. Mutat Res 443:95–110, 1999.

168. Alberts DS, Einspahr J, Rees-McGee S, et al. Effects of dietary wheat bran fiber on rectal epithelial cell proliferation in patients with resection for colorectal cancers. J Natl Cancer Inst 82:1280–1285, 1990.

169. DeCosse JJ, Miller HH, Lesser ML. Effect of wheat fiber and vitamins C and E on rectal polyps in patients with familial adenomatous polyposis. J Natl Cancer Inst 81:1290–1297, 1989.

170. Rooney PS, Hunt LM, Clarke PA, et al. Wheat fibre, lactulose and rectal mucosal proliferation in individuals with a family history of colorectal cancer. Br J Surg 81:1792–1794, 1994.

171. Alberts DS, Ritenbaugh C, Story JA, et al. Randomized, double-blinded, placebo-controlled study of effect of wheat bran fiber and calcium on fecal bile acids in patients with resected adenomatous colon polyps. J Natl Cancer Inst 88:81–92, 1996.

172. Alberts DS, Einspahr J, Ritenbaugh C, et al. The effect of wheat bran fiber and calcium supplementation on rectal mucosal proliferation rates in patients with resected adenomatous colorectal polyps. Cancer Epidemiol Biomarkers Prev 6:161–169, 1997.

173. Martinez ME, Reid ME, Guillen-Rodriguez J, et al. Design and baseline characteristics of study participants in the Wheat Bran Fiber trial. Cancer Epidemiol Biomarkers Prev 7:813–816, 1998.

174. Earnest DL, Sampliner RE, Roe DJ, et al. Progress report: the Arizona phase III study of the effect of wheat bran fiber on recurrence of adenomatous colon polyps. Am J Med 106:43S–45S, 1999.

175. Alberts DS, Martinez ME, Roe DJ, et al. Lack of effect of a high-fiber cereal supplement on the recurrence of colorectal adenomas. Phoenix Colon Cancer Prevention Physicians' Network. N Engl J Med 342: 1156–1162, 2000.

176. Faivre J, Couillault C, Kronborg O, et al. Chemoprevention of metachronous adenomas of the large bowel: design and interim results of a randomized trial of calcium and fibre. ECP Colon Group. Eur J Cancer Prev 6:132–138, 1997.

177. Bonithon-Kopp C, Kronborg O, Giacosa A, et al. Calcium and fibre supplementation in prevention of colorectal adenoma recurrence: a randomised intervention trial. European Cancer Prevention Organisation Study Group. Lancet 356:1300–1306, 2000.

178. Newmark HL, Wargovich MJ, Bruce WR. Colon cancer and dietary fat, phosphate, and calcium: a hypothesis. J Natl Cancer Inst 72:1323–1325, 1984.

179. Martinez ME, Willett WC. Calcium, vitamin D, and colorectal cancer: a review of the epidemiologic evidence. Cancer Epidemiol Biomarkers Prev 7:163–168, 1998.

180. Bostick RM, Potter JD, Fosdick L, et al. Calcium and colorectal epithelial cell proliferation: a preliminary randomized, double-blinded, placebo-controlled clinical trial. J Natl Cancer Inst 85:132–141, 1993.

181. Bostick RM. Human studies of calcium supplementation and colorectal epithelial cell proliferation. Cancer Epidemiol Biomarkers Prev 6: 971–980, 1997.

182. Bergsma-Kadijk JA, van 't Veer P, Kampman E, Burema J. Calcium does not protect against colorectal neoplasia. Epidemiology 7:590–597, 1996.

183. Hyman J, Baron JA, Dain BJ, et al. Dietary and supplemental calcium and the recurrence of colorectal adenomas. Cancer Epidemiol Biomarkers Prev 7:291–295, 1998.

184. Alder RJ, McKeown-Eyssen G, Bright-See E. Randomized trial of the effect of calcium supplementation on fecal risk factors for colorectal cancer. Am J Epidemiol 138:804–814, 1993.

185. Lupton JR, Steinbach G, Chang WC, et al. Calcium supplementation modifies the relative amounts of bile acids in bile and affects key aspects of human colon physiology. J Nutr 126:1421–1428, 1996.

186. Lipkin M, Newmark H. Effect of added dietary calcium on colonic epithelial-cell proliferation in subjects at high risk for familial colonic cancer. N Engl J Med 313:1381–1384, 1985.

187. Rozen P, Fireman Z, Fine N, et al. Oral calcium suppresses increased rectal epithelial proliferation of persons at risk of colorectal cancer. Gut 30:650–655, 1989.

188. Barsoum GH, Hendrickse C, Winslet MC, et al. Reduction of mucosal

crypt cell proliferation in patients with colorectal adenomatous polyps by dietary calcium supplementation. Br J Surg 79:581–583, 1992.

189. Wargovich MJ, Isbell G, Shabot M, et al. Calcium supplementation decreases rectal epithelial cell proliferation in subjects with sporadic adenoma. Gastroenterology 103:92–97, 1992.

190. Thomas MG, Thomson JP, Williamson RC. Oral calcium inhibits rectal epithelial proliferation in familial adenomatous polyposis. Br J Surg 80:499–501, 1993.

191. Steinbach G, Lupton J, Reddy BS, et al. Effect of calcium supplementation on rectal epithelial hyperproliferation in intestinal bypass subjects. Gastroenterology 106:1162–1167, 1994.

192. Holt PR, Atillasoy EO, Gilman J, et al. Modulation of abnormal colonic epithelial cell proliferation and differentiation by low-fat dairy foods: a randomized controlled trial. JAMA 280:1074–1079, 1998.

193. Gregoire RC, Stern HS, Yeung KS, et al. Effect of calcium supplementation on mucosal cell proliferation in high risk patients for colon cancer. Gut 30:376–382, 1989.

194. Stern HS, Gregoire RC, Kashtan H, et al. Long-term effects of dietary calcium on risk markers for colon cancer in patients with familial polyposis. Surgery 108:528–533, 1990.

195. Bostick RM, Fosdick L, Wood JR, et al. Calcium and colorectal epithelial cell proliferation in sporadic adenoma patients: a randomized, double-blinded, placebo-controlled clinical trial. J Natl Cancer Inst 87:1307–1315, 1995.

196. Baron JA, Tosteson TD, Wargovich MJ, et al. Calcium supplementation and rectal mucosal proliferation: a randomized controlled trial. J Natl Cancer Inst 87:1303–1307, 1995.

197. Armitage NC, Rooney PS, Gifford KA, et al. The effect of calcium supplements on rectal mucosal proliferation. Br J Cancer 71:186–190, 1995.

198. Cats A, Kleibeuker JH, van der Meer R, et al. Randomized, double-blinded, placebo-controlled intervention study with supplemental calcium in families with hereditary nonpolyposis colorectal cancer. J Natl Cancer Inst 87:598–603, 1995.

199. Weisgerber UM, Boeing H, Owen RW, et al. Effect of longterm placebo controlled calcium supplementation on sigmoidal cell proliferation in patients with sporadic adenomatous polyps. Gut 38:396–402, 1996.

200. Karagas MR, Tosteson TD, Greenberg ER, et al. Effects of milk and milk products on rectal mucosal cell proliferation in humans. Cancer Epidemiol Biomarkers Prev 7:757–766, 1998.

201. Duris I, Hruby D, Pekarkova B, et al. Calcium chemoprevention in colorectal cancer. Hepatogastroenterology 43:152–154, 1996.

202. Hofstad B, Almendingen K, Vatn M, et al. Growth and recurrence of colorectal polyps: a double-blind 3-year intervention with calcium and antioxidants. Digestion 59:148–156, 1998.

203. Baron JA, Beach M, Mandel JS, et al. Calcium supplements for the prevention of colorectal adenomas. Calcium Polyp Prevention Study Group. N Engl J Med 340:101–107, 1999.

204. Biasco G, Paganelli GM, Brandi G, et al. Chemoprevention of colorectal cancer: role of antioxidant vitamins. Eur J Cancer Prev (Suppl 1) 3:87–91, 1992.

205. Riboli E, Slimani N, Kaaks R. Identifiability of food components for cancer chemoprevention. IARC Sci Publ 139:23–31, 1996.

206. Enger SM, Longnecker MP, Chen MJ, et al. Dietary intake of specific carotenoids and vitamins A, C, and E, and prevalence of colorectal adenomas. Cancer Epidemiol Biomarkers Prev 5:147–153, 1996.

207. Tseng M, Murray SC, Kupper LL, Sandler RS. Micronutrients and the risk of colorectal adenomas [published erratum appears in Am J Epidemiol 1997;146(9):788]. Am J Epidemiol 144:1005–1014, 1996.

208. Patterson RE, White E, Kristal AR, et al. Vitamin supplements and cancer risk: the epidemiologic evidence. Cancer Causes Control 8:786–802, 1997.

209. Whelan RL, Horvath KD, Gleason NR, et al. Vitamin and calcium supplement use is associated with decreased adenoma recurrence in patients with a previous history of neoplasia. Dis Colon Rectum 42:212–217, 1999.

210. Shamberger RJ, Tytko SA, Willis CE. Antioxidants and cancer. Part VI. Selenium and age-adjusted human cancer mortality. Arch Environ Health 31:231–235, 1976.

211. Knekt P, Aromaa A, Maatela J, et al. Serum vitamin E, serum selenium and the risk of gastrointestinal cancer. Int J Cancer 42:846–850, 1988.

212. Knekt P, Aromaa A, Maatela J, et al. Serum selenium and subsequent risk of cancer among Finnish men and women. J Natl Cancer Inst 82:864–868, 1990.

213. Clark LC, Hixson LJ, Combs GFJ, et al. Plasma selenium concentration predicts the prevalence of colorectal adenomatous polyps. Cancer Epidemiol Biomarkers Prev 2:41–46, 1993.

214. Nelson RL, Davis FG, Sutter E, et al. Serum selenium and colonic neoplastic risk. Dis Colon Rectum 38:1306–1310, 1995.

215. Zheng Y, Kramer PM, Olson G, et al. Prevention by retinoids of azoxymethane-induced tumors and aberrant crypt foci and their modulation of cell proliferation in the colon of rats. Carcinogenesis 18:2119–2125, 1997.

216. Zheng Y, Kramer PM, Lubet RA, et al. Effect of retinoids on AOM-induced colon cancer in rats: modulation of cell proliferation, apoptosis and aberrant crypt foci. Carcinogenesis 20:255–260, 1999.

217. Cahill RJ, O'Sullivan KR, Mathias PM, et al. Effects of vitamin antioxidant supplementation on cell kinetics of patients with adenomatous polyps. Gut 34:963–967, 1993.

218. Greenberg ER, Baron JA, Tosteson TD, et al. A clinical trial of antioxidant vitamins to prevent colorectal adenoma. Polyp Prevention Study Group. N Engl J Med 331:141–147, 1994.

219. Hennekens CH, Buring JE, Manson JE, et al. Lack of effect of long-term supplementation with beta carotene on the incidence of malignant neoplasms and cardiovascular disease. N Engl J Med 334:1145–1149, 1996.

220. Lee IM, Cook NR, Manson JE, et al. Beta-carotene supplementation and incidence of cancer and cardiovascular disease: the Women's Health Study. J Natl Cancer Inst 91:2102–2106, 1999.

221. Malila N, Virtamo J, Virtanen M, et al. The effect of alpha-tocopherol and beta-carotene supplementation on colorectal adenomas in middle-aged male smokers. Cancer Epidemiol Biomarkers Prev 8:489–493, 1999.

222. Albanes D, Malila N, Taylor PR, et al. Effects of supplemental alpha-tocopherol and beta-carotene on colorectal cancer: results from a controlled trial (Finland). Cancer Causes Control 11:197–205, 2000.

223. No authors listed. The effect of vitamin E and beta carotene on the incidence of lung cancer and other cancers in male smokers. The Alpha-Tocopherol, Beta Carotene Cancer Prevention Study Group. N Engl J Med 330:1029–1035, 1994.

224. Omenn GS, Goodman GE, Thornquist MD, et al. Effects of a combination of beta carotene and vitamin A on lung cancer and cardiovascular disease. N Engl J Med 334:1150–1155, 1996.

225. Bussey HJ, DeCosse JJ, Deschner EE, et al. A randomized trial of ascorbic acid in polyposis coli. Cancer 50:1434–1439, 1982.

226. Paganelli GM, Biasco G, Brandi G, et al. Effect of vitamin A, C, and E supplementation on rectal cell proliferation in patients with colorectal adenomas. J Natl Cancer Inst 84:47–51, 1992.

227. McKeown-Eyssen G, Holloway C, Jazmaji V, et al. A randomized trial of vitamins C and E in the prevention of recurrence of colorectal polyps. Cancer Res 48:4701–4705, 1988.

228. Roncucci L, Di Donato P, Carati L, et al. Antioxidant vitamins or lactulose for the prevention of the recurrence of colorectal adenomas. Colorectal Cancer Study Group of the University of Modena and the Health Care District 16. Dis Colon Rectum 36:227–234, 1993.

229. Hercberg S, Preziosi P, Briancon S, et al. A primary prevention trial using nutritional doses of antioxidant vitamins and minerals in cardiovascular diseases and cancers in a general population: the SU.VI.MAX study—design, methods, and participant characteristics. SUpplementation en VItamines et Mineraux AntioXydants. Control Clin Trials 19:336–351, 1998.

230. Hercberg S, Preziosi P, Galan P, et al. The SU.VI.MAX Study: a primary prevention trial using nutritional doses of antioxidant vitamins and minerals in cardiovascular diseases and cancers. SUpplementation on Vitamines et Mineraux AntioXydants. Food Chem Toxicol 37:925–930, 1999.

231. Bonelli L, Conio M, Picasso M, et al. Chemoprevention of metachronous adenomas of the large bowel: a double-blind randomized trial of antioxidants. In: 3rd United European Gastroenterology Week, Oslo, Abstract Book. 1994, A61.

232. Rexrode KM, Lee IM, Cook NR, et al. Baseline characteristics of participants in the Women's Health Study. J Womens Health Gend Based Med 9:19–27, 2000.

233. Moertel CG, Fleming TR, Creagan ET, et al. High-dose vitamin C versus placebo in the treatment of patients with advanced cancer who have had no prior chemotherapy. A randomized double-blind comparison. N Engl J Med 312:137–141, 1985.

234. Clark LC, Combs GFJ, Turnbull BW, et al. Effects of selenium supplementation for cancer prevention in patients with carcinoma of the skin. A randomized controlled trial. Nutritional Prevention of Cancer Study Group [published erratum appears in JAMA 1997;277(19):1520]. JAMA 276:1957–1963, 1996.

235. Benito E, Stiggelbout A, Bosch FX, et al. Nutritional factors in colorectal cancer risk: a case–control study in Majorca. Int J Cancer 49:161–167, 1991.

236. Freudenheim JL, Graham S, Marshall JR, et al. Folate intake and carcinogenesis of the colon and rectum. Int J Epidemiol 20:368–374, 1991.

237. Meyer F, White E. Alcohol and nutrients in relation to colon cancer in middle-aged adults. Am J Epidemiol 138:225–236, 1993.

238. Ferraroni M, La Vecchia C, D'Avanzo B, et al. Selected micronutrient intake and the risk of colorectal cancer. Br J Cancer 70:1150–1155, 1994.

239. Glynn SA, Albanes D, Pietinen P, et al. Colorectal cancer and folate status: a nested case–control study among male smokers. Cancer Epidemiol Biomarkers Prev 5:487–494, 1996.

240. Lashner BA, Heidenreich PA, Su GL, et al. Effect of folate supplementation on the incidence of dysplasia and cancer in chronic ulcerative colitis. A case–control study. Gastroenterology 97:255–259, 1989.

241. Lashner BA, Provencher KS, Seidner DL, et al. The effect of folic acid supplementation on the risk for cancer or dysplasia in ulcerative colitis. Gastroenterology 112:29–32, 1997.

242. Boutron-Ruault MC, Senesse P, Faivre J, et al. Folate and alcohol intakes: related or independent roles in the adenoma–carcinoma sequence? Nutr Cancer 26:337–346, 1996.

243. Chen J, Giovannucci EL, Hunter DJ. MTHFR polymorphism, methyl-replete diets and the risk of colorectal carcinoma and adenoma among U.S. men and women: an example of gene–environment interactions in colorectal tumorigenesis. J Nutr 129:560S–564S, 1999.

244. Kelloff GJ, Boone CW, Sigman CC, Greenwald P. Chemoprevention of colorectal cancer. In: Young GP, Rozen P, Levin B (eds): Prevention and Early Detection of Colorectal Cancer. W.B. Saunders, London, 1996, pp 115–139.

245. Kruis W, Forstmaier G, Scheurlen C, Stellaard F. Effect of diets low and high in refined sugars on gut transit, bile acid metabolism, and bacterial fermentation. Gut 32:367–371, 1991.

246. Burley VJ. Sugar consumption and cancers of the digestive tract. Eur J Cancer Prev 6:422–434, 1997.

247. Nehlig A, Debry G. Coffee and cancer: a review of human and animal data. World Rev Nutr Diet 79:185–221, 1996.

248. Ekbom A. Review: substantial coffee consumption was associated with a lower risk of colorectal cancer in the general population. Gut 44:597, 1999.

249. Baron JA, Greenberg ER, Haile R, et al. Coffee and tea and the risk of recurrent colorectal adenomas. Cancer Epidemiol Biomarkers Prev 6: 7–10, 1997.

250. Bushman JL. Green tea and cancer in humans: a review of the literature. Nutr Cancer 31:151–159, 1998.

251. Hartman TJ, Tangrea JA, Pietinen P, et al. Tea and coffee consumption and risk of colon and rectal cancer in middle-aged Finnish men. Nutr Cancer 31:41–48, 1998.

252. Kune GA, Vitetta L. Alcohol consumption and the etiology of colorectal cancer: a review of the scientific evidence from 1957 to 1991. Nutr Cancer 18:97–111, 1992.

253. Blot WJ. Alcohol and cancer. Cancer Res 52:2119s–2123s, 1992.

254. Longnecker MP, Orza MJ, Adams ME, et al. A meta-analysis of alcoholic beverage consumption in relation to risk of colorectal cancer. Cancer Causes Control 1:59–68, 1990.

255. Nyren O, Bergstrom R, Nystrom L, et al. Smoking and colorectal cancer: a 20-year follow-up study of Swedish construction workers. J Natl Cancer Inst 88:1302–1307, 1996.

256. Knekt P, Hakama M, Jarvinen R, et al. Smoking and risk of colorectal cancer. Br J Cancer 78:136–139, 1998.

257. Terry MB, Neugut AI. Cigarette smoking and the colorectal adenoma-carcinoma sequence: a hypothesis to explain the paradox. Am J Epidemiol 147:903–910, 1998.

258. Baron JA, Sandler RS, Haile RW, et al. Folate intake, alcohol consumption, cigarette smoking, and risk of colorectal adenomas. J Natl Cancer Inst 90:57–62, 1998.

259. Cordain L, Latin RW, Behnke JJ. The effects of an aerobic running program on bowel transit time. J Sports Med Phys Fitness 26:101–104, 1986.

260. Regensteiner JG, Mayer EJ, Shetterly SM, et al. Relationship between habitual physical activity and insulin levels among nondiabetic men and women. San Luis Valley Diabetes Study. Diabetes Care 14:1066–1074, 1991.

261. Martinez ME, Heddens D, Earnest DL, et al. Physical activity, body mass index, and prostaglandin E2 levels in rectal mucosa. J Natl Cancer Inst 91:950–953, 1999.

262. Colditz GA, Cannuscio CC, Frazier AL. Physical activity and reduced risk of colon cancer: implications for prevention. Cancer Causes Control 8:649–667, 1997.

263. Sporn MB, Dunlop NM, Newton DL, Smith JM. Prevention of chemical carcinogenesis by vitamin A and its synthetic analogs (retinoids). Fed Proc 35:1332–1338, 1976.

264. Kelloff GJ, Crowell JA, Steele VE, et al. Progress in cancer chemoprevention. Ann N Y Acad Sci 889:1–13, 1999.

265. Benner SE, Pajak TF, Lippman SM, et al. Prevention of second primary tumors with isotretinoin in patients with squamous cell carcinoma of the head and neck: long-term follow-up. J Natl Cancer Inst 86:140–141, 1994.

266. Hawk E, Viner JL, Lawrence JA. Biomarkers as surrogates for cancer development. Curr Oncol Rep 2:242–250, 2000.

267. Hawk E, Lubet R, Limburg P. Chemoprevention in hereditary colorectal cancer syndromes. Cancer 86:2551–2563, 1999.

268. Lupulescu A. Prostaglandins, their inhibitors and cancer. Prostaglandins Leukot Essent Fatty Acids 54:83–94, 1996.

269. Williams CS, Mann M, DuBois RN. The role of cyclooxygenases in inflammation, cancer, and development. Oncogene 18:7908–7916, 1999.

270. Smalley WE, Griffin MR. The risks and costs of upper gastrointestinal disease attributable to NSAIDs. Gastroenterol Clin North Am 25:373–396, 1996.

271. Eberhart CE, Coffey RJ, Radhika A, et al. Up-regulation of cyclooxygenase 2 gene expression in human colorectal adenomas and adenocarcinomas. Gastroenterology 107:1183–1188, 1994.

272. Oshima M, Dinchuk JE, Kargman SL, et al. Suppression of intestinal polyposis in Apc delta716 knockout mice by inhibition of cyclooxygenase 2 (COX-2). Cell 87:803–809, 1996.

273. Dannenberg AJ, Zakim D. Chemoprevention of colorectal cancer through inhibition of cyclooxygenase-2. Semin Oncol 26:499–504, 1999.

274. Ahnen DJ. Colon cancer prevention by NSAIDs: what is the mechanism of action? Eur J Surg (Suppl) 582:111–114, 1998.

275. Wechter WJ, Murray EDJ, Kantoci D, et al. Treatment and survival study in the C57BL/6J-APC(Min)/+(Min) mouse with R-flurbiprofen. Life Sci 66:745–753, 2000.

276. Craven PA, DeRubertis FR. Effects of aspirin on 1,2-dimethylhydrazine-induced colonic carcinogenesis. Carcinogenesis 13:541–546, 1992.

277. Pence BC, Dunn DM, Zhao C, et al. Chemopreventive effects of calcium but not aspirin supplementation in cholic acid–promoted colon carcinogenesis: correlation with intermediate endpoints. Carcinogenesis 16:757–765, 1995.

278. Williamson SL, Kartheuser A, Coaker J, et al. Intestinal tumorigenesis in the Apc1638N mouse treated with aspirin and resistant starch for up to 5 months. Carcinogenesis 20:805–810, 1999.

279. Caignard A, Martin M, Reisser D, et al. Effects of cimetidine and indomethacin on the growth of dimethylhydrazine-induced or transplanted intestinal cancers in the rat. Br J Cancer 50:661–665, 1984.

280. Barnes CJ, Hardman WE, Cameron IL, Lee M. Aspirin, but not sodium salicylate, indomethacin, or nabumetone, reversibly suppresses 1,2-methylhydrazine-induced colonic aberrant crypt foci in rats. Dig Dis Sci 42:920–926, 1997.

281. Danzi M, Ferulano GP, Abate S, Califano G. Enhancement of colonic cancer by indomethacin treatment in dimethylhydrazine pretreated rats. Carcinogenesis 5:287–289, 1984.

282. Ritland SR, Leighton JA, Hirsch RE, et al. Evaluation of 5-aminosalicylic acid (5-ASA) for cancer chemoprevention: lack of efficacy against nascent adenomatous polyps in the Apc(Min) mouse. Clin Cancer Res 5:855–863, 1999.

283. Nigro ND, Bull AW, Boyd ME. Inhibition of intestinal carcinogenesis in rats: effect of difluoromethylornithine with piroxicam or fish oil. J Natl Cancer Inst 77:1309–1313, 1986.

284. Reddy BS, Nayini J, Tokumo K, et al. Chemoprevention of colon carcinogenesis by concurrent administration of piroxicam, a nonsteroidal antiinflammatory drug with D,L-α-difluoromethylornithine, an ornithine decarboxylase inhibitor, in diet. Cancer Res 50:2562–2568, 1990.

285. Rao CV, Tokumo K, Rigotty J, et al. Chemoprevention of colon carcinogenesis by dietary administration of piroxicam, α-difluoromethylornithine, 16 α-fluoro-5-androsten-17-one, and ellagic acid individually and in combination. Cancer Res 51:4528–4534, 1991.

286. Li H, Schut HA, Conran P, et al. Prevention by aspirin and its combination with α-difluoromethylornithine of azoxymethane-induced tumors, aberrant crypt foci and prostaglandin E2 levels in rat colon. Carcinogenesis 20:425–430, 1999.

287. Jacoby RF, Cole CE, Tutsch K, et al. Chemopreventive efficacy of combined piroxicam and difluoromethylornithine treatment of Apc mutant Min mouse adenomas, and selective toxicity against Apc mutant embryos. Cancer Res 60:1864–1870, 2000.

288. Torrance CJ, Jackson PE, Montgomery E, et al. Combinatorial chemoprevention of intestinal neoplasia. Nat Med 6:1024–1028, 2000.

289. Agarwal B, Rao CV, Bhendwal S, et al. Lovastatin augments sulindac-induced apoptosis in colon cancer cells and potentiates chemopreventive effects of sulindac. Gastroenterology 117:838–847, 1999.

290. Kune GA, Kune S, Watson LF. Colorectal cancer risk, chronic illnesses, operations, and medications: case control results from the Melbourne Colorectal Cancer Study. Cancer Res 48:4399–4404, 1988.

291. Rosenberg L, Palmer JR, Zauber AG, et al. A hypothesis: nonsteroidal anti-inflammatory drugs reduce the incidence of large-bowel cancer. J Natl Cancer Inst 83:355–358, 1991.

292. Suh O, Mettlin C, Petrelli NJ. Aspirin use, cancer, and polyps of the large bowel. Cancer 72:1171–1177, 1993.

293. Logan RF, Little J, Hawtin PG, Hardcastle JD. Effect of aspirin and non-steroidal anti-inflammatory drugs on colorectal adenomas: case–control study of subjects participating in the Nottingham faecal occult blood screening programme. BMJ 307:285–289, 1993.

294. Muscat JE, Stellman SD, Wynder EL. Nonsteroidal antiinflammatory drugs and colorectal cancer. Cancer 74:1847–1854, 1994.

295. Müller AD, Sonnenberg A, Wasserman IH. Diseases preceding colon cancer. A case–control study among veterans. Dig Dis Sci 39:2480–2484, 1994.

296. Peleg I, Maibach HT, Brown SH, Wilcox CM. Aspirin and nonsteroidal anti-inflammatory drug use and the risk of subsequent colorectal cancer. Arch Intern Med 154:394–399, 1994.

297. Pinczowski D, Ekbom A, Baron J, et al. Risk factors for colorectal cancer in patients with ulcerative colitis: a case–control study. Gastroenterology 107:117–120, 1994.

298. Martinez ME, McPherson RS, Levin B, Annegers JF. Aspirin and other nonsteroidal anti-inflammatory drugs and risk of colorectal adenomatous polyps among endoscoped individuals. Cancer Epidemiol Biomarkers Prev 4:703–707, 1995.

299. Bansal P, Sonnenberg A. Risk factors of colorectal cancer in inflammatory bowel disease. Am J Gastroenterol 91:44–48, 1996.

300. Peleg I, Lubin MF, Cotsonis GA, et al. Long-term use of nonsteroidal antiinflammatory drugs and other chemopreventors and risk of subsequent colorectal neoplasia. Dig Dis Sci 41:1319–1326, 1996.

301. Reeves MJ, Newcomb PA, Trentham-Dietz A, et al. Nonsteroidal anti-inflammatory drug use and protection against colorectal cancer in women. Cancer Epidemiol Biomarkers Prev 5:955–960, 1996.

302. La Vecchia C, Negri E, Franceschi S, et al. Aspirin and colorectal cancer. Br J Cancer 76:675–677, 1997.

303. Neugut AI, Rosenberg DJ, Ahsan H, et al. Association between coronary heart disease and cancers of the breast, prostate, and colon. Cancer Epidemiol Biomarkers Prev 7:869–873, 1998.

304. Rosenberg L, Louik C, Shapiro S. Nonsteroidal antiinflammatory drug use and reduced risk of large bowel carcinoma. Cancer 82:2326–2333, 1998.

305. Sandler RS, Galanko JC, Murray SC, et al. Aspirin and nonsteroidal anti-inflammatory agents and risk for colorectal adenomas. Gastroenterology 114:441–447, 1998.

306. Smalley W, Ray WA, Daugherty J, Griffin MR. Use of nonsteroidal anti-inflammatory drugs and incidence of colorectal cancer: a population-based study. Arch Intern Med 159:161–166, 1999.

307. Bucher C, Jordan P, Nickeleit V, et al. Relative risk of malignant tumors in analgesic abusers. Effects of long-term intake of aspirin. Clin Nephrol 51:67–72, 1999.

308. Collet JP, Sharpe C, Belzile E, et al. Colorectal cancer prevention by non-steroidal anti-inflammatory drugs: effects of dosage and timing. Br J Cancer 81:62–68, 1999.

309. Langman MJ, Cheng KK, Gilman EA, Lancashire RJ. Effect of anti-inflammatory drugs on overall risk of common cancer: case–control study in general practice research database. BMJ 320:1642–1646, 2000.

310. Breuer-Katschinski B, Nemes K, Rump B, et al. Long-term use of non-steroidal antiinflammatory drugs and the risk of colorectal adenomas. The Colorectal Adenoma Study Group. Digestion 61:129–134, 2000.

311. Paganini-Hill A, Hsu G, Ross RK, Henderson BE. Aspirin use and incidence of large-bowel cancer in a California retirement community. J Natl Cancer Inst 83:1182–1183, 1991.

312. Paganini-Hill A. Aspirin and colorectal cancer: the Leisure World cohort revisited. Prev Med 24:113–115, 1995.

313. Sturmer T, Glynn RJ, Lee IM, et al. Aspirin use and colorectal cancer: post-trial follow-up data from the Physicians' Health Study. Ann Intern Med 128:713–720, 1998.

314. Greenberg ER, Baron JA, Freeman DHJ, et al. Reduced risk of large-bowel adenomas among aspirin users. The Polyp Prevention Study Group. J Natl Cancer Inst 85:912–916, 1993.

315. Schreinemachers DM, Everson RB. Aspirin use and lung, colon, and breast cancer incidence in a prospective study. Epidemiology 5:138–146, 1994.

316. Giovannucci E, Egan KM, Hunter DJ, et al. Aspirin and the risk of colorectal cancer in women. N Engl J Med 333:609–614, 1995.

317. Garcia-Rodriguez LA, Huerta-Alvarez C. Reduced incidence of colorectal adenoma among long-term users of nonsteroidal antiinflammatory drugs: a pooled analysis of published studies and a new population-based study. Epidemiology 11:376–381, 2000.

318. Garcia-Rodriguez LA, Huerta-Alvarez C. Reduced risk of colorectal cancer among long-term users of aspirin and nonaspirin nonsteroidal antiinflammatory drugs. Epidemiology 12:88–93, 2001.

319. Waddell WR, Loughry RW. Sulindac for polyposis of the colon. J Surg Oncol 24:83–87, 1983.

320. Labayle D, Fischer D, Vielh P, et al. Sulindac causes regression of rectal polyps in familial adenomatous polyposis. Gastroenterology 101:635–639, 1991.

321. Giardiello FM, Hamilton SR, Krush AJ, et al. Treatment of colonic and rectal adenomas with sulindac in familial adenomatous polyposis. N Engl J Med 328:1313–1316, 1993.

322. Nugent KP, Farmer KC, Spigelman AD, et al. Randomized controlled trial of the effect of sulindac on duodenal and rectal polyposis and cell proliferation in patients with familial adenomatous polyposis. Br J Surg 80:1618–1619, 1993.

323. Winde G, Schmid KW, Brandt B, et al. Clinical and genomic influence of sulindac on rectal mucosa in familial adenomatous polyposis. Dis Colon Rectum 40:1156–1168; discussion 1168–1159, 1997.

324. Tonelli F, Valanzano R, Dolara P. Sulindac therapy of colorectal polyps in familial adenomatous polyposis. Dig Dis 12:259–264, 1994.

325. Niv Y, Fraser GM. Adenocarcinoma in the rectal segment in familial polyposis coli is not prevented by sulindac therapy. Gastroenterology 107:854–857, 1994.

326. Thorson AG, Lynch HT, Smyrk TC. Rectal cancer in FAP patient after sulindac [letter]. Lancet 343:180, 1994.

327. Lynch HT, Thorson AG, Smyrk T. Rectal cancer after prolonged sulindac chemoprevention. A case report. Cancer 75:936–938, 1995.

328. Giardiello FM, Spannhake EW, DuBois RN, et al. Prostaglandin levels in human colorectal mucosa: effects of sulindac in patients with familial adenomatous polyposis. Dig Dis Sci 43:311–316, 1998.

329. Hixson LJ, Earnest DL, Fennerty MB, Sampliner RE. NSAID effect on sporadic colon polyps. Am J Gastroenterol 88:1652–1656, 1993.

330. Ladenheim J, Garcia G, Titzer D, et al. Effect of sulindac on sporadic colonic polyps. Gastroenterology 108:1083–1087, 1995.

331. Matsuhashi N, Nakajima A, Fukushima Y, et al. Effects of sulindac on sporadic colorectal adenomatous polyps. Gut 40:344–349, 1997.

332. Gann PH, Manson JE, Glynn RJ, et al. Low-dose aspirin and incidence of colorectal tumors in a randomized trial. J Natl Cancer Inst 85:1220–1224, 1993.

333. Piazza GA, Alberts DS, Hixson LJ, et al. Sulindac sulfone inhibits azoxymethane-induced colon carcinogenesis in rats without reducing prostaglandin levels. Cancer Res 57:2909–2915, 1997.

334. Reddy BS, Kawamori T, Lubet RA, et al. Chemopreventive efficacy of sulindac sulfone against colon cancer depends on time of administration during carcinogenic process. Cancer Res 59:3387–3391, 1999.

335. Mahmoud NN, Boolbol SK, Dannenberg AJ, et al. The sulfide metabolite of sulindac prevents tumors and restores enterocyte apoptosis in a murine model of familial adenomatous polyposis. Carcinogenesis 19:87–91, 1998.

336. van Stolk R, Stoner G, Hayton WL, et al. Phase I trial of exisulind (sulindac sulfone, FGN-1) as a chemopreventive agent in patients with familial adenomatous polyposis. Clin Cancer Res 6:78–89, 2000.

337. McCracken JD, Wechter WJ, Liu Y, et al. Antiproliferative effects of the enantiomers of flurbiprofen. J Clin Pharmacol 36:540–545, 1996.

338. Wechter WJ, Kantoci D, Murray EDJ, et al. R-flurbiprofen chemoprevention and treatment of intestinal adenomas in the APC(Min)/+ mouse model: implications for prophylaxis and treatment of colon cancer. Cancer Res 57:4316–4324, 1997.

339. Crofford LJ, Lipsky PE, Brooks P, et al. Basic biology and clinical application of specific cyclooxygenase-2 inhibitors. Arthritis Rheum 43:4–13, 2000.

340. Takahashi M, Fukutake M, Yokota S, et al. Suppression of azoxymethane-induced aberrant crypt foci in rat colon by nimesulide, a selective inhibitor of cyclooxygenase 2. J Cancer Res Clin Oncol 122:219–222, 1996.

341. Reddy BS, Rao CV, Seibert K. Evaluation of cyclooxygenase-2 inhibitor for potential chemopreventive properties in colon carcinogenesis. Cancer Res 56:4566–4569, 1996.

342. Fukutake M, Nakatsugi S, Isoi T, et al. Suppressive effects of nimesulide, a selective inhibitor of cyclooxygenase-2, on azoxymethane-induced colon carcinogenesis in mice. Carcinogenesis 19:1939–1942, 1998.

343. Kawamori T, Rao CV, Seibert K, Reddy BS. Chemopreventive activity of celecoxib, a specific cyclooxygenase-2 inhibitor, against colon carcinogenesis. Cancer Res 58:409–412, 1998.

344. Yoshimi N, Kawabata K, Hara A, et al. Inhibitory effect of NS-398, a selective cyclooxygenase-2 inhibitor, on azoxymethane-induced aber-

rant crypt foci in colon carcinogenesis of F344 rats. Jpn J Cancer Res 88:1044–1051, 1997.

345. Yoshimi N, Shimizu M, Matsunaga K, et al. Chemopreventive effect of N-(2-cyclohexyloxy-4-nitrophenyl)methane sulfonamide (NS-398), a selective cyclooxygenase-2 inhibitor, in rat colon carcinogenesis induced by azoxymethane. Jpn J Cancer Res 90:406–412, 1999.

346. Reddy BS, Hirose Y, Lubet R, et al. Chemoprevention of colon cancer by specific cyclooxygenase-2 inhibitor, celecoxib, administered during different stages of carcinogenesis. Cancer Res 60:293–297, 2000.

347. Oshima M, Murai N, Kargman S, et al. Chemoprevention of intestinal polyposis in the Apcδ716 mouse by rofecoxib, a specific cyclooxygenase-2 inhibitor. Cancer Res 61:1733–1740, 2001.

348. Dolara P, Caderni G, Tonelli F. Nimesulide, a selective anti-inflammatory cyclooxygenase-2 inhibitor, does not affect polyp number and mucosal proliferation in familial adenomatous polyposis. Scand J Gastroenterol 34:1168, 1999.

349. Steinbach G, Lynch PM, Phillips RK, et al. The effect of celecoxib, a cyclooxygenase-2 inhibitor, in familial adenomatous polyposis. N Engl J Med 342:1946–1952, 2000.

350. Rao KV, Detrisac CJ, Steele VE, et al. Differential activity of aspirin, ketoprofen and sulindac as cancer chemopreventive agents in the mouse urinary bladder. Carcinogenesis 17:1435–1438, 1996.

351. Aronow WS. Antiplatelet agents in the prevention of cardiovascular morbidity and mortality in older patients with vascular disease. Drugs Aging 15:91–101, 1999.

352. Hennekens CH. Update on aspirin in the treatment and prevention of cardiovascular disease. Am Heart J 137:S9–S13, 1999.

353. Flynn BL, Theesen KA. Pharmacologic management of Alzheimer disease part III: nonsteroidal antiinflammatory drugs—emerging protective evidence? Ann Pharmacother 33:840–849, 1999.

354. Okolicsanyi L, Lirussi F, Strazzabosco M, et al. The effect of drugs on bile flow and composition. An overview. Drugs 31:430–448, 1986.

355. Campagnoli C, Biglia N, Cantamessa C, et al. Effect of progestins on IGF-I serum level in estrogen-treated postmenopausal women. Zentralbl Gynakol 119:7–11, 1997.

356. Grodstein F, Newcomb PA, Stampfer MJ. Postmenopausal hormone therapy and the risk of colorectal cancer: a review and meta-analysis. Am J Med 106:574–582, 1999.

357. Potter JD, Bostick RM, Grandits GA, et al. Hormone replacement therapy is associated with lower risk of adenomatous polyps of the large bowel: the Minnesota Cancer Prevention Research Unit Case–Control Study. Cancer Epidemiol Biomarkers Prev 5:779–784, 1996.

358. Jacobson JS, Neugut AI, Garbowski GC, et al. Reproductive risk factors for colorectal adenomatous polyps (New York City, NY, United States). Cancer Causes Control 6:513–518, 1995.

359. Peipins LA, Newman B, Sandler RS. Reproductive history, use of exogenous hormones, and risk of colorectal adenomas. Cancer Epidemiol Biomarkers Prev 6:671–675, 1997.

360. Chen MJ, Longnecker MP, Morgenstern H, et al. Recent use of hormone replacement therapy and the prevalence of colorectal adenomas. Cancer Epidemiol Biomarkers Prev 7:227–230, 1998.

361. Pegg AE, Shantz LM, Coleman CS. Ornithine decarboxylase as a target for chemoprevention. J Cell Biochem Suppl 22:132–138, 1995.

362. Rozhin J, Wilson PS, Bull AW, Nigro ND. Ornithine decarboxylase activity in the rat and human colon. Cancer Res 44:3226–3230, 1984.

363. Hixson LJ, Garewal HS, McGee DL, et al. Ornithine decarboxylase and polyamines in colorectal neoplasia and mucosa. Cancer Epidemiol Biomarkers Prev 2:369–374, 1993.

364. Meyskens FLJ, Gerner EW. Development of difluoromethylornithine (DFMO) as a chemoprevention agent. Clin Cancer Res 5:945–951, 1999.

365. Erdman SH, Ignatenko NA, Powell MB, et al. APC-dependent changes in expression of genes influencing polyamine metabolism, and consequences for gastrointestinal carcinogenesis, in the Min mouse. Carcinogenesis 20:1709–1713, 1999.

366. Tempero MA, Nishioka K, Knott K, Zetterman RK. Chemoprevention of mouse colon tumors with difluoromethylornithine during and after carcinogen treatment. Cancer Res 49:5793–5797, 1989.

367. Kingsnorth AN, King WW, Diekema KA, et al. Inhibition of ornithine decarboxylase with 2-difluoromethylornithine: reduced incidence of dimethylhydrazine-induced colon tumors in mice. Cancer Res 43:2545–2549, 1983.

368. Tutton PJ, Barkla DH. Comparison of the effects of an ornithine decarboxylase inhibitor on the intestinal epithelium and on intestinal tumors. Cancer Res 46:6091–6094, 1986.

369. Saydjari R, Townsend CMJ, Barranco SC, Thompson JC. Differential sensitivity of pancreatic and colon cancer to cyclosporine and α-difluoromethylornithine in vivo. Invest New Drugs 6:265–272, 1988.

370. Zhang SZ, Luk GD, Hamilton SR. Alpha-difluoromethylornithine-induced inhibition of growth of autochthonous experimental colonic tumors produced by azoxymethane in male F344 rats. Cancer Res 48:6498–6503, 1988.

371. Luk GD, Zhang SZ, Hamilton SR. Effects of timing of administration and dose of difluoromethylornithine on rat colonic carcinogenesis. J Natl Cancer Inst 81:421–427, 1989.

372. Pereira MA, Khoury MD. Prevention by chemopreventive agents of azoxymethane-induced foci of aberrant crypts in rat colon. Cancer Lett 61:27–33, 1991.

373. Tsunoda A, Shibusawa M, Tsunoda Y, et al. Reduced growth rate of dimethylhydrazine-induced colon tumors in rats. Cancer Res 52:696–700, 1992.

374. McGarrity TJ, Peiffer LP. Selenium and difluoromethylornithine additively inhibit DMH-induced distal colon tumor formation in rats fed a fiber-free diet. Carcinogenesis 14:2335–2340, 1993.

375. Wargovich MJ, Chen CD, Jimenez A, et al. Aberrant crypts as a biomarker for colon cancer: evaluation of potential chemopreventive agents in the rat. Cancer Epidemiol Biomarkers Prev 5:355–360, 1996.

376. Kulkarni N, Zang E, Kelloff G, Reddy BS. Effect of the chemopreventive agents piroxicam and D,L-α-difluoromethylornithine on intermediate biomarkers of colon carcinogenesis. Carcinogenesis 13:995–1000, 1992.

377. Singh J, Kelloff G, Reddy BS. Effect of chemopreventive agents on intermediate biomarkers during different stages of azoxymethane-induced colon carcinogenesis. Cancer Epidemiol Biomarkers Prev 1:405–411, 1992.

378. Heby O. DNA methylation and polyamines in embryonic development and cancer. Int J Dev Biol 39:737–757, 1995.

379. Singh J, Kulkarni N, Kelloff G, Reddy BS. Modulation of azoxymethane-induced mutational activation of ras protooncogenes by chemopreventive agents in colon carcinogenesis. Carcinogenesis 15:1317–1323, 1994.

380. Ajani JA, Ota DM, Grossie VBJ, et al. Evaluation of continuous-infusion α-difluoromethylornithine therapy for colorectal carcinoma. Cancer Chemother Pharmacol 26:223–226, 1990.

381. Abeloff MD, Rosen ST, Luk GD, et al. Phase II trials of α-difluoromethylornithine, an inhibitor of polyamine synthesis, in advanced small cell lung cancer and colon cancer. Cancer Treat Rep 70:843–845, 1986.

382. Boyle JO, Meyskens FLJ, Garewal HS, Gerner EW. Polyamine contents in rectal and buccal mucosae in humans treated with oral difluoromethylornithine. Cancer Epidemiol Biomarkers Prev 1:131–135, 1992.

383. Love RR, Carbone PP, Verma AK, et al. Randomized phase I chemoprevention dose-seeking study of α-difluoromethylornithine. J Natl Cancer Inst 85:732–737, 1993.

384. Meyskens FLJ, Emerson SS, Pelot D, et al. Dose de-escalation chemoprevention trial of α-difluoromethylornithine in patients with colon polyps. J Natl Cancer Inst 86:1122–1130, 1994.

385. Meyskens FLJ, Gerner EW, Emerson S, et al. Effect of α-difluoromethylornithine on rectal mucosal levels of polyamines in a randomized, double-blinded trial for colon cancer prevention. J Natl Cancer Inst 90:1212–1218, 1998.

386. Love RR, Jacoby R, Newton MA, et al. A randomized, placebo-controlled trial of low-dose α-difluoromethylornithine in individuals at risk for colorectal cancer. Cancer Epidemiol Biomarkers Prev 7:989–992, 1998.

387. Saydjari R, Townsend CMJ, Barranco SC, Thompson JC. Effects of cyclosporine and α-difluoromethylornithine on the growth of mouse colon cancer in vitro. Life Sci 40:359–366, 1987.

388. Watabe J, Bernstein H. The mutagenicity of bile acids using a fluctuation test. Mutat Res 158:45–51, 1985.

389. Martinez JD, Stratagoules ED, LaRue JM, et al. Different bile acids exhibit distinct biological effects: the tumor promoter deoxycholic acid induces apoptosis and the chemopreventive agent ursodeoxycholic acid inhibits cell proliferation. Nutr Cancer 31:111–118, 1998.

390. Ochsenkuhn T, Bayerdorffer E, Meining A, et al. Colonic mucosal proliferation is related to serum deoxycholic acid levels. Cancer 85:1664–1669, 1999.

391. Earnest DL, Holubec H, Wali RK, et al. Chemoprevention of azoxymethane-induced colonic carcinogenesis by supplemental dietary ursodeoxycholic acid. Cancer Res 54:5071–5074, 1994.

392. Narisawa T, Fukaura Y, Terada K, Sekiguchi H. Inhibitory effects of ursodeoxycholic acid on N-methylnitrosourea-induced colon carcinogenesis and colonic mucosal telomerase activity in F344 rats. J Exp Clin Cancer Res 18:259–266, 1999.

393. Guldutuna S, Zimmer G, Imhof M, et al. Molecular aspects of membrane stabilization by ursodeoxycholate. Gastroenterology 104:1736–1744, 1993.

# Chapter 53

# Molecular Biology of Colorectal Cancer

## LI-KUO SU

The development of colorectal cancer from normal epithelial cells is a multistep process. A molecular genetic model proposed more than a decade ago has been proven to be a major genetic pathway for colorectal tumorigenesis.[1,2] It is clear that the alteration of many genes, including both proto-oncogenes and tumor suppressor genes, is involved in this complex process of tumorigenesis. Several of these genes have been identified and their functions elucidated. In addition, other molecular alterations that may contribute to the development of colorectal cancer have been discovered.

## The Major Genetic Pathway

### APC Tumor Suppressor Gene

Inactivation of the adenomatous polyposis coli (*APC*) gene is the genetic alteration that initiates the development of most colorectal tumors. The *APC* gene is mutated somatically in most colorectal tumors and in germline of patients with familial adenomatous polyposis (FAP).

Familial adenomatous polyposis is an autosomal dominant inherited disease that predisposes patients to colorectal cancer. Patients with FAP usually develop hundreds to thousands of benign colorectal polyps in their second or third decades of life. If these polyps are not removed, some of them will progress to malignancy. A genetic locus for FAP was revealed by the identification of an interstitial deletion on chromosome 5q in an FAP patient.[3] Linkage analyses confirmed this observation and further localized the FAP locus to the 5q21–22 region.[4–6] Molecular genetic analyses of sporadic colorectal tumors suggested that the development of sporadic colorectal tumors was initiated by somatic mutations of the gene for FAP.[7–9]

Combination studies involving both sporadic colorectal tumors and patients with FAP led to the isolation of the *APC* gene.[10–13] The importance of *APC* as a tumor suppressor gene in colorectal tumorigenesis has been demonstrated by the identification of germline mutations in FAP patients and somatic mutations in colorectal tumors.[10–17] Almost all identified *APC* mutations cause truncations of the APC protein. Consistent with Knudson's two-hit hypothesis that both alleles of a tumor suppressor gene are inactivated in cancer,[18] inactivation of both alleles of *APC* has been demonstrated in sporadic colorectal tumors and colorectal tumors from FAP patients. The tumor suppressor function of *APC* has also been demonstrated in several mouse models. Multiple intestinal neoplasia (*Min*) mice were derived from an *N*-ethyl-*N*-nitrosourea-treated founder mouse and carried a nonsense germline mutation in the *Apc* gene.[19,20] Two other mouse strains carrying germline *Apc* mutations were generated by gene-knockout techniques.[21,22] These three strains of mouse all exhibit a phenotype similar to that seen in human FAP patients, i.e., they develop multiple intestinal tumors at a young age. Inactivation of both *Apc* alleles was found in adenomas from *Min* mice containing as few as only two dysplastic crypts.[23] In another mouse model, intestinal tumors could be found 4 weeks after both *Apc* alleles were inactivated in adult mice.[24] These results show that inactivation of *APC* is the initiating genetic event for colorectal tumorigenesis.

While patients with typical FAP develop hundreds to thousands of colorectal polyps beginning at a young age, patients with attenuated FAP develop fewer colorectal tumors at an older age. Initially, there was controversy about whether attenuated FAP was a subtype of FAP and about the role of *APC* in attenuated FAP.[25,26] It is now clear, however, that attenuated FAP is caused by germline mutations in *APC*.[27–29] Mounting evidence has shown that individuals with a germline mutation of *APC* in its first four coding exons, its alternatively spliced region of exon 9, or its 3′ half of coding region usually develop attenuated FAP.[28,30–34] However, there can be significant variation in the phenotype of individuals carrying the same germline mutation,[34,35] but the reason for this phenotype variation is not clear.

A germline *APC* mutation *I1307K* found mainly in Ashkenazi Jews has recently been shown to increase colon cancer risk in its carriers about twofold.[36–41] This mutation is a single nucleotide alteration that changes codon 1307 of *APC* from ATA (coding for isoleucine) to AAA (coding for lysine). This nucleotide change itself does not appear to affect the tumor suppressor function of *APC*. However, this single nucleotide alteration changes the DNA sequence around codon 1307 from $(A)_3T(A)_4$ to $(A)_8$. This stretch of eight adenosines appears to significantly increase mutations in this region and cause a frame shift of the *I1307K* allele of *APC*.[36,40,42] Carriers of *APCI1307K* have an increased risk for developing colon cancer because the *I1307K* allele mutates more easily than the wild-type *APC* does.

The way in which *APC* exerts its tumor suppressor function was not obvious when the gene was first identified. The *APC* gene encodes a 10.5 kb mRNA that translates to a protein of 2843 amino acids. The APC protein has been shown to interact with many cellular proteins. It is now believed that APC's association with β-catenin and promotion of the degradation of β-catenin are most relevant to its tumor suppressor function.[43–46] Mammalian β-catenin had been studied for its association with the E-cadherin family of cell adhesion molecules and its importance in cell–cell interaction.[47–49] It is now known that β-catenin has another function in the cell nucleus. β-Catenin was shown to interact with T-cell factor (TCF), also known as lymphoid enhancer-binding factor (LEF), and translocate into the nucleus to form a transcription-active complex. Perturbation of this complex formation profoundly affected the development of *Xenopus* embryos.[50,51] Human β-catenin was then shown to interact with TCF-4 in colon cancer cell lines and to regulate transcription activity of promoters containing the TCF-binding sequence.[52,53] Much evidence has been gathered to support the hypothesis that regulation of β-catenin is the major tumor suppression activity of *APC*. Somatic mutations of the β-catenin gene have been identified in both human and rodent colorectal tumors that do not have the *APC* mutation.[53–57] These somatic mutations are all in a region of β-catenin known to be important for regulating its stability. Several of these mutant β-catenins were shown to be resistant to APC-mediated degradation. In addition, transgenic mice expressing stable β-catenin mutants developed intestinal tumors.[58]

A picture of how APC regulates β-catenin degradation has emerged. APC binds not only β-catenin but also glycogen synthase kinase-3β (GSK3β) and Axin.[59–61] A model has been proposed that APC and Axin serve as a scaffold to bring β-catenin and GSK3β close to each other and facilitate the phosphorylation of β-catenin by GSK3β.[62,63] The β-catenin mutants found in colorectal cancers all have mutations at the region that is critical for β-catenin to be phosphorylated by GSK3β. APC and Axin themselves are also phosphorylated by GSK3β, enhancing their binding of β-catenin. The phosphorylated β-catenin is bound by β-TrCP,[64–66] the first step for the ubiquitination of β-catenin. The ubiquitinated β-catenin is then degraded by proteasome. Mutant APC proteins, almost all of which are truncated, cannot form this multiprotein complex and therefore cannot properly regulate the degradation of β-catenin. The resulting excessive β-catenin can then associate with TCF and translocate into the nucleus, where the β-catenin/TCF-4 complex activates the expression of genes that promote tumorigenesis.

Several genes whose expressions are regulated by the β-catenin/ TCF-4 complex have been identified. The c-*MYC* oncogene and *PPARδ*, which encodes peroxisome proliferator-activated receptor δ, were identified as β-catenin/TCF-4 regulated genes because the expression of each was reduced when wild-type *APC* was expressed in a colon cancer cell line that expressed only endogenous mutant *APC*.[67,68] The high frequency and early expression of matrix metalloproteinase-7 (MMP-7), also known as matrilysin, during both human and mouse intestinal tumorigenesis led to the discovery that the expression of both human and mouse *MMP-7* was regulated by the β-catenin/TCF-4 complex.[69,70] Direct regulation of the expression of these genes by the β-catenin/TCF-4 complex was confirmed by the identification of TCF-4–binding sites at the promoters of these genes. In addition, cyclin D1 was identified as a β-catenin/TCF-4–regulated gene because sequence analysis of its promoter identified a TCF-4–binding sequence.[71,72] The expression of reporter genes regulated by promoters of these genes was increased or decreased when the transcription activity of β-catenin/TCF-4 was manipulated to increase or decrease, respectively. Mutation of potential TCF-4–binding sites in these promoters resulted in the reduction of transcription of reporter genes controlled by these promoters. Furthermore, the protein levels of MYC, PPARδ, and cyclin D1 were reduced when β-catenin/TCF-4 transcription activity was reduced by the expression of the wild-type *APC* or a dominant negative mutant of TCF-4 that interfered with the activity of the β-catenin/TCF-4 complex.

In experimental systems, overexpression of c-*MYC* transforms cells in culture and induces tumorigenesis in animals. Furthermore, overexpression of c-*MYC* has been identified in many human neoplasms.[73,74] c-*MYC* has been shown to be important for many different aspects of cell biology, including proliferation, apoptosis, and differentiation. MYC protein is a transcription factor and controls cell growth by regulating the expression of many genes.[75] c-*MYC* oncogene is frequently overexpressed at mRNA and protein levels in both early and late stages of colorectal tumors.[76–78] Although the overexpression of c-*MYC* in other types of neoplasms often resulted from rearrangements or amplifications of the c-*MYC* gene, gross alteration of the c-*MYC* gene was rarely found in colorectal tumors. The identification of c-*MYC* as a target gene for β-catenin/TCF-4 provides a mechanistic explanation for the overexpression of c-*MYC* in colorectal cancer and a clue to the tumor suppressor function of *APC*.

PPARδ, a member of the nuclear receptor superfamily, functions as a ligand-dependent, sequence-specific transcription factor.[79–81] The mechanism by which PPARδ contributes to colorectal tumorigenesis is not yet known. However, the identification of *PPARδ* as a target gene of β-catenin/TCF-4 provides an intriguing link between nonsteroidal anti-inflammatory drugs (NSAIDs) and colorectal tumorigenesis. Numerous studies have shown that NSAIDs reduce colorectal tumorigenesis in both humans and mice.[82–84] The inhibition of cyclooxygenase (COX) activity by NSAIDs has been suggested as the mechanism for their tumor suppression activity. However, there are many observations that are inconsistent with this suggestion (see discussion in Hart et al.[65]). It was shown that sulindac and indomethacin, two NSAIDs, suppressed the transcription activity of PPARδ.[68] Therefore, if the deregulation of PPARδ activity contributed to colorectal tumorigenesis, the inhibition of PPARδ's activity by NSAIDs could suppress colorectal tumorigenesis.

Matrix metalloproteases (MMPs) have been strongly implicated in tumor invasion and metastasis.[85,86] However, there are many differences between MMP-7 and other MMPs, and evidence suggests that MMP-7 is also important for the growth of early-stage tumors. Unlike most other MMPs, which are expressed at the stroma, MMP-7 was shown to be expressed in colon cancer epithelial cells. Also different from most other MMPs, which are expressed at late stages of colorectal tumorigenesis, MMP-7 was shown to be expressed in colorectal adenomas.[87] Increased and decreased expressions of MMP-7 in human colon cancer cell lines were shown to enhance and reduce, respectively, the tumorigenicity of these cell lines in mice.[88] Furthermore, Min mice that did not express MMP-7 developed fewer and smaller intestinal tumors than those expressing MMP-7.[89] The identification of MMP-7 as a target gene for β-catenin/TCF-4 regulated transcription could explain the early and epithelial expression of MMP-7 in colorectal cancer development. This finding is also consistent with the suggestion that MMP-7 contributes to colorectal tumorigenesis.

The importance of cyclin D1 in cell cycle regulation led to the investigation of whether its expression was controlled by β-catenin/TCF-4.[71,72,90] As mentioned earlier, evidence presented by two different laboratories strongly supports the idea that the expression of cyclin D1 is regulated by β-catenin/TCF-4. This evidence includes the presence of a TCF-binding sequence in the promoter of the cyclin D1 gene, the regulation of the promoter activity of cyclin D1 gene by β-catenin/TCF-4, and the requirement of the TCF-binding sequence in the promoter for its activity to be regulated by β-catenin/TCF-4. Moreover, the level of cyclin D1 protein in cells increased or decreased when the activity of β-catenin/TCF-4 in those cells was enhanced or reduced, respectively. These results could explain how cyclin D1 is overexpressed in some colorectal tumors. The correlation between activated β-catenin/TCF-4 activity and the overexpression of cyclin D1 during colorectal tumorigenesis may not be straightforward. It has been documented that cyclin D1 is overexpressed in colorectal adenomas and carcinomas. However, only 20% to 50% of colorectal tumors were shown to overexpress cyclin D1,[91–94] even though almost all earliest-stage colorectal tumors have mutations in either APC or β-catenin. Therefore, although overexpression of cyclin D1 may contribute to the progression of colorectal tumors, it is less clear whether the overexpression of cyclin D1 resulting from activation of β-catenin/TCF-4 activity is critical for the initiation of colorectal tumorigenesis.

### ras Oncogenes

ras genes are among the earliest identified human proto-oncogenes. Different ras genes encode three very similar proteins: H-Ras, K-Ras, and N-Ras.[95,96] Point mutations altering codons 12, 13, or 61 of H-ras and N-ras have been found in about 50% of human colorectal tumors.[1,97,98] There is a low incidence of mutations in small adenomas but a high incidence in large adenomas and carcinomas.[1] It has also been shown that in some adenomas, the codon 12 mutation of K-ras occurs in some areas while the wild-type ras occurs in other areas of the same tumor. In contrast, this type of heterogeneity in the K-ras mutation was not found in carcinomas.[99] These results strongly indicate that most ras mutations occur after adenomas are formed but before they progress to carcinoma.

Ras belongs to a superfamily of small GTPases.[100,101] Wild-type Ras normally binds guanosine diphosphate (GDP) and is inactive. Upon receiving activation signals, such as those from activated growth factor receptors, Ras releases GDP and binds guanosine triphosphate (GTP), a process facilitated by guanine nucleotide exchange factors. Ras becomes active when it binds to GTP and activates its effectors, such as RAF and phosphatidylinositol 3-kinase. Ras is deactivated when the bound GTP is hydrolyzed to become GDP, a process enhanced by GTPase-

activating proteins (GAPs). Transforming Ras mutants have greatly reduced both intrinsic and GAP-mediated GTPase activity.[100–104] The functional role of amino acids 12 and 61 of Ras in GAP-activated GTPase activity became better understood when the three-dimensional structure of the Ras–GAP complex was elucidated. These amino acids were shown to be critical to forming the catalytic active site.[105]

The functional importance of mutant Ras in human colon cancers has been demonstrated. The growth rate in vitro and the tumorigenicity in nude mice of two human colon cancer cell lines were shown to be significantly reduced when the mutant ras alleles in these cell lines were inactivated.[106] ras mutation by itself, however, does not appear to be sufficient for neoplastic transformation. ras mutations were found at a very high frequency in human colon aberrant crypt foci. However, aberrant crypt foci that did not have the APC mutation were nondysplastic, whereas the only dysplastic aberrant crypt focus was found to have both APC and ras mutations.[107–110] These results, and those described earlier, strongly indicate that although mutation of ras alone can cause aberrant crypt proliferation, lesions that contain only the ras mutation do not progress to tumors. Mutant ras can, however, promote tumor progression in lesions initiated by APC mutations.

### p53 Tumor Suppressor Gene

The p53 gene was believed to be an oncogene because of its ability to cooperate with other oncogenes to transform cells. Results of several investigations in the late 1980s demonstrated that p53 genes previously used to transform cells were mutants and that wild-type p53 was actually a tumor suppressor gene.[111–115] One of these earliest pieces of evidence in this regard was the identification of somatic mutations of p53 in human colon cancers.[111] Mutations of the p53 tumor suppressor gene have since been found in most human cancers.[116,117] Mutations of p53 occur late during colorectal tumor development. Loss of heterozygosity (LOH) of chromosome 17p, where p53 resides, occurs frequently in colon cancer but rarely in adenomas.[1] In addition, overexpression of p53, indicative of p53 mutations, is found much more often in colorectal carcinomas than in adenomas.[118–121]

p53 has been shown to contribute to many cellular processes, including cell cycle regulation, genomic stability, and apoptosis.[122,123] The p53 protein normally has a very short half-life in cells. When induced by stresses such as DNA damage, inappropriate proliferation signals, or depletion of nutrient and/or oxygen, p53 protein is phosphorylated and becomes stable. The p53 protein is a transcription factor with sequence-specific DNA-binding activity.[124,125] Many genes whose expression is regulated by p53 have been identified, and many of their functions could contribute to the broad cellular functions of p53.[122,126] Almost all mutant p53 proteins derived from cancers have altered sequence-specific DNA-binding and transcription activities.[124,125,127,128] Through X-ray crystallography we have learned that amino acid residues that were frequently mutated in tumors were critical for either p53–DNA interaction or maintaining appropriate p53 conformation.[129]

### Chromosome 18q

A high incidence of LOH of the long arm of chromosome 18 has been found in advanced colorectal cancer.[1,9,130] The LOH indicates that one or more tumor suppressor genes are present in this chromosome region and that inactivation of these genes leads to the progression of colon cancer. Several potential tumor suppressor genes in this region have been identified: *DCC* (deleted in colorectal cancer),[131] *SMAD4* (also known as *DPC4*),[132] and *SMAD2* (also known as *MADR2, JV18-1*)[133,134] (for nomenclature of SMAD family see Derynck et al.[135]). It has been difficult to determine which of these genes is the most important tumor suppressor gene targeted for LOH. One reason for this is that the region of 18q with LOH is large and contains at least two of these genes. The other reason is that somatic mutations of these genes are rare in colon cancer.[133,134,136–139] Nevertheless, two studies showed that LOH at 18q is strongly correlated with lower survival rates in patients with stage II colorectal cancer.[140,141] In another study, this correlation was not seen but the survival rate of stage II colon cancer patients was remarkably high.[142]

The results from several studies have strongly indicated that *DCC* and *SMAD4* play important roles in colon cancer progression. *DCC* was isolated by positional cloning from chromosome 18q[131] and shown to encode a transmembrane protein that is highly expressed on the surface of axons and differentiated intestinal epithelial cells.[143] It was later shown that *DCC* encodes a receptor for netrin-1 and is important for the development of the nervous system.[144–146] The function of *DCC* in normal colorectal epithelial cell development and in colorectal cancer progression remains unclear. However, colorectal cancers with LOH at chromosome 18q usually do not express DCC.[143,147] More importantly, reduced expression of DCC in colorectal cancer is correlated with a poor prognosis.[147,148]

*SMAD4* encodes a protein that plays a critical role in the transforming growth factor (TGF)-β signal transduction pathway.[149,150] *SMAD4* was isolated as a tumor suppressor gene for pancreatic cancer, and a high incidence of somatic mutations of *SMAD4* has been found in pancreatic cancers.[132] Although somatic mutations of *SMAD4* have been found in only 10% to 30% of colorectal cancers, there is a higher incidence of somatic mutations of *SMAD4* in advanced colon cancer than in early-stage colon cancer.[137,139,151] Moreover, intestinal tumors that developed in mice carrying a germline mutation in the *Apc* gene were more likely to progress to malignant tumors in mice also carrying mutant *Smad4* than in mice carrying wild-type *Smad4*.[152] These results strongly suggest that inactivation of *SMAD4* contributes to the progression of colorectal cancer. In addition, germline mutations of *SMAD4* have been found in patients with juvenile polyposis, an autosomal dominant disease that predisposes patients to hamartomatous polyposis and gastrointestinal cancer.[153,154]

## Genomic Stability

### Microsatellite Instability

Microsatellites are short-repeat DNA sequences. Although the term *microsatellite* was initially used to describe CA dinucleotide repeats, it can be used to describe repeats of one to five nucleotides of any base composition. Similar to other genetic materials, microsatellites are stably inherited. Microsatellites have become very powerful tools for genetic studies, such as linkage analysis and LOH analysis, because of their special characteristics: they appear to be widely distributed in the genome, most of them are polymorphic, and they can be easily detected and typed.[155–158] Although microsatellites are normally stably inherited, they become highly unstable in cells that lack DNA mismatch repair capacity. This instability occurs in some sporadic colon cancers and in most colon cancers in patients with hereditary nonpolyposis colorectal cancer (HNPCC).

Also known as Lynch syndrome, HNPCC is an autosomal dominant inherited disorder that predisposes patients to colorectal cancer.[159–162] In 1993, an HNPCC gene was shown by linkage analysis to be on chromosome 2.[163] However, because there were well-characterized HNPCC patients whose disease did not show linkage to the gene on chromosome 2, it was clear that HNPCC could be caused by mutations in other genes. This was confirmed almost immediately by the identification of a second HNPCC gene at chromosome 3.[164] At about the same time, investigators discovered an unexpected genetic feature in most colorectal tumors from HNPCC patients and in 10% to 20% of all colorectal tumors: these tumors appeared to have new alleles in addition to their germline alleles at several microsatellite markers.[165–167] Various investigators referred to this feature as replication error (RER), mutator mutation phenotype (MMP), or microsatellite instability (MSI). Intriguingly, similar phenotypes were observed in yeast when any one of a number of genes important for DNA mismatch repair was mutated.[168] The role of mismatch repair genes in HNPCC was confirmed by the identification of human DNA mismatch repair genes *hMSH2* and *hMLH1* as the HNPCC genes on chromosomes 2 and 3, respectively.[169–172] Studies of many HNPCC families showed that *hMSH2* and *HMLH1* were the two major genes responsible for HNPCC. However, germline mutations in three other mismatch repair genes (*hPMS1, hPMS2,* and *hMSH6*) have also been found in patients with HNPCC or HNPCC-like disease.[173–176] Similar to other tumor suppressor genes and consistent with Knudson's two-hit hypothesis, both alleles of a mismatch repair gene are mutated in a tumor. The deficiency of DNA mismatch repair activity in human colon cancer cell lines showing MSI was confirmed by several different assays.[177]

A model for DNA mismatch repair has emerged from studies of bacteria, yeast, and mammalian cells.[178] In mammalian cells, MSH2 protein associates with MSH6 and MSH3 proteins to form MutSα and MutSβ complexes, respectively. Depending on the size of the mismatch, one of these complexes detects and binds to the mismatch region. MLH1 associates with PMS2 or PMS1 to form MutLα and MutLβ complexes, respectively. These MutL complexes interact with the MutS complexes bound on mismatch sites and recruit other proteins that are necessary for removing the mismatch and synthesizing correct DNA sequences. The central roles of MSH2 and MLH1 in forming MutS and MutL complexes, respectively, and the potential overlapping in functions between MSH3 and MSH6 and between PMS proteins could explain why the most HNPCCs are caused by germline mutations of either the *hMSH2* or *hMLH1* gene.

Because MSI sporadic colon cancers and colon tumors from HNPCC patients have a similar MSI phenotype, it was surprising that somatic mutations of mismatch repair genes were found in only a small numbers of MSI sporadic colon cancers.[179–181] Several recent studies showed that, instead of mutations in the coding region of *hMSH2* and *hMLH1* genes, the promoter of *hMLH1* was hypermethylated in the majority of MSI sporadic colorectal tumors and the hMLH1 protein was not expressed in those tumors.[182–185] The silencing of *hMLH1* by hypermethylation has the same result as mutation of both alleles of the gene, i.e., there is no functional hMLH1 protein, and, therefore, the cell is deficient in mismatch repair capacity. The hypermethylation has not been found in the promoter of *hMSH2*.

It has been hypothesized that HNPCC patients are predisposed to colorectal cancer because somatic mutations of genes important for colorectal tumorigenesis occur at higher rates once the cells become deficient in DNA mismatch repair capacity.[169,170]

It has since been shown that genes coding for TGF-β type II receptor, insulin-like growth factor II receptor, proapoptotic protein BAX, cell cycle regulator E2F-4, and mismatch repair proteins MSH3 and MSH6 are mutated in HNPCC or MSI sporadic colon cancer.[186–192] Mutations of these genes occur at microsatellite-like sequences within these genes, and mutations of both alleles of a gene have been identified in some tumors.

## Chromosome Instability

Aneuploidy is common in cancer, including colorectal cancer. Aneuploidy can be caused by one or a few abnormal chromosome segregations or by persistent abnormality in chromosome segregation during the tumor development. In the former scenario, chromosomes segregate normally in most cell divisions during tumor development, but abnormal chromosome segregation in one or a few cell divisions during this long process leads to aneuploidy. In the latter case, abnormal chromosome segregation occurs almost every time cells divide.[193] Using fluorescence in situ hybridization, it was shown that colon cancer cell lines that were aneuploid had persistent abnormality in chromosome segregation.[194] Intriguingly, of the eight human colon cancer cell lines that were investigated, only one had both MSI and chromosome instability while the other seven had either MSI or chromosome instability. Cell fusion experiments showed that the fusion of a chromosome-unstable cell with a chromosome-stable cell resulted in a chromosome-unstable hybrid. Therefore, in contrast to MSI, which is a recessive trait, the chromosome instability appeared to be a dominant trait.[194] The observation that MSI colon cancer cell lines are usually chromosome-stable is consistent with findings that HNPCC and MSI colon cancers are more likely to be diploid and less likely to have LOH.[167,195,196] Although a major function of p53 is maintaining genome integrity, the chromosome stability of colon cancer cells does not directly correlate with the p53 status of these cells.[194] The chromosome instability in some colon cancers appears to be caused by mutations in a mitotic checkpoint gene, *hBUB1*. Consistent with chromosome instability being a dominant trait, expression of mutant BUB1 converted a colon cancer cell line that displayed chromosome stability to one that displayed chromosome instability.[197] However, the molecular basis for the chromosome instability in most colon cancers remains unknown.

## Other Molecular Alterations

### COX-2

Cyclooxygenase, also known as prostaglandin-endoperoxidase or prostaglandin H synthase, catalyzes the conversion of arachidonic acid to prostaglandin $H_2$. Two different genes encode two different cyclooxygenases, COX-1 and COX-2. COX-1 is expressed constitutively at a constant level in many tissues and is involved in many physiologic functions. COX-2 is responsible for inflammatory processes, and its expression is induced by several stimuli.[198,199] The expression of *COX-2* has been shown to be increased in human colorectal tumors and in murine intestinal tumors.[200–205] The molecular mechanism for overexpression of *COX-2* during colorectal tumorigenesis is not understood. As described earlier, NSAIDs have been found to reduce colorectal tumorigenesis in both human and murine.[83,84] Although NSAIDs could inhibit gastrointestinal tumorigenesis by a COX-2-independent mechanism, several studies have shown that a COX-2-specific inhibitor can reduce colorectal tumorigenesis in FAP patients

and in mice.[206–208] In addition, mice that do not express COX-2 because of homozygous *Cox-2* gene knockout develop fewer and smaller intestinal polyps than those in mice carrying either one or two copies of the wild-type *Cox-2* gene.[209] These results indicate that COX-2 contributes to colorectal tumorigenesis.

### SRC Oncogene

The specific activity of pp60$^{c\text{-}SRC}$ has been shown to increase during colorectal tumorigenesis.[210–214] pp60$^{c\text{-}SRC}$ is the protein product of the proto-oncogene *SRC* and is a protein tyrosine kinase. The kinase activity of pp60$^{c\text{-}SRC}$ is highly regulated and is induced by many growth factors. The importance of pp60$^{c\text{-}SRC}$ in many cellular functions has been well documented.[215] Recently, pp60$^{c\text{-}SRC}$ has been shown to be also essential for the induction of human vascular endothelial growth factor (VEGF) by hypoxia.[216,217] The specific activity of pp60$^{c\text{-}SRC}$ was shown to be higher in colorectal polyps than in normal tissue. The specific activity of pp60$^{c\text{-}SRC}$ is further increased in colorectal carcinomas and in liver metastases from colorectal cancer. Reduction of the pp60$^{c\text{-}SRC}$ level in a colorectal cancer cell line reduced the proliferation of these cells in vitro and, to an even greater extent, the tumorigenicity of these cells in mice.[218] These cells expressed a reduced level of VEGF in cell culture under hypoxic conditions compared to that of their parental cells. Furthermore, tumors formed by these cells had reduced vascularization compared with tumors induced by the parental cells.[219,220] The mechanism for the increased pp60$^{c\text{-}SRC}$ enzyme activity during colorectal tumorigenesis is not clear. A recent report showed that a truncating mutation at codon 531 of *SRC* existed in a significant portion of the colorectal cancers examined and that the mutant pp60$^{c\text{-}SRC}$ had increased enzyme activity as well as transforming activity.[221] However, this specific mutation was not found in 479 advanced-stage colorectal cancers in a separate study.[222]

### DNA Methylation

Most of the cytosine at CG dinucleotides is methylated in most human somatic cells.[223] Global hypomethylation of genomic DNA was observed in human colorectal adenomas, a result suggesting that the hypomethylation occurred early during colorectal tumorigenesis.[224,225] Reduction of DNA methylase activity, however, was shown to decrease intestinal tumorigenesis in *Min* mice.[226] One possible explanation that reconciles these conflicting observations is that although colorectal tumorigenesis is facilitated by global DNA hypomethylation, it is also promoted by hypermethylation at specific genetic loci. Methylation could be a mechanism in addition to mutation to inactivate tumor suppressor genes.[227] As described earlier, MSI in most sporadic colorectal tumors is caused by the lack of *hMLH1* expression due to hypermethylation at its promoter. Silencing of other tumor suppressor genes in other types of human cancers has been documented.[227] Techniques have been developed and applied to identify genes that are preferentially methylated in human colon cancer.[227–229] A subtype of colorectal tumors with CIMP (CpG island methylator phenotype) has been proposed on the basis of results of one such investigation.[228]

### Gene Expression

The expression levels of many genes may differ between colorectal cancer and normal colorectal epithelial cells. Some of these changes result directly or indirectly from the gene mutations described above. For example, the increased expression of c-*MYC* is the direct consequence of the increased transcription activity of the β-catenin/TCF complex caused by mutations of either *APC* or β-catenin. The MYC protein itself is a transcription factor, and it can increase the expression of many other genes. The alteration of DNA methylation in colorectal tumors could also decrease the expression of many genes. Traditionally, expression levels of a gene that is potentially important for colorectal tumorigenesis are compared between colon cancer and normal colon epithelium to determine whether expression is altered in colon cancer. New techniques have been developed to identify genes whose expression is different between two cell populations.[230–233] A profile of the difference in gene expression between normal colon epithelium and colon cancer has been reported using one of these new techniques.[234]

## Alternative Genetic Pathways?

Although there is a high incidence of mutations of *ras* and *p53* genes in human colon cancer, it is clear that these mutations do not occur in every case. It is possible that colon cancers that do not have *ras* or *p53* mutations do have mutations in other genes whose products participate in the same functional pathway as that of Ras or p53. This pattern is similar to cases of colorectal tumors that do not have inactivating *APC* mutations but do have activating mutations in the β-catenin gene; APC and β-catenin participate in the same functional pathway for regulating colon epithelial cell growth. However, there has been no strong evidence to support this hypothesis, and the possibility that colorectal tumors could progress along a different pathway cannot be ruled out.

It is possible that a potential alternative pathway is the major pathway for the progression of a group of colorectal tumors. Although mutations of *ras* and *p53* have been found in MSI colorectal tumors, there is evidence that mutations of these genes occur less frequently in these tumors than in those without MSI.[166,192,195,235,236] Differences in mutation rates of *ras* and *p53* between CIMP⁺ and CIMP⁻ colorectal tumors have also been suggested.[237] Several studies have shown that HNPCC patients with colon cancer have a higher survival rate than that of patients with similar stages of sporadic colon cancer.[238–240] While the less aggressive behavior of colon cancer in HNPCC patients may be the consequence of the MSI of these tumors as suggested, the possibility that this is the consequence of chromosome stability or of progression of these tumors along a different pathway cannot be ruled out.[170,241,242]

## References

1. Vogelstein B, Fearon ER, Hamilton SR, et al. Genetic alterations during colorectal-tumor development. N Engl J Med 319:525–532, 1988.
2. Fearon ER, Vogelstein B. A genetic model for colorectal tumorigenesis. Cell 61:759–767, 1990.
3. Herrera L, Kakati S, Gibas L, Pietrzak E, Sandberg AA. Gardner syndrome in a man with an interstitial deletion of 5q. Am J Med Genet 25:473–476, 1986.
4. Bodmer WF, Bailey CJ, Bodmer J, et al. Localization of the gene for familial adenomatous polyposis on chromosome 5. Nature 328:614–616, 1987.
5. Leppert M, Dobbs M, Scambler P, et al. The gene for familial polyposis coli maps to the long arm of chromosome 5. Science 238:1411–1413, 1987.
6. Meera Khan P, Tops CM, v.d. Broek M, et al. Close linkage of a highly polymorphic marker (D5S37) to familial adenomatous polyposis (FAP) and confirmation of FAP localization on chromosome 5q21–q22. Hum Genet 79:183–185, 1988.
7. Solomon E, Voss R, Hall V, et al. Chromosome 5 allele loss in human colorectal carcinomas. Nature 328:616–619, 1987.
8. Vogelstein B, Fearon ER, Hamilton SR, et al. Genetic alterations during colorectal-tumor development. N Engl J Med 319:525–532, 1988.
9. Vogelstein B, Fearon ER, Kern SE, et al. Allelotype of colorectal carcinomas. Science 244:207–211, 1989.
10. Kinzler KW, Nilbert MC, Su L-K, et al. Identification of FAP locus genes from chromosome 5q21. Science 253:661–665, 1991.
11. Nishisho I, Nakamura Y, Miyoshi Y, et al. Mutations of chromosome 5q21 genes in FAP and colorectal cancer patients. Science 253:665–669, 1991.
12. Groden J, Thliveris A, Samowitz W, et al. Identification and characterization of the familial adenomatous polyposis coli gene. Cell 66:589–600, 1991.
13. Joslyn G, Carlson M, Thliveris A, et al. Identification of deletion mutations and three new genes at the familial polyposis locus. Cell 66:601–613, 1991.
14. Miyoshi Y, Ando H, Nagase H, et al. Germ-line mutations of the *APC* gene in 53 familial adenomatous polyposis patients. Proc Natl Acad Sci USA 89:4452–4456, 1992.
15. Miyoshi Y, Nagase H, Ando H, et al. Somatic mutations of the *APC* gene in colorectal tumors: mutation cluster region in the APC gene. Hum Mol Genet 1:229–233, 1992.
16. Powell SM, Zilz N, Beazer-Barclay Y, et al. *APC* mutations occur early during colorectal tumorigenesis. Nature 359:235–237, 1992.
17. Miyaki M, Konishi M, Kikuchi-Yanoshita R, et al. Characteristics of somatic mutation of the adenomatous polyposis coli gene in colorectal tumors. Cancer Res 54:3011–3020, 1994.
18. Knudson AG Jr. Hereditary cancer, oncogenes, and antioncogenes. Cancer Res 45:1437–1443, 1985.
19. Moser AR, Pitot HC, Dove WF. A dominant mutation that predisposes to multiple intestinal neoplasia in the mouse. Science 247:322–324, 1990.
20. Su L-K, Kinzler KW, Vogelstein B, et al. Multiple intestinal neoplasia caused by a mutation in the murine homolog of the *APC* gene. Science 256:668–670, 1992.
21. Fodde R, Edelmann W, Yang K, et al. A targeted chain-termination mutation in the mouse *Apc* gene results in multiple intestinal tumors. Proc Natl Acad Sci USA 91:8969–8973, 1994.
22. Oshima M, Oshima H, Kitagawa K, et al. Loss of *Apc* heterozygosity and abnormal tissue building in nascent intestinal polyps in mice carrying a truncated *Apc* gene. Proc Natl Acad Sci USA 92:4482–4486, 1995.
23. Levy DB, Smith KJ, Beazer-Barclay Y, et al. Inactivation of both *APC* alleles in human and mouse tumors. Cancer Res 54:5953–5958, 1994.
24. Shibata H, Toyama K, Shioya H, et al. Rapid colorectal adenoma formation initiated by conditional targeting of the *Apc* gene. Science 278:120–123, 1997.
25. Lynch HT, Smyrk T, Lanspa SJ, et al. Flat adenomas in a colon cancer–prone kindred. J Natl Cancer Inst 80:278–282, 1988.
26. Stella A, Resta N, Gentile M, et al. Exclusion of the *APC* gene as the cause of a variant form of familial adenomatous polyposis (FAP). Am J Hum Genet 53:1031–1037, 1993.
27. Lynch HT, Smyrk TC, Watson P, et al. Hereditary flat adenoma syndrome: a variant of familial adenomatous polyposis? Dis Colon Rectum 35:411–421, 1992.
28. Spirio L, Olschwang S, Groden J, et al. Alleles of the *APC* gene: an attenuated form of familial polyposis. Cell 75:951–957, 1993.
29. Lynch HT, Smyrk T, McGinn T, et al. Attenuated familial adenomatous polyposis (AFAP). A phenotypically and genotypically distinctive variant of FAP. Cancer 76:2427–2433, 1995.
30. van der Luijt RB, Vasen HF, Tops CM, et al. *APC* mutation in the alternatively spliced region of exon 9 associated with late-onset familial adenomatous polyposis. Hum Genet 96:705–710, 1995.
31. van der Luijt RB, Meera Khan P, Vasen HF, et al. Germline mutations in the 3′ part of APC exon 15 do not result in truncated proteins and are associated with attenuated adenomatous polyposis coli. Hum Genet 98:727–734, 1996.
32. Young J, Simms LA, Tarish J, et al. A family with attenuated familial adenomatous polyposis due to a mutation in the alternatively spliced region of APC exon 9. Hum Mutat 11:450–455, 1998.
33. Friedl W, Meuschel S, Caspari R, et al. Attenuated familial adenomatous polyposis due to a mutation in the 3′ part of the *APC* gene. A clue for understanding the function of the APC protein. Hum Genet 97:579–584, 1996.
34. Soravia C, Berk T, Madlensky L, et al. Genotype–phenotype correlations in attenuated adenomatous polyposis coli. Am J Hum Genet 62:1290–1301, 1998.

35. Brensinger JD, Laken SJ, Luce MC, et al. Variable phenotype of familial adenomatous polyposis in pedigrees with 3′ mutation in the *APC* gene. Gut 43:548–552, 1998.

36. Laken SJ, Petersen GM, Gruber SB, et al. Familial colorectal cancer in Ashkenazim due to a hypermutable tract in *APC*. Nat Genet 17:79–83, 1997.

37. Rozen P, Shomrat R, Strul H, et al. Prevalence of the *I1307K APC* gene variant in Israeli Jews of differing ethnic origin and risk for colorectal cancer. Gastroenterology 116:54–57, 1999.

38. Woodage T, King SM, Wacholder S, et al. The *APCI1307K* allele and cancer risk in a community-based study of Ashkenazi Jews. Nat Genet 20:62–65, 1998.

39. Gryfe R, Di Nicola N, Lal G, Gallinger S, Redston M. Inherited colorectal polyposis and cancer risk of the *APC I1307K* polymorphism. Am J Hum Genet 64:378–384, 1999.

40. Gruber SB, Petersen GM, Kinzler KW, Vogelstein B. Cancer, crash sites, and the new genetics of neoplasia. Gastroenterology 116:210–212, 1999.

41. Drucker L, Shpilberg O, Neumann A, et al. Adenomatous polyposis coli *I1307K* mutation in Jewish patients with different ethnicity: prevalence and phenotype. Cancer 88:755–760, 2000.

42. Gryfe R, Di Nicola N, Gallinger S, Redston M. Somatic instability of the *APC I1307K* allele in colorectal neoplasia. Cancer Res 58:4040–4043, 1998.

43. Su L-K, Vogelstein B, Kinzler KW. Association of the APC tumor suppressor protein with catenins. Science 262:1734–1737, 1993.

44. Rubinfeld B, Souza B, Albert I, et al. Association of the *APC* gene product with beta-catenin. Science 262:1731–1734, 1993.

45. Munemitsu S, Albert I, Souza B, Rubinfeld B, Polakis P. Regulation of intracellular beta-catenin levels by the adenomatous polyposis coli (APC) tumor-suppressor protein. Proc Natl Acad Sci USA 92:3046–3050, 1995.

46. Kinzler KW, Vogelstein B. Lessons from hereditary colorectal cancer. Cell 87:159–170, 1996.

47. Kemler R. From cadherins to catenins: cytoplasmic protein interactions and regulation of cell adhesion. Trends Genet 9:317–321, 1993.

48. Tsukita S, Nagafuchi A, Yonemura S. Molecular linkage between cadherins and actin filaments in cell–cell adherens junctions. Curr Opin Cell Biol 4:834–839, 1992.

49. Gumbiner BM. Proteins associated with the cytoplasmic surface of adhesion molecules. Neuron 11:551–564, 1993.

50. Behrens J, von Kries JP, Kuhl M, et al. Functional interaction of beta-catenin with the transcription factor LEF-1. Nature 382:638–642, 1996.

51. Molenaar M, van de Wetering M, Oosterwegel M, et al. XTcf-3 transcription factor mediates beta-catenin–induced axis formation in *Xenopus* embryos. Cell 86:391–399, 1996.

52. Korinek V, Barker N, Morin PJ, et al. Constitutive transcriptional activation by a β-catenin–Tcf complex in APC−/− colon carcinoma. Science 275:1784–1787, 1997.

53. Morin PJ, Sparks AB, Korinek V, et al. Activation of β-catenin–Tcf signaling in colon cancer by mutations in β-catenin or *APC*. Science 275:1787–1790, 1997.

54. Sparks AB, Morin PJ, Vogelstein B, Kinzler KW. Mutational analysis of the APC/β-catenin/Tcf pathway in colorectal cancer. Cancer Res 58:1130–1134, 1998.

55. Dashwood RH, Suzui M, Nakagama H, Sugimura T, Nagao M. High frequency of β-catenin (*Ctnb1*) mutations in the colon tumors induced by two heterocyclic amines in the F344 rat. Cancer Res 58:1127–1129, 1998.

56. Takahashi M, Fukuda K, Sugimura T, Wakabayashi K. Beta-catenin is frequently mutated and demonstrates altered cellular location in azoxymethane-induced rat colon tumors. Cancer Res 58:42–46, 1998.

57. Suzui M, Ushijima T, Dashwood RH, et al. Frequent mutations of the rat β-catenin gene in colon cancers induced by methylazoxymethanol acetate plus 1-hydroxyanthraquinone. Mol Carcinog 24:232–237, 1999.

58. Harada N, Tamai Y, Ishikawa T, et al. Intestinal polyposis in mice with a dominant stable mutation of the β-catenin gene. EMBO J 18:5931–5942, 1999.

59. Rubinfeld B, Albert I, Porfiri E, et al. Binding of GSK3β to the APC–β-catenin complex and regulation of complex assembly. Science 272:1023–1026, 1996.

60. Behrens J, Jerchow BA, Wurtele M, et al. Functional interaction of an axin homolog, conductin, with β-catenin, APC, and GSK3β. Science 280:596–599, 1998.

61. Hart MJ, de los Santos R, Albert IN, Rubinfeld B, Polakis P. Downregulation of β-catenin by human Axin and its association with the *APC* tumor suppressor, β-catenin and GSK3 β. Curr Biol 8:573–581, 1998.

62. Polakis P. The oncogenic activation of beta-catenin. Curr Opin Genet Dev 9:15–21, 1999.

63. Peifer M, Polakis P. Wnt signaling in oncogenesis and embryogenesis—a look outside the nucleus. Science 287:1606–1609, 2000.

64. Kitagawa M, Hatakeyama S, Shirane M, et al. An F-box protein, FWD1, mediates ubiquitin-dependent proteolysis of β-catenin. EMBO J 18:2401–2410, 1999.

65. Hart M, Concordet JP, Lassot I, et al. The F-box protein β-TrCP associates with phosphorylated β-catenin and regulates its activity in the cell. Curr Biol 9:207–210, 1999.

66. Liu C, Kato Y, Zhang Z, et al. β-Trcp couples β-catenin phosphorylation-degradation and regulates *Xenopus* axis formation. Proc Natl Acad Sci USA 96:6273–6278, 1999.

67. He TC, Sparks AB, Rago C, et al. Identification of c-*MYC* as a target of the *APC* pathway. Science 281:1509–1512, 1998.

68. He TC, Chan TA, Vogelstein B, Kinzler KW. PPARδ is an APC-regulated target of nonsteroidal anti-inflammatory drugs. Cell 99:335–345, 1999.

69. Crawford HC, Fingleton BM, Rudolph-Owen LA, et al. The metalloproteinase matrilysin is a target of β-catenin transactivation in intestinal tumors. Oncogene 18:2883–2891, 1999.

70. Brabletz T, Jung A, Dag S, Hlubek F, Kirchner T. Beta-catenin regulates the expression of the matrix metalloproteinase-7 in human colorectal cancer. Am J Pathol 155:1033–1038, 1999.

71. Tetsu O, McCormick F. Beta-catenin regulates expression of cyclin D1 in colon carcinoma cells. Nature 398:422–426, 1999.

72. Shtutman M, Zhurinsky J, Simcha I, et al. The cyclin D1 gene is a target of the β-catenin/LEF-1 pathway. Proc Natl Acad Sci USA 96:5522–5527, 1999.

73. Marcu KB, Bossone SA, Patel AJ. myc function and regulation. Annu Rev Biochem 61:809–860, 1992.

74. Nesbit CE, Tersak JM, Prochownik EV. *MYC* oncogenes and human neoplastic disease. Oncogene 18:3004–3016, 1999.

75. Dang CV. c-*Myc* target genes involved in cell growth, apoptosis, and metabolism. Mol Cell Biol 19:1–11, 1999.

76. Erisman MD, Rothberg PG, Diehl RE, et al. Deregulation of c-*myc* gene expression in human colon carcinoma is not accompanied by amplification or rearrangement of the gene. Mol Cell Biol 5:1969–1976, 1985.

77. Sikora K, Chan S, Evan G, et al. c-*myc* oncogene expression in colorectal cancer. Cancer 59:1289–1295, 1987.

78. Finley GG, Schulz NT, Hill SA, et al. Expression of the *myc* gene family in different stages of human colorectal cancer. Oncogene 4:963–971, 1989.

79. Lemberger T, Desvergne B, Wahli W. Peroxisome proliferator-activated receptors: a nuclear receptor signaling pathway in lipid physiology. Annu Rev Cell Dev Biol 12:335–363, 1996.

80. Michalik L, Wahli W. Peroxisome proliferator-activated receptors: three isotypes for a multitude of functions. Curr Opin Biotechnol 10:564–570, 1999.

81. Vamecq J, Latruffe N. Medical significance of peroxisome proliferator-activated receptors. Lancet 354:141–148, 1999.

82. Smalley WE, DuBois RN. Colorectal cancer and nonsteroidal anti-inflammatory drugs. Adv Pharmacol 39:1–20, 1997.

83. Taketo MM. Cyclooxygenase-2 inhibitors in tumorigenesis (part II). J Natl Cancer Inst 90:1609–1620, 1998.

84. Taketo MM. Cyclooxygenase-2 inhibitors in tumorigenesis (part I). J Natl Cancer Inst 90:1529–1536, 1998.

85. Wilson CL, Matrisian LM. Matrilysin: an epithelial matrix metalloproteinase with potentially novel functions. Int J Biochem Cell Biol 28:123–136, 1996.

86. Chambers AF, Matrisian LM. Changing views of the role of matrix metalloproteinases in metastasis. J Natl Cancer Inst 89:1260–1270, 1997.

87. Newell KJ, Witty JP, Rodgers WH, Matrisian LM. Expression and localization of matrix-degrading metalloproteinases during colorectal tumorigenesis. Mol Carcinog 10:199–206, 1994.

88. Witty JP, McDonnell S, Newell KJ, et al. Modulation of matrilysin levels in colon carcinoma cell lines affects tumorigenicity in vivo. Cancer Res 54:4805–4812, 1994.

89. Wilson CL, Heppner KJ, Labosky PA, Hogan BL, Matrisian LM. Intestinal tumorigenesis is suppressed in mice lacking the metalloproteinase matrilysin. Proc Natl Acad Sci USA 94:1402–1407, 1997.

90. Sherr CJ. Cancer cell cycles. Science 274:1672–1677, 1996.

91. Bartkova J, Lukas J, Strauss M, Bartek J. The PRAD-1/cyclin D1 oncogene product accumulates aberrantly in a subset of colorectal carcinomas. Int J Cancer 58:568–573, 1994.

92. Arber N, Hibshoosh H, Moss SF, et al. Increased expression of cyclin D1 is an early event in multistage colorectal carcinogenesis. Gastroenterology 110:669–674, 1996.

93. Maeda K, Chung Y, Kang S, et al. Cyclin D1 overexpression and prognosis in colorectal adenocarcinoma. Oncology 55:145–151, 1998.

94. Zhang T, Nanney LB, Luongo C, et al. Concurrent overexpression of cyclin D1 and cyclin-dependent kinase 4 (Cdk4) in intestinal adenomas from multiple intestinal neoplasia (Min) mice and human familial adenomatous polyposis patients. Cancer Res 57:169–175, 1997.

95. Barbacid M. ras genes. Annu Rev Biochem 56:779–827, 1987.

96. Lowy DR, Willumsen BM. Function and regulation of ras. Annu Rev Biochem 62:851–891, 1993.

97. Bos JL, Fearon ER, Hamilton SR, et al. Prevalence of ras gene mutations in human colorectal cancers. Nature 327:293–297, 1987.

98. Forrester K, Almoguera C, Han K, Grizzle WE, Perucho M. Detection of high incidence of K-ras oncogenes during human colon tumorigenesis. Nature 327:298–303, 1987.

99. Shibata D, Schaeffer J, Li ZH, Capella G, Perucho M. Genetic heterogeneity of the c-K-ras locus in colorectal adenomas but not in adenocarcinomas. J Natl Cancer Inst 85:1058–1063, 1993.

100. Bourne HR, Sanders DA, McCormick F. The GTPase superfamily: a conserved switch for diverse cell functions. Nature 348:125–132, 1990.

101. Bourne HR, Sanders DA, McCormick F. The GTPase superfamily: conserved structure and molecular mechanism. Nature 349:117–127, 1991.

102. Boguski MS, McCormick F. Proteins regulating Ras and its relatives. Nature 366:643–654, 1993.

103. Rebollo A, Martinez AC. Ras proteins: recent advances and new functions. Blood 94:2971–2980, 1999.

104. Pincus MR, Brandt-Rauf PW, Michl J, Carty RP, Friedman FK. ras-p21-induced cell transformation: unique signal transduction pathways and implications for the design of new chemotherapeutic agents. Cancer Invest 18:39–50, 2000.

105. Scheffzek K, Ahmadian MR, Kabsch W, et al. The Ras–RasGAP complex: structural basis for GTPase activation and its loss in oncogenic Ras mutants. Science 277:333–338, 1997.

106. Shirasawa S, Furuse M, Yokoyama N, Sasazuki T. Altered growth of human colon cancer cell lines disrupted at activated Ki-ras. Science 260:85–88, 1993.

107. Pretlow TP, Brasitus TA, Fulton NC, Cheyer C, Kaplan EL. K-ras mutations in putative preneoplastic lesions in human colon. J Natl Cancer Inst 85:2004–2007, 1993.

108. Smith AJ, Stern HS, Penner M, et al. Somatic APC and K-ras codon 12 mutations in aberrant crypt foci from human colons. Cancer Res 54:5527–5530, 1994.

109. Jen J, Powell SM, Papadopoulos N, et al. Molecular determinants of dysplasia in colorectal lesions. Cancer Res 54:5523–5526, 1994.

110. Yamashita N, Minamoto T, Ochiai A, Onda M, Esumi H. Frequent and characteristic K-ras activation and absence of p53 protein accumulation in aberrant crypt foci of the colon. Gastroenterology 108:434–440, 1995.

111. Baker SJ, Fearon ER, Nigro JM, et al. Chromosome 17 deletions and p53 gene mutations in colorectal carcinomas. Science 244:217–221, 1989.

112. Hinds P, Finlay C, Levine AJ. Mutation is required to activate the p53 gene for cooperation with the ras oncogene and transformation. J Virol 63:739–746, 1989.

113. Finlay CA, Hinds PW, Levine AJ. The p53 proto-oncogene can act as a suppressor of transformation. Cell 57:1083–1093, 1989.

114. Malkin D, Li FP, Strong LC, et al. Germ-line p53 mutations in a familial syndrome of breast cancer, sarcomas, and other neoplasms. Science 250:1233–1238, 1990.

115. Srivastava S, Zou ZQ, Pirollo K, Blattner W, Chang EH. Germ-line transmission of a mutated p53 gene in a cancer-prone family with Li-Fraumeni syndrome. Nature 348:747–749, 1990.

116. Nigro JM, Baker SJ, Preisinger AC, et al. Mutations in the p53 gene occur in diverse human tumour types. Nature 342:705–708, 1989.

117. Hollstein M, Sidransky D, Vogelstein B, Harris CC. p53 mutations in human cancers. Science 253:49–53, 1991.

118. Scott N, Bell SM, Sagar P, et al. p53 expression and K-ras mutation in colorectal adenomas. Gut 34:621–624, 1993.

119. Darmon E, Cleary KR, Wargovich MJ. Immunohistochemical analysis of p53 overexpression in human colonic tumors. Cancer Detect Prev 18:187–195, 1994.

120. Kaklamanis L, Gatter KC, Mortensen N, et al. p53 expression in colorectal adenomas. Am J Pathol 142:87–93, 1993.

121. Ohue M, Tomita N, Monden T, et al. A frequent alteration of p53 gene in carcinoma in adenoma of colon. Cancer Res 54:4798–4804, 1994.

122. Levine AJ. p53, the cellular gatekeeper for growth and division. Cell 88:323–331, 1997.

123. Burns TF, El-Deiry WS. The p53 pathway and apoptosis. J Cell Physiol 181:231–239, 1999.

124. Kern SE, Kinzler KW, Bruskin A, et al. Identification of p53 as a sequence-specific DNA-binding protein. Science 252:1708–1711, 1991.

125. El-Deiry WS, Kern SE, Pietenpol JA, Kinzler KW, Vogelstein B. Definition of a consensus binding site for p53. Nat Genet 1:45–49, 1992.

126. Yu J, Zhang L, Hwang PM, et al. Identification and classification of p53-regulated genes. Proc Natl Acad Sci USA 96:14517–14522, 1999.

127. Bargonetti J, Friedman PN, Kern SE, Vogelstein B, Prives C. Wild-type but not mutant p53 immunopurified proteins bind to sequences adjacent to the SV40 origin of replication. Cell 65:1083–1091, 1991.

128. Pietenpol JA, Tokino T, Thiagalingam S, et al. Sequence-specific transcriptional activation is essential for growth suppression by p53. Proc Natl Acad Sci USA 91:1998–2002, 1994.

129. Cho Y, Gorina S, Jeffrey PD, Pavletich NP. Crystal structure of a p53 tumor suppressor–DNA complex: understanding tumorigenic mutations. Science 265:346–355, 1994.

130. Law DJ, Olschwang S, Monpezat JP, et al. Concerted nonsyntenic allelic loss in human colorectal carcinoma. Science 241:961–965, 1988.

131. Fearon ER, Cho KR, Nigro JM, et al. Identification of a chromosome 18q gene that is altered in colorectal cancers. Science 247:49–56, 1990.

132. Hahn SA, Schutte M, Hoque AT, et al. DPC4, a candidate tumor suppressor gene at human chromosome 18q21.1. Science 271:350–353, 1996.

133. Riggins GJ, Thiagalingam S, Rozenblum E, et al. Mad-related genes in the human. Nat Genet 13:347–349, 1996.

134. Eppert K, Scherer SW, Ozcelik H, et al. MADR2 maps to 18q21 and encodes a TGFβ-regulated MAD-related protein that is functionally mutated in colorectal carcinoma. Cell 86:543–552, 1996.

135. Derynck R, Gelbart WM, Harland RM, et al. Nomenclature: vertebrate mediators of TGFβ family signals. Cell 87:173, 1996.

136. Cho KR, Oliner JD, Simons JW, et al. The DCC gene: structural analysis and mutations in colorectal carcinomas. Genomics 19:525–531, 1994.

137. Thiagalingam S, Lengauer C, Leach FS, et al. Evaluation of candidate tumour suppressor genes on chromosome 18 in colorectal cancers. Nat Genet 13:343–346, 1996.

138. Takagi Y, Kohmura H, Futamura M, et al. Somatic alterations of the DPC4 gene in human colorectal cancers in vivo. Gastroenterology 111:1369–1372, 1996.

139. Miyaki M, Iijima T, Konishi M, et al. Higher frequency of Smad4 gene mutation in human colorectal cancer with distant metastasis. Oncogene 18:3098–3103, 1999.

140. Jen J, Kim H, Piantadosi S, et al. Allelic loss of chromosome 18q and prognosis in colorectal cancer. N Engl J Med 331:213–221, 1994.

141. Martinez-Lopez E, Abad A, Font A, et al. Allelic loss on chromosome 18q as a prognostic marker in stage II colorectal cancer. Gastroenterology 114:1180–1187, 1998.

142. Carethers JM, Hawn MT, Greenson JK, Hitchcock CL, Boland CR. Prognostic significance of allelic lost at chromosome 18q21 for stage II colorectal cancer. Gastroenterology 114:1188–1195, 1998.

143. Hedrick L, Cho KR, Fearon ER, et al. The DCC gene product in cellular differentiation and colorectal tumorigenesis. Genes Dev 8:1174–1183, 1994.

144. Chan SS, Zheng H, Su MW, et al. UNC-40, a C. elegans homolog of DCC (deleted in colorectal cancer), is required in motile cells responding to UNC-6 netrin cues. Cell 87:187–195, 1996.

145. Kolodziej PA, Timpe LC, Mitchell KJ, et al. frazzled encodes a Drosophila member of the DCC immunoglobulin subfamily and is required for CNS and motor axon guidance. Cell 87:197–204, 1996.

146. Keino-Masu K, Masu M, Hinck L, et al. Deleted in colorectal cancer (DCC) encodes a netrin receptor. Cell 87:175–185, 1996.

147. Saito M, Yamaguchi A, Goi T, et al. Expression of DCC protein in colorectal tumors and its relationship to tumor progression and metastasis. Oncology 56:134–141, 1999.

148. Shibata D, Reale MA, Lavin P, et al. The DCC protein and prognosis in colorectal cancer. N Engl J Med 335:1727–1732, 1996.

149. Massague J. TGF-β signal transduction. Annu Rev Biochem 67:753–791, 1998.

150. Zhou S, Buckhaults P, Zawel L, et al. Targeted deletion of Smad4 shows it is required for transforming growth factor beta and activin signaling in colorectal cancer cells. Proc Natl Acad Sci USA 95:2412–2416, 1998.

151. Koyama M, Ito M, Nagai H, Emi M, Moriyama Y. Inactivation of both alleles of the DPC4/SMAD4 gene in advanced colorectal cancers: iden-

tification of seven novel somatic mutations in tumors from Japanese patients. Mutat Res 406:71–77, 1999.

152. Takaku K, Oshima M, Miyoshi H, et al. Intestinal tumorigenesis in compound mutant mice of both *Dpc4* (*Smad4*) and *Apc* genes. Cell 92: 645–656, 1998.

153. Howe JR, Roth S, Ringold JC, et al. Mutations in the *SMAD4/DPC4* gene in juvenile polyposis. Science 280:1086–1088, 1998.

154. Houlston R, Bevan S, Williams A, et al. Mutations in *DPC4* (*SMAD4*) cause juvenile polyposis syndrome, but only account for a minority of cases. Hum Mol Genet 7:1907–1912, 1998.

155. Litt M, Luty JA. A hypervariable microsatellite revealed by in vitro amplification of a dinucleotide repeat within the cardiac muscle actin gene. Am J Hum Genet 44:397–401, 1989.

156. Weber JL, May PE. Abundant class of human DNA polymorphisms which can be typed using the polymerase chain reaction. Am J Hum Genet 44:388–396, 1989.

157. Weissenbach J. A second generation linkage map of the human genome based on highly informative microsatellite loci. Gene 135:275–278, 1993.

158. Weissenbach J. Microsatellite polymorphisms and the genetic linkage map of the human genome. Curr Opin Genet Dev 3:414–417, 1993.

159. Lynch HT, Smyrk TC, Watson P, et al. Genetics, natural history, tumor spectrum, and pathology of hereditary nonpolyposis colorectal cancer: an updated review. Gastroenterology 104:1535–1549, 1993.

160. Marra G, Boland CR. Hereditary nonpolyposis colorectal cancer: the syndrome, the genes, and historical perspectives. J Natl Cancer Inst 87:1114–1125, 1995.

161. Lynch HT, de la Chapelle A. Genetic susceptibility to non-polyposis colorectal cancer. J Med Genet 36:801–818, 1999.

162. Vasen HF, Watson P, Mecklin JP, Lynch HT. New clinical criteria for hereditary nonpolyposis colorectal cancer (HNPCC, Lynch syndrome) proposed by the International Collaborative group on HNPCC. Gastroenterology 116:1453–1456, 1999.

163. Peltomaki P, Aaltonen LA, Sistonen P, et al. Genetic mapping of a locus predisposing to human colorectal cancer. Science 260:810–812, 1993.

164. Lindblom A, Tannergard P, Werelius B, Nordenskjold M. Genetic mapping of a second locus predisposing to hereditary non-polyposis colon cancer. Nat Genet 5:279–282, 1993.

165. Aaltonen LA, Peltomaki P, Leach FS, et al. Clues to the pathogenesis of familial colorectal cancer. Science 260:812–816, 1993.

166. Ionov Y, Peinado MA, Malkhosyan S, Shibata D, Perucho M. Ubiquitous somatic mutations in simple repeated sequences reveal a new mechanism for colonic carcinogenesis. Nature 363:558–561, 1993.

167. Thibodeau SN, Bren G, Schaid D. Microsatellite instability in cancer of the proximal colon. Science 260:816–819, 1993.

168. Strand M, Prolla TA, Liskay RM, Petes TD. Destabilization of tracts of simple repetitive DNA in yeast by mutations affecting DNA mismatch repair. Nature 365:274–276, 1993.

169. Fishel R, Lescoe MK, Rao MR, et al. The human mutator gene homolog *MSH2* and its association with hereditary nonpolyposis colon cancer. Cell 75:1027–1038, 1993.

170. Leach FS, Nicolaides NC, Papadopoulos N, et al. Mutations of a *mutS* homolog in hereditary nonpolyposis colorectal cancer. Cell 75:1215–1225, 1993.

171. Bronner CE, Baker SM, Morrison PT, et al. Mutation in the DNA mismatch repair gene homologue *hMLH1* is associated with hereditary nonpolyposis colon cancer. Nature 368:258–261, 1994.

172. Papadopoulos N, Nicolaides NC, Wei YF, et al. Mutation of a *mutL* homolog in hereditary colon cancer. Science 263:1625–1629, 1994.

173. Nystrom-Lahti M, Wu Y, Moisio AL, et al. DNA mismatch repair gene mutations in 55 kindreds with verified or putative hereditary nonpolyposis colorectal cancer. Hum Mol Genet 5:763–769, 1996.

174. Nicolaides NC, Carter KC, Shell BK, et al. Genomic organization of the human *PMS2* gene family. Genomics 30:195–206, 1995.

175. Miyaki M, Konishi M, Tanaka K, et al. Germline mutation of *MSH6* as the cause of hereditary nonpolyposis colorectal cancer. Nat Genet 17:271–272, 1997.

176. Akiyama Y, Sato H, Yamada T, et al. Germ-line mutation of the *hMSH6/GTBP* gene in an atypical hereditary nonpolyposis colorectal cancer kindred. Cancer Res 57:3920–3923, 1997.

177. Parsons R, Li GM, Longley MJ, et al. Hypermutability and mismatch repair deficiency in RER+ tumor cells. Cell 75:1227–1236, 1993.

178. Buermeyer AB, Deschenes SM, Baker SM, Liskay RM. Mammalian DNA mismatch repair. Annu Rev Genet 33:533–564, 1999.

179. Liu B, Nicolaides NC, Markowitz S, et al. Mismatch repair gene defects in sporadic colorectal cancers with microsatellite instability. Nat Genet 9:48–55, 1995.

180. Borresen AL, Lothe RA, Meling GI, et al. Somatic mutations in the *hMSH2* gene in microsatellite unstable colorectal carcinomas. Hum Mol Genet 4:2065–2072, 1995.

181. Moslein G, Tester DJ, Lindor NM, et al. Microsatellite instability and mutation analysis of *hMSH2* and *hMLH1* in patients with sporadic, familial and hereditary colorectal cancer. Hum Mol Genet 5:1245–1252, 1996.

182. Cunningham JM, Christensen ER, Tester DJ, et al. Hypermethylation of the hMLH1 promoter in colon cancer with microsatellite instability. Cancer Res 58:3455–3460, 1998.

183. Herman JG, Umar A, Polyak K, et al. Incidence and functional consequences of hMLH1 promoter hypermethylation in colorectal carcinoma. Proc Natl Acad Sci USA 95:6870–6875, 1998.

184. Kane MF, Loda M, Gaida GM, et al. Methylation of the hMLH1 promoter correlates with lack of expression of hMLH1 in sporadic colon tumors and mismatch repair-defective human tumor cell lines. Cancer Res 57:808–811, 1997.

185. Veigl ML, Kasturi L, Olechnowicz J, et al. Biallelic inactivation of *hMLH1* by epigenetic gene silencing, a novel mechanism causing human MSI cancers. Proc Natl Acad Sci USA 95:8698–8702, 1998.

186. Markowitz S, Wang J, Myeroff L, et al. Inactivation of the type II TGF-β receptor in colon cancer cells with microsatellite instability. Science 268:1336–1338, 1995.

187. Parsons R, Myeroff LL, Liu B, et al. Microsatellite instability and mutations of the transforming growth factor beta type II receptor gene in colorectal cancer. Cancer Res 55:5548–5550, 1995.

188. Souza RF, Appel R, Yin J, et al. Microsatellite instability in the insulin-like growth factor II receptor gene in gastrointestinal tumours. Nat Genet 14:255–257, 1996.

189. Rampino N, Yamamoto H, Ionov Y, et al. Somatic frameshift mutations in the *BAX* gene in colon cancers of the microsatellite mutator phenotype. Science 275:967–969, 1997.

190. Souza RF, Yin J, Smolinski KN, et al. Frequent mutation of the E2F-4 cell cycle gene in primary human gastrointestinal tumors. Cancer Res 57:2350–2353, 1997.

191. Malkhosyan S, Rampino N, Yamamoto H, Perucho M. Frameshift mutator mutations. Nature 382:499–500, 1996.

192. Fujiwara T, Stolker JM, Watanabe T, et al. Accumulated clonal genetic alterations in familial and sporadic colorectal carcinomas with widespread instability in microsatellite sequences. Am J Pathol 153:1063–1078, 1998.

193. Lengauer C, Kinzler KW, Vogelstein B. Genetic instabilities in human cancers. Nature 396:643–649, 1998.

194. Lengauer C, Kinzler KW, Vogelstein B. Genetic instability in colorectal cancers. Nature 386:623–627, 1997.

195. Konishi M, Kikuchi-Yanoshita R, Tanaka K, et al. Molecular nature of colon tumors in hereditary nonpolyposis colon cancer, familial polyposis, and sporadic colon cancer. Gastroenterology 111:307–317, 1996.

196. Bocker T, Schlegel J, Kullmann F, et al. Genomic instability in colorectal carcinomas: comparison of different evaluation methods and their biological significance. J Pathol 179:15–19, 1996.

197. Cahill DP, Lengauer C, Yu J, et al. Mutations of mitotic checkpoint genes in human cancers. Nature 392:300–303, 1998.

198. Dubois RN, Abramson SB, Crofford L, et al. Cyclooxygenase in biology and disease. FASEB J 12:1063–1073, 1998.

199. Vane JR, Bakhle YS, Botting RM. Cyclooxygenases 1 and 2. Annu Rev Pharmacol Toxicol 38:97–120, 1998.

200. Eberhart CE, Coffey RJ, Radhika A, et al. Up-regulation of cyclooxygenase 2 gene expression in human colorectal adenomas and adenocarcinomas. Gastroenterology 107:1183–1188, 1994.

201. Kargman SL, O'Neill GP, Vickers PJ, et al. Expression of prostaglandin G/H synthase-1 and -2 protein in human colon cancer. Cancer Res 55:2556–2559, 1995.

202. DuBois RN, Radhika A, Reddy BS, Entingh AJ. Increased cyclooxygenase-2 levels in carcinogen-induced rat colonic tumors. Gastroenterology 110:1259–1262, 1996.

203. Kutchera W, Jones DA, Matsunami N, et al. Prostaglandin H synthase 2 is expressed abnormally in human colon cancer: evidence for a transcriptional effect. Proc Natl Acad Sci USA 93:4816–4820, 1996.

204. Sano H, Kawahito Y, Wilder RL, et al. Expression of cyclooxygenase-1 and -2 in human colorectal cancer. Cancer Res 55:3785–3789, 1995.

205. Williams CS, Luongo C, Radhika A, et al. Elevated cyclooxygenase-2 levels in *Min* mouse adenomas. Gastroenterology 111:1134–1140, 1996.

206. Steinbach G, Lynch PM, Phillips RK, et al. The effect of celecoxib, a cyclooxygenase-2 inhibitor, in familial adenomatous polyposis. N Engl J Med 342:1946–1952, 2000.

207. Kawamori T, Rao CV, Seibert K, Reddy BS. Chemopreventive activity of celecoxib, a specific cyclooxygenase-2 inhibitor, against colon carcinogenesis. Cancer Res 58:409–412, 1998.

208. Reddy BS, Hirose Y, Lubet R, et al. Chemoprevention of colon cancer by specific cyclooxygenase-2 inhibitor, celecoxib, administered during different stages of carcinogenesis. Cancer Res 60:293–297, 2000.

209. Oshima M, Dinchuk JE, Kargman SL, et al. Suppression of intestinal polyposis in Apc δ716 knockout mice by inhibition of cyclooxygenase 2 (COX-2). Cell 87:803–809, 1996.

210. Bolen JB, Veillette A, Schwartz AM, DeSeau V, Rosen N. Activation of pp60c-src protein kinase activity in human colon carcinoma. Proc Natl Acad Sci USA 84:2251–2255, 1987.

211. Cartwright CA, Kamps MP, Meisler AI, Pipas JM, Eckhart W. pp60c-src activation in human colon carcinoma. J Clin Invest 83:2025–2033, 1989.

212. Cartwright CA, Meisler AI, Eckhart W. Activation of the pp60c-src protein kinase is an early event in colonic carcinogenesis. Proc Natl Acad Sci USA 87:558–562, 1990.

213. Talamonti MS, Roh MS, Curley SA, Gallick GE. Increase in activity and level of pp60c-src in progressive stages of human colorectal cancer. J Clin Invest 91:53–60, 1993.

214. Termuhlen PM, Curley SA, Talamonti MS, Saboorian MH, Gallick GE. Site-specific differences in pp60c-src activity in human colorectal metastases. J Surg Res 54:293–298, 1993.

215. Thomas SM, Brugge JS. Cellular functions regulated by Src family kinases. Annu Rev Cell Dev Biol 13:513–609, 1997.

216. Mukhopadhyay D, Tsiokas L, Zhou XM, et al. Hypoxic induction of human vascular endothelial growth factor expression through c-Src activation. Nature 375:577–581, 1995.

217. Schlessinger J. New roles for Src kinases in control of cell survival and angiogenesis. Cell 100:293–296, 2000.

218. Staley CA, Parikh NU, Gallick GE. Decreased tumorigenicity of a human colon adenocarcinoma cell line by an antisense expression vector specific for c-Src. Cell Growth Differ 8:269–274, 1997.

219. Fleming RY, Ellis LM, Parikh NU, et al. Regulation of vascular endothelial growth factor expression in human colon carcinoma cells by activity of src kinase. Surgery 122:501–507, 1997.

220. Ellis LM, Staley CA, Liu W, et al. Down-regulation of vascular endothelial growth factor in a human colon carcinoma cell line transfected with an antisense expression vector specific for c-src. J Biol Chem 273:1052–1057, 1998.

221. Irby RB, Mao W, Coppola D, et al. Activating SRC mutation in a subset of advanced human colon cancers. Nat Genet 21:187–190, 1999.

222. Daigo Y, Furukawa Y, Kawasoe T, et al. Absence of genetic alteration at codon 531 of the human c-src gene in 479 advanced colorectal cancers from Japanese and Caucasian patients. Cancer Res 59:4222–4224, 1999.

223. Bird A. The essentials of DNA methylation. Cell 70:5–8, 1992.

224. Goelz SE, Vogelstein B, Hamilton SR, Feinberg AP. Hypomethylation of DNA from benign and malignant human colon neoplasms. Science 228:187–190, 1985.

225. Feinberg AP, Gehrke CW, Kuo KC, Ehrlich M. Reduced genomic 5-methylcytosine content in human colonic neoplasia. Cancer Res 48:1159–1161, 1988.

226. Laird PW, Jackson-Grusby L, Fazeli A, et al. Suppression of intestinal neoplasia by DNA hypomethylation. Cell 81:197–205, 1995.

227. Jones PA, Laird PW. Cancer epigenetics comes of age. Nat Genet 21:163–167, 1999.

228. Toyota M, Ahuja N, Ohe-Toyota M, et al. CpG island methylator phenotype in colorectal cancer. Proc Natl Acad Sci USA 96:8681–8686, 1999.

229. Toyota M, Ho C, Ahuja N, et al. Identification of differentially methylated sequences in colorectal cancer by methylated CpG island amplification. Cancer Res 59:2307–2312, 1999.

230. Hubank M, Schatz DG. Identifying differences in mRNA expression by representational difference analysis of cDNA. Nucl Acids Res 22:5640–5648, 1994.

231. Velculescu VE, Zhang L, Vogelstein B, Kinzler KW. Serial analysis of gene expression. Science 270:484–487, 1995.

232. Duggan DJ, Bittner M, Chen Y, Meltzer P, Trent JM. Expression profiling using cDNA microarrays. Nat Genet 21:10–14, 1999.

233. Cole KA, Krizman DB, Emmert-Buck MR. The genetics of cancer—a 3D model. Nat Genet 21:38–41, 1999.

234. Zhang L, Zhou W, Velculescu VE, et al. Gene expression profiles in normal and cancer cells. Science 276:1268–1272, 1997.

235. Losi L, Ponz de Leon M, Jiricny J, et al. K-ras and p53 mutations in hereditary non-polyposis colorectal cancers. Int J Cancer 74:94–96, 1997.

236. Olschwang S, Hamelin R, Laurent-Puig P, et al. Alternative genetic pathways in colorectal carcinogenesis. Proc Natl Acad Sci USA 94:12122–12127, 1997.

237. Toyota M, Ohe-Toyota M, Ahuja N, Issa JP. Distinct genetic profiles in colorectal tumors with or without the CpG island methylator phenotype. Proc Natl Acad Sci USA 97:710–715, 2000.

238. Sankila R, Aaltonen LA, Jarvinen HJ, Mecklin JP. Better survival rates in patients with MLH1-associated hereditary colorectal cancer. Gastroenterology 110:682–687, 1996.

239. Lin KM, Shashidharan M, Ternent CA, et al. Colorectal and extracolonic cancer variations in MLH1/MSH2 hereditary nonpolyposis colorectal cancer kindreds and the general population. Dis Colon Rectum 41:428–433, 1998.

240. Watson P, Lin KM, Rodriguez-Bigas MA, et al. Colorectal carcinoma survival among hereditary nonpolyposis colorectal carcinoma family members. Cancer 83:259–266, 1998.

241. Shibata D, Peinado MA, Ionov Y, Malkhosyan S, Perucho M. Genomic instability in repeated sequences is an early somatic event in colorectal tumorigenesis that persists after transformation. Nat Genet 6:273–281, 1994.

242. Bodmer W, Bishop T, Karran P. Genetic steps in colorectal cancer. Nat Genet 6:217–219, 1994.

# Chapter 54

# Familial Colorectal Cancer Syndromes

THOMAS C. SMYRK AND HENRY T. LYNCH

Is cancer hereditary? This question has been asked by physicians and patients for hundreds of years. Molecular genetic research demonstrates that the answer is unequivocally yes for a subset of cancers. Indeed, more than 40 germline mutations have been identified as etiologic for cancer susceptibility,[1] and new links between mutations and cancer syndromes are made almost monthly. Colorectal cancer (CRC) has been a particularly fruitful area of study for molecular geneticists, and we now enter an era during which CRC patients and the clinicians who care for them will harvest the benefits of molecular research.

The annual incidence of CRC in the United States is 129,400.[2] If even 5% of those cancers have a primary hereditary basis, then 6500 new CRCs each year are amenable to prevention or early diagnosis if the hereditary predisposition is recognized and managed appropriately. This 5% estimate is conservative; the known hereditary syndromes account for approximately the same percentage of CRCs, and it is very likely that new, more subtle genetic contributors to CRC risk (in the form of high-prevalence, low-penetrance mutations) will be discovered. One example of the latter is the variant of the adenomatous polyposis coli (*APC*) gene described by Laken and colleagues.[3] The variant gene features a missense mutation (T → A transversion) that causes a substitution of lysine for isoleucine at codon 1307 (I1307K). Protein function is not affected, but the transversion changes the base sequence from (A)3T(A)4 to (A)8, resulting in an unstable tract at risk for somatic mutations. Laken found the variant gene in 6% of Jews of eastern European (Ashkenazi) descent; early indications are that it roughly doubles one's risk for CRC.[4] Gruber and colleagues[5] suggest that more high-prevalence, low-penetrance mutations remain to be discovered and that this type of cancer susceptibility accounts for a substantial fraction of all CRC.

This chapter will review the classification, diagnosis, and management of the established hereditary syndromes that have CRC as an integral malignancy (Table 54–1).

## General Principles in Familial Colorectal Cancer Syndromes

Some general comments on the value of family history and the judicious use of genetic testing apply to all hereditary syndromes. The importance of obtaining a complete family history hardly needs repeating: family history is the most widely available, least invasive, and most cost-efficient test for finding hereditary CRC syndromes; genetic testing plays a confirmatory role in some settings and may be used to screen at-risk individuals in others, but mass screening for genetic susceptibility to CRC is problematic, both ethically and economically, and is likely to remain so for some time. A complete family history will include information about tumors of all anatomic sites, since the syndromes discussed in this chapter can have extracolonic manifestations. In some hereditary nonpolyposis colorectal cancer (HNPCC) families, for example, female mutation carriers are at a higher lifetime risk for endometrial cancer than for CRC.[6] A patient with CRC might report endometrial cancer in several relatives but deny a family history of CRC, leading the unwary physician to miss a potential HNPCC family. Of course, the family history will be useful only if the person taking the history is conversant with the ever-expanding litany of familial cancer syndromes, a daunting task. An excellent short review has been published by the Mayo Familial Cancer Program.[7]

If the family history suggests the possibility of a hereditary CRC syndrome, genetic testing may be indicated. The importance of genetic counseling, both before and after genetic testing

**Table 54-1** Hereditary form of colorectal cancer

| Type | Inheritance Pattern | Gene | Polyps | Cancer | Noncancer Features | Screening | Surtical Management and/or Prophylaxis | Pre-symptomatic DNA Testing | Genetic Counseling |
|---|---|---|---|---|---|---|---|---|---|
| Familial adenomatous polyposis (FAP) | AD | *APC* gene at chromosome 5q, mutation distal to 5' | Adenomatous, often start in distal colon/ rectum; usually >100 polyps; adenomas may occur in small bowel; gastric polyps common, usually fundic gland polyps | CRC, average age at onset 39 years; many cases in teens and twenties; cancer of small bowel; stomach particularly in (Japan), pupillary thyroid cancer, periampullary carcinoma, sarcoma, brain tumor | Gardner's variant— epidermoid cysts of skin, osteomas of mandible, congenital hypertrophy of the retinal pigment epithelium; desmoid tumors (intraabdominal) do not metastasize but may kill by direct extension and may be initiated by surgery (dissected surfaces); adrenal adenomas | If positive for *APC* germline mutation: baseline flexible sigmoidoscopy at age 10–12 years and annually thereafter; upper endoscopy every 1–3 years starting when colonic polyps first appear; screen remaining rectal segment (annually) after surgical prophylaxis; if at risk but not tested for *APC*: follow same strategy; if eventually found to be *APC* negative: baseline sigmoidoscopy at age 15–20 years and, if sigmoidoscopy is negative, revert to general population screening recommendations | Prophylactic subtotal colectomy with low ileorectal anastomosis when phenotype (florid polyposis) identified; consider rectal mucosectomy with ileal pouch anal anastomosis if too many rectal polyps to manage or if compliance for rectal segment follow-up is poor; consider chemoprevention with sulindac (while reducing polyps, cancer may still occur) | Test for *APC* germline mutation as early as age 10–12 years | Initiate in pre-teens, include parents |
| Attenuated familial adenomatous polyposis coli (AFAP) | AD | *APC* gene at chromosome 5q, mutation proximal to 5' | Ordinary adenomas but also flat adenomas with proximal colonic predominance; may be few (5–10), sometimes >100 | CRC with average age at onset 55 years; occasional periampullary carcinoma | Fundic gland polyps in stomach; adenomas in duodenum | Colonoscopy and upper endoscopy, beginning at age 20 years and annually for *APC* germline-positive patients or every 2 years if at genetic risk but not tested for *APC* | Prophylactic subtotal colectomy if too many polyps to manage; consider chemoprevention with sulindac | Test for *APC* germline mutation at age 20 years | Initiate at age 20 years, include parents |

| Syndrome | Inheritance | Gene | Polyp features | Cancer | Other features | Screening | Surgery | Gene variant | Initiate |
|---|---|---|---|---|---|---|---|---|---|
| Ashkenazi Jewish I1307K mutation | AD | I1307K mutation in APC | Occasional adenomatous colonic polyps | CRC, "young" age at onset but average age of onset not known | None known | Full colonoscopy, starting at age 30–35 years in gene carriers | Standard CRC surgery | Ashkenazi APC mutation | Initiate at age 25 years |
| Turcot's syndrome (HNPCC, FAP) | AD | Both FAP (APC) and HNPCC, hPMS2, hMLH1, mutation variants | Multiple colonic adenomas, but may not be florid | CRC and central nervous system, particularly brain tumors; in APC (FAP families) cerebellar medulloblastomas; in hMLH1 and hPMS2 (HNPCC families) glioblastoma multiforme | Rare examples of multiple café-au-lait spots and pigmented nevi but not clear if truly integral to the syndrome | Baseline flexible sigmoidoscopy at age 10–12 years and annual flexible sigmoidoscopy thereafter; consider CT scan or MRI of brain | Prophylactic subtotal colectomy if colonic polyps present, as in FAP; in HNPCC variant, colonoscopy | Two DNA variants: (1) APC gene with predominance of cerebellar medulloblastoma. (2) hMLH1 or hPMS2, with predominance of glioblastoma multiforme | Initiate at age 10–12 years, include parents |
| Juvenile polyposis coli | AD | Protein tyrosine phosphate gene (PTEN) SMAD4/DPC4 | Diffuse hamartomatous polyps (may have adenomatous component) in colon, but may occur in small bowel and stomach | CRC | Children may manifest diarrhea (may be severe) | Initiate colonoscopy at age 10–12 years | Prophylactic subtotal colectomy when phenotype present with too many polyps to manage | Tyrosine phosphate gene (PTEN) | Initiate in pre-teens, include parents |
| Peutz-Jeghers syndrome | AD | Gene encoding serine threonine kinase (STK11) on chromosome 19p13.3 LKB1/STK11 | Peutz-Jeghers polyps (may have adenomatous features) in stomach, small bowel, and colon | Stomach, small bowel, colon, sex cord tumors of ovary and testes | Mucocutaneous melanin pigmentation | Baseline colonoscopy and upper endoscopy, initiate at age 20 years; flexible sigmoidoscopy annually thereafter | Consider prophylactic subtotal colectomy if too many polyps to manage and if mixed adenomatous features | Serine threonine kinase (STK11) on chromosome 19p13.3 | Initiate in teens, include parents |
| Hereditary mixed polyposis syndrome (HMPS) | AD | Unknown; possible site on chromosome 6q | Atypical colonic juvenile polyps, adenomatous and hyperplastic polyps; usually <15 colon polyps | CRC | None known | Colonoscopy, initiate at age 20 years, every 2–3 years thereafter | Polypectomy; consider prophylactic colectomy if polyps too many to manage | None known | Initiate in teens |

(continued)

**Table 54-1** Hereditary form of colorectal cancer (*Continued*)

| Type | Inheritance Pattern | Gene | Polyps | Cancer | Noncancer Features | Screening | Surtical Management and/or Prophylaxis | Pre-symptomatic DNA Testing | Genetic Counseling |
|---|---|---|---|---|---|---|---|---|---|
| Discrete colonic adenomatous polyps and CRC of Burt | AD; may be similar to pattern of some familial CRC | Unknown | Occasional (never florid) adenomatous colonic polyps | CRC, average age in accord with population expectations | None known | Initiate baseline flexible sigmoidoscopy at age 40 and every 3 years thereafter | Standard surgical procedure for CRC | None known | Initiate at age 25–30 years |
| Hereditary nonpolyposis colorectal cancer (HNPCC) | AD | Germline mutations of any of the mismatch repair genes: *hMSH2* at chromosome 2p; *hMLH1* at chromosome 3p; *hPMS1* at chromosome 2q; *hPMS2* at chromosome 7q | Occasional colonic adenomas that are on average larger and more villous and at younger age than in general population. Colonic polyps no more frequent than in general population | CRC most common, with proximal predominance and an excess of synchronous and metachronous CRC. Others include cancer of the endometrium, ovary, small bowel, and stomach, and transitional-cell carcinoma of the ureter and renal pelvis. Average age of cancer onset is 44 years; may show rapid progression from adenoma to CRC | Muir-Torre syndrome variant shows cancer features of HNPCC but includes sebaceous adenomas, sebaceous epitheliomas, basal cell epitheliomas with sebaceous differentiation, meibomian gland carcinomas, and sebaceous carcinomas; single or multiple keratoacanthomas | Colonoscopy, initiate at age 20–25 years, annually for germline mutation carriers; every other year when mutation studies are lacking; endometrial aspiration biopsy at the same time as colonoscopy | Subtotal colectomy for initial CRC; consider option of prophylactic subtotal colectomy for germline carriers; consider prophylactic total abdominal hysterectomy and bilateral salpingo-oophorectomy for patients with initial CRC who do not want future pregnancies | Test for germ-line mutations no earlier than age 18–20 years | Initiate at age 18 years, prior to any consideration for gene testing |
| Familial CRC | Empirical risk 3-fold increase for CRC in patients with one or more first-degree relatives with CRC; likely multifactorial and/or low penetrant genes | Unknown | In accord with population expectations | CRC, comparable to general population for age of onset and colonic location | None | Baseline flexible sigmoidoscopy at age 35, repeat every 3 years; if two first-degree relatives affected or one at age <50 years, risk is 4- to 6-fold increased, and full colonoscopy every 3–5 years is indicated | Standard surgical procedure for CRC | None known | Initiate at age 30–35 years |

| Inflammatory bowel disease (ulcerative colitis [UC] and Crohn's disease) | Unknown; possible AD in some families; polygenic also likely | Tentative findings of linkage to chromosomes 16 (IBD$_1$) and 12 (IBD$_2$) | Pseudopolyps (non-adenomatous) | CRC; lymphoma of gastrointestinal tract | UC: arthritis, pyoderma gangrenosum, annular erythemas, and vascular thromboses, sclerosing cholangitis CD: features similar to UC but small bowel involvement prominent; may involve colon | UC: colonoscopy, annual in patients with chronic pancolitis of ≥8 years duration; check for high-grade dysplasia of colonic mucosa CD: BE may help; X-ray of small bowel may show rigidity, narrowing submucosal edema, or stenosis, inflammation, "cobblestoned appearance." May see clinical and genetic overlap in UC and CD | Subtotal colectomy for CRC; consider prophylactic subtotal colectomy for patients with persistent high-grade dysplasia of colonic mucosa in UC. Proctocolectomy if IBD mandates | None known | Initiate at age 18–20 years |
|---|---|---|---|---|---|---|---|---|---|

(Adapted with permission from Lynch et al., Eur J Cancer 31A:1039–1046, 1995.)

Abbreviations: AD, autosomal dominant; BE, barium enema; CD, Crohn's disease; CRC, colorectal cancer; FAP, familial adenomatous polyposis; HNPCC, hereditary nonpolyposis colorectal cancer; IBD, inflammatory bowel disease; UC, familial ulcerative colitis.

HNPCC registry at Roswell Park Cancer Institute and found multiple CRC in 25. Twenty of the 93 (21.5%) had metachronous tumors; 7 (7.5%) had synchronous CRC. Two of the 7 (28.6%) patients with synchronous CRC also developed a metachronous CRC. It is important to be aware that even after a subtotal colectomy is performed, the rectum remains vulnerable. Rodriguez-Bigas and co-workers[68] have shown the incidence of rectal carcinoma in patients with HNPCC after total abdominal colectomy to be 12% over 12 years. Despite the tendency toward multiple CRCs in HNPCC patients, several studies have documented improved survival in HNPCC vs. stage-matched controls.[69,70]

We are continuing to learn about the extracolonic tumor spectrum in HNPCC. Table 54–4 lists the extracolonic tumors for which HNPCC patients are at increased risk. Molecular studies may expand that list. For example, breast cancer does not appear to occur at a significantly higher frequency in patients with HNPCC,[47,71,72] but the observation that MSI is considerably more common in breast cancers from HNPCC family members than in sporadic breast cancer[73] suggests that breast cancer is an integral tumor in HNPCC, albeit perhaps one with lower penetrance than others.[74]

Mutation-based studies have also highlighted the particularly high risk for endometrial carcinoma. Froggatt and colleagues[75] studied age-related risks from colorectal, endometrial, and ovarian carcinomas in eight HNPCC families from Newfoundland with a specific hMSH2 mutation (nt943 + 3 A → T). The risk of colorectal cancer was higher ($P < 0.01$) in males than females (0.63 vs. 0.30 and 0.85 vs. 0.44 at ages 50 and 60 years, respectively) and females had a high risk of endometrial cancer (0.5 at age 60) and premenopausal ovarian cancer (0.2 at age 50). Dunlop and colleagues[6] also studied female MMR gene mutation carriers in HNPCC and found that their risk for endometrial carcinoma exceeded that for CRC. Vasen and colleagues[76] found the lifetime risk of endometrial cancer to be 61% for hMSH2 and 42% for hMLH1 mutation carriers.

Gastric carcinoma is another extracolonic manifestation of HNPCC that deserves special mention because it seems to illustrate interaction between genes and environment. The worldwide decline in gastric cancer has been paralleled by a decreasing prevalence of gastric cancer in HNPCC families. In addition, most gastric cancers in HNPCC are of the intestinal type,[77] the histologic type that has declined in the general population, and is thought to be influenced by environmental factors.

Hereditary nonpolyposis colorectal cancer with only colonic involvement can be subclassified as Lynch syndrome I, and HNPCC with colonic and extracolonic tumors, as Lynch syndrome II (Fig. 54–2). There is some genetic rationale for this clinical division since extracolonic cancers are more common in families with hMSH2 mutations than in those with hMLH1 mutations.[76,78,79] Some of the variety in clinical presentation may also result from the type of mutation that has occurred. Jäger and colleagues,[80] for example, described five Danish families with a splice donor mutation of hMLH1 that resulted in a silenced allele. Mutation carriers had a high risk for CRC, but the ratio of CRC to extracolonic cancer in those 5 families was 23:2, compared with 91:44 in families with other mutations.

Extracolonic tumors seem to be characteristic of families with hMSH6 mutations, suggesting that this genotype may also contribute to Lynch syndrome II phenotypes. Miyaki and co-workers[81] were the first to describe a family with germline hMSH6 mutations. Affected individuals had cancers of the colon, endometrium, ovary, and pancreas, with cancers of the endometrium and ovary predominating. Wijnen and colleagues[82] studied 214 putative HNPCC kindreds that did not have the hMSH2 or hMLH1 mutations. Nine different truncating hMSH6 pathogenic germline mutations were identified in 10 of these families. The ratio of CRC to endometrial cancer in these families was 31:22. In addition to the truncating mutations, six missense hMSH6 mutations of unknown significance were detected in 11 families. The clinical features of these families differed from those of the families with hMSH6 truncating mutations in that CRCs outnumbered extracolonic cancers at a ratio of 29 to 4.

## Diagnosis

The diagnosis of HNPCC starts with pedigree analysis. Prior to 1990, descriptive criteria were still emerging and were highly variable in the literature, leading to considerable confusion as to what constituted HNPCC. Concern about this problem led to the development of the Amsterdam criteria:[83] at least three relatives

**Table 54–4** Hereditary nonpolyposis colorectal cancer phenotypes

| Phenotypic Feature | Comment |
| --- | --- |
| Colonic adenomas | HNPCC is a "nonpolyposis," but adenomas do occur, age at onset for adenomatous is possibly younger than that for sporadic adenomas; may be more likely than sporadic adenomas to progress to carcinoma[92] |
| Colorectal carcinoma | Predominantly found in proximal colon (70%); early onset (age, 45 years); multiple CRCs[66] |
| Endometrial carcinoma | May be more common than CRC in female germline mutation carriers[76] |
| Gastric carcinoma | Declining incidence in HNPCC[76] |
| Pancreatic carcinoma | Described in some families[160] |
| Ovarian carcinoma<br>Cancer of small bowel<br>Hepatobiliary cancer<br>Urinary tract carcinoma | Relative risk for cancer increases significantly for each organ site but is highly variable within and between families[71] |
| Breast cancer | Molecular evidence suggests that breast cancer is integral[73] |
| Glioblastoma multiforme | Some "Turcot's syndrome" families are actually HNPCC families[23] |
| Skin lesions<br>  Sebaceous adenoma<br>  Sebaceous carcinoma<br>  Keratoacanthomas | Muir-Torre syndrome is a subset of HNPCC[90,161,162] |

Abbreviations: CRC, colorectal cancer; HNPCC, hereditary nonpolyposis colorectal cancer.

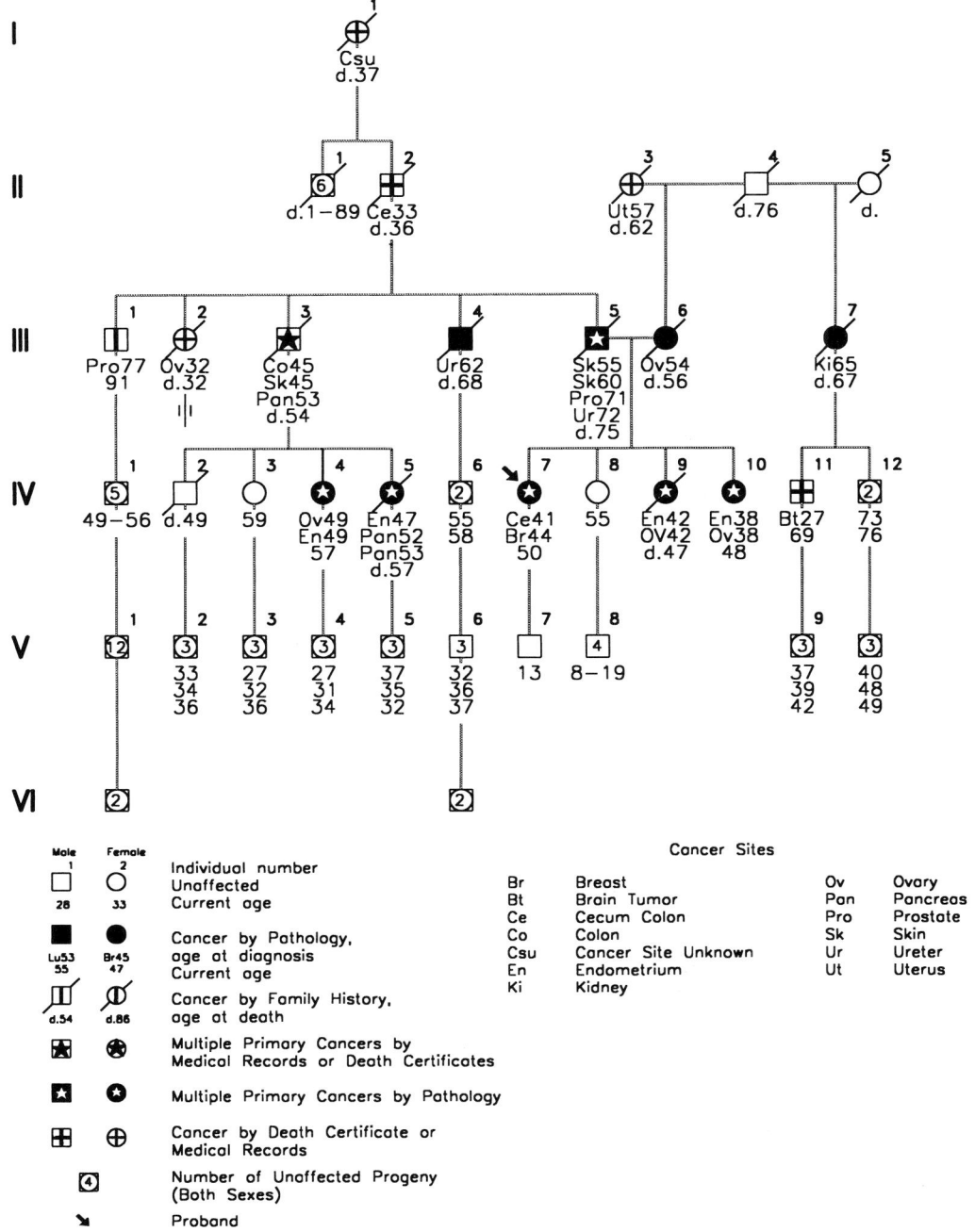

**Figure 54-2** Updated pedigree of a family showing early-onset synchronous carcinoma of the endometrium and ovary in two sisters, early-onset carcinoma of the cecum in the proband, and a pattern of cancer distribution in the paternal lineage consonant with Lynch syndrome II.

(Adapted from Lynch HT, Cavalieri JR, Lynch JF, Casey MJ. Gynecologic cancer clues to Lynch syndrome II diagnosis: a family report. Gynecol Oncol 44:198–203, 1992.)

should have CRC; one should be a first-degree relative of the other two; at least two successive generations should be affected; at least one CRC should be diagnosed before age 50; FAP should be excluded; and tumors should be verified by pathologic examination.

The Amsterdam criteria, while highly successful, had limitations, particularly the failure to consider extracolonic cancers in the diagnosis. New criteria (Table 54–5) were developed by the International Collaborative Group on Hereditary Nonpolyposis Colorectal Cancer (ICG-HNPCC).[84] These criteria are not meant

to replace the Amsterdam criteria. Rather, the ICG-HNPCC recommends that *both* the Amsterdam criteria and the new criteria be utilized to identify putative HNPCC families.[84]

The contribution of physical findings to the diagnosis is limited. The cutaneous signs of Muir-Torre syndrome (sebaceous adenomas, carcinomas, and keratoacanthomas) represent, so far as we know, the only premonitory signs of HNPCC.[85–88] Muir-Torre syndrome demonstrates an autosomal dominant inheritance pattern exactly like that found in HNPCC[89–91] and shows the same cancer spectrum as that in Lynch syndrome II (Fig. 54–3).

**Table 54–5** International Collaborative Group on Hereditary Nonpolyposis Colorectal Cancer definition of hereditary nonpolyposis colorectal cancer (Lynch Syndrome)

Familial clustering of colorectal and/or endometrial cancer
Associated cancers: cancer of the stomach, ovary, ureter/renal pelvis, brain, small bowel, hepatobiliary tract, and skin (sebaceous tumors)
Development of cancer at an early age
Development of multiple cancers
Features of colorectal cancer: *(1)* predilection for proximal colon; *(2)* improved survival; *(3)* multiple colorectal cancers; *(4)* increased proportion of mucinous tumors, poorly differentiated tumors, and tumors with marked host-lymphocytic infiltration and lymphoid aggregation at the tumor margin
Features of colorectal adenoma: *(1)* number of adenomas vary from one to a few; *(2)* increased proportion of adenomas with a villous growth pattern; and *(3)* probably rapid progression from adenoma to carcinoma
High frequency of MSI (MSI-high)
Immunohistochemistry: loss of MLH1, MSH2, or MSH protein expression
Germline mutation of MMR genes (*MSH2, MLH1, MSH6, PMS1, PMS2*)

MMR, mismatch repair; MSI, microsatellite instability. (Adapted with permission from Vasen et al., Gastroenterology 116:1453–1456, 1999.[84])

As indicated by its name, HNPCC is not a polyposis, so the clinician cannot rely on multiple gastrointestinal polyps as a clue to the diagnosis. Adenomas do occur in HNPCC patients. Jass[92] has shown that colonic adenomas in patients with HNPCC have an earlier age of onset, are larger, and are more likely to show villous features and severe dysplasia than adenomas in the general population. Thus, a large villous adenoma in a young adult might prompt a more careful look into that patient's family history.

The histologic appearance of CRC can sometimes be a clue to the diagnosis of HNPCC. It has been recognized for over a decade that CRCs in this setting are often mucinous or poorly differentiated.[93,94] With the discovery that germline mutations of DNA MMR genes are responsible for HNPCC has come the realization that colon cancers (whether hereditary or sporadic) with defective DNA MMR have MSI. These so-called MSI-high CRCs have characteristic features that pathologists can recognize. One such characteristic is solid, non–gland-forming growth by cells with round, fairly regular nuclei. We have designated this pattern "undifferentiated medullary carcinoma," in deference to earlier descriptions of the same tumor by Gibbs[95] as "undifferentiated carcinoma" and by Jessurun and colleagues[96] as "medullary carcinoma." The clinicopathologic features of undifferentiated medullary carcinoma were thoroughly described by Ruschoff and co-workers.[97]

A second characteristic of MSI-high colon cancers is morphologic evidence of host lymphoid response. This can take the form of lymphoid aggregates in tissue adjacent to tumor (Crohn's-like reaction) or lymphocytes intimately admixed with tumor cells (tumor-infiltrating lymphocytes). The Crohn's-like reaction, popularized by Graham and Appelman[98] as a marker of improved prognosis in HNPCC, is usually, but not always, reported to be more common in HNPCC and other MSI-high CRCs.[94,98,99] Tumor-infiltrating lymphocytes (TILs) have even more promise as a marker of MSI-high status. This phenomenon, first linked to sporadic MSI-high CRC by investigators from the Mayo Clinic,[100] was used to great effect by Jass and colleagues[101] in algorithms for recognizing sporadic MSI-high CRC. In our experience, TILs are significantly more common in colon cancers from HNPCC patients than from sporadic controls.[102] In

fact, TILs are the single best marker for MSI-high status that we have seen; when TILs are present in a CRC, that tumor is almost invariably MSI-high. Since roughly 15% of all CRCs are MSI-high, the finding of undifferentiated medullary histology, Crohn's-like reaction, or TILs does not necessarily prove HNPCC, but the presence of MSI-high–type histology should prompt a review of the family history.

The role of genetic testing is not as well defined for HNPCC as it is for FAP. An excellent summary of the current state of the art, current difficulties, and future directions is provided by Terdiman and co-workers[103] The difficulties are partly technical: there are multiple candidate genes to test and hundreds of different mutations within those genes. The HNPCC mutations are less likely than FAP mutations to result in truncated proteins, making truncated protein assays less sensitive in HNPCC. A full-scale mutational analysis of DNA MMR genes is an expensive and labor-intensive effort.

A bigger obstacle to the uniform application of genetic testing in HNPCC is continuing debate about whom to test. Two general approaches have been advocated, one based on clinical criteria and one based on molecular criteria. The clinical approach would reserve genetic testing for patients meeting the Amsterdam criteria, ICG-HNPCC criteria, or some less stringent clinical benchmark (e.g., onset of CRC at less than 35 years of age, multiple synchronous CRC). The molecular approach would screen *all* CRCs for the presence of MSI and then proceed to genetic testing for all MSI-high CRCs or a subset selected on the basis of clinical criteria.

There is a third possible approach, one that begins with pathologic criteria. Jass and colleagues[101] have demonstrated that clinicopathologic criteria are sensitive and specific for MSI-high CRC. Our own experience is the same; as noted above, TILs seem to be an excellent marker of MSI-high status. If these findings are reproducible, then pathologic assessment of MSI-high features is an essentially free screening test for MSI because the pathologist is already performing a histologic review of resected CRC. If pathology suggests that a given CRC is MSI-high, clinical review of the patient's family history can direct the decision about gene testing.

## Surveillance and Management

The natural history of HNPCC determines surveillance and management strategies (Table 54–6). Given the early age of CRC onset and the disease's predilection for the proximal colon, we initiate colonoscopy at age 25. We believe colonoscopy should be repeated yearly. In our own experience, 10% of patients had a CRC within 5 years of a colon resection or a negative colonoscopy.[104] Others have reported CRC at intervals of less than 2 years.[105] Theoretical considerations (small numbers of adenomas in HNPCC, but high risk for CRC) suggest that adenomas in HNPCC may be more aggressive than sporadic adenomas.[106,107]

In a study by Finnish investigators,[108] one group of HNPCC patients chose regular colonoscopic screening, while another refused surveillance. The authors removed 22 adenomas from the group under surveillance, preventing an estimated 7.4% cancers when compared to the group that refused surveillance. Järvinen et al.[109] updated this HNPCC cohort with an evaluation of the efficacy of screening in a controlled trial of colonoscopies and polypectomies over 15 years. They studied the incidence of CRC and survival in two cohorts of at-risk members of 22 HNPCC-prone families. They provided colonic screening at three-year

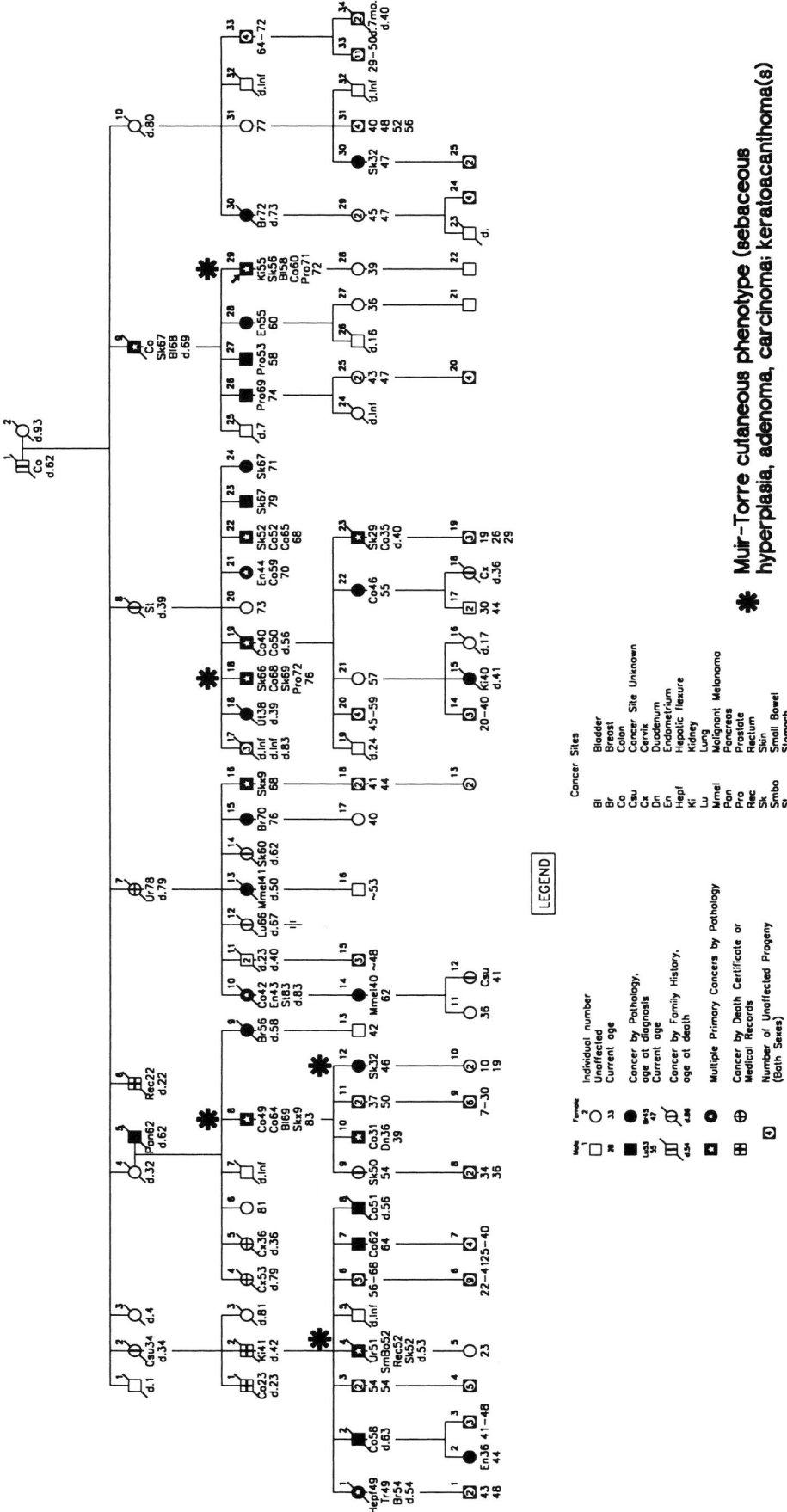

**Figure 54-3** Pedigree of family with tumor spectrum consonant with Muir-Torre cutaneous phenotype in association with Lynch syndrome II variant. (Adapted from Lynch HT, Fusaro RM, Roberts L, Voorhees GJ, Lynch JF. Muir-Torre syndrome in several members of a family with a variant of the cancer family syndrome. Br J Dermatol 113:295–301, 1985.)

**Table 54-6** Surveillance and management of hereditary nonpolyposis colorectal cancer

| Procedures | Comment |
|---|---|
| Genetic counseling | Educate patient and family members about natural history of the disease, genetics, emotional factors, economic factors, and concerns about insurance and/or employment discrimination |
| Colonoscopy | Initiate at age 20 to 25; perform annually if carrier of deleterious germline mutation, otherwise biannually |
| Gynecologic sonography (endometrium/ovary) | Start ultrasound of the endometrium/ovaries at age 30 to 35 and repeat annually |
| Gastric/small bowel endoscopy | Initiate upper endoscopy at age 30; repeat annually if family history of gastric or small bowel cancer, otherwise biannually |
| Surgical prophylaxis | Consider subtotal colectomy for germline mutation carriers, for patients showing poor compliance with screening, and for patients with strong emotional concerns and a poor quality of life caused by fear, anxiety, and apprehension of cancer; consider prophylactic TAH-BSO for women who present with CRC and who do not desire future pregnancies |

CRC, colorectal cancer; HNPCC, hereditary nonpolyposis colorectal cancer; TAH-BSO, total abdominal hysterectomy and bilateral salpingo-oophorectomy.

intervals for 133 subjects and compared them with 119 control subjects who had no screening. Findings disclosed the following:

CRC developed in 8 screening subjects (6%) compared with 19 control subjects (16%; $P = 0.014$). The CRC rate was reduced by 62%. In mutation-positive subjects alone, the CRC rates were 18% in screened subjects and 41% in controls ($P = 0.02$). The decrease resulted from the removal of adenomas in 13 mutation-positive individuals (30%) and in 6 subjects with unknown mutation status (40%). All CRCs in the study were local, causing no deaths, compared with 9 deaths caused by CRC in the controls. The overall death rates were 10 vs. 26 subjects in the study and control groups ($P = 0.003$), 4 vs. 12 in mutation-positive subjects ($P = 0.05$).

Thus, this study showed that colonoscopic screening every 3 years more than halved the risk of CRC and prevented some CRC deaths. Overall mortality was decreased by about 65% in the Lynch syndrome families.

Surveillance for extracolonic cancers is directed primarily at the endometrium and ovary. We recommend endometrial ultrasound and endometrial aspiration studies beginning at age 30 and repeated annually. Transvaginal ovarian ultrasound and CA-125 analysis may be helpful for ovarian cancer surveillance; however, the patient must realize the limitations of these procedures, given the anatomic location of the ovaries. Screening for other extracolonic cancers is assessed on a case-by-case basis, depending on which lesions have occurred in excess in the particular family.

Is there a role for prophylactic subtotal colectomy and/or prophylactic total abdominal hysterectomy and bilateral salpingo-oophorectomy (TAH-BSO) in HNPCC germline mutation carriers? A patient from an HNPCC kindred with an *hMSH2* or *hMLH1* germline mutation has an approximately 85% to 90% lifetime risk for CRC. A female mutation carrier has a lifetime risk of 40% to 60% for endometrial carcinoma and 10% to 15% for ovarian cancer. Given this background, the choice between intensive surveillance and prophylactic surgery needs to be discussed in depth during the genetic counseling process. Prophylactic surgery may be a prudent option for a patient who is likely to show poor compliance with screening or who is unusually apprehensive about his or her lifetime risk in the face of the germline mutation. In many ways, prophylactic surgery in HNPCC patients is not significantly different from the well-accepted prophylactic surgical approach in FAP. In FAP patients, the average age of CRC onset is 39 years; in HNPCC, it is about 44 years. Colorectal cancer occurs at approximately the same frequency in

germline carriers of the two syndromes. The only difference is that in FAP we have the florid polyposis phenotype to guide us.

### Genetic Counseling

Genetic counseling for all types of hereditary cancer must include education for the patient about the hereditary cancer syndrome manifested in his or her family. The disorder's natural history, available screening methods, and, when appropriate, prophylactic surgery options should all be discussed. The pros and cons of DNA testing should be discussed prior to collecting blood specimens and repeated at the time of disclosure of the results. Patients must also be advised about the possibility of insurance or employment discrimination. When a germline mutation is discovered, the possibility of variable phenotypic expression and reduced penetrance should be discussed.

An example of such genetic counseling in an extended Lynch syndrome II family with *hMSH2* mutation illustrates these concerns.[110] Regardless of whether patients were found to be positive or negative for the *hMSH2* germline mutation, counseling revealed considerable emotional stress. The main concerns of the patients centered on reproductive issues, potential transmission of the deleterious gene to progeny, and discrimination by insurance companies and/or employers. Those who were positive for the *hMSH2* germline mutation had many concerns about their lifetime cancer risk. More than half of those patients who were found to harbor the *hMSH2* mutation considered the option of prophylactic subtotal colectomy. At-risk family members sought genetic risk assessment primarily for the benefit of their children and secondarily for their own benefit.

Lerman et al.[111] interviewed 208 adult male and female members of four extended HNPCC families by telephone. The authors found that the presence of depression symptoms "significantly reduced rates of HNPCC test use (odds ratio [OR], 0.34; 95% confidence interval [CI], 0.17–0.66). Although rates of test use were identical between men and women, the presence of depression symptoms resulted in a fourfold decrease in test use among women (OR, 0.25; 95% CI, 0.08–0.80) and a smaller, nonsignificant reduction among men (OR, 0.49; 95% CI, 0.19–1.27)." Lower levels of formal education were also a barrier to test acceptance.

We recently described a Gypsy family with the Muir-Torre syndrome and an *hMSH2* germline mutation.[112] Genetic counseling proved extremely difficult, largely because of family members' lack of belief that we were interested in helping them. We tried to focus on their cutaneous signs, emphasizing the strong correlation between these stigmata and cancer expression. Genetic counseling in this situation was not unlike convincing patients who have florid colonic adenomas and who are members of an FAP family that the polyposis phenotype is directly associated with colorectal carcinoma vulnerability. We continue to follow this Gypsy family, but their compliance with our cancer surveillance recommendations remains poor.

## Hamartomatous Polyposis Syndromes

### Peutz-Jeghers Syndrome

Descriptions of Peutz-Jeghers syndrome (PJS) date to 1921, when Peutz described three Dutch siblings with pigmented spots, colicky abdominal pain, rectal bleeding, and multiple intestinal polyps.[113] Jeghers and colleagues later described the syndrome in the English literature.[114] The incidence of PJS is unknown; it is thought to be about one-tenth as common as FAP.[115] The inheritance pattern is autosomal dominant.

Peutz-Jeghers syndrome has been mapped to a locus on chromosome 19p13.3.[116,117] The gene responsible for the syndrome encodes a serine threonine kinase, STK11 (also known as LKB1).[116] Abnormal (i.e., inactive) forms of this kinase may lead to defective control of cellular growth and differentiation. Not all familial cases of PJS can be linked to 19p13.3, leading to speculation that there is a second locus for the syndrome.[118,119]

The diagnosis of PJS requires histologic confirmation of a hamartomatous, Peutz-Jeghers–type polyp. Because such polyps can be seen in individuals who do not have PJS, clinical diagnosis also requires at least two of the following: small bowel polyposis; family history of PJS; or pigmented macules on buccal mucosa, lips, fingers, and toes.[120] Genetic testing for the syndrome is being developed.[121]

Characteristic melanotic skin pigmentation is seen in 95% of individuals with PJS. The cutaneous lesions are dark brown or black macules located in the perioral region, buccal mucosa, hands, and feet. They appear during the first few years of life, increase in intensity up to puberty, and then gradually fade.

The hamartomatous polyps of PJS are distinctive, with thick bundles of smooth muscle arranged in a branching pattern. The mucosa atop this smooth muscle scaffold is often thickened and inflamed. Mucosa may be displaced into the submucosa, leading to a mistaken diagnosis of carcinoma. Overdiagnosis of malignancy can be avoided in this situation if one takes note of the lamina propria accompanying the displaced glands and recognizes the lack of cytologic atypia. Adenomas, hyperplastic polyps, and mixtures of the two have all been reported in PJS patients.

Peutz-Jeghers polyps have been found in the entire gastrointestinal tract. The small bowel is the site affected most often, but the stomach and colon can also be involved; esophageal polyps are rare. A large study from the Mayo Clinic found gastric polyps in 24% of PJS patients, small intestinal polyps in 96%, colonic polyps in 26%, and rectal polyps in 24%.[122] The polyps are almost always multiple but tend to number in the dozens rather than the hundreds. Peutz-Jeghers polyps have also been described in respiratory mucosa and the urinary tract. One member of the Dutch family originally studied by Peutz suffered from severe nasal polyposis and eventually developed a nasal carcinoma.[123] Unfortunately, the histologic features of the nasal polyps were not recorded, and the tissue is no longer available for review.

Several studies (summarized in Table 54–7) have demonstrated convincingly that PJS increases risk for malignancy. In a retrospective look at 31 PJS patients, Giardiello and colleagues[120] found a relative cancer risk 18 times that of the general population. Malignancies involved pancreas (4), breast (2), stomach (2), colon (2), lung (2), endometrium (1), ovary (1), and multiple myeloma (1). Spigelman et al.[124] reported that 72 retrospectively studied PJS patients were 13 times more likely than the general population to develop a malignancy. The tumors involved the colon, stomach, small intestine, ovary, fallopian tube, thyroid, and lung. Investigators from the Mayo Clinic[125] found a relative cancer risk of 9.9 in 34 PJS patients, with cancers of the colon (7), breast (6), lung (3), and cervix (2) predominating. The Mayo Clinic group also found a particularly high incidence of breast and gynecologic cancers, contributing to a relative cancer risk of 18.5 in women vs. 6.2 in men.

The study of the Dutch family originally described by Peutz has been updated, and the findings further demonstrate that PJS is not a benign condition.[123] Of 22 affected individuals, 7 developed carcinoma (3 colon, 1 stomach, 1 gastrointestinal not otherwise specified, 1 breast, and 1 nasal cavity). All patients with malignancy were dead of their disease before age 50.

While the gastrointestinal polyps are hamartomatous, there is strong evidence that they are often the source of gastrointestinal malignancy. Dysplastic and malignant changes in Peutz-Jeghers polyps are well described,[126] and half of the gastrointestinal cancers in Spigelman et al.'s study[124] were associated with residual hamartomatous polyps. Molecular evidence also supports the concept of a hamartoma–(adenoma)–carcinoma sequence. Wang and colleagues,[127] for example, described allelic loss of STK11 in carcinomas of the breast, colon, and cervix, a colonic adenoma, and hamartomatous polyps. Gruber and colleagues[128] de-

**Table 54–7** Cancer risk in Peutz-Jeghers Syndrome

| Study | Cancer Prevalence | Relative Risk | Comment |
|---|---|---|---|
| Giardiello et al.[120] | 15 of 31 patients | 18 | Colon, pancreas, stomach, breast, lung, endometrium, ovary, multiple myeloma |
| Spigelman et al.[124] | 16 of 72 patients | 13 | Colon, stomach, small bowel, ovary, fallopian tube, thyroid, lung |
| Boardman et al.[125] | 18 of 34 patients | 9.9 | Relative risk higher for women (18.5 vs 6.2); colon, breast, lung, cervix most common |
| Westerman et al.[123] | 7 of 22 patients | — | All cancer patients dead of disease by age 50; colon, stomach, nasal cavity, gastrointestinal not otherwise specified, breast |

scribed allelic loss of chromosome 19p markers near STK11 in 70% of hamartomas and carcinomas from PJS patients.

Several distinctive tumors deserve special mention. Nearly every female PJS patient will have ovarian involvement by a sex cord tumor with annular tubules (SCTAT). In this setting, the tumors are bilateral in at least two-thirds of cases (in contrast to SCTAT in the sporadic setting, which is almost always unilateral). In PJS patients, SCTAT is often an incidental finding during surgery for gastrointestinal symptoms. Males may develop a testicular tumor roughly corresponding to ovarian SCTAT—feminizing Sertoli cell tumor—but it is less common than the ovarian tumor. An unusual form of cervical cancer, minimal deviation adenocarcinoma (adenoma malignum), is also characteristic of PJS. This rare tumor accounts for 1% to 3% of all cervical adenocarcinomas (though in one series it affected 4 of 27 women with PJS).[129]

The surveillance protocol advocated by the St. Mark's Polyposis Registry[130] includes yearly hemoglobin analysis and yearly ultrasound examination of the pelvis in females and of the pancreas in all patients. A testicular ultrasound examination should also be done in males who have feminizing features. Biannual upper and lower endoscopy with small bowel X-ray is recommended. Regular mammography and cervical smears are critical surveillance measures. Tomlinson and Houlston[131] suggest that upper endoscopy, colonoscopy, and small bowel X-ray begin in the second decade of life, and that mammography begin at age 25.

The gastrointestinal polyps in patients with PJS may be associated with bleeding, obstruction, or intussusception. Conservative removal (snare polypectomy) is favored over segmental resection of bowel to avoid development of a short bowel syndrome.

## Familial Juvenile Polyposis

The evaluation of patients with juvenile polyps can be difficult. As shown in Table 54–8, polyps with similar histology can be seen in several different settings. Sporadic juvenile polyps are relatively common (one autopsy study of patients under 21 years of age reported a prevalence of 1%).[132] Usually solitary, the polyps are innocuous and do not increase risk for cancer of the colon,[133,134] despite the fact that dysplasia has been described in as many as 35% of apparently sporadic juvenile polyps.[135] The discovery of multiple juvenile polyps in a patient without a family history of polyposis can create a diagnostic dilemma; thus, various numbers in the range of 5 to 10 have been proposed as an upper limit for the number of sporadic juvenile polyps. Genetic testing will undoubtedly play a role in the evaluation of

**Table 54–8** Juvenile polyposis syndromes with similar histology in a variety of settings

| Condition | Comment |
|---|---|
| Sporadic juvenile polyps | Common in colon and rectum; usually solitary; usually pedunculated |
| Cronkhite-Canada syndrome | Acquired nonfamilial condition with polyps throughout the gut; polyps are often described as hyperplastic but may be indistinguishable from sessile juvenile polyps |
| Familial juvenile polyposis | Juvenile polyps, almost always multiple and usually sessile |
| Hereditary mixed polyposis syndrome | Juvenile polyps, alone or with hyperplastic and adenomatous areas, are the histologic hallmark of this putative syndrome |

such patients in the future. Multiple polyps with a histology similar to that of juvenile polyps may be seen in the Cronkhite-Canada syndrome, an acquired, nonfamilial condition comprising gastrointestinal polyps, onycholysis, alopecia, and skin hyperpigmentation.[136] Even when there are multiple juvenile polyps and a family history of polyposis, the diagnosis of juvenile polyposis must be made with care since Cowden's syndrome and its allelic congeners have similar polyps but put a very different spectrum of organs at risk for carcinoma.

Juvenile polyposis was first described as a distinct entity by McColl and colleagues in 1964.[137] The familial connection was made by Sachatello and colleagues,[138] who described a kindred with three generations of affected individuals. The inheritance pattern is autosomal dominant. Two variants have been described: a rare, usually fatal juvenile polyposis of infancy accompanied by diarrhea, protein-losing enteropathy, and alopecia; and the more common juvenile polyps of childhood. Extraintestinal anomalies have been reported in association with juvenile polyps; these include hydrocephalus, thyroglossal duct cyst, tetralogy of Fallot, coarctation of the aorta, idiopathic hypertrophic subaortic stenosis, and malrotation of the gut.

Molecular biologists have made dramatic progress in understanding juvenile polyposis, first linking it to a locus on chromosome 18q21,[139] then identifying germline mutations in familial juvenile polyposis (FJP) families in a component of the TGF-β signaling pathway, *SMAD4*.[140,141] Genetic testing is expected to change the way at-risk patients are screened and managed. It will also allow better classification of juvenile polyposis syndromes and help resolve several unanswered questions: Is the infantile form of juvenile polyposis allelic with the more common form, or is it an acquired disease akin to a childhood Cronkhite-Canada syndrome? Are the congenital anomalies described in the literature truly a manifestation of FJP, or do they represent missed cases of Cowden's syndrome or other genetic conditions?

The clinical diagnosis of FJP is based on histologic confirmation of a juvenile polyp, plus the presence of polyposis (i.e., more than 5 to 10 polyps) *or* a family history of polyposis. Even then, FJP is a diagnosis of exclusion; Cowden's syndrome must be ruled out. As noted above, genetic testing will almost certainly supplement clinical judgment in the classification of the hamartomatous polyposis syndromes.

Histologically, the juvenile polyp is dominated by an expanded, inflamed lamina propria. Dilated crypts are scattered irregularly in this background. The crypt epithelium is bland in uncomplicated juvenile polyps, but dysplasia can be present and should be sought by the pathologist. Slender smooth muscle fibers course through the lamina propria, but in contrast to the Peutz-Jeghers polyp, are not a prominent feature. The surface epithelium is often eroded, accounting for the frequent occurrence of rectal bleeding. In the sporadic setting, juvenile polyps are often pedunculated. As noted above, FJP, Cronkhite-Canada syndrome, and Cowden's syndrome can have histologically similar polyps. In the syndrome of juvenile polyposis, juvenile polyps may be found in the colorectum (98%), stomach (14%), duodenum (2%), and jejunum and ileum (7%).[142,143] Juvenile polyps of the stomach are histologically indistinguishable from hyperplastic polyps.

Patients with FJP are at increased risk for CRC. The cumulative lifetime risk estimated by Järvinen is 50%,[144] an estimate that compares remarkably well with an estimate from the University of Iowa describing a large FJP kindred in which 16 of 29 (55%) affected individuals developed gastrointestinal cancer.[145]

Eleven members of the Iowa kindred had colon cancer, and six had gastric cancer.

Individuals who have FJP need regular endoscopic surveillance. Scott-Conner and colleagues[143] recommend upper and lower gastrointestinal endoscopy every 3 years as long as no lesions are detected. Small numbers of polyps can be managed by polypectomy; in these cases, endoscopy should be repeated every year, if polyps persist. If there are multiple polyps in the colon, subtotal colectomy is recommended. Multiple gastric polyps, particularly if dysplasia is present, should prompt consideration of gastrectomy.

Children with large numbers of polyps present a difficult management problem. Colectomy is the prudent choice, but we believe regular colonoscopy with removal of the largest polyps until puberty is also an option.

### Cowden's Syndrome

Cowden's syndrome (CS) was described by Lloyd and Dennis in 1963.[146] The syndrome is characterized by multiple hamartomas, particularly involving the skin, and increased risk for carcinoma of the breast and thyroid. Colorectal cancers have been described in this syndrome, but the risk for them is unproven. The syndrome is discussed here because CS can be confused with juvenile polyposis.

Germline mutations of the tumor suppressor gene *PTEN* on chromosome 10q23 have been implicated in Cowden's syndrome.[147,148] Female mutation carriers have a 30% lifetime risk for breast cancer. Thyroid adenomas and carcinomas also occur to excess. Other reported associated cancers include cancers of the colon, kidney, endometrium, skin (melanoma and Merkel cell carcinoma), and lung. Benign lesions seen frequently in affected individuals are lipomas, giant fibroadenomas of the breast, and hemangiomas. Patients with dysplastic cerebellar gangliocytoma may be subclassified as having Lhermitte-Duclos disease.

Clinically, the diagnosis of Cowden's syndrome is suggested by the presence of skin lesions, breast or thyroid cancer, macrocephaly, and gastrointestinal hamartomas. The International Cowden Syndrome Consortium has published operational criteria for the diagnosis.[7]

Surveillance should include frequent breast examination and annual mammography beginning at age 20. Prophylactic mastectomy is a consideration in female mutation carriers. Surveillance for thyroid masses is also recommended. The value of colonoscopy in affected patients is unproven.

Another hamartomatous polyposis syndrome, Bannayan-Riley-Ruvalcaba (BRR) syndrome (Ruvalcaba-Myhre syndrome), also maps to chromosome 10q23,[149] and germline mutations of *PTEN* have been identified in these patients.[150] Cowden's and BRR syndromes have partial clinical overlap. The hallmarks of the BRR syndrome are multiple lipomas, macrocephaly, and pigmented macules of the glans penis. Both syndromes are thought to be different presentations of a single syndrome.[151,152] The cancer risk associated with the BRR syndrome is unknown.

### Hereditary Mixed Polyposis Syndrome

In 1996, Thomas and colleagues[153] described a large family exhibiting atypical juvenile polyps, colonic adenomas, hyperplastic colonic polyps, and colorectal carcinomas. Polyps and cancer risk were inherited in an autosomal dominant manner. Genetic linkage analysis mapped the locus for the condition to chromosome 6q. The phenotype of hereditary mixed polyposis syndrome (HMPS) was carefully described by the same group in a later publication.[154] Thirteen individuals from this large family have developed colorectal cancer; with a median age of 47 years at diagnosis.

Hereditary mixed polyposis syndrome illustrates the difficulty of classifying polyposis syndromes by phenotype and the potential value of molecular studies. Given the variety of polyps that have been described in juvenile polyposis patients—hamartomatous, adenomatous, hyperplastic, and mixtures of all three—it would be difficult to argue from phenotype alone that HMPS is not a variant of juvenile polyposis. Genetic linkage of HMPS to chromosome 6q, however, suggests that a different gene is involved. If the gene can be identified and germline mutations can be documented in affected patients, HMPS will be confirmed as a new hereditary syndrome. Then, careful clinicopathologic studies might disclose differences between HMPS and FJP in terms of polyp distribution, cancer risk, and extraintestinal manifestations and lead to surveillance and management recommendations that differ between the two.

## Conclusion

Hereditary colorectal cancer is genetically and phenotypically heterogeneous. Mutations in one gene (*APC*) can produce a range of phenotypes, mutations in different genes with similar functions (the various DNA mismatch repair genes) are responsible for one syndrome, and mutations in different genes with different functions (*SMAD4* and *PTEN*) cause syndromes with overlapping phenotypes. Clinically, both FAP and HNPCC have their "typical" presentations, but the reader should be aware that one's first contact with an FAP family might be a patient with one adenoma and one's first contact with an HNPCC family might be a patient with endometrial cancer. Gene–environment interactions and the effect of modifier genes add complexity to an already complex field. Molecular biology will provide many new insights, but careful clinical observation remains as important as ever.

What does the future hold? As Collins[155] notes, we have learned the location of approximately half of the 80,000 or more genes that constitute the human genome. Furthermore, he states that "about 15% of the 3 billion bits of DNA code that spell out instructions for every function a human body carries out is now available in public databases. In just 12 months, a highly useful working draft of 90% of the genome will be available, and by 2003, the full DNA sequence of the human will give us unprecedented opportunities to observe and understand the literal Book of Life."[155]

The benefits for those affected by and treating hereditary colon cancer syndromes should be enormous. Better classification, by using genotype in conjunction with phenotype, is already a reality for some syndromes. Early identification of gene carriers is possible now for some syndromes and will undoubtedly become possible for others, thus allowing targeted surveillance and prophylaxis. Finally, understanding the function of the culprit genes will lead to treatments designed to counteract their deleterious effects and possibly even restore their wild-type genetic function.

### References

1. Vogelstein B, Kinzler KW (eds). The Genetic Basis of Human Cancer. McGraw-Hill, New York, 1998.
2. Landis SH, Murray T, Bolden S, Wingo PA. Cancer statistics, 1999. Cancer J Clin 49:8–31, 1999.

3. Laken SJ, Petersen GM, Gruber SB, et al. Familial colorectal cancer in Ashkenazim due to a hypermutable tract in *APC*. Nat Genet 17:79–83, 1997.

4. Rozen P, Shomrat R, Strul H, et al. Prevalence of the I1307K *APC* gene variant in Israeli Jews of differing ethnic origin and risk for colorectal cancer. Gastroenterology 116:54–57, 1999.

5. Gruber SB, Petersen GM, Kinzler KW, Vogelstein B. Cancer, crash sites, and the new genetics of neoplasia. Gastroenterology 116:210–212, 1999.

6. Dunlop MG, Farrington SM, Carothers AD, et al. Cancer risk associated with germline DNA mismatch repair gene mutations. Hum Mol Genet 6:105–110, 1997.

7. Lindor NM, Greene MH, and Mayo Familial Cancer Program. The concise handbook of family cancer syndromes. J Natl Cancer Inst 90:1039–1071, 1998.

8. American Society of Clinical Oncology. Statement of the American Society of Clinical Oncology: genetic testing for cancer susceptibility. J Clin Oncol 14:1730–1736, 1996.

9. Lynch HT. Dynamic Genetics Counseling for Clinicians. C.C. Thomas, Springfield, IL, 1969.

10. Belchetz LA, Bert T, Bapat BV, Cohen Z, Gallinger S. Changing causes of mortality in patients with familial adenomatous polyposis. Dis Colon Rectum 39:384–387, 1996.

11. Bulow S. Familial polyposis coli. Dan Med Bull 34:1–15, 1987.

12. Luschka H. Ueber polypose Vegetationen der gesammten Dickdarmschleimhaut. Arch Pathol Anat Physiol Klin Med 20:133–142, 1861.

13. Sklifosovski NV. Polyadenoma tractus intestinalis. Vrach 2:55–57, 1881.

14. Cripps WH. Two cases of disseminated polyps of the rectum. Trans Pathol Soc Lond 33:165–168, 1882.

15. Smith T. Three cases of multiple polypi of the lower bowel occurring in one family. Saint Bartholomews Hosp Rep 23:225–229, 1887.

16. Handford H. Disseminated polypi of the large intestine becoming malignant: strictures (malignant adenoma) of the rectum and of the splenic flexure of the colon; secondary growths in the liver. Trans Pathol Soc Lond 41:133–137, 1890.

17. Lockhart-Mummery P. Cancer and heredity. Lancet i:427–429, 1925.

18. Herrera L, Kakati S, Gibas L, Pietrzak E, Sandberg AA. Gardner syndrome in a man with an interstitial deletion of 5q. Am J Med Genet 25:473–476, 1986.

19. Bodmer WF, Bailey CJ, Bodmer J, et al. Localization of the gene for familial adenomatous polyposis on chromosome 5. Nature 328:614–616, 1987.

20. Leppert M, Dobbs M, Scambler P, et al. The gene for familial polyposis coli maps to the long arm of chromosome 5. Science 238:1411–1413, 1987.

21. Laken SJ, Papadopoulos N, Petersen GM, et al. Analysis of masked mutations in familial adenomatous polyposis. Proc Natl Acad Sci USA 96:2322–2326, 1999.

22. Gardner EJ, Richards RC. Multiple cutaneous and subcutaneous lesions occurring simultaneously with hereditary polyposis and osteomatosis. Am J Hum Genet 5:139–147, 1953.

23. Hamilton SR, Liu B, Parsons RE, et al. The molecular basis of Turcot's syndrome. N Engl J Med 332:839–847, 1995.

24. Tomlinson IPM, Neale K, Talbot IC, et al. A modifying locus for familial adenomatous polyposis may be present on chromosome 1p35–36. J Med Genet 33:268–273, 1996.

25. Lynch HT, Smyrk T, Lanspa SJ, et al. Flat adenomas in a colon cancer–prone kindred. J Natl Cancer Inst 80:278–282, 1988.

26. Muto T, Kamiya J, Sawada T, et al. Small "flat adenoma" of the large bowel with special reference to its clinical pathologic features. Dis Colon Rectum 28:847–851, 1985.

27. Lynch HT, Smyrk TC, Watson P, et al. Hereditary flat adenoma syndrome: a variant of familial adenomatous polyposis? Dis Colon Rectum 35:411–421, 1992.

28. Spirio L, Otterud B, Stauffer D, et al. Linkage of a variant or attenuated form of adenomatous polyposis coli to the adenomatous polyposis coli (*APC*) locus. Am J Hum Genet 51:92–100, 1992.

29. Spirio L, Olschwang S, Groden J, et al. Alleles of the *APC* gene: an attenuated form of familial polyposis. Cell 75:951–957, 1993.

30. Leppert M, Burt R, Hughes J, et al. Genetic analysis of an inherited predisposition to colon cancer in a family with a variable number of adenomatous polyps. N Engl J Med 322:904–908, 1990.

31. Lynch HT, Smyrk T, McGinn T, et al. Attenuated familial adenomatous polyposis (AFAP): a phenotypically and genotypically distinctive variant of FAP. Cancer 76:2427–2433, 1995.

32. Gardner RJM, Kool D, Edkins E, et al. The clinical correlates of a 3′ truncating mutation (codons 1982–1983) in the adenomatous polyposis coli gene. Gastroenterology 113:326–331, 1997.

33. Hughes LJ, Michels VV. Risk of hepatoblastoma in familial adenomatous polyposis. Am J Med Genet 43:1023–1025, 1992.

34. Hawk E, Lubet R, Limburg P. Chemoprevention in hereditary colorectal cancer syndromes. Cancer 86:2551–2563, 1999.

35. Wallace MH, Phillips RKS. Upper gastrointestinal disease in patients with familial adenomatous polyposis. Br J Surg 85:742–750, 1998.

36. Marcial MA, Villafana M, Hernandez-Denton J, Colon-Pagan JR. Fundic gland polyps: prevalence and clinicopathologic features. Am J Gastroenterol 88:1711–1713, 1993.

37. Choudhry U, Boyce HW, Coppola D. Proton pump inhibitor–associated gastric polyps: a retrospective analysis of their frequency, and endoscopic, histologic and ultrastructural characteristics. Am J Clin Pathol 110:615–621, 1998.

38. Domizio P, Talbot IC, Spigelman AC, Williams CB, Phillips RKS. Upper gastrointestinal pathology in familial adenomatous polyposis: results from a prospective study of 102 patients. J Clin Pathol 43:738–743, 1990.

39. Goodman AJ, Dundas SAC, Scholefield JH, Johnson BF. Gastric carcinoma and familial adenomatous polyposis. Int J Colorectal Dis 3:201–203, 1988.

40. Zwick A, Munir M, Ryan CK, et al. Gastric adenocarcinoma and dysplasia in fundic gland polyps of a patient with attenuated adenomatous polyposis coli. Gastroenterology 113:659–663, 1997.

41. Hofgärtner WT, Thorp M, Ramus MW, et al. Gastric adenocarcinoma associated with fundic gland polyps in a patient with attenuated familial adenomatous polyposis. Am J Gastroenterol 94:2275–2281, 1999.

42. Arvanitis ML, Jagelman DG, Fazio VN, Lavery IC, McGannon E. Mortality in patients with familial adenomatous polyposis. Dis Colon Rectum 33:639–642, 1990.

43. Gurbuz AK, Giardiello FM, Petersen GM, et al. Desmoid tumours in familial adenomatous polyposis. Gut 35:377–381, 1994.

44. Rodriguez-Bigas MA, Mahoney MC, Karakousis CP, Petrelli NJ. Desmoid tumors in patients with familial adenomatous polyposis. Cancer 74:1270–1274, 1994.

45. Warthin AS. Heredity with reference to carcinoma. Arch Intern Med 12:546–555, 1913.

46. Lynch HT, Shaw MW, Magnuson CW, Larsen AL, Krush AJ. Hereditary factors in cancer: study of two large Midwestern kindreds. Arch Intern Med 117:206–212, 1966.

47. Itoh H, Houlston RS, Harocopos C, Slack J. Risk of cancer death in first-degree relatives of patients with hereditary nonpolyposis cancer syndrome (Lynch type II): a study of 130 kindreds in the United Kingdom. Br J Surg 77:1367–1370, 1990.

48. Jass JR, Stewart SM, Schroeder D, Lane MR. Screening for hereditary nonpolyposis colorectal cancer in New Zealand. Eur J Gastroenterol Hepatol 4:523–527, 1992.

49. Vasen HF, Hartog Jager FCA, Menko FH, Nagengast FM. Screening for hereditary nonpolyposis colorectal cancer: a study of 22 kindreds in the Netherlands. Am J Med 86:278–281, 1989.

50. Ponz de Leon M, Sassatelli R, Sacchetti C, Zanghieri G, Scalmati A, Roncucci L. Familial aggregation of tumors in the 3-year experience of a population-based colorectal cancer registry. Cancer Res 49:4344–4348, 1989.

51. Abusamra H, Maximova S, Bar-Meir S, Krispin M, Rotmensch HH. Cancer family syndrome of Lynch. Am J Med 83:981–983, 1987.

52. Mecklin J-P, Jarvinen HJ, Peltokallio P. Cancer family syndrome: genetic analysis of 22 Finnish kindreds. Gastroenterology 30:328–333, 1986.

53. Mecklin JP. Frequency of hereditary nonpolyposis colorectal carcinoma. Gastroenterology 93:1021–1025, 1987.

54. Boland CR, Troncale FJ. Familial colonic cancer without antecedent polyposis. Ann Intern Med 100:700–701, 1984.

55. Peltomäki P, Aaltonen L, Sistonen P, et al. Genetic mapping of a locus predisposing to human colorectal cancer. Science 260:810–812, 1993.

56. Lindblom A, Tannergard P, Werelius B, Nordenskjold M. Genetic mapping of a second locus predisposing to hereditary nonpolyposis colorectal cancer. Nat Genet 5:279–282, 1993.

57. Fishel R, Lescoe MK, Rao MRS, et al. The human mutator gene homolog *MSH2* and its association with hereditary nonpolyposis colon cancer. Cell 75:1027–1038, 1993.

58. Leach FS, Nicolaides NC, Papadopoulos N, et al. Mutations of a *mutS* homolog in hereditary nonpolyposis colorectal cancer. Cell 75:1215–1225, 1993.

59. Bronner CE, Baker SM, Morrison PT, et al. Mutation in the DNA mismatch repair gene homologue *hMLH1* is associated with hereditary nonpolyposis colon cancer. Nature 368:258–261, 1994.

60. Papadopoulos N, Nicolaides NC, Wei Y-F, et al. Mutation of a *mutL* homolog in hereditary colon cancer. Science 263:1625–1629, 1994.

61. Lu S-L, Kawabata M, Imamura T, et al. HNPCC associated with germ-line mutation in the TGF-β type II receptor gene. Nat Genet 19:17–18, 1998.

62. Mecklin J-P, Järvinen HJ, Hakkiluoto A, et al. Frequency of hereditary nonpolyposis colorectal cancer: a prospective multicenter study in Finland. Dis Colon Rectum 38:588–593, 1995.

63. Aaltonen LA, Salovaara R, Kristo P, et al. Incidence of hereditary non-polyposis colorectal cancer and the feasibility of molecular screening for the disease. N Engl J Med 338:1481–1487, 1998.

64. Lynch HT, Drouhard T, Lanspa S, et al. Mutation of an *mutL* homo-logue in a Navajo family with hereditary nonpolyposis colorectal cancer. J Natl Cancer Inst 86:1417–1419, 1994.

65. Weber TK, Chin H-M, Rodriguez-Bigas M, et al. Novel *hMLH1* and *hMSH2* germline mutations in African Americans with colorectal cancer. JAMA 281:2316–2320, 1999.

66. Lynch HT, Smyrk TC, Watson P, et al. Genetics, natural history, tumor spectrum, and pathology of hereditary nonpolyposis colorectal cancer: an updated review. Gastroenterology 104:1535–1549, 1993.

67. Box JC, Rodriguez-Bigas MA, Weber TK, Petrelli NJ. Clinical implications of multiple colorectal carcinomas in hereditary nonpolyposis colorectal carcinoma. Dis Colon Rectum 42:717–721, 1999.

68. Rodriguez-Bigas MA, Vasen HFA, Pekka-Mecklin J, et al. Rectal cancer risk in hereditary nonpolyposis colorectal cancer after abdominal colectomy. Ann Surg 225:202–207, 1997.

69. Sankila R, Aaltonen LA, Jarvinen HJ, Mecklin J-P. Better survival rates in patients with *MLH1*-associated hereditary colorectal cancer. Gastro-enterology 110:682–687, 1996.

70. Watson P, Lin K, Rodriguez-Bigas MA, et al. Colorectal carcinoma survival among hereditary nonpolyposis colorectal cancer family members. Cancer 83:259–266, 1998.

71. Watson P, Lynch HT. Extracolonic cancer in hereditary nonpolyposis colorectal cancer. Cancer 71:677–685, 1993.

72. Nelson CL, Sellers TA, Rich SS, Potter JD, McGovern PG, Kushi LH. Familial clustering of colon, breast, uterine, and ovarian cancers as assessed by family history. Genet Epidemiol 10:235–244, 1993.

73. Risinger JI, Barrett JC, Watson P, Lynch HT, Boyd J. Molecular genetic evidence of the occurrence of breast cancer as an integral tumor in patients with the hereditary nonpolyposis colorectal cancer syndrome. Cancer 77:1836–1843, 1996.

74. Boyd J, Rhei E, Federici MG, et al. Male breast cancer in the hereditary nonpolyposis colorectal cancer syndrome. Breast Cancer Res Treat 53:87–91, 1999.

75. Froggatt NJ, Green J, Brassett C, et al. A common *MSH2* mutation in English and North American HNPCC families: origin, phenotypic expression, and sex specific differences in colorectal cancer. J Med Genet 36:97–102, 1999.

76. Vasen HFA, Wijnen JT, Menko FH, et al. Cancer risk in families with hereditary nonpolyposis colorectal cancer diagnosed by mutation analysis. Gastroenterology 110:1020–1027, 1996.

77. Aarnio M, Salovaara R, Aaltonen LA, Mecklin J-P, Järvinen HJ. Features of gastric cancer in hereditary non-polyposis colorectal cancer syndrome. Int J Cancer 74:551–555, 1997.

78. Lin KM, Shashidharan M, Thorson AG, et al. Cumulative incidence of colorectal and extracolonic cancers in *MLH1* and *MSH2* mutation carriers of hereditary nonpolyposis colorectal cancer. J Gastrointest Surg 2:67–71, 1998.

79. Lin KM, Shashidharan M, Ternent CA, et al. Colorectal and extra-colonic cancer variations in *MLH1/MSH2* hereditary nonpolyposis colo-rectal cancer kindreds and the general population. Dis Colon Rectum 41:428–433, 1998.

80. Jäger AC, Bisgaard ML, Myrhoj T, Bernstein I, Rehfeld JF, Nielsen FC. Reduced frequency of extracolonic cancers in hereditary nonpolyposis colorectal cancer families with monoallelic *hMLH1* expression. Am J Hum Genet 61:129–138, 1997.

81. Miyaki M, Konishi M, Tanaka K, et al. Germline mutation of *MSH6* as the cause of hereditary nonpolyposis colorectal cancer. Nat Genet 17:271–272, 1997.

82. Wijnen J, de Leeuw W, Vasen H, van der Klift H, Møller P, Stormorken A. Familial endometrial cancer in female carriers of *MSH6* germline mutations. Nat Genet 23:142–144, 1999.

83. Vasen HFA, Mecklin J-P, Meera Khan P, Lynch HT. The International Collaborative Group on Hereditary Nonpolyposis Colorectal Cancer (ICG-HNPCC). Dis Colon Rectum 34:424–425, 1991.

84. Vasen HFA, Watson P, Mecklin J-P, Lynch HT, and ICG-HNPCC. New clinical criteria for hereditary nonpolyposis colorectal cancer (HNPCC, Lynch syndrome) proposed by the International Collaborative Group on HNPCC. Gastroenterology 116:1453–1456, 1999.

85. Lynch HT, Smyrk T. Hereditary nonpolyposis colorectal cancer (Lynch syndrome): an updated review. Cancer 78:1149–1167, 1996.

86. Kruse R, Rütten A, Lamberti C, et al. Muir-Torre phenotype has a frequency of DNA mismatch-repair-gene mutations similar to that in hereditary nonpolyposis colorectal cancer families defined by the Amsterdam criteria. Am J Hum Genet 63:63–70, 1998.

87. Cohen PR, Kohn SR, Kurzrock R. Association of sebaceous gland tumors and internal malignancy: the Muir-Torre syndrome. Am J Med 90:606–613, 1991.

88. Esche C, Kruse R, Lamberti C, et al. Muir-Torre syndrome: clinical features and molecular genetic analysis. Br J Dermatol 136:913–917, 1997.

89. Lynch HT, Lynch PM, Pester J, Fusaro RM. The cancer family syndrome: rare cutaneous phenotypic linkage of Torre's syndrome. Arch Intern Med 141:607–611, 1981.

90. Lynch HT, Lynch PM, Pester JA, Fusaro RM. Sebaceous neoplasia and visceral cancer (Torre's syndrome) and its relationship to the cancer family syndrome. In: Lynch HT, Fusaro RM (eds): Cancer-Associated Genodermatoses. Van Nostrand Reinhold, New York, 1982, pp 366–393.

91. Tanner MM, Tirkkonen M, Kallioniemi A, et al. Increased copy number at 20q13 in breast cancer: the critical region and exclusion of candidate genes. Cancer Res 54:4257–4260, 1994.

92. Jass JR. Colorectal adenoma progression and genetic change: is there a link? Ann Med 27:301–306, 1995.

93. Mecklin J-P, Jarvinen HJ. Clinical features of colorectal carcinoma in cancer family syndrome. Dis Colon Rectum 29:160–164, 1986.

94. Jass JR, Smyrk TC, Stewart SM, Lane MR, Lanspa SJ, Lynch HT. Pathology of hereditary non-polyposis colorectal cancer. Anticancer Res 14:1631–1634, 1994.

95. Gibbs NM. Undifferentiated carcinoma of the large intestine. Histopathology 1:77–84, 1977.

96. Jessurun MR, Manivel JC. Cecal, poorly differentiated adenocarcinomas, medullary-type [abstract]. Mod Pathol 5:43A, 1992.

97. Ruschoff J, Dietmaier W, Luttges J, et al. Poorly differentiated colonic adenocarcinoma, medullary type. Am J Pathol 150:1815–1825, 1997.

98. Graham DM, Appelman HD. Crohn's-like lymphoid reaction and colorectal carcinoma: a potential histologic prognosticator. Mod Pathol 3:332–335, 1990.

99. Smyrk TC, Lynch HT, Watson PA, Appelman HD. Histologic features of hereditary nonpolyposis colorectal carcinoma. In: Utsunomiya J, Lynch HT (eds): Hereditary Colorectal Cancer. Springer-Verlag, Tokyo, 1990, pp 357–362.

100. Thibodeau SN, French AJ, Roche PC, et al. Altered expression of *hMSH2* and *hMLH1* in tumors with microsatellite instability and genetic alterations in mismatch repair genes. Cancer Res 56:4836–4840, 1996.

101. Jass JR, Do K-A, Simms LA, et al. Morphology of sporadic colorectal cancer with DNA replication errors. Gut 42:673–679, 1998.

102. Smyrk TC, Watson P, Lin K, Kapler C, Lynch HT. Tumor-infiltrating lymphocytes in hereditary nonpolyposis colorectal cancer (HNPCC) [abstract]. Mod Pathol 12:85A, 1999.

103. Terdiman JP, Conrad PG, Sleisenger MH. Genetic testing in hereditary colorectal cancer: indications and procedures. Am J Gastroenterol 94:2344–2356, 1999.

104. Lanspa SJ, Jenkins JX, Cavalieri RJ, et al. Surveillance in Lynch syndrome: how aggressive? Am J Gastroenterol 89:1978–1980, 1994.

105. Vasen HFA, Nagengast FM, Khan PM. Interval cancers in hereditary non-polyposis colorectal cancer (Lynch syndrome). Lancet 345:1183–1184, 1995.

106. Jass JR, Stewart SM, Stewart J, Lane MR. Hereditary nonpolyposis colorectal cancer—morphologies, genes and mutations. Mutat Res 310:125–133, 1994.

107. Jass JR, Cottier DS, Pokos V, Parry S, Winship IM. Mixed epithelial polyps in association with hereditary non-polyposis colorectal cancer providing an alternative pathway of cancer histogenesis. Pathology 29:28–33, 1997.

108. Järvinen HJ, Mecklin J-P, Sistonen P. Screening reduces colorectal cancer rate in families with hereditary nonpolyposis colorectal cancer. Gastroenterology 108:1405–1411, 1995.

109. Järvinen HJ, Aarnio M, Mustonen H, et al. Controlled 15-year trial on screening for colorectal cancer in families with hereditary nonpolyposis colorectal cancer. Gastroenterology 118:829–834, 2000.

110. Lynch HT, Lemon S, Smyrk T, et al. Genetic counseling in hereditary nonpolyposis colorectal cancer: an extended family with *MSH2* mutation. Am J Gastroenterol 91:2489–2493, 1996.

111. Lerman C, Hughes C, Trock BJ, et al. Genetic testing in families with hereditary nonpolyposis colon cancer. JAMA 281:1618–1622, 1999.

112. Lynch HT, Leibowitz R, Smyrk T, et al. Colorectal cancer and the Muir-Torre syndrome in a Gypsy family: a review. Am J Gastroenterol 94: 575–580, 1999.

113. Peutz JL. A very remarkable case of familial polyposis of mucous membrane of intestinal tract accompanied by peculiar pigmentations of skin and mucous membrane [in Dutch]. Nederlands Tijdschrift voor Geneeskunde 10:134–146, 1921.

114. Jeghers H, McKusick VA, Katz KH. Generalized intestinal polyposis and melanin spots of the oral mucosa, lips and digits: a syndrome of diagnostic significance. N Engl J Med 241:993–1005, 1949.

115. Burt RW, Bishop DT, Cannon LA, Dowdle MA, Lee RE, Skolnick MH. Dominant inheritance of adenomatous colonic polyps and colorectal cancer. N Engl J Med 312:1540–1544, 1985.

116. Jenne DE, Reimann H, Nezu J, et al. Peutz-Jeghers syndrome is caused by mutations in a novel serine threonine kinase. Nat Genet 18:38–44, 1998.

117. Hemminki A, Tomlinson I, Markie D, et al. Localization of a susceptibility locus for Peutz-Jeghers syndrome to 19p using comparative genomic hybridization and targeted linkage analysis. Nat Genet 15:87–90, 1997.

118. Olschwang S, Markie D, Seal S, et al. Peutz-Jeghers disease: most, but not all, families are compatible with linkage to 19p13.3. J Med Genet 35:42–44, 1998.

119. Mehenni H, Blouin J-L, Radhakrishna U, et al. Peutz-Jeghers syndrome: confirmation of linkage to chromosome 19p13.3 and identification of a potential second locus, on 19q13.4. Am J Hum Genet 61:1327–1334, 1997.

120. Giardiello FM, Welsh SB, Hamilton SR, et al. Increased risk of cancer in the Peutz-Jeghers syndrome. N Engl J Med 316:1511–1514, 1987.

121. Wang Z-J, Churchman M, Avizienyte E, et al. Germline mutations of the LKB1 (STK11) gene in Peutz-Jeghers patients. J Med Genet 36: 365–368, 1999.

122. Bartholomew LG, Dahlin DC, Waugh JGM. Intestinal polyposis associated with mucocutaneous melanin pigmentation (Peutz-Jeghers syndrome). Gastroenterology 32:434–451, 1957.

123. Westerman AM, Entius MM, de Baar E, et al. Peutz-Jeghers syndrome: 78-year follow-up of the original family. Lancet 353:1211–1215, 1999.

124. Spigelman AD, Murray V, Phillips RKS. Cancer and the Peutz-Jeghers syndrome. Gut 30:1588–1590, 1989.

125. Boardman LA, Thibodeau SN, Schaid DJ, et al. Increased risk for cancer in patients with the Peutz-Jeghers syndrome. Ann Intern Med 128: 896–899, 1998.

126. Perzin KH, Bridge MF. Adenomatous and carcinomatous changes in hamartomatous polyps of the small intestine (Peutz-Jeghers syndrome): report of a case and review of the literature. Cancer 49:971–983, 1982.

127. Wang ZJ, Ellis I, Zauber P, et al. Allelic imbalance at the LKB1 (STK11) locus in tumours from patients with Peutz-Jeghers' syndrome provides evidence for a hamartoma–(adenoma)–carcinoma sequence. J Pathol 188:9–13, 1999.

128. Gruber SB, Entius MM, Petersen GM, et al. Pathogenesis of adenocarcinoma in Peutz-Jeghers syndrome. Cancer Res 58:5267–5270, 1998.

129. Young RH, Welch WR, Dickersin GR, Scully RE. Ovarian sex cord tumor with annular tubules: review of 74 cases including 27 with Peutz-Jeghers syndrome and four with adenoma malignum of the cervix. Cancer 50:1384–1402, 1982.

130. Spigelman AD, Arese P, Phillips RKS. Polyposis: the Peutz-Jeghers syndrome. Br J Surg 82:1311–1314, 1995.

131. Tomlinson IP, Houlston RS. Peutz-Jeghers syndrome. J Med Genet 34: 1007–1011, 1997.

132. Helwig EB. Adenomas of the large intestine in children. Am J Dis Child 72:289–295, 1946.

133. Nugent KP, Talbot IC, Hodgson SV, Phillips RK. Solitary juvenile polyps: not a marker for subsequent malignancy. Gastroenterology 105: 698–700, 1993.

134. Lynch HT, Smyrk T, Lynch J, Lanspa S, McGinn T, Cavalieri RJ. Genetic counseling in an extended attenuated familial adenomatous polyposis kindred. Am J Gastroenterol 91:455–459, 1996.

135. Coffin CM, Dehner LP. What is a juvenile polyp? An analysis based on 21 patients with solitary and multiple polyps. Arch Pathol Lab Med 120:1032–1038, 1996.

136. Cronkhite LW, Canada WJ. Generalized gastrointestinal polyposis: an unusual syndrome of polyposis, pigmentation, alopecia, and onychotrophia. N Engl J Med 252:1011–1015, 1955.

137. McColl I, Bussey HJR, Veale AMO, Morson BC. Juvenile polyposis coli. Proc R Soc Med 57:896–897, 1964.

138. Sachatello CR, Pickren JW, Grace JT. Generalized juvenile gastrointestinal polyposis: a hereditary syndrome. Gastroenterology 58:699–708, 1970.

139. Howe JR, Ringold JC, Summers RW, Mitros FA, Nishimura DY, Stone EM. A gene for familial juvenile polyposis maps to chromosome 18q21.1. Am J Hum Genet 62:1129–1136, 1998.

140. Howe JR, Ringold JC, Hughes JH, Summers RW. Direct genetic testing for Smad4 mutations in patients at risk for juvenile polyposis. Surgery 126:162–170, 1999.

141. Howe JR, Roth S, Ringold JC, et al. Mutations in the SMAD4/DPC4 gene in juvenile polyposis. Science 280:1086–1088, 1998.

142. Desai DC, Neal KF, Talbot IC, Hodgson SV, Phillips RK. Juvenile polyposis. Br J Surg 82:14–17, 1995.

143. Scott-Conner CEH, Hausmann M, Hall TJ, Skelton DS, Anglin BL, Subramony C. Familial juvenile polyposis: patterns of recurrence and implications for surgical management. J Am Coll Surg 181:407–413, 1995.

144. Järvinen HJ. Juvenile gastrointestinal polyposis. Prob Gen Surg 10: 749–757, 1993.

145. Howe JR, Mitros FA, Summers RW. The risk of gastrointestinal carcinoma in familial juvenile polyposis. Ann Surg 5:751–756, 1998.

146. Lloyd KMI, Dennis M. Cowden's disease: a possible new symptom complex with multiple system involvement. Ann Intern Med 58:136–142, 1963.

147. Liaw D, Marsh DJ, Li J, et al. Germline mutations of the PTEN gene in Cowden disease, an inherited breast and thyroid cancer syndrome. Nat Genet 16:64–67, 1997.

148. Lynch ED, Ostermeyer EA, Lee MK, et al. Inherited mutations in PTEN that are associated with breast cancer, Cowden disease, and juvenile polyposis. Am J Hum Genet 61:1254–1260, 1997.

149. Zigman AF, Lavine JE, Jones MC, Boland CR, Carethers JM. Localization of the Bannayan-Riley-Ruvalcaba syndrome gene to chromosome 10q23. Gastroenterology 113:1433–1437, 1997.

150. Marsh DJ, Dahia PLM, Zheng Z, et al. Germline mutations in PTEN are present in Bannayan-Zonana syndrome. Nat Genet 16:333–334, 1997.

151. Arch EM, Goodman BK, Van Wesep RA, et al. Deletion of PTEN in a patient with Bannayan-Riley-Ruvalcaba syndrome suggests allelism with Cowden disease. Am J Med Genet 71:489–493, 1997.

152. Celebi JT, Tsou HC, Chen F, et al. Phenotypic findings of Cowden syndrome and Bannayan-Zonana syndrome in a family associated with a single germline mutation in PTEN. J Med Genet 36:360–364, 1999.

153. Thomas HJW, Whitelaw SC, Cottrell SE, et al. Genetic mapping of the hereditary mixed polyposis syndrome to chromosome 6q. Am J Hum Genet 58:770–776, 1996.

154. Whitelaw SC, Murday VA, Tomlinson IPM, et al. Clinical and molecular features of the hereditary mixed polyposis syndrome. Gastroenterology 112:327–334, 1997.

155. Collins FS. Shattuck Lecture—medical and societal consequences of the Human Genome Project. N Engl J Med 341:28–37, 1999.

156. Caspari R, Olschwang S, Moslein G, et al. Familial adenomatous polyposis: mutation at codon 1309 and early onset of colon cancer. Lancet 343:629–632, 1994.

157. Caspari R, Olschwang S, Friedl W, et al. Familial adenomatous polyposis: desmoid tumours and lack of ophthalmic lesions (CHRPE) associated with APC mutations beyond codon 1444. Hum Mol Genet 4: 337–340, 1995.

158. Eccles DM, van der Luijt R, Breukel C, et al. Hereditary desmoid disease due to a frameshift mutation at codon 1924 of the APC gene. Am J Hum Genet 59:1193–1201, 1996.

159. Brensinger JD, Laken SJ, Luce MC, et al. Variable phenotype of familial adenomatous polyposis in pedigrees with 3′ mutation in the APC gene. Gut 43:548–552, 1998.

160. Lynch HT, Voorhees GJ, Lanspa SJ, McGreevy PS, Lynch JF. Pancreatic carcinoma and hereditary nonpolyposis colorectal cancer: a family study. Br J Cancer 52:271–273, 1985.

161. Lynch HT, Fusaro RM, Roberts L, Voorhees GJ, Lynch JF. Muir-Torre syndrome in several members of a family with a variant of the cancer family syndrome. Br J Dermatol 113:295–301, 1985.

162. Lynch HT, Fusaro RM. Muir-Torre syndrome: heterogeneity, natural history, diagnosis, and management. Prob Gen Surg 10:1–14, 1993.

# Chapter 55

# Pathology and Natural History of Colorectal Cancer

GRANT STEMMERMANN AND CECILIA FENOGLIO-PREISER

Sporadic carcinoma of the large bowel is commonly encountered among individuals in prosperous, industrialized countries. It is the second most common cancer in American women, after breast cancer; and the third most common cancer in American men, following cancer of the prostate and lung.[1,2] Only lung cancer surpasses it as a cause of cancer death in the United States.[2] In contrast, colorectal cancer is much less common in undeveloped countries, either as an incident event or as a cause of death. People migrating to the United States from low-risk countries quickly acquire the high risk of the host country,[3,4] as do the inhabitants of countries that evolve from a developing status to economic prosperity. For example, the annual age-adjusted colorectal cancer incidence rate per 100,000 for men in Miyagi, Japan, rose from 11.3 to 41.6 in only 20 years between 1972 and 1992,[1,5] so that the Japanese rates now exceed those of the United Kingdom. These trends strongly suggest that environmental factors play a key role in the development of cancer of the large bowel, although well-recognized colorectal cancer syndromes have been linked to specific germline mutations. The environmental and genetic associations of this common cancer make it a model for the molecular events that characterize the induction of solid tumors. This chapter will summarize the epidemiology, pathology, pathogenesis, and behavior of large bowel cancer and its precursors.

## Colorectal Anatomy

The incidence of large bowel cancer shows wide variation from subsite to subsite, and cancers in different subsites not only are associated with different risk factors but also display differences in behavior. The subdivisions of the large intestine include the cecum, vermiform appendix, ascending colon, transverse colon, descending colon, sigmoid colon, rectosigmoid colon, and rec-

tum. Many studies reduce these subdivisions into three subsets: right colon, including the colon from the cecum to the splenic flexure; left colon, including the descending, sigmoid, and rectosigmoid segments; and rectum. This segregation does not reflect differences in ethnic-specific subsite incidence patterns in the United States, as shown in Table 55–1.[6] The Japanese show the highest overall rates, with cancers of the sigmoid, rectosigmoid, and rectum accounting for the difference. African Americans have the lowest overall incidence but show the highest age-adjusted incidence of tumors involving the segments from the hepatic flexure through the descending colon (12.1/100,000), compared with whites (9.4), Chinese Americans (7.0), and Japanese Americans (6.3). Age- and gender-dependent influences on subsite incidence in two large registries (Connecticut and Denmark) suggest etiologic differences between the origin of cancers of the ascending colon and cecum and that of the remainder of the colon in women, and between men and women for cancers of the sigmoid colon and rectum.[7,8] The basis for these differences has not been established, but differences in the type or concentration of fecal carcinogens have been proposed, as well as differences in subsite susceptiblity to neoplastic change. At least one inherited risk, hereditary nonpolyposis colon cancer (HNPCC), is associated with proximal right-sided tumors.[9] A Japanese study indicates that the localization of cancer in the different large bowel subsites is clearly related to the surface area of the mucosa exposed to fecal carcinogens.[10] When assessed on this basis, the relative incidence per unit area is highest in the rectum (21.0), followed by the cecum (7.0), the sigmoid colon (4.8) and ascending colon (2.5), descending colon (1.7), and transverse colon (1.0). The same study shows wide individual variation in the surface area of each subsite, suggesting that individual risk may depend on the extent of mucosa exposed to carcinogens. Finally, it has been suggested that cancers of the

**Table 55-1** Age-adjusted annual U.S. incidence rates, colorectal cancer, males, SEER registries, 1973–1977

| Colorectal Subsite | White[a] | African American[b] | Chinese[c] | Japanese[d] |
|---|---|---|---|---|
| Cecum/appendix | 7.3 | 8.1 | 5.1 | 6.1 |
| Ascending colon | 4.2 | 4.1 | 2.8 | 3.8 |
| Hepatic flexure | 1.0 | 1.4 | 0.4 | 1.1 |
| Transverse colon | 4.1 | 4.6 | 2.1 | 1.7 |
| Splenic flexure | 1.2 | 2.1 | 0.4 | 1.2 |
| Descending colon | 3.1 | 4.0 | 4.1 | 2.3 |
| Sigmoid colon | 13.8 | 10.2 | 17.9 | 19.4 |
| Rectosigmoid colon | 5.7 | 3.8 | 6.6 | 12.0 |
| Rectum | 13.3 | 9.5 | 17.0 | 16.1 |
| Large Bowel, NOS | 2.0 | 2.3 | 1.0 | 1.0 |
| Total | 55.8 | 50.1 | 57.4 | 64.7 |

NOS, not otherwise specified; SEER, Surveillance, Epidemiology, and End Results.

[a]All SEER registries.

[b]Detroit, Atlanta, and New Orleans.

[c]Chinese Americans in San Francisco.

[d]Japanese Americans in Hawaii.

right colon, whether sporadic or inherited, are genetically more stable than cancers of the sigmoid colon or rectum.[11]

The distribution of adenomatous polyps, which are recognized precursors of sporadic colorectal cancers, generally parallels the distribution of their malignant counterparts. Both are most common in the sigmoid and rectosigmoid colon, and in the cecum and ascending colon.[12,13] Moreover, the gross configuration of some colorectal tumors is also subsite dependent. For example, lesions that have been identified as flat or depressed adenomas and cancers appear to have a predilection for the right colon,[14] whereas large villous adenomas are most commonly encountered at the opposite extremes of the bowel, in the cecum and rectum.

## Epidemiology

### Geographic Pathology

The wide international differences in colorectal cancer incidence are shown in Figure 55–1.[15] Countries in the five regions with the highest incidence of colorectal cancer are well developed, prosperous, and heavily industrialized. The nations in the five regions with the lowest incidence of these tumors are undeveloped and have economies based on the production of raw materials or agricultural products. The level of economic development between these extremes can be roughly gauged from the colorectal cancer incidence rates. Conspicuous differences are also evident in the occurrence of cancer of the colon and rectum in the United States, with the highest colorectal mortality rates concentrated in the industrialized states of the northeast and north central regions.[16] This distribution is independent of gender or ethnicity. Other countries also show significant regional differences in colorectal cancer mortality. In China, a country with relatively low rates of colorectal cancer, the highest rates are concentrated in Jiangsu and Zhejiang provinces, where a close correlation exists between schistosomiasis and large bowel cancer.[17]

Colorectal cancer shares similar geographic and temporal associations with other diseases and has inverse associations with others. For example, populations at high risk for colorectal cancer frequently also show high rates of coronary heart disease and breast cancer, but relatively low rates of cerebrovascular disease

and stomach cancer. Migrants from countries with high rates of stomach cancer retain that risk into old age, but quickly acquire the risk of colorectal cancer. The patterns of disease in the children and grandchildren of migrants come to resemble the patterns of disease of the host country. Thus, Japanese who migrated to Hawaii experience increased rates of coronary heart disease, at a level midway between the rates of Japan and the United States, and higher rates of colorectal cancer than those of the host population.[18]

### Demography

The age-specific incidence and mortality rates of sporadic colorectal cancers in the United States rise steeply after age 50, as shown in Figure 55–2.[2] The male-to-female incidence ratio is

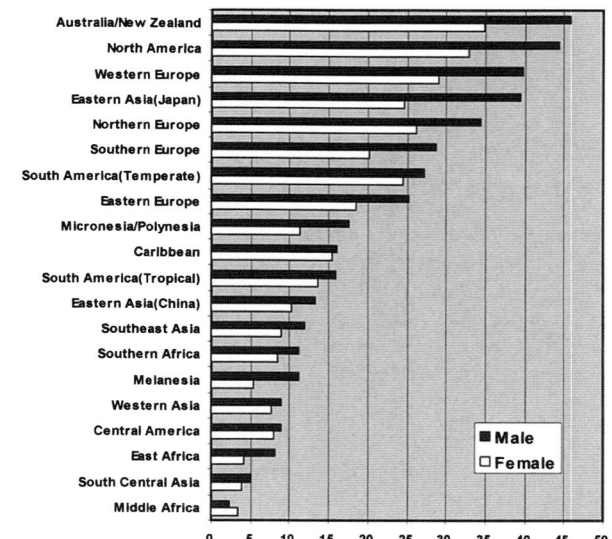

**Figure 55-1** Worldwide, age-standardized incidence rates for colorectal cancer.

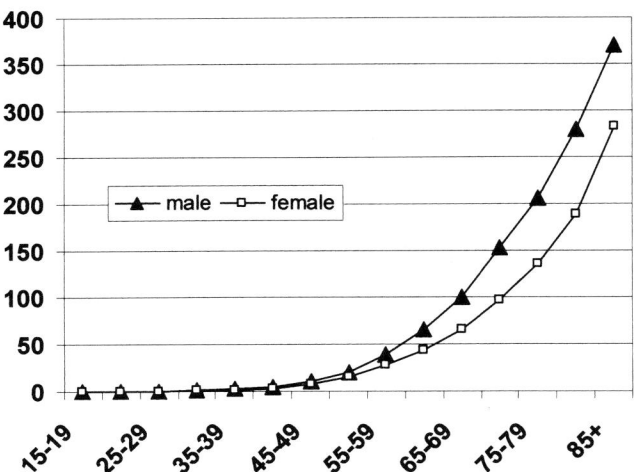

**Figure 55-2** Age-specific male and female incidence rates for colorectal cancer in the United States, all ethnic groups combined.

1.44, and the mortality ratio is 1.47. The age-adjusted incidence of colorectal cancer was fairly stable between 1973 and 1989 for U.S. white Americans of both genders, as was rectal cancer incidence among African American men and women. However, the age-adjusted incidence and mortality rates for colon cancer rose among African American men during this time frame as follows: the 1973 incidence in this group was 31.3, compared to 48.0 in 1989, and the mortality rate rose from 20.9 in 1973 to 28.4 in 1989. The late age of onset of most colorectal cancers, the distinct geographic patterns of high risk, and the upsurge in incidence rates among migrants and African Americans suggests a strong environmental influence on the development of this cancer. It is possible, however, that the good nutrition and hygiene available to people in prosperous Western societies enables many to live to the seventh, eighth, and ninth decades of life, when the vast majority of these cancers are diagnosed.

## Environmental Factors

The shifts in cancer and coronary heart disease incidence among migrants suggest that national dietary practices might account for the postmigration increase in both diseases. Burkitt[19] observed that blacks in Kenya and Uganda seldom acquired diseases that are common in Europe and North America. This led him to propose the concept of "Western diseases," which he attributed to a diet deficient in plant fiber and unrefined carbohydrate, but with excess energy from fats and refined carbohydrate.[19] Among these diseases he included colorectal cancer, the adenomatous polyps from which cancer develops, diverticulosis, obesity, coronary heart disease, and diabetes mellitus. Burkitt believed that fiber protected the large bowel mucosa from carcinogens by increasing fecal mass and decreasing bowel transit time. This hypothesis was supported by correlative studies indicating that the proportions of animal fat and protein are higher in high-risk countries and that carbohydrate and fiber constitute a larger share of the diet in low-risk countries.[20,21] This hypothesis has generated a large number of case–control and cohort studies that have attempted to confirm these findings directly. However, no consistent direct or inverse relations between macronutrients (fat, protein, carbohydrate) and large bowel cancer have been identified.[21–24] For ex-

ample, a prospective study of Hawaiian Japanese men, who are at particularly high risk of colorectal cancer, used a 24-hour recall examination to assess the dietary practices in apparently healthy men. This study showed an inverse relation between fat intake and the subsequent development of colorectal cancer,[23] whereas a large prospective study of women in the Nurses Health Study found a direct association with fat intake, which no longer remained after controlling for meat intake.[22,24] The inconsistencies among these studies probably arise from differences in the methods used to assess past and present patterns of food consumption and from the inability to assess the effect of small differences in food intake in homogenous populations.[22] Existing data suggest that vegetables are associated with lower risk, but fiber does not account for this association.[21]

The most consistent environmental variable associated with colorectal cancer is a positive balance between energy consumption over expenditure.[21] Obesity, weight gain since age 25, and sedentary occupation are consistently and directly associated with colon cancer risk but not with rectal cancer. Physical activity and its surrogate marker, a low resting pulse,[25] inversely relate to colon cancer.[26] These findings help to explain the rise in colorectal cancer rates that accompanies urbanization and improved socioeconomic status.[27] They may also explain the regional differences in colorectal cancer risk that have been observed in the United States.[16] However, the mechanism that explains the protective effect of physical activity and negative energy balance is still unclear.

Alcohol intake has been directly associated with rectal cancer in a large number of studies.[28] The toxic effects of alcohol metabolism on the rectal mucosa have been suggested as a possible mechanism. The relationship between alcohol and colon cancer is inconsistent. When a direct association is present, it is strongest when based on the percent of daily energy intake.[29] That alcohol may play a role in colon cancer as well as in rectal cancer is suggested by its direct association with colonic adenomas in most studies.[22] This effect may result from alcohol's displacement of protective micronutrients in the diet.

Meat consumption is associated with increased risk of colon cancer, but this may be related to the generation of mutagenic heterocyclic amines on the surface of meat cooked at high temperatures,[30] rather than on meat's fat or protein content.[21] It has been proposed that dietary calcium might be protective against colorectal cancer, but both prospective and cross-sectional studies have been inconsistent in this respect.[21,22] It is possible that the increase in risk associated with a low calcium intake may be confined to the sigmoid colon in patients whose calcium intake is insufficient to support the needs of an expanded bone mass. The calcium intake of Japanese subjects in Hawaii is very low when compared to white Americans, perhaps because of inherited lactase deficiency. The calcium intake level in Hawaiian Japanese is the same as in Japan, but because these individuals are taller than indigenous Japanese, their expanded bone mass amplifies their calcium deficit. Although no association has been found between calcium intake and overall colon cancer in these people, an inverse dose-dependent association exists between calcium intake and cancer of the sigmoid colon, an effect that is enhanced in the tallest individuals.[31] Calcium homeostasis is maintained by reabsorption in the proximal colon if calcium intake is low. As a result, feces may be devoid of calcium on reaching the sigmoid colon. Other micronutrients that may be protective against large bowel cancer include folate and methionine, particularly among individuals with a high alcohol intake.[32]

Several other environmental factors have been clearly associated with an increased risk of colorectal cancer. These account for only a small proportion of the large bowel cancers in high-risk societies. The most common of these factors is inflammatory bowel disease (IBD)[33]—ulcerative colitis and Crohn's disease. Areas with the highest incidence of IBD (Western Europe, North America) also experience the highest rates of sporadic colorectal cancer. The cumulative risk of colorectal cancer increases with the duration of the ulcerative colitis, with a range of 7%–45% at 25 to 35 years.[34,35] Other, less common environmental risk factors include therapeutic radiation,[36] schistosomiasis,[37] and the presence of a ureterosigmoidostomy.[38]

The increased risk of cancer induction with IBD, and perhaps with schistosomiasis as well, may result from the generation of nitric oxide (NO) by activated macrophages, neutrophils, and T cells.[39] Nitric oxide has the potential to induce genomic damage directly by nitrosative deamination of DNA[40] and NO-releasing compounds are mutagenic in the *Salmonella typhosa* system.[41] The association with ureterosigmoidostomy has been attributed to the activation of fecal carcinogens by urine, although, as in IBD, the reacting cells that characterize chronic inflammation might also explain this association.

## Genetic Changes and Inherited Colorectal Cancer Risk

Several inherited syndromes are associated with increased risk of colorectal cancer. Although these syndromes account for only a minority of colorectal cancers, discovery of the molecular abnormalities that generate these tumors helps us to understand the stepwise induction of sporadic cancers as well. A detailed description of the molecular pathology of colorectal cancer can be found in Chapter 53. A brief summary follows here.

The development of invasive colorectal cancer is a multistep process that begins with adenoma and ends with metastatic disease (Fig. 55–3) and, finally, the death of the patient. As originally proposed by Vogelstein and co-workers,[42,43] this progression involves four genetic events (Fig. 55–4), including activation

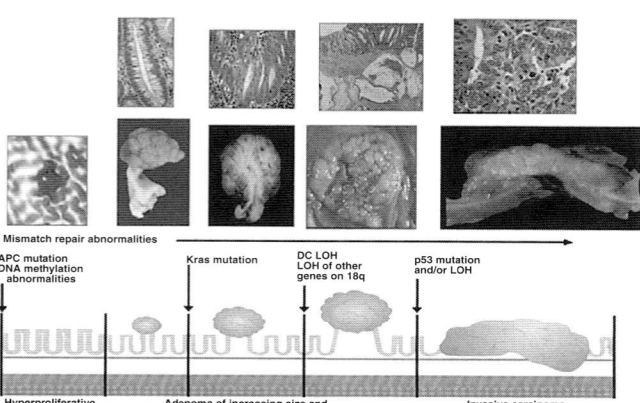

Mismatch repair abnormalities

APC mutation
DNA methylation
abnormalities

Kras mutation

DC LOH
LOH of other
genes on 18q

p53 mutation
and/or LOH

Hyperproliferative
epithelium

Adenoma of increasing size and
degree of dysplasia

Invasive carcinoma

**Figure 55–3** Colon cancer progression model. The lesions with each step are shown above the diagram. From left to right: aberrant crypt focus, tubular adenoma, gross and microscopic appearance; adenoma showing high-grade dysplasia, gross and microscopic; invasive, mucoid cancer, gross and microscopic; invasive, poorly differentiated cancer, gross and microscopic.

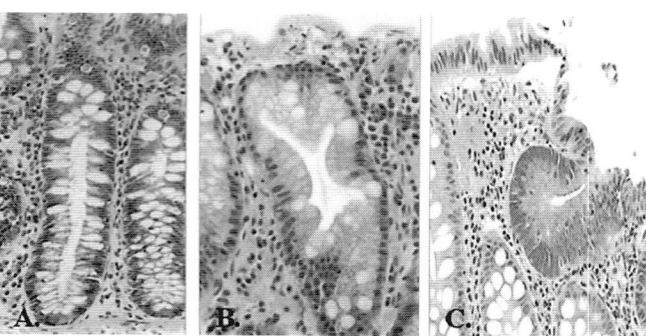

**Figure 55–4** *A:* Expanded replication zones, early ACF. The constituent cells are not neoplastic but show nuclear enlargement and occasional loss of cytoplasmic mucus. *B:* Hyperplastic ACF. The epithelium of a single gland shows the characteristic serrate configuration of these lesions. *C:* Adenomatous ACF. A small infolding of dysregulated epithelium involves the superficial aspects of a single mucosal gland.

of *ras* oncogenes and inactivation of tumor suppressor genes on chromosomes 5q, 17p, and 18q. The ras proteins may play a role in signal transduction and mutations in this gene are found in 50% of colon cancers, in adenomas, and, as recently described, in some hyperplastic polyps as well.[44] The *p53* gene on chromosome 17p is a tumor suppressor that binds DNA. Mutations that inactivate the *p53* gene occur in 85% of colorectal cancers. The deleted in colon cancer (*DCC*) gene at chromosome 18q22 is found in 70% of colorectal cancers.[45,46] The tumor suppressor gene on chromosome 5q has been termed the *APC* gene.[47] Mutations in this gene are found in 80% of somatic colorectal cancers and underlie familial adenomatosis (FAP). Subsequently, other pathways for colorectal tumorgenesis have been proposed, as new mutations continue to be identified. For example, germline mutations in DNA mismatch are found in the familial cancers comprising hereditary nonpolyposis colon cancer (HNPCC).[48] The five most common HNPCC mutations are found on chromosomes 2p, 2q, 3p, and 7p. The great majority of cancers in HNPCC cases show microsatellite instability (MSI), a feature of some sporadic cancers as well. Studies of sporadic cancers indicate that the presence or absence of MSI, or whether MSI is identified in one locus (MSI-L) or more than one locus (MSI-H), may have biologic significance. Tumors with MSI-H show fewer metastases at the time of diagnosis,[49] and loss of one DNA repair gene (O-6-methylguanine DNA methyltransferase [MGMT]) occurs much more often in MSI-L cancers than in MSI-H or MSI-stable cancers. Finally, most colorectal cancers exhibit replication errors with genetic instability if they develop before age 35, even in the absence of HNPCC. Only a small minority of colorectal cancers that appear after age 35 do so.[50] Germline mutations have been identified in some, but not all, of these patients. It would appear, therefore, that the mechanisms that underlie colorectal cancers in young patients differ from those of older patients.[50]

Two basic types of inherited colorectal cancer exist, each with several subtypes. The presence of preexisting polyps is a dominant feature of one type, whereas polyps are inconspicuous in the second type. The most common hereditary syndromes are summarized in Table 55–2. Familial adenomatosis may present in several ways, depending on the location of the mutation within the gene. Adenomatous polyps may carpet the entire length of the large bowel in classical FAP, or they may number up to 50

**Table 55-2** Syndromes showing increased risk of colorectal cancer

| Syndrome | Age | Polyps (n) | Inheritance | Cancer at Other Sites | Subsite |
|----------|-----|-----------|-------------|----------------------|---------|
| FAP | <39 | >100 | AD | Ampulla, CNS | None |
| AAPC | 55 | 1–50 | AD | Ampulla, thyroid, small bowel | Proximal to splenic flexure |
| HNPCC (L I) | <50 | — | AD | — | Proximal to splenic flexure |
| HNPCC (L II) | <50 | — | AD | Ovary, stomach, endometrium, breast | Proximal to splenic flexure |
| Li-Fraumeni | 45 | | AD | Breast, osteosarcoma, adrenal cortex, leukemia | None |
| BRCA 1 | 70 | — | AD | Breast | None |

AAPC, attenuated adenomatous polyposis; AD, autosomal dominant; FAP, familial adenomatous polyposis; HNPCC, hereditary non-polyposis colon cancer; LI, II, Lynch I, II.

in attenuated adenomatous polyposis coli (AAPC). Patients with FAP also may develop tumors at sites other than the colon. Polyps are especially common in the proximal duodenum and adjacent to the ampulla of Vater, with subsequent development of cancer at these sites. This occurs so often among FAP patients who have had a prophylactic colectomy that it justifies the use of periodic screening endoscopy to discover treatable lesions. Mesenchymal expression of mutations in the FAP gene may help to identify this condition, or may complicate its treatment. Thus, osteomas of the jaw and the presence of unerupted teeth are markers for this syndrome,[51] whereas retroperitoneal or abdominal wall desmoid tumors commonly occur in FAP patients after surgery.[52] Although the desmoid tumors do not metastasize, they have a tendency to recur and may show relentless local progression.

Hereditary nonpolyposis colorectal cancer is a familial cancer syndrome, defined by the presence among first-degree relatives of at least one patient under age 50 years and cancers in two succeeding generations. The cancers may be confined to the large bowel (Lynch I syndrome) or may involve a variety of other tumor sites as well (Lynch II syndrome).[9] These sites include ovary, endometrium, stomach, small bowel, and the renal pelvis/ureteral urothelium. The colorectal cancers in HNPCC patients favor the proximal right colon, are often diploid, and are often multiple. Although these tumors are often poorly differentiated mucinous cancers, they have a more favorable prognosis than sporadic cancers. They are also characterized by a conspicuous host lymphocyte reaction, both within the tumor and adjacent to it.

Colorectal cancers are components of two other familial cancer syndromes but are not the most commonly expressed tumors in either syndrome. The Li-Fraumeni syndrome results from germline mutations in the *TP53* gene and is expressed by the development of cancers at multiple sites in children and young adults.[53] Soft tissue sarcomas, osteosarcomas, brain tumors, leukemias, and adrenocortical carcinomas predominate in this autosomal dominant condition. A recent review of published cases of 738 Li-Fraumeni cancers in 185 kindreds identified 402 cancers in carriers of this gene. Seven of these were colorectal cancers (1.7%), with an average age at diagnosis of 33 years. The first-degree relatives of these patients, who have a 50% chance of having the mutation, experienced 296 cancers, of which 12 were colorectal cancers (4.1%), with an average age at diagnosis of 45 years.[54] Mutations in the *BRCA1* gene on chromosome 17q21 account for approximately 40%–50% of inherited breast cancers, and patients in families with this autosomal dominant mutation show an estimated relative risk of 4.11 (95% confidence interval [CI], 2.36–7.15) of developing colorectal cancer.[55]

## Pathology

### Anatomic Precursors

The earliest precursor of colorectal cancer is the aberrant crypt focus (ACF) (Fig. 55–4), first described in the colon mucosa of mice treated with the carcinogen azomethane.[56] Similar lesions have been identified in the human large bowel mucosa. Because ACF may have the histologic appearance of hyperplastic polyps[57,58] or may show the histologic features of adenomas[57] (Fig. 55–4), it is reasonable to assume that these foci represent the earliest manifestations of these two lesions.

Hyperplastic polyps, once considered to be non-neoplastic mucosal excrescences of the large bowel mucosa, have recently been found to share some features with neoplasms—clonality and *ras* gene mutations.[44] These findings might explain the close association of these lesions with colorectal cancer risk.[12,13] One variant of these polyps, mixed hyperplastic/adenomatous polyps, suggests that they may evolve into adenomas. The typical hyperplastic polyps seldom exceed 5 mm in diameter and are most common in the distal sigmoid colon and rectum. They are characterized by slower replication rates than those in normal colonic glands and an apparent hypermaturity of the surface cells.[59]

Adenomatous polyps are recognized colorectal cancer precursors, and the probability of finding cancer in an adenomatous polyp is proportional to its size.[60] Whatever their gross configuration, they are characterized by two distinctive biologic deviations from the normal large bowel mucosa,[61,62] as shown in

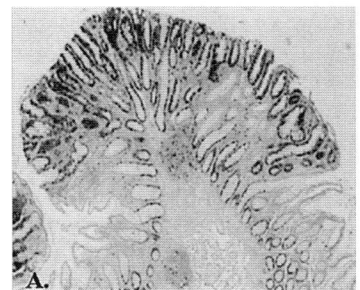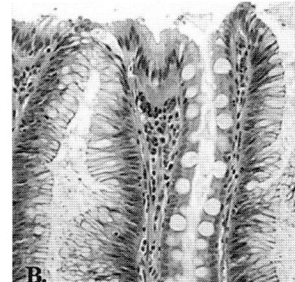

**Figure 55-5** *A:* Adenomatous polyp showing superficial replication, as demonstrated by the K-67 immunostain. *B:* Junction of adenomatous epithelium with normal mucosa. Note the enlarged nuclei and their loss of basal polarity. Mucus goblets are reduced size, and absorption cells are no longer apparent.

Figure 55–5: *(1)* dysregulated proliferation, manifested by an upward shift in the replication compartment, such that markers for replicating cells and mitoses may be found from the surface to the base of affected glands; and *(2)* failure to fully differentiate as they move from the crypt to the surface. The cells of adenomas resemble crypt cells and fail to develop into mature goblet cells.

Different gross and histologic variations of adenomas are recognized (Fig. 55–6) and the polyp's configuration also influences the level of risk of carcinoma. These include, in increasing order of cancer risk; tubular adenoma, tubulovillus adenoma, villus adenoma, and flat, or depressed, adenoma.

Tubular adenomas form spherical mucosal elevations that may be pedunculated or sessile. They maintain their cryptal architecture but are lined by dysplastic cells. Markers for cell turnover indicate that replication of the glandular epithelium is not limited to crypts but is found along the entire length of the gland and on the surface. Indeed, extremely small tubular adenomas may involve only the upper one-third of the mucosa.

*Villous adenomas* consist of long, finger-like fronds lined with dysplastic epithelium. This epithelium is supported by a slender vascular core and usually shows greater degrees of dysplastic change than the epithelium of tubular adenomas. Villous adenomas are much larger than tubular adenomas, occasionally measuring more than 10 cm in diameter. Large villous adenomas often show areas of malignant change and show a predilection for the proximal and distal ends of the large bowel, with 23% arising in the cecum and 55% arising in the rectum.

*Tubulovillous* adenomas are a mixture of villous and tubular components and tend to be intermediate in size between tubular and villous adenomas. *Flat* or *depressed adenomas* may have a serrated appearance and are most common in the right colon. They are often composed of glandular epithelium showing high-grade dysplasia and are more likely to show areas of malignant change than are elevated lesions of the same size. Flat or depressed adenomas may be very difficult to detect by endoscopy unless the mucosa is sprayed with dye.

Whatever forms adenomas assume, they can include neuroendocrine elements. One study found argyophilic neuroendodrine cells in 129 (59%) of 218 adenomas, and immunohistochemical studies identified a variety of products among them. In some cases, neuroendocrine cells are scattered through the adenomas

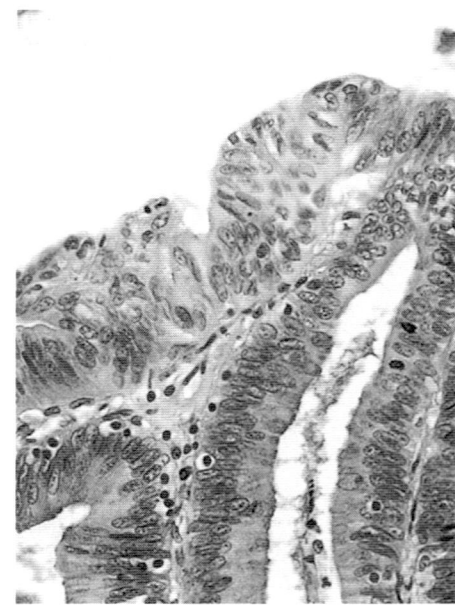

**Figure 55–7** Dysplastic surface epithelium in case of inflammatory bowel disease. Compare the dysplastic epithelium with the adjacent nondysplastic epithelium with respect to the loss of nuclear polarity, the nuclear pleomorphism, and altered nuclear-to-cytoplasmic ratio.

in patterns similar to that found in the normal colon. In other cases they are very numerous and appear to be a component of the neoplasm.[63] The presence of neuroendocrine cells in an adenoma does not correlate with clinical behavior. It does, however, explain the presence of these elements in carcinomas, and it is consistent with the concept of the entodermal derivation of neuroendocrine cells.

The mucosal changes that precede cancer induction in IBD are more subtle than the dysplasia of adenomatous polyps that evolve into sporadic or inherited cancers. The classification of IBD mucosal histology identifies three categories: negative for dysplasia, indefinite for dysplasia, and positive for dysplasia (Fig. 55–7).[64] The dysplastic mucosa roughly resembles the dysplasia found in sporadic adenomas, with the exception that it rarely forms grossly visible lesions. The diagnosis of indefinite for dysplasia is made when the cytological changes exceed those expected to result from regeneration in response to inflammation but are insufficient to merit a diagnosis of dysplasia. The exuberant reparative changes encountered in long-standing IBD may be extremely difficult to distinguish from dysplasia. Several markers have been used to identify mucosal dysplasia, including cell cycle proliferation markers such as Ki-67. Deregulation of the proliferative cell pool is indicated if Ki-67–positive cells are found in surface as well as crypt cells.[65] Immunohistochemical stains that identify mutations in the *p53* gene are often positive in the later stages of colorectal neoplasms. These stains have been used to identify areas of mucosal dysplasia in IBD,[66] but the basal portions of apparently nondysplastic mucosa may show labeling with this marker, whereas dysplastic mucosa may not. The subtlety of the neoplastic changes associated with ulcerative colitis is highlighted by the fact that even invasive tumors may not be identified on gross inspection of resected specimens but are discovered only after microscopic examination of a large number of random sections.

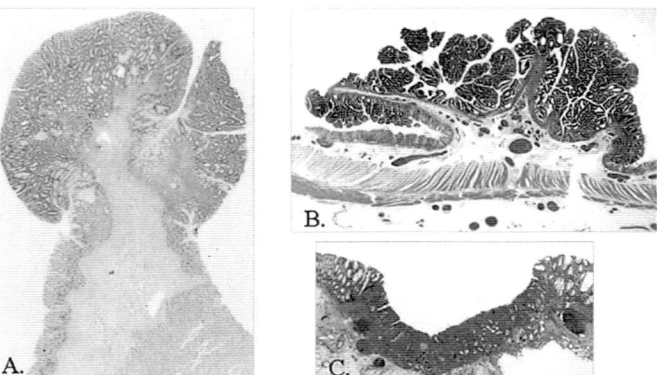

**Figure 55–6** Variation in the structure of adenomatous polyps. *A:* Pedunculated, tubular adenoma. *B:* Villus adenoma showing exuberant exophytic growth. *C:* Depressed adenoma.

## Colorectal Carcinoma

Only tumors that penetrate the muscularis mucosae are considered to be malignant at this site. This is in contrast to malignancy-defining invasion in the stomach and esophagus, where invasion into the lamina propria is sufficient for a diagnosis of invasive malignancy. The gross appearance of colorectal cancer may be papillary, exophytic, ulcerating, flat, or infiltrating. These growth patterns determine the symptoms produced by the cancer. Flat lesions may be entirely asymptomatic, whereas bleeding is most likely in exophytic and ulcerating cancers. Infiltrating tumors cause intestinal obstruction. Many cancers exhibit more than one of these growth patterns. Flat, grossly inconspicuous cancers are not uncommon among patients with HNPCC and IBD. The location of a colorectal cancer may also influence its gross appearance. Cancers of the cecum and ascending colon are more likely to be exophytic and show abundant mucus production than are more distal cancers. Cancers of the transverse and descending colons are often infiltrating in type and may produce annular constrictions. Late-stage cancers may adhere to and invade contiguous structures, producing fistulas into the urinary bladder, the vagina, or the small bowel.

The occurrence of multiple colorectal carcinomas in the same person is not unusual. Estimates of the frequency of multiplicity show considerable variation in most clinical studies, and synchronous multicentricity is more common than metachronous cases in these reports. Population-based cohort studies may achieve a more accurate estimate of these frequencies and proportions. Thus, an Italian study, covering the years 1984–1992, found 1298 colorectal cancer patients in a population of 265,227. Fifty-three of these (4%) patients had multicentric tumors, including 33 synchronous cases (2.5%) and 20 (1.5%) metachronous cases.[67] In this study, patients with multiple cancers were more likely to have a family history compatible with HNPCC than patients with single cancers. The proportion of metachronous cases increases with the duration of observation in population-based studies of older patients. For example, in an analysis of data from the Japan Hawaii Cancer Study in the 20 years from 1972 to 1992, 862 patients with colorectal cancer were identified among 12,339 Hawaiian Japanese men who were born between 1895 and 1925. Of these, 55 (6.4%) had multicentic tumors, 25 (2.9%) of which were synchronous and 30 (3.5%) were metachronous (unpublished observations). Both studies found that patients with multiple colorectal cancers are more likely to have associated adenomatous polyps than patients with single tumors. The Italian study also showed that the second tumor in metachronous cases was more likely to have a higher Dukes stage and less favorable prognosis than were single cancers.[67]

The majority of colorectal cancers form recognizable glands,[68] but vary from well- to poorly differentiated in their histologic patterns. Cytologic and histologic grading is helpful in assessing the prognosis of patients with these cancers. There is a broad spectrum of histologic variation among these tumors (Figs. 55–8 and 55–9A), and in some cases the whole spectrum of differentiation may be found in one cancer. In well-differentiated tumors, 95% of the cancer shows recognizable glandular formation. In poorly differentiated cancers, less than 50% of the tumor forms recognizable glands. Moderately differentiated cancers, which account for the majority of colorectal cancers, lie between these two groups. The least differentiated cancers may appear as solid sheets of cells that form no recognizable structures.

A minority of colorectal cancers deviate from these characteristic histologic growth patterns. Mucinous cancers are the most

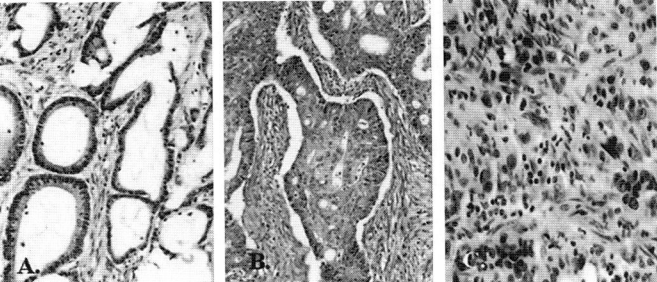

**Figure 55–8** Examples of different levels of differentiation, colorectal cancer. *A:* Well differentiated; *B:* moderately differentiated; *C:* poorly differentiated.

common of these, and they present in two forms: colloid carcinomas (Fig. 55–9B) and signet ring cancers (Fig. 55–9C). Colorectal cancers that develop in young patients and in patients with HNPCC are often mucinous in type. Colloid cancers are characterized by the formation of large mucus lakes that penetrate locally along tissue planes. The epithelium of these tumors may be well differentiated and may constitute such an inconspicuous component of the tumor mass that it may be difficult to find. Signet ring cell cancers are much less common than colloid cancers, tend to occur in young patients, and may be very aggressive. Their descriptive name is derived from the characteristic compression of the nucleus by accumulations of mucus in the cytoplasm. These tumor cells are not cohesive and are supported by a desmoplastic stroma. Advanced signet ring tumors may present in the form of a linitis plastica similar to that associated with diffuse cancers of the stomach. Indeed, they must be differentiated from diffuse gastric cancers that often metastasize to pelvic organs, including the distal colon and rectum.

Less common variants of large bowel carcinoma include adenosquamous carcinomas, small cell carcinoma (Fig. 55–9D), carcinosarcomas, and carcinomas with embryonal components.

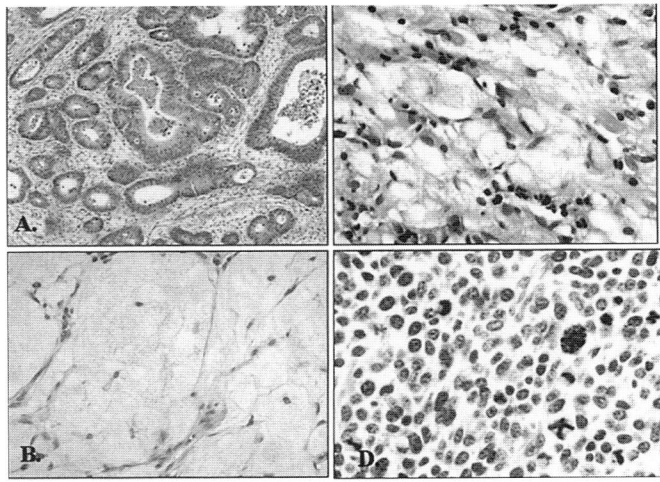

**Figure 55–9** *A:* The histologic pattern of a common form of colorectal cancer. Compare this with some less common variants: *B:* Colloid cancer characterized by abundant extracellular mucus and inconspicuous, bland epithelium. *C:* Signet ring cancer with cancer cells showing nuclei crowded to the periphery of the cells by cytoplasmic mucus. *D:* Small cell cancer with scanty cytoplasm, small oval to round nuclei, and frequent mitoses.

Even in aggregate, these less common tumors constitute such a small proportion of colorectal carcinomas that they have little effect on the incidence or mortality of large bowel cancer.

Pure squamous colorectal cancer is very uncommon, and the presence of a squamous component in an adenocarcinoma is a form of metaplasia derived from a pluripotent intestinal stem cell. The relative proportions of glandular and squamous components vary widely in these cancers. These tumors are most commonly encountered in the right colon and in cancers arising against a background of IBD. When the squamous component of an adencarcinoma appears to be benign, the cancer is termed an *adenoacanthoma.*

Small cell carcinomas may arise anywhere in the large bowel but tend to be most common in the right colon of older patients. In both structure and behavior, they resemble small cell cancers of the lung. Ultrastucturally, these carcinomas contain the membrane-bound core granules that are features of neuroendocrine cells. Small cell cancers are extremely aggressive, metastasize widely, and may show extensive areas of necrosis. Small cell cancer of the lung often metastasizes to the gastrointestinal tract, and it may be difficult to determine whether a large bowel cancer of this type is primary or secondary.

Choriocarcinomas of the colorectum are uncommon. Although many colorectal adenocarcinomas elaborate human chorionic gonadotropin (hCG), the term *choriocarcinoma* should be limited to those cancers that contain recognizable trophoblastic elements. Typically, these cancers are composed of both epithelial and trophoblastic components, and immunostains for hGC label both cell types. Choriocarcinomas may have a grossly hemorrhagic appearance. These are very aggressive tumors that commonly metastasize to the liver. Patients with this tumor may have very high levels of circulating hCG, and post-treatment blood level assays of this product can serve as a useful prognostic marker.

Carcinosarcomas of the large bowel are adenocarcinomas that contain areas of osseous, cartilagenous, rhabdoid, or simple spindle cell metaplasia. Because their sarcomatous components stain positively for epithelial as well as mesenchymal immunohistochemical markers, it is likely that they are derived from pluripotent intestinal stem cells. These cancers are very aggressive and have a poor prognosis.

As noted above, cancers in different subsites of the large bowel may have distinctive structural and behavioral characteristics. This is particularly true of the appendix, which is the source of less than 1% of large bowel cancers. Approximately 40% of these cancers are mucinous cystadenocarcinomas. These cancers, like mucoid cancers in other parts of the bowel, may produce large mucus lakes with inconspicuous, fairly bland neoplastic epithelium. They may obstruct the lumen of the appendix, which subsequently enlarges to form a mucocele. The continuing production of mucus may result in penetration of the appendiceal wall and dissemination into the peritoneal cavity, or pseudomyxoma peritonei. Patients who present with pseudomyxoma peritonei also may also have a cancer derived from the ovary or from other parts of the bowel, but the appendix must always be considered as a potential source of such cancers. All of the other forms of large bowel cancer may appear in the appendix, including typical adenocarcinoma and signet ring cancers. Appendiceal cancers of all types may be asymptomatic until late in the course of the disease, but the mucinous cystadencarcinomas have a less favorable prognosis than that of other types.

The extent of the lymphocyte infiltration of the cancer and the presence of Crohn's-type lymphocytic infiltration in the tissues bordering the cancer (Fig. 55–10) have both been linked to

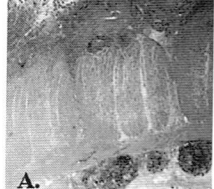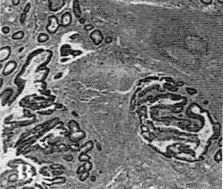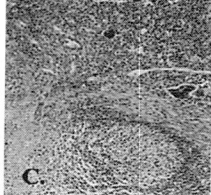

**Figure 55–10** Examples of host reaction to colorectal cancer. *A:* Crohn's-type lymphocytic infiltrate in the non-neoplastic tissues bordering the cancer. These consist of B cells. *B:* Low-power view of cancer showing infiltrating lymphocytes in supporting stroma. *C:* High-power view of dense collections of lymphocytes in stroma. Many of these cells are T cells.

tumor stage and survival.[69,70] Other histologic variables that influence the stage of these cancers include vascular and lymphatic invasion (Fig. 55–11).

The Dukes system of staging rectal cancer was one of the earliest attempts to assess the anatomic extent of any cancer. The system has been repeatedly modified over time, and the TNM system, based on extent of primary tumor (T), regional lymph node metastasis (N), and distant metastasis (M), now used by the American Joint Committee on Cancer (AJCC) and the World Health Organization (WHO) constitutes its latest refinement.[71] The TNM classification of colorectal cancer is summarized in Table 55–3. The TNM stage 1 corresponds to the original Dukes type A tumors, TNM stage 2 equates with Dukes type B tumors, and TNM stage 3 corresponds to Dukes type C tumors. The Dukes system had no equivalent for TNM stage 4. The Surveillance, Epidemiology, and End Results (SEER) registries that publish population-based survival studies in the United States separate all tumors into three categories: localized (equivalent to TNM stages 1 and 2), regional (equivalent to TNM stage 3), and distant (equivalent to TNM stage 4). The N component of the TNM system and the designation of regional disease in the SEER system each depend on adequate sampling of the regional lymph nodes. This raises the issue as to how the term *adequate* is defined. Thus routine histologic sampling of these nodes may miss micrometastases that can be identified with immunohistochemial stains for epithelial elements. These stains, in turn, may miss tumor-associated products that can be detected by a carcinoembryonic antigen (CEA)-specific nested reverse-transcriptase polymerase chain reaction (RT-PCR).[72] The latter technique detected micrometastases in nodes from 14 of 26 patients that

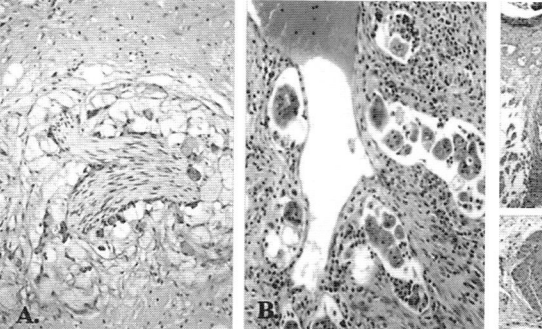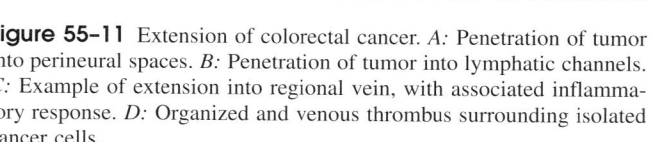

**Figure 55–11** Extension of colorectal cancer. *A:* Penetration of tumor into perineural spaces. *B:* Penetration of tumor into lymphatic channels. *C:* Example of extension into regional vein, with associated inflammatory response. *D:* Organized and venous thrombus surrounding isolated cancer cells.

**Table 55-3** TNM classification of colorectal cancers

| Stage | Description |
|---|---|
| *Primary Tumor (T)* | |
| Tx | Primary tumor cannot be assessed |
| T0 | No evidence of primary tumor |
| Tis | Carcinoma in situ: intraepithelial or invasion of lamina propria |
| T1 | Tumor invades submucosa |
| T2 | Tumor invades muscularis propria |
| T3 | Tumor invades through muscularis propria into subserosa or into nonperitonealized pericolic or perirectal tissues |
| T4 | Tumor directly invades other organs or structures and/or perforates visceral peritoneum |
| *Regional Lymph Nodes (N)* | |
| Nx | Regional lymph nodes cannot be assessed |
| N0 | No regional lymph node metastases |
| N1 | Metastases to 1-3 lymph nodes |
| N2 | Metastases in 4 or more lymph nodes |
| *Distant Metastases (M)* | |
| Mx | Distant metastases cannot be assessed |
| M0 | No distant metastases |
| M1 | Distant metastasis |

| | Stage Grouping | | |
|---|---|---|---|
| Stage | T | N | M |
| Stage 0 | Tis | N0 | M0 |
| Stage 1 | T1 | N0 | M0 |
| | T2 | N0 | M0 |
| Stage 2 | T3 | N0 | M0 |
| | T4 | N0 | M0 |
| Stage 3 | Any T | N1 | M0 |
| | Any T | N2 | M0 |
| Stage 4 | Any T | Any N | M1 |

### Distant Metastasis (M)

- MX Presence of distant metastasis cannot be assessed
- M0 No distant metastasis
- M1 Distant metastasis

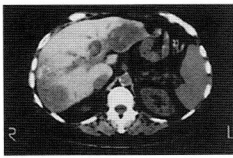

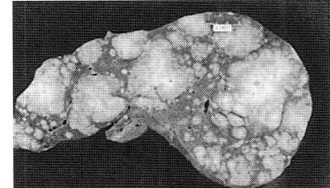
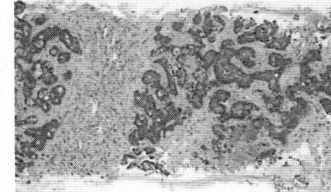

**Figure 55-12** Liver metastases from colorectal cancer as seen with computerized axial tomography scan imaging, on gross inspection and microscopically. The liver is the most common, and usually the first, metastatic site of this cancer.

showed no evidence of tumor with standard hematoxylin and eosin–stained slides.[72] Although the tumors associated with and without PCR-detected micrometastases were similar in size and differentiation, the observed survivals were 36% and 75%, respectively ($P = 0.03$). Application of this procedure on a grand scale may not be feasible at this time, but this observation clearly needs confirmation with much larger numbers. If the observation is confirmed, modification of the N component of the TNM system[73] may be warranted.

Colorectal cancer metastases develop through a sequence of interrelated steps,[74] and clinically relevant lesions must complete all of the steps. Spread to distant sites requires penetration of vascular channels, resulting in either lymphatic or hematogenous spread. An international review of 1541 colorectal cancers at autopsy demonstrated that hematogenous metastases from large bowel cancer evolve as a cascade, appearing first in the liver (Fig. 55-12), then the lungs, and finally in other organs.[75] Purely hematogenous spread is, however, the exception rather than the rule. This analysis showed that 73% of the 1244 cases with regional lymph node metastases had distant metastases, compared with only 26% of cases without regional node involvement. Identification of cancer cells in the regional veins or lymphatic channels in patients with resected colorectal cancers is associated with a poor prognosis in most studies, but the relationship is often weakened on multivariate analysis.[73] These disparate results may result, in part, from the fact that not all circulating cancer cells give rise to metastases. Although vascular invasion is a critical

step in the metastatic process, the development of distant lesions depends on the viability of the cancer cells after they penetrate the vascular channels and on their ability to survive in a new location.[74] Technical problems that arise from differences in the number of cases analyzed in various studies, as well as the number of sections examined in each case, also contribute to these inconsistencies.[73]

Some infiltrating colorectal cancers penetrate perineural spaces, an occurrence that is associated with a poor prognosis in many studies.[73] Although several molecular and oncogenic markers have been proposed to supplement the TNM staging system, none has been sufficiently well studied to be designated as a general oversight procedure.[73]

The tumor component (T) of the TNM system is difficult to apply to rectal cancer because the rectum has no serosal surface. These tumors often recur locally after resection, and the likelihood of recurrence is increased if the tumor has penetrated close to the line of resection. Sophisticated imaging techniques now allow us to estimate the depth of invasion toward the outer, or radial, margin of the rectum. Involvement of the radial margin is used to identify patients whose cancers may merit neoadjuvant treatment prior to definitive surgery. With or without neoadjuvant therapy, scrupulous histologic examination of the radial margin of resected specimens is necessary to accurately assess the prognosis of patients with rectal cancer.

The stage of colorectal cancer is the most important predictor of survival, but ethnicity also influences the probability of survival. The SEER data for the years 1983–1987 are shown in Table 55-4.[2] Patients of all ages, both genders, and all ethnic groups show a 5-year relative survival rate of 88.9% with localized tumors, 57.5% for regional tumors, and 5.9% for cancers with distant involvement. Neither age nor gender is associated

**Table 55-4** 5-Year relative survival with colorectal cancer, SEER registries, all ages, both genders, 1983–1987

| Stage | All Races (%) | Whites (%) | African Americans (%) |
|---|---|---|---|
| All Stages | 57.4 | 58.3 | 47.5 |
| Localized | 88.9 | 89.7 | 82.4 |
| Regional | 57.5 | 58.2 | 49.2 |
| Distant | 5.9 | 6.0 | 4.8 |
| Unstaged | 30.9 | 31.7 | 28.5 |

with significant differences in survival, but whites have better survival than African Americans at all stages. This database also showed an increase in 5-year survival from 49.4% for the years 1974–1976 to 57.5% for the years 1983–1988 ($P < 0.05$), a trend that probably reflects improved diagnosis and treatment of this cancer. An independent study of Japanese Americans in the SEER registry shows better survival than that among either whites or African Americans.[76] The basis for these ethnic differences has not been established.

Histopathologic factors that have been related to poor prognosis include an infiltrative invasive edge, as opposed to an expansile margin. Signet ring tumors and those that produce large amounts of mucus often present at a late stage and have a poor prognosis. High microvessel density has been interpreted as an adverse prognostic factor because of the need for neovascularization to support tumor growth.[77] As noted above, the presence of lymphocytes in the cancer (predominantly T cells) and groups of B-cell follicles at the outer margin of the tumor are associated with lower-stage tumors and with a favorable 5-year survival. Numerous genetic markers have been assessed to determine their effect on survival, but until these markers are evaluated in large, prospective, population-based studies, their independent weight will be difficult to gauge. Among the more promising of these is the observation that colorectal cancers of the MSI-H type have fewer metastases and a better prognosis than microsatellite-stable tumors.[49]

## Future Prospects

In view of the relatively stable incidence trends for colorectal cancer, and with improved management, we should expect to see gradually decreasing mortality rates from this cancer. This trend could be offset, however, by an increasing numbers of people who live past age 70. Nonetheless, preventive efforts may blunt the surge in the number of patients with colorectal cancer that might follow these demographic changes. The recent observations that cyclooxygenase (COX) plays a part in colon tumorgenesis and that COX-2 inhibitors cause regression in polyp size and number in patients with FAP[78] suggest that these drugs might be effective in preventing sporadic cancer as well.[79] Increased periodic endoscopic screening of high-risk patients to identify and remove adenomas may also contribute to a future decline in the incidence and mortality from this cancer.

## References

1. Parkin DM, Whelan SL, Ferlay J, Raymond J, Young J. Cancer in Five Continents, Vol. VII, IARC Publication No. 143. IARC, Lyon, 1997.
2. Miller BA, Ries LAG, Hankey B, Kosary CL, Edwards BK. Cancer Statistics Review 1973–1989. NIH Publication 92-2789. National Cancer Institute, Bethesda, 1992, pp I.25–26.
3. Stemmermann GN, Nomura AMY, Kolonel L. Cancer among Japanese Americans in Hawaii. In: Kurihara M (ed): Changing Cancer Patterns and Topics in Cancer Epidemiology, Gann Monograph on Cancer Research 33. Gann, Tokyo, 1987, pp 99–108.
4. Thomas DB, Karagas MR. Migrant studies. In: Schottenfeld D, Fraumeni J (eds): Cancer Epidemiology and Prevention, 2nd ed. Oxford University Press, New York, 1996, pp 236–254.
5. Waterhouse J, Muir C, Correa P, Powell J. Cancer in Five Continents, Vol III. IARC Publication No. 15. IARC, Lyon, 1976.
6. Young JL, Percy CL, Asire AJ. Surveillance, Epidemiology, and End Results. NCI Monograph 57. U.S. Department of Health and Human Services, National Institutes of Health, Bethesda MD, 1981.
7. Dubrow R, Bernstein J, Holford TR. Age–period–cohort modelling of large bowel cancer incidence by anatomic subsite and sex in Connecticut. Int J Cancer 53:907–13, 1993.
8. Dubrow R, Johansen C, Skov T, Holford TR. Age–period–cohort modelling of large bowel cancer incidence by anatomic subsite and sex in Denmark. Int J Cancer 58:324–329, 1994.
9. Lynch HT, Smyrk TC, Watson P, et al. Genetic, natural history, tumor spectrum, and pathology of hereditary non-polyposis colorectal cancer: an updated review. Gastroenterology 104:1535–1539, 1993.
10. Sadohiro S, Ohmura T, Saito T, Suzuki S. Relation between length and surface area of each segment of the large intestine and the incidence of colorectal cancer. Cancer 68:84–87, 1991.
11. Bullfill JA. Colorectal cancer: evidence of distinct genetic categories based on proximal and distal location. Ann Intern Med 113:779–788, 1990.
12. Stemmermann GN, Yatani R. Diverticulosis and polyps of the large intestine. Cancer 31:1260–1270, 1973.
13. Sato E. Adenomatous polyps of large intestine in autopsy and surgical material. Gann 65:295–306, 1974.
14. Hamilton SR. Flat adenomas: what you can't see can hurt you. Radiology 187:309, 1993.
15. Parkin DM, Pisani P, Ferlay J. Estimates of world-wide cancer incidence of 23 major cancers. Int J Cancer 80:577–591, 1999.
16. Devesa SS, Grauman DJ, Blot WJ, Pennello GA, Hoover RN, Fraumeni JF. Atlas of Cancer Mortality in the United States. NIH Publication No. 99-4564. National Institutes of Health, Bethesda MD, 1999, pp 116–133.
17. Li J-Y. Investigation of geographic patterns of cancer mortality in China. In: Third Symposium on Epidemiology and Cancer Registries in the Pacific Basin. NIH Publication No. 82-2438. National Institutes of Health, 1982, Washington DC, pp 17–42.
18. Haenszel W, Kurihara M. Studies in Japanese migrants: mortality from cancer and other diseases among Japanese in the United States. J Natl Cancer Inst 40:43–68, 1968.
19. Burkitt D. Surgical diseases of the large bowel and other related diseases. In: Trowell HC, Burkitt DP (eds): Western Diseases: Their Emergence and Prevention. Edward Arnold, London, 1981, pp 33–43.
20. Kagan A, Harris B, Winkelstein W, Johnson KG, et al. Epidemiologic studies of heart disease and stroke in Japanese living in Japan, Hawaii, and California. J Chron Dis 27:3455–3464, 1974.
21. Potter JD. Nutrition and colon cancer. Cancer Causes Control 7:127–146, 1996.
22. Schottenfeld D, Winawer SJ. Cancer of the large intestine. In: Schottenfeld D and Fraumeni JF (eds): Cancer Epidemiology and Prevention, 2nd ed. Oxford University Press, New York, 1996, pp 813–840.
23. Stemmermann GN. Geographic epidemiology of colorectal cancer: the role of dietary fat. In: Seitz HK, Wright NA, Simanoski UA (eds): Colorectal Cancer: From Pathogenesis to Prevention. Springer-Verlag, Berlin, 1989, pp 1–43.
24. Willett WC, Stampfer MJ, Colditz GA, et al. Relation of meat, fat, and fiber intake to the risk of colon cancer in a prospective study among women. N Engl J Med 323:1664–1672, 1990.
25. Clausen JP. Effect of physical training on cardiovascular adjustments to exercise in man. Phys Rev 58:779–915, 1977.
26. Persky V, Dyer AR, Leonas J, et al. Heart rate: a risk factor for cancer? Am J Epidemiol 114:477–487, 1981.
27. Tajima K, Hirose K, Nakagawa N, Kuroishi T, Tominaga S. Urban–rural difference in the trend of colorectal cancer mortality with special reference to the subsites of colon in Japan. Jpn, J Cancer Res 76:717–728, 1985.
28. Jensen OM, Paine SL, McMichael AJ, Ewertz M. Alcohol. In: Schottenfeld D, Fraumeni JF (eds): Cancer, Epidemiology and Prevention, 2nd ed. Oxford University Press, New York, 1996, pp 290–318.
29. Stemmermann GN, Nomura AMY, Chyou P, et al. Prospective study of alcohol intake and large bowel cancer. Dig Dis Sci 35:1414–1420, 1990.
30. Nagao M, Sugimura T. Carcinogenic factors in food with relevance to colon cancer development. Mutat Res 290:43–51, 1993.
31. Stemmermann GN, Nomura AMY, Chyou PH. The influence of dairy and non-dairy calcium on subsite large bowel cancer risk. Dis Colon Rectum 33:190–194, 1990.
32. Giovannuci E, Rimm EB, Ascherio A, Stampfer MJ, Colditz GA, Willett WC. Alcohol, low methionine–low folate diets and risk of colon cancer in men. J Natl Canc Inst 87:265–273, 1995.
33. Heimann TM, Oh SC, Martinelli G, et al. Colorectal carcinoma associated with ulcerative colitis: a study of prognostic indicators. Am J Surg 164:13–20, 1992.
34. Katzka I, Brody RS, Morris E, et al. Assessment of colorectal cancer risk in patients with ulcerative colitis. Gastroenterology 85:22–29, 1983.
35. Podolsky DK. Inflammatory bowel disease. N Engl J Med 325:1008–1016, 1991.
36. Greenwald R, Barkin JS, Hensley GT, Kalser MH. Cancer of the colon as a late sequel of pelvic radiation. Am J Gastroenterol 69:196–198, 1978.
37. Ming-Chai C, Chi-Yuan C, Pei-Yu C, Jen-Chun H. Evolution of colorectal cancer in schistosomiasis. Cancer 46:1661–1675, 1980.

38. Harford FJ, Fazio VW, Epstein LM, Hewitt CB. Rectosigmoid carcinoma occurring after ureterosigmoidoscopy. Dis Colon Rectum 27:321–327, 1984.

39. Kirk SJ, Rizan MC, Barbul A. Cloned murine T-lymphocytes synthesize a molecule with the biologic characteristics of nitric oxide. Biophys Res Commun 173:660–665, 1990.

40. Wink DA, Kasprzak KS, Maragos CM, et al. DNA deaminating ability and genotoxicity of nitric oxide and its progenitors. Science 254:1001–1003, 1991.

41. Arroyo PL, Hatch-Pigott V, Mower HF. Mutagenicity of nitric oxide and its inhibition by antioxidants. Mutat Res 281:193–202, 1992.

42. Fearon ER, Vogelstein B. A genetic model for colorectal carcinoma. Cell 61:759–767, 1990.

43. Vogelstein B, Kinzler KW. The multistep nature of cancer. Trends Genet 9:138–147, 1993.

44. Otori K, Oda Y, Hasebe K, Mukai K, et al. High frequency of K-ras mutations in human colorectal hyperplastic polyps. Gut 40:660–663, 1997.

45. Vogelstein B, Fearon ER, Hamilton S, et al. Genetic alterations during colorectal tumor development. N Engl J Med 319:525–532, 1988.

46. Ilas M, Tomlinson IPM. Genetic pathways in colorectal cancer. Histopathology 28:389–399, 1996.

47. Groden J, Thliveris A, Samowitz W, et al. Identification and characterization of the familial adenomatous polyposis gene. Cell 66:589–600, 1991.

48. Boland CR. Hereditary nonpolyposis colon cancer. In: Vogelstein B, Kinzler KW (eds): The Genetic Basis of Human Cancer. McGraw Hill, New York, 1997, pp 333–346.

49. Whitehall VLJ, Walsh MD, Young J, Leggett BA, Jass J. Methylation of O-6-methylguanine DNA methyltranferase characterizes a subset of colorectal cancer with low-level DNA microsatellite instability. Cancer Res 61:827–830, 2001.

50. Liu B, Farrington SM, Peterson GM, et al. Genetic instability occurs in the majority of young patients with colorectal cancer. Nat Med 1:348–352, 1995.

51. Utsunomiya J, Nakamura T. The occult osteomatous changes in the mandible of patients with familial polyposis coli. Br J Surg 62:45–51, 1975.

52. Jarvinen HJ. Desmoid disease as part of familial adenomatosis coli. Acta Chir Scand 153:379–382, 1987.

53. Li FP, Fraumeni JF Jr. Soft tissue sarcomas, breast cancer and other neoplasms: a familial cancer syndrome? Ann Intern Med 71:747–752, 1969.

54. Nichols KE, Malkin D, Garber JE, Fraumeni JF Jr, Li FP. Germ-line p53 mutations predispose to a wide spectrum of early onset cancers. Cancer Epidemiol Biomarkers Prev 10:83–87, 2001.

55. Ford D, Easton DF, Bishop DT, Narod SA, Goldgar D. Breast cancer linkage consortium: risk of cancer in BRCA 1 mutation carriers. Lancet 343:962–965, 1994.

56. McLellan EA, Bird RP. Aberrant crypts: potential preneoplastic lesions in the murine colon. Cancer Res 48:6187–6192, 1988.

57. Gregorio CD, Losi L, Fante R, et al. Histology of aberrant crypt foci in the human colon. Histopathology 30:328–334, 1997.

58. Araki K, Ogata T, Kobayashi M, Yatani R. A morphological study on the histogenesis of human colorectal hyperplastic polyps. Gastroenterology 109:1468–1474, 1995.

59. Hayashi T, Stemmermann GN, Yatani R, Apostol J. The pathogenesis of hyperplastic polyps of the colon: ultrastructure and in vitro cell kinetics. In: Farber E, Kawachi T, Nagayo T, et al. (eds): Pathophysiology of Carcinogenesis in Digestive Organs. University Park Press, Baltimore, 1977, pp 323–333.

60. Grinnell RS, Lane N. Benign and malignant adenomatous polyps and papillary adenomas of the colon and rectum: an analysis of 1856 tumors in 1335 patients. Int Abst Surg 106:519–538, 1958.

61. Fenoglio CM, Kaye GI, Pascal RR, Lane N. Defining the precursor tissue of ordinary large bowel carcinoma: implications for cancer prevention. Pathol Annu 12:87–116, 1977.

62. Kaye GI, Fenoglio CM, Pascal R, Lane N. Comparative electron microscopic features of normal, hyperplastic and adenomatous colon epithelium. Gastroenterology 64:926–945, 1973.

63. Van den Ingh HF, Van den Broek LJ, Verhofstad AAJ. Neuroendocrine cells in colorectal adenomas. J Pathol 148:231–233, 1986.

64. Riddell RH, Goldman H, Ransonhoff DE, et al. Dysplasia in inflammatory bowel disease: standardized classification with clinical application. Hum Pathol 14:931–968, 1983.

65. Noffsinger AE, Miller MA, Cusi MV, Fenoglio-Preiser CM. The pattern of cell proliferation in neoplastic and nonneoplastic lesions of ulcerative colitis. Cancer 78:2307–2372, 1996.

66. Noffsinger AE, Belli JM, Miller MA, Fenoglio-Preiser CM. A unique basal pattern of p53 expression in ulcerative colitis is associated with mutation in the p53 gene. Histopathology 39:482–492, 2001.

67. Fante R, Roncucci L, Di Gregorio C, et al. Frequency and clinical features of multiple tumors of the large bowel in the general population and in patients with hereditary colorectal cancer. Cancer 17: 2013–2021, 1996.

68. Fenoglio-Preiser CM, Noffsinger A, Stemmermann GN, et al. Carcinomas and other epithelial and neuroendocrine tumors of the large intestine. In: Gastrointestinal Pathology—An Atlas and Text, 2nd ed. Lippincott-Raven, Philadelphia, 1999, pp 909–1068.

69. Harrison JC, Dean PJ, El-Zeky F, Van der Zwaag R. Impact of the Crohn's-like lymphoid reaction on staging of right-sided colon cancer. Hum Pathol 26:31–38, 1995.

70. Jass JR, Love SB, Northover JMA. A new prognostic classification of rectal cancer. Lancet 1:1303–1306, 1987.

71. Fleming ID, Cooper JS, Henson DE, et al. AJCC Cancer Staging Manual, 5th ed. Lippincott-Raven, Philadelphia, 1992, pp 83–93.

72. Liefers GJ, Cleton-Jansen AM, Cornelis JH, et al. Micrometastases and survival in stage II colorectal cancer. N Engl J Med 339:223–228, 1998.

73. Compton C, Fenoglio-Preiser CM, Pettigrew N, Fielding LP. American Joint Committee on Cancer Prognostic Factors Consensus Conference. Colorectal Working Group. Cancer 88:1739–1757, 2000.

74. Gutman M, Fidler IJ. Biology of human colon cancer metastasis. World J Surg 19:226–234, 1995.

75. Weiss L, Grundman E, Torhorst J, et al. Haematogenous metastatic patterns in colonic carcinoma: an analysis of 1541 autopsies. J Pathol 150: 195–203, 1986.

76. Hirohata T, Nomura AMY, Rellahan W, et al. Survival patterns from large bowel cancer in Hawaii. Hawaii Med J 36:343–347, 1977.

77. Warren RS, Yuan H, Matil MR, et al. Regulation by vascular endothelial growth factor of human colon cancer tumorigenesis in a mouse model of experimental liver metastasis. J Clin Invest 95:1789–1797, 1995.

78. Giardello FM, Hamilton SR, Krush AJ, et al. Treatment of colonic and rectal adenoma with sulindac in familial adenomatous polyposis. N Engl J Med 328:1313–1316, 1993.

79. Sheehan KM, Sheahan K, O'Donoghue DP, et al. The relationship between cyclooxygenase-2 expression and colorectal cancer. JAMA 282: 1254–1257, 1999.

# Chapter 56

## Clinical Aspects and Management of Colon Adenocarcinoma: Diagnostic and Staging Procedures

ROBERT R. CIMA AND RONALD BLEDAY

Approximately 1.2 million new cases of invasive cancers, excluding skin cancer, were diagnosed in the United States in 2001.[1] Colon cancer accounted for nearly 48,000 deaths in the United States in 1999.[1] When combined with rectal cancer, colorectal cancer is the third most common cause of cancer deaths in men, behind lung cancer and prostate cancer and in women, behind lung cancer and breast cancer. Early detection of colon cancer often translates into a lower stage of disease and improved chances for survival. This chapter discusses the modalities most commonly used to diagnose and appropriately stage colon cancer. The use of these modalities to screen populations at risk for colon cancer is discussed in Chapter 52.

### History and Physical Examination

Most patients with colon cancer are asymptomatic at the time of diagnosis. Patients who present with symptoms and signs indicative of colon cancer usually have more advanced disease. Patients may present with abdominal pain, pelvic pain, back pain, changes in bowel habits, changes in stool caliber, passage of blood per rectum, nausea, vomiting, fatigue, anorexia, or weight loss.

Taking a thorough medical history can allow appropriate risk stratification of the patient. The American Cancer Society has defined three risk categories for colon cancer.[2] Individuals at low risk have no symptoms referable to colonic process, have no family history of colon cancer among their first-degree relatives, and are least 50 years of age. Individuals at moderate risk have at least one first-degree relative with a colon cancer, have a personal history of colonic polyps, or have had a prior colonic malignancy. Individuals at high risk may have a known genetic syndrome that predisposes them to develop colon cancer or a personal history of an inflammatory bowel disorder. Choices of screening and evaluation should be based on the risk stratification of the individual patient and the clinical presentation.

Physical examination will not often help in either the diag-

nosis or staging of a colon cancer. However, the examination should include a general examination aimed at identifying other medical conditions that may contribute to the presenting symptoms or that may require further evaluation before any surgical procedure. Again, most patients with colon cancer do not show signs of the disease upon physical examination unless there is advanced disease. In such cases, a palpable abdominal mass may be present or a mass may be found upon rectal examination. Digital rectal examination may reveal fecal occult blood. Abdominal distension may result from a partial or a complete obstruction or from ascites. Hepatomegaly may be detected in cases of substantial metastatic disease.

### Laboratory Tests

Laboratory tests are usually nonspecific in evaluating cases of possible colon cancer. However, laboratory tests are useful in excluding other disease processes that may underlie constitutional symptoms. In cases of unexplained microcytic anemia the colon should always be evaluated for bleeding from a polyp or tumor. Liver function tests are nonspecific because they may show no abnormalities even in the presence of hepatic metastases. Changes in clotting time often occur late after extensive replacement of the liver by metastatic disease. The role of the tumor marker carcinembryonic antigen (CEA) in colorectal cancer screening and surveillance is still being defined.[3–5] Most physicians agree that CEA is nonspecific and too expensive for use as a screening tool. However, a considerable amount of literature indicates that an elevated preoperative CEA is a prognostic indicator of poor outcomes in patients with colon cancer.[5]

### Digital Rectal Examination

Currently the American Cancer Society recommends an annual digital rectal examination for low-risk patients beginning at the age of 40 years. This examination should be performed along with part of a comprehensive medical history and physical examination. The main purpose of this digital rectal examination is to detect low rectal lesions and, in men, to examine the prostate gland. The examination may also reveal other anal canal or rectal pathologies that account for false-positive occult blood test.

## Fecal Occult Blood Test

The most commonly used screening test for colon and rectal cancer is the fecal occult blood test (FOBT). The most extensively studied FOBT, the guaiac impregnated slide test, detects hemoglobin pseudoperoxidase activity in stool samples. Clinicians using this test to screen patients for colon and rectal cancer must be aware of the many reasons for both false-positive and false-negative readings. False-positive results are most commonly caused by non-neoplastic sources, while false-negative results are associated with intermittently bleeding or nonbleeding polyps or tumors. Ingestion of foods that contain pseudoperoxidase, such as red meat, melons, broccoli, cabbage, and potatoes, can also cause false-positive results. The use of vitamin C supplements can result in false-negative results. Although the use of oral supplemental iron was also thought to cause false-negative results, a recent study did not find any significant interference.[6] Only an estimated 30% of cancers and large polyps bleed enough to be detected by FOBT. All the major studies that have evaluated FOBT have use two slides prepared from each of three consecutive stool samples; the utility of FOBT using a single stool sample obtained during a digital rectal examination has not been thoroughly assessed. In addition, workers debate whether the slide should be rehydrated; a practice that increases the sensitivity but also the false-positive rates of FOBT.

Because of its availability and relative ease of use, FOBT is widely used to screen patients for colon and rectal cancer. However, the reliability of this test depends largely on whether the evaluator employs the correct method of obtaining a sample. Also, some physicians are reluctant to offer further diagnostic tests with only one or two positive cards. These limitations have led to major difficulties in the widespread acceptance of FOBT as a diagnostic and screening tool.

The utility of FOBT as a screening test for colon and rectal cancer in asymptomatic individuals at moderate risk has been evaluated in five large trials.[7–11] The positive predictive value of FOBT ranged from 20% to 60%. In all the trials, the stages of colon cancers detected in the screened population were lower than those in the unscreened population. However, only one trial showed a lower mortality rate in the annually screened group than that in the unscreened group. The 13-year follow-up period revealed a 33% lower cumulative mortality rate in the screened population than that in the unscreened group.

## Modalities Used to Evaluate the Colonic Mucosa

Colon cancer screening and detection are based on the evaluation of colonic mucous. The purpose of the evaluation is to determine whether colonic polyps are present. Most physicians agree that most colon cancers develop from adenomatous polyps. Polyps are histologically classified as either non-neoplastic or neoplastic. Neoplastic polyps are most commonly adenomas, and it is believed that most colonic carcinomas arise within adenomas. The time course for adenoma-to-carcinoma sequence is generally thought to be 5–10 years. Several findings support the adenoma-to-carcinoma hypothesis. Adenomas are distributed in the colon in a pattern similar to that of colon cancers but occur 5–10 years before these cancers. Many colon cancers occur adjacent to the remnants of polyps. Finally, patients who have undergone endoscopic removal of polyps have a lower incidence of carcinomas than those who have not undergone this procedure.

There are two types of non-neoplastic polyps: hyperplastic polyps and hamartomas. While histologically benign, hyperplastic polyps can contain areas of adenomatous changes, a finding that warrants their removal by polypectomy. If biopsy of a small rectal or sigmoid polyp shows adenomatous changes, the entire colon should be evaluated by colonoscopy.

The most common neoplastic polyps found in the colon are adenoms. Autopsy studies have reported that adenomas are present in 20%–60% of patients with colon or rectal cancer.[12–15] In a study of average-risk, asymptomatic patients, adenomas were found upon colonoscopy in 20%–40% of patients.[16–18] Adenomas are divided into three histologic types: tubular adenomas, villous adenomas, and tubulovillous adenomas. Data from the National Polyp Study and St. Mark's Hospital show that approximately 75%–85% of adenomas are tubular, 8%–15% are tubulovillous, and 5%–10% are villous.[19,20] Tubular adenomas usually form a stalk, while villous adenomas have a broad base. The size of an adenoma often correlates with the histology of the polyp. In the St. Mark's experience, 76% of tubular adenomas were less than 1 cm in diameter, 20% were 1–2 cm, and only 4% were greater than 2 cm. In contrast, only 14% of villous adenomas were less than 1 cm in diameter, while more than 60% were larger than 2 cm. Both villous histology and increased polyp size are associated with an increased risk of cancer within the polyp. Regardless of size, approximately 5% of tubular adenomas harbor a malignancy, while nearly 40% of villous adenomas show evidence of cancer. Also, as the size of the polyp increases, so does its potential for malignancy. Only 1% of polyps less than 1 cm in diameter show evidence of malignant transformation, while 50% of polyps greater than 2 cm in diameter have areas of carcinoma. Therefore, barium studies and endoscopic evaluation of the colon are designed to detect polypoid lesions early in the adenoma-to-carcinoma sequence to prevent the transformation of a polyp into a cancer or to deter cancers at an early stage.

## Barium Single-Contrast and Double-Contrast Studies

For years, the barium enema was the method of choice for evaluating the colonic mucous and anatomy. Multiple reports have documented that the sensitivity of contrast studies is comparable to that of endoscopic evaluation of the colon. However, the most important factor in the usefulness of contrast studies is the expertise of the radiologist. For the single-contrast enema, barium is instilled in the rectum under fluoroscopic observation. This technique is useful in evaluating the gross anatomy of the colon and lumen caliber, determining the distensibility of colonic segments, and detecting intraluminal masses or masses causing extrinsic compression. Postevacuation films allow colonic mucous to be evaluated more thoroughly for small ulcerations and polyps. In a double-contrast study, a combination of high-density barium and air is instilled into the rectum, and radiographs are taken with the patient in a series of standard positions. As the patient is moved, the barium settles in the most dependent areas of the colons. A polyp on the dependent surface of the colon appears as a filling defect, while a polyp on the nondependent surface is highlighted with barium against an air interface.

The usefulness of either the single- or the double-contrast method depends upon the expertise of the person performing the study. Only one large single-institution study has compared the sensitivity levels of the two methods. Johnson and colleagues[21] at the Mayo Clinic performed nearly 97,000 colonic barium single- or double-contrast studies over a 5.5-year period. These studies identified 1140 colorectal cancers in 1084 patients. The authors concluded that both methods were equally sensitive with a 4.8% error rate for a single-contrast study and a 4.7% error rate for the double contrast study.

The role of barium studies in the screening for colon cancer is controversial when compared to the sensitivity of endoscopy. Again, the use of this modality depends upon the patient's risk factors for colonic polyps or cancer. Current American Cancer Society screening guidelines recommend that barium studies be used only in individuals at low risk for colon or rectal cancer and that these individuals be screened every 5–10 years after the age of 50. After reviewing the data on the sensitivity of both single- and double-contrast barium studies, Glick et al.[22] reported that these studies have a 70% to 90% sensitivity for detecting colonic polyps greater than 1 cm in diameter, a finding suggesting that most polyps that might harbor a malignancy would be detected. Proponents of barium studies point out that this method offers several advantages over endoscopy, including a lower rate of complications associated with the procedure and lower cost. However, detection of a polyp greater than 1 cm in diameter or of multiple polyps by barium studies would require subsequent endoscopic biopsy to rule out malignancy, thus necessitating another step in the diagnostic work-up.

## Endoscopy

The most common reason to study the colonic mucous is to determine whether polyps are present. While double-contrast barium studies and colonoscopy are approximately equal in their ability to detect polyps 1 cm or greater in diameter, flexible sigmoidoscopy and colonoscopy have the added advantage of serving as both a diagnostic tool and a therapeutic intervention. The mere presence of a polyp or its appearance, as determined by either a barium study or an endoscopy, does not correlate with malignant potential of the polyp. Endoscopic biopsy is needed to make a definitive tissue diagnosis.

Flexible sigmoidoscopy is used to evaluate the distal colon and rectum. This method offers several advantages over barium studies and colonoscopy. First, flexible sigmoidoscopy does not require any sedation. Second, the method does not require any special diet or an extensive preprocedure bowel preparation; usually, the patient only requires a few enemas just before the procedure. The sigmoidoscope is advanced into the distal 60–70 cm of the colon. The mucous is evaluated while the instrument is slowly withdrawn from the colon. Minimal insufflation of air is performed during the insertion. During the withdrawal, the colon can be distended with air to allow careful inspection of the mucous. Polyps may be removed or biopsied during the procedure.

Many workers consider video endoscopy the gold standard for evaluating the colonic mucous. However, under certain circumstances, the sensitivity of endoscopy may be no better than that of a contrast study. Rex and colleagues[23] reported that unless the endoscopy is performed by a gastroenterologist trained in endoscopy, the sensitivity of this technique to detect for polyps and cancer is no better than that of either single-contrast or double-contrast barium studies.[23] Furthermore, even when performed by experienced endoscopists, video endoscopy is associated with a significant miss rate for polyp detection. Rex and colleagues[24]

found that the miss rate for adenomas in patients who had two colonoscopies on the same day ranged from 20% to 30%. The miss rate was 24% when same endoscopist performed both colonoscopies. Importantly, the miss rate for adenomas greater than 1 cm in diameter was less than 6%, which means the likelihood of missing a cancerous adenoma is relatively low. As previously stated, the main advantages of endoscopy are its high sensitivity of detection and its ability to perform both diagnostic and therapeutic interventions with a relatively low complications rate. However, because the sensitivity of endoscopy is operator-dependent, the sensitivity of this modality as a screening method maybe limited.

## Virtual Colonoscopy

As computerized axial tomography (CAT) scan technology and software have advanced, the resolution of the image provided by this method has likewise improved dramatically. The advent of the helical scanner and the improvements in computer graphics have allowed two-dimensional axial images provided by CAT scans to be reconstructed in a three-dimensional format. Early results in a few centers using specific protocols have shown that this method has a sensitivity comparable to that of colonoscopic evaluation by an experienced endoscopist.[25,26] In a report by Fenlon et al.,[25] patients at high risk for colonic polyps or cancers had a standard bowel preparation followed by a helical computed tomography (CT) scan performed after insufflation of air into the colon and the administrtion of glucagon to minimize colonic peristalsis and spasm. Immediately following the scan, the patients underwent colonoscopy. Among 100 patients at high risk, virtual colonoscopy enabled the visualization of the entire colon in 87 patients while the endoscopy enabled the viewing of the entire colon in 89 patients. Virtual colonoscopy had a 71% sensitivity to detect all polyps and a 91% sensitivity to detect polyps at least 1 cm in diameter.[25] As technology improves, the use of virtual colonoscopy to screen individuals at high risk may reduce the need for frequent endoscopy. However, like barium studies, virtual colonscopy does not offer the diagnostic and therapeutic intervention provided by endoscopy.

## Staging of Colon Cancer

The purpose of staging any cancer is to describe the anatomic extent of the lesion. Staging aids in planning treatment, evaluating response to treatment, comparing the results of various treatment regimens, and determining prognosis. The growing knowledge of the molecular biology of colon cancer and the use of molecular biologic techniques to identify molecular evidence of metastatic disease will undoubtedly change how colon cancer is staged in the next decade. The current mechanism for staging colon cancer relies heavily on radiologic and pathologic staging. Staging by clinical examination is often only useful in identifying patients with far-advanced metastatic disease, which is relatively uncommon.

Radiologic evaluation plays many roles in the staging of colon cancer. The most commonly used radiologic study after the diagnosis of colon cancer is the abdominal and pelvic CAT scan. Often a preoperative scan for a colon cancer is unnecessary because this technique would provide little new information that would change the operative approach. Patients diagnosed with colon cancer almost always undergo operative exploration and resection of the colonic primary tumor. In a retrospective analysis of patients who obtained preoperative CAT scans, McAndrew and Saba[27] reported that only 3 out of 67 patients had incidental findings that led to changes in the surgical approach. However, a preoperative CAT scan may be useful if clinical examination suggests that the tumor is large or involves adjacent abdominal structures. The presurgical identification of hepatic metastases does not alter the management of the initial surgery. Furthermore, the identification of large or multiple hepatic metastatic lesions does not necessitate a combined colonic and anatomic hepatic resection. Studies that have evaluated this combination have clearly shown that attempts to remove hepatic metastases at the time of the primary colonic resection should be limited to only very peripheral hepatic lesions that can be removed in a nonanatomic fashion. Such lesions can be seen and felt and thus do not require preoperative localization.

The role of the CAT scan in preoperative staging of colon cancer has changed since the introduction of this technique. Preliminary case reports and small series found that CAT scans were highly accurate in staging colon cancer. Freeny and colleagues[28] reviewed preoperative CAT scans and found that they correctly staged only 47% in 103 patients with colorectal cancers. Among patients with the incorrectly staged disease, the cancer was upstaged in 83% of cases after the operative specimen was evaluated. The main disadvantage of CAT in staging colon cancer is that this technique is ineffective in the identification of involved lymph nodes. The accepted size for a suspicious lymph node on CAT is a node greater than 1 cm in diameter. Using a CAT scan, it is difficult to identify mesenteric lymph nodes that are often involved only with microscopic tumor deposits. With this limitation, the ability of CAT scans to distinguish between pathologic stage B and C lesions is extremely hard. In the review by McAndrew and Saba[27] CAT scans correctly identified lymph node involvement in only 19% of cases.

Recent changes in CAT scan technology and techniques may improve the staging accuracy. The use of air insufflation of water enemas has been reported to enhance the accuracy of CAT scans in staging colon cancers. Harvey and colleagues[26] used helical CAT scans with colonic air insufflation to preoperatively evaluate patients with known or strongly suspected colon carcinomas. All patients subsequently either underwent endoscopic biopsy or surgical resection for pathologic confirmation of the lesion.

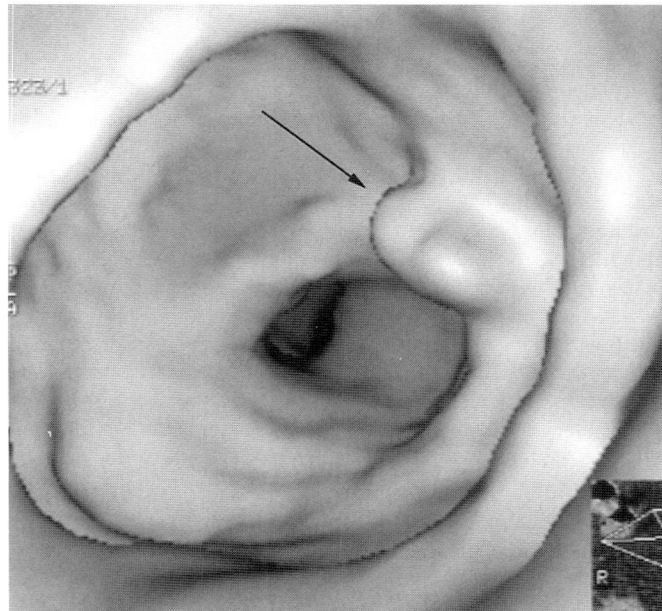

**Figure 56–1** Endoluminal image showing a 1.2-cm polyp (arrow) within the descending colon using virtual CT colonography (virtual colonoscopy). The finding was confirmed by colonoscopy.

Among 46 patients, the colon cancer was identified in 38 patients and was correctly staged 79% of the time. The sensitivity for serosal infiltration was 100% while the specificity was 33%. However, the sensitivity for lymph node involvement was only 56%. As experience with virtual colonoscopy increases, the accuracy of the staging may also be increased. Morrin and colleagues[29] recently reported their experience and found that they correctly identified pericoloic lymph nodes with pathologically proved metastatic disease in 81% of the patients studied.[29] Examples of the images generated by virtual colonoscopy are shown in Figures 56–1 and 56–2.

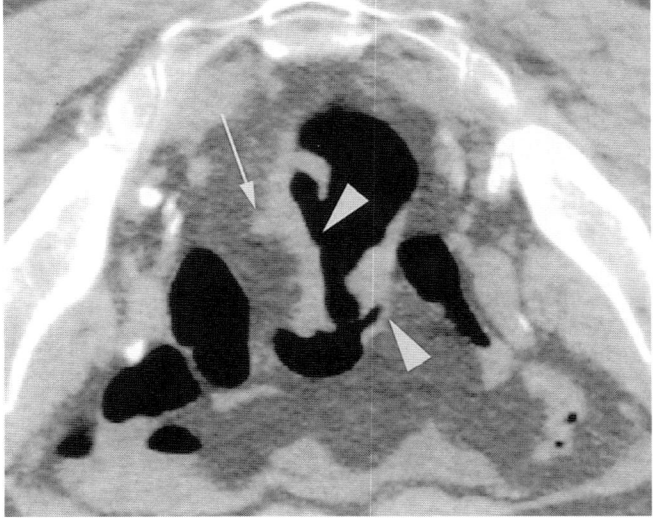

A

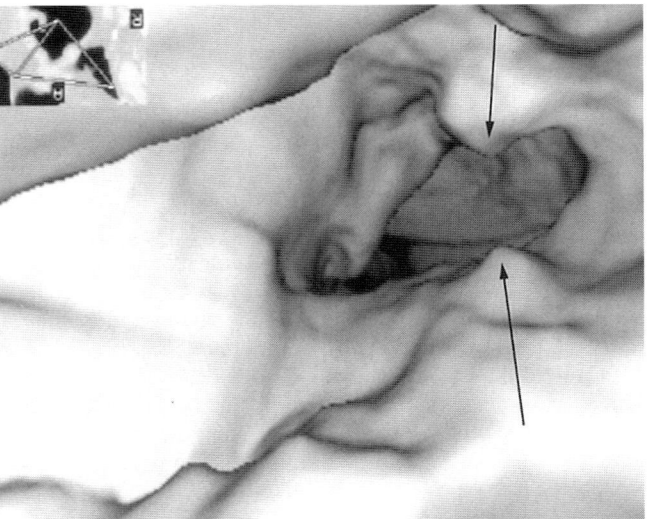

B

**Figure 56–2** *A:* Axial prone CT scan through the sigmoid colon shows a distal sigmoid mass with circumferential thickening of the colon wall (arrowheads). In addition, there is stranding in the pericolic tissues with an 8-mm lymph node identified just lateral to the sigmoid mass (arrow).

The appearance is consistent with a sigmoid carcinoma with transserosal spread and pericolic lymphadenopathy (T3, N1 or Dukes C1 cancer). *B:* Endoluminal view showing heaped-up margins of the cancer with luminal narrowing (arrows).

## Other Modalities

Endoluminal colonoscopic ultrasound is another radiologic modality being used to stage colon cancer. Similar to the use of the rectal ultrasound for staging rectal cancer, colonoscopic ultrasound provides an accurate picture of the local extent of disease. In a review of the literature on colonic endoluminal ultrasound, Rosch and Classen[30] reported that the technique offers a staging accuracy of 75%–85%. In a more recent study, the sensitivity of this method for local staging of colon cancer was 92%, but the sensitivity for staging of lymph nodes was only 65%.[31] While reports suggest that endoluminal colonoscopic ultrasound is highly accurate in staging colon cancer, the utility of this modality in colon cancer is different from that in rectal cancer. The main difference is that in rectal cancer, the identification of a higher stage of disease preoperatively often leads to preoperative adjuvant therapy thought to improve local regional control and perhaps survival. Currently, there is no preoperative adjuvant therapy for colon cancer. Thus, preoperative identification of the pathologic stage of a colon cancer would not change the sequence of therapy. Future advances in therapy may make better use of information provided by endoluminal ultrasound.

## Staging Systems

The most important aspect of colon cancer staging is its role in determining the prognosis. While radiographic staging may provide some information on the extent of cancer, decisions regarding treatment plans will continue to be based on pathologic evaluation of resection specimens. The number and site of lymph nodes involved in colon cancer affect survival rates. The numerous staging systems that have been developed to stratify the extent of disease all consider either the number or the location of the involved lymph nodes. Currently, the most widely accepted staging system for colon cancer in the United States is the TNM classification system. In this system, stage III disease is defined by the presence of lymph node metastasis (N) and is subdivided into three subgroups by the number of lymph nodes involved with metastatic cancer. N1 disease involves one to three lymph nodes; N2 disease involves at least four lymph nodes; and N3 disease involves any number of lymph nodes along a named vascular trunk.

Because accurate staging of lymph nodes affects prognosis, the choice of the method of pathologic analysis of the resection specimen is vital. In a recent study by Ratto and colleagues,[32] the use of conventional pathologic analysis was compared wit thorough dissection of the lymph nodes. The authors found that conventional analysis of pathologic specimens significantly underestimated the extent of metastatic disease. Patients in whom disease is understaged on the basis of conventional pathologic analysis may not be considered for adjuvant therapy. This problem worsens as new technology is used to analyze lymph nodes, as in breast cancer and melanoma. Immunohistochemical staining of microscopically negative lymph nodes may identify molecular evidence of tumor deposits of unknown clinical importance. As these new technologies are analyzed, the system of staging colon cancer may be further refined to predict more accurately disease recurrence and patient survival.

## Summary

If diagnosed early, colon cancer is one of the more preventable cancers. During the second half of the twentieth century, epidemiological studies identified specific age groups and other populations at risk for the development of colon cancer. There are multiple effective diagnostic tools that, when applied properly, can detect colon cancer at an earlier stage of disease and thus improve the chances for survival. A careful history and other tests are used to stratify patients by their risk for developing colon cancer. Changes in radiologic techniques and advances in pathologic analysis of the primary tumors or lymph nodes in resected specimens may enhance the accuracy of the staging of colon cancer and therefore allow for a more appropriate use of adjuvant treatments.

## References

1. Landis SH, Murray T, Bolden S, Wingo PA. Cancer Statistics, 1999. CA Cancer J Clin 49:8–31, 1999.
2. American Cancer Society. Cancer Facts and Figures. American Cancer Society Publication No. 5008–5096, 1996.
3. Slentz K, Senagore A, Hibbert J, et al. Can preoperative and postoperative CEA predict survival after colon cancer resection? Am Surg 60:528–532, 1994.
4. Wolf RF, Cohen AM. The miniscule benefit of serial carcinoembryonic antigen monitoring after effective curative treatment for primary colorectal cancer. J Am Coll Surg. 185:60–64, 1997.
5. Harrison LE, Guillem JG, Paty P, Cohen AM. Preoperative carcinoembryonic antigen predicts outcomes in node-negative colon cancer patients: a multivariate analysis of 572 patients. J Am Coll Surg 185:55–59, 1997.
6. Anderson GD, Yuellig TR, Krone RE Jr. An investigation into the effects of oral iron supplementation on in vivo Hemoccult stool testing. Am J Gastroenterol 85:558–561, 1990.
7. Mandel JS, Bond JH, Church TR, et al. Reducing mortality from colorectal cancer by screening for fecal occult blood. N Engl J Med. 328:1365–1371, 1993.
8. Kronborg O, Fenger C, Olsen J, et al. Randomised study of screening for colorectal cancer with faecal-occult-blood test. Lancet 348:1467–1471, 1996.
9. Hardcastle JD, Chamberlain JO, Robinson MHE, et al. Randomised controlled trial of faecal-occult-blood screening for colorectal cancer. Lancet 348:1472–1477, 1996.
10. Kewnter J, Bjork S, Haglind E, et al. Results of screening, rescreening, and follow-up in a prospective randomized study for detection of colorectal cancer by fecal occult blood testing. Scand J Gastroenterol 29:468–473, 1994.
11. Winawer SJ, Zauber AG, O'Brien MJ, et al. Screening for colorectal cancer with fecal occult blood testing and sigmoidoscopy. J Natl Cancer Inst 85:1311–1318, 1993.
12. Bombi JA. Polyps of the colon in Barcelona, Spain: an autopsy study. Cancer 61:1472–1476, 1988.
13. Vatn MH, Stalsberg H. The prevalence of polyps of the large intestine in Oslo: an autopsy study. Cancer 49:819–825, 1982.
14. Arminski TC, McLean DW. Incidence and distribution of adenomatous polyps of the colon and rectum based on 1,000 autopsy examinations. Dis Colon Rectum 7:249–261, 1964.
15. Rickert RR, Auerbach O, Garfinkel L, et al. Adenomatous lesions of the large bowel: an autopsy study. Cancer 43:1847–1857, 1979.
16. Winawer SJ, Zauber AG, O'Brien MJ, et al. The National Polyp Study: design, method, and characteristics of patients with newly diagnosed polyps. Cancer 70:1236–1245, 1992.
17. Disario JA, Foutch PG, Mai HD, et al. Prevalence and malignant potential of colorectal polyps in asymptomatic, average-risk men. Am J Gastroenterol 86:941–945, 1991.
18. Rex DK, Lehman GA, Hawes RH, et al. Screening colonoscopy in asymptomatic average risk persons with negative fecal occult blood tests. Gastroenterology 100:64–67, 1991.
19. O'Brien MJ, Winawer SJ, Zauber AG, et al. The National Polyp Study: patient and polyp characteristics associated with high-grade dysplasia in colorectal adenomas. Gastroenterology 98:371–379, 1990.
20. Muto T, Bussey HJR, Morson BC. The evolution of cancer of the colon and rectum. Cancer 36:2251–2270, 1975.
21. Johnson CD, Listrup DM, Fish NM, et al. Barium enema: detection of colonic lesions in a community population. AJR Am J Roentgenol 140:1143–1149, 1983.
22. Glick S, Wagner JL, Johnson CD. Cost-effectiveness of double-contrast barium enema in screening for colorectal cancer. AJR Am J Roentgenol 170:629–636, 1998.

23. Rex DK, Rahmani EY, Haseman JH, et al. Relative sensitivity of colonoscopy and barium enema for detection of colorectal cancer in clinical practice. Gastroenterology 112:17–23, 1997.

24. Rex DK, Cutler CS, Lemmel GT, et al. Colonoscopic miss rates of adenomas determined by back to back colonoscopies. Gasteroenterology 112:24–28, 1997.

25. Fenlon, HM, Nunes DP, Schroy PC, et al. A comparison of virtual and conventional colonoscopy for the detection of colorectal polyps. N Engl J Med 341:1496–1503, 1999.

26. Harvey CJ, Amin Z, Hare CMB, et al. Helical CT pneumocolon to assess colonic tumors: radiologic–pathologic correlation. AJR Am J Roentgenol 170:1439–1443, 1998.

27. McAndrew MR, Saba AK. Efficacy of routine preoperative computed tomography scans in colon cancer. Am Surg 65:205–208, 1999.

28. Freeny PC, Marks WM, Ryan JA, Bolen JW. Colorectal carcinoma evaluation with CT: preoperative staging and detection of postoperative recurrence. Radiology 158:347–353, 1986.

29. Morrin MM, Farrell R, Raptopoulos V, et al. Role of virtual computed tomographic colonography in patients with colorectal cancers and obstructing colorectal lesions. Dis Colon Rectum 43:303–311, 2000.

30. Rosch T, Classen M. Colonoscopic ultrasonography. Semin Colon Rectal Surg 3:49–56, 1992.

31. Norton SA, Thomas MG. Staging of rectosigmoid neoplasia with colonoscopic endoluminal ultrasonography Br J Surg 86:942–946, 1999.

32. Ratto C, Sofo L, Ippoliti M, et al. Accurate lymph-node detection in colorectal specimens resected for cancer is of prognostic significance. Dis Colon Rectum 42:143–158, 1999.

course of 5-FU at the same dosage was repeated 6 weeks later. The 5-year overall survival for the 308 patients who were resected with curative intent was 58.5% for those receiving chemotherapy and 49.4% for those treated with surgery alone. Although the results did appear to suggest a trend toward improved survival with chemotherapy, these differences did not reach statistical significance. Furthermore, in a somewhat larger trial, 522 patients who underwent resection with curative intent were randomized to either observation or postoperative 5-FU, this time with a longer duration of therapy.[46,47] This trial demonstrated no significant difference in overall 5-year survival between the two treatment arms, with 48.9% for the group receiving chemotherapy and a 44.2% for the group treated with surgery alone.

Several early studies were reported in which 5-FU was given by oral administration.[48,49] Such an approach would not be favored now, given the knowledge that there are large interpatient differences in the absorption and metabolism of orally administered 5-FU. In one such report, 421 patients with resected stage II or III colorectal cancer were entered on a randomized placebo-controlled trial of oral 5-FU at a dose of 5 mg/kg/day for 3 months, or placebo for the same time period.[49] No significant differences in either disease-free or overall survival between the two groups were seen.

In 1984 the Gastrointestinal Tumor Study Group (GITSG) reported the results of a four-arm trial in patients with stage II and III colon cancers.[50] Patients were randomized to either postoperative BCG, postoperative 5-FU plus BCG, postoperative 5-FU plus semustine, or no postoperative therapy. A total of 621 patients were randomized, 572 of whom were considered evaluable. With a median follow-up of 5½ years, no significant differences were observed in terms of either recurrence-free survival or overall survival rates between any of the four treatment arms.

A recurrent problem in many of these early adjuvant trials was that of a relatively small number of patients in each treatment arm. This made identification of any possible subtle benefits impossible. In 1988, a large meta-analysis of adjuvant trials in colorectal cancer was reported.[51] This meta-analysis included all randomized trials of adjuvant therapy in colorectal cancer that contained a surgery-only control arm and were published in English through 1986. Seventeen such trials, involving approximately 4700 patients, were included. It should be noted that many of these trials employed what would now be regarded as less than ideal doses and/or schedules of 5-FU. Analysis of these trials indicated a very small, nonsignificant benefit of therapy in terms of overall survival, with a mortality odds ratio (OR) of 0.83 in favor of therapy (95% confidence interval [CI], 0.70 to 0.98). Overall, this meta-analysis suggested that a modest benefit might be achievable with chemotherapy, but that larger studies would be needed to detect such a minimal difference.

## Large-Scale Randomized Trials: Dawn of the Modern Era of Adjuvant Therapy

The National Surgical Adjuvant Breast and Bowel Project (NSABP) cooperative group was the first to report a large-scale, randomized trial that showed a statistically significant survival advantage for colon cancer patients receiving adjuvant chemotherapy. In a study of 1166 Dukes' B and C colon carcinoma patients randomized to receive either methyl-CCNU plus vincristine plus fluorouracil (MOF), BCG, or no further therapy,[52] the patients treated with surgery alone were at 1.29 times the risk of developing a treatment failure and 1.31 times the risk of dying compared to patients receiving chemotherapy ($P = 0.02$ and

$P = 0.05$, respectively). There was no survival advantage for patients receiving BCG. Of significant concern, however, was the finding that three patients receiving this MOF chemotherapy regimen developed acute leukemia and three additional patients in this group developed myelodysplastic syndrome, presumably secondary to the methyl-CCNU.

### Fluorouracil plus Levamisole

Because of encouraging preliminary data,[53] the North Central Cancer Treatment Group (NCCTG) conducted a three-arm study that randomly assigned Dukes $B_2$ and C patients to surgery followed by either 5-FU plus levamisole, levamisole alone, or no further treatment.[19] Levamisole is a veterinary anthelminthic. In vitro evidence had suggested that levamisole might enhance the immunization of animals against *Brucella abortus.* The possibility that levamisole might therefore function as an immunostimulant led to its investigation of it as an anticancer agent.[54,55] The results from this trial were encouraging,[56] leading to a large-scale confirmatory trial,[57–59] conducted through the National Cancer Institute (NCI) intergroup mechanism.

In this trial, known as Intergroup 0035, a total of 929 eligible patients with Dukes' C colon cancer and 318 patients with transmural, node-negative (Dukes' B2) disease were treated. Results are summarized in Table 57–4. Of the node-positive (Dukes' C) patients treated with surgery alone, 44% remained alive and disease-free at 5 years, as compared with 61% of patients who received 5-FU and levamisole. This difference, which represents a 39% reduction in mortality, was highly statistically significant ($P < 0.0001$).

The results for adjuvant treatment for Dukes B2, node-negative disease were less encouraging, and failed to show a statistically significant benefit for treatment of this patient population.[59] Seventy-nine percent of patients receiving chemotherapy and 71% of patients on the observation arm were free of recurrence at 7 years follow-up. This difference was not statistically significant ($P = 0.10$). The 7-year survival was 72% for. each arm of the study.

On the basis of the results of Intergroup 0035, the NCI issued a consensus statement in 1990 establishing adjuvant chemotherapy as the standard of care for patients with node-positive resected colon cancer, in the absence of medical or psychiatric contraindications to such treatment.[60]

The mechanism by which levamisole functions in the treatment of cancer is not at all clear. It has not been consistently

**Table 57–4** Intergroup-0035: Long-term follow-up results of adjuvant 5-fluorouracil plus levamisole[23,24]

| Stage/Treatment | Patients (n) | Recurrence-free Survival[a] (%) | Overall Survival[a] (%) |
|---|---|---|---|
| Stage III 5-FU/levamisole | 304 | 61 | 60 |
| Stage III Surgery alone | 315 | 44 | 47 |
| Stage II 5-FU/levamisole | 159 | 79 | 72 |
| Stage II Surgery alone | 159 | 71 | 72 |

5-FU, 5-Fluorouracil.

[a]Median follow-up for Dukes' C patients is 6.5 years. The median follow-up for Dukes' B2 patients is 7 years.

demonstrated that levamisole has a detectable effect on the immune system at the concentrations which are achieved clinically.[61,62] Although it has been suggested that levamisole may simply potentiate 5-FU by inhibiting intracellular phosphatases involved in its degradation,[63] this effect cannot be demonstrated at the concentrations achieved clinically.[64] One report indicated that levamisole may stimulate the expression of major histocompatibility complex (MHC) class 1 antigens on the surface of colon cancer cells grown in vitro.[65] The authors of this report speculate that this antigen expression could possibly make the cancer cells more vulnerable to detection by the immune system. While this speculation is intriguing, it would seem premature to accept this as the mechanism of action for levamisole. It is not known whether an increase in MHC class 1 antigen expression to levamisole occurs in vivo, and whether this would, in fact, lead to a clinically significant improvement in immune function.[62]

Thus the mechanism of action for levamisole remains unknown. In fact, the possibility exists that levamisole may not be an active agent at all.[66] It is possible that the large-scale trials of 5-FU and levamisole simply had adequate numbers of patients and adequate treatment duration to permit detection of a modest clinical benefit of 5-FU.

## Fluorouracil Plus Leucovorin

Over the past decade, 5-FU plus leucovorin, on one of a variety of schedules, has been the most commonly used drug regimen for treatment of unresectable metastatic colorectal cancer.[67] Several randomized trials comparing various schedules of 5-FU and leucovorin have shown equivalency.[68,69] A number of investigators have evaluated 5-FU/leucovorin regimens for the adjuvant treatment of colon cancer. The National Surgical Adjuvant Breast and Bowel Project (NSABP) C-03 study compared 1 year of treatment with either 5-FU and leucovorin or the MOF regimen (methyl-CCNU, vincristine, and 5-FU). This MOF regimen had been shown to be superior to observation in the NSABP C-01 trial. The C-03 study found superior disease-free survival for patients receiving weekly 5-FU plus high-dose leucovorin.[70]

The other early report of activity from 5-FU plus high-dose leucovorin came from the International Multicenter Pooled Analysis of Colon Cancer Trials (IMPACT). This study was a combined analysis of three nearly identical trials conducted in Italy, Canada, and France.[71] A total of 1493 patients were randomly assigned to postoperative chemotherapy or to surgery alone. This trial was open to Dukes' B and C patients, and the majority (56%) were staged as Dukes' B. The 3-year event-free survival for Dukes' C patients was 44% with surgery alone vs. 62% for patients randomized to postoperative chemotherapy. The initially reported difference in Dukes' B patients was substantially smaller, with 76% and 79% of surgery-only and chemotherapy patients, respectively, remaining event-free at 3 years. A more recent update of these 1016 Dukes' B2 patients in fact showed no significant increase in either event-free or overall survival for patients receiving adjuvant 5-FU/leucovorin.[72] The authors concluded that "this data set does not support the routine use of 5-FU plus leucovorin in all patients with B2 colon cancer."

Subsequently, several important trials addressing the role of leucovorin in the adjuvant treatment of colon cancer have been reported. The NSABP C-04 trial[73] randomly assigned Dukes' B and C patients to receive either 5-FU plus high-dose leucovorin for 1 year, the same 5-FU plus leucovorin schedule with oral levamisole (50 mg orally three times daily for 3 days, every other week), or 5-FU plus levamisole for 1 year of therapy. This trial

**Table 57–5** Results of adjuvant 5-fluouracil plus leucovorin or levamisole, NSABP CO-4 trial

| | 5-FU + LV (%) | | 5-FU + LEV (%) | | RR[a] | |
|---|---|---|---|---|---|---|
| Stage | DFS | Survival | DFS | Survival | DFS | Survival |
| All patients | 65 | 74 | 60 | 70 | 0.84 | 0.85 |
| Dukes' B | 75 | 84 | 71 | 81 | 0.78 | 0.71 |
| Dukes' C | 57 | 67 | 53 | 63 | 0.87 | 0.90 |

DFS, 5-year disease-free survival; 5-FU, 5-fluorouracil; LEV, levamisole; LV, leucovorin; NSABP, National Surgical Adjuvant Breast and Bowel Project; RR, relative risk.
[a]Overall risk of an event or death for 5-FU + LV patients relative to 5-FU + LEV.

randomized a total of 2151 patients. The 5-year disease-free survival for 5-FU/leucovorin was 65%, vs. 60% for the 5-FU/levamisole group ($P = 0.04$). The 5-year overall survival difference approached but did not achieve statistical significance ($P = 0.07$). The addition of levamisole to 5-FU/leucovorin conferred no additional advantage. Results are shown in Table 57–5.

In another major trial that has been reported in abstract form, the North Central Cancer Treatment Group (NCCTG) and the National Cancer Institute of Canada (NCIC) compared treatment with 5-FU plus levamisole, with or without leucovin, for 6 or 12 months, in a two by two design.[74] The results of this trial indicate that 12 months of chemotherapy was not superior to 6 months. Furthermore, the addition of leucovorin to 5-FU/levamisole offered no significant benefit (Table 57–6).

Perhaps the most definitive trial to date, which has established the current standard of care, is the Intergroup trial INT-0089. This trial randomized patients to one of four treatment arms: 5-FU plus levamisole for 52 weeks; 5-FU plus weekly high-dose leucovorin for 32 weeks (5-FU 500 mg/m$^2$ and leucovorin 500 mg/m$^2$ weekly for 6 weeks, repeated every 8 weeks for 4 cycles); 5-FU plus low-dose leucovorin on a daily $\times$ 5 schedule (5-FU 425 mg/m$^2$ and leucovorin 20 mg/m$^2$ for 5 consecutive days, repeated every 28 days for 6 cycles); or the same schedule of 5-FU plus low-dose leucovorin with levamisole added. The two 5-FU/leucovorin arms were comparable for efficacy, and were comparable in efficacy to the longer regimen of 5-FU/levamisole. The 5-FU/leucovorin/levamisole arm was statistically superior to 5-FU/levamisole, but was not superior to 5-FU/leucovorin. Results are shown in Table 57–7. The authors concluded that levamisole does not appear to be a mandatory component of the treatment regimen, and either of the 5-FU/leucovorin regimens studied can be considered the current standard of care for adjuvant treatment of stage III patients.[75]

**Table 57–6** Results of adjuvant 5-fluorouracil plus levamisole, with or without leucovorin, NCIC/NCCTG trial[76]

| Chemotherapy | Duration (Months) | 5-Year Disease-Free Survival (%) | 5-Year Overall Survival (%) |
|---|---|---|---|
| 5-FU/LV/Lev | 6 | 63 | 70 |
| 5-FU/Lev | 6 | 58 | 60 |
| 5-FU/LV/Lev | 12 | 57 | 63 |
| 5-FU/Lev | 12 | 63 | 68 |

5-FU, 5-fluorouracil; Lev, levamisole; LV, leucovorin; NCCTG, North Central Cancer Treatment Group; NCIC, National Cancer Institute of Canada.

**Table 57-7** Results of adjuvant 5-fluorouracil plus levamisole and/or leucovorin, intergroup trial INT-0089[77]

| | 5-year Disease-Free Survival (%) | 5-year Overall Survival (%) |
|---|---|---|
| 5-FU/low-dose leucovorin (daily × 5 schedule) | 60 | 66 |
| 5-FU/high-dose leucovorin (weekly schedule) | 59 | 65 |
| 5-FU/levamisole | 56 | 63 |
| 5-FU/leucovorin/levamisole | 60 | 67 |

5-FU, 5-fluorouracil.

## Current State of Adjuvant Treatment

Taken together, where do all of these trials leave us in terms of current recommendations for treatment? At the time of this writing, the evidence is overwhelming that both disease-free and overall survival can be substantially improved in stage III patients with adjuvant 5-FU-based chemotherapy. Either of the 5-FU/leucovorin regimens used in the INT-0089 study (see Table 57-7) would seem most appropriate for standard treatment.

The issue of treatment for stage II patients remains far more controversial. Most trials have had insufficient numbers of patients with stage II disease to have sufficient power to detect modest differences. Trials such as the INT-0035 have been flatly negative, with a 7-year survival of 72% in each arm (5-FU/levamisole vs. surgery alone).[59] The IMPACT trials also failed to show a benefit for adjuvant treatment of stage II patients.[72] Other trials have demonstrated very modest benefits for treatment of stage II patients.[73] A pooled analysis of four trials from the NSABP claimed to demonstrate a role for adjuvant treatment of stage II patients,[76] however, as discussed in an editorial accompanying the study, the authors used highly unorthodox statistical methods to support their conclusions.[77]

At present we lack the necessary information to make a definitive statement regarding adjuvant treatment of stage II patients. Much of the literature would appear to support the conclusions of the IMPACT investigators that "studies in B2 colon cancer designed with a no-treatment control arm should be considered appropriate."[72] Certain prognostic factors, however, have been correlated with higher risk for recurrence in patients with Dukes' B2 tumors. These factors have included obstruction of the bowel lumen or perforation of the bowel wall by tumor.[78] Analysis of risk factors for recurrence in the intergroup 5-FU plus levamisole trial confirmed perforation to be an independent risk factor, but did not find obstruction to correlate with higher risk for recurrence. Other potential risk factors that are less well established include an elevated preoperative CEA, a poorly differentiated histology, or a high S-phase fraction. Data have been reported indicating that the presence of an 1 Sq deletion in colorectal tumors may correlate with a poor prognosis.[79] Patients with stage II colon cancer and one or more of the above risk factors are at higher risk for recurrence. What is not clear is whether adjuvant therapy in these high-risk Dukes' B2 patients can reduce that risk. In the absence of definitive data, clinical judgement and full patient education regarding the available data on this matter must be employed. It would appear to be reasonable to offer adjuvant chemotherapy to Dukes' B2 patients with established high-risk prognostic factors who are also appropriately informed and selected.

## Investigational Approaches

### Portal Vein Infusion

The liver is the most common site for distant metastases of colorectal cancer,[38,39,80] with up to half of all relapsing patients presenting with hepatic metastases as their first site of failure. This pattern would not be unexpected, as the cancer cells are able to access the liver via the portal venous system, along the same channels used by nutrients traveling from the bowel to the liver.[81,82] While tumors greater than 1 cm in diameter derive most of their blood supply from the hepatic artery, tumors less than 5 mm obtain their blood supply from both the hepatic and portal circulations.[83,84] The delivery of chemotherapy directly into the portal vein would therefore be a reasonable approach to explore for the administration of adjuvant treatment.

Early phase I studies of this approach showed that 5-FU could be safely administered intraportally. In fact, due to the extraction, or "first-pass clearance" of 5-FU by the liver,[85] substantially higher doses of 5-FU can be safely given by intraportal infusion than by intravenous infusion. A preliminary report of a small randomized trial[86] of systemic vs. intraportal 5-FU appeared encouraging. However, a follow-up report of that same trial, which included a larger number of patients, showed a benefit only for Dukes' B patients.[87]

A more substantial randomized trial was reported by the NSABP C-02 trial.[88] In this trial, 1158 patients with Dukes' A, B, or C colon cancers were randomly assigned to either a 7-day intraportal infusion of 5-FU (600 mg/m$^2$/day) or to surgery alone. Contrary to what might have been expected, the incidence of hepatic metastases was not significantly different between the two treatment groups. A small but statistically significant advantage in disease-free survival (74% vs. 64% at 4 years) was demonstrated for the group receiving intraportal chemotherapy.

The Swiss Group for Clinical Cancer Research (SAKK) obtained a similar result.[89,90] In this trial, 533 patients were randomized to receive either intraportal postoperative chemotherapy or surgery alone. The chemotherapy regimen consisted of a single 2-hour infusion of mitomycin C (10 mg/m$^2$) followed immediately by a 7-day infusion of 5-FU at a dose of 500 mg/m$^2$/day, with both drugs administered intraportally. Again there was no difference in the incidences of hepatic metastases between the two groups. The 5-year disease-free and overall survival rates were modestly improved, however, in those patients who received the intraportal treatment (57% vs. 48% and 66% vs. 55%, respectively).

Ten randomized studies evaluating portal vein infusion were combined in a meta-analysis involving over 4000 patients.[91] This analysis revealed only a modest (4%) improvement in 5-year overall survival for the patients receiving portal infusion. At present, the use of intraportal adjuvant chemotherapy should be regarded as having unproven benefit, and its use should be limited to investigational settings.

### Intraperitoneal Chemotherapy

Studies on the patterns of clinical failure in patients with colorectal cancer following resection[39] as well as studies using planned second-look laparotomy[92,93] have demonstrated both the liver and the peritoneal surfaces to be at particularly high risk for metastases. There is a strong rationale for postoperative intraperitoneal chemotherapy. First, this approach delivers extremely high concentrations of chemotherapy directly onto the peritoneal surfaces. In addition, because the peritoneal cavity is drained by portal lymphatics into the portal vein, intraperitoneal administration of chemotherapy delivers high concentrations of drug to the portal vein.[94,95] Animal studies support this approach. Intraperitoneal administration of 5-FU reduced the incidence of macroscopic peritoneal tumor growth and hepatic metastases compared to untreated controls in a rat model. Systemic 5-FU in this model resulted in no reduction in peritoneal metastases compared to the untreated controls.[95] Because floxuridine and, to a lesser extent, 5-FU have a high first-pass clearance through the liver, these drugs are good potential candidates for intraperitoneal administration. As shown by pharmacologic investigations of intraperitoneal 5-FU and floxuridine, hepatic clearance of these agents results in intraperitoneal concentrations 200- to 400-fold higher than those found systemically.[94,96]

A small randomized trial of systemic vs. intraperitoneal chemotherapy following resection of colon cancer did show a decrease in peritoneal metastases in the group receiving intraperitoneal chemotherapy. No differences in overall survival or in the incidence of hepatic metastases were noted, however.[97] This study was limited by its small size and the fact that initiation of chemotherapy up to 2 full months following surgery was permitted. Such delays in treatment could increase the chance of spread of tumor outside of the peritoneal cavity and might permit the establishment of hepatic micrometastases with substantial hepatic arterial blood supply.

A nonrandomized pilot trial investigated the combination of immediate postoperative intraperitoneal floxuridine and leucovorin plus systemic 5-FU and levamisole.[98] Patients received intraperitoneal therapy twice daily for 3 consecutive days every other week for three cycles. Levamisole was begun orally with the second intraperitoneal cycle, and systemic 5-FU by bolus injection daily × 5 was given starting with the beginning of the third intraperitoneal cycle. These systemic doses of 5-FU given concurrently with intraperitoneal chemotherapy were escalated in a phase I dose escalation schema. On day 29 after the start of 5-FU, weekly 5-FU and every-other-week levamisole were started and continued to complete 1 year of therapy. This combined intraperitoneal and systemic treatment was well tolerated, with no apparent increase in perioperative morbidity. At a median follow-up of 24 months, 24 of 28 patients were alive and free of disease.

A randomized trial somewhat larger than the randomized study discussed above compared intraperitoneal plus systemic 5-FU plus leucovorin to systemic 5-FU plus levamisole.[99] A total of 241 patients with high-risk stage II or stage III colon cancer were randomized. No benefit was seen for the stage II patients after a median follow-up of 4 years. However, among the 196 eligible patients with stage III disease, an estimated 43% reduction in mortality was seen. This trial is still relatively small, but the results are encouraging, and suggest that the use of intraperitoneal strategies may be useful in the adjuvant therapy of colon cancer. Further investigations of this approach will be needed, however, to better evaluate its utility and safety.

## Monoclonal Antibodies

The relatively large molecular size of monoclonal antibodies may interfere with efficient transport of these agents into solid tumor tissue.[100] One means of dealing with this problem could be to target small-volume minimal residual disease. A patient who has

undergone a complete resection of all gross tumor but who is at risk for microscopic residual disease presents an optimal minimal residual disease situation. On the basis of this rationale, several investigators have explored the use of monoclonal antibody therapies in the adjuvant setting in colon cancer.

Diagnostically, it has been demonstrated that monoclonal antibodies can be used to identify micrometastases in bone marrow specimens taken from colorectal cancer patients[101] and that the presence of these bone marrow metastases correlates with a poor clinical prognosis.[102] Therapeutically, a murine monoclonal IgG$_{2a}$ antibody directed against the 17-1A epitope has been developed that has in vitro the ability to induce antibody-dependent cellular cytotoxicity[103–105] and to inhibit growth of human colon cancer xenografts in nude mice.[106]

Early clinical trials of this antibody were undertaken first in patients with advanced metastatic disease. These studies reported several instances of minor tumor regressions, and no major toxicities were reported.[107] Having demonstrated both tolerable toxicity and evidence of clinical activity, investigators then began randomized trials to evaluate this antibody in the adjuvant setting.[108] One hundred sixty-six patients were entered into the trial and randomized to receive either monoclonal antibody treatment or surgery alone. Patients in the adjuvant treatment group received 500 mg of 17-1A antibody 2 weeks after surgery by 1 hour intravenous infusion, followed by four 100 mg infusions given at 4-week intervals.

With a median follow-up of 7 years and 98% of patients followed for more than 5 years, 57% of the patients who received monoclonal antibodies were alive, while the surviving percentage of patients receiving surgery alone was 37%. This raw difference of 20 percentage points represents a 32% reduction in mortality (95% CI, 8%–51%). Caution must be used in interpreting these data because of the relatively small sample size. Nevertheless, these initial results are encouraging, and large-scale phase III testing of this antibody is currently in progress.

## Antitumor Vaccines

When the immune system fails to recognize a cancer cell as foreign or is unable to destroy that cell, clinical malignancy develops. Strategies for vaccination therefore attempt to stimulate the patient's immune system to recognize and eradicate tumor cells; however, these cells have necessarily already escaped immune surveillance. While using the immune system to control or destroy tumors is intellectually appealing, it has thus far proved to be difficult to accomplish. As discussed above, large immunologic effector cells and antibodies penetrate poorly into large tumor masses. However, small-volume micrometastases, as would be found in the adjuvant setting, would be a more practical target for immunologic attack.

In theory, the optimal target for immune therapy would be a tumor-specific antigen which is unique to, and always expressed on, tumor cells, and which is never expressed by nonmalignant cells. Thus far, no such perfect tumor-specific antigen has been found. In the absence of this, several strategies have been pursued.

In one approach, investigators have tried to identify an antigen with a high frequency of expression on tumor cells and a relatively low frequency of expression on normal cells. Since CEA is a tumor-associated antigen in many adenocarcinomas, including many colorectal cancers, considerable effort has been focused on raising anti-CEA antibodies. These efforts have been largely frustrated because cancer patients appear to be relatively immune-tolerant to CEA. One promising approach to circumventing this problem has been the development of an anti-idiotype monoclonal antibody vaccine, which biologically and serologically mimicks CEA.[109] Preliminary data indicate that anti-CEA antibody responses can be elicited, and large-scale phase III trials of this agent in resected colorectal cancer patients are planned.

Other work has focussed on other potential immunologic targets. The blood group–related epitopes Tn and sialylated Tn (sTn), which are expressed on mucins of many epithelial tumors, including colorectal carcinomas, are one target that is being explored. Investigators have developed vaccines from partially desialylated ovine submaxillary gland mucin (modified OSM), which contains both Tn and sTn determinants. In a small preliminary clinical trial, cohorts of patients were selected for treatment with either modified OSM, modified OSM plus the immunologic adjuvant DETOX, or modified OSM plus BCG (bacillus. Calmette-Guerin).[110] The goal of this study was to determine if antibody titers to Tn and sTn could be raised by these vaccinations. While none of the six patients receiving modified OSM alone developed antibodies, four of eight patients receiving modified OSM plus DETOX and five of six patients receiving modified OSM plus BCG demonstrated marked increases in antibody titers. Further investigations into this approach are ongoing, using more potent immune adjuvants. Efforts are also being made to augment Tn and sTn by covalent attachment of immunogenic carrier proteins, to make these epitopes more immunogenic.

Active specific immunotherapy (ASI) is a different approach to immunologic stimulation. In this approach, patients receive immunizations with a combination of BCG and a preparation of their own irradiated tumor cells. It has been demonstrated that irradiation of the tumor cells destroys the cell's ability to proliferate, but does not destroy its immunogenic stimulatory capacity. A small preliminary randomized trial involving only 80 patients with either colon or rectal cancer has been reported.[111] No overall survival benefit for the immunized patients was shown. However, a retrospective subset analysis did show a statistically significant improvement in survival for the immunized colon cancer patients only. This trial is limited by its small size (only 47 colon cancer patients), the retrospective nature of the subset analyses, and other substantial problems in methodology.[112]

More recently, a somewhat larger trial of ASI in colon cancer patients has been reported.[113] This trial randomized 83 stage III patients and 170 stage II patients to receive ASI or surgery alone. Median follow-up was 5.3 years, but the range was from 8 months to 9 years. There was no significant benefit seen in the stage III patients, with 15 recurrences in the treated population and 17 recurrences in the control population ($P = 0.52$). In the stage II patients, 23 patients recurred, with 10 recurrences in the treated population. Recurrence-free survival for stage II patients was superior for the treated group ($P = 0.032$); however, disease-specific survival and overall survival and overall survival were not statistically significantly improved ($P = 0.09$ and $P = 0.149$, respectively). Although further maturation of these data and/or additional, larger trials may be useful, at this time the results would appear to be insufficient to support a recommendation of ASI as standard therapy in resected colon cancer.

## New Chemotherapies

After years of relative stagnation with 5-FU and its biomodulation, the world of colon cancer therapy has seen several agents enter clinical practice and/or clinical trials that have demonstrated substantial antitumor activity in the metastatic setting. Irinotecan plus 5-FU/leucovorin has been shown to have superior activity to 5-FU/leucovorin alone.[114,115] Similarly, oxaliplatin plus 5-FU/leucovorin has been shown to have activity superior to that of 5-FU/leucovorin alone.[116] Both irinotecan/5-FU/leucovorin and oxaliplatin/5-FU/leucovorin combination therapies have now entered randomized clinical trials against 5-FU/leucovorin alone in resected stage III colon cancer. The oral fluorinated pyrimidines UFT and capecitabine have also demonstrated usefulness in stage IV colorectal cancer, with antitumor activity similar to that of 5-FU/leucovorin, but with decreased toxicities.[117–119] These agents have also entered clinical trials in the adjuvant setting. It should be emphasized that until the results of these clinical trials are known, use of these newer agents in the adjuvant treatment of colon cancer remains strictly investigational.

## Conclusions

Important advances have been made in the surgical management of colon cancer and in our understanding of the role of adjuvant chemotherapy for this disease. Current standard regimens of 5-FU and leucovorin have been shown convincingly to reduce the incidence of recurrences and to prolong overall survival in patients with resected stage III disease. Although patients with stage II disease have a better overall prognosis than those with stage III, the relative merits of adjuvant treatment in these patients remains controversial. Despite the advances that have been made, far too many patients with resected colon cancer ultimately relapse and die of their disease. Thus, there remains a pressing need for continued development of improved adjuvant treatments. Through carefully designed and conducted clinical trials, the roles of new agents and new technologies in adjuvant therapy are continuing to be aggressively investigated. Considering the strong scientific and clinical rationales behind these agents and technologies, there is every reason to be optimistic regarding the prospects for continued therapeutic improvements. Participation of eligible patients in these clinical trials must be actively encouraged. Only in this way will we be able to continue to expand on the progress that has been made thus far.

## References

1. Hida J, Yasutomi M, Maruyama T, Fujimoto K, Uchida T, Okuno K. The extent of lymph node dissection for colon carcinoma: the potential impact on laparoscopic surgery [see comments]. Cancer 80:188–192, 1997.
2. Turnbull RB Jr, Kyle K, Watson FR, Spratt J. Cancer of the colon: the influence of the no-touch isolation technic on survival rates. Ann Surg 166:420–427, 1967.
3. Wiggers T, Jeekel J, Arends JW, et al. No-touch isolation technique in colon cancer: a controlled prospective trial. Br J Surg 75:409–415, 1988.
4. Hayashi N, Egami H, Kai M, Kurusu Y, Takano S, Ogawa M. No-touch isolation technique reduces intraoperative shedding of tumor cells into the portal vein during resection of colorectal cancer. Surgery 125:369–374, 1999.
5. Sales JP, Wind P, Douard R, Cugnenc PH, Loric S. Blood dissemination of colonic epithelial cells during no-touch surgery for rectosigmoid cancer [letter]. Lancet 354:392, 1999.
6. Joosten JJ, Strobbe LJ, Wauters CA, Pruszczynski M, Wobbes T, Ruers TJ. Intraoperative lymphatic mapping and the sentinel node concept in colorectal carcinoma [see comments]. Br J Surg 86:482–486, 1999.
7. Saha S, Wiese D, Badin J, et al. Technical details of sentinel lymph node mapping in colorectal cancer and its impact on staging. Ann Surg Oncol 7:120–124, 2000.
8. Gall FP, Tonak J, Altendorf A. Multivisceral resections in colorectal cancer. Dis Colon Rectum 30:337–341, 1987.
9. Izbicki JR, Hosch SB, Knoefel WT, Passlick B, Bloechle C, Broelsch CE. Extended resections are beneficial for patients with locally advanced colorectal cancer. Dis Colon Rectum 38:1251–1256, 1995.

10. Rowe VL, Frost DB, Huang S. Extended resection for locally advanced colorectal carcinoma [see comments]. Ann Surg Oncol 4:131–136, 1997.

11. Koea J, Conlon K, Paty P, Guillem J, Cohen A. Pancreatic and/or duodenal resection for advanced carcinoma of the right colon: is it justified? Dis Colon Rectum 43:460–465, 2000.

12. Mulcahy HE, Toner M, Patchett SE, Daly L, O'Donoghue DP. Identifying stage B colorectal cancer patients at high risk of tumor recurrence and death. Dis Colon Rectum 40:326–331, 1997.

13. McGregor JR, O'Dwyer PJ. The surgical management of obstruction and perforation of the left colon. Surg Gynecol Obstet 177:203–208, 1993.

14. Stephenson BM, Shandall AA, Farouk R, Griffith G. Malignant left-sided large bowel obstruction managed by subtotal/total colectomy. Br J Surg 77:1098–1102, 1990.

15. Murray JJ, Schoetz DJ Jr, Coller JA, Roberts PL, Veidenheimer MC. Intraoperative colonic lavage and primary anastomosis in nonelective colon resection. Dis Colon Rectum 34:527–531, 1991.

16. Single-stage treatment for malignant left-sided colonic obstruction: a prospective randomized clinical trial comparing subtotal colectomy with segmental resection following intraoperative irrigation. The SCOTIA Study Group. Subtotal Colectomy versus On-table Irrigation and Anastomosis [see comments]. Br J Surg 82:1622–1627, 1995.

17. Kiefhaber P, Kiefhaber K, Huber F. Preoperative neodymium-YAG laser treatment of obstructive colon cancer. Endoscopy 18(Suppl 1):44–46, 1986.

18. Tejero E, Fernandez-Lobato R, Mainar A, et al. Initial results of a new procedure for treatment of malignant obstruction of the left colon. Dis Colon Rectum 40:432–436, 1997.

19. Wholey MH, Levine EA, Ferral H, Castaneda-Zuniga W. Initial clinical experience with colonic stent placement. Am J Surg 175:194–197, 1998.

20. MacKeigan JM, Ferguson JA. Prophylactic oophorectomy and colorectal cancer in premenopausal patients. Dis Colon Rectum 22:401–405, 1979.

21. Morrow M, Enker WE. Late ovarian metastases in carcinoma of the colon and rectum. Arch Surg 119:1385–1388, 1984.

22. O'Brien PH, Newton BB, Metcalf JS, Rittenbury MS. Oophorectomy in women with carcinoma of the colon and rectum. Surg Gynecol Obstet 153:827–830, 1981.

23. Graffner HO, Alm PO, Oscarson JE. Prophylactic oophorectomy in colorectal carcinoma. Am J Surg 146:233–235, 1983.

24. Young-Fadok TM, Wolff BG, Nivatvongs S, Metzger PP, Ilstrup DM. Prophylactic oophorectomy in colorectal carcinoma: preliminary results of a randomized, prospective trial. Dis Colon Rectum 41:277–283; discussion 283–285, 1998.

25. Enker WE, Dragacevic S. Multiple carcinomas of the large bowel: a natural experiment in etiology and pathogenesis. Ann Surg 187:8–11, 1978.

26. Evers BM, Mullins RJ, Matthews TH, Broghamer WL, Polk HC Jr. Multiple adenocarcinomas of the colon and rectum. An analysis of incidences and current trends. Dis Colon Rectum 31:518–522, 1988.

27. Langevin JM, Nivatvongs S. The true incidence of synchronous cancer of the large bowel. A prospective study. Am J Surg 147:330–333, 1984.

28. Arenas RB, Fichera A, Mhoon D, Michelassi F. Incidence and therapeutic implications of synchronous colonic pathology in colorectal adenocarcinoma. Surgery 122:706–709; discussion 709–710, 1997.

28a. Passman MA, Pommier RF, Vetto JT. Synchronous colon primaries have the same prognosis as solitary colon cancers. Dis Colon Rectum 39:329–334, 1996.

29. Buess G, Kipfmuller K, Hack D, Grussner R, Heintz A, Junginger T. Technique of transanal endoscopic microsurgery. Surg Endosc 2:71–75, 1988.

30. Steele RJ, Hershman MJ, Mortensen NJ, Armitage NC, Scholefield JH. Transanal endoscopic microsurgery—initial experience from three centres in the United Kingdom. Br J Surg 83:207–210, 1996.

31. Milsom JW, Kim SH. Laparoscopic versus open surgery for colorectal cancer. World J Surg 21:702–705, 1997.

32. Stage JG, Schulze S, Moller P, et al. Prospective randomized study of Laparoscopic versus open colonic resection for adenocarcinoma [see comments]. Br J Surg 84:391–396, 1997.

33. Milsom JW, Bohm B, Hammerhofer KA, Fazio V, Steiger E, Elson P. A prospective, randomized trial comparing Laparoscopic versus conventional techniques in colorectal cancer surgery: a preliminary report [see comments]. J Am Coll Surg 187:46–54; discussion 54–55, 1998.

34. Stocchi L, Nelson H. Laparoscopic colectomy for colon cancer: trial update. J Surg Oncol 68:255–267, 1998.

35. Cohen AM, Tremiterra S, Candela F, Thaler HT, Sigurdson ER. Prognosis of node-positive colon cancer. Cancer 67:1859–1861, 1991.

36. Minsky BD. Additional pathologic prognostic factors. In: Cohen AM, Winawer SJ (eds): Cancer of the Colon, Rectum, and Anus. New York: McGraw-Hill, 1995, xxii, 1154, [8] of plates.

37. Harrison LE, Guillem JG, Paty P, Cohen AM. Preoperative carcinoembryonic antigen predicts outcomes in node-negative colon cancer patients: a multivariate analysis of 572 patients. J Am Coll Surg 185:55–59, 1997.

38. Willett CG, Tepper JE, Cohen AM. Failure patterns following curative resection of colonic carcinoma. Ann Surg 200:685–690, 1984.

39. Minsky BD, Mies C, Rich TA, Recht A, Chaffey JT. Potentially curative surgery of colon cancer: Patterns of failure and survival. J Clin Oncol 6:106–118, 1986.

40. Mrazek R, Economou S, McDonald GO, Slaughter DP, Cole WH. Prophylactic and adjuvant use of nitrogen mustard in the surgical treatment of cancer. Ann Surg 150:745–755, 1959.

41. Holden GA, Dixon WJ, Kuzma JW. The use of triethylene thiophosphoramide as an adjuvant to the surgical treatment of colorectal carcinoma. Ann Surg 165:481–489, 1967.

42. Grossi CE, Nealon TF Jr, Rousselot LM. Adjuvant chemotherapy in resectable cancer of the colon and rectum. Surg Clin North Am 52:925–933, 1972.

43. Li MC, Ross ST. Chemoprophylaxis for patients with colorectal cancer: prospective study with five-year follow-up. JAMA 235:2825–2828, 1976.

44. Mavligit GM, Burgess MA, Seibert GB, Jubert AV, McBride CM, Gehan EA, et al. Prolongation of postoperative disease-free interval and survival in human colorectal cancer by B.C.G. or B.C.G. plus 5-fluorouracil. Lancet 1:871–876, 1976.

45. Dwight RW Humphrey EW, Higgins GA, Keehn RJ. FUDR as an adjuvant to surgical treatment of large bowel cancer. J Surg Oncol 5:243–250, 1973.

46. Higgins GA, Humphrey EW, Juler GL, et al. Adjuvant chemotherapy in the surgical treatment of large bowel cancer. Cancer 38:1461, 1976.

47. Higgins GA, Dwight RW, Smith JV, et al. Fluorouracil as an adjuvant to surgery in carcinoma of the colon. Arch Surg 102:339, 1971.

48. Lawrence W Jr, Terz JJ, Horsley S III, Donaldson M, Lovett WL, Brown PW, Ruffner BW, Regelson W. Chemotherapy as an adjuvant to surgery for colorectal cancer. Ann Surg 181:616–623, 1975.

49. Hafstrom L, Rudenstam CM, Domellof L. A randomized trial of oral 5-fluorouracil versus placebo as adjuvant therapy in colorectal cancer Dukes B and C: results after 5 years observation time. Br J Surg 72:138–141, 1985.

50. Gastrointestinal Tumor Study Group. Adjuvant therapy of colon cancer: results of a prospectively randomized trial. N Engl J Med 310:737–742, 1984.

51. Buyse M, Zeleniuch-Jacquotte A, Chalmers TC. Adjuvant therapy of colorectal cancer. Why we still don't know. JAMA 259:3571–3578, 1988.

52. Wolmark N, Fisher B, Rockette H, Redmond C, Wickerham DL, Fisher ER, et al. Postoperative adjuvant chemotherapy or BCG for colon cancer: results from NSABP Protocol CO-1. J Natl Cancer Inst 80:30–36, 1988.

53. Verhaegen H, DeCree J, DeCock W, et al. Levamisole therapy in patients with colorectal cancer. In: Terry WD, Rosenberg SA (eds): Immunotherapy of Human Cancer. Elsevier, New York, 1982, pp 225–229.

54. Chirigos MA, Amery WK. Combined levamisole therapy: an overview of its protective effects. In: Terry WD, Rosenberg SA (eds): Immunotherapy of Human Cancer. Raven Press, New York, 1978, pp 181–195.

55. Renoux G. The general immunopharmacology of levamisole. Drugs 20:89–99, 1980.

56. Laurie JA, Moertel CG, Fleming TR, Wiend HS, Leigh JE, Rubin J, et al. Surgical adjuvant therapy of large bowel carcinoma: an evaluation of levamisole and the combination of levamisole and fluorouracil. J Clin Oncol 7:1447–1456, 1989.

57. Moertel CG, Fleming TR, Macdonald JS, Haller DG, Laurie JA, Goodman PJ, et al. Levamisole and fluorouracil for adjuvant therapy of resected colon carcinoma. N Engl J Med 322:352–358, 1990.

58. Moertel CG, Fleming TR, Macdonald JS, Haller DG, Laurie JA, Tangen CM, et al. Fluorouracil plus levamisole as effective adjuvant therapy after resection of stage III colon carcinoma: a final report. Ann Intern Med 122:321–326, 1995.

59. Moertel CG, Fleming TR, Macdonald JS, Haller DG, Laurie JA, Tangen CM, et al. Intergroup study of fluorouracil plus levamisole as adjuvant therapy for stage II/Dukes' B2 colon cancer. J Clin Oncol 13:2936–2943, 1995.

60. NIH Consensus Conference. Adjuvant therapy for patients with colon and rectal cancer. JAMA 264:1444–1450, 1990.

61. Stevenson HC, Green I, Hamilton JM. Levamisole: known effects on the immune system, clinical results, and future applications to the treatment of cancer. J Clin Oncol 9:2052–2066, 1991.

62. Takimoto CH. Enigma of fluorouracil and levamisole. J Natl Cancer Inst 87:471–473, 1995.

63. Kovach JS, Svingen PA, Schaid DJ. Levamisole potentiation of fluorouracil antiproliferative activity mimicked by orthovanadate, an inhibitor of tyrosine phosphatase. J Natl Cancer Inst 84:515–519, 1992.

64. Grem JL, Allegra CJ. Toxicity of levamisole and 5-fluorouracil in human clon carcinoma cells. J Natl Cancer Inst 81:1413–1417, 1989.

65. Abdalla EE, Blair GE, Jones RA, Sue-Ling HM, Johnston D. Mechanism of synergy of levamisole and fluorouracil: induction of human leucocyte antigen class I in a colorectal cancer cell line. J Natl Cancer Inst 87:489–496, 1995.

66. Mayer RJ. Does adjuvant therapy work in colon cancer? N Engl J Med 322:399–401, 1990.

67. Moertel CG. Chemotherapy of colorectal cancer. N Engl J Med 330:1136–1142, 1994.

68. Poon MA, O'Connell MJ, Wieand HS, et al. Biochemical modulation of fluorouracil with leucovorin. Confirmatory evidence of improved therapeutic efficacy in advanced colorectal cancer. J Clin Onco 19:1967–1972, 1991.

69. Buroker TR, O'Connell MJ, Wieand HS, et al. Randomized comparison of two schedules of fluorouracil and leucovorin in the treatment of advanced colorectal cancer. J Clin Oncol 12:14–20, 1994.

70. Wolmark N, Rockette H, Fisher B, Wickerman DL, Redmond C, Fisher ER, et al. The benefit of leucovorin-modulated fluorouracil as postoperative adjuvant therapy for primary colon cancer: results from National Surgical Adjuvant Breast and Bowel Project Protocol C0-3. J Clin Oncol 11:1879–1887, 1993.

71. International Multicenter Pooled Analysis of Colon Cancer Trials Investigators. Efficacy of adjuvant fluorouracil and folinic acid in colon cancer. Lancet 345:939–44, 1995.

72. International Multicenter Pooled Analysis of B2 Colon Cancer Trials (IMPACT B2) Investigators. Efficacy of adjuvant fluorouracil and folinic acid in B2 colon cancer. J Clin Oncol 17:1356–1363, 1999.

73. Wolmark N, Rockette H, Mamounas EP, Jones J, Wieand S, Wickerham DL, Bear HD, Atkins JN, Dimitrov NV, Glass AG, Fisher, ER Fisher B. Clinical trial to assses the relative efficacy of fluorouracil and leucovorin, fluoruracil and levamisole, and fluorouracil, leucovorin, and levamisole in patients with Dukes' B and C carcinoma of the colon: results from National Surgical Adjuvant Breast and Bowel Project C-04. J Clin Oncol 17:3553–3559, 1999.

74. O'Connell MJ, Laurie JA, Kahn M, Fitzgibbons RJ Jr, Erlichman C, Shepard L, Moertel CG, Kocha WI, Pazdur R, Wieand HS, Rubin J, Vukov AM, donohue JH, Krook JE, Figueredo A. Prospectively randomized trial of postoperative adjuvant chemotherapy in patients with high-risk colon cancer. J Clin Oncol 16:295–300, 1998.

75. Haller DG, Catalano PJ, MacDonald JS, Mayer RJ. Fluorouracil (FU), leucovorin (LV), and levamisole (LEV) adjuvant therapy for colon cancer: five-year final report of INT-0089. Proc Am Soc Clin Oncol 17:256a, 1998.

76. Mamounas E, Wieand S, Wolmark N, Bear HD, Atkins JN, Sog K, Jones J, Rockette H. Comparative efficacy of adjuvant chemotherapy in patients with Dukes' B versus Dukes' C colon cancer: results from four national surgical adjuvant breast and bowel project adjuvant studies (C-O1, C-02, C-03, C-04). J Clin Oncol 17:1349–1355, 1999.

77. Harrington DP. The tea leaves of small trials. J Clin Oncol 17:1336–1338, 1999.

78. Willet CG, Tepper JE, Cohen AM. Obstructive and perforative colonic carcinoma: patterns of failure. J Clin Oncol 3:379–384, 1985.

79. Jen J, Kim H, Piantadosi S, et al. Allelic loss of chromosome 18q and prognosis in colorectal cancer. N Engl J Med 331:213–221, 1994.

80. Weiss L, Grundmann E, Torhorst J. Haematogenous metastatic patterns of colonic carcinoma: an analysis of 1541 necropsies. J Pathol 150:195–199, 1986.

81. Dukes CE. Discussion on major surgery in carcinoma of the rectum, with and without colostomy, excluding the anal canal and including the rectosigmoid. Proc R Soc Med 50:1031–1043, 1957.

82. Fisher ER, Turnbull RB. The cytologic demonstration and significance of tumor cells in the mesenteric venous blood in patients with colorectal carcinoma. Surg Gynecol Obstet 100:102–108, 1955.

83. Ackerman NB. The blood supply of experimental liver metastases. IV. Changes in vascularity with increasing tumor growth. Surgery 75:589–597, 1974.

84. Basserman R. Changes of vascular pattern of tumors and surrounding tissue during different phases of metastatic growth. Cancer Res 100:256–264, 1986.

85. Almersjo O, Brandberg A, Gustavsson B. Concentration of biologically active 5-fluorouracil in the general circulation during continuous portal infusion in man. Cancer Lett 1975 1:113.

86. Taylor I, Rowling JT, West C. Adjuvant cytotoxic liver perfusion for colorectal cancer. Br J Surg 66:833–837, 1979.

87. Taylor I, Machin D, Mullee M, Trotter G, Cooke T, West C. A randomized controlled trial of adjuvant portal vein cytotoxic perfusion in colorectal cancer. Br J Surg 72:359–363, 1985.

88. Wolmark N, Rockette H, Wickerman DL, Fisher B, Redmond C, Fisher ER, et al. Adjuvant therapy of Dukes' A, B, and C adenocarcinoma of the colon with portal vein fluorouracil hepatic infusion: preliminary results of National Surgical Adjuvant Breast and Bowel Project Protocol C-02. J Clin Oncol 8:1466–1475, 1990.

89. Weber W, Laffer U, Metzger U. Adjuvant portal liver infusion with 5-fluorouracil and mitomycin in colorectal cancer. Anticancer Res 13(5C):1839–1840, 1993.

90. Swiss Group for Clinical Cancer Research. Long-term results of single course of adjuvant intraportal chemotherapy for colorectal cancer. Lancet 345:349–352, 1995.

91. Liver Infusion Meta-analysis Group. Portal vein chemotherapy for colorectal cancer: a meta-analysis of 4,000 patients in 10 studies. J Natl Cancer Inst 98:497–505, 1997.

92. Gunderson LL, Sosin H. Areas of failure found at reoperation (second or symptomatic look) following "curative surgery" for adenocarcinoma of the rectum: clinicopathologic correlation and implications for adjuvant therapy. Cancer 34:1278–1292, 1974.

93. Tong D, Russel AH, Dawson LE, Wisbeck W. Second laparotomy for proximal colon cancer: sites of recurrence and implications for adjuvant therapy. Am J Surg 145:382–386, 1983.

94. Speyer JL, Sugarbaker PH, Collins JM, Dedrick RL, Klecker RW Jr, Meyers CE. Portal levels and hepatic clearance of 5-fluorouracil after intraportal administration in humans. Cancer Res 41:1916–1922, 1981.

95. Archer SG, McCulloch RK, Gray BN. A comparative study of the pharmacokinetics of continuous portal vein infusion versus intraperitoneal infusion of 5-fluorouracil. Reg Cancer Treat 2:105–111, 1989.

96. Speyer JL, Collins JM, Dedrick RL, Brennan MF, Buckpit AR, Londer H, et al. Phase I and pharmacological studies of 5-fluorouracil administered intraperitoneally. Cancer Res 40:567–572, 1980.

97. Sugarbaker PH, Gianola FJ, Speyer JC, Wesley R, Barofsky I, Meyers CE. Prospective randomized trial of intravenous versus intraperitoneal 5-fluorouracil in patients with advanced primary colon or rectal cancer. Surgery 98:414–421, 1985.

98. Kelsen DP, Saltz L, Cohen AM, Yao TJ, Enker W, Tong W, et al. A phase I trial of immediate postoperative intraperitoneal floxuridine and leucovorin plus systemic 5-fluorouracil and levamisole after resection of high-risk colon cancer. Cancer 74:2224–2233, 1994.

99. Scheithauer W, Komek GV, Maczell A, Kamer J, Salem G, Greiner R, Burger D, Stoger F, Ritschel J, Kovats E, Vischer HM, Schneeweiss B, Depisch D. Combined intravenous and intraperitoneal chemotherapy with fluorouracil + leucovorin vs fluorouracil + levamisole for adjvant therapy of resected colon cancer. Br J Cancer 77:1349–1354, 1998.

100. Jain RK. Physiological barriers to delivery of monoclonal antibodies and other macromolecules in tumors. Cancer Res 50:2741–2751, 1990.

101. Riethmuller G, Johnson GP. Monoclonal antibodies in the detection and therapy of micrometastatic epithelial cancers. Curr Opin Immunol 4:647–655, 1992.

102. Lindemann F, Schlimok G, Dirschedl P, Witte J, Riethmuller G. Prognostic significance of micrometastatic tumor cells in bone marrow of colorectal cancer patients. Lancet 340:685–689, 1992.

103. Herlyn M, Steplewski Z, Herlyn D, Koprowski H. Colorectal carcinoma-specific antigen: detection by means of monoclonal antibodies. Proc Natl Acad Sci USA 76:1438–1442, 1979.

104. Herlyn D, Koprowsky H. IgG2a monoclonal antibodies inhibit human tumor growth through interaction with effector cells. Proc Nat Acad Sci USA 79:4761–4765, 1982.

105. Gottlinger HG, Funke 1, Johnson JP, Gokel JM, Riethmuller G. The epithelial cell surface antigen 17-1 A, a target for antibody-mediated tumour therapy: its biochemical nature, tissue distribution and recognition by different monoclonal antibodies. Int J Cancer 38:27–53, 1986.

106. Herlyn DM, Steplewski Z, Herlyn MF, Koprowski H. Inhibition of growth of colorectal carcinoma in nude mice by monoclonal antibody. Cancer Res 40:717–721, 1980.

107. Mellstedt H, Frodin JJE, Masuccci G. The therapeutic use of monoclonal antibodies in colorectal carcinoma. Semin Oncol 2:462–477, 1991.

108. Riethmuller G, Schneider-Gadicke E, Schlimok G, Schmiegel W, Raab R, Hoffken K, et al. Randomized trial of monoclonal antibody for adjuvant therapy of resected Dukes C colorectal carcinoma. Lancet 343: 1177–1183, 1994.

109. Foon KA, John WJ, Chakraborty M, Ruma D, Teitelbaum A, Garrison J, Kashala O, Chatterjee SK, Bhattacharya-Chatterjiee M. Clinical and immune responses in resected colorectal cancer patients treated with anti-idiotype monoclonal antibody vaccine that mimics carcinoembryonic antigen. J Clin Oncol 17:2889–2895, 1999.

110. O'Boyle KP, Zamore R, Adluri S, Cohen A, Kefeny N, Welt S, et al. Immunization of colorectal cancer patients with modified ovine submaxillary gland mucin and adjuvants induces IgM and IgG antibodies to Sialylated Tn. Cancer Res 52:5663–5667, 1992.

111. Hoover HC, Brandhorst JS, Peters LC, Surdyke MG, Takeshita Y, Madariaga J, et al. Adjuvant active specific immunotherapy for human colorectal cancer: 6.5-year median follow-up of a phase II prospectively randomized trial. J Clin Oncol 11:390–399, 1993.

112. Moertel CG. Vaccine adjuvant therapy for colorectal cancer: "very dramatic" or ho-hum? J Clin Oncol 11:385–386, 1993.

113. Vermorken JB, Claessen AM, van Tinteren H, Gail HE, Ezinga R, Meijer S, Scheper RJ, Meijer CJ, Bloemena E, Ransom JH, Hanna MG Jr, Pinedo HM. Active specific immunotherapy for stage II and stage III human colon cancer: a randomized trial. Lancet 353: 345–350, 1999.

114. Saltz LB, Locker PK, Pirotta N, Elfring GL, Miller LL. Weekly irinotecan (CPT-11), leucovorin (LV), and fluorouracil (FU) is superior to daily × 5 LV/FU in patients (PTS) with previously untreated metastatic colorectal cancer (CRC). Proc Am Soc Clin Oncol 18:233a, 1999.

115. Douillard JY, Cunningham D, Roth AD, et al. A randomized phase III trial comparing irinotecan (IRI) + 5FU/folinic acid (FA) to the same schedule of 5FU/FA patients (pts) with metastatic colorectal cancer (MCRC) as front line chemotherapy (CT). Proc Am Soc Clin Oncol 18:233a, 1999.

116. De Gramont A, Figer M, Seymour M, Homerin N, le Bail J, Cassidy C, et al. A randomized trial of leucovorin and fluorouracil with or without oxaliplatin in advanced colorectal cancer. Proc Am Soc Clin Oncol 17:257a, 1998.

117. Douillard JY, Hoff PM, Skillings JR, Eisenberg P, Davidson N, Harper P, Vincent MD, Lembersky BC, Thompson S, Maniero A, Benner SE. Multicenter phase III study of uracil/tegafur and oral leucovorin versus fluorouracil and leucovorin in patients with previously untreated metastatic colorectal cancer. J Clin Oncol 20:3605–3616, 2002.

118. Cartwright TH, Cohn A, Varkey JA, Chen YM, Szatrowski TP, Cox JV, Schulz JJ. Phase II study of oral capecitabine in patients with advanced or metastatic pancreatic cancer. J Clin Oncol 20:160–164, 2002.

119. Van Cutsem E, Twelves C, Cassidy J, Allman D, Bajetta E, Boyer M, Bugat R, Findlay M, Frings S, Jahn M, McKendrick J, Osterwalder B, Perez-Manga G, Rosso R, Rougier P, Schmiegel WH, Seitz JF, Thompson P, Vieitez JM, Weitzel C, Harper P, Xeloda Colorectal Cancer Study Group. Oral capecitabine compared with intravenous fluorouracil plus leucovorin in patients with metastatic colorectal cancer: results of a large phase III study. J Clin Oncol 19:4093–4096, 2001.

# Clinical Aspects and Management of Rectal Adenocarcinoma: Diagnostic and Staging Procedures

SANDEEP LAHOTI

In the United States, colorectal cancer is the fourth most common cancer and the second leading cause of cancer death. Annually, approximately 129,000 new cases of colorectal cancer are diagnosed, with 57,000 associated deaths.[1] Without preventive action, approximately 6% of Americans will develop colorectal cancer sometime in their lives. Unfortunately, at the time of diagnosis, more than half of these patients have either locally advanced disease (5-year survival rate, 50%) or metastatic disease (5-year survival rate, 10%). In several large, randomized trials, the early diagnosis of colorectal cancer was associated with a 15%–30% decrease in colorectal cancer-related mortality.[2–4] This chapter discusses the diagnostic and staging modalities available for rectal cancer.

## Diagnosis

### Clinical Picture and Digital Rectal Examination

Rectal adenocarcinomas, like adenocarcinomas of the colon, tend to be slow-growing and may be present for as long as 5 years before symptoms appear. Persons with asymptomatic disease may have occult blood loss from their tumors, with the bleeding rate increasing with tumor size and degree of ulceration.[5] Other symptoms of rectal cancer are also similar to those of colon cancer and are related to the anatomic site to some extent. Cancers of the proximal colon usually grow larger before producing symptoms than those of the left colon. Constitutional symptoms of anorexia, weight loss, and microcytic anemia tend to occur more commonly with right-sided cancers. Because the left colon has a narrower lumen, cancers of the left colon present more often with obstructive symptoms than do cancers of the right colon. Urgency, tenesmus, and a change in bowel habits such as diarrhea or constipation are also seen with cancer of the left colon.

Hematochezia or a coating of blood over the surface of the stool is common with left colon and rectal cancers.

Extracolonic symptoms are uncommon and usually arise when there is metastatic disease or local spread to surrounding organs. Such features include symptoms related to fistulas to the bladder or vagina or obstructive jaundice due to liver metastases. Rectal cancers may also invade surrounding nerves, resulting in perineal or sacral pain. These symptoms are nonspecific and usually occur late in the disease process. Physical examination is also usually not useful in detecting symptoms until late in the disease process. Patients with large tumor burden may appear cachetic or may have manifestations of metastatic disease such as hepatomegaly. The most revealing part of the physical examination may be the digital rectal exam (DRE). Masses of the mid or distal rectum can usually be palpated; however, the sensitivity of this examination will naturally depend on the length of the examining finger.

### Barium Enema

Barium enema (BE) radiography can be performed with barium alone (single-contrast) or with air instilled after the barium has been evacuated (dual-contrast or air-contrast). The air-contrast barium enema (ACBE) visualizes the colonic mucosa better than the single-contrast method and should be chosen over single-contrast BE if used as a screening test.

Despite their ability to visualize the entire colon, barium enemas have poor sensitivity for detecting cancer and polyps. Results from several studies suggest that the sensitivity of ACBE is 50%–80% for polyps less than 1 cm, 70%–90% for polyps greater than 1 cm, and 55%–85% for Dukes' A and B cancers.[6–9] Additionally, 5%–10% of BE examinations are unsatisfactory, necessitating a repeat examination or a colonoscopy.[10–12] False-positive rates for BE as high as 10% for large polyps and 50% for small polyps have also been reported.[8,11,13]

If a BE is used as a screening test, it should be combined with a flexible sigmoidoscopy because overlapping bowel loops may present adequate visualization of the rectosigmoid colon on a BE. Although some radiologists no longer recommend sigmoidoscopy with the improved double-contrast BE technique,[14–16] a large randomized trial showed that almost 25% of cancers and an equal number of large polyps in the rectosigmoid colon could be missed by ACBE.[17]

### Endoscopic Examination

Currently, an endoscopic examination of the colon is the most accurate method for diagnosing rectal cancer (Color Fig. 58–1; see separate color insert). An inherent advantage over BE is that biopsies of any visualized abnormalities can be obtained. While flexible sigmoidoscopy and colonoscopy should have similar accuracy rates for diagnosing rectal cancers, a colonoscopy is generally preferred because it allows the examiner to evaluate the proximal colon for any synchronous polyps or cancer.

Although colonoscopy is considered to be the gold standard,[18] it is not foolproof. Studies have shown that the cecum is reached in only 80%–95% of procedures, leaving some portion of colon unexamined in 5%–20% of cases.[19–21] In a prospective study in which 90 patients underwent back-to-back colonoscopies by two experienced endoscopists, the endoscopist missed small polyps in 15% of cases and rarely missed large polyps.[6] In a recent retrospective study, 6 out of 346 cases of colorectal cancers were missed as a result of inaccurate depth of insertion in 5 patients and nonidentification of a rectal lesion in another patient.[22] Nevertheless, a colonoscopic examination is believed to be the best method for visualizing the colon and rectum.

## Staging

Preoperative staging is crucial for determining the approach in the treatment of rectal cancer. In the last two decades, the treatment of rectal cancer has evolved from a single treatment to multiple options based on the disease stage at diagnosis. The techniques of radical resection and reconstruction have been refined, the role and results of local excisions are better defined, and neoadjuvant treatment has decreased the rate of local recurrence and has improved survival rates.[23–26] The correct staging of rectal lesions helps to determine the appropriate surgical management and to identify those patients who would benefit from preoperative adjuvant therapy.

The staging of rectal cancer involves identifying the depth of tumor (T) penetration through the rectal wall and the presence or absence of diseased lymph nodes (N) and detecting distant metastases (M). The preoperative staging of rectal cancer is based on the TNM system of classification. There are various modalities for staging rectal cancer, including DRE, endoscopic ultrasonography, computed tomography (CT), and magnetic resonance imaging (MRI). Each method has its own strengths and limitations. Optimally, a combination of staging methods should be used to mitigate these limitations.

### Local Staging

#### Digital rectal examination

As mentioned previously, most rectal tumors can be detected on DRE. An assessment of local tumor spread can also be obtained during a DRE by judging tumor fixity.[27] Accuracy rates ranging from 44% to 83% have been reported for the assessment of local tumor spread using this technique, with accuracy rates increasing with clinical experience.[28] However, DRE cannot differentiate between inflammatory and malignant fixation, and this can lead to overstaging. Also, substantial proportions of rectal tumors lie beyond the reach of digital palpation, and there is significant interobserver variation. Finally, nodal involvement cannot be determined via DRE.

### Endorectal ultrasonography

Wild and Reid first performed rectal ultrasonography in 1956,[29] but it was not until the 1980s that the images were of sufficient quality to be clinically useful for imaging rectal cancer. Initial studies used nonoptical rigid probes. The probe was inserted blindly into the rectum, and then imaging was performed. Over the last decade, use of flexible endoscopes into which the ultrasound transducer is incorporated has increased. These flexible echoendoscopes were primarily designed for imaging the upper gastrointestinal tract but they can also be used for imaging rectal lesions (Figs. 58–2 and 58–3).

Endorectal ultrasonography of the rectal wall, with either the rigid or flexible probe, demonstrates five alternating hyper- and hypoechoic layers.[30,31] The histologic correlation of the echolayers is as follows: first layer, hyperechoic interface between water and the mucosa; second-layer, hypoechoic mucosa and muscularis mucosa; third layer, hyperechoic submucosa plus the interface between the submucosa and muscularis propria; fourth layer, hypoechoic muscularis propria minus the interface between the submucosa and the muscularis propria; and fifth layer, hyperechoic interface between the muscularis propria and perirectal fat.

Multiple studies have assessed the use of endorectal ultrasonography for the staging of rectal carcinoma. The accuracy in determining T stage has ranged from 75% to 92% (Table 58–1), with sensitivity being affected by tumor stage.[32–49] In a meta-analyis of 11 studies, the sensitivity for staging T1–T4 tumors was 84%, 76%, 96%, and 76%, respectively.[50] Overstaging, which is a particular problem with T2 tumors, accounts for two-thirds of inaccurately staged rectal cancers.[43] Sonographically, peritumoral inflammatory infiltrate is indistinguishable from malignant

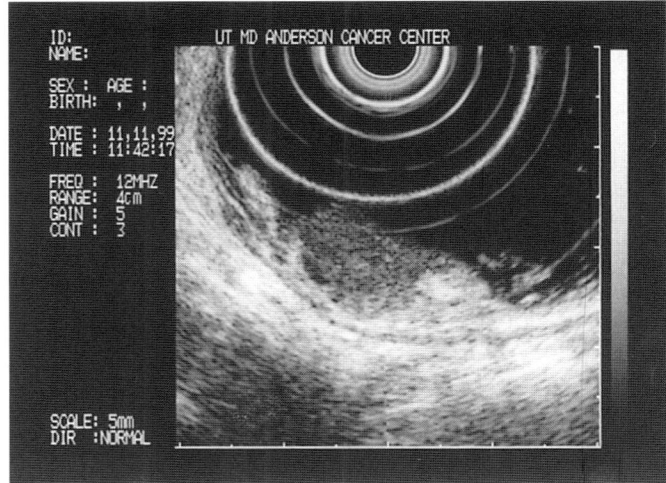

**Figure 58–2** Endorectal sonogram displaying a T1 rectal cancer. The lesion extends into the submucosa but does not involve the muscularis propria.

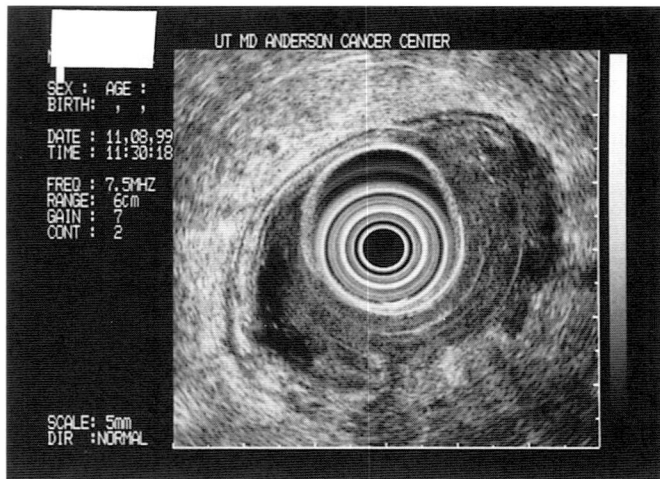

**Figure 58–3** Endorectal sonogram of the lesion displayed in Figure 58–1. The T3 lesion extends through the muscularis propria.

tissue, which can lead to overstaging.[36] Understaging can also occur and is believed to be due to the presence of microscopic cancer infiltration that is beyond the resolution of the equipment.[43] In addition, 14% of stenotic tumors may not be adequately staged because the endosonography's scope cannot traverse the stenosis.[51] The degree of operator experience[33,38,50] and the level of tumor in the rectum, with reduced accuracy rates for tumors lower in the rectum,[38,42] are other factors that can influence the accuracy of tumor staging with endorectal ultrasonography.

Endorectal ultrasonography is less accurate for lymph node staging than for tumor staging as it can be difficult to identify tumor deposits within lymph nodes. The characteristics of a lymph node are unlikely to be sufficiently altered to allow detection if only a small deposit or a micrometastasis is present. Sonographic detection is more likely if the whole node is replaced by tumor or the node is enlarged secondary to the metastasis. Endorectal ultrasonography also cannot differentiate

**Table 58–1** Studies demonstrating accuracy of rectal ultrasonography in staging rectal cancer, 1990–1999

| Study | Patients (n) | T Stage (%) | N Stage (%) |
|---|---|---|---|
| Jochem et al., 1990[32] | 50 | 80 | 72 |
| Hildebrandt et al., 1990[53] | 113 | — | 78 |
| Orrom et al., 1999[33] | 75 | 75 | 88 |
| Tio et al., 1991[34] | 61 | 80 | 62 |
| Boyce et al., 1992[35] | 45 | 89 | 79 |
| Katsura et al., 1992[36] | 120 | 92 | — |
| Cho et al., 1993[37] | 76 | 82 | — |
| Herzog et al., 1993[38] | 118 | 89 | 80 |
| Glaser et al., 1993[39] | 154 | 86 | 81 |
| Kaneko et al., 1996[40] | 38 | 76 | — |
| Nielsen et al., 1996[41] | 100 | 85 | — |
| Sailer et al., 1997[42] | 154 | 78 | — |
| Akasu et al., 1997[43] | 164 | 82 | 77 |
| Osti et al., 1997[44] | 63 | 83 | 66 |
| Heneghan et al., 1997[45] | 39 | 85 | 52 |
| Kuntz et al., 1997[46] | 31 | 85 | 90 |
| Massari et al., 1998[47] | 75 | 91 | 76 |
| Hamada et al., 1998[48] | 33 | 82 | 87 |
| Norton and Thomas, 1999[49] | 121 | 92 | 65 |

between inflammatory and metastatic lymph nodes. Some sonographic features of lymph nodes suggestive of malignant involvement are round shape, poor echogenicity, and size greater than 5 mm.[52,53] On the basis of sonographic size alone, 50%–70% of detected nodes greater than 0.5 cm in diameter will be involved, whereas less than 20% of nodes smaller than 4 mm will be involved.[54] Some investigators have considered any visualized lymph node adjacent to an area of tumor to be involved.[55] Overall, the reported accuracy of endorectal ultrasonography for staging lymph nodes ranges from 62% to 83%.[32–35,38,39,43–49,53] (Table 58–1). Sonographic ultrasound–guided biopsy can be performed to confirm involvement of suspicious nodes.

## Computed tomography

The primary utility for CT in the local staging of rectal cancer is to demonstrate local extension into adjacent organs, which is effectively shown with obliteration of tissue planes between the viscera.[56] T staging using CT is based on the thickness of the rectal wall and irregularity of the outer margin of the wall (Fig. 58–4). Computed tomography is unable to depict the various layers of the bowel wall or microscopic invasion of the fat surrounding the rectum, thereby limiting its accuracy for T staging.[56] Like endorectal ultrasonography, CT scanning cannot accurately assess nodal staging. Lymph node size and shape and the separability of lymph nodes from the primary tumor determine nodal staging.[57] A nodal diameter of greater than 1 cm is considered consistent with malignant involvement, as is a distorted nodal shape. Small metastases that are within a node but that do not change the size or shape of the node will not be detected on CT since the internal architecture of lymph nodes is

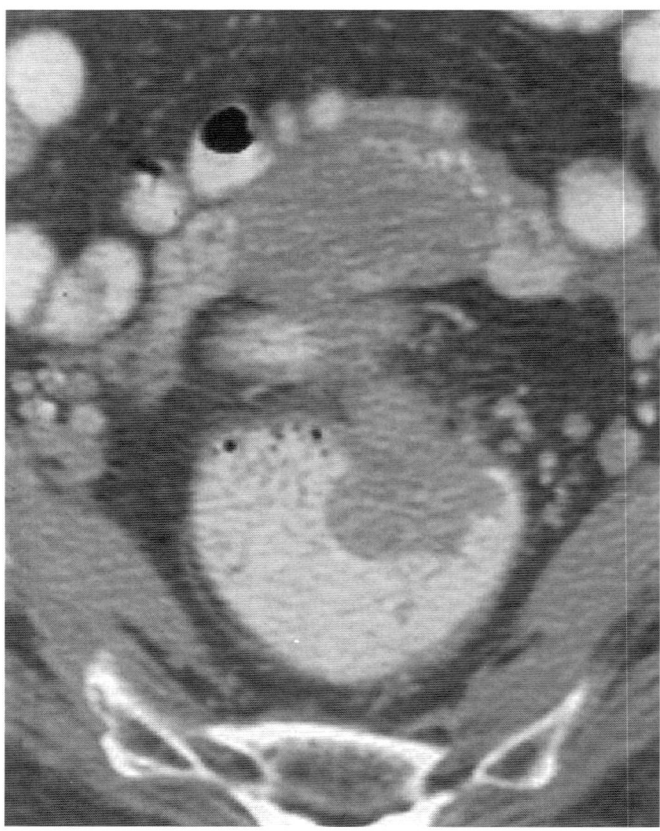

**Figure 58–4** Computed tomography scan using rectal barium contrast demonstrating a T3 lesion.

**Table 58-2** Studies comparing accuracy of staging primary rectal carcinoma rectal ultrasonography and computed tomography

| Study | Patients (n) | T Stage (%) Accuracy in Determining | | N Stage (%) Accuracy in Determining | |
|---|---|---|---|---|---|
| | | US | CT | US | CT |
| Romano et al., 1985[105] | 23 | 87 | 83 | — | — |
| Beynon et al., 1986[30] | 44 | 91 | 82 | — | — |
| Kramann and Hildebrandt, 1986[106] | 29 | 93 | 79 | — | — |
| Beynon et al., 1989[54] | 46 | — | — | 87 | 57 |
| Holdsworth et al., 1988[107] | 36 | 86 | 94 | 61 | 70 |
| Rifkin et al., 1989[55] | 81 | 91 | 75 | 80 | 72 |
| Waizer et al., 1989[108] | 68 | 76 | 66 | — | — |
| Rotte et al., 1989[109] | 30 | 84 | 76 | — | — |
| Pappalardo et al., 1990[110] | 14 | 93 | 86 | 86 | 57 |
| Akasu et al., 1990[111] | 41 | 80 | 46 | 78 | 66 |
| Goldman et al., 1991[112] | 32 | 81 | 52 | — | — |
| Herzog et al., 1993[38] | 87 | 91 | 75 | 80 | — |
| Osti et al., 1997[44] | 63 | 83 | 74 | 66 | 57 |
| Kim et al., 1999[78] | 89 | 81 | 65 | 64 | 57 |

CT, computed tomography; US, ultrasound.

not demonstrated with CT.[56] While initial reports of the use of CT for tumor staging were encouraging, those results were due to most patients in early studies having advanced disease.[57] The limitations of CT have only become clear in more recent studies. Recent trials of CT staging have reported accuracies for tumor staging between 46% and 94% and for lymph node staging between 57% and 72% (Table 58–2). Computed tomography is more accurate in showing extensive invasion of surrounding tissue than in demonstrating local adenopathy or minimal pericolonic tumor extension, as evidenced by results of a study that demonstrated that the accuracy of CT staging increased from 17% for Dukes' B lesions to 81% for Dukes' D lesions.[58] Studies that have compared CT with endorectal ultrasonography have consistently shown endorectal ultrasonography to be more accurate for local tumor and lymph node staging (Table 58–2).

## Magnetic resonance imaging

Magnetic resonance imaging with a body coil appears generally to have the same limitations as those of CT.[57] Assessment of T stage can be a problem because MRI with a body coil cannot depict the various layers of the bowel wall or microscopic invasion of the fat surrounding the rectum[56] (Fig. 58–5). Determining nodal involvement by means of MRI with a body coil can also be a problem because nodes do not have characteristic MRI features associated with malignant involvement. Nodal involvement on MRI is determined according to size criteria alone. Therefore, small metastases or micrometastases that do not change the lymph node size are not detected (Fig. 58–6). In studies using a body coil, the overall accuracy of MRI for preoperative staging of rectal cancer has ranged from 59% to 95% and the accuracy for nodal staging, from 39% to 95%.[59–70] The usefulness of MRI for staging rectal cancer has substantially improved with the development of endorectal coils. Use of endorectal coils with MRI (EMRI) allows the identification of three distinct rectal wall layers: an inner layer corresponding to the mucosa and submucosa, a middle layer representing the muscularis propria, and an outer layer comprising the serosa and perirectal fat.[71] It also allows a more consistent degree of accuracy, with T-stage accuracy ranging from 66% to 91% and N-stage accuracy ranging from 72% to 79%.[72–78] In trials directly comparing endorectal ultrasound and EMRI results, have been comparable in terms of local staging accuracy (Table 58–3); however, endorectal ultrasound is faster and less expensive.

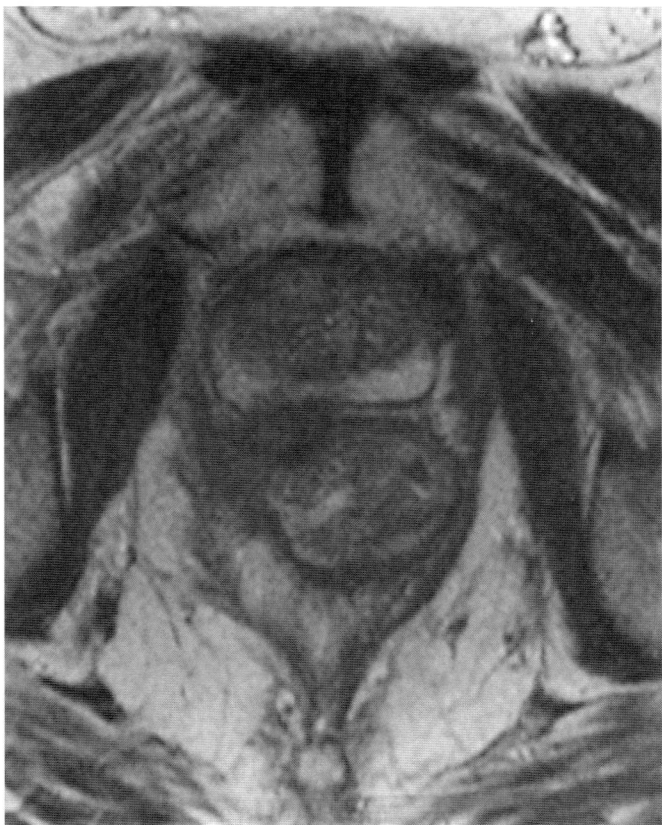

**Figure 58-5** T2-weighted MR image demonstrating a T4 rectal cancer with extension into the prostate.

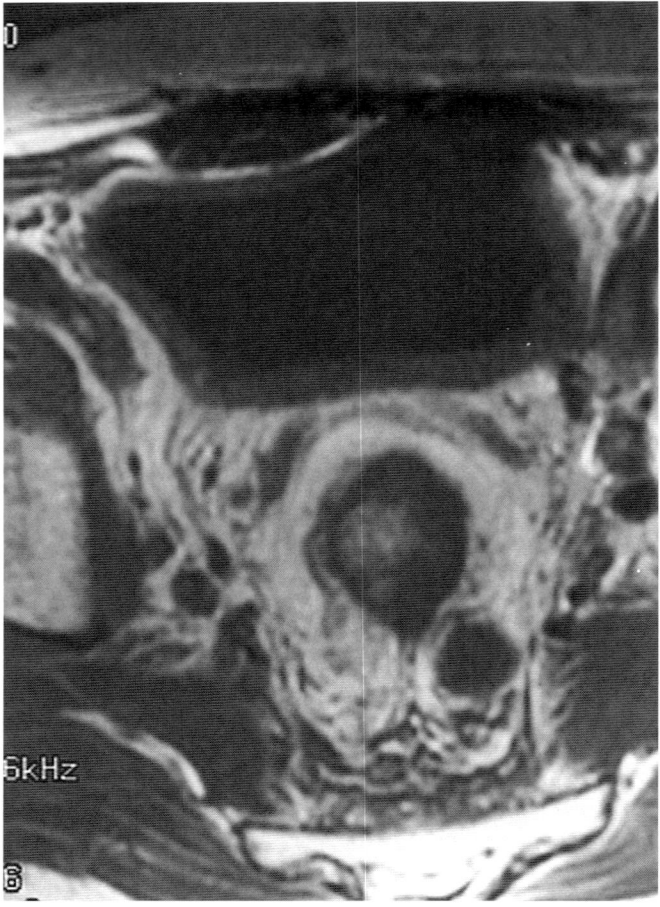

**Figure 58–6** T1-weighted MR image demonstrating a T3 rectal cancer with adjacent metastatic lymph node (N1).

### Distant Staging

While the appropriate extent of preoperative imaging to assess metastatic spread of tumor is unclear, a contrast-enhanced abdominal CT is often recommended. Findings on CT can frequently change clinical management. In a series of 158 patients, abdominal CT detected abnormalities that deferred clinical management in 35% of cases.[79] A CT scan allows visualization of the liver, the

primary site of metastatic spread of rectal carcinoma, along with an assessment of involvement of other intraabdominal organs or peritoneal carcinomatosis. The addition of a contrast agent improves the sensitivity for detecting liver metastases. The use of CT during arterial portography has a reported accuracy approaching 95% for detection of hepatic metastases.[80–82] It is often employed during preoperative planning when ablation or resection of hepatic metastases is contemplated. However, the logistics, costs, and additional risks associated with arterial catheter placement preclude the use of CT arterial portography for routine metastatic surveillance. Spiral CT is more accurate than conventional CT for detecting peritoneal carcinomatosis.[56]

The efficacy of MRI with the use of standard body coils has similar efficacy to that of contrast-enhanced CT in the detection of liver metastases.[83,84] Magnetic resonance imaging is also beneficial for detecting and characterizing liver lesions as benign cysts, hemangiomas, or metastases. With the recent development of liver-specific contrast agents and the advent of new pulse sequences, MRI could now replace CT as a means of evaluation for metastatic liver disease.

Currently, the role of radioimmunoscintigraphy and positron emission tomography (PET) in the staging of rectal cancer is not yet defined. Radioimmunoscintigraphy with a variety of radioisotopes, antibodies, and antigen targets has been used for imaging colorectal cancer. Several studies have found it to be of limited usefulness in the primary detection of colorectal cancer, with a diagnostic accuracy ranging from 74% to 96%.[85–91] However, it may be useful for the detection of occult metastases.[92–96] Micrometastases may be detected via radioimmunoguided surgery (RIGS), an intraoperative procedure in which a surgeon uses a handheld gamma probe to identify tumor sites.[97–99]

Positron emission tomography relies on the accelerated rate of glucose metabolism in malignant tumor cells and the demonstration of this metabolic rate with isotopes tagged to deoxyglucose.[100] In one small study of 16 patients, PET was compared with CT for the detection of primary and recurrent colorectal cancer.[101] Although PET had a higher sensitivity (90%) than that of CT (60%), CT had a higher specificity (100% vs. 66%). The predictive accuracy for the detection of colorectal cancer was 83% for PET and 56% for CT. Most investigations of the use of PET for colorectal cancer have focused on the detection of recurrent or residual disease.[102–104] Data supporting a role for PET in the preoperative staging of rectal cancer are lacking.

Investigation of metastatic spread outside the abdomen is gen-

**Table 58–3** Studies comparing accuracy of staging primary rectal carcinoma with rectal ultrasonography and magnetic resonance imaging

| Study | Coil Type | (n) | T Stage (%) Accuracy in Determining | | N Stage (%) Accuracy in Determining | |
|---|---|---|---|---|---|---|
| | | | US | MRI | US | MRI |
| Waizer et al., 1991[62] | Body | 13 | 85 | 77[a] | — | — |
| Thaler et al., 1994[69] | Body | 34 | 88 | 82 | 80 | 60 |
| Joosten et al., 1995[75] | Endorectal | 15 | 66 | 66 | — | — |
| Meyenberg et al., 1995[113] | Endorectal | 21 | 83 | 40 | — | — |
| Zagoria et al., 1997[76] | Endorectal | 10 | 70 | 80 | — | — |
| Kulling et al., 1998[77] | Endorectal | 13 | 85 | 77 | 62 | 62 |
| Kim et al., 1999[78] | Endorectal | 89 | 81 | 81 | 64 | 63 |

MRI, magnetic resonance imaging; US, ultrasound.

[a]Overall accuracy as opposed to separate T and N staging.

erally limited to chest radiography. The colon should also be evaluated for synchronous tumors, and this is usually done via colonoscopy.

## Summary

The signs and symptoms of rectal cancer can be nonspecific. Currently, our best test for diagnosis is an endoscopic evaluation of the colon; a colonoscopy is preferred because it also allows evaluation of the proximal colon for any synchronous lesions. The preoperative assessment of the colon has increased in importance as therapy is individualized on basis of disease stage. The presence of distant intraabdominal metastases is best evaluated by contrast-enhanced CT, although MRI with recently developed scanning techniques and contrast agents may play an increasing role in the future. Endorectal ultrasound should be performed for local staging of rectal cancer in cases in which distant metastases are not evident.

## References

1. Landis SH, Murray T, Bolden S, Wingo PA. Cancer statistics, 1999. CA Cancer J Clin 49:8–31;1999.
2. Mandel JS, Bond JH, Church TR, et al. Reducing mortality from colorectal cancer by screening for fecal occult blood. Minnesota Colon Cancer Control Study [published erratum appears in N Engl J Med 1993; 329:672]. N Engl J Med 328:1365–1371, 1993.
3. Hardcastle JD, Chamberlain JO, Robinson MH, et al. Randomized controlled trial of a faecal-occult-blood screening for colorectal cancer. Lancet 384:1472–1477, 1996.
4. Kronborg O, Ferger C, Olsen J, Jorgensen OD, Sondergaard O. Randomized study of screening for colorectal cancer with faecal-occult-blood test. Lancet 384:1467–1471, 1996.
5. Bresalier RS, Kim YS. Malignant neoplasms of the large intestine. In: Feldman M, Scharschmidt BF, Sleisenger MH (eds): Sleisenger & Fordtran's Gastrointestinal and Liver Disease, 6th ed. W.B. Saunders, Philadelphia, 1998, pp 1906–1942.
6. Hixson LJ, Femerty MB, Sampliner RE, McGee D, Garewal H. Prospective study of the frequency and size distribution of polyps missed by colonoscopy. J Natl Cancer Inst 82:1769–1772, 1990.
7. Fork FT. Double contrast enema and colonoscopy in polyp detection. Gut 22:971–977, 1990.
8. Steine S, Stordahl A, Lunde OC, Loken K, Laerum E. Double contrast barium enema versus colonoscopy in the diagnosis of neoplastic disorders: aspects of decision-making in general practice. Fam Pract 10: 288–291, 1993.
9. Hixson LJ, Fennerty MB, Sampliner RE, Garewal HS. Prospective blinded trial of the colonoscopic miss-rate of large colorectal polyps. Gastrointest Endosc 37:125–127, 1991.
10. Bloomfield JA. Reliability of barium enema in detecting colonic neoplasia. Med J Aust 2:631–633, 1981.
11. Jaramillo E, Slezak P. Comparison between double-contrast barium enema and colonoscopy to investigate lower gastrointestinal bleeding. Gastrointest Radiol 17:81–83, 1992.
12. Brewster NT, Grieve DC, Saunders JH. Double-contrast barium enema and flexible sigmoidoscopy for routine colonic investigation. Br J Surg 8:445–447, 1994.
13. Jensen J, Kewenter J, Aszteely M, Iycke G, Wojciechowski J. Double-contrast barium enema and flexible rectosigmoidoscopy: a reliable diagnostic combination for detection of colorectal neoplasm. Br J Surg 77:270–272, 1990.
14. Evers K, Laufer I, Gordon RL, Kressel HY, Herlinger H, Gohel VK. Double contrast enema examination for detection of rectal cancers. Radiology 140:635–639, 1981.
15. Reilly J, Rusin L, Theuerkauf F. Colonoscopy: its role in cancer of the colon and rectum. Dis Colon Rectum 25:532–538, 1982.
16. Thoeni R, Menuck L. Comparison of barium enema and colonoscopy in the detection of small colonic polyps. Radiology 124:631–635, 1977.
17. Kewenter J, Brevinge G, Engaras B, Haglind E. The yield of flexible sigmoidoscopy and double contrast barium enema in the diagnosis of neoplasms of large bowel in patients with a positive hemoccult test. Endoscopy 27:159–163, 1995.
18. Burke CA, Van Stolk RV. Colorectal cancer screening: making sense of the different guidelines (review). Clev Clin J Med 66:303–311, 1999.
19. Lieberman DA, Smith FW. Screening for colon malignancy with colonoscopy. Am J Gastroenterol 86:946–951, 1991.
20. Rex DK, Lehman GA, Hawes RH, Ulbright TM, Smith JJ. Screening colonoscopy in asymptomatic average-risk persons with negative fecal occult blood tests. Gastroenterology 100:64–67, 1991.
21. Godreau CJ. Office-based colonoscopy in a family practice. Fam Pract Res J 12:313–320, 1992.
22. Miller BJ, Cohen JR, Theile DE, Schache DJ, Ku JK. Diagnostic failure in colonoscopies for malignant disease. Aust N Z J Surg 68:331–333, 1998.
23. Loggie BW. Surgical concepts in the treatment of colorectal cancer [review]. Semin Roentgenol 31:111–117, 1996.
24. Rich TA, Skibber JM, Ajani JA, et al. Preoperative infusional chemoradiation therapy for stage T3 rectal cancer. Int J Radiat Oncol Biol Phys 32:1025–1029, 1995.
25. Krook JE, Moertel CG, Gunderson LL, et al. Effective surgical adjuvant therapy for high-risk rectal carcinoma. N Engl J Med 324:709–715, 1991.
26. Swedish Rectal Cancer Group. Improved survival with preoperative radiotherapy in rectal cancer. N Engl J Med 336:980–987, 1997.
27. Mason AY. President's Address: rectal cancer: the spectrum of selective surgery. Proc R Soc Med 69:237–244, 1976.
28. Nicholls RJ, Galloway DJ, Mason AY, Boyle P. Clinical local staging of rectal cancer. Br J Surg 72(Suppl):S51–S52, 1985.
29. Wild JJ, Reid JM. Diagnostic use of ultrasound. Br J Phys Med 19: 248–257, 1956.
30. Beynon J, Foy DM, Temple LN, Channer JL, Virjee J, Mortensen NJ. The endosonic appearance of normal colon and rectum. Dis Colon Rectum 29:810–813, 1986.
31. Kimmey MB, Martin RW, Haggitt RC, Wang KY, Franklin DW, Silverstein FE. Histologic correlates of gastrointestinal ultrasound images. Gastroenterology 96:433–441, 1989.
32. Jochem RJ, Reading CC, Dozois RR, et al. Endorectal ultrasonographic staging of rectal carcinoma. Mayo Clin Proc 65:1571–1577, 1990.
33. Orrom WJ, Wong WD, Rothenberger DA, Jensen LL, Goldberg SM. Endorectal ultrasound in the preoperative staging of rectal tumors. A learning experience. Dis Colon Rectum 33:654–659, 1990.
34. Tio TL, Coene PP, van Delden OM, Tytgat GN. Colorectal carcinoma: preoperative TNM classification with endosonography. Radiology 179: 165–170, 1991.
35. Boyce GA, Sivak MV, Lavery IC, et al. Endoscopic ultrasound in the pre-operative staging of rectal cancer. Gastrointest Endosc 38:468–471, 1992.
36. Katsura Y, Yamada K, Ishizawa T, Yoshinaka H, Shimazu H. Endorectal ultrasonography for the assessment of wall invasion and lymph node metastasis in rectal cancer. Dis Colon Rectum 35:362–368, 1992.
37. Cho E, Nakajima M, Yasuda K, Ashihara T, Kawai K. Endoscopic ultrasonography in the diagnosis of colorectal cancer invasion. Gastrointest Endosc 39:521–527, 1993.
38. Herzog U, von Flue M, Tondelli P, Schuppisser JP. How accurate is endorectal ultrasound in the preoperative staging of rectal cancer? Dis Colon Rectum 36:127–134, 1993.
39. Glaser F, Kuntz C, Schlag P, Herfarth C. Endorectal ultrasound for control of preoperative radiotherapy of rectal cancer. Ann Surg 217:64–71, 1993.
40. Kaneko K, Boku N, Hosokawa K, et al. Diagnostic utility of endoscopic ultrasonography for preoperative rectal cancer staging estimation. Jpn J Clin Oncol 26:30–35, 1996.
41. Nielsen MB, Qvitzau S, Pedersen JF, Christiansen J. Endosonography for preoperative staging or rectal tumors. Acta Radiol 37:799–803, 1996.
42. Sailer M, Leppert R, Bussen D, Fuchs KH, Thiede A. Influence of tumor position on accuracy of endorectal ultrasound staging. Int J Colorectal Dis 40:1180–1186, 1997.
43. Akasu T, Sugihara K, Moriya Y, Fujita S. Limitations and pitfalls of transrectal ultrasonography for staging of rectal cancer. Int J Colorectal D 40:S10–S15, 1997.
44. Osti MF, Padovan FS, Pirolli C, et al. Comparison between transrectal ultrasonography and computed tomography with rectal inflation of gas in preoperative staging of lower rectal cancer. Eur Radiol 7:26–30, 1997.
45. Heneghan JP, Salem RR, Lange RC, Taylor KJ, Hammers LW. Transrectal sonography in staging rectal carcinoma: the role of gray-scale, color-flow, and doppler imaging analysis. AJR Am J Roentgenol 169: 1247–1252, 1997.

# Clinical Aspects and Management of Rectal Adenocarcinoma
## Management Options: Resectable Rectal Carcinoma

GEOFFREY A. PORTER AND JOHN M. SKIBBER

Improving the management of resectable rectal cancer involves the optimization of patient outcomes through *(1)* a detailed understanding of the pathology of rectal cancer and its relation to surgical techniques; *(2)* multidisciplinary management; *(3)* organ and function conservation; *(4)* analysis of outcomes based on quality of life as well as morbidity, recurrence, and survival; and *(5)* treatment selection based on biologic factors. Selection of the best route to accomplish these goals is guided by the extent of disease at presentation. Advances in management involve both clinical and translational research issues.

The goal of the treatment of rectal carcinoma is cure or local control of disease with maintenance of an acceptable quality of life. The biology of a particular patient's tumor is the most important factor in overall outcome. Adequate surgical removal of the tumor is the major treatment factor affecting local control and cure. The adequacy of the surgical removal of the tumor and overall outcome can be influenced by the use of adjuvant radiation and chemotherapy. The principles of surgical management of rectal cancer are *(1)* removal of the primary tumor with adequate margins of normal tissue, *(2)* treatment of the draining lymphatics, and *(3)* restoration of function. Appropriate adjuvant therapies can enhance local control, reduce systemic recurrence, and increase organ preservation. Our focus is on the management at each stage of resectable rectal cancer. In this chapter, we describe the management of early, localized rectal cancer and resectable rectal cancers with locoregional spread.

Accomplishment of the stated goals of rectal cancer management is easier for upper and middle rectal cancers than for low rectal cancers. In patients with low rectal cancer, abdominoperineal resection (APR) has been the gold standard of management. However, APR requires a permanent colostomy, which adversely affects the patient's quality of life. Advances in rectal cancer management and surgical techniques have improved our ability to achieve oncologic control and optimal patient function without APR, even in patients with low rectal cancers.

## Surgical Approaches and Techniques

### Local Excision

Full-thickness local excision can be effective in the treatment of selected early low rectal cancers. Local excision is used as curative therapy for patients who have superficial tumors, and it is used as alternative therapy in medically compromised patients and in those who refuse standard therapy. Patient selection is paramount to using these techniques successfully and requires an understanding of the limitations of the techniques and the biology of T1/T2 rectal cancer.

Transanal excision is the most common method of local excision. Selection factors based on tumor size and degree of circumferential involvement predict the potential for a successful transanal excision. Both adequate dilatation of the anus and a good light source are essential, and exposure is aided by the use of specialized perianal retractors. The excision is begun by marking a margin of normal tissue around the lesion. This margin must be greater than 1 cm. The bowel wall is then cut with cautery. The local excision is performed in a full-thickness manner, meaning that the deep plane of dissection should be within the perirectal fat. The defect is closed in a primary fashion to avoid subsequent scarring.

A posterior proctotomy (or Kraske's procedure) is useful for large posterior lesions and provides better access to more proximal lesions than does transanal excision. In this procedure, a posterior longitudinal incision is made just above the anus to the inferior border of the gluteus maximus. The coccyx is removed and the underlying levator muscles are divided longitudinally in the midline. This permits excellent exposure for mobilization of the rectum and allows either a full-thickness local excision or a sleeve resection.[1] A transsphincteric excision (Bevan's or York-Mason) involves an approach similar to that of the posterior proctotomy except that the anal sphincter is divided posteriorly in the midline. It is critical to identify and reconstruct each portion of the sphincter complex, but if these are done, functional problems can be minimized.[2]

The choice of technique for local excision is dictated by tumor characteristics and the surgeon's ability to expose the tumor and control the margins of excision. The transanal approach generally has less morbidity. Posterior approaches have the advantage of better exposure of larger lesions but are associated with a higher rate of fistula formation and the potential for tumor seeding of the posterior wound. Whichever method is selected, the full-thickness excision must have at least 1-cm margins of normal tissue surrounding the tumor. An inadequate margin is a predictor of failure.[3] Piecemeal or submucosal excision is not considered adequate surgical treatment of invasive rectal cancer. Fragmentation of the tumor is associated with an increased incidence of local recurrence. If the lesion cannot be adequately resected by local excision, then a more standard locoregional surgical approach should be used. In a curative case, the patient should be counseled to consider local excision as a form of definitive biopsy, especially when transmural penetration or adverse histologic characteristics are found in the local excision specimen. In most instances, these patients should undergo more extensive surgery.

The criteria used to select patients for local excision are intended to make a negative-margin, full-thickness local excision technically feasible and to ensure a low risk of lymph node metastasis (Table 59-1). Physical assessment, computed tomography (CT), and endorectal ultrasonography are helpful in the preoperative evaluation. Imaging findings can be used to select patients for local excision procedures by determining the depth of tumor penetration into the rectal wall and the presence of enlarged lymph nodes. Most patients with rectal cancer do not meet the criteria for treatment by local excision alone because of the size or extent of the tumor.

Curative surgical treatment for rectal cancer requires tumor excision with margins of normal tissue and treatment of the lymph nodes draining the tumor site. Local excision alone meets only the first requirement. Factors that can help identify patients who are at low risk for lymphatic metastasis include small tumors, absence of lymphatic and vascular invasion, well- or moderately differentiated tumor, and absence of clinical or radiologic evidence of enlarged lymph nodes. The assumed low risk in patients treated with local excision alone is accepted, because such procedures do not involve resection of the mesorectal lymph nodes. However, many of the classic criteria can be unreliable predictors of lymphatic involvement.

The major factor predicting patient survival and perirectal lymph node metastasis is the depth of penetration of the primary tumor. In 1966, Morson[5] reported that lymphatic metastasis arose

**Table 59-1** Indications for local excision of rectal cancer

Tumor <3 cm in greatest dimension
Invades only the submucosa or superficial muscularis
Favorable pathologic grade

From Nivatvongs S, Wolff BG. Technique of per anal excision for carcinoma of the low rectum. World J Surg 16:447–450, 1992.[4]

from 10% of tumors confined to the submucosa, 12% of tumors invading the muscularis propria, and 58% of tumors extending beyond the bowel wall. Others have found a higher incidence of lymphatic metastasis in association with T2 rectal carcinoma. In a study of tumors treated by radical resection, the incidence of lymphatic metastasis was 12% for T1 tumors and 22% for T2 tumors.[6] The incidence of lymphatic metastasis increased in the presence of lymphatic or blood vessel invasion or poorly differentiated tumors. Nelson et al.[7] reported that 29% of patients with lesions smaller than 2 cm in diameter had evidence of lymph node metastasis. Thus, selection for local excision based on the classic indications will lead to inadequate treatment of a significant number of patients with lymphatic involvement. This makes the addition of adjuvant therapy to local excision a logical choice.

The incidence of lymph node metastasis in patients with T1 tumors approximates the recurrence rate for T1 cancers treated by local excision alone. Some studies describe a 3% to 10% rate of local recurrence after excision alone.[8] Survival rates in patients with T1 rectal carcinomas treated with local excision alone or radical resection are 90% to 100%.[9] Local excision alone is a reasonable treatment for T1 carcinoma of the rectum if the tumor meets the previous selection criteria. A caveat is that blood vessel or lymphatic invasion is a significant predictor of lymph node involvement and poor survival. In such cases, either standard surgical therapy involving total mesorectal excision or, if the patient refuses or cannot tolerate standard surgical therapy, the use of adjuvant therapy after local excision should be considered.

In patients with T2 rectal carcinomas, the risk of lymph node metastasis is 10% to 30%.[5,6] However, local excision procedures preclude lymph node excision. Studies show higher local recurrence rates for tumors involving the muscularis propria that are treated with local excision alone, possibly because of the failure to treat these lymphatic metastasis. Recurrence rates range from 17% to 24% in patients with T2 tumors. Survival rates are 78% to 82% with excision alone. In patients with T2 carcinomas of the rectum, the risk of lymph node metastasis in the mesorectum must be addressed by either resection of the mesorectum during proctectomy or, if a local excision is done, the addition of concomitant chemotherapy and radiation therapy to reduce the incidence of pelvic recurrence.

Many studies, mostly retrospective and single-institution, have examined the results of local excision alone in the management of T1/T2 rectal cancer. In a review of all published series of reasonable follow-up in which this approach was used, Graham et al.[8] found the combined local recurrence rate for T1 lesions to be 5% (range 0%–12%) and for T2 lesions, 18% (range 8%–27%). The clinically significant rate of local recurrence, especially compared with lower rates of local recurrence in historical series of similar patients treated with APR (0%–10%),[9-11] has driven multiple studies examining the use of both postoperative radiotherapy and postoperative chemoradiation after local excision in selected patients.

In one of the first series with an adequately long follow-up, Bailey et al.[12] reported their experience with local excision between 1978 and 1988. Of the 64 study patients, 34 (54%) received postoperative radiotherapy, and 2 of those (5.9%) had local recurrences. The crude 5-year survival rate in this series was 74.3% and the 5-year disease-specific survival rate, 90.3%. This study provided some of the first indirect evidence regarding the long-term efficacy of adjuvant radiotherapy and demonstrated the need for long-term follow-up to determine accurate rates of survival and local recurrence.

In a similar report from the Massachusetts General and Emory University Hospitals, 52 patients were treated with local excision alone, while 47 patients were given postoperative adjuvant radiotherapy.[13] Although the patients chosen to receive postoperative radiotherapy were at higher risk of local failure because they had higher-stage lesions than the patients treated with local excision alone (70% T2 vs. 15% T2, respectively), 5-year local recurrence–free survival (LRFS) and disease-free survival (DFS) rates were significantly better in the patients who received adjuvant therapy (LRFS 10% vs. 28%; DFS 74% vs. 66%). The median follow-up in this study was 51 months. The authors also reported trends, although not statistically significant, toward improved survival and less local recurrence in a subgroup of patients given 5-fluorauracil–based chemotherapy in addition to adjuvant radiotherapy. The authors concluded that adjuvant chemoradiation should be offered to all T2 patients undergoing local excision as well as all T1 patients with high-risk histologic features (advanced grade or lymphatic/vascular invasion).

A prospective series from The University of Texas M. D. Anderson Cancer Center reported excellent local control rates for 46 patients treated with local excision and postoperative chemotherapy or radiation therapy.[14] T3 tumors were also treated in this way in patients who were medically compromised or refused standard therapy. All tumors were less than 5 cm from the anal verge and smaller than 4 cm. All patients underwent negative-margin, full-thickness excisions via a transanal, transsphincteric, or posterior approach to the rectum. Postoperative radiation therapy (53 Gy) was given through posterior and two lateral fields. 5-Fluorouracil was given concomitantly during radiotherapy to eight patients with T3 lesions. The overall survival rate at 3 years was 93%. Table 59–2 shows the pattern of treatment failure by the American Joint Committee on Cancer (AJCC) T stage. Local recurrence–free survival at 3 years was 90%. None of the patients with T1 tumors demonstrated treatment failure. One of the patients with a T2 tumor and vascular and lymphatic invasion had simultaneous local and distant failure. Three of the 15 patients with T3 tumors had local failure as a component of their disease recurrence. T1 and T2 rectal carcinomas could be adequately controlled by this program of local excision and postoperative radiation, but not T3 tumors. An update of the M. D. Anderson Cancer Center experience with local excision seems to support these findings, with 4-year LRFS rates of 95%, 80%, and 73% for T1, T2, and T3 tumors, respectively.[3] Multivariate analysis found that only tumor stage and margin status were independent predictors for local recurrence.

Perhaps the best data regarding the modern-day approach to local excision for T1/T2 rectal cancer come from the initial results of a Cancer and Leukemia Group (CALG) prospective phase II trial.[15] This study enrolled patients who met the usual criteria for the local excision of distal rectal cancer: mobile tumors confirmed up to the rectal wall (T1/T2), less than 4 cm in size, less

**Table 59-3** Patterns of local recurrence after local excision with and without the use of postoperative radiotherapy

| Series | Patients (n) | Local Recurrence (n) | Local Recurrence >2 Years after Surgery n (%) |
|---|---|---|---|
| *Local Excision Alone* | | | |
| Chakravarti et al.[13] | 52 | 10 | 2 (20) |
| Bailey et al.[12] | 28 | 2 | 1 (50) |
| Willett et al.[16] | 40 | 6 | 1 (17) |
| Biggers et al.[17] | 141 | 36 | 4 (11) |
| *Local Excision + Postoperative Radiotherapy* | | | |
| Chakravarti et al.[13] | 47 | 8 | 6 (75) |
| Bailey et al.[12] | 34 | 2 | 1 (50) |
| Willett et al.[16] | 26 | 4 | 2 (50) |

than 40% of the bowel wall circumference in size, and with no evidence of lymph node involvement. Patients were registered after a negative-margin, full-thickness local excision. Patients with T1 tumors received no further treatment, while patients with T2 tumors received adjuvant chemoradiation therapy. Recognizing the impracticality of using a randomized clinical trial to directly compare local excision with more radical locoregional procedures, the authors conducted this phase II trial with three main goals:

1. To determine whether survival of patients with T1 and T2 adenocarcinoma of the rectum who are treated with limited, sphincter-sparing surgery is comparable to that of historical controls treated with APR
2. To assess the locoregional recurrence rate of rectal cancer as a function of tumor stage
3. To assess the toxicity of combining limited, sphincter-sparing surgery with postexcisional radiation and concurrent chemotherapy in the treatment of stage T2 low-lying adenocarcinomas of the rectum.

A total of 110 eligible patients completed the study protocol (59 with T1 tumors and 51 with T2 tumors). The 6-year overall and disease-free survival rates were 85% and 78%. Overall, nine patients (2 T1, 7 T2) had local recurrence of disease, and four of them died of the disease. Perioperative morbidity was minimal. Although further follow-up is necessary to confirm these findings, the authors concluded that this treatment approach is reasonable in this carefully selected group of patients.

Patterns of disease recurrence provide some biological insight into the effectiveness of local excision in patients with T1/T2 tumors treated with or without postoperative adjuvant therapy. Table 59–3 shows the timing of local recurrence in selected large series of patients who did or did not receive postoperative radiotherapy. As the data suggest, postoperative radiotherapy seems to result in a shift toward later local failure when compared with local excision alone. In the combined experience of Massachusetts General and Emory University Hospitals, the median time to local recurrence was 13.5 months for patients treated with local excision alone and 55 months for patients treated with postoperative radiotherapy.[13] This finding not only emphasizes the clinical importance of extended follow-up in these patients but also reinforces the need for any studies in which local excision and postoperative radiation are used to provide long-term follow-up.

In examining outcome among any groups of rectal cancer patients treated with local excision, regardless of the use of adjuvant therapy, two critical questions must be addressed:

1. How often can locoregional recurrence be treated effectively with further surgery?
2. How effective is such surgery?

**Table 59-2** Patterns of failure by American Joint Committee on Cancer T stage of disease after local excision and adjuvant therapy

| | T1 (n = 16) | T2 (n = 15) | T3 (n = 15) | Total (n = 46) |
|---|---|---|---|---|
| Local recurrence only | 0 | 0 | 2 | 2 (4%) |
| Distant recurrence only | 0 | 0 | 4 | 4 (7%) |
| Combined recurrence | 0 | 1 | 1 | 2 (4%) |

From Ota DM, Skibber JM, Rich TA. M. D. Anderson Cancer Center experience with local excision and multimodality therapy for rectal cancer. Surg Clin North Am 1:147–152, 1992.

**Table 59-4** Surgical salvage of locoregional recurrence after local excision of T1/T2 rectal carcinoma

| Series | Patients (n) | LR[a] (n) | Salvaged[b] n (%) | Salvage Procedure | Outcome |
|---|---|---|---|---|---|
| Chakravarti et al.[13] | 99 | 18 | 10 (56) | 9 APR | 5 DOD |
| | | | | 1 Exenteration | 3 DOC |
| | | | | | 2 NED |
| Wong et al.[18] | 25 | 6 | 5 (83) | 4 APR | 3 DOD |
| | | | | 1 Exenteration | 2 NED |
| Steele et al.[15] | 59 (T1) | 3 | 2 (67) | All APRE | 1 DOD |
| | 51 (T2) | 7 | 7 (100) | All APR | 3 DOD |
| | | | | | 4 NED |
| Bailey et al.[12] | 53 | 4 | 3 (75) | 2 APR | 1 DOD |
| | | | | 1 LE | 2 NED |
| Bleday et al.[19] | 48 | 4 | 3 (75) | All APR | 1 DOD |
| | | | | | 1 AWD |
| | | | | | 1 NED |
| Valentini et al.[20] | 21 | 3 | 2 (67) | All APR | 1 DOD |
| | | | | | 1 NED |
| Taylor et al.[21] | 47 | 17 | 7 (50) | 5 APR | 3 DOD |
| | | | | 2 LE | 1 AWD |
| | | | | | 3 NED |
| Bouvet et al.[3] | 90 | 11 | 5 (45) | All APR | All ED |

Abbreviations: APR, abdominoperineal resection; AWD, alive with disease; DOC, dead of other causes; DOD, dead of disease; LE, local excision; NED, no evidence of disease.

[a]Local recurrences (LR) alone and combined with distant recurrences.

[b]Number of potentially curative (margin-negative) salvage procedures.

[c]Five patients had T3 tumors.

Unfortunately, the published experience addressing these two questions is based on small numbers of patients who had recurrent disease after local excision, and thus it is difficult to make definitive conclusions. Results of attempted salvage patients with local recurrence after local excision (with or without adjuvant therapy) are summarized in Table 59–4. In these combined series comprising 493 patients, 73 patients suffered local failure either alone or in combination with distant disease. In 44 (60%) of these patients, a potentially curative, margin-negative salvage procedure had been performed, most often by APR. Of these 44 patients, 21 (48%) had no evidence of disease at varying lengths of follow-up. Salvage seems to be possible in more than half of patients with isolated local failure after local excision; however, more than 50% of those patients will eventually die of their disease. Therefore, it appears that the argument for a liberal approach to selecting patients for local excision based on good salvage potential in patients whose disease recurs is not supported by the literature.

Baron et al.[22] examined the issue of salvage after local excision at the Memorial Sloan-Kettering Cancer Center. They compared the outcome in 21 patients who had undergone local excision followed by immediate APR or low anterior resection (LAR) for tumors with adverse histological features with the outcome in 21 patients who underwent local excision followed by salvage LAR or APR at the time of clinical local recurrence. Disease-free survival was significantly improved in the patients undergoing immediate LAR or APR (94.1% vs. 55.5%, $P < 0.05$), a finding that again emphasizes that salvage after local excision does not seem to be an optimal strategy.

Alternative forms of local therapy for T1 and T2 rectal cancer have been reported, including endocavitary irradiation, fulguration, cryosurgery, and Nd:YAG laser therapy.[23] Of these modalities, endocavitary irradiation has received the most attention. In Papillon's[24] initial experience with this technique in 1972, the local recurrence rate was 7% and the 5-year overall survival rate was 72% among a selected, low-risk group of patients. The potential advantage of endocavitary irradiation over external beam radiotherapy is the ability to deliver a higher dose of radiation in a more concentrated fashion to the tumor. Both Papillon and others have subsequently reported similar results, again among highly selected low-risk patients.[25–27] Birnbaum et al.[28] identified "ideal" characteristics of rectal lesions for treatment by combination endocavitary and external beam irradiation (Table 59–5). Among 72 patients, they found that recurrence was significantly less likely in those patients with "ideal" tumors/than in those with non-ideal tumors (15% vs. 48%, $P = 0.01$). These authors stressed the importance of careful clinical and endorectal ultrasound staging to identify patients ideally suited to this treatment approach.

Transanal endoscopic microsurgery (TEM), in which either submucosal excision (for adenomas) or full-thickness excision (for invasive carcinomas) is performed though an operating rectoscope, has recently emerged as an option for the local treatment of rectal cancer.[29,30] Proponents of this approach claim that it allows improved exposure over the transanal approach without the small, but undeniable, risk of fecal fistula or sphincter dysfunction of the posterior or transsphincteric proctotomy. In a recent series, local recurrence occurred in 2 of 16 patients (12.5%)

**Table 59-5** Ideal characteristics of rectal cancer lesions for combination endocavitary and external beam radiation

Well or moderately differentiated
Mobile
Not ulcerated
<3 cm in diameter
<12 cm from the anal verge

From Birnbaum EH, Ogunbiyi OA, Gagliardi G, et al: Selection criteria for treatment of rectal cancer with combined external and endocavitary radiation. Dis Colon Rectum 42:727–733, 1994.

with T1 lesions undergoing TEM.[29] However, the authors of this series thought that TEM alone was not appropriate treatment for T2 lesions. Further follow-up and experience are required to establish a role for TEM.

Patients with T3 carcinoma of the rectum are considered at high risk for local recurrence, lymph node metastasis, and distant metastasis. Reported series show that local excision alone for T3 carcinomas results in an unacceptably high recurrence rate. Trials of adjuvant chemotherapy and radiation therapy used with radical surgical treatment for these high-risk tumors have demonstrated that patients benefit from the addition of chemotherapy and radiation therapy. The use of chemotherapy and radiation therapy in patients with T3 rectal cancers undergoing local excision also improves local control when compared with excision alone. However, this control is not equivalent to the control that can be obtained by more radical surgical procedures and adjuvant therapy. Patients with T3 tumors who are selected for local excision often are poor candidates for more extensive surgical procedures because of comorbid disease, and their options are therefore limited. It would seem reasonable to use adjuvant chemotherapy and radiation therapy in addition to local excision in patients with T3 rectal cancer.

Neoadjuvant therapy in patients with T3 rectal carcinomas can decrease the size and penetration of these lesions and sterilize regional lymph nodes. This is an important consideration because most patients with T3 rectal cancer will not be candidates for local excision strictly on the basis of lesion size. Preoperative chemoradiation therapy can reduce the incidence of positive lymph nodes in patients with T3 carcinomas and can result in a significant rate of complete pathologic responses. Despretz et al.[31] reported results in 25 patients with rectal cancer treated with preoperative external radiation therapy (35 Gy) followed by local excision and brachytherapy. Local recurrence developed in 5 of the 25 patients. Mohiuddin et al.[32] reported results in 14 patients who underwent preoperative radiation (45 Gy) followed by full-thickness excision; local recurrence developed in 3 patients. In general, complete response rates are higher in patients treated with preoperative chemotherapy and radiation therapy than in those treated with preoperative radiation therapy alone. We are examining our own experience with patients undergoing chemoradiation therapy and subsequent local excision of T3 tumors. This approach seems to be technically feasible but should be considered only for patients with T3 tumors who are not candidates for a more standard surgical approach.

For patients with T3 carcinomas, it seems that postoperative chemotherapy and radiation are required after local excision. The preoperative use of chemotherapy and radiation therapy to downstage the disease and permit a more satisfactory local excision may be feasible. Since this approach has not yet been validated, it should be considered only for medically compromised patients with T3 rectal cancer.

In summary, radical locoregional resection remains the surgical treatment of choice for many patients with T1 or T2 adenocarcinoma of the rectum. However, with careful selection, patients can be reasonably treated with local excision. Moreover, some patients who undergo local excision for T1 low rectal cancer and have no adverse prognostic characteristics can avoid subsequent adjuvant therapy. For patients with T1 tumors with adverse pathologic characteristics (vascular or lymphatic invasion) or T2 tumors, the increased risk of lymph node metastasis seems to justify the use of adjuvant radiation therapy if local excision is used, although validation of this approach awaits further follow-up of patients in the current national registry. Patients with

adverse characteristics found on local excision should undergo standard surgical therapy.

## Locoregional Resection for Rectal Cancer

Patients with stage II or III rectal cancer (60%–80% of patients with rectal cancer) have tumors that are large and biologically aggressive. Disease at this stage carries a higher risk of local and systemic recurrence after treatment. Accordingly, strategies have been developed to address these issues through locoregional resection and multimodality therapy. However, adequate surgical resection and choice of technique are the most critical treatment factors determining patient outcome.

The surgical management of stage II and III tumors is based on the following issues: (1) the importance of the lateral spread of rectal cancer in local tumor recurrence; (2) the need for total mesorectal excision to minimize pelvic recurrence; (3) restoration of function by coloanal anastomosis after resection of low rectal cancers; and (4) optimization of bowel function and quality of life after low rectal anastomosis. Surgical management cannot be separated from the use of preoperative or postoperative chemoradiation for most patients with stage II or III rectal cancer, as will be discussed later in this chapter.

The risk of spread to local lymph nodes and the risk of local recurrence increase as tumor penetration of the rectal wall increases. This has led to the development of operations such as the APR that achieve tumor-free proximal and distal tissue margins and remove the upward pathways of lymphatic spread from rectal cancer.[33] The distal margin has been shown to be adequate when it is 2 cm from the edge of the tumor.[34,35] However, more recently, the work of Quirke and others has dramatically demonstrated the importance of lateral tumor spread in the local recurrence of resected rectal cancers.[36–38]

The pelvis confines the rectum by its bony sidewalls, with major blood vessels, pelvic organs, lymph nodes, and nerves encroaching on the circumference of the rectum and mesorectum. While all of these confining structures are important to functional well-being, they allow little room for obtaining wide margins of normal tissue around a transmural rectal tumor, especially when the tumor is located anteriorly. Among patients with local recurrence, tumor involvement at the circumferential margin of resection has been found in 85% of cases.[36] While distal margins are measured in centimeters, circumferential margins are often measured in millimeters. Because of problems in obtaining adequate exposure in the low pelvis and surrounding structures, circumferential margins around rectal cancers can be highly variable and minimal. In this regard, surgeon experience and surgical technique play key roles in the prevention of local recurrence. Controlled sharp dissection must be done with close attention to these margins. Involvement of the circumferential margins can result from direct spread, mesenteric implants, vascular or lymphatic invasion, or cancer-bearing lymph nodes.[37] Tumor involvement of the circumferential margins of resection is frequently due to spread in the mesorectum distal to the tumor (Table 59–6).[38] This factor is an important cause of involvement of the radial margin. If luminal resection margins are limited to 2 cm beyond the tumor, then it becomes critical to completely resect the mesorectum beyond this limit to eliminate this source of local recurrence. The long-term outcome is poor in the presence of a positive circumferential margin.[38]

Understanding the importance of the circumferential clearance of rectal tumors has affected the accepted surgical procedures for the management of rectal cancer. The mesorectum is

**Table 59–6** Importance of distal mesorectal spread in producing an involved radial margin

| Curative Resection Specimens (n = 20) | Distal Mesorectal Spread | Involvement of Radial Margin |
|---|---|---|
| 16 | Negative | 2 (13%) |
| 4 | Positive | 2 (50%) |

From Adam IJ, Mohamdee MO, Martin IG, et al. Role of circumferential involvement in the local recurrence of rectal cancer. Lancet 344:707–711, 1994.

the extension of the large bowel mesentery along the posterior wall of the rectum. This blood vessel– and lymph node–bearing structure is enveloped by the fascia propria of the rectum. Total mesorectal excision by full mobilization of the rectum along anatomic planes has been demonstrated to be effective in the surgical management of rectal cancer.[39] Dissection is carried out along areolar planes that allow for hemostasis, identification of important nerves, and prevention of violation of the visceral fascia investing the mesorectum. This type of surgical resection for rectal cancer minimizes the potential for an inadequate circumferential margin and thereby reduces the possibility of local recurrence.

McAnena and co-workers described the long-term outcome of 57 patients treated by this approach.[39] The mean follow-up was 4.8 years. Local recurrence was seen in only 3.5% of the patients, and overall 5-year survival rate was 81%. While these are commendable data, it should be noted that 31% of these patients had Dukes' A lesions, who experience local and distant failure less often than patients with Dukes' B and C lesions. It should also be noted that "serious" postoperative complications occurred in 17% of patients and that the diverting colostomies were not closed in six patients. In a subsequent larger review of their experience with total mesorectal excision for rectal cancer, MacFarlane and colleagues[40] studied 135 patients with Dukes' B and C rectal cancers who were treated with surgery only, by one surgeon (Heald), over a 13-year period with a mean of follow-up of 7.5 years. None of these patients received adjuvant radiation or chemotherapy, yet there was only a 5% local recurrence rate. Further long-term follow-up of a larger group of patients confirmed these findings by finding a 10-year local recurrence rate of 4% and a 10-year disease-free survival rate of 78%, although a slightly somewhat more liberal approach to adjuvant therapy has been recently adopted by Heald.[41] These results compare favorably with the results from the North Central Cancer Treatment Group study that forms the basis for current recommendations for adjuvant therapy in the United States.[42]

In North America, similar results have been obtained with high rates of local recurrence-free survival when a total mesorectal excision is done by meticulous sharp dissection along the pelvic sidewalls. Enker's report[43] on this subject called for full rectal mobilization along anatomic planes to obtain complete mesorectal excision. In a series of 42 men who underwent sphincter-preserving surgery for low rectal cancer with this technique, only one had local recurrence (median follow-up of 20 months). Moreover, potency was preserved in 88% of the patients. In this study, meticulous sharp dissection accomplished the goals of total circumferential clearance of the tumor and preservation of sexual function.

Lymphatic drainage of the rectum not only runs proximally along the inferior mesenteric vessels but also follows the middle rectal vessels to the lateral pelvic sidewall and into iliac nodes.

Wide pelvic lymphadenectomy has been proposed for the treatment of rectal cancer. Although there is little doubt that the presence of metastasis in such lymph nodes is a highly significant negative prognostic factor, there is no evidence to support a therapeutic benefit of the routine addition of extensive lymphadenectomy to standard locoregional procedures.[44–46] As the morbidity of this procedure is significant, with most patients suffering urinary dysfunction and impotence, pelvic lymphadenectomy cannot be recommended in any resectable rectal cancer surgical algorithm.

Both Heald and Enker have questioned the need for adjuvant radiation and chemotherapy when total mesorectal excision is performed on T3, N0, M0 rectal cancers. This controversial point may be answered through a proposed European trial involving surgeons trained in this technique. Fielding[47] reported on a 1995 conference that discussed the application of the surgical techniques proposed by Heald. Two issues were identified regarding the use of proper surgical technique to reduce the local recurrence of rectal cancer. Fielding states that it is "abundantly clear that in Europe and North America only a minority of patients with rectal cancer are treated by surgeons highly skilled in total mesorectal excision."[47] The answer by Norwegian surgeons has been to remove rectal cancer surgery from routine surgical teaching and to concentrate training in total mesorectal excision among specialized "gastrointestinal surgeons." In addition, they propose that the surgical specimens obtained by such surgeons be audited. Furthermore, in a region of Sweden where all rectal cancer surgery has been concentrated in one colorectal unit, survival seems to have improved and local recurrence rates have dropped.[48] Such an approach would be highly controversial in the United States given existing concerns over the fragmentation of general surgical training and current practice patterns.

Over the past 5 years, several studies have suggested that the surgeon's experience is an important prognostic factor in rectal cancer. In a population-based study of 683 patients, Porter and colleagues[49] found a significant local recurrence and survival advantage among the patients of surgeons with colorectal surgery fellowship training or surgeons with a higher caseload. In addition, a greater rate of sphincter preservation for low rectal cancer was also found to be associated with these surgeon groups. Other studies suggest that hospital volume, hospital type (university vs. community), and surgeon experience influence survival and recurrence outcomes.[50–52] These differences likely relate to technical factors, such as the difficulty of total mesorectal excision, that are difficult to identify even prospectively. What to do with these findings is a source of significant controversy.

Heald asserts that systemic micrometastasis in rectal cancer patients arise from local recurrence due to inadequate surgical clearance of the primary tumor.[53] He proposes a reduction in the use of systemic adjuvant therapy based on this concept. This idea directly conflicts with the studies that form the basis for adjuvant therapy recommendations in the United States. It also conflicts with the concept of the early systemic spread of biologically aggressive rectal cancer producing micrometastasis that are present at the time of the locoregional treatment of primary rectal cancers.

When a surgeon performs a total mesorectal excision as proposed by Heald and Enker to reduce local recurrence and improve survival in rectal cancer, the decision as to which surgical procedure to use remains. In general, three operative procedures can be performed, all of which conform to the principles of total mesorectal excision: LAR, APR, and total proctectomy with coloanal anastomosis (CAA). For rectal cancer patients, a major component of quality of life is sphincter preservation. This is simple to accomplish in middle and upper rectal cancers, for which LAR allows adequate removal of the tumor and surrounding lymphatics and end-to-end anastomosis. In patients with low rectal cancers that do not involve the levators or sphincters, the anus can still be spared by proctectomy and coloanal anastomosis. Preoperative chemoradiation may facilitate this. However, patients with levator or sphincter involvement are best managed by APR and permanent colostomy.

Low anterior resection involves the transabdominal resection of the rectum and mesorectum above the level of the levator ani complex. After complete mobilization of the rectum en bloc with the mesorectum, the rectum is divided at least 2 cm below the distal edge of the tumor (Figure 59–1). Although the length of mesorectal excision will exceed this, there is evidence that total mesorectal excision is not required for upper rectal cancers. Reconstruction of the rectum is then carried out between the completely mobilized left colon and the remaining rectal stump. The use of LAR in middle and selected low rectal cancer has increased over the past 30 years for two main reasons. First, the double-stapled technique has permitted an easier and lower anastomosis, with leak rates (clinical or radiographic) similar to or better than those obtained with handsewn techniques.[54–56] Second, although 5 cm was previously thought to be the minimum acceptable distal margin, acceptance of a 2-cm distal margin has allowed lower tumors to be resected by LAR.[34,35]

Abdominoperineal resection involves a combined transabdominal and perineal approach to complete resection of the rectum, mesorectum, levator muscles, and anus with formation of a permanent colostomy. The rectum and mesorectum are mobilized via an abdominal approach. A perineal approach is used to widely resect the levator complex and anus along with an appropriate margin of perianal skin. A permanent end colostomy is carried out. As sphincter preservation (by LAR and proctectomy with

CAA) has become increasingly popular both technically and oncologically, the overall proportion of rectal cancer patients undergoing APR has decreased.[48] However, APR remains the only surgical option for many patients with rectal cancer, specifically those with sphincter complex involvement, deep pelvic fixation, or limited preoperative sphincter function.

Although LAR and APR are the traditional methods of locoregional resection in rectal cancer, proctectomy with CAA has emerged as a well-accepted surgical option in carefully selected patients. This approach can spare patients a permanent colostomy while still producing good functional and cancer-related outcomes. A recent review of 117 patients from the Mayo and Cleveland Clinics provides a perspective on the utility of proctectomy and CAA for patients with low rectal cancer.[57] The patients were treated over a 10-year period (1981 to 1991). The median distance of the tumor from the anal verge was 6 to 7 cm. The technique that was used required complete mobilization of the rectum to the levators, transanal transection of the rectum, complete mobilization of the left colon, and endoanal anastomosis. The authors recommended loop ileostomy for most patients. The effectiveness of this procedure in preventing local recurrence was demonstrated by the low local recurrence rate of 7%. However, it should be noted that 46% of the patients in this series had stage I disease. This point is important when assessing the wider applicability of this technique. Fecal continence was satisfactory in 78% of cases, and overall bowel function seemed to be improved in patients who had a colonic J pouch reservoir created for the CAA. There were no surgery-related deaths. Early and late complications were related mainly to the anastomosis leaking (10%) and healing with a stricture (21%). The role of adjuvant therapy in the 43% of patients receiving radiation or chemotherapy could not be assessed.

A CAA is really an extension of a properly done LAR. The proctectomy is extended down to the level of the upper anal canal and levators. Lateral ligaments are divided with attention to obtaining an adequate radial margin and preserving the pelvic autonomic nerves. Performing the posterior aspect of the dissection initially may facilitate the more difficult anterior dissection. The dissection results in the complete exposure of the pelvic floor and complete excision of the mesorectum. The fully mobilized rectum can then be considered for amputation by either a transanal technique or transection at the upper end of the anal canal with a stapler. The reconstruction consists of delivering the mobilized left colon to the anal canal and performing an anastomosis with full-thickness sutures through the colon and internal sphincter. Alternatively, a stapled anastomosis may be done. A diverting stoma is then usually created. We tend to use a diverting ileostomy, which allows adequate fecal division.

Several groups have reported on patients who had a 6- to 10-cm colonic J pouch reservoir constructed with no additional risk or compromise of the anastomosis.[58] This technique is done in hopes of increasing the volume of the neorectum and thereby decreasing stool frequency. The formation of the colon pouch has been compared with the straight CAA in randomized clinical trials. Physiologic measures and short-term outcomes seem to be improved with the pouch, although these findings are disputed by some.[59,60] However, these differences in function may disappear with time.[61] It has also been suggested that a colonic J pouch may leak less because of improved vascular supply to the apex of the pouch.[62] In general, we try to use such a pouch in most patients undergoing CAA, although its use may be limited in patients with an inadequate length of colon or a small pelvis and a thick mesentery.

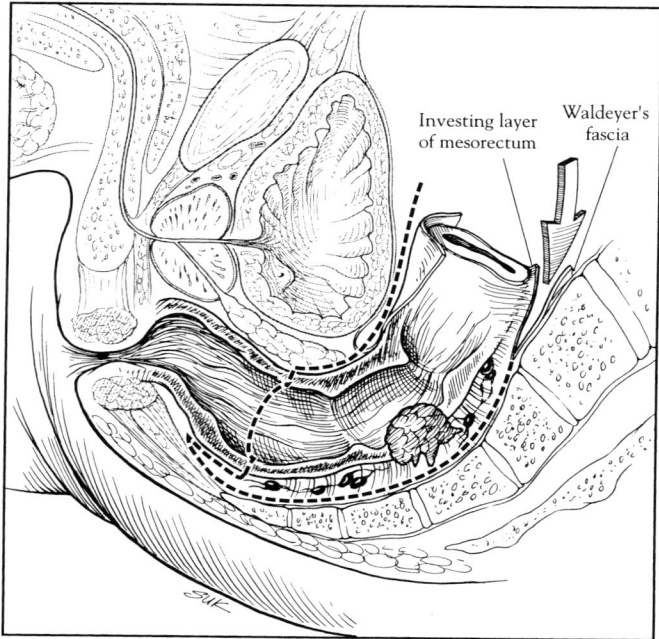

**Figure 59–1** Plane of dissection in total mesorectal excision. Note the plane is between the investing fascia of the mesorectum and Waldeyer's fascia. This entire dissection should be done in a sharp manner.

The results of a properly done CAA seem to be oncologically equivalent to those of APR in properly selected patients. Normal anorectal function returns in all but about 5% to 10% of patients. Pelvic infection rates are about 6%. Anal sphincter tone is usually preserved, and sensation and reflex inhibition of the anal sphincters can be retained.

Major long-term postoperative problems after CAA are related to rectal capacitance and compliance and manifest as urgency and frequency of bowel movements. These symptoms gradually improve over the 9 to 10 months after closure of the temporary stoma. Complete fecal continence is usually achieved in 85% to 100% of patients. Occasional soiling due to the inability to differentiate between gas and stool may occur in 10% of patients. In a series from the Mayo Clinic described by Drake and colleagues,[63] patients who had a CAA for malignancies had a stool frequency of 2.6 per 24 hours, and only 1 of 19 patients was incontinent.

Results from the Mayo and Cleveland Clinics study are similar to those of others describing proctectomy and CAA for rectal cancer.[64] In the absence of cancer recurrence or gross incontinence, patients are usually satisfied with the results, and the need for conversion to a permanent colostomy is rare. However, avoiding pelvic sepsis during the postoperative period is critical to reduce the risk of anal stricture, which is often untreatable and results in unsatisfactory function. Thus, proctectomy and CAA can be done on selected patients, with low local recurrence rates, acceptable functional results, and low mortality. While complication rates can be significant, the ability to preserve the sphincter when the only alternative is a permanent colostomy seems worthwhile in studies of long-term outcome.

There have been numerous studies comparing the oncologic results of APR with those of sphincter-preserving procedures (LAR or proctectomy with CAA). In a randomized clinical trial by the Gastrointestinal Tumor Study Group intended to examine the benefit of adjuvant therapy in rectal cancer, patients who underwent APR had a higher recurrence rate than did patients undergoing LAR ($P < 0.05$).[65] However, this probably reflected the presence of larger, more advanced tumors in the patients undergoing APR. Several other studies involving large numbers of rectal cancer patients have shown no significant differences in local recurrence or survival rates between patients undergoing APR and those undergoing sphincter preservation.[66–68] In summary, there is no evidence that, in appropriately selected patients, sphincter-preserving locoregional procedures compromise oncologic outcome.

## Adjuvant Therapy

The first adjuvant therapy in rectal cancer to be assessed for efficacy was postoperative radiotherapy. Both the Gastrointestinal Tumor Study Group and the National Adjuvant Breast and Bowel Project performed randomized clinical trials and found decreased local recurrence rates, but not improved survival, in stage II and III rectal cancer patients receiving postoperative radiotherapy compared with patients undergoing surgery alone.[65,69]

The addition of chemotherapy to postoperative radiotherapy seemed logical in an effort to influence the development of systemic disease. Indeed, current standards of care for high-risk (stage II and III) rectal cancer in the United States are based on a study conducted by the North Central Cancer Treatment Group.[42] Reported in 1991 by Krook and colleagues, this large, randomized trial for high-risk (stage II and III) rectal cancer patients compared postoperative fluorouracil and radiation with postoperative radiation alone. Reduced local recurrence, systemic recurrence, and cancer-related death as well as improved overall survival were seen in patients randomly assigned to receive chemotherapy in addition to postoperative radiotherapy. It appears that the improvement in local control accrued from the direct cytotoxic effects of the chemotherapy as well as from fluorouracil's radiation-sensitizing effects on residual microscopic disease in the pelvis. Clearly, the reduction in distant metastasis was the major factor in the overall improvement in survival; however, the effect of preventing pelvic recurrence on a patient's quality of life cannot be overlooked.

The next major step in adjuvant therapy for rectal cancer came from a report from an intergroup trial testing the role of protracted or continuous intravenous infusion of fluorouracil combined with radiation therapy as postoperative therapy. The rationale for this protocol was based on in vitro studies indicating that optimal cytotoxicity was obtained by continuous exposure of tumor cells to fluorouracil after irradiation.[70] A pilot study by Rich and co-workers[71] showed the regimen to be well tolerated during radiation therapy. In a trial of 680 patients, significant reductions were seen in overall rates of tumor relapse and distant metastasis.[18] Survival was significantly increased in those who received the protracted infusion of fluorouracil during irradiation. The protracted infusion did not appear to reduce the rate of local recurrence; however, analysis may have been hampered by the small number of local recurrences seen in the study.

As stated at the National Institutes of Health Consensus Conference (1990), a standard approach has emerged as the most widely used in North America.[72] This approach involves six cycles of 5-fluorouracil–based chemotherapy with concurrent pelvic radiotherapy (45–50 Gy) to all stage II and III rectal cancer patients following resection. The most significant advantage of this approach over a neoadjuvant approach is that stage is already known; thus patients with T1–2 N0 M0 tumors may be spared additional treatment.

## Neoadjuvant Therapy

The potential advantages of neoadjuvant over adjuvant therapy for resectable stage II and III rectal cancer can be classified as biological (improved tissue oxygenation, reduced potential for tumor implantation resulting from surgery), physical (no postsurgical fixation of the small bowel in the pelvis), and functional (ability to shrink the tumor and increased likelihood of sphincter preservation).[73] However, any randomized clinical trial comparing the postoperative and neoadjuvant approaches with adjuvant therapy is extremely difficult to conduct owing to the effect of preoperative treatment on pathologic staging and the difficulty of patient recruitment because of preexisting physician and patient biases.

Although there have been many randomized clinical trials comparing preoperative radiation with surgery alone, most of these trials did not use radiotherapy dosing strategies currently considered appropriate.[74–76] Among the studies taking a reasonable approach to radiotherapy, local recurrence seemed to be reproducibly reduced with preoperative radiotherapy compared to surgery alone.[77,78] However, more recently, the Swedish Rectal Cancer Study showed a significant improvement in local recurrence and survival with the use of a short course of radiotherapy vs. surgery alone.[79] Notably, patients in this trial did not receive chemotherapy, and the delivery of radiotherapy (25 Gy, given over 5 days beginning 1 week preoperatively) differed substantially from the delivery strategy traditionally used in North America (45–50 Gy, given over 25–30 days beginning 4–6 weeks preoperatively). Further follow-up from this study is needed to assess the risk of late toxicity due to the high-dose-per-fraction Swedish approach. A French study that examined the issue of interval between completion of radiotherapy and surgery found that a longer period was beneficial in terms of response and sphincter preservation.[80]

As previously described, there are many recent reports of highly selected patients with low rectal cancer undergoing sphincter preservation. However, it is uncertain whether this approach can or should be applied to the more common cases of stage III low rectal cancer. Efforts to widen the role of sphincter-preserving surgery to include those previously requiring APR have used preoperative radiation and, more recently, concurrent neoadjuvant chemoradiation.

Minsky and colleagues[64] reported on the efficacy and toxicity of preoperative radiation with proctectomy and CAA for low rectal cancer in patients who otherwise would have required an APR. Twenty-two patients with a diagnosis of invasive resectable T2 or T3, primary adenocarcinoma of the distal rectum (median distance from anal verge, 4 cm) were treated. All were believed to require APR as a standard operative approach. External beam radiation therapy was given to a total dose of 50.4 Gy. Four to 5 weeks later, resection was performed in 21 of the 22 patients. Ninety percent of those who had resection had a CAA as well. Ten percent of patients had a complete response. Therapy was well tolerated, and the anatomic leak rate was only 6%. Eighty-nine percent had a good or excellent functional result. Local failure alone occurred in 5%. These data reveal acceptable local control, survival, and functional results in selected patients treated with preoperative radiation therapy and proctectomy with CAA as an alternative to APR.

Numerous other single-institution reports have described similar results. For example, outstanding sphincter-preserving results in the treatment of low rectal cancers after preoperative radiation have been described by Marks and co-workers at Thomas Jefferson University.[81] They demonstrated long-term adequate sphincter function in 91% of patients, with local recurrence rates of less than 13%.

Preoperative radiation therapy does not appear to increase the morbidity of sphincter-preservation procedures. Bowel habits and sphincter function after preoperative therapy and surgery have been acceptable. This management approach to stage II and III rectal carcinomas whose distal edge is located 3 to 7 cm from the anal verge will be applicable to many more patients than will local excision techniques.

Considerable "downstaging" can occur after preoperative radiation or chemoradiation; however, this term is something of a misnomer. Radiation alone has produced complete pathologic response rates of 10% to 17%.[73,75,76] Concurrent preoperative chemoradiation has produced complete response rates of 20% to 30%.[82] Among patients who had tumors less than 7 cm from the anal verge and who underwent preoperative chemoradiation, Janjan and co-workers[83] found a high rate of sphincter preservation in patients who had a complete response compared with those who did not (53% vs. 38%). However, the meaning of a pathologic complete response for a patient in long-term follow-up is unclear, although preliminary evidence suggests that it may be a prognostic factor for improved survival.[84] Moreover, the absence of mucosal tumor clearly does not assure a complete response since residual tumor may be found within or beyond the rectal wall or within lymph nodes in the absence of residual mu-

cosal tumor.[82,84] Among 41 patients with partial or complete primary tumor response to preoperative chemoradiation, 9 (16%) were found to have metastatic disease in mesorectal lymph nodes.[84] Thus, the clinical tumor shrinkage induced by preoperative therapy does not necessarily "downstage" the disease. Obviously, shrinking the tumor may allow achievement of acceptable negative margins and may facilitate sphincter preservation. However, at this time the definition of "acceptable" margins after preoperative treatment is unclear and will require clinical trials and study.

Notably, preoperative chemoradiation can be given on an outpatient basis with virtually no increase in surgical complications. Preoperative chemoradiation therapy has been demonstrated to be less toxic than postoperative chemoradiation.[85] Minsky et al. reported that when identical chemoradiation regimens were given preoperatively or postoperatively, significantly fewer patients experienced grade 3 or 4 toxic effects when the adjuvant treatment was given preoperatively. In this study,[85] 13% of patients treated preoperatively experienced gastrointestinal toxicity, whereas 48% of patients treated postoperatively had grade 3 or 4 gastrointestinal or genitourinary toxic effects.

Rich and colleagues[86] reported on the outcome of 77 patients treated with preoperative chemoradiation therapy who then underwent resection of low rectal T3 cancers staged by ultrasonography.[86] The preoperative treatment was continuous-infusion fluorouracil (300 mg/m$^2$/day) given with daily irradiation (45 Gy in 25 fractions over 5 weeks). Surgery was performed 6 weeks later. Sphincter preservation was accomplished in 67% of these patients, in whom the mean distance of the tumor from the anal verge was 5 cm. A complete pathologic response was found in 29% and local recurrence in 4% of cases. Acute, perioperative, and late complications of treatment were not increased relative to historical data on the use of radiation alone.

Two other studies bring up issues regarding the functional outcome of sphincter preservation and the use of adjuvant therapy. Quality of life after rectal cancer treatment can be greatly affected by bowel function regardless of whether or not a stoma is present. If function is poor after sphincter-preserving surgery, then the patient's quality of life may be impaired more than if a permanent colostomy is present.[87] This issue will need to be addressed in future clinical studies. Kollmorgen and co-workers[88] studied the long-term effects of chemoradiation therapy on bowel function when this adjuvant therapy was given postoperatively. One hundred patients were studied after extensive exclusions were made to minimize confounding variables affecting outcomes. The group of patients that did not receive postoperative treatment uniformly had fewer problems with bowel function. In contrast, clustering of bowel movements, stool frequency, and fecal soiling were all increased when the reconstructed rectum was postoperatively irradiated (Table 59–7). As is clear from this study, long-term detrimental effects on bowel function can result from postoperative chemoradiation.

Further support for this conclusion can be drawn from the results of a study by Paty and colleagues on the functional outcomes of CAA for rectal cancer.[89] Postoperative radiation significantly increased the frequency of stools and significantly impaired the pattern of evacuation. These results imply that for patients who need adjuvant chemoradiation, it may be advantageous to deliver this therapy preoperatively. By not irradiating the rectal pouch used for reconstruction, subsequent problems with rectal compliance causing symptoms of urgency and frequency may be avoided. This issue is being addressed in current

**Table 59-7** Long-term effect of postoperative chemoradiation therapy on bowel function in rectal cancer patients

| Postoperative Therapy | Median Bowel Movements per Day (n) | Patients (%) | | | |
|---|---|---|---|---|---|
| | | Clustering of Bowel Movements | Occasional | Frequent | Urgency |
| None | 2 | 3 | 7 | 0 | 19 |
| Chemoradiation | 7 | 42 | 39 | 17 | 17 |

From Kollmorgen CF, Meagher AP, Wolff BG, Pemberton JH, Martenson JA, Illstrup DM. The long-term effects of adjuvant postoperative chemoradiotherapy for rectal carcinoma on bowel function. Ann Surg 220:676–682, 1994.

trials of preoperative and postoperative chemoradiation for low rectal cancer being done in the United States in which both quality of life and bowel function are being studied.

Sphincter preservation during multivisceral resections for locally advanced rectal cancer can be performed in patients who have involvement of adjacent pelvic organs. For this procedure, the surgeon must be prepared to resect adherent pelvic viscera or bone since "separating" adherent tumor from the sacrum or bladder is an assurance of local failure. Almost all patients who require multivisceral resections are treated preoperatively with radiation therapy or chemoradiation therapy, because of the limited ability to obtain negative margins in the confines of the pelvis even with multivisceral resections. The use of neoadjuvant therapy has markedly reduced local recurrence rates and improved sphincter-preservation rates even for fixed tumors. Selected patients may benefit from intraoperative radiation therapy or brachytherapy.[90]

Preoperative chemoradiotherapy does not appear to increase the morbidity of resection in patients with locally advanced rectal cancer.[91] The rectum can be reconstructed after multivisceral resections for rectal cancers without fear of compromising the oncologic outcome.[92] Resection of adjacent organs such as the bladder or uterus in addition to a large portion of the rectum leaves the pelvis quite empty. This added exposure is a double-edged sword; although the increased area in which to work in the pelvis increases the surgeon's ability to create a technically satisfactory anastomosis, the large empty space may contribute to postoperative pelvic infection or subsequent small bowel obstructions. One of the ways to fill this pelvic space is to reconstruct the rectum with either a remaining rectal stump or a coloanal anastomosis. Well-vascularized nonirradiated tissues such as the omentum or a rectus muscle flap may be placed in the pelvis to further fill the space and improve healing of the irradiated pelvic tissues. Such pelvic reconstruction can be performed safely with good functional results.[93]

In summary, adjuvant therapy has become an important tool in the management of stage II and III rectal cancer. Postoperative radiotherapy reduces the risk of local recurrence and, when combined with 5-fluorouracil–based chemotherapy, both improve survival and reduces local recurrence. Low-dose preoperative radiotherapy is ineffective, but moderate-dose radiotherapy in biologically similar regimens (45–50 Gy over 5–6 weeks or 25 Gy over 1 week) reduces local recurrence and may improve survival, although long-term follow-up for side effects of the high-dose-per-fraction technique is still required. Preoperative radiotherapy is more likely to be completed as planned and appears to be more efficacious and less morbid.[85,94] The ideal chemotherapeutic regimen, particularly in a neoadjuvant setting, has yet to be established, as many current recommendations are based on

experience with postoperative chemoradiation. Standard guidelines regarding the choice of preoperative vs. postoperative chemoradiation await the results of two ongoing randomized trials, although accrual to such trials is very difficult.

## References

1. Hargrove WC III, Gertner MH, Fitts WT Jr. The Kraske operation for carcinoma of the rectum. Surg Gynecol Obstet 148:931–937, 1979.
2. Bevan AD. Carcinoma of the rectum: treatment by local excision. Dis Colon Rectum 29:906–911, 1986.
3. Bouvet M, Milas M, Giacco G, et al. Predictors of recurrence after local excision and postoperative chemoradiation therapy of adenocarcinoma of the rectum. Ann Surg Oncol 6:26–32, 1999.
4. Nivatvongs S, Wolff BG. Technique of per anal excision for carcinoma of the low rectum. World J Surg 16:447–450, 1992.
5. Morson BC. Factors influencing the prognosis of early cancer of the rectum. Proc R Soc Med 59:607–608, 1966.
6. Minsky BD, Rich T, Recht A, Harvey W, Mies C. Selection criteria for local excision with or without adjuvant radiation therapy for rectal cancer. Cancer 63:1421–1429, 1989.
7. Nelson JC, Numr AN, Thomford N. Criteria for the selection of early carcinomas of the rectum. Arch Surg 122:533–536, 1987.
8. Graham RA, Gainsey L, Jessup JM. Local excision of rectal carcinoma. Am J Surg 160:306–312, 1990.
9. McDermott FT, Hughes ESR, Phil E, Johnson WR, Price AB. Local recurrence after potentially curative resection for rectal cancer in a series of 1008 patients. Br J Surg 72:34–37, 1985.
10. Sticca RP, Rodriguez-Gibas M, Penetrante RB, et al. Curative resection for stage I rectal cancer: natural history, prognostic factors, and recurrence patterns. Cancer Invest 14:491–497, 1996.
11. Wilson S, Beahrs O. The curative treatment of carcinoma of the sigmoid, rectosigmoid, and rectum. Ann Surg 183:556–563, 1976.
12. Bailey RH, Huval WV, Max E. Local excision of carcinoma of the rectum for cure. Surgery 111:555–561, 1990.
13. Chakravarti N, Compton CC, Shellitop C, et al. Long-term follow-up of patients with rectal cancer managed by local excisions with and without adjuvant irradiation. Ann Surg 230:49–54, 1999.
14. Ota DM, Skibber JM, Rich TA. M. D. Anderson Cancer Center experience with local excision and multimodality therapy for rectal cancer. Surg Clin North Am 1:147–152, 1992.
15. Steele GD, Herndon JE, Bleday R, et al. Sphincter–Sparing treatment of distal rectal cancer. Ann Surg Oncol 6:433–441, 1999.
16. Willett CG, Tepper JE, Donnelly S, et al. Patterns of failure following local excision and local excision and postoperative radiation therapy for invasive rectal adenocarcinoma. J Clin Oncol 7:1003–1008, 1989.
17. Biggers O, Beart RW, Ilstrup JM. Local excision of rectal cancer. Dis Colon Rectum 29:374–377, 1986.
18. Wong CS, Stern H, Cummings BJ. Local excision and postoperative radiation therapy for rectal carcinoma. Int J Radiat Oncol Biol Phys 25:669–675, 1993.
19. Bleday R, Breen E, Jessup JM, et al. Prospective evaluation of local excision for small rectal cancers. Dis Colon Rectum 40:388–392, 1997.
20. Valentini V, Morganti AG, DeSantis M, et al. Local excision and external beam radiotherapy in early rectal cancer. Int J Radiat Oncol Biol Phys 35:759–764, 1996.
21. Taylor RH, Hay JH, Larsson SN. Transanal local excision of selected low rectal cancers. Am J Surg 175:360–363, 1998.

22. Baron, PL, Enker WE, Zakowski MF, Urmacher C. Immediate vs. salvage resection after local treatment for early rectal cancer. Dis Colon Rectum 38:177–181, 1995.

23. Crile G, Turnbull RB. Role of electrocoagulation in the treatment of carcinoma of the rectum. Surg Gynecol Obstet 135:391–397, 1972.

24. Papillon J. Endocavitary irradiation of early rectal cancers for cure: a series of 123 cases. Proc R Soc Med 66:1179–1181, 1973.

25. Hull TLL, Saxton JP. Endocavitary irradiation: an option in select patients with rectal cancer. Dis Colon Rectum 37:391–398, 1994.

26. Myerson RJ, Ualz BJ, Kodner IJ, Fleshman J, Fri RD, Konefal JB. Endocavitary radiation therapy for rectal cancer: results with and without external beam. Endocurie/Hyperthermia Oncol 5:195–199, 1989.

27. Papillon JB. Endocavitary irradiation in the conservative treatment of adenocarcinoma of the rectum. World J Surg 20:644–650, 1992.

28. Birnbaum EH, Ogunbiyi OA, Gagliardi G, et al. Selection criteria for treatment of rectal cancer with combined external and endocavitary radiation. Dis Colon Rectum 42:727–733, 1994.

29. Saclarides TJ. Transanal endoscopic microsurgery: a single surgeon's experience. Arch Surg 133:595–599, 1998.

30. Buess G, Kipfmuller K, Ibald R, et al. Clinical results of transanal endoscopic microsurgery. Surg Endosc 2:235–250, 1988.

31. Despretz J, Otmezguine Y, Grimard L, Calitchi E, Julien M. Conservative management of tumors of the rectum by radiotherapy and local excision. Dis Colon Rectum 33:113–116, 1990.

32. Mohiuddin M, Marks G, Bannon J. High-dose preoperative radiation and full thickness local excision: a new option for selected T3 distal rectal cancers. Int J Radiat Oncol Biol Phys 30:845–849, 1994.

33. Miles WE. A method of performing abdomino-perineal excision for carcinoma of the rectum and of the terminal portion of the pelvic colon (1908). CA Cancer J Clin 2:716–720, 1971.

34. Wolmark N, Fisher B. An analysis of survival and treatment failure following abdominoperineal and sphincter saving resection in Dukes B and C rectal carcinoma: report of the NSAABP clinical trials. National Surgical Adjuvant Breast and Bowel Project. J Natl Cancer Inst 80:21–29, 1988.

35. Pollett WG, Nicholls RJ. The relationship between the extent of distal clearance and survival and local recurrence rates after curative anterior resection for carcinoma of the rectum. Ann Surg 198:159–163, 1983.

36. Quirke P, Durdy P, Dixon MF, et al. Local recurrence of rectal adenocarcinoma due to inadequate surgical resection: histopathological study of lateral tumor spread and surgical excision. Lancet 2:996–999, 1986.

37. Quirke P, Scott N. The pathologist's role in the assessment of local recurrence in rectal carcinoma. Surg Oncol Clin North Am 1:1–17, 1992.

38. Adam IJ, Mohamdee MO, Martin IG, et al. Role of circumferential involvement in the local recurrence of rectal cancer. Lancet 344:707–711, 1994.

39. McAnena OJ, Heald RJ, Lockhart-Mummery HE. Operative and functional results of total mesorectal excision with ultra-low anterior resection in the management of carcinoma of the lower one-third of the rectum. Surg Gynecol Obstet 170:517–521, 1990.

40. MacFarlane JK, Ryall RDH, Heald RJ. Mesorectal excision for rectal cancer. Lancet 341:457–460, 1993.

41. Heald RJ, Moran BJ, Ryall RD, Sexton R, MacFarlane JK. Rectal cancer: the Basingstoke experience of total mesorectal excision, 1978–1997. Arch Surg 133:894–898, 1998.

42. Krook JE, Moertel CG, Gunderson LL, et al. Effective surgical adjuvant therapy in high risk rectal carcinoma. N Engl J Med 324:709–715, 1991.

43. Enker WE. Potency, cure, and local control in the operative treatment of rectal cancer. Arch Surg 127:1396–1402, 1992.

44. Moreira LF, Hizuta A, Iwagaki H, et al. Lateral lymph node dissection for rectal carcinoma below the pentanol reflection. Br J Surg 81:293–296, 1994.

45. Hojo K, Koyama Y, Moriya Y. Lymphatic spread and its prognostic value in patients with rectal cancer. Am J Surg 144:350–354, 1982.

46. Glass RE, Ritchie JK, Thompson HR, Mumm CV. The results of surgical treatment of cancer of the rectum by radical resection and extended abdoiliac lymphadenectomy. Br J Surg 72:599–602, 1985.

47. Fielding LP. Optimizing surgical treatment of rectal cancer. Lancet 340:113–116, 1995.

48. Dahlberg M, Glimelius B, Pahlman L. Changing strategy for rectal cancer is associated with improved outcome. Br J Surg 86:379–384, 1999.

49. Porter GA, Soskolne CL, Yakimets WW, Newman SC. Surgeon–related factors and outcome in rectal cancer. Ann Surg 227:157–167, 1998.

50. Holm T, Johansson H, Cedermark B, et al. Influence of hospital- and surgeon-related factors on outcome after treatment of rectal cancer with and without preoperative radiotherapy. Br J Surg 84:657–663, 1997.

51. Hermanek P, Wiebelt H, Staimmer D, Riedle S. Prognostic factors of rectum carcinoma–experience of the German multicentre study SBCRC. Tumori 81:60–64, 1995.

52. Simons AJ, Ker R, Groshen S, et al. Variations in the treatment of rectal cancer: the influence of hospital type and caseload. Dis Colon Rectum 40:641–646, 1997.

53. Heald RJ, Husband EM, Ryall RD. The mesorectum in rectal cancer surgery—the clue to pelvic recurrence? Br J Surg 69:613–616, 1982.

54. Steichen FM, Rauitch MM. History of mechanical devices and instruments for suturing. Curr Probl Surg 19:1–52, 1982.

55. Beart RW Jr, Kelly KA. Randomized prospective evaluation of the EEA stapler for colorectal anastomoses. Am J Surg 141:143–147, 1981.

56. Docherty JG, McGreggor JR, Akyol AM, Murray GD, Galloway DJ. Comparison of manually constructed and stapled anastomoses in colorectal surgery. West of Scotland and Highland Anastomosis study. Ann Surg 221:176–184, 1995.

57. Cavaliere F, Pemberton JH, Cosimelli M, Fazio VW, Beast RW. Coloanal anastomosis for rectal cancer: long-term results at the Mayo and Cleveland Clinics. Dis Colon Rectum 38:807–812, 1995.

58. Lazorthes F, Fages P, Chiotasso P, Lemozy J, Bloom E. Resection of the rectum with construction of a colonic reservoir and coloanal anastomosis for carcinoma of the rectum. Br J Surg 73:136–138, 1986.

59. Hallbook O, Pahlman K, Kroj M, et al. Randomized comparison of straight and colonic J pouch after low anterior resection. Ann Surg 224:58–65, 1996.

60. Seow-choen F, Goh HS. Prospective randomized trial comparing J colonic pouch-anal amastomosis and straight coloanal reconstruction. Br J Surg 82:608–610, 1995.

61. Dehni N, Tiret E, Singland JD, et al. Long-term functional outcome after low anterior resection: comparison of low colorectal anastomosis and colonic J-pouch-anal anastomosis. Dis Colon Rectum 41:558–563, 1998.

62. Hallbook O, Johansson KS, Odahl R. Laser doppler blood flow measurement in rectal resection for carcinoma: comparison between the straight and colonic J pouch reconstruction. Br J Surg 83:389–392, 1996.

63. Drake DB, Pemberton JH, Beast RW, Dozois RR, Wolff BG. Coloanal anastomosis in the management of benign and malignant rectal disease. Ann Surg 205:600–605, 1989.

64. Minsky BD, Cohen AM, Enker WE, Sigurdson E. Phase I/II trial of preoperative radiation therapy and coloanal anastomosis in distal invasive resectable rectal cancer. Int J Radiat Oncol Biol Phys 23:387–392, 1992.

65. Gastrointestinal Tumor Study Group. Prolongation of the disease-free interval in surgically treated rectal carcinoma. N Engl J Med 312:1465–1472, 1985.

66. Paty PB, Enker WE, Cohen AM, Lauwers GY. Treatment of rectal cancer by low anterior resection with coloanal anastomosis. Ann Surg 219:365–373, 1994.

67. Zaheer S, Pemberton JH, Farouk R, et al. Surgical treatment of adenocarcinoma of the rectum. Ann Surg 227:800–811, 1998.

68. Williams NS, Johnston D. Survival and recurrence after sphincter saving resection and abdominoperineal resection for carcinoma of the middle third of the rectum. Br J Surg 71:278–282, 1984.

69. Fisher B, Wolmark N, Rockette H, et al. Postoperative adjuvant chemotherapy or radiation therapy for rectal cancer: results from NSABP protocol R-01. J Natl Cancer Inst 80:21–29, 1988.

70. Byfield JE, Calabro-Jones P, Klisak I, Kulhanian G. Pharmacologic requirements for obtaining sensitization of human tumor cells in vitro to combined 5-fluorouracil for ftorafur and X-rays. Radiat Oncol Biol Phys 8:1923–1933, 1982.

71. Rich TA, Lokich JJ, Chaffey JT. A pilot study of protracted venous infusion of 5-fluorouracil and concomitant radiation therapy. J Clin Oncol 3:402–406, 1985.

72. NIH Consensus Conference. Adjuvant therapy for patients with colon and rectal cancer. JAMA 264:1444–1450, 1990.

73. Cohen AM, Minsky BD, Schilsky RL. Cancer of the rectum. In: DeVita VT, Hellman S, Rosenberg SA (eds): Cancer: Principles and Practice of Oncology, 5th ed. Lippincott Raven, Philadelphia, 1997, pp 1197–1234.

74. Duncan W. Adjuvant radiotherapy in rectal cancer: the MRC trials. Br J Surg 72:559, 1985.

75. Rider WD, Palmer JA, Mahoney LJ, Robertson CT. Preoperative irradiation in operable cancer of the rectum: report of the Toronto Trial. Can J Surg 20:335–342, 1977.

76. Roswit B, Higgin GA Jr, Keehn R. Preoperative irradiation for carcinoma of the rectum and rectosigmoid colon: report of a National Veterans Administration randomized study. Cancer 35:1597–1602, 1975.

77. Gerard A, Buyse M, Nordlinger B, et al. Preoperative radiotherapy as adjuvant treatment in rectal cancer: Final results of a randomized study of the European Organization for Research and Treatment of Cancer (EORTC). Ann Surg 706:606–613, 1988.

78. Cedarmark B. The Stockholm II trial on preoperative short-term radiotherapy in operable rectal carcinoma: a prospective randomized trial. Proc Am Soc Clin Oncol 13:198, 1994.

79. Swedish Rectal Cancer Trial. Improved survival with preoperative radiotherapy in resectable rectal cancer. N Engl J Med 336:980–987, 1997.

80. Gerard JP. The use of radiotherapy for patients with low rectal cancer: an overview of the Lyon experience. Aust N Z J Surg 64:457–463, 1994.

81. Marks G, Mohuiddin M, Eitan A, Masoni L, Rakinic J. High-dose preoperative radiation and radical-sphincter preserving surgery for rectal cancer. Arch Surg 126:1534–1540, 1991.

82. Meterissian S, Skibber JM, Rich TA, et al. Patterns of residual disease after preoperative chemoradiation in ultrasound T3 rectal carcinoma. Ann Surg Oncol 1:111–116, 1994.

83. Janjan NA, Khoo, Abbruzzese J, et al. Tumor downstaging and sphincter preservation with preoperative chemoradiation in locally advanced rectal cancer: the M. D. Anderson Cancer Center experience. Int J Radiat Oncol Biol Phys 44:1027–1038, 1999.

84. Fleming J, Hunt K, Feig B, et al. Primary tumor response to preoperative chemoradiation does not ensure the absence of regional lymph node metastasis in patients with locally advanced rectal cancer (abstract 2082). Proceedings of 40th Meeting of the Society of Surgery of the Alimentary Tract, Orlando, FL, May 16–19, 1999.

85. Minsky BD, Cohen AM, Kemeny N, et al. Combined modality therapy of rectal cancer: decreased acute toxicity with the preoperative approach. J Clin Oncol 10:1218–1224, 1992.

86. Rich TA, Skibber JM, Ajani JA, et al. Preoperative infusional chemoradiation therapy for stage T3 rectal cancer. Int J Radiat Oncol Biol Phys 32:1025–1029, 1995.

87. Sprangers MAG, Taal BG, Aaronson NK, te Velde A. Quality of life in colorectal cancer: stoma vs nonstoma patients. Dis Colon Rectum 38:361–364, 1995.

88. Kollmorgen CF, Meagher AP, Wolff BG, Pemberton JH, Martenson JA, Illstrup DM. The long-term effects of adjuvant postoperative chemoradiotherapy for rectal carcinoma on bowel function. Ann Surg 220:676–682, 1994.

89. Paty PB, Enker WE, Cohen AM, Minsky BI, Friedlander-Kar H. Long-term functional results of coloanal anastomosis for rectal cancer. Am J Surg 167:90–95, 1994.

90. Weinstein GD, Rich TA, Shumate CR, et al. Preoperative infusional chemoradiation and surgery with or without an electron beam intraoperative boost for advanced primary rectal cancer. Int J Radiat Oncol Biol Phys 32:197–204, 1995.

91. Shumate CR, Rich TA, Skibber JM, Ajani JA, Ota DM. Preoperative chemotherapy and radiation therapy for locally advanced primary and recurrent rectal cancer: a report of surgical morbidity. Cancer 7:3690–3695, 1993.

92. Lowy AM, Rich TA, Skibber JM, Dubrow RA, Curley SA. Preoperative infusional chemoradiation, selective intraoperative radiation and resection for locally advanced pelvic recurrence of colorectal adenocarcinoma. Ann Surg 223:177–185, 1996.

93. deHaas WG, Miller MJ, Kroll WJ, et al. Perineal wound closure with the rectus abdominous flap following tumor ablation. Ann Surg Oncol 1:101–103, 1993.

94. Frykholm GJ, Glimelius B, Pahlman L. Preoperative on postoperative irradiation in adenocarcinoma of the rectum: final treatment results of a randomized trial and an evaluation of late secondary effects. Dis Colon Rectum 36:564–572, 1993.

# Chapter 60

# Clinical Aspects and Management of Rectal Adenocarcinoma
## *Management Options: Unresectable Rectal Carcinoma*

BRUCE D. MINSKY

In patients with primary, resectable (T3) rectal cancer, a significant improvement in local control and survival can be achieved with the use of radiation therapy plus 5-fluorouracil (5-FU)–based chemotherapy (combined-modality therapy).[1–3] It is more difficult to obtain these same results for patients with more advanced disease. For locally advanced or unresectable rectal cancers, collectively defined as T4 disease, there is no uniform way to determine resectability. Depending on the series, the tumor can vary from a tethered or "marginally resectable" cancer to a fixed cancer with adherence to, or direct invasion of, adjacent organs or vital structures. This has prognostic implications, since patients with gross invasion of tumor into vital pelvic structures may be approached in a palliative rather than a curative fashion. The definition of resectability also depends on whether the assessment is based on radiographic criteria, a clinical office examination, examination under anesthesia, or examination at the time of surgery. For example, tumors thought to be unresectable at the time of clinical or radiographic examination may be found to be more mobile when the patient is relaxed under anesthesia. There are also prognostic differences between primary and recurrent tumors, and many series do not report the results separately. The heterogeneity of the disease and absence of a uniform definition of resectability may explain some of the variation in results seen among the series.

Selected patients with primary unresectable disease may be cured with initial radical surgery such as a pelvic exenteration. These include patients with tumors invading the prostate, the base of the bladder, or the uterus where the disease can be resected en bloc with negative margins. Midline posterior tumors adherent to or invading the distal sacrum may be resectable for cure with an extended abdominoperineal resection (APR) that includes the sacrum. Even though these extensive cancers may be resected with negative margins with an exenteration, they still re-

quire combined-modality therapy to improve local control. In patients with recurrent unresectable disease, the tumor is commonly more locally extensive than indicated by physical and radiographic examinations. With the exception of a limited recurrence at the suture line, initial surgery in this group of patients will likely leave residual disease. Therefore, patients with primary or recurrent unresectable disease should receive preoperative combined modality therapy.

Physical examination, computed tomography (CT) scan, magnetic resonance imaging (MRI), and cystoscopy all have a role in staging the disease in these patients. Involvement of the sciatic notch, as indicated by symptoms or pelvic imaging, predicts a situation unlikely to be helped by surgery. With CT or MRI, recurrent pelvic tumor, especially following an APR, is difficult to differentiate from scar. Positron emission imaging (PET) may offer a more accurate assessment.[4]

## Preoperative Radiation Therapy

Since surgery commonly leaves residual disease in the pelvis in patients with T4 disease, the standard approach has been preoperative pelvic radiation therapy. Given the increased complete response[5] and resection[6] rates seen when 5-FU–based chemotherapy is added to adjuvant radiation in the preoperative setting, as well as the improvement in local control in the postoperative setting,[3] most patients with T4 disease receive combined-modality therapy. The primary goals of preoperative therapy are to convert an unresectable cancer into a resectable one and decrease the incidence of local failure.

The optimal use of preoperative radiation therapy requires full doses (45–50.4 Gy) using conventional fractionation (1.8–2.0 Gy/fraction) and, to achieve optimal downstaging, a 4- to 6-week delay between the completion of radiation and surgery.

The discussion below will be limited to series that meet these criteria.

In a seminal report from the Massachusetts General Hospital (MGH) of 25 patients with recurrent or primary unresectable cancer, complete resection with negative margins was possible in 64% following preoperative radiation therapy.[7] Despite negative margins, the incidence of local failure was 38%. The nine patients who were unable to undergo a complete resection were dead of disease within 28 months.

The British Medical Research Council completed a randomized trial of preoperative radiation therapy (40 Gy in 20 fractions) vs. surgery alone for 279 patients with clinical T4 primary rectal cancer.[8] Patients who received preoperative radiation had a significant decrease in local failure (36% vs. 46%, $P = 0.04$) and distant failure (35% vs. 48%, $P = 0.02$). There was an improvement in median survival (31 months vs. 24 months, $P = $ NS) but no difference in survival (32% vs. 28%). The 36% local failure rate following preoperative radiation is consistent with the MGH data and supports the need for additional treatment such as intraoperative radiation therapy.

As one would predict, the results of therapy in patients with primary disease are more favorable than in those with recurrent disease. In the MGH series, the rate of complete resection with negative margins was 59% for patients with primary cancers[9] compared with 44% for those with recurrent cancers.[10] Limiting the analysis to the most favorable group of patients (i.e., those with primary cancers and negative margins), the 5-year actuarial local failure rate was 29% and disease-free survival was 60%. Therefore, even in this most favorable group, local failure is still almost 30%. At the University of Florida, in the 48% of patients who were able to undergo a complete resection with negative margins, the local failure rate was 55% and the 5-year determinate survival was 20%.[11,12] Tobin and colleagues[13] reported a local failure rate of 20% and 5-year survival of 60% in 85 patients treated with preoperative radiation. At Memorial Sloan-Kettering Cancer Center, 58% of patients underwent a complete resection with negative margins following preoperative radiation, and the local failure rate was 25%.[14]

Tethered cancers have the most favorable outcome of all T4 cancers. In a separate report from the MGH, the results for 28 patients with tethered rectal cancers treated with preoperative radiation were presented.[15] "Tethered" cancers were defined as the partial tumor mobility by digital exam consistent with extensive perirectal spread and adherence but not fixation to unresectable structures. Although a complete resection with negative margins was possible in 93% of cases, the local failure rate was 24%. Tobin et al.[13] reported a local failure rate of 14% and a 5-year survival of 68% in 49 patients with tethered cancers treated with preoperative radiation.

In conclusion, following full-dose preoperative radiation, most series report that over 90% of patients with tethered disease and 48% to 64% of patients with unresectable disease will be converted to a resectable status. However, despite complete resection and negative margins, the local failure rate will vary, depending on the degree of tumor fixation, from 24% to 55%.

## Enhancing the Outcome of Preoperative Radiation Therapy

A major limitation of pelvic radiation therapy is that in many cases the dose required to achieve an adequate level of local control exceeds the tolerance of the surrounding normal tissues. In an attempt to improve the results of preoperative radiation, a number of approaches have been used. The most promising have included intraoperative radiation therapy (IORT) and the addition of systemic chemotherapy.

### Intraoperative Radiation Therapy

The primary advantage of IORT is that radiation can be delivered at the time of surgery to the site with the highest risk of local failure (the tumor bed) while decreasing the dose to the surrounding normal tissues. Intraoperative radiation therapy can be delivered by two techniques: electron beam and brachytherapy. With the electron-beam technique, the radiation is delivered by a linear accelerator and, with the use of a cone, is directed to the tumor bed. When the IORT is finished, the cone is removed and the surgery is completed.

Brachytherapy is delivered by using either a low-dose rate or high-dose rate (HDR) technique. The low-dose method involves implantation of radioactive sources with either removable iridium-192 afterloading catheters or iodine-125 or palladium-103 permanent seeds.[16] The permanent seeds can be sutured or implanted directly into the tumor. As an alternative, they can be placed in an absorbable mesh, which is then sutured to the tumor bed.[17] Most of the low-dose brachytherapy experience has been in patients with gross residual disease. Low-dose brachytherapy has also been used as an alternative to electron-beam IORT in patients with negative tumor margins.[18,19] High-dose rate brachytherapy utilizes a flexible multichannel applicator that conforms to the tumor bed. Once the applicator is positioned, an iridium-192 source is programmed to deliver a uniform dose to the area at risk at a dose rate similar to that used for electron-beam IORT.[19,20]

A technical advantage of brachytherapy is that, because of anatomic or technical constraints, there are virtually no clinical situations in which IORT cannot be delivered.[19] In contrast, anatomic or technical constraints prevented the delivery of electron-beam IORT in 10% of patients in the M. D. Anderson series[21] and in 9% of patients in the MGH series with recurrent[22] and primary unresectable disease.[23]

The results of IORT depend on whether the patient has primary unresectable or recurrent disease and whether the margins of resection are negative or there is microscopic or gross residual disease. The discussion below will be limited to patients who, in general, receive preoperative pelvic radiation with or without 5-FU–based chemotherapy. In general, most patients receive 45–50.4 Gy to the pelvis and 10–20 Gy IORT via either electron beam or with a flexible HDR applicator. The lower IORT doses are most commonly used for patients with negative tumor margins and the higher doses are used for patients with microscopic or gross residual disease.

#### Primary unresectable disease

The largest experience and longest median follow-up of patients receiving preoperative therapy followed by IORT has been reported by the MGH (Table 60–1).[23] In that series, local failure in patients with negative margins decreased from 18% without IORT to 11% with IORT. In patients with positive margins, local failure decreased from 83% without IORT to 43% with IORT if there was gross residual disease, and to 32% with IORT if there is microscopic residual disease. For all patients in the series (with or without IORT), the 5-year disease-free survival was 63% for patients with negative margins and 32% for patients with positive margins. These results underscore the importance of delivering preoperative therapy to help achieve the most complete

**Table 60-1** Selected series of patients with primary locally advanced/unresectable rectal cancer with or without intraoperative radiation therapy

| Series | Patients (n) | Follow-up (Months) | Preoperative Treatment[a] | IORT | Local Failure Margins — Negative | Local Failure Margins — Patients (n) | Local Failure Margins — Positive | Local Failure — Total | Survival Margins — Negative | Survival Margins — Positive | Survival — Total |
|---|---|---|---|---|---|---|---|---|---|---|---|
| Mayo Clinic[24] | 61 | 18 minimum | 45–55 Gy ± 5-FU / 10–20 Gy IORT | Yes | 18 6% crude / 7% 5-year | 19 (micro) / 16 (gross) | 5% crude / 16% 5-year / 25% crude / 27% 5-year | 13% crude | — | Gross 21% 5-year | 46% 5-year |
| MGH[23] | 145 | 41 median | 45–50.4 Gy ± 5-FU ± 10–20 Gy IORT | Yes | 45 11% 5-year | 21 (micro) / 7 (gross) / 28 total | 32% 5-year / 43% 5-year / 35% 5-year | DFS | 63% 5-year DFS | 32% 5-year | — |
| Heidelberg[25] | 40 | 18 median | 41.4 Gy + 5-FU / 10–18 Gy IORT | No / Yes | 66 18% 5-year | 6 total | 83% 5-year | — / 91% DFS | — / — | — / — | — |
| Memorial Sloan-Kettering[19] | 18 | 18 median | 50.4 Gy + 5-FU/LV / 10–20 Gy HDR IORT | Yes | 8% 2-year | | 62% 2-year | 19% 2-year | 77% 2-year DFS | 38% 2-year DFS | 69% 2-year |
| New England Deaconess[26] | 27 | 24 median | 50.4 Gy ± 5-FU / 12.5–17 Gy orthovoltage IORT | Yes | — | | — | 27% crude | — | — | 41% NED |
| Munich[20] | 19 | — | 39.6 Gy BID + 5-FU / 15 Gy HDR IORT | Yes | — | | — | 10% crude | — | — | — |

Abbreviations: BID, twice a day radiation; DFS, disease free survival; 5-FU, 5-fluorouracil; HDR, high-dose rate; IORT, intraoperative radiation therapy; LV, leucovorin; micro, microscopic; MGH, Massachusetts General Hospital; NED, no evidence of disease.

[a]In most patients.

resection as possible. If negative margins cannot be obtained, then microscopic residual disease is still preferable to gross residual disease. Reports from the Mayo Clinic[24] and Memorial Sloan Kettering[19] had similar local failure rates in patients with negative margins (7% and 8%, respectively). Other series from Munich,[20] Heidelberg,[25] and the New England Deaconess Hospital[26] have also been reported.

### Recurrent disease

In the setting of recurrent disease, the largest experience with IORT is that of the Mayo Clinic.[27] In contrast to the series of patients treated for primary unresectable disease, those series of patients with recurrent disease had less uniform treatment programs, including some who received prior pelvic radiation[22,27] and some who were treated with IORT alone.[19,28] Selected series are seen in Table 60–2.

At the Mayo Clinic, 119 patients received, in general, 50.4–54 Gy preoperatively followed by 7.5–20 Gy electron-beam IORT.[27] The higher IORT doses were used in patients with residual disease. For patients with negative tumor margins, the crude local failure rate was 6%. This increased to 18% for patients with microscopic residual disease and 25% for patients with gross residual disease. The 5-year actuarial local failure rates were 27% for patients with microscopic disease and 45% for patients with gross residual disease. For all patients in the series the overall 5-year survival was 20%. The M. D. Anderson,[21] Memorial Sloan-Kettering,[19,29] and the French IORT groups[30] reported similar local failure rates for all patients (36%, 37%, and 31%, respectively). In another series of 25 patients selected to receive IORT, the 5-year survival was 21%.[31]

In contrast, the results from the MGH were not as favorable.[22] The MGH reported a 5-year actuarial local failure rate of 89% for patients with gross residual disease and 70% for the total patient group. The 5-year disease-free survival was 21% for patients with negative margins and only 7% for those with positive margins. Investigators from Eindhoven also reported that compared with patients with negative or microscopic positive margins, patients with gross residual disease had significantly lower rates of 3-year actuarial local control (21% vs. 79%, P = 0.01), disease-free survival (11% vs. 54%, P = 0.0008), and overall survival (35% vs. 74%, P < 0.05).[32] The Memorial Sloan-Kettering series had a 2-year survival of 0% among patients with positive margins,[19,29] whereas the Heidelberg series had a 4-year disease-free survival of 29%.[33] In contrast to patients with recurrent disease who have negative or microscopically positive margins, it is unclear if those with positive margins benefit from aggressive therapy.

### Complications of electron-beam intraoperative radiation therapy

Initial reports of neuropathy, vasculitis, bone necrosis, and ureteral injury in canines who received IORT came from Gillette et al.[34,35] In two canine series, hyperthermia increased the neurological complications of IORT.[36,37] In another canine series, IORT induced secondary malignancies in 15% of cases, most of which occurred at doses greater than 25 Gy.[38]

As the IORT data have matured, similar morbidity rates have been reported in humans. The incidence of toxicity depends on whether the patient has primary or recurrent cancer. In the MGH IORT experience, the incidence of complications was higher in patients with recurrent disease (10% soft tissue or sacral injury and 10% pelvic neuropathy) than in those with primary disease (2% sacral necrosis or ureteral obstruction).[9,10] In the Eindhoven series, 16% of patients developed neuropathy, however, the neuropathy was grade 3 in only 3% of cases.[32]

Higher complication rates have been reported from the Mayo Clinic.[39] In patients with primary or recurrent colorectal cancer, the incidence of peripheral neuropathy was 32%. The symptoms of pain, numbness, and tingling resolved in 40% of patients. Weakness resolved in only 13%. Ureteral obstruction or hydronephrosis was seen in 63% of patients who had no evidence of ureteral obstruction at presentation. Although there was no relationship between the incidence of complications and the external-beam dose, the incidence of complications increased with the IORT dose.

In contrast to the situation in patients who undergo adjuvant therapy for resectable rectal cancers, it is difficult to clearly separate treatment-related complications from disease-related complications in patients with unresectable primary and/or recurrent rectal cancers. The total incidence ranges from 15% to 50% in most series and is highest in patients with the most advanced disease (recurrent unresectable). Complications such as delayed healing, an increase in infection, fistula formation, and neuropathy may be the result of recurrent tumor, aggressive surgery, radiation, or a combination of these. In a trial by the Radiation Therapy Oncology Group (RTOG 85-08), the 2-year actuarial risk of significant complications in 42 patients with advanced or recurrent rectal cancer who received IORT as a component of their therapy was 16%.[40] However, compared with a nonrandomized group of patients who underwent surgery without IORT, patients who received IORT had no significant increase in acute surgical complications.[41]

In summary, data from phase I/II trials suggest that the addition of IORT to preoperative radiation therapy with or without chemotherapy provides better local control than preoperative therapy alone. The results in the subset of patients with recurrent cancer and/or residual disease are still not optimal. Unfortunately, no phase III trials of IORT are in progress.

## Preoperative Combined-Modality Therapy

The encouraging results seen in patients with resectable rectal cancer who receive adjuvant postoperative combined-modality therapy[1–3] have resulted in a shift to preoperative combined-modality therapy. Determination of whether preoperative combined-modality therapy is more effective than preoperative radiation therapy in patients with T3 resectable disease is being addressed in an ongoing randomized trial from the European Organization for Research and Treatment of Cancer (EORTC). This trial will determine if bolus 5-FU/leucovorin administered either preoperatively and/or postoperatively is superior to preoperative radiation therapy alone.

There are a number of potential advantages of preoperative combined-modality therapy for the treatment of rectal cancer. First, nonrandomized data from Memorial Sloan-Kettering suggest that patients who receive such therapy are able to tolerate higher chemotherapy doses and experience significantly lower acute toxicity than those who receive postoperative combined modality therapy.[42]

Second, in patients with unresectable disease, the addition of chemotherapy to preoperative radiation therapy increases the downstaging and resectability rates.[5] Frykholm et al.[43] reported an enhanced resectability rate in patients with unresectable rectal cancer who received preoperative radiation therapy and 5-FU, methotrexate, plus leucovorin rescue compared to patients who received radiation alone (71% vs. 34%). Enhanced resectability

**Table 60-2** Selected series of patients with recurrent rectal cancer: intraoperative radiation therapy with or without pre- or postoperative therapy

| Series | Patients (n) | Follow-up (Months) | Preoperative Treatment[a] | Local Failure — Margins: Patients (n) Negative | Negative | Patients (n) Positive | Positive | Total | Survival — Margins: Negative | Positive | Total |
|---|---|---|---|---|---|---|---|---|---|---|---|
| Mayo Clinic[27] | 119 | — | 50.4–54 Gy 7.5–20 Gy IORT Some postop EBRT | 17 | 6% crude | 40 (micro) 65 (gross) | 18% crude 27% 5-year 25% crude 40% 5-year | 20% crude 37% 5-year | — | — | 20% 5-year — |
| MGH[22] | 41 | 31 median | 50.4 Gy ± 5-FU 10–20 Gy IORT Some prior EBRT | 27 | 58% 5-year (or micro) | 14 (gross) | 89% 5-year | 70% 5-year DFS | 21% 5-year DFS | 7% 5-year | 16% 5-year |
| Heidelberg[33] | 31 | 28 median | 41.4 Gy (22 preop) mean 13.7 Gy IORT | 14 | 21% crude 22% 4-year | 9 (micro) 8 (gross) | 33% crude 39% 4-year 37% crude 40% 4-year | 29% crude | 71% 4-year DFS | 29% 4-year DFS | 48% 4-year (DFS) 58% 4-year |
| Memorial Sloan-Kettering[19] | 46 | 18 median | (16) 50.4 Gy ± 5-FU/LV 10–20 Gy HDR IORT (25) 10–20 Gy IORT alone | — | 18% 2-year | — | 81% 2-year | 37% 2-year DFS | 71% 2-year DFS | 0% 2-year | 47% 2-year |
| New England Deaconess[26] | 13 | 24 median | 50.4 Gy ± 5-FU 12.5–17 Gy orthovoltage IORT | — | | — | | 73% | — | — | 27% NED |
| French IORT Group[30] | 73 | 30 median | (30) 39 Gy ± 5-FU 10–15 Gy IORT (43) 10–15 Gy IORT alone | — | | — | | 31% 3-year (57% margins–) | — | — | 31% 3-year |
| M. D. Anderson Cancer Center[21] | 43[b] | 26 median | 45 Gy + 5-FU ± CDDP 10–20 Gy IORT | — | | — | | 36% | — | — | 3 7% 5-year (DFS) 58% 5-year |
| Eindhoven[32] | 37 | 37 mean | (17) 50.4 Gy preop 10 Gy IORT (5) 30 Gy reirradiation 15 Gy IORT (15) 17.5 Gy IORT | 15 | 13% crude | 8 (micro) 14 (gross) | 13% crude 43% crude | 24% crude 40% 3-year | — | — | 32% 3-year (DFS) 58% 3-year |

Abbreviations: DFS, disease free survival; EBRT, external-beam pelvic radiation therapy; 5-FU, 5-fluorouracil; HDR, high-dose rate intraoperative radiation therapy; IORT, intraoperative radiation; MGH, Massachusetts General Hospital; micro, microscopic.

[a]In most patients.

[b]Excluding 10 patients with multifocal or extrapelvic disease.

is an important end point, since patients with initially unresectable rectal cancer who have microscopic or gross residual disease have higher local failure and lower survival rates than those patients who undergo a complete resection with negative margins.[23,24,27]

The third advantage of treating rectal cancer with preoperative combined-modality therapy is that there is no delay in starting systemic therapy. The metastatic burden is smaller, and few drug-resistant cells are likely to be present.[44]

The fourth advantage is that sphincter preservation is more likely. For patients with clinically resectable disease, the primary goals of preoperative therapy are local control and sphincter preservation. In contrast, for patients with unresectable disease, the primary goals are local control and increasing the chance of a complete resection with negative margins. However, sphincter preservation is still possible in such patients.

Series assessing the ability of preoperative therapy to convert an operation from an APR to a sphincter-sparing procedure are limited to patients with T2–3 clinically resectable disease. This requires a pretreatment prospective clinical assessment. The operating surgeon examines the patient prior to the start of preoperative therapy and determines the type of operation required. In this setting, sphincter preservation rates of approximately 75% have been reported.[45] None of the series that include patients with T4 disease have used a preoperative assessment. Therefore, it is not possible to accurately determine the impact of preoperative therapy on enhancing sphincter preservation in the subset of patients with T4 disease.

The presence of T4 disease is not, by itself, a contraindication to sphincter preservation. Sphincter preservation rates following preoperative therapy in patients with primary unresectable disease are 29% at the MGH[23] and 50% at Memorial Sloan-Kettering;[46] the rate in patients with recurrent disease at the M. D. Anderson is 48%.[21] However, in patients who undergo more aggressive approaches, including extensive pelvic operations and IORT, function results may not be satisfactory.[47]

A large experience with preoperative radiation therapy at the Thomas Jefferson University has been reported.[48] In tumors located in the distal 2 cm of the rectum, 91% of patients had sphincter-preserving surgery, and 86% had "satisfactory" functional results. Since this trial included patients with early-stage disease (T1) as well as patients with unresectable (T4) disease, the results are not comparable with those in other series that include only patients with T4 disease.

There have been a number of phase I/II trials of preoperative combined modality therapy in patients with T4 disease.[19–27,30,33,46,49–52] Some included patients with T3 disease, thereby making interpretation of the local control and survival results difficult.[12,48,53] Most of these trials have used 45–50.4 Gy of pelvic radiation at 1.8–2.0 Gy/fraction plus two cycles of concurrent 5-FU–based chemotherapy with bolus 5-FU/leucovorin or continuous infusion 5-FU, followed by surgery and an additional four cycles of postoperative chemotherapy. Most of these studies have been discussed above in the section on IORT (Tables 60–1 and 60–2). Some have used methotrexate[54] or interferon.[55] Marsh et al.[12] have combined chronobiologically shaped 5-FU infusion with preoperative radiation therapy. Phase I/II trials examining the use of newer chemotherapeutic agents,[56] such as Tomudex,[56–59] oral UFT/leucovorin,[60] CPT-11,[61,62] oxaliplatin, and capecitabine with preoperative radiation therapy are in progress. Whether any of these combinations will be more effective than 5-FU–based therapy remains to be determined.

## Correlation of Response of Primary Tumor and Outcome

Most studies involving patients with T3 disease suggest that with an increase in the response rate of the primary tumor comes a corresponding increase in the ability to perform sphincter-preserving surgery. Yet, the degree to which response rate predicts outcome and the decision as to whether the subset of patients who achieve a complete response still require radical surgery are controversial. Furthermore, most studies do not report the results for patients with T3 and T4 disease separately, thereby making the data difficult to interpret.

Kaminsky-Forrett et al.[63] studied 88 patients who had clinical T3–4 rectal cancers and received preoperative radiation therapy with or without 5-FU/leucovorin. They noted a decrease in local failure (4% vs.15%) and a significant increase in 5-year cancer-specific survival (100% vs. 45%, $P = 0.01$) in patients who achieved a complete or near-complete response (pathologic stage T0–2 N0 disease) compared with those who achieved less of a response (pathologic stage T3–4 and/or N1–2).[63] In a series of 315 patients with clinical T3–4 disease who received preoperative radiation, Ahmad and colleagues[64] reported a 5-year actuarial local control rate of 96% and a 91% survival rate in the subset of 49 who achieved a complete response. Similar data were reported by Guillem et al.[65]

Two studies have examined whether surgery is still necessary following a complete response, and they have reported conflicting results. Habr-Gama and colleagues[66] treated 118 patients with clinical T1–3 rectal cancers with preoperative 50.4 Gy + 5-FU/leucovorin.[66] Of the 36 patients who achieved a biopsy-proven complete response, 30 did not undergo surgery. With a median follow-up of 36 months, 28 (93%) remained without evidence of disease. In a smaller series from Rossi et al.,[66a] 16 patients (13 with T4 tethered disease) received similar preoperative treatment. If they then achieved a biopsy-proven complete response, they received an additional boost of 20–30 Gy via brachytherapy. The six patients (38%) who had a complete response remained without evidence of disease for a median of only 11 months.

Although the results from Habr-Gama and colleagues are intriguing, their analysis did not include patients with T4 disease. Radical surgery following preoperative adjuvant therapy remains the standard of care. In the subset of patients who either have medically inoperable disease or refuse radical surgery, local excision may be an alternative.[67]

### Predicting Response to Preoperative Therapy Using Tumor Markers

A variety of tumor markers have been identified that may help predict tumors that will respond favorably to preoperative therapy (Table 60–3). Using the knowledge that rapidly dividing cells are more sensitive to radiation, Willett et al.[68] analyzed the proliferative index in patients with T4 disease who received preoperative radiation therapy with or without 5-FU. Tumors with a higher proliferation index had a higher response rate to preoperative therapy, and following radiation, there was a corresponding reduction in the proliferative index.[69] In a follow-up study, the authors reported that the addition of 5-FU to preoperative radiation therapy decreased the levels of three markers of proliferation (mitotic counts, Ki-67, and PCNA) compared with radiation therapy alone.[70]

In a series reported by Rich[71] of 50 patients treated with preoperative combined-modality therapy, tumors that had a low

**Table 60-3** Molecular predictors of response to preoperative therapy in rectal cancer[a]

| Series | Patients (n) | Clinical Stage | Preoperative Therapy | CR (%) | Findings |
|---|---|---|---|---|---|
| Desai et al.[74] | 23 | T3–4 | RT | 9 | ↑ Downstaging with normal p53 and/or PCNA negative |
| Fu et al.[117] | 49 | T1–3 | RT | 4 | ↑ Downstaging, ↑ local failure, and ↓ survival with mutated p53 and normal p21 |
| Sakakura et al.[118] | 28 | T3–4 | CMT + hyperthermia | — | ↑ Downstaging with ↑ apoptotic index, highest correlation with wild-type p53 |
| Scott et al.[119] | 24 | T3–4 | CMT | 25 | ↑ Apoptotic index with ↑ CR, no relationship to p53 or bcl-2 |
| Tannapfel et al.[120] | 32 | T3–4 | CMT | — | ↑ Apoptotic index following preop CMT, Q proliferative capacity (Ki67, PCNA) following CMT (this did not predict the CR rate) |
| Luna-Perez et al.[121] | 26 | T3–4 | CMT | 15 | ↑ CR with normal p53 vs. mutated p53 |
| Willett et al.[70] | 153 | T3–4 | RT ± CMT | 12 | ↑ Downstaging with ↑ growth fraction (↑ mitotic count, Ki-67, and PCNA) |
| Nehls et al.[122] | 100 | T1–3 | RT | — | No change in p53 expression pre- vs. post-RT |
| Adell et al.[123] | 148 | T1–4 | RT | — | In p53-negative patients, decreased local failure; in p53-positive patients, no benefit |

Abbreviations: CMT, combined modality therapy (radiation therapy + chemotherapy); CR, pathologic complete response; RT, radiation therapy; ↑, increased; ↓, decreased.

[a]All analyses were performed by immunohistochemistry on paraffin-fixed tissues.

spontaneous apoptosis index and were positive for BCL-2 staining had lower rates of downstaging. In 167 patients treated with preoperative radiation, there was a significant increase in downstaging in well-differentiated cancers.[72] Using residual tumor cell density rather than stage as a measure of disease, this difference did not reach statistical significance. By univariate analysis, patients with a pathologic complete response had a nonsignificant improvement in survival. Berger and associates[73] found that well-differentiated tumors had a greater degree of downstaging than did moderately or poorly differentiated tumors.

Desai and colleagues[74] reported a higher incidence of recurrence but less downstaging in PCNA-positive rectal cancers. By multivariate analysis, Neoptolemos and associates[75] showed that this index did not add to the prognostic value of the Dukes' staging system. The proliferative index may be useful in predicting the response to preoperative therapy, however, given the conflicting data, additional experience is needed.

In conclusion, although some tumor markers may be predictive of response, the decision to use preoperative therapy should not be based solely on their presence or absence. The development of tumor markers that can help predict response and prognosis remains an active area of investigation.[76]

### Intraoperative or Postoperative Radiation Therapy for Residual Disease

For a variety of reasons, some patients with unresectable cancer do not receive preoperative therapy or, despite a preoperative assessment of resectability, are not able to undergo a complete resection. In this setting, does IORT and/or postoperative pelvic radiation therapy have any benefit? As previously discussed, the interpretation of treatment results is complicated because many studies combine patients with primary and recurrent cancers as well as patients with gross and microscopic residual disease. Patients are randomly selected to receive chemotherapy, and some

series include patients with metastatic disease. The discussion below will be limited to those series in which patients had disease limited to the pelvis.

For patients whose disease has failed to respond to prior pelvic radiation, the therapeutic options are limited. The standard therapy is usually palliative surgery or systemic chemotherapy. The response rate with chemotherapy may be reduced in a pelvis that has received full-dose radiation. Is there a role for more aggressive treatment? A variety of aggressive options for patients whose disease failed prior pelvic radiation are available (Table 60–4). Although these are investigational approaches, they may offer an improvement in local control in selected patients.

### Subtotal Resection and Postoperative Radiation Therapy

At the Mayo Clinic, 17 patients with rectal cancer received postoperative radiation therapy (40–60 Gy).[77] Six received concurrent 5-FU–based chemotherapy. For the total patient group, the local failure rate was 76%, and the 5-year actuarial survival was 24%. The seven patients with gross residual disease had a higher local failure rate (86% vs. 70%) and lower survival rate (14% vs. 30%) than those of the 10 patients with microscopic residual disease. There was no clear dose–response curve; only one patient, however, received ≥56 Gy.

A separate report from the Mayo Clinic presented the results of a palliative (subtotal) resection for locally recurrent rectal cancer in 106 patients.[78] 5-FU was administered to 48% of these patients. In the subset of 34 patients with gross residual disease who received IORT and postoperative therapy, the 3-year survival was 44%. However, despite the encouraging survival rate, 40% experienced local failure and 60% experienced distant failure. Univariate analysis revealed a significant improvement in survival in those patients who had microscopic vs. gross residual disease, received IORT, had a limited number of sites of tu-

**Table 60-4** Aggressive surgical plus radiotherapeutic salvage techniques in patients with unresectable and/or recurrent rectal cancer

| Series | Patients (n) | Treatment | Median Follow-up (Months) | Margins | Local Failure (%) | Survival |
|---|---|---|---|---|---|---|
| USC/Mayo Clinic[124] | 30 | Surgery + brachytherapy | 27 | (20) Gross (8) Microscopic (2) Negative | 62% 34% 0% | 23% NED |
| Mayo Clinic[125] | 16 | Sacral resection + IORT | 18 | — | 25% | 48% 2-year |
| Thomas Jefferson University | 39 | Preoperative 36 Gy (reirradiation) + surgery | 36 | — | 55% 5-year | 24% 5-year 45 months median |
| Ohio State University[126] | 26[a] | Surgery + IORT | 28 | — | 77% 4-year | 36% 4-year 23 months median |
| Memorial Sloan-Kettering[16] | 36 | Surgery + brachytherapy | 24 | Gross | 44% | 25% 4-year |
| Memorial Sloan-Kettering[19] | 46 | HDR IORT[b] + surgery | 17.5 | — | 37% 2-year | 47% 2-year |

Abbreviations: HDR, high-dose rate; IORT, intraoperative radiation therapy; NED, no evidence of disease.

[a]Only 69% with prior external beam radiation therapy.

[b]Includes 16 patients who received preoperative radiation but not prior pelvic radiation.

mor fixation, and had a higher performance status. These data suggest that even in patients with locally recurrent residual disease, an aggressive approach should be considered.

Other reports have included both patients with cancers of the rectum and colon as well as patients with primary disease and patients with recurrent disease. In a MGH series, patients received somewhat higher doses of radiation (60–70 Gy) than did patients in the Mayo Clinic series who received external-beam alones.[79] Seven patients in the MGH series received electron-beam IORT. For the total group, the local failure rate was 42% and the 5-year disease-free survival was 18%. The 23 patients with gross residual disease had a higher local failure rate (57% vs. 30%) and a significantly lower survival rate (4% vs. 42%) than did the 30 patients with microscopic residual disease. The improvement in local control in these patients compared to that in the patients in the Mayo Clinic series may have been related to the higher radiation doses. There was no clear dose–response curve in patients with gross disease. However, patients with microscopic residual disease who received <60 Gy did have a higher incidence of local failure than those who received ≥60 Gy (38% vs. 26%).

Another factor that may have an impact on the local failure rate is the volume of gross residual disease. This is consistent with the experience from the MGH[22,23] and the Mayo Clinic[24,27] IORT series, in which patients with gross residual disease had lower survival and higher local failure rates than patients with microscopic residual disease (Tables 60–1 and 60–2).

The dose of radiation needed to treat potential microscopic residual disease (following a complete resection) is 45 to 50.4 Gy. This is within the tolerance of the surrounding normal tissues. However, when biopsy-proven microscopic or gross residual disease is present (following a subtotal resection), the dose of radiation required is higher. Even in situations where the small bowel can be excluded from the external-beam radiation field, other surrounding normal tissues in the pelvis limit the dose to 60 to 65 Gy, which may be inadequate to control large volumes of gross residual tumor. Therefore, it is not surprising that the results for patients with residual disease who receive postoperative radiation therapy are disappointing. The obvious advantage of preoperative therapy is that it decreases the primary tumor volume, thereby allowing maximum surgery and IORT.

## Reirradiation Followed by Surgery

Lingareddy and colleagues[80] reported the use of reirradiation in a selected group of 39 patients with a local recurrence who had received prior pelvic radiation (Table 60–4). These patients received a median dose of 36 Gy through limited lateral fields plus continuous-infusion 5-FU. A partial pelvic field was treated, and the bladder and small bowel were excluded as much as possible from the radiation field. After a median follow-up of 3 years, the 5-year actuarial local failure rate was 55% and survival was 24%. In highly selected patients, retreatment with limited fields may be an option, however, this approach should be considered experimental.

## External-Beam Radiation Therapy Alone

Although the best results are seen in patients who are able to have radical surgery as a component of their therapy, there are patients who do not undergo surgery because their tumors are medically inoperable, they present with extensive unresectable disease grossly invading bone, they have received prior pelvic radiation, or they refuse surgery. In general, these patients are treated with external-beam radiation therapy with or without chemotherapy.[14,80–86]

The largest reported series is 519 patients from Princess Margaret Hospital and has a median survival of 14 months and 5-year survival of 5% (Table 60–5).[84] In the subset of patients in whom high doses of radiation (≥50 Gy) were delivered, the median survival was 24 months and the 5-year survival was 13%. Other selected series have had similar results (14% survival at 3 years[80] and 31% survival at 2 years).[85] These series, however, have had shorter follow-up and fewer patients. In a subset of patients without metastatic disease who received >46 Gy, Overgaard and colleagues reported a 2-year survival of 30%.[87] A 3-year survival of 30% was reported from Minsky and associates.[14]

Pelvic radiation also provides very effective palliation. In the subset of 84 patients who received >45 Gy in the series from Princess Margaret Hospital, the following presenting symptoms were palliated by 6–8 weeks following the completion of radiation: pain (89%), bleeding (79%), neurologic (52%), mass effect (71%), discharge (50%), urologic (22%), and other (42%).[84] In a series from Thomas Jefferson University, complete plus partial

**Table 60-5** Nonsurgical palliative radiotherapeutic options in patients with unresectable or inoperable rectal cancer

| Series | Treatment | Patients (n) | Subset | Median Follow-up (Months) | Local Failure | Survival (%) | Definition of Palliation | Palliation of Patients with Symptoms at Presentation (%) | | | | | |
|---|---|---|---|---|---|---|---|---|---|---|---|---|---|
| | | | | | | | | Pain | Bleeding | Neuro | Mass | Discharge | Total |
| Princess Margaret Hospital[84] | 20–60 Gy ± 5-FU | 519 | Total | — | 93% 5-year | 5% 5-year | 6–8 weeks s/p EBRT | 78 | 68 | 27 | 53 | 44 | — |
| | >45 Gy ± 5-FU | 84 | — | — | — | — | 6–8 weeks s/p EBRT | 89 | 79 | 52 | 71 | 50 | — |
| | ≥50 Gy ± 5-FU | 74 | — | — | 85% 5-year | 13% 5-year | — | — | — | — | — | — | — |
| | ≥50 Gy ± 5-FU | 42 | Resect but refused[a] | — | — | 21% 5-year | — | — | — | — | — | — | — |
| Thomas Jefferson University[80] | Reirradiation with 30.6 Gy ± 5-FU (failed EBRT) | 52 | Total | 16 | — | 14% 3-year | Complete | 65 | 100 | — | 24 | — | — |
| | | | | | | | Partial | 28 | — | — | 64 | — | — |
| | | | | | | | Total | 93 | 100 | — | 88 | — | — |
| | | | | | | | Duration (months) | 9 | 10 | — | 8 | — | — |
| | | | | | | | Until death | 33 | 100 | — | 20 | — | — |
| Centre Hospitalier Lyon Sud[86] | Intracavitary + 39 Gy accelerated EBRT ± brachytherapy | 29 | Total | 46 | 38% | 68% 5-year | | — | — | — | — | — | — |
| Peter McCallum Cancer Institute[85] | 50–60 Gy | 39 | Radically treated | 49 | — | 31% 2-year | Complete | — | — | — | — | — | 33 |
| | | | | | | | Partial | — | — | — | — | — | 52 |
| | | | | | | | Total | — | — | — | — | — | 85 |

Abbreviations: EBRT, external-beam radiation therapy; 5-FU, 5-fluorouracil; Neuro, neurological symptoms; s/p, status post.

[a]Patients with potentially resectable tumors who refused surgery.

symptomatic relief was achieved in the following categories: pain (65% + 28%), bleeding (100%), and mass effect (24% + 64%).[80] The duration of palliation was 8–10 months.

Even in elderly patients, pelvic radiation offers effective palliation. Valentini et al.[88] delivered combined-modality therapy (38–45 Gy plus mitomycin C and continuous-infusion 5-FU) to a group of 17 patients with a median age of 79 (range: 75–90). Symptomatic relief was obtained in four of four patients with pelvic pain and five of six patients with rectal bleeding. The 18% incidence of grade 3+ toxicity was similar to that reported for the general population who receive preoperative combined modality therapy.

These data suggest that patients with advanced rectal cancers that are medically inoperable should be treated aggressively with pelvic radiation therapy as a component of their therapy. It offers not only a defined cure rate but a high degree of palliation of symptoms.

### Postoperative Radiation Therapy and Chemotherapy

Two randomized trials of postoperative combined modality therapy vs. radiation alone have been conducted: one by the RTOG and another by the Eastern Cooperative Oncology Group (ECOG). In the RTOG trial, 129 patients with residual, primary unresectable, or recurrent rectal cancer were randomized to receive either radiation therapy plus concurrent 5-FU followed by maintenance 5-FU/MeCCNU, or radiation therapy alone.[89] Some patients received IORT. There was no significant difference in the estimated actuarial 2-year survival rate between patients who received combined-modality therapy and those who received radiation therapy alone (44% vs. 36%). Of the patients with gross residual disease, on either arm, 25% had no evidence of disease, 6% had disease that was locally controlled, and 50% died with some component of local failure.

The ECOG randomized 30 patients with recurrent, residual, or primary inoperable rectal cancer to receive postoperative continuous-course radiation therapy or split-course radiation therapy plus 5-FU followed by maintenance 5-FU/MeCCNU.[90] The median survival in both arms was 17 months. The five patients with primary inoperable cancer (considered gross residual) had the shortest 2-year survival (0%) compared with the 16 patients with recurrent disease (25%) or the 9 patients with residual disease (54%).

Therefore, postoperative combined-modality therapy, as designed and delivered in these two randomized trials, did not have a significant impact on survival compared with postoperative radiation therapy alone in this subset of patients. Other chemotherapeutic agents and schedules are being investigated.

### Intraoperative Radiation Therapy Alone for Gross Residual Disease

Some patients with recurrent rectal cancer have clinically unresectable gross residual pelvic disease and, because they received prior full-dose pelvic radiation therapy, would require an attempt at resection without the benefit of pre- and/or postoperative radiation therapy. Furthermore, when IORT is not available, this group of patients is commonly approached in a palliative fashion because surgery alone will not control gross residual disease.

The results of a study of 36 patients with recurrent rectal cancer who had gross residual disease remaining in the pelvis fol-

lowing biopsy alone or subtotal resection were reported from Memorial Sloan-Kettering.[16] After a median follow-up of 24 months, the local failure rate was 44%, and the 4-year actuarial survival was 25% (Table 60–4). The local control rate was dependent on the volume of residual disease. With brachytherapy, the tumor volume is proportional to the volume of the implant. The local failure rate was lower in those patients who underwent subtotal resection than in those who underwent a biopsy alone (33% vs. 66%), and lower in those with an iodine-125 implant volume of <40 cm[3] than in those receiving ≥40 cm[3] (39% vs. 100%). Severe treatment-related complications were seen in 11% of patients whose tumors were locally controlled.

The experience with electron-beam IORT in this group of patients is more limited. Calvo et al.[91] reported on a subgroup of five patients with gross residual or recurrent colorectal cancer who received 10–80 Gy via electron-beam IORT.[91] All patients had tumors that were >4 cm. After a median follow-up of 11 months, the incidence of local failure was 40%. Complications included one case of pelvic abscess, two cases of pelvic pain, and one case of lower extremity neuropathy. The more recent trial by Martinez-Monge and co-workers[92] included patients with extrapelvic disease, therefore, it will not be discussed.

In summary, the limited data suggest that IORT with electrons or brachytherapy does not improve the ultimate survival rate in this group of patients. However, it does offer reasonable local control (56% to 60%) with acceptable morbidity. Since local control in and of itself is an important end point in the treatment of rectal cancer, it is appropriate to continue to evaluate IORT as part of an overall aggressive approach in patients with residual disease who are unable to receive pelvic radiation therapy.

## Investigational Approaches

A number of investigational approaches have been employed in an attempt to improve the treatment results in patients with both resectable and unresectable rectal cancers as well as in patients with other pelvic malignancies. These approaches include neutron beam radiation, hyperthermia, radiosensitizers, radioprotectors, three-dimensional treatment planning, and altered radiation fractionation schemes.

### Neutron Beam Radiation Therapy

The theoretical advantages of using neutrons over more conventional photon radiation include increased sensitivity of hypoxic cells to radiation and more advantageous radiation repair and sensitivity characteristics of normal tissues. The results of two randomized trials comparing neutron and photon therapy in patients with unresectable and/or recurrent rectal cancers were reported by Duncan and colleagues.[93] A total of 35 patients received neutrons via a variety of techniques and doses. Not only were there no significant differences in local control or survival, but patients who received neutrons experienced higher acute and late grade 3+ skin toxicity. The preferential absorption of neutrons in fat may have contributed to the complications seen in the skin and subcutaneous tissues. Similar severe and fatal complications were reported in a series of 25 patients with advanced rectal cancer treated by Batterman.[94] In light of these findings and despite the theoretical advantages, there is little interest in the treatment of rectal cancer with neutrons.

## Hyperthermia

Hyperthermia, in conjunction with radiation, has been used mostly as a palliative modality in rectal cancer.[95–99] The rationale for its use is based on an in vitro synergistic interaction of radiation and hyperthermia. The use of this combination in patients with various pelvic and abdominal malignancies has been studied in a phase I/II trial by the RTOG.[100] The acute and long-term toxicities were acceptable; however, in 68% of the patients, the hyperthermia had to be discontinued because it caused discomfort. Hyperthermia has been reported to increase the neurological complications of patients receiving IORT.[36,37]

## Radiosensitizers

Randomized clinical trials in patients with rectal cancer have clearly shown that 5-FU is a radiosensitizer. When compared with radiation alone, the combination of 5-FU with adjuvant postoperative radiation therapy in patients with resectable disease significantly decreases local failure.[1–3] Various mechanisms for 5-FU–mediated radiosensitization have been proposed, however, none alone explains all the interactions.[101] Nonrandomized data from Rhomberg et al.[102] suggest that razoxane may improve local control and median survival in patients who receive radiation for inoperable recurrent rectal cancer. Trials of other radiosensitizers have not shown a clear benefit.

## Radioprotectors

The benefit of radioprotectors is controversial. Five randomized trials examined the efficacy of various compounds to decrease bowel toxicity. These trials have included such compounds as butyric acid to decrease chronic radiation proctitis,[103] sucralfate enemas to decrease acute radiation proctitis,[104] olsalazine to decrease acute enteritis,[105] and mesalazine to decrease acute radiation enteritis.[106] All of these randomized trials have been negative. In a randomized trial of 73 patients with pelvic malignancies, the addition of 5-aminosalicylic acid (5-ASA) increased rather than decreased acute radiation toxicity. Diarrhea was more frequent in patients who received radiation plus 5-ASA than in those receiving radiation alone (91% vs. 74%, $P = 0.07$).[107]

Liu and colleugues[108] performed a randomized trial of pelvic radiation therapy (2.25 Gy/fraction to 45 Gy) with or without the radioprotector WR-2721 in patients with inoperable or unresectable rectal cancer. The incidence of RTOG long-term grade 3+ gastrointestinal, genitourinary, and skin toxicity was 3% in patients who received radiation therapy alone, compared to 0% in those who received radiation therapy plus WR-2721. A separate trial by Montana and colleagues[109] showed no benefit from a topical application of WR-2721 to the rectal mucosa. These data suggest that WR-2721 does not offer radioprotection in patients with rectal cancer who receive pelvic radiation therapy.

## Three-Dimensional Radiation Treatment Planning

Innovative techniques using three-dimensional (3-D) treatment planning are being investigated. In a study by the Photon Treatment Planning Collaborative Working Group, the most important contribution of 3-D treatment planning in rectal cancer was the ability to plan and localize the target and normal tissues at all levels of the treatment volume rather than using the traditional method of planning with only a single central transverse slice

and simulation films.[110] There was also a slight improvement in dosimetry when there were no constraints on the type of planning (i.e., when noncoplanar beams were used). A randomized trial of conformal vs. conventional radiation therapy in 266 evaluable patients with pelvic malignancies has been reported by Tait and co-workers.[111] Although the volume of normal tissue volumes in the radiation field decreased with conformal vs. conventional treatment (689 cm$^3$ vs. 792 cm$^3$), there was no difference in the level of symptoms or in the medication prescribed.

Investigators in Uppsala examined six patients with rectal cancer who underwent both proton and conventional photon treatment planning.[112] Dose–volume histogram analysis showed that protons offered only a marginal benefit in sparing normal tissues.

## Altered Radiation Fractionation Approaches

Various fractionation programs have evolved whose goal is enhancing tumor cell damage by radiation without increasing normal tissue injury.[113] The repair of subcellular injury, regeneration, cell cycle redistribution, and reoxygenation are all factors at the cellular level contributing to differences in how various normal tissues and tumors respond to fractionated radiation. Hyperfractionation and accelerated fractionation schemes take advantage of some of these factors. Their late effects should be the same as or, more likely, less than those of conventional fractionation schemes. A phase I trial from Lausanne of postoperative accelerated hyperfractionation (1.6 Gy twice a day [BID] to 48 Gy) reported acceptable acute toxicity.[114] Recent data from the Lausanne investigators suggest that BID radiation is better tolerated when delivered preoperatively than postoperatively.[115] Bozzetti and colleagues[116] reported a pathologic complete response rate of only 9% in 59 patients with ultrasound stage T2–3 disease who preoperatively received 1.5 Gy BID to 45 Gy.

The major limitation of accelerated hyperfractionation is acute normal tissue toxicity. Since it is unlikely that these altered fractionation schemes can be combined with adequate doses of systemic chemotherapy, Movsas and colleagues[50] limited the hyperfractionated portion to the boost. In their phase I trial of preoperative combined-modality therapy, patients received conventional pelvic radiation plus continuous infusion 5-FU followed by a boost of escalating doses of hyperfractionated radiation (1.2 Gy BID). Provided the small bowel was excluded after the total dose reached 52.3 Gy, the recommended dose level for this approach was 61.8 Gy. In a randomized trial of patients receiving radiation therapy for pelvic malignancies, 3-D conformal radiation therapy decreased the volume of normal tissue in the field but did not decrease acute toxicity.[111]

## Approach to Patients with Synchronous Metastatic Disease

A subset of patients with rectal cancer present with unresectable disease and synchronous extrapelvic disease. Since the natural history of these patients is dependent on a variety of factors such as the volume and site(s) of metastatic disease and, in those with recurrent disease, the disease-free interval, treatment recommendations are individualized and there is no standard of care. The management of these patients is discussed in greater detail in Chapter 61. At Memorial Sloan-Kettering, the general approach is to deliver preoperative combined-modality therapy both as a therapeutic measure and to help identify those patients who may benefit from an aggressive surgical approach. If, following the completion of therapy, there has been a response at both the primary and metastatic tumor site(s), then the patient is evaluated, on a case-by-case basis, for resection of the primary tumor and distant metastasis.

## References

1. Gastrointestinal Tumor Study Group. Prolongation of the disease-free interval in surgically treated rectal carcinoma. N Engl J Med 312:1465–1472, 1985.
2. Gastrointestinal Tumor Study Group. Adjuvant therapy of colon cancer: results of a prospectively randomized trial. N Engl J Med 310:737–743, 1984.
3. Krook JE, Moertel CG, Gunderson LL, Wieand HS, Collins RT, Beart RW, et al. Effective surgical adjuvant therapy for high-risk rectal carcinoma. N Engl J Med 324:709–715, 1991.
4. Takeuchi O, Saito N, Koda K, Sarashina H, Nakajima N. Clinical assessment of positron emission tomography for the diagnosis of local recurrence in colorectal cancer. Br J Surg 86:932–937, 1999.
5. Minsky BD, Cohen AM, Kemeny N, Enker WE, Kelsen D, Reichman B, et al. Enhancement of radiation induced downstaging of rectal cancer by 5-FU and high dose leucovorin chemotherapy. J Clin Oncol 10:79–84, 1992.
6. Minsky BD, Cohen A, Enker W, Kelsen D, Kemeny N, Ilson D, et al. Preoperative 5-FU, low dose leucovorin, and concurrent radiation therapy for rectal cancer. Cancer 73:273–280, 1994.
7. Dosoretz DE, Gunderson LL, Hedberg S, Hoskins B, Blitzer PH, Shipley W, et al. Preoperative irradiation for unresectable rectal and rectosigmoid carcinomas. Cancer 52:814–818, 1983.
8. Medical Research Council Rectal Cancer Working Party. Randomised trial of surgery alone versus radiotherapy followed by surgery for potentially operable, locally advanced rectal cancer. Lancet 348:1605–1610, 1996.
9. Willett CG, Shellito PC, Tepper JE, Eliseo R, Convery K, Wood WC. Intraoperative electron beam radiation therapy for primary locally advanced rectal and rectosigmoid carcinoma. J Clin Oncol 9:843–849, 1991.
10. Willett CG, Shellito PC, Tepper JE, Eliseo R, Convery K, Wood WC. Intraoperative electron beam radiation therapy for recurrent locally advanced rectal or rectosigmoid carcinoma. Cancer 67:1504–1508, 1991.
11. Mendenhall WM, Bland KI, Pfaff WW, Million RR, Copeland EM, III. Initially unresectable rectal adenocarcinoma treated with preoperative irradiation and surgery. Ann Surg 205:41–44, 1987.
12. Marsh RW, Chu NM, Vauthey JN, Mendenhall WM, Lauwers GY, Bewsher C, et al. Preoperative treatment of patients with locally advanced unresectable rectal adenocarcinoma utilizing continuous chronobiologically shaped 5-fluorouracil infusion and radiation therapy. Cancer 78:217–225, 1996.
13. Tobin RL, Mohiuddin M, Marks G. Preoperative irradiation for cancer of the rectum with extrarectal fixation. Int J Radiat Oncol Biol Phys 21:1127–1132, 1991.
14. Minsky BD, Cohen AM, Enker WE, Harrison LB, Sigurdson E. Radiation therapy for unresectable rectal cancer. Int J Radiat Oncol Biol Phys 21:1283–1289, 1991.
15. Willett CG, Shellito PC, Rodkey GV, Wood WC. Preoperative irradiation for tethered rectal carcinoma. Radiother Oncol 21:141–142, 1991.
16. Minsky BD, Cohen AM, Enker WE, Harrison LB, Fass D, Sigurdson E. Intraoperative brachytherapy alone in incompletely resected recurrent rectal cancer. Radiother Oncol 21:115–120, 1991.
17. Dibiase SJ, Rosenstock JG, Shabason L, Corn BW. Tumor bed brachytherapy with a mesh template: an accessible alternative to intraoperative radiotherapy. J Surg Oncol 66:104–109, 1997.
18. Minsky BD, Kemeny N, Cohen AM, Enker WE, Kelsen DP, Reichman B, et al. Preoperative high-dose leucovorin/5-fluorouracil and radiation therapy for unresectable rectal cancer. Cancer 67:2859–2866, 1991.
19. Harrison LB, Minsky BD, Enker WE, Mychalczak B, Guillem J, Paty PB, et al. High dose rate intraoperative radiation therapy (HDR-IORT) as part of the management strategy for locally advanced primary and recurrent rectal cancer. Int J Radiat Oncol Biol Phys 42:325–330, 1998.
20. Huber FT, Stepan R, Zimmermann F, Fink U, Molls M, Siewert JR. Locally advanced rectal cancer: resection and intraoperative radiotherapy using the flab method combined with preoperative or postoperative radiochemotherapy. Dis Colon Rectum 39:774–779, 1996.
21. Lowy AM, Rich TA, Skibber JM, Dubrow RA, Curley SA. Preoperative infusional chemoradiation, selective intraoperative radiation, and resection for locally advanced pelvic recurrence of colorectal adenocarcinoma. Ann Surg 223:177–185, 1996.
22. Wallace HJ III, Willett CG, Shellito PC, Coen JJ, Hoover HC. Intraoperative radiation therapy for locally advanced recurrent rectal or rectosigmoid cancer. J Surg Oncol 60:122–127, 1995.
23. Nakfoor BM, Willett CG, Shellito PC, Kaufman DS, Daly WJ. The impact of 5-fluorouracil and intraoperative electron beam radiation therapy on the outcome of patients with locally advanced primary rectal and rectosigmoid cancer. Ann Surg 228:194–200, 1998.
24. Gunderson LL, Nelson H, Martenson JA, Cha S, Haddock M, Devine R, et al. Locally advanced primary colorectal cancer: intraoperative electron and external beam irradiation ± 5-FU. Int J Radiat Oncol Biol Phys 37:601–614, 1997.
25. Kallinowski F, Eble MJ, Buhr HJ, Wannenmacher M, Herfarth CH. Intraoperative radiotherapy for primary and recurrent rectal cancer. Eur J Surg Oncol 21:191–194, 1995.
26. Kim HK, Jessup JM, Beard CJ, Bornstein B, Cady B, Stone MD, et al. Locally advanced rectal carcinoma: pelvic control and morbidity following preoperative radiation therapy, resection, and intraoperative radiation therapy. Int J Radiat Oncol Biol Phys 38:777–783, 1997.
27. Gunderson LL, Nelson H, Martenson JA, Cha S, Haddock M, Devine R, et al. Intraoperative electron and external beam irradiation with or without 5-fluorouracil and maximum surgical resection for previously unirradiated, locally recurrent colorectal cancer. Dis Colon Rectum 39:1379–1395, 1996.
28. Grinnell RS. The lymphatic and venous spread of carcinoma of the rectum. Ann Surg 116:200–215, 1942.
29. Alekitar KM, Zelefsky MJ, Paty PB, Guillem J, Saltz LB, Cohen AM, et al. High dose rate intraoperative brachytherapy for recurrent colorectal cancer. Int J Radiat Oncol Biol Phys 48:219–226, 2000.
30. Bussieres E, Gilly FN, Rouanet P, Mahe MA, Roussel A, Delannes M, et al. Recurrences of rectal cancers: results of a multimodal approach with intraoperative radiation therapy. Int J Radiat Oncol Biol Phys 34:49–56, 1995.
31. Hashiguchi Y, Sekine T, Sakamoto H, Tanaka Y, Kazumoto T, Kato S, et al. Intraoperative irradiation after surgery for locally recurrent rectal cancer. Dis Colon Rectum 42:886–893, 1999.
32. Mannaerts GHH, Martijn H, Crommelin MA, Stultiens GNM, Dries W, Repelaraer van Driel OJ, et al. Intraoperative electron beam radiation therapy for locally recurrent rectal carcinoma. Int J Radiat Oncol Biol Phys 45:297–308, 1999.
33. Eble MJ, Lehnert T, Treiber M, Latz D, Herfarth C, Wannenmacher M. Moderate dose intraoperative and external beam radiotherapy for locally recurrent rectal carcinoma. Radiother Oncol 49:169–174, 1998.
34. Gillette EL, Powers BE, McChesney SL, Park RD, Withrow SJ. Response of aorta and branch arteries to experimental intraoperative irradiation. Int J Radiat Oncol Biol Phys 17:1247–1255, 1989.
35. McChesney-Gillette SL, Gillette EL, Powers BE, Park RD, Withrow SJ. Ureteral injury following experimental intraoperative irradiation. Int J Radiat Oncol Biol Phys 17:791–798, 1989.
36. Vujaskovic Z, Gillette SM, Powers BE, Stukel TA, LaRue SM, Gillette EL, et al. Effects of intraoperative irradiation and intraoperative hyperthermia on canine sciatic nerve: neurologic and electrophysiologic study. Int J Radiat Oncol Biol Phys 34:125–131, 1995.
37. Vujaskovic Z, Powers BE, Paardekoper G, Gillette SM, Gillette EL, Colaacchio TA. Effects of intraoperative irradiation (IORT) and intraoperative hyperthermia (IOHT) on canine sciatic nerve: histopathological and morphometric studies. Int J Radiat Oncol Biol Phys 43:1103–1109, 1999.
38. Johnstone PAS, Laskin WB, DeLuca AM, Barnes M, Kinsella TJ, Sindelar WF. Tumors in dogs exposed to experimental intraoperative radiotherapy. Int J Radiat Oncol Biol Phys 34:853–857, 1996.
39. Gunderson LL, O'Connell MJ, Dozois RR. The role of intraoperative irradiation in locally advanced primary and recurrent rectal adenocarcinoma. World J Surg 16:495–501, 1992.
40. Lanciano RM, Calkins AR, Wolkov HB, Buzydlowski J, Noyes RD, Sause W, et al. A phase I/II study of intraoperative radiotherapy in advanced unresectable or recurrent carcinoma of the rectum: a Radiation Therapy Oncology Group (RTOG) study. J Surg Oncol 53:20–29, 1993.
41. Noyes RD, Weiss SM, Krall JM, Sause WT, Owens JR, Wolkov HB, et al. Surgical complications of intraoperative radiation therapy: the Radiation Therapy Oncology Group experience. J Surg Oncol 50:209–215, 1993.
42. Minsky BD, Cohen AM, Enker WE, Kemeny N, Kelsen DP, Reichman B, et al. Combined modality therapy of rectal cancer: decreased acute toxicity with the preoperative approach. J Clin Oncol 10:1218–1224, 1992.

43. Frykholm G, Glimelius B, Pahlman L. Preoperative irradiation with and without chemotherapy (MFL) in the treatment of primary non-resectable adenocarcinoma of the rectum. Results from two consecutive studies. Eur J Clin Oncol 11:1535–1541, 1989.

44. Kelsen DP, Hilaris B, Martini N. Neoadjuvant chemotherapy and surgery of cancer of the esophagus. Semin Surg Oncol 2:170–176, 1986.

45. Wagman R, Minsky BD, Cohen AM, Guillem JG, Paty PB. Sphincter preservation with preoperative radiation therapy and coloanal anastomosis: long term follow-up. Int J Radiat Oncol Biol Phys 42:51–57, 1998.

46. Minsky BD, Cohen A, Enker W, Kelsen D, Kemeny N, Ilson D, et al. Pre-operative 5-FU, low dose leucovorin, and radiation therapy for locally advanced/unresectable rectal cancer. Int J Radiat Oncol Biol Phys 37:289–295, 1997.

47. Shibata D, Guillem JG, Lanouette NM, Paty P, Minsky B, Harrison L, et al. Functional and quality of life outcomes in patients with rectal cancer after combined modality therapy, intraoperative radiation therapy, and sphincter preservation. Dis Colon Rectum 43:752–758, 2000.

48. Mohiuddin M, Regine WF, Marks GJ, Marks JW. High-dose preoperative radiation and the challenge of sphincter-preservation surgery for cancer of the distal 2 cm of the rectum. Int J Radiat Oncol Biol Phys 40:569–574, 1998.

49. Chen ET, Mohiuddin M, Brodovsky H, Fishbein G, Marks J. Downstaging of advanced rectal cancer following combined preoperative chemotherapy and high dose radiation. Int J Radiat Oncol Biol Phys 30:169–175, 1994.

50. Movsas B, Hanlon A, Lanciano R, Scher RM, Weiner LM, Sigurdson ER, et al. Phase I dose escalating trial of hyperfractionated pre-operative chemoradiation for locally advanced rectal cancer. Int J Radiat Oncol Biol Phys 42:43–50, 1998.

51. Videtic GMM, Fischer BJ, Perera FE, Bauman GS, Kocha WI, Taylor M, et al. Preoperative radiation with concurrent 5-fluorouracil continuous infusion for locally advanced unresectable rectal cancer. Int J Radiat Oncol Biol Phys 42:319–324, 1998.

52. Sofo L, Ratto C, Doglietto GB, Valentini V, Trodella L, Ippoliti M, et al. Intraoperative radiation therapy in integrated treatment of rectal cancers. Results of phase II study. Dis Colon Rectum 39:1396–1403, 1996.

53. Janjan NA, Abbruzzese J, Pazdur R, Khoo R, Cleary K, Dubrow RA, et al. Prognostic implications of response to preoperative infusional chemoradiation in locally advanced rectal cancer. Radiother Oncol 51:153–160, 1999.

54. Minsky BD, Conti J, Cohen AM, Kelsen DP, Saltz L, Guillem J, et al. Acute toxicity of neoadjuvant bolus 5-FU/methotrexate and leucovorin rescue followed by continuous infusion 5-FU plus preoperative radiation therapy for rectal cancer. Radiat Oncol Investig 4:90–97, 1996.

55. Perera F, Fisher B, Kocha W, Plewes E, Taylor M, Vincent M. A phase I pilot study of pelvic radiation and alpha-2A interferon in patients with locally advanced or recurrent rectal cancer. Int J Radiat Oncol Biol Phys 37:297–303, 1997.

56. Botwood N, James R, Vernon C, et al. A phase I study of "Tomudex" (raltitrexed) with radiotherapy (RT) as adjuvant treatment in patients (pt) with operable rectal cancer [abstract]. Proc Am Soc Clin Oncol 17:277a, 1998.

57. James RD, Price P, Valentini V. Raltitrexed (Tomudex) concomitant with radiotherapy as adjuvant treatment for patients with rectal cancer: preliminary results of phase I studies. Eur J Cancer 35:S19–S22, 1999.

58. Valentini V, Morganti AG, Fiorentino G, et al. Chemoradiation with raltitrexed (Tomudex) and concomitant preoperative radiotherapy has potential in the treatment of stage II/III resectable rectal cancer [abstract]. Proc Am Soc Clin Oncol 18:257a, 1999.

59. James RD, Price P, Smith M. Raltitrexed (Tomudex) plus radiotherapy is well tolerated and warrants further investigation in patients with advanced inoperable/recurrent rectal cancer [abstract]. Proc Am Soc Clin Oncol 18:288a, 1999.

60. Feliu J, Calvillo J, Escribano A, et al. Neoadjuvant therapy of rectal carcinoma with UFT-folinic acid (LV) plus radiotherapy [abstract]. Proc Am Soc Clin Oncol 18:239a, 1999.

61. Mitchell E, Ahmad N, Fry RD, et al. Combined modality therapy of locally advanced or recurrent adenocarcinoma of the rectum: preliminary report of a phase I trial of chemotherapy (CT) with CPT-11, 5-FU, and concomitant irradiation (RT) [abstract]. Proc Am Soc Clin Oncol 18:247a, 1999.

62. Minsky BD, O'Reilly E, Wong D, et al. Daily low-dose irinotecan (CPT-11) plus pelvic irradiation as preoperative treatment of locally advanced rectal cancer [abstract]. Proc Am Soc Clin Oncol 18:266a, 1999.

63. Kaminsky-Forrett MC, Conroy T, Luporsi E, Peiffert D, Lapeyre M, Boissel P, et al. Prognostic implications of downstaging following preoperative radiation therapy for operable T3–T4 rectal cancer. Int J Radiat Oncol Biol Phys 42:935–941, 1998.

64. Ahmad NR, Nagle DA, Topham A. Pathologic complete response predicts long-term survival following preoperative radiation therapy for rectal cancer [abstract]. Int J Radiat Oncol Biol Phys 39:284, 1997.

65. Guillem JG, Ruo L, Tickoo S, et al. Prognostic significance of extent of rectal cancer response to preoperative radiation therapy (RT) +/− chemotherapy [abstract]. Proc Am Soc Clin Oncol 19:245a, 2000.

66. Habr-Gama A, de Souza PM, Ribeiro U, Nadalin W, Gansl R, H.S.e Sousa A, et al. Low rectal cancer: impact of radiation and chemotherapy on surgical treatment. Dis Colon Rectum 41:1087–1096, 1998.

66a. Rossi BM, Nakogawa WT, Novoes PE, et al. Radiation and chemotherapy instead of surgery for low infiltrative rectal adenocarcinoma: a prospective trial. Ann Surg Oncol 5:113–118, 1998.

67. Ahmad NR, Nagle DA. Preoperative radiation therapy followed by local excision. Semin Radiat Oncol 8:36–38, 1998.

68. Willett CG, Warland G, Coen J, Shellito PC, Compton CC. Rectal cancer: the influence of tumor proliferation on response to preoperative irradiation. Int J Radiat Oncol Biol Phys 32:57–61, 1995.

69. Willett CG, Warland G, Hagan MP, Daly WJ, Coen J, Shellito PC, et al. Tumor proliferation in rectal cancer following preoperative irradiation. J Clin Oncol 13:1417–1424, 1995.

70. Willett CG, Hagan M, Daley W, Warland G, Shellito PC, Compton CC. Changes in tumor proliferation of rectal cancer induced by preoperative 5-fluorouracil and irradiation. Dis Colon Rectum 41:62–67, 1998.

71. Rich TA. Infusional chemoradiation for operable rectal cancer: post-, pre-, or nonoperative management? Oncology 11:295–315, 1997.

72. Rich TA, Sinicrope F, Stephens C, et al. Downstaging of T3 rectal cancer after preoperative infusional chemoradiation is correlated with spontaneous apoptosis index and BCL-2 staining [abstract]. Int J Radiat Oncol Biol Phys 36:259, 1996.

73. Berger C, de Muret A, Garaud P, Chapet S, Bourlier P, Reynaud-Bougnoux A, et al. Preoperative radiotherapy (RT) for rectal cancer: predictive factors of tumor downstaging and residual tumor density (RTCD): prognostic implications. Int J Radiat Oncol Biol Phys 37:619–627, 1997.

74. Desai GR, Myerson RJ, Higashikubo R, Birnbaum E, Fleshman J, Fry R, et al. Carcinoma of the rectum: possible cellular predictors of metastatic potential and response to radiation therapy. Dis Colon Rectum 39:1090–1096, 1996.

75. Neoptolemos JP, Oates GD, Newbold KM, Robson AM, McConkey C, Powell J. Cyclin/proliferation cell nuclear antigen immunohistochemistry does not improve the prognostic power of Dukes' or Jass' classifications for colorectal cancer. Br J Surg 82:184–187, 1995.

76. Nicholl ID, Dunlop MG. Molecular markers of prognosis in colorectal cancer. J Natl Cancer Inst 91:1267–1269, 1999.

77. Schild SE, Martenson JA, Gunderson LL, Dozois RR. Long-term survival and patterns of failure after postoperative radiation therapy for subtotally resected rectal adenocarcinoma. Int J Radiat Oncol Biol Phys 16:459–463, 1989.

78. Suzuki K, Gunderson LL, Devine RM, Weaver AM, Dozois RR, Ilstrup DM, et al. Intraoperative irradiation after palliative surgery for locally recurrent rectal cancer. Cancer 75:939–952, 1995.

79. Allee PE, Tepper JE, Gunderson LL, Munzenrider JE. Postoperative radiation therapy for incompletely resected colorectal carcinoma. Int J Radiat Oncol Biol Phys 17:1171–1176, 1989.

80. Lingareddy V, Ahmad NR, Mohiuddin M. Palliative reirradiation for recurrent rectal cancer. Int J Radiat Oncol Biol Phys 38:785–790, 1997.

81. Papillon J, Berard PH. Endocavitary irradiation in the conservative treatment of adenocarcinoma of the low rectum. World J Surg 16:451–457, 1992.

82. Kodner IJ, Shemesh EI. Radiation therapy as definitive treatment for adenocarcinoma of the rectum. Surgery 114:850–860, 1993.

83. Brierley JD, Cummings BJ, Wong CS, Keane TJ, O'Sullivan B, Catton CN, et al. Adenocarcinoma of the rectum treated by radical external radiation therapy. Int J Radiat Oncol Biol Phys 31:255–259, 1995.

84. Wong CS, Cummings BJ, Brierley JD, Catton CN, McLean M, Catton P, et al. Treatment of locally recurrent rectal carcinoma—results and prognostic factors. Int J Radiat Oncol Biol Phys 40:427–435, 1998.

85. Guiney MJ, Smith JG, Worotniuk V, Ngan S, Blakey D. Radiotherapy treatment for isolated loco-regional recurrence of rectosigmoid cancer following definitive surgery: Peter McCallum Cancer Institute experience: 1981–1990. Int J Radiat Oncol Biol Phys 38:1019–1025, 1997.

86. Gerard JP, Roy P, Coquard R, Barbet N, Romestaing P, Ayzac L, et al. Combined curative radiation therapy alone in (T1) T2–3 rectal adenocarcinoma: a pilot study of 29 patients. Radiother Oncol 38:131–137, 1996.

87. Overgaard M, Overgaard J, Sell A. Dose–response relationship for radiation therapy of recurrent, residual, and primarily inoperable colorectal cancer. Radiother Oncol 1:217–225, 1984.

88. Valentini V, Morganti AG, Luzi S, Mantello G, Mantini G, Salvi G, et al. Is chemoradiation feasible in elderly patients? A study of 17 patients with anorectal carcinoma. Cancer 80:1387–1392, 1997.

89. Rominger CJ, Gelber RD, Gunderson LL, Conner N. Radiation therapy alone or in combination with chemotherapy in the treatment of residual or inoperable carcinoma of the rectum and rectosigmoid or pelvic recurrence following colorectal surgery. Radiation Therapy Oncology Group study (76-16). Am J Clin Oncol 8:118–127, 1985.

90. Danjoux CE, Gelber RD, Catton GE, Klaassen DJ. Combination chemoradiotherapy for residual, recurrent, or inoperable carcinoma of the rectum: ECOG Study (EST 3276). Int J Radiat Oncol Biol Phys 11:765–771, 1985.

91. Calvo FA, Algarra SM, Azinovic I, Santos M, Escude L, Hernandez JL, et al. Intraoperative radiotherapy for recurrent and/or residual colorectal cancer. Radiother Oncol 15:133–140, 1989.

92. Martinez-Monge R, Nag S, Martin EW. Three different intraoperative radiation modalities (electron beam, high-dose-rate brachytherapy, and iodine-125 brachytherapy) in the adjuvant treatment of patients with recurrent colorectal adenocarcinoma. Cancer 86:236–247, 1999.

93. Duncan W, Arnott SJ, Jack WJL, Orr JA, Kerr GR, Williams JR. Results of two randomized trials of neutron therapy in rectal adenocarcinoma. Radiother Oncol 8:191–198, 1987.

94. Battermann JJ. Results of d+T fast neutron irradiation on advanced tumors of the bladder and rectum. Int J Radiat Oncol Biol Phys 8:2159–2164, 1982.

95. Nishimura Y, Hiraoka M, Akuta K, Jo S, Nagata Y, Masunaga SI, et al. Hyperthermia combined with radiation therapy for primarily unresectable and recurrent colorectal cancer. Int J Radiat Oncol Biol Phys 23:759–768, 1992.

96. Graf R, Wust P, Gellermann J, et al. Phase II trial of radiation therapy with 45 Gy, 5-fluorouracil (5-FU), and mitomycin-C (MMC) in patients with anal cancer - a rationale to add regional hyperthermia [abstract]. Int J Radiat Oncol Biol Phys 36:296, 1996.

97. Furuta K, Konishi F, Kanazawa K, Saito K, Sugawara T. Synergistic effects of hyperthermia in preoperative radiochemotherapy for rectal carcinoma. Dis Colon Rectum 40:1303–1312, 1997.

98. Ohno S, Tomoda M, Tomisaki S, Kitamura K, Mori M, Maehara Y, et al. Improved surgical results after combining preoperative hyperthermia with chemotherapy and radiotherapy for patients with carcinoma of the rectum. Dis Colon Rectum 40:401–406, 1997.

99. Ichikawa D, Yamaguchi T, Yoshioka Y, Sawai K, Takahashi T. Prognostic evaluation of preoperative combined treatment for advanced cancer in the lower rectum with radiation, intraluminal hyperthermia, and 5-fluorouracil suppository. Am J Surg 171:346–350, 1996.

100. Emami B, Myerson RJ, Scott C, Gibbs F, Lee C, Perez CA. Phase I/II study, combination of radiotherapy and hyperthermia in patients with deep-seated malignant tumors: report of a pilot study by the Radiation Therapy Oncology Group. Int J Radiat Oncol Biol Phys 20:73–79, 1991.

101. Pu AT, Robertson JM, Lawrence TS. Current status of radiation sensitization by fluoropyrimidines. Oncology 9:707–714, 1995.

102. Rhomberg W, Eiter H, Hergan K, Schneider B. Inoperable recurrent rectal cancer: results of a prospective trial with radiation therapy and razoxane. Int J Radiat Oncol Biol Phys 30:419–425, 1994.

103. Talley NA, Chen F, King D, Jones M, Talley NJ. Short-chain fatty acid in the treatment of radiation proctitis. A randomized, double-blind, placebo-controlled, cross-over pilot trial. Dis Colon Rectum 40:1046–1050, 1997.

104. O'Brien PC, Franklin CI, Dear KBG, Hamilton CC, Poulsen M, Joseph DJ, et al. A phase III double-blind randomised study of rectal sucralfate suspension in the prevention of acute radiation proctitis. Radiother Oncol 45:117–123, 1997.

105. Martenson JA, Hyland G, Moertel CG, Mailliard JA, O'Fallon JR, Collins RT, et al. Olsalizine is contraindicated during pelvic radiation therapy: results of a double-blind randomized clinical trial. Int J Radiat Oncol Biol Phys 35:299–303, 1996.

106. Resbeut M, Marteau P, Cowen D, et al. A randomized double blind placebo controlled multicenter study of mesalazine for the prevention of acute radiation enteritis. Radiother Oncol 44:59–63, 1997.

107. Baughan CA, Canney PA, Buchanan RB, Pickering RM. A randomized trial to assess the efficacy of 5-aminosalicylic acid for the prevention of radiation enteritis. Clin Oncol 5:19–24, 1993.

108. Liu T, Liu Y, He S, Zhang Z, Kligerman MM. Use of radiation with or without WR-2721 in advanced rectal cancer. Cancer 69:2820–2825, 1992.

109. Montana GS, Anscher MS, Mansbach II CM, Daly N, Delannes M, Clarke-Pearson D, et al. Topical application of WR-2721 to prevent radiation-induced proctosigmoiditis. Cancer 69:2826–2830, 1992.

110. Shank B, LoSasso T, Brewster L, Burman C, Cheng E, Chu JCH, et al. Three-dimensional treatment planning for post-operative treatment of rectal carcinoma. Int J Radiat Oncol Biol Phys 21:253–265, 1991.

111. Tait DM, Nahum AE, Meyer LC, Law M, Dearnaley DP, Horwich A, et al. Acute toxicity in pelvic radiotherapy; a randomised trial of conformal versus conventional treatment. Radiother Oncol 42:121–136, 1997.

112. Isacsson U, Montelius A, Jung B, Glimelius B. Comparative treatment planning between proton and X-ray therapy in locally advanced rectal cancer. Radiother Oncol 41:263–272, 1996.

113. Withers HR. Biological basis for altered fractionation schemes. Cancer 55:2086–2095, 1985

114. Coucke PA, Cuttat JF, Mirimanoff RO. Adjuvant postoperative accelerated hyperfractionated radiotherapy in rectal cancer: a feasibility study. Int J Radiat Oncol Biol Phys 27:885–889, 1993.

115. Coucke PA, Sartorelli B, Cuttat JF, Jeanneret W, Gillet M, Mirimanoff RO. The rationale to switch from postoperative hyperfractionated accelerated radiotherapy to preoperative hyperfractionated accelerated radiotherapy in rectal cancer. Int J Radiat Oncol Biol Phys 32:181–188, 1995.

116. Bozzetti F, Baratti D, Andreola S, Zucali R, Schiavo M, Spinelli P, et al. Preoperative radiation therapy for patients with T2–T3 carcinoma of the middle-to-lower rectum. Cancer 86:398–404, 1999.

117. Fu CG, Tominaga O, Nagawa H, Nita ME, Masaki T, Ishimaru G, et al. Role of p53 and p21/WAF1 detection in patient selection for preoperative radiotherapy in rectal cancer patients. Dis Colon Rectum 41:58–74, 1998.

118. Sakakura C, Koide K IDWT, Kimura A, Taniguchi H, Hagiwara A, Yamaguchi T, et al. Analysis of histologic therapeutic effect, apoptosis rate and p53 status after combined treatment with radiation, hyperthermia, and 5-fluorouracil suppositories for advanced rectal cancers. Br J Cancer 77:159–166, 1998.

119. Scott N, Hale A, Deakin M, Hand P, Adab FA, Hall C, et al. A histopathological assessment of the response of rectal adenocarcinoma to combination chemoradiotherapy: relationship to apoptotic activity, p53, and bcl-2 expression. Eur J Surg Oncol 24:169–173, 1998.

120. Tannapfel A, Nusslein S, Fietkau R, Katalinic A, Kockerling F, Wittekind C. Apoptosis, proliferation, bax, bcl-2, and p53 status prior to and after preoperative radiochemotherapy for locally advanced rectal cancer. Int J Radiat Oncol Biol Phys 41:585–591, 1998.

121. Luna-Perez P, Arriola EL, Cuadra Y, Alvarado I, Quintero A. p53 protein overexpression and response to induction chemoradiation therapy in patients with locally advanced rectal adenocarcinoma. Ann Surg Oncol 5:203–208, 1998.

122. Nehls O, Klump B, Holzmann K, Lammering G, Borchard F, Gruenagel HH, et al. Influence of p53 status on prognosis in preoperatively irradiated rectal carcinoma. Cancer 85:2541–2548, 1999.

123. Adell G, Sun XF, Olle S, Klintenberg C, Sjodahl R, Nordenskjold B. p53 status: an indicator for the effect of preoperative radiotherapy of rectal cancer. Radiother Oncol 51:169–174, 1999.

124. Goes RN, Beart RW, Simons AJ, Gunderson LL, Grado G, Streeter O. Use of brachytherapy in management of locally recurrent rectal cancer. Dis Colon Rectum 40:1177–1179, 1997.

125. Magrini S, Nelson H, Gunderson L, Sim FH. Sacropelvic resection and intraoperative electron irradiation in the management of recurrent anorectal cancer. Dis Colon Rectum 39:1–9, 1996.

126. Nag S, Martinez-Monge R, Mills J, Bauer C, Grecula J, Nieroda C, et al. Intraoperative high-dose rate brachytherapy in recurrent metastatic colorectal carcinoma. Ann Surg Oncol 5:16–22, 1998.

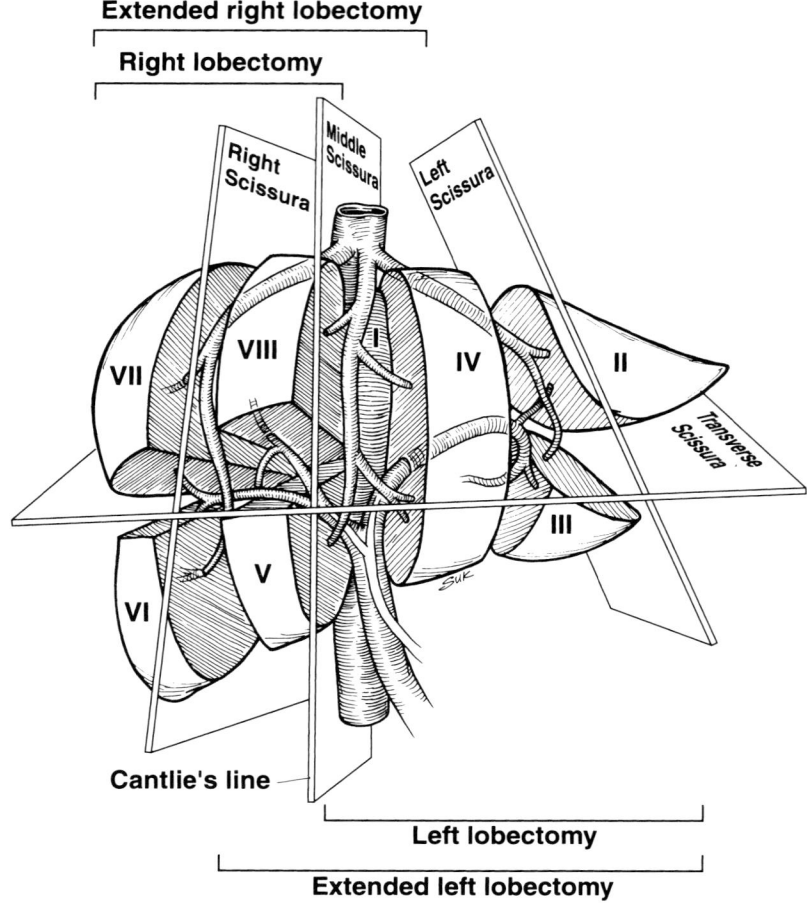

**Figure 61-2** The liver is divided into eight segments on the basis of Couinaud's anatomical studies. The hepatic veins and the umbilical fissure define the resection lines for major hepatic resections.

is to eliminate all metastases with negative resection margins. Under intermittent vascular inflow occlusion (the Pringle maneuver), the hepatic parenchyma is divided with an ultrasonic dissector. Bleeding from small vessels is controlled with electrocautery, while larger vessels and biliary radicals are individually sutured and ligated. The argon-beam coagulator may also be useful to obtain final hemostasis.[18]

## Surgical Results and Factors Affecting Survival

Liver resection is now a well-controlled procedure, with a complication rate of ≤30%. The perioperative mortality rate for resection of hepatic colorectal metastasis at major centers is now approaching 0%. Perioperative morbidity and mortality rates and survival rates after hepatic resection for colorectal metastasis are presented in Table 61-2.[19-27] Factors affecting survival are presented in Table 61-3.[8,28-30] Factors most consistently associated with recurrence are (1) positive resection margin, (2) discovery of liver metastasis synchronous with the primary cancer, and (3) primary tumor with one or more positive lymph node(s).

In the past, the resection of hepatic colorectal metastases was not performed in patients with more than three or four lesions[31] or lesions within 1 cm of major vessels (the vena cava or main hepatic veins). The number of metastases is no longer considered to be as important a predictor of long-term survival as pre-

viously thought. Indeed, the excision of all demonstrable tumors with clear resection margins has been shown to be of much greater importance.[32] Although a resection margin of 1 cm or more is desirable, occasionally this cannot be achieved for technical reasons. Provided the margin is microscopically tumor-free, long-term survival and cure are possible (although somewhat reduced) with margins of less than 1 cm (overall 5- and 10-year survival rates, 37% and 21%, respectively, with a 1- to 9-mm margin, vs. 43% and 28%, respectively, with a ≥10-mm margin).[32] An anticipated close resection margin does not, therefore, constitute a contraindication to resection.

The presence of hilar metastases has traditionally been considered extrahepatic disease and therefore a contraindication for surgical intervention. Nakamura and colleagues[32] published results from their 20-year experience with hepatectomy for colorectal cancer metastases. In this review, 43 of 79 patients who underwent liver resection for colorectal metastases underwent hepatoduodenal, retropancreatic, and celiac lymph node dissection. Of these 43 patients, 7 had histologically confirmed positive lymph nodes. Two of these seven patients survived for more than 5 years. Beckurts and associates[33] reported on 126 patients who underwent hepatectomy and hepatoduodenal lymphadenectomy for colorectal liver metastases. In this series, the 5-year survival rates were 0% for lymph node-positive patients and 22% for lymph node-negative patients. Thus, most patients with positive

**Table 61-2** Morbidity, mortality, and survival after hepatic resection of colorectal metastases

| Study | Patients | Morbidity | Mortality 30 Days | Mortality Total | 5-Year Survival (%) | Median Survival (months) |
|---|---|---|---|---|---|---|
| Adson et al., 1984[19] | 141 | — | — | 4 | 25 | 21 |
| Ringe et al., 1990[20] | 119/157 | 10 | 5 | — | 27 | 35 |
| Doci et al., 1991[21] | 100 | 11 | — | 5 | 30 | — |
| Herfarth and Hohenberger, 1992[22] | 161 | 31 | — | 3 | 20–30 | 28 |
| Rosen et al., 1992[23] | 280 | — | — | 4[a] | 25 | — |
| Sugihara et al., 1993[24] | 109 | — | 2 | — | 48 | — |
| Gozzetti et al., 1994[25] | 108 | 21 | 1 | — | 28 | — |
| Gayowski et al., 1994[26] | 204 | — | 0 | 1 | 32 | 33 |
| Scheele et al., 1996[27] | 376/471 | 16 | 5 | 6 | 39 | 41 |

[a]Sixty-day mortality.

lymph nodes do not benefit from hepatectomy for colorectal metastases, and lymph node positivity remains a contraindication to resection.

Other factors that may increase the risk of recurrence after the resection of liver metastases include symptomatic disease, the presence of satellitosis (metastases around the main metastatic nodule within the same segment or within 2 cm and less than 50% of the size of the main metastasis), and a high preoperative CEA level.[34] The performance of an anatomic resection has also been shown to be a significant factor related to overall and tumor-free survival.[35] The performance of such "anatomic resections" has been facilitated by the widespread availability of intraoperative ultrasound, which allows for the precise delineation of the vascular anatomy within individual segments. This strategy is supported by two pathologic studies indicating that colorectal metastases spread intrahepatically along the portal triads.[35,36]

## Results of Reresection

The most common sites of recurrence following resection of hepatic colorectal metastases are the liver and lung.[37] Several groups have now reported successful repeat liver metastasis resections.[38–44] In one published series, the median survival was 34 months and the 5-year survival rate was 32% for 170 consecutive patients undergoing repeat hepatic resection.[43] In small series involving patients with isolated liver and lung metastases, the resection of metastases from both sites has been reported with favorable results.[45–47] DeMatteo and colleagues[48] recently reported on 81 patients who underwent both liver and lung resections for metastatic colorectal carcinoma. Most (87%) of the lung resections in this highly selected group were wedge excisions. The median actuarial survival once a patient had both liver and lung metastases resected was 3.8 years.

With repeat liver or lung resection providing an option for cure, follow-up evaluation after the resection of colorectal metastases is justified. Routine follow-up should include an office visit 2 weeks after hospital discharge. A CEA level that was elevated preoperatively should return to normal 6 weeks after surgery. Office visits with liver function studies and assessment of CEA levels should thereafter be repeated every 3 months. Patients should undergo abdominal and pelvic CT and chest X-rays every 4 to 6 months and a colonoscopy the first year after colon resection and every 3 years thereafter if the baseline colonoscopy is negative. This rigorous schedule should be continued for up to 7 years, based on the long-term follow-up data of the disease-free survival after liver resection (Fig. 61–1).

## Novel Treatment Approaches

### Cryoablation

Cryoablation is a local ablative technique for the treatment of unresectable primary and metastatic disease to the liver. This method uses a vacuum-insulated cryoprobe, cooled by liquid nitrogen, to rapidly freeze and thaw the liver tumor. The cryprobe is inserted into the tumor with the aid of intraoperative ultrasound, allowing for controlled freezing and thawing of the tumor. Cryoablation preserves the normal liver parenchyma, while tumor cells are destroyed without resection. Cryoablation causes tissue destruction by several mechanisms: (1) intracellular freezing, (2) extracellular freezing that causes vascular thrombosis, (3) electrolyte shifting that causes intracellular dehydration and cell death, and (4) induction of hypoxic mediated cell death.

A number of studies have demonstrated the safety of this technique.[49] Although mortality rates of 0% to 4% have been reported,[49] major procedure-related complications have occurred. These include hypothermia, biliary fistula, intrahepatic and subphrenic abscess, coagulopathy, and pyrexia.[50]

**Table 61-3** Predictors of recurrence after hepatic resection of colorectal metastases

| Study | Positive Margin | Synchronous Tumor | Node-Positive Primary | Size >10 cm | Metastases | Bilobar |
|---|---|---|---|---|---|---|
| Gayowski et al., 1994[26] | Yes | Yes | Yes | No | Yes | Yes |
| Scheele et al., 1995[6] | Yes | Yes | Yes | Yes | No | No |
| Jamison et al., 1997[8] | No | — | No | No | No | — |
| Jenkins et al., 1997[28] | Yes | Yes | — | — | No | — |
| Ambiru et al., 1999[29] | Yes | — | Yes | — | Yes | — |
| Fong et al., 1999[30] | Yes | — | Yes | — | Yes | No |

Cryoablation is associated with a high recurrence rate, both in the liver and at extrahepatic sites. Seifert and Morris[51] analyzed 85 patients who were not candidates for resection and who underwent complete cryoablation of colorectal liver metastases over a 7-year period. At a median follow-up of 22 months, local recurrence at the cryosite was observed in 33% of patients, liver recurrence in 65%, and extrahepatic recurrence in 56%. Multivariate analysis indicated that metastasis size greater than 3 cm was the only independent factor associated with local recurrence. Seifert hypothesized that this phenomenon was due to the inability to achieve an adequate decrease in temperature farther away from the cryoprobe. A similar pattern of failure was found by Ravikumar and colleagues,[52] who studied 32 patients with liver tumors, including 24 patients with colorectal metastases. In this study, 28% of patients remained disease-free after a median follow-up of 24 months. Of the patients with recurrence, 32% had recurrence in the liver only; 54%, in the liver and at extrahepatic sites; and 14%, at extrahepatic sites only. Of the patients with recurrence in the liver only, 9% had recurrence at the treatment site.

To identify prognostic factors that may improve the results of cryoablation, Seifert and Morris[53] also analyzed 116 patients who underwent cryosurgery for metastatic colorectal cancer. The following factors were found to be independently associated with a favorable outcome: a low presurgical serum CEA level, metastases of less than 3 cm diameter, the absence of extrahepatic disease, absence of nodal involvement, complete cryoablation, and good or moderate differentiation of the primary tumor. In this series, 37% of patients remained alive at a follow-up of 23 months. The median survival was 26 months, with a 5-year survival rate of 13%.

Cryoablation has been combined with resection when the margin is involved or suboptimal <1 cm). Seifert and Morris[53] performed cryotherapy of the resection edge in 44 patients after liver resection for colorectal liver metastases with an involved or inadequate resection margin. The reasons for performing cryoablation included an involved resection margin in 24 patients and a close margin (<1 cm) in another 20 patients. At a median follow-up of 19 months, 16 patients were alive and disease-free, and 26 patients, 15 of whom died, developed a recurrence. Nineteen patients developed recurrences that involved the liver, but only five (9%) of these recurrences were at the resection edge. The median overall and disease-free survival were 33 months and 23 months, respectively.

Cryoablation has been combined with surgical resection for limited bilobar hepatic colorectal metastases. Johnson and associates[54] compared seven patients who underwent cryoablation alone to seven patients who underwent combined resection and cryoablation of the contralateral lobe. In the cryoablation-alone group, five of seven patients had a recurrence at the cryosite, whereas only two patients in the combined-therapy group had a recurrence. All recurrences occurred in tumors located centrally near major vascular structures. Therefore, the investigators in that study recommended using cryotherapy as an adjunct to resection for small, contralateral, peripherally located tumors after standard surgical techniques have been used to remove centrally located tumors.

Hepatic cryoablation can be used as a local ablative technique when surgery is not possible. Unfortunately, because many of the patients in these cases have tumors with unfavorable biology, cryotherapy is associated with a high recurrence rate (9% to 33%) and a decreased survival rate (5-year survival, 13%) when compared to resection. In selected patients, cryoablation, especially when combined with resection, may improve local disease control and may allow a greater proportion of patients with liver metastases to undergo potentially curative treatment.

### Radiofrequency ablation

Radiofrequency ablation (RFA) is the newest technique used for the local ablation of tumors not amenable to resection. This technique is performed percutaneously as an interventional radiologic procedure or intraoperatively laparoscopically or as part of a laparotomy. An RFA needle is placed inside the substance of the tumor, as in cryosurgery, under radiographic (i.e., CT or ultrasound) guidance. The needle array is deployed, and thermal energy is generated. The cell membranes are destroyed, and the intracellular proteins degenerate as the temperature exceeds 45°C to 50°C.

Curley and colleagues[55] recently reported a series involving 123 patients with primary or metastatic hepatic malignancies treated with RFA. Of these patients, 50% (61) had hepatic colorectal metastases. Small (<3 cm) peripheral tumors were treated by percutaneous ultrasound-guided RFA in 31 patients, and the remaining patients were treated during an open operative procedure. To prevent bile duct injuries, patients with tumors near the main right or left bile ducts were excluded from the study. Patients were still considered for RFA in cases in which the tumor abutted a major portal or hepatic branch or the vena cava. In this series, there were no treatment-related deaths, and the complication rate was 2.4%. After a median follow-up of 15 months, only 1.8% of tumors had recurred at the RFA site. Unfortunately, 27.6% of patients had recurrence at distant sites. The tumors in two of the three cases with local recurrences were >6 cm in diameter. The only complications in this series were one perihepatic abscess and one hemorrhage into the treated tumor.

Solbiati and colleagues[56] also reported on 29 patients with 44 liver metastases, most from colorectal cancer, who were treated with percutaneous RFA. At a median follow-up of 18 months, the disease-free survival rate was 33% and the overall survival rate was 89%. Progression of disease at the RFA site was seen in 34% of treated lesions. This is in contrast to the 1.8% local recurrence reported by Curley and associates.[55] All of the patients in the study by Solbiati and colleagues were treated percutaneously, whereas only 25% of the patients in the study by Curley and associates series were treated in this manner. Curley and associates used the percutaneous technique only in patients with isolated peripheral lesions, whereas Solbiati and colleagues used the percutaneous technique in patients with multiple central lesions. This difference in approach may directly impact the ability to achieve complete tumor destruction.

Preliminary data indicate that RFA can be used as a local ablative technique in cases in which the patient is not a surgical candidate. Unfortunately, the rate of extrahepatic recurrences is high because patients remain at risk for systemic failure. Radiofrequency ablation should further be investigated as part of prospective studies because current studies provide only short-term follow-up data. At M. D. Anderson Cancer Center, RFA is now being used as part of a protocol that combines RFA and the placement of a hepatic artery infusion pump in an effort to minimize intrahepatic recurrences following ablation alone.

### Portal vein embolization

Preoperative portal vein embolization (PVE) is an option in selected patients prior to extended liver resection if there is concern regarding possible postoperative liver failure or complications due to a small liver remnant volume. The rationale for this technique is to induce hypertrophy of the future liver remnant (FLR).

The first clinical report demonstrating this technique was by Kinoshita and colleagues in 1986.[57] In this study, 21 patients with a diagnosis of hepatocellular carcinoma underwent preoperative PVE and hepatic artery embolization. Postembolization CT scans and operative findings confirmed hypertrophy of the contralateral liver. Kawasaki and colleagues[58] reported on five patients with metastatic colorectal cancer who underwent preoperative right PVE to allow extended right hepatectomy in conjunction with wedge resections of the left lateral segment. Embolizations were performed from 9 days to 8 months prior to surgical resection, and the mean survival was 47 months.

The material used for PVE is *(1)* ethiodized oil (Ultrafluid Lipiodol; Laboratoire Guerbet, Aulnay-Sous-Bois, France) with cyanoacrylate (NBCA/Histoacryl; B. Braum AG, Melsungen, Germany); *(2)* a combination of gelatin (Gelfoam; Upjohn Co., Kalamazoo, MI), thrombin, and Gianturco coils (Cook, Inc., Bloomington, IN); or *(3)* alcohol. No specific substance has emerged as superior to the others in terms of safety and efficacy. Portal vein embolization may be performed either by percutaneous ultrasonographically guided puncture of a portal vein radicle or by an open operative technique in which the ileocolic vein is cannulated. Portal vein embolization is well tolerated and in noncirrhotic livers induces a 25% to 80% increase in the absolute volume of the nonembolized liver (Fig. 61–3). Four to 6 weeks are usually required to enable adequate hypertrophy in normal livers. After this period, surgical resection can be planned. Complications with this technique are few and include bleeding, hemobilia, and possible propagation of the thrombus. Accessing the ipsilateral lobe may avoid these problems, since the instrumented lobe is eventually resected.

General indications for PVE are based on the size of the FLR and the extent of the proposed procedure. Currently, there is no consensus as to the safe minimal size for the FLR. In a series by Vauthey and associates,[59] FLRs were calculated in 20 patients prior to an extended right lobectomy. In 12 patients who underwent PVE, there was a significant increase in the FLR (26% vs. 36%, $P < 0.01$). Fifteen patients eventually underwent resection; of these, those who had FLRs of 25% or less had an increase in the length of hospital stay and postoperative complication rate.

Portal vein embolization is most useful as part of a multimodality approach that includes neoadjuvant chemotherapy and surgery. The neoadjuvant studies of Elias and colleagues[60] and Bismuth and colleagues[61] both included patients who underwent preoperative PVE to increase the size of the FLR.

## Summary

Surgical resection remains the only treatment that leads to long-term survival and occasionally the cure of patients with hepatic colorectal metastases. The 5-year survival rates of patients who undergo surgical resection are 30% to 40%. Because of this, a surgeon experienced in hepatic resections should always be consulted to evaluate patients with hepatic colorectal metastases. In recent years, the indications for resection have been extended, and the only absolute contraindications are extrahepatic disease or an anticipated incomplete resection. Multimodality treatments incorporating systemic and regional chemotherapy along with surgical resection are being investigated. In patients who have undergone liver resection, close follow-up is important because reresection remains an option in selected patients. Patients who do not meet the criteria for surgical resection and do not have extrahepatic disease should be included in protocols investigating combined regional (hepatic artery chemotherapy) and ablative therapies (RFA or cryoablation).

## Regional Chemotherapy in Colorectal Cancer

As described in the beginning of this chapter, the liver is the main site of metastasis in cases of colorectal cancer. In one necropsy series, 43.6% of 1541 colorectal cancer patients died with evidence of liver metastases, with almost half those having exclusively liver involvement.[62] Most patients with liver involvement will die of hepatic failure.[63] The first randomized trials employ-

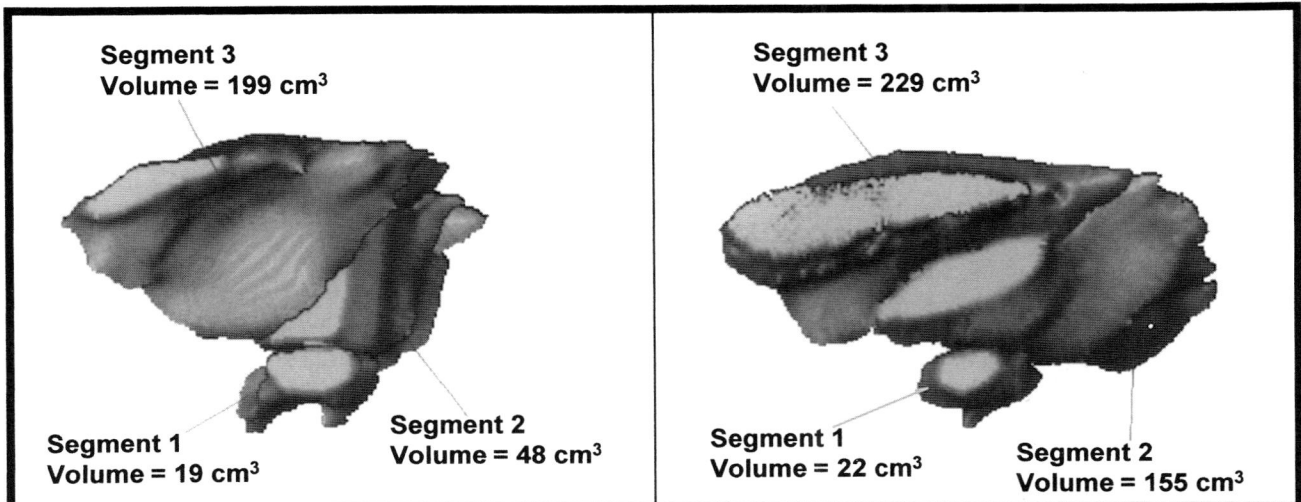

**Figure 61–3** Preoperative three-dimensional reconstruction of future liver remnant (FLR) prior to extended right lobectomy (segments 1, 2, and 3) before *(left)* and after *(right)* portal vein embolization. The FLR increased from 266 cm³ to 406 cm³ in 6 weeks. (Reproduced with permission from Vauthey JN, et al. Standardized measurement of the future liver remnant prior to extended liver resection: methodology and clinical associations. Surgery 127:512–519, 2000.)

ing hepatic regional chemotherapy in an attempt to control hepatic metastases and prolong life were reported in 1979.[64,65]

The goal for hepatic regional chemotherapy has been the delivery of high doses of chemotherapy to the liver while avoiding systemic side effects. Hepatic exposure to 5-fluorouracil (5-FU) and 5-fluoro-2-deoxyurdiine (FUDR) may be increased 100 and 400 times, respectively, when these drugs are given as a hepatic arterial infusion (HAI) rather than as a systemic intravenous (SIV) infusion.[66,67] As a result of high rates of hepatic extraction, particularly with FUDR,[68] higher response rates are expected and systemic exposure is reduced by 20% to 50%,[69] potentially reducing systemic toxicity.[70]

Investigators have used both arterial and portal venous approaches to regional delivery. According to perfusion studies of liver necropsy specimens, colorectal metastases receive over 80% of their blood from the hepatic arterial circulation.[71] By contrast, only subclinical metastases of submillimetric size are fed by significant amounts of portal venous blood.[72] Similarly, Sigurdson and colleagues[73] used tritium-labeled FUDR and demonstrated that HAI achieved significantly greater tumor drug levels than portal vein infusion (PVI) (12.4 nmol/g vs. 0.8 nmol/g, $P < 0.01$).[73] These facts prompted the study of HAI therapy in metastatic disease and the use of PVI as adjuvant therapy.[74]

## Regional Chemotherany: Surgical Techniques

Investigators have significant experience with HAI therapy and the technique has been well described.[2,75–78] Although the hepatic artery catheter can be placed angiographically and used with success,[79] high rates of bleeding and catheter thrombosis have marginalized this method,[74] and surgery is typically employed. The patient's anatomy is frequently defined using angiography so that accessory hepatic arteries and anatomic variations may be identified. Branches to the duodenum and stomach are ligated to prevent gut perfusion and ulceration, and accessory hepatic arteries are ligated to limit nondrug arterial flow. Cholecystectomy is standardly performed during the procedure. The gastroduodenal artery is cannulated near the junction of the common hepatic artery. Fluorescein dye and a technetium 99m macroaggregated albumin scan are employed to visualize liver perfusion and a misperfused stomach or duodenum. Subcutaneous implantable or extracorporeal portable pumps are attached to the catheter.

The placement of catheters for PVI is less onerous, with either the umbilical vein remnant or a mesenteric vein being employed. The catheter is usually placed at the time of resection of the primary tumor. Venography can be employed to ensure function.

## Regional Chemotherapy: Toxicity

Immediate postoperative complications with HAI or PVI include catheter thrombosis and pump-pocket hematoma. Later, although thrombosis and pump-pocket infection can occur, drug toxicities play an increasing a role in HAI. Apart from mechanical or thrombotic events, late complications in PVI are generally limited to the systemic effects of chemotherapy. Hepatitis occurs in over half of patients treated with HAI, the rate of hepatitis varying with its definition, but it usually necessitates only altered dosing. Duodenal or gastric inflammation and ulceration occur in 20% to 40% of cases[80] and have been fatal. Biliary tract toxicity can also be serious. Cholecystectomy is universally recommended for HAI therapy because of the risk of cholecystitis.[81] Biliary stricture, occurring in up to 23% of patients in randomized trials,[76] often requires stenting and may be fatal.

Three methods have been employed to try to reduce HAI-related toxicity: chronomodulation, dexamethasone infusion, and alternating infusions of FUDR and 5-FU. To improve drug tolerance, Focan and colleagues[82] employed chronomodulation, a method of altering infusion rates over a 24-hour period to match enzyme activity levels, in patients with unresectable liver metastases. In this phase II randomized study, chronomodulation did allow higher dosing of combined HAI FUDR and SIV 5-FU with comparable toxicity. However, response rates were not improved, possibly because more modulated patients had previously received cytotoxic therapy.

With the understanding that biliary toxicity can limit drug dosing, Kemeny and associates[83] undertook a trial employing dexamethasone in 50 patients with unresectable liver metastases. Patients were randomly allotted to receive HAI FUDR 0.3 mg/kg/day for 14 of each 28 days with or without 20 mg of dexamethasone over the same period. There was a modest trend toward an improvement in planned dose given for the dexamethasone group, but this was only significant in the fifth of 6 months (42% vs 19%, $P = 0.05$). Bilirubin was elevated to 200% of baseline in 9% of dexamethasone-treated patients compared to 30% of non–dexamethasone-treated patients, but this was not statistically significant and was not accompanied by a decrease in the frequency of sclerosing cholangitis (0% vs. 6%, respectively). While not a primary end point, response rates differed between the patient groups, with 71% responding in the dexamethasone group and 40% responding in the group receiving FUDR alone ($P = 0.03$). The results of this study suggest that dexamethasone may improve optimal dosing.

In a phase II study, Stagg and associates[84] used alternating HAI FUDR (0.1 mg/kg/day for days 1–8) and SIV bolus 5-FU (15 mg/kg/day on days 15, 22, and 29) in a 35-day cycle designed to limit the respective drug toxicities. The doses used for each drug were less than the doses used in other studies for the same agents used alone. None of the 64 patients had treatment termination secondary to drug toxicity, and the overall response rate of 50% is comparable to response rates in other studies. Like other efforts to limit toxicity, alternate drug dosing requires greater study.

## Hepatic Intraarterial Chemotherapy in Unresectable Liver Metastases

Although response rates have been encouraging, trials comparing HAI to SIV therapy have not consistently shown that HAI therapy provides a survival advantage. To address the power limitations of these studies, two meta-analyses have examined HAI therapy in patients with unresectable hepatic metastases. The majority of these patients had not received previous systemic chemotherapy.

The Meta-Analysis Group in Cancer[85] analyzed seven randomized studies[76,86–91] that compared HAI to SIV chemotherapy, using individual data from six of these studies and using the overall data in the study by Hohn and colleagues[87] only for response analysis (Table 61–4). All HAI arms employed FUDR. Two of the seven studies[76,91] allowed ad libitum treatment in the intravenous group, meaning that not all of these patients were treated. These two studies were not used to compare response rates, although they were included in the survival analyses.

In total, the analysis included 654 patients, with 73% of patients having a primary colon cancer and 27% a primary rectal cancer. Tumor response was seen in 41% of patients allocated to HAI (complete response [CR], 3%; partial response [PR], 38%)

**Table 61-4** Hepatic Intraarterial Infusion: Phase III Studies

| Study | Treatment Regimen | Patients (n) | Response Rate (%) | Survival, Duration, or Rate |
|-------|-------------------|--------------|-------------------|------------------------------|
| *Unresectable Disease* | | | | |
| N. Kemeny et al.[83] | HAI FUDR/dexa | 25 | 71* | MS, 23 months |
| | HAI FUDR | 25 | 40* | MS, 15 months |
| Hohn et al.[87] | HAI FUDR | 67 | 42* | MS, 503 days |
| | SIV FUDR | 76 | 10* | MS, 484 days |
| N. Kemeny et al.[88] | HIA FUDR | 48 | 50* | MS, 17 months |
| | SIV FUDR | 51 | 20* | MS, 12 months |
| Martin et al.[89] | HIA FUDR | 33 | 48* | MS, 12.6 months |
| | SIV 5-FU | 36 | 21* | MS, 10.5 months |
| Chang et al.[86] | HAI FUDR | 32 | 62* | 2 years, 22% |
| | SIV FUDR | 32 | 17* | 2 years, 15% |
| Rougier et al.[76] | HAI FUDR | 81 | 43[b] | 1 year, 64%* |
| | ±SIV 5-FU | 82 | 9 | 1 year, 44%* |
| Allen-Mersh et al.[91] | HAI FUDR | 51 | NA | MS, 405 days* |
| | ±SIV chemotherapy | 49 | NA | MS, 226 days* |
| Wagmant et al.[93a] | HAI FUDR | 31 | 55 | MS, 13.8 months |
| | SIV 5-FU/HAI FUDR | 10 | 20 | MS, 11.6 months |
| Grage et al.[64] | HAI 5-FU | 31 | 34 | MS, 10.3 months |
| | SIV 5-FU | 30 | 23 | MS, 13.3 months |
| Hunt et al.[95] | Embolization | 22 | NA | MS, 8.7 months |
| | HAI 5-FU/microspheres | 19 | NA | MS, 13 months |
| | No treatment | 20 | NA | MS, 9.6 months |
| Safi et al.[96] | HAI/SIV FUDR | 41 | 52 | 2 yr, 43% |
| | HAI FUDR | 23 | 48 | 2 years, 55% |
| Lorenz and Muller[70] | HAI 5-FU/LV | 57 | 45* | MS, 9.2 months |
| | HAI FUDR | 54 | 43.2* | MS, 5.9 months |
| | SIV 5-FU/LV | 57 | 19.7* | MS, 6.6 months |
| N. Kemeny et al.[97] | HAI FMB | 46 | 47 | MS, 19.1 months |
| | HAI FUDR | 49 | 33 | MS, 14 months |
| *Resectable Disease* | | | | |
| Lorenz et al.[100] | HIA 5-FU/LV | 108 | NA | MS, 34.5 months |
| | Resection only | 111 | NA | MS, 40.8 months |
| M. Kemeny et al.[101] | HAI FUDR/SIV 5-FU | 32 | NA | 2 years, 80% |
| | Resection only | 45 | NA | 2 years, 79% |
| N. Kemeny et al.[78] | HAI FUDR/dexa plus SIV 5-FU/±LV | 74 | NA | 2 years, 86%* |
| | SIV 5-FU/± LV | 82 | NA | 2 years, 72%* |

Abbreviations: dexa, dexamethasone; 5-FU, 5-fluorouracil; FMB, fluorodeoxyuridine, mitomycin, and carmustine; FUDR, fluorodeoxyuridine; HAI, hepatic artery infusion; LV, leucovorin; MS, median survival; NA, not applicable or unavailable; SIV, systemic intravenous; ±, with or without.

*$P \leq 0.05$ [a]Other arms not shown. [b]Not intention to treat. Significance unspecified. (Data from Landis SH, Murray T, Bolden S, Wingo PA. Cancer statistics, 1999. Ca: a Cancer Journal for Clinicians 49:8–31, 1999.[1])

compared to 14% of patients allocated to intravenous systemic therapy (CR, 2%; PR, 12%), with a response odds ratio (OR) of 0.25 (95% confidence interval [CI], 0.16–0.40) for systemic therapy. The mean response durations were 38 weeks in the HAI group and 32 weeks in the SIV group.

As impressive as this was, it did not translate into a clear survival advantage for the HAI group. Survival for all trials, effectively comparing HAI to SIV or ad libitum therapy, did show an advantage for HAI therapy, with a survival hazard ratio of 0.73 (95% CI, 0.61–0.88) for the HAI group. However, comparing HAI to SIV and excluding the ad libitum trials, the hazard ratio was 0.81 (95% CI, 0.62–1.05; $P = 0.14$), with comparative median survivals of 16 months in the HAI group and 12.2 months in the SIV group. The advantage was lost.

Two caveats must be mentioned. First, the study by Hohn and colleagues,[87] with 143 patients, was excluded from the survival analysis, diminishing its power. Second, some patients in the SIV

group were allowed to cross over to HAI if their SIV treatment was not successful. This involved 31 of 51 patients in the trial of N. Kemeny and associates,[88] and six of six patients in that of M. Kemeny and associates.[90] Crossover also occurred in the opposite direction. This crossover limits the ability to discern a statistical difference between the two treatments.

In the second meta-analysis, Hannantas and colleagues[92] examined similar trials[76,86–89,93] using whole study data, with a total of 579 patients. Again, in the HAI arms FUDR was administered, and systemic treatment arms included 5-FU or FUDR. The meta-analysis excluded the study by Allen-Mersh and associates[91] because the non-HAI group required no treatment. At the same time, however, it included the study by Rougier and associates,[76] a study that contained an ad libitum control arm, in which only 50% of the 82 patients received any SIV therapy. In addition, 24 (30%) of 81 patients in the HAI group received systemic 5-FU therapy upon failure, leading to gross differences in treatment intensity. At 1 year, the absolute survival difference was 12.9% ($P = 0.002$) in favor of HAI, and at 2 years the difference was 7.5% ($P = 0.026$). Exclusion of the study by Rougier and associates[76] resulted in a 1-year survival advantage of 10% ($P = 0.04$), although this advantage was lost at 2 years (6% advantage, $P = 0.12$). The improved survival found in this meta-analysis may have hinged on the addition of the study by Hohn and associates[87] as well as the additional numbers provided by the study by Wagman and associates.[93] Note that the Meta-Analysis Group in Cancer study did use individual data, which may be a superior method of analysis.[94]

Other trials not included in the above meta-analyses have examined HAI in patients with unresectable disease and no previous chemotherapy exposure. In one of the earliest randomized studies, Grage and colleagues,[64] compared 31 patients receiving HAI 5-FU with 30 patients receiving systemic 5-FU. After the initial 2 weeks of HAI 5-FU therapy, however, both groups received the same intravenous maintenance therapy. Response rates and median survival differences were not statistically significant.

In a similar cohort, Hunt and colleagues[95] found no survival difference between patients receiving hepatic artery embolization (22 patients), treatment with hepatic arterial injection with 5-FU–impregnated microspheres (19 patients), or no treatment (20 patients).

On the premise that extrahepatic relapse is common, Safi and colleagues[96] compared FUDR administered by HAI and SIV routes to FUDR administered by HAI only. Twenty of the 43 patients in the HAI-only treatment group were acquired from a nonrandomized pilot study, and the combined treatment group was composed of only 21 patients. No statistically significant difference was found between groups with respect to response rate, survival, or the appearance of extrahepatic metastases.

In the only randomized trial using HAI leucovorin with 5-FU, Lorenz and Muller[70] studied a multicenter cohort of 168 patients with unresectable liver metastases. Patients were randomized to HAI 5-FU and leucovorin (infusion of 1 g/m$^2$/day of 5-FU and bolus of 200 mg/m$^2$/day of leucovorin for 5 of each 28 days), SIV 5-FU and leucovorin infusion (as HAI but 800 mg/m$^2$/day 5-FU), or HAI FUDR (0.2 mg/kg/day for 14 of 28 days for three cycles and then reduced to 0.15 mg/kg/day). The primary end point was time to disease progression, which occurred after 9.2 months, 6.6 months, and 5.9 months, respectively. This result was significantly different only between the HAI 5-FU and leucovorin and the HAI FUDR groups ($P = 0.0332$). Response rates were in line with other randomized trials (45% for HAI 5-FU/leucovorin, 19.7% for SIV 5-FU/leucovorin, and 43.2% for HAI FUDR). Median survival times were not statistically different (18.7 months, 17.6 months, and 12.7 months, respectively) except in a subgroup of patients with less than 25% of liver replacement (23.3 months, 13.4 months, and 21.7 months, respectively, $P$ value not given). Interestingly, extrahepatic recurrence was decreased in patients receiving HAI 5-FU and leucovorin ($P = 0.01$) or SIV 5-FU and leucovorin ($P = 0.025$) compared to those receiving HAI FUDR (12.5% vs. 18.3% vs. 40.5%, respectively). In results that further support systemic cytotoxic exposure, patients receiving either HAI or SIV 5-FU and leucovorin had greater rates of grade 3 or 4 stomatitis and nausea and vomiting, or of any grade of skin toxicity or diarrhea. Overall, grade 3 or 4 toxicity was present in 67.5% of HAI 5-FU and leucovorin–treated patients, 66.2% of SIV 5-FU and leucovorin–treated patients, and 29.7% of HAI FUDR-treated patients. Two patients died of biliary sclerosis in the HAI FUDR group; the 30-day mortality rate was 6.3% in the HAI group overall vs. 1.8%

in the SIV-treated group. This study confirms the response rate advantage of HAI treatment. It also reaffirms the systemic effects of treatment with 5-FU and leucovorin, regardless of the route of delivery. This study was not powered to detect a survival benefit and could not show an overall advantage for any treatment arm.

To take advantage of other cytotoxic agents that have demonstrated responses in metastatic colorectal cancer, Kemeny and associates[97] studied 95 patients who had previously received cytotoxic therapy and had unresectable liver metastases. Patients received either FUDR alone (0.3 mg/kg/day for 14 of 28 days) or the same dosage of FUDR with mitomycin and carmustine, the latter two given alternatively every fourth week (10 mg/m$^2$ and 150 mg/m$^2$, respectively). Overall response rates and survival times were not significantly different. A post hoc analysis found a better response rate to combined chemotherapy in patients who had progressed on systemic chemotherapy (47% vs. 23%, $P = 0.035$). This study demonstrated that patients previously treated with systemic chemotherapy responded to HAI therapy.

Finally, in a small percentage of some series, investigators have noted that HIA chemotherapy can render previously unresectable disease operable, with the hope for prolonged survival.[98,99]

In summary, HAI chemotherapy has shown improved response rates over systemic chemotherapy alone, with 41% vs. 14% in one meta-analysis. Good response rates are also seen after failed systemic chemotherapy. The likelihood of a survival advantage with HAI therapy is less clear. Although there is a suggestion of improvement, the possible benefits are obscured by small patient numbers and methodological difficulties.

## Hepatic Intraarterial Chemotherapy in Resectable Liver Metastases

While most of the HAI studies have examined patient cohorts with unresectable disease, Lorenz and colleagues[100] studied the impact of HAI 5-FU and folinic acid compared with that of no additional treatment in patients with resected liver metastases. An interim analysis of 226 accrued patients revealed no survival difference, and the trial was aborted. In a similar postresection cohort, M. Kemeny and associates[101] examined 32 patients randomized to HAI FUDR and systemic infusional 5-FU and 45 patients randomized to no further treatment and found no significant survival difference. In contrast, N. Kemeny and associates[78] found an improved survival in 74 patients randomized to HAI FUDR plus dexamethasone and systemic 5-FU plus or minus leucovorin compared to survival in 82 patients randomized to the systemic treatment only. At 2 years, the actuarial survival rates were 90% vs. 70%, respectively ($P < 0.001$), and the progression-free survival rates were 57% vs. 42%, respectively ($P = 0.07$). The patients in the study by N. Kemeny and associates had more extensive hepatic resections than did the patients in the study by Lorenz and associates, with fewer wedge resections and more lobectomies, and had an apparent greater use of next-line treatment. This suggests a difference in the studies' cohorts or in the aggressiveness of treatment, either of which could alter outcomes. Additional studies will be needed in this area for clarification.

## Hepatic Intraarterial Chemotherapy: Other Studies

Researchers have examined numerous other aspects of regional therapy in predominantly noncontrolled studies in attempts to improve outcomes. To increase local dosing intensity, some investigators have employed the technically demanding method of isolated liver perfusion. In this scheme, the liver is isolated intraoperatively and connected to an extracorporeal circuit, allowing intense cytotoxic dosing. To date, phase I and II trials have shown some responses, but the limited data and demanding surgery restrict this treatment to trials.[102-105]

Chemoembolization is a method of generating tumor ischemia and prolonging cytotoxic exposure. Martinelli and colleagues[106] randomized 24 patients to undergo chemoembolization with polyvinyl alcohol (PVA) or PVA impregnated with 5-FU and interferon (IFN)-$\alpha_2$a and found an overall response rate of 25%, with a median survival of 9.3 months. Five patients suffered bleeding duodenal ulcers, one requiring surgery. In the small study by Hunt and associates[95] noted above, chemoembolization demonstrated no benefit over embolization alone or no further treatment. Other investigators have employed microspheres loaded with yttrium.[107] As yet, however, there is insufficient information to condone the use of this treatment outside of trials.[105,108]

Patt and associates[109] combined immunotherapy with chemotherapy using HAI. Forty-eight patients with 5-FU and leucovorin-refractory liver metastases were infused with IFN-$\alpha_2$b (5 MU/m$^2$ over 6 hours) and 5-FU (1500 mg/m$^2$ over 18 hours) for 5 days of each week for 4 to 5 weeks. Of 45 evaluable patients, 3 patients (6.7%) had complete remissions and 12 (26.7%) had partial remissions. Also, despite a World Health Organization (WHO) grade 3 or 4 mucositis rate of 40% and granulocytopenia rate of 42%, there was no similarly graded hepatobiliary toxicity. Complication rates were similar to those in HAI chemotherapy trials.

Okuno and colleagues[110] employed weekly HAI interleukin-2 (IL-2) (1.4–2.1 MU), 5-FU (250 mg), and mitomycin C (2–4 mg) in 18 patients with resectable liver metastases. Toxicity was limited to cholangitis in one patient and common transient fevers. The 5-year survival rate after 6 months of therapy was 75%.

Other investigators have used tumor necrosis factor $\alpha$ (TNF-$\alpha$) and melphalan in phase I studies with isolated liver perfusion. The high complication and hepatic toxicity rates suggest that this treatment has limited potential.[111,112]

## Hepatic Intraarterial Chemotherapy: Quality of Life

In a rare study of the effect of HAI on the quality of life, Earlam and colleagues,[113] examined 135 patients with unresectable liver metastases. Patients were treated with typical HAI (FUDR 0.2 mg/kg/day daily for 14 days each 28 days), continuous systemic infusional chemotherapy (leucovorin 30 mg/m$^2$/day and 5-FU 450 mg/m$^2$/day for 5 days monthly), or only symptomatic control. The patient data for the SIV arm were taken from a separate randomized trial. The patients treated with symptomatic control had higher levels of anxiety, but only during the first month. Those treated with systemic therapy had increased symptom scores for sore mouth and tingling hands and feet during therapy compared with the scores for symptomatic control patients. No overall difference in quality of life was detected between patients who received HAI therapy and those who received SIV therapy, or between patients who received HAI therapy and those who received only symptom control.

In the original study from which the Earlam HAI data were derived, Allen-Mersh and associates[91] noted that control patients had a median survival of 226 days, of which a short median of 12 days was spent with an abnormal physical-symptom score. Differences between control patients and those who received HAI therapy could not be detected.

## Hepatic Intraarterial Chemotherapy: Costs

The Meta-Analysis Group in Cancer used data gathered from their meta-analysis on HAI chemotherapy (see above) to perform a cost-effectiveness analysis with 1995 U.S. dollar values and data collected from Stanford University Medical Center (Palo Alto, CA) and Henri Mondor Hospital (Paris, France ).[114] Societal costs were excluded. With a mean gain in life expectancy of 3.2 months for patients who underwent HAI, the cost per life-year benefit of HAI was $72,300 in Palo Alto and $73,635 in Paris. Using data from patients seen between 1988 and 1995, Durand-Zaleski and associates[115] analyzed the cost-effectiveness of HAI, SIV chemotherapy, and symptom control, taking societal costs into account. When comparing HAI to SIV chemotherapy, the cost per life-year gained was £31,892, whereas SIV chemotherapy resulted in a cost per life-year of £41,527 over that of symptom control. These figures are in the upper range for the acceptable costs of a therapy.

## Portal Vein Infusion

In 1997, the Liver Infusion Meta-Analysis Group published a meta-analysis[116] of 10 studies[65,117-123] that was based on individual patient data to evaluate the benefit of PVI of chemotherapy. This analysis was important because only two of the included studies could independently demonstrate improvement in survival.[65,117] To be included in the meta-analysis, trials had to be randomized to an arm of continuous postoperative adjuvant PVI of cytotoxic chemotherapy or an arm with no further treatment and had to have commenced before 1987. Individual data were obtained from 10 of 11 eligible trials. In line with intention-to-treat principles, all randomized patients were included and mortality rates were calculated on the basis of results from some patients who were actually excluded from trials following randomization and surgery, after hepatic metastases or other ineligibility criteria were found. This may account for the fact that a mortality benefit found in one trial[121] was not found in the pooled individual data taken from this trial for the meta-analysis.

In general, PVI treatment consisted of infusion of 0.5 to 0.6 mg/m$^2$/day of 5-FU for 7 consecutive days following surgery. Two studies also employed mitomycin C (10 or 12 mg/m$^2$ on day 1).[120,121] Three of the studies included an additional control arm of 7 days PVI of heparin[119,120,124] and one included a control arm of 24 hours PVI of urokinase.[122] One study, referred to as the Australasia study, included a further control arm of systemic infusional 5-FU.

The meta-analysis, which included 3499 patients, compared the PVI treatment group to the group that received no further treatment. For all 10 trials, the annual relative risk reduction in mortality was 13.6% ($P = 0.006$). When the investigators excluded the earliest trial,[65,117] which had a never-again matched 39% relative risk reduction ($P = 0.008$), the reduction fell to 11% ($P = 0.04$). Life-table estimates suggest that survival curves do not diverge until some years after treatment, with an eventual 6-year absolute survival difference of 4.7% ($P = 0.006$). Excluding the earliest trial, this number again fell, this time to 3.6% ($P = 0.04$). When the analysis was stratified for disease stage, and stage D patients (8.2% of the PVI group and 7.2% of the nontreated group) were excluded, the absolute survival benefit at 5 years was 6.0% ($P = 0.001$), which highlights the risk for the effect of stage migration. No stage taken individually demonstrated statistical improvement in survival.

When PVI of cytotoxic therapy was compared with PVI of heparin or urokinase, a pooling of the four relevant studies revealed a 20% relative risk reduction in mortality ($P = 0.04$). By contrast, the Australasia study, which included both portal venous and systemic venous chemotherapy arms, showed no statistical difference in survival.

In terms of liver recurrence, 2 of the 10 trials demonstrated an independent statistically significant decrease in the liver as the site of first recurrence.[117,122] However, the overall heterogeneity of the trials was significant ($P = 0.0003$), precluding reliance on the pooled result (a 28.2% relative risk reduction).

In an update of a study[126] not included in this meta-analysis, Weber and colleagues[125] examined 469 patients with operable colorectal cancer. Similar to the above trials, PVI patients received 5-FU (0.5 g/m$^2$/day for 7 days postoperatively) and mitomycin C (l0 mg/m$^2$ at 24 hours postoperatively). After a close median follow-up of 5.8 years, the actuarial 5-year survival rate was significantly improved (69% vs. 59%, $P = 0.048$). In a similar vein, Kimura and colleagues[127] employed PVI 5-FU and mitomycin for 14 days followed by 6 months of oral 5-FU (150 mg/day), compared with SIV 5-FU and mitomycin in similar doses. After 5 years of follow-up in 110 patients, there was no difference in recurrence rates (19% vs. 26%, respectively).

More recently, James and associates[128] randomized 3681 patients to receive either 7 days of adjuvant PVI of 5-FU (1 g/day) plus heparin (5000 U/day) or no further treatment. Additionally, patients with rectal cancer were randomized to receive radiation (option of either preoperative 20–25 Gy in 4–5 fractions or postoperative 45 Gy in 20 fractions) or no radiation. Preliminary results at a median follow-up duration of 4 years demonstrated a nonstatistically significant estimated survival benefit of 2.5% at 5 years ($P = 0.20$). This magnitude of benefit is in line with that of the meta-analysis. A 5-year median follow-up in the radiation arms also showed a nonstatistically significant advantage for radiation treatment.

Labianca and associates[129] reported preliminary results of an important trial of 1094 patients who received PVI 5-FU (500 mg/m$^2$/day) and heparin (5000 UI/day) for 7 days, systemic peripheral L-folinic acid (100 mg/m$^2$ daily × 5) and 5-FU (370 mg/m$^2$ daily × 5) every 28 days for 6 months, or a combination of these treatments. The median follow-up was only 35 months, but there was no evidence of altered outcome.

Considering all PVI data, one finds a possible 5% 5-year survival benefit. Annual relative risk reductions may be in the range of 10%–15%. Interestingly, hepatic recurrences were not clearly reduced. Furthermore, there is an insufficient number of trials comparing PVI to systemic therapy. This suggests the possibility that the benefit of PVI may be derived from its systemic effects, a question the study by Labianca and associates[129] should help answer. If 7 days of PVI proved to be equivalent to 6 months of SIV chemotherapy, patient convenience and overall costs might be improved. Without further direct comparison, it is difficult to recommend PVI over conventional systemic therapy.

## Systemic Therapy

Even though the liver remains the main site for metastatic spread from colorectal cancer, other organs are commonly affected. The lungs and the peritoneum are commonly involved, and other sites such as the bones and the central nervous system can be affected. Patients who are treated with local therapies for liver metastasis commonly experience a recurrence of disease and die of extrahepatic metastasis.

The development of active chemotherapy regimens for colorectal cancer has been difficult, and only a handful of agents have demonstrated enough activity to be used in clinical practice. The last decade has witnessed the arrival of several new agents with the promise of changing this scenario, and three drugs have been approved by the Food and Drug Administration (FDA) for treatment of colorectal cancer since 1996. It would be beyond the scope of this chapter to list every single agent being studied for use against colorectal cancer, and we will concentrate on the agents that have been approved by regulatory agencies or that are in advanced stages of development

### 5-Fluorouracil

Since its synthesis by Heidelberger and colleagues[130] in 1957, 5-fluorouracil (5-FU) has been the most extensively used therapeutic agent for the treatment of colorectal cancer. The mechanism of action of 5-FU depends on three active metabolites: 5-fluorodeoxyuridine monophosphate (FdUMP), 5-fluorodeoxyuridine triphosphate (5-FdUTP), and fluorouracil triphosphate (FUTP). The intracellular conversion of 5-FU to FdUMP inhibits the enzyme thymidydilate synthase (TS), leading to the inhibition of DNA synthesis and the induction of apoptosis.[131] The binding of 5-FdUMP to TS is optimized in the presence of 5,10-methylenetetrahydrofolate (THF), resulting in a more sustained inhibition of TS. The conversion of 5-FU to 5-FUTP results in incorporation of this nucleotide into RNA, causing abnormal RNA processing, whereas the formation of 5-FdUTP leads to misincorporation into DNA, resulting in DNA strand breaks. The extent to which any of these pathways predominates in human tumors is unknown and is likely to vary across tumor types and with different 5-FU administration schedules or types of biochemical modulation applied.

While anabolism is clearly critical in the conversion of 5-FU to the active nucleotides FdUMP, FUTP, and FdUTP, catabolism controls the amount of 5-FU available for anabolism and thus occupies an important position in the overall metabolism of 5-FU. Dihydropyrimidine dehydrogenase (DPD) is the initial rate-limiting enzyme in pyrimidine catabolism, converting over 85% of clinically administered 5-FU to 5-FUH2, an inactive metabolite, in an enzymatic step that is effectively irreversible. An understanding of these metabolic pathways provides opportunities to optimize fluoropyrimidine chemotherapy by selecting those tumors most likely to respond to therapy. In addition, new fluoropyrimidine modulators and prodrugs have been developed that may enhance the effectiveness of 5-FU.

Because of the limited antitumor activity of single-agent 5-FU, various biochemical modulators and administration schedules have been investigated in patients with advanced colorectal cancer. Some of the modulators studied include folinic acid (FA), also known as leucovorin, methotrexate (MTX), trimetrexate (TMX), interferon (IFN), $N$-(phosphonacetyl)-L-aspartic acid (PALA), and levamisole.

Since the 1980s, the combination of 5-FU and FA has been considered the standard treatment for advanced colorectal cancer. Poon and colleagues[132] showed that combined 5-FU/FA increases the response rate and the time to treatment failure, prolongs survival, and improves quality of life compared with 5-FU alone. A seven-arm phase II trial by the Southwest Oncology Group (SWOG)[133] suggested that infusional 5-FU produced the most favorable toxicity spectrum and the longest survival compared with the six other 5-FU regimens, warranting further investigation in phase III trials. This trial by the SWOG randomly allocated 620 patients with advanced colorectal cancer to receive one of the following treatments: bolus 5-FU, bolus 5-FU with either low-dose or high-dose FA, protracted infusion of 5-FU with or without low-dose FA, or high-dose 24-hour infusiona1

5-FU with or without PALA. Confirmed response rates ranged from 13% to 24%. At a median follow-up duration of 37 months, there was minimal difference among the seven regimens with respect to progression-free survival. However, there was a trend toward longer survival for patients who received the low-dose continuous-infusion and the 24-hour-infusion 5-FU regimens; patients who received PALA plus high-dose infusional 5-FU had shorter survival durations. Overall survival ranged from 13 to 15 months for all treatments.

Two published meta-analyses addressed the effect of 5-FU treatment on objective tumor response and survival in advanced colorectal cancer. One study[134] compared 5-FU and FA with 5-FU alone; the other[135] compared 5-FU via continuous infusion with 5-FU via bolus administration. Both meta-analyses confirmed that the 5-FU/FA and 5-FU continuous infusion produced better objective response rates (23% vs. 11%, $P < 10^{-7}$ and 22% vs. 14%, $P = 0.0002$, respectively). Combined 5-FU/FA provided no survival advantage over 5-FU alone ($P = 0.57$).[134] An evaluation of individual prognostic factors demonstrated that patients with a good performance status or metastases confined to the liver had significantly better survival ($P < 10^{-9}$ and $P = 0.046$, respectively). The overall survival was significantly higher for patients who received continuous-infusion 5-FU ($P = 0.04$), although the median survival times were close.[135] Multivariate analysis showed that patients with good performance status had improved tumor response and survival ($P < 0.0001$, $P < 0.0001$, respectively), and that patients with rectal cancer at the primary tumor site had improved survival compared with those with colon cancer ($P = 0.0003$). The combination of 5-FU and FA increases the efficacy of 5-FU with tolerable adverse effects, while achieving symptom palliation.

Until recently, the most widely used regimens for the treatment of patients with metastatic colorectal cancer were the Mayo Clinic regimen,[132] which uses low-dose FA with 5-FU bolus for 5 days once every month, and the Gastrointestinal Tumor Study Group (GITSG) regimen[136] (developed by the Roswell Park Cancer Institute), which consists of a 2-hour infusion of high-dose FA with 5-FU bolus once a week for 6 weeks, every 8 weeks. It is unclear which dose of FA is necessary for a clinically effective modulation of bolus 5-FU. Preclinical data indicate that in the case of single-bolus dose of 5-FU, as given in the GITSG protocol, a high dose of FA is necessary to achieve sufficient polyglutamation and stable formation of the inhibitory ternary complex of 5-FdUMP/THF/TS. In contrast, with daily 5-FU, as in the Mayo Clinic protocol, a daily low dose of FA can achieve the same effect. Both regimens have served as control arms for phase III trials investigating new fluoropyrimidines or combinations with new agents.[137]

Despite a meta-analysis[138] that included eight randomized clinical trials with 1178 patients demonstrating improved response rates and survival for combined 5-FU/MTX over 5-FU alone (OR, 0.87; $P = 0.024$), 5-FU/MTX is rarely used in clinical practice. The reason for this could be that 5-FU/MTX confers only a modest improvement in efficacy compared to 5-FU/FA. In addition, MTX must be administered 24 hours before 5-FU, creating an inconvenience for the patient.

Trimetrexate also potentiates the cytotoxicity of 5-FU.[139] Conti and associates[140] demonstrated a 20% response rate in heavily pretreated advanced colorectal cancer patients, while Blanke and associates[141] reported an overall response rate of 42% in 36 untreated patients.[142] On the basis of two randomized trials,[142a,142b] investigators concluded that the addition of TMX to a weekly regimen of 5-FU/LV did not improve the outcome for patients with advanced colorectal cancer.

In summary, 5-FU plays a major role in the treatment of colorectal cancer. Intravenous bolus 5-FU plus FA still remains a viable option for the treatment of this disease. Although a protracted infusion of 5-FU is superior to 5-FU in terms of response rate, time to progression, and toxicity profile, this modality has a major impact on the patient's quality of life, with minimal improvement in overall survival.

## Oral Fluoropyrimidines

Oral fluoropyrimidines were developed as an alternative, simplified strategy for achieving protracted exposure to 5-FU chemotherapy. Their advantages include fewer catheter-related complications, schedule flexibility, and reductions in professional health-care resources, administration costs, and toxicity-related hospitalizations.[143] Oral 5-FU has not gained widespread clinical acceptance because of its erratic absorption in the gastrointestinal tract, with over 85% of the drug being converted by DPD to inactive metabolites. The circadian pattern[144–146] and the wide variation of DPD activity among individuals[147,148] and tumors[149] are responsible for much of the variability in pharmacokinetics, oral bioavailability, toxicity, and efficacy following administration of 5-FU.

Two methods have been studied to circumvent catabolism of 5-FU by DPD, allowing for oral dosing of 5-FU. One was to design oral 5-FU precursors such as tegafur plus uracil (UFT) and capecitabine (Xeloda), which are absorbed as intact molecules via the gastrointestinal tract and then converted into 5-FU. The other was to develop DPD-inactivating agents, such as eniluracil, that would allow reliable absorption of orally administered 5-FU.

### Capecitabine

Capecitabine (Xeloda) resulted from an effort to develop an oral, tumor-selective fluoropyrimidine carbamate that exploits the higher levels of thymidine phosphorylase observed in tumors than in normal tissue and plasma. The drug is absorbed from the gut as an intact molecule and is not affected by the thymidine phosphorylase present in the intestine. In the liver and tumor tissue, capecitabine is converted to doxifluridine and then to 5-FU by thymidine phosphorylase. Dose-limiting toxic effects observed with capecitabine are diarrhea, vomiting, and hand-foot (palmarplantar erythrodysesthesia) syndrome.[150] The results of two phase III trials[151,152] comparing capecitabine at 2500 mg/m$^2$/day for 2 weeks every 3 weeks to intravenous 5-FU at 425 mg/m$^2$ plus FA at 20 mg/m$^2$/day for 5 days every 4 weeks as first-line treatment for metastatic colorectal cancer (Table 61–1) showed that the most common treatment-related grade 3 and 4 toxicities associated with capecitabine were hand-foot syndrome and diarrhea, whereas the most common grade 3 and 4 toxicities with 5-FU/FA were neutropenia, diarrhea, and stomatitis. Survival (median, 12.9 months in each group) and time to progression (median, 4.6 and 4.7 months with capecitabine and 5-FU/FA, respectively) were equivalent. Investigators in both studies concluded that the oral administration of capecitabine resulted in a higher response rate and a more favorable toxicity profile than those of 5-FU biomodulation. Capecitabine is now FDA approved for the management of patients with metastatic colorectal cancer.

### UFT (tegafur plus uracil)

UFT is a combination in a 4:1 molar ratio of tegafur, a 5-FU prodrug metabolized primarily by hepatic microsomal enzymes, and uracil, a competitive inhibitor of DPD. Tegafur has demonstrated modest antitumor activity as a single agent.[153,154] Because of marked gastrointestinal toxicity and lethargy during intensive intravenous schedules, however, the clinical development of tegafur in the United States was halted. Japanese clinical investigators concentrated on prolonged oral schedules of the drug, observing only mild toxicities.[155] The biomodulation of tegafur with uracil results in an enhanced concentration of 5-FU in tumors and an improved antitumor effect.[156,157] Schedule-dependent toxicities observed in phase I trials with single-agent UFT included neutropenia in patients who received a 5-day schedule and diarrhea in those who received a 28-day schedule. Because of the extensive clinical experience with the biochemical modulation of 5-FU by FA, further development of UFT examined in combination with oral FA was examined. The dose-limiting toxicity of this combination administered for 28 consecutive days every 35 days was diarrhea. The recommended dose for phase II trials was 300 to 350 mg/m$^2$/day of UFT plus 150 mg/day of FA.[158–161]

The results of two multinational phase III trials[162,163] comparing a combination of UFT plus oral FA, also known as ORZEL, to intravenous 5-FU and FA as the initial treatment for patients with metastatic colorectal cancer were reported. In the first trial,[162] which included 816 patients, UFT (300 mg/m$^2$/day) and FA (75 mg or 90 mg/day) were administered orally for 28 days every 35 days, and 5-FU (425 mg/m$^2$/day) and FA (20 mg/m$^2$/day) were given intravenously for 5 days every 28 days. The study demonstrated that the two combinations were equally efficacious (overall response rates of 12% for the UFT plus FA and 15% for the 5-FU plus FA). While producing survival rates equivalent to those of 5-FU/LV, ORZEL treatment had a lower incidence of side effects, requiring less use of antibiotics, growth factors, and antiemetics. In the second trial,[163] 380 patients were randomized to receive either intravenous 5-FU plus FA or ORZEL, with regimens similar to those in the first study, except that the 5-FU/FA was administered every 35 days and all the patients received 90 mg/day of FA. The study demonstrated equivalent median times to progression and survival durations. The ORZEL treatment provided an equally effective but safer and more convenient oral alternative to the standard intravenous 5-FU/FA regimen. ORZEL is being evaluated in the adjuvant treatment of patients with stage II and III colon cancer and as a radiosensitizing agent.[154,164,165]

## Eniluracil

Eniluracil is an irreversible inactivator of DPD.[166] When oral 5-FU is administered concurrently with eniluracil, the bioavailability of 5-FU is markedly improved.[167] The dose-limiting toxicity of this combination was neutropenia, which was schedule-dependent.[168] In a multicenter phase II study of metastatic colorectal cancer using a dose of 1 mg/m$^2$ 5-FU plus 10 mg/m$^2$ eniluracil given orally twice daily for 28 days followed by 7 days of rest, the observed treatment-related toxicities were unexpectedly low. Subsequently, the doses of both agents were increased to 1.15 mg/m$^2$ 5-FU and 11.5 mg/m$^2$ eniluracil twice daily for 28 days. An overall response rate of 29% was observed, with 57% of patients having stable disease after two courses of therapy.[169,170] Phase III trials comparing the combination of oral 5-FU and eniluracil with the intravenous 5-FU/LV in previously untreated patients with metastatic colorectal cancer have been completed but unfortunately the results were not very encouraging.[170a]

## Irinotecan

Irinotecan (CPT -11), a semisynthetic soluble derivative of the plant alkaloid camptothecin, acts by inhibiting topoisomerase 1.[171] The dose-limiting toxicity observed in phase I trials of irinotecan were diarrhea and neutropenia.[172–174] Other toxicities included nausea, vomiting, alopecia, and early cholinergic-like syndrome that may include diarrhea. Two schedules were selected for phase II trials in patients with metastatic colorectal cancer: 350 mg/m$^2$ once every 3 weeks, in Europe, and 125–150 mg/m$^2$ every week for 4 weeks followed by 2 weeks of rest, in the United States. The response rates in the phase II trials of patients with metastatic colorectal cancer were between 19% and 32%[174,175] for patients in whom irinotecan was used as the first-line treatment and between 13% and 25% in 5-FU–refractory patients.[176,177]

To accurately define irinotecan's clinical benefit in the treatment of refractory colorectal cancer, two randomized phase III trials were conducted, primarily in Europe. Rather than focusing on surrogate end points of response rate and time to progression, these trials examined clinical end points such as irinotecan's effect on survival, quality of life, and amelioration of disease-related symptoms.

The first study[178] compared irinotecan at 350 mg/m$^2$ as a 90-minute infusion every 3 weeks (189 patients) to best supportive care (BSC) (90 patients). With a median follow-up of 13 months, the median survival was 9.2 months for irinotecan-treated patients, compared with 6.5 months for the patients treated with BSC alone ($P = 0.0001$). The 1-year overall survival rate was 36.2% for the irinotecan-treated patients vs. 13.8% for those who received BSC. All significant quality-of-life scores, with the exception of diarrhea, favored the irinotecan group.

The second prospective randomized phase III trial[179] compared irinotecan at 350 mg/m$^2$ as a 90-minute infusion every 3 weeks (133 patients) with one of three infusional 5-FU regimens (134 patients) as second-line treatment for patients with metastatic colorectal cancer. With a median follow-up of 15 months, the median survival duration was 10.8 months for the irinotecan group compared with 8.5 months for the 5-FU group ($P = 0.035$), and 1-year survival rates were 45% and 32%, respectively. Quality-of-life variables and control of disease-related symptoms in the two groups were comparable. On the basis of these two trials, irinotecan has become the standard treatment for patients with metastatic colorectal carcinoma whose disease progressed or recurred following 5-FU.

Irinotecan has also been investigated in combination with 5-FU plus FA (IFL) in two phase III trials[180,181] comparing 5-FU plus FA to IFL for initial treatment of metastatic colorectal cancer. In the U.S. trial,[180] the overall response rate and the median time to treatment failure were better in the IFL group (49% and 5.0 months, respectively) than in the 5-FU plus FA group (27% and 3.8 months, respectively) ($P < 0.001$ and $P < 0.05$, respectively). Similarly, in the European trial,[181] the response rate and the median progression-free survival were better in the three-drug combination arm compared with the standard-treatment arm: 39% vs. 22% and 8.1 vs. 4.3 months, respectively. Matured survival data presented to the FDA's Oncology Drug Advisory Committee (ODAC) showed a survival benefit for the patients who received the combination of 5-FU, FA, and irinotecan. The FDA has approved irinotecan as first-line therapy in combination with 5-FU and leucovorin (FA) for patients with metastatic colorectal cancer. It is also approved for patients whose disease has recurred or progressed after initial 5-FU–based therapy. Given these encouraging results, randomized trials are being conducted in the adjuvant setting.

## Oxaliplatin

Oxaliplatin is a novel third-generation diaminocyclohexane platinum agent that acts mainly by forming DNA adducts.[182,183] Unlike cisplatin and carboplatin, oxaliplatin is active against colorectal cancer.[184] The dose limiting toxicity of this agent is peripheral sensory neuropathy, believed to be dose-related and reversible upon discontinuation of the drug. The renal and auditory toxicities observed with the other available platinum compounds are not seen with oxaliplatin.[185–187] In previously untreated patients with advanced colorectal carcinoma, oxaliplatin at 130 mg/m$^2$ every 3 weeks produced response rates and survival durations comparable to those of 5-FU plus leucovorin or irinotecan as the first-line treatment.[188] In 5-FU–refractory patients, the results with oxaliplatin were similar to those achieved with irinotecan in the same setting.[189] In these trials, the incidence and severity of peripheral sensory neuropathy correlated with increasing cumulative doses of oxaliplatin. Other toxicities, all of which were mild to moderate, included diarrhea, nausea, and vomiting. Synergy between 5-FU and oxaliplatin was initially demonstrated in preclinical models and has been confirmed in clinical trials. In patients with advanced colorectal cancer who have not previously undergone chemotherapy, the combination of chronomodulated 5-FU (700 to 1000 mg/m$^2$/day), oxaliplatin (25 mg/m$^2$/day), and leucovorin (300 mg/m$^2$/day), administered for 4 days every 14 days, produced a 67% response rate and a median survival in excess of 19 months.[190] The potential benefit of oxaliplatin when added to 5-FU/LV as the first-line therapy for patients with advanced colorectal cancer was subsequently evaluated in phase III randomized trials.

Giacchetti and colleagues[191] compared chronomodulated 5-FU/LV with or without short-infusion oxaliplatin every 3 weeks in 200 patients with advanced colorectal carcinoma. The response rates after three cycles were 12% (95% CI, 6% to 20%) with chronomodulated 5-FU/LV alone and 34% (95% CI, 24%–44%) with 5-FU/LV plus oxaliplatin ($P < 0.01$). The progression-free survival was longer (8.9 months vs. 5.2 months) in the oxaliplatin arm, and the overall survival times were comparable (17.6 months vs. 19.4 months) between the two arms. This survival equivalence was attributed to the crossover of 57 patients to the oxaliplatin/5-FU/FA treatment upon progression in the control arm, with performance of metastasectomy in more than 20% of patients after crossover. In another study, de Gramont and colleagues[192] randomized 420 patients to receive bimonthly 5-FU/FA with or without oxaliplatin 85 mg/m$^2$ on day 1. The response rate was significantly higher in the oxaliplatin arm (50.7% vs. 22.3%, $P = 0.0001$). Progression-free survival was also improved in the oxaliplatin arm (8.2 months vs. 6.2 months, $P = 0.0001$); however, oxaliplatin did not significantly impact survival (16.0 months vs. 14.7 months).

Oxaliplatin plus 5-FU/FA (FOLFOX) has also shown promising results in patients with advanced colorectal carcinoma refractory to 5-FU. The FOLFOX regimens, consisting of flat-rate infusions of oxaliplatin combined with 5-FU (continuous infusion with or without a bolus) and FA, were systematically studied in this patient population by de Gramont and associates.[193–195] The overall response rates ranged between 20% and 53%, the median progression-free survival times were 5.0 to 6.2 months, and the median overall survival times were 10 to 15 months. The most common grade 3 and 4 toxicities were myelosuppression (neutropenia in 9% to 40% of patients and thrombocytopenia in 2% to 15% of patients), peripheral sensory neuropathy (7% to 16%), and gastrointestinal toxicity. Recent reports of the FOLFOX regimens[195,196] showed that patients who received 85 mg/m$^2$ or more oxaliplatin had a higher response rate and a longer progression-free survival time than those of patients who received less than 85 mg/m$^2$ oxaliplatin (39% vs. 19%, $P = 0.03$, and 28 weeks vs. 26 weeks, $P = 0.02$, respectively). Other trials of ox-

aliplatin plus other widely used 5-FU–based regimens have confirmed the activity of this combination in advanced 5-FU–refractory colorectal cancer.[197]

A three-arm randomized intergroup clinical trial (N9741) for the initial treatment of advanced colorectal cancer was conducted and a planned interim analysis was performed in April 2002.[197a] The treatment arms were IFL, FOLFOX4, and irinotecan and oxaliplatin. FOLFOX4 is oxaliplatin at 85 mg/m$^2$ administered as a 2-hour infusion on day 1; FA at 200 mg/m$^2$ administered as a 2-hour infusion on days 1 and 2; followed by a loading dose of 5-FU, 400 mg/m$^2$ IV bolus, then 600 mg/m$^2$ 5-FU administered by an ambulatory pump over 22 hours days 1 and 2. The patients accrued to the IFL and FOLFOX4 arms formed the basis of the study analysis. There were 264 and 267 patients accrued to the IFL and FOLFOX4 regimens, respectively, with a minimum follow-up for these patients of 1 year. The analysis demonstrated that outcomes for patients receiving FOLFOX4 were significantly better than those for patients with the standard IFL arm. There was a significantly better time to tumor progression for FOLFOX4 than for IFL (8.8 months vs. 6.9 months; $P = 0.0009$), higher response rate (38% vs. 29%; $P = 0.03$), and improved overall survival (18.6 months vs. 14.1 months; $P = 0.002$). The 1-year survival rate was 71% for patients who received FOLFOX4 compared to 58% among those who received IFL. The toxicity profile was also less severe in patients receiving FOLFOX4. On the basis of this analysis, accrual to all arms of the N9741 protocol except FOLFOX4 was discontinued.

In August 2002, the FDA approved oxaliplatin for use in combination with infusional 5-FU plus FA for the treatment of patients with colorectal cancer whose disease has recurred or progressed during or within 6 months of completion of first-line therapy with the combination of bolus 5-FU plus FA and irinotecan. This approval was based on a clinical trial demonstrating that patients treated with FOLFOX4 had an increased response rate compared to patients given infusional 5-FU plus FA or oxaliplatin alone. The study was a multicenter, randomized, three-arm controlled study conducted in the United States and Canada that compared the efficacy and safety of oxaliplatin in combination with an infusional schedule of 5-FU plus FA to that with the same dose and schedule of 5-FU plus FA alone or with single-agent oxaliplatin. A total of 821 patients with advanced colorectal cancer that had relapsed or progressed during or within 6 months of first-line therapy with bolus 5-FU plus FA and irinotecan were enrolled in the trial. Patients were randomized to FOLFOX4 as described above, to 5-FU plus FA administered as described above, or to oxaliplatin at 85 mg/m$^2$ administered as a 2-hour infusion. Cycles were repeated every 2 weeks. A planned interim analysis for response rate was conducted after 459 patients were enrolled. The number of patients analyzed in each arm were 152 for FOLFOX4, 151 for oxaliplatin alone, and 156 for 5-FU plus FA. The response rate was 9%, 1%, and 0% ($P = 0.0002$) with a median time to progression of 4.6 months, 1.6 months, and 2.7 months, respectively, for each arm as listed above. At the time of approval, the data on the effects of the combination on survival were immature.

The results of phase II trials analyzing the combination of oxaliplatin with irinotecan in patients with advanced colorectal carcinoma refractory to 5-FU have also been reported.[198] The overall response rates for patients who received different doses and schedules were 44% and 42%, with stable disease present in 35% and 36% of patients. The median time to progression was 7.5 months in both studies. The results of these trials suggest that the combination of oxaliplatin and irinotecan may be an effective salvage therapy in 5-FU–refractory patients.

## Raltitrexate

Raltitrexate (Tomudex) is the first of the specific thymidine synthase (TS) inhibitors to undergo extensive clinical evaluation. The pattern of toxicity associated with raltitrexate is different from that with 5-FU/FA, with a lower incidence of severe mucositis and leukopenia than with 5-FU/FA.[199,200] In a phase II trial,[201] the response rate for 176 patients with colorectal cancer who received raltitrexate was 25.6. Two large phase III trials[202,203] initiated in Europe compared raltitrexate and 5-FU/FA in patients with metastatic colorectal cancer who had not undergone chemotherapy. There were no significant differences in response rates, times to progression, or median survival times between the patients who received raltitrexate and those who received 5-FU/FA. A third trial,[204] performed in North America, found similar response rates between the treatment arms, but the survival was significantly shorter for patients treated with raltitrexate than for those treated with 5-FU/FA (9.7 months vs. 12.7 months, respectively, $P = 0.01$). In a more recent multicenter randomized trial[205] comparing raltitrexate and two 5-FU–based regimens, preliminary results showed no significant differences between the three regimens in terms of response rates and median survival durations. However, although the 5-FU–based regimens were broadly equivalent on all major endpoints, raltitrexate was inferior in terms of treatment-related deaths, progression-free survival, and predefined quality-of-life parameters.

The results of trials investigating the combination of raltitrexate with other agents in patients with advanced disease have recently been reported. In a dose-escalating study of raltitrexate combined with 5-FU,[206] a high proportion of patients achieved disease stabilization and the median survival time was 16.2 months. Another phase II trial evaluated the efficacy of and patient tolerance associated with raltitrexate and oxaliplatin administered every 3 weeks in 57 previously untreated patients.[207] An interim analysis of 20 evaluable patients showed a response rate of 40%, with an additional 10% of patients having stable disease.

## Newer Agents

Our new and greater understanding of the molecular biology of colorectal cancer allows the development of targeted therapies. Some promising examples include the newer antiangiogenesis drugs, the farnesyl transferase inhibitors, the monoclonal antibodies, the tyrosine kinase inhibitors, and vaccines. After decades of having only 5-FU to study, clinical researchers of colorectal cancer find themselves busy with the pleasant work of sorting through an array of newer therapies in search of the best treatments for this dreadful disease.

## References

1. Landis SH, Murray T, Bolden S, Wingo PA. Cancer statistics, 1999. CA Cancer J Clin 49:8–31, 1999.
2. Venook AP. Update on hepatic intra-arterial chemotherapy. Oncology (Huntingt) 11:947–957, 1997.
3. Vauthey JN, Marsh RDW, Cendan JC, Chu NM, Copeland EM. Arterial therapy of hepatic colorectal metastases. Br J Surg 83:447–455, 1996.
4. Silen W. Status of hepatic resection for metastases from colorectal carcinoma. Presented at the First Shanghai International Symposium on Gastrointestinal Cancers, November 1988.
5. Silen W. Hepatic resection for metastases from colorectal carcinoma is of dubious value. Arch Surg 124:1021–1022, 1989.
6. Scheele J, Stang R, Altendorf-Hofmann A, Paul M. Resection of colorectal liver metastases. World J Surg 19:59–71, 1995.
7. D'Angelica M, Brennan MF, Fortner JG, Cohen AM, Blumgart LH, Fong Y. Ninety-six five-year survivors after liver resection for metastatic colorectal cancer. J Am Coll Surg 185:554–559, 1997.
8. Jamison RL, Donohue JH, Nagorney DM, Rosen CB, Harmsen WS, Ilstrup DM. Hepatic resection for metastatic colorectal cancer results in cure for some patients. Arch Surg 132:505–510, 1997.
9. Hamm B, Vogl TJ, Branding G, et al. Focal liver lesions: MR imaging with Mn-DPDP—initial clinical results in 40 patients. Radiology 182:167–174, 1992.
10. Seneterre E, Taourel P, Bouvier Y, et al. Detection of hepatic metastases: ferumoxides-enhanced MR imaging versus unenhanced MR imaging and CT during arterial portography. Radiology 200:785–792, 1996.
11. Vauthey JN. Liver imaging. A surgeon's perspective. Radiol Clin North Am 36:445–457, 1998.
12. Yonekura Y, Benua RS, Brill AB, et al. Increased accumulation of 2-deoxy-2-[$^{18}$F]fluoro-D-glucose in liver metastases from colon carcinoma. J Nucl Med 23:1133–1137, 1982.
13. Vitola JV, Delbeke D, Meranze SG, Mazer MJ, Pinson CW. Positron emission tomography with F-18-fluorodeoxyglucose to evaluate the results of hepatic chemoembolization. Cancer 78:2216–2222, 1996.
14. Beets G, Penninckx F, Schiepers C, et al. Clinical value of whole-body positron emission tomography with [$^{18}$F]fluorodeoxyglucose in recurrent colorectal cancer. Br J Surg 81:1666–1670, 1994.
15. Lai DT, Fulham M, Stephen MS, et al. The role of whole-body positron emission tomography with [$^{18}$F]fluorodeoxyglucose in identifying operable colorectal cancer metastases to the liver. Arch Surg 131:703–707, 1996.
16. Couinaud C. Le Foie. Etudes Anatomiques et Chirugicales. Masson, Paris, 1957.
17. Goldsmith N, Woodburne R. The surgical anatomy pertaining to liver resection. Surg Gynecol Obstet 105:310–318, 1957.
18. Bilimoria M, Vauthey J. Technique of extended hepatic resection. In: Koeckerling F (ed): Liver Surgery. Thieme Verlag, New York, pp 171–178, 2001.
19. Adson MA, van Heerden JA, Adson MH, Wagner JS, Ilstrup DM. Resection of hepatic metastases from colorectal cancer. Arch Surg 119:647–651, 1984.
20. Ringe B, Bechstein WO, Raab R, Meyer HJ, Pichlmayr R. Leberresektion bei 157 Patienten mit colorectalen Metastasen. Chirurg 61:272–279, 1990.
21. Doci R, Gennari L, Bignami P, Montalto F, Morabito A, Bozzetti F. One hundred patients with hepatic metastases from colorectal cancer treated by resection: analysis of prognostic determinants. Br J Surg 78:797–801, 1991.
22. Herfarth C, Hohenberger P. Synchrone resektion von lebermetastasen kolorektaler Karzinome. Langenbecks Arch Surg 66–72, 1992.
23. Rosen CB, Nagorney DM, Taswell HF, et al. Perioperative blood transfusion and determinants of survival after liver resection for metastatic colorectal carcinoma. Ann Surg 216:493–504, 1992.
24. Sugihara K, Hojo K, Moriya Y, Yamasaki S, Kosuge T, Takayama T. Pattern of recurrence after hepatic resection for colorectal metastasis. Br J Surg 80:1032–1035, 1993.
25. Gozzetti G, Mazziotti A, Grazi GL, Jovine E, Frena A. Undici anni di esperienza nella terapia chirurgica delle metastasi epatiche da tumori colo-rettali. Chir Ital 46:30–36, 1994.
26. Gayowski TJ, Iwatsuki S, Madariaga JR, et al. Experience in hepatic resection for metastatic colorectal cancer: analysis of clinical and pathologic risk factors. Surgery 116:703–710, 1994.
27. Scheele J, Altendorf-Hofmann A, Stangl R, Schmidt K. Chirurgische Resektion kolorektaler Lebermetastasen: Goldstandard für solitare und radikal resektable Herde. Swiss Surg Suppl 4:4–17, 1996.
28. Jenkins LT, Millikan KW, Bines SD, Staren ED, Doolas A. Hepatic resection for metastatic colorectal cancer. Am Surg 63:605–610, 1997.
29. Ambiru S, Miyazaki M, Isono T, et al. Hepatic resection for colorectal metastases: analysis of prognostic factors. Dis Colon Rectum 42:632–639, 1999.
30. Fong Y, Fortner J, Sun RL, Brennan MF, Blumgart LH. Clinical score for predicting recurrence after hepatic resection for metastatic colorectal cancer: analysis of 1001 consecutive cases. Ann Surg 230:309–318, 1999.
31. Craig J, Peters R, Edmondson H. Metastatic tumors. In: Hartmann W, Sobin L (eds): Tumors of the Liver and Intrahepatic Bile Ducts. Atlas of Tumor Pathology, Series 2. Armed Forces Institute of Pathology, Washington, DC, 1989, pp 256–267.
32. Nakamura S, Suzuki S, Konno H. Resection of hepatic metastases of colorectal carcinoma: 20 years' experience. J Hepatobiliary Pancreat Surg 6:16–22, 1999.
33. Beckurts KT, Holscher AH, Thorban S, Bollschweiler E, Siewert JR. Significance of lymph node involvement at the hepatic hilum in the resection of colorectal liver metastases. Br J Surg 84:1081–1084, 1997.

34. Scheele J, Stangl R, Altendorf-Hofmann A, Gall FP. Indicators of prognosis after hepatic resection for colorectal secondaries. Surgery 110: 13–29, 1991.

35. Yamamoto J, Sugihara K, Kosuge T, et al. Pathologic support for limited hepatectomy in the treatment of liver metastases from colorectal cancer. Ann Surg 221:74–78, 1995.

36. Shirabe K, Takenaka K, Gion T, et al. Analysis of prognostic risk factors in hepatic resection for metastatic colorectal carcinoma with special reference to the surgical margin. Br J Surg 84:1077–1080, 1997.

37. Hughes KS, Rosenstein RB, Songhorabodi S, et al. Resection of the liver for colorectal carcinoma metastases. A multi-institutional study of long-term survivors. Dis Colon Rectum 31:1–4, 1988.

38. Griffith KD, Sugarbaker PH, Chang AE. Repeat hepatic resections for colorectal metastases. Surgery 107:101–104, 1990.

39. Lange JF, Leese T, Castaing D, Bismuth H. Repeat hepatectomy for recurrent malignant tumors of the liver. Surg Gynecol Obstet 169:119–126, 1989.

40. Andersson R, Tranberg KG, Bengmark S. Reresection of colorectal liver secondaries: a preliminary report. J Hepatobiliary Pancreat Surg 2: 69–72, 1990.

41. Stone MD, Cady B, Jenkins RL, McDermott WV, Steele GD Jr. Surgical therapy for recurrent liver metastases from colorectal cancer. Arch Surg 125:718–721, 1990.

42. Fortner JG. Recurrence of colorectal cancer after hepatic resection. Am J Surg 155:378–382, 1988.

43. Fong Y, Blumgart LH, Cohen A, Fortner J, Brennan MF. Repeat hepatic resections for metastatic colorectal cancer. Ann Surg 220:657–662, 1994.

44. Fernandez-Trigo V, Shamsa F, Sugarbaker PH. Repeat liver resections from colorectal metastasis. Repeat Hepatic Metastases Registry. Surgery 117:296–304, 1995.

45. Goya T, Miyazawa N, Kondo H, Tsuchiya R, Naruke T, Suemasu K. Surgical resection of pulmonary metastases from colorectal cancer. 10-year follow-up. Cancer 64:1418–1421, 1989.

46. Yano T, Hara N, Ichinose Y, Yokoyama H, Miura T, Ohta M. Results of pulmonary resection of metastatic colorectal cancer and its application. J Thorac Cardiovasc Surg 106:875–879, 1993.

47. Gough DB, Donohue JH, Trastek VA, Nagorney DM. Resection of hepatic and pulmonary metastases in patients with colorectal cancer. Br J Surg 81:94–96, 1994.

48. DeMatteo R, Minnard E, Kemeny N, et al. Outcome after resection of both liver and lung metastasis in patients with colorectal cancer. Proc Am Soc Clin Oncol 18:249a, 1999.

49. Gagne D, Roh M. Cryosurgery for hepatic malignancies. In: Curley S (ed): Liver Cancer. Springer, New York, 1998, pp 173–200.

50. Onik G, Rubinsky B, Zemel R, et al. Ultrasound-guided hepatic cryosurgery in the treatment of metastatic colon carcinoma. Preliminary results. Cancer 67:901–907, 1991.

51. Seifert JK, Morris DL. Indicators of recurrence following cryotherapy for hepatic metastases from colorectal cancer. Br J Surg 86:234–240, 1999.

52. Ravikumar TS, Kane R, Cady B, Jenkins R, Clouse M, Steele G Jr. A 5-year study of cryosurgery in the treatment of liver tumors. Arch Surg 126:1520–1523, 1991.

53. Seifert JK, Morris DL. Cryotherapy of the resection edge after liver resection for colorectal cancer metastases. Aust N Z J Surg 68:725–728, 1998.

54. Johnson LB, Krebs TL, Van Echo D, et al. Cytoablative therapy with combined resection and cryosurgery for limited bilobar hepatic colorectal metastases. Am J Surg 174:610–613, 1997.

55. Curley SA, Izzo F, Delrio P, et al. Radiofrequency ablation of unresectable primary and metastatic hepatic malignancies: results in 123 patients. Ann Surg 230:1–8, 1999.

56. Solbiati L, Goldberg SN, Ierace T, et al. Hepatic metastases: percutaneous radio-frequency ablation with cooled-tip electrodes. Radiology 205:367–373, 1997.

57. Kinoshita H, Sakai K, Hirohashi K, Igawa S, Yamasaki O, Kubo S. Preoperative portal vein embolization for hepatocellular carcinoma. World J Surg 10:803–808, 1986.

58. Kawasaki S, Makuuchi M, Kakazu T, et al. Resection for multiple metastatic liver tumors after portal embolization. Surgery 115:674–677, 1994.

59. Vauthey J, Chaoui A, Do K, et al. Standardized measurement of the future liver remnant prior to extended liver resection: methodology and clinical associations. Surgery 127:512–519, 2000.

60. Elias D, Lasser P, Rougier P, Ducreux M, Bognel C, Roche A. Frequency, technical aspects, results, and indications of major hepatectomy after prolonged intra-arterial hepatic chemotherapy for initially unresectable hepatic tumors. J Am Coll Surg 180:213–219, 1995.

61. Bismuth H, Adam R, Levi F, et al. Resection of nonresectable liver metastases from colorectal cancer after neoadjuvant chemotherapy. Ann Surg 224:509–520, 1996.

62. Weiss L, Grundmann E, Torhorst J, et al. Haematogenous metastatic patterns in colonic carcinoma: an analysis of 1541 necropsies. J Pathol 150:195–203, 1986.

63. Goslin R, Steele G Jr, Zamcheck N, Mayer R, MacIntyre J. Factors influencing survival in patients with hepatic metastases from adenocarcinoma of the colon or rectum. Dis Colon Rectum 25:749–754, 1982.

64. Grage TB, Vassilopoulos PP, Shingleton WW, et al. Results of a prospective randomized study of hepatic artery infusion with 5-fluorouracil versus intravenous 5-fluorouracil in patients with hepatic metastases from colorectal cancer: a Central Oncology Group study. Surgery 86:550–555, 1979.

65. Taylor I, Rowling J, West C. Adjuvant cytotoxic liver perfusion for colorectal cancer. Br J Surg 66:833–837, 1979.

66. Ensminger WD, Gyves JW. Clinical pharmacology of hepatic arterial chemotherapy. Semin Oncol 10:176–182, 1983.

67. Ensminger WD, Gyves JW. Regional chemotherapy of neoplastic diseases. Pharmacol Ther 21:277–293, 1983.

68. Ensminger WD, Rosowsky A, Raso V, et al. A clinical–pharmacological evaluation of hepatic arterial infusions of 5-fluoro-2′-deoxyuridine and 5-fluorouracil. Cancer Res 38:3784–3792, 1978.

69. Chen HS, Gross JF. Intra-arterial infusion of anticancer drugs: theoretic aspects of drug delivery and review of responses. Cancer Treat Rep 64: 31–40, 1980.

70. Lorenz M, Muller HH. Randomized, multicenter trial of fluorouracil plus leucovorin administered either via hepatic arterial or intravenous infusion versus fluorodeoxyuridine administered via hepatic arterial infusion in patients with nonresectable liver metastases from colorectal carcinoma. J Clin Oncol 18:243–254, 2000.

71. Breedis C, Young G. The blood supply of neoplasms in the liver. Am J Pathol 30:969, 1954.

72. Archer SG, Gray BN. Vascularization of small liver metastases. Br J Surg 76:545–548, 1989.

73. Sigurdson ER, Ridge JA, Kemeny N, Daly JM. Tumor and liver drug uptake following hepatic artery and portal vein infusion. J Clin Oncol 5:1836–1840, 1987.

74. Kemeny N, Fata F. Arterial, portal, or systemic chemotherapy for patients with hepatic metastasis of colorectal carcinoma. J Hepatobiliary Pancreat Surg 6:39–49, 1999.

75. Venook AP, Stagg RJ, Lewis BJ. Regional chemotherapy for colorectal cancer metastatic to the liver. Oncology (Huntingt) 2:19–26, 1988.

76. Rougier P, Laplanche A, Huguier M, et al. Hepatic arterial infusion of floxuridine in patients with liver metastases from colorectal carcinoma: long-term results of a prospective randomized trial. J Clin Oncol 10: 1112–1118, 1992.

77. Kemeny NE, Ron IG. Hepatic arterial chemotherapy in metastatic colorectal patients. Semin Oncol 26:524–535, 1999.

78. Kemeny N, Huang Y, Cohen AM, et al. Hepatic arterial infusion of chemotherapy after resection of hepatic metastases from colorectal cancer. N Engl J Med 341:2039–2048, 1999.

79. Thirlwell MP, Hollingsworth LM, Herba MJ, Boileau G, Boos G, MacFarlane JK. Ambulatory hepatic artery infusion chemotherapy for cancer of the liver. Am J Surg 151:585–589, 1986.

80. Rougier P. Are there indications for intraarterial hepatic chemotherapy or isolated liver perfusion? The case of liver metastases from colorectal cancer. Recent Results Cancer Res 147:3–12, 1998.

81. Ottery FD, Scupham RK, Weese JL. Chemical cholecystitis after intrahepatic chemotherapy. The case for prophylactic cholecystectomy during pump placement. Dis Colon Rectum 29:187–190, 1986.

82. Focan C, Levi F, Kreutz F, et al. Continuous delivery of venous 5-fluorouracil and arterial 5-fluorodeoxyuridine for hepatic metastases from colorectal cancer: feasibility and tolerance in a randomized phase II trial comparing flat versus chronomodulated infusion. Anticancer Drugs 10:385–392, 1999.

83. Kemeny N, Seiter K, Niedzwiecki D, et al. A randomized trial of intrahepatic infusion of fluorodeoxyuridine with dexamethasone versus fluorodeoxyuridine alone in the treatment of metastatic colorectal cancer. Cancer 69:327–334, 1992.

84. Stagg RJ, Venook AP, Chase JL, et al. Alternating hepatic intra-arterial floxuridine and fluorouracil: a less toxic regimen for treatment of liver metastases from colorectal cancer. J Natl Cancer Inst 83:423–428, 1991.

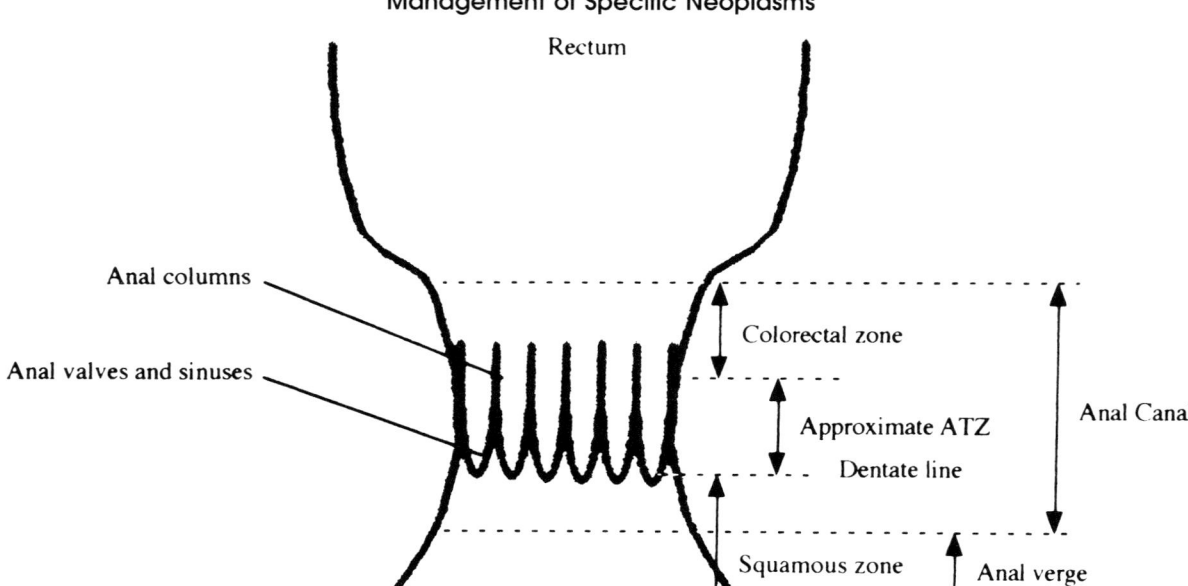

**Figure 62-1** The anal canal with anatomic and histologic landmarks. ATZ, anal transition zone.

## Molecular Biology of Anal Epithelial Neoplasia: Central Role of HPV

It is now well established that HPV is the causative agent of genital warts and plays a central role in the pathogenesis of anal cancer and precancer.[9] Many different HPVs have been identified and are categorized as high risk (types 16, 18, 45, and 56), intermediate risk (types 31, 33, 35, 39, 51, and 52), or low risk (types 6, 11, 42, 43, and 44) on the basis of the frequency with which they are found in invasive genital tract cancers.[10] The low-risk HPV types 6 and 11 are commonly found in condylomata.[11] A high percentage of invasive anal cancers have been found to

contain the same HPV types found in cervical carcinoma[12–14] (Table 62–1), and there is a strong association between a clinical history of cervical neoplasia, genital/anal warts, and invasive squamous cell carcinoma.[11,12,15–18] Women with a history of cervical neoplasia are at an elevated risk for anal neoplasia and carcinoma.[19]

The presence of high-risk HPV types is associated with decreased levels of the tumor suppressor genes *p53* (wild type) and *Rb*. This is thought to be secondary to the HPV E6 and E7 viral proteins, respectively, which bind the tumor suppressor proteins and inactivate them by either increased degradation or sequestration.[9,13] The E6 and E7 proteins of HPV types 16 and 18 are

**Table 62-1** World Health Organization sites and classification of anal carcinomas along with human papillomavirus association[32]

| Anatomic Site and Classification of Anal Carcinoma | HPV Association | Study |
|---|---|---|
| *Anal Canal* | | |
| Squamous cell carcinoma (cloacogenic) | + | Frisch et al., 1997[49] |
|     Large cell, keratinizing | | |
|     Large cell, nonkeratinizing (transitional) | | |
|     Basaloid | | |
| Adenocarcinoma | | |
|     Rectal type | − | Frisch et al., 1997;[49] Higgins et al., 1991[110] |
|     Anal gland | −/+ | Higgins et al., 1991;[110] Koulos et al., 1991[111] |
|     Anorectal fistula | ND | |
| Small cell carcinoma | ND | |
| Undifferentiated | ND | |
| *Anal Margin* | | |
| Squamous cell carcinoma | + | Frisch et al., 1999[112] |
| Giant condyloma (verrucous carcinoma) | + | Poletti et al., 1993[113] |
| Basal cell carcinoma (of skin) | − | Boxman et al., 2000[62] |
| Bowen's disease (carcinoma in situ) | + | Frisch et al., 1999[112] |
| Paget's disease | − | Brainard, 2000[70] |

Abbreviations: HPV, human papillomavirus; ND, no data; +, present; −, absent.

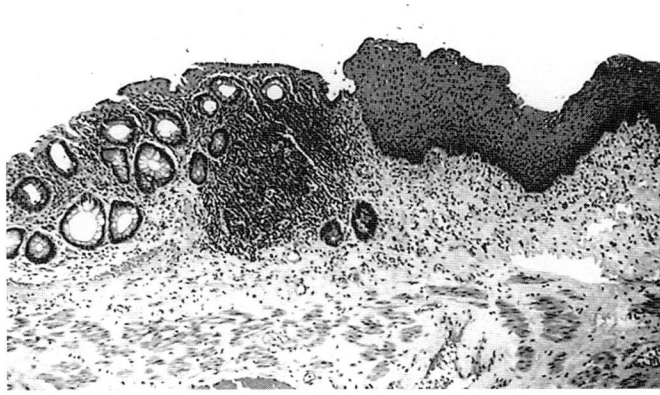

**Figure 62–2** The anal squamocolumnar junction (anal transition zone) showing the colonic type mucosa (left side) and squamous mucosa (right side) (×100).

associated with the ability to transform cells in vitro, but the E6 or E7 proteins from low-risk HPV types 6 and 11 are not, probably because the proteins from the low-risk HPV types do not bind the tumor suppressor proteins.[9,20] This inactivation of regulatory proteins leads to disruption of the cell cycle, chromosomal instability, and abnormalities thought to be responsible for malignant transformation.[21]

Mutations in the *p53* gene and overexpression of the c-*myc* oncogene have been implicated in the progression of AIN,[22,23] and elevated levels of mutant *p53* have been found in greater than 50% of invasive anal carcinomas.[22]

Anal carcinoma is also associated with abnormalities in chromosome 11 (11q22) and in the short arm of chromosome 3 (3p22);[24] amplification of 3q is seen in anal dysplasia.[21] Such abnormalities of chromosome 3 are associated with high-risk HPV types, especially type 16.[25]

## Definitions and Classification of Anal Neoplastic Lesions

Anal neoplasia is classified as invasive cancer or intraepithelial neoplasia, which is thought to be the precursor to invasive disease.[26] Invasive anal cancer is considered to be present when the neoplastic cells have penetrated the basement membrane and infiltrated into the underlying stroma. In AIN, the abnormal cells are contained above the basement membrane. While most anal malignancies are carcinomas (epithelium-derived tumors), other malignancies, such as melanoma and lymphoma, rarely arise within the anal canal.

Traditionally, to classify invasive anal carcinomas, pathologists have used confusing terminology that took into account the kind of epithelium from which the tumor was considered to have arisen (cloacogenic, nonkeratinizing squamous, and keratinizing squamous) or specific morphologic features of the tumor. For example, cancers were classified as either keratinizing or nonkeratinizing, transitional (if they resembled urothelium), basaloid (if they resembled basal cells and had peripheral palisading), or mucoepidermoid (if mucinous microcysts were present).[27] The term *cloacogenic carcinoma* was previously used nonspecifically to refer to both the basaloid and the large-cell nonkeratinizing squamous cell carcinomas. The World Health Organization (WHO) classification scheme, which is simplified but does contain some of these terms, is shown in Table 62–1.

Currently, there is a good deal of evidence that many of the traditional classifications have little basis. A recent study by Fenger and colleagues[28] showed that the subdivision of epidermoid anal squamous carcinomas advocated by the WHO has a markedly low inter- and intrapathologist reproducibility.[29] Other studies have shown that there is no or minimal prognostic significance to separating anal squamous cell carcinomas into the more common variants.[27,29,30] Keratin-expression profiles differ among the so-called variants, but these differing keratin profiles are also seen in the metaplastic epithelium of the transition zone.[31]

These studies, along with others demonstrating that most anal carcinomas (with the exception of adenocarcinomas and small cell tumors) are HPV related (Table 62–1), suggest that a reevaluation of the current classification scheme is necessary. A more logical approach may be to classify all HPV-related carcinomas together while continuing to indicate whether tumors appear to be located in the anal margin or canal, since this does appear to have some clinical relevance.

## Squamous Cell Carcinoma

### Clinical Features

Squamous cell carcinoma and its variants are the most common tumors of the anal canal and anal margin, accounting for over 70% of tumors in this region.[14] Most anal tumors arise within the anal canal instead of the anal margin.[7,32] Anal canal carcinomas are thought to be more common in women, with the female-to-male ratio ranging from 2:1 to 4:1.[29,31] Anal margin carcinomas are more common in men, with a male-to-female ratio of approximately 4:1.[29,31] The peak incidence in both groups occurs around the fifth or sixth decade of life.[14,29] The associated risk factors for anal carcinoma include a history of receptive anal intercourse, male homosexuality, smoking, a history of cervical dysplasia, independent carcinomas of the lower genital tract (such as cervical carcinoma), condyloma acuminatum, and immunosuppression related to organ transplantation or HIV.[7,8,33,34]

The clinical presentation of anal carcinoma is nonspecific. Most patients (70%–80%) are first diagnosed with benign anorectal conditions.[7] Presentation can be characterized by anal bleeding (50% of patients), pain (40%), an anal mass (25%), and/or pruritis (15%), but approximately 25% of patients are asymptomatic.[8,35] Because the symptoms of anal carcinoma are nonspecific, patients tend to present late with large tumors.

The gross appearance of anal canal tumors is deceptive and does not help in the histologic typing of the tumors (Fig. 62–3). They can be flat, raised, annular, ulcerated, and/or polypoid, with a mean size at presentation of 3 to 4 cm, and they may obscure the point of origin.[7,36] Most anal canal tumors arise at or below the dentate line and then either grow upward into the rectum or outward into the perianal tissues.[35,36] Involvement of the perianal skin may be superficial with only surface ulceration, mimicking a benign condition; in other cases, a deeply ulcerated neoplasm is present.

### Histology

Histologically, squamous cell carcinoma of the anal canal is most commonly characterized by invasive tumor islands and nests with peripheral palisading of the cells and central eosinophilic necrosis (Fig. 62–4). Foci of keratinization can be present. These tumors are sometimes composed of cells with decreased amounts of cytoplasm compared with the large cell carcinomas and re-

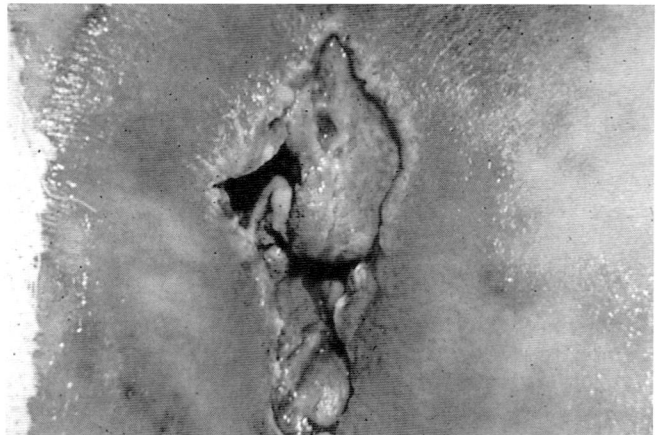

**Figure 62–3** Clinical presentation of advanced anal carcinoma.

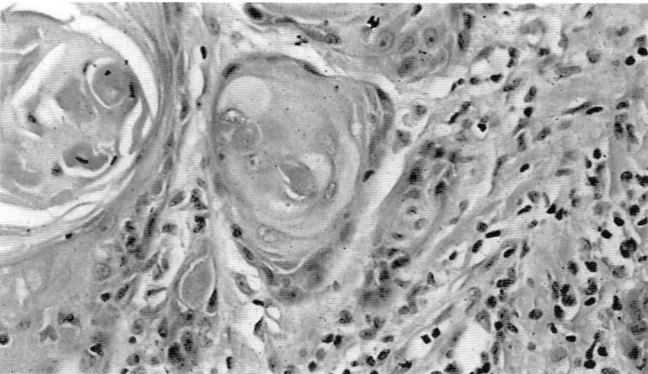

**Figure 62–5** Invasive keratinizing squamous cell carcinoma with large whorls of keratinization (×400).

semble basal cells of the epithelium, hence the designation *basaloid squamous cell carcinoma.*

Keratinizing squamous cell carcinoma, which is more common in the anal margin, is characterized by invasive nests of large cells with prominent keratinization and hyperchromatic nuclei with large nucleoli (Fig. 62–5). Nonkeratinizing, or transitional, squamous cell carcinoma has similar histologic features but lacks the prominent keratinizing component. The nonkeratinizing form has in the past been inappropriately called *transitional carcinoma* because of its superficial resemblance to transitional (urothelial) carcinoma of the bladder. Necrosis can be prominent.

Other variants of squamous cell carcinoma include squamous cell carcinoma with mucinous microcysts (formerly designated *mucoepidermoid carcinoma*), the pseudoadenoid cystic pattern, and the pseudosarcomatous patterns.[36,37]

## Treatment

Currently, the most common treatment approach for anal canal tumors is a combination of radiation therapy and chemotherapy, sometimes followed by local or abdominoperineal resection for more advanced tumors.[14,38] Abdominoperineal resection has significant morbidity, with loss of the anal sphincter requiring a permanent colostomy, and an operative mortality rate of around 5%.[7] Local excision is adequate for small tumors (less than 2 cm) that do not involve the dentate line.[7]

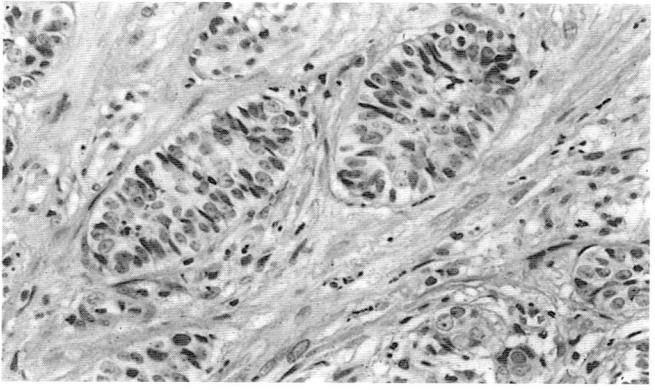

**Figure 62–4** The typical histologic appearance of invasive anal squamous cell carcinoma with invasive nests of tumor showing peripheral palisading (×400).

The treatment differs for anal margin tumors. About 60% of anal margin tumors are amenable to local excision, and advanced cases respond well to radiation therapy and chemotherapy, which can achieve local cure in 80% to almost 100% of patients.[7]

## Prognosis

Factors that have been clearly associated with prognosis include the size of the tumor, depth of invasion, extent of local spread, nodal status, and location of the tumor at presentation; the prognostic value of histologic subtyping is minimal and, as mentioned, not reproducible.[27–30] The size of the tumor at presentation appears to be one of the most important prognostic factors, with most tumors 2 cm or less being amenable to cure.[8]

The TNM staging system for anal carcinoma and the staging criteria of Boman and colleague,[30] which emphasize the depth of invasion, are shown in Table 62–2. The depth of tumor invasion is an important prognostic factor, with tumors confined to the anal epithelium or subepithelial connective tissues having a significantly better prognosis than those with penetration into the muscle or adjacent pelvic tissues.[30]

Anal margin tumors tend to have a better prognosis than anal canal tumors. Anal margin tumors have higher cure rates, probably due to earlier presentation with smaller tumors, easier accessibility, and the possibility of cure through local excision rather than abdominoperineal resection.[7,29,31]

The overall 5-year survival rate for patients with anal canal squamous cell carcinoma is 60%–80% for patients undergoing combined radiation therapy and chemotherapy and around 60% for those undergoing abdominoperineal resection.[7] The 5-year survival rate for patients with anal margin carcinoma varies from 65% to almost 100%, depending on the study.[7] Locoregional recurrence of carcinoma in both groups portends a poor prognosis,[7,35] although salvage abdominoperineal resection after combined radiation therapy and chemotherapy can prolong survival.[14] Inguinal lymph node involvement at presentation is associated with a poor prognosis, with a 5-year survival rate of less than 20%.[7]

## Giant Condyloma/Verrucous Carcinoma (Buschke-Loewenstein Tumor)

Giant condyloma/verrucous carcinoma is a rare entity of the anorectal region. Grossly, giant condyloma and verrucous carcinoma present as a single large, warty, exophytic, cauliflower-like growth. HPV types 6, 11, and 16, as well as others, have been

**Table 62-2** TNM staging system[a] and staging system of Boman et al.[30] for anal canal tumors

| TNM | | Boman et al. |
|---|---|---|
| *Primary Tumor (T)* | | *Stage A* |
| Tx | Primary tumor cannot be assessed | Tumor confined to epithelium and |
| T0 | No evidence of primary tumor | subepithelial connective tissue |
| Tis | Carcinoma in situ (AIN III/Bowen's disease) | *Stage B* |
| T1 | <2 cm in greatest dimension | |
| T2 | 2–5 cm in greatest dimension | Tumor penetration into muscle or |
| T3 | >5 cm in greatest dimension | adjacent pelvic tissues |
| T4 | Tumor of any size with invasion of adjacent organ | B1    Invasion of internal sphincter |
| | | B2    Invasion of external sphincter |
| *Regional Lymph Nodes (N)* | | B3    Invasion of adjacent pelvic tissues |
| Nx | Regional lymph nodes cannot be assessed | *Stage C* |
| N0 | No regional lymph node metastases | |
| N1 | Metastasis in perirectal lymph nodes(s) | Metastasis to regional lymph nodes |
| N2 | Metastasis in unilateral internal iliac and/or | (inguinal or pelvic) |
| | inguinal lymph node(s) | *Stage D* |
| N3 | Metastasis in perirectal and inguinal lymph nodes | |
| | and/or bilateral internal iliac lymph nodes and/or | Unresectable regional tumor or distant |
| | inguinal lymph nodes | metastasis |
| *Distant Metastasis (M)* | | |
| Mx | Presence of distant metastasis cannot be assessed | |
| M0 | No distant metastasis | |
| M1 | Distant metastasis | |

[a]According to International Union Against Cancer (UICC).[114]

detected in giant condyloma and verrucous carcinoma.[39–42] Histologically, giant condyloma resembles condyloma acuminata and is composed of extremely well-differentiated squamous epithelium that invades the stroma in a pushing (rather than diffuse) fashion. Giant condyloma and verrucous carcinoma seem to be similar entities, with giant condyloma and verrucous carcinoma forming a continuum.[43,44] Giant condyloma is often associated with dysplasia, carcinoma, or both.[32] Some authors advocate designating all cases of giant condyloma verrucous carcinoma, but the issue is still controversial.[32,45] Others suggest screening for high-risk HPV types to decide on the management of giant condyloma, although the absence of high-risk HPV types does not exclude the possibility of invasive carcinoma within giant condyloma.[46] These tumors have a high rate of recurrence (66%), especially in patients with a long history of disease, and a high rate of malignant transformation (56%), but almost no risk for distant metastasis.[47] In a study by Chu and colleagues,[47] radical surgery led to cure in 61% of patients, whereas chemotherapy with or without local excision led to cure in only 25% of patients.[47]

### Adenocarcinoma

Adenocarcinoma of the anus comprises from 8% to 19% of anal tumors.[7,14] Three major types of anal adenocarcinoma are rectal type adenocarcinoma, anal gland adenocarcinoma, and adenocarcinoma associated with anal fissures (most commonly mucinous adenocarcinomas).

### Rectal Type Adenocarcinoma

Rectal type adenocarcinoma is the most common adenocarcinoma in the anal canal and usually arises within the upper zone lined by colorectal type mucosa (Fig. 62–6). The etiology is similar to that for colorectal carcinomas, with frequent mutations in

p53.[48] There is no association between rectal type adenocarcinoma and HPV.[49] Rectal adenocarcinomas can spread into the anal region, making the distinction between rectal and anal adenocarcinomas difficult.[32] Histologically, rectal type adenocarcinomas are identical to colorectal adenocarcinomas.[36]

### Anal Gland Adenocarcinoma

Anal gland adenocarcinoma is extremely uncommon and is composed of small acini and tubules lined by cuboid cells with scant mucin production that infiltrate the stroma. These are thought to arise from the anal glands that open onto the mucosal surface; usually the overlying mucosa is intact.[32] The etiology is unknown. The difficulty in diagnosing anal gland carcinoma lies in finding a definite transition from anal gland to invasive carcinoma,[36] although rare case reports document the presence of anal gland dysplasia in association with invasive adenocarcinoma.[50–52]

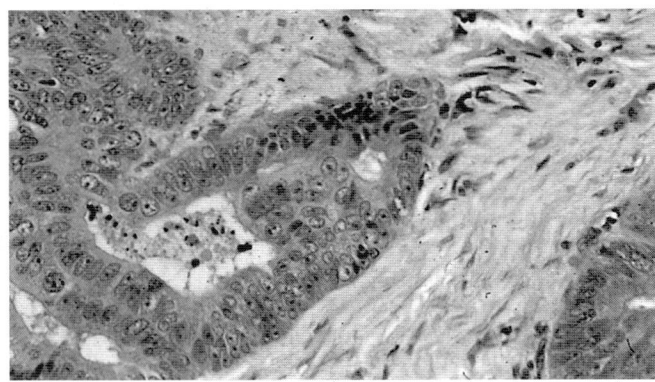

**Figure 62-6** Colorectal type adenocarcinoma occurring in the anal canal (×400).

## Adenocarcinoma Associated with Anal Fissures

Adenocarcinomas of the anus associated with fistula tend to be mucinous ("colloid") adenocarcinomas and most often arise in patients with a long history of anal and perianal disease.[53] In most cases, there is little involvement of the overlying rectal and anal mucosa. Microscopically, there is abundant mucin within cystic spaces lined by columnar neoplastic epithelium. Signet ring cells, which can diffusely infiltrate the underlying tissue, may be present.[53] The origin of these tumors is controversial, with theories postulating that they arise from the anal glands, develop within the fistula itself, or may be from congenital duplication of the hindgut.[36]

### Treatment and Prognosis

Traditionally, anal adenocarcinoma has been treated by abdominoperineal resection with or without additional combined radiation therapy and chemotherapy,[14] although some investigators now advocate combined radiation therapy and chemotherapy prior to surgery.[54] Klas and associates[14] reported an overall 5-year survival rate of 63% for patients with adenocarcinoma treated by surgery with or without adjuvant chemotherapy/radiation therapy. This survival rate may have been secondary to the fact that most of their patients presented with small tumors (<5 cm), and larger tumors were treated either pre- or postoperatively with combined chemotherapy/radiation therapy. Other studies have found a markedly poor prognosis, mostly secondary to advanced stage at diagnosis.[54,55] In a study by Basik and colleagues,[55] patients had a median survival time of 29 months after treatment.

## Malignant Melanoma

Extracutaneous malignant melanoma is rare, but it accounts for approximately 10% of primary anal malignancies other than adenocarcinoma.[36] A recent study by Cagir and associates[56] showed that the overall incidence of anorectal melanoma has increased, with this increase being most marked in young men (<45 years old) in the San Francisco area; indirect evidence implicates HIV as a risk factor in the development of anorectal melanoma.[56] Ethnic groups with a low risk for cutaneous melanoma have no such advantage with anorectal melanoma (i.e., sun exposure is not a risk factor for anorectal melanoma).[57] Patients often present complaining of pain, bleeding, a mass, or "hemorrhoids," sometimes present for long periods of time.[58] Anorectal melanomas can arise anywhere from the anal verge to the colorectal zone of the anal canal.[36] These tumors can be flat or pedunculated, and most contain abundant melanin pigment, sometimes with an adjacent junctional (or in situ) component.[58] They can be mistaken for hemorrhoids or a primary rectal tumor if they extend into the colorectal zone.[35] Histologically, anorectal melanoma resembles melanoma at other body sites, composed of large pleomorphic cells with large nuclei, prominent nucleoli, and abundant melanin, although many other patterns have been described.[36] The diagnosis is readily confirmed by immunohistochemical reactivity for S-100 protein and HMB-45. The prognosis is directly related to the tumor size and depth of invasion and is generally extremely poor since most patients present with extensive local or disseminated disease.[31,56,59] The 5-year survival rate was 33% in the study by Klas and colleagues;[14] the mean survival was 22 months in the Quan study.[59] Most authors now advocate local excision with adjuvant therapy rather than radical surgery because of the uniformly poor prognosis regardless of treatment modality and the morbidity associated with abdominoperineal resection.[14,58]

## Small Cell Carcinoma

Small cell carcinoma of the anus is an uncommon virulent malignancy of the anus. No studies have been done on the etiology of small cell carcinoma of the anus, although cervical small cell carcinomas are associated with HPV and with loss of Rb expression.[60] Histologically, small cell carcinoma of the anus resembles small cell carcinoma at other sites in the body. The cells form large, solid nests of tumor with central necrosis and have scanty amounts of cytoplasm and nuclei with coarse, grainy chromatin. The differential diagnosis for small cell carcinoma of the anus includes basaloid squamous cell carcinoma. Immunohistochemically, however, basaloid squamous cell carcinoma is positive for high-molecular-weight cytokeratins and carcinoembryonic antigen, whereas small cell carcinoma is positive for neuroendocrine markers (chromogranin, neurofilament, and neuron-specific enolase).[61] Most patients with small cell carcinoma of the anus present with advanced disease, and the 5-year survival rates are dismal; in one study, only one of seven patients survived 5 years.[30] This patient underwent an abdominoperineal resection, but most patients present with unresectable disease.[36]

## Basal Cell Carcinoma (of Skin)

Basal cell carcinoma occurs usually in the perianal skin and sometimes in the anal margin; in rare cases, it encroaches on the anal canal. Basal cell carcinoma of the skin is associated with sun exposure and mutations in the *PATCHED* gene; most data suggest that there is no significant association with HPV.[62–64] Basaloid squamous cell carcinoma of the anus should be excluded since it is more common in this anatomic region and associated with a much worse prognosis than that of basal cell carcinoma.[65] Histologically, basal cell carcinoma is composed of large nests of basaloid cells, often with clefting between the surrounding stroma and the tumor nests. Necrosis is unusual. These tumors are low grade with an excellent prognosis and can be cured by local excision or radiation.[65]

## Paget's Disease

Paget's disease is a rare disease of the anus that is most often found in the perianal region, but it can be found in the anal canal and the anal verge.[66] The disease is more common in women than men.[66] Strictly defined, it is an in situ malignant neoplasm of the intraepidermal portion of apocrine glands, with or without associated dermal involvement.[67] Paget's disease can, however, represent the intraepidermal spread of an associated adenocarcinoma of anal or rectal origin.[36,68,69] Approximately 50% of cases of anal Paget's disease are associated with an underlying malignancy, which can be synchronous or develop many years later.[36,67] Paget's disease is not associated with HPV, although it can be associated with squamous proliferative lesions.[70] On examination, Paget's disease is usually an erythematous, ulcerated, eczematoid lesion, and patients often complain of itching or tenderness. Histologically, Paget's disease reveals malignant-appearing cells with large nuclei, prominent nucleoli, and pale cytoplasm sprinkled throughout the epidermis or mucosa (Fig. 62–7). The most common treatment is local excision, with a recurrence rate of approximately 61%.[66] Recurrences are amenable to re-excision and the 5-year survival rate for patients without visceral malignancies is similar to that for age-matched controls.[66] Those cases associated with visceral malignancies have a poor prognosis.[68] The two types of Paget's disease can be differentiated immunohistochemically. Paget's disease arising from

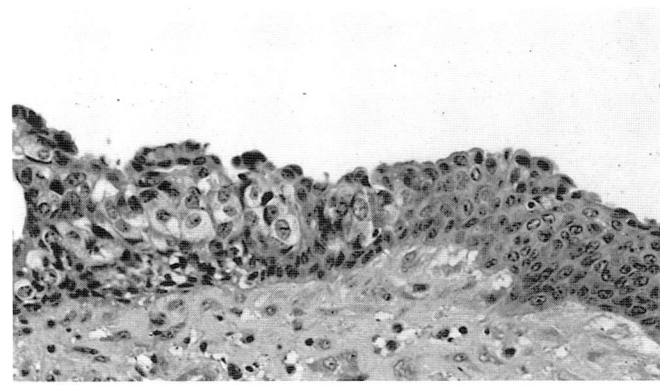

**Figure 62-7** Paget's disease of the anal canal. Note the pale cells sprinkled throughout the metaplastic squamous (transitional) mucosa (left side) (×400).

the skin marks with antibodies to cytokeratin-7 and gross cystic disease fluid protien-15 (GCDFP-15) but not cytokeratin-20, whereas Paget's disease arising from visceral malignancies marks with antibodies to cytokeratin-7 and cytokeratin-20 but is negative for GCDFP-15.[68]

## Lymphoma

Primary anal lymphoma is extremely rare in the general population, but the incidence of anal lymphoma is markedly increased in people with HIV or acquired immune deficiency syndrome (AIDS). Most patients with anorectal lymphoma present in the sixth decade of life, except for patients with HIV or AIDS, who usually present in the third or fourth decade and whose tumors are usually associated with the Epstein-Barr virus.[71] Anal lymphomas are usually low-grade, small-cell types in non-AIDS patients and mostly high-grade B-cell lymphomas in patients with HIV or AIDS.[71] The prognosis for anorectal lymphoma in patients with HIV is poor, with a less than 50% 1-year survival rate.[72]

## Anal Intraepithelial Neoplasia

Lesions in which the abnormal cells remain contained above the basement membrane are referred to as *anal intraepithelial neoplasia* (AIN). Traditionally, these lesions have been classified as AIN 1, AIN 2, and AIN 3/anal carcinoma in situ (AIS). AIN 1 is the morphologic expression of what is generally self-limited HPV infection, or condyloma (see below). It is currently believed that AIN 3/AIS is the immediate precursor of invasive anal cancer. However, considerably less data are available concerning the relationship between AIN 3 and invasive anal cancer than for the relationship between cervical intraepithelial neoplasia (CIN) 3 and invasive cervical cancer. Anal intraepithelial neoplasia has been noted to be present in the adjacent mucosa in most cases (70%–84%) of invasive anal squamous cell carcinoma.[73,74] Other neoplasms, such as anal melanoma or anal adenocarcinoma, are not associated with AIN.[53] Histologically, CIN and AIN are indistinguishable and have similar HPV types implicated as etiologic agents, with HPV type 16 being present in most high-grade AIN lesions.[11,75,76]

AIN 3 is an incidental finding in about 0.2% to 2.3% of hemorrhoidectomy specimens.[77,78] The average age of patients with AIN 3 lesions is less than that of patients with anal carcinoma.

Risk factors for the development of AIN include a history of sexually transmitted diseases, genital warts, cervical neoplasia, internal anal warts, receptive anal sex, male homosexuality, HIV infection, and immunosuppression.[19,33,79–82] Dysplasia is seen with increased frequency in incidental surgical specimens from homosexual men.[83]

Clinically, AIN can present with bleeding, pruritis, and burning, although often patients are asymptomatic, especially when lesions are flat and located in the anal canal rather than at the anal verge.[84,85] Grossly, the lesions can appear erythematous and/or have the appearance of a typical wart. Sometimes dysplasia manifests as flat white patches of epithelium, similar to that seen in the female genital tract, although it can be present in otherwise normal-appearing mucosa.[85,86]

Histologically, the grading of AIN is similar to the grading system for cervical neoplasia.[79] In AIN 1, the immature dysplastic squamous cells are confined to the lower third of the epithelium, with more superficial layers often showing koilocytotic atypia with the typical crinkled hyperchromatic nucleus and perinuclear halo (Fig. 62–8). Often the basal layer is hyperchromatic with a disordered arrangement. These changes can be seen in condyloma as well as in flat mucosa. In AIN 2, the lower two-thirds of the epithelium is replaced with the atypical immature squamous cells, but there is some maturation of the cells in the upper third of the epithelium. In AIN 3 (carcinoma in situ), the epithelium is completely replaced with immature neoplastic cells (Fig. 62–9). The neoplastic cells are often overlapping and crowded, with mitosis present above the basal layer. Bowen's disease is the perianal skin equivalent of AIN 3, with similar associations to HPV and anal carcinoma.[36,84] Recent studies have revealed considerable interobserver variation in the histologic grading of AIN, even for high-grade AIN, and have suggested a simplified version of grading AIN as either low-grade or high-grade lesions.[87]

The treatment of high-grade AIN/carcinoma in situ is controversial. Some clinicians recommend complete surgical excision with histologically negative margins, while others advocate ablative therapy with a laser or cryotherapy.[84] Anal intraepithelial neoplasia is difficult to eradicate by either method, however, as it has a high tendency to recur.[88,89] Given the low incidence of progression to invasive carcinoma, some even recommend ob-

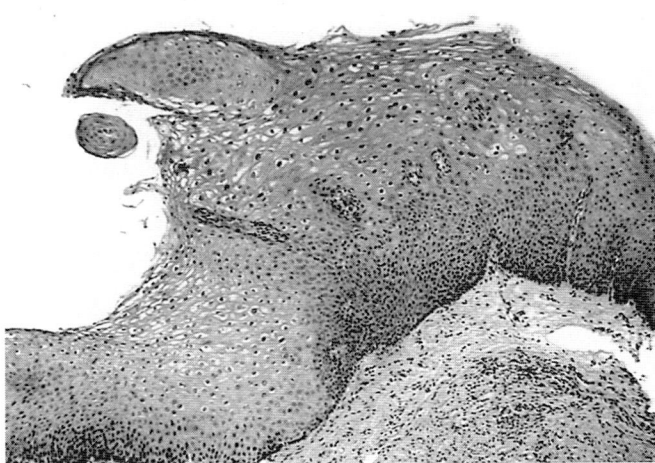

**Figure 62-8** Low-grade anal intraepithelial neoplasia (AIN I) with the more superficial cells showing the typical koilocytic changes associated with HPV infection (dark irregular nuclei and perinuclear halos) (×100).

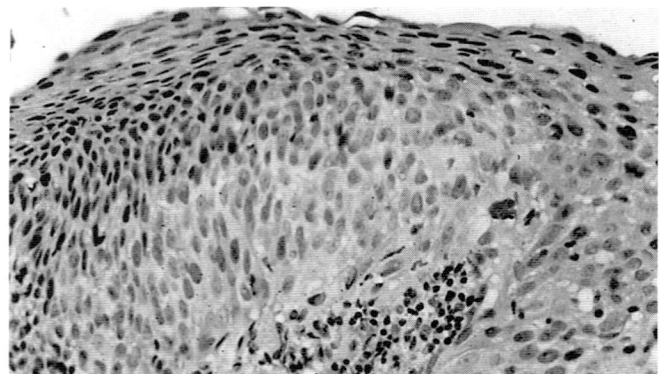

**Figure 62-9** High-grade anal intraepithelial neoplasia. There is replacement of almost the entire thickness of the epithelium by immature dysplastic cells (×400).

servation alone, especially for diffuse disease that would require extensive surgery.[84] Low-grade AIN can be managed by routine follow-up, because spontaneous regression of these lesions can occur over time.[90]

## Condylomata

The term *condyloma acuminata* is a common clinical term used to describe genital warts. Condyloma acuminata are raised, whitish lesions with papillary excrescences that can be seen on physical examination of the anal verge.[81] The lesions are frequently multifocal and may reach considerable size. Condylomata often present as new bumps or growths on the perianal skin, and some patients report itching, burning, pain, or bleeding.[91] Internal condylomata occur in the anal canal and can occur above the dentate line. They are not visible without the aid of anoscopy and can affect over 50% of people with external warts.[9] While internal condylomata are asymptomatic most of the time, patients may present with bleeding.[92] Condylomata can have a variety of appearances, from discrete warts to wart rings encircling the anal canal.[93] The gross appearance of condylomata cannot be used to distinguish between lesions with and without high-grade dysplasia; therefore, a biopsy is necessary to rule out high-grade dysplasia.[93,94]

Histologically, condylomata reveal papillary fronds lined by thickened, often hyperkeratotic, squamous epithelium, usually with some evidence of koilocytotic atypia (Fig. 62–8). Sometimes koilocytes are absent, possibly secondary to resolution of the viral infection.[95] Moderate- to high-grade dysplasia can be seen in condylomata and usually is associated with male homosexuality, disease above the dentate line, and/or immunosuppression.[94] More recent data from ongoing studies show that internal condylomata are much more often associated with high-grade dysplasia than external condylomata (29% vs. 7%, respectively) (CM Surawitcz, unpublished data, 1999).

The therapy for condylomata is similar to that for AIN, although excision is often recommended for large or obstructing lesions.

## Natural History of Anal Intraepithelial Neoplasia

Studies have documented the progression of low-grade AIN to high-grade AIN[26,82] and the progression from normal mucosa to

high-grade AIN.[96] Also, AIN 3/AIS tends to occur at a younger age (late fourth decade) than anal carcinoma.[79,88,89] However, longitudinal studies such as those documenting the progression of cervical neoplasia to invasive carcinoma are not available for anal disease. Only scattered case reports and small series document the progression of AIN 3 to invasive squamous carcinoma.[76,80,97,98] In a study by Scholefield and colleagues[90] of 70 patients with AIN, eight patients developed invasive carcinomas over the 4-year study period, apparently as a result of progression of high-grade AIN.[90] However, it has been estimated that only 2%–6% of cases of AIN 3 progress to invasive cancer.[84] More research is needed to define the natural history of AIN and the factors contributing to its progression to invasive anal carcinoma.

## Anal Cytology

Anal pap smears have been introduced as a screening tool for AIN, similar to cervical pap smears and screening for cervical neoplasia. Several studies have shown that anal cytology is effective in detecting and monitoring the development or progression of anal lesions.[26,98,99] Anal cytology screening of homosexual men who presented to a genitourinary clinic by revealed previously undiagnosed anal squamous lesions in 31% of patients.[100] Goldie and colleagues[101] found that in men with HIV, a biannual anal pap, if begun early in HIV infection, could result in an incremental cost-effectiveness ratio of $13,000 per quality-adjusted life-year saved.[101] This underscores the importance of anal cytology screening in at-risk populations.

The grading of anal cytology is similar to that of the cervix and is divided into unsatisfactory specimens, negative, atypical, low-grade squamous intraepithelial neoplasia, and high-grade squamous intraepithelial lesions (SIL). Two hundred well-visualized cells are necessary for the smears to be considered adequate. Glandular cells help to indicate whether the anal transition zone was sampled or not, although according to Palefsky and colleagues,[102] the presence or absence of glandular cells does not affect the utility of the anal smear in detecting dysplasia.[102] Low-grade SIL often have features of HPV infection, with enlarged hyperchromatic nuclei and a perinuclear halo. High-grade SIL show a higher nucleus-to-cytoplasm ratio, with irregular hyperchromatic nuclei (Fig. 62–10) and may have features of keratinization.

The sensitivity of cytology in detecting anal lesions is unknown but appears to be similar to that of cervical cytology, with

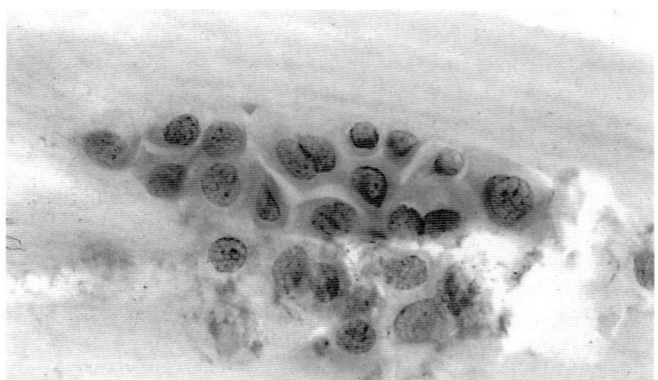

**Figure 62-10** Appearance of high-grade anal intraepithelial neoplasia on an anal pap smear with a markedly high nucleus-to-cytoplasm ratio and hyperchromatic, slightly irregular nuclei (oil, ×1000).

estimates for detection of high-grade AIN ranging in different studies from 36% to 98%.[75,93,102] Cytology is useful in screening for anal squamous lesions, especially since cytology can detect AIN in visually normal mucosa.[85] However, as in the cervix, if there is a clinically detectable lesion, biopsies should be obtained to rule out dysplasia. Anal cytology should only be used as a screening tool concurrently with anoscopy and biopsy.

## Human Immunodeficiency Virus and Anal Neoplasia

The increased risk of anal carcinoma in patients with iatrogenic immunosuppression is well known,[103] thus, it is not suprising that the incidence of anal neoplasia is increased in patients with HIV infection,[81] especially those with marked immunosuppression.[104] Infection with HPV is known to have a more aggressive course, to be refractory to treatment, and to recur more frequently in men and women with HIV,[105] and numerous studies have shown that all HPV types are more common in patients who are HIV positive than in those who are HIV negative.[93,96,106,107] The prevalence of AIN is higher overall among patients with HIV, and HIV-positive men with CD4 counts below 500 show a 2.9-fold increased risk for AIN.[106,107] The risk of progression to high-grade SIL has been shown to be associated with HIV infection, especially in patients with CD4 counts less than 500.[26,96,99] The exact role of HIV in HPV-associated neoplasia is uncertain, but most researchers believe that the immunosuppressive effects of HIV infection, rather than a direct effect of HIV itself, leads to an enhanced expression of HPV infection and an increase in HPV-induced epithelial abnormalities.[107,108] Other possible theories for the role of HIV in HPV-associated neoplasia include increased expression of HPV viral E6 and E7 proteins secondary to secreted HIV-1 proteins[109] and decreased specific T-cell proliferative response to HPV-16 E6 or E7 peptides.[21]

## References

1. Melbye M, Rabkin C, Frisch M, Biggar RJ. Changing patterns of anal cancer incidence in the United States, 1940–1989. Am J Epidemiol 139:772–780, 1994.
2. Frisch M, Melbye M, Moller H. Trends in incidence of anal cancer in Denmark. BMJ 306:419–422, 1993.
3. Daling JR, Weiss NS, Hislop TG, et al. Sexual practices, sexually transmitted diseases, and the incidence of anal cancer. N Engl J Med 317:973–977, 1987.
4. Qualters JR, Lee NC, Smith RA, Aubert RE. Breast and cervical cancer surveillance, United States, 1973–1987. Mor Mortal Wkly Rep CDC Surveill Summ 41:1–7, 1992.
5. Goedert JJ, Cote TR, Virgo P, et al. Spectrum of AIDS-associated malignant disorders. Lancet 351:1833–1839, 1998.
6. Fenger C: Anal canal. In: Sternberg SS (ed): Histology for Pathologists, 2nd ed. Lippincott-Raven, Philadelphia, 1997, pp 551–571.
7. Deans GT, McAleer JJ, Spence RA. Malignant anal tumours. Br J Surg 81:500–508, 1994.
8. Ryan DP, Compton CC, Mayer RJ. Carcinoma of the anal canal. N Engl J Med 342:792–800, 2000.
9. Kuypers JM, Kiviat NB. Anal papillomavirus infections. In: Surawicz C, Owen R (eds): Gastrointestinal and Hepatic Infections, 1st ed. W.B. Saunders Company, Philadelphia, 1995, pp 279–285.
10. Lorincz AT, Reid R, Jenson AB, Greenberg MD, Lancaster W, Kurman RJ. Human papillomavirus infection of the cervix: relative risk associations of 15 common anogenital types. Obstet Gynecol 79:328–337, 1992.
11. Duggan MA, Boras VF, Inoue M, McGregor SE, Robertson DI. Human papillomavirus DNA determination of anal condylomata, dysplasias, and squamous carcinomas with in situ hybridization. Am J Clin Pathol 92:16–21, 1989.
12. Palmer JG, Scholefield JH, Coates PJ, et al. Anal cancer and human papillomaviruses. Dis Colon Rectum 32:1016–1022, 1989.
13. Scheffner M, Werness BA, Huibregtse JM, Levine AJ, Howley PM. The E6 oncoprotein encoded by human papillomavirus types 16 and 18 promotes the degradation of p53. Cell 63:1129–1136, 1990.
14. Klas JV, Rothenberger DA, Wong WD, Madoff RD. Malignant tumors of the anal canal: the spectrum of disease, treatment, and outcomes. Cancer 85:1686–1693, 1999.
15. Hill SA, Coghill SB. Human papillomavirus in squamous carcinoma of anus [letter]. Lancet 2:1333, 1986.
16. Gal AA, Saul SH, Stoler MH. In situ hybridization analysis of human papillomavirus in anal squamous cell carcinoma. Mod Pathol 2:439–443, 1989.
17. Kiyabu MT, Shibata D, Arnheim N, Martin WJ, Fitzgibbons PL. Detection of human papillomavirus in formalin-fixed, invasive squamous carcinomas using the polymerase chain reaction. Am J Surg Pathol 13:221–224, 1989.
18. Palefsky JM, Holly EA, Gonzales J, Berline J, Ahn DK, Greenspan JS. Detection of human papillomavirus DNA in anal intraepithelial neoplasia and anal cancer. Cancer Res 51:1014–1019, 1991.
19. Moscicki AB, Hills NK, Shiboski S, et al. Risk factors for abnormal anal cytology in young heterosexual women. Cancer Epidemiol Biomarkers Prev 8:173–178, 1999.
20. Crum CP. The female genital tract. In: Cotran RS, Kumar V, Collins T, Robbins SL (eds): Robbins Pathologic Basis of Disease, 6th ed. W.B. Saunders, Philadelphia, 1999, p 1049.
21. Palefsky JM. Anal squamous intraepithelial lesions: relation to HIV and human papillomavirus infection. J Acquir Immune Defic Syndr 21 (Suppl 1):S42–S48, 1999.
22. Ogunbiyi OA, Scholefield JH, Smith JH, Polacarz SV, Rogers K, Sharp F. Immunohistochemical analysis of p53 expression in anal squamous neoplasia. J Clin Pathol 46:507–512, 1993.
23. Ogunbiyi OA, Scholefield JH, Rogers K, Sharp F, Smith JH, Polacarz SV. C-myc oncogene expression in anal squamous neoplasia. J Clin Pathol 46:23–27, 1993.
24. Muleris M, Salmon RJ, Girodet J, Zafrani B, Dutrillaux B. Recurrent deletions of chromosomes 11q and 3p in anal canal carcinoma. Int J Cancer 39:595–598, 1987.
25. Heselmeyer K, Schrock E, du Manoir S, et al. Gain of chromosome 3q defines the transition from severe dysplasia to invasive carcinoma of the uterine cervix. Proc Natl Acad Sci USA 93:479–484, 1996.
26. Palefsky JM, Holly EA, Hogeboom CJ, et al. Virologic, immunologic, and clinical parameters in the incidence and progression of anal squamous intraepithelial lesions in HIV-positive and HIV-negative homosexual men. J Acquir Immune Defic Syndr Hum Retrovirol 17:314–319, 1998.
27. Dougherty BG, Evans HL. Carcinoma of the anal canal: a study of 79 cases. Am J Clin Pathol 83:159–164, 1985.
28. Fenger C, Frisch M, Jass JJ, Williams GT, Hilden J. Anal cancer subtype reproducibility study. Virchows Arch 436:229–233, 2000.
29. Shepherd NA, Scholefield JH, Love SB, England J, Northover JM. Prognostic factors in anal squamous carcinoma: a multivariate analysis of clinical, pathological and flow cytometric parameters in 235 cases. Histopathology 16:545–555, 1990.
30. Boman BM, Moertel CG, O'Connell MJ, et al. Carcinoma of the anal canal. A clinical and pathologic study of 188 cases. Cancer 54:114–125, 1984.
31. Williams GR, Talbot IC. Anal carcinoma—a histological review. Histopathology 25:507–516, 1994.
32. Jass JR, Sobin LH, Morson BC. Histological Typing of Intestinal Tumours. Springer-Verlag, Berlin, 1989.
33. Daling JR, Weiss NS, Klopfenstein LL, Cochran LE, Chow WH, Daifuku R. Correlates of homosexual behavior and the incidence of anal cancer. JAMA 247:1988–1990, 1982.
34. Daling JR, Sherman KJ, Hislop TG, et al. Cigarette smoking and the risk of anogenital cancer. Am J Epidemiol 135:180–189, 1992.
35. Rosai J. Anus. In: Rosai J (ed): Ackerman's Surgical Pathology, 8th ed. Mosby, St. Louis, 1996, pp 805–814.
36. Fenger C. Anal neoplasia and its precursors: facts and controversies. Semin Diagn Pathol 8:190–201, 1991.
37. Kuwano H, Iwashita A, Enjoji M. Pseudosarcomatous carcinoma of the anal canal. Dis Colon Rectum 26:123–128, 1983.
38. Miller EJ, Quan SH, Thaler HT. Treatment of squamous cell carcinoma of the anal canal. Cancer 67:2038–2041, 1991.
39. Noel JC, Vandenbossche M, Peny MO, et al. Verrucous carcinoma of the penis: importance of human papillomavirus typing for diagnosis and therapeutic decision. Eur Urol 22:83–85, 1992.
40. Kibrite A, Zeitouni NC, Cloutier R. Aggressive giant condyloma acuminatum associated with oncogenic human papilloma virus: a case report. Can J Surg 40:143–145, 1997.

41. Kato N, Ueno H, Tanaka H, Nishikawa T. Human papillomavirus type 6 associated Buschke-Loewenstein tumor (giant condyloma acuminatum). J Dermatol 20:773–778, 1993.

42. Pilotti S, Donghi R, D'Amato L, et al. HPV detection and p53 alteration in squamous cell verrucous malignancies of the lower genital tract. Diagn Mol Pathol 2:248–256, 1993.

43. Bogomoletz WV, Potet F, Molas G. Condylomata acuminata, giant condyloma acuminatum (Buschke-Lowenstein tumour) and verrucous squamous carcinoma of the perianal and anorectal region: a continuous precancerous spectrum? Histopathology 9:155–169, 1985.

44. Bertram P, Treutner KH, Rubben A, Hauptmann S, Schumpelick V. Invasive squamous-cell carcinoma in giant anorectal condyloma (Buschke-Lowenstein tumor). Langenbecks Arch Chir 380:115–118, 1995.

45. Dogan G, Oram Y, Hazneci E, Ozen S, Karincaoglu Y, Ciralik H. Three cases of verrucous carcinoma. Australas J Dermatol 39:251–254, 1998.

46. Haycox CL, Kuypers J, Krieger JN. Role of human papillomavirus typing in diagnosis and clinical decision making for a giant verrucous genital lesion. Urology 53:627–630, 1999.

47. Chu QD, Vezeridis MP, Libbey NP, Wanebo HJ. Giant condyloma acuminatum (Buschke-Lowenstein tumor) of the anorectal and perianal regions. Analysis of 42 cases. Dis Colon Rectum 37:950–957, 1994.

48. Jakate SM, Saclarides TJ. Immunohistochemical detection of mutant P53 protein and human papillomavirus-related E6 protein in anal cancers. Dis Colon Rectum 36:1026–1029, 1993.

49. Frisch M, Glimelius B, van den Brule AJ, et al. Sexually transmitted infection as a cause of anal cancer. N Engl J Med 337:1350–1358, 1997.

50. Yeong ML, Wood KP, Scott B, Yun K. Synchronous squamous and glandular neoplasia of the anal canal. J Clin Pathol 45:261–263, 1992.

51. Hagihara P, Vazquez MD, Parker JC Jr, Griffen WO. Carcinoma of anal-ductal origin: report of a case. Dis Colon Rectum 19:694–701, 1976.

52. Behan WM, Burnett RA. Adenocarcinoma of the anal glands. J Clin Pathol 49:1009–1011, 1996.

53. Fenger C. Anal canal tumors and their precursors. Pathol Annu 23(Pt 1):45–66, 1988.

54. Anthony T, Simmang C, Lee EL, Turnage RH. Perianal mucinous adenocarcinoma. J Surg Oncol 64:218–221, 1997.

55. Basik M, Rodriguez-Bigas MA, Penetrante R, Petrelli NJ. Prognosis and recurrence patterns of anal adenocarcinoma. Am J Surg 169:233–237, 1995.

56. Cagir B, Whiteford MH, Topham A, Rakinic J, Fry RD. Changing epidemiology of anorectal melanoma. Dis Colon Rectum 42:1203–1208, 1999.

57. Miller BJ, Rutherford LF, McLeod GR, Cohen JR. Where the sun never shines: anorectal melanoma. Aust N Z J Surg 67:846–848, 1997.

58. Wanebo HJ, Woodruff JM, Farr GH, Quan SH. Anorectal melanoma. Cancer 47:1891–1900, 1981.

59. Quan SH. Anal cancers. Squamous and melanoma. Cancer 70(5 Suppl):1384–1389, 1992.

60. Herrington CS, Graham D, Southern SA, Bramdev A, Chetty R. Loss of retinoblastoma protein expression is frequent in small cell neuroendocrine carcinoma of the cervix and is unrelated to HPV type. Hum Pathol 30:906–910, 1999.

61. Wick MR, Weatherby RP, Weiland LH. Small cell neuroendocrine carcinoma of the colon and rectum: clinical, histologic, and ultrastructural study and immunohistochemical comparison with cloacogenic carcinoma. Hum Pathol 18:9–21, 1987.

62. Boxman IL, Russell A, Mulder LH, Bavinck JN, Schegget JT, Green A. Case-control study in a subtropical Australian population to assess the relation between non-melanoma skin cancer and epidermodysplasia verruciformis human papillomavirus DNA in plucked eyebrow hairs. The Nambour Skin Cancer Prevention Study Group. Int J Cancer 86:118–121, 2000.

63. Wicking C, Smyth I, Bale A. The hedgehog signalling pathway in tumorigenesis and development. Oncogene 18:7844–7851, 1999.

64. Rosso S, Joris F, Zanetti R. Risk of basal and squamous cell carcinomas of the skin in Sion, Switzerland: a case–control study. Tumori 85:435–442, 1999.

65. Nielsen OV, Jensen SL. Basal cell carcinoma of the anus—a clinical study of 34 cases. Br J Surg 68:856–857, 1981.

66. Sarmiento JM, Wolff BG, Burgart LJ, Frizelle FA, Ilstrup DM. Paget's disease of the perianal region—an aggressive disease? Dis Colon Rectum 40:1187–1194, 1997.

67. Goldman S, Ihre T, Lagerstedt U, Svensson C. Perianal Paget's disease: report of five cases. Int J Colorectal Dis 7:167–169, 1992.

68. Nowak MA, Guerriere-Kovach P, Pathan A, Campbell TE, Deppisch LM. Perianal Paget's disease: distinguishing primary and secondary lesions using immunohistochemical studies including gross cystic disease fluid protein-15 and cytokeratin 20 expression. Arch Pathol Lab Med 122:1077–1081, 1998.

69. Kubota K, Akasu T, Nakanishi Y, Sugihara K, Fujita S, Moriya Y. Perianal Paget's disease associated with rectal carcinoma: a case report. Jpn J Clin Oncol 28:347–350, 1998.

70. Brainard JA, Hart WR. Proliferative epidermal lesions associated with anogenital Paget's disease. Am J Surg Pathol 24:543–552, 2000.

71. Ioachim HL, Antonescu C, Giancotti F, Dorsett B, Weinstein MA. EBV-associated anorectal lymphomas in patients with acquired immune deficiency syndrome. Am J Surg Pathol 21:997–1006, 1997.

72. Place RJ, Huber PJ, Simmang CL. Anorectal lymphoma and AIDS: an outcome analysis. J Surg Oncol 73:1–4; discussion 5, 2000.

73. Fenger C, Nielsen VT. Precancerous changes in the anal canal epithelium in resection specimens. Acta Pathol Microbiol Immunol Scand A 94:63–69, 1986.

74. Beckmann AM, Daling JR, Sherman KJ, et al. Human papillomavirus infection and anal cancer. Int J Cancer 43:1042–1049, 1989.

75. Sonnex C, Scholefield JH, Kocjan G, et al. Anal human papillomavirus infection: a comparative study of cytology, colposcopy and DNA hybridisation as methods of detection. Genitourin Med 67:21–25, 1991.

76. Scholefield JH, Hickson WG, Smith JH, Rogers K, Sharp F. Anal intraepithelial neoplasia: part of a multifocal disease process. Lancet 340:1271–1273, 1992.

77. Grodsky L. Unsuspected anal cancer discovered after minor anorectal surgery. Dis Colon Rectum 10:471–478, 1967.

78. Fenger C, Nielsen VT. Dysplastic changes in the anal canal epithelium in minor surgical specimens. Acta Pathol Microbiol Scand A 89:463–465, 1981.

79. Fenger C, Nielsen VT. Intraepithelial neoplasia in the anal canal. The appearance and relation to genital neoplasia. Acta Pathol Microbiol Immunol Scand A 94:343–349, 1986.

80. Tilston P. Anal human papillomavirus and anal cancer. J Clin Pathol 50:625–634, 1997.

81. Palefsky J. Human papillomavirus infection among HIV-infected individuals. Implications for development of malignant tumors. Hematol Oncol Clin North Am 5:357–370, 1991.

82. Palefsky JM, Holly EA, Gonzales J, Lamborn K, Hollander H. Natural history of anal cytologic abnormalities and papillomavirus infection among homosexual men with group IV HIV disease. J Acquir Immune Defic Syndr 5:1258–1265, 1992.

83. Nash G, Allen W, Nash S. Atypical lesions of the anal mucosa in homosexual men. JAMA 256:873–876, 1986.

84. Cleary RK, Schaldenbrand JD, Fowler JJ, Schuler JM, Lampman RM. Perianal Bowen's disease and anal intraepithelial neoplasia: review of the literature. Dis Colon Rectum 42:945–951, 1999.

85. Surawicz CM, Critchlow C, Sayer J, et al. High-grade anal dysplasia in visually normal mucosa in homosexual men: seven cases. Am J Gastroenterol 90:1776–1778, 1995.

86. Laverty CR, Russell P, Hills E, Booth N. The significance of non-condylomatous wart virus infection of the cervical transformation zone. A review with discussion of two illustrative cases. Acta Cytol 22:195–201, 1978.

87. Carter PS, Sheffield JP, Shepherd N, et al. Interobserver variation in the reporting of the histopathological grading of anal intraepithelial neoplasia. J Clin Pathol 47:1032–1034, 1994.

88. Marchesa P, Fazio VW, Oliart S, Goldblum JR, Lavery IC. Perianal Bowen's disease: a clinicopathologic study of 47 patients. Dis Colon Rectum 40:1286–1293, 1997.

89. Sarmiento JM, Wolff BG, Burgart LJ, Frizelle FA, Ilstrup DM. Perianal Bowen's disease: associated tumors, human papillomavirus, surgery, and other controversies. Dis Colon Rectum 40:912–918, 1997.

90. Scholefield JH, Ogunbiyi OA, Smith JH, Rogers K, Sharp F. Treatment of anal intraepithelial neoplasia. Br J Surg 81:1238–1240, 1994.

91. Koutsky LA, Kiviat NB. Genital human papillomavirus. In: Holmes KK (ed): Sexually Transmitted Diseases, 3rd ed. McGraw-Hill, New York, 1999, pp 347–359.

92. Metcalf A. Anorectal disorders. Five common causes of pain, itching, and bleeding. Postgrad Med 98:81–84, 87–89, 92–94, 1995.

93. Surawicz CM, Kirby P, Critchlow C, Sayer J, Dunphy C, Kiviat N. Anal dysplasia in homosexual men: role of anoscopy and biopsy. Gastroenterology 105:658–666, 1993.

94. Metcalf AM, Dean T. Risk of dysplasia in anal condyloma. Surgery 118:724–726, 1995.

95. Rock B, Shah KV, Farmer ER. A morphologic, pathologic, and virologic study of anogenital warts in men. Arch Dermatol 128:495–500, 1992.

96. Critchlow CW, Surawicz CM, Holmes KK, et al. Prospective study of high grade anal squamous intraepithelial neoplasia in a cohort of homosexual men: influence of HIV infection, immunosuppression and human papillomavirus infection. AIDS 9:1255–1262, 1995.

97. Ogunbiyi OA, Scholefield JH, Robertson G, Smith JH, Sharp F, Rogers K. Anal human papillomavirus infection and squamous neoplasia in patients with invasive vulvar cancer. Obstet Gynecol 83:212–216, 1994.

98. Sayers SJ, McMillan A, McGoogan E. Anal cytological abnormalities in HIV-infected homosexual men. Int J STD AIDS 9:37–40, 1998.

99. Lacey HB, Wilson GE, Tilston P, et al. A study of anal intraepithelial neoplasia in HIV positive homosexual men. Sex Transm Infect 75:172–177, 1999.

100. Haye KR, Maiti H, Stanbridge CM. Cytological screening to detect subclinical anal human papillomavirus (HPV) infection in homosexual men attending genitourinary medicine clinic. Genitourin Med 64:378–382, 1988.

101. Goldie SJ, Kuntz KM, Weinstein MC, Freedberg KA, Welton ML, Palefsky JM. The clinical effectiveness and cost-effectiveness of screening for anal squamous intraepithelial lesions in homosexual and bisexual HIV-positive men. JAMA 281:1822–1829, 1999.

102. Palefsky JM, Holly EA, Hogeboom CJ, Berry JM, Jay N, Darragh TM. Anal cytology as a screening tool for anal squamous intraepithelial lesions. J Acquir Immune Defic Syndr Hum Retrovirol 14:415–422, 1997.

103. Sillman FH, Sentovich S, Shaffer D. Ano-genital neoplasia in renal transplant patients. Ann Transplant 2:59–66, 1997.

104. Melbye M, Cote TR, Kessler L, Gail M, Biggar RJ. High incidence of anal cancer among AIDS patients. The AIDS/Cancer Working Group. Lancet 343:636–639, 1994.

105. Northfelt DW, Palefsky JM. Human papillomavirus-associated anogenital neoplasia in persons with HIV infection. AIDS Clin Rev 241–259, 1992.

106. Palefsky JM, Holly EA, Ralston ML, et al. Anal squamous intraepithelial lesions in HIV-positive and HIV-negative homosexual and bisexual men: prevalence and risk factors. J Acquir Immune Defic Syndr Hum Retrovirol 17:320–326, 1998.

107. Kiviat NB, Critchlow CW, Holmes KK, et al. Association of anal dysplasia and human papillomavirus with immunosuppression and HIV infection among homosexual men. AIDS 7:43–49, 1993.

108. Caussy D, Goedert JJ, Palefsky J, et al. Interaction of human immunodeficiency and papilloma viruses: association with anal epithelial abnormality in homosexual men. Int J Cancer 46:214–219, 1990.

109. Vernon SD, Hart CE, Reeves WC, Icenogle JP. The HIV-1 tat protein enhances E2-dependent human papillomavirus 16 transcription. Virus Res 27:133–145, 1993.

110. Higgins GD, Uzelin DM, Phillips GE, Pieterse AS, Burrell CJ. Differing characteristics of human papillomavirus RNA-positive and RNA-negative anal carcinomas. Cancer 68:561–567, 1991.

111. Koulos J, Symmans F, Chumas J, Nuovo G. Human papillomavirus detection in adenocarcinoma of the anus. Mod Pathol 4:58–61, 1991.

112. Frisch M, Fenger C, van den Brule AJ, et al. Variants of squamous cell carcinoma of the anal canal and perianal skin and their relation to human papillomaviruses. Cancer Res 59:753–757, 1999.

113. Poletti PA, Halfon A, Marti MC. Papillomavirus and anal carcinoma. Int J Colorectal Dis 13:108–111, 1998.

114. Hermanek P, Sobin LH, and International Union Against Cancer. TNM Classification of Malignant Tumours. Springer-Verlag, Berlin, 1987.

or four photon field beam arrangements, or a direct perineal field with photon or electrons with the patient in the prone position.

An alternative technique, recommended if the planned dose of radiation is to exceed 50 Gy, is to start with a three-field beam arrangement with a posterior field and two lateral fields (Fig. 63–2). The superior and inferior borders of the posterior and lateral fields are similar to the superior and inferior borders used with the anterior/posterior technique. The lateral borders on the posterior field are flared out to capture the inguinal nodes. We highly recommend that CT scans be used to delineate the location of the entire inguinal node region.[35] The integration of three-dimensional imaging to plan the treatment of anal cancer allows a reduction in the amount of bladder and small bowel included in the treatment fields (Color Fig. 63–3; see separate color insert).

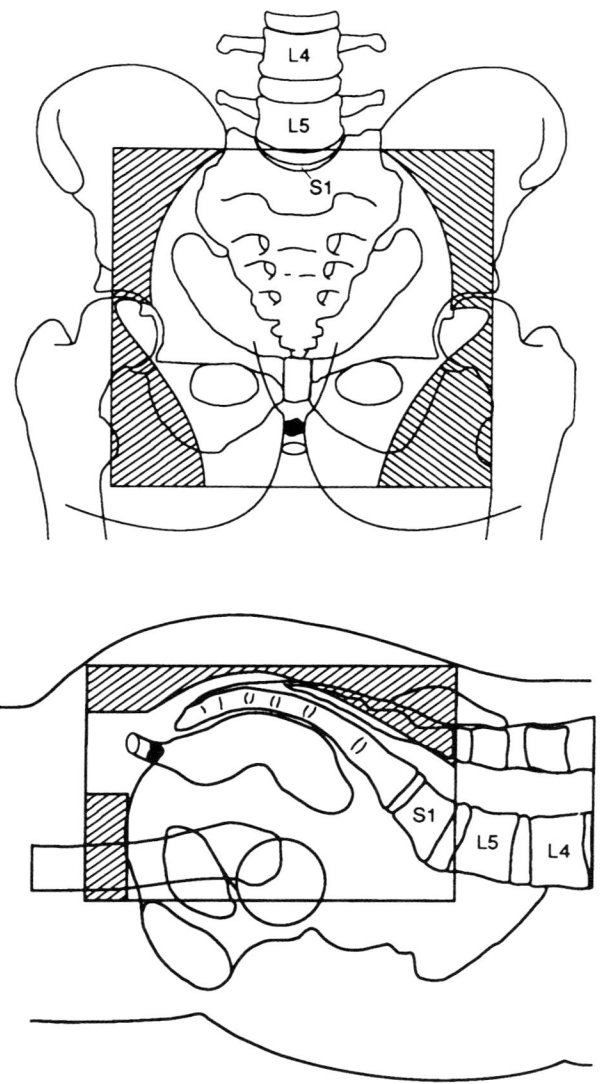

**Figure 63–2** Diagrams of three-field (posterior and opposed lateral) arrangement for a patient with early-stage squamous cell cancer of the anus (T2 N0 M0). Note the flare-out of the lateral borders of the posterior field to encompass the inguinal nodes. The dose delivered to the inguinal nodes from this three-field approach is approximately 35% of the prescribed dose, thus requiring an electron boost to deliver the full dose to this area. (Used with permission from Minsky BD. Anal canal cancer. In: Leibel SA, Phillips TL (eds): Textbook of Radiation Oncology, 1st ed. W.B. Saunders, Philadelphia, p 703, 1998.)

Debate continues regarding whether the entire inguinal node region must be treated. The Radiation Therapy Oncology Group (RTOG) protocols advocate treating only the medial inguinal lymph nodes in patients with no evidence of metastases to the inguinal region, and extending the fields to encompass the lateral inguinal lymph nodes if metastasis is present. However, this approach makes it difficult to clearly delineate the medial from the lateral inguinal nodes. Inclusion of the entire inguinal node region is reasonable when radiation is given in a combined-modality approach, since the morbidity is modest following radiation doses less than 50 Gy.

Brachytherapy has been used more consistently in Europe than in the United States, especially for the earlier-stage anal cancers.[37–39] Papillon pioneered the use of interstitial brachytherapy in the management of anal cancer.[24,31] However, despite the excellent control rates in patients with early-stage disease, the risk of nodal failure and the problems with anal canal and rectal necrosis in larger cancers have diminished enthusiasm for this approach.

Following radiation therapy, approximately 10% of patients experience late complications that necessitate surgical intervention. These complications can include decreased anal sphincter tone resulting in incontinence, chronic bladder irritation with urgency, impotence, perianal and perineal skin dermatitis and pruritis, and edema of the genitalia. With the use of conformal radiation beam arrangements to the boost fields and the optimization of combined modality regimens, the risks of both acute and late morbidity are expected to decrease.

## Chemoradiation Therapy

Despite reasonable results achieved using either external beam radiation therapy or abdominoperineal resection, the need for more effective or less morbid treatments has stimulated interest in combined modality therapy. The initial report by Nigro and colleagues[40] in 1974 described the use of external beam radiotherapy (30 Gy in 15 fractions) with mitomycin C 10–15 mg/m$^2$ on the first day of therapy. 5-fluorouracil (5-FU) at 1000 mg/m$^2$ was administered as a continuous venous infusion daily for 4 days for two cycles that commenced on days 1 and 29. All three patients initially treated with this therapy showed complete pathologic response of their primary tumors, which were initially greater than 2 cm in diameter. Subsequent reports by the same investigators showed that chemoradiation achieved an 89% pathologic complete regression rate and an overall 5-year survival rate of 80%, despite the fact that one-third of the tumors were greater that 4 cm in diameter.[41,42] Surgery was performed only as a salvage procedure in cases in which viable tumor was found on biopsy 6–8 weeks after completion of chemoradiation.

Since these compelling results were reported, numerous phase II trials and single-arm, single-institution experiences have yielded similar results.[28,41,43,44] Table 63–4 summarizes the results of studies reporting on more than 50 patients.[28,41,42,44] However, several variables, such as differing chemotherapy and radiotherapy regimens, inconsistency in the reporting of tumor staging (made more complicated by changes in AJCC staging criteria) and differing tumor locations, make it difficult to compare these studies. Nevertheless, the low mortality and high survival rates and the preservation of the anal sphincter have resulted in widespread adoption of this form of therapy despite the initial absence of randomized clinical trials comparing surgery with chemoradiation.

Large national and international cooperative groups have conducted prospective randomized trials comparing radiation alone

**Table 63-4** Selected phase II trials of combined-modality therapy of epidermoid carcinoma of the anus

| Study | Chemotherapy | RT Dose (Gy) | Patients (n) | APR (%) | Survival % (Years) |
|---|---|---|---|---|---|
| Nigro et al., 1989[42] | 5-FU 1000 mg/m$^2$/day $\times$ 4 days, 2 cycles MMC 10–15 mg/m$^2$, day 1 only | 30 | 104 | 30 | 83 (5) |
| Sischy 1989[43] | 5-FU 1000 mg/m$^2$/day $\times$ 4 days, 2 cycles MMC 10 mg/m$^2$, day 2 | 40 | 79 | 10 | 73 (3) |
| Cummings et al., 1991[28] | 5-FU 1000 mg/m$^2$/day $\times$ 4 days, 2 cycles MMC 10 mg/m$^2$, days 1, 43 split course | 48–50 | 53 | 9 | 76 (5)[a] |
| Cummings et al., 1991[28] | 5-FU 1000 mg/m$^2$/day $\times$ 4 days, 2 cycles split course | 48–50 | 66 | 26 | 64 (5) |
| Tanum et al., 1991[44] | 5-FU 1000 mg/m$^2$/day $\times$ 4 days MMC 10–15 mg/m$^2$, day 1 | 50 | 94 | 18 | 72 (5) |

APR, abdominoperineal resection; 5-FU, 5-fluorouracil; MMC, mitomycin C; RT, radiation therapy.

[a]Pooled results between studies.

to chemoradiation (Table 63–5).[45–47] The United Kingdom Coordinating Committee for Cancer Research (UKCCCR) trial randomly allocated 585 patients to either external beam radiotherapy (45 Gy in 20 to 25 fractions, depending on institutional practice) alone or with 5-FU (750 mg/m$^2$ daily for 5 days or 1000 mg/m$^2$ daily for 4 days by continuous venous infusion, starting on days 1 and 29) and mitomycin C (12 mg/m$^2$ on day 1 only).[45] Reduced doses were recommended for elderly patients (over age 80 years) and for those with intercurrent illness. Patients with epidermoid carcinoma of the anal margin or anal canal were eligible. However, patients with small tumors believed to be suitable for excision (i.e., stage T1 N0 M0) were excluded from the study. Twenty-four percent of patients had palpable lymphadenopathy. Since local control of disease was the primary end point of the study, patients with metastatic disease were also included. Tumor response was assessed 6 weeks after completion of therapy; surgery for salvage therapy was considered if the patient achieved less than 50% tumor regression and the tumor was deemed resectable. For patients with a partial response (50% to <100% response) to primary therapy, boost irradiation (15 Gy in 6 fractions with electrons or photons, or iridium-192 implant) was recommended. Assessment of clinical response 6 weeks after completion of therapy indicated a numerically greater rate of complete and partial responses in the combined modality arm than in the group treated with radiation alone ($P = 0.08$). However, a comparison of the two groups after a median follow-up of 42 months showed that the combined-modality arm had significantly lower rates of local failure (39% vs. 61%, $P < 0.0001$) and cause-specific death from anal cancer (28% vs. 39%, $P =$

0.02) even though the chemoradiation arm contained a slightly higher percentage of stage T4 and node-palpable tumors. Overall survival rates of the two treatment arms was not significantly different, likely because of the successful surgical salvage treatment. The incidence of early toxicity was higher in patients receiving combined modality therapy than in those treated with radiation alone. Six patients died from toxicity of chemotherapy. The two treatment arms had similar rates of morbidity after surgical salvage. This UKCCCR trial demonstrated that combined chemoradiation was more effective than radiation therapy alone in achieving local control of anal cancers. However, the study has been criticized for the inclusion of patients with known metastatic disease and for the inconsistent application of radiation therapy, chemotherapy, and salvage treatment with surgery.

In a similar trial in 103 patients, the European Organization for Research and Treatment of Cancer (EORTC) confirmed the efficacy of combined chemoradiation over radiation therapy alone.[46] Chemotherapy in the combined-modality arm consisted of 5-FU at 750 mg/m$^2$ daily for 5 days commencing on days 1 and 29 and mitomycin C at 15 mg/m$^2$ on day 1 only. As in the UKCCCR study, patients with either anal canal or anal margin tumors were eligible. Initial doses of radiation were similar to those used in the UKCCCR trial. Following a 6-week rest, a boost dose of 15 Gy was administered to complete responders and 20 Gy to partial responders. Response was assessed on the basis of clinical findings; a biopsy after radiotherapy was not routinely performed. The boost was administered as photons, electrons, or $^{192}$Ir implant. Salvage surgery was recommended in cases of inadequate response to primary therapy, defined as tumor progres-

**Table 63-5** Randomized clinical trials of combined-modality therapy in epidermoid carcinoma of the anus

| Cooperative Group | Study Arm | RT Dose (Gy) | Patients (n) | Local Failure Rate % (Years) | Overall Survival % (Years) |
|---|---|---|---|---|---|
| UKCCR, 1996[45] | 5-FU/MMC/RT | 45 | 292 | 39 (3) | 65 (3) |
| | RT | 45 | 285 | 61 (3) | 58 (3) |
| Bartelink, 1997[46] | 5-FU/MMC/RT | 45 + 15–20 | 51 | 29 (3) | 56 (5)[a] |
| | RT | 45 + 15–20 | 52 | 48 (3) | 56 (5)[a] |
| RTOG/ECOG[47] | 5-FU/MMC/RT | 45–50 0.4 $\pm$ 0.9 | 146 | 9 (4)[b] | 78 (4) |
| | 5-FU/RT | 45–50 0.4 $\pm$ 0.9 | 145 | 22 (4)[b] | 71 (4) |

5-FU, 5-fluorouracil; MMC, mitomycin C; RT, radiation therapy; RTOG/ECOG, Radiation Therapy Oncology Group/Eastern Cooperative Oncology Group; UKCCR, United Kingdom Coordinating Committee for Cancer Research.

[a]Pooled results between arms.

[b]Colostomy rate.

sion or no tumor response measured 6 weeks from the completion of radiation therapy. The complete response rate was higher in the chemoradiation group than in the radiation-only group (80% vs. 54%, respectively, $P = 0.01$). The rate of locoregional recurrence was significantly lower and the rates of progression-free and event-free survival were higher in the chemoradiation group. Overall survival rates were comparable, although more patients were colostomy-free in the combined modality arm than in the radiation-only arm (48% vs. 24%, respectively, at 2 years, $P = 0.002$). As expected, the rate of acute toxicity following chemoradiation was higher than that seen following radiation alone.

While chemoradiation is the preferred therapy for most cancers of the anal region, investigators continue to debate the optimal chemotherapy regimen. Investigators at the Princess Margaret Hospital reported that the inclusion of mitomycin C in the chemotherapy regimen improved results in a series of single-arm studies.[28,48] However, the risk-to-benefit ratio of mitomycin C was still questioned.[49] Mitomycin C is a myelotoxic agent that occasionally causes pulmonary, cardiac, and mucosal and skin injury as well as rarer conditions such as microangiopathic hemolytic anemia and hemolytic uremic syndrome. To determine the importance of mitomycin C in the chemotherapy regimen for epidermoid anal carcinoma, the Eastern Clinical Oncology Group (ECOG) and the Radiation Therapy Oncology Group (RTOG) conducted a randomized trial.[47] Between 1988 and 1991, 310 patients were randomly allocated to receive either combined-modality treatment consisting of radiation therapy (45 Gy in 25 fractions; 50.4 Gy for N1 disease) and 5-FU at 1000 mg/m$^2$/day by continuous venous infusion for 4 days commencing on days 1 and 29, or the same regimen plus mitomycin C at 10 mg/m$^2$ on days 1 and 29. Patients underwent a full-thickness biopsy of the primary site 4 to 6 weeks after completion of therapy. On the basis of a single-arm experience,[50] patients with either positive biopsies or persistent palpable lymphadenopathy underwent further radiotherapy (9 Gy in five fractions) with concurrent salvage chemotherapy (5-FU as above starting on day 1 of salvage radiotherapy plus cisplatin at 100 mg/m$^2$ infused over 4–6 hours on day 2). Abdominoperineal resection was recommended for patients with a positive biopsy 3 to 4 weeks following completion of therapy. With a median follow-up of 3.5 years, the 6-week negative biopsy rate for the mitomycin C/5-FU arm was higher than that in the 5-FU–only arm (92.2% vs. 86%, respectively) but the results were not statistically different ($P = 0.14$). Disease-free survival was significantly better in the mitomycin C–containing arm (76% vs. 53%, $P = 0.0003$). However, overall survival rates were not different in the two arms, with only an insignificantly prolonged survival in the mitomycin C–containing arm (78% vs. 71%, $P = 0.31$). Acute treatment-related hematologic toxicity was significantly higher in the mitomycin C arm, and more life-threatening toxicities occurred in mitomycin C–treated patients. Of the four patients who died as a result of therapy, three were in the mitomycin C–containing arm. All four patients died of neutropenic sepsis.

Updated results of the RTOG/EORTC study were presented in abstract form in 1998.[51] Five years of follow-up data showed that mitomycin C improved rates of local control and colostomy-free survival, regardless of the stage of disease. However, rates of costomy-free survival among mitomycin C–treated patients remained low both for T3/T4 primary tumors (55%) and for node-positive disease (37%), suggesting the continued need for improved therapy. This RTOG/EORTC trial demonstrates the important role of mitomycin C in reducing local failure in patients treated with chemoradiation. The trial also demonstrates the toxicity inherent in combined-modality therapy, particularly mitomycin C–related enhancement of myelosupression, and the need for careful patient selection and management.

Replacement of mitomcycin C with cisplatin may enhance the efficacy of the chemotherapeutic regimen but may also increase the hematologic toxicity, particularly in patients with human immunodeficiency virus (HIV) disease, thus this also requires prospective evaluation. The RTOG is conducting a randomized phase III study to compare 5-FU, mitomcyin C, and radiation therapy; 5-FU, mitomycin C, and radiation therapy; and 5-FU, cisplatin, and radiation therapy in treatment of primary cancers of the anal canal greater than 2 cm in diameter. Patients are being stratified by gender, clinical nodal status, and diameter of the primary tumor.

The single-arm and randomized clinical trials cited above clearly demonstrate the efficacy of chemoradiation therapy in the treatment of patients with synchronous lymphandenopathy. Multivariant analysis shows, however, that the presence of palpable nodal disease is a significant risk factor for relapse after definitive primary therapy.[46,47,51] Seventeen percent of patients in the RTOG/EORTC intergroup trial had nodal disease. While patient numbers are too small to definitively address the role of mitocycin C in node-positive patients, only 5 of 25 patients receiving radiation, 5-FU, and mitomycin C required surgery, as did 9 of 25 patients who received radiation and 5-FU, for an overall colostomy rate of 28% for node-positive patients.[47] Colostomy-free survival for node-positive patients receiving 5-FU and mitomycin C was 37% at 5 years, compared with 41% for node-positive patients receiving only 5-FU.[51] In contrast, surgical series demonstrated poor long-term local control (15%) achieved with abdominoperineal resection and inguinal lymphadenectomy with or without postoperative radiotherapy.[24,25]

The role of primary chemoradiation for adenocarcinomas of the anal region is controversial. Joon and colleagues[52] reported 14 patients with adenocarcinoma of the anus treated with radiation alone or in combination with chemotherapy. Surgery was limited to either incisional or excisional biopsy. With a median follow-up of 6.6 years, none of the six patients treated with curative intent have had disease recurrence.

The studies clearly show that combined-modality therapy is an effective sphincter-sparing procedure that should be offered to all patients with epidermoid anal canal tumors without distant metastases. Except for cases of T1 tumors, chemoradiation is clearly superior to either surgery or radiation therapy alone. The addition of mitomycin C to 5-FU is superior to 5-FU alone as a concurrent chemoradiation approach.

### Anal Cancer in HIV-Positive Patients

Combined-modality therapy for the treatment of anal cancer in patients who are HIV positive should be administered with caution. Several reports have demonstrated enhanced acute toxicities in HIV-positive patients undergoing combined-modality therapy, with many unable to complete the prescribed course of treatment.[53,54] However, combined-modality approaches appear feasible in the subset of HIV-positive patients with CD4 counts greater than 200. Hoffman and colleagues[55] reported that among 17 HIV-positive patients with anal cancer, all nine patients with CD4 counts of 200 or more achieved local tumor control with chemoradiation. Four of the nine patients needed treatment breaks of approximately 2 weeks. Of the eight patients who had pretreatment CD4 counts less than 200, seven were treated with chemoradiation. A high morbidity rate was observed with this combined-modality approach, with four patients requiring hospitalization for toxicities, including intractable diarrhea and moist desquamation. Despite eventual local control in six patients with CD4 counts less than 200, four patients ultimately required colostomy either for a therapy-related complication or for salvage. Peddada and colleagues[56] suggested lowering the radiation doses to reduce late toxicities in HIV-positive patients. Other options include reducing the size of the radiation fields and modifying the chemotherapy regimen, such as omitting mitomycin C.

## Management of Anal Cancer in the Elderly

Anal cancers are not uncommon in the elderly population. Workers have questioned whether the treatment of anal cancer in the elderly patients should be similar to the approach for younger persons with the same stage of disease. Allal and colleagues[57] investigated the feasibility of combined-modality treatment of patients aged 75 years or older with anal carcinoma. Radiation therapy was administered to 47 patients, of whom 21 received concomitant chemotherapy. Radiation was administered in a split course, with an initial median dose of 39.6 Gy, followed by an interval of 43 days median and then either brachytherapy or an external beam boost (median boost dose 20 Gy). Chemotherapy was started on day 1 and generally consisted of one cycle of mitomycin C (median dose 9.5 mg/m$^2$) and a 96-hour infusion of 5-FU (median dose 600 mg/ m$^2$/day). Forty patients (85%) completed treatment. Acute toxicity resulted in a shortening of the planned course of irradiation in two patients and an unplanned treatment break in 11 patients (four in the radiation-alone group and seven in the combined modality group). Grade 2 and 3 acute reactions were observed in 43% and 54% of patients, respectively. Two-thirds of patients receiving combined-modality therapy experienced grade 3 reactions, compared with one-third in the radiation-only group. Among patients receiving combined modality therapy, grade 2 or 3 leukopenia and fatigue were observed in 25% and 58% of patients, respectively. Although five patients who experienced grade 3 or 4 late complications were all treated with combined-modality therapy, the actuarial 5-year local control and overall survival rates were better in the combined-modality group.

## Nonsurgical Salvage Regimens

Experience suggests that approximately 50% of patients with anal cancer are cured by salvage abdominoperineal resection.[18,25,45,58–59] Although abdominoperineal resection is the standard salvage treatment for tumor recurrence or persistence following chemoradiation, nonsurgical salvage regimens are also being developed. Flam and colleagues[47,50] described a salvage regimen based on 5-FU and cisplatin that was incorporated in the RTOG/EORTC intergroup trial. Of the 22 patients undergoing salvage chemoradiation, 12 were rendered biopsy-negative complete responders; 6 of the 12 are disease-free survivors. Interestingly, 70% of patients in the UKCCCR study who had only a partial response immediately following combined-modality therapy achieved disease-free status during follow-up.[45] This finding emphasizes the importance of watchful waiting in the first 6–8 weeks following combined-modality therapy. Data from Princess Margaret Hospital suggest that anal cancers regress slowly, with complete regression taking up to 1 year.[60]

## Perianal Cancer

Epidermoid carcinoma of the anal margin is an uncommon tumor that is usually localized and that rarely extends to underlying soft tissues. Metastases to distant organs are uncommon. Most anal margin cancers are amenable to local excision with a 1-cm margin and most local recurrences can be re-excised. For tumors encompassing more than one-half the circumference of the anus, abdominoperineal excision has traditionally been recommended.[25]

Although large series are lacking, the use of radiotherapy alone has achieved good results.[61,62] Anal margin carcinomas were eligible for entry into both the UKCCCR and the EORTC randomized trials, but the small number of patients with anal margin carcinoma precludes definitive comment on the efficacy of chemoradiation over radiotherapy alone or excision alone for these patients.[45,46] For small tumors, local excision appears to be the most efficient management option. Radiotherapy with or without brachytherapy is acceptable treatment for most localized tumors. The results of chemoradiation for cancers of the anal canal suggest that this therapy is appropriate for large tumors of the anal margin and for patients with nodal disease, but clinicians should appreciate that the available data supporting such treatment are limited.

## Treatment of Locally Advanced or Metastatic Disease

Because many patients with bulky tumors or lymphadenopathy cannot undergo sphincter preservation, the Cancer and Leukemia Group B (CALGB) performed a phase II trial in patients with T3 or T4 primary tumors or bulky lymphadenopathy (N2/N3).[63] In the study (reported in abstract form only), 45 patients received continuous infusion of 5-FU (1000 mg/m$^2$ daily for 5 days) with cisplatin (100 mg/m$^2$ on day 1) on weeks 1 and 5, followed by external beam radiotherapy (45 Gy) on weeks 9 through 17, with a 19-day break in treatment after 30.6 Gy. The 5-FU and mitomycin C therapy was repeated, concurrent with radiotherapy, on weeks 9 and 15. If residual disease was found after primary therapy, salvage therapy similar to that employed in the ECOG/RTOG intergroup trial was administered. Induction chemotherapy alone resulted in complete clinical and radiographic regression of disease in 8 patients and a partial response in 21 patients, for a 64% rate of response to initial systemic therapy. Upon completion of primary therapy, 80% of patients had achieved complete tumor regression. With a median follow-up of 21 months, 67% of patients remain disease-free and 56% are colostomy- and disease-free. Although induction chemotherapy demonstrates promising response rates for anal carcinoma, similar to those achieved for squamous cell carcinomas of other sites such as head and neck, such gains may not translate into improvements in survival and local control. Indeed, a report by Miller and associates[64] employing 5-FU and mitomycin C prior to radiotherapy but without concurrent chemoradiation yielded inferior results in a single-arm study. A randomized, controlled clinical trial is clearly warranted.

Few data have been accumulated on the treatment of metastatic epidermoid anal carcinoma, mainly because the disease is rare and primary treatment is successful in most patients. The literature does contain case reports of patients successfully treated with agents and regimens effective against other squamous cell carcinomas of other origins; these regimens include doxorubicin, cisplatin alone or with 5-FU, bleomycin, and vincristine with or

**Table 65-4** Procedures used to evaluate islet cell tumors

| Test | Purpose | Brief Description | Interpretation |
|------|---------|------------------|----------------|
| Secretin test | Diagnose gastrinoma | Infuse secretin (2 U/kg) as intravenous bolus with measurement of serum gastrin at 0, 2, 5, 10, and 15 minutes | Normal response is <50% increase of serum gastrin over basal value |
| Calcium stimulation | Diagnose gastrinoma | 15 mg calcium/kg in 500 ml normal saline infused over 3 hours. Measure serum gastrin at 0, 1, 2, and 3 hours | Normal response is <50% increase of serum gastrin over basal value |
| Meal stimulation test for pancreatic polypeptide and gastrin | Diagnostic test for gastrinomas in MEN-1 | Consume 560-kcal meal rich in carbohydrates (66 g) and low in protein (18 g) and fat (22 g) over 20 minutes with measurement of serum gastrin and pancreatic polypeptide at 0, 10, 20, and 60 minutes | Normal response is a serum pancreatic polypeptide or gastrin level less than 2 times the basal level. False-positive rate, approximately 12% |
| Selective arterial calcium injection with hepatic venous sampling | Localize hormone secreting tumor, most commonly insulinoma, to specific pancreatic arterial distribution | Selective injection of calcium into specific pancreatic arteries with sampling of hepatic venous effluent for insulin or other peptides after each injection | An increase in the hepatic venous (0, 30, 60, and 120 seconds) serum peptide (insulin) concentration after selective arterial injection indicates a likely tumor in the distribution of the artery |

MEN-1, multiple endocrine neoplasia type 1.

three times a day),[48,78] phenytoin (300 to 600 mg/day),[42] or propanolol.[79]

Glucagon, the major hormone released in response to hypoglycemia, has also been used in the control of tumor-induced hypoglycemia. It stimulates hepatic glucose production by inducing glycogenolysis and gluconeogenesis. Prolonged infusion of glucagon through a portable pump on an outpatient basis has been successfully used in five patients with hypoglycemia.[52]

## Gastrinomas

Zollinger and Ellison[80] first described the gastrinoma syndrome in 1955 in two patients with recurrent peptic ulcer disease (PUD), gastric acid hypersecretion, and an islet cell tumor of the pancreas. Several years later, Gregory and co-workers[81] showed that these tumors produce a potent stimulator of gastric acid secretion. The same group discovered that this substance is produced

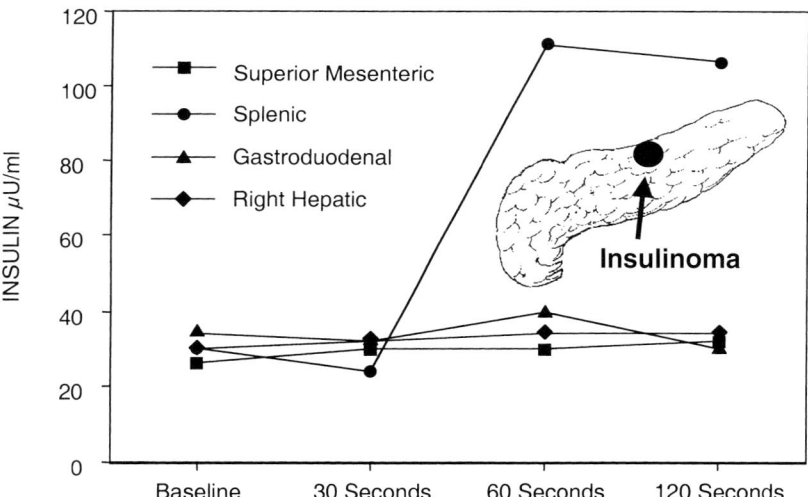

**Figure 65-3** Selective injection of calcium into the superior mesenteric, splenic, and gastroduodenal arteries with measurement of insulin in timed specimens obtained from the hepatic vein. In this patient, there is a pronounced increase in the hepatic venous insulin concentration following injection of a calcium solution into the splenic artery. During a surgical exploratory procedure, an insulinoma (indicated in the inset) was identified in the distribution of the splenic artery. This approach provides additional evidence regarding the localization of a pancreatic islet tumor and may provide direction to the surgeon during a pancreatic exploration in which there is a failure to localize the tumor by other radiographic techniques.

**Table 65-5** Causes of hypergastrinemia other than gastrinomas

Acid-reducing drugs
Pernicious anemia (achlorydria)
Antral G-cell hyperplasia
Gastric outlet obstruction
Retained gastric antrum syndrome

by the antral cells of the stomach and named it *gastrin*.[82] The clinical features of the Zollinger-Ellison syndrome (ZES) in patients during the 1950s and early 1960s were characterized by extensive gastric, duodenum, and small bowel ulceration and metastasis of the gastrinoma to the liver in one-third to one-half of cases. The development of the gastrin radioimmunoassay (RIA) and improvement in imaging by widespread application of arteriography in the late 1960s provided the opportunity for preoperative diagnosis of tumors.[83] The recognition that secretin[84] and later calcium[85,86] stimulate a brisk rise of serum gastrin provided a tool for earlier diagnosis. Secretin, a small peptide, normally inhibits gastrin secretion by the antral G cells but is stimulatory in gastrinoma cells.[87] This test made it possible to differentiate hypergastrinemia caused by gastrin-producing tumors from hypergastrinemia of other causes (Table 65–5). The initial treatment for ZES was total gastrectomy; in fact, during the 1950s and 1960s, more patients died from complications of PUD than from metastatic tumor. The introduction of histamine $H_2$ receptor antagonists in the mid-1970s and proton-pump inhibitors in the subsequent decades has made it possible to control PUD with certainty in most patients. The management of gastrinoma has gone through several phases. Gastrectomy was the therapy recommended by Zollinger, in large part because resection of large tumors with metastases was difficult and there was no effective therapy to prevent acid secretion. Subsequently, the ability to diagnose the tumors preoperatively by measurement of basal or stimulated gastrin levels led to a period during which surgical resection of pancreatic tumors was common. The disappointment over surgical cure rates and the subsequent introduction of $H_2$ receptor antagonists and proton-pump inhibitors resulted in a shift of the pendulum to medical therapy. In recent years, the management has returned to a surgical paradigm with the recognition that duodenal carcinoid-like tumors, not previously recognized, cause most ZES. Their recognition and removal have improved patient outcomes.

## Clinical Features

Zollinger-Ellison syndrome can occur sporadically or in association with MEN-1. Gastrinomas are the most common functional islet cell tumors in patients with MEN-1, and 20% of patients presenting with ZES have MEN-1.[88,89] The most common symptom is epigastric pain resulting from one or more duodenal or jejunal ulcers. Complications such as gastric or duodenal perforation are also frequent in these patients. The second most common symptom is diarrhea (40%), which is the only presenting complaint in 20% of patients.[89] The diarrhea is caused by malabsorption caused by the excessive gastric acid delivery to the intestine. The failure of intestinal bicarbonate to neutralize gastric acid leads to acid-mediated damage to intestinal mucosa, inactivation of pancreatic enzymes, and bile salt precipitation leading to steatorrhea. Other gastrointestinal symptoms such as heartburn, dysphagia, and esophagitis are also common.

## Diagnosis

Table 65–6 shows clinical situations in which the diagnosis of ZES should be suspected. The initial screening test should be a fasting serum gastrin level. This should be performed after discontinuation (for at least 1 week) of all $H_2$ blockers and proton-pump inhibitors. A fasting serum gastrin level of more than 1000 pg/ml combined with evidence of excessive gastric acid production is predictive of gastrinoma. Most patients with ZES present with a serum gastrin level between 150 and 1000 pg/ml.[90] This basal level of gastrin is not diagnostic, and further testing is necessary to exclude other causes of hypergastrinemia (Table 65–4).

Achlorhydria caused by pernicious anemia or pharmacologic agents that inhibit acid secretion is a common cause of an elevated serum gastrin. Achlorhydria can be excluded by measuring gastric acid output or by measuring the gastric pH level. Patients with ZES have gastric pH levels at or lower than 2. The basal gastric acid output is more than 15 mEq/hour in patients with ZES and greater than 5 mEq/hour in patients who have previously undergone surgery to treat PUD. Other less common causes of hypergastrinemia associated with gastric acid hypersecretion include antral G-cell hyperplasia, gastric outlet obstruction, and the so-called retained gastric antrum syndrome. The later condition results from placement of antral tissue in a location where it is not bathed by gastric acid during a Billroth II gastrojejunostomy. The secretin test is useful for differentiating between these causes of hypergastrinemia. Patients with ZES will respond to secretin infusion with an increase in serum gastrin within 10 minutes to greater than 200 pg/ml from the basal level.[91,92] The test is performed in the fasting state several days following discontinuation of all acid-reducing medications. A bolus of secretin (2 U/kg) is given intravenously. Serum gastrin is then measured at baseline and at 2, 5, 10, and 15 minutes (Table 65–4). Unfortunately, secretin has been taken off the market in the United States. Other provocative tests include the calcium, bombesin, and meal tests.[92–97] Calcium, in particular, is a useful alternative (Table 65–4). In normal subjects or those with duodenal ulcer disease, a calcium infusion (4 mg elemental calcium as calcium gluconate over 3 hours) will stimulate the serum gastrin to a value less than 100 pg/ml, whereas those with gastrinomas have an average increase to 800 pg/ml.[85]

Most gastrinomas occur in the *gastrinoma triangle*, defined as the confluence of the cystic and common bile ducts superiorly, the second and third parts of the duodenum inferiorly, and the neck and body of the pancreas medially (Fig. 65–4). This is an area thought to derive predominantly from the ventral pancreatic bud during development (Fig. 65–5). Other tumor types commonly found in this region include pancreatic polypeptide-secreting tumors (PPomas) and somatostatinomas. In contrast, glucagonomas and insulinomas, tumors that occur most commonly in the body and tail of the pancreas, are thought to be derived from the dorsal pancreatic bud (Fig. 65–5).[98–102] Gastri-

**Table 65-6** Clinical manifestations suggestive of Zollinger-Ellison Syndrome

Recurrent or persistent peptic ulcer disease
Multiple ulcers in an unusual location (e.g., jejunum)
Peptic ulcer disease with secretory diarrhea
Complications of peptic ulcer disease (e.g., perforation, bleeding)
Family history of peptic ulcer disease, primary hyperparathyroidism or nephrolithiasis

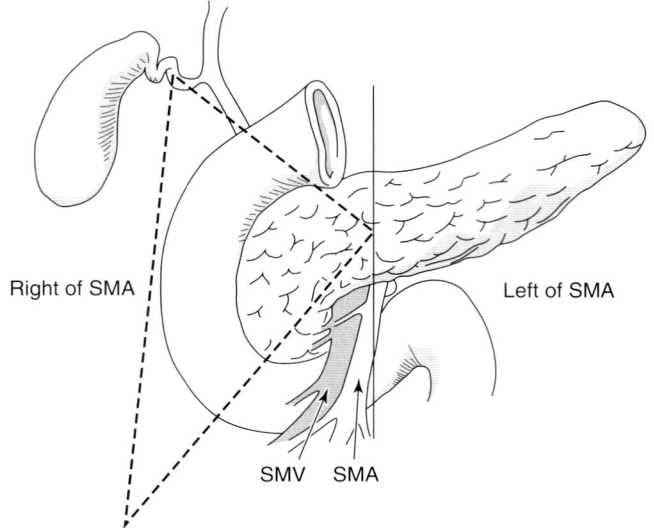

**Figure 65–4** The gastrinoma triangle. The retroperitoneal structures, showing the pancreas, duodenum, extrahepatic biliary system, superior mesenteric artery (SMA), and superior mesenteric vein (SMV). The anatomic areas to the right and left of the SMA are shown separated by a solid vertical line drawn through the neck of the pancreas. The gastrinoma triangle is depicted (dashed lines) to the right of the SMA. (Reproduced from Howard TJ, Sawicki M, Lewin KJ, et al. Pancreatic polypeptide immunoreactivity in sporadic gastrinoma: relationship to intraabdominal location. Pancreas 11:350–356, 1993.)

nomas may occur in the duodenal wall,[103,104] lymph nodes,[105–107] or in other extrapancreatic locations.[108–110]

In the MEN-1 syndrome, duodenal gastrinomas are much more common than pancreatic gastrinomas.[99,111] In addition, gastrinomas in MEN-1 are frequently very small, submucosal, and multicentric. Other unusual sources of primary gastrinomas previously reported include the liver, spleen, ovary, heart, and lymph nodes.[105,112,113]

Gastrinomas are frequently malignant, and approximately 30% of patients present with liver metastases. Metastasis is more common in pancreatic gastrinomas than in extrapancreatic gastrinomas. Metastatic disease most commonly involves the liver, but it can also involve the lungs, heart, bone, and adrenal glands. Since the advent of early biochemical diagnosis, most patients present with small gastrinomas. Early diagnosis is beneficial; the 10-year survival rate is 85% in patients with localized disease but only 30% in patients with metastatic disease.[89,114]

It is important for an individual patient to meet strict biochemical criteria that include excess acid production and evidence of abnormal gastrin production before initiating studies to localize the tumor. A cardinal rule in the current localization of gastrinoma is that these tumors are frequently small, may be located in the gastrinoma triangle or pancreas, and may be multiple. Localization studies will be discussed separately. It will suffice to say that early diagnosis may identify the tumor(s) prior to any abnormal imaging study. In these cases, increasingly more common, surgical experience and the use of intraoperative localization techniques such as ultrasound provide the greatest opportunity for a curative procedure.[115]

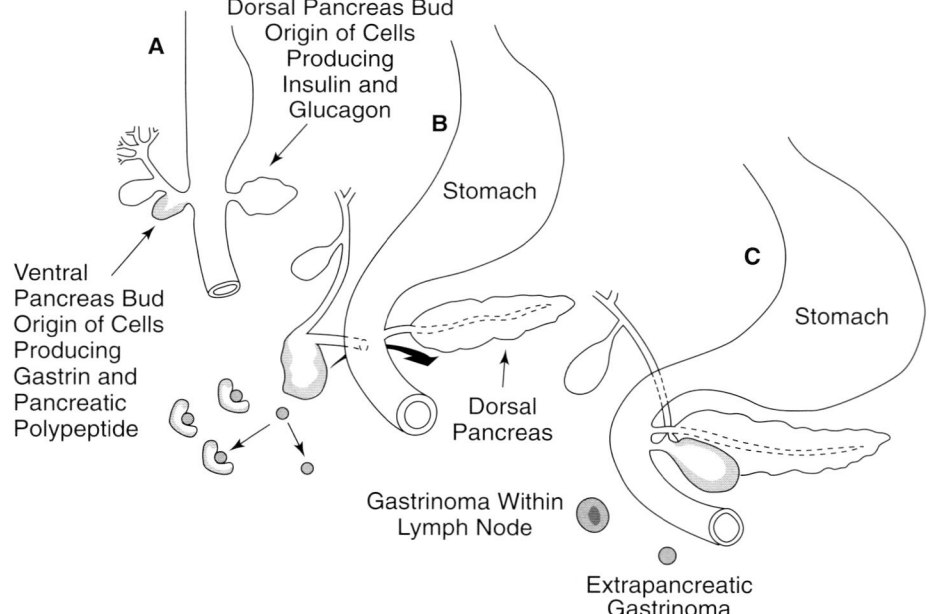

**Figure 65–5** Hypothetical embryologic events that occur in the upper gastrointestinal tract during the fifth to sixth week of intrauterine development, i.e., ventral pancreatic bud outpouching (*A*); dorsal migration of ventral pancreatic bud, with theoretical cellular dispersion into extrapancreatic sites and developing nodal tissue (*B*); and completed rotation in adult, with the development of gastrinoma within lymph nodes or extrapancreatic gastrinoma (*C*). The location of gastrinomas and pancreatic polypeptide producing tumors is superimposable, suggesting an origin from the ventral pancreatic bud. In contrast, the distribution of insulinomas and glucagonomas suggests an origin from the dorsal pancreatic bud. (Modified with permission from Passaro E, Howard TJ, Sawicki MP, Watt PC, Stabile BE. The origin of sporadic gastrinomas within the gastrinoma triangle: a theory. Arch Surg 133:13–16, 1998.)

## Treatment

In patients with ZES, the treatment goal is to avoid complications of PUD and to surgically excise the tumor when possible. In patients with sporadic gastrinoma without metastatic disease, surgery should be performed with the intent to cure. In a prospective study of 124 patients with no radiological evidence of metastases who were followed for almost 9 years, patients who underwent surgical resection of a tumor had a much lower incidence of liver metastases (3%) than did patients treated medically (23%),[116] a finding that argues for a surgical approach in early ZES.[117,118]

H$_2$ receptor blockers (i.e., cimetidine, famotidine, nizatidine, and ranitidine) and proton-pump inhibitors (i.e., omeprazole, lansoprazole) can effectively alleviate the symptoms of ZES by reducing gastric acid hypersecretion. The proton-pump inhibitors inhibit acid secretion by irreversibly binding to the hydrogen/potassium ATPase present on the surface of parietal cells. In the case of omeprazole, patients are started on a dose of 20 mg twice a day; the dose is then adjusted to achieve a gastric acid output less than 10 mEq/hour in patients with no previous PUD surgery or less than 5 mEq/hour in patients with previous surgery.[89] Patients with gastrinoma require a much higher dose than patients with PUD (i.e., up to 120 mg/day of omeprazole, with a mean dose of 80 mg/day).[119] Symptomatic relief of PUD symptoms is not the best indicator of adequate gastric acid control. Gastric acid output should be measured and maintained lower than 10 mEq/hour to promote healing of intestinal, gastric, and esophageal mucosa.[89]

A potential risk of long-term use of proton-pump inhibitors is the development of hypergastrinemia and gastric carcinoid tumors. The concern about carcinoid development was first raised after gastric carcinoids were identified in rats treated for long periods with omeprazole.[120,121] Gastric carcinoid tumors are known to occur in patients with autoimmune atrophic gastritis and achlorhydria.[122–124] The presumed mechanism for carcinoid development in this condition and in patients treated with proton-pump inhibitors is a failure or interference of the normal suppressive feedback loop of gastric acid on gastrin production by the antral G cell. The resultant increased gastrin production stimulates proliferation of the enterochromaffin-like (carcinoid) cells, which normally stimulate acid production by production of histamine.

There have been reports of development of gastric carcinoid tumors with lymph node metastasis in MEN-1 patients treated with omeprazole.[89] Since gastric carcinoid tumors occur normally in this group of patients, it is unclear whether these tumors were caused by omeprazole. In other long-term studies in patients with reflux esophagitis[125] and a 4-year prospective study of 40 patients with ZES, there was no evidence of gastric carcinoids,[126,127] which suggests that it is the molecular defect in MEN-1 that promotes development of gastric carcinoid tumors. Nevertheless, prudence suggests that patients treated long term with any acid-reducing medication should have periodic gastric endoscopy to exclude development of a carcinoid tumor.[89]

The management of ZES in patients with MEN-1 is more complex than in patients with sporadic gastrinomas. The role of surgery is controversial, since MEN-1 patients frequently develop multiple islet cell tumors, and recurrent tumor formation in pancreatic tissue remaining from the primary operative procedure is common. Therefore, surgical resection is often not curative unless the entire pancreas and duodenum are removed. Most surgeons balance the long-term risks of diabetic complications associated with total pancreatectomy with the need to effectively treat the disease by performance of a subtotal pancreatectomy with careful examination of the duodenum and gastrinoma triangle for carcinoid-like tumors. If a second surgical procedure is required, it is often 10–15 years later, delaying the onset of diabetes. The rationale for delaying such surgery is based on the belief, not entirely validated by prospective studies, that small islet cell tumors (<1 cm) are less likely to metastasize. Total pancreatectomy and careful examination of the duodenum with excision of any identified tumors may be appropriate in kindreds with MEN-1 where there is a high incidence of islet cell malignancy. Another indication for surgery is the presence of islet cell tumors greater than 2 cm in diameter, since these tumors are most likely to metastasize to the liver.[89] Tumors within the pancreatic head can be enucleated; tumors within the body and tail can be resected by distal or subtotal pancreatectomy.[89] The duodenal wall should be carefully explored, since MEN-1 patients frequently have multiple tumors in this area.[99,128–131] Most patients with ZES and MEN-1 syndrome should be treated with H$_2$ receptor blockers or proton-pump inhibitors because these agents can effectively control clinical manifestations of ZES. However, patients so treated should be carefully monitored by frequent endoscopic examination and biopsy of the gastric mucosa to exclude the development of gastric carcinoids.[89,132,133]

## Vipomas

In 1958, Verner and Morrison[134] described a patient who presented with watery diarrhea, hypokalemia, and an islet cell tumor. The syndrome they described has been variously given the names Verner-Morrison syndrome, the pancreatic cholera syndrome, or the **W**atery **D**iarrhea, **H**ypokalemia, and **A**chloridria (or hypochloridria) (WDHA) syndrome.[135,136] In the early 1970s, patients with this syndrome were found to have hypersecretion of VIP[137,138] with high plasma and tumor levels of VIP.[137] Vasoactive intestinal peptide is a 28–amino acid peptide that binds to a specific receptor on intestinal epithelial cells and stimulates cAMP production, leading to fluid and electrolyte secretion into the lumen.[139,140] This peptide is also a strong inhibitor of gastric acid secretion, which likely causes achloridria in patients with vipomas. In experiments in humans, VIP infusion resulted in a shift from the absorption of intestinal water and electrolyte to their secretion, leading to secretory diarrhea.[141]

In addition to VIP, vipomas frequently secrete other substances, including prostaglandin E$_2$, peptide histidine methionine (PHM), calcitonin, pancreatic polypeptide, and neurotensin. All of these may contribute to the clinical manifestations of vipoma.[140,142–144] Indeed, the failure of VIP infusions to stimulate the profound watery diarrhea found in Verner-Morrison patients suggests that other factors besides VIP contribute to the diarrhea.[145]

### Clinical features

Vipomas most commonly develop in the pancreas, 75% of them in the pancreatic tail.[146] However, these are not the only tumors that produce this clinical syndrome or produce VIP. Others include colon carcinoma, pheochromocytoma, hepatoma, bronchogenic carcinomas, and adrenal tumors.[147] Patients with vipomas usually present with large tumors (>3 cm) and with liver metastasis (approximately 50% of cases). The hallmark of this syndrome is watery diarrhea (stool volume >3 L/day). It is considered to be a secretory diarrhea in that it persists after fasting and produces an odorless stool having a low stool osmolal gap. Because the diarrhea depletes sodium, potassium, chloride and bicarbonate, patients present with volume depletion, hypokalemia, hypochloridria, and severe metabolic acidosis. Some patients may also present with hypercalcemia,[148,149] which is thought to be mediated by one of the secretory products of this tumor. Vasoactive intestinal peptide, PTH-RP, and PTH (in patients with MEN-1) have been suggested as candidates for this effect.[150,151]

## Diagnosis

Vipoma should be suspected in any patient with chronic, unexplained secretory diarrhea. Other causes of secretory diarrhea include infectious enterocolitis (due to enterotoxigenic *Escherichia coli* or to *Vibrio cholera*), microscopic or collagenous colitis, factitious diarrhea due to surreptitious use of laxatives, bile salt malabsorption due to ileal resection, or carcinoid syndrome. Stool analysis for osmolality, sodium, and potassium is nonspecific but can confirm a secretory diarrhea. The osmolality of the stool can be calculated by adding the concentrations of sodium and potassium and then multiplying by 2 to account for unmeasurable anions. An osmolal gap can then be calculated by subtracting the measured stool osmolality (as determined by the laboratory) from the calculated osmolality. A secretory diarrhea has an osmolal gap less than 50 mosm/kg. Besides having a high-volume secretory diarrhea, patients with Verner-Morrison syndrome will often have a high level of serum VIP. Localization of a vipoma is usually not a problem since patients often present with large tumors that are detectable by an abdominal CT scan or by somatostatin receptor scintigraphy.

## Treatment

Management of a patient with Verner-Morrison syndrome combines several approaches. Surgical removal of the tumor, where possible, is the primary therapy. In patients with unresectable or metastatic tumor, the goal is to control the diarrhea, replace fluid and electrolyte losses, and correct the base-acid disorder. The bicarbonate and potassium deficit should be assessed. The patient should first receive 2 L of normal saline (154 mEq $Na^+$/L) to achieve hemodynamic stability and then half-normal saline mixed with 44 mEq (1 ampoule) sodium bicarbonate to correct the metabolic acidosis. Potassium and magnesium should be replaced intravenously as needed.

Octreotide is the treatment of choice for controlling VIP secretion and the resulting diarrhea.[152–154] The usual dose is 50 to 100 μg, three times a day. The recent introduction of long-acting octreotide or lanreotide provides more convenient alternatives if effective. In our experience, a few patients have required an octreotide drip for the control of acute diarrhea. The introduction of somatostatin analogues for the treatment of Verner-Morrison syndrome improved outcomes substantially. Prior to their use, patients died frequently within a year from overwhelming fluid and electrolyte abnormalities or from complications of combined chemotherapy and high-dose glucocorticoid therapy (the only other effective therapy to reduce diarrhea). During the past decade, survival has improved substantially by combining somatostatin analogue therapy, judicious use of corticosteroids, chemotherapy, and arterial embolization of metastatic tumor. Survival periods of 15–17 years have been described by Nguyen et al.[155] and have been observed in our own practice. Surgical debulking of dominant hepatic metastasis may reduce morbidity associated with VIP production, although it is generally not indicated if there is diffuse metastatic disease. There is one report of hepatic transplantation resulting in long-term survival, although in this case primary therapy focused on cytotoxic chemotherapy and octreotide treatment.[156]

## Somatostatinomas

The somatostatinoma syndrome, first reported[157] in 1977, consists of diabetes mellitus, diarrhea (steatorrhea), cholelithiasis, indigestion, and hypochlorhydria associated with a pancreatic or duodenal tumor. The syndrome is also called an "inhibitory syndrome" because the clinical manifestations are secondary to the suppressive effects of somatostatin on secretion of hormones such as insulin, glucagon, cholecystokinin, VIP, motilin, and secretin.

One hundred seventy-three cases of somatostatinomas have been reported in the literature.[158] Pancreatic somatostatinomas and duodenal somatostatinomas are equally common, and only a few (<5%) originate from other sites (i.e., lung, jejunum, colon, rectum, thyroid, stomach, cystic duct). The pancreatic tumors arise more commonly in the head than in tail of the pancreas; most duodenal tumors arise in the ampulla of Vater.[159–166] The duodenal tumors tend to be smaller, and symptoms related to their local effects (e.g., biliary obstruction) tend to be more common than symptoms of somatostatin hypersecretion. In contrast to pancreatic somatostatinomas, duodenal somatostatinomas are frequently associated with von Recklinghausen's disease (50%), but rarely associated with the somatostatinoma syndrome.[159–161,163,167–170]

Both pancreatic and duodenal somatostatinomas have malignant potential. In about half of the cases, the patient presents with metastatic disease, a finding that reduces long-term survival. Metastasis or local invasion occurs most commonly in liver and lymph nodes. Other sites of metastasis include bone, kidney, adrenal gland, skin, peritoneum, and brain[171,172] In addition to somatostatin, the pancreatic tumors produce additional hormonally induced clinical manifestations that include hypoglycemia (insulin),[173,174] marked diarrhea (calcitonin),[175] and Cushing's syndrome (ACTH).[176] Somatostatinomas are less commonly associated with MEN-1 (6%), but when they are, the tumors tend to be multiple and benign.[158]

The diagnosis of a pancreatic somatostatinoma is made by the presence of the clinical syndrome and an elevated plasma somatostatin level. The tumors are usually large enough to be easily identifiable by imaging studies. Duodenal somatostatinomas, unlike duodenal carcinoid-like tumors producing ZES, are difficult to diagnose because they produce no typical clinical symptoms and are infrequently associated with elevations of plasma somatostatin levels. Diagnosis of duodenal somatostatinoma may not occur until there are obstructive symptoms or metastatic disease.

The treatment of somatostatinomas includes surgical resection and local or systemic chemotherapy for metastatic disease.

# Parathyroid Hormone–Related Peptide-Secreting Tumors

The association of hypercalcemia with islet cell tumors is well established. The differential diagnosis of hypercalcemia in a patient with an islet cell tumor includes hyperparathyroidism (MEN-1), hypercalcemia associated with Verner-Morrison syndrome, and production of PTH-rp by the tumor or somatostatinoma.[148,149,177] The identification of PTH-rp as a cause of humoral hypercalcemia led to the recognition that islet cell carcinomas frequently produce this peptide and that there is a subgroup of patients whose tumors produce only PTH-rp.[178] These patients have high serum PTH-rp levels, and their tumors contain high levels of PTH-rp peptide and RNA, as shown by immunohistochemical analysis and in situ hybridization.[179] These tumors, called *PTH-rpomas*, are frequently large (5–18 cm in diameter) and vascular.[178] They commonly involve the tail of the pancreas and, in more than 90% of cases, are associated with liver metastases.[178] The primary treatment is surgical resection followed by systemic chemotherapy to treat residual, metastatic disease. The major cause of morbidity and mortality in patients with these large but slowly growing tumors is hypercalcemia. Standard therapy for hypercalcemia (intravenous hydration, furosemide, bisphosphonates, plicamycin, gallium nitrate, calcitonin, corticosteroids)[180] is effective in the short term, but the patient either becomes resistant or develops renal (plicamycin and gallium) or hepatic (plicamycin) toxicity that limits their use. The development of PTH-rp–specific antagonists, monoclonal antibodies specific for inactivation of PTH-rp, or osteoprotegerin-like analogues that interfere with osteoclast differentiation offer hope for improving outcomes in these patients in the future.[181]

### Growth Hormone or Growth Hormone–Releasing Hormone–Secreting Islet Cell Tumors

Acromegaly is most commonly caused by a GH-secreting pituitary adenoma. However, acromegaly may also result from ectopic production of GH[182] or GHRH.[183–185] Patients with GH- or GHRH-secreting islet cell tumors usually present with acromegalic features, elevated plasma GH and IGF-1 levels, a normal-sized pituitary gland on MRI, and a large pancreatic mass. In these patients the diurnal rhythm of GH secretion is lost along with the ability to respond to thyroid-releasing hormone (TRH) and GHRH stimulation tests,[186] a point that differentiates these patients from those with GH-producing pituitary tumors. The clinical features of acromegaly and elevated plasma GH and IGF-1 levels normalize after successful resection of the islet cell tumor.[182,187] Somatostatin analogues can be used to treat patients with residual disease, although it has been suggested that they are less effective in this context than in patients with GH-producing pituitary tumors.[182]

### Nonfunctional Islet Cell Tumors

About 50% of all islet cell carcinomas are deemed nonfunctional because there is no clinical syndrome associated with the hypersecretion of hormones by such tumors. These tumors either produce no identifiable hormone or they produce hormones that do not cause clinical syndromes (i.e., pancreatic polypeptide [PPomas] or neurotensin [neurotensinomas]).[186] In 60% to 90% of cases, they produce chromogranin A, a marker of neuroendocrine differentiation. The nonfunctioning islet cell tumors are usually large at presentation since the patient's presenting symptoms are usually due to the tumor mass and not to a hormonal syndrome. An exception occurs in patients with MEN-1, whose biochemical screening includes the measurement of pancreatic polypeptide. The treatment for nonfunctional islet cell tumors is surgical resection and systemic chemotherapy if the tumor is unresectable or invasive.

### Regional and Systemic Treatment of Metastatic Islet Cell Carcinomas

#### Surgery

Surgical resection is the treatment of choice for neuroendocrine tumors of the gastrointestinal tract. If the tumor is not localized or unresectable, further intervention is necessary. Control of symptoms related to hormonal hypersecretion is extremely important, as it will allow the patient to tolerate treatment aimed at controlling the tumor mass. Palliative surgery may help control the clinical syndrome and should be attempted in patients who present with metastatic disease. Frequently, the reduction in tumor load will lead to a significant reduction in hormonal levels and better control of the clinical syndrome. Surgical options in patients with metastatic disease include resection or cryoablation of liver metastases and liver transplantation. Further control of the clinical syndrome and growth of the tumor can be obtained by systemic chemotherapy, hepatic artery embolization with or without local chemotherapy, and local radiotherapy.

#### Chemotherapy

Several trials have examined chemotherapeutic regimens for gastrointestinal neuroendocrine tumors (Table 65–7). The drugs used have included streptozocin, doxorubicin, 5-fluorouracil, dacarbazine, and cyclophosphamide. Patients with pancreatic islet cell carcinomas tend to respond better than patients with intestinal neuroendocrine tumors (30% to 70% compared with 0% to 26%).[154,188,189]

Streptozocin is currently the chemotherapeutic agent of choice for treatment of metastatic islet cell tumors.[190] The overall rate of response to streptozocin alone ranges from 36% to 65%. When streptozocin is given in combination with other agents, the response rate is higher. Moertel and colleagues[191] reported that the overall rate of response to streptozocin plus 5-fluorouracil was 63% compared with a rate of 36% for streptozocin alone. In another study by the same group,[189] the overall rate of response to streptozocin in combination with doxorubicin was 69%. The combined regimen of streptozocin plus doxorubicin was well tolerated, increased the median duration of response to 20 months, and resulted in a survival advantage. Rivera and Ajani[192] evaluated the response to streptozocin, doxorubicin, and 5-fluorouracil in 11 patients with metastatic islet cell carcinoma. Six of the 11 patients achieved a partial response, one had a minor response, two had stable disease, and two had progressive disease. The median survival was higher for responders (21 months) than for nonresponders (14.5 months). Because the addition of 5-fluorouracil to streptozocin and doxorubicin did not result in significantly better responses, the current first-line therapy for metastatic islet cell carcinoma is streptozocin and doxorubicin. In all of these trials, most patients who responded to treatment had partial responses marked by biochemical improvement and reduction of the tumor mass. Complete responses were seen in 0% to 30% of cases, but in most of these cases the disease tended to recur.[188,189,191,192] Therefore, the only curative treatment available for islet cell carcinoma appears to be surgery.

One important practical question is when to start the chemotherapy. Because islet cell carcinomas are indolent, there is no clear survival benefit of early therapy, and the interval of disease progression is variable in each patient, current recommendations suggest starting treatment when patients are symptomatic or when there is clear progression of the disease after a period of observation.

Another chemotherapeutic agent tested against islet cell carcinomas is interferon (IFN-α).[193,194] In initial studies, nude BALB/c mice were injected with human neuroendocrine pancreatic tumor cells and then treated with IFN-α alone or in combination with other drugs. The result was a significant antitumor effect. In patients with neuroendocrine tumors, however, the results have not been so encouraging; clinical responses have been seen

**Table 65–7** Selected reports of systemic chemotherapy in islet cell carcinoma

| Study | Total Patients (n) | Tumor Type (n) | Chemotherapy Drug/Patients Treated (n) | Objective Response (%) |
|---|---|---|---|---|
| Moertel et al., 1980[191] (Mayo Clinic) | 84 | Insulinoma (15), gastrinoma (12), vipoma (1), glucagonoma (3), PTH-rpomas (2), nonfunctioning (43), others (10) | STZ (41)<br>STZ + 5-FU (43) | 36<br>63 |
| Moertel et al., 1992[189] (Mayo Clinic) | 105 | Gastrinoma (26), insulinoma (6), vipoma (4), glucagonoma (4), hypercalcemia (7), nonfunctional (55), others (14) | STZ + 5-FU (33)<br>STZ + DOXO (36)<br>CZT (33) | 45<br>69<br>30 |
| Rivera et al., 1998[192] (MDACC) | 12 | Islet cell carcinoma | STZ + 5-FU + DOXO (12) | 54.5 |
| Moertel et al., 1991[197] (Mayo Clinic) | 45 (divided into three groups) | Islet cell carcinoma (14), anaplastic neuroendocrine carcinoma (18) carcinoid tumor (13) | Cisplatin + etoposide (45) | 14<br>67<br>0 |
| Ramanathan et al., 2001[198] (Univ. Pittsburgh, ECOG) | 50 | Islet cell carcinoma | DTIC (50) | 34 |
| Ansell et al., 2001[199] (Mayo Clinic) | 24 | Islet cell carcinoma (9), anaplastic neuroendocrine carcinoma (1), carcinoid tumor (14) | High-dose paclitaxel (24) | 8% (overall response), grade 4 hematologic toxicity (50%) |
| Cheng and Saltz, 1999[269] (MSKCC) | 16 | Islet cell carcinoma | STZ + DOXO (16) | 6 |
| Kim et al., 1999[205] (MDACC) | 14 | Islet cell carcinoma | STZ + 5-FU + HAE (14) | 50% (tumor response), 90% (biochemical response) |

Abbreviations: CZT, chlorozotocin; DOXO, doxorubicin; DTIC, dacarbazine; ECOG, Eastern Cooperative Oncology Group; 5-FU, 5-fluorouracil; HAE, hepatic artery embolization; MDACC, M. D. Anderson Cancer Center; MSKCC, Memorial Sloan-Kettering Cancer Center; STZ, streptozocin.

in about 47% of patients, with tumor regression in 12%–15%.[190] The main side effects of treatment with IFN-α are fatigue, myalgia, weight loss, and anemia. The effect of IFN-α is comparable to that of octreotide, i.e., minimal tumoricidal activity but stabilization of the disease in a significant percentage of patients. Therefore, in patients in whom other therapeutic options have failed, IFN-α therapy to stabilize disease status may be considered.[195]

Despite significant advances in the diagnosis and identification of the different islet cell tumors and their hormonal syndromes, almost no advance has been made in improving the outcome (i.e., survival rate) of patients with malignant, invasive disease. Most patients with unresectable islet cell carcinoma die of the disease since therapies other than surgical resection do not result in cure. Therefore, more therapeutic modalities are needed to treat unresectable disease. Angiogenesis inhibitors are good candidates since islet cell tumors are very vascular. In fact, in a recent study using a mouse model of pancreatic islet cell carcinogenesis, a variety of antiangiogenesis drugs significantly reduced the tumor burden by 60% to 80%.[196] Recent trials with different chemotherapeutic agents such as paclitaxel, cisplatin, etoposide, and dacarbazine (DTIC) have failed to demonstrate significant activity against islet cell carcinomas in general.[197–199] One exception is the use of DTIC in glucagonomas, which are reported to respond frequently to this drug.[200,201]

## Hepatic Artery Embolization

Hepatic artery embolization with or without infusion of simultaneous chemotherapy has been used to manage hepatic metastasis with some success. This procedure is never curative but is useful for reducing the severity of certain hormonal syndromes or improving overall hepatic function with subsequent improvements in the quality of life for patients. The rationale for hepatic artery embolization is that metastatic tumors most commonly derive their vascular supply from the hepatic artery, whereas hepatic parenchyma has a dual circulation from the hepatic artery and portal circulation. The portal vein supplies approximately 75% of the normal liver's blood supply, whereas the hepatic artery supplies most of the blood to hepatic neoplasms. Therefore, hepatic artery embolization preferentially affects the blood supply to the tumor while having little effect on the normal liver parenchyma. The embolization is usually performed with particulate embolic materials such as Ivalon or Gelfoam. Within approximately 72 hours, intrahepatic collateral vessels reconstitute the hepatic arterial circulation. Because occlusion of larger, more central blood vessels results in the formation of collateral vessels, the embolization of smaller and more peripheral blood vessels is preferable.[202,203] To maximize the ischemic effect on the tumor, the vascular bed supplying the tumor is repeatedly and selectively occluded.

Most of the experience with hepatic artery embolization was obtained in patients with metastatic carcinoid tumors; however, this treatment has been proven to be just as useful in patients with metastatic islet cell carcinomas.[202,204] In their experience with sequential hepatic embolization in 22 patients with islet cell tumors metastatic to the liver, Ajani and colleagues[204] performed a total of 97 embolizations (a median of four embolizations per patient). A partial response (defined as a 50% or greater reduction in tumor volume) was documented in 12 patients, a minor response (defined as a less than 50% reduction in tumor volume) in 4, only symptomatic improvement in 5, and no benefit in 1 patient. Objective responses were usually seen after the second embolization. Most patients also showed improvement of the hormonal syndrome due to a significant decrease in hormone levels.

Hepatic artery embolization is often effective for reduction of VIP or insulin production, reducing diarrhea or hypoglycemia, respectively. It is less effective for treatment of clinical manifestations caused by gastrin or PTH-rp. In our experience, there has been clinical improvement in occasional cases following hepatic artery embolization for patients with no obvious hormonal syndrome. Explanations or hypotheses to explain this improvement include the reduction in tumor mass, improvement in hepatic cell function, or the reduction of a high-output type of cardiac dysfunction that develops in patients with extensive hepatic metastasis.

Chemoembolization of the hepatic artery produced results similar to those of hepatic embolization with Ivalon or Gelfoam alone. In one series, 20 patients (17 patients with carcinoid tumors and 3 with islet cell tumors) underwent repetitive hepatic artery embolization using encapsulated cisplatin. Of the 18 patients that were evaluated, 6 had a partial response, 8 had a minor response, and 4 had no response. Twelve patients showed a 50% reduction in symptoms.[203]

It is important to exercise caution in the application of this technique. Patients with poor hepatic function or poor performance status should be excluded, since deaths related to hepatic failure or peritoneal inflammation have occurred. Most commonly, embolization is staged, with embolization of a hepatic lobe or subsegment of a lobe performed in different hospitalizations. There have been several deaths in patients treated with hepatic embolization. Retrospective analysis of these deaths revealed that, in all cases, the patients had extensive liver metastases involving more than 50% of the liver parenchyma, serum lactic dehydrogenase (LDH) levels greater than 425 mU/ml, serum glutamic oxaloacetic transaminase (SGOT) levels greater than 100 mU/ml, and bilirubin levels greater than 2 mg/dl. Therefore, hepatic embolization should either not be used or used judiciously (e.g., only subsegmental embolization should be performed) in patients with these risk factors.[202]

After embolization, patients may experience nausea, vomiting, fever, and abdominal discomfort. These symptoms are accompanied by leukocytosis and elevated liver function. A transient but clinically significant consequence of this treatment is the release of hormones into the circulation, which frequently worsens the hormonal syndrome. The symptoms can often be effectively controlled by octreotide for certain hormones. We frequently pretreat patients who have a hormonal secretory process affected by somatostatin with an octreotide infusion at a dosage of 20 to 50 μg/hour. The response to hepatic artery embolization usually lasts less than 5 months, and the best results occur when the embolization is followed by systemic chemotherapy.[205]

### Clinical Use of Somatostatin Analogues

The main function of somatostatin is to inhibit various hormones, although a number of studies have suggested that it also functions as an antiproliferative agent.[206] Because somatostatin binds to specific membrane receptors on target cells, the presence of somatostatin receptors on target tissues is critical to its action. Most islet cell tumors express large numbers of somatostatin receptors,[207] which fall into at least five different subtypes.[208]

Though somatostatin binds to all five subtypes, the somatostatin analogue octreotide binds with highest affinity to subtypes 2 and 5 and with less affinity to subtype 3. Most human endocrine pancreatic tumors, including nonfunctioning islet cell tumors, express subtype 2 receptors; insulinomas tend to express subtype 3 receptors.[207,209]

Octreotide is a synthetic eight–amino acid peptide that has a much longer half-life (113 minutes) than somatostatin (approximately 3 minutes).[190,208] It has been used both as a radiodiagnostic tool for localization of tumors and as treatment for hormonal syndromes. Its diagnostic use was illustrated in a European multicenter study of somatostatin receptor scintigraphy (SRS). Using SRS, researchers effectively identified 100% of glucagonomas, 88% of vipomas, 73% of gastrinomas, and 82% of nonfunctioning tumors.[210] Only 46% of insulinomas were detected in the study, with the low detection rate attributted to the lower concentration of somatostatin receptor subtype 2 in these tumors.[210]

Octreotide is very useful for the control of symptoms related to hormonal hypersecretion, thereby improving the quality of life of patients with these symptoms. It has been shown to be extremely helpful in patients with vipomas, in whom diarrhea, hypokalemia, and acidosis caused by overproduction of VIP can be life threatening. It has also been shown to control or reduce the clinical features associated with the glucagonoma syndrome. Octreotide is also useful in controlling symptoms of ZES, although acid-reducing drugs (e.g., proton-pump inhibitors) remain the medical treatment of choice in such patients. Conversely, octreotide is not very helpful in controlling the hypoglycemia seen in patients with insulinomas because these tumors do not express significant amounts of somatostatin receptor subtype 2 and because octreotide can suppress the activity of counterregulatory hormones such as GH. Octreotide is also useful in treating patients with GHRH-producing islet cell tumors but is of little value in treating patients with somatostatinomas.[149,211–223]

## Genetic Syndromes Associated with Islet Cell Tumors

There are four primary genetic syndromes to consider when evaluating tumors of the neuroendocrine gastrointestinal tract. These syndromes include MEN-1, von Hippel-Lindau, NF-1, and tuberous sclerosis (Table 65–2). Each of these disorders evolves from loss of tumor suppressor gene function. The first three clinical syndromes and their genetic abnormalities will be described below.

### Multiple Endocrine Neoplasia Type 1

Multiple endocrine neoplasia type 1 is an autosomal dominant disorder characterized by hyperplasia of the parathyroid glands (hyperparathyroidism) in 90% of affected individuals, by islet cell tumors in 75% to 81%, and by pituitary adenomas in 10% to 65%. This genetic syndrome accounts for approximately 25% of all islet cell tumors. It is important to identify these patients, as they, and potentially other family members, are at great risk of developing other neoplastic manifestations. The clinical manifestations of islet cell tumors in MEN-1 are similar to those of sporadic tumors; however, unlike sporadic tumors, in MEN-1 they are typically multiple, which makes their cure by surgical resection difficult. Sporadic islet cell tumors, by contrast, are more likely than MEN-1 tumors to be malignant (70% vs. 30% to 50%), perhaps because the tumors in MEN-1 are most commonly detected earlier by screening.

In 1988, the gene responsible for causing the familial disorder was mapped to chromosome 11q13 by linkage analysis and a loss of heterozygosity (LOH) was demonstrated at this locus in MEN-1 tumors.[224] Nearly 10 years passed before the mutations within a single gene were identified.[225] Positional cloning via meiotic recombination and tumor LOH studies narrowed the candidate region to less than 300 kb, at which point the entire genomic interval was sequenced.[225] A search of expressed sequences within this region led to the identification of the *MEN1* gene. In the original report by Chandrasekharappa and colleagues,[225] a single gene in the region was found to contain 12 different mutations in 14 probands of 15 affected MEN-1 families. This gene, now called the *MEN1* gene, is composed of 10 exons that produce a 2.8 kb transcript encoding the 610–amino acid protein termed *menin*.[225]

The identity of the *MEN1* gene was quickly confirmed, and over 173 unique mutations of this gene have been described.[226] The kinds of mutations observed are similar to those observed for the *p53* tumor suppressor gene. Mutations are distributed throughout the protein-coding region, and a large number of others affect RNA splicing.[227] The majority of mutations result in premature truncation of the protein (loss of function) due to frameshift (insertions, deletions) and nonsense mutations. Missense mutations are thought to involve important functional areas of the gene, but the way in which menin functions as a tumor suppressor is not entirely clear. Menin appears to be sublocalized to the cell nucleus. Menin has been shown to bind specifically to the transcription factor JunD, thereby preventing its interaction with its cognate transcriptional complex.[228] More recent studies have also documented interaction of menin with NF-κB and Pem, both transcriptional factors, although the physiologic relevance of these interactions is unknown.[229,230]

The distribution of mutations across the coding region of the *MEN1* gene makes mutational analysis in MEN-1 families unpredictable and tedious. This, coupled with the low frequency of the disorder, has relegated genetic screening predominantly to research laboratories. Commercial sites offering MEN-1 testing are listed at http://www.genetests.org. An additional complication is that there are still a number of MEN-1 kindreds without an identifiable *MEN1* mutation. The range for mutation detection varies from 50% to 100% (average 77%) in known MEN-1 kindreds and it has been suggested that a second *MEN1* gene may exist.[231–234] The question of the value of genetic testing in patients with de novo MEN-1 has been addressed in small series. Approximately 64% (55 of 86 patients) with clearly defined de novo MEN-1 (three manifestations without a family history) have mutations. In contrast, in patients who present with two of three manifestations of MEN-1 without a family history, a low percentage have identifiable *MEN1* mutations, which suggests that genetic testing in this group does not have great value.[235] In another series,[236] an examination of 27 sporadic gastrinomas found a high incidence of LOH at the *MEN1* gene locus (93%) and a somatic mutation frequency of 33%, but only a single patient was found to harbor a germline mutation. Similarly, an examination of 12 sporadic insulinomas found *MEN1* gene somatic mutations in two tumors, neither of which were found to be germline.[237] These findings are somewhat surprising because retrospective phenotypic estimates in patients with sporadic islet cell tumors suggest that a diagnosis of MEN-1 should be considered, particularly in patients with gastrinomas and insulinomas where 5% to 25% of cases are found to be a part of the genetic syndrome MEN-1. Collectively, these studies clearly implicate the *MEN1* gene in the pathogenesis of these tumor types, but raise questions regarding the value of genetic screening for familial disease in patients with apparently sporadic disease.

## Von Hippel–Lindau Disease

Von Hippel-Lindau (VHL) disease is an autosomal dominant neoplastic disorder characterized by renal cell carcinoma (RCC), retinal and cerebellar hemangioblastomas, pancreatic cysts, pheochromocytomas, and papillary cystadenoma of the epididymis.[160,168,238,239]

Pancreatic islet cell tumors are observed in approximately 12%–17% of VHL patients, typically those between the ages of 20–35 years, and are often found in association with pheochromocytoma.[35] The majority of these pancreatic tumors are nonfunctional and frequently malignant, therefore meriting prompt surgical intervention.[240]

The tumor suppressor gene responsible for VHL was identified in 1993 by positional cloning of DNA sequences from chromosome 3p25.[241] The *VHL* gene is composed of three exons spanning approximately 12.4 kb; however, with only a 213–amino acid protein coding region, the task of genetic screening has been straightforward and is commercially available (www.genetests.org). As a result, more than 500 VHL kindreds have been analyzed, and germline mutations have been found in most of these families.[226,242] *VHL* mutations, like those found in *MEN1*, have been extremely heterogeneous and are distributed throughout the coding sequence; the majority are deletion, frameshift, or nonsense mutations that lead to inactivation of the *VHL* gene by producing a truncated and nonfunctional protein. However, approximately 15% to 20% of patients have large germline deletions or rearrangements that are detectable only by Southern analysis.[243] While there is no clear-cut association of specific mutations with islet tumors, missense mutations have been associated with an increased susceptibility to pheochromocytoma.[244]

The VHL protein itself has diverse functions and appears to be involved in several key cell proliferation pathways. A search for proteins that interact with VHL identified specific associations with elongin B and elongin C, proteins that play an important role in gene transcription elongation. Interaction of VHL with the elongins and the Cul-2 protein is thought to specifically inhibit transcription elongation of hypoxia-inducible mRNAs.[245] In support of this idea, the elongin-interacting domain mapped to a region of the VHL protein that is frequently mutated in patients. In the cytoplasm, the elongin family members play an equally important role. The Cul-2 protein is also part of the E3 ubiquitin ligase complex. Therefore, an additional function of VHL is to mediate the degradation of yet unidentified proteins involved in cell cycle regulation for ubiquitin-mediated proteolysis.[246,247] Finally, VHL protein can also interact with fibronectin and is required for the assembly of a fibronectin matrix.[248] Thus, the VHL tumor suppressor protein appears to have a role in regulation of angiogenesis, extracellular matrix formation, and the cell cycle.

Although somatic *VHL* gene mutations have also been identified in sporadic tumors, including renal cell carcinomas and pheochromocytomas,[249,250] the role of this gene in the development of sporadic pancreatic tumors is unclear. An examination of pancreatic neuroendocrine tumors[251] and microcystic adenomas[252] derived from individuals with known *VHL* gene mutations has clearly demonstrated the LOH at the *VHL* locus. However, a study of sporadic pancreatic endocrine tumors derived from 43 patients showed surprising results.[253] Although there was a high incidence of LOH at the *VHL* gene locus (31%), DNA sequencing of the other copy of the *VHL* gene showed no mutations. These findings suggest that the *VHL* gene does not play a role in the development of pancreatic endocrine tumors and that a second tumor suppressor gene exists nearby on chromosome 3p. These results suggest that, in the absence of other features of VHL disease, screening for VHL mutations is of little value in patients with pancreatic tumors, although no large study has been conducted. From a practical standpoint, there are no reports of pancreatic tumors occurring in VHL kindreds in the absence of other tissue involvement.

## Neurofibromatosis

Islet cell tumors and duodenal somatostatinomas have been rarely associated with neurofibromatosis type 1 (NF-1). Neurofibromatosis type 1, also referred to as *von Recklinghausen's disease*, can involve any organ system; however, clinical diagnosis is made on the basis of the presence of common manifestations. These include café-au-lait macules, neurofibromas, axillary or inguinal freckling, optic nerve glioma, and Lisch nodules (iris hamartomas).[254,255] Gastrointestinal involvement in NF-1 disease occurs in three principal forms: hyperplasia of the submucosal and myenteric nerve plexuses and mucosal ganglioneuromatosis; gastrointestinal stromal tumors; and of specific concern here, somatostatin-producing carcinoids of the periampullary region of the duodenum that contain psammoma bodies and which may be associated with pheochromocytoma.[256]

Duodenal endocrine tumors, in general, are uncommon, accounting for less than 2% of all gastrointestinal endocrine tumors. However, approximately 50% of all duodenal somatostatinomas are found in association with von Recklinghausen's NF-1.[167,168,257–259] Most somatostatinomas (70%) occur in the pancreas (see earlier section),[260] and the finding of a duodenal somatostatinoma should raise the question of NF-1. Furthermore, clinical presentation of duodenal somatostatinomas is rarely associated with somatostatinoma syndrome (diarrhea, diabetes, cholelithiasis). As a result, duodenal somatostatinomas seldom produce a recognizable syndrome and typically go undiagnosed until they are identified as a result of biliary obstruction or serendipitously.

The *NF1* gene was originally mapped to chromosome 17 by Barker and colleagues[261] in 1987. The genetic region containing the gene was further narrowed by the discovery of chromosomal rearrangements in NF-1 patients involving the 17q11.2 region.[262,263] The first mutations and partial characterization of the *NF1* gene were reported by two independent groups in 1990.[264,265] Complete characterization of the *NF1* gene locus was hampered by the size of the gene. The 60-exon gene spans approximately 335 kb of genomic DNA, producing a mRNA of approximately 12 kb. The open reading frame of the gene, named *neurofibromin*, predicts a protein of 2818 amino acids with homology to the catalytic domain of GTPase-activating proteins.[266] Neurofibromin, through its GTPase activity, inhibits p21 *ras* activity; inactivating mutations of neurofibromin lead to uncontrolled p21 *ras* activation of the MAPK signaling pathway[267] and are thought to cause tumors through this mechanism. The vast majority of *NF1* mutations are either nonsense or frameshift mutations, predicting a premature truncation of the neurofibromin, consistent with the supposed tumor suppressor function.[268]

An important question to consider in the context of this section is whether specific NF1 gene mutations can serve to predict those NF-1 patients most likely to develop duodenal somatostatinomas. Unfortunately, routine genetic analysis of the *NF1* gene has been hampered by the large size of the gene. Although over 200 unique genetic defects and mutations have been reported, the genetic defects present in most NF-1 patients, including those presenting with duodenal somatostatinomas, remain unknown.[268] There is no genotype–phenotype correlation. It is also unclear whether to perform *NF1* genetic analysis in patients presenting with duodenal somatostatinomas. A comparison of patients with somatostatinomas with and without associated NF-1 found no differences in clinical features or histologic changes of the tumor, except that production of hormonally active peptides occurs more frequently in the context of NF-1.[168] From a clinical standpoint, this would argue against the value of genetic testing, especially when one considers that the key indicators of NF-1 (neurofibromas) are typically present at the time of duodenal somatostatinoma discovery. However, the important question of whether loss of *NF1* function plays a key role in the development of duodenal somatostatinomas remains unanswered.

## References

1. Wermers RA, Fatourechi V, Wynne AG, Kvols LK, Lloyd RV. The glucagonoma syndrome. Clinical and pathologic features in 21 patients. Medicine 75:53–63, 1996.
2. Krejs GJ. Gastrointestinal endocrine tumors. Am J Med 82 (Suppl 5B): 1–3, 1987.
3. Whitwam JG. APUD cells and the apudomas. A concept relevant to anaesthesia and endocrinology. Anaesthesia 32:879–888, 1977.
4. Gould VE. Neuroendocrinomas and neuroendocrine carcinomas: APUD cell system neoplasms and their aberrant secretory activities. Pathol Annu 12:33–62, 1997.
5. Becker SW, Kahn D, Rothman S. Cutaneous manifestations of internal malignant tumors. Arch Dermatol Syphiligr 45:1069–1080, 1942.
6. McGavran MH, Unger RH, Recant L, et al. A glucagon-secreting α-cell carcinoma of the pancreas. N Engl J Med 274:1408–1413, 1966.
7. Wilkinson DS. Necrolytic migratory erythema with carcinoma of the pancreas. Trans St Johns Hosp Dermatol Soc 59:244–250, 1973.
8. Sweet RD. A dermatosis specifically associated with a tumor of pancreatic α cells. Br J Dermatol 90:301–308, 1974.
9. Henry JG, Xue N, Kinder BK, Inzucchi SE. A 73-year-old man with hyperglycemia, skin rashes, anemia and weight loss. J Clin Endocrinol Metab 81:2428–2433, 1996.
10. Bloom SR, Polak JM. The glucagonoma syndrome. Adv Exp Med Biol 106:183–194, 1978.
11. Frankton S, Bloom SR. Gastrointestinal endocrine tumours. Glucagonomas. Baillieres Clin Gastroenterol 10:697–705, 1996.
12. Wynick D, Hammond PJ, Bloom SR. The glucagonoma syndrome. Clin Dermatol 11:93–97, 1993.
13. Bloom SR, Polak JM. Glucagonomas, VIPomas and somatostatinomas. Clin Endocrinol Metab 9:285–297, 1980.
14. Wermers RA, Fatourechi V, Kvols LK. Clinical spectrum of hyperglucagonemia associated with malignant neuroendocrine tumors. Mayo Clin Proc 71:1030–1038, 1996.
15. Bloom SR, Polak JM. Glucagonoma syndrome. Am J Med 82:25–36, 1987.
16. Kheir SM, Omura EF, Grizzle WE, Herrera GA, Lee I. Histologic variation in the skin lesions of the glucagonoma syndrome. Am J Surg Pathol 10:445–453, 1986.
17. Huang W, Williams CM, McNeely MC. A persistent periorificial eruption. Necrolytic migratory erythema (NME) (glucagonoma). Arch Dermatol 133:909, 1997.
18. Blackford S, Wright S, Roberts DL. Necrolytic migratory erythema without glucagonoma: the role of dietary essential fatty acids. Br J Dermatol 125:460–462, 1991.
19. Stacpoole PW. The glucagonoma syndrome: clinical features, diagnosis, and treatment. Endocrine Rev 2:347–361, 1981.
20. Holmes A, Kilpatrick C, Proietto J, Green MD. Reversal of a neurologic paraneoplastic syndrome with octreotide (Sandostatin) in a patient with glucagonoma. Am J Med 91:434–436, 1991.
21. von Schenck H, Thorell JI, Berg J, et al. Metabolic studies and glucagon gel filtration pattern before and after surgery in a case of glucagonoma syndrome. Acta Med Scand 205:155–162, 1979.
22. Prinz RA, Badrinath K, Banerji M, Sparagana M, Dorsch TR, Lawrence AM. Operative and chemotherapeutic management of malignant glucagon-producing tumors. Surgery 90:713–719, 1981.

23. Smith AP, Doolas A, Staren ED. Rapid resolution of necrolytic migratory erythema after glucagonoma resection. J Surg Oncol 61:306–309, 1996.

24. Khandekar JD, Oyer D, Miller HJ, Vick NA. Neurologic involvement in glucagonoma syndrome: response to combination chemotherapy with 5-fluorouracil and streptozotocin. Cancer 44:2014–2016, 1979.

25. Halban PA, Weir G. Islet cell hormones: production and degradation. In: Becker KL (ed): Principles and Practice of Endocrinology and Metabolism, Vol 1. J.B. Lippincott, Philadelphia, 1995, pp 1191–1198.

26. Roggli VL, Judge DM, McGavran MH. Duodenal glucagonoma: a case report. Hum Pathol 10:350–353, 1979.

27. Gleeson MH, Bloom SR, Polak JM, et al. An endocrine tumor in kidney affecting small bowel structure, motility and absorptive function. Gut 12:773–782, 1971.

28. Makowka L, Tzakis AG, Mazzaferro V, et al. Transplantation of the liver for metastatic endocrine tumors of the intestine and pancreas. Surg Gynecol Obstet 168:107–111, 1989.

29. Alsina AE, Bartus S, Hull D, Rosson R, Schweizer RT. Liver transplant for metastatic neuroendocrine tumor. J Clin Gastroenterol 12:533–537, 1990.

30. Arnold JC, O'Grady JG, Bird GL, Calne RY, Williams R. Liver transplantation for primary and secondary hepatic apudomas. Br J Surg 76:248–249, 1989.

31. Altimari AF, Bhoopalam N, O'Dorsio T, Lange CL, Sandberg L, Prinz RA. Use of a somatostatin analog (SMS 201-995) in the glucagonoma syndrome. Surgery 100:989–996, 1986.

32. Banting FG, Best CH. The internal secretion of the pancreas. J Lab Clin Med 7:251–266, 1922.

33. Wilder RM, Allan FN, Power MH, Robertson HE. Carcinoma of the islands of the pancreas: hyperinsulinism and hypoglycemia. JAMA 89:348–355, 1927.

34. Howland G, Campbell WR, Maltby EJ, Robinson WL. Dysinsulinism: convulsions and coma due to islet cell tumor of the pancreas with operation and cure. JAMA 93:674–679, 1929.

35. Jensen RT. Pancreatic endocrine tumors: recent advances. Ann Oncol 10 (Suppl 4):170–176, 1999.

36. Eriksson B, Oberg K, Skogseid B. Neuroendocrine pancreatic tumors. Clinical findings in a prospective study of 84 patients. Acta Oncol 28:373–377, 1989.

37. Clarke M, Crofford OB, Graves HA Jr, Scott HW Jr. Functioning β cell tumors (insulinomas) of the pancreas. Ann Surg 175:956–974, 1972.

38. Chang HY, Huang HS, Lin JD, Huang BY, Huang MJ, Jeng LB. Insulinoma—clinical experience in ten cases. Chang Keng I Hsueh Tsa Chih 17:28–38, 1994.

39. Boukhman MP, Karam JH, Shaver J, Siperstein AE, Duh QY, Clark OH. Insulinoma—experience from 1950 to 1995. West J Med 169:98–104, 1998.

40. Atkinson AB, Hadden DR, Kennedy TL, Montgomery DA, McIlrath E, Weaver JA. Insulinomas in Northern Ireland between 1960 and 1980. A review of 16 cases. Ulster Med J 50:21–32, 1981.

41. Stefanini P, Carboni M, Patrassi N, De Bernardinis G, Negro P. Problems of the management of insulinomas. Review of 132 cases treated with medical measures. Acta Diabetol Latina 11:71–77, 1974.

42. Fajans SS, Floyd JC Jr. Diagnosis and medical management of insulinomas. Annu Rev Med 30:313–329, 1979.

43. Service FJ. Insulinoma and other islet-cell tumors. Cancer Treat Res 89:335–346, 1997.

44. Service FJ, Dale AJ, Elveback LR, Jiang NS. Insulinoma: clinical and diagnostic features of 60 consecutive cases. Mayo Clin Proc 51:417–429, 1976.

45. Service FJ, McMahon MM, O'Brien PC, Ballard DJ. Functioning insulinoma—incidence, recurrence, and long-term survival of patients: a 60-year study. Mayo Clin Proc 66:711–719, 1991.

46. Danforth DN Jr, Gorden P, Brennan MF. Metastatic insulin-secreting carcinoma of the pancreas: clinical course and the role of surgery. Surgery 96:1027–1037, 1984.

47. Dizon AM, Kowalyk S, Hoogwerf BJ. Neuroglycopenic and other symptoms in patients with insulinomas. Am J Med 106:307–310, 1999.

48. Grant CS. Insulinoma. Surg Oncol Clin North Am 7:819–844, 1998.

49. Grant CS. Gastrointestinal endocrine tumours. Insulinoma. Baillieres Clin Gastroenterol 10:645–671, 1996.

50. Service FJ. Hypoglycemias. Compr Ther 2:27–31, 1976.

51. Gerich JE. Hypoglycemia. In: DeGroot LJ (ed): Endocrinology, 4th ed. W.B. Saunders, Philadelphia, 2001, pp 921–940.

52. Hoff AO, Vassilopoulou-Sellin R. The role of glucagon administration in the diagnosis and treatment of patients with tumor hypoglycemia. Cancer 82:1585–1592, 1998.

53. Service FJ. Hypoglycemic disorders. N Engl J Med 332:1144–1152, 1995.

54. Stefanini P, Carboni M, Patrassi N, Basoli A. Beta-islet cell tumors of the pancreas: results of a study on 1,067 cases. Surgery 75:597–609, 1974.

55. Grama D, Eriksson B, Martensson H, et al. Clinical characteristics, treatment and survival in patients with pancreatic tumors causing hormonal syndromes. World J Surg 16:632–639, 1992.

56. Kaplan EL, Lee CH. Recent advances in the diagnosis and treatment of insulinomas. Surg Clin North Am 59:119–129, 1979.

57. Service FJ, O'Brien PC, McMahon MM, Kao PC. C-peptide during the prolonged fast in insulinoma. J Clin Endocrinol Metab 76:655–659, 1993.

58. Turner RC, Heding LG. Plasma proinsulin, C-peptide and insulin in diagnostic suppression tests for insulinomas. Diabetologia 13:571–577, 1977.

59. Yki-Jarvinen H, Pelkonen R, Koivisto VA. Failure to suppress C-peptide secretion by euglycaemic hyperinsulinaemia: a new diagnostic test for insulinoma? Clin Endocrinol Oxf 23:461–466, 1985.

60. Lorenzi M, Gerich JE, Karam JH, Forsham PH. Failure of somatostatin to inhibit tolbutamide-induced insulin secretion in patients with insulinomas: a possible diagnostic tool. J Clin Endocrinol Metabol 40:1121–1124, 1975.

61. Doolas A. Steps in the diagnosis of three functioning endocrine tumors. Surg Clin North Am 51:195–210, 1971.

62. Seckl MJ, Mulholland PJ, Bishop AE, et al. Hypoglycemia due to an insulin-secreting small-cell carcinoma of the cervix. N Engl J Med 341:733–736, 1999.

63. Doherty GM, Doppman JL, Shawker TH, et al. Results of a prospective strategy to diagnose, localize, and resect insulinomas. Surgery 110:989–996; discussion 996–987, 1991.

64. Pasieka JL, McLeod MK, Thompson NW, Burney RE. Surgical approach to insulinomas. Assessing the need for preoperative localization. Arch Surg 127:442–447, 1992.

65. Menegaux F, Schmitt G, Mercadier M, Chigot JP. Pancreatic insulinomas. Am J Surg 165:243–248, 1993.

66. Grant CS, Charboneau JW, Reading CC, James EM, Galiber A. Insulinoma: the value of intraoperative ultrasonography. Wien Klin Wochensch 100:376–380, 1988.

67. Angelini L, Bezzi M, Tucci G, et al. The ultrasonic detection of insulinomas during surgical exploration of the pancreas. World J Surg 11:642–647, 1987.

68. Thompson GB, Service FJ, van Heerden JA, et al. Reoperative insulinomas, 1927 to 1992: an institutional experience. Surgery 114:1196–1204; discussion 1205–1196, 1993.

69. Thompson GB, van Heerden JA, Grant CS, Carney JA, Ilstrup DM. Islet cell carcinomas of the pancreas: a twenty-year experience. Surgery 104:1011–1017, 1988.

70. Grant CS. Surgical aspects of hyperinsulinemic hypoglycemia. Endocrinol Metab Clin North Am 28:533–554, 1999.

71. Lo CY, Chan FL, Tam SC, Cheng PW, Fan ST, Lam KS. Value of intra-arterial calcium stimulated venous sampling for regionalization of pancreatic insulinomas. Surgery 128:903–909, 2000.

72. Brandle M, Pfammatter T, Spinas GA, Lehmann R, Schmid C. Assessment of selective arterial calcium stimulation and hepatic venous sampling to localize insulin-secreting tumours. Clin Endocrinol Oxf 55:357–362, 2001.

73. Hiramoto JS, Feldstein VA, LaBerge JM, Norton JA. Intraoperative ultrasound and preoperative localization detects all occult insulinomas. Arch Surg 136:1020–1025, discussion 1025–1026, 2001.

74. Hearn PR, Ahmed M, Woodhouse NJ. The use of SMS 201–995 (somatostatin analogue) in insulinomas. Additional case report and literature review. Hormone Res 29:211–213, 1988.

75. Gama R, Marks V, Wright J, Teale JD. Octreotide exacerbated fasting hypoglycaemia in a patient with a proinsulinoma; the glucostatic importance of pancreatic glucagon. Clinl Endocrinol Oxf 43:117–120, 1995.

76. Fajans SS, Floyd JCJ, Thiffault CA. Further studies on diazoxide suppression of insulin release from abnormal and normal islet tissue in man. Ann N Y Acad Sci 150:261–280, 1968.

77. Goode PN, Farndon JR, Anderson J, et al. Diazoxide in the management of patients with insulinoma. World J Surg 10:586–592, 1986.

78. De Marinis L, Barbarino A. Calcium antagonists and hormone release: effects of verapamil on insulin release in normal subjects and patients with islet-cell tumor. Metabolism 29:599–604, 1980.

79. Scandrelli C, Zaccaria M, De Palo C, et al. The effect of propanolol on hypoglycemia. Observations in five insulinoma patients. Diabetalogica 5:297–301, 1978.

80. Zollinger RM, Ellison EH. Primary peptic ulceration of the jejunum associated with islet cell tumors of the pancreas. Ann Surg 142:709–728, 1955.

81. Gregory RA, Tracy JH, French JM, et al. Extraction of gastrin-like substance from the pancreatic tumor in a case of Zollinger-Ellison syndrome. Lancet 1:1045–1048, 1960.

82. Gregory RA, Grossman MI, Tracy JH, et al. Native of gastrin secretagogue in Zollinger-Ellison tumors. Lancet 2:543–544, 1964.

83. McGuigin JE, Trudeau WL. Immunological measurement of elevated levels of gastrins in the serum of patients with pancreatic tumors of the Zollinger-Ellison variety. N Engl J Med 278:1308–1313, 1968.

84. Isenberg JI, Walsh JH, Passaro E Jr, Moore EW, Grossman MI. Unusual effect of secretin on serum gastrin, serum calcium, and gastric acid secretion in a patient with suspected Zollinger-Ellison syndrome. Gastroenterology 62:626–631, 1972.

85. Deveney CW, Deveney KS, Jaffe BM, Jones RS, Way LW. Use of calcium and secretin in the diagnosis of gastrinoma (Zollinger-Ellison syndrome). Ann Intern Med 87:680–686, 1977.

86. Vezzadini C, Poggioli R, Casoni I, Vezzadini P. Use of calcium provocative test in the diagnosis of gastroenteropancreatic endocrine tumors. Panminerva Med 38:255–258, 1996.

87. McGuigin JE, Wolfe MM. Secretin injection test in the diagnosis of gastrinoma. Gastroenterology 79:1324–1327, 1989.

88. Norton JA, Cornelius MJ, Doppman JL, Maton PN, Gardner JD, Jensen RT. Effect of parathyroidectomy in patients with hyperparathyroidism, Zollinger-Ellison syndrome, and multiple endocrine neoplasia type I: a prospective study. Surgery 102:958–966, 1987.

89. Norton JA. Gastrinoma: advances in localization and treatment. Surg Oncol Clin North Am 7:845–861, 1998.

90. Delvalle J, Yamada T. Zollinger-Ellison syndrome. In: Yamada T (ed): Textbook of Gastroenterology. J.B. Lippincott, Philadelphia, 1995, p 1430.

91. Slaff JL, Howard JM, Maton PN, et al. Prospective assessment of provocative gastrin tests in 81 consecutive patients with Zollinger-Ellison sindrome. Gastroenterology 90:1637–1643, 1986.

92. Frucht H, Howard JM, Slaff JI, et al. Secretin and calcium provocative tests in the Zollinger-Ellison syndrome. A prospective study. Ann Intern Med 111:713–722, 1989.

93. Frucht H, Howard JM, Stark HA, et al. Prospective study of the standard meal provocative test in Zollinger-Ellison syndrome. Am J Med 87:528–536, 1989.

94. Basso N, Passaro E Jr. Calcium-stimulated gastric secretion in the Zollinger-Ellison syndrome. Arch Surg 101:399–402, 1970.

95. Basso N, Passaro E, Lezoche E, Mennini G, Speranza V. La stimulation de la secretion gastrique apres infusion de calcium dans le syndrome de Zollinger-Ellison. J Chir 103:493–498, 1972.

96. Basso N, Lezoche E, Materia A, Passaro E Jr, Speranza V. Studies with bombesin in the Zollinger—Ellison syndrome. Br J Surg 68:97–100, 1981.

97. Passaro E Jr, Basso N, Walsh JH. Calcium challenge in the Zollinger-Ellison syndrome. Surgery 72:60–67, 1972.

98. DeLellis RA, Gagel RF, Kaplan MM, Curtis LE. Gastrinoma of duodenal G-cell origin. Cancer 38:201–208, 1976.

99. Pipeleers-Marichal M, Somers G, Willems G. Gastrinomas in the duodenums of patients with multiple endocrine neoplasia type 1 and the Zollinger-Ellison syndrome. N Engl J Med 322:723–727, 1990.

100. Passaro E Jr, Howard TJ, Sawicki MP, Watt PC, Stabile BE. The origin of sporadic gastrinomas within the gastrinoma triangle: a theory. Arch Surg 133:13–16; discussion 17, 1998.

101. Stabile BE, Morrow DJ, Passaro E Jr. The gastrinoma triangle: operative implications. Am J Surg 147:25–31, 1984.

102. Norton JA, Doppman JL, Jensen RT. Curative resection in Zollinger-Ellison syndrome. Results of a 10-year prospective study. Ann Surg 215:8–18, 1992.

103. Delcore R Jr, Cheung LY, Friesen SR. Characteristics of duodenal wall gastrinomas. Am J Surg 160:621–623; discussion 623–624, 1990.

104. Thompson NW, Pasieka J, Fukuuchi A. Duodenal gastrinomas, duodenotomy, and duodenal exploration in the surgical management of Zollinger-Ellison syndrome. World J Surg 17:455–462, 1993.

105. Arnold WS, Fraker DL, Alexander HR, Weber HC, Norton JA, Jensen RT. Apparent lymph node primary gastrinoma. Surgery 116:1123–1129; discussion 1129–1130, 1994.

106. Sawady J, Mendelsohn G. Extrapancreatic gastrinoma with pancreatic islet cell hyperplasia. Arch Pathol Lab Med 113:536–538, 1989.

107. Kitagawa M, Hayakawa T, Kondo T, et al. Gastrinoma in a mesenteric lymph node. Am J Gastroenterol 84:660–662, 1989.

108. Norton JA, Doppman JL, Collen MJ, et al. Prospective study of gastrinoma localization and resection in patients with Zollinger-Ellison syndrome. Ann Surg 204:468–479, 1986.

109. Liu TH, Zhong SX, Chen YF, et al. Gastric gastrinoma. Chin Med J (Engl) 102:774–782, 1989.

110. Thompson NW, Vinik AI, Eckhauser FE, Strodel WE. Extrapancreatic gastrinomas. Surgery 98:1113–1120, 1985.

111. Pipeleers-Marichal M, Donow C, Heitz PU, Kloppel G. Pathologic aspects of gastrinomas in patients with Zollinger-Ellison syndrome with and without multiple endocrine neoplasia type I. World J Surg 17: 481–488, 1993.

112. Maton PN, Mackem SM, Norton JA, Gardner JD, O'Dorisio TM, Jensen RT. Ovarian carcinoma as a cause of Zollinger-Ellison syndrome. Natural history, secretory products, and response to provocative tests. Gastroenterology 97:468–471, 1989.

113. Gibril F, Curtis LT, Termanini B, et al. Primary cardiac gastrinoma causing Zollinger-Ellison syndrome. Gastroenterology 112:567–574, 1997.

114. Norton JA, Doherty GM, Fraker DL, et al. Surgical treatment of localized gastrinoma within the liver: a prospective study. Surgery 124:1145–1152, 1998.

115. Norton JA. Intraoperative methods to stage and localize pancreatic and duodenal tumors. Ann Oncol 10 (Suppl) 4:182–184, 1999.

116. Fraker DL, Norton JA, Alexander HR, Venzon DJ, Jensen RT. Surgery in Zollinger-Ellison syndrome alters the natural history of gastrinoma. Ann Surg 220:320–328; discussion 328–330, 1994.

117. Gauger PG, Thompson NW. Early surgical intervention and strategy in patients with multiple endocrine neoplasia type 1. Best Pract Res Clin Endocrinol Metab 15:213–223, 2001.

118. Simeone DM, Scheiman JM, Thompson NW. The "serendipitous" surgical cure of the Zollinger-Ellison syndrome in a patient with multiple endocrine neoplasia type 1 despite an unsuspected diagnosis of either disease. J Clin Gastroenterol 32:268–271, 2001.

119. Frucht H, Maton PN, Jensen RT. Use of omeprazole in patients with Zollinger-Ellison syndrome. Dig Dis Sci 36:394–404, 1991.

120. Larsson H, Carlsson E, Mattsson H, et al. Plasma gastrin and gastric enterochromaffin-like cell activation and proliferation. Studies with omeprazole and ranitidine in intact and antrectomized rats. Gastroenterology 90:391–399, 1986.

121. Freston JW. Omeprazole, hypergastrinemia, and gastric carcinoid tumors. Ann Intern Med 121:232–233, 1994.

122. Sculco D, Bilgrami S. Pernicious anemia and gastric carcinoid tumor: case report and review. Am J Gastroenterol 92:1378–1380, 1997.

123. Anonymous. Case records of the Massachusetts General Hospital. Weekly clinicopathological exercises. Case 9-1997. A 39-year-old woman with pernicious anemia and a gastric mass. N Engl J Med 336: 861–867, 1997.

124. Perasso A, Ciancamerla G, Testino G, et al. Multiple gastric carcinoid in type A gastritis: clinical findings and therapeutic proposal. J Clin Gastroenterol 13:607–609, 1991.

125. Klinkenberg-Knol EC, Festen HP, Jansen JB, et al. Long-term treatment with omeprazole for refractory reflux esophagitis: efficacy and safety. Ann Intern Med 121:161–167, 1994.

126. Maton PN, Lack EE, Collen MJ, et al. The effect of Zollinger-Ellison syndrome and omeprazole therapy on gastric oxyntic endocrine cells. Gastroenterology 99:943–950, 1990.

127. Maton PN, Vinayek R, Frucht H, et al. Long-term efficacy and safety of omeprazole in patients with Zollinger-Ellison syndrome: a prospective study. Gastroenterology 97:827–836, 1989.

128. Norton JA, Fraker DL, Alexander HR, et al. Surgery to cure the Zollinger-Ellison syndrome. N Engl J Med 341:635–644, 1999.

129. Thompson NW. Current concepts in the surgical management of multiple endocrine neoplasia type 1 pancreatic-duodenal disease. Results in the treatment of 40 patients with Zollinger-Ellison syndrome, hypoglycaemia or both. J Intern Med 243:495–500, 1998.

130. Farley DR, van Heerden JA, Grant CS, Thompson GB. Extrapancreatic gastrinomas. Surgical experience. Arch Surg 129:506–511; discussion 511–502, 1994.

131. Thompson NW. Management of pancreatic endocrine tumors in patients with multiple endocrine neoplasia type 1. Surg Oncol Clin North Am 7:881–891, 1998.

132. Cadiot G, Lehy T, Mignon M. Gastric endocrine cell proliferation and fundic argyrophil carcinoid tumors in patients with the Zollinger-Ellison syndrome. Acta Oncol 32:135–140, 1993.

133. Cadiot G, Lehy T, Ruszniewski P, Bonfils S, Mignon M. Gastric endocrine cell evolution in patients with Zollinger-Ellison syndrome. In-

fluence of gastrinoma growth and long-term omeprazole treatment. Dig Dis Sci 38:1307–1317, 1993.

134. Verner JV, Morrison AB. Islet cell tumor and a syndrome of refractory watery diarrhea and hypokalemia. Am J Med 25:374–380, 1958.

135. Matsumoto KK, Peter JB, Schultze RG, et al. Watery diarrhea and hypokalemia associated with pancreatic islet cell adenoma. Gastroenterology 50:231–242, 1966.

136. Krejs GJ. VIPoma syndrome. Am J Med 82:37–48, 1987.

137. Bloom SR, Polak JM, Pearse AGE. Vasoactive intestinal peptide and watery-diarrhea syndrome. Lancet 2:14–16, 1973.

138. Said SI, Mutt V. Potent peripheral and splanchnic vasodilator peptide from normal gut. Nature 225:863–864, 1970.

139. Bloom SR, Yiangou Y, Polak JM. Vasoactive intestinal peptide secreting tumors. Pathophysiological and clinical correlations. Ann N Y Acad Sci 527:518–527, 1988.

140. Meriney DK. Pathophysiology and management of VIPoma: a case study. Oncol Nurs Forum 23:941–948; quiz 949–950, 1996.

141. Krejs GJ. Effect of vasoactive intestinal peptide in man. Ann N Y Acad Sci 527:501–507, 1988.

142. Bloom SR, Christofides ND, Delamarter J, Buell G, Kawashima E, Polak JM. Diarrhoea in VIPoma patients associated with cosecretion of a second active peptide (peptide histidine isoleucine) explained by single coding gene. Lancet 2:1163–1165, 1983.

143. Bloom SR, Lee YC, Lacroute JM, et al. Two patients with pancreatic apudomas secreting neurotensin and VIP. Gut 24:448–452, 1983.

144. Brunt LM, Mazoujian G, O'Dorisio TM, Wells SA Jr. Stimulation of vasoactive intestinal peptide and neurotensin secretion by pentagastrin in a patient with VIPoma syndrome. Surgery 115:362–369, 1994.

145. Kane MG, O'Dorisio TM, Krejs GJ. Production of secretory diarrhea by intravenous infusion of vasoactive intestinal polypeptide. N Engl J Med 309:1482–1485, 1983.

146. Perry RR, Vinik AI. Clinical review 72: diagnosis and management of functioning islet cell tumors. J Clin Endocrinol Metab 80:2273–2278, 1995.

147. Said SI, Faloona GR. Elevated plasma and tissue levels of vasoactive intestinal polypeptide in the watery-diarrhea syndrome due to pancreatic, bronchogenic and other tumors. N Engl J Med 293:155–160, 1975.

148. Hirose S, Kobayashi K, Kajikawa K, Sawabu N. A case of watery diarrhea, hypokalemia and hypercalcemia associated with nonulcerogenic islet cell tumor of the pancreas. Am J Gastroenterol 64:382–386, 1975.

149. Venkatesh S, Vassilopoulou-Sellin R, Samaan NA. Somatostatin analogue: use in the treatment of VIPoma with hypercalcemia. Am J Med 87:356–357, 1989.

150. Hohmann EL, Levine L, Tashjian AH Jr. Vasoactive intestinal peptide stimulates bone resorption via a cyclic adenosine 3′,5′-monophosphate-dependent mechanism. Endocrinology 112:1233–1239, 1983.

151. Wu TJ, Lin CL, Taylor RL, Kvols LK, Kao PC. Increased parathyroid hormone–related peptide in patients with hypercalcemia associated with islet cell carcinoma. Mayo Clin Proc 72:1111–1115, 1997.

152. O'Dorisio TM, Mekhjian HS, Gaginella TS. Medical therapy of VIPomas. Endocrinol Metab Clin N Am 18:545–556, 1989.

153. O'Dorisio TM, Gaginella TS, Mekhjian HS, Rao B, O'Dorisio MS. Somatostatin and analogues in the treatment of VIPoma. Ann N Y Acad Sci 527:528–535, 1988.

154. Eriksson B, Oberg K. An update of the medical treatment of malignant endocrine pancreatic tumors. Acta Oncol 32:203–208, 1993.

155. Nguyen HN, Backes B, Lammert F, et al. Long-term survival after diagnosis of hepatic metastatic VIPoma: report of two cases with disparate courses and review of therapeutic options. Dig Dis Sci 44:1148–1155, 1999.

156. Hengst K, Nashan B, Avenhaus W, et al. Metastatic pancreatic VIPoma: deteriorating clinical course and successful treatment by liver transplantation. Z Gastroenterol 36:239–245, 1998.

157. Ganda OP, Weir GC, Soeldner JS, et al. "Somatostatinoma": a somatostatin-containing tumor of the endocrine pancreas. N Engl J Med 296:963–967, 1977.

158. Soga J, Yakuwa Y. Somatostatinoma/inhibitory syndrome: a statistical evaluation of 173 reported cases as compared to other pancreatic endocrinomas. J Exp Clin Cancer Res 18:13–22, 1999.

159. Chen RS, Tang CK, Lee JY, Kurland CL. Duodenal somatostatin-containing tumor with psammoma bodies. Hum Pathol 16:517–519, 1985.

160. Chetty R, Essa A. Heterotopic pancreas, periampullary somatostatinoma and type I neurofibromatosis: a pathogenetic proposal. Pathology 31:95–97, 1999.

161. Dayal Y, Doos WG, O'Brien MJ, Nunnemacher G, DeLellis RA, Wolfe HJ. Psammomatous somatostatinomas of the duodenum. Am J Surg Pathol 7:653–665, 1983.

162. Fincher RK, Christensen ED, Tsuchida AM. Ampullary somatostatinoma in a patient with Merkel cell carcinoma. Am J Gastroenterol 94:1955–1957, 1999.

163. Marcial MA, Pinkus GS, Skarin A, Hinrichs HR, Warhol MJ. Ampullary somatostatinoma: psammomatous variant of gastrointestinal carcinoid tumor—an immunohistochemical and ultrastructural study. Report of a case and review of the literature. Am J Clin Pathol 80:755–761, 1983.

164. O'Brien TD, Chejfec G, Prinz RA. Clinical features of duodenal somatostatinomas. Surgery 114:1144–1147, 1993.

165. Sawady J, Katzin WE, Mendelsohn G, Aron DC. Somatostatin-producing neuroendocrine tumor of the ampulla (ampullary somatostatinoma). Evidence of prosomatostatin production. Am J Clin Pathol 97:411–415, 1992.

166. Stamm B, Hedinger CE, Saremaslani P. Duodenal and ampullary carcinoid tumors. A report of 12 cases with pathological characteristics, polypeptide content and relation to the MEN I syndrome and von Recklinghausen's disease (neurofibromatosis). Virchows Arch A Pathol Anat Histopathol 408:475–489, 1986.

167. Dayal Y, Tallberg KA, Nunnemacher G, DeLellis RA, Wolfe HJ. Duodenal carcinoids in patients with and without neurofibromatosis. A comparative study. Am J Surg Pathol 10:348–357, 1986.

168. Mao C, Shah A, Hanson DJ, Howard JM. Von Recklinghausen's disease associated with duodenal somatostatinoma: contrast of duodenal versus pancreatic somatostatinomas. J Surg Oncol 59:67–73, 1995.

169. Swinburn BA, Yeong ML, Lane MR, Nicholson GI, Holdaway IM. Neurofibromatosis associated with somatostatinoma: a report of two patients. Clin Endocrinol 28:353–359, 1988.

170. Taccagni GL, Carlucci M, Sironi M, Cantaboni A, Di Carlo V. Duodenal somatostatinoma with psammoma bodies: an immunohistochemical and ultrastructural study. Am J Gastroenterol 81:33–37, 1986.

171. Abe T, Oshida K, Matsumoto K, Iida M, Sanno N. Brain metastasis from malignant pancreatic somatostatinoma. Case report. J Neurosurg 85:681–684, 1996.

172. Konomi K, Chijiiwa K, Katsuta T, Yamaguchi K. Pancreatic somatostatinoma: a case report and review of the literature. J Surg Oncol 43:259–265, 1990.

173. Pipeleers D, Couturier E, Gepts W, Reynders J, Somers G. Five cases of somatostatinoma: clinical heterogeneity and diagnostic usefulness of basal and tolbutamide-induced hypersomatostatinemia. J Clin Endocrinol Metabol 56:1236–1242, 1983.

174. Wright J, Abolfathi A, Penman E, Marks V. Pancreatic somatostatinoma presenting with hypoglycaemia. Clin Endocrinol Oxf 12:603–608, 1980.

175. Krejs GJ, Orci L, Conlon JM, et al. Somatostatinoma syndrome. Biochemical, morphologic and clinical features. N Engl J Med 301:285–292, 1979.

176. Kovacs K, Horvath E, Ezrin C, Sepp H, Elkan I. Immunoreactive somatostatin in pancreatic islet-cell carcinoma accompanied by ectopic A.C.T.H. syndrome [letter]. Lancet 1:1365–1366, 1977.

177. Stavri GT, Pritchard GA, Williams EJ, Stamatakis JD. Somatostatinoma of the pancreas with hypercalcemia: a case report. Eur J Surg Oncol 18:298–300, 1992.

178. Mao C, Carter P, Schaefer P, et al. Malignant islet cell tumor associated with hypercalcemia. Surgery 117:37–40, 1995.

179. Ratcliffe WA, Bowden FP, Dunne FP, et al. Expression and processing of parathyroid hormone–related protein in a pancreatic endocrine cell tumour associated with hypercalcemia. Clin Endocrinol 40:679–686, 1993.

180. Body JJ. Current and future directions in medical therapy: hypercalcemia. Cancer 88:3054–3058, 2000.

181. Morony S, Capparelli C, Lee R, et al. A chimeric form of osteoprotegerin inhibits hypercalcemia and bone resorption induced by IL-1β, TNF-α, PTH, PTHrP, and 1, 25(OH)2D3. J Bone Miner Res 14:1478–1485, 1999.

182. Ezzat S, Ezrin C, Yamashita S, Melmed S. Recurrent acromegaly resulting from ectopic growth hormone gene expression by a metastatic pancreatic tumor. Cancer 71:66–70, 1993.

183. Berger G, Trouillas J, Bloch B, et al. Multihormonal carcinoid tumor of the pancreas. Secreting growth hormone–releasing factor as a cause of acromegaly. Cancer 54:2097–2108, 1984.

184. Guillemin R, Brazeau P, Bohlen P, Esch F, Ling N, Wehrenberg WB. Growth hormone–releasing factor from a human pancreatic tumor that caused acromegaly. Science 218:585–587, 1982.

185. Bohlen P, Brazeau P, Esch F, Ling N, Wehrenberg WB, Guillemin R. Human growth hormone releasing factor and somatostatin from two pancreatic tumors: isolation and characterization. Regul Pept 6:343–353, 1983.

186. Krejs GJ. Non-insulin-secreting tumors of the gastroenteropancreatic system. In: Wilson JD (ed): Williams Textbook of Endocrinology, 9th ed. W.B. Saunders, Philadelphia, 1998, pp 1663–1674.

187. Caplan RH, Koob L, Abellera RM, Pagliara AS, Kovacs K, Randall RV. Cure of acromegaly by operative removal of an islet cell tumor of the pancreas. Am J Med 64:874–882, 1978.

188. Engstrom PF, Lawin PT, Moertel CG, et al. Streptozotocin plus fluorouracil versus doxorubicin therapy for metastatic carcinoid tumors. J Clin Oncol 2:1255, 1984.

189. Moertel CG, Lefkopoulo M, Lipsitz S, et al. Streptozocin-doxorubicin, streptozocin-fluorouracil, or chlorozotocin in the treatment of advanced islet cell carcinoma. N Engl J Med 326:519–523, 1992.

190. Miller CA, Ellison C. Therapeutic alternatives in metastatic neuroendocrine tumors. Surg Oncol Clin North Am 7:863–878, 1998.

191. Moertel CG, Hanley JA, Johnson LA. Streptozocin alone compared with streptozocin plus fluorouracil in the treatment of advanced islet-cell carcinoma. N Engl J Med 303:1189–1194, 1980.

192. Rivera E, Ajani JA. Doxorubicin, streptozocin, and 5-fluorouracil chemotherapy for patients with metastatic islet-cell carcinoma. Am J Clin Oncol 21:36–38, 1998.

193. Eriksson B, Oberg K, Alm G, et al. Treatment of malignant endocrine pancreatic tumours with human leucocyte interferon. Lancet 2:1307–1309, 1986.

194. Andreyev HJN, Scott-Mackie P, Cunningham D, et al. Phase II study of continuous infusion fluorouracil and interferon alpha-2b in the palliation of malignant neuroendocrine tumors. J Clin Oncol 13:1486, 1995.

195. Veenhof CH. Pancreatic endocrine tumours, immunotherapy and gene therapy: chemotherapy and interferon therapy of endocrine tumours. Ann Oncol 10 Suppl 4:185–187, 1999.

196. Bergers G, Javaherian K, Lo K-M, Folkman J, Hanahan D. Effects of angiogenesis inhibitors on multistage carcinogenesis in mice. Science 284:808–812, 1999.

197. Moertel CG, Kvols LK, O'Connell MJ, Rubin J. Treatment of neuroendocrine carcinomas with combined etoposide and cisplatin. Evidence of major therapeutic activity in the anaplastic variants of these neoplasms. Cancer 68:227–232, 1991.

198. Ramanathan RK, Cnaan A, Hahn RG, Carbone PP, Haller DG. Phase II trial of dacarbazine (DTIC) in advanced pancreatic islet cell carcinoma. Study of the Eastern Cooperative Oncology Group-E6282. Ann Oncol 12:1139–1143, 2001.

199. Ansell SM, Pitot HC, Burch PA, Kvols LK, Mahoney MR, Rubin J. A phase II study of high-dose paclitaxel in patients with advanced neuroendocrine tumors. Cancer 91:1543–1548, 2001.

200. Marynick SP, Fagadau WR, Duncan LA. Malignant glucagonoma syndrome: response to chemotherapy. Ann Intern Med 93:453–454, 1980.

201. Kurose T, Seino Y, Ishida H, et al. Successful treatment of metastatic glucagonoma with dacarbazine [letter]. Lancet 1:621–622, 1984.

202. Carrasco CH, Charnsangavej C, Ajani J, Samaan NA, Richli W, Wallace S. The carcinoid syndrome: palliation by hepatic artery embolization. AJR Am J Roentgenol 147:149–154, 1986.

203. Diamandidou E, Ajani JA, Yang DJ, et al. Two-phase study of hepatic artery vascular occlusion with microencapsulated cisplatin in patients with liver metastases from neuroendocrine tumors. AJR Am J Roentgenol 170:339–344, 1998.

204. Ajani JA, Carrasco CH, Charnsangavej C, Samaan NA, Levin B, Wallace S. Islet cell tumors metastatic to the liver: effective palliation by sequential hepatic artery embolization. Ann Intern Med 108:340–344, 1988.

205. Kim YH, Ajani JA, Carrasco CH, et al. Selective hepatic arterial chemoembolization for liver metastases in patients with carcinoid tumor or islet cell carcinoma. Cancer Invest 17:474–478, 1999.

206. Paran H, Paran D. Angiogenesis and tumor growth. N Engl J Med 334:921, 1996.

207. Reubi JC, Hacki WH, Lamberts SW. Hormone-producing gastrointestinal tumors contain a high density of somatostatin receptors. J Clin Endocrinol Metabol 65:1127–1134, 1987.

208. Lamberts SW, van der Lely AJ, de Herder WW, Hofland LJ. Octreotide. N Engl J Med 334:246–254, 1996.

209. Reubi JC. Somatostatin receptors as markers for endocrine tumors. JAMA 257:3277, 1987.

210. Krenning EP, de Jong M, Kooij PP, et al. Radiolabelled somatostatin analogue(s) for peptide receptor scintigraphy and radionuclide therapy. Ann Oncol 10 Suppl 2:S23–29, 1999.

211. Boden G, Ryan IG, Eisenschmid BL, Shelmet JJ, Owen OE. Treatment of inoperable glucagonoma with the long-acting somatostatin analogue SMS 201-995. N Engl J Med 314:1686–1689, 1986.

212. Vinik AI, Tsai ST, Moattari AR, Cheung P, Eckhauser FE, Cho K. Somatostatin analogue (SMS 201-995) in the management of gastroenteropancreatic tumors and diarrhea syndromes. Am J Med 81:23–40, 1986.

213. Maton PN, Gardner JD, Jensen RT. Use of long-acting somatostatin analog SMS 201-995 in patients with pancreatic islet cell tumors. Dig Dis Sci 34:28S–39S, 1989.

214. Lamberts SW. Somatostatin analogs in the management of gastrointestinal tumors. Hormone Res 29:118–120, 1988.

215. Krausz Y, Bar-Ziv J, de Jong RB, et al. Somatostatin-receptor scintigraphy in the management of gastroenteropancreatic tumors. Am J Gastroenterol 93:66–70, 1998.

216. Anderson JV, Bloom SR. Neuroendocrine tumours of the gut: long-term therapy with the somatostatin analogue SMS 201-995. Scand J Gastroenterol 119:115–128, 1986.

217. Williams G, Anderson JV, Williams SJ, Bloom SR. Clinical evaluation of SMS 201-995. Long-term treatment in gut neuroendocrine tumours, efficacy of oral administration, and possible use in non-tumoural inappropriate TSH hypersecretion. Acta Endocrinol Suppl 286:26–36, 1987.

218. Trautmann ME, Neuhaus C, Lenze H, et al. The role of somatostatin analogs in the treatment of endocrine gastrointestinal tumors. Horm Metab Res 27:24–27, 1993.

219. Arnold R, Frank M, Kajdan U. Management of gastroenteropancreatic endocrine tumors: the place of somatostatin analogues. Digestion 55 (Suppl 3):107–113, 1994.

220. Maton PN. Use of octreotide acetate for control of symptoms in patients with islet cell tumors. World J Surg 17:504–510, 1993.

221. Clements D, Elias E. Regression of metastatic vipoma with somatostatin analogue SMS 201-995 [letter]. Lancet 1:874–875, 1985.

222. Koelz A, Kraenzlin M, Gyr K, et al. Escape of the response to a long-acting somatostatin analogue (SMS 201-995) in patients with VIPoma. Gastroenterology 92:527–531, 1987.

223. Juby LD, Burke DA, Axon AT. Somatostatin analogue SMS 201-995 long-term therapy for vipoma. Postgrad Med J 63:287–289, 1987.

224. Larsson C, Skogseid B, Oberg K, Nakamura Y, Nordenskjold M. Multiple endocrine neoplasia type 1 gene maps to chromosome 11 and is lost in insulinoma. Nature 332:85–87, 1988.

225. Chandrasekharappa SC, Guru SC, Manickam P, et al. Positional cloning of the gene for multiple endocrine neoplasia-type 1. Science 276:404–407, 1997.

226. Krawczak M, Cooper DN. The human gene mutation database. Trends Genet 13:121–122, 1997.

227. Mutch MG, Dilley WG, Sanjurjo F, et al. Germline mutations in the multiple endocrine neoplasia type 1 gene: evidence for frequent splicing defects. Hum Mutat 13:175–185, 1999.

228. Agarwal SK, Guru SC, Heppner C, et al. Menin interacts with the AP1 transcription factor JunD and represses JunD-activated transcription. Cell 96:143–152, 1999.

229. Heppner C, Bilimoria KY, Agarwal SK, et al. The tumor suppressor protein menin interacts with NF-κB proteins and inhibits NF-κB-mediated transactivation. Oncogene 20:4917–4925, 2001.

230. Lemmens IH, Forsberg L, Pannett AA, et al. Menin interacts directly with the homeobox-containing protein Pem. Biochem Biophys Res Commun 286:426–431, 2001.

231. Agarwal SK, Kester MB, Debelenko LV, et al. Germline mutations of the MEN1 gene in familial multiple endocrine neoplasia type 1 and related states. Hum Mol Genet 6:1169–1175, 1997.

232. Cote GJ, Lee JE, Evans DB, et al. Five novel mutations in the familial multiple endocrine neoplasia type 1 (MEN1) gene. Mutations in brief no. 188. Online. Hum Mutat 12:219, 1998.

233. Teh BT, Kytola S, Farnebo F, et al. Mutation analysis of the MEN1 gene in multiple endocrine neoplasia type 1, familial acromegaly and familial isolated hyperparathyroidism. J Clin Endocrinol Metab 83:2621–2626, 1998.

234. Guo SS, Sawicki MP. Molecular and genetic mechanisms of tumorigenesis in multiple endocrine neoplasia type-1. Mol Endocrinol 15:1653–1664, 2001.

235. Dackiw AP, Cote GJ, Fleming JB, et al. Screening for MEN1 mutations in patients with atypical endocrine neoplasia. Surgery 126:1097–1103; discussion 1103–1094, 1999.

With extensive colonization, the follicles may no longer be easily recognized. However, with special stains for follicular dendritic cells, which can be demonstrated by their reactivity with CD21, the presence of follicular centers can be confirmed. The neoplastic lymphoid cells typically invade epithelial structures to form lymphoepithelial lesions (Figs. 66–3 and 66–4). The typical centrocyte-like B-cell lymphocytic infiltrate, together with the presence of gastric epithelial destruction caused by an invasion of the glandular and foveolar epithelium by the neoplastic B cells (the lymphoepithelial lesions), are the most important histological criteria for establishing a diagnosis of low-grade MALT lymphoma. The destruction of the epithelia by the neoplastic lymphoid cells can be clearly demonstrated by the use of cytokeratin stains that react with residual epithelial structures (Fig. 66–4). Confirmation that the lymphoid infiltrate is composed of B cells is obtained by immunostains with B-cell markers such as CD20 (Color Fig. 66–5; see separate color insert). The infiltrating tumor-associated T cells are a minor cellular subset in the infiltrate and can be distinguished by immunoreactivity with CD3 antibodies. Differential diagnosis from other extranodal low-grade lymphomas, including small lymphocytic lymphomas, mantle cell lymphomas, follicular lymphomas, and lymphoplasmacytic lymphomas, is best achieved examining immunochemical properties. Low-grade MALT lymphomas are CD5 and CD10 negative and may be positive for CD23 and CD43. Unlike MALT lymphomas, small lymphocytic lymphomas and mantle cell lymphomas are CD5 positive, and follicular lymphomas are usually CD10 positive. Lymphoplasmacytoid lymphomas and MALT lymphomas share some immunochemical features, and the diagnosis essentially rests on the morphological features.[4,7,37]

The diagnosis and therapeutic management of low-grade gastric MALT lymphomas are often based exclusively on the evaluation of biopsy material. Diagnostic accuracy in gastric lymphomas based solely on biopsies is limited but can be significantly improved by using immunohistochemistry and molecular biological techniques.[42] Appropriate tissue sampling is very important for accurate diagnosis. Although specific guidelines are not available, extensive sampling is important for ensuring accurate representation of mucosal lesions associated with the lymphoma as well as for assessing coexisting gastritis or other *H. pylori*–associated complications.[16] The Houston Gastritis Workshop recommended taking a total of five stomach biopsies (two from the gastric corpus, two from the gastric antrum, and one from the incisura angularis) and additional biopsies from suspicious areas.[16] During follow-up of patients with low-grade MALT lymphoma, Wotherspoon and colleagues[25] routinely took biopsies from both the gastric corpus and the antrum (one biopsy from the gastric corpus and five from the gastric antrum).

### Florid Chronic *H. pylori* Gastritis vs. Low-Grade Mucosa-Associated Lymphoid Tissue Lymphoma

The diagnosis of low-grade MALT lymphoma is sometimes difficult to establish in endoscopic biopsy samples where simple florid lymphoid response to *H. pylori* infection and a rare, suspicious, small lymphoepithelial lesion constitutes the only findings. Repeated evaluation and more extensive biopsy sampling may help confirm the diagnosis. In addition, evaluation of monoclonality, which supports the presence of a neoplastic process, may be used. However, the accuracy of polymerase chain reaction (PCR) methods in the assessment of MALT lymphomas has not been fully established. The PCR amplification of specific IgH

gene rearrangements as a means of demonstrating monoclonality works equally well with DNA extracted from frozen and paraffin-embedded tissues. While some studies indicate that *H. pylori* gastritis appears mainly as a benign polyclonal condition, with single or dominant bands seen only in 1.3% of the samples of gastritis examined,[43] others detected a clonal band in 38% of patients with *H. pylori*–chronic active gastritis.[44] Weston and colleagues[45] determined the sensitivity and specificity of heavy-chain clonality in the detection of gastric lymphoma, finding values of 73.3% and 45.7%, respectively. On the basis of these values, the authors concluded that determination of monoclonality by PCR is not acceptable for confirming the diagnosis of gastric lymphoma, as it is too sensitive, detecting minute populations of clonal lymphocytes that occur in benign diseases as well as larger populations of clonal lymphocytes associated with malignant gastric lymphoproliferative diseases.[45] The general view is that PCR is not specific enough to assess clonality; therefore, PCR remains at the investigational level in this setting. Southern blot gene rearrangement testing is a more specific method for determining clonality in the evaluation of gastric lymphocytic infiltrates but is not feasible with small endoscopic biopsies because of the limited amount of DNA available from small biopsy fragments. The addition of molecular markers associated with malignancy may eventually be useful in the diagnostic work-up of gastric lymphoid lesions, but these methods are still being evaluated. Molecular methods that might be used in clinical applications include cytogenetic abnormalities such as trisomy 3,[46] reduced levels of bcl-2, t(11;18)(q21;q21), and nuclear BCL10 expression in higher-grade disease.[35,47]

### Low- and High-Grade Gastric Mucosa-Associated Lymphoid Tissue Lymphomas

High-grade lymphoma may develop from low-grade MALT lymphomas.[6,9,27,48] In a series of 60 gastric lymphomas, Hsi and colleagues[48] found a spectrum of disease, from pure low-grade MALT lymphomas to mixed low- and high-grade lesions and pure high-grade lymphomas.[48] High-grade lymphomas were classified in three groups on the basis of the presence or absence of a low-grade component and lymphoepithelial lesions (LELs): (*1*) high-grade MALT lymphomas appearing in low-grade MALT lymphomas (LG/HG MALT lymphomas); (*2*) large cell lymphoma with LELs composed of large cells (high-grade LELs) but without a low-grade component (HG MALT lymphomas); and (*3*) diffuse large cell lymphoma without a low-grade MALT lymphoma component or LELs (DLCL). Twenty-two lymphomas were classified as low-grade MALT lymphomas, 16 as LG/HG MALT lymphomas, 10 as HG MALT lymphomas, and 12 as DLCL.[48] De Jong and co-workers[9] characterized a group of MALT lymphomas containing variable amounts of a higher-grade component. Importantly, low-grade MALT lymphomas with a large cell component composing 1%–10% of the infiltrate showed significantly worse prognosis than pure low-grade MALT lymphomas. At least one-third of all high-grade MALT lymphomas are secondary, since low-grade foci can be found elsewhere in the stomach.[27,49] Peng and others[50] examined low- and high-grade gastric MALT lymphoma components from the same patient to determine whether a genetic link between the two lesions could be established. PCR and sequence analyses were performed to identify clone-specific rearranged IgH gene sequences. In each case electrophoresis confirmed that the PCR products from the two components were identical in size. Direct sequencing revealed common clone-specific IgH gene rearrangements in both lesions, providing genetic evidence for a clonal link. These results support the notion that high-grade MALT lymphomas generally evolve from low-grade clones.[50]

## Clinical Features of Gastric Mucosa-Associated Lymphoid Tissue Lymphomas

Low-grade gastric MALT lymphomas usually occur in patients older than 50 years but can affect patients of a broad age range.[6] A few cases of gastric MALT lymphoma associated with *H. pylori* infection have been reported in immunocompetent children.[51,52] The mean ages reported in several studies were 56 years,[53] 59.5 years,[37] and 58.6 years,[48] and ranged from 18–76 years,[53] 16–88 years,[48] and 18–76 years.[37]

Interestingly, the ages of patients at diagnosis of high-grade MALT lymphomas appear to be higher than those of patients at diagnosis of low-grade MALT lymphomas, supporting the notion that high-grade MALT lymphomas may progress from lower-grade lesions.[53] In a study reported by Hoshida and colleagues[53] the mean age at diagnosis of low-grade MALT lymphoma was 57.6 years, compared with 65.5 years for high-grade MALT lymphoma. No strong correlation with gender has been found, with studies reporting either that the disease affects similar numbers of men and women,[6,25] or that men are diagnosed slightly more frequently.[7,27]

The presenting symptoms of gastric MALT lymphoma are usually those of nonspecific dyspepsia.[54] The presence of an abdominal mass or severe abdominal pain is rare.[7] Endoscopic examination usually reveals evidence of chronic gastritis and sometimes the presence of erosions or one or multiple ulcers.[54] Gastric MALT lymphoma may be multifocal and most often involves the gastric antrum but it may occur in any area of the stomach, including the gastric cardia.[6] Low-grade MALT lymphomas are usually diagnosed at stage IE, and only a small proportion at stage II$_{E1}$ involve gastric lymph nodes.[7,53] Extraabdominal dissemination is also rare.[7] Compared with lower-grade MALT lymphomas, the higher-grade MALT lymphomas more frequently present as a tumor mass and are more frequently larger.[53]

## Clinical Management of Gastric Mucosa-Associated Lymphoid Tissue Lymphomas

### *H. pylori* eradication and regression of low-grade mucosa-associated lymphoid tissue lymphomas

The evidence linking *H. pylori* infection with the development of gastric MALT lymphoma includes data showing that *H. pylori* eradication in patients with low-grade MALT lymphomas results in regression of the lymphoma in most cases. Therefore, the therapeutic approaches to gastric MALT lymphomas should address the presence of *H. pylori* infection. Other factors that determine the therapeutic approach are tumor grade and stage of the disease. Most studies have reported that eradication of *H. pylori* alone causes more than 70% of cases diagnosed as low-grade MALT lymphomas to regress or indeed to be cured (Table 66–1).[25,27,29,55,56] The complete disappearance of MALT lymphoma after successful eradication of *H. pylori* infection was described for the first time by Wotherspoon and co-workers in five of six patients.[25] Two years later, Bayerdorffer and colleagues,[27] reported the outcome of gastric MALT lymphoma in 33 *H. pylori*–infected patients. Four to eight months after eradi-

**Table 66–1** Regression of mucosa-associated lymphoid tissue lymphoma after *H. pylori* eradication

| Study | Complete Regression (%) | Partial Regression (%) | Follow-up Period (Months) |
|---|---|---|---|
| Sackmann et al.[55] | 54 | 23 | 2–20 |
| Steinbach et al.[29] | 50 | 29 | 18–70 |
| Weston et al.[56] | 56 | 23 | 3–73 |
| Nobre-Leitao et al.[96] | 100 | None | Up to 7 |
| Pinotti et al.[86] | 67 | Not Assessed | Up to 60 |
| Bayerdorffer et al.[27] | 70 | 12 | 6.5–18 |
| Wotherspoon et al.[25] | 100 | None | 4–10 |

cation of *H. pylori*, 70% of the patients had complete remission, 12% showed partial regression, and 18% did not show any changes.[27] Another study reported the results from 84 patients with low-grade gastric MALT lymphoma in stage IE treated with a dual regimen to eradicate *H. pylori*.[57] Complete remission was observed in 68 (81%) of the cases, and partial remission was found in 4 patients. The remaining 12 patients did not respond after *H. pylori* eradication and were offered an alternative treatment protocol.[57] Neubauer and co-workers found[58] that 40 of 50 patients with *H. pylori* infection achieved complete remission of low-grade MALT lymphomas after eradication, but 5 patients subsequently relapsed.[58] The median time of continuous complete remission for the 40 patients was 15.4 months. Among six patients whose lymphomas did not respond to eradication of *H. pylori,* four had high-grade lymphomas upon surgery. Interestingly, PCR assessment of B-cell monoclonality during follow-up showed continued detection of monoclonality in 22 of 31 patients in complete remission,[58] a finding also reported by other studies.[27,59] In the study by Bayerdorffer and colleagues,[27] 18% of the lymphomas that regressed still displayed B-cell monoclonal patterns upon PCR.[27] In addition, there have been several case reports of low-grade MALT lymphoma regression after eradication *of H. pylori*.[60,61] The follow-up of six patients with superficially invasive low-grade MALT lymphoma after *H. pylori* eradication reported by Isaacson and others[59] shows that in most cases of *H. pylori*–associated, superficially invasive gastric MALT lymphoma, eradication of *H. pylori* is followed by prolonged disease-free remission. However, complete remission may be delayed up to 1 year or more.[59] Therefore, it appears that the use of antibiotics to eradicate *H. pylori* removes a growth stimulus from gastric MALT lymphoma. However, because the antibiotic therapy fails to remove the neoplastic B-cell clone, the monoclonal clone may re-expand. However, in the absence of concomitant reinfection with *H. pylori,* this event might be self-limiting.[59] Finally, some workers have reported the intriguing findings of complete disappearance of some cases of extragastric MALT lymphoma, such as those localized in the salivary gland, small intestine, and rectum, following treatment for *H. pylori* infection.[62–64] The implications of these findings are that *H. pylori* could have a systemic effect by providing the initial stimulus for clonal expansion of the lymphoid response. Additional studies are needed to address this interesting possibility. While complete regression of *H. pylori*–positive MALT lymphoma can be detected as early as 4 weeks after the end of treatment to eradicate *H. pylori,* a smaller proportion of cases undergo partial regression or do not regress even after long follow-up periods.[27] Relapses appear to be infrequent and may or may not be associated with *H. pylori* reinfection.[59,65] In a report of 97 patients with complete remission, Stolte and colleagues[65] reported seven recurrences, which included one case of high-grade lymphoma, one case associated with *H. pylori* reinfection, and five cases that recurred without reinfection. Some cases may appear to have recurred when in fact the lesions were overlooked at earlier follow-up examinations, since MALT lymphoma can be multifocal. Echoendoscopy may also be helpful to evaluate staging of the lymphoma lesions and to predict the response to therapy by eradication of *H. pylori*.[55] Sackmann and colleagues[55] sought to determine whether echoendoscopy could predict the outcome of treatment of low-grade MALT lymphoma by eradication of *H. pylori*. Interestingly, they found that 12 of 14 patients with lymphoma restricted to the mucosa or submucosa (stage $I_{E1}$) at echoendoscopy showed complete regression of MALT lymphoma, in contrast with none of the 10 patients with higher-stage lymphoma. In stage $I_{E1}$ patients, the rates of complete regression of MALT lymphoma were 60% at 6 months, 79% at 12 months, and 100% at 14 months, respectively.[55]

## *H. pylori* Eradication Protocols

Until recently, specific recommendations for *H. pylori* eradication were limited to peptic ulcer disease.[66] However, at the Digestive Health Initiative (DHI) International Update Conference on *H. pylori* held in the United States in 1997, recommendations for *H. pylori* testing and treatment were broadened.[67] *H. pylori* testing and eradication of the infection were also recommended after resection of early gastric cancer and for low-grade MALT lymphoma.[67] Furthermore, at the European *Helicobacter Pylori* Study Group meeting held in Maastricht, The Netherlands, the indications for eradication of *H. pylori* were further expanded to include *H. pylori*–positive patients with low-grade gastric MALT lymphoma, with further recommendations that the disease be managed in specialized centers.[68] The meeting participants reached a consensus that treatment regimens should be simple and well tolerated and should achieve eradication rates of over 80% on an intention-to-treat basis. The group strongly recommended that eradication treatment include a triple therapy with a proton-pump inhibitor (PPI) and two of the following antibiotics: clarithromycin, a nitroimidazole (metronidazole or tinidazole), and amoxicillin.[68]

Available protocols for *H. pylori* eradication use a combination of antimicrobial agents and either a PPI or ranitidine bismuth citrate.[69,70] Despite the combinatorial effect of drugs in regimens used to treat *H. pylori* infection, the cure rates are at best between 80% and 95%.[69,71] Antimicrobial resistance and lack of patient compliance are the most important factors influencing poor outcome.[69,71–74]

Currently, the most widely used therapies to eradicate *H. pylori* consist of a PPI (or ranitidine bismuth citrate) plus two antibiotics (clarithromycin, metronidazole, amoxicillin, and tetra-

cycline). In general, the best results are achieved by administering the three drugs twice a day for 10 to 14 days, at the dosages indicated in Table 66–2.[69,75,76] The accepted definition of cure is that there is no evidence of *H. pylori* after a period of at least 4 weeks after ending the antimicrobial therapy.[69,77]

Follow-up endoscopies with biopsy sampling are required for patients who have a diagnosis of low-grade MALT lymphoma and who receive *H. pylori* eradication as the first-line treatment to evaluate the MALT lymphoma lesions and to determine whether *H. pylori* has been eradicated.

## Treatment Approaches for Gastric Mucosa-Associated Lymphoid Tissue Lymphoma

Treatment options for gastric MALT lymphomas are determined by the stage and grade of the lesions and by specific institutional preferences. The options include surgery, radiotherapy, and chemotherapy, in addition to *H. pylori* eradication if *H. pylori* infection is diagnosed.

As discussed above, long-term follow-up studies showed that after *H. pylori* eradication, low-grade MALT lymphomas that reached complete remission were all in stage IE, limited to the gastric mucosa and submucosa (stage $I_{E1}$). In contrast, complete regression was not achieved in tumors that extended beyond the submucosa (stage $I_{E2}$), in lymphomas at stage II or higher and in high-grade lymphomas.[55,59,65,78] After *H. pylori* therapy, prolonged follow-up is recommended and should include endoscopy and multiple biopsies.[55,65,78] The follow-up schemes for low-grade MALT lymphoma after *H. pylori* eradication have varied among studies. In the protocol followed by Bayerdorffer and colleagues,[78] the first follow-up endoscopy after treatment was performed 4 weeks after the therapy, to determine whether *H. pylori* eradication was successful and to assess the activity of gastritis and the evolution of the MALT lymphoma lesions. After eradication was documented, *H. pylori*–negative patients were examined every 4 weeks until complete histological regression of the lymphoma lesions was documented. Thereafter, the patients underwent endoscopy every 6 months.[78] Therefore, for stage $I_{E1}$ low-grade MALT lymphomas, the use of *H. pylori* eradication to induce lymphoma regression, followed by long-term follow-up, appears to be a reasonable approach. An alternative for low-grade MALT lymphomas refractory to antibiotic therapy is radiotherapy alone.[1] Other alternatives are the use of chlorambucil alone or the combined-modality therapy used in localized aggressive lymphomas.[1]

Currently, the treatment modalities recommended for MALT lymphomas at stage $I_{E2}$ and II and for high-grade tumors in stages II and I include surgical resection by total or subtotal gastrectomy, chemotherapy, or radiotherapy. Each of these therapies may be used according to several different protocols, reviewed by

**Table 66–2** Common treatment protocols for *H. pylori* infection[69,75,76]

| Bismuth Subsalicylate–Based Triple Therapy | Proton Pump Inhibitor–Based Triple Therapy | Ranitidine Bismuth Citrate–Based Triple Therapy |
|---|---|---|
| Bismuth subsalicylate, 525 mg qid | Lansoprazole, 30 mg, or omeprazole, 20 mg bid | Ranitidine bismuth citrate, 400 mg bid |
| Metronidazole, 250 mg qid | Clarithromycin, 500 mg bid | Clarithromycin, 500 mg bid |
| Tetracycline, 500 mg qid | Metronidazole, 500 mg bid, or amoxicillin, 1000 mg bid | Metronidazole, 500 mg bid, or amoxicillin, 1000 mg bid |

Crump and colleagues.[1] Combination chemotherapy is the standard approach for disseminated disease (stages III and IV). If coexisting *H. pylori* infection is diagnosed, eradication should be attempted even for high-grade lesions and tumors that extend beyond the gastric submucosa. This intervention should be taken because *H. pylori* provides a stimulus for the development of additional low-grade lesions and because *H. pylori* infection is a risk factor in the development of gastric carcinoma.[79–81] Cases of coexisting MALT lymphoma and adenocarcinomas have indeed been reported.[82–84]

### Prognosis of Gastric Mucosa-Associated Lymphoid Tissue Lymphoma

Clinically, MALT lymphomas are indolent neoplasms. At the time of diagnosis, low-grade MALT lymphomas are usually at stage IE or IIE, and dissemination is slow.[85] The 5-year projected overall survival of patients with primary low-grade MALT lymphoma of the stomach reported by Pinotti and colleagues[86] was 82%. The clinical features with greatest prognostic significance for localized primary gastric MALT lymphoma are the initial stage at diagnosis,[53,87] the absolute tumor size, and the histological grade of the lymphoma.[9,85–87] It is becoming increasingly recognized that MALT lymphomas undergo progression from a phase that consists of pure low-grade MALT lymphoma, followed by lesions that contain increasing amounts of a high-grade component, and finally cases in which no low-grade component can be identified. The presence of a high-grade component makes the prognosis of these lymphomas substantially worse. For example, de Jong and colleagues[9] found that low-grade MALT lymphomas that contained a diffuse large cell component ranging from 1% to 10% of the infiltrate (group B) had a significantly worse prognosis than that of pure low-grade MALT lymphomas (group A). Patients with pure low-grade MALT lymphomas (group A) had a 10-year disease-specific survival rate of 90%, whereas patients with low-grade MALT lymphomas with a high-grade component (group B) had a disease-specific survival rate of 74%.[9,88] Patients with tumors with a blastic component greater than 10% and those with no obvious low-grade component had similarly adverse prognosis, with 10-year survival of approximately 45%.[9]

### Mucosa-Associated Lymphoid Tissue–Type Intestinal Lymphomas

Most B-cell lymphomas of the small intestine and colorectum are MALT lymphomas,[7,89,90] which occur less frequently in the intestine than in the stomach. Approximately one-third of the GI MALT lymphomas occur in the jejunum ileum, and these tumors are extremely rare in the colon.[2] In a study by Domizio and colleagues,[90] two-thirds of the patients were men, and the peak incidence was in the seventh decade of life. Recent studies show that MALT lymphomas are the most frequent lymphomas of the small bowel. In a study of 80 small intestinal lymphomas by Nakamura and co-workers,[89] 21 cases (26%) were diagnosed as low-grade B-cell lymphoma (15 marginal zone B-cell lymphomas of MALT type, 2 mantle cell lymphomas, and 4 follicle center lymphomas), 46 cases (58%) were diagnosed as high-grade B-cell lymphomas (19 large cell lymphomas with a low-grade MALT component, 17 diffuse large cell lymphomas without MALT features, 7 Burkitt lymphomas, and 3 lymphoblastic lymphomas), and 13 cases (16%) were diagnosed as T-cell lymphomas. In a study of small bowel intestinal lymphomas by Dom-

izio and colleagues,[90] 66% were primary B-cell lymphomas and 34% were T-cell lymphomas. Of the B-cell lymphomas, 62% were diffuse high-grade lymphomas, 20% were low-grade MALT lymphomas, 11% were lymphomas with both low- and high-grade components, and 7% were other low-grade types. Of the T-cell lymphomas, 83% were high-grade lymphomas, and 49% were enteropathy-associated lymphomas.[90]

The histological features of intestinal MALT lymphomas are similar to those of MALT lymphomas that arise in the stomach, but in general, lymphoepithelial lesions and the presence of a low-grade component occur less frequently in the intestine than in the stomach. Features of high-grade transformation are more frequent in intestinal MALT lymphomas than in the stomach.[6]

### Clinical Features of Intestinal Mucosa-Associated Lymphoid Tissue Lymphoma

Common presenting features of primary small bowel lymphoma are abdominal pain, weight loss, small bowel obstruction, and acute abdomen.[90] Most tumors occur as single lesions. The mesenteric lymph nodes are usually involved (stage IIE), but dissemination outside the abdomen is unusual at the time of diagnosis.[7] The coexistence of small bowel lymphoma and gastric MALT lymphoma has been described in isolated cases.[7] In the group of patients reviewed by Domizio and colleagues,[90] B-cell lymphomas were annular or polypoid masses in the distal and terminal ileum, while most T-cell lymphomas were ulcerated plaques or strictures in the proximal small bowel. The literature includes several case reports of marginal B-cell lymphoma of MALT type presenting as multiple lymphomatous polyposis of the gastrointestinal tract. These lymphomas presented with multiple mucosal polyps affecting variable lengths of colonic and small bowel mucosa.[91–94] Cases in which MALT lymphoma of the duodenum formed multiple polypoid lesions have also been described.[95]

### Clinical Management and Prognosis of Intestinal Mucosa-Associated Lymphoid Tissue Lymphoma

The optimal management of GI lymphomas has not been determined by prospective randomized clinical trials.[1] However, segmental resection of the involved bowel and associated lymphatics is usually recommended.[1] Resection is potentially curative if complete excision of the lymphoma is achieved and if only contiguous nodes are involved (stage IE or IIE). Surgical resection followed by adjuvant chemotherapy is warranted when the patient is considered a surgical candidate.[2] If curative resection is not feasible, palliative resection followed by combination chemotherapy is usually recommended. Radiation provides effective palliation for extensive unresectable disease. For patients with disseminated disease in whom complete tumor resection is not feasible, chemotherapy followed by radiotherapy is recommended.[1]

The prognosis of intestinal MALT lymphoma is worse than that of the gastric counterpart, with 5-year survival rates of 44%–75% for low-grade tumors and 25%–37% for high-grade tumors.[49,90] The 5-year survival rate for patients with unresectable intestinal MALT lymphoma is less than 25%. Relapses have been reported to occur more than 5 years after resection.[49] Adverse prognostic features include perforation, high-grade histology, multiple tumors, colorectal and/or gastric involvement, diffuse infiltration, high-grade histology, and advanced stage.[89,90]

## Summary

The definition, current understanding of pathogenesis, clinical features and staging systems, and the therapeutic approaches for GI MALT lymphoma were discussed in this chapter. Future studies are needed to better define the role of *H. pylori* infection and other as yet unknown stimuli that might trigger the development of these neoplasms in the gut. More studies are also required to identify novel treatment modalities with higher response rates in this group of relatively indolent lymphomas.

## References

1. Crump M, Gospodarowicz M, Shepherd FA. Lymphoma of the gastrointestinal tract. Semin Oncol 26:324–337, 1999.
2. Papachristodoulou A, Misiakos E, Kouraklis G, Androulaki A, Gogas J. Surgical treatment of gastrointestinal B-cell mucosa-associated tissue lymphomas. South Med J 90:723–728, 1997.
3. Weingrad DN, Decosse JJ, Sherlock P, et al. Primary gastrointestinal lymphoma: a 30-year review. Cancer 49:1258–1265, 1982.
4. Chan JK, Banks PM, Cleary ML, et al. A revised European-American classification of lymphoid neoplasms proposed by the International Lymphoma Study Group. A summary version. Am J Clin Pathol 103:543–560, 1995.
5. Banks PM, Isaacson PG. MALT lymphomas in 1997. Where do we stand? Am J Clin Pathol 111:S75–83, 1999.
6. Isaacson PG. Gastrointestinal lymphomas of T- and B-cell types. Mod Pathol 12:151–158, 1999.
7. Isaacson PG, Norton AJ. Malignant lymphoma of the gastrointestinal tract. In: Isaacson PG (ed): Extranodal Lymphomas. Churchill Livingstone, Edinburgh, pp. 15–65, 1994.
8. Zinzani PL, Magagnoli M, Ascani S, et al. Nongastrointestinal mucosa-associated lymphoid tissue (MALT) lymphomas: clinical and therapeutic features of 24 localized patients. Ann Oncol 8:883–886, 1997.
9. de Jong D, Boot H, van Heerde P, Hart GA, Taal BG. Histological grading in gastric lymphoma: pretreatment criteria and clinical relevance. Gastroenterology 112:1466–1474, 1997.
10. Carbone PP, Kaplan HS, Musshoff K, Smithers DW, Tubiana M. Report of the Committee on Hodgkin's Disease Staging Classification. Cancer Res 31:1860–1861, 1971.
11. Musshoff K. Prognostic and therapeutic implications of staging in extranodal Hodgkin's disease. Cancer Res 31:1814–1827, 1971.
12. Gray GM, Rosenberg SA, Cooper AD, et al. Lymphomas involving the gastrointestinal tract. Gastroenterology 82:143–152, 1982.
13. Parsonnet J, Hansen S, Rodriguez L, et al. *Helicobacter pylori* infection and gastric lymphoma. N Engl J Med 330:1267–1271, 1994.
14. Parker SL, tong T, Bolden S, et al. Cancer Statistics 1997. CA Cancer J Clin 1:5–27, 1997.
15. Genta RM, Robason GO, Graham DY. Simultaneous visualization of *Helicobacter pylori* and gastric morphology: a new stain. Hum Pathol 25:221–226, 1994.
16. Dixon MF, Genta RM, Yardley JH, Correa P. Classification and grading of gastritis. The updated Sydney system. International Workshop on the Histopathology of Gastritis, Houston 1994. Am J Surg Pathol 20:1161–1181, 1996.
17. Doglioni C, Wotherspoon AC, Moschini A, de Boni M, Isaacson PG. High incidence of primary gastric lymphoma in northeastern Italy. Lancet 339:834–835, 1992.
18. Wotherspoon AC, Ortiz-Hidalgo C, Falzon MR, Isaacson PG. *Helicobacter pylori*–associated gastritis and primary B-cell gastric lymphoma. Lancet 338:1175–1176, 1991.
19. Eidt S, Stolte M, Fischer R. *Helicobacter pylori* gastritis and primary gastric non-Hodgkin's lymphomas. J Clin Pathol 47:436–439, 1994.
20. Genta RM, Hamner HW, Graham DY. Gastric lymphoid follicles in *Helicobacter pylori* infection: frequency, distribution, and response to triple therapy. Hum Pathol 24:577–583, 1993.
21. Stolte M, Eidt S. Lymphoid follicles in antral mucosa: immune response to *Campylobacter pylori*? J Clin Pathol 42:1269–1271, 1989.
22. Genta RM, Hamner HW. The significance of lymphoid follicles in the interpretation of gastric biopsy specimens. Arch Pathol Lab Med 118:740–743, 1994.
23. Enno A, O'Rourke JL, Howlett CR, et al. MALToma-like lesions in the murine gastric mucosa after long-term infection with *Helicobacter felis*. A mouse model of *Helicobacter pylori*–induced gastric lymphoma. Am J Pathol 147:217–222, 1995.
24. Enno A, O'Rourke J, Braye S, Howlett R, Lee A. Antigen-dependent progression of mucosa-associated lymphoid tissue (MALT)-type lymphoma in the stomach. Effects of antimicrobial therapy on gastric MALT lymphoma in mice. Am J Pathol 152:1625–1632, 1998.
25. Wotherspoon AC, Doglioni C, Diss TC, et al. Regression of primary low-grade B-cell gastric lymphoma of mucosa-associated lymphoid tissue type after eradication of *Helicobacter pylori*. Lancet 342:575–577, 1993.
26. Carlson SJ, Yokoo H, Vanagunas A. Progression of gastritis to monoclonal B-cell lymphoma with resolution and recurrence following eradication of *Helicobacter pylori*. JAMA 275:937–939, 1996.
27. Bayerdorffer E, Neubauer A, Rudolph B, et al. Regression of primary gastric lymphoma of mucosa-associated lymphoid tissue type after cure of *Helicobacter pylori* infection. MALT Lymphoma Study Group. Lancet 345:1591–1594, 1995.
28. Roggero E, Zucca E, Pinotti G, et al. Eradication of *Helicobacter pylori* infection in primary low-grade gastric lymphoma of mucosa-associated lymphoid tissue. Ann Intern Med 122:767–769, 1995.
29. Steinbach G, Ford R, Glober G, et al. Antibiotic treatment of gastric lymphoma of mucosa-associated lymphoid tissue. An uncontrolled trial. Ann Intern Med 131:88–95, 1999.
30. Regimbeau C, Karsenti D, Durand V, et al. Low-grade gastric MALT lymphoma and *Helicobacter heilmannii* (*Gastrospirillum hominis*). Gastroenterol Clin Biol 22:720–723, 1998.
31. Hussell T, Isaacson PG, Crabtree JE, Spencer J. The response of cells from low-grade B-cell gastric lymphomas of mucosa-associated lymphoid tissue to *Helicobacter pylori*. Lancet 342:571–574, 1993.
32. Hussell T, Isaacson PG, Crabtree JE, Spencer J. *Helicobacter pylori*–specific tumour-infiltrating T cells provide contact dependent help for the growth of malignant B cells in low-grade gastric lymphoma of mucosa-associated lymphoid tissue. J Pathol 178:122–127, 1996.
33. Greiner A, Knorr C, Qin Y, et al. Low-grade B cell lymphomas of mucosa-associated lymphoid tissue (MALT-type) require CD40-mediated signaling and Th2-type cytokines for in vitro growth and differentiation. Am J Pathol 150:1583–1593, 1997.
34. Isaacson PG. Gastric MALT lymphoma: from concept to cure. Ann Oncol 10:637–645, 1999.
35. Liu H, Ye H, Dogan A, et al. T(11;18)(q21;q21) is associated with advanced mucosa-associated lymphoid tissue lymphoma that expresses nuclear BCL10. Blood 98:1182–1187, 2001.
36. Willis TG, Jadayel DM, Du MQ, et al. Bcl10 is involved in t(1;14) (p22;q32) of MALT B cell lymphoma and mutated in multiple tumor types. Cell 96:35–45, 1999.
37. Yoshino T, Akagi T. Gastric low-grade mucosa-associated lymphoid tissue lymphomas: their histogenesis and high-grade transformation. Pathol Int 48:323–331, 1998.
38. Gaidano G, Capello D, Gloghini A, et al. Frequent mutation of bcl-6 proto-oncogene in high grade, but not low grade, MALT lymphomas of the gastrointestinal tract. Haematologica 84:582–588, 1999.
39. Driessen A, Tierens A, Ectors N, et al. Primary diffuse large B cell lymphoma of the stomach: analysis of somatic mutations in the rearranged immunoglobulin heavy-chain variable genes indicates antigen selection. Leukemia 13:1085–1092, 1999.
40. Matolcsy A, Nagy M, Kisfaludy N, Kelenyi G. Distinct clonal origin of low-grade MALT-type and high-grade lesions of a multifocal gastric lymphoma. Histopathology 34:6–8, 1999.
41. Isaacson PG, Spencer J. Malignant lymphoma of mucosa-associated lymphoid tissue. Histopathology 11:445–462, 1987.
42. Strecker P, Eck M, Greiner A, et al. Diagnostic value of stomach biopsy in comparison with surgical specimen in gastric B-cell lymphomas of the MALT type. Pathologe 19:209–213, 1998.
43. de Mascarel A, Dubus P, Belleannee G, Megraud F, Merlio JP. Low prevalence of monoclonal B cells in *Helicobacter pylori* gastritis patients with duodenal ulcer. Hum Pathol 29:784–790, 1998.
44. El-Zimaity HM, El-Zaatari FA, Dore MP, et al. The differential diagnosis of early gastric mucosa-associated lymphoma: polymerase chain reaction and paraffin section immunophenotyping. Mod Pathol 12:885–893, 1999.
45. Weston AP, Banerjee SK, Horvat RT, et al. Specificity of polymerase chain reaction monoclonality for diagnosis of gastric mucosa-associated lymphoid tissue (MALT) lymphoma: direct comparison to Southern blot gene rearrangement. Dig Dis Sci 43:290–299, 1998.
46. Wotherspoon AC, Finn TM, Isaacson PG. Trisomy 3 in low-grade B-cell lymphomas of mucosa-associated lymphoid tissue. Blood 85:2000–2004, 1995.
47. Nakamura S, Akazawa K, Kinukawa N, Yao T, Tsuneyoshi M. Inverse correlation between the expression of bcl-2 and p53 proteins in primary gastric lymphoma. Hum Pathol 27:225–233, 1996.

48. Hsi ED, Eisbruch A, Greenson JK, et al. Classification of primary gastric lymphomas according to histologic features. Am J Surg Pathol 22: 17–27, 1998.

49. Radaszkiewicz T, Dragosics B, Bauer P. Gastrointestinal malignant lymphomas of the mucosa-associated lymphoid tissue: factors relevant to prognosis. Gastroenterology 102:1628–1638, 1992.

50. Peng H, Du M, Diss TC, Isaacson PG, Pan L. Genetic evidence for a clonal link between low and high-grade components in gastric MALT B-cell lymphoma. Histopathology 30:425–429, 1997.

51. Mezlini A, Kchir N, Chaabouni M, Ben Rejeb A, Ben Ayed F. Primary gastric MALT lymphoma in children. Report of 2 cases. Arch Anat Cytol Pathol 47:38–43, 1999.

52. Gianni L, Tassinari D, Sartori S, Rinaldi P, Ravaioli A. Gastric, duodenal and rectal multifocal MALT lymphoma: the possible co-existence of two different cell populations. Eur J Cancer 34:1640–1641, 1998.

53. Hoshida Y, Kusakabe H, Furukawa H, et al. Reassessment of gastric lymphoma in light of the concept of mucosa-associated lymphoid tissue lymphoma: analysis of 53 patients. Cancer 80:1151–1159, 1997.

54. Taal BG, Boot H, van Heerde P, et al. Primary non-Hodgkin lymphoma of the stomach: endoscopic pattern and prognosis in low versus high grade malignancy in relation to the MALT concept. Gut 39:556–561, 1996.

55. Sackmann M, Morgner A, Rudolph B, et al. Regression of gastric MALT lymphoma after eradication of *Helicobacter pylori* is predicted by endosonographic staging. MALT Lymphoma Study Group. Gastroenterology 113:1087–1090, 1997.

56. Weston AP, Banerjee SK, Horvat RT, et al. Prospective long-term endoscopic and histologic follow-up of gastric lymphoproliferative disease of early stage IE low-grade B-cell mucosa-associated lymphoid tissue type following *Helicobacter pylori* eradication treatment. Int J Oncol 15: 899–907, 1999.

57. Thiede C, Morgner A, Alpen B, et al. What role does *Helicobacter pylori* eradication play in gastric MALT and gastric MALT lymphoma? Gastroenterology 113:S61–S64, 1997.

58. Neubauer A, Thiede C, Morgner A, et al. Cure of *Helicobacter pylori* infection and duration of remission of low-grade gastric mucosa-associated lymphoid tissue lymphoma. J Natl Cancer Inst 89:1350–1355, 1997.

59. Isaacson PG, Diss TC, Wotherspoon AC, et al. Long-term follow-up of gastric MALT lymphoma treated by eradication of *H. pylori* with antibodies. Gastroenterology 117:750–751, 1999.

60. Yoshikane H, Yokoi T, Hidano H, et al. Regression of superficial gastric MALT lymphoma with unsuccessful eradication therapy for *Helicobacter pylori* infection. J Gastroenterol 32:812–816, 1997.

61. Tanahashi T, Tatsumi Y, Sawai N, et al. Regression of atypical lymphoid hyperplasia after eradication of *Helicobacter pylori*. J Gastroenterol 32: 543–547, 1997.

62. Alkan S, Karcher DS, Newman MA, Cohen P. Regression of salivary gland MALT lymphoma after treatment for *Helicobacter pylori*. Lancet 348:268–269, 1996.

63. Fischbach W, Tacke W, Greiner A, Konrad H, Muller H. Regression of immunoproliferative small intestinal disease after eradication of *Helicobacter pylori*. Lancet 349:31–32, 1997.

64. Inoue S, Matsumoto T, Iida M, et al. Regression of gastric lymphoma of mucosa-associated lymphoid tissue by *Helicobacter pylori* eradication: endoscopic observation. Gastrointest Endosc 46:377–379, 1997.

65. Stolte M, Morgner A, Meining A, et al. Early and long-term results of *Helicobacter pylori* cure of MALT lymphoma—what are the pitfalls? In: Hunt RH, Tytgat G (eds): *Helicobacter pylori*. Basic Mechanisms to Clinical Cure. Kluwer Academic Publishers, Dordrecht, pp 373–380, 2000.

66. NIH Consensus Conference. *Helicobacter pylori* in peptic ulcer disease. NIH Consensus Development Panel on *Helicobacter pylori* in Peptic Ulcer Disease. Jama 272:65–69, 1994.

67. Peura D. The report of the Digestive Health Initiative International Update Conference on *Helicobacter pylori*. Gastroenterology 113:S4–S8, 1997.

68. Group EHPS. Current European concepts in the management of *Helicobacter pylori* infection. The Maastricht Consensus Report. Gut 41: 8–13, 1997.

69. Genta RM, Graham DY. Diagnosis and treatment of *Helicobacter pylori* infection. In: Graham DY, Genta RM, Dixon MF (eds): Gastritis. Lippincott Williams & Wilkins, Philadelphia, PA, 1999, 189–201.

70. Bazzoli F, Zagari RM, Fossi S, et al. Short-term low-dose triple therapy for the eradication of *Helicobacter pylori*. Eur J Gastroenterol Hepatol 4:773–777, 1994.

71. van der Hulst RWM, Keller JJ, Raws EA, Tytgat GNJ: Treatment of *Helicobacter pylori* infection in humans: a review of the world literature. Helicobacter 1:6–19, 1996.

72. Graham DY, Lew GM, Malaty HM, et al. Factors influencing the eradication of *Helicobacter pylori* with triple therapy. Gastroenterology 102: 493–496, 1992.

73. Dore MP, Piana A, Carta M, et al. Amoxycillin resistance is one reason for failure of amoxycillin-omeprazole treatment of *Helicobacter pylori* infection. Aliment Pharmacol Ther 12:635–639, 1998.

74. Dore MP, Leandro G, Realdi G, Sepulveda AR, Graham DY. Effect of pretreatment antibiotic resistance to metronidazole and clarithromycin on outcome of *Helicobacter pylori* therapy: a meta-analytical approach. Dig Dis Sci 45:68–76, 2000.

75. Hopkins RJ. Current FDA-approved treatments for *Helicobacter pylori* and the FDA approval process. Gastroenterology 113:S126–S130, 1997.

76. Sepulveda AR, Dore MP, Bazzoli F. Chronic gastritis (www.emedicine. com). Emedicine 2, 2001.

77. Hopkins RJ, Girardi LS, Turney EA. Relationship between *Helicobacter pylori* eradication and reduced duodenal and gastric ulcer recurrence: a review. Gastroenterology 110:1244–1252, 1996.

78. Bayerdorffer E, Miehlke S, Neubauer A, Stolte M. Gastric MALT-lymphoma and *Helicobacter pylori* infection. Aliment Pharmacol Ther 11 Suppl 1:89–94, 1997.

79. Yamaoka Y, Kodama T, Kashima K, Graham DY, Sepulveda AR. Variants of the 3′ region of the *cagA* gene in *Helicobacter pylori* isolates from patients with different *H. pylori*–associated diseases. J Clin Microbiol 36:2258–2263, 1998.

80. Graham DY. *Helicobacter pylori* infection in the pathogenesis of duodenal ulcer and gastric cancer: a model. Gastroenterology 113:1983–1991, 1997.

81. Sepulveda AR. Molecular testing of *Helicobacter pylori*–associated chronic gastritis and premalignant gastric lesions: clinical implications. J Clin Gastroenterol 32:377–382, 2001.

82. Baron BW, Bitter MA, Baron JM, Bostwick DG. Gastric adenocarcinoma after gastric lymphoma. Cancer 60:1876–1882, 1987.

83. von Herbay A, Schreiter H, Rudi J. Simultaneous gastric adenocarcinoma and MALT-type lymphoma in *Helicobacter pylori* infection. Virchows Arch 427:445–450, 1995.

84. Montalban C, Castrillo JM, Lopez-Abente G, et al. Other cancers in patients with gastric MALT lymphoma. Leuk Lymphoma 33:161–168, 1999.

85. Montalban C, Castrillo JM, Abraira V, et al. Gastric B-cell mucosa-associated lymphoid tissue (MALT) lymphoma. Clinicopathological study and evaluation of the prognostic factors in 143 patients. Ann Oncol 6:355–362, 1995.

86. Pinotti G, Zucca E, Roggero E, et al. Clinical features, treatment and outcome in a series of 93 patients with low-grade gastric MALT lymphoma. Leuk Lymphoma 26:527–537, 1997.

87. Dworkin B, Lightdale CJ, Weingrad DN, et al. Primary gastric lymphoma. A review of 50 cases. Dig Dis Sci 27:986–992, 1982.

88. de Jong D, Aleman BM, Taal BG, Boot H. Controversies and consensus in the diagnosis, work-up and treatment of gastric lymphoma: an international survey. Ann Oncol 10:275–280, 1999.

89. Nakamura S, Matsumoto T, Takeshita M, et al. A clinicopathologic study of primary small intestine lymphoma: prognostic significance of mucosa-associated lymphoid tissue-derived lymphoma. Cancer 88:286–294, 2000.

90. Domizio P, Owen RA, Shepherd NA, Talbot IC, Norton AJ. Primary lymphoma of the small intestine. A clinicopathological study of 119 cases. Am J Surg Pathol 17:429–442, 1993.

91. Yatabe Y, Nakamura S, Nakamura T, et al. Multiple polypoid lesions of primary mucosa-associated lymphoid-tissue lymphoma of colon. Histopathology 32:116–125, 1998.

92. Rabaud C, May T, Canton P. Acquired Willebrand's syndrome in a patient with gastric MALT lymphoma. Presse Med 26:769, 1997.

93. Ugljesic M, Jankovic S, Petrovic M, Radosevic N, Markovic M. Diffuse involvement of the gastrointestinal tract with MALT lymphoma. Endoscopy 29:S37, 1997.

94. Breslin NP, Urbanski SJ, Shaffer EA. Mucosa-associated lymphoid tissue (MALT) lymphoma manifesting as multiple lymphomatosis polyposis of the gastrointestinal tract. Am J Gastroenterol 94:2540–2545, 1999.

95. Ohtsuka T, Kodama K, Nishikata F, et al. Mucosa-associated lymphoid tissue lymphoma of the duodenum forming multiple polypoid lesions: report of a case. Surg Today 29:557–559, 1999.

96. Nobre-Leitao C, Lage P, Cravo M, et al. Treatment of gastric MALT lymphoma by *Helicobacter pylori* eradication: a study controlled by endoscopic ultrasonography. Am J Gastroenterol 93:732–736, 1998.

# Chapter 67

# Low- and High-Grade Lymphomas

### FERNANDO CABANILLAS AND BARBARA PRO

Non-Hodgkin's lymphomas (NHLs) comprise a heterogeneous group of malignant neoplasms arising mostly in lymph node tissue but sometimes at extranodal sites. These extranodal NHLs are referred to as *primary extranodal lymphomas*. The incidence of NHLs has been rising steadily over the last two to three decades. According to Surveillance, Epidemiology, and End Results (SEER) data for the period from 1974 to 1988, the incidence of nodal NHL increased 1.7% to 2.5% per year and the incidence of extranodal NHL, 3.0% to 6.9% per year.[1,2]

The gastrointestinal (GI) tract is the most common site of extranodal NHL, accounting for 30% to 45% of all extranodal NHLs and for 4% to 20% of all NHLs.[3,4] In Western countries, the highest incidence of GI lymphoma is in the stomach (55% to 70%), followed by the small intestine (20% to 35%) and colorectum (5% to 10%); in the Middle East, the highest incidence is in the small intestine.

Multiple risk factors for the pathogenesis of GI lymphomas have been reported. These include *Helicobacter pylori* infection, immunodeficiency states, celiac disease, and inflammatory bowel disease.

Primary GI lymphoma does not represent a single disease but several clinicopathologic entities, some of which arise exclusively in the GI tract. The histologic classification of lymphomas has been evolving over the years to include new diseases identified using immunologic and genetic techniques. In the last 40 years, many classification systems have been used that were primarily designed for node-based lymphomas. However, because of the distinguishing features of GI lymphomas, the application of these classifications has been questioned.

A workshop was organized during the Fifth International Conference on Malignant Lymphomas (Lugano, Italy, June 1993) to discuss the problems of evaluating patients with GI lymphomas.[5] In that workshop, recommendations were made to adopt the histologic classification proposed by Isaacson after the recognition of mucosa-associated lymphoid tissue (MALT) lymphoma as a distinct entity (Table 67–1).

The Ann Arbor system was initially designed to stage Hodgkin's disease but is commonly applied to NHLs including extranodal presentations. In GI lymphomas, a second and more commonly used system is based on Musshoff's modification of the Ann Arbor staging system (Table 67–2).[6]

Primary GI lymphoma needs to be distinguished from secondary involvement of the GI tract by nodal disease, particularly in patients presenting with disseminated disease. Dawson et al.[7] initially defined primary lymphoma of the GI tract according to the following strict criteria: GI tract lesion with or without regional nodal involvement, no mediastinal node involvement, no tumor in the spleen or liver, and a normal white blood cell count. The definition has been subsequently revised and extended to include a wider variety of cases. Currently, a primary GI tract lymphoma is defined as a GI tract lesion that is the only or predominant one and/or causes the patient's presenting symptoms.

## Primary Gastric Large Cell Lymphoma

Although the stomach is the most common site of GI lymphomas, primary gastric lymphoma (PGL) is rare. It comprises 2% to 7% of all gastric malignancies. The significant geographic variation in the incidence of the disease probably reflects the varying prevalence of etiologic factors. A cooperative British-Italian study reported that the incidence of PGL in an area of northeastern Italy was 13 times higher than that in similar communities in the United Kingdom and was associated with a higher rate of infection by *H. pylori* (87% vs. 50% to 60%).[8] The role of *H. pylori* infection in gastric MALT lymphoma is well recognized, but its importance in other histologic subtypes remains

**Table 67-1** Pathological classification of gastrointestinal lymphomas

*B cell*

Mucosa-associated lymphoid tissue (MALT) type
  Low grade
  High grade with or without evidence of a low-grade component
Immunoproliferative small intestinal disease (IPSID)
  Low grade
  High grade with or without evidence of a low-grade component
Mantle cell
Burkitt's and Burkitt-like
Other types corresponding to nodal counterparts

*T cell*

Enteropathy-associated T-cell lymphoma (EATCL)
Other types not associated with enteropathy

to be determined.[9,10] This section will discuss only gastric large cell NHL; gastric MALT lymphoma is discussed in Chapter 66.

The presenting symptoms of PGL are nonspecific and resemble those of benign conditions and gastric adenocarcinoma. These symptoms are epigastric pain, weight loss, nausea, and vomiting. The fever and night sweats more characteristic of nodal presentations are uncommon in gastric lymphoma.[11] Primary gastric lymphoma commonly involves the middle and distal third of the stomach; multifocal and diffuse involvement is common. The disease occurs in slightly more men than women. The median age at presentation is 60 years.

Initial evaluation should include a complete physical examination including ear, nose, and throat examination; routine laboratory studies including lactic dehydrogenase (LDH) and β2 microglobulin; radiographic studies; upper GI tract endoscopy; and bone marrow aspiration and biopsy. Currently, a histologic diagnosis can be determined by endoscopy in more than 90% of cases. Furthermore, progressive advances in technology and expertise now allow adequate evaluation of extent of disease via endoscopic ultrasonography and contrast radiographic studies. Therefore, staging laparotomy is no longer recommended, and surgery is indicated for diagnosis only in emergency cases, when patients present with GI tract bleeding, obstruction, or perforation.

Although a few cases of T-cell lymphoma have been reported, most cases of PGL are of B-cell origin.[12] The most common histologic subtypes are B-cell lymphomas of the MALT type and diffuse large cell lymphomas. When a differential diagnosis including benign conditions is difficult, gene rearrangement studies for light- and heavy-chain restriction can identify the presence of monoclonality, a typical feature of malignant lymphoproliferative disorders.

**Table 67-2** Modified Ann Arbor Staging Classification for Gastrointestinal Lymphomas

| Stage | Description |
|---|---|
| Stage I | Lymphoma confined to gastrointestinal tract (single primary site or multiple noncontiguous lesions) |
| Stage II | Nodal involvement on one side of diaphragm |
| Stage II$_1$ | Involvement of contiguous lymph nodes |
| Stage II$_2$ | Involvement of noncontiguous, subdiaphragmatic lymph nodes |
| Stage III | Involvement of lymph nodes on both sides of diaphragm |
| Stage IV | Involvement of one or more extralymphatic organs or tissues |

Adapted from Musshoff K. Klinische Stadieneinteilung der nicht-Hodgkin Lymphome. Strahlentherapie 153:218–221, 1977.[6]

In the past, the standard of care for patients with early-stage PGL (stage I or II) was surgical resection followed by radiation therapy, chemotherapy, or both. Surgery was considered the only curative modality for patients with limited disease. Partial gastrectomy was recommended even for patients with more advanced disease to avoid the risk of GI bleeding and perforation during chemotherapy. Now, a more conservative approach is gaining support for several reasons. First, the risk of bleeding or perforation during primary chemotherapy has been overestimated. In the most recent and largest series, the incidence of hemorrhage was 0% to 6%, whereas the incidence of perforation was 0% to 2%.[13,14] Patients at high risk of GI complications can be easily identified by endoscopic ultrasonography. Risk factors associated with GI bleeding are large ulcerative lesions, depth of infiltration of the gastric wall, and thrombocytopenia. High-risk patients should be carefully monitored during the initial treatment or considered for surgical resection.

In recent years, an increasing number of studies have suggested that the addition of chemotherapy improves the results of surgery. In some series, the use of primary chemotherapy, radiation therapy, or combined modalities has produced results similar to those obtained with surgery and adjuvant treatment. In a series of 119 patients with stage I and II disease, treatment with radiation therapy alone or combined with surgery produced similar 5-year survival rates (71% vs. 82%).[11] In a prospective randomized study, 75 patients were assigned to receive surgery alone, surgery followed by chemotherapy, or preoperative radiation followed by surgery and chemotherapy. Survival at 3 years was 100% in patients treated with radiation, surgery, and adjuvant chemotherapy vs. 51% in the group treated with surgery alone.[15] Aviles and colleagues[16] reported on the effectiveness of chemotherapy as a single modality in a prospective nonrandomized trial; 28 patients received chemotherapy alone and 24 patients underwent surgical resection followed by chemotherapy. There was no difference in survival between the two groups. The policy at The University of Texas M. D. Anderson Cancer Center has been to treat stage I and II PGL conservatively, using a combined chemoradiation therapy program.

In a series of 34 patients treated with four cycles of chemotherapy followed by radiation therapy and then followed by up to eight additional cycles of chemotherapy, the 5-year survival and the event-free survival rates were 73% and 62%, respectively.[17] In a recent randomized study in patients with localized NHLs, chemoradiation therapy was superior to chemotherapy alone, and the duration of chemotherapy was significantly reduced when involved-field radiation was used.[18] Although this series was not limited to gastric lymphomas, the results are probably applicable to PGL. Further studies are needed to evaluate the optimal treatment schedule and the role of consolidation radiotherapy in early-stage PGL.

For patients with advanced disease (stage III or IV), the recommended treatment is systemic chemotherapy. The standard regimen includes cyclophosphamide, doxorubicin, vincristine, and prednisone (CHOP). Patients with adverse prognostic features (i.e., bulky disease, elevated LDH and β2 microglobulin levels, advanced age, poor performance status) who receive conventional treatment have a poor outcome and should be considered for investigational studies of more intensive regimens.

## Small Bowel Lymphoma

Approximately 20% to 35% of primary GI lymphomas arise in the small bowel. Distinct clinicopathologic entities include the

Western type, the immunoproliferative small intestinal disease (IPSID), or Mediterranean type, enteropathy-associated T-cell lymphoma (EATCL), and Burkitt's lymphoma.

### Western Type

Most intestinal lymphomas observed in Western countries occur in men in their sixth to seventh decades. Common presenting features include abdominal pain, weight loss, changes in bowel habits, and bowel obstruction. Approximately 10% of patients present with perforation.[19] Radiographic findings are nonspecific and include dilatation and thickening of the distal small bowel on follow-through examination. The diagnosis is often made at laparotomy. Very few cases are diagnosed preoperatively by endoscopy. Most small bowel lymphomas of the Western type are intermediate grade and common histologic subtypes are diffuse large B-cell lymphoma and immunoblastic lymphoma. Poor prognostic factors include advanced stage, high-grade histology, perforation, and multiple tumors. The initial treatment is usually surgical resection followed by chemotherapy, radiation therapy, or combined-modality therapy.

The experience at M. D. Anderson Cancer Center, as recently reported by Ha and colleagues,[20] suggests that postoperative chemotherapy and radiation therapy reduce the risk of distant metastases and local recurrence, respectively. In a series of 61 patients with primary small bowel lymphoma, 46 underwent complete surgical resection of the primary tumor, and 9 patients underwent only partial resection. The predominant histologic subtypes were diffuse large cell lymphoma (55%) and follicular lymphoma (21%). All but four patients received postoperative treatment consisting of chemotherapy alone (47%), radiation therapy alone (29%), or chemotherapy and radiation therapy combined (29%). As shown by analysis of the patterns of recurrence, chemotherapy reduced the risk of recurrence outside the abdominopelvic cavity, whereas radiation therapy appeared to produce better local control.[20]

### Immunoproliferative Small Intestinal Disease

Mediterranean B-cell lymphoma, also known as IPSID, occurs mainly in the Middle East and North Africa.[21] Patients are usually in their second or third decade of life, have low socioeconomic status, and live in areas of poor sanitation and hygiene. The main presenting symptom is malabsorption. Physical examination often reveals peripheral edema, clubbing, and an abdominal mass. In contrast to Western lymphoma, which usually involves only one segment of the small bowel, IPSID involves the entire small intestine. Barium X-rays of IPSID show diffuse dilatation of the duodenum, jejunum, and proximal ileum. Endoscopy reveals several abnormalities including thickened folds, nodules, and ulcers.[22] Bacterial overgrowth and intestinal parasitosis, usually caused by giardia, are common. Laboratory tests indicate the abnormal presence of an IgA heavy-chain protein, called $\alpha$-chain protein ($\alpha$-CP), in serum, urine, saliva, or intestinal secretions.[23] The pathogenetic theory is that chronic antigenic stimulation leads to the clonal proliferation of B lymphocytes that produce IgA heavy chains. Early-stage IPSID, like *H. pylori*–associated gastric MALT lymphoma, may regress after treatment with antibiotics (e.g., tetracycline, metronidazole-ampicillin). In the few series of patients treated with antibiotics, response rates have ranged from 33% to 71%.[24,25] At more advanced stages, the prognosis is very poor and significantly worse

than that of other low-grade B-cell lymphomas. The 5-year survival rates are as low as 23%.[26] Combination chemotherapy with an anthracycline-based regimen is frequently used.

### Enteropathy-Associated T-Cell Lymphoma

The association between celiac disease and intestinal lymphoma is well documented. Compared with patients without celiac disease, patients with celiac disease have a 200 times higher risk of developing lymphoma of the small bowel. As shown by immunohistochemical and molecular studies, lymphomas arising in association with malabsorptive states are of T-cell origin. To describe these tumors, O'Farrelly and co-workers have introduced the term *enteropathy-associated T-cell lymphoma* (EATCL).[27,28]

Approximately 50% of cases of patients with EATCL present with an intestinal perforation. The jejunum is the most frequently involved site and multifocal disease is found in the most cases (Fig. 67–1). The frequency of intestinal recurrences is very high, and the prognosis is extremely poor. In a series of 119 cases of primary lymphoma of the small intestine, Domizio and colleagues reported a 5-year survival rate of 75% for patients with low-grade B-cell lymphoma but only 25% for patients with T-cell lymphomas.[19]

### Burkitt's Lymphoma

Burkitt's lymphoma is a common childhood lymphoma, accounting for up to one-third of pediatric lymphomas in the United States. The classic endemic African form frequently involves the jaw and other facial bones. The nonendemic form often involves the GI tract. Patients usually present with abdominal pain, nausea, vomiting, GI bleeding, and intussusception; intestinal perforation is rare (Fig. 67–2). The ileocecal region is commonly involved, and in about 25% of patients a palpable mass is present in the right iliac fossa.

The primary treatment modality is combination chemotherapy.[29] The regimens most commonly used include cyclophosphamide, vincristine, methotrexate, and doxorubicin, with or without prednisone. Central nervous system (CNS) prophylaxis is recommended for all patients regardless of stage. Patients with localized disease have an excellent prognosis and cure rates as high as 100%. Bone marrow involvement and CNS disease are associated with worse outcome. However, improved results in advanced-stage disease have recently been achieved by using high-dose ara-C and methotrexate.

## Colorectal Lymphoma

Colorectal lymphomas are extremely rare, accounting for only 5% to 10% of all GI lymphomas. The main presenting symptoms are blood in the stool, abdominal pain, and changes in bowel habits. Diffuse large cell lymphoma is the most common histologic subtype. Most patients present with limited disease (stage I or II).[30] The initial treatment is usually surgical resection followed by chemotherapy, radiation therapy, or both.[30,31] Involved-field radiation therapy alone has been used successfully to treat MALT lymphoma of the rectum.[32]

## Multiple Lymphomatous Polyposis

Multiple lymphomatous polyposis (MLP) is an uncommon type of GI lymphoma characterized by multiple polypoid lesions

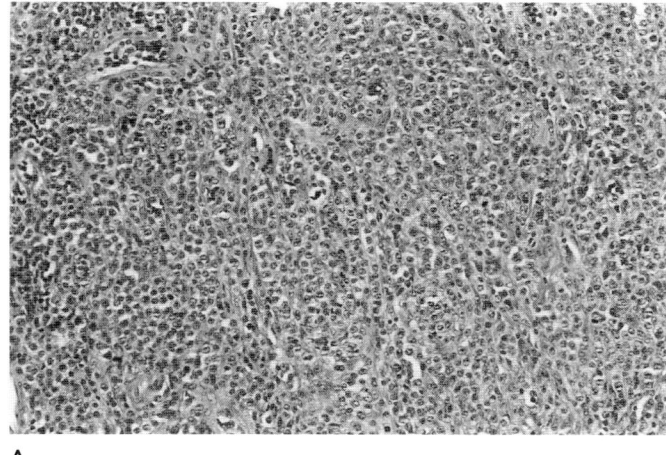

A

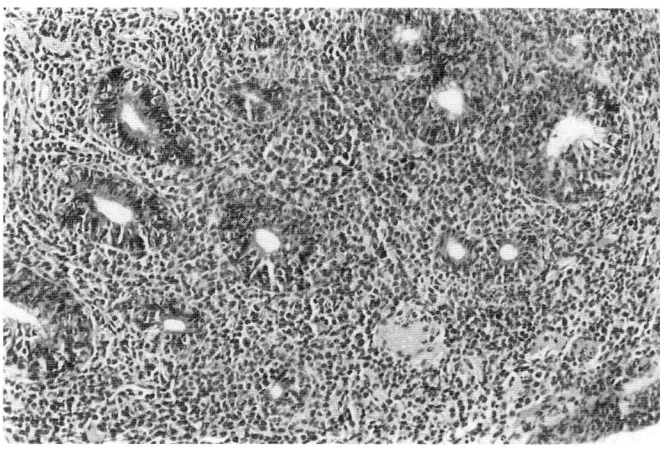

B

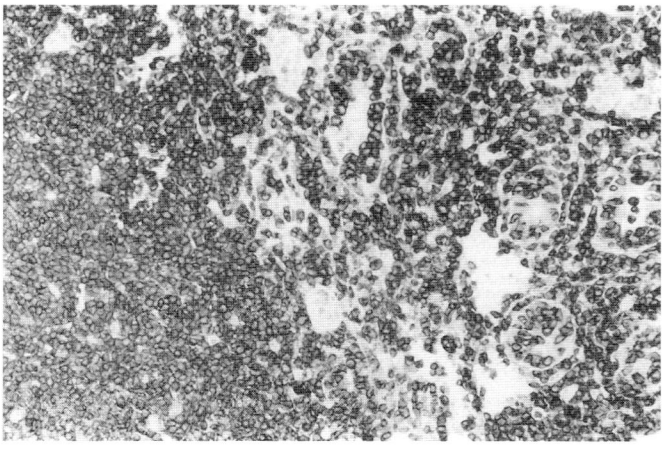

C

**Figure 67-1** *A:* A 68-year-old man with intestinal T-cell lymphoma in mucosa and submucosa of small intestine (segmental resection). *B:* Same patient as A. Mucosal biopsy of colon demonstrates epitheliotropism of neoplastic lymphocytes. *C:* Immunoperoxidase staining demonstrates CD3 positivity in neoplastic lymphocytes. (Photomicrographs courtesy of Dr. John T. Manning, M. D. Anderson Cancer Center.)

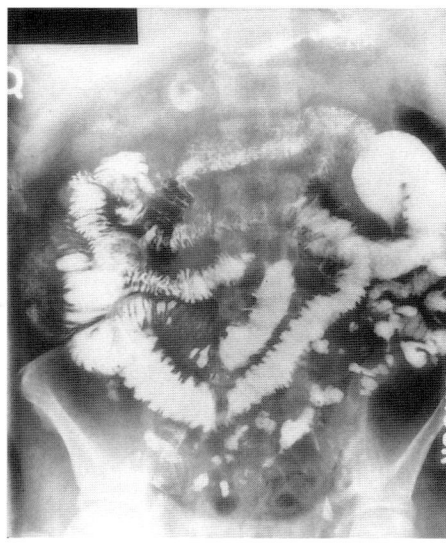

**Figure 67-2** Small bowel obstruction in a patient with Burkitt's lymphoma. In the United States, small bowel is the most common extranodal site of presentation for Burkitt's lymphoma. Note in the left upper quadrant the dilated loop of small bowel ending sharply and forming the "bird's beak" sign typical of this tumor.

involving long segments of the GI tract. The term was first introduced in 1961 by Cornes and colleagues to describe a heterogeneous group of polypoid lymphomas involving the GI tract at multiple foci.[33] More recently, MLP has been recognized as a distinct entity that in most cases represents the GI presentation of mantle cell lymphoma. Occasionally, follicular lymphoma can produce a similar picture at presentation.

Mantle cell lymphoma usually presents as a systemic disorder involving the lymph nodes, bone marrow, spleen, and GI tract. The tumor cells express mature B-cell markers (CD19, CD20) and CD5, a T-cell-associated antigen normally expressed by a subpopulation of B cells in the mantle zone of lymph nodes. The genetic hallmark of mantle cell lymphoma is translocation of the *bcl-1* gene on chromosome 11 and the Ig heavy-chain gene on chromosome 14. Cytogenetic and molecular studies have shown *bcl-1* gene rearrangement in many cases of MLP.[34,35]

The clinical features of MLP are similar to those of mantle cell lymphoma. The mean age at diagnosis is 61 years, and there is a strong male predominance (88%).[36] The most common presenting symptoms are weight loss, fatigue, diarrhea, abdominal pain, and GI bleeding. Although any part of the GI tract can be involved, there is usually a dominant mass involving the ileocecal region (Fig. 67-3). On endoscopy, MLP appears as small nodular or polypoid lesions ranging in size from 2 mm to several centimeters.

In most cases, patients present with advanced disease. The most frequently involved sites are the bone marrow, peripheral lymph nodes, Waldeyer's ring, and liver. The prognosis for MLP is significantly worse than for low-grade GI lymphomas (i.e., the MALT or follicular types); the median survival is less than 3 years. Patients treated with anthracycline-based regimens frequently experience relapse in a pattern similar to that for mantle cell lymphoma. A recent study suggests that the hyper-CVAD/ MTX-ara-C regimen (fractionated cyclophosphamide, doxorubicin, vincristine, and dexamethasone alternated with high-dose

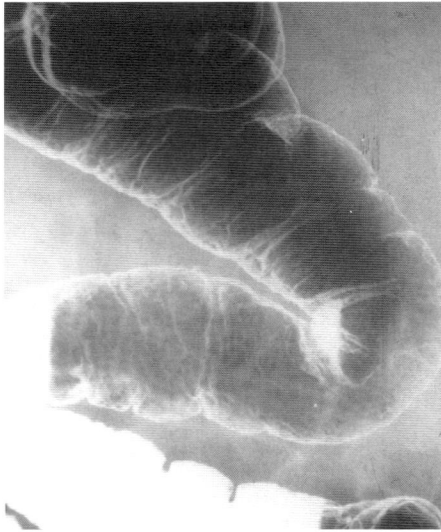

**Figure 67–3** Barium enema in a patient with mantle cell lymphoma and multiple lymphomatous polyposis. Note the numerous small filling defects (polyps) present throughout the colon. (Photograph courtesy of Dr. Luis Baez.)

methotrexate and cytarabine) followed by high-dose chemoradiotherapy and stem cell transplant may improve the outcome of patients with mantle cell lymphoma.[37] The published reports on high-dose chemotherapy and autologous transplantation in MLP have shown encouraging results.[38,39]

## Gastrointestinal Lymphoma in the HIV-Positive Patient

Non-Hodgkin's lymphoma is the second most common malignancy observed in individuals infected with the human immunodeficiency virus (HIV), and it is recognized as an AIDS-defining illness.[40] Lymphoma is usually a late complication of HIV infection, occurring in the setting of significant immunosuppression. In 1991, the U.S. Centers for Disease Control (CDC) reported that 3.4% of patients who developed AIDS had NHL as their initial AIDS-defining illness.[41] The pathogenesis of HIV-related lymphoma is probably multifactorial. Chronic hyperproliferation of B lymphocytes is commonly observed in HIV-infected individuals. Although there is no evidence of a direct role of HIV in this malignant transformation, HIV is thought to be involved indirectly, by either stimulating the release of numerous cytokines and growth factors or allowing infection by other viruses such as the Epstein-Barr virus (EBV).

Increased levels of IL-6 and IL-10 gene expression have been observed in AIDS-associated NHLs. Both cytokines function as autocrine growth factors in lymphomas.[42,43] The role of oncogene mutations, particularly those resulting in deregulation of c-myc, is also under investigation. Rearrangements of c-myc have been observed in approximately 60% to 80% of AIDS-associated NHLs and differences have been observed in different pathologic subtypes.[44] The role of EBV in the development of systemic AIDS-related lymphomas remains to be defined. Although evidence of latent EBV infection is present in nearly all cases of primary CNS lymphoma, 40% to 60% of patients with systemic disease do not have EBV DNA sequences in their tumors.[45]

Unlike Kaposi's sarcoma, which occurs primarily in homosexual and bisexual men, NHL can occur in all groups at risk

for HIV infection. HIV-associated lymphomas are usually high grade, are of B-cell lineage, and commonly arise in extranodal sites. The most common histologic subtypes are immunoblastic and small noncleaved cell, Burkitt's and Burkitt's-like.[46–48]

The GI tract is the second most common site of extranodal presentation, occurring in 10% to 28% of cases.[48] B symptoms are common and more than 90% of patients present with widespread disease. The different areas of the GI tract appear equally involved, but a higher incidence at unusual sites, including anus and rectum, has been observed.

The staging evaluation should include computed tomography (CT) of the chest, abdomen, pelvis, and brain; gallium-67 scanning; bone marrow biopsy; and, when clinically indicated, a GI series and endoscopy. Because asymptomatic leptomeningeal disease is present in approximately 20% of patients with AIDS-associated lymphoma, lumbar puncture should be part of the initial staging evaluation.[49]

Chemotherapy is the mainstay of treatment of AIDS-associated lymphoma. However, as described below, the optimal treatment regimen remains to be defined. AIDS-associated lymphoma frequently occurs late in the course of HIV infection, when systemic disease is advanced and HIV-related bone marrow suppression exacerbates the myelosuppression induced by chemotherapy. Thus, a significant factor in the poor outcome of patients with AIDS-associated NHL is the poor tolerance of chemotherapy due to functional impairment of the bone marrow reserve and to the presence of multiple opportunistic infections. Moreover, chemotherapy can interfere with the continued use of concurrent myelosuppressive antiretroviral agents such as zidovudine.

Several studies have investigated the effectiveness of various dose-intensive chemotherapy regimens (Table 67–3). Despite high response rates, the incidence of myelosuppression and infectious complications is very high, the duration of response extremely short, and the median survival only 5–6 months.[50–52] Imrie and co-workers[53] reported the results of a retrospective analysis of 31 patients with HIV-associated GI lymphoma. Twenty-seven patients were treated with systemic chemotherapy, 24 of whom were evaluable for response and toxicity. Most patients received either CHOP (cyclophosphamide, doxorubicin, vincristine, and prednisone) or a modified VACOP-B regimen (Adriamycin, etoposide, vincristine, cyclophosphamide, bleomycin, prednisone, and intrathecal cytarabine). A complete response was observed in only 38% of patients and a partial response in 46%. Hematologic toxicity was significant; 81% of

**Table 67–3** AIDS-Lymphoma: treatment results

| Regimen | Patients Evaluated (n) | CR (%) | OI (%) | Median Survival (Months) | Study |
|---|---|---|---|---|---|
| Pro-MACE-MOPP | 15 | 20 | 27 | 5.0 | 51 |
| HD Ara-C + HD MTX + others | 9 | 33 | 78 | 6.0 | 50 |
| COMET-A | 38 | 58 | 28 | 5.2 | 52 |
| Low-dose M-BACOD + IT Ara-C | 35 | 46 | 20 | 6.5 | 49 |

Abbreviations: COMET-A, cyclophosphamide, vincristine, methotrexate, etoposide, high-dose cytosine arabinoside; CR, complete response; HD Ara-C, high-dose cytosine arabinoside; HD MTX, high-dose methotrexate; IT Ara-C, intrathecal cytosine arabinoside; M-BACOD, methotrexate, bleomycin, doxorubicin, cyclophosphamide, vincristine, dexamethasone; OI, opportunistic infections; Pro-MACE-MOPP, prednisone, methotrexate, doxorubicin, cyclophosphamide, etoposide, nitrogen mustard, vincristine, procarbazine, prednisone.

patients required a dose reduction because of myelosuppression. The median duration of response was 5 months. Thirty-five percent of patients died of treatment-related toxicity or AIDS complications. Bone marrow involvement and a performance status of >2 on the ECOG scale were associated with shorter survival.[53] More recently, several studies have explored the feasibility and efficacy of less aggressive regimens. Kaplan and colleagues[54] reported the first controlled clinical trial comparing low-dose with standard-dose chemotherapy. HIV-seropositive patients were randomly assigned to receive either a standard-dose regimen of methotrexate, bleomycin, doxorubicin, cyclophosphamide, vincristine, and dexamethasone (M-BACOD) plus granulocyte-macrophage colony-stimulating factor (GM-CSF) or a low-dose regimen of M-BACOD plus GM-CSF only when clinically indicated. Although no significant difference in overall or disease-free survival was noted, fewer hematologic toxic effects were observed in patients treated on the low-dose regimen.[54]

Further studies will be necessary to evaluate whether the use of new antiretroviral agents and the better supportive therapy now available for HIV-infected patients will permit the use of more intensive chemotherapy and improve the outcome of HIV-related NHL.

## References

1. Devesa SS, Fears T. Non-Hodgkin's lymphoma time trends: United States and international data. Cancer Res 52(Suppl):5432s–5440s, 1992.
2. Devesa SS, Silverman DT, Young JL Jr, et al. Cancer incidence and mortality trends among whites in the United States. 1947–84. J Natl Cancer Inst 79:701–770, 1987.
3. Hermann R, Panahon AM, Barcos MP, Walsh D, Stutzmann L. Gastrointestinal involvement in non-Hodgkin's lymphoma. Cancer 46:215–222, 1980.
4. Freeman C, Berg JW, Cutler SJ. Occurrence and prognosis of extranodal lymphomas. Cancer 29:252–260, 1972.
5. Rohatiner A, d'Amore F, Coiffier B, et al. Report on a workshop convened to discuss the pathological and staging classifications of gastrointestinal tract lymphoma. Ann Oncol 5:397–400, 1994.
6. Musshoff K. Klinische Stadieneinteilung der nicht-Hodgkin Lymphome. Strahlentherapie 153:218–221, 1977.
7. Dawson IMP, Cornes JS, Morson BC. Primary malignant lymphoid tumors of the intestinal tract: report of 37 cases with a study of factor influencing prognosis. Br J Surg 49:80–89, 1961.
8. Doglioni C, Wotherspoon AC, Moschini A, et al. High incidence of primary gastric lymphoma in northeastern Italy. Lancet 339:834–835, 1992.
9. Wotherspoon AC, Ortiz-Hildago C, Falzon MR, Isaacson PG. *Helicobacter pylori*–associated gastritis and primary B-cell gastric lymphoma. Lancet 338:1175–1176, 1991.
10. Parsonnet J, Hansen S, Rodriguez L, et al. *Helicobacter pylori* infection and gastric lymphoma. N Engl J Med 330:1267–1271, 1994.
11. Taal BG, Burgers JMV, van Heerde P, Hart AAM, Somers R. The clinical spectrum and treatment of primary non-Hodgkin's lymphoma of the stomach. Ann Oncol 4:839–846, 1993.
12. Sueoka N, Inokushi K, Nishigaki H, et al. Genotype configuration in a case of primary gastric lymphoma with T-cell phenotype. Cancer Genet Cytogenet 101:103–108, 1998.
13. Bozzetti F, Audisio RA, Giardini R, Gennari L. Role of surgery in patients with primary non-Hodgkin's lymphoma of the stomach: an old problem revisited. Br J Surg 80:1101–1106, 1993.
14. Burgers JMV, Taal BG, van Heerde P, et al. Treatment results of primary stage I and II non-Hodgkin's lymphoma of the stomach. Radiother Oncol 11:319–326, 1988.
15. Shchepotin IB, Stephen D, Evans RT, et al. Primary non-Hodgkin's lymphoma of the stomach: three radical modalities of treatment in 75 patients. Ann Surg Oncol 3:277–284, 1996.
16. Aviles A, Diaz-Maqueo JC, de la Torre A, et al. Is surgery necessary in the treatment of primary gastric non-Hodgkin's lymphoma? Leuk Lymphoma 5:365–369, 1991.
17. Maor MH, Velasquez WS, Fuller LM, Silvermintz KB. Stomach conservation in stages IE and IIE gastric non-Hodgkin's lymphoma. J Clin Oncol 8:266–271, 1990.
18. Miller TP, Dahlberg S, Cassady JR. Chemotherapy alone compared with chemotherapy plus radiotherapy for localized intermediate- and high-grade non-Hodgkin's lymphoma. N Engl J Med 339:21–26, 1998.
19. Domizio P, Owen RA, Shepherd NA, Talbot IC, Norton AJ. Primary lymphoma of the small intestine: a clinicopathological study of 119 cases. Am J Surg Pathol 17:429–442, 1993.
20. Ha CS, Cho MJ, Allen PK, Fuller LM, Cabanillas F, Cox JD. Primary non-Hodgkin lymphoma of the small bowel. Radiology 211:183–187, 1999.
21. Al-Mondhiri H. Primary lymphoma of the small intestine: East–West contrast. Am J Hematol 22:89–105, 1986.
22. Halphen M, Najjr T, Jaafoura H, et al. Diagnostic value of upper intestinal fiber endoscopy in primary small intestinal lymphoma: a prospective study by the Tunisian-French Intestinal Lymphoma Group. Cancer 58:2140–2145, 1986.
23. Seligmann M, Rambaud JC. Alpha-chain disease: an immunoproliferative disease of the secretory immune system. Ann N Y Acad Sci 409:478–485, 1983.
24. Banisadre M, Feridoon A, Modtajabai A, Dutz W, Navab F. Immunoproliferative small intestinal disease and primary small intestinal lymphoma: relation to alpha chain protein. Cancer 56:1384–1391, 1985
25. Ben-Ayed F, Halphen M, Najjar T, et al. Treatment of alpha chain disease: result of a prospective study in 21 Tunisian patients by the Tunisian-French Intestinal Lymphoma Study Group. Cancer 63:1251–1256, 1989.
26. Al-Bahrani ZR, Al-Mohindri H, Bakir F, et al. Clinical and pathologic subtypes of primary intestinal lymphoma: experience with 132 patients over a 14-year period. Cancer 52:1666–1672, 1983.
27. Chott A, Dragosics B, Radaszkiewicz T. Peripheral T-cell lymphomas of the intestine. Am J Pathol 141:1361–1371, 1992.
28. O'Farrelly C, Feighery C, O'Brian DS, et al. Humoral response to wheat protein in patients with coeliac disease and enteropathy associated T-cell lymphoma. BMJ 293:908–910, 1986.
29. Magrath IT. Small noncleaved cell lymphoma (Burkitt's and Burkitt-like lymphomas). In: Magrath IT (ed): The Non-Hodgkin's Lymphomas. Arnold, London, 1997, pp 781–811.
30. Cho MJ, Ha CS, Allen PK, Fuller LM, Cabanillas F, Cox JD. Primary non-Hodgkin lymphoma of the large bowel. Radiology 205:535–539, 1997.
31. Gospodarowicz MK, Sutcliffe SB. The extranodal lymphomas. Semin Radiat Oncol 5:281–300, 1995.
32. Crump M, Gospodarowicz M, Shepherd FA. Lymphoma of the gastrointestinal tract. Semin Oncol 26:324–337,1999.
33. Cornes JS. Multiple lymphomatous polyposis of the gastrointestinal tract. Cancer 14:249–257, 1961.
34. Smir BN, Ramaika CA, Cho CG, et al. Molecular evidence links lymphomatous polyposis of the gastrointestinal tract with mantle cell lymphoma. Hum Pathol 26:1282–1285, 1995.
35. Kumar S, Krenacs L, Otsuki T, et al. bcl-1 rearrangement and cyclin D1 protein expression in multiple lymphomatous polyposis. Am J Clin Pathol 105:736–743, 1996.
36. O'Briain DS, Kennedy MJ, Daly PA, et al. Multiple lymphomatous polyposis of the gastrointestinal tract: a clinicopathologically distinctive form of non-Hodgkin's lymphoma of B-cell centrotypic type. Am J Surg Pathol 13:691–699, 1989.
37. Khouri IF, Romaguera J, Kantarjian H, et al. Hyper-CVAD and high dose methotrexate/cytarabine followed by stem-cell transplantation: an active regimen for aggressive mantle-cell lymphoma. J Clin Oncol 16:3803–3809, 1998.
38. Ruskone-Fourmestraux A, Delmer A, Lavergne A, et al. Multiple lymphomatous polyposis of the gastrointestinal tract: prospective clinico-pathologic study of 31 cases. Groupe D'etude des Lymphomes Digestifs. Gastroenterology 112:7–16, 1997.
39. Mahe B, Moreau A, Moreau PH, Le Tortorec S, Harousseau JL, Milpied N. High-dose radiochemotherapy followed by autologous stem cell transplantation in four patients with multiple lymphomatous polyposis. Cancer 75:2742–2746, 1995.
40. Centers for Disease Control. Revision of the case definition of acquired immunodeficiency syndrome for national reporting—United States. Ann Intern Med 103:402–403, 1985.
41. Beral V, Peterman T, Berkelman R, Jaffe H. AIDS-associated non-Hodgkin's lymphoma. Lancet 337:805–809, 1991.
42. Nakajima K, Martinez-Maza O, Hirano T, et al. Induction of IL-6 (B-cell stimulatory factor-2/IFN-β-2) production by human immunodeficiency virus. J Immunol 142:531–536, 1989.
43. Benjamin D, Knobloch TJ, Abrams J, Dayton MA. Human B-cell IL-10: B-cell lines derived from patients with AIDS and Burkitt's lymphoma constitutively secrete large quantities of IL-10 [abstract]. Blood 78:384a, 1991.

44. Subar M, Neri A, Inghirami G, Knowles DM, Dalla-Favera R. Frequent c-*myc* oncogene activation and infrequent presence of Epstein-Barr virus genome in AIDS-associated lymphoma. Blood 72:667–671, 1988.

45. MacMahon EME, Glass JD, Hayward ST, et al. Epstein Barr virus in AIDS-related primary central nervous system lymphoma. Lancet 338: 969–973, 1991.

46. Levine AM. Acquired immunodeficiency syndrome–related lymphoma. Blood 80:8–20, 1992.

47. Strauss DJ. HIV-associated lymphomas. Curr Opin Oncol 9:450–454, 1997.

48. Levine AM, Gill PS, Meyer PR, et al. Retrovirus and malignant lymphoma in homosexual men. JAMA 254:1921–1925, 1985.

49. Levine AM, Wernz JC, Kaplan L, et al. Low-dose chemotherapy with central nervous system prophylaxis and azidothymidine maintenance in AIDS-related lymphoma: a prospective multi-institutional trial. JAMA 266:884–888, 1991.

50. Gill PS, Levine AM, Krailo M, et al. AIDS-related malignant lymphoma: results of prospective treatment trials. J Clin Oncol 5:1322–1328, 1987.

51. Dugan M, Subar M, Odajnyk C, et al. Intensive, multiagent chemotherapy for AIDS-related diffuse large cell lymphoma [abstract]. Blood 68: 124a, 1986.

52. Kaplan LD, Abrams DI, Feigal E, et al. AIDS-associated non-Hodgkin's lymphoma in San Francisco. JAMA 261:719–724, 1989.

53. Imrie KR, Sawka CA, Kutas G, et al. HIV-associated lymphoma of the gastrointestinal tract: the University of Toronto AIDS–Lymphoma Study Group experience. Leuk Lymphoma 16:343–349, 1995.

54. Kaplan LD, Straus JD, Testa MA, et al. Low-dose compared with standard-dose m-BACOD chemotherapy for non-Hodgkin's lymphoma associated with immunodeficiency virus infection. N Engl J Med 336: 1641–1648, 1997.

# Section 11

## Sarcomas of the Gastrointestinal Tract

# Chapter 68

# Epidemiology, Pathology, Molecular Biology, and Natural History of Gastrointestinal Sarcomas

MALCOLM M. BILIMORIA, RUSSELL S. BERMAN, AND RAPHAEL E. POLLOCK

There are approximately 7000 new cases of sarcoma each year, the vast majority of which involve the extremities.[1] Sarcomas can involve any of the visceral organs within the abdominal cavity but most commonly involve the gastrointestinal (GI) tract. Three percent of all sarcomas, or about 150 cases each year, are GI sarcomas.[2] This chapter will discuss GI sarcomas, highlighting the biologic and pathologic aspects as well as the natural history of these unusual tumors.

## Epidemiology

Most GI sarcomas develop during the fourth to sixth decade of life (median age at presentation, 55 years). There is a slight female-to-male predominance (1.4:1), but no apparent ethnic, geographic, or racial predisposition to this disease.[3] The male-to-female ratio stated above holds for sarcomas at all GI sites except esophagus.[4] There is no known familial predisposition to development of this disease, but there is a well-described syndrome that includes GI sarcomas.

Carney's syndrome is a triad of GI sarcomas, pulmonary chondromas, and extraadrenal paragangliomas that occurs in young women, thus a genetic etiology may play a role in the development of these tumors.[5] The GI sarcomas that develop as part of the syndrome are predominantly gastric and display a relatively indolent course when compared with that of GI sarcomas not associated with the syndrome. The pulmonary chondromas that arise after the development of the GI sarcomas are particularly troubling for the clinician as the chondromas have often been misinterpreted as pulmonary metastases from the GI sarcoma. This triad occurs in the absence of familial disease, implicating an as-yet uncharacterized somatic mutational etiology. An association between diseases of genetic aberration and GI sarcomas, however, has been seen. The development of non-neural stromal tumors of the GI tract, often of low-grade malignant potential, has been noted in patients with neurofibromatosis.[6]

Although no occupational exposure has been noted as an etiology for GI sarcomas in humans, there are known carcinogens with respect to the rat model. Gastric sarcomas were induced in rats given N-methyl-N¹-nitro-N-nitrosoguanidine (MNNG) with sodium taurochlorate.[7] The sarcomas that developed were primarily gastric, and they were associated with gastric adenocarcinomas in 16% of cases. Interestingly, rats given MNNG orally without sodium taurochlorate did not develop GI sarcomas but rather developed gastric adenocarcinomas.[8,9] Pathologic evaluation in these instances showed less epithelial damage when MNNG was given without sodium taurochlorate. Some authors have concluded that damage to the normal mucosal barrier of the stomach must occur to allow MNNG to effectively cause GI sarcoma formation. This theory has been supported by experiments noting the development of GI sarcomas when MNNG is given in conjunction with aspirin, which is known to erode the gastric epithelial barrier.[10] Likewise, Wistar rats given MNNG with hot water appeared to develop esophageal sarcomas.[11] The hot water is believed to damage the esophageal epithelium enough to allow MNNG-induced sarcoma formation.

Certain infections in dogs have been associated with esophageal fibrosarcomas; however, no corresponding relationship has been noted in humans.[12] Gastrointestinal sarcomas have been noted in humans who have received radiation to the abdomen for the treatment of other malignancies, but an appreciable increase in risk has not been clearly demonstrated.[13]

Gastrointestinal sarcomas are associated with other primary tumors. Shiu and co-workers[14] noted that 27% of GI sarcomas were associated with other malignancies usually developing some years after the diagnosis of the GI sarcoma. Over 50% of the associated malignancies were adenocarcinomas of GI origin. This observation indicates that clinicians must maintain a high index of suspicion for secondary malignancies and close follow-up for their patients with GI sarcomas.

## Pathology

Sarcomas of the GI tract were first described by Golden and Stout[15] in 1949. Martin and co-workers[16] were the first to note the smooth muscle origin of some of these tumors. Stout described a bizarre form of smooth muscle proliferation and introduced the term *leiomyoblastoma*. Since then, improvements in pathology and clarification of the pathologic terms have led to a classification system that emphasizes the stromal description of the tumor (Table 68–1). The classification is generally divided into two parts based on features of differentiation. Some pathologists have further divided gastrointestinal stromal tumors (GIST) into gastrointestinal stromal sarcomas (GISS) representing those tumors with clear malignant features and GIST representing tumors of undetermined malignant potential.[17] Fortunately, recent reports largely use the term *GIST* to describe all stromal tumors with even the slightest dedifferentiation and in essence have combined *GIST* and *GISS* into a single classification referred to in the literature as *GIST*. Thus, the term *GI sarcomas* will be used in this chapter to describe all GIST with any evidence of malignant dedifferentiation.

A large part of the confusion regarding the nomenclature of these tumors stems from their relative rarity, which has allowed only a handful of pathologists to gain any significant experience with these tumors. Gastrointestinal sarcomas account for 1%–2% of all gastric tumors and 0.1% of all colorectal tumors.[18]

Tumor cells are spindle shaped with scant cytoplasm and hyperchromatic nuclei. Mitotic figures are common; a mitotic count of greater than 10 per 50 high-power field often defines a high-grade tumor and less than 10, a low-grade tumor.[19] This definition, however, remains controversial, as others have advocated five mitoses per 50 high-power field as an arbitrary measure of tumor grade.[20,21] Cellularity often corresponds with the tumor grade, as it is often high in high-grade tumors and low in low-grade tumors. Tumor necrosis is noted in high-grade tumors, but is usually absent in low-grade tumors.

Immunohistochemistry is an important modality in obtaining an accurate histologic diagnosis of GI sarcomas. Ueyama and co-workers[20] found that 92% of all GI sarcomas stained positive for muscle-specific actin (HHF35). Correspondingly, a positive reaction for S-100 denotes a tumor of Schwann cell origin. Although defining the cells of origin for GI sarcomas is of interest, the information does not appear to help in determining the

aggressiveness of these tumors. Pike and associates[22] found that most GI stromal tumors stained positive for desmin but that there was no difference in the positive reactions between more benign and malignant tumors. Saul and colleagues[23] also noted that immunoreactivity appeared to have no effect on determining whether the tumors are benign or malignant.

Nuclear atypia has been useful in distinguishing benign from malignant GI tumors. In general, tumors with greater than 5–10 mitoses per 50 high-power field are associated with nuclear atypia; patients with such tumors have a poor prognosis when compared with patients who have no nuclear atypia or fewer than 5–10 mitoses per 50 high-power field.[20]

## Molecular Biology

Advances in molecular biology have allowed researchers to gain a better understanding of the mechanisms behind sarcoma growth. Unfortunately, the rarity of GI sarcomas results in limited human tumor samples, which are needed to further investigate the driving forces behind sarcoma development, growth, and metastasis. Experiments involving human cell culture and sarcoma animal models, however, have shed some light on these complex mechanisms.

One of the most common genetic mutations seen in sarcomas involves the tumor suppressor gene *p53*. An estimated 30%–50% of all sarcomas harbor a *p53* mutation.[24] The precise role of *p53* mutations in sarcoma carcinogenesis remains uncertain, particularly in light of the fact that 50% or more of these tumors are without *p53* mutations. It is clear, however, that mutations of *p53* are more common in metastatic than in primary and high-grade or low-grade sarcomas.[25] In addition, *p53* mutated sarcomas are associated with significantly decreased overall survival when compared with sarcomas without *p53* mutations, which suggests that *p53* mutations play a tumorigenic role in aggressive sarcomas.[26]

Transfection of wild-type *p53* into human sarcoma cell lines that contain *p53* mutations has given insight into the role of *p53* in these tumors. The restoration of wild-type *p53* has been shown to inhibit cell proliferation in sarcoma cell lines and decrease tumorgenicity in a mouse tumor model.[27] The tumor suppressive effects appear to remain dependent on the overall expression of wild-type *p53*. Cells expressing low levels of wild-type *p53* show moderate suppression compared with cells expressing high levels of *p53*, which display much greater tumor suppression.

More recently, researchers have found aberrations not in a p53 pathway but in the closely related Rb–cyclin D pathway. It is clear that p53 works as a transcription factor that recognizes specific DNA fragments that flank important genes throughout the human genome. One of these genes is a protein whose function is to inhibit cyclin–cyclin-dependent kinases and thereby prevent phosphorylation of downstream targets. One of these downstream targets is pRb, whose function, when properly phosphorylated, is to prevent cells from entering the S phase of the cell cycle.[28] Dei Tos and co-workers[29] studied p53 and Rb–cyclin D pathways in human leiomyosarcoma specimens and found that mutations in the *p53* gene could only be seen in approximately 20% of cases. Aberrations of the Rb–cyclin D pathway, however, were noted in greater than 90% of cases, suggesting that one of the molecular defects that drives these tumors involves a pathway downstream from the often implicated p53 pathway. Continued research into p53 and Rb–cyclin D pathways may provide further insight into mechanisms of growth and metastasis.

While research into the role of *p53* in sarcoma tumor growth continues, researchers have found other molecular defects not seen in normal tissues. Hirota and colleagues[30] recently found

**Table 68–1** Classification of stromal tumors of the gastrointestinal tract

*Tumors with Well-developed Features of Differentiation*

Leiomyoma
Schwannoma
Glomus tumor
Neurofibroma/ganglioneuroma

*Gastrointestinal Sarcomas*[a]

GI sarcomas with primitive or incomplete myoid differentiation
GI sarcomas with primitive or incomplete neural differentiation
GI sarcomas with primitive or incomplete autonomic nerve differentiation (plexoma)
GI sarcomas with mixed neural/myoid differentiation

[a]Includes gastrointestinal stromal tumors (GIST) and gastrointestinal stromal sarcomas (GISS).

that point mutations of c-*kit* were present in 83% of GI sarcomas studied. In addition, when c-*kit* is transfected into Ba/F3 murine lymphoid cell lines, it exerts transformation of this cell line.[30]

Telomerase activity in GI sarcomas has also been studied in hopes of gaining insight into the molecular mechanisms of sarcoma carcinogenesis. Telomerase is a ribonucleoprotein that supplies telomeric DNA to the telomere. Its activity is suppressed in normal cells where progressive shortening of the telomere occurs at each cell division, eventually leading to programmed cell death.[31] Telomerase activity has been noted in 80%–90% of all cancers, which suggests that telomerase activity or its regulation in it plays an important role in carcinogenesis and tumor progression.[32,33] One study found that positive telomerase activity was more often seen in metastatic GI sarcomas than in primary GI sarcomas and that patients whose primary GI sarcomas demonstrated telomerase activity had a significantly decreased overall survival.[34] Other poor prognostic factors such as larger tumor size and increased numbers of mitoses were also associated with positive telomerase activity.

Milas and associates[35] investigated the relationship between telomerase activity and *p53* status to determine whether telomerase activity is affected by *p53* mutations. They found no association between telomerase activity and *p53* status, suggesting that the tumor suppresser effects of *p53* and the cell cycle–regulating effects of telomerase work independently in sarcoma cells.

## Natural History

### Esophageal Sarcomas

Esophageal sarcomas are so rare that their characterization in the literature comes largely from case reports. These sarcomas are primarily of smooth muscle origin (leiomyosarcoma) or fibrous origin (fibrosarcoma), with isolated reports of osteosarcomas and chondrosarcomas.[36–38] They appear to arise most commonly in the distal two-thirds of the esophagus and present in association with dysphagia (90%), weight loss (30%), regurgitation (20%), and retrosternal pain (20%).[3,39,40] The diagnosis is usually made by means of an upper barium study or endoscopic evaluation and biopsy. Computed tomography (CT) and endoscopic ultrasound are important in determining local invasion.

Surgery is the main therapeutic option; approximately 75% of tumors are amenable to complete resection (removal of all gross disease). Unfortunately, cure rates remain low (30% 5-year survival in most retrospective reports).[3,39] Several older reports note long-term survival after radiotherapy alone; however, it is not clear if the tumors reported were of low malignant potential and would have grown slowly even without radiation.[41,42]

### Gastric Sarcomas

Patients with gastric sarcomas present initially with vague symptoms including pain (20%–63%), anorexia (33%–45%), GI bleeding (36%–50%), and weight loss (20%–42%).[43,44] Approximately 10% of gastric sarcomas are found as a result of diagnostic evaluations for apparently unrelated conditions, most commonly at the time of esophagoduodenoscopy to rule out ulcer disease.

As expected, laboratory studies are nonspecific. Mild leukocytosis in conjunction with a microcytic anemia is often seen. Carcinoembryonic antigen (CEA) levels are normal even with extensive disease. Upper GI barium studies usually reveal a smooth-walled lesion marked by central ulceration. Endoscopy is useful in visualizing the lesion, but biopsies are conclusive in only 40% of cases.[43] Computed tomography is helpful in determining not only whether there is evidence of local invasion of adjacent organs but also whether liver metastases are present.

The percentage of patients presenting with metastatic disease varies from 19% in a series from Memorial Sloan-Kettering Cancer Center to 35% in a series from The University of Texas M. D. Anderson Cancer Center.[45,46] The most common sites of metastases include liver (60%), peritoneal surfaces (30%), and lung (10%). Gastric sarcomas, like GI sarcomas in general, rarely metastasize to lymph nodes; several large series demonstrate no positive lymph nodes.[44–46] Primary therapy involves surgical resection without attention to extensive lymphadenectomy. In one series, the 5-year survival for patients undergoing complete resection vs. incomplete resection was 40% vs. 0%, respectively.[46] The goal of resection, therefore, is clearly centered on complete excision with negative margins. Wedge resections or partial gastrectomies are viable options, as no survival advantage has been noted for more extensive resections.[47,48]

Survival for patients with gastric sarcomas is no different from that for patients with sarcomas elsewhere in the GI tract; the 5-year survival is approximately 30%.[44–46] As for patients with GI sarcomas at other sites, the prognosis for patients with gastric sarcomas is dependent on the grade of their sarcomas. Lindsay and co-workers[49] found a 5-year survival of 55% for patients with low-grade GI sarcomas versus and 12% for those with high-grade GI sarcomas. Likewise, Evans[19] noted a 5-year survival of 85% for patients with low-grade tumors and 5% for those with high-grade gastric and small bowel sarcomas[18] (Table 68–2).

**Table 68–2** Literature review of 5-year survival by tumor location and grade

| Study | Patients (n) | Tumor Location | 5-year Survival (%) |
|---|---|---|---|
| Shiu et al.[48] | | | |
| Grade not specified | 41 | Gastric | 54 |
| Lindsay et al.[49] | | | |
| Low grade | 10 | Gastric | 55 |
| High grade | 25 | Gastric | 12 |
| Akwari et al.[21] | | | |
| Low grade | 27 | Small bowel | 50 |
| High grade | 41 | Small bowel | 15 |
| Shiu et al.[14] | | | |
| Grade not specified | 18 | Small bowel | 37 |
| Evans[19] | | | |
| Low grade | 8 | Small bowel | 85 |
| High grade | 21 | Small bowel | 5 |
| Akwari et al.[21] | | | |
| Low grade | 10 | Colorectal | 50 |
| High grade | 4 | Colorectal | 0 |
| Meijer et al.[57] | | | |
| Low grade | 12 | Colorectal | 90 |
| High grade | 17 | Colorectal | 25 |
| Dougherty et al.[58] | | | |
| Low grade | 22 | All GI sites | 80 |
| High grade | 30 | All GI sites | 10 |
| Ng et al.[45] | | | |
| Low grade | 36 | All GI sites | 40 |
| High grade | 45 | All GI sites | 19 |
| Conlon et al.[46] | | | |
| Low grade | 12 | All GI sites | 65 |
| High grade | 26 | All GI sites | 10 |

## Small Bowel Sarcomas

Sarcomas comprise approximately 17% of all small bowel malignancies.[1] The small bowel subdivisions are involved in proportion to their length: one-third of small bowel sarcomas affect the jejunum and one-third affect the ileum. Adenocarcinoma of the small bowel is much more common than sarcoma in all segments except for Meckel's diverticulum, where sarcomas comprise 44% of all tumors.[50] For unknown reasons, sarcomas of the small bowel have been associated with metachronous malignancies at a rate of approximately 20%.[51]

Symptoms of small bowel sarcomas are usually nonspecific; pain and bleeding are seen in slightly more than 50% and a palpable mass, in only 20% of patients.[3] Unusual presentations have included hyperemesis from a β-chain human chorionic gonadotropin (β-HCG) producing sarcoma and small bowel torsion from a sarcoma of Meckel's diverticulum.[52,53]

An upper GI series with small bowel follow-through will identify an intraluminal lesion in 50% of cases.[14] Larger lesions can be detected by CT scan, while bleeding lesions can be detected by the tumor "blush" noted at angiography. Surgery is again the main treatment option and results in removal of all gross disease in approximately 60% of cases.[54]

Most studies have found that the actual GI location of a sarcoma has little bearing on overall survival. One study, however, found that patients with small bowel sarcomas had a slightly worse prognosis than that of patients with sarcomas at all other sites; however, the number of small bowel sarcomas in the series was low (4 vs. 34 sarcomas at other GI locations).[46] Five-year survival rates in most series are similar to those for other GI sarcomas: 50%–85% for patients with low-grade tumors and 5–15% for those with high-grade tumors (Table 68–2).[18,54] Median survival depends on the presence of localized disease (46 months) or metastatic disease (19 months).[54] As for gastric sarcomas, the site of failure is most often the liver or peritoneal surfaces.

## Colorectal Sarcomas

Sarcomas of the colon account for less than 0.1% of all colorectal malignancies.[55] Within the colon, the cecum appears to be a predominant site; rectal sarcomas are even more common, as they outnumber colonic sarcomas 2 to 1.[56] Presenting symptoms include pain (36%), bleeding (24%), and change in bowel habits (22%).[57] Colonoscopy with biopsy usually confirms the diagnosis, although negative biopsies are more common for these tumors than for colorectal adenocarcinoma.[56]

Curative surgery is less likely for colorectal sarcomas, as only 44% of such tumors are associated with complete excision. As with the other GI sarcomas, high-grade tumors are associated with a worse 5-year survival, with a 25% 5-year survival for high-grade tumors and a 90% 5-year survival for low-grade tumors (Table 68–2).[57,58] Pelvic CT and magnetic resonance imaging scans are particularly helpful in delineating local extent of disease in rectal sarcomas. Local failure remains a significant problem, with local recurrence noted in 25% of patients.[57] Approximately 33% of patients with resectable colorectal sarcomas will develop metastatic disease, primarily in the liver or peritoneum.[58]

Clinicians must be aware of a rare but well-documented paraneoplastic syndrome that can arise not only in patients with colorectal sarcomas but also in patients with GI sarcomas at any site. Hypoglycemia can occur in patients with GI sarcomas and is believed to be secondary to secretion of an insulin-like growth factor.[59,60] More recently, Hoff and Sellin[61] have advocated using a glucagon stimulation test to confirm the diagnosis. The best treatment for sarcoma-induced hypoglycemia is resection of the tumor. Patients with unresectable GI sarcomas have been treated with continuous glucagon infusions, usually through an implantable pump, resulting in symptomatic relief of their hypoglycemia.

## Recurrent Gastrointestinal Sarcomas

A continuing problem with treatment of GI sarcomas is their propensity to recur despite removal of all gross disease. Ng and associates[45] analyzed the extent of disease in 100 patients who died as a result of their GI sarcomas. They found that 89% had peritoneal disease and 78% had liver metastases at the time of death. Extraabdominal metastases were noted in only 28% of patients, with metastases to the lungs accounting for most of these.

Interestingly, it appears that recurrent disease in the liver develops irrespective of the prognostic factors associated with the primary tumor, while peritoneal recurrences are highly dependent on prognostic factors such as tumor grade and tumor size.[45] Patients with recurrent disease in the liver or on peritoneal surfaces when present in isolation can benefit from surgical resection if complete removal is possible. This is in contrast to patients with extraabdominal metastases, who should be offered resection more judiciously since this condition often represents a more biologically advanced disease state than intraabdominal metastases. A disease-free interval of greater than 18 months is associated with prolonged survival after metastatectomy.[45]

## References

1. Barclay THC, Schapira DV. Malignant tumors of the small intestine. Cancer 51:878–881, 1983.
2. Ranchod M, Kempson RL. Smooth muscle tumors of the gastrointestinal tract: a pathologic analysis of 100 cases. Cancer 39:255–262, 1977.
3. Licht JD, Weissmann LB, Antman K. Gastrointestinal sarcomas. Semin Oncol 15:181–188, 1988.
4. Martin JD, Grisamore JM. Leiomyosarcoma of the esophagus. Surg Gynecol Obstet 107:238–242, 1958.
5. Carney JA. The triad of gastric epitheliod leiomyosarcomas, pulmonary chondromas and extra-adrenal paragangliomas: a five-year review. Medicine 62:159–169, 1983.
6. Schaldenbrand JD, Appleman HD. Solitary solid stromal gastrointestinal tumors in von Recklinghausen's disease with minimal smooth muscle differentiation. Hum Pathol 15:229–232, 1984.
7. Cohen A, Geller SA, Horowitz I, et al. Experimental models for gastric leiomyosarcoma. Cancer 53:1088–1092, 1984.
8. Saito T, Sasaki M, Iwaamatsu M, Tamada R, Inokuchi K. Experimental gastric carcinoma induced by N-methyl-N'-nitro-N-nitrosoguanidine. J Cancer Res Clin Oncol 97:51–62, 1980.
9. Sugar J, Szentirmay Z, Kralovansky J. Pathologic features of N-methyl-N'-nitro-N-nitrosoguanidine–induced neoplastic and preneoplastic lesions of rat stomach. IARC Sci Publ 31:667–675, 1980.
10. Weisburger JH, Williams GM. Metabolism of chemical carcinogens. In: Becker FF (ed): Cancer: A Comprehensive Treatise, 2nd ed. Plenum Press, New York, 1982, pp 241–243.
11. H. Yioris N, Ivankovis S, Lehmert T. Effect of thermal injury and oral administration of N-methyl-N'-nitro-N-nitrosoguanidine on the development of esophageal tumors in Wistar rats. Oncology 41:36–38, 1984.
12. Bailey WS. Spirocerca lupi: a continuing injury. Parasitology 58:3–22, 1972.
13. Lieber MR, Winans CS, Griem ML, et al. Sarcomas arising after radiotherapy for peptic ulcer disease. Dig Dis Sci 30:593–599, 1985.
14. Shiu MH, Farr GH, Quan SHG, et al. Myosarcomas of the small and large bowel: a clinicopathologic study. J Surg Oncol 24:67–72, 1983.
15. Stout AP. Bizarre smooth muscle tumors of the stomach. Cancer 15:400–409, 1962.
16. Martin JF, Bazin P, Feroldi J, Cabanne F. Tumeurs myoides intramurales de l'estomac—considerations microscopiques a propos de 6 cas. Ann Anat Pathol 5:484–497, 1960.

17. Suster S. Gastrointestinal stromal tumors. Semin Diagn Pathol 13:297–313, 1996.
18. McGrath PC, Neifeld JP, Lawerence W, et al. Gastrointestinal sarcomas: analysis of prognostic factors. Ann Surg 207:706–710, 1987.
19. Evans HL. Smooth muscle tumors of the gastrointestinal tract. Cancer 56:2242–2250, 1985.
20. Ueyama T, Guo KJ, Hashimoto H, Daimaru Y, Enjoji M. A clinicopathologic and immunohistochemical study of gastrointestinal stromal tumors. Cancer 69:947–955, 1991.
21. Akwari OE, Dozois RR, Weiland LH, et al. Leiomyosarcoma of the large and small bowel. Cancer 42:1375–1384, 1978.
22. Pike A, Lloyd RV, Appleman H. Cell markers in gastrointestinal stromal tumors: an immunohistochemical study. Hum Pathol 19:830–834, 1988.
23. Saul SH, Rast ML, Brooks JJ. The immunohistochemistry of gastrointestinal tumors: evidence supporting an origin from smooth muscle. Am J Surg Pathol 11:464–473, 1987.
24. Toguchida J, Yamaguchi T, Ritchie B, et al. Mutation spectrum of the *p53* gene in bone and soft tissue sarcomas. Cancer Res 52:6194–6199, 1992.
25. Latres E, Drobnjak M, Pollack D, et al. Chromosome 17 and *p53* mutations in adult soft tissue sarcomas. Am J Pathol 145:345–355, 1994.
26. Drobnjak M, Latres E, Pollack D, et al. Prognostic implications of p53 nuclear overexpression and high proliferation index of Ki-67 in adult soft tissue sarcomas. J Natl Cancer Inst 86:549–554, 1994.
27. Pollack R, Lang A, Ge T, Sun D, Tan M, Yu D. Wild-type *p53* and a *p53* temperature-sensitive mutant suppress human soft tissue sarcoma by enhancing cell cycle control. Clin Cancer Res 4:1985–1994, 1998.
28. Hunter T, Pines J. Cyclins and cancer. II. Cyclin D and CDK inhibitors come of age. Cell 79:573–582, 1994.
29. Dei Tos AP, Maestro R, Doglioni C, et al. Tumor suppressor genes and related molecules in leiomyosarcoma. Am J Pathol 148:1037–1048, 1996.
30. Hirota S, Isozaki K, Yasuhiro M, et al. Gain-of-function mutations of c-*kit* in human gastrointestinal stromal tumors. Science 279:577–580, 1998.
31. Kim NW, Piatyszek MA, Prowse KR, Harley CB, West MD, Ho PL. Specific association of human telomerase activity with immortal cells and cancer. Science 266:2011–2015, 1994.
32. Hiyama K, Hiyama E, Ishioka S, Yamakido M, Inai K, Gazdar AF. Telomerase activity in small-cell and non–small-cell lung cancer. J Natl Cancer Inst 87:895–902, 1995.
33. Hiyama E, Yokoyama T, Tatsumoto N, Hiyama K, Imamura Y, Murakami Y. Telomerase activity in gastric cancer. Cancer Res 55:3258–3262, 1955.
34. Sakurai S, Fukayama M, Kaizaki Y, et al. Telomerase activity in gastrointestinal stromal tumors. Cancer 83:2060–2066, 1998.
35. Milas M, Yu D, Sun DT, Pollock RE. Telomerase activity of sarcoma cell lines and fibroblasts is independent of p53 status. Clin Cancer Res 4:1573–1579, 1998.
36. Bloch 1NIJ, Iozzo RV, Edmunds LH, et al. Polypoid synovial sarcoma of the esophagus. Gastroenterology 92:229–233, 1987.
37. McIntyre M, Webb JW, Browning JCP. Osteosarcoma of the esophagus. Hum Pathol 13:680–684, 1982.
38. Wolfel DA. Leiomyosarcoma of the esophagus. Am J Radiol 89:127–131, 1963.
39. Camishion RC, Gibbon JH, Templeton JV. Leiomyosarcoma of the esophagus. Ann Surg 53:951–956, 1961.
40. Ranier WG, Bras A. Leiomyosarcomas of the esophagus: review of the literature and report of three cases. Surgery 58:343–347, 1963.
41. Goodner JT, Miller TR, Watson WL. Sarcomas of the esophagus. Am J Radiol 89:132–139, 1963.
42. Athanasoulis CA, Aral IM. Leiomyosarcoma of the esophagus. Gastroenterology 54:271–274, 1968.
43. Lee JSY, Nascimento AG, Farnell MB, et al. Epithelioid gastric stromal tumors (leiomyoblastomas): a study of fifty-five cases. Surgery 118:653–660, 1995.
44. Grant CS, Kim CH, Farrugia G, et al. Gastric leiomyosarcoma: prognostic factors and surgical management. Arch Surg 126:985–990, 1991.
45. Ng EH, Pollock RE, Romsdahl MM. Prognostic implications of patterns of failure for gastrointestinal leiomyosarcomas. Cancer 69:1334–1341, 1992.
46. Conlon KC, Casper ES, Brennan MF. Primary gastrointestinal sarcomas: analysis of prognostic variables. Ann Surg Oncol 2:26–31, 1995.
47. Kimura H, Yonemura Y, Kadoya N, et al. Prognostic factors in primary gastrointestinal leiomyosarcoma: a retrospective study. World J Surg 15:771–777, 1991.
48. Shiu MH, Farr GH, Papachristou DN, et al. Myosarcomas of the stomach: natural history, prognostic factors, and management. Cancer 49:177–187, 1982.
49. Lindsay PC, Ordonez N, Raaf JH. Gastric leiomyosarcoma: clinical and pathological review of fifty patients. J Surg Oncol 18:399–421, 1981.
50. Coit DG. Cancer of the small intestine. In: DeVita VT, Hellman S, Rosenberg SA (eds): Cancer—Principles and Practice of Oncology, 5th ed. J.B. Lippincott, Philadelphia, 1997, pp 1128–1143.
51. Lee YM. Leiomyosarcoma of the gastrointestinal tract: general pattern and recurrence. Cancer Treat Rev 10:91–101, 1983.
52. Meredith RF, Wagman LD, Piper JA, et al. Beta-chain human chorionic gonadotropin-producing leiomyosarcoma of the small intestine. Cancer 58:131–135, 1986.
53. Weinstein EC, Dockerty MB, Waugh JM. Neoplasm of Meckel's diverticulum. Int Abstr Surg 116:103–111, 1963.
54. Ng EH, Pollock RE, Munsell MF, Atkinson EN, Romsdahl MM. Prognostic factors influencing survival in gastrointestinal leiomyosarcomas: implications for surgical management and staging. Ann Surg 215:68–77, 1992.
55. Khalfia AA, Bong WL, Rao VK, Williams MJ. Leiomyosarcoma of the rectum: report of a case and review of the literature. Dis Colon Rectum 31:34–35, 1986.
56. Astarjiam NA, Tseng CH, Keating JA, et al. Leiomyosarcomas of the colon: report of a case. Dis Colon Rectum 20:139–143, 1977.
57. Meijer S, Peretz T, Gaynor JJ, et al. Primary colorectal sarcoma: a retrospective review and prognostic factor study of 50 consecutive patients. Arch Surg 125:1163–1168, 1990.
58. Dougherty MJ, Compton C, Talbert M, Wood WC. Sarcomas of the gastrointestinal tract: separation into favorable and unfavorable prognostic groups by mitotic count. Ann Surg 214:569–574, 1991.
59. Immerman SC, Sener SF, Khandekar JD. Causes and evaluation of tumor-induced hypoglycemia. Arch Surg 117:905–908,1982.
60. Samaan NA, Pham FK, Sellin RV, et al. Successful treatment of hypoglycemia using glucagon in a patient with an extrahepatic tumor. Ann Int Med 113:404–406, 1990.
61. Hoff AO, Sellin RV. The role of glucagon administration in the diagnosis and treatment of patients with tumor hypoglycemia. Cancer 82:1585–1592, 1998.

# Chapter 69

# Clinical Aspects and Management of Gastrointestinal Sarcomas

## *Management Options: Potentially Resectable Gastrointestinal Sarcomas*

JANICE N. CORMIER AND PETER W.T. PISTERS

Gastrointestinal (GI) stromal tumors (GISTs), of which leiomyosarcomas represent a subset, have presented a diagnostic and therapeutic dilemma for decades. The complexity of defining these tumors is magnified by the rarity of their occurrence (accounting for only 0.1% to 3% of all GI malignancies) and by their anatomic heterogeneity (esophagus to anorectum). Most of the available data come from retrospective single-institution analyses of small series of patients treated over long periods. In addition, the variability in the histopathologic spectrum of these tumors and the uncertainty in their classification make accurate characterization of the risk of recurrence for individual patients difficult.

Surgery remains the primary treatment modality for localized and even locally advanced GI leiomyosarcomas (LMS), as this group of tumors has been particularly resistant to standard antisarcoma chemotherapy regimens. Several reports have addressed outcome after surgical resection of GI LMS.[1–4] These findings will be summarized in this chapter.

### Pathologic Classification

The histopathologic criteria for determining the malignant potential of GISTs have been poorly defined until relatively recently. Consequently, earlier series have often included a broad spectrum of lesions, including GI mesenchymal tumors of histologic type other than LMS, such as benign leiomyoma.[5] Several morphologic features have been found to be valuable in determining the malignant potential of GISTs.[6–10] Suster[7] proposed several morphologic criteria for determining malignancy, including tumor size larger than 5 cm, infiltration of adjacent structures, presence of tumor necrosis, increased nucleus/cytoplasm ratio, mitotic rate more than 1 to 5 per 10 high-power ($10\times$) field, and infiltration of overlying mucosa. In Suster's study, high-

grade tumors were defined by the extent and number of malignant features present; the presence of two or more malignant features within a single lesion was regarded as an indication of aggressive potential. Of these features, the most reliable and reproducible variable for histologic grading has been mitotic count; the presence of 2 to 5 mitoses per 10 high-power ($10\times$) field has been consistently associated with an increased risk for distant metastasis.[7,8]

### Clinical Presentation

#### Symptoms

Patients who have GI LMS often present with nonspecific GI symptoms, the nature of which depends on the site of the primary tumor. For example, in a series from Memorial Sloan-Kettering Cancer Center, early satiety and dyspepsia were associated with upper GI primary tumors, whereas tenesmus and altered bowel habits were common for tumors of the lower GI tract.[11,12] In another series that included 50 patients with colorectal LMS, 36% presented with abdominal pain, 24% with GI bleeding, and 22% with change in bowel habits.[13]

Several investigators have reported on the clinical presentation of GI LMS.[12,14] In a report of 80 patients with a variety of smooth muscle tumors of the upper and lower GI tract, the most common presenting symptoms and signs were GI bleeding (44%), abdominal mass (38%), and abdominal pain (21%).[9] Among 38 patients from Memorial Sloan-Kettering with GI LMS, 92% presented with symptoms including abdominal pain (63%), anorexia (45%), weight loss (42%), fatigue (32%), GI bleeding (either occult bleeding or hematochezia, 45%), or an abdominal mass (34%).[11] Interestingly, no patient in these series presented with visceral perforation, which likely reflects the fact that few patients are referred to a tertiary care center for emergency manifestations of malignancy. In contrast, other investigators have reported that 30% to 50% of patients with GI LMS present with surgical emergencies such as perforated viscus or life-threatening bleeding.[15,16] In a report limited to patients with small bowel tumors, Shiu et al.[12] noted that most of these patients presented with symptoms of abdominal pain, GI hemorrhage, tumor-related intestinal perforation (4 of 18 patients), intestinal obstruction, or an abdominal mass. This variability in clinical presentation likely relates to the referral-based (rather than the population-based) nature of the patient populations, the limitations of retrospective data collection, and the anatomic and histopathologic variability of these tumors.

## Radiographic and Endoscopic Findings

Establishing a preoperative diagnosis of GI LMS is often difficult. Radiologic assessment including computed tomography (CT) of the abdomen and pelvis can be useful in some cases to determine the tumor's anatomic location, size, and relationship to adjacent viscera. In a series from Memorial Sloan-Kettering, abnormalities on CT scans were noted for 97% of patients with GI LMS.[11] Patients with localized disease frequently present with a medium to large intraabdominal mass without radiographic evidence of regional lymph node metastases (which would be typical in patients with an adenocarcinoma of comparable size and anatomic location) (Fig. 69–1). In patients with advanced disease, CT scanning can demonstrate disseminated intraabdominal masses without the concomitant ascites and infiltration of tissue planes usually associated with locally advanced adenocarcinoma (Fig. 69–2).

Endoscopy, either esophagogastroduodenoscopy or colonoscopy, has become the mainstay for evaluating symptoms related to the GI tract. For tumors involving the stomach, upper endoscopy with endoscopic ultrasonography and biopsy can frequently distinguish adenocarcinoma from gastric LMS. This distinction is clinically significant because the extent of resection (gastrectomy vs. local excision) and the need for regional lymph node dissection are different for these two conditions. However, this technique may not be sufficient to distinguish LMS from its benign counterpart, leiomyoma. In two series, preoperative endoscopic biopsy of gastric tumors provided a histologic diagnosis in only 50% of patients.[11,17]

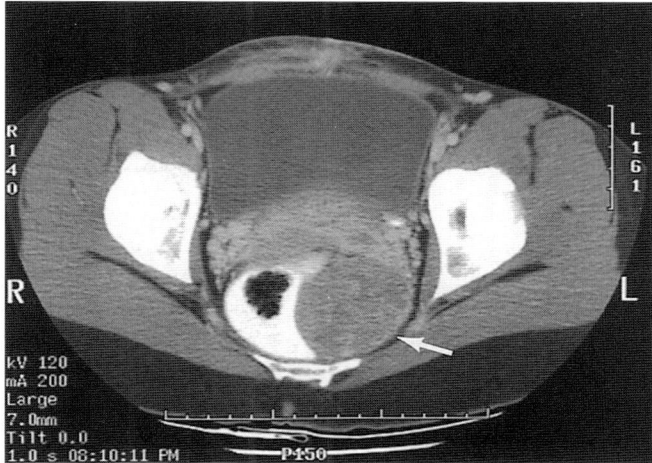

**Figure 69–2** Computed tomography scan from a 35-year-old woman with disseminated intraabdominal masses (sarcomatosis) originating from small bowel leiomyosarcoma that had been resected 6 months before. Large tumor implants in the pelvis (the largest of which is marked with an arrow) have displaced the uterus and rectum without direct invasion.

## Surgical Options for Localized and Locally Advanced Disease

Preoperative evaluation of patients with suspected GI LMS includes CT staging and endoscopic evaluation with tissue biopsy whenever feasible. This information assists in preoperative planning and provides an opportunity for referral of patients to centers with expertise in performing en bloc tumor resection if the staging evaluation reveals a locally advanced mass.

### Gastric Tumors

The results of treatment of gastric LMS were once thought to be better than those for LMS at other GI sites.[6] Overall 5-year survival rates after potentially curative resection for gastric LMS have ranged from 32% to 63%.[14,18] As is true for LMS at other GI sites, high-grade histology and large tumor size (>5 cm) adversely affect prognosis.

Table 69–1 summarizes results from five studies of surgical resection for gastric stromal tumors.[2,6,17,19,20] As is common for retrospective reports covering extended periods, the series included a heterogeneous group of gastric stromal tumors, occasionally including benign leiomyomas. In one study, benign tumors constituted most of the reported cases and were included in the analysis of disease-specific survival.[6] Inclusions such as these make comparison of survival data among series quite difficult and have led to the probably false impression that gastric LMS has a more favorable prognosis than LMS arising elsewhere in the GI tract.

For localized disease, the therapeutic benefit of total gastrectomy over local excision has long been debated. Although a prospective trial has never been conducted, several retrospective studies have failed to show significant survival differences related to the extent of surgical resection.[2,6,17,20] In a series of 53 patients with gastric LMS from the Mayo Clinic, wide local ex-

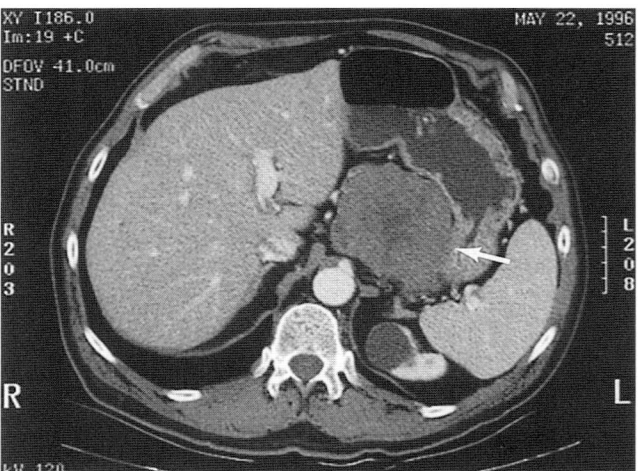

**Figure 69–1** Computed tomography scan of a 59-year-old patient with a 10.5-cm gastrointestinal leiomyosarcoma arising from the posterior gastric fundus (arrow) without associated regional adenopathy.

**Table 69-1** Summary of clinical reports of gastric stromal tumors[a]

| Factor | M. D. Anderson, 1980[19] | M. D. Anderson, 1981[20] | Mayo Clinic, 1991[2] | Roswell Park, 1994[17] | Lahey Clinic, 1996[6] |
|---|---|---|---|---|---|
| GI stromal tumors | 43 | 50 | 53 | 32 | 46 |
| Gastric LMS | 43 | 50 | 53 | 30 | 9 |
| Operation performed | | | | | |
|    Wedge resection | NR | 20 | 30 | 11 | 19 |
|    Formal gastrectomy | NR | 23 | 22 | 18 | 21 |
|    Other | NR | 7 | 1 | 3 | 6 |
| Complete resection | 29 (67%) | 34 (68%) | 45 (85%) | 21 (66%) | |
| Adjacent organs resected | | | 15 (28%) | 12 (38%) | |
| Recurrences (distant + local) | 46% (local only) | NR | 19 (36%) | NR | NR |
| Median survival | | | | | |
|    After curative resection | 34 months | 44 months | NR | 40 months | NR |
|    After palliative resection | 14.5 months | NR | NR | 8 months | NR |
| 5-year overall survival | NR | 19% | NR | 26% | NR |
|    After curative resection | 38% | 32% | 61% | 34% | 95% |
|    After palliative resection | NR | NR | NR | 10% | 60% |

Abbreviations: GI, gastrointestinal; LMS, leiomyosarcomas; NR, not reported. [a]Units are numbers of patients unless otherwise indicated,

cision was performed in 30 patients (57%); distal subtotal gastrectomy, in 16 patients (30%); total gastrectomy, in 2 patients (4%); and esophagogastrectomy, in 4 patients (8%).[2] The overall rate of potentially curative resection was 85% and the 5-year survival rate for the patients who underwent curative resection was 61%. Again, large tumor size and high-grade histology were shown to be adverse prognostic factors. Isolated local recurrence occurred in only three patients, two of whom had large, high-grade tumors, one of which ruptured during resection. The only patient with an isolated local recurrence who may have benefited from initial gastrectomy remained disease-free 5 years after local excision of the recurrence. The authors concluded that among patients who underwent curative resection, the type of operation was not significantly associated with survival after adjustments were made for histologic grade and tumor size.[2]

On the basis of the existing literature and the relative infrequency of local recurrence compared to that of distant recurrences, the general recommendation for surgical management of gastric LMS is that if resection with a microscopically negative surgical margin can be achieved with partial gastrectomy or wedge resection, then those techniques are reasonable alternatives to total gastrectomy. However, there may be cases in which local excision presents technical challenges to the surgeon owing to tumor location or size. For example, achieving an adequate proximal surgical margin may not be possible for gastric LMS located near the gastroesophageal junction without a total or proximal subtotal gastrectomy. Large LMS arising from the stomach that invade or are inseparable from adjacent organs should be resected en bloc with the adjacent involved viscera to ensure satisfactory gross and microscopic surgical margins.

Lymphatic spread is not the primary route of metastasis. Lymphatic spread has been reported in only 0% to 16% of cases of GI LMS.[2,14,17,20,21] In the series from Bedikian et al.,[19] none of the 29 patients who had curative gastrectomy had perigastric lymph node metastases. As discussed later in this chapter, most recurrent disease appears with systemic metastases as the first site of failure rather than locoregional failure.[4] Consequently, routine lymphadenectomy is not recommended as part of the resection for gastric LMS.

## Small Bowel and Large Bowel Tumors

Segmental resection of the small or large intestine is the standard treatment for GI LMS arising from these sites. For tumors in the jejunum, ileum, or colon, the tumor is excised with the involved segment of intestine and its mesentery, without any formal mesenteric lymphadenectomy.[21] For patients undergoing complete excision of LMS in the small or large bowel, 5-year survival rates range between 40% and 50%.[8,10,14,22]

In another series from Memorial Sloan-Kettering involving 38 patients with GIST involving the small or large intestine,[21] tumors that were intraluminal, small, and noninvasive could be successfully treated by excision or segmental bowel resection, producing a 5-year survival rate of 86%. Ten (71%) of 14 patients with small GI sarcomas (defined as tumors with a diameter of up to 5 cm) survived 5 years compared with 4 (27%) of 15 patients with larger GI sarcomas (>5 cm). The authors of this study concluded that small, noninvasive sarcomas of the small intestine and colon can be treated by segmental resection of bowel with a wedge excision of mesentery, but that complete resection of large tumors and those invading adjacent organs usually requires a more extensive surgical procedure that frequently involves multiorgan resection.[21]

The duodenum is a unique segment of the GI tract because of its anatomic relationship to the head of the pancreas and distal common bile duct. Local excision of duodenal sarcomas may be possible for very small tumors located on the antimesenteric surface of the duodenum. However, pancreaticoduodenectomy is usually required for large tumors or those involving the head of the pancreas (Fig. 69–3).[1,21]

## Rectal Tumors

For LMS originating in the rectum, the surgical approach is again based on the anatomic location and size of the tumor. Meijer et al.[13] reviewed the experience of 50 patients with primary colorectal sarcoma at Memorial Sloan-Kettering. In 32 cases, the primary tumor was located in the rectum, and 18 tumors involved the colon. Of the rectal lesions, 15 were treated by abdomino-

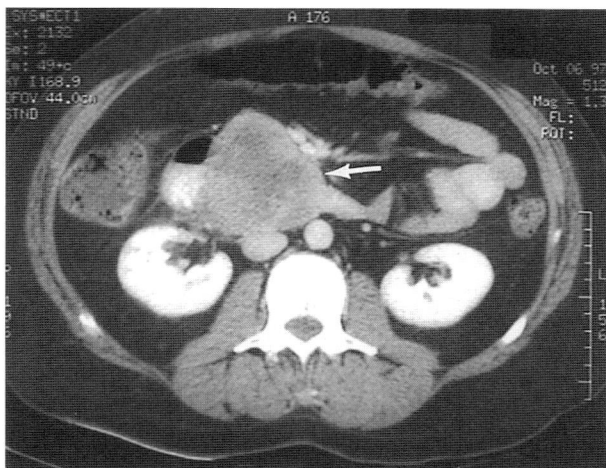

**Figure 69-3** Contrast-enhanced CT scan of a 10-cm gastrointestinal stromal tumor (arrow) arising from the third portion of the duodenum with extension into the uncinate process and inferior pancreatic head. Resection was accomplished by extended pancreaticoduodenectomy.

perineal resection, and 12 were treated with local excision. As has been found for LMS at other anatomic sites, the extent of surgery had no discernible effect on outcome.

For small lesions in the lower rectum, a transanal resection may allow negative-margin resection. Large or locally invasive lesions may require more extensive operations for complete tumor extirpation (Fig. 69–4).[1,13] In the series of GI stromal tumors discussed earlier,[21] 8 of 17 patients with rectal LMS required an abdominoperineal resection, and 3 of 17 patients had lesions that necessitated total pelvic exenteration for tumor clearance.

## Recurrent Disease

Recurrences are common after resection of GI LMS and can occur many years after initial treatment. In one series, 69% of patients who underwent a complete resection died of recurrent dis-

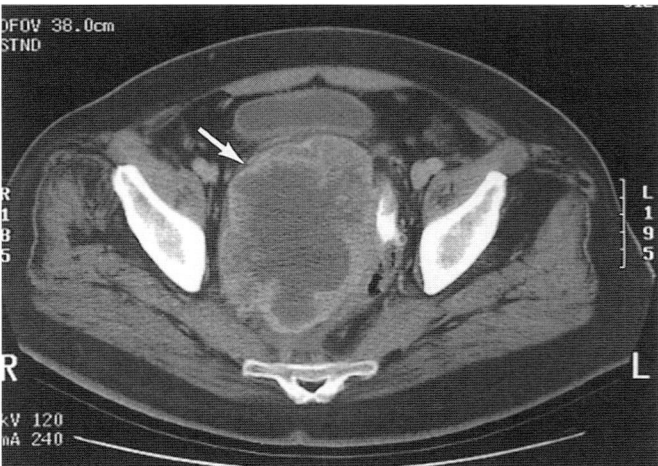

**Figure 69-4** Computed tomography scan with rectal contrast demonstrating a 12.0 × 8.5 cm pelvic mass in a 50-year-old man. The mass was resected en bloc by total pelvic exenteration. Pathologic examination revealed origin from the rectum.

ease.[23] The predominant pattern of failure is peritoneal recurrence or liver metastases.[24,25] In a study by Ng and colleagues[4] from The University of Texas M. D. Anderson Cancer Center, 50% of patients with GI LMS had liver metastases as the first site of recurrence. For other forms of soft tissue sarcoma, the pulmonary parenchyma is the most common site of first failure.

Regional recurrence in the peritoneum (sarcomatosis) is the other predominant site of failure after complete surgical resection. Patients with high-grade tumors, incomplete tumor resections, or tumors that before or during surgery rupture are at higher risk for regional recurrences.[9,10,14] The median survival time for these patients has been reported to be 18 to 24 months. In a recent report examining the outcome of 19 patients with sarcomatosis originating from GIST, the 2-year overall survival rate was 37%, and the median time from the diagnosis of sarcomatosis to death was 14 months.[26] Of 37 patients with sarcomatosis of various histologic types in one study, those with low-volume disease (<5 cm tumor diameter or <10 peritoneal nodules) had a 2-year survival rate of 75% compared with only 14% for patients with larger-volume disease (>5 cm tumor or >50 peritoneal nodules).[26]

Some patients with isolated liver metastases from visceral LMS can benefit from hepatic resection. Eleven patients underwent resection of isolated LMS metastases at Johns Hopkins University.[23] The median overall survival time for these patients after resection was 39 months; of the six patients who underwent a complete resection, five were alive at a median follow-up of 53 months. In another recent report of 26 patients with hepatic metastases from gastrointestinal LMS, the median survival time in the subset of 15 patients who underwent resection with negative tumor margins was 32 months, with a 5-year actuarial survival rate of 20%.[24] These authors concluded that hepatic resection may be appropriate for carefully selected patients with isolated hepatic recurrence. Surgical resection may be an effective treatment for isolated recurrences at other distant sites as well.[3]

## Outcome

Table 69–1 summarizes five studies of patients with GISTs of gastric origin.[2,6,17,19,20] The rate of potentially curative resection for gastric LMS in these series ranged from 66% to 85%, with an overall 5-year survival rate of approximately 25%. The 5-year survival rate after curative resection was 32% to 61%, excluding the study noted earlier that involved with predominantly benign tumors.[6]

Table 69–2 summarizes the published experience for the entire spectrum of GISTs.[1,3,5,9–11,13,14,18,21,25,27] The 5-year survival rate for all patients with GISTs has ranged from 20% to 45% and has reached 75% for early-stage tumors that were completely excised. In the two largest series, the actuarial 5-year survival rate for all patients ranged from 28% to 35%.[10,25] Again, patients with complete resections had better overall survival rates than those who underwent an incomplete resection.

## Prognostic Factors

Gastrointestinal LMS vary widely in their clinical behavior. Of the various prognostic factors that have been analyzed, the clinicopathologic factor most consistently shown to affect survival has been tumor grade. To date, the most important and reproducible morphologic feature identified in determining tumor grade for LMS has been the mitotic rate.[7,8,22,28] To assess the

**Table 69-2** Summary of clinical reports on gastrointestinal stromal tumors[a]

| Factor | Memorial Sloan-Kettering, 1982[21] | Cleveland Clinic, 1982[27] | Medical College of Virginia, 1987[14] | China, 1988[5] | Memorial Sloan-Kettering, 1990[13] | Japan, 1991[3] | M. D. Anderson, 1992[10] | Roswell Park, 1995[1] | Memorial Sloan-Kettering, 1995[11] | Taiwan, 1996[9] | New Orleans, 1998[18] | Memorial Sloan-Kettering, 2000[25] |
|---|---|---|---|---|---|---|---|---|---|---|---|---|
| GI stromal tumors | 38 | 28 | 51 | 160 | 50 | 36 | 191 | 39 | 38 | 80 | 12 | 200 |
| LMS | 34 | 28 | 44 | 87 | 49 | 36 | 191 | 37 | 35 | 45 | 0 | |
| *Site* | | | | | | | | | | | | |
| Esophagus | 0 | 0 | 3 | 1 | 0 | 2 | 0 | 0 | 0 | 1 | 0 | 2 |
| Stomach | 0 | 0 | 26 | 34 | 0 | 18 | 72 | 0 | 20 | 32 | 7 | 78 |
| Small bowel | 18 | 28 | 14 | 37 | 0 | 16 | 79 | 32 | 9 | 33 | 3 | 63 |
| Large bowel | 3 | 0 | 5 | 3 | 32 | 0 | 22 | 4 | 2 | 2 | 1 | 11 |
| Rectum | 17 | 0 | 3 | 12 | 18 | 0 | 0 | 3 | 7 | 12 | 1 | 21 |
| Other | | | | | | | 18 | | | | | 25 |
| Complete resection | 20 (53%) | 22 (79%) | 30 (59%) | NR | 32 (64%) | 27 (75%) | 99 (52%) | 6 (15%) | 27 (71%) | 36 (45%) | 11 (92%) | 80 (40%) |
| *Stage at Presentation* | | | | | | | | | | | | |
| I | NR | NR | NR | NR | NR | NR | NR | 2 | NR | NR | 7 | NR |
| II | NR | NR | NR | NR | NR | NR | NR | 3 | NR | NR | 2 | NR |
| III | NR | NR | NR | NR | NR | NR | NR | 1 | NR | NR | 0 | NR |
| IVA | NR | NR | NR | NR | NR | NR | NR | | NR | NR | 2 | NR |
| IVB | NR | NR | NR | NR | NR | NR | NR | 28 | NR | NR | 0 | NR |
| Not known | | | | | | | | 6 | | | 1 | |
| Overall 5-year survival rate | 44% | 45% | 40% | 43% | NR | NR | 28% | 20% | 28% | 20% | NR | 35% |
| 5-year survival rate with curative resection | 65% | NR | 63% | NR | 62% | 75% | 48% | NR | NR | 20% | NR | 54% |

GI, gastrointestinal; LMS, leiomyosarcomas; NR, not reported.

[a]Units are numbers of patients unless otherwise indicated.

**Table 69–3** Overall stage-specific 5-year survival rates of 109 patient with gastrointestinal leiomyosarcoma according to the M. D. Anderson Cancer Center staging classification

| Tumor Stage | TGM Classification | Patients n (%) | Overall 5-Year Survival Rates (%) |
|---|---|---|---|
| I | T1 G1 M0 | 10 (7) | 75 |
| II | T2 G1 M0 | 12 (9) | 52 |
| III | T1–2 G2 M0, or T3 any G M0 | 47 (34) | 28 |
| IVA | M1 or residual disease after surgery | 46 (33) | 12 |
| IVB | T4 | 24 (17) | 7 |

Abbreviations: T1, localized, <5 cm; T2, localized, ≥5 cm; T3, contiguous organ invasion or peritoneal implants, any size; T4, tumor ruptured, any size. G1, low grade; G2, high grade. M0, no metastases; M1, metastases present. Modified from Ng et al.,[10] with permission.

contribution of various pathologic factors, investigators from M. D. Anderson evaluated the surgical specimens from 56 patients with LMS and 10 years of follow-up. Expert pathologic review demonstrated that other histologic variables such as cellularity, nuclear pleomorphism, and tumor necrosis did not provide significant additional prognostic information beyond that provided by mitotic rate alone.

Most investigators evaluating prognostic factors in patients with GI LMS have found high-grade histology to be an adverse prognostic factor for survival.[1,6,9–12,14] The median survival duration for patients with low-grade tumors was 33 to 43 months, compared with 15 to 36 months for those with high-grade tumors.[1,10,11] In a recent report from Memorial Sloan-Kettering of 27 patients who underwent complete tumor resection, those with low-grade tumors had a 5-year survival rate of 72%, compared with only 18% for those with high-grade tumors.[11]

Tumor size is also a well-known prognostic factor; the most commonly used cut-off is 5 cm. Patients with tumors smaller than 5 cm survive longer (median, 68 months) than patients with tumors larger than 10 cm.[1,9,21]

Another factor associated with adverse prognosis is tumor rupture. Tumor rupture places patients at increased risk for early regional recurrence.[4,10] Patients whose tumors rupture before or during surgical resection, even if all gross disease is removed, have event-free outcomes similar to those of patients who undergo incomplete resection, with median survival time of only 17 months.[4,10] In one study, patients with sarcomatosis or visceral metastases had median survival times of 23 and 19 months.[10] In another series in which 74% of patients presented with sarcomatosis, the median survival time from diagnosis was only 7.4 months.[1]

The prognostic significance of tumor extension to adjacent viscera is less certain. Several authors have reported that tumor invasion into adjacent organs eventually proves fatal despite extended en bloc resections.[9,12,14,19,21] However, other authors have concluded that the need for resection of contiguous organs did not adversely affect survival if the primary tumor was completely excised.[10,11] The overall therapeutic recommendation for patients with tumor extension to adjacent organs, like that for patients with isolated hepatic metastases, is that en bloc resection of locally advanced disease may be reasonable in otherwise healthy patients with good performance status, particularly in the absence of effective nonsurgical therapies.

Ng and colleagues[10] proposed a staging system for GI LMS based on their prognostic factor analysis (Table 69–3). In this system, the determinants of stage are tumor size (T), including adjacent organ invasion, and tumor rupture; tumor grade (G); and metastases (M). Using this classification, Ng and colleagues were able to stratify overall 5-year survival rates by stage: stage I, 75%; stage II, 52%; stage III, 28%; stage IVA, 12%; and stage IVB, 7% (Fig. 69–5).[10]

### Recent Therapeutic Advances

The distinctive molecular features of GISTs have been better characterized over the last 5 years. These tumors are thought to arise from a pacemaker cell within the gastrointestinal tract known as the interstitial cell of Cajal.[29,30] The interstitial cells of Cajal and GIST cells express the hematopoietic progenitor cell marker CD34 and the growth factor receptor c-Kit (CD117).[31–33] c-Kit is a transmembrane glycoprotein receptor with an internal tyrosine kinase component that when activated triggers a cascade of intracellular signals regulating cell growth and survival.[34–36]

c-Kit expression has emerged as an important defining feature of GISTs. Treatment with imatinib (Gleevec, ST1571), a selective c-Kit inhibitor, has resulted in impressive clinical responses in a large percentage of patients with advanced GISTs. Mutations of c-Kit are common in GISTs, and most of the mutations result from an in-frame deletion or a point mutation in exon 11 (the juxtamembrane domain). These mutations, which occur predominantly in malignant GISTs,[37] lead to ligand-independent activation of the tyrosine kinase of c-Kit.[31] The re-

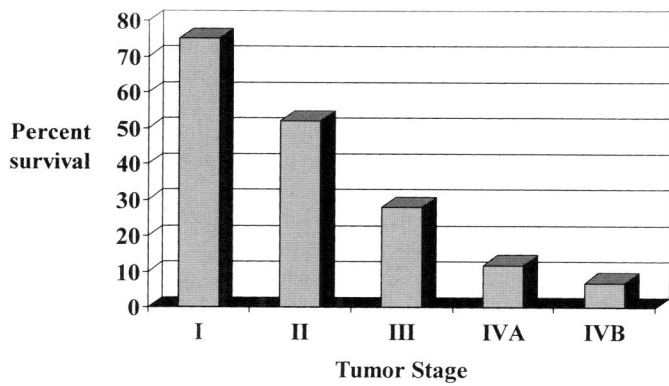

**Figure 69–5** Stage-specific 5-year survival rates for 139 patients who underwent surgery for gastrointestinal leiomyosarcoma at M. D. Anderson Cancer Center. (From Ng et al.,[10] with permission.)

famide and growth factors in chemotherapy-naive patients with soft-tissue sarcomas. Sarcoma 1(3,4):198, 1997.

21. Edmonson J, Marks R, Buckner J, Mahoney M. Contrast of response to D-MAP + sargramostim between patients with advanced malignant gastrointestinal stromal tumors and patients with other advanced leiomyosarcomas. Proc Am Soc Clin Oncol 18:541a, 1999.

22. Patel SR, Jenkins J, Papadopoulos NE, Burgess MA, Plager C, Pisters PWT, Feig BW, Hunt K, Pollack A, Zagars G, Pollock RE, Benjamin RS. Preliminary results of a two-arm phase 2 trial of gemcitabine in patients with gastrointestinal leiomyosarcomas and other soft-tissue sarcomas [abstract 2091]. Proc Am Soc Clin Oncol 18:541a, 1999.

23. Mavligit GM, Zukiwski AA, Salem PA, Lamki L, Wallace S. Regression of hepatic metastases from gastrointestinal leiomyosarcoma after hepatic arterial chemoembolization. Cancer 68:321–323, 1991.

24. Mavligit GM, Zukwiski AA, Ellis LM, Chuang VP, Wallace S. Gastrointestinal leiomyosarcoma metastatic to the liver. Durable tumor regression by hepatic chemoembolization infusion with cisplatin and vinblastine. Cancer 75:2083–2088, 1995.

25. Holtz D, Bilimoria M, Mirza N, et al. Recent experience with sarcomatosis: low volume disease predicts for improved survival. Proceedings of the 5th Annual Scientific Meeting of the Connective Tissue Oncology Society, Washington, D.C., 1999.

26. Eilber FC, Rosen G, Forscher C, Nelson SD, Dorey FJ, Eilber FR. Surgical resection and intraperitoneal chemotherapy for recurrent abdominal sarcomas. Ann Surg Oncol 6:645–650, 1999.

27. Tuveson DT, Fletcher CDM, Singer S, et al. STI571 inactivation of the GIST c-KIT oncoprotein: biological and clinical implications. Oncogene 20:5054–5058, 2001.

28. Joensuu H, Roberts PJ, Sarlomo-Rikala M, et al. Effect of the tyrosine kinase inhibitor STI571 in a patient with a metastatic gastrointestinal tumor. N Engl J Med 344:1052–1056, 2001.

29. Van Oosterom AT, Judson I, Verweij J, et al. STI 571, an active drug in metastatic gastrointestinal stromal tumors, an EORTC phase 1 study. Lancet 358:1421, 2001.

30. Judson IR, Verweij J, van Oosterom A, et al. Imatinib, an active agent for GIST but not for other soft-tissue sarcoma subtypes not characterized for KIT and PDGF-R expression—results of an EORTC phase 2 study [abstract 1608]. Proc Am Soc Oncol 21:403a, 2002.

31. von Mehren M, Blanke CD, Joensuu H, et al. Evaluation of the safety and efficacy of an oral molecularly targeted therapy STI 571, in patients with unresectable or metastatic gastrointestinal stromal tumors expressing C-KIT (CD 117) [abstract 1609]. Proc Am Soc Oncol 21:403a, 2002.

32. Demetri GD, von Mehren M, Blanke CD, et al. Efficacy and safety of imatinib mesylate in advanced gastrointestinal stromal tumors. N Engl J Med 347:472–480, 2002.

# Part III

# Palliative Care of Patients with Gastrointestinal Malignancy

# Chapter 71

# Nutritional Support of Patients with Gastrointestinal Malignancies

FLORIAN STRASSER AND EDUARDO BRUERA

Malnutrition is a frequent problem in patients with gastrointestinal malignancies and is distressing for both the patients and their families.[1] Because many malnutrition-associated symptoms, such as anorexia and asthenia, are silent symptoms, unlike pain or shortness of breath, the importance of malnutrition is often underestimated, and malnutrition is underdiagnosed.[2] Malnutrition can be categorized as primary (metabolic) or secondary (starvation) cachexia, which often occur together. Because their respective treatments frequently differ, it is important to distinguish between these two types of cachexia. *Primary cachexia* is a paraneoplastic, metabolic cancer anorexia–cachexia syndrome (ACS), whereas *secondary cachexia* is a condition resulting from impaired nutritional intake secondary to obstacles in the gastrointestinal tract or other disorders of gastrointestinal function. To highlight the complexity of nutritional issues in patients with cancer, the term *malnutrition/cachexia* will be used in this chapter. Its management involves multiple health-care professionals participating in the decision making.

This chapter will focus on malnutrition/cachexia in patients with advanced disease because this disorder occurs with higher frequency and has a greater impact during the later stages of cancer, although some suggestions will be made about the nutritional approach at the earlier stages of illness.

## Definition of Malnutrition/Cachexia

*Malnutrition/cachexia* is usually defined by the presence of weight loss. An involuntary weight loss of more than 5% of the patient's pre-illness weight or more than 5% within the previous 6 months is considered to be clinically significant.[3] Other parameters, such as hypoalbuminemia, anorexia, asthenia,[4,5] chronic nausea,[6,7] changes in body image, reduced caloric intake, or a clinical judgment of reduced muscle and fat mass, can serve as criteria for the presence of malnutrition/cachexia.[3] These additional criteria can help detect malnutrition/cachexia in patients with relevant fluid retention (pleural effusion, ascites, edema), where the extent of weight loss due to malnutrition/cachexia is masked by the accumulation of fluids.[8] No standardized criteria are currently available for either diagnosing malnutrition/cachexia or differentiating primary from secondary cachexia in patients with advanced cancer.

## Epidemiology of Malnutrition/Cachexia

Weight loss affects the vast majority of patients with neoplastic disease, and occurs in more than 80% of patients with terminal-stage disease.[9] The classic study by DeWys and colleagues[10] showed that 54% of 3074 patients who had various different tumors and who were recruited by the Eastern Cooperative Oncology Group (ECOG) for chemotherapy trials experienced weight loss (46% of patients had 0% weight loss; 22% of patients had 0% to 5% weight loss; 17% of patients had 5% to 10% weight loss; 15% of patients had >10% weight loss). The weight loss was assessed by patient interviews for the 6 months before study entry and was expressed as a percentage determined on the basis of the patient's weight before illness (except in cases of pancreatic cancer, in which weight loss was assessed for the previous 2 months).[10] Numerous other studies have documented high frequencies of weight loss, ranging from 24% to 83%, at the time of the diagnosis of cancer—i.e., before chemotherapy or surgery[11–14]—and increasing frequency with more advanced disease.[15–17] However, the reported frequencies vary widely, even in cases of an individual primary tumor.[13]

In patients with advanced pancreatic cancer, for example, the frequencies reported in recently published phase II and phase III studies were 36% (*n* [patients at enrollment] = 25),[18] 47% (*n* =

in various wasting conditions, including cancer cachexia, sepsis, and fasting.[107] Data from experimental cachexia models show increased expression of both ubiquitine protein $E_2$ and proteasome subunits.[99,108,109] This process is independent of the amount of protein consumed.

Lipid-mobilizing factor has been demonstrated in the serum and urine of patients with cancer cachexia. Experimentally, it caused the immediate release of glycerol when animals were intubated with epididymal adipodicytes,[110–112] and clinically correlated with both the extent of weight loss[113] and the patient's response to chemotherapy.[114] Lipid-mobilizing factor is believed to counteract the two major proposed mechanisms of the decrease in body lipids in patients with cancer cachexia—mainly, the inhibition of the clearing enzyme lipoprotein lipase, which prevents adipocytes from extracting fatty acids from plasma lipoproteins for storage, and the direct stimulation of triglyceride hydrolysis in adipocytes by activation of triglyceride lipase.

The role of cortisol in the propagation of malnutrition/cachexia is not well established. The infusion of cortisol can cause protein loss, acute-phase protein response, increased energy expenditure, and glucose intolerance,[115,116] and elevated levels of cortisone and glucagon have been shown in patients with cancer.[117–121] Data from an in vivo study in a mouse model showed no improvement in weight loss during treatment with mifepristone/RU38486, an anticortisol medication.[122]

## Mechanism of anorexia

The pathogenesis of anorexia, or reduction in appetite, and the relationship between anorexia and weight loss are matters of further investigation. Anorexia can occur without weight loss, but also with other clinical features of malnutrition/cachexia.[123] Whether anorexia and weight loss are different presentations of the same syndrome or different pathogenetic mechanisms needs to be revealed. As discussed above, proinflammatory cytokines can have anorexic effects (e.g., hormones in the hypothalamus may contribute to anorexia, since serotonergic activity in the hypothalamus can be anorectic). One study found that levels of free tryptophan, the precursor of serotonin, were increased in cancer patients and were associated with reduced food intake.[124] Neuropeptide-Y levels are probably lower in anorectic cancer patients than in healthy control subjects. Experimental data from tumor-bearing rats failed to show that neuropeptide-Y injected in the the hypothalamic region could simulate feeding.[125] The significance of leptin, a hormone produced by fat tissue and that suppresses appetite and increases energy expenditure to maintain weight stability, is unclear. Leptin is the primary signal through which the hypothalamus senses nutritional state and modulates food intake and energy balance. Leptin reduces food intake by down-regulating appetite-stimulating factors, primarily neuropeptide-Y4, and by up-regulating appetite-reducing neuropeptides, such as melanocyte-stimulating hormones. Leptin levels are increased in some models of inflammation.[126,127] Initial data in patients with cancer and weight loss, however, showed low levels of leptin.[128] A recent study showed that cannabinoid CB1 receptor knockout mice eat less than their wild-type littermates do, and the CB1 antagonist SR141716A reduces food intake in wild-type but not knockout mice. Findings that defective leptin signaling is associated with elevated hypothalamic but not cerebellar levels of endocannabinoids (in obese *db/db* and *ob/ob* mice and Zucker rats) and that acute treatment of normal rats and *ob/ob* mice with leptin reduces anandamide and 2-arachidonoyl glycerol in the hypothalamus indicate that endocannabinoids in the hypothalamus may tonically activate CB1 receptors to maintain food intake and form part of the neural circuitry regulated by leptin.[129] These findings support the idea that endocannabinoids are involved in the pathogenesis of anorexia.

## Chronic nausea and autonomic failure

Chronic nausea, early satiety, and anorexia can be manifestations of autonomic failure, which can occur as a consequence of malnutrition/cachexia, but also represent a probably distinct paraneoplastic syndrome in patients with advanced cancer and can occur as an adverse effect of neurotoxic treatments or neuropathic conditions, such as diabetes mellitus or spinal cord compression. Whether the gastrointestinal (chronic nausea), cardiovascular (postural hypotension and fixed heart rate[130]), and constitutional (asthenia and chronic fatigue[131]) symptoms of autonomic insufficiency represent the same underlying mechanism remains unknown.

## Mechanism of asthenia

Asthenia can be an important symptom in the context of primary cachexia, especially if it is perceived more as weakness than loss of energy (reflecting decreased muscle function rather than psychological fatigue).[132] Considering the many factors that influence asthenia, a less clear distinction between primary asthenia and secondary asthenia than that between primary cachexia and secondary cachexia can be made. Primary asthenia is found to be cancer related, resulting from metabolic paraneoplastic mechanism; in contrast, secondary asthenia is caused by many factors other than cachexia.[133] In patients with breast cancer, a poor correlation between asthenia and nutritional status was found.[134] The pathogenesis of asthenia is beyond the scope of this chapter.

## Hypogonadotropic hypogonadism/ growth hormone deficiency

Chronic (inflammatory) diseases can be associated with complex neuroendocrine alterations.[135,136] Endogenous opioids play an important role in the regulation of gonadotropins (i.e., lueteinizing hormone [LH]) and in the neuromodulation of growth hormone (GH) and thyroid stimulating hormone (TSH).[137] In patients with nonmalignant chronic pain (mainly resulting from failed back surgery), long-term intrathecal administration (27 ± 16 months) of opioids was associated with the development of hypogonadotropic hypogonadism, as well as central hypocorticism and GH deficiency.[138] The administration of GH to patients with noncancer cachexia (cardiac cachexia,[139,140] aging,[141] chronic obstructive pulmonary disease[142]) increased lean body mass, and GH replacement in patients with HIV-wasting improved function.[143] Because of concerns that GH might stimulate tumor growth, no clinical trials of GH to treat patients with cancer cachexia have been reported. Several studies of anabolic steroids have shown increases in fat-free mass in patients with HIV-wasting,[144] end-stage renal disease,[145] and chronic obstructive pulmonary disease.[146] Low testosterone levels were found in HIV patients, and testosterone replacement therapy was beneficial.[147–149] In summary, data from studies involving noncancer wasting conditions suggest that hormonal abnormalities are important in cancer cachexia. In patients with cancer ACS, such hormonal abnormalities may be hidden behind the effects of predominant inflammatory alterations and tumor-related cachectic factors.

## Taste alterations

Whether taste alterations are an independent symptom in the context of progressive cancer, or whether they are sequelae of paraneoplastic treatment or of complications in the oral cavity is controversial. There is a positive correlation between weight loss and the presence of the normal taste sensation.[150] The role of zinc deficiency in taste alterations requires further research. Plasma zinc levels in patients with bronchial carcinoma and leukemic cells in the blood of patients with leukemia are lower than they are in healthy patients and in normal blood cells, respectively.[151]

### Secondary Cachexia

Several conditions leading to impaired caloric intake or loss of nutrients occur in patients suffering from cancer and can be categorized into one of four groups (Table 71–1): *(1)* impaired oral intake (e.g., stomatitis, dysphagia, odynophagia, bowel obstruction, vomiting, severe constipation,[152] intractable pain, severe dyspnea, severe depression, delirium, and social obstacles); *(2)* impaired gastrointestinal absorption (e.g., malabsorption, exocrine pancreatic insufficiency, and chronic severe diarrhea); *(3)* catabolism (e.g., hyperthyroidism, chronic and acute infection, and chronic active inflammation); and *(4)* significant loss of proteins (e.g., loss of bodily fluids [i.e., frequent puncture of ascites or pleural fluid], and nephrotic syndrome).

#### Gastrointestinal surgery

Patients undergoing gastrointestinal surgery (e.g., esophagectomy, gastrectomy, gastrointestinal bypass, pancreatoduodenectomy, and colectomy) are at risk for developing secondary cachexia and starvation. The patient's weight can usually be maintained after the postoperative phase using nutritional supplements or enteral or parenteral nutrition (see below). In cases in which progressive cancer causes ACS or complications such as infection, spinal cord injury potentiating autonomic failure, symptomatic brain metastasis, and hypercalcemia, the impairment of gastrointestinal integrity increases the risk of malnutrition/cachexia.

### Most Common Causes of Malnutrition/Cachexia

The mechanisms leading to malnutrition/cachexia vary during the trajectory of illness. At diagnosis, the most common causes of malnutrition/cachexia are the metabolic and local effects of the tumor. During antineoplastic treatments, the therapy commonly causes weight loss and other symptoms. In the context of progressive, advanced cancer, the disease causes metabolic and localized effects; psychosocial factors emerge, and treatments such as opioids or antidepressants may lead to malnutrition/cachexia (Fig. 71–1).

### Summary

In summary, the following issues are relevant in the pathogenesis of ACS:

- The difference between primary (metabolic) and secondary (starvation) malnutrition/cachexia is important to determine.
- Primary cachexia is a paraneoplastic metabolic syndrome with increased metabolism in the context of chronic inflammation.
- Alterations in the cytokine milieu play a major role in the perpetuation of metabolic, neuroendocrine, and symptomatic manifestations of primary cachexia.
- Primary cachexia increases muscle proteolysis but also acute-phase protein synthesis. Nutrients can increase protein synthesis but not proteolysis.

- Cachectic factors, such as PIF and LMF produced by the tumor, play an increasing role in mediating malnutrition/cachexia.
- The symptoms anorexia and asthenia correlate incompletely with weight loss and represent metabolic syndromes that are probably distinguishable.

### Assessment of Malnutrition/Cachexia

Probably the most important diagnostic test in the evaluation of malnutrition is clinical suspicion. Because malnutrition/cachexia is a silent syndrome, it is paramount to assess actively.

The assessment of a patient's nutritional status includes evaluation of different domains, as mentioned below, and there is wide variation in what is meant by nutritional status, ranging from pure anthropometrics to function to quality of life. Nutritional assessment using laboratory and technical data alone has failed to consistently identify patients at risk for nutritionally mediated complications and symptomatic impact.[153] Clinical judgment as a basis for assessing nutritional status was equivalent to objective measurements in a study involving 59 patients admitted to a surgical ward.[154] These results led to the development of the subjective global assessment (SGA) tool, which was predictive of nutrition-associated complications of patients undergoing gastrointestinal surgery. The SGA has been valuable for predicting nutrition-related complications in different populations, such as geriatric patients[155] and patients with chronic renal failure,[156] AIDS,[157] and cancer.[158] A study that included 87 patients with gastrointestinal and urologic tumors showed that level of food intake, problems with eating, physical activity, and muscle wastage during the 6 months preceeding the assessment contributed to the SGA classification by weight loss. Survival was found to be significantly higher in SGA A than in SGA B+C ($P < 0.001$). Another study on patients with liver transplantation failed to show a prognostic effect of the SGA on survival.[159]

To optimally care for patients with advanced cancer and their families, it is paramount to acknowledge the emotional impact of anorexia, weight loss, and declining function.[160] Although pathophysiologically, anorexia is probably an epiphenomenon of, instead of a primary mechanism leading to, malnutrition/cachexia, anorexia both independent and in combination with weight loss affects quality of life to a major extent. Declining function as a consequence of malnutrition/cachexia is a major contributor to discomfort for patients and their families. As with pain, declining function and malnutrition need no longer to be accepted as an indispensable sequel of advanced cancer.[161]

### Components of Malnutrition/Cachexia Assessment

The following factors are included in the comprehensive assessment of malnutrition/cachexia:

1. Body composition, anthropometrics, and weight (all static assessments)
2. Functional tests, including muscle function (dynamic assessments)
3. Symptomatic impact of nutritional status on quality of life
4. Caloric intake and appetite
5. Causes of secondary cachexia
6. Extent of primary cachexia
7. Immunologic status, anergy.

### Body Composition and Anthropometrics: Static Assessments

Assessment of body composition requires a thorough, careful history of the patient's *weight* and a skillful weight measurement

---

tus and questionnaire), symptomatic impact (assessed by an easy screening tool evaluating appetite, seum albumin levels, and, in the future, PIF) as well as thorough exclusion or documentation of causes of secondary cachexia will reach a high level of quality. Most sophisticated tests are still investigational and do not yet clearly improve the assessment.

### Nutritional Support for Patients Undergoing Chemotherapy and Radiation Therapy

Supplemental enteral nutrition and nutritional counseling,[189,191] as well as parenteral nutrition,[193] have failed to show benefits in terms of response rates, survival, treatment tolerance, and side using standardized scales and avoiding variability due to clothing. Weight loss should be quantified as a percentage based on weight lost during the previous 2 or 6 months as well on pre-illness weight, and assessment of voluntary weight loss should be done. The presence of fluid retention needs to be assessed as

## Functional Assesments

The results of grip strength,[171] which is a dynamometric assessment, have shown this technique to be a prognostic tool in postoperative surgical patients.[172,173] In a recent study,[174]dynamometric measurements were used as one of the main outcome

effects for patients receiving standard-dose chemotherapy and standard radiation therapy.[194] Although total parenteral nutrition (TPN) could increase the nutritional intake of these patients, it was associated with an increased mortality rate, even when catheter-related septicemia was excluded.[195,196] It has been recommended that nutritional support be indicated for patients with cancer who have severe, treatment-associated gastrointestinal toxic effects that preclude oral intake for more than 10 days and for patients with a normal life expectancy whose inability to eat is the principal impediment to normal functioning.[197] The final position paper from the American College of Physicians in 1989 concluded that, in patients with cancer, "parenteral nutritional support was associated with net harm, and no condition should be defined in which such treatment appeared to be of benefit."

Any type of nutritional support may, however, benefit patients undergoing bone marrow transplantation, who suffer from relevant gastrointestinal toxic effects, such as enteropathic mucocitis or esophagitis associated with the antineoplastic treatment. Parenteral nutrition improved overall survival, disease-free survival, and time to relapse, but did not improve results concerning engraftment, duration of hospitalization or the incidence of bacteriemia, or graft-versus-host disease.[198]

### Nutritional Support for Surgery Patients

The data supporting the perioperative administration of supplemental nutrition are conflicting because of various factors: the durations of nutritional support vary by study; the stage of disease and nutritional status of the patients vary; the studies involve small numbers of patients and in many cases lack randomization and untreated control groups; and patients differ in nutritional status before surgery, or the duration of nutrition was inadequate.[196,199,200] Several large trials of preoperative parenteral nutrition showed significant improvements in energy intake but no improvements in nutritional measurements or functional outcome; unfortunately, these studies also showed increased complication rates and a trend toward shorter survival duration.[201–203] Nutritional support for 7–10 days prior to surgery may reduce postoperative complications.[187,188,204] Malnourished patients should continue receiving nutritional support postoperatively, and if the gastrointestinal tract cannot be used for tube feeding, parenteral nutrition should be started immediately after surgery but changed to enteral nutrition as soon as possible.

### Nutritional Support for Patients with Terminal Cancer

In patients with primary cachexia due to progressive cancer, invasive artificial nutrition is usually not beneficial[205] and may negatively affect the patient's quality of life.[206,207] The European Association for Palliative Care published guidelines on the use of artificial nutrition vs. hydration in patients with terminal cancer.[208] It was concluded that the controversy surrounding the benefit of nutritional therapy arose in part from the definition of terminal cancer patients as a groups with different needs, expectations, and potential for medical intervention, as well as the difficulties to predict the patient's life expectancy and likely responses to nutritional support.

### Counseling

In avoiding nutritional support for patients with progressive cachexia one should be mindfull of the severe psychosocial distress to many patients and their families, as well as the profound philosophical and, in some cases, religious connotations. Therefore, it is important to adequately counsel patients and their families and to address the anxiety of family members arising from the idea that their relative is "starving to death." Reframing the family's understanding of cachexia as a condition associated with metabolic abnormalities due to the cancer instead of death by starvation is a useful strategy. It is helpful for the family to understand that the administration of more food to the patient will not result in additional fat or increase overall muscle synthesis because of the generally irreversible underlying abnormalities. This reframing can decrease the level of emotional distress in both the patients and their families and can help preserve the social benefits of meal times. When progressive disease occurs and oral intake is likely to decrease to almost nothing, adequate mouth care and small amounts of ice chips or sips of cold beverages may be adequate for some patients. In patients with symptoms related to dehydration, the use of hypodermoclysis can be very useful in maintaining adequate hydration of the patient at home, with little cost and minimal invasiveness.[209]

### Expected survival

In patients with terminal disease, nutritional support needs to be considered when the patient's estimated life expectancy with the underlying disease is longer than the average life expectancy with starvation. Healthy adults die from starvation after a nitrogen loss of 35% of the ideal weight, i.e., after 60–75 days, despite adequate adipose reserves, because protein mass is the major determinant of starvation.[210] No similar data about patients with advanced cancer are available, because this patient population is very heterogeneous. Patients with progressive, terminal cancer die from starvation after an estimated 15–30 days. The average rate of nitrogen loss in a healthy adult, 3 g/day, increases to 15–20 g/day for a patient with systemic inflammatory response syndrome, such as sepsis or severe trauma, leading to a 30% reduction of muscular mass after 10–13 days and of body cell mass after 20 days.[211]

The predicted survival time of patients with advanced cancer is accurate in only 20% to 70% of cases, even if estimated by experienced health-care professionals. Physicians overestimate survival time by a factor 2–5, and accurate survival predictions are more likely for very ill patients.[212,213] Nutritional support may to some extent counteract factors that may predict survival (i.e., causes of secondary cachexia, such as dysphagia), complicating the clinical decision making.

In summary, the determination of whether nutritional support is indicated for a patient with cancer is based on proper evaluation of the patient for primary or secondary cachexia. The greater the number of underlying metabolic paraneoplastic alterations that are present, the less nutritional intervention is of benefit. Even a reversal of the decrease in protein synthesis has been shown not to decrease proteolysis resulting from aggressive nutritional treatments but only to increase protein turnover.[214]

### Nutritional Principles

As mentioned above, the patient has to be assessed to allow a decision-making process, including some crucial questions:

- Does the gut work?
- How long is the foreseen period of nutritional support (duration)?
- Is the patient under risk for aspiration?
- How is the patient's cognition?

If the gut works, use it

Extended periods of quiescence of the bowel, with or without parenteral nutrition, should be avoided, if possible, for several reasons:[215]

1. Various stressors have an impact on translocation of intestinal bacteria and endotoxins.
2. The gut plays an essential role in the systemic immune competence.
3. Within days of stopping enteral stimulation by food, a significant mucosal atrophy occurs, with decreases in villous height and number and in the rate of mucosal cell turnover. This atrophy results partly from the decrease in gut tropic hormones levels that occurs without intestinal stimulation and absence of specific gut nutrition, such as glutamine and short-chain fatty acids.[216]
4. These data support the concept that, as soon as possible, oral intake should be achieved.

## Nutritional requirements

The nutritional requirements of patients with cancer who most often have a combination of mixed primary and secondary cachexia are not well established.

**Water** The right water is needed: less free extracellular water, more sodium-bound, "functional" water. In patients with advanced cancer, a careful balance has to be maintained between overhydration, which can be harmful to some patients (e.g., those with ascites, chronic heart failure, peripheral edema associated with thrombosis or hypalbuminemia, and dehydration). Dehydration perpetuates constipation and its sequelae, such as arterial hypotension, causing a propensity for falls in the context of the common autonomic failure, increased opioid toxicity, and a lower threshold for delirium, among other conditions. The administration of carbohydrates (i.e., glucose and insulin) can counteract the loss of extracellular fluid by inhibiting renal sodium excretion.

The effects of glucose-based TPN on positive water and sodium balance have also been demonstrated in patients with cancer.[217] In patients with advanced cancer, the clearance of free water is often decreased. Hyponatremia occurs in about 4% of patients with advanced cancer.[218] Antidiuretic hormone (ADH) levels can be increased, by production of the tumor as a paraneoplastic disease; in response to a myriad of pharmacologic compounds, including many anticonvulsants, antineoplastic agents, and opioids; or as a physiologic reaction to the loss of intracellular water secondary to wasting. Syndrome of inappropriate secretion of antidiuretic hormone (SIADH) accounts only for about a third of the cases of hyponatraemia; another third is caused by sodium depletion. In patients with advanced cancer and protein malnutrition, the urea load to the kidney is decreased, and the invisible water loss caused by physical activity is decreased,[219] whereas the level of synthesis of endogenous water is maintained by the oxidation of carbohydrates and fat during fasting states.

**Energy** Most patients with progressive, advanced cancer are hypermetabolic. The discrepancy in reported resting energy expenditure (REE) may be partly explained by the calculation of REE on the basis of unit of body cell mass instead of frank weight. Physical activity contributes an average of 25% to total energy expenditure whereas digestion contributes an average of 5%. Therefore, the basal energy expenditure is calculated to be about 1 kcal/kg/hour. If the patient's nutritional status is to be recovered, the patient's nutrition needs to increase substantially.

**Proteins** The stimated daily protein supply is 1 to 2 g proteins/kg/day, provided that the blood level nitrogen values remain in the normal range.

**Lipids** A high lipid/glucose ratio (50:50) is typically desired because of the concern that glucose may increase tumor growth.

**Carbohydates** Because some tissues, such as those of the central nervous system, erythrocytes, renal medulla, and bone marrow, are preferably glucose-dependent, an appropriate amount of glucose must be delivered to the tissues to prevent gluconeogenesis (i.e., the conversion of amino acids resulting from the breakdown of protein to glucose in the liver). A total of 100 g of protein is necessary to produce 56 g of glucose. A dose of 200–400 g of glucose per day should be sufficient to produce a protein-sparing effect and reduce gluconeogenesis. However, patients with inflammatory conditions, which often occur as part of the cancer ACS, the required glucose levels may be significantly increased.

## Enteral vs. Parenteral Nutrition

Parenteral nutrition has no proven benefits over enteral nutrition in patients with a functional bowel. Both enteral and parenteral nutrition have advantages and disadvantages (Table 71–4). Enteral nutrition is much cheaper than parenteral nutrition and can be easily administered at home.

Enteral nutrition can be maintained in cases in which the oral route cannot be used. The morbidity associated with enteral nutrition is in most cases due to aspiration, pneumonia, and diarrhea. The risk of aspiration is increased for patients with delayed gastric emptying but can be reduced by frequent aspiration of the gastric contents in the first days after starting the enteral infusion so that gastric stasis can be detected. The establishment of a gastrostomy by endoscopic or ultrasonographic methods makes a nasogastric tube unnecessary in most patients and substantially increases the patient's comfort level. As the disease progress, the gastrointestinal tract in patients with (total) bowel obstruction can be drained. Complications associated with enteral nutrition are bloating, infection, and bleeding.

Parenteral nutrition can be used to maintain nutrition in cases in which oral and enteral nutrition are not appropriate. There is

**Table 71–4** Common complications of enteral and parenteral nutrition

*Enteral Nutrition*

Aspiration
    Avoid gastric placement, consider jejunal tube
    Lower osmolality, decrease rate/hour
    Consider metoclopramide
    Lower osmolality of formula, change formula
Diarrhea
Constipation
Dehydration
Electrolyte alterations
Hyperglycemia
Occlusion or clogging of feeding tube
Nasal irrigation
Tube displacement

*Parenteral Nutrition*

Central venous access complications
    Pneumothorax
    Malposition
    Thrombosis
Infections
Volume overload
Glucose, and electrolyte imbalance
Excessive $CO_2$ production

no evidence, however, that parenteral nutrition improves survival duration in patients with end-stage cancer. Parenteral nutrition is associaetd with many complications, such as catheter-related pneumothorax, sepsis, thrombosis, bleeding, hepatic dysfunction, and fluid and electrolyte imbalance, and it costs 10 times more than enteral nutrition. The maintenance of parentral nutrition in the patient's home requires acquisition and preparation of the formula, maintenance of intravenous access and sterility, and compliance with the administration of solutions every day. Because of associated complications, the ineffectivity in most patients with advanced cancer, and the difficulty associated with maintaining parenteral nutrition in the patient's home, the use of parenteral nutrition does not have a major role in advanced cancer care except in selected patients.

The decision of whether to pursue nutritional support and whether to use nutritional supplements or enteral or parenteral nutrition should be discussed in depth with the patient and the patient's family. It is important to negotiate and define end points and to review frequently how well these goals are being met; the results should be discussed with both the patient and family. It is foreseeable that the discontinuation of nutritional support will lead to misunderstanding and more psychosocial distress, thus decisions about nutritional support should be shared with both the patient and the patient's family in a progressive manner.[33,220,221]

## Enteral nutrition

The presence of primary and secondary cachexia and the stage of the disease are factors in determining whether enteral nutrition is indicated. Patients generally prefer oral nutrition to enteral nutrition. Enteral nutrition is appropriate despite an intact oral pathway in a few types of cases. The first involves patients with incomplete stenosis of the upper gastrointestinal tract who can tolerate only very frequent and small amounts of food. In these patients, the distal end of the tube can be positioned below the obstruction, and nutrition can be delivered at the normal rate. The second type of case involves patients with severe early satiety, despite treatment with prokenetics, or with partial gastric outlet obstruction. In these patients, the slow and continuous administration of the nutrition solution improves absorptive capacity. The third type of case involves application of specific nutrition solutions that may not be tolerated orally, especially in patients with taste abnormalities or those with severe fatigue or irreversible cognitive impairment.[222]

**Choosing enteral access** The route selected for enteral access depends on the condition of the gastrointestinal tract, the presence and site of gastrointestinal obstructions, the estimated duration of the feeding, and the risk of pulmonary aspiration.

If possible, nutrition is administered in the stomach, since the complete digestion and absorption through this route better reflect physiologic intake. The use of hyperosmolar formula, as well as continuous or bolus feeding, reduces the time required to administer the enteral nutrition.[223] A planned duration of less than 30 days for enteral nutrition is sometimes considered to be an indication for a nasoenteral tube instead of a gastrostomy, although this must be negotiated with the patient. Small, flexible nasoenteral tubes and biocompatible materials for the tubes have improved patients' tolerance. The diameter of the tube must be chosen in relation to the planned formula because the viscosity and osmolality of the formula determine the smallest diameter possible without clogging.[224] In cases in which aspiration is a risk, a more distal placement of the tip of the tube can reduce

that risk since the pyloric sphincter and ligament of Treitz provide protection against aspiration.[225]

Nasoenteric tubes can be placed at bedside in patients whose upper gastrointestinal tract is not obstructed, by turning the patient in the correct position. The use of prokinetic agents (such as metoclopramide or erythromycin) before tube placement increases the percentage of cases in which the tube successfully passes into the duodenum to 90%.[226] Fluoroscopic or endoscopic guidance may be necessary when the patient has malignant obstruction or neurologic dysphagia.[227] Before starting the administration of nutrition, the tube tip position should be checked (by auscultation of injected air, aspiration of gastric acid, or X-ray) to avoid pulmonary feeding.

Typical local complications of nasoenteric tubes are epistaxis, nasal mucosal irritation, or ulceration, piriformis sinus perforation, and otitis media. Perforation in the esophagus or gastric or duodenal segments and intubation of the lungs are other complications. Gastrointestinal bleeding and cardiac complications such as arrhythmia or myocardial infarction are additional risks.

Enteral access may also be obtained using a gastrostomy. Requirements for a gastrostomy are normal duodenal transit and the absence of a risk of aspiration. Surgical placement of the gastrostomy is seldom done; the most frequently used procedures are endoscopic (i.e., percutaneous endoscopic gastrostomy [PEG]) or radiologic (i.e., percutaneous fluoroscopic gastrostomy [PFG]). The most serious complications of PEG or PFG are intraabdominal leaks from the stomach and deep stromal infections. The morbidity and mortality rates vary. Although the mortality rate is considered to be less than 1%, it is highly dependent on the experience and skill of the health-care professional performing the intervention. A wide range of complications (e.g., large amounts of ascites or interposition of the liver or transverse colon between the stomach and the abdominal wall) is associated with gastrostomy, especially in cancer patients.

An ileostomy is indicated in patients at high risk for pulmonary aspiration and in patients with delayed gastric emptying, chronic intermittent vomiting, gastroesophageal reflux, previous partial or total gastrectomy, and neuromuscular dysfunction resulting from injury to the spinal cord or head. Various techniques for performing an ileostomy or a gastrectomy are available, including a mini-laparectomy jejunostomy, percutaneous endoscopic or fluoroscopic ileostomy, and transgastric ileostomy. Because jejunostomy carries a substantial risk of complications and death, a feeding jejunostomy should be performed only if clearly indicated in patients with a high potential for long-term use or patients in whom a gastrostomy is not feasible.[228]

**Feeding regimens and enteral formulations** The enteral regimen reported to improve the nutritional status of patients with cancer is 35 kcal/kg/day, and the free water requirement is about 35 ml/kg/day. Both natural enteral formulations, which have a risk of bacterial contamination and/or enzymatic degradation, and artificial enteral formulations, which have been designed for many different situations or diseased states, are available.

Artificial formulations include the polymeric formulation and the elemental diet. The polymeric formulation contains carbohydrates, fats, and proteins in complex forms, all of which require some degree of digestion and absorption. The elemental diets are a mixture of small particles, such as maltodextrins, free amino acids or dipeptides, and easily absorbed fats, such as medium-chain triglyceride oil. The polymeric formula can be hypocaloric, normocaloric, or hypercaloric, as well as hyperproteic, and formulas are available with or without fibers.

A standard diet is polymeric, normocaloric, and lactose-free, with or without fibers. This diet generally provides 100–120 calories per 100 ml (carbohydrates account for 50%–60% of total energy; fats, 30%–40%, and amino acids, 12%–20%), with osmolarity ranging from 220 to 350 mOsm/L. The addition of fibers such as laxatives can be useful in some patients. Dietary fibers are contraindicated in patients with opioid-associated constipation, however, because of the high incidence of fecal impaction, but soluble fibers can be important to maintain the trophic status of the bowel mucosa, especially in the colon.[229,230] Elemental diets have a high osmolarity and are used for patients with severely reduced digestive and absorptive capacity, although they are seldom used in cancer patients. Elemental diet formulae specific for renal failure (a highly concentrated formula with low levels of protein, phosphorus, magnesium, potassium, and sodium), hepatic failure (a formula that contains branched-chain amino acids and a low level of aromatic amino acid), and pulmonary failure (a formula with a high amount of fat to limit $CO_2$ production) are available.

**Methods of delivering enteral nutrition** Enteral nutrition can be delivered by bolus, with the use of gravity, or with the assistance of a pump. Feeding to the stomach can be done both by bolus or gravity; feeding to the jejunum, however, should be performed with the help of a peristaltic pump, and therefore, intermittent feeding is not possible with jejunal feeding. In cases in which the stomach can act as a reservoir, feeding is more physiologic and allows the patient to have free intervals for daily activity. Continuous feeding may be administred overnight; artificial formulations are generally used because the feeding tube has a small diameter and the natural formula presents a high risk of obstruction. Solutions with limited osmolarity ($<$350 mOsm) are used to minimize irritation of the mucosa. The rate of administration is begun at 20 ml/hour and progressively increased to a maximum of 80 ml/hour.

**Complications associated with tube feeding** The most common complications associated with tubal feeding are mechanical. One mechanical complication is tubal obstruction, which occurs more often in small enteric tubes or jejunostomies. This complication can be prevented by carefully washing the tubes with 20 ml of water every 6–8 hours and always after each meal or discontinuation of the feeding or after meals. The tube can be unclogged with various materials, such as hot water, peroxide water, Coca-Cola, or pancreatic enzymes.

A second mechanical complication is dislodging of the tube. A dislodged tube should be replaced within a few days to avoid the closure of the enteral stoma.

The most serious and feared complication associated with tube feeding is aspiration pneumonia. Patients who have aspirated previously and patients with altered consciousness, gastroporesis, and tubes in the second or third part of the duodenum are at risk for aspiration pneumonia. To minimize the risk of this complication the patient should be kept in a semirecumbent position at the initial delivery of formula, which should be delivered at a slow (40 ml/hour) rate or with a small bolus.

Diarrhea, the most common complication of tubal feeding, has a multifactoral etiology.[231] Diarrhea is associated with hyperosmolar formulations and high delivery rates. Antibiotic treatment and acid-suppressive medication (e.g., protone blockers, $H_2$ antagonist) alter the intestinal microflora. Bacterial overgrowth can also cause diarrhea. Lactose intolerance and formula contamination should be considered as a possible cause of diarrhea.

Peristomal infection is a local complication, which seldom requires replacement of the tubes.

As with oral feeding, regular assessment of the bowel history and a high clinical suspicion for constipation are necessary, as is monitoring of metabolic complications such as dehydration, electrolyte imbalances, and nutritional trace element or vitamin deficiencies.

The administration of drugs through feeding tubes has become easier, since many important medications are now available in elixirs or allow crushing and mixing with water. Those medications which require gastric milieu are suboptimally absorbed when administered through a jejunal tube. Sustained-release medications and enteric-coated preparations lose their sustained-release characteristics when they are crushed. A new long-term sustained-release opioid comes in capsules with little bullets, each of which has sustained-release properties. Enteral formula may be incompatible with other medications, especially syrups with a high alcoholic content, which may coagulate the formula.

## Parenteral nutrition

Parenteral nutrition (PEN) can be administered in small volumes and as a continous infusion over 24 hour. In many cases, patients do not realize that they are receiving several thousand calories per day. Parenteral nutrition is passive nutrition and can be administred to patients in any condition.

Glucose is the only carbohydrate energy source available for PEN; it can be administered in concentrations of 20% to 60%. One gram of glucose provides 3.7 kcal. Glucose should not be used as the sole source of energy, however, because this has been associated with essential fatty acid deficiency, fatty liver infiltration, and increased $CO_2$. The infusion rate of glucose should not exceed 5 mg/kg/minute (or 500 mg/kg/hour) or 4–5 g/kg/day to prevent metabolic alterations.

Lipids are the most dense energy substrates, with 1 g yielding about 9 kcal. Fats are administered in the form of a lipid emulsion, which contains a triglyceride core surrounded by a phospholipid layer (i.e., soya lethicin or egg), at a concentration of about 20% to 30%. Since fat emulsions are isotonic, they can be given through a peripheral vein. The infusion rate of lipid emulsions should not exceed 100 mg/kg/hour, or 2g/kg/day. Modern mixed emulsions (MCT/LCT) can be administered in higher concentrations (150 mg/kg/hour) and enable the addition of other lipds, such as omega-3 fatty acids.

Amino acids (AAs), 1 g of which yields only 4 kcal, are administered to provide substrate for protein synthesis. The energy requirments are fullfilled with glucose and lipids, respectively. The infusion rate of AAs is the same as for lipid emulsion, i.e., it should not exceed 100 mg/kg/hour, or 2g/kg/day. Typical AA solutions contain concentrations of 5% to 15% of AA, and contain 40%–50% of essential AA and 50%–60% of nonessential AA.

**Infusion techniques** The use of a single bag to deliver PEN should be encouraged for several reasons: lower cost, lower risk of contamination, increased level of safety and ease of administration, probably reduced risk of metabolic complications, and probably improved use of nutrients. It is important to monitor the stability of calcium, inorganic phosphate, and lipid emulsion. Because the addition of fat emulsion lessens vein irritation by reducing the osmolarity of the nutrition formula, the administration of TPN via peripheral veins is possible. Solutions should be prepared using the laminar flow technique. The schedule of administration (i.e., continous infusion with volumetric pumps vs. cyclic administration, mainly overnight) must be targeted to the patient, and the patient's autonomy must be taken into account.

The TPN regimen must be designed according to the patient's nutritional requirements, instead of the capacity and tolerance of the vein, and therefore a central venous catheter (CVC) should be scheduled for any planned nutritional support. However, there are no clear advantages for any type of CVC, whether a long-line from the antecubital fossa, subcutaneous tunnelization, or port-à-cath. The latter two possibilities are probably less associated with infectious side effects. A multilumen catheter should be avoided if there are no indications other than TPN, because of the higher infection rates. Catheters should not be changed routinely without a specific indication. It is crucial to maintain a high level of care and sterility, and the CVC should not be used if it is not necessary (private catheter for nutrition only). During the change of dressing of the CVC, surgical sterility should be achieved, using the same techniques as in the operating room, with adequate scrubbing and antiseptics. There is no standard practice for CVC flushing. Normally the CVC is flushed after each use with 0.9% saline, without heparin. However, to fix a nonfunctioning CVC, a heparin lock (of 100 IU/ml) is advisable. The CVC needs to be clamped properly to prevent air embolism, back flow, and subsequent CVC thrombosis. The best way to enable good CVC access is not to touch; if it requires handling, strict antiseptic rules should be followed.

**Complications and contraindications of total parenteral nutrition** Mechanical complications associated with TPN include pneumothorax, malpositioning of the catheter, and thrombosis of the central vein. Metabolic complications include volume overload, hyperglycemia, hypoglycemia, electrolyte imbalance, essential micronutrient deficiencies, long-term hepatic steatosis, cholelithiasis, excessive $CO_2$ production, and long-term metabolic bone disease. The most feared complications are contamination of the catheter and sepsis. To avoid complications, it is crucial to have a protocol for regular monitoring of PEN, a nutritional support team,[232] and meticulous catheter management. Infectious disease principles apply, with avoidance of prophylactic antibiotics and appropriate cultivation prior to empiric antibiotic treatments.

## Immunonutrition

Immunonutrition is a new form nutrition that adds immuno-modulating agents to the nutritional formulae. In several recent prospective randomized, clinical trials in more than 1000 patients admitted to intensive care units (ICUs) (trauma, gastrointestinal surgery, sepsis, and mixed ICU patients), the administration of immunonutrition has improved outcomes.[233] A meta-analysis of 11 randomized trials found that nutritional support supplemented with key nutrients significantly reduced the risk of infectious complications and the overall length of hospital stay, in both patients with critical illnesses and those with gastrointestinal cancer.[234]

Almost all trials have used omega-3 essential fatty acids at a dose of 3–6 g/day with a mixture of eicosapentaenoic acid (EPA) and docosahexaenoic acid (DHA). Omega-3 fatty acids, specifically EPA, play a role in modulating immunologic responses or the metabolic alterations secondary to inflammation. Omega-3 fatty acids are believed to counteract the prostaglandin E2- and 15-HETE-mediated effects. These reactions not only have been

up-regulated in cancer cachexia but are also involved in inflammation secondary to trauma, surgery, or other ICU conditions.

Part of the key nutrients is always L-arginine, which is regarded as a nonessential AA, but is known to stimulate several hormones, including GH, prolactin, insulin-like growth factor, glucagon, somatostatin, and norepinephrin.[235] Arginine is also a precursor of nitric oxide, which is involved in a wide variety of processes, including cytoxic activity of immune cells, secretory functions, regulation of blood flow, and gastrointestinal motility. In renal models of sepsis, arginine improved survival and likely improved wound healing.[236]

Most immunonutrition preparations also include glutamine, which is primarily synthesized in skeletal muscle. Although glutamine is the most abundant AA, it is now considered to be conditionally essential in several illness states. Glutamine is the primary energy source for enterocytes, but neither the small nor the large intestine can synthesize enough amounts of glutamine.[237] Glutamine is also required for macrophage and lymphocyte function and is a precursor for nucleotide synthesis. Clinical data show that, compared with standard preparation, glutamine supplementation can reduce the rate of infections and shorten the hospital stay for patients who undergo a bone marrow transplantation.[238,239] Glutamine supplementation has also been shown to improve irinotecan-induced diarrhea.[240]

Most immunonutrition diets contain nucleotides, which are crucial for the synthesis of RNA and DNA and the competence of the energy transfer system. However, the effect of single-agent nucleotides remains unknown.

In patients with primary cachexia, the value of immunonutrition vs. pharmacologic treatment using omega-3 fatty acids, or more specifically EPA, has not been shown.

## Treatment of Primary Cachexia

Complete reversal of primary cachexia is achievable only by eliminating the tumor mass. Unfortunately, this is not possible in most patients with advanced malignancies. Therefore, reasonable goals of clinical management include improving the patient's general comfort; easing symptoms such as anorexia, chronic nausea, asthenia, and psychological distress related to changes in body image; and improving the patient's level of function. Because the frequency and intensity of the symptoms of primary cachexia vary by patient (mostly because of more severe coexisting symptoms), symptomatic interventions for malnutrition/cachexia should be based on individual and, in many cases, dynamic treatment goals.

### Antineoplastic treatment

Antineoplastic treatments have been assessed on the basis of the classical oncologic outcome measurements of response rate, survival, toxicity, and adverse effects,[241,242] as well as their effects on symptoms associated with cancer. However, the indication for antineoplastic treatments to alleviate symptoms and improve quality of life, and the monitoring of patients undergoing these treatments, regardless of whether a symptomatic benefit is achieved, are difficult. Even though several of the phase III studies assessing chemotherapy for patients with advanced cancer were carefully designed, several factors might have contributed to biased conclusions regarding symptomatic end points. For several reasons, the control arms were not placebo controlled, therefore the high symptomatic placebo effect of many interventions in patients with advanced cancer, which reached 30% to 50% improvement of several symptoms such as pain,[243] anorexia,[244] and tiredness, could have contributed to a biased interpretation of the symptomatic benefit. The effectiveness and quality of the accompagnying symptom-control interventions, often referred to as "best supportive care," have not been controlled for in most trials, mostly because of a lack of prospective definitions and of trained palliative-care teams. Nevertheless, an antineoplastic treatment that is carefully tailored and monitored can improve symptoms and newer antineoplastic treatments aiming for stabilization,[245] instead of reduction of the cancer, will strenghten this approach.

### Pharmacological treatment

Pharmacologic treatment of patients with primary cachexia attempts to manipulate the metabolic alterations, with the main purpose being to improve the patient's symptoms instead of influence the natural course of the disease.[246] The purpose of pharmacologic treatment of patients with primary cachexia is to antagonize the main symptoms, anorexia, chronic nausea, and asthenia. Unfortunately, with the three current available therapies (corticosteroids, progestins, and prokinetics), only a minority of patients experience a significant body weight gain and therefore the psychological distress associated with a negative body image is not reduced by pharmacological interventions. Other interventions, such as hydrazine sulphate and cyproheptadine, have been found to be of no or very limited usefulness. As we learn more about the metabolic changes associated with primary cachexia, several new drugs (e.g., anticytokines), or older drugs reevaluated for new uses (e.g., thalidomide) are being assessed for their effect in patients with primary cachexia.

### Established treatments

Currently, there is enough evidence to support the use of three pharmacological treatments in primary cachexia.

**Prokinetics** Of the prokinetic drugs, metoclopramide is the best studied agent. The roles of the other prokinetic drugs, such as domperidone as well as newer agents such as the 5-HT$_4$-agonists, remain to be clarified. Metoclopramide is an antidopaminergic drug that exhibits some 5-HT$_3$-antagonistic and 5-HT$_4$-agonistic activity and exerts effective central antiemetic and gastric emptying properties. Patients who complain of chronic nausea and early satiety profit the most from metoclopramide.[6,247–250] Chronic nausea associated with autonomic failure and opioid therapy is among the conditions most likely to respond to metoclopramide; the use of oral or subcutaneous metoclopramide treatment can result in significantly improved appetite and food intake.[251,252] Dose-limiting side effects of metoclopramide, especially when used in combination with haloperidol, are extrapyramidal symptoms.

**Corticosteroids** Dexamethasone, methylprednisolone, and prednisolone have been evaluated in at least five double-blind, randomized, controlled trials that demonstrated the effects of different types and dosages of corticosteroids on symptoms of patients with cancer cachexia.[253–257] Most research has shown that the effect of these agents on factors such as appetite, food intake, sensation of well-being, and performance status is limited to a maximum of approximately 4 weeks. Most studies have failed to show that these agents significantly improve weight. The best type and dose of corticosteroid have not been established, but most authors have used prednisone at doses ranging from 20 mg to 40 mg or equivalent. The mechanism of the drug's effect on appetite, energy, and sense of well-being is unclear; it may be related to central euphoric activity, modulation of prostaglandin metabolism, or cytokine inhibition. Despite the wide range of side effects and the caution advised by some authors, the use of corticosteroids in patients with advanced cancer is becoming widely accepted.[258] Because of their short-lasting but substantial improvement of symptoms, these drugs can be used in patients with an expected short survival duration for whom weight gain is not a likely outcome.

**Progestational drugs** The observation that treatment with progestational drugs as therapy for hormone-responsive tumors resulted in significant weight gain in patients both with and without tumor response prompted investigations of megestrol acetate and medroxyprogesterone for the treatment of anorexia/cachexia. More than a dozen randomized controlled trials have found that megestrol acetate can improve appetite, caloric intake, and nutritional variables in patients with advanced cancer.[259,260] Similar findings have been reported for patients with AIDS-wasting.[261] Megestrol acetate given in doses ranging from 160 to 1600 mg has demonstrated a dose-related benefit. At lower doses appetite improves and with higher doses caloric intake increases, a body weight gain (mostly fat) can be achieved, and the sensation of well-being can be improved. An optimal dose integrating these effects is approximately 800 mg/day.[262] The adverse effects are probably related to dosage and the number of tablets taken. Because high doses of the medication may be expensive, it is justifiable to start the patient on a lower dosage (300 mg to 480 mg/d1y) and to titrate the dose upward on the basis of clinical response. Recent studies involving terminally ill patients have demonstrated that compared with placebo, lower doses of megestrol (160 to 480 mg/day) result in rapid (<1 week) improvement in symptoms (i.e., appetite, fatigue, and general sense of well-being) without any significant change in nutritional status.[263] Thus, the data suggest that megestrol acetate improves symptoms by mechanisms other than weight gain. Studies conducted on medroxyprogesterone acetate have also demonstrated that this drug improves symptoms and aspects of nutritional status.[264]

The mechanisms of action of megestrol acetate and medroxyprogesterone acetate in appetite stimulation and weight gain observed in cachectic patients may be related to central appetite stimulation, anabolic effects, glucocorticoid activity, or cytokine modulation.[265] Recent research suggests that medroxyprogesterone acetate can induce appetite by stimulating neuropeptide-Y and may hinder the activity of some cytokines such as IL-1, IL-6, and TNF-α.[266]

Both megestrol acetate and medroxyprogesterone can induce thromboembolic phenomena—breakthrough bleeding, peripheral edema, hyperglycemia, hypertension and Cushing's syndrome, alopecia, adrenal suppression, and adrenal insufficiency, particularly if the drug is abruptly discontinued.[267] In most clinical trials, patients rarely need to stop these drugs because of related side effects. Adverse effects that limit the use of megestrol acetate and medroxyprogesterone include thromboembolic disease, glucose intolerance, fluid overload, and hypertension.[268] One study that involved patients receiving antineoplastic therapy for non–small cell lung cancer showed that megestrol acetate therapy might decrease survival and increase the rate of thromboembolic disease.[269]

### Other drugs

**Hydrazine sulfate** In a pilot study of hydrazine sulfate, which was developed as an inhibitor of gluconeogenesis (by

**Table 71-5** Established pharmacologic treatments for primary cachexia

| Beneficial Effects on: | Effect of Treatment by Drug | | |
|---|---|---|---|
| | Corticosteroids | Progestins | Metoclopramide |
| Weight gain | | | |
| Nonfluid | − | + | − |
| Lean body mass | − | − | − |
| Anorexia | + | + + | + |
| Chronic nausea | + | + | + + |
| Early satiety | − | ? | + |
| Fatigue/asthenia | + | + | − |
| Performance status | + | ? | − |
| Quality of life, sense of well-being | + | + | − |

Abbreviations: −, no effect; +, mild effect; + +, strong effect; ?, disputed effect.

tisense of NF-κB, anti–IL-6 receptor antibodies, anti-TNF antibodies, soluble TNF-receptors), antioxidants, insulin-sensitizing agents, lipid modulators (e.g., activators of lipoprotein lipase, L-carnitine), anabolic cytokines (e.g., IL-15), and cannabinoid-receptor antagonists.[322–324]

## Summary of Pharmacologic Treatment of Primary Cachexia

The established pharmacologic treatments for primary cachexia are listed in Table 71–5. A summary of these treatments is given below:

- The individual symptomatic goals guide the decision for treatment.
- Antineoplastic treatments can provide symptomatic relief.
- Level I evidence shows that corticosteroids, progestins, and metoclopramide are effective in primary cachexia.
- Corticosteroids improve appetite and, in many cases, quality of life for a few weeks.
- Progestins improve appetite at low doses, cause nonfluid weight gain at higher doses, and, in some cases, influence quality of life.

- Metoclopramide alleviates chronic nausea and anorexia in the context of early satiety and probably autonomic failure.
- Several promising drugs, such as omega-3 fatty acids, thalidomide, cannabinoids, ATP, and betamimetics, are under clinical experimental evaluation.

## Decision Making and Perspectives

Nutrition has to be tailored to the needs of individual patients and their families, taking into account psychosocial factors and the patient's need for specific nutrients. Management of nutritional issues has in recent years shifted from a more nutrition-based approach to an integrative approach, in which outcomes such as improvement of function and symptomatic benefit are of increasing importance. With increased emphasis on individualized goals of antineoplastic treatments, the decision making for nutritional support requires careful discussion with both the patient and the patient's family (Fig. 71–3).

A careful assessment and the better definition of the underlying mechansim of weight loss in an individual patient allows more efficient interventions for both nutritional support and treatment for primary cachexia. Several new agents for the treatment of primary cachexia have reached the stage of randomized controlled trials. The mechanisms of action at different levels differ by agent and include appetite stimulation through the central nervous system, a reduction in cytokine production, a reduction in production of proteolytic or lipolytic factors by the tumor, and modulating effects on muscles and protein breakdown. The targeting of interventions at multiple different sites of action will allow the development of combined therapies for the management of cancer anorexia–cachexia and malnutrition. Because the different syndromes associated with weight loss (i.e., anorexia, asthenia, and even primary cachexia) have not yet been appropriately characterized, the methodology chosen for future trials constitutes the best way to assess the intensity of anorexia, asthenia, and other symptoms, as well as caloric intake, nutritional status, function, and well-being.

This emerging body of research strongly suggests that it is possible to interfere with cancer malnutrition/cachexia at multi-

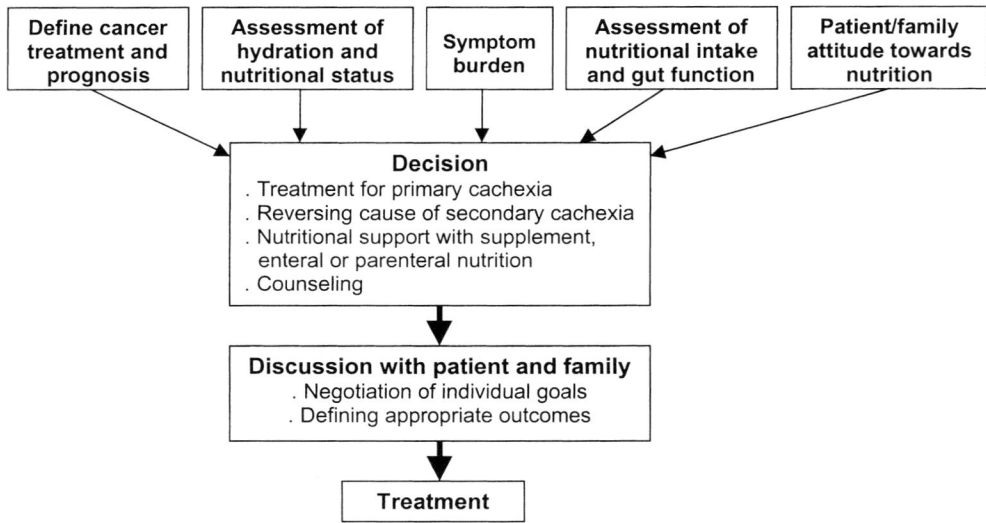

**Figure 71-3** Management of malnutrition/cachexia: decision making.

ple levels other than by decreasing tumor mass. The ultimate objective is to eliminate the concept of cachexia as a normal and inevitable consequence of advanced cancer.

## References

1. Hockley JM, Dunlop R, Davies RJ. Survey of distressing symptoms in dying patients and their families in hospital and the response to a symptom control team. BMJ (Clin Res Ed) 296(6638):1715–1717, 1988.
2. Velikova G, Wright P, Smith AB, et al. Self-reported quality of life of individual cancer patients: concordance of results with disease course and medical records. J Clin Oncol 19:2064–2073, 2001.
3. Bruera E, Fainsinger R. Clinical management of cachexia and anorexia. In: Doyle D, Hanks GWC, MacDonald N (eds): Oxford Textbook of Palliative Medicine, 2nd ed. Oxford University Press, Oxford, 1998, pp 548–556.
4. MacDonald N, Alexander HR, Bruera E. Cachexia–anorexia–asthenia. J Pain Symptom Manage 10:151–155, 1995.
5. Watanabe S, Bruera E. Anorexia and cachexia, asthenia, and lethargy. Hematol Oncol Clin North Am 10:189–206, 1996.
6. Pereira J, Bruera E. Chronic nausea. In: Bruera E, Higginson I (eds): Cachexia–Anorexia in Cancer Patients. Oxford University Press, Oxford, 1996, pp 23–37.
7. Bruera E, Catz Z, Hooper R, Lentle B, MacDonald N. Chronic nausea and anorexia in advanced cancer patients: a possible role for autonomic dysfunction. J Pain Symptom Manage 2:19–21, 1987.
8. Strasser F. Impact of fluid retention on evaluation of cancer cachexia [abstract 33]. Support Care Cancer 8:249, 2000.
9. Bruera E, MacDonald RN. Nutrition in cancer patients: an update and review of our experience. Issues in symptom control. Part 3. J Pain Symptom Manage 3:133–140, 1988.
10. DeWys WD, Begg C, Lavin PT, et al. Prognostic effect of weight loss prior to chemotherapy in cancer patients. Eastern Cooperative Oncology Group. Am J Med 69:491–497, 1980.
11. Muller JM, Brenner U, Dienst C, Pichlmaier H. Preoperative parenteral feeding in patients with gastrointestinal carcinoma. Lancet 1(8263):68–71, 1982.
12. Andreyev HJ, Norman AR, Oates J, Cunningham D. Why do patients with weight loss have a worse outcome when undergoing chemotherapy for gastrointestinal malignancies? Eur J Cancer 34:503–509, 1998.
13. Terwee CB, Nieven Van Dijkum EJ, Gouma DJ, et al. Pooling of prognostic studies in cancer of the pancreatic head and periampullary region: the Triple-P study. Triple-P study group. Eur J Surg 166:706–712, 2000.
14. Portenoy RK, Thaler HT, Kornblith AB, et al. Symptom prevalence, characteristics and distress in a cancer population. Qual Life Res 3:183–189, 1994.
15. Reuben DB, Mor V, Hiris J. Clinical symptoms and length of survival in patients with terminal cancer. Arch Intern Med 148:1586–1591, 1988.
16. O'Gorman P, McMillan DC, McArdle CS. Longitudinal study of weight, appetite, performance status, and inflammation in advanced gastrointestinal cancer. Nutr Cancer 35:127–129, 1999.
17. Curtis EB, Krech R, Walsh TD. Common symptoms in patients with advanced cancer. J Palliat Care 7:25–29, 1991.
18. Rauch DP, Maurer CA, Aebi S, et al. Activity of gemcitabine and continuous infusion fluorouracil in advanced pancreatic cancer. Oncology 60:43–48, 2001.
19. Hoffman K, Glimelius B. Evaluation of clinical benefit of chemotherapy in patients with upper gastrointestinal cancer. Acta Oncol 37:651–659, 1998.
20. Ulrich-Pur H, Kornek GV, Raderer M, et al. A phase II trial of biweekly high dose gemcitabine for patients with metastatic pancreatic adenocarcinoma. Cancer 88:2505–2511, 2000.
21. Martin JL, Harvey HA, Lipton A, Martin R. Combined chemoradiotherapy for unresectable pancreatic cancer. Am J Clin Oncol 22:309–314, 1999.
22. Feliu J, Lopez Alvarez MP, Jaraiz MA, et al. Phase II trial of gemcitabine and UFT modulated by leucovorin in patients with advanced pancreatic carcinoma. The ONCOPAZ Cooperative Group. Cancer 89:1706–1713, 2000.
23. Burch PA, Block M, Schroeder G, et al. Phase III evaluation of octreotide versus chemotherapy with 5-fluorouracil or 5-fluorouracil plus leucovorin in advanced exocrine pancreatic cancer: a North Central Cancer Treatment Group study. Clin Cancer Res 6:3486–3492, 2000.
24. Cantore M, Pederzoli P, Cornalba G, et al. Intra-arterial chemotherapy for unresectable pancreatic cancer. Ann Oncol 11:569–573, 2000.
25. David AK, Vaughn DJ, Holroyde CP, Armstead B, Haller DG. A phase II trial of 5-fluorouracil, leucovorin, and interferon α 2A (IFN-α 2a) in metastatic pancreatic carcinoma: a Penn Cancer Clinical Trials Group (PCCTG) trial. Am J Clin Oncol 23:37–39, 2000.
26. Berlin JD, Adak S, Vaughn DJ, et al. A phase II study of gemcitabine and 5-fluorouracil in metastatic pancreatic cancer: an Eastern Cooperative Oncology Group Study (E3296). Oncology 58:215–218, 2000.
27. Burris H, Storniolo AM. Assessing clinical benefit in the treatment of pancreas cancer: gemcitabine compared to 5-fluorouracil. Eur J Cancer 33(Suppl 1):S18–S22, 1997.
28. Burris HA 3rd, Moore MJ, Andersen J, et al. Improvements in survival and clinical benefit with gemcitabine as first-line therapy for patients with advanced pancreas cancer: a randomized trial J Clin Oncol 15:2403–2413, 1997.
29. Cascinu S, Silva RR, Barni S, et al. A combination of gemcitabine and 5-fluorouracil in advanced pancreatic cancer, a report from the Italian Group for the Study of Digestive Tract Cancer (GISCAD). Br J Cancer 80:1595–1598, 1999.
30. Vainio A, Auvinen A. Prevalence of symptoms among patients with advanced cancer: an international collaborative study. Symptom Prevalence Group. J Pain Symptom Manage 12:3–10, 1996.
31. Dunlop R. Clinical epidemiology of cancer cachexia. In: Bruera E, Higginson I (eds): Cachexia–Anorexia in Cancer Patients. Oxford University Press, Oxford, 1996, pp 76–82.
32. Verweij J, Nooter K, Stoter G. Principles of systemic therapy of cancer. In Cavalli F, Hansen H, Kaye SB (eds): Textbook of Medical Oncology, 2nd ed. Martin Dunitz Ltd, London, 2000, pp 67–98.
33. Bruera E, Sweeney C. Cachexia and asthenia in cancer patients. Lancet Oncol 1:138–147, 2000.
34. Gullo L, Migliori PT, Casadei R, Marrano D. Do early symptoms of pancreatic cancer exist that can allow an earlier diagnosis? Pancreas 22:210–213, 2001.
35. Walsh D, Donnelly S, Rybicki L. The symptoms of advanced cancer: relationship to age, gender, and performance status in 1,000 patients. Support Care Cancer 8:175–179, 2000.
36. Donnelly S, Walsh D, Rybicki L. The symptoms of advanced cancer: identification of clinical and research priorities by assessment of prevalence and severity. J Palliat Care 11:27–32, 1995.
37. Komurcu S, Nelson KA, Walsh D. The gastrointestinal symptoms of advanced cancer. Support Care Cancer 9:32–39, 2001.
38. Vigano A, Bruera E, Jhangri GS, Newman SC, Fields AL, Suarez-Almazor ME. Clinical survival predictors in patients with advanced cancer. Arch Intern Med 160:861–868, 2000.
39. Loprinzi CL, Laurie JA, Wieand HS, et al. Prospective evaluation of prognostic variables from patient-completed questionnaires. North Central Cancer Treatment Group. J Clin Oncol 12:601–607, 1994.
40. Reuben DB, Mor V, Hiris J. Clinical symptoms and length of survival in patients with terminal cancer. Arch Intern Med 148:1586–1591, 1988.
41. Llobera J, Esteva M, Rifa J, Benito E, Terrasa J, Rojas C, et al. Terminal cancer. Duration and prediction of survival time. Eur J Cancer 36:2036–2043, 2000.
42. Bruera E, Carraro S, Roca E, Cedaro L, Chacon R. Association between malnutrition and caloric intake, emesis, psychological depression, glucose taste, and tumor mass. Cancer Treat Rep 68:873–876, 1984.
43. Ingham J, Portenoy R. Cachexia in context: the interactions among anorexia, pain, and other symptoms. In Bruera E, Higginson I (eds): Cachexia–Anorexia in Cancer Patients. Oxford University Press, Oxford, 1996, pp 158–171.
44. Klein S, Kinney J, Jeejeebhoy K, et al. Nutrition support in clinical practice: review of published data and recommendations for future research directions. Summary of a conference sponsored by the National Institutes of Health, American Society for Parenteral and Enteral Nutrition, and American Society for Clinical Nutrition. Am J Clin Nutr 66:683–706, 1997.
45. Laviano A, Meguid MM. Nutritional issues in cancer management. Nutrition 12:358–371, 1996.
46. Koretz RL. Parental nutrition: is it oncologically logical? (review). J Clin Oncol 2:534–538, 1984.
47. Creutzberg EC, Schols AM, Weling-Scheepers CA, Buurman WA, Wouters EF. Characterization of nonresponse to high caloric oral nutritional therapy in depleted patients with chronic obstructive pulmonary disease. Am J Respir Crit Care Med 161(3 Pt 1):745–752, 2000.
48. Theologides A, Ehlert J, Kennedy BJ. The calorie intake of patients with advanced cancer. Minn Med 59:526–529, 1976.
49. Nelson KA, Walsh D, Sheehan FA. The cancer anorexia–cachexia syndrome. J Clin Oncol 12:213–225, 1994.

50. Body JJ. The syndrome of anorexia–cachexia. Curr Opin Oncol 11: 255–260, 1999.

51. Bruera E. ABC of palliative care. Anorexia, cachexia, and nutrition. BMJ 315(7117):1219–1222, 1997.

52. Brennan MF. Uncomplicated starvation versus cancer cachexia. Cancer Res 37(7 Pt 2):2359–2364, 1977.

53. Fearon KC, Preston T. Body composition in cancer cachexia. Infusionstherapie 17(Suppl 3):63–66, 1990.

54. Heymsfield SB, McManus CB. Tissue components of weight loss in cancer patients. A new method of study and preliminary observations. Cancer 55(1 Suppl):238–249, 1985.

55. Tisdale MJ. Wasting in cancer. J Nutr 129(1S Suppl):243S–246S, 1999.

56. Jaskowiak NT, Alexander HR. The pathophysiology of cancer cachexia. In Doyle D, Hanks GWC, MacDonald N (eds): Oxford Textbook of Palliative Medicine, 2nd ed. Oxford University Press, New York, 1998, pp 534–548.

57. Zylicz Z, Schwantje O, Wagener DJ, Folgering HT. Metabolic response to enteral food in different phases of cancer cachexia in rats. Oncology 47:87–91, 1990.

58. Falconer JS, Fearon KC, Plester CE, Ross JA, Carter DC. Cytokines, the acute-phase response, and resting energy expenditure in cachectic patients with pancreatic cancer. Ann Surg 219:325–331, 1994.

59. Tayek JA. A review of cancer cachexia and abnormal glucose metabolism in humans with cancer. J Am Coll Nutr 11:445–456, 1992.

60. Heber D, Chlebowski RT, Ishibashi DE, Herrold JN, Block JB. Abnormalities in glucose and protein metabolism in noncachectic lung cancer patients. Cancer Res 42:4815–4819, 1982.

61. Shaw JH, Wolfe RR. Glucose and urea kinetics in patients with early and advanced gastrointestinal cancer: the response to glucose infusion, parenteral feeding, and surgical resection. Surgery 101:181–191, 1987.

62. Vlassara H, Spiegel RJ, San Doval D, Cerami A. Reduced plasma lipoprotein lipase activity in patients with malignancy-associated weight loss. Horm Metab Res 18:698–703, 1986.

63. Melville S, McNurlan MA, Calder AG, Garlick PJ. Increased protein turnover despite normal energy metabolism and responses to feeding in patients with lung cancer. Cancer Res 50:1125–1131, 1990.

64. Pisters PW, Pearlstone DB. Protein and amino acid metabolism in cancer cachexia: investigative techniques and therapeutic interventions. Crit Rev Clin Lab Sci 30:223–272, 1993.

65. Baumann H, Gauldie J. The acute phase response [review]. Immunol Today 15:74–80, 1994.

66. Attaix D, Combaret L, Tilignac T, Taillandier D. Adaptation of the ubiquitin-proteasome proteolytic pathway in cancer cachexia [review]. Mol Biol Rep 26:77–82, 1999.

67. Williams A, Sun X, Fischer JE, Hasselgren PO. The expression of genes in the ubiquitin-proteasome proteolytic pathway is increased in skeletal muscle from patients with cancer. Surgery 126:744–749, 1999.

68. Guttridge DC, Mayo MW, Madrid LV, Wang CY, Baldwin AS Jr. NF-κB-induced loss of MyoD messenger RNA: possible role in muscle decay and cachexia. Science 289(5488):2363–2366, 2000.

69. Mitch WE, Price SR. Transcription factors and muscle cachexia: is there a therapeutic target? Lancet 357(9258):734–735, 2001.

70. Tisdale MJ. Biomedicine. Protein loss in cancer cachexia. Science 289(5488):2293–2294, 2000.

71. Bozzetti F, Gavazzi C, Ferrari P, Dworzak F. Effect of total parenteral nutrition on the protein kinetics of patients with cancer cachexia. Tumori 86:408–411, 2000.

72. Barber MD, Fearon KC, McMillan DC, Slater C, Ross JA, Preston T. Liver export protein synthetic rates are increased by oral meal feeding in weight-losing cancer patients. Am J Physiol Endocrinol Metab 279(3):E707–E714, 2000.

73. Staal-van den Brekel AJ, Schols AM, Dentener MA, ten Velde GP, Buurman WA, Wouters EF. The effects of treatment with chemotherapy on energy metabolism and inflammatory mediators in small-cell lung carcinoma. Br J Cancer 76:1630–1635, 1997.

74. Torelli GF, Meguid MM, Moldawer LL, et al. Use of recombinant human soluble TNF receptor in anorectic tumor-bearing rats. Am J Physiol 277(3 Pt 2):R850–R855, 1999.

75. Costelli P, Carbo N, Tessitore L, et al. Tumor necrosis factor-alpha mediates changes in tissue protein turnover in a rat cancer cachexia model. J Clin Invest 92:2783–2789, 1993.

76. Socher SH, Martinez D, Craig JB, Kuhn JG, Oliff A. Tumor necrosis factor not detectable in patients with clinical cancer cachexia. J Natl Cancer Inst 80:595–598, 1988.

77. Maltoni M, Fabbri L, Nanni O, et al. Serum levels of tumour necrosis factor alpha and other cytokines do not correlate with weight loss and anorexia in cancer patients. Support Care Cancer 5:130–135, 1997.

78. Thompson MP, Cooper ST, Parry BR, Tuckey JA. Increased expression of the mRNA for hormone-sensitive lipase in adipose tissue of cancer patients. Biochim Biophys Acta 1180:236–242, 1993.

79. Scuderi P, Sterling KE, Lam KS, et al. Raised serum levels of tumour necrosis factor in parasitic infections. Lancet 2(8520):1364–1365, 1986.

80. Kaliman P, Canicio J, Testar X, Palacin M, Zorzano A. Insulin-like growth factor-II, phosphatidylinositol 3-kinase, nuclear factor-κB and inducible nitric-oxide synthase define a common myogenic signaling pathway. J Biol Chem 274:17437–17344, 1999.

81. Cahlin C, Korner A, Axelsson H, Wang W, Lundholm K, Svanberg E. Experimental cancer cachexia: the role of host-derived cytokines interleukin (IL)-6, IL-12, interferon-gamma, and tumor necrosis factor alpha evaluated in gene knockout, tumor-bearing mice on C57 Bl background and eicosanoid-dependent cachexia. Cancer Res 60:5488–5493, 2000.

82. Fujita J, Tsujinaka T, Yano M, et al. Anti-interleukin-6 receptor antibody prevents muscle atrophy in colon-26 adenocarcinoma-bearing mice with modulation of lysosomal and ATP-ubiquitin-dependent proteolytic pathways. Int J Cancer 68:637–643, 1996.

83. Strassmann G, Fong M, Kenney JS, Jacob CO. Evidence for the involvement of interleukin 6 in experimental cancer cachexia. J Clin Invest 89:1681–1684, 1992.

84. Espat NJ, Auffenberg T, Rosenberg JJ, et al. Ciliary neurotrophic factor is catabolic and shares with IL-6 the capacity to induce an acute phase response. Am J Physiol 271(1 Pt 2):R185–R190, 1996.

85. Yasumoto K, Mukaida N, Harada A, et al. Molecular analysis of the cytokine network involved in cachexia in colon 26 adenocarcinoma-bearing mice. Cancer Res 55:921–927, 1995.

86. Scott HR, McMillan DC, Crilly A, McArdle CS, Milroy R et al. The relationship between weight loss and interleukin 6 in non–small-cell lung cancer. Br J Cancer 73:1560–1562, 1996.

87. Matthys P, Dijkmans R, Proost P, et al. Severe cachexia in mice inoculated with interferon-γ-producing tumor cells. Int J Cancer 49:77–82, 1991.

88. Costelli P, Llovera M, Lopez-Soriano J, et al. Lack of effect of eicosapentaenoic acid in preventing cancer cachexia and inhibiting tumor growth. Cancer Lett 97:25–32, 1995.

89. Khan S, Tisdale MJ. Catabolism of adipose tissue by a tumour-produced lipid-mobilising factor. Int J Cancer 80:444–447, 1999.

90. Hussey HJ, Tisdale MJ. Effect of a cachectic factor on carbohydrate metabolism and attenuation by eicosapentaenoic acid. Br J Cancer 80:1231–1235, 1999.

91. Tisdale MJ. Biology of cachexia. J Natl Cancer Inst 89(23):1763–1773, 1997.

92. Tisdale MJ. Metabolic abnormalities in cachexia and anorexia [review]. Nutrition 16:1013–1014, 2000.

93. Smith KL, Tisdale MJ. Mechanism of muscle protein degradation in cancer cachexia. Br J Cancer 68:314–318, 1993.

94. Smith KL, Tisdale MJ. Increased protein degradation and decreased protein synthesis in skeletal muscle during cancer cachexia. Br J Cancer 67:680–685, 1993.

95. Belizario JE, Katz M, Chenker E, Raw I. Bioactivity of skeletal muscle proteolysis-inducing factors in the plasma proteins from cancer patients with weight loss. Br J Cancer 63:705–710, 1991.

96. Todorov P, Cariuk P, McDevitt T, Coles B, Fearon K, Tisdale M. Characterization of a cancer cachectic factor. Nature 379(6567):739–742, 1996.

97. Todorov PT, Deacon M, Tisdale MJ. Structural analysis of a tumor-produced sulfated glycoprotein capable of initiating muscle protein degradation. J Biol Chem 272:12279–12288, 1997.

98. Cariuk P, Lorite MJ, Todorov PT, Field WN, Wigmore SJ, Tisdale MJ. Induction of cachexia in mice by a product isolated from the urine of cachectic cancer patients. Br J Cancer 6:606–613, 1997.

99. Lorite MJ, Thompson MG, Drake JL, Carling G, Tisdale MJ. Mechanism of muscle protein degradation induced by a cancer cachectic factor. Br J Cancer 78:850–856, 1998.

100. Lorite MJ, Cariuk P, Tisdale MJ. Induction of muscle protein degradation by a tumour factor. Br J Cancer 76:1035–1040, 1997.

101. Smith HJ, Lorite MJ, Tisdale MJ. Effect of a cancer cachectic factor on protein synthesis/degradation in murine C2C12 myoblasts: modulation by eicosapentaenoic acid. Cancer Res 59:5507–5513, 1999.

102. De Blaauw I, Heeneman S, Deutz NE, von Meyenfeldt MF. Increased whole-body protein and glutamine turnover in advanced cancer is not matched by an increased muscle protein and glutamine turnover. J Surg Res 68:44–55, 1997.

103. Wigmore SJ, Todorov PT, Barber MD, Ross JA, Tisdale MJ, Fearon KC. Characteristics of patients with pancreatic cancer expressing a novel cancer cachectic factor. Br J Surg 87:53–58, 2000.

104. Rodemann HP, Goldberg AL. Arachidonic acid, prostaglandin E2 and F2 alpha influence rates of protein turnover in skeletal and cardiac muscle. J Biol Chem 257:1632–1638, 1982.

105. Hasselgren PO, Zamir O, James JH, Fischer JE. Prostaglandin E2 does not regulate total or myofibrillar protein breakdown in incubated skeletal muscle from normal or septic rats. Biochem J 270:45–50, 1990.

106. Barrett R, Hyde SA, Scott OM, Dubowitz V. Changes in center of gravity in boys with Duchenne muscular dystrophy. Muscle Nerve 11:1157–1163, 1988.

107. Goll DE, Thompson VF, Taylor RG, Christiansen JA. Role of the calpain system in muscle growth [review]. Biochimie 74:225–237, 1992.

108. Baracos VE, DeVivo C, Hoyle DH, Goldberg AL. Activation of the ATP–ubiquitin–proteasome pathway in skeletal muscle of cachectic rats bearing a hepatoma. Am J Physiol 268(5 Pt 1):E996–E1006, 1995.

109. Temparis S, Asensi M, Taillandier D, et al. Increased ATP–ubiquitin–dependent proteolysis in skeletal muscles of tumor-bearing rats. Cancer Res 54:5568–5573, 1994.

110. Kitada S, Hays EF, Mead JF. A lipid mobilizing factor in serum of tumor-bearing mice. Lipids 15:168–174, 1980.

111. Masuno H, Yamasaki N, Okuda H. Purification and characterization of a lipolytic factor (toxohormone-L) from cell-free fluid of ascites sarcoma 180. Cancer Res 41:284–288, 1981.

112. Beck SA, Tisdale MJ. Production of lipolytic and proteolytic factors by a murine tumor-producing cachexia in the host. Cancer Res 47:5919–5923, 1987.

113. Groundwater P, Beck SA, Barton C, Adamson C, Ferrier IN, Tisdale MJ. Alteration of serum and urinary lipolytic activity with weight loss in cachectic cancer patients. Br J Cancer 62:816–821, 1990.

114. Beck SA, Groundwater P, Barton C, Tisdale MJ. Alterations in serum lipolytic activity of cancer patients with response to therapy. Br J Cancer 62:822–825, 1990.

115. Bessey PQ, Watters JM, Aoki TT, Wilmore DW. Combined hormonal infusion simulates the metabolic response to injury. Ann Surg 200:264–281, 1984.

116. Watters JM, Bessey PQ, Dinarello CA, Wolff SM, Wilmore DW. Both inflammatory and endocrine mediators stimulate host responses to sepsis. Arch Surg 121:179–190, 1986.

117. Schaur RJ, Fellier H, Gleispach H, Fink E, Kronberger L. Tumor host relations. I. Increased plasma cortisol in tumor-bearing humans compared with patients with benign surgical diseases. J Cancer Res Clin Oncol 93:281–285, 1979.

118. Schaur RJ, Semmelrock HJ, Schauenstein E, Kronberger L. Tumor host relations. II. Influence of tumor extent and tumor site on plasma cortisol of patients with malignant diseases. J Cancer Res Clin Oncol 93:287–292, 1979.

119. Burt ME, Aoki TT, Gorschboth CM, Brennan MF. Peripheral tissue metabolism in cancer-bearing man. Ann Surg 198:685–691, 1983.

120. Knapp ML, al-Sheibani S, Riches PG, Hanham IW, Phillips RH. Hormonal factors associated with weight loss in patients with advanced breast cancer. Ann Clin Biochem 28(Pt 5):480–486, 1991.

121. Holroyde CP, Skutches CL, Boden G, Reichard GA. Glucose metabolism in cachectic patients with colorectal cancer. Cancer Res 44(12 Pt 1):5910–5913, 1984.

122. Llovera M, Garcia-Martinez C, Costelli P, et al. Muscle hypercatabolism during cancer cachexia is not reversed by the glucocorticoid receptor antagonist RU38486. Cancer Lett 99:7–14, 1996.

123. Grosvenor M, Bulcavage L, Chlebowski RT. Symptoms potentially influencing weight loss in a cancer population. Correlations with primary site, nutritional status, and chemotherapy administration. Cancer 63:330–334, 1989.

124. Cangiano C, Testa U, Muscaritoli M, et al. Cytokines, tryptophan and anorexia in cancer patients before and after surgical tumor ablation. Anticancer Res 14(3B):1451–1455, 1994.

125. Chance WT, Balasubramaniam A, Thompson H, Mohapatra B, Ramo J, Fischer JE. Assessment of feeding response of tumor-bearing rats to hypothalamic injection and infusion of neuropeptide Y. Peptides 17:797–801, 1996.

126. Grunfeld C, Zhao C, Fuller J, Pollack A, Moser A, Friedman J, Feingold KR. Endotoxin and cytokines induce expression of leptin, the ob gene product, in hamsters. J Clin Invest 97:2152–2157, 1996.

127. Sarraf P, Frederich RC, Turner EM, et al. Multiple cytokines and acute inflammation raise mouse leptin levels: potential role in inflammatory anorexia. J Exp Med 185:171–175, 1997.

128. Simons JP, Schols AM, Campfield LA, Wouters EF, Saris WH. Plasma concentration of total leptin and human lung-cancer–associated cachexia. Clin Sci (Colch) 93:273–277, 1997.

129. Di Marzo V, Goparaju SK, Wang L, et al. Leptin-regulated endocannabinoids are involved in maintaining food intake. Nature 410 (6830):822–825, 2001.

130. Bruera E, Chadwick S, Fox R, Hanson J, MacDonald N. Study of cardiovascular autonomic insufficiency in advanced cancer patients. Cancer Treat Rep 70:1383–1387, 1986.

131. Rowe PC, Bou-Holaigah I, Kan JS, Calkins H. Is neurally mediated hypotension an unrecognised cause of chronic fatigue? Lancet 345 (8950):623–624, 1995.

132. Glaus A. Fatigue and cachexia in cancer patients. Support Care Cancer 6:77–78, 1998.

133. Neuenschwander H, Bruera E. Asthenia–Cachexia. In: Bruera E, Higginson I (eds): Cachexia–Anorexia in Cancer Patients. Oxford University Press, Oxford, 1996, pp 57–75.

134. Bruera E, Brenneis C, Michaud M, et al. Association between asthenia and nutritional status, lean body mass, anemia, psychological status, and tumor mass in patients with advanced breast cancer. J Pain Symptom Manage 4:59–63, 1989.

135. Grinspoon S, Corcoran C, Lee K, et al. Loss of lean body and muscle mass correlates with androgen levels in hypogonadal men with acquired immunodeficiency syndrome and wasting. J Clin Endocrinol Metab 81:4051–4058, 1996.

136. Grinspoon S, Corcoran C, Miller K, et al. Body composition and endocrine function in women with acquired immunodeficiency syndrome wasting. J Clin Endocrinol Metab 82:1332–1337, 1997.

137. Morley JE: The endocrinology of the opiates and opioid peptides [review]. Metabolism. 30:195–209, 1981.

138. Abs R, Verhelst J, Maeyaert J, et al. Endocrine consequences of long-term intrathecal administration of opioids. J Clin Endocrinol Metab 85:2215–2222, 2000.

139. Isgaard J, Bergh CH, Caidahl K, Lomsky M, Hjalmarson A, Bengtsson BA. A placebo-controlled study of growth hormone in patients with congestive heart failure. Eur Heart J 19:1704–1711, 1998.

140. Osterziel KJ, Strohm O, Schuler J, et al. Randomised, double-blind, placebo-controlled trial of human recombinant growth hormone in patients with chronic heart failure due to dilated cardiomyopathy. Lancet 351(9111):1233–1237, 1998.

141. Papadakis MA, Grady D, Black D, et al. Growth hormone replacement in healthy older men improves body composition but not functional ability. Ann Intern Med 124:708–716, 1996.

142. Burdet L, de Muralt B, Schutz Y, Pichard C, Fitting JW. Administration of growth hormone to underweight patients with chronic obstructive pulmonary disease. A prospective, randomized, controlled study. Am J Respir Crit Care Med 156:1800–1806, 1997.

143. Schambelan M, Mulligan K, Grunfeld C, et al. Recombinant human growth hormone in patients with HIV-associated wasting. A randomized, placebo-controlled trial. Serostim Study Group. Ann Intern Med 125:873–882, 1996.

144. Strawford A, Barbieri T, Neese R, et al. Effects of nandrolone decanoate therapy in borderline hypogonadal men with HIV-associated weight loss. J Acquir Immune Defic Syndr Hum Retrovirol 20:137–146, 1999.

145. Johansen KL, Mulligan K, Schambelan M. Anabolic effects of nandrolone decanoate in patients receiving dialysis: a randomized controlled trial. JAMA 281:1275–1281, 1999.

146. Ferreira IM, Verreschi IT, Nery LE et al. The influence of 6 months of oral anabolic steroids on body mass and respiratory muscles in undernourished COPD patients. Chest 114:19–28, 1998.

147. Miller K, Corcoran C, Armstrong C, et al. Transdermal testosterone administration in women with acquired immunodeficiency syndrome wasting: a pilot study. J Clin Endocrinol Metab 83:2717–2725, 1998.

148. Bhasin S, Storer TW, Javanbakht M, et al. Testosterone replacement and resistance exercise in HIV-infected men with weight loss and low testosterone levels. JAMA 283:763–770, 2000.

149. Bhasin S, Storer TW, Asbel-Sethi N, et al. Effects of testosterone replacement with a nongenital, transdermal system, Androderm, in human immunodeficiency virus-infected men with low testosterone levels. J Clin Endocrinol Metab 83:3155–3162, 1998.

150. DeWys WD, Walters K. Abnormalities of taste sensation in cancer patients. Cancer 36:1888–1896, 1975.

151. Davies IJ, Musa M, Dormandy TL. Measurements of plasma zinc. II. In malignant disease. J Clin Pathol 21:363–365, 1968.

152. Mancini I, Bruera E. Constipation in advanced cancer patients. Support Care Cancer 6:356–364, 1998.

153. Jeejeebhoy KN, Detsky AS, Baker JP. Assessment of nutritional status. J Parenter Enteral Nutr (5 Suppl):193S–196S, 1990.

154. Baker JP, Detsky AS, Wesson DE, et al. Nutritional assessment: a comparison of clinical judgement and objective measurements. N Engl J Med 306:969–972, 1982.

155. Dearman K, Replogle WH, Cora VL, Meeks M, Canada T. Use of subjective global assessment to identify nutrition-associated complications and death in geriatric long-term care facility residents. J Am Coll Nutr 19:570–577, 2000.

156. Lawson JA, Lazarus R, Kelly JJ. Prevalence and prognostic significance of malnutrition in chronic renal insufficiency. J Renal Nutr 11:16–22, 2001.

157. Niyongabo T, Melchior JC, Henzel D, Bouchaud O, Larouze B. Comparison of methods for assessing nutritional status in HIV-infected adults. Nutrition 15:740–743, 1999.

158. Persson C, Sjoden PO, Glimelius B. The Swedish version of the patient-generated subjective global assessment of nutritional status: gastrointestinal vs. urological cancers. Clin Nutr 18:71–77, 1999.

159. Figueiredo F, Dickson ER, Pasha T, et al. Impact of nutritional status on outcomes after liver transplantation. Transplantation 70:1347–1352, 2000.

160. Higginson I, Winget C. Psychological impact of cancer cachexia on the patient and family. In: Bruera E, Higginson I (eds): Cachexia–Anorexia in Cancer Patients. Oxford University Press, Oxford, 1996, pp 172–183.

161. Bruera E, Higginson I. Preface. In: Bruera E, Higginson I (eds): Cachexia–Anorexia in Cancer Patients. Oxford University Press, Oxford, 1996, pp. v–vi.

162. Durnin JV, Womersley J. Body fat assessed from total body density and its estimation from skinfold thickness: measurements on 481 men and women aged from 16 to 72 years. Br J Nutr 32:77–97, 1974.

163. Conlisk EA, Haas JD, Martinez EJ, Flores R, Rivera JD, Martorell R. Predicting body composition from anthropometry and bioimpedance in marginally undernourished adolescents and young adults. Am J Clin Nutr 55:1051–1060, 1992.

164. Simons JP, Schols AM, Westerterp KR, ten Velde GP, Wouters EF. The use of bioelectrical impedance analysis to predict total body water in patients with cancer cachexia. Am J Clin Nutr 61:741–745, 1995.

165. Presta E, Wang J, Harrison GG, Bjorntorp P, Harker WH, Van Itallie TB. Measurement of total body electrical conductivity: a new method for estimation of body composition. Am J Clin Nutr 37:735–739, 1983.

166. Sarhill N, Walsh D, Nelson K, Homsi J, Komurcu S. Bioelectrical impedance, cancer nutritional assessment, and ascites. Support Care Cancer 8:341–343, 2000.

167. Loprinzi CL, Schaid DJ, Dose AM, Burnham NL, Jensen MD. Body-composition changes in patients who gain weight while receiving megestrol acetate. J Clin Oncol 11:152–154, 1993.

168. Mazess RB, Barden HS, Bisek JP, Hanson J: Dual-energy X-ray absorptiometry for total-body and regional bone-mineral and soft-tissue composition. Am J Clin Nutr 51:1106–1112, 1990.

169. Roubenoff R, Kehayias JJ, Dawson-Hughes B, Heymsfield SB. Use of dual-energy X-ray absorptiometry in body-composition studies: not yet a "gold standard" [review]. Am J Clin Nutr 58:589–591, 1993.

170. Pichard C, Kyle UG. Body composition measurements during wasting diseases [review]. Curr Opin Clin Nutr Metab Care 1:357–361, 1998.

171. Windsor JA, Hill GL. Grip strength: a measure of the proportion of protein loss in surgical patients. Br J Surg 75:880–882, 1988.

172. Hunt DR, Rowlands BJ, Johnston D. Hand grip strength—a simple prognostic indicator in surgical patients. JPEN J Parenter Enteral Nutr 9:701–704, 1985.

173. Klidjian AM, Foster KJ, Kammerling RM, Cooper A, Karran SJ. Relation of anthropometric and dynamometric variables to serious postoperative complications. BMJ 281(6245):899–901, 1980.

174. Agteresch HJ, Dagnelie PC, van der Gaast A, Stijnen T, Wilson JH. Randomized clinical trial of adenosine 5′-triphosphate in patients with advanced non–small-cell lung cancer. J Natl Cancer Inst 92:321–328, 2000.

175. Jatoi A, Loprinzi CL, Sloan J, Goldberg RM. Is ATP (adenosine 5′-triphosphate), like STP, a performance-enhancing additive for the tanks of cancer patients? J Natl Cancer Inst 92:290–291, 2000.

176. Kaasa T, Wessel J, Darrah J, Bruera E. Inter-rater reliability of formally trained and self-trained raters using the Edmonton Functional Assessment Tool. Palliat Med 14:509–517, 2000.

177. Mendoza TR, Wang XS, Cleeland CS, et al. The rapid assessment of fatigue severity in cancer patients: use of the Brief Fatigue Inventory. Cancer 85:1186–1196, 1999.

178. Bruera E, Kuehn N, Miller MJ, Selmser P, Macmillan K. The Edmonton Symptom Assessment System (ESAS): a simple method for the assessment of palliative care patients. J Palliat Care 7:6–9, 1991.

179. Portenoy RK, Thaler HT, Kornblith AB, et al. The Memorial Symptom Assessment Scale: an instrument for the evaluation of symptom prevalence, characteristics and distress. Eur J Cancer 30A:1326–1336, 1994.

180. Yellen SB, Cella DF, Webster K, Blendowski C, Kaplan E. Measuring fatigue and other anemia-related symptoms with the Functional Assessment of Cancer Therapy (FACT) measurement system. J Pain Symptom Manage 13:63–74, 1997.

181. Chang VT, Hwang SS, Hulsen I, Alejandro Y, Hankinson MT, Kasimis B. Functional assessment of appetite cachexia therapy (FAACT) in patients with advanced cancer. Am Soc Clin Oncol 2000. Abstract 2395 p 608a.

182. Burke M, Bryson EI, Kark AE. Dietary intakes, resting metabolic rates, and body composition in benign and malignant gastrointestinal disease. BMJ 280(6209):211–215, 1980.

183. Bruera E, Chadwick S, Cowan L, Drebit D, Hanson J, MacDonald N, van Konkelenberg Y. Caloric intake assessment in advanced cancer patients: comparison of three methods. Cancer Treat Rep 70:981–983, 1986.

184. Deutsch JC. Normal digestive physiology and the evaluation of digestive function [review]. Semin Oncol 25(2 Suppl 6):4–11, 1998.

185. Chandra RK. Nutrition, immunity, and infection: present knowledge and future directions. Lancet 1(8326 Pt 1):688–691, 1983.

186. Barber MD, Fearon KC, Delmore G, Loprinzi CL. Should cancer patients with incurable disease receive parenteral or enteral nutritional support? Eur J Cancer 34:279–285, 1998.

187. Klein S, Koretz RL. Nutrition support in patients with cancer: what do the data really show? Nutr Clin Pract 9:91–100, 1994.

188. Koretz RL. Parental nutrition: is it oncologically logical? [review]. J Clin Oncol 2:534–538, 1984.

189. Evans WK, Nixon DW, Daly JM, et al. A randomized study of oral nutritional support versus ad lib nutritional intake during chemotherapy for advanced colorectal and non–small-cell lung cancer. J Clin Oncol 5:113–124, 1987.

190. Seligman PA, Fink R, Massey-Seligman EJ. Approach to the seriously ill or terminal cancer patient who has a poor appetite. Semin Oncol 25(2 Suppl 6):33–34, 1998.

191. Ovesen L, Allingstrup L, Hannibal J, Mortensen EL, Hansen OP. Effect of dietary counseling on food intake, body weight, response rate, survival, and quality of life in cancer patients undergoing chemotherapy: a prospective, randomized study. J Clin Oncol 11:2043–2049, 1993.

192. Pencharz PB. Aggressive oral, enteral or parenteral nutrition: prescriptive decisions in children with cancer. Int J Cancer Suppl 11:73–75, 1998.

193. Parenteral nutrition in patients receiving cancer chemotherapy. American College of Physicians. Ann Intern Med 110:734–736, 1989.

194. Klein S, Simes J, Blackburn GL. Total parenteral nutrition and cancer clinical trials. Cancer 58:1378–1386, 1986.

195. McGeer AJ, Detsky AS, O'Rourke K. Parenteral nutrition in cancer patients undergoing chemotherapy: a meta-analysis. Nutrition 6:233–240, 1990.

196. Hill AD, Daly JM. Current indications for intravenous nutritional support in oncology patients. Surg Oncol Clin North Am 4:549–563, 1995.

197. Souba WW. Nutritional support. N Engl J Med 336:41–48, 1997.

198. Weisdorf SA, Lysne J, Wind D, et al. Positive effect of prophylactic total parenteral nutrition on long-term outcome of bone marrow transplantation. Transplantation 43:833–838, 1987.

199. Detsky AS, Baker JP, O'Rourke K, Goel V. Perioperative parenteral nutrition: a meta-analysis [review]. Ann Intern Med 107:195–203, 1987.

200. Detsky AS. Parenteral nutrition—is it helpful? N Engl J Med 325:573–575, 1991.

201. Perioperative total parenteral nutrition in surgical patients. The Veterans Affairs Total Parenteral Nutrition Cooperative Study Group. N Engl J Med 325:525–532, 1991.

202. Sandstrom R, Drott C, Hyltander A, et al. The effect of postoperative intravenous feeding (TPN) on outcome following major surgery evaluated in a randomized study. Ann Surg 217:185–195, 1993.

203. Brennan MF, Pisters PW, Posner M, Quesada O, Shike M. A prospective randomized trial of total parenteral nutrition after major pancreatic resection for malignancy. Ann Surg 220:436–441, 1994.

204. Heys SD, Gough DB, Eremin O. Is nutritional support in patients with cancer undergoing surgery beneficial? Eur J Surg Oncol 22:292–297, 1996.

205. Winter SM. Terminal nutrition: framing the debate for the withdrawal of nutritional support in terminally ill patients [review]. Am J Med 109:723–726, 2000.

206. Torelli GF, Campos AC, Meguid MM. Use of TPN in terminally ill cancer patients. Nutrition 15:665–667, 1999.

207. Tchekmedyian NS, Zahyna D, Halpert C, Heber D. Assessment and maintenance of nutrition in older cancer patients [review]. Oncology (Huntingt) 6(2 Suppl):105–111, 1992.

208. Bozzetti F, Amadori D, Bruera E, et al. Guidelines on artificial nutrition versus hydration in terminal cancer patients. European Association for Palliative Care. Nutrition 12:163–167, 1996.

209. Bruera E, Legris MA, Kuehn N, Miller MJ. Hypodermoclysis for the administration of fluids and narcotic analgesics in patients with advanced cancer. J Pain Symptom Manage 5(4):218–20, 1990.

210. Cherel Y, Robin JP, Heitz A, Calgari C, Le Maho Y. Relationships between lipid availability and protein utilization during prolonged fasting. J Comp Physiol [B] 162:305–313, 1992.

211. Kotler DP, Tierney AR, Wang J, Pierson RN Jr. Magnitude of body-cell-mass depletion and the timing of death from wasting in AIDS. Am J Clin Nutr 50:444–447, 1989.

212. Vigano A, Dorgan M, Bruera E, Suarez-Almazor ME. The relative accuracy of the clinical estimation of the duration of life for patients with end of life cancer. Cancer 86:170–176, 1999.

213. Christakis NA, Lamont EB. Extent and determinants of error in doctors' prognoses in terminally ill patients: prospective cohort study. BMJ 320(7233):469–472, 2000.

214. Bozzetti F, Gavazzi C, Mariani L, Crippa F. Artificial nutrition in cancer patients: which route, what composition? [review]. World J Surg 23:577–583, 1999.

215. Duggan C, Nurko S. "Feeding the gut": the scientific basis for continued enteral nutrition during acute diarrhea [review]. J Pediatr 131:801–808, 1997.

216. Ottery FD. Rethinking nutritional support of the cancer patient: the new field of nutritional oncology [review]. Semin Oncol 21:770–778, 1994.

217. Gray GE, Meguid MM. Can total parenteral nutrition reverse hypoalbuminemia in oncology patients? Nutrition 6:225–228, 1990.

218. Berghmans T, Paesmans M, Body JJ. A prospective study on hyponatraemia in medical cancer patients: epidemiology, aetiology and differential diagnosis. Support Care Cancer 8:192–197, 2000.

219. Bruera E, Belzile M, Watanabe S, Fainsinger RL. Volume of hydration in terminal cancer patients. Support Care Cancer 4:147–150, 1996.

220. Tchekmedyian NS. Pharmacoeconomics of nutritional support in cancer. Semin Oncol 25(2 Suppl 6):62–69, 1998.

221. Mercadante S. Parenteral versus enteral nutrition in cancer patients: indications and practice [review]. Support Care Cancer 6:85–93, 1998.

222. Shike M. Nutrition therapy for the cancer patient [review]. Hematol Oncol Clin North Am 10:221–234, 1996.

223. Guenter P, Susan J, Jacobs DO, Rombeau JL. Administration and delivery of interal nutrition. In: Rombeau JL, Caldwell MD (eds): Clinical Nutrition/Enteral Nutrition, 2nd ed. W.B. Saunders, Philadelphia, 1993, pp 512–536.

224. Daly JM, Torosian MH. Nutritional support. In: DeVita DT, Hellman S, Rosenberg SA (eds): Cancer Principles and Practice of Oncology, 4th ed. J.B. Lippincott, Philadelphia, 1993, pp 2480–2501.

225. Saunders C, Nishikawa R, Wolfe B. Surgical nutrition: a review. J R Coll Surg Edinb 38:195–204, 1993.

226. Lord LM, Weiser-Maimone A, Pulhamus M, Sax HC. Comparison of weighted vs unweighted enteral feeding tubes for efficacy of transpyloric intubation. JPEN J Parenter Enteral Nutr 17:271–273, 1993.

227. Gutierrez ED, Balfe DM. Fluoroscopically guided nasoenteric feeding tube placement: results of a 1-year study. Radiology 178:759–762, 1991.

228. Adams MB, Seabrook GR, Quebbeman EA, Condon RE. Jejunostomy. A rarely indicated procedure. Arch Surg 121:236–238, 1986.

229. Lin HC, Zhao XT, Chu AW, Lin YP, Wang L. Fiber-supplemented enteral formula slows intestinal transit by intensifying inhibitory feedback from the distal gut. Am J Clin Nutr 65:1840–1844, 1997.

230. Kapadia SA, Raimundo AH, Grimble GK, Aimer P, Silk DB. Influence of three different fiber-supplemented enteral diets on bowel function and short-chain fatty acid production. JPEN J Parenter Enteral Nutr 19:63–68, 1995.

231. Silk DA, Payne-Jame JJ. Complications of enteral nutrition. In: Rombeau JL, Caldwell MD (eds): Clinical Nutrition. Enteral and Tube Feeding. W.B. Saunders, Philadelphia, 1990, pp 510–531.

232. Litterman TO. Efficacy and safety of total parenteral nutrition. Nutrition 6:319–328, 1990.

233. Zaloga TP. Immune-enhancing enteral diets: worth the beef? Crit Care Med 26:1143–1146, 1998.

234. Heys SD, Walker LG, Smith I, Eremin O. Enteral nutritional supplementation with key nutrients in patients with critical illness and cancer: a meta-analysis of randomized controlled clinical trials. Ann Surg 229:467–477, 1999.

235. Barton RG. Immune-enhancing enteral formulas: are they beneficial in critically ill patients? [review]. Nutr Clin Pract 12:51–62, 1997.

236. Gianotti L, Alexander JW, Pyles T, Fukushima R. Arginine-supplemented diets improve survival in gut-derived sepsis and peritonitis by modulating bacterial clearance. The role of nitric oxide. Ann Surg 217:644–653, 1993.

237. James LA, Lunn PG, Middleton S, Elia M. Distribution of glutaminase and glutamine synthetase activities in the human gastrointestinal tract. Clin Sci (Colch) 94:313–319, 1998.

238. Ziegler TR, Young LS, Benfell K, et al. Clinical and metabolic efficacy of glutamine-supplemented parenteral nutrition after bone marrow transplantation. A randomized, double-blind, controlled study. Ann Intern Med 116:821–828, 1992.

239. Schloerb PR, Skikne BS. Oral and parenteral glutamine in bone marrow transplantation: a randomized, double-blind study. JPEN J Parenter Enteral Nutr 23:117–122, 1999.

240. Savarese D, Al-Zoubi A, Boucher J. Glutamine for irinotecan diarrhea J Clin Oncol 18:450–451, 2000.

241. Effects of vinorelbine on quality of life and survival of elderly patients with advanced non–small-cell lung cancer. The Elderly Lung Cancer Vinorelbine Italian Study Group. J Natl Cancer Inst 91:66–72, 1999.

242. Cunningham D, Pyrhonen S, James RD, et al. Randomised trial of irinotecan plus supportive care versus supportive care alone after fluorouracil failure for patients with metastatic colorectal cancer. Lancet 352(9138):1413–1418, 1998.

243. Turner JA, Deyo RA, Loeser JD, Von Korff M Fordyce WE. The importance of placebo effects in pain treatment and research [review]. JAMA 271:1609–1614, 1994.

244. Pearce JM. The placebo enigma [review]. Q J Med 88:215–220, 1995.

245. Korn EL, Arbuck SG, Pluda JM, Simon R, Kaplan RS, Christian MC. Clinical trial designs for cytostatic agents: are new approaches needed? J Clin Oncol 19:265–272, 2001.

246. Gagnon B, Bruera E. A review of the drug treatment of cachexia associated with cancer. Drugs 55:675–688, 1998.

247. Bruera E, Seifert L, Watanabe S, et al. Chronic nausea in advanced cancer patients: a retrospective assessment of a metoclopramide-based antiemetic regimen. J Pain Symptom Manage 11:147–153, 1996.

248. Shivshanker K, Bennett RW Jr, Haynie TP. Tumor-associated gastroparesis: correction with metoclopramide. Am J Surg 145:221–225, 1983.

249. Bruera ED, MacEachern TJ, Spachynski KA, et al. Comparison of the efficacy, safety, and pharmacokinetics of controlled release and immediate release metoclopramide for the management of chronic nausea in patients with advanced cancer. Cancer 74:3204–3211, 1994.

250. Bruera E, Belzile M, Neumann C, Harsanyi Z, Babul N, Darke A. A double-blind, crossover study of controlled-release metoclopramide and placebo for the chronic nausea and dyspepsia of advanced cancer. J Pain Symptom Manage 19:427–435, 2000.

251. Nelson KA, Walsh TD. Metoclopramide in anorexia caused by cancer-associated dyspepsia syndrome (CADS). J Palliat Care 9:14–18, 1993.

252. Bruera E, MacEachern T, Spachynski K, et al. Comparison of the efficacy, safety and pharmacokinetics of controlled release and immediate release metoclopramide for the management of chronic nausea in patients with advanced cancer. Cancer 74:3204–3211, 1994.

253. Moertel CG, Schutt AJ, Reitemeier RJ, Hahn RG. Corticosteroid therapy of preterminal gastrointestinal cancer. Cancer 33:1607–1609, 1974.

254. Willox JC, Corr J, Shaw J, Richardson M, Calman KC, Drennan M. Prednisolone as an appetite stimulant in patients with cancer. BMJ (Clin Res Ed) 288(6410):27, 1984.

255. Bruera E, Roca E, Cedaro L, Carraro S, Chacon R. Action of oral methylprednisolone in terminal cancer patients: a prospective randomized double-blind study. Cancer Treat Rep 69:751–754, 1985.

256. Della Cuna GR, Pellegrini A, Piazzi M. Effect of methylprednisolone sodium succinate on quality of life in preterminal cancer patients: a placebo-controlled, multicenter study. The Methylprednisolone Preterminal Cancer Study Group. Eur J Cancer Clin Oncol 25:1817–1821, 1989.

257. Popiela T, Lucchi R, Giongo F. Methylprednisolone as palliative therapy for female terminal cancer patients. The Methylprednisolone Female Preterminal Cancer Study Group. Eur J Cancer Clin Oncol 25:1823–1829, 1989.

258. Ettinger AB, Portenoy RK. The use of corticosteroids in the treatment of symptoms associated with cancer [review]. J Pain Symptom Manage 3:99–103, 1988.

259. Jatoi A, Kumar S, Sloan JA, Nguyen PL. On appetite and its loss. J Clin Oncol 18:2930–2932, 2000.

260. Maltoni M, Nanni O, Scarpi E, Rossi D, Serra P, Amadori D. High-dose progestins for the treatment of cancer anorexia–cachexia syn-

drome: A systematic review of randomised clinical trials. Ann Oncol 12:289–300, 2001.

261. Muurahainen N, Mulligan K. Clinical trials update in human immunodeficiency virus wasting [review]. Semin Oncol 25(2 Suppl 6):104–111, 1998.

262. Loprinzi CL, Michalak JC, Schaid DJ, et al. Phase III evaluation of four doses of megestrol acetate as therapy for patients with cancer anorexia and/or cachexia. J Clin Oncol 11:762–767, 1993.

263. Beller E, Tattersall M, Lumley T, et al. Improved quality of life with megestrol acetate in patients with endocrine-insensitive advanced cancer: a randomised placebo-controlled trial. Australasian Megestrol Acetate Cooperative Study Group. Ann Oncol 8:277–283, 1997.

264. Simons JP, Aaronson NK, Vansteenkiste JF, et al. Effects of medroxyprogesterone acetate on appetite, weight, and quality of life in advanced-stage non–hormone-sensitive cancer: a placebo-controlled multicenter study. J Clin Oncol 14:1077–1084, 1996.

265. Mantovani G, Maccio A, Lai P, Massa E, Ghiani M, Santona MC. Cytokine activity in cancer-related anorexia/cachexia: role of megestrol acetate and medroxyprogesterone acetate. Semin Oncol 25(2 Suppl 6): 45–52, 1998.

266. Mantovani G, Maccio A, Esu S, et al. Medroxyprogesterne acetate reduces the production of cytokines and serotonin involved in anorexia/cachexia and emesis by peripheral blood mononuclear cells of cancer patients [abstract]. Biochem Soc Trans 25:296, 1997.

267. Leinung MC, Liporace R, Miller CH. Induction of adrenal suppression by megestrol acetate in patients with AIDS. Ann Intern Med 122:843–845, 1995.

268. Ottery FD, Walsh D, Strawford A. Pharmacologic management of anorexia/cachexia. Semin Oncol 25(2, Suppl 6):35–44, 1998.

269. Rowland KM, Loprinzi CL, Shw EG, et al: Randomised double-blind placebo-controlled trial of cisplatin and etoposide plus megestrol acette/placebo in extensive stage small cell lung cancer: A North America Cancer Treatment Group study. J Clin Oncol 14:135–141, 1996.

270. Loprinzi CL, Kuross SA, O'Fallon JR et al. Randomised placebo-controlled evaluation on hydrazine sulphate in patients with advanced colorectal cancer. J Clin Oncol 12:1121–1125, 1994.

271. Loprinzi CL, Goldberg RM, Su JQ, et al. Placebo-controlled trial of hydrazine sulphate in patients with newly diagnosed non–small-cell lung cancer. J Clin Oncol 12:1126–1129, 1994.

272. Kosty MP, Fleishman SB, Herndon JE, et al. Cisplsatin, vinblastine, and hydrazine sulphate in advanced non–small-cell lung cancer; a randomized placebo-controlled double-blind phase III study of the cancer and leukaemia group B. J Clin Oncol 12:1113–1120, 1994.

273. Kardinal CG, Loprinzi CL, Schaid DJ, et al. A controlled trial of cyproheptadine in cancer patients with anorexia and/or cachexia. Cancer 65:2657–2662, 1990.

274. Dezube BJ, Sherman ML, Fridovich-Keil JL, Allen-Ryan J, Pardee AB: Down-regulation of tumor necrosis factor expression by pentoxifylline in cancer patients: a pilot study. Cancer Immunol Immunother 36:57–60, 1993.

275. Combaret L, Ralliere C, Taillandier D, Tanaka K, Attaix D. Manipulation of the ubiquitin-proteasome pathway in cachexia: pentoxifylline suppresses the activation of 20S and 26S proteasomes in muscles from tumor-bearing rats. Mol Biol Rep 26:95–101,1999.

276. Goldberg RM, Loprinzi CL, Mailliard JA, et al. Pentoxifylline for treatment of cancer anorexia and cachexia? A randomized, double-blind, placebo-controlled trial. J Clin Oncol 13:2856–2859, 1995.

277. Lundholm K, Gelin J, Hyltander A, et al: Anti-inflamatory treatment may prolong survival in undernourished patients with metastatic solid tumours. Cancer Res 54:5602–5606, 1994.

278. Wigmore SJ, Falconer JS, Plester CE, et al. Ibuprofen reduces energy expenditure and acute-phase protein production compared with placebo in pancreatic cancer patients. J Cancer 2:185–188, 1995.

279. Beal JE, Olson R, Laubenstein L, et al. Dronabinol as a treatment for anorexia associated with weight loss in patients with AIDS. J Pain Symptom Manage 10:89–97, 1995.

280. Regelson W, Butler JR, Schulz J, et al. Tetrahydrocannbinol as an effective antidepressant and appetite-stimulating agent in advanced cancer patients. In: Braude MC, Szara S (eds): The Pharmacology of Marihuana: A Monograph of the National Institute of Drug Abuse, Raven, New York, 1976, pp 763–776.

281. Plasse TF, Gorter RW, Krasnow SH, Lane M, Shepard KV, Wadleigh RG. Recent clinical experience with dronabinol. Pharmacol Biochem Behav 40: 695–700, 1991.

282. Nelson K, Walsh D, Deeter P, Sheehan F. A phase II study of δ-9-tetrahydrocannabinol for appetite stimulation in cancer-associated anorexia. J Palliat Care 10:14–18, 1994.

283. Kirkham TC, Williams CM. Synergistic efects of opioid and cannabinoid antagonists on food intake. Psychopharmacology (Berl) 153(2): 267–270, 2001.

284. Hengge UR, Baumann M, Maleba R, Brockmeyer NH, Goos M. Oxymetholone promotes weight gain in patients with advanced human immunodeficiency virus (HIV-1) infection. Br J Nutr 75:129–138, 1996.

285. Grinspoon S, Corcoran C, Anderson E, et al. Sustained anabolic effects of long-term androgen administration in men with AIDS wasting. Clin Infect Dis 28:634–636, 1999.

286. Loprinzi CL, Kugler JW, Sloan JA, et al. Randomized comparison of megestrol acetate versus dexamethasone versus fluoxymesterone for the treatment of cancer anorexia/cachexia. J Clin Oncol 17:3299–3306, 1999.

287. Evans WJ, Roubenoff R, Shevitz A. Exercise and the treatment of wasting: aging and human immunodeficiency virus infection [review]. Semin Oncol 25(2 Suppl 6):112–122, 1998.

288. Sheffield-Moore M. Androgens and the control of skeletal muscle protein synthesis [review]. Ann Med 32:181–186, 2000.

289. Bartlett DL, Stein TP, Torosian MH. Effect of growth hormone and protein intake on tumor growth and host cachexia. Surgery 117:260–267, 1995.

290. Tayek JA, Brasel JA. Failure of anabolism in malnourished cancer patients receiving growth hormone: a clinical research center study. J Clin Endocrinol Metab 80:2082–2087, 1995.

291. Wang W, Iresjo BM, Karlsson L, Svanberg E. Provision of rhIGF-I/IGFBP-3 complex attenuated development of cancer cachexia in an experimental tumor model. Clin Nutr 19:127–132, 2000.

292. Fang CH, Li BG, Sun X, Hasselgren PO. Insulin-like growth factor I reduces ubiquitin and ubiquitin-conjugating enzyme gene expression but does not inhibit muscle proteolysis in septic rats. Endocrinology 141:2743–2751, 2000.

293. Corral LG, Haslett PA, Muller GW, et al. Differential cytokine modulation and T cell activation by two distinct classes of thalidomide analogues that are potent inhibitors of TNF-α. J Immunol 163:380–386, 1999.

294. Peukman V, Fisch M, Bruera E. Potential novel uses of thalidomide, focus on palliative care. Drugs 60:273–292, 2000.

295. Bruera E, Neumann CM, Pituskin E, Calder K, Ball G, Hanson J. Thalidomide in patients with cachexia due to terminal cancer: preliminary report. Ann Oncol 10:857–859, 1999.

296. Thomas DA, Kantarjian HM: Current role of thalidomide in cancer treatment [review]. Curr Opin Oncol 12:564–573, 2000.

297. Raje N, Anderson K. Thalidomide—a revival story. N Engl J Med 341: 1606–1609, 1999.

298. Neri B, de Leonardis V, Gemelli MT, et al. Melatonin as biological response modifier in cancer patients. Anticancer Res 18(2B):1329–1332, 1998.

299. Lissoni P, Paolorossi F, Tancini G, et al. Is there a role for melatonin in the treatment of neoplastic cachexia? Eur J Cancer 32A:1340–1343, 1996.

300. Costelli P, Garcia-Martinez C, Llovera M, et al. Muscle protein waste in tumor-bearing rats is effectively antagonized by a β 2-adrenergic agonist (clenbuterol). Role of the ATP-ubiquitin–dependent proteolytic pathway. J Clin Invest 95:2367–2372, 1995.

301. Chance WT, Zhang X, Zuo L, Balasubramaniam A. Reduction of gut hypoplasia and cachexia in tumor-bearing rats maintained on total parenteral nutrition and treated with peptide YY and clenbuterol. Nutrition 14:502–507, 1998.

302. Carbo N, Lopez-Soriano J, Tarrago T, at al.: Comparative effects of β2-adrenergic agonists on muscle waste associated with tumour growth. Cancer Lett 115:113–118, 1997.

303. Choo J, Horän M, Little R, Rothwell N. Effects of the β 2-adrenoceptor agonist, clenbuterol, on muscle atrophy due to food deprivation in the rat. Metabolism 39:647–650, 1990.

304. Maltin CA, Delday MI, Watson JS. Clenbuterol, a beta-adrenoceptor agonist, increases relative muscle strength in orthopaedic patients. Clin Sci (Colch) 84:651–654, 1993.

305. Meydani SN, Lichtenstein AH, Cornwall S, et al. Immunologic effects of national cholesterol education panel step-2 diets with and without fish-derived N-3 fatty acid enrichment. J Clin Invest 92:105–113, 1993.

306. Endres S, Ghorbani R, Kelley VE, et al. The effect of dietary supplementation with n-3 polyunsaturated fatty acids on the synthesis of interleukin-1 and tumor necrosis factor by mononuclear cells. N Engl J Med 320:265–271, 1989.

307. Wigmore SJ, Fearon KC, Maingay JP, Ross JA. Down-regulation of the acute-phase response in patients with pancreatic cancer cachexia receiving oral eicosapentaenoic acid is mediated via suppression of interleukin-6. Clin Sci (Colch) 92:215–221, 1997.

308. Wigmore SJ, Ross JA, Falconer JS, et al. The effect of polyunsaturated fatty acids on the progress of cachexia in patients with pancreatic cancer. Nutrition 12 (Suppl 1):S27–S30, 1996.

309. Wigmore SJ, Fearon KC, Ross JA. Modulation of human hepatocyte acute phase protein production in vitro by n-3 and n-6 polyunsaturated fatty acids. Ann Surg 225:103–111, 1997.

310. Barber MD, McMillan DC, Preston T, Ross JA, Fearon KC. Metabolic response to feeding in weight-losing pancreatic cancer patients and its modulation by a fish-oil-enriched nutritional supplement. Clin Sci (Colch) 98:389–399, 2000.

311. Hellerstein MK, Wu K, McGrath M, et al. Effects of dietary n-3 fatty acid supplementation in men with weight loss associated with the acquired immune deficiency syndrome: relation to indices of cytokine production. J Acquir Immune Defic Syndr Hum Retrovirol 11:258–270, 1996.

312. Beck SA, Smith KL, Tisdale MJ. Anticachectic and antitumor effect of eicosapentaenoic acid and its effect on protein turnover. Cancer Res 51:6089–6093, 1991.

313. Wigmore SJ, Barber MD, Ross JA, Tisdale MJ, Fearon KC. Effect of oral eicosapentaenoic acid on weight loss in patients with pancreatic cancer. Nutr Cancer 36:177–184, 2000.

314. Barber MD, Ross JA, Voss AC, et al. The effect of an oral nutritional supplement enriched with fish oil on weight-loss in patients with pancreatic cancer. Br J Cancer 81:80–86, 1999.

315. Gogos CA, Ginopoulos P, Salsa B, Apostolidou E, Zoumbos NC, Kalfarentzos F. Dietary omega-3 polyunsaturated fatty acids plus vitamin E restore immunodeficiency and prolong survival for severely ill patients with generalized malignancy: a randomized controlled trial. Cancer. 82:395–402, 1998.

316. Hellerstein MK, Wu K, McGrath M, et al. Effects of dietary n-3 fatty acid supplementation in men with weight loss associated with the acquired immune deficiency syndrome: relation to indices of cytokine production. J Acquir Immun Defic Syndr Hum Retrovirol 11:258–270, 1996.

317. Haskell CM, Wong M, Williams A, Lee LY. Phase I trial of extracellular adenosine 5′-triphosphate in patients with advanced cancer. Med Pediatr Oncol 27:165–173, 1996.

318. Haskell CM, Mendoza E, Pisters KM, Fossella FV, Figlin RA. Phase II study of intravenous adenosine 5′-triphosphate in patients with previously untreated stage IIIB and stage IV non–small cell lung cancer. Invest New Drugs 16:81–85, 1998.

319. Agteresch HJ, Dagnelie PC, Rietveld T, van den Berg JWO, Wilson JHP. Beneficial effects of adenosine triphosphate on nutritional status of lung cancer patients: a randomized clinical trial [abstract]. Clin Nutr 18:49, 1999.

320. Agteresch HJ, Dagnelie PC, Rietveld T, van den Berg JW, Danser AH, Wilson JH. Pharmacokinetics of intravenous ATP in cancer patients. Eur J Clin Pharmacol 56:49–55, 2000.

321. Agteresch HJ, Leij-Halfwerk S, Van Den Berg JW, Hordijk-Luijk CH, Wilson JH, Dagnelie PC. Effects of ATP infusion on glucose turnover and gluconeogenesis in patients with advanced non–small-cell lung cancer. Clin Sci (Colch) 98:689–695, 2000.

322. MacDonald N. Cachexia-anorexia workshop: introduction [review]. Nutrition 16:1007–1008, 2000.

323. MacDonald N. Workshop summary and conclusions [review]. Nutrition 16:1019–1020, 2000.

324. Kotler DP. Cachexia [review]. Ann Intern Med 133:622–634, 2000.

# Chapter 72

# Management of Obstructive Complications of Upper Gastrointestinal Tract: Esophagus, Stomach, and Biliary Tree

ANDREW Q. GIAP AND KENNETH J. CHANG

Despite extensive advances in diagnostic and treatment strategies, the 5-year survival rate of patients with esophageal, gastric, and biliary cancer remains unchanged. Most patients who present in an advanced stage are not candidates for curative resection. The principal goals of therapeutic intervention are oftentimes palliative therapy for malignant obstruction and maintaining the highest possible level of independence and quality of life. Traditional approaches to palliative therapy have included surgery, chemotherapy, and radiation. However, recent technologic advances have placed endoscopic modalities at the forefront of palliative treatments. High-risk palliative surgery for gastrointestinal malignancy is increasingly being replaced by local tumor-repressive methods, such as stent insertion and tissue ablative therapies. Endoscopy has evolved from a tool used to provide tissue diagnosis to one used as an integral part of staging, with endoscopic ultrasound, and as treatment of early-stage tumors, with endoscopic mucosal resection, photodynamic therapy, or the Nd:YAG laser. However, a major milestone of endoscopy is its role in the palliative treatment of advanced esophageal, gastric, and biliary cancer. A variety of traditional endoscopic techniques including dilatation, laser, and rigid endoprosthesis have proved effective over the years. More recent advances include intratumoral injection therapy, photodynamic therapy, and self-expanding metal stents.

This chapter reviews the most current endoscopic modalities, along with their limitations and guidelines. Emphasis on patient selection based on functional status, life expectancy, tumor characteristics (such as stage, location, and shape), and local expertise in these endoscopic procedures are also discussed.

## Malignant Dysphagia

Prognosis of patients with carcinomas of the esophagus and cardia is generally poor, with an overall 5-year survival rate of only 7% to 11%.[1] At the time of diagnosis more than 50% of patients are beyond cure, and palliation is their only option.[2] Relief of dysphagia is the primary aim of any palliative technique. In addition, progressive dysphagia due to local obstruction or incessant coughing from a tracheobronchoesophageal fistula frequently causes patient distress, and malnutrition and may also need to be addressed.

Palliative therapies for advanced esophageal cancer include surgery, radiation therapy, chemotherapy, endoscopic procedures, or a combination of these treatments. Surgery probably provides the most effective palliation of dysphagia but is associated with high morbidity and mortality rates, and hence is precluded in many patients with concomitant medical problems.[3–5] Radiation therapy and chemotherapy are rarely used alone to provide palliation. Endoscopy alone or in combination with other techniques may be used to provide palliation. Various endoscopic palliative modalities, such as dilatation, laser, and rigid endoprosthesis, have been available for many years. However, intratumoral injection therapy, photodynamic therapy, and self-expanding metal stents (SEMS) represent significant recent advances in endoscopic palliation of malignant esophageal obstruction.

## Dilatation

For many years, esophageal dilatation has been an integral part of most palliative treatment programs as either a sole or an adjunctive therapy. Dilatation can maintain luminal patency in most patients. Other advantages include simplicity, economy, widespread availability of equipment, short procedure time, and relative safety. In one series, 24 of 26 patients resumed a regular or soft diet with little morbidity and no mortality after undergoing repeated dilatation.[6] In addition, dilatation is an essential adjunct to other endoscopic modalities, such as stent placement, thermal treatment, and photodynamic therapy. The disadvantages of dilatation are related to the short-term relief of dysphagia, necessitating repeated dilatations, and up to a 5% risk of perforation.[7]

The dilating equipment most commonly used consists of polyvinyl dilators (Savary-Gilliard type or American type), metal olives (Eder-Puestow type), hydrostatic balloons, Key-Med advanced dilators, and mercury-filled rubber bougies (Maloney type or Hurst type).[8,9]

To ensure safety, malignancies should be dilated over a guidewire with endoscopic guidance. When the malignant lesion cannot be passed with an endoscope, both endoscopic and fluoroscopic control may be needed.[8] For tight or tortuous malignant strictures, many clinicians use lubricated polyvinyl tapered dilators (such as the Savary-Gilliard type) over a taut guidewire under fluoroscopic control to ensure that the dilator has passed. Once the tight stricture has been initially dilated in this fashion, other techniques may be employed.

Although endoscopic through-the-scope hydrostatic balloon dilators were initially met with some enthusiasm, many clinicians found them unpredictable and less effective in cases of tight, irregular malignant strictures. Recently marketed dilators of this type have shown some improvement, but further studies are needed.

Mercury-filled rubber bougies that are inserted blindly should be used only in a malignant stricture that has already been dilated over a guidewire. It is also frequently recommended that, if used, these dilators should be fluoroscopically guided.

As a sole palliative technique, dilatation usually requires multiple repeat procedures and has been shown to be safe and effective. In patients with very advanced cancer and a short life expectancy, a few endoscopic dilations may be the safest and least expensive palliative modality.

## Stents

Endoscopic implantation of stents, especially the newer generation of SEMS, has emerged as an effective palliative modality for inoperable esophageal cancer. Stent placement offers rapid and usually long-lasting relief of dysphagia and is the method of choice for bronchoesophageal fistulas.[10]

Stent insertion is indicated when dilatation becomes ineffective or too difficult for the patient or the physician or when the required frequency of dilatation becomes unacceptable. In addition, stent implantation is reserved for patients with long circumferential stenoses, rapidly growing tumors, and extraluminal neoplasms leading to compression of the esophageal lumen and recurrent cancer after initial treatment with surgery, radiotherapy, chemotherapy, or laser photocoagulation.[11]

Endoscopic stent placement is contraindicated in uncooperative, unmotivated patients and in circumstances in which the quality of life cannot be improved. This measure is also relatively contraindicated in strictures that are soft, noncircumferential, or angulated, precluding the anchorage of the prosthetic device. Because of the risks of poor tolerance, dislocation, and persistent dysphagia, endoscopic stents, especially conventional plastic endoprostheses, should also be avoided in malignant strictures within 2 cm of the upper esophageal sphincter.

## Conventional Plastic Esophageal Stents

Older, conventional plastic esophageal stents, such as the Wilson Cook, Atkinson, and Celestin prostheses, are seldom used now but are still commercially available in a variety of different materials, elasticities, and funnel shapes with different shaft diameters and channel sizes. Implantation of plastic stents is technically successful in more than 90% of patients with intrinsic or extrinsic obstruction of the upper or middle one-third of the esophagus.[11] Following stent placement, most patients can tolerate solid and semisolid food.[12–16] Results are less favorable for lesions of the lower esophagus and gastric cardia.[17] Angulation at this site may cause blockage of the upper end of the prosthesis, resulting in pressure necrosis that may predispose the patient to bleeding, perforation, or the formation of a mediastinal fistula, whereas the distal end may become obstructed owing to compression of the gastric wall.[11]

Using either endoscopic or radiologic guidance, plastic stents are placed into a malignant stricture following tumor dilatation. Stents are usually pushed into position with a pusher tube after being loaded onto an endoscope or inner guiding tube that has been placed across the stricture. The repositioning or removal of a plastic stent can usually be achieved with a repositioner, which has a balloon at its tip to hold the prosthesis. Specially designed prostheses with self-inflating, foam-covered cuffs can be used to seal refractory esophagorespiratory fistulas and iatrogenic esophageal perforations and to tamponade massive bleeding from esophageal tumors.[18,19]

Although effective and inexpensive, rigid plastic stents have fallen out of favor because of the difficulty in placement, the risk of migration, and the high perforation rate. Plastic stent implantation often requires dilatation of the malignant stricture to a large diameter (i.e., up to 48) prior to insertion, thereby predisposing the patient to the risk of esophageal perforation.[20] In a retrospective study of 400 patients in The Netherlands, early complications of the use of rigid stents included bleeding in 1%, perforation in 7%, and migration within 4 weeks in 15% of patients.[21] Late complications included migration after 4 weeks in 8%, stent obstruction in 6%, and pressure necrosis in 3% of cases.[21] Many other studies have illustrated that stent placement achieves effective relief of dysphagia and closing of esophagorespiratory fistulas, but not without a significant perforation rate ranging from 5% to 10%.[17,22–25]

## Self-Expanding Metal Stents

Self-expanding metal stents made of various types of wire mesh have been gaining favor as a very effective palliative tool in malignant esophageal obstruction. One advantage of these stents is that, compared with rigid plastic stents, SEMS can be compressed into a smaller-diameter delivery device assigned to facilitate their placement. They have a thin wall and can expand to a diameter of 20 mm. The metal mesh engages the tumor with radial outward force, locking the stent in place and decreasing the risk of migration. Disadvantages include higher cost, difficulty in repositioning or removing the stent once employed, and tumor ingrowth resulting in reocclusion. However, the recent development of metal stents with Teflon coatings has reduced the problem of tumor ingrowth, thus minimizing the risk of reocclusion.

Similar to plastic prostheses, numerous SEMS are commercially available. Self-expanding metal stents are offered in various types of metal, designs, types of coating, and specifications. Current available SEMS include the Esophacoil stent (Instent, Eden Prairie, MN), the Ultraflex stent (Boston Scientific, Natick, MA), and the Wallstent (Schneider Europe, Bulach, Switzerland). Also available are three types of Z-stents: the Esophageal-Z Stent (Wilson-Cook, Winston-Salem, NC), the Cook Z-Stent (William Cook Europe, Bjaeverskov, Denmark) and the Song Esophageal Endoprosthesis (Solco Intermed Co., South Korea).

**Table 72–1** Malignant dysphagia

| Endoscopic Modality | Suitable Candidates |
| --- | --- |
| Dilatation | Advanced cancer; short life expectancy (requiring few endoscopic dilatations) |
| Self-expanding metal stent (SEMS) | Exophytic tumor at middle one-third of esophagus; tracheoesophageal fistulas |
| Nd:YAG laser | Exophytic, intraluminal tumor <5 cm in length at upper middle or distal esophagus; scope passage required |
| Bipolar electrocoagulation | Circumferential, infiltrating tumor <5 cm in length; scope passage required |
| Argon-plasma coagulation (APC) | Limited data; experimental technique |
| Photodynamic therapy (PDT) | Circumferential, flat, angulated, and infiltrating tumor >5 cm in length; in upper, middle, or lower one-third of the esophagus, gastroesophageal junction, or in an anastomotic site; scope passage not required |
| Alcohol and injections of other sclerosants | Limited data; experimental technique |

## Malignant Gastric Outlet Obstruction

In most patients, malignant gastric outlet obstructions are caused by gastric, pancreatic, or biliary cancers. Patients typically present late in the clinical course of their disease with early satiety, nausea, vomiting, and weight loss. Historically, surgical gastroenterostomy and enterostomy have been the standard treatments for malignant stenoses of the proximal small bowel. Unfortunately, surgical intervention is associated with significant morbidity and mortality, contingent in part on the functional status of the patient.[89–91] Therefore, endoscopic palliative treatments with periodic bougienage or SEMS in patients at high risk for surgical complications have been offered as an alternative therapy. Alternatively, comfort care measures alone may be reasonable in patients who are at high risk for complications or who have stage IV disease.

### Balloon Dilatation

Endoscopic treatment of benign gastric outlet obstruction by balloon dilatation has been advocated as an alternative to surgery.[92–94] However, since the introduction of $H_2$ blockers and *Helicobacter pylori* eradication, benign gastric outlet obstruction has become less prevalent, and the incidence of malignancy as the cause has reportedly increased.[95–97] Moreover, recent studies have reported a low 16% rate of long-term sustained efficacy of endoscopic balloon dilation for pyloric stenoses and a high recurrent rate.[98,99] To date, no literature is available on the utility of this procedure as a palliative treatment for malignant gastric outlet obstruction.

### Stents

Expandable metallic prostheses are being used in various gastrointestinal stenoses. However, experience using self-expanded metallic stents for gastric outlet and proximal small bowel obstructions is limited. Duodenal prostheses have been used since 1992 to relieve gastric outlet obstructions in postsurgical patients.[100–102] The first use of a metallic stent for an inoperable malignant pyloric stenosis in a patient without previous surgical intervention was reported in 1993 by Song and colleagues.[103] In a recent study by Nevitt and colleagues,[104] stent insertions were technically successful and clinical improvement, defined as increased oral intake, was seen in seven (87.5%) of eight patients with a mean survival of 5 months. In a prospective evaluation, Soetikno and colleagues[105] showed that Wallstent placement afforded palliative relief of malignant gastric outlet obstruction in 9 of 12 patients. Despite the available technology for insertion of expandable stents into a variety of malignant stenotic locations, various problems remain. First, many of the delivery systems are too short to pass from the mouth to the duodenum. Second, the gastric antrum is at such an acute angle to the esophageal axis or the axis of the gastric body that it has been difficult to insert a stent with the introducer currently available.[104] Moreover, the use of esophageal stents has inherent problems such as tumor ingrowth and overgrowth, although these complications are theoretically amenable to re-stenting and/or endoscopic thermal treatment. Bleeding, perforation, formation of granulation tissue at the edges of the prosthesis, and food impaction are other potential complications. In addition, it may be necessary to stent the biliary and/or pancreatic ducts prior to stenting the second portion of the duodenum.

### Percutaneous Endoscopic Jejunostomy and Endoscopic Gastrojejunostomy

Gauderer and Ponsky[106,107] first described the technique of percutaneous endoscopic gastrostomy (PEG) almost two decades ago. Enteral feeding through PEG has increasingly been used in homes, hospitals, and other institutions. However, PEG has two major limitations: a risk of aspiration in up to 30% of patients and prohibition of enteral feeding in gastric outlet obstruction.[108–110] To overcome these limitations, percutaneous endoscopic gastrojejunostomy (PEGJ), in which a jejunostomy tube is placed through the gastrostomy tube, has been attempted. However, the use of smaller J-tube diameters in some studies yielded discouraging results due to frequent clogging and migration of the feeding tube back into the stomach.[111–114] Other workers have advocated direct percutaneous endoscopic jejunostomy (PEJ), reporting success rates as high as 86%.[115–117] However, the direct method of creating a stoma into the jejunum is technically more demanding, requiring a high degree of precision in localizing the jejunal puncture site.[116] Recently, a few other variations of PEGJ techniques using a larger J-tube caliber have yielded more encouraging results. We have described a novel technique of introducing the larger jejunostomy tube (12 Fr) via a thin-scope technique using a guidewire under fluoroscopic guidance to ensure placement of the tube beyond the ligament of Treitz.[118] Since the initial report applying this technique, we have achieved placement of the jejunostomy tube at or beyond the ligament of Treitz in 23 (92%) of 25 consecutive patients, including 8 patients with malignant gastric outlet obstruction. Therefore, PEGJ and direct PEJ can facilitate enteral feeding in patients with malignant outlet obstruction.

While PEGJ enables simultaneous gastric drainage and enteral feeding, it does not allow the patient to resume oral intake of solid food. We usually employ PEGJ for patients with end-stage tumors or as a temporary measure that can be readily removed.

## Summary

In patients who are surgical candidates with greater than 6 months expected survival, a surgical palliative bypass is the most reasonable approach. For those who have a much shorter expected survival or who are not surgical candidates, endoscopic approaches should be considered—either stent placement or PEGJ (Table 72–2). In the future, novel endoscopic techniques to perform gastrojejunostomy laparoscopic should be developed to bypass these gastric outlet obstructions.

## Malignant Biliary Obstruction

Malignant obstruction of the biliary tree is curable by surgical resection in less than 20% of cases.[119] A retrospective study of 165 patients with malignant biliary obstruction by Schmassman and colleagues[120] reported that 66% had pancreatic cancer, 14% had metastatic cancer, and the remaining 20% had bile duct or gallbladder cancer. Since most patients are not eligible for resection with curative intent, the palliation of jaundice and pruritus and the prevention of ascending cholangitis should be the primary objectives.[121] These goals can be achieved with endoscopic–radiologic drainage of the bile flow or with surgical biliary–enteric bypass.

### Stents

Since Soehendra and Rejinders-Frederix[122] first described endoscopic biliary stenting in 1980, endoscopic insertion of a biliary endoprosthesis across a biliary stricture as a result of inoperable malignancy has become a well-recognized method of palliation, with a success rate of over 90%.[123–126] This measure efficiently relieves jaundice and generally improves the comfort and nutritional status during the patient's remaining life.[127] In a large, randomized trial, endoscopic biliary stenting compared favorably with percutaneous transhepatic drainage, incurring a lower complication rate and a lower 30-day mortality rate.[128] Biliary bypass surgery has proved an effective alternative to stenting, and the two methods have achieved similar long-term survival rates in several randomized trials.[127,129] However, endoscopic drainage via stenting has a lower procedure-related mortality rate and usually results in a shorter hospital stay and therefore a more favorable cost-effectiveness ratio.[130]

The most commonly used endoprostheses are made of polyethylene and are 10 Fr or 11.5 Fr in diameter. They are inexpensive and can easily be exchanged as long as duodenal intubation with a large channel duodenoscope remains possible. The success rate of plastic stent insertion is about 90% and is higher in patients with distal tumors.[131] The major disadvantage of these endoprostheses is their inevitable obstruction, which occurs as a result of bacterial colonization and sludge formation in 30% of stents within 3 months and in up to 70% of stents within 6 months after insertion, with a median patency of 4 to 5 months.[132] The rate of stent occlusion is higher for stents placed for a hilar as opposed to a more distal obstruction.[131] Obstruction is generally evidenced by recurrence of jaundice and/or cholangitis; the latter condition makes endoscopic stent exchange urgent. Early, prophylactic exchange of endoprostheses has been advocated to prevent cholangitis.[133]

Early postprocedural complications, which have occurred in 10% to 20% of patients in most studies, are related to the sphincterotomy or to the insertion of the stent itself.[134] The most frequent early postprocedural complication, cholangitis, is reported to occur in as many as 10% to 15% of patients and is probably due to the introduction of bacteria during the procedure into the stagnant bile proximal to the stricture.[135]

A major advancement in stent technology was the development of the metal expandable stent. The technical success rate of insertion and relief of obstruction is over 95%, with few immediate complications.[136,137] However, erosion of biliary metal stents through the duodenal wall with resultant hemorrhage has been reported.[138,139] Self-expanding metal stents are much more expensive than plastic stents. However, compared with the traditional polyethylene stents, SEMS have a larger diameter (8 to 10 mm or 25 to 31 Fr) and thus are able to achieve pallation of the malignant stricture with significantly longer stent patency.[136,140–143] One randomized study demonstrated that the initial cost of metal stents was more than offset in the long term by a significant decrease in hospital costs as compared with those associated with plastic stent exchanges.[140] However, the median patency of metal stents was found to be much lower than the median survival time of patients, suggesting that these expensive stents may have benefited only a small minority of patients. In a recent randomized study, Prat and colleagues[144] demonstrated that the general use of metallic stents was the least expensive and the prophylactic exchange of plastic stents was the most costly option in patients surviving more than 6 months. In a report of a multivariate analysis that showed that tumors less than 30 mm in diameter correlated with a median survival of 6.6 months, the same group asserted that metallic stents should be reserved for inoperable tumors of less than 30 mm and that larger tumors are effectively palliated with plastic stents.[145]

### Photodynamic Therapy

Photodynamic therapy has also been recently applied to relieve obstructive tumors of the biliary tract. The photosensitizer Photofrin has been demonstrated to accumulate preferentially in bile duct neoplasms, reaching peak values during the first 2

**Table 72–2** Malignant gastric outlet obstruction

| Endoscopic Modality | Suitable Candidates |
| --- | --- |
| Stents | Limited experience using self-expanded metallic stents for gastric outlet and proximal small bowel obstructions |
| Percutaneous endoscopic jejunostomy (PEJ) or endoscopic gastrojejunostomy (PEGJ) | Nonsurgical; short life expectancy; patient is unable to eat solids with this modality |

**Table 72–3** Malignant biliary obstruction

| Endoscopic Modality | Suitable Candidates |
| --- | --- |
| Plastic stent | Tumors >30 mm in diameter |
| Self-expanding metal stent (SEMS) | Tumor <30 mm in diameter |
| Photodynamic therapy | May be useful in bilar lesions; limited data (PDT) |

days.[146] Ortner and colleagues[147] evaluated the effect of PDT on cholestasis, quality of life, and survival time in patients with non-resectable Bismuth type III or IV cholangiocarcinoma. The study provided promising evidence that PDT was effective in providing biliary drainage and improving quality of life in nine patients with nonresectable disseminated Bismuth type III and IV cholangiocarcinomas.[147] Moreover, a comparison of the patients' survival times with current published data seemed to showed that PDT prolonged survival.[147] These encouraging preliminary results indicate that larger studies with longer follow-up times are needed to further evaluate and confirm the efficacy of this novel technique.

## Summary

Malignant biliary obstruction can be effectively palliated with the use of endoscopically placed plastic or self-expanding metal stents. Considerations between surgical and endoscopic bypass include expected patient survival and surgical risk. Photodynamic therapy may be an alternative in bilar lesions where stenting is more difficult (Table 72–3).

## References

1. Parker SL, Tong T, Bolden S, Wingo PA. Cancer statistics, 1996. CA Cancer J Clin 46:5–2, 1996.
2. Watson A. Self-expanding metal esophageal endoprostheses: which is best? Eur J Gastroenterol Hepatol 10:363–365, 1998.
3. Holscher AH, Bollschweiler E, Schneider PM, Siewert JR. Prognosis of early esophageal cancer. Comparison between adeno- and squamous cell carcinoma. Cancer 76:178–186, 1995.
4. Moghissi K. Surgical resection for stage I cancer of the oesophagus and cardia. Br J Surg 79:935–937, 1992.
5. Watson A. Operable esophageal cancer: current results from the West. World J Surg 18:361–366, 1994.
6. Heit HA, Johnson LF, Siegel SR, Boyce HW Jr. Palliative dilation for dysphagia in esophageal carcinoma. Ann Intern Med 89:629–631, 1978.
7. Lundell L, Leth R, Lind T, et al. Palliative endoscopic dilatation in carcinoma of the esophagus and esophagogastric junction. Acta Chir Scand 155:179–184, 1989.
8. Tytgat GN. Dilation therapy of benign esophageal stenoses. World J Surg 13:142–148, 1989.
9. Tytgat GN. Endoscopic therapy of esophageal cancer: possibilities and limitations. Endoscopy 22:263–267, 1990.
10. May A, Ell C. Palliative treatment of malignant esophagorespiratory fistulas with Gianturco-Z stents. A prospective clinical trial and review of the literature on covered metal stents. Am J Gastroenterol 93:532–535, 1998.
11. Neuhaus H. The use of stents in the management of malignant esophageal strictures. Gastrointest Endosc Clin North Am 8:503–519, 1998.
12. De Palma GD, di Matteo E, Romano G, et al. Plastic prosthesis versus expandable metal stents for palliation of inoperable esophageal thoracic carcinoma: a controlled prospective study. Gastrointest Endosc 43:478–482, 1996.
13. Gasparri G, Casalegno PA, Camandona M, et al. Endoscopic insertion of 248 prostheses in inoperable carcinoma of the esophagus and cardia: short-term and long-term results. Gastrointest Endosc 33:354–356, 1987.
14. Knyrim K, Wagner HJ, Bethge N, Keymling M, Vakil N. A controlled trial of an expansile metal stent for palliation of esophageal obstruction due to inoperable cancer. N Engl J Med 329:1302–1307, 1993.
15. Liakakos TK, Ohri SK, Townsend ER, Fountain SW. Palliative intubation for dysphagia in patients with carcinoma of the esophagus. Ann Thorac Surg 53:460–463, 1992.
16. Spinelli P, Cerrai FG, Dal Fante M, et al. Endoscopic treatment of upper gastrointestinal tract malignancies. Endoscopy 25:675–678, 1993.
17. Spinelli P, Cerrai FG, Ciuffi M, et al. Endoscopic stent placement for cancer of the lower esophagus and gastric cardia. Gastrointest Endosc 40:455–457, 1994.
18. Sargeant IR, Thorpe S, Bown SG. Cuffed esophageal prosthesis: a useful device in desperate situations in esophageal malignancy. Gastrointest Endosc 38:669–675, 1992.
19. Lux G, Wilson D, Wilson J, Demling L. A cuffed tube for the treatment of oesophago-bronchial fistulae. Endoscopy 19:28–30, 1987.
20. Kozarek RA, Raltz S, Brugge WR, et al. Prospective multicenter trial of esophageal Z-stent placement for malignant dysphagia and tracheoesophageal. Gastrointest Endosc 44:562–567, 1996.
21. van den Brandt-Gradel V, den Hartog Jager FC, Tytgat GN. Palliative intubation of malignant esophagogastric obstruction. J Clin Gastroenterol 9:290–297, 1987.
22. Boyce HW Jr. Medical management of esophageal obstruction and esophageal-pulmonary fistula. Cancer 50:2597–2600, 1982.
23. den Hartog Jager FC, Bartelsman JF, Tytgat GN. Palliative treatment of obstructing esophagogastric malignancy by endoscopic positioning of a plastic prosthesis. Gastroenterology 77:1008–1014, 1979.
24. Richter JM, Hilgenberg AD, Christensen MR, et al. Endoscopic palliation of obstructive esophagogastric malignancy. Gastrointest Endosc 34:454–458, 1988.
25. Sridhar KS, Barreras L, Saldana MJ, Manten H. Respiratory tract fistulae in recurrent aerodigestive cancers after chemotherapy. Cancer 61:247–251, 1988.
26. Grund KE, Storek D, Becker HD. Highly flexible self-expanding meshed metal stents for palliation of malignant esophagogastric obstruction. Endoscopy 27:486–494, 1995.
27. Song HY, Do YS, Han YM, et al. Covered, expandable esophageal metallic stent tubes: experiences in 119 patients. Radiology 193:689–695, 1994.
28. Saxon RR, Barton RE, Katon RM, et al. Treatment of malignant esophagorespiratory fistulas with silicone-covered metallic Z stents. J Vasc Interv Radiol 6:237–242, 1995.
29. Saxon RR, Morrison KE, Lakin PC, et al. Malignant esophageal obstruction and esophagorespiratory fistula: palliation with a polyethylene-covered Z-stent. Radiology 202:349–54, 1997.
30. Weigert N, Neuhaus H, Rosch T, et al. Treatment of esophagorespiratory fistulas with silicone-coated self-expanding metal stents. Gastrointest Endosc 41:490–496, 1995.
31. Ell C, Hochberger J, May A, Fleig WE, Hahn EG. Coated and uncoated self-expanding metal stents for malignant stenosis in the upper GI tract: preliminary clinical experiences with wallstents. Am J Gastroenterol 89:1496–1500, 1994.
32. Ell C, May A, Hahn E. Gianturco-Z stents in the palliative treatment of malignant esophageal obstruction and esophagotracheal. Endoscopy 27:495–500, 1995.
33. Kinsman KJ, DeGregorio BT, Katon RM, et al. Prior radiation and chemotherapy increase the risk of life-threatening complications after insertion of metallic stents for esophagogastric malignancy. Gastrointest Endosc 43:196–203, 1996.
34. Neuhaus H, Hoffmann W, Dittler HJ, Niedermeyer HP, Classen M. Implantation of self-expanding esophageal metal stents for palliation of malignant dysphagia. Endoscopy 24:405–410, 1992.
35. Siersema PD, Hop WC, Dees J, Tilanus HW, van Blankenstein M. Coated self-expanding metal stents versus latex prostheses for esophagogastric cancer with special reference to prior radiation and chemotherapy: a controlled, prospective study. Gastrointest Endosc 47:113–120, 1998.
36. Ng TM, Spencer GM, Sargeant IR, Thorpe SM, Bown SG. Management of strictures after radiotherapy for esophageal cancer. Gastrointest Endosc 43:584–590, 1996.
37. Raijman I, Siddique I, Lynch P. Does chemoradiation therapy increase the incidence of complications with self-expanding coated stents in the management of malignant esophageal strictures? Am J Gastroenterol 92:2192–2196, 1997.
38. Cwikiel W, Stridbeck H, Tranberg KG, et al. Malignant esophageal strictures: treatment with a self-expanding nitinol stent. Radiology 187:661–665, 1993.
39. Vermeijden JR, Bartelsman JF, Fockens P, Meijer RC, Tytgat GN. Self-expanding metal stents for palliation of esophagocardial malignancies. Gastrointest Endosc 41:58–63, 1995.

40. Watkinson AF, Ellul J, Entwisle K, Mason RC, Adam A. Esophageal carcinoma: initial results of palliative treatment with covered self-expanding endoprostheses. Radiology 195:821–827, 1995.

41. Ell C, Riemann JF, Lux G, Demling L. Palliative laser treatment of malignant stenoses in the upper gastrointestinal tract. Endoscopy 18:21–26, 1986.

42. Krasner N, Barr H, Skidmore C, Morris AI. Palliative laser therapy for malignant dysphagia. Gut 28:792–798, 1987.

43. Maunoury V, Brunetaud JM, Cochelard D, et al. Endoscopic palliation for inoperable malignant dysphagia: long-term follow-up. Gut 33:1602–1607, 1992.

44. Vanmoerkerke I, Rutgeerts P, Vantrappen G. The role of laser therapy in the palliative treatment of esophageal cancer. J Belge Radiol 74:401–406, 1991.

45. Fleischer D, Sivak MV Jr. Endoscopic Nd:YAG laser therapy as palliation for esophagogastric cancer. Parameters affecting initial outcome. Gastroenterology 89:827–831, 1985.

46. Lightdale CJ, Zimbalist E, Winawer SJ. Outpatient management of esophageal cancer with endoscopic Nd:YAG laser. Am J Gastroenterol 82:46–50, 1987.

47. Naveau S, Chiesa A, Poynard T, Chaput JC. Endoscopic Nd-YAG laser therapy as palliative treatment for esophageal and cardial cancer. Parameters affecting long-term outcome. Dig Dis Sci 35:294–301, 1990.

48. Cello JP, Gerstenberger PD, Wright T, Melnick J, Meiselman MS. Endoscopic neodymium-YAG laser palliation of nonresectable esophageal malignancy. Ann Intern Med 102:610–612, 1985.

49. Mellow MH, Pinkas H. Endoscopic therapy for esophageal carcinoma with Nd:YAG laser: prospective evaluation of efficacy, complications, and survival. Gastrointest Endosc 30:334–339, 1984.

50. Rutgeerts P, Vantrappen G, Broeckaert L, et al. Palliative Nd:YAG laser therapy for cancer of the esophagus and gastroesophageal junction: impact on the quality of remaining life. Gastrointest Endosc 34:87–90, 1988.

51. Spinelli P, Dal Fante M, Mancini A. Endoscopic palliation of malignancies of the upper gastrointestinal tract using Nd:YAG laser: results and survival in 308 treated patients. Lasers Surg Med 11:550–555, 1991.

52. Lightdale CJ, Heier SK, Marcon NE, et al. Photodynamic therapy with porfimer sodium versus thermal ablation therapy with Nd:YAG laser for palliation of esophageal cancer: a multicenter randomized trial. Gastrointest Endosc 42:507–512, 1995.

53. Buset M, des Marez B, Baize M, et al. Palliative endoscopic management of obstructive esophagogastric cancer: laser or prosthesis? Gastrointest Endosc 33:357–361, 1987.

54. Loizou LA, Grigg D, Atkinson M, Robertson C, Bown SG. A prospective comparison of laser therapy and intubation in endoscopic palliation for malignant dysphagia. Gastroenterology 100:1303–1310, 1991.

55. Ell C, May A. Self-expanding metal stents for palliation of stenosing tumors of the esophagus and cardia: a critical review. Endoscopy 29:392–398, 1997.

56. Alexander GL, Wang KK, Ahlquist D, et al. Does performance status influence the outcome of Nd:YAG laser therapy of proximal esophageal tumors? Gastrointest Endosc 40:451–454, 1994.

57. Jensen DM, Machicado G, Randall G, Tung LA, English-Zych S. Comparison of low-power YAG laser and BICAP tumor probe for palliation of esophageal cancer strictures. Gastroenterology 94:1263–1270, 1988.

58. Johnston JH, Fleischer D, Petrini J, Nord HJ. Palliative bipolar electrocoagulation therapy of obstructing esophageal cancer. Gastrointest Endosc 33:349–353, 1987.

59. Fleischer D. A comparison of endoscopic laser therapy and BICAP tumor probe therapy for esophageal cancer. Am J Gastroenterol 82:608–612, 1987.

60. Gossner L, Ell C. Malignant strictures. Thermal treatment. Gastrointest Endosc Clin North Am 8:493–501, 1998.

61. Heindorff H, Wojdemann M, Bisgaard T, Svendsen LB. Endoscopic palliation of inoperable cancer of the oesophagus or cardia by argon electrocoagulation. Scand J Gastroenterol 33:21–23, 1998.

62. Saidi RF, Marcon NE. Nonthermal ablation of malignant esophageal strictures. Photodynamic therapy, endoscopic intratumoral injections, and novel modalities. Gastrointest Endosc Clin North Am 8:465–491, 1998.

63. Forbes IJ, Cowled PA, Leong AS, et al. Phototherapy of human tumours using haematoporphyrin derivative. Med J Aust 2:489–493, 1980.

64. Hayata Y, Kato H, Okitsu H, Kawaguchi M, Konaka C. Photodynamic therapy with hematoporphyrin derivative in cancer of the upper gastrointestinal tract. Semin Surg Oncol 1:1–11, 1985.

65. McCaughan JS Jr, Hicks W, Laufman L, May E, Roach R. Palliation of esophageal malignancy with photoradiation therapy. Cancer 54:2905–2910, 1984.

66. Ell C, Gossner L. Photodynamic therapy: its potential for the treatment of gastrointestinal malignancies and precancerous conditions [editorial]. Endoscopy 26:262–264, 1994.

67. Fisher AM, Murphree AL, Gomer CJ. Clinical and preclinical photodynamic therapy. Lasers Surg Med 17:2–31, 1995.

68. Moore JV, West CM, Whitehurst C. The biology of photodynamic therapy. Phys Med Biol 42:913–935, 1997.

69. Orth K, Ruck A, Stanescu A, Beger HG. Intraluminal treatment of inoperable oesophageal tumours by intralesional photodynamic therapy with methylene blue [letter]. Lancet 345:519–520, 1995.

70. Heier SK, Rothman KA, Heier LM, Rosenthal WS. Photodynamic therapy for obstructing esophageal cancer: light dosimetry and randomized comparison with Nd:YAG laser therapy. Gastroenterology 109:63–72, 1995.

71. Okunaka T, Kato H, Conaka C, et al. Photodynamic therapy of esophageal carcinoma. Surg Endosc 4:150–153, 1990.

72. Reed CE. Comparison of different treatments for unresectable esophageal cancer. World J Surg 19:828–835, 1995.

73. Likier HM, Levine JG, Lightdale CJ. Photodynamic therapy for completely obstructing esophageal carcinoma. Gastrointest Endosc 37:75–78, 1991.

74. McCaughan JS Jr, Nims TA, Guy JT, et al. Photodynamic therapy for esophageal tumors. Arch Surg 124:74–80, 1989.

75. Schweitzer VG, Bologna S, Batra SK. Photodynamic therapy for treatment of esophageal cancer: a preliminary report. Laryngoscope 103:699–703, 1993.

76. Jin M, Yang B, Zhang W, Wang Y. Photodynamic therapy for upper gastrointestinal tumours over the past 10 years. Semin Surg Oncol 10:111–113, 1994.

77. McCaughan JS Jr, Ellison EC, Guy JT, et al. Photodynamic therapy for esophageal malignancy: a prospective twelve-year study. Ann Thorac Surg 62:1005–1110, 1996.

78. Raijman I, Lalor E, Marcon NE. Photodynamic therapy for tumor ingrowth through an expandable esophageal stent. Gastrointest Endosc 41:73–74, 1995.

79. Scheider DM, Siemens M, Cirocco M, et al. Photodynamic therapy for the treatment of tumor ingrowth in expandable esophageal stents. Endoscopy 29:271–274, 1997.

80. Otani T, Tatsuka T, Kanamaru K, Okuda S. Intramural injection of ethanol under direct vision for the treatment of protuberant lesions of the stomach. Gastroenterology 69:123–129.

81. Nwokolo CU, Payne-James JJ, Silk DB, Misiewicz JJ, Loft DE. Palliation of malignant dysphagia by ethanol-induced tumour necrosis. Gut 35:299–303, 1994.

82. Payne-James JJ, Spiller RC, Misiewicz JJ, Silk DB. Use of ethanol-induced tumor necrosis to palliate dysphagia in patients with esophagogastric cancer. Gastrointest Endosc 36:43–46, 1990.

83. Chung SC, Leong HT, Choi CY, Leung JW, Li AK. Palliation of malignant esophageal obstruction by endoscopic alcohol injection. Endoscopy 26:275–277, 1994.

84. Loscos JM, Calvo E, Alvarez-Sala JL, Espinos D. Treatment of dysphagia and massive hemorrhage in esophageal carcinoma by ethanol injection [letter]. Endoscopy 25:544, 1993.

85. Maiwand MO, Homasson JP. Cryotherapy for tracheobronchial. Clin Chest Med 16:427–443, 1995.

86. Johnston CM, Schoenfeld LP, Mysore JV, Dubois A. Endoscopic spray cryotherapy: a new technique for mucosal ablation in the esophagus. Gastrointest Endosc 50:86–92, 1999.

87. Karcz D, Popiela T, Szczepanik AM, et al. Preoperative endoscopic intratumoral application of tumor necrosis factor alpha in patients with locally advanced resectable gastric cancer [letter]. Endoscopy 26:369–370, 1994.

88. Mukai M, Kubota S, Morita S, Akanuma A. A pilot study of combination therapy of radiation and local administration of OK-432 for esophageal cancer. Five-year survival and local control rate. Cancer 75:2276–2280, 1995.

89. Weaver DW, Wiencek RG, Bouwman DL, Walt AJ. Gastrojejunostomy: is it helpful for patients with pancreatic cancer? Surgery 102:608–613, 1987.

90. Meijer S, De Bakker OJ, Hoitsma HF. Palliative resection in gastric cancer. J Surg Oncol 23:77–80, 1983.

91. Smith JW, Brennan MF. Surgical treatment of gastric cancer. Proximal, mid, and distal stomach. Surg Clin North Am 72:381–399, 1992.

92. Lindor KD, Ott BJ, Hughes RW Jr. Balloon dilatation of upper digestive tract strictures. Gastroenterology 89:545–548, 1985.

93. Kozarek RA, Botoman VA, Patterson DJ. Long-term follow-up in patients who have undergone balloon dilation for gastric outlet obstruction. Gastrointest Endosc 36:558–561, 1990.

94. Kozarek RA. Dilation therapy for gastric outlet obstruction. Are balloons a bust? [editorial]. J Clin Gastroenterol 17:2–4, 1993.

95. Johnson CD, Ellis H. Gastric outlet obstruction now predicts malignancy. Br J Surg 77:1023–1024, 1990.

96. Shone DN, Nikoomanesh P, Smith-Meek MM, Bender JS. Malignancy is the most common cause of gastric outlet obstruction in the era of $H_2$ blockers. Am J Gastroenterol 90:1769–1770, 1995.

97. Awan A, Johnston DE, Jamal MM. Gastric outlet obstruction with benign endoscopic biopsy should be further explored for malignancy. Gastrointest Endosc 48:497–500, 1998.

98. Lau JY, Chung SC, Sung JJ, et al. Through-the-scope balloon dilation for pyloric stenosis: long-term results. Gastrointest Endosc 43:98–101, 1996.

99. Kuwada SK, Alexander GL. Long-term outcome of endoscopic dilation of nonmalignant pyloric stenosis. Gastrointest Endosc 41:15–17, 1995.

100. Topazian M, Ring E, Grendell J. Palliation of obstructing gastric cancer with steel mesh, self-expanding endoprostheses. Gastrointest Endosc 38:58–60, 1992.

101. Kozarek RA, Ball TJ, Patterson DJ. Metallic self-expanding stent application in the upper gastrointestinal tract: caveats and concerns. Gastrointest Endosc 38:1–6, 1992.

102. Truong S, Bohndorf V, Geller H, Schumpelick V, Gunther RW. Self-expanding metal stents for palliation of malignant gastric outlet obstruction. Endoscopy 24:433–435, 1992.

103. Song HY, Yang DH, Kuh JH, Choi KC. Obstructing cancer of the gastric antrum: palliative treatment with covered metallic stents. Radiology 187:357–358, 1993.

104. Nevitt AW, Vida F, Kozarek RA, Traverso LW, Raltz SL. Expandable metallic prostheses for malignant obstructions of gastric outlet and proximal small bowel. Gastrointest Endosc 47:271–276, 1998.

105. Soetikno RM, Lichtenstein DR, Vandervoort J, et al. Palliation of malignant gastric outlet obstruction using an endoscopically placed Wallstent. Gastrointest Endosc 47:267–270, 1998.

106. Gauderer MW, Ponsky JL, Izant RJ Jr. Gastrostomy without laparotomy: a percutaneous endoscopic technique. J Pediatr Surg 15:872–875, 1980.

107. Ponsky JL, Gauderer MW, Stellato TA. Percutaneous endoscopic gastrostomy. Review of 150 cases. Arch Surg 118:913–914, 1983.

108. Hassett JM, Sunby C, Flint LM. No elimination of aspiration pneumonia in neurologically disabled patients with feeding gastrostomy. Surg Gynecol Obstet 167:383–388, 1988.

109. Steffes C, Weaver DW, Bouwman DL. Percutaneous endoscopic gastrostomy. New technique—old complications. Am Surg 55:273–277, 1989.

110. Burtch GD, Shatney CH. Feeding gastrostomy. Assistant or assassin? Am Surg 51:204–207, 1985.

111. Lewis BS. Perform PEJ, not PED. Gastrointest Endosc 36:311–313, 1990.

112. DiSario JA, Foutch PG, Sanowski RA. Poor results with percutaneous endoscopic jejunostomy. Gastrointest Endosc 36:257–260, 1990.

113. Henderson JM, Strodel WE, Gilinsky NH. Limitations of percutaneous endoscopic jejunostomy. J Parenter Enteral Nutr 17:546–550, 1993.

114. Kaplan DS, Murthy UK, Linscheer WG. Percutaneous endoscopic jejunostomy: long-term follow-up of 23 patients. Gastrointest Endosc 35:403–406, 1989.

115. Shike M, Wallach C, Likier H. Direct percutaneous endoscopic jejunostomies. Gastrointest Endosc 37:62–65, 1991.

116. Shike M, Latkany L, Gerdes H, Bloch AS. Direct percutaneous endoscopic jejunostomies for enteral feeding. Gastrointest Endosc 44:536–540, 1996.

117. Shike M, Latkany L. Direct percutaneous endoscopic jejunostomy. Gastrointest Endosc Clin North Am 8:569–580, 1998.

118. Chaurasia OP, Chang KJ. A novel technique for percutaneous endoscopic gastrojejunostomy tube placement. Gastrointest Endosc 42:165–168, 1995.

119. Boring CC, Squires TS, Tong T, Montgomery S. Cancer statistics, 1994. CA Cancer J Clin 44:7–26, 1994.

120. Schmassmann A, von Gunten E, Knuchel J, et al. Wallstents versus plastic stents in malignant biliary obstruction: effects of stent patency of the first and second stent on patient compliance and survival. Am J Gastroenterol 91:654–659, 1996.

121. Magistrelli P, Masetti R, Coppola R, et al. Changing attitudes in the palliation of proximal malignant biliary obstruction. J Surg Oncol Suppl 3:151–153, 1993.

122. Soehendra N, Reynders-Frederix V. Palliative bile duct drainage—a new endoscopic method of introducing a transpapillary drain. Endoscopy 12:8–11, 1980.

123. Shepherd HA, Royle G, Ross AP, et al. Endoscopic biliary endoprosthesis in the palliation of malignant obstruction of the distal common bile duct: a randomized trial. Br J Surg 75:1166–1168, 1988.

124. Andersen JR, Sorensen SM, Kruse A, Rokkjaer M, Matzen P. Randomised trial of endoscopic endoprosthesis versus operative bypass in malignant obstructive jaundice. Gut 30:1132–1135, 1989.

125. Kozarek RA. Endoscopy in the management of malignant obstructive jaundice. Gastrointest Endosc Clin North Am 6:153–176, 1996.

126. Soehendra N, Binmoeller KF, Grimm H. Endoscopic therapy for biliary obstruction. World J Surg 16:1066–1073, 1992.

127. Ballinger AB, McHugh M, Catnach SM, Alstead EM, Clark ML. Symptom relief and quality of life after stenting for malignant bile duct obstruction. Gut 35:467–470, 1994.

128. Speer AG, Cotton PB, Russell RC, et al. Randomised trial of endoscopic versus percutaneous stent insertion in malignant obstructive jaundice. Lancet 2(8550):57–62, 1987.

129. Smith AC, Dowsett JF, Russell RC, Hatfield AR, Cotton PB. Randomised trial of endoscopic stenting versus surgical bypass in malignant low bileduct obstruction. Lancet 344(8938):1655–1660, 1994.

130. Dowsett JF, Vaira D, Hatfield AR, et al. Endoscopic biliary therapy using the combined percutaneous and endoscopic technique. Gastroenterology 96:1180–1186, 1989.

131. Cheung KL, Lai EC. Endoscopic stenting for malignant biliary obstruction. Arch Surg 130:204–207, 1995.

132. Sung JJ, Chung SC. Endoscopic stenting for palliation of malignant biliary obstruction. A review of progress in the last 15 years. 40:1167–1173, 1995.

133. Frakes JT, Johanson JF, Stake JJ. Optimal timing for stent replacement in malignant biliary tract obstruction. Gastrointest Endosc 39:164–167, 1993.

134. Cotton PB, Lehman G, Vennes J, et al. Endoscopic sphincterotomy complications and their management: an attempt at consensus. Gastrointest Endosc 37:383–393, 1991.

135. Motte S, Deviere J, Dumonceau JM, et al. Risk factors for septicemia following endoscopic biliary stenting. Gastroenterology 101:1374–1381, 1991.

136. Huibregtse K, Carr-Locke DL, Cremer M, et al. Biliary stent occlusion—a problem solved with self-expanding metal stents? European Wallstent Study Group. Endoscopy 24:391–394, 1992.

137. Vitale GC, Larson GM, George M, Tatum C. Management of malignant biliary stricture with self-expanding metallic stent. Surg Endosc 10:970–973, 1996.

138. Ee H, Laurence BH. Haemorrhage due to erosion of a metal biliary stent through the duodenal wall. Endoscopy 24:431–432, 1992.

139. Marano BJ Jr, Bonanno CA. Metallic biliary endoprosthesis causing duodenal perforation and acute upper gastrointestinal bleeding [letter]. Gastrointest Endosc 40:257–258, 1994.

140. Davids PH, Groen AK, Rauws EA, Tytgat GN, Huibregtse K. Randomised trial of self-expanding metal stents versus polyethylene stents for distal malignant biliary obstruction. Lancet 340(8834–8835):1488–1492, 1992.

141. Knyrim K, Wagner HJ, Pausch J, Vakil N. A prospective, randomized, controlled trial of metal stents for malignant obstruction of the common bile duct. Endoscopy 25:207–212, 1992.

142. Cotton PB. Metallic mesh stents—is the expanse worth the expense? [editorial]. Endoscopy 24:421–423, 1992.

143. O'Brien S, Hatfield AR, Craig PI, Williams SP. A three-year follow-up of self-expanding metal stents in the endoscopic palliation of long-term survivors with malignant biliary obstruction. Gut 36:618–621, 1995.

144. Prat F, Chapat O, Ducot B, et al. A randomized trial of endoscopic drainage methods for inoperable malignant strictures of the common bile duct. Gastrointest Endosc 47:1–7, 1998.

145. Prat F, Chapat O, Ducot B, et al. Predictive factors for survival of patients with inoperable malignant distal biliary strictures: a practical management guideline. Gut 42:76–80, 1998.

146. Pahernik SA, Dellian M, Berr F, et al. Distribution and pharmacokinetics of Photofrin in human bile duct cancer. Photochem Photobiol B 47:58–62, 1998.

147. Ortner MA, Liebetruth J, Schreiber S, et al. Photodynamic therapy of nonresectable cholangiocarcinoma. Gastroenterology 114:536–542, 1998.

# Chapter 73

# Management of Obstructive Complications of Lower Gastrointestinal Tract: Colon and Rectum

YASSER AL-ANTABLY AND SANDEEP LAHOTI

The most common cause of colonic obstruction in the United States is adenocarcinoma, representing about 50% of large bowel obstruction.[1] Between 8% to 25% of patients with colorectal adenocarcinoma present with obstructions.[2–4] Of all malignant obstructive lesions, 60%–75% are located in the left colon.[5–7]

The highest risk of obstruction is with tumors located at the splenic flexure or in the descending colon, followed by the sigmoid colon, and the least risk, with tumors in the ascending colon and rectum.[2,4,8] Tumors on the right side of the colon are more likely to grow in the form of a fungating mass projecting into the lumen, while tumors in the left colon tend to infiltrate the colonic wall. This pattern might help explain the lower incidence of obstruction in the right colon.[9] Other contributing factors for the decreased incidence of right colonic obstruction include its larger diameter, as well as the liquid state of the stools in that side of the colon.

Patients presenting with obstructive cancer tend to have a higher incidence of Dukes' D stage, nodal involvement, liver metastasis, and peritoneal involvement.[2,5,10] These patients have significantly lower survival rates.[4,5,11] The effect of bowel obstruction on survival is influenced by location. Bowel obstruction involving the right colon is associated with significantly decreased disease-free survival, independent of nodal status or tumor encirclement.[11]

## Clinical Presentation

Large bowel obstruction usually has an insidious onset,[12] but it is occasionally abrupt, occurring within hours or days.[13] Crampy abdominal pain is the most common complaint of patients with bowel obstruction.[13] Pain can be described as gaseous distention or bloating, and is usually poorly localized. Constipation is a prominent feature of colonic obstruction, and patients often complain of complete obstipation and inability to pass gas. Patients can also present with diarrhea or small loose stools.[13] Nausea and vomiting are usually late symptoms, and usually indicate an incompetent ileocecal valve.

Abdominal examination usually reveals abdominal distention, with diffuse, ill-localized tenderness. The abdomen is tympanitic on percussion, and bowel sounds are usually present. Rarely, a mass can be palpated on abdominal or rectal examination.[12] Other findings might be related to metastatic disease, including hepatosplenomegaly and ascites. Presence of peritoneal signs, including absence of bowel sounds, is an ominous sign and usually indicates bowel perforation.

## Diagnostic Studies

Plain abdominal X-rays are usually the first step in diagnosing a large bowel obstruction. Supine, left lateral decubitus, and upright films of the abdomen, as well as posteroanterior and lateral chest films are important for diagnosing and localizing colonic obstruction and ruling out bowel perforation.[13,14] The colon will be distended above the level of obstruction, with absence of gas below the level of obstruction. Occasionally, air-fluid levels can be seen. However, the diagnosis of large bowel obstruction can sometimes be difficult with plain X-ray films alone.[12] Water-soluble contrast enema may be necessary for correct diagnosis and for differentiating obstruction from Olgivie's syndrome. Chapman et al.[15] compared plain radiographs with contrast enemas for the diagnosis of large bowel obstruction. Plain X-rays had a sensitivity of 84% and specificity of 72%, while contrast enema had a sensitivity of 96% and specificity of 98%. A contrast enema may also help differentiate complete from partial obstruction, which would dictate urgency and the method of definitive treatment. To avoid barium impaction at or above the site of obstruction, a water-soluble contrast enema is preferred to barium enema.

Computed tomography (CT) scanning has been used in evaluating patients with large bowel obstruction, but its value appears limited to patients with intussusception or diverticular abscess.[15]

Proctosigmoidoscopy can also be used to demonstrate the malignant nature of distally obstructive colonic lesions.[16] Colonoscopy should be avoided in complete colonic obstruction, as air insufflation might exacerbate colonic distention and precipitate perforation.

## Management of Malignant Obstruction of the Large Bowel

Patients with large bowel obstruction are usually elderly and acutely ill. Management of such patients mandates immediate resuscitation, followed by definitive treatment.

### Resuscitation

Patients with large bowel obstruction are usually dehydrated and occasionally have electrolyte imbalance, particularly if they have experienced prolonged vomiting. Aggressive intravenous fluid resuscitation with appropriate crystalloids and correction of electrolyte imbalance should be initiated immediately. Monitoring of fluid balance, including nasogastric tube placement and aspiration of upper gastrointestinal contents, is particularly important in patients with protracted nausea and vomiting. Enemas might help to partially relieve a distal large bowel obstruction.

### Definitive Management

Palliative management of such patients depends on several factors, including comorbid conditions, the patient's ability to withstand surgery, site of colonic obstruction, and the degree of obstruction. There are several modalities for managing patients with malignant obstruction of the colon, including surgical resection, palliative colostomy, cecostomy, dilation, laser ablation, and self-expandable stents.

### Surgical Management

Surgical management of malignant obstruction of the colon depends on the location of obstruction, i.e., proximal or distal. Proximal colon includes the cecum, ascending colon, hepatic flexure, and the transverse colon. Distal colon includes the splenic flexure through the rectum.

#### Proximal colonic obstruction

In patients with malignant obstruction of the colon proximal to the splenic flexure, right hemicolectomy and ileocolic anastomosis have been considered the standard treatment since the mid-1960s.[3,12,14,17] The risk of a one-stage surgery in these situations, including anastomosic leak and in-hospital mortality, is comparable to that in patients without obstruction.[3] However, if a patient is severely ill or has already developed peritonitis and cannot withstand surgery, then proximal diverting loop ileostomy or ileostomy with exteriorization of proximal colon will be the immediate procedure of choice to stabilize the patient's situation.[14]

#### Distal colonic obstruction

In contrast to surgical management of right colonic malignant obstruction, the surgical management of left colonic malignant obstruction has been more controversial. The surgical options for left colonic malignant obstruction include initial decompression, either via cecostomy[18–20] or proximal colostomy,[20] followed by staged resection or immediate resection with or without primary anastomosis. For many years, the three-stage procedure (diverting colostomy, resection of tumor, and colostomy closure) was the primary method used.[21–23] However, this procedure has fallen out of favor because of increased operative mortality and morbidity,[21,24] longer hospital stay,[22–24] and overall lower survival, compared with primary resection.[21,25,26] Also, a large percentage of these patients do not undergo subsequent colostomy closure.[23,27] This procedure is still used in special circumstances, such as when the patient is unstable during surgery.[28]

Recently, the majority of left colonic obstructions due to malignancy have been managed by primary resection with immediate[24,29–34] or delayed[25,35] anastomosis. Whether an immediate or delayed anastomosis should be performed is a matter of debate. For many decades, surgical attitudes have been influenced by unfavorable experiences in the early twentieth century with primary anastomosis to treat the obstructed bowel.[26,36,37] However, the introduction of intraoperative lavage[38] has helped to decrease the complications associated with an immediate anastomosis. Several case series have demonstrated that primary resection with immediate anastomosis can be safely performed, with complication rates similar to those of staged procedures.[24,30–32] An advantage of resection with primary anastomosis is that it reduces the length of hospital stay compared with the total hospital stay for a staged procedure.[24] A disadvantage of resection with delayed anastomosis is the presence of a colostomy, which, in a large percentage of patients, is not subsequently reversed.[23,27] Presently, resection with delayed anastomosis is a good option for patients with risk factors (e.g., perforated left colon cancer, poor nutritional status, immunosuppression) that preclude a primary anastomosis.[14]

The extent of the resection—i.e., subtotal colectomy vs. segmental resection—is also a matter of controversy. Distal colocolic or colorectal anastomoses are considered to be more susceptible to leakage than ileocolic or ileorectal anastomoses.[27] Differences in fecal material consistency, collagen metabolism,[39–41] and blood supply,[39,40] particularly when left colonic obstruction is present, are possible contributing factors.

Several studies have demonstrated that subtotal colectomy with ileocolic anastomosis is a reasonable alternative to intraoperative lavage and primary colonic anastomosis.[42–45] However, a subtotal colectomy does require the sacrifice of an extended colonic segment, a sacrifice that would not be necessary to treat the underlying cancer. The only randomized trial comparing the two alternatives showed no difference in mortality or morbidity but subtotal colectomy resulted in a significantly increased postoperative bowel frequency.[46] At present, segmental resection with anastomosis is the preferred option except in patients with a right-sided concomitant tumor, ischemia of the right colon, or serosal tears of the cecum, in which case a subtotal colectomy may be indicated.[14]

### Nonsurgical Management

Emergency surgery for obstructive lesions of the colorectum is associated with high morbidity and mortality. A significant number of patients with colorectal malignant obstruction are elderly and have other comorbid conditions putting them at high operative risk. Relieving colonic obstruction, even on a temporary basis, would provide a window of opportunity to stabilize these patients and allow colonic preparation for a more elective surgery.

Also, patients with advanced malignancy, with distant or extensive local metastasis, would benefit from nonsurgical relief of their colorectal obstruction as a palliative measure. Laser ablation and colonic stents are two of the more commonly used nonsurgical procedures to establish lumen patency in obstructed colonic lesions.

## Laser photoablation

Laser energy has been used for curative and palliative therapy in the gastrointestinal tract. Laser is best utilized for palliation in patients with locally advanced or metastatic colorectal tumors, or those patients with underlying medical problems precluding surgery. Laser therapy could also be used to reestablish lumen patency preoperatively in patients with malignant obstruction of the colon.[47–49] Malignancies of the rectosigmoid are most suited for endoscopic laser therapy because of easy accessibility, easy preparation with enemas, and the retroperitoneal location of the rectosigmoid that reduces the risk of free perforation.[50] However, laser photoablation has occasionally been used for treatment of right-colonic lesions.[47] In most published reports, neodymium: yttrium aluminum garnet (Nd:YAG) was used,[47,49,51–55] however, argon laser photocoagulation has also been used.[55]

Success of laser therapy for recanalization of the obstructed colonic lumen can be achieved in 86%–100% of patients[47,49,51–55] (Fig. 73–1). Occasionally, mechanical dilation by means of a balloon or forceps debulking may be performed prior to laser ablation.[51,53,54] Once the obstruction has been relieved, most patients are followed in an outpatient setting with repeated laser treatment every 3–4 weeks to maintain lumen patency.

Although there is extensive worldwide experience with endoscopic laser therapy demonstrating its safety and efficacy, multiple complications have been reported. Perforation has been reported in 0%–8%,[47,49,50–55] bleeding in up to 2.7%,[52,55] stenosis in 1.7%,[55] and mortality (mostly secondary to perforation) in up to 2.7%.[52,55] Other disadvantages of laser therapy include the high cost of the initial laser equipment, production of smoke during photoablation, and damage to the endoscope. The latter two problems can be solved by using a dual-channel endoscope for smoke suctioning and by being attentive to the position of the laser fiber tip during the procedure. However, the initial high cost of the laser equipment remains an obstacle to widespread use of endoscopic laser therapy, particularly with the advent and increasing use of expandable metallic stents for the same purpose.

## Self-expandable metallic stents

Placement of self-expandable metallic stents is a relatively new nonsurgical method for relieving colorectal obstruction. In 1992,

Keen and Orsay[56] reported the successful use of a 24 Fr thoracotomy tube as a "stent" in relieving colonic obstruction in a 70-year-old woman with obstructing tumor of the rectum. The patient was successfully stabilized and had a mechanical colonic preparation followed by elective low anterior resection with primary rectosigmoid anastomosis.

In the same year, Spinelli et al.[57] reported on the use of self-expanding stainless steel mesh stents in the palliative treatment of 13 patients with rectal tumors. Endoscopy was used for placement of the stents and was successful in 12 of the 13 patients.

In 1994, Tejero et al.[58] reported the placement of a self-expanding esophageal Wallstent (Schneider) in two patients with obstructing sigmoid cancer. The stents were placed under fluoroscopic guidance using a Superstiff guidewire (Cook) that was introduced through the anus with the help of a Berenstein catheter (Bard). These two patients were also successfully stabilized and mechanically prepared for elective sigmoid resection with colorectal anastomosis.

Several case series have been reported since then[59–75] in which self-expanding stents were used for palliation or in preparation for surgery in patients with distal obstructing lesions in the colon. The majority of patients had colorectal malignancy; however, a few had colorectal compression or infiltration by other malignancies, particularly ovarian and prostatic carcinomas.[64,65,68,71] All reported studies involved patients with distal colonic obstruction, except for one case report by Campbell et al.[75] involving a successful stent placement in the proximal transverse colon. All reported cases of colonic stent placement involved using fluoroscopy as an essential tool for localizing the obstructing lesion, confirming stent placement in the appropriate position before deployment, confirming patency of the stent after deployment, and detecting post-stent placement complications, including perforation.

Endoscopy has also been used in several studies to assist in placing the guidewire through the tumor, to confirm distal position of the stent before deployment, and confirm optimal position and patency of the stent after deployment[60,62–66,68,69,72,73] (Fig. 73–2). Success rates of placing the self-expandable metallic stents vary from 63% to 100%.[61–74] Most case series reported a success rate of 90% or greater.

Initially, different types of stents were used to relieve colonic obstruction. These included the esophageal Wallstent (Schneider),[58,59,63,65,67] Gianturco stent (Cook),[61] Ultraflex knitted nitinol stent (Microvasive),[64,66,68] EsophaCoil (InStent),[60,64,66,68] biliary Wallstent (Schneider),[64,68] and tracheobronchial Wallstent (Schneider).[71] Currently, Wallstent enteral endoprothesis (Schneider) is being designed, produced, and marketed specifically for the use in the colon. It has a diameter of 22 mm and is available in 6- and 9-cm lengths. The Wallstent is made of a nonferromagnetic metallic alloy and thus does not interfere or cause artifact with CT or MRI imaging.[61,76]

While the placement of colonic stents is usually successful, they can be associated with complications, such as colonic perforation, stent migration, stent obstruction, rectal bleeding, and abdominal or anorectal pain.

**Colonic perforation**  This is the most serious complication of stent placement. It has been reported in 3%–16% of patients.[62,64,68,73,74] Some of the perforations were believed to be related to balloon dilation of the stent[64] after placement or were due to the guidewire.[64] Some of the perforations were silent and were discovered only at surgery.[70,74] All patients should have a plain abdominal X-ray and possibly a gastrografin enema fol-

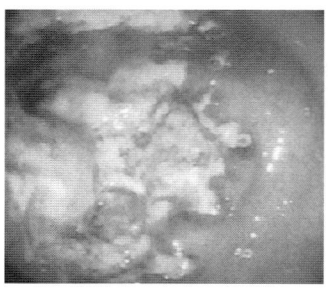 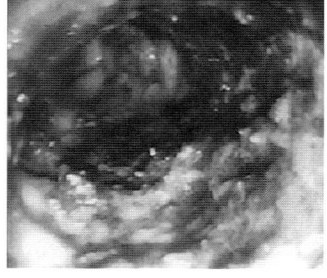

**A**          **B**

**Figure 73-1**  *A:* Contact laser being applied for palliation of obstruction due to malignancy. *B:* Reestablishment of a patent colonic lumen after laser therapy.

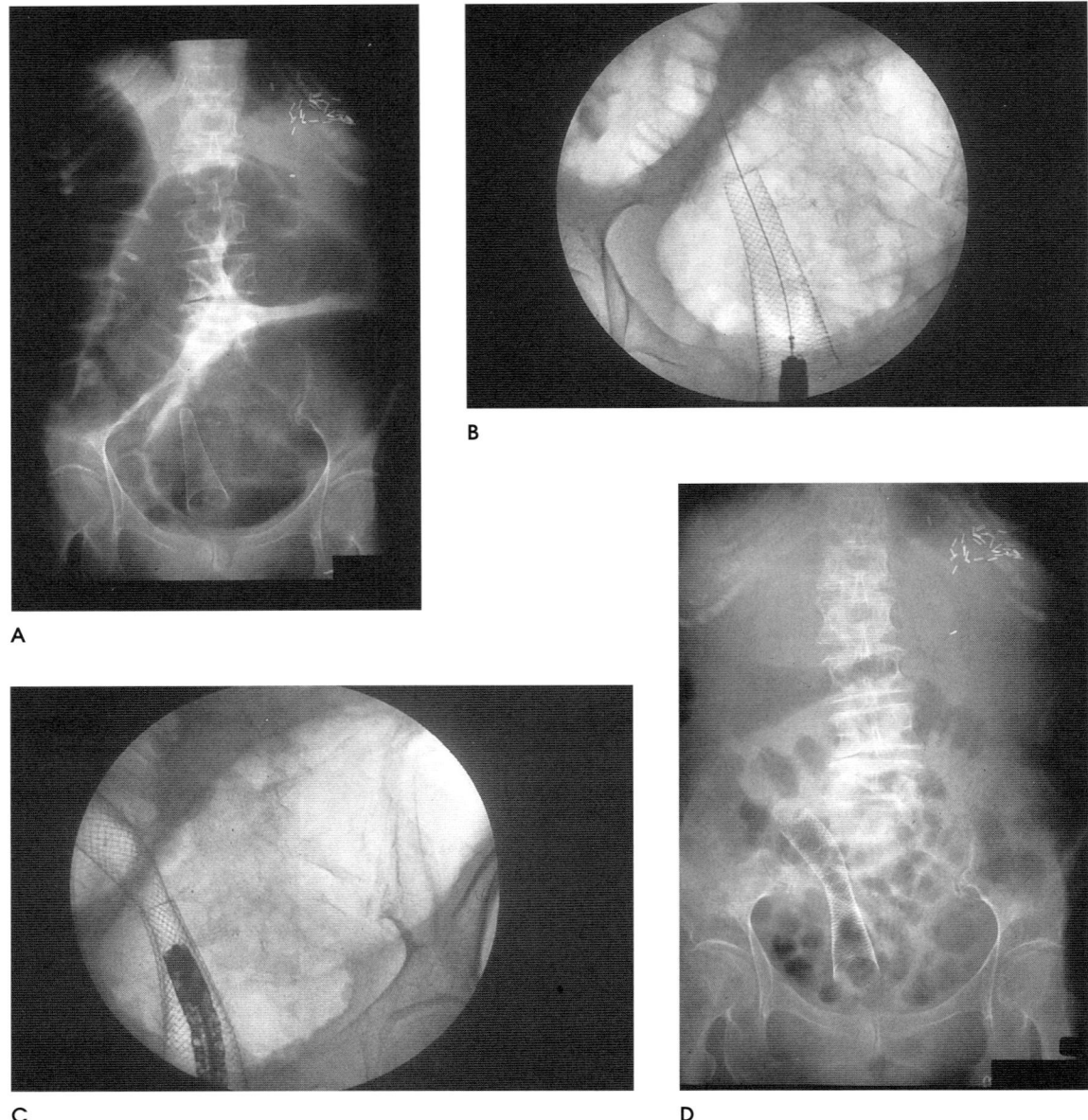

**Figure 73-2** *A:* Abdominal X-ray with dilated loops of large bowel due to distal obstruction. A colonic stent was placed that did not completely bridge the obstruction. *B:* A guidewire being passed through the initial stent under fluoroscopic and endoscopic guidance. *C:* A deployed second stent with complete bridging of the obstruction. *D:* Postprocedure abdominal film several days later demonstrating adequate decompression.

lowing colonic stent placement to rule out perforation. Patients with colonic stents should be investigated carefully if they develop abdominal pain, and perforation should always be ruled out. If perforation develops after stent placement, management depends on the clinical picture. If the patient is stable, with minimal symptoms and no signs of sepsis, conservative management with NPO and intravenous antibiotics can be tried. Otherwise, surgical repair is usually necessary.

**Stent migration** This has been reported to occur in 6%–10% of patients.[62,64,68–73] Most stent migrations occur within the first 24 hours but can occur days later.[64] Migration of a stent can be related to the small diameter of the stent[68] or to shrinkage of the tumor by chemotherapy or radiotherapy.[64–68] Migrated stents have been removed by flexible sigmoidoscopy and biopsy for-

ceps,[68] or by using a long, curved, blunt Kelly clamp to collapse migrated stents and, through gentle rotation, bring it out of the rectum.[71] Gastrografin contrast study should be performed following removal of a stent to ensure absence of perforation.

**Stent obstruction** Obstruction of the stent can occur secondary to tumor growth[65,66,68,73] or due to stool impaction.[65] Stool impaction will usually resolve with enemas; however, patients should be placed on laxatives to prevent such impactions. Laser vaporization,[66,73] argon plasma coagulation, or placement of another stent inside the original stent[68] can be used to treat patients with obstruction of the stent secondary to tumor ingrowth.

**Rectal bleeding** This complication is usually mild and self-limiting. It might be caused by the manipulation of the guidewire and catheters during the procedure. It has been reported in a few cases.[61,62,65,74]

**Abdominal or anorectal pain** Pain is usually mild and does not require specific treatment.[62,74]

The only known contraindication for colonic stent placement is the presence of colonic perforation.[61] Rectal examination should be avoided in patients with known colonic stents, as the Wallstent has sharp barbs at both ends and can cause injury to the fingers of the examining physician.[76] Also, resected surgical specimens with stents should be handled with extreme caution by surgeons and pathologists.

## References

1. Greenlee HB, Pienkos EJ, Vanderbilt PC, et al. Acute large bowel obstruction: comparison of county, Veterans Administration, and community hospital populations. Arch Surg 108:470–476, 1974.
2. Korenaga D, Hiroaki U, Kazuyuki M, Kusumoto T, Baba, H, Shigeaki T, Moriguchi S, Sugimachi K. Prognostic factors in Japanese patients with colorectal cancer: the significance of large bowel obstruction—univariate and multivariate analysis. J Surg Oncol 47:188–192, 1991.
3. Phillips RK, Hittinger R, Fry JS, Fielding LP. Malignant large bowel obstruction. Br J Surg 72:296–302, 1985.
4. Kaufman Z, Eiltch E, Dinbar A. Completely obstructive colorectal cancer. J Surg Oncol 41:230–235, 1989.
5. Papachristodoulou A, Zografos G, Markopoulos CH, Fotiadis C, Gogas J, Sechas M, Skalkeas G. Obstructive colonic cancer. J R Coll Surg Edinb 38:296–298, 1993.
6. Kyllonen LE. Obstruction and perforation complicating colorectal carcinoma. Acta Chir Scand 153:607–614, 1987.
7. Leitman IM, Sullivan JD, Brams D, DeCosse JJ. Multivariate analysis of morbidity and mortality from the initial surgical management of obstructing carcinoma of the colon. Surg Gynecol Obstet 174:513–518, 1992.
8. MacKenzie S, Thomson SR, Baker LW. Management options in malignant obstruction of the left colon. Surg Gynecol Obstet 174:337–345, 1992.
9. Fitchett C, Hoffman G. Obstructing malignant lesions of the colon. Gastrointestinal and hepatobiliary malignancies. Surg Clin North Am 66:807–820, 1986.
10. Barillari P, Aurello P, De Angelis R, Valabrega S, Ramacciato G, D'Angelo F, Fegiz G. Management and survival of patients affected with obstructive colorectal cancer. Int Surg 77:251–255, 1992.
11. Wolmark N, Wieand S, Rockette H, Fisher B, Glass A, Walter L, Lerner H, Cruz A, Volk H, Shibata H, Evans J, Prager D, and other NSABP Investigators. The prognostic significance of tumor location and bowel obstruction in Dukes' B and C colorectal cancer. Ann Surg 6:743–752, 1983.
12. Matheson NA. Management of obstructed and perforated large bowel carcinoma. Baillieres Clin Gastroentrol 3:671–697, 1989.
13. Jackson BR. The diagnosis of colonic obstruction. Dis Colon Rectum 25:603–609, 1982.
14. Lopez-Kostner F, Hool GR, Lavery IC. Management and causes of acute large-bowel obstruction. Surg Clin North Am 77:1265–1290, 1997.
15. Chapman AH, McNamara M, Porter G. The acute contrast enema in suspected large bowel obstruction: value and technique. Clin Radiol 46:273, 1992.
16. Turnage RH, Bergen PC. Intestinal obstruction and ileus: In Feldman M, Sleisenger M, Scharschmidt B (eds): Sleisinger and Fordtran's Gastrointestinal and Liver Disease: Pathophysiology, Diagnosis, Management, Vol. 2, 6th ed. W. B. Saunders Philadelphia, 1998, pp 1799–1810.
17. Glashan RW, John HT. Experience with carcinoma of the large bowel. Br J Surg 52:573–577, 1965.
18. Brewer, MS, Brewer RJ. Tube cecostomy for obstructing cancer of the left colon. KMA J 91:14–16, 1993.
19. Balslev I, Hans-Eric J, Nielsen J. The place of cecostomy in the relief of obstructive carcinoma of the colon. Dis Col Rectum 13:207–210, 1970.
20. Halay F, Syphax B, Leffal LD Jr. Diagnosis and management of acute large bowel obstruction. J Natl Med Assoc 63:362–364, 1971.
21. Sjodahl R, Franzen T, Nystrom PO. Primary versus staged resection for acute obstructing colorectal carcinoma. Br J Surg 79:685–688, 1992.
22. Gandrup P, Lund L, Balslev I. Surgical treatment of acute malignant large bowel obstruction. Eur J Surg 158:427–430, 1992.
23. Gutman M, Kaplan O, Skornick Y, Greif F, Kahn P, Rozin RR. Proximal colostomy: still an effective emergency measure in obstructing carcinoma of the large bowel. J Surg Oncol 41:210–212, 1989.
24. Tan SG, Nambiar R. Left colonic cancer: primary or staged? Aust N Z J Surg 65:728–731, 1995.
25. Fieldings LP, Wells BW. Survival after primary and after staged resection for large bowel obstruction caused by cancer. Br J Surg 61:16–18, 1974.
26. Irvin TT, Greaney MG. The treatment of colonic cancer presenting with intestinal obstruction. Br J Surg 64:741–744, 1977.
27. Deans GT, Krukowski ZH, Irwin ST. Malignant obstruction of the left colon. Br J Surg 81:1270–1276, 1994.
28. Gutman M, Kaplan O, Skornick Y, Greif F, Kahn P, Rozin R. Proximal colostomy: still an effective emergency measure in obstructing carcinoma of the large bowel. J Surg Oncol 41:210–212, 1989.
29. Dorudi S, Wilson NM, Heddle RM. Primary restorative colectomy in malignant left-sided large bowel obstruction. Ann R Coll Surg Engl 72:393–395, 1990.
30. Tan SG, Nambiar R, Rauff A, Goh HS. Primary resection and anastomosis in obstructed descending colon due to cancer. Arch Surg 126:748–751, 1991.
31. Poon RTP, Law WL, Chu KW, Wong J. Emergency resection and primary anastomosis for left-sided obstruction colorectal carcinoma in the elderly. Br J Surg 85:1539–1542, 1998.
32. Stewart J, Diament RH, Brennan TG. Management of obstructing lesions of the left colon by resection, on-table lavage, and primary anastomosis. Surgery 114:502–505, 1993.
33. Nyam DCNK, Seow-Choen F, Leong AFPK, Ho YH. Colonic decompression without on-table irrigation for obstructing left-sided colorectal tumors. Br J Surg 83:786–787, 1996.
34. White CM, Macfie J. Immediate colectomy and primary anastomosis for acute obstruction due to carcinoma of the left colon and rectum. Dis Colon Rectum 28:155–157, 1985.
35. Huddy SPJ, Shorthouse AJ, Marks CG. The surgical treatment of intestinal obstruction due to left-sided carcinoma of the colon. Ann R Coll Surg Engl 70:40–43, 1988.
36. Dutton JW, Hreno A, Hampson LG. Mortality and prognosis of obstructing carcinoma of the large bowel. Am J Surg 131:36–41, 1976.
37. Glenn F, McSherry CK. Obstruction and perforation in colorectal cancer. Ann Surg 173:983–992, 1971.
38. Dudley HAF, Radcliffe AG, McGeehan D. Intraoperative irrigation of the colon to permit primary anastomosis. Br J Surg 67:80–81, 1980.
39. Ohtani H, Sasano N. Microvascular changes in the stroma of human colonrectal carcinomas: ultrastructural histochemical study. Jpn J Cancer Res 80:360–365, 1989.
40. Papanicolaou G, Ahn YK, Nikas DJ, Fielding LP. Effect of large bowel obstruction on colonic blood flow. An experimental study. Dis Colon Rectum 32:673–679, 1990.
41. Agrez MV, Chua FK. The role of colon fibroblast in malignant large bowel obstruction—an experimental in vitro model. Br J Cancer 62:567–572, 1990.
42. Halevy A, Levi J, Orda R. Emergency subtotal colectomy: a new trend for treatment of obstructing carcinoma of the left colon. Ann Surg 210:220–223, 1989.
43. Klatt GR, Martin WH, Gillespie JT. Subtotal colectomy with primary anastomosis without diversion in the treatment of obstructing carcinoma of the left colon. Am J Surg 141:577–578, 1981.
44. Deutsch AA, Zelikovski A, Sternberg A, Reiss R. One–stage subtotal colectomy with anastomosis for obstructing carcinoma of the left colon. Dis Colon Rectum 26:227–230, 1983.
45. Morgan WP, Jenkins N, Lewis P, Aubrey G. Management of obstructing carcinoma of the left colon by extended right hemicolectomy. Am J Surg 149:327–329, 1985.
46. Ross S. Single-stage treatment for malignant left-sided colonic obstruction: a prospective randomized clinical trail comparing subtotal colectomy with segmented resecton following intraoperative irrigation. Br J Surg 82:1622–1627, 1995.
47. Kiefhaber, P. Keifhaber K, Huber F. Preoperative neodymium-YAG laser treatment of obstructive colon cancer. Endoscopy 18(Suppl 1):44–46, 1986.
48. Eckhauser M. Imbembo A, Mansour E. The role of pre-resection laser recanalization for obstructing carcinoma of the colon and rectum. Surgery 106:710–717, 19889.
49. Eckhauser ML, Mansour EG. Endoscopic laser therapy for obstructing and/or bleeding colorectal carcinoma. Am Surg 58:358–363, 1992.

50. Ginsberg GG, Fleischer DE. Endoscopic therapy for sessile lesions. In: Yamada T (ed): Textbook of Gastroenterology, 2nd ed. J.B. Lippincott, Philadelphia, 1995, pp 3011–3038.

51. Walfisch S. Stern H, Ball S. Use of Nd-YAG laser ablation in colorectal obstruction and palliation in high-risk patients. Dis Colon Rectum 32: 1060–1064, 1989.

52. Daneker GW Jr, Carlson GW, Hohn DC, Lynch P, Roubein L, Levin B. Endoscopic laser recanalization is effective for prevention and treatment of obstruction in sigmoid and rectal cancer. Arch Surg 126:1348–1352, 1991.

53. Arrigoni A, Pennazio M, Spandre M, Rossini FP. Emergency endoscopy: recanalizatio of intestinal obstruction caused by colorectal cancer. Gastrointest Endosc 40:576–580, 1994.

54. Rau BK, Harikrishnan KM, Krishna S. Nd-YAG Laser therapy for palliation of obstructed colorectal carcinomas. Indian J Cancer 31:240–243, 1994.

55. Mathus-Vliegen EMH, Tytgat GNJ. Laser ablation and palliation in colorectal malignancy. Gastrointest Endosc 32:393–396, 1986.

56. Keen RR, Orsay CP. Rectosigmoid stent for obstructing colonic neoplasms. Dis Colon Rectum 35:912–913, 1992.

57. Spinelli P, Dal Fante M, Mancini A. Self-expanding mesh stent for endoscopic palliation of rectal obstructing tumors: a preliminary report. Surg Endosc 6:72–74, 1992.

58. Tejero E, Mainar A, Fernandez L, Tobio R, De Gregorio MA. New procedure for the treatment of colorectal neoplastic obstructions. Dis Colon Rectum 37:1158–1159, 1994.

59. Tejero E, Mainar A, Fernandez L, Tieso A, Cuezva JF, San Jose A. New procedure for relief of malignant obstruction of the left colon. Br J Surg 85:34–35, 1995.

60. Vandervoort J, Weiss EJ, Somnay K, Tham TCK, Wong RCK, Carr-Locke DL. Self-expanding metal stent for obstructing adenocacinoma of the sigmoid. Gastrointest Endosc 6:739–741, 1996.

61. Mainar A, Tejero E, Maynar M, Ferral H, Castaneda-Zuniga W. Colorectal obstruction: treatment with metallic stents. Radiology 198:761–764, 1996.

62. Saida Y, Sumiyama Y, Nagao, J, Takase M. Stent endoprosthesis for obstucting colorectal cancers. Dis Colon Rectum 39:552–555, 1996.

63. Aquise M, Tejero E, Mainar A. A new option in the treatment of complete and acute obstruction due to colorectal cancer. Endoscopy 29:229, 1997.

64. Canon CL, Baron TH, Morgan DE, Dean PA, Koehler RE. Treatment of colonic obstruction with expandable metal stents: radiologic features. AJR Am J Roentgenol 168:199–205, 1997.

65. Tejero E, Fernandez-Lobato R, Mainar A, Montes C, Pinto I, Fernandez L, Jorge E, Lozano R. Initial results of a new procedure for treatment of malignant obstruction of the left colon. Dis Colon Rectum 40:432–436, 1997.

66. Dohmoto M, Hunerbein M, Schlag PM. Application of rectal stents for palliation of obstructing rectosigmoid cancer. Surg Endosc 11:758–761, 1997.

67. Turegano-Fuentes F, Echenagusia-Belda A, Simo-Muerza G, Camunez F, Munoz-Jimenez F, Del Valle Hernandez E, Quintans-Rodriguez A. Transanal self-expanding metal stents as an alternative to palliative colostomy in selected patients with malignant obstruction of the left colon. Br J Surg 85:232–235, 1998.

68. Baron TH, Dean PA, Yates MR, Canon C, Koehler RE. Expandable metal stents for the treatment of colonic obstruction: techniques and outcomes. Gastrointest Endosc 47:277–286, 1998.

69. Soonawalla Z, Thakur K, Boorman P, Macfarlane P, Sathananthan N, Parker M. Use of self-expanding metallic stents in the management of obstruction of the sigmoid colon. AJR Am J Roentgenol 171:633–636, 1998.

70. Wallis F, Campbell KL, Eremin O, Hussey JK. Self-expanding metal stents in the management of colorectal carcinoma—a preliminary report. Clin Radiol 53:251–254, 1998.

71. Wholey MH, Levine EA, Ferral H, Castaneda-Zuniga W. Initial clinical experience with colonic stent placement. Am J Surg 175:194–197, 1998.

72. Choo IW, Do YS, Suh SW, Chun H, Choo SW, Park HS, Kang SK, Kim SK. Malignant colorectal obstruction: treatment with a flexible covered stent. Radiology 206:415–421, 1998.

73. Tack J, Gevers A, Rutgeerts P. Self-expandable metallic stents in the palliation of rectosigmoidal carcinoma: a follow-up study. Gastrointest Endosc 48:267–271, 1998.

74. Mainar A, De Gregorio MA, Tejero E, Tobio R, Alfonso E, Pinto I, Herrera M, Femandez JA. Acute colorectal obstruction: treatment with self-expandable metallic stents before scheduled surgery—results of a multicenter study. Radiology 210:65–69, 1999.

75. Campbell KL, Hussey JK, Eremin O. Expandable metal stent application in obstructing carcinoma of the proximal colon: report of a case. Dis Colon Rectum 40:1391–1393, 1997.

76. Lopera JE, Ferral H, Wholey M, Maynar M, Castaneda-Zuniga W. Treatment of colonic obstruction with metalic stents: indication, technique, and complications. AJR Am J Roentgenol 169:1285–1290, 1997.

# Chapter 74

# Pain Management

AHMED ELSAYEM AND EDUARDO BRUERA

Each year more than one million Americans are diagnosed with cancer, and approximately half of them die of their disease.[1] Pain is one of the most common symptoms associated with cancer, affecting an estimated 50% of all cancer patients and approximately 70% of those with advanced disease.[2] The prevalence of pain in patients with common gastrointestinal malignancies is outlined in Table 74–1.

In 1973, Marks and Sachar[3] conducted a survey on the use of pain therapy in the teaching ward of a teaching hospital in the United States. The authors found that pain was not controlled in more than two-thirds of the patients. The opioid doses often were too low, the interval between doses was too long, prn (as needed) orders were abused, and the health-care staff had an exaggerated fear of patients becoming addicted. This initial report led to a growing awareness that the majority of cancer patients died with unrelieved pain.[4]

During the last 15 years, the World Health Organization (WHO) and other cancer and pain societies have launched major cancer pain educational programs.[4–6] These strategies have resulted in a major improvement in the management of cancer pain[7] and an increase in the worldwide use of opioid analgesic.[6,8]

By some estimates, 90% of cancer pain should be effectively controlled by following the WHO guidelines. Evidence suggests, however, that cancer pain is still undertreated.[8] In a study of more than 1000 patients treated at centers affiliated with the Eastern Cooperative Oncology Group, pain was reported by two-thirds of patients, and it was severe enough to impair function in more than one-third. Poor pain assessment, advanced age, good performance status, and female gender were predictors of inadequate pain control in this study.[8] Table 74–2 highlights the major causes of poor pain control. The purpose of this chapter is to discuss the prevalence, assessment, and management of pain among patients with gastrointestinal malignancies.

## Causes and Classification of Pain

In most patients with advanced cancer, chronic pain is attributable to the primary or metastatic cancer's direct stimulation of afferent nerve structures. Pain associated with direct tumor involvement occurs in 65%–85% of patients with advanced cancer.[9] Cancer therapy accounts for pain in approximately 15%–25% of patients receiving chemotherapy, surgery, or radiation therapy.[10] Finally, 3%–10% of cancer patients have pain caused by non-cancer-related problems. In these patients, the pain syndromes reflect those most commonly observed in the general population.

Most patients with advanced cancer have multiple causes and sites of pain. In one survey, 81% of patients reported two or more distinct pain complaints, and 34% reported three distinct pains.[11] Primary tumors that commonly metastasize to bone, such as breast or prostate cancers, are more often associated with pain (60%–80%) than are lymphomas and leukemias.[6] Although fewer than 15% of patients with nonmetastatic disease report pain, 80% or more of terminally ill patients with widely disseminated cancer experience pain requiring treatment.[11]

Pain may be described by its temporal course (acute or chronic) or by its pathophysiologic mechanism and character (nociceptive or neuropathic). Nociceptive pain is further divided into somatic or visceral.

Nociceptive pain results from the activation of nociceptive receptors in tissues and organs, whereas neuropathic pain is the result of injury to the peripheral or central nervous system. Somatic pain (for example, bone metastasis) usually is well local-

**Table 74–1** Frequency of pain in advanced cancer patients with gastrointestinal malignancies

| Primary Site | Prevalence % (range) |
| --- | --- |
| Esophagus | 87 (80–93) |
| Stomach | 78 (67–93) |
| Pancreas | 81 (72–95) |
| Colorectal | 70 (47–95) |
| Liver | 70 (65–100) |

Adapted from Bonica JJ. Bonica's Management of Pain, 3rd ed. Loeser JD (ed). Lippincott Williams and Wilkins, Philadelpia, 2001, p 427.

ized and tender to pressure, and is often perceived as a dull background aching.[12] Visceral pain from deep-seated structures is less well localized and often involves referred pain to cutaneous sites. Visceral pain may be a deep aching or a throbbing pain that may be sharp if the organ capsules are involved (for example, liver) or colicky if hollow viscera are obstructed (for example, colon).

Neuropathic pain arises from damage to neural structures. Its distribution is along a dermatome, and the pain is described as burning with sensory changes such as allodynia or hyperalgesia (for example, dysesthetic pain in postherpetic neuralgia). Occasionally neuropathic pain is a shooting, lancinating pain (for example, glossopharyngeal or trigeminal neuralgia).[12]

Patients with advanced cancer generally have chronic constant pain intermittently punctuated by acute breakthrough pain. Patients may also have acute pain following a surgical procedure, such as laparotomy, or chemotherapy-related mucositis. Table 74–3 illustrates different pathophysiologic mechanisms of pain. Incidental pain is usually acute and triggered by certain maneuvers, such as swallowing in esophageal cancer, defecation in rectal cancer, or movement in spinal metastasis. Some cancers are associated with more than one type of pain; for example, the pancreatic cancer pain syndrome[13] may be visceral from pancreatic gland and duodenal infiltration, somatic from retroperitoneal and parietal peritoneum involvement, and neuropathic secondary to radiculopathy from retroperitoneal spread or lumbosacral plexopathy. Moreover, the degree of pain associated with surgical laparotomy and mucocytis from chemotherapy cannot be overemphasized.

## Pain Assessment

Lack of knowledge in pain assessment by clinicians and nurses has been blamed for poor pain control in cancer patients.[14–18] Adequate and appropriate treatment of pain in patients with advanced cancer begins with a thorough initial assessment of the patient and the pain. Figure 74–1 summarizes steps in the production of pain. Unfortunately, neither step 1 (nociception) or step 2 (perception) can be measured at the present time. Therefore, all our assessments for pain intensity are based on the patients' expression of pain.

**Table 74–2** Factors contributing to poor pain control

Inadequate assessment
Inadequate knowledge about pain by health-care professional
Excessive concern about side effects of pain medications
Misinformation about opioid tolerance and dependence issues
Poorly accessible or unavailable pain management services
Legislative and regulatory barriers by national or regional governments

Unlike pain in other medical conditions, cancer pain is complicated by the high level of distress from the lethal threat of the disease and from its associated pain. Many patients and their families believe this pain is untreatable, a misconception that leads to significant emotional suffering.[19]

## Essential Components of the Initial Assessment

### Detailed history and physical examination

The initial assessment of pain should reveal information about the onset, duration, location, severity, character, aggravating and relieving factors, and previous treatment and side effects of medication. The physical exam should focus on mood and affect, areas of tenderness, and palpable masses. A detailed neurological exam should be conducted.

### Psychological distress

Cancer pain increases psychological distress, disturbs sleep and social life, and compromises quality of life.[20–24] The emotional suffering experienced by cancer patients manifests itself as fear, anxiety, and depression and may result in increased pain expression.[19,25] Consequently, patients often exhaust personal and psychological resources to cope with this threat.[26]

### Investigations

Laboratory tests and diagnostic imaging should be obtained if indicated by the history and physical examination. Renal function should be assessed before opioids are prescribed because most opioids are renally excreted, and active metabolites can accumulate and become neurotoxic under conditions of renal insufficiency.

Repeat assessments should be performed at regular intervals and whenever pain changes or new pain appears.

## Assessment of Pain in Three Steps

Pain assessment can be broken down into the following three steps.

Step 1: Determine the probable type and origin of the pain, as outlined above.

Step 2: Measure the intensity of the pain and record concurrent symptoms. It is crucial to assess and monitor the pain intensity. Visual analogue scales, verbal scales, numerical scales, or more complex pain questionnaires are simple and reliable tools.[27] The most important aspect of effective pain assessment and monitoring is the graphic display of pain intensity in the patient's chart. Years ago it became apparent that a regular graphic display of patient vital signs helped make abnormalities that required correction quite visible. Regular inclusion of laboratory results and X-rays in the medical record also makes visible a number of factors not readily accessible to physical examination. The appropriate recording of pain and other symptoms accomplishes a similar task: making an unseen phenomenon visible, moreover, it assists the health-care team in the overall planning and monitoring of quality of care.[11,27] Figure 74–2 summarizes bedside tools for assessment of pain intensity. Some tests, such as the Edmonton Symptom Assessment Scale,[27,28] allow graphic display of multiple symptoms simultaneously.

Step 3: Conduct multidimensional pain assessment.

In the past, cancer pain and hospice groups relied on a more unidimensional assessment based on the assumption that 100% of a given patient's expression of pain was due to nociception and was therefore treatable with analgesic drugs. This simplistic

**Table 74–3** Types of pain

| Types | Subtype | Example | Characteristics |
|---|---|---|---|
| Somatic | Bone | Metastatic esophageal or pancreatic cancer | Localized, constant, aching |
| | Soft tissue | Retroperitoneal tumor, ascites | Localized, waxing and waning |
| Visceral | Hollow organ | Colon/stomach | Diffuse, squeezing and crampy |
| | Capsular | Liver | Constant, could be sharp |
| Neuropathic | Deafferentation | Sacral plexopathy | Burning, continuous |
| | Lancinating | Trigeminal neuralgia | Tingling, sharp, of short duration |

approach could result in massive doses of opioids and, in turn, in opioid-related toxicity and excessive reliance on pharmacological approaches to pain control.

Instead, pain expression should be interpreted as a multidimensional construct. Table 74–4 summarizes the multidimensional assessment necessary to interpret pain. In a given patient, a pain intensity score of 8 out of 10 can be the result of nociception plus a certain level of somatization, coping chemically, and mild delirium. A multidimensional assessment can help differentiate the relative contributions of the different dimensions of pain to the patient's expression, thereby assisting in the planning of care.

A positive history of alcoholism or drug abuse indicates that the patient is at a higher risk of seeking chemical means of coping. Alcoholism occurs in 5%–15% of the general population and in approximately 20% of hospitalized patients.[29] Unfortunately, the diagnosis is not made in more than two-thirds of patients.[29,30] Four-item questionnaires, such as the CAGE assessment, are a simple and usually accurate diagnostic tool.[30] A history of alcoholism is a major prognostic factor for the development of opioid dose escalation and opioid-related neurotoxicity.[31] However, when cancer patients undergo regular screening for alcoholism and are provided with multidimensional and multidisciplinary support, both pain intensity and overall opioid use do not significantly differ between alcoholic patients and those with no history of alcoholism.[32]

Somatization, either as a primary coping strategy or as a result of affective disorders such as anxiety or depression, is also an independent predictive factor for a poor outcome among patients with cancer pain.[31] The appropriate assessment and management of affective disorders with both pharmacological and nonpharmacological techniques, and appropriate counseling of patients with a history of somatization can improve symptom control and patient satisfaction with care.

Cognitive failure is a common complication among patients with advanced cancer.[33] Cognitive failure makes the assessment of pain intensity and other dimensions of pain difficult. In addition, cognitive failure can be aggravated by pharmacological interventions. Therefore, cognitive function should be assessed regularly using tools such as the Mini-Mental State Examination.[33]

## Association Between Pain and Other Symptoms

Pain is only one of many symptoms experienced by cancer patients.[32] As a result, pain must be assessed within the context of other symptoms for a number of reasons. For example, pain may not be the symptom that is having the greatest effect on a patient's quality of life at a given point in time. The experience of pain may affect the perception and expression of other symptoms, and vice versa, resulting in misinterpretation of symptoms and inappropriate management. Also, pain treatment may lead directly to a worsening of other symptoms, such as opioid-related nausea, constipation, somatization, and delirium. The Edmonton Symptom Assessment System[32] is an example of an organized approach to serial measurement of multiple symptoms. This tool involves the completion of a panel of visual analogue scales on a regular basis by the patient or by a nurse if the patient is cognitively impaired. The challenge of the multidimensional pain assessment is therefore not only to discern the various components of pain expression but also to integrate that construct into the broader and more complex model of overall patient distress.

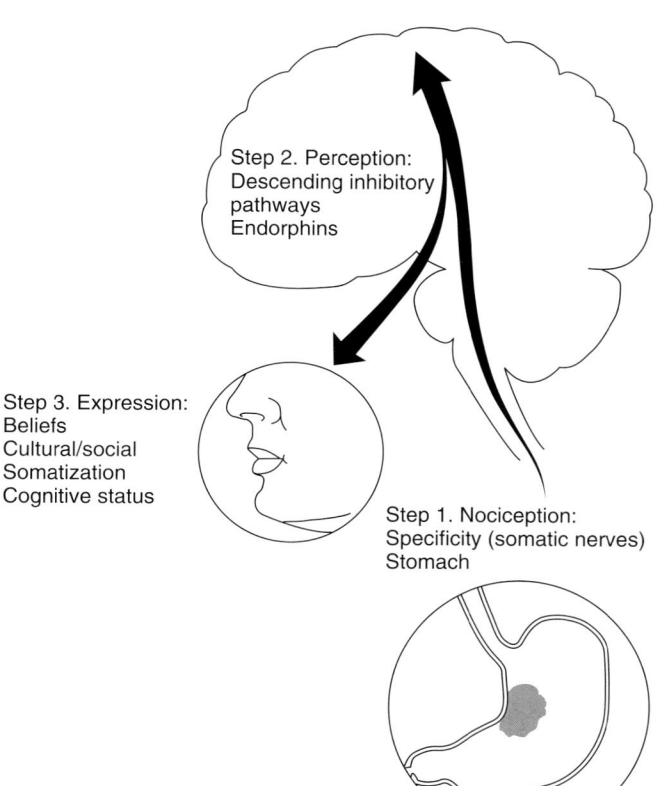

Step 2. Perception: Descending inhibitory pathways Endorphins

Step 3. Expression: Beliefs Cultural/social Somatization Cognitive status

Step 1. Nociception: Specificity (somatic nerves) Stomach

**Figure 74–1** Steps in the production of pain.

## Management of Cancer Pain

Pain management is an integral part of the comprehensive care of cancer patients.[34] Successful management depends on the physician's ability to assess the patient and the pain, identify the pain syndrome, formulate a treatment plan, and discuss it with

- Visual Analogue Scale (10 cm)

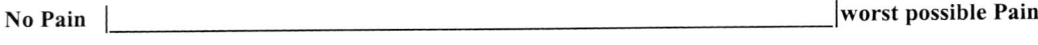

No Pain |_____|worst possible Pain

- Simple descriptive Pain intensity Scale

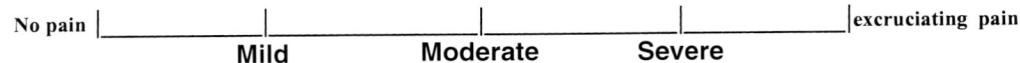

No pain |_____|_____|_____|_____|excruciating pain
　　　　　　**Mild**　　　　　**Moderate**　　　**Severe**

- Numerical Rating Scale

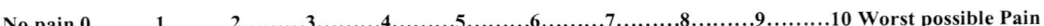

No pain 0.........1.........2.........3.........4.........5.........6.........7.........8.........9.........10 Worst possible Pain

**Figure 74-2** Simple bedside tools for the assessment of pain intensity.

the patient and family. Most cancer patients respond to simple oral medications. In more complex cases in which suffering and psychosocial distress complicate pain perception, a multidisciplinary approach is required.

Pharmacological treatment is the main approach to cancer pain. Specific treatment of infection, drainage of an abscess, and other interventions may reduce the pain intensity and obviate the need for escalating doses of opioids. Ultimately, this will save the patient from experiencing unnecessary side effects. Other specific modalities such as stenting or dilatation[35–38] for obstruction or anethesiological procedures such as celiac plexus block[39–42] may be indicated in patients with certain gastrointestinal malignancies. In the following sections we will discuss general support measures and pharmacological and nonpharmacological approaches to pain management in this patient population.

### General Support Measures and Patient Education

Patients should receive appropriate counseling and information regarding their pain and the factors that influence it. The physician should set a realistic goal for pain management and discuss the goal with the patient. For most patients, pain intensity can be reduced to a tolerable level but may not disappear completely. Cost of treatment and possible side effects should be discussed

**Table 74-4** Multidimensional assessment of pain in cancer patients

Cause (cancer, cancer treatment, unrelated to cancer)
Intensity (visual analogue scale, numerical, verbal etc.)
Alcoholism/drugs (CAGE questionnaire, etc.)
Psychosocial distress (somatization)
Cognitive function (MMSQ, etc.)
Mechanism (neuropathic, non-neuropathic)
Nature (continuous, incidental)
Other related symptoms (ESAS, etc.)

ESAS, Edmonton Symptom Assessment System; MMSQ, Mini-Mental State Questionnaire. (From Bruera E, Neumann CM. Cancer pain. In: Mitchell M (ed): Pain 1999—An Updated Review (Refresher Course Syllabus). IASP Press, Seattle, 1999, with permission.)

in advance. This approach will enhance compliance and improve patient satisfaction with the treatment.

As in other aspects of health care, good communication increases satisfaction and enhances compliance. Two important myths to dispel with the patient and family are those related to addiction and tolerance. Many patients fear that taking opioids for cancer pain will make them addicts, but there is strong evidence to the contrary.[4,5] Many patients also fear that if they receive full opioid doses now, tolerance will develop and make pain uncontrollable in the future. Appropriate counseling of patients and families on these issues and on expected side effects, such as constipation, sedation, and nausea, and their management will increase patient compliance.

### Pharmacological Management

In 1984 the WHO proposed a simple analgesic ladder for the pharmacological management of cancer pain.[43] Experience with the application of this ladder in several countries worldwide has shown that the simple principles of escalating nonopioid to strong opioid analgesics is safe and effective. In addition to the WHO guidelines, a number of other excellent guidelines have been published.[5,6] Figure 74–3 summarizes the WHO analgesic ladder.

#### Nonopioid analgesics

Acetaminophen or nonsteroidal anti-inflammatory drugs (NSAIDs) are effective analgesics for patients with mild cancer pain, and they can be combined with opioids in patients with moderate to severe pain.[4–6,44] Because acetaminophen does not inhibit prostaglandin synthesis, it does not affect platelet function or cause significant renal or gastrointestinal toxicity. Therefore, it is easier to use alone or in combination with opioids in patients with advanced cancer. Commercial preparations containing codeine or oxycodone and acetaminophen are among the most widely prescribed analgesics for cancer pain. The major side effect of acetaminophen is its hepatotoxic effect. As a result, liver function should be assessed periodically, and the cumulative dose should not exceed 4 g/day. Hepatotoxicity can occur at a lower dose with concomitant alcohol use. The risk also is increased in malnourished patients and in those on chronic anticonvulsant therapy.[45–47]

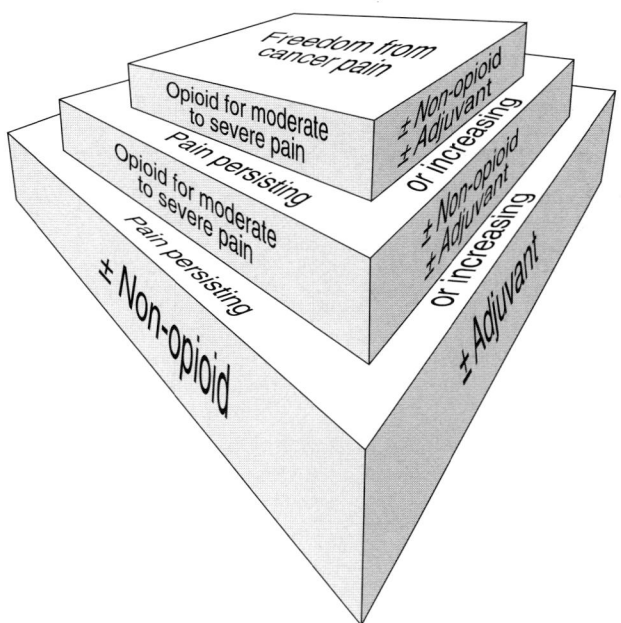

**Figure 74-3** Summary of the World Health Organization analgesic ladder.

**Table 74-5** Opioid treatment of cancer pain

Educate the patient regarding myths about addiction, tolerance, and side effects.
Set a realistic goal.
Oral route is the first choice; consider another route if this route is not available.
Administer around the clock. Start with small doses and titrate individually.
Allow for extra doses for rescue analgesia. Consider slow release when the patient is stable.
Prevent nausea and constipation by concomitant use of antiemetics and laxatives.
Consider adjuvant drugs to manage side effects or a specific pain syndrome.
Consider opioids as only one part of the total pain management plan.
Reassess and evaluate for toxicity.

The majority of nonopioid analgesics are NSAIDs. Their effect on the inflammatory process is a key component of their analgesic property. In addition to their well-demonstrated peripheral effects, NSAIDs recently have been found to have central effects at both the spinal and supraspinal level.

The main limitations of NSAIDs are their relatively flat dose–response curve and the risk of gastrointestinal, renal, and bleeding side effects. These effects are related to the inhibition of cyclooxygenase (COX). A new generation of COX-2 inhibitors was introduced recently.[48] These include agents such as celecoxib and rofecoxib. Both agents have a lower occurrence of toxicity than conventional NSAIDs and they are effective alone or in combination with opioid analgesics. Long-term efficacy and safety have not been established in cancer patients.[49] Because not enough studies have compared the efficacy and safety of different NSAIDs for cancer pain, no clear evidence exists that one type of NSAID is more effective than others in this patient population.

## Opioids

Opioids remain the mainstay in the treatment of cancer pain. Opioids interrupt pain perception at different levels in the central nervous system,[50] including disruption of the transmission of nociception at the spinal cord level. Opioids also activate descending inhibitory systems that modulate pain perception at the level of the basal ganglia. Moreover, opioids alter response to nociception at the level of the limbic system, decreasing the affective response to nociception.[51] Table 74–5 summarizes the general principles of opioid treatment of cancer pain.

**Routes of opioid delivery** The oral route of administration is preferable for most patients because this approach is safe, effective, and convenient and and is easy to use in the home setting.[52,53] However, 80% of patients with cancer pain will require an alternative route before death.[54] The development of alternative routes for systemic opioid delivery has been a major factor in facilitating home management of cancer pain.

The intravenous route gives rapid effect with bolus administration. It is suitable for immediate postoperative pain control and for times when the gastrointestinal route is not available because of vomiting, dysphagia, or severe mucositis or bowel obstruction. The most significant disadvantage of this route is the need for hospital admission and the possibility of infectious complications.

Patient-controlled analgesia (PCA) is a safe and effective mode of opioid administration.[53] The opioids can be given intravenously, subcutaneously, or through the epidural space. Some patients report better control of their postoperative pain when they use this modality compared with regular opioid administration or continuous infusion.[54]

The subcutaneous route is another safe and effective mode of opioid administration.[55,56] Subcutaneous opioids can be given intermittently, either by the patient or a family member, with a preloaded syringe or portable device.[57] Blood levels of opioids are comparable with subcutaneous and intravenous administration.[58] A single subcutaneous site can be used for an average of 7 days.[59] Complications with this route are infrequent and consist of redness, leakage, and swelling. These complications rarely require treatment other than changing the administration site.[59,60]

Rectal administration of opioids has been investigated for the short-term treatment of acute pain.[61] Despite interpersonal variation in bioavailability,[62,63] most patients achieve good pain control at relatively low doses. The disadvantages of rectally administered opioids in chronic cancer patients include the need for repeated administration and its associated discomfort and the lack of a range of doses that can be given by this route.

Several studies have shown that the transdermal route (e.g., fentanyl) also is effective for cancer pain.[64] The drug transfers slowly from the patch and forms a reservoir under the skin that releases the drug at a uniform level for up to 72 hours.[65] Because of the slowly declining plasma concentration after the patch is removed and the considerable delay in reaching steady-state plasma levels, treatment with the fentanyl patch should be limited to cancer patients whose pain is stable and will require relatively low-dose opioids. In this latter group of patients, the fentanyl patch provides a useful alternative when the oral route is unacceptable.

A transmucosal route of opioid delivery recently became available. Oral fentanyl lozenges, made in a candy form and absorbed directly through the oral mucosa, are effective in managing acute incidental pain.[66,67]

**Table 74-6** Opioid analgesics most frequently recommended for cancer pain

| Type of Opioid | Name of Opioid | Common Route | Equivalent Price[a] | Other Routes |
|---|---|---|---|---|
| Weak | Codeine | PO | — | IV, SC |
| Weak | Dextropropoxyphene | PO | — | — |
| Strong | Morphine | PO | 1 | IV, SC, Supp |
| Strong | SR Morphine | PO | 5 | — |
| Strong | Hydromorphone | PO | 3 | IV, SC, Supp |
| Strong | Oxycodone | PO | 3.6 | SC[b] |
| Strong | SR Oxycodone | PO | 6.5 | — |
| Strong | Fentanyl | TD | 6.5 | TM, IV |
| Strong | Methadone | PO | 0.15 | IV, Supp |
| Strong | Diamorphine[b] | IV | — | SC |

[a]Approximate relative price when using a daily dose equivalent to morphine 100 mg by mouth. [b]Not available in the United States.

IV, intravenous; PO, oral; SC, subcutaneous; SR, slow release; Supp, Suppository; TD, transdermal; TM, transmucosal.

**Specific opioids** Several systems are used to classify opioids. One system classifies the agents according to their addiction potential as weak or strong. Other classification systems use an agonist–antagonist approach. Table 74–6 summarizes the most commonly recommended opioids for cancer pain.

The so-called *weak opioids* have a flat dose-response curve and are often subjected to fewer prescribing restrictions. A typical example of this group of drugs is codeine.[4,5] Weak opioids are often combined with acetaminophen or aspirin. As the cancer disease advances, oral administration of the more potent opioids provides excellent pain relief for most patients.

Among *strong opioids*, morphine has been considered the treatment of choice. However, other opioid agonists, such as oxycodone and hydromorphone, exhibit similar pharmacokinetic and pharmacodynamic properties.[4,5] Morphine can be given orally, intravenously, subcutaneously, and rectally and it is available in immediate-release and sustained-release forms. A typical starting dose of immediate-release morphine is 5–10 mg every 4 hours in patients who have not previously taken opioids. When a patient is switched from another opioid (usually codeine or oxycodone) to morphine, it is important to calculate the equianalgesic dose in order to determine which morphine-equivalent doses are the threshold for pain control. The starting dose may be insufficient, and relatively rapid titration may be needed, particularly if pain is severe. When the effective dose of short-acting morphine has been established, patients can be maintained on this preparation indefinitely, or a slow-release preparation can be administered every 12 hours. Slow-release preparations provide constant plasma levels of the drug for long periods of time, making them more suitable for patients with advanced cancer.[68] In some countries, once-a-day slow-release morphine preparations are available.

Hydromorphone is a semisynthetic derivative of morphine that is approximately five to six times as potent. It is well absorbed from the gastrointensinal tract. Hydromorphone can be given through the same routes as those used for morphine, but it is particularly valuable subcutaneously because of its high solubility.[69] The drug usually is given in immediate-release form every 4 hours. Sustained-release preparations given every 12 hours are available in some countries.[70]

Oxycodone is available either as a single-entity preparation or in combination with aspirin or acetaminophen.[71] It is usually given orally but intravenous preparations are available in some countries. A slow-release preparation, which can be given every 12 hours, is available.

Fentanyl is available in most countries as a transdermal patch with a duration of effectiveness of approximately 3 days. The drug is metabolized by the liver and has high lipid solubility. Elevation of body temperature increases the rate of transdermal absorption.[72] Fentanyl can also be given intravenously.

Methadone has a long duration of action, making it suitable for patients with advanced cancer. However, its half-life is unpredictable and can range from 13 to 100 hours.[73,74] Methadone also interacts with many medications prescribed for advanced-cancer patients. As a result, this medicine must be used with care. Nonetheless, methadone is a unique drug with good bioavailability when given orally. It is inexpensive, has no active metabolites, and has a lower incidence of associated constipation.[75] Moreover, methadone is excreted through the fecal route, making it a suitable drug for patients with renal insufficiency.[75] Methadone can also be given intravenously. The subcutaneous route is not recommended because of local skin irritation.[76] Custom-made methadone capsules or suppositories (administered three times daily)[77] have been shown to be effective and relatively inexpensive.[77]

The opioid agonist–antagonist analgesics have established efficacy in the control of acute pain, especially procedure-related pain. Their use in chronic cancer pain, however, is limited by the possibility of precipitous withdrawal in the patient who has been taking morphine-type drugs, by their analgesic ceiling effects (when the higher drug dose does not provide additional pain relief), and, in the case of pentazocine, by the production of a relatively high proportion of disturbing psychotomimetic effects.

Meperidine should not be used on a chronic basis because of the production of a neurotoxic metabolite, normeperidine, which can cause central nervous system excitatory side effects.[4,5,44]

It is important to remember that there may be large individual differences in the required dose of opioid, depending on such factors as the patient's prior opioid history, activity level, and metabolism. In addition to a regular opioid dose, patients need to have access to extra rescue doses of opioids for episodes of pain exacerbation. These extra doses of rapid-release opioid traditionally have been assumed to be approximately 10% of the daily opioid dose. The patient's report of pain severity and pain relief and the monitoring of opioid-induced side effects are the best guidelines for opioid titration.

**Side effects** A number of side effects are associated with the use of opioids for cancer pain. In most patients, these side effects can be easily managed through patient education and reassurance about the usually transient nature of sedation and nausea, careful selection of route and dose, and use of additional drugs, such as antiemetics and laxatives. Table 74–7 summarizes the main side effects of opioids. Sedation, constipation, and nausea are the three most common side effects.

Daytime *sedation* or mild mental clouding commonly occur at the beginning of opioid treatment or after a significant increase in dose. These effects usually disappear in a few days.[78] However, some patients experience more prolonged sedation that does not respond to a change in dose or even the type of opioid. In these patients, adding low-dose methylphenidate or other psychostimulants may improve daytime arousal and concentration.[79] The central depressant effects of opioids are exacerbated by the administration of hypnotics such as benzodiazepines or consumption of alcohol.

**Table 74–7** Common side effects of opioids

| Problem | Suggested Intervention |
|---|---|
| Sedation | May improve spontaneously with continued use. If it persists, consider psychostimulant (e.g., methylphenidate) |
| Nausea | Start metoclopramide at 10 mg every 4 hours around the clock for 3 days as needed |
| Constipation | Start laxative concomitantly (e.g., Senokot-S) |
| Pruritis | Give antihistamine |
| Cognitive failure | Consider opioid rotation (see below) |
| Respiratory depression | Reduce the opioid dose for mild depression. If moderate or severe, treat with naloxone. |

Probably constipation is the most common adverse effect of opioids (Fig. 74–4). Opioids act at multiple sites in the gastrointestinal tract to produce a decrease in both peristalsis and intestinal secretions. Because tolerance to the constipatory effects of opioids develops very slowly, most patients will require regular laxative treatment for the duration of the opioid therapy. In recent years, oral preparations of naloxone or naltrexone have been tried as a means of preventing and managing particularly severe cases of constipation. Because these drugs have limited systemic absorption, they are potentially capable of controling opioid-induced constipation with minimal withdrawal effects or pain exacerbation. Clinical trials are attempting to define the role of these drugs.[80]

More than half of patients given opioids experience nausea. In most patients, nausea resolves rapidly with continued use of the medications. Nausea is caused primarily by stimulation of the chemoreceptor trigger zone in the medulla and by delayed gastric emptying. Antiemetics such as metoclopramide are effective against these two mechanisms of opioid-induced nausea and emesis and are often successful in treating or preventing this symptom.[81]

Opioids have a direct depressant effect on the respiratory center in the brain stem. They decrease the minute ventilation and

depress the response of medullary centers to carbon dioxide.[82] Pain counteracts this effect and stimulates respiration. Patients usually develop tolerance to the respiratory effect of opioids after continuous use. Respiratory depression occurs when large doses of opioids are given frequently, or when regular doses are given to debilitated patients.[82] Mild respiratory depression responds to dose reduction. More severe cases may require administration of the opioid antagonist naloxone.[74] Naloxone should be given in small bolus doses of 0.1 mg at a time until an improved level of consciousness is observed. High-dose boluses of naloxone can precipitate severe withdrawal, increased pain, or even grand mal seizures. Occasionally patients with a high circulating blood level of an opioid need a continuous infusion of naloxone until the opioids are metabolized or eliminated.[74]

Central nervous system side effects consist of both an exacerbation of the more common depressant toxicities, such as sedation and cognitive failure, or the triggering of a number of excitatory side effects, such as hallucinosis, agitated delirium, myoclonus, grand mal seizures, and, in extreme cases, hyperalgesia.[83,84]

Figure 74–5 summarizes the putative mechanism for opioid-induced neurotoxicity (OIN). Some metabolites, such as morphine- or hydromorphone-6-glucuronides, are capable of binding to the opioid receptor, thereby inducing some of the traditional depressant side effects. Other metabolites, such as morphine- or hydromorphone-3-glucuronide, normorphine, and probably others, are capable of causing excitatory side effects by nonopioid mechanisms. Because these metabolites are all the result of liver metabolism and renal elimination, decreased glomerular filtration can aggravate OIN.

Table 74–8 summarizes the diagnosis, management, and prevention of OIN. Specifically, hyperactivity and the presence of one or more symptoms of delirium in patients with a history of high opioid dose, prolonged administration, borderline cognition, or decreased glomerular filtration (renal failure, dehydration, or drugs such as NSAIDs) can indicate OIN. This complication is managed by changing the type of opioid (to facilitate the elimination of both parent drug and active metabolites), attempting to increase renal elimination by hydration and discontinuation of potentially neurotoxic drugs, eliminating drugs that can aggravate delirium (e.g., benzodiazepines, tricyclic antidepressants), and addressing symptoms. If severe agitation, hallucinations, or delusions are observed, haloperidol may be required temporarily. In extreme cases, a subcutaneous infusion of midazolam may be required for sedation while opioid rotation and hydration take place.

Once the acute episode of OIN has been resolved, it is important to consider risk factors for future episodes, such as somatization, chemical coping, or tolerance, and to reevaluate dosing. Primary care physicians, other health professionals, and family members should be advised about the possibility of this problem recurring in the future.

Other less common side effects of opioids include sweating, vertigo, pruritus, and urinary retention. As a result of international educational efforts, cancer patients today are exposed to higher doses of opioids for longer periods of time than ever before. Probably as a result of this increased exposure, a number of new opioid toxicities have been described. Pulmonary edema has been seen in addicts treated for overdoses, but it also can be observed in cancer patients undergoing rapid opioid titration for uncontrolled pain.[83]

**Opioid rotation** If an opioid or its active metabolites are causing OIN, rotation of the opioid may help alleviate the problem. Several studies have shown that this is a safe and reliable

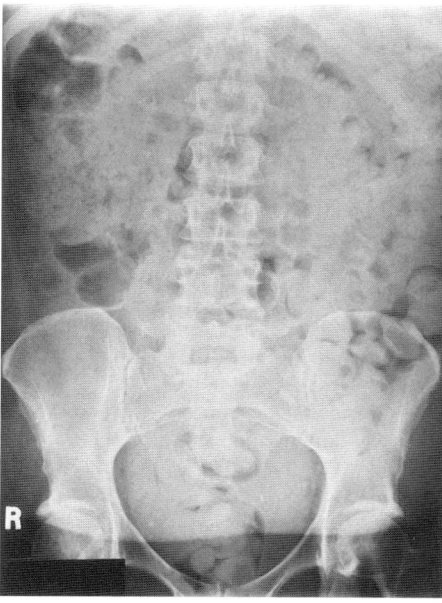

**Figure 74–4** Severe constipation in a cancer patient on opioids.

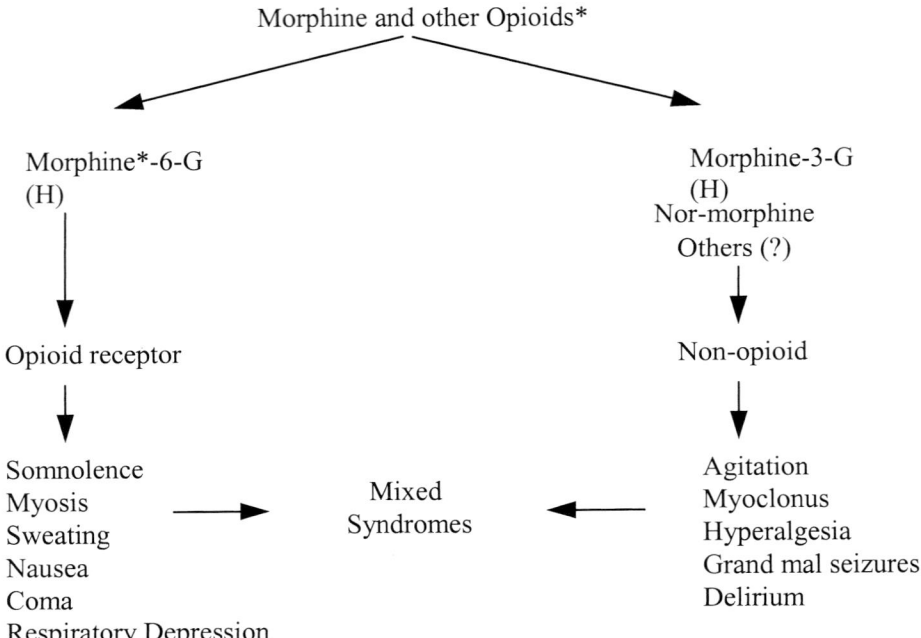

* other opioids with known active metabolites include Hydromorphone, Fentanyl,

diamorphine, Oxycodone and propoxyphene.

**Figure 74-5** Putative mechanism for opioid-induced neurotoxicity. *Other opioids with known active metabolites include hydromorphone, fentanyl, diamorphine, oxycodone, and propoxyphene. (Adapted from Cavalli F, Hansen HH, Kaye SB. Textbook of Medical Oncology, 2nd ed. Martin Dunitz, London, 1997, with permission.)

method of decreasing neurotoxicity while maintaining analgesia.[83,84] The ideal alternative opioid is yet to be determined. In patients who develop OIN while on morphine, a trial of another opioid agonist, such as hydromorphone, oxycodone, or fentanyl, usually is effective. The reverse usually is effective as well. If OIN develops after rotation among the first-line agonists, a second-line opioid, such as methadone or parenteral fentanyl, can be used. Methadone has the advantages of low cost, lack of active metabolites, excellent oral bioavailability, and N-methyl-D-aspartate (NMDA) receptor antagonism. (Excitability amino acids such as NMDA are implicated in opioid tolerance and neuropathic pain.) However, methadone also has the disadvantage of a long and variable half-life and a poorly defined equianalgesic dose compared with morphine or hydromorphone.[73] When opioid rotation is considered, most clinicians will change the dose of one opioid for another, following guidelines such as those summarized in Table 74–9. These guidelines are based on studies comparing single doses of opioids in volunteers or patients with postoperative pain who are generally receiving low overall doses of opioids. In these patients, the traditional view has been that the dose ratio between the newer and older opioid is independent of total opioid dose (e.g., 10 mg of morphine = 2 mg of hydromorphone; 100 mg of morphine = 20 mg of hydromorphone). The traditional view also assumes that dose ratio is the same in both directions of the rotation (e.g., 10 mg of morphine = 2 mg of hydromorphone, and 2 mg of hydromorphone = 10 mg morphine). Finally, it assumes minimal interpersonal variability in the ratios (Table 74–8). Recent studies of a number of opioid agonists have revealed major differences in dose ratio in different patient populations. With some opioids, such as methadone, the dose ratio changes dramatically according to the previous total opioid dose. For example, the morphine/methadone ratio usually is 5:1 or less in patients receiving less than 150 mg of total morphine before rotation, compared with 15:1 or more in patients re-

**Table 74-8** Opioid-induced neurotoxicity

*Symptoms and Signs*

Visual and tactile hallucinations
Severe sedation
Delirium
Myoclonus

*Predisposing Factors*

Prolonged use of high-dose opioids
Renal failure and dehydration
Poor prognostic factors for pain control (e.g., alcoholism, somatization, and incidental pain)

*Management*

Hydration to increase elimination of metabolites
Opioid rotation
Stop psychoactive medications (e.g., benzodiazepines and antidepressants)
Consider symptomatic treatment of agitation (e.g., haloperidol)
Recognize and manage reasons for opioid escalation
Reassess frequently
Family counseling

**Table 74–9** Conversion from another opioid to morphine

a. Total amount of opioid that effectively control pain in 24 hours.
b. Multiply by conversion factor in table below. Give 30% less of the new opioid to avoid partial cross tolerance.
c. Divide the number of doses per day.

| Opioid[a] | From Parenteral Opioid to Parenteral Morphine | From Same Parenteral Opioid to Oral Opioid | From Oral Opioid to Oral Morphine | From Oral Morphine to Oral Opioid |
|---|---|---|---|---|
| Morphine | 1 | 2.5 | 1 | 1 |
| Hydromorphone | 5 | 2 | 5 | 0.2 |
| Meperidine | 0.13 | 4 | 0.1 | 10 |
| Levorphanol | 5 | 2 | 5 | 0.2 |
| Codeine | — | — | 0.15 | 7 |
| Oxycodone | — | — | 1.5 | 0.7 |
| Hydrocodone | — | — | 0.15 | 7 |

[a]Methadone has a variable equianalgesic dose, therefore, it was not included in this table. **Caution:** There is wide interpersonal variation in equianalgesic doses. Personalized titration and frequent monitoring are required.

ceiving more than 500 mg of morphine per day before rotation.[85] The dose ratio often is not the same in both directions; therefore, different ratios may need to be used when patients change from morphine to hydromorphone as opposed to hydromorphone to morphine.[86] Finally, the results of most studies agree that patients with cancer pain who are receiving chronic opioid analgesia display large interpersonal variability in dose ratio.

This emerging body of evidence suggests that currently available equianalgesic dose guidelines often are inappropriate for cancer pain. Newer tables will need to incorporate more complex ratios with wider margins of variability. In the meantime, opioid rotations should use relatively lower doses of the new opioid and should be accompanied by frequent patient monitoring for both side effects and analgesia.

### Pain in Special Situations

Some patients present with very complex pain syndromes. Two of these specific syndromes are related to incidental pain and neuropathic pain. *Incidental pain* is defined as pain that is suddenly and severely aggravated as a result of movements, swallowing, defecation, or urination. Pain control usually is excellent if the patient remains immobile or refrains from performing the pain-causing maneuver.[87] The frequency of painful episodes ranges from just a few each day to several hundred per day. The dose of opioid capable of maintaining good analgesia during rest is insufficient during incidental pain, and a significant increase in dose results in unacceptable toxicity, mostly sedation, during the period between pain episodes.[87] Attempts should be made to increase the local control of the incidental pain episodes through techniques such as radiation therapy, orthopedic procedures, or neurosurgical procedures such as percutaneous cordotomy. Bisphosphonates, are useful in relieving bone pain—both the continuous and the incidental components.[88]

A recent study suggests that adding methylphenidate permits an increase in the maximal tolerated opioid dose and decreases pain and sedation in patients who had reached their dose-limiting dose for incidental pain.[89]

*Neuropathic pain* usually is pain resulting from damage to the central or peripheral nervous system. Although there is strong debate on this subject,[90,91] some evidence suggests that patients with neuropathic pain require higher doses of opioids and are less likely to achieve good pain control with the standard WHO approach.[90] These patients often require adjuvant drugs, typically centrally acting drugs such as tricyclic antidepressants for deafferentation pain, or carbamazepine, clonazepam, or baclofen for lancinating pain.[92] These patients also often require several trials of different centrally acting drugs in combination with opioid analgesics and corticosteroids.

### Adjuvant Drugs

Adjuvant analgesic drugs are commonly used in advanced-cancer patients for multiple purposes. These include enhancement of analgesia initiated by another medication (typically an opioid), their own additional analgesic effect, and/or treatment of opioid-induced side effects. Adjuvant drugs have remained popular despite limited clinical studies strongly confirming their role in managing cancer-related pain. Table 74–10 summarizes some of the more commonly used adjuvant drugs. Most cancer patients receive at least one adjuvant drug.[93] As shown in Table 74–10, most adjuvant drugs are used for difficult pain syndromes, including neuropathic and bone pain.

Among the agents frequently used to manage neuropathic pain, tricyclic antidepressants, systemic local anesthetics, and baclofen traditionally have been used for dysesthetic pain, whereas anticonvulsants such as gabapentin, carbamazepine, and phenytoin have been used more often to manage lancinating pain.[92] These agents are rarely effective in more than 30% of patients.

**Table 74–10** Adjuvant drugs for cancer pain

*Neuropathic Pain*

Anticonvulsants, e.g., gabapentin
Tricyclic antidepressant
Corticosteroids
Selective serotonin reuptake inhibitors
N-methyl-D-aspartate antagonists (ketamine, dextromethorphan, and others)
Baclofen

*Bone Pain*

Bisphosphonates

*Muscle Spasm*

Cyclobenzaprine
Baclofen

Unfortunately, very few controlled trials have compared many of these agents. Therefore, the choice of first-line drugs should be based on safety, potential interaction with other agents, and the experience of different clinicians.

Corticosteroids are strong analgesics, especially in cerebral and spinal tumors. The mechanism of action is poorly understood, but it could be attributable to their anti-inflammatory effect and their role in antagonizing the cytokines associated with tumor involvement. Moreover, corticosteroids have excellent antiemetic activity, and they stimulate appetite and elevate mood.[94]

In the case of bone pain, bisphosphonates are effective in reducing pain in lytic bone metastases, as well as in decreasing the number of adverse events, such as fractures, need for radiation therapy, and hypercalcemia.[95]

In recent years, activation of the NMDA receptor by endogenous ligands such as excitatory amino acids has been found to promote pain and hyperalgesia. Three old drugs, ketamine, dextromethorphan, and methadone, are competitive NMDA receptor antagonists. The first two drugs are potentially useful agents that are capable of potentiating opioid analgesia. Randomized, controlled trials are needed to better define the role of ketamine and dextromethorphan as adjuvants to opioid analgesics. The dual effect on opioid receptors and NMDA receptors might explain the reduced level of cross-tolerance between methadone and other opioid agonists.

In some circumstances, using an adjuvant medication has the potential to cause problems. Because the majority of adjuvant drugs have central nervous system effects, the most frequent interactions between different adjuvant drugs or between an adjuvant medication and opioids involve central side effects. A number of simple measures can assist clinicians in preventing excessive toxicity from adjuvant drugs:

- Identify opioids as the first-line treatment for the majority of cancer pain syndromes and attempt to properly titrate dosages with the most effective type and route of opioid before adding adjuvant drugs.
- Add one adjuvant drug at a time to avoid combined or enhanced side effects.
- Use an effective (high) dose of the selected adjuvant drug to rapidly determine its effectiveness in controlling pain or side effects.
- Define outcome measures at the start of treatment. For example, psychostimulants may be used to potentiate the opioid analgesic effect, decrease opioid-induced sedation, and/or treat depression, hypoactive-hyperalert delirium, and somatization, but the dose and latency period may be quite different for each expected outcome.
- Discontinue the adjuvant drug quickly if it is ineffective.
- Always monitor sedation and cognition.

## Nonpharmacological Management

Appropriate multidimensional assessment and pharmacological treatment result in excellent pain control for the majority of cancer patients. However, some patients continue to have severe pain that does not respond fully to pharmacological treatment, or the effective pharmacological treatment results in intolerable toxicity. Nonpharmacological interventions should be considered for these patients.

Table 74–11 summarizes nonpharmacological methods. Some of these approaches should be universal, such as appropriate counseling of patients and families. Other approaches, including transcutaneous nerve stimulation, relaxation/imagery, or physiotherapy can be attempted in most patients because of the techniques' relatively limited side effects and cost. Finally, when pharmacological and less invasive nonpharmacological ap-

**Table 74–11** Nonpharmacological methods of treating cancer pain

Counseling (spiritual and/or social)
Physical therapy and occupational therapy
Relaxation techniques (music therapy)
Acupuncture
Orthopedic, neurosurgical and anesthesiological procedures
Transcutaneous electrical nerve stimulation
Radiation therapy

proaches are not effective, several other interventional techniques can be attempted. These include radiation therapy and anesthesiologic and neurosurgical procedures. Insertion of a biliary stent percutaneously or during endoscopic retrograde cholangiopancreatography is a common method of relieving pain associated with obstructive jaundice.[35] Dilatation, stent placement, and laser are frequently used to palliate the pain associated with obstruction in advanced esophageal and rectal malignancies.[36–38] Finally, celiac plexus block has been shown to reduce the intensity of severe visceral nociceptive pain associated with advanced pancreatic, stomach, and hepatic malignancies.[39–41] Polani and associates[42] compared the efficacy of celiac plexus block to pharmacological therapy and found statistically significant improvements in pain in the immediate postoperative period with celiac plexus block but no long-term difference. Although traditionally these techniques have been used to relieve pain of non-neuropathic origin, several investigators have recognized that many of these invasive procedures can also be helpful to patients with intractable neuropathic pain syndrome.[96]

Radiation therapy should always be considered in patients with painful bony metastases. Single large fractions may be as effective as multiple fractions and may reduce patient discomfort and cost.[97] Among anesthesiological techniques, the most commonly used procedures include celiac plexus block in patients with abdominal malignancies, and epidural and intrathecal administration of opioids and local anesthetics in patients with intractable pain in the lower half of the leg or those who cannot tolerate systemic opioids because of severe toxicity.[96]

Percutaneous cordotomy is the most popular neurosurgical approach.[98] This procedure is minimally invasive and achieves effective analgesia in more than 80% of patients, particularly when applied to unilateral pain in the lower half of the body. Among patients with pathological or impending fractures, orthopedic procedures, such as internal fixation or vertebroplasty, can be very beneficial in reducing pain and increasing mobility.

## Conclusion

Pain is very common in patients with gastrointestinal malignancies, and its management is an integral part of the integral plan of these patients' cancer care. Clinicians should be knowledgeable about the different types of pain syndromes, patient assessment for pain and other symptoms, and different modalities of pain treatment. Although some patients can be treated with simple measures, the majority of cancer patients will require opioids to control their pain at some point in the disease process. Therefore, physicians who treat cancer patients should thoroughly understand this class of medications, including routes of administration and possible side effects. Finally, physicians should educate patients and family members about the assessment and treatment of cancer pain. Appropriate discussion of the importance of regular versus "as-needed" treatment and the myth of addiction will increase treatment compliance and ultimately improve pain control.

## References

1. Foley KM. The treatment of cancer pain. N Engl J Med 313:84–95, 1985.
2. Bonica, JJ. Treatment of cancer pain: current status and future needs. In: Fields HL, Dubner R, Cervero F (eds): Advances in Pain Research and Therapy, Vol 9. Proceedings of the Fourth World Congress on Pain. Raven Press, New York, 1985, pp 589–616.
3. Marks RM, Sachar EJ. Undertreatment of medical inpatients with narcotic analgesics. Ann Intern Med 78:173–181, 1973.
4. World Health Organization Expert Committee report. Cancer Pain Relief and Palliative Care. Technical Series 804. World Health Organization, Geneva, 1990, p 19.
5. U.S. Department of Health and Human Services: Management of Cancer Pain. Clinical Practice Guidelines. AHCPR Publications, Rockville, MD, No. 94–0592, 1994.
6. World Health Organization Cancer Pain Relief, 2nd ed. World Health Organization, Geneva, Switzerland, 1996.
7. Bruera E, Schoeller T. Changing patterns of cancer pain management. Perspect Pain Manag 1:4–8, 1992.
8. Cleeland CS, Gonin R, Hatfield AK, et al. Pain and its treatment in outpatients with metastatic cancer. N Engl J Med 330:592–596, 1994.
9. Foley KM. Pain syndromes in patients with cancer. In: Bonica JJ, Ventafridda V (eds): Advances in Pain Research and Therapy, 59. Raven Press, New York, 1979, pp 59–75.
10. Higginson IJ. Innovations in assessment: epidemiology and assessment of pain in advanced cancer. In: Jansen TS, Turner JA, Wiesenfeld-Hallen Z (eds): Proceedings of the 8th World Congress on Pain: Progress in Pain Research and Management, Vol 8. IASP Press, Seattle, 1997, pp 707–716.
11. Foley KM. Supportive care and quality of life. In: De Vita VT, Hellman S, Rosenberg SA (eds): Cancer Principles and Practice of Oncology, 5th ed. Lippincott-Raven, Philadelphia, 1997, pp 2807–2841.
12. Nguyen P, Zekry H, Bruera E. Cancer pain assessment and palliative care management. Oncology 3:135–140, 2000.
13. Caraceni A, Portenoy RK. Pain management in patients with pancreatic carcinoma. Cancer 78:639–653, 1996.
14. Lame F, Colleau SM, Brasseur L, et al. Multicentre study of cancer pain and its treatment in France. BMJ 310:1034–1037, 1995.
15. Rawal N, Hylander J, Arner S. Management of terminal cancer pain in Sweden: a nationwide survey. Pain 54:169–179, 1993.
16. Kaasalainen V, Vainio A, Ali-Melkkila T. Development in the treatment of cancer pain in Finland: the third nationwide survey. Pain 70:175–183, 1997.
17. Lame F, Fontaine A, Brasseur L, et al. France: status of cancer pain and palliative care. J Pain Symptom Manage 12:106–108, 1996.
18. Laudico AV. The Philippines: status of cancer pain and palliative care. J Pain Symptom Manage 12:99–101, 1996.
19. Twycross R. Pain Relief in Advanced Cancer. Churchill Livingstone, London, 1994.
20. McCaffery M. Pain contol. Barriers to the use of available information. World Health Organization Expert Committee on Cancer Pain Relief and Active Supportive Care. Cancer 70:1438–1449, 1992.
21. Zech DF, Grond S, Lynch J, et al. Validation of World Health Organization Guidelines for cancer pain relief: a 10-year prospective study. Pain 63:65–76, 1995.
22. Sloan PA, Donnelly MB, Schwartz RW, et al. Cancer pain assessment and management by housestaff. Pain 67:475–481, 1996.
23. Sheidler VR, McGuire DB, Grossman SA, et al. Analgesic decision-making skills of nurses. Oncol Nurs Forum 19:1531–1534, 1992.
24. Von Roenn JH, Cleeland CS, Gonin R, et al. Physician attitudes and practice in cancer pain management. A survey from the Eastern Cooperative Oncology Group. Ann Intern Med 119:121–126, 1993.
25. Allende S, Carvell HC. Mexico: status of cancer pain and palliative care. J Pain Symptom Manage 12:118–120, 1996.
26. Sun WZ, Hou WY, Li JH. Republic of China: status of cancer pain and palliative care. J Pain Symptom Manage 12:127–129, 1996.
27. Bruera E, Kuehn N, Miller MJ, Selmser P, Macmillan K. The Edmonton symptom assessment system (ESAS): a simple method for the assessment of palliative care patients. J Palliat Care 7:6–9, 1991.
28. Chang VT, Hwang SS, Feuerman M. Validation of the Edmonton Symptom Assessment Scale. Cancer 88:2164–2171, 2000.
29. Moore R, Bone L, Geller B, et al. Prevalence, detection and treatment of alcoholism in hospitalized patients. JAMA, 261:403–407, 1989.
30. Bruera E, Moyano J, Seifert L, Fainsinger RL, Hanson J, Suarez-Almazor M. The frequency of alcoholism among patients with pain due to terminal cancer. J Pain Symptom Manage 10:599–603, 1995.
31. Bruera E, Schoeller T, Wenk R, et al. A prospective multicenter assessment of the Edmonton Staging System for cancer pain. J Pain Symptom Manage 10:348–355, 1995.
32. Bruera E, MacDonald S. Audit methods: the Edmonton Symptom Assessment System. In: Higginson I (ed): Clinical Audit in Palliative Care. Radcliffe Medical Press, Oxford, 1993 pp 61–77.
33. Pereira J, Hanson J, Bruera E. The frequency and clinical course of cognitive impairment in patients with terminal cancer. Cancer 79:835–842, 1997.
34. Levy MH. Supportive oncology: forward. Semin Oncol 21:699–700, 1994.
35. Spinelli P, Dal Fante M, Mancim A. Self-expanding mesh stent for endoscopic palliation of rectal obstructing tumors: a preliminary report. Surg Endosc 6:72–74, 1992.
36. Anderson ID, Manson SM, Martin DF, et al. Relief of metastatic biliary obstruction by stent placement: is it worthwhile? Surg Oncol 2:113–117, 1993.
37. Lightdale CJ. Self-expanding metal stents for esophageal and gastric cancer: a new opening [editorial]. Gastrointest Endosc 38:86–88, 1992.
38. Garcia C, Collins T, Ide S, et al. Nd:YAG laser as a therapeutic option in the management of gastrointestinal cancer. Del Med J 65:369–373, 1993.
39. Ward EM, Rorie DK, Narss LA, et al. The celiac ganglia in man: normal anatomic variations. Anesth Analg 58:461–465, 1979.
40. De Cicco M, Matovic M, Balestreri L, et al. Single-needle celiac plexus block: is needle tip position critical in patients with no regional anatomic distortions? Anesthesiology 87:1301–1308, 1997.
41. Eisenberg E, Carr DB, Chalmers TC. Neurolytic celiac plexus block for treatment of cancer pain: a meta-analysis. Anesth Analog 80:290–295, 1995.
42. Polani E, Finco G, Gottin L, et al. Prospective randomized double-blind trial of neurolytic celiac plexus block in patients with pancreatic cancer. Br J Surg 85:199–201, 1998.
43. World Health Organization Expert Committee. Cancer Pain Relief and Palliative Care. Technical Series 804. World Health Organization. Geneva, 1990.
44. Principles of Analgesic Use in the Treatment of Acute Pain and Chronic Cancer Pain: A Concise Guide to Medical Practice. American Pain Society, Skokie, IL, 1992.
45. Whitcomb DC, Block GD. Association of acetaminophen hepatotoxicity with fasting and ethanol use. JAMA 272:1845–1850, 1994.
46. Kaysen GA, Pond SM, Roper MN, et al. Combined hepatic and renal injury in alcoholics during therapeutic use of acetaminophen. Arch Intern Med 145:2019–2023, 1985.
47. Buckley N, Whyte I, Dawson A. Long-term anticonvulsant therapy worsens outcome in paracetamol-induced fulminant hepatic failure [letter]. Hum Exp Toxicol 12:411–412, 1993.
48. Lane NE. Pain management in osteoarthritis: the role of COX-2 inhibitors. J Rheumatol 24(Suppl 49):20–24, 1997.
49. Jenkins C, Bruera E. Nonsteroidal anti-inflammatory drugs as adjuvant analgesics in cancer patients. Palliat Med 13:183–196, 1999.
50. Duggan AW, North RA. Electrophysiology of opioids. Pharmacol Rev 35:219–281, 1983.
51. Benedetti C. Neuroanatomy and biochemistry of antinociception. In Bonica JJ, Ventafridda V (eds): Advances in Pain Research and Therapy, Vol 2. Raven Press, New York, 1979, pp 31–44.
52. Fainsinger R, Bruera E, Miller MJ, Hanson J, MacEachern T. Symptom control during the last week of life on a palliative care unit. J Palliat Care 7:5–11, 1991.
53. Ripamonti C, Bruera E. Current status of patient controlled analgesia in cancer patients. J Oncol 11:373–384, 1997.
54. Bollish SJ, Collins CL, Hirking DM, et al. Efficacy of patient-controlled versus conventional analgesia for postoperative pain. Clin Pharmacokinet 4:48, 1985.
55. Ventafridda V, Spoldi E, Caraceni A, et al. The importance of continuous SC morphine administration for cancer pain control. Pain Clin 1:47–56, 1986.
56. Kerr I, Sone M, DeAngelis C, et al. Continuous narcotic infusion with patient-controlled analgesia for chronic cancer pain in outpatients. Ann Intern Med 108:554–557, 1988.
57. Bruera E. Subcutaneous administration of opioids in the management of cancer pain. In: Foley K, Ventafridda V (eds): Advances in Pain Research and Therapy, Vol. 16. Raven Press, New York, 1990, pp 203–218.

58. Shen R, Arieli S. Administration of potassium by subcutaneous infusion in elderly patients. BMJ 285:1167–1168, 1982.

59. Waldmann C, Eason J, Rambohul E, et al. Serum morphine levels: a comparison between continuous subcutaneous and intravenous infusion in postoperative patients. Anesth Analg 39:768–771, 1984.

60. Brenneis C, Michaud M, Bruera E, et al. Local toxicity during subcutaneous infusion of narcotics: a prospective study. Cancer Nurs 10:172–176, 1987.

61. Brook-Williams P, Hoover LH. Morphine suppositories for intractable pain. CMAJ 126:14, 1982.

62. Johsson T, Christensen CB, Jordening H, et al. The bioavailability of rectally administered morphine. Pharmacol Toxicol 62:203–205, 1988.

63. Moolenaar F, Visser J, Leuvermann A, et al. Bioavailability of morphine from suppositories. Int J Pharmacol 45:161–164, 1988.

64. Miser AW, Narang PK, Dothage JA, et al. Transdermal fentanyl for pain control in patients with cancer. Pain 37:15–21, 1989.

65. Alexander-Williams JM, Rowbotham DJ. Novel routes of opioid administration. Br J Aneasth 81:3–7, 1998.

66. Peng PWH, Sandier AN. A review of the use of fentanyl analgesia in the management of acute pain in adults. Anesthesiology 90:576–599, 1999.

67. Siddal PJ, Cousins MJ. Pain mechanisms and management: an update. Clin Exp Pharmacol Physiol 22:679–688, 1999.

68. Gourlay GK. Sustained relief of chronic pain: pharmacokinetics of sustained-release morphine. Clin Pharmacokinet 35:173–190, 1998.

69. Moulin DE, Kreeft JH, Murray-Parsons N, et al. Comparison of continuous subcutaneous and intravenous hydromorphone infusions for management of cancer pain. Lancet 45:11–17, 1991.

70. Hays H, Hagen N, Thirlwell M, et al. Comparative clinical efficacy and safety of immediate-release and controlled-release hydromorphone for chronic severe cancer pain. Cancer 74:1808–1816, 1994.

71. Glare PA, Walsh TD. Dose-ranging study of oxycodone for chronic pain in advanced cancer. J Clin Oncol 973–978, 1993.

72. Alexander-Williams JM, Rowbotham DJ. Novel routes of opioid administration. Br J Anaesth 81:3–7, 1998.

73. Ripamonti C, Zecca E, Bruera E. An update on the clinical use of methadone for cancer pain. Pain 70:109–115, 1997.

74. Fainsinger R, Schoeller T, Bruera E. Methadone in the management of cancer pain: a review. Pain 52:137–147, 1993.

75. Sweeney C, Bruera E. New role for old drugs: methadone. Prog Palliat Med 9:8–10, 2001.

76. Bruera E, Fainsinger R, Moore M, et al. Local toxicity with subcutaneous methadone. Experience of two centers. Pain 45:141–143, 1991.

77. Bruera E, Watanabe S, Fainsinger RL, et al. Custom-made capsules and suppositories of methadone for patients on high-dose opioids for cancer pain. Pain 62:141–146, 1995.

78. Bruera E, Macmillan K, Hanson J, MacDonald RN. The cognitive effects of the administration of narcotic analgesics in patients with cancer pain. Pain 39:13–16, 1989.

79. Bruera E, Brenneis C, Paterson AHG, MacDonald RN. Use of methyl-phenidate as an adjuvant to narcotic analgesics in patients with advanced cancer. J Pain Symptom Manage 4:3–6, 1989.

80. Mancini I, Bruera E. Constipation in advanced cancer patients. Support Care Cancer 6:356–364, 1998.

81. Pereira J, Bruera E. Chronic nausea. In: Bruera E, Higginson I (eds): Cachexia–Anorexia in Cancer Patients. Oxford University Press, Oxford, 1996, pp 23–37.

82. Miyoshi H, Leckband S. Systemic opioid analgesics. In: Loeser J, Butler S, Chapman C, Turk D (eds): Bonica's Management of Pain, 3rd ed. Lippincott Williams & Wilkins, Philadelphia, 2001, pp 1682–1709.

83. Bruera E, Miller MJ. Non-cardiogenic pulmonary edema after narcotic treatment for cancer pain. Pain 39:297–300, 1989.

84. Ripamonti C, Bruera E. CNS adverse effects of opioids in cancer patients. Guidelines for treatment. CNS Drugs 8:21–37, 1997.

85. Ripamonti C, De Conno F, Groff L, et al. Equianalgesic dose/ratio between methadone and other opioid agonists in cancer pain: comparison of two clinical experiences. Ann Oncol 9:79–83, 1998.

86. Lawlor P, Turner K, Hanson J, Bruera E. Dose ratio between morphine and hydromorphone in patients with cancer pain: a retrospective study. Pain 72:79–85, 1997.

87. Portenoy RK, Hagen NA. Breakthrough pain definition, prevalence and characteristics. Pain 41:273–281, 1990.

88. Ernst DS, MacDonald RN, Paterson AHG, Jensen J, Brasher P, Bruera E. A double-blind crossover trial of intravenous clodronate in metastatic bone pain. J Pain Symptom Manage 7:4–11, 1992.

89. Bruera E, Fainsinger R, MacEachern T, Hanson J. The use of methylphenidate in patients with incident cancer pain receiving regular opiates. A preliminary report. Pain 50:75–77, 1992.

90. Portenoy RK, Foley KM, Inturrisi CE. The nature of opioid responsiveness and its implications for neuropathic pain: new hypotheses derived from studies of opioid infusions. Pain 43:273–286, 1990.

91. Arner G, Meyerson BA. Lack of analgesic effect of opioids on neuropathic and idiopathic forms of pain. Pain 33:11–23, 1988.

92. Bruera E, Ripamonti C. Adjuvants to opioid analgesics. In: Patt R (ed): Cancer Pain. J.B. Lippincott, Philadelphia, 1993, pp 142–159.

93. Oneschuk D, Bruera E. The dark side of adjuvant analgesic drugs. Prog Palliat Care 5:5–13, 1997.

94. Bruera E, Roca E, Cedaro L, Carraro S, Chacon R. Action of oral methylprednisolone in terminal cancer patients: a prospective randomized double blind study. Cancer Treat Rep 69:751–754, 1985.

95. Pereira J, Mancini I, Walker P. The role of bisphosphonates in malignant bone pain: a review. J Palliat Care 14:14–22, 1998.

96. Crammond T. Invasive techniques for neuropathic pain in cancer. In: Bruera E, Portenoy RK (eds): Topics in Palliative Care, Vol. 2. Oxford University Press, New York, 1998, pp 63–90.

97. Hoskin, PJ. Radiotherapy in symptom management. In: Doyle D, Hanks GWC, MacDonald N (eds): Oxford Textbook of Palliative Medicine. Oxford University Press, Oxford, 1998, pp 267–282.

98. Arbit E, Bilsky MH. Neurosurgical approaches in palliative care. In Doyle D, Hanks GWC, MacDonald N (eds): Oxford Textbook of Palliative Medicine. Oxford University Press, Oxford, 1998, pp 414–420.

# Index

Page numbers followed by f and t indicate figures and tables, respectively.